PEDRETTI'S

OCCUPATIONAL THERAPY

Practice Skills for Physical Dysfunction

PEDRETTI'S

OCCUPATIONAL THERAPY

Practice Skills for Physical Dysfunction

SIXTH EDITION

Heidi McHugh Pendleton, PhD, OTR/L, FAOTA

Professor
Department of Occupational Therapy
San Jose State University
San Jose, California

Winifred Schultz-Krohn, PhD, OTR/L, BCP, SWC, FAOTA

Associate Professor
Department of Occupational Therapy
San Jose State University
San Jose, California

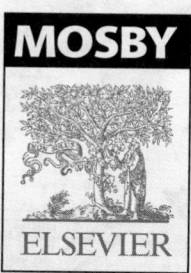

MOSBY

ELSEVIER

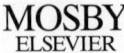

MOSBY
ELSEVIER

11830 Westline Industrial Drive
St. Louis, Missouri 63146

PEDRETTI'S OCCUPATIONAL THERAPY: ISBN-13: 978-0-323-03153-0
PRACTICE SKILLS FOR PHYSICAL DYSFUNCTION ISBN-10: 0-323-03153-6
Copyright © 2006 by Mosby, Inc., an affiliate of Elsevier Inc.

Notice

Previous editions copyrighted 1981, 1985, 1990, 1996, 2001

ISBN-13: 978-0-323-03153-0
ISBN-10: 0-323-03153-6
Chapter 31 © 2005 by Cathy Runyan OTR/L (www.RecoveringFunction.com)

Publishing Director: Linda Duncan
Editor: Kathy Falk
Developmental Editor: Melissa Kuster Deutsch
Publishing Services Manager: Julie Eddy
Project Manager: Rich Barber
Designer: Julia Dummitt

Printed in the United States

Last digit is the print number: 9 8 7 6 5 4 3

Michelle Pressman Abrams, MS, OTR/L
Therapist
Department of Occupational/Hand Therapy
NovaCare Rehabilitation
Phoenix, Arizona

Carole Adler, BA, OTR/L, ATP
Rehab Case Manager, Spinal Cord Injury
Santa Clara Valley Medical Center
San Jose, California

Denis Anson, MS, OTR/L
Director of Research and Development
Assistive Technology Research Institute
College Misericordia
Dallas, Pennsylvania

Deborah Bolding, MS, OTR/L, CHT, BCP
Clinical Education Coordinator
Rehabilitation Services
Stanford Hospital and Clinics
Palo Alto, California

Estelle B. Breines, PhD, OTR, FAOTA
President
Geri-Rehab, Inc.
Lebanon, New Jersey
Executive Director
Developmental Rehabilitation Services
Lebanon, New Jersey

Ann Burkhardt, OTD, OTR/L, FAOTA
Director and Associate Professor
Division of Occupational Therapy
Long Island University
Brooklyn, New York
Professional Associate
Occupational Therapy Assistant Program
Mercy College
Dobbs Ferry, New York

Sandra E. Burnett, MA, OTR/L, MFT
Professor, ADA/504 Compliance Officer
Disabled Student Program
Santa Monica Community College District
Santa Monica, California

Gordon Umphred Burton, PhD, OTR
Emeritus Professor and Chair
Department of Occupational Therapy
San Jose State University
San Jose, California

Michael W.K. Chan, MBA, OTR/L, OT (C)
Assistant Professor
School of Health Sciences
Eastern Michigan University
Ypsilanti, Michigan

Cynthia Cooper, MFA, MA, OTR/L, CHT
Director of Hand Therapy in Arizona
NovaCare Rehabilitation
Phoenix, Arizona

Elizabeth DePoy, PhD, MSW, OTR
Professor
Department of Occupational Therapy
University of Maine
Orono, Maine

Lisa Deshaies, OTR/L, CHT
Adjunct Clinical Faculty
Department of Occupational Science &
Occupational Therapy
University of Southern California
Los Angeles, California
Occupational Therapy Clinical Specialist
Occupational Therapy Department
Rancho Los Amigos National Rehabilitation Center
Downey, California

Joyce M. Engel, PhD, OTR/L
Professor
Department of Rehabilitation Medicine
Occupational Therapy Division
University of Washington
Seattle, Washington

Jeffrey Englander, MD
Project Director
Rehabilitation Research Center for
Traumatic Brain Injury
Santa Clara Medical Center
San Jose, California

Anne Fisher, ScD, OTR, FAOTA
Professor
Umeå University
Institution for Community Medicine
and Rehabilitation
Division of Occupational Therapy
Umeå University
Umeå, Sweden
Adjunct Professor
Department of Occupational Therapy
Colorado State University
Ft. Collins, Colorado

Diane Foti, MS, OTR/L
Clinical Specialist
Kaiser Permanente
Union City, California

Alison Hewitt George, MS, OTR/L
Lecturer
Department of Occupational Therapy
San Jose State University
San Jose, California

Glen Gillen, EdD, OTR, BCN
Assistant Professor
Programs in Occupational Therapy
Columbia University
New York, New York

Lynn Gitlow, PhD, OTR/L, ATP
Director
Department of Occupational Therapy
Husson College
Bangor, Maine

Carolyn Glogoski, Ph.D., OTR/L
Associate Professor
Department of Occupational Therapy
Eastern Michigan University
Ypsilanti, Michigan

Jennifer S. Glover, MS, OTR/L
Area Director
Genesis Rehabilitation Services
Windsor, Connecticut

Luella Grangaard, MS, OTR/L, CHT
Manager, Occupational Therapy
Rehabilitation Services
Eisenhower Medical Center
Rancho Mirage, California

Denise Haruko Ha, OTR/L
Occupational Therapist
Occupational Therapy Vocational Services
Rancho Los Amigos National
Rehabilitation Center
Downey, California

Karen Nelson Jenks, MS, ORT/L, SWC
Clinical Administrator
Services for Brain Injury
San Jose, California

Judy M. Jourdan, MSA, OTR
Therapy Manager
Memorial Home Care
South Bend, Indiana

Lisa M. Kanazawa, MS, OTR/L
Consultant
Rebuilding Together Diablo Valley
Danville, California

Mary C. Kasch, OTR/L, CHT, FAOTA
Executive Director
Hand Therapy Certification Commission
Rancho Cordova, California

Denise D. Keenan, OTR, CHT
Adjunct Faculty
Department of Occupational Therapy
University of Utah
Salt Lake City, Utah
Senior Hand Therapist
Rehabilitation Services
Intermountain Health Care, Inc
Salt Lake City, Utah

Amy Phillips Killingsworth, MA, OTR/L
Professor
Department of Occupational Therapy
San Jose State University
San Jose, California

Barbara L. Kornblau, JD, OT/L, FAOTA, DAAPM, ABDA, CCM, CDMS
Professor
Departments of Occupational Therapy,
Public Health, Law
Nova Southeastern University
Fort Lauderdale, Florida
Attorney and Counselor at Law
Private Practice
Miami, Florida

Donna Lashgari, MS, OTR/CHT
Rehabilitation Manager
Stanford University Hospitals and Clinics
Palo Alto, California

Sonia Lawson, PhD, OTR/L
Assistant Professor
Department of Occupational Therapy and
Occupational Science
Towson University
Towson, Maryland

Susan M. Lillie, BS, OTR/L, CDRS
Supervisor, Adaptive Driving
Evaluation Program
Therapy Services
Santa Clara Valley Medical Center
San Jose, California

Maureen Michele Matthews, OT/L
Outpatient Program Manager
Therapy Services
Santa Clara Valley Medical Center
San Jose, California

Guy McCormack, PhD, OTR/L, FAOTA
Chair
Department of Occupational Therapy
School of Heath Professions
University of Missouri—Columbia
Columbia, Missouri

Rochelle McLaughlin, MS, OTR/L
Administrative Analyst Specialist
San Jose State University
San Jose, California
Occupational Therapist
Rehabilitation Research Center
Santa Clara Valley Medical Center
San Jose, California

Nancy Vandewiele Milligan, PhD, OTR
Occupational Therapy Program
Wayne State University
Detroit Michigan

Jill J. Page, OTR/L
Industrial Rehabilitation Consultant
Ergoscience, Inc.
Birmingham, Alabama

Shawn C. Phipps, MS, OTR/L
Occupational Therapy Supervisor
Department of Occupational Therapy
Rancho Los Amigos National Rehabilitation Center
Downey, California
Clinical Instructor and Lecturer
Occupational Therapy Program
Department of Health and Human Sciences
California State University Dominguez Hills
Carson, California

Michael A. Pizzi, PhD, OTR/L, FAOTA
Wellness Coach, CEO
Wellness Lifestyles, Inc.
New York, New York

Sara A. Pope-Davis, MOT, OTR
Occupational Therapist
Memorial Outpatient Therapy Services
Memorial Hospital and Health System
South Bend, Indiana

Linda Anderson Preston, MS, OTR/L, BCN
Clinical Specialist
Patricia Neal Outpatient Therapy Center
Roane Medical Center
Harriman, Tennessee

Sandra Utley Reeves, OTR/L
Occupational Therapist
Department of Rehabilitation Services
Shands Hospital at the University of Florida
Gainesville, Florida

S. Maggie Reitz, PhD, OTR/L, FAOTA
Chairperson and Professor
Department of Occupational Therapy and Occupational
Science
Towson University
Towson, Maryland

Pamela Richardson, PhD, OTR/L, FAOTA
Associate Professor
Department of Occupational Therapy
San Jose State University
San Jose, California

Pamela S. Roberts, MSHA, OTR/L, SCFES, CPHQ, FAOTS
Manager, Rehabilitation and Neurology
Department of Rehabilitation and Division of Neurology
Cedars-Sinai Medical Center
Los Angeles, California

Charlotte Brasic Royeen, PhD, OTR, FAOTA
Dean, Doisy College of Health Sciences
Professor of Occupational Therapy and Occupational
Science
Saint Louis University
St. Louis, Missouri

Cathy Runyan, OTR/L
NDT Adult Hemiplegia Instructor
Recovering Function
San Jose, California

Marjorie E. Scaffa, PhD, OTR, FAOTA
Chair
Department of Occupational Therapy
University of South Alabama
Mobile, Alabama

Amy Schmidt, MS, PAM, OTR/L
Occupational Therapy Supervisor
Department of Occupational and Recreation Therapy
Neurology and Adult Brain Injury Services
Ranchos Los Amigos National Rehabilitation Center
Downey, California

Kathleen Barker Schwartz, EdD, OTR/L, FAOTA
Professor
Department of Occupational Therapy
San Jose State University
San Jose, California

Jerilyn (Gigi) Smith, MS, OTR/L
Fieldwork Director, Lecturer
Department of Occupational Therapy
San Jose State University
San Jose, California

Marti Southam, Ph.D., OTR/L, FAOTA
Associate Professor, Chairperson
Department of Occupational Therapy
San Jose State University
San Jose, California

Michelle Tipton-Burton, MS, OTR/L
Therapy Director
Day Treatment Program
Santa Clara Valley Medical Center
San Jose, California

J. Martin Walsh, OTR/L, CHT
Manager of Examination Services
Hand Therapy Certification Commission
Rancho Cordova, California

Mary Warren, MS, OTR/L, FAOTA
Assistant Professor, Director Graduate Certificate in Low
Vision Rehabilitation
Department of Occupational Therapy
University of Alabama at Birmingham
Birmingham, Alabama

Christine M. Wietlisbach, MPA, OTR/L, CHT, CWS
Instructor
Occupational Therapy Program
Loma Linda University
Loma Linda, California
Occupational Therapist
Hand Clinic
Department of Physical Rehabilitation
Eisenhower Medical Center
Rancho Mirage, California

Lynn Yasuda, MSEd, OTR/L, FAOTA
Honorary Clinical Faculty
Department of Occupational Science and Occupational
Therapy
University of Southern California
Los Angeles, California
Occupational Therapy Education Consultant and Research
Occupational Therapist
Occupational Therapy and Rehabilitation Engineering
Center
Rancho Los Amigos National Rehabilitation Center
Downey, California

*We wish to dedicate this sixth edition
of Pedretti's Occupational Therapy: Practice Skills for Physical Dysfunction
to Lorraine Williams Pedretti,
whose thoughtfulness, love of her profession, and dedication to the education
of her students provided the impetus to embark on the daunting task of writing
and editing an original textbook (and ensuing editions) for evaluation and treatment
of adults with physical disabilities. As academic colleagues of Professor Pedretti,
we were inspired by her example and challenged to accept the responsibility to continue
in her footsteps to contribute to the advancement of the profession.
It is our hope that our efforts have honored her example and lived up to her faith in us.*

*We would also like to dedicate this edition to occupational therapy students
(past, present, and future) who are the future of our wonderful profession:
may you find the happiness and fulfillment
that we have as proud occupational therapists.*

FOREWORD

It is a privilege to write the foreword to the sixth edition of *Pedretti's Occupational Therapy: Practice Skills for Physical Dysfunction*. I was the book's original author and primary editor of the five previous editions. The book had its inception in 1981. It has been widely used by occupational therapy students in the United States and abroad for the past 25 years. Over this time, it has enjoyed a reputation as a textbook that was written in a practical and comprehensible way, covering the essential theoretical and practical information needed for clinical practice. As editions progressed, the text evolved and expanded to keep pace with changes in the rapidly growing body of knowledge and expanding areas of clinical practice in occupational therapy. It is very gratifying for me to know that this book will continue to be an important resource for students, occupational therapy educators, and clinicians in the profession.

I was very pleased that my professional colleagues at San Jose State University, Dr. Heidi McHugh Pendleton and Dr. Winifred Schultz-Krohn, agreed to become editors of the sixth edition. Dr. Pendleton, who was my student many years ago, joined the faculty of San Jose State University in 1987 after many years of clinical practice working with clients with physical dysfunction. It was gratifying to witness her professional and academic development, to observe her numerous professional achievements, and to see her earn the doctorate in the field. Dr. Winifred Schultz-Krohn came to San Jose State University in 1996 with excellent credentials and qualifications. She has many years of clinical practice in pediatrics, is a board-certified pediatric occupational therapist, and has previous academic experience. She has extensive education and expertise in neurological dysfunction. She continued her outstanding academic achievements and earned her doctorate since joining the faculty at San Jose State University. These editors are professional and academic leaders in the field. They have published numerous articles and book chapters and have received many professional awards and recognitions. They have clinical and academic expertise and a wealth of professional knowledge that makes them eminently qualified for the editorial roles they have undertaken. They have done an excellent job in authoring chapters and coordinating the preparation of the sixth edition.

These editors have assembled a roster of excellent contributors: leaders and experts in the occupational therapy profession who are well qualified to write on their respective subjects. As the profession grew and changed, the content and format of the textbook evolved to reflect the changes. Therefore, more contributors were invited to participate in the preparation of each edition. There are 57 contributors in the sixth edition, and 25 of those are new contributors.

The content of the sixth edition reflects the substantive changes that have occurred in occupational therapy philosophy and practice since the previous edition in 2001. The content of this edition has been restructured and is based on the new Occupational Therapy Practice Framework, with more emphasis on evidence-based practice and client-centered practice. The content reflects new research and theories, new techniques, and current trends in the profession. This fresh new approach includes case studies, clinical reasoning skills, ethical questions and concerns, factors of cultural diversity, and practice notes that are threaded throughout the book. There are four new chapters, and there is new information on prevention and wellness. The enhanced content will teach the student essential clinical reasoning skills and provoke thinking about potential ethical and cultural considerations in treatment. In this edition, there is even more comprehensive coverage of physical dysfunction than in previous editions. Especially exciting within this sixth edition is the accompanying Evolve website for students and instructors. This development brings this textbook into the electronic information age and has great potential for independent study by students and as a resource for occupational therapy educators.

Writing and editing a textbook is no small task. It takes a great deal of time, patience, and persistence. It involves dealing with numerous people—several editors, contributors, vendors, models, photographers, and artists. The process takes from 2 to 3 years to complete. When I was editor, I often asked myself why I continued to do it. But once the product is in hand, much of the difficulty is forgotten. It is always gratifying to see the finished product and to give thanks to all of those whose work and contributions made it possible. Unfortunately, no edition is forever. After a few years, it is time to produce another edition! So we do it again, to keep our precious production alive and moving forward as a vital resource in the field of occupational therapy. At some point, we must say, "No, I cannot do this again." I was so fortunate that my worthy colleagues agreed to adopt this textbook and keep the production going when I reached that place. I am very grateful that they have produced this excellent work, and so pleased that it will continue to be associated with the occupational therapy program of excellence at San Jose State University.

Lorraine Williams Pedretti, M.S., OTR/Ret
Professor Emeritus
San Jose State University

PREFACE

It was a great honor to be asked to assume the editorship of the sixth edition of *Pedretti's Occupational Therapy: Practice Skills for Physical Dysfunction.* To follow in the footsteps of the inimitable Lorraine Pedretti was at once an awesome responsibility and a rewarding journey. The opportunity to work with authors, each a leading expert in his or her field, was an unparalleled experience of the exceptional ability of stellar occupational therapists to organize their time and unselfishly devote their scholarship to the education of future generations of the profession.

Since the publication of the fifth edition, there have been changes within the profession and within the clinical practice of occupational therapy for clients with physical dysfunction. Many of those changes served to shape the approach we took to the new edition and are reflected within the context of each of the chapters. Our mission and intention was to embrace these changes and continue to honor the primacy of occupation that has been the foundation of this textbook for the past several editions.

The sixth and latest edition is framed and guided by the Occupational Therapy Practice Framework: Domain and Process (OTPF), designed to describe the focus and dynamic process of the profession. Key to the OTPF is its view of the overarching goal of occupational therapy; that is, engagement in occupation to support participation in life. This conceptualization of the importance of occupation is emphasized throughout the text. Two chapters are devoted to explicating this new model, and the language and the concepts that comprise the model are incorporated into each of the remaining chapters. The concepts of process and practice, evaluation and intervention, performance skills and patterns, contexts and activity demands, client factors, and intervention applications are all thoroughly illustrated throughout.

To honor the centrality of the client to occupational therapy practice, the chapters begin with case studies, which are then threaded throughout, guiding the reader through the information and relating the content to the specific case descriptions. Thus, the reader is able to experience the clinical reasoning and decision-making skills of the expert clinicians who authored the chapters. Authors of individual chapters were asked to follow the initial presentation of their case studies by crafting several probative or "critical thinking" questions that would peak the readers' curiosity, further motivating their attention to and questioning of the chapter content and consequently facilitating the learning process.

Direct answers to these critical thinking questions are provided either within or at the end of each of the chapters.

This textbook, written for an intended audience of master's degree occupational therapy students and as a reference for practicing occupational therapists, has always been acknowledged for its practical application and focus on practice. Theory and evidence-based content are presented in each chapter and then applied using case descriptions as a foundation for practice. Occupational therapy's role in health and wellness, as well as prevention, is addressed throughout the text. Similarly, occupational therapy's commitment to the importance of considering cultural and ethnic diversity is reflected in every chapter.

New features provided by the publisher's editorial staff are the OT Practice Notes and the Ethical Considerations boxes that are highlighted throughout many of the chapters. The information contained in these boxes (pulled from the chapter content) conveys ideas that are relevant to students' future practice areas and thoughts about some of the possible ethical dilemmas and decisions with which they might be confronted. New support materials include the Evolve website, which includes both a link to student-related materials as well as an instructor link with access to the *Instructor's Resource Manual* (also available in printed and CD-ROM version) and a test bank.

During the process of editing this book, including the stages of envisioning and designing the contents and format, selecting the authors, and reading and giving input to their work, we were guided by our commitment to honoring the occupational welfare of our clients, particularly adults with physical disabilities, through excellent preparation of their future occupational therapists. To that end we sought preeminent authors, those who not only had recognition for expertise in their topic area, but who also embraced the primary importance of occupation to their practice and scholarship. Our goal was to engender excitement in the reader for occupational therapy in the area of physical dysfunction, while providing cutting-edge information and promoting models of best practice. Our extensive and rewarding clinical and academic careers in the profession of occupational therapy and our experiences with hard-working and inspiring clients and students served as the inspiration for our best efforts, which we trust are evident in this book.

Heidi McHugh Pendleton
Winifred Schultz-Krohn

ACKNOWLEDGMENTS

We would like to thank the authors, past and present, for their exceptional contributions and willingness to continue the tradition of excellence that has come to be associated with the Pedretti book. The impressive list of authors for the sixth edition continues the Pedretti reputation for including nationally and internationally known experts in their topic areas and disciplines. We are fortunate to feature contributions from many new authors and included among them are administrators, educators, researchers, and master clinicians.

We would also like to acknowledge the superb contribution of the dedicated editors and staff at Elsevier. We are especially grateful to Kathy Falk, Senior Editor, and Melissa Kuster, Developmental Editor, who patiently and painstakingly mentored us through our first foray into the long and arduous editing process. They are simply outstanding! Our thanks go to Rich Barber, project manager, who, with exceptional attention to detail, made sure that the final product reflected the efforts of all involved.

To those publishers and vendors who permitted us to use material from their publications, we extend our sincere gratitude. Photographers and artists, and the clients and models who posed for photographs are gratefully acknowledged. Michelle Tipton Burton and Monica Bascio were particularly generous in finding just the right photographs to capture the importance of occupation to participation in life – we thank you!

Finally, we would like to extend heartfelt appreciation to our colleagues, friends, and families, without whose help and support this accomplishment could not have been achieved. Special expressions of thank you go to the faculty and staff at San Jose State, who could be counted upon for their support and good wishes during this process.

Heidi McHugh Pendleton extends her gratitude to her husband, Forrest Pendleton (for immeasurable love and support without which this endeavor could never have succeeded) and to her sisters, Deirdre McHugh and Kathleen McHugh (for a lifetime of support). Her love and appreciation go to all of her nieces, nephews, and stepson, including Dar, Jim, Nicky, Elizabeth, Jimmy D, Megan, Kelsey, Jamie, Jessica, and Katie—their love and enthusiasm make everything possible.

Winifred Schultz-Krohn extends a huge thank you to her always supportive, ever-patient husband, Kermit Krohn. His tireless love made the project possible. She is also very grateful for the support and encouragement received by her brother Tom Schultz, his wife Barb Fraser, and niece Sarah, her sister Donna Friedrich, husband Don, nephew Brian, sister Nancy Yamasaki, and husband Bryan, and her parents, Don and Eleanor Schultz.

The co-editors would like to thank each other—great friends at the beginning of the process—we were able to be there for each other, make our own unique contributions, and ultimately sustain our friendship throughout the process, emerging even better friends in the joy of our accomplishment.

CONTENTS

PART V The Occupational Therapy Process: Implementation of Intervention

PART VI Intervention Applications

OCCUPATIONAL THERAPY

Practice Skills for Physical Dysfunction

Overview: Occupational Therapy Foundations for Physical Dysfunction

1

The Occupational Therapy Practice Framework and the Practice of Occupational Therapy for People with Physical Disabilities

HEIDI McHUGH PENDLETON
WINIFRED SCHULTZ-KROHN

KEY TERMS

Occupational therapy practice framework	International classification of functioning, disability, and health	Areas of occupation	Activity demands
Domain		Performance skills	Client factors
Process	Occupation	Performance patterns	Evaluation
		Contexts	

LEARNING OBJECTIVES

After studying this chapter the student or practitioner will be able to do the following:

1. Briefly describe the history of the evolution of the Occupational Therapy Practice Framework.
2. Describe the need for the OTPF in the practice of occupational therapy (OT) for persons with physical disabilities.
3. Describe the fit between the OTPF and the ICF and how they inform and enhance the occupational therapist's understanding of physical disability.
4. Describe the elements of the OTPF including domain and process and the relationship of each to the other.

5. List and describe the components that comprise the occupational therapy domain and give examples of each.
6. List and describe the components that comprise the occupational therapy process and give examples of each.
7. Briefly describe the occupational therapy intervention levels and give an example of each as it might be used in a physical disability practice setting.

CHAPTER OUTLINE

The occupational therapy practice framework: overview
   History of the evolution of the OTPF
   Need for the OTPF
   Fit between the OTPF and the ICF
The OTPF: description

The occupational therapy domain
The occupational therapy process
Strategies for learning the OTPF
The OTPF: its use in this book
Summary

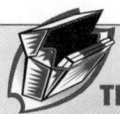

THREADED CASE STUDY: KENT AND KAREN, PART 1

Kent is a highly skilled and very competent occupational therapist with over 25 years of clinical experience working in a large rehabilitation center with adult clients who have physical disabilities. He is currently the supervising occupational therapist on the spinal cord injury (SCI) unit. Through his reading of occupational therapy (OT) publications, attendance at conferences and workshops, and his interactions with his OT staff and interning OT students, he has become increasingly aware of the emergence of the Occupational Therapy Practice Framework (OTPF). Initially he was annoyed that, among the many challenges to his professional time and efforts, he would now have to learn, yet again, a new "language" in order to provide competent intervention. He secretly expressed feelings such as "why fix something that isn't broken?" However, he reluctantly acknowledged the necessity for the change, is impressed by what he has learned so far, and is convinced that he can no longer postpone delving in and really learning and implementing the OTPF into his clinical practice.

Throughout his practice Kent has found it helpful to relate new or novel occupational therapy information he is learning to the relevant circumstances that are experienced by either him or one of his clients, and consequently considers the impact the new information might have on either his own life or that of his client.

While learning the OTPF (also referred to as the Framework) he decided to keep in mind one of his most recently admitted clients, Karen, a 25-year-old administrative assistant for a busy law office, who incurred a cervical SCI and now has C6 functional quadriplegia that necessitates using a wheelchair for mobility. By keeping Karen in mind, Kent expects not only to learn the Framework but to also reinforce his new knowledge by putting it to immediate use in his practice.

Critical Thinking Questions

As you read through the chapter, keep in mind the challenges that learning the OTPF and integrating it into practice will pose for Kent. Think of strategies that you might recommend or use yourself to learn and integrate the information into your practice. Also, consider the objectives for the chapter outlined above as well as the following questions:

1. Why was there a need for the OTPF and how does it fill that need?
2. How might the specific information being presented about the OTPF apply to Kent or Karen?
3. Are there tools that Kent and other OT practitioners can use that will facilitate learning the OTPF and integrating it into practice?

THE OCCUPATIONAL THERAPY PRACTICE FRAMEWORK: OVERVIEW

Many changes have occurred in the practice of *occupational therapy* (OT) for persons with physical disabilities since the publication of the last edition of *Occupational Therapy: Practice Skills for Physical Dysfunction* in 2001. Occupational therapy practice settings are increasingly moving away from traditional healthcare environments, such as the hospital and rehabilitation center, and gradually moving more toward the home and community milieu. The provision of occupational therapy service has become more client-centered and the concept of occupation is increasingly and proudly named as both the preferred intervention and the desired outcome of the services. Clinicians, researchers, and scholars have sought to implement evidence-based practice by learning more about the benefits of occupation to not only remediate problems after the onset of physical disability, but to also anticipate and prevent physical disability and promote wellness. Not surprisingly, economic concerns have severely shortened the amount of time allotted for OT services, thus necessitating more deliberate and resourceful decisions about how these services can most effectively be delivered.

In response to these changes, and many other practice advances, came a change, or evolution, in the language with which occupational therapists describe what they do and how they do it. This change resulted in a document called the **Occupational Therapy Practice Framework** (OTPF), a tool developed by the profession to more clearly articulate and enhance the understanding of what OT practitioners do (occupational therapy **domain**) and how they do it (occupational therapy **process**). The intended beneficiaries of the OTPF were envisioned as including not only OT practitioners (an internal audience) but also the recipients of OT services (called clients), other healthcare professionals, and those providing reimbursement for OT services (comprising an external audience).

The OTPF was developed and thoroughly articulated in the "Occupational Therapy Practice Framework: Domain and Process,"[1] which was published in the *American Journal of Occupational Therapy* (*AJOT*) in 2002. This is an important document every OT practitioner will want to have and reference frequently. It can be downloaded from the American Occupational Therapy Association (AOTA) web site by selecting AJOT Online and the November/December 2002 issue. Another helpful tool for learning the OTPF is the introductory article in the same *AJOT* issue by Youngstrom entitled "The Occupational Therapy Practice Framework: The Evolution of Our Professional Language."[17]

It is not the intention of the current chapter to supplant this comprehensive document but, rather, to describe and increase the reader's understanding of the OTPF and its relationship to the practice of occupational therapy with adults who have physical disabilities. To achieve this, the chapter begins with a discussion of the history of the OTPF followed by sections describing the need for the OTPF and the fit between the OTPF and the World Health Organization's (WHO) International Classification of Function and Disability (ICF). Next, a detailed description of the Framework is presented with emphasis on fully explicating the domain of occupational therapy through examples from the case study and introducing the occupational therapy process, which will be discussed more thoroughly in a subsequent chapter on application of the OTPF to physical dysfunction. The types of occupational therapy intervention proposed by the Framework are examined and illustrated by examples typically employed in physical disabilities practice settings. The chapter concludes with suggestions and strategies for learning the OTPF and an overview of how the Framework is integrated as a unifying thread throughout the remaining chapters in the book.

HISTORY OF THE EVOLUTION OF THE OTPF

In 1999, the Commission on Practice (COP) of the AOTA was charged with reviewing the *Uniform Terminology for Occupational Therapy*, third edition (UT-III).[2] Under the leadership of Chair, Mary Jane Youngstrom, MS, OTR, FAOTA, the COP sought feedback from numerous and varied OT practitioners, scholars, and leaders in the profession regarding the continued suitability of the UT-III to determine whether to update the document or to rescind it. Previous editions of the UT in 1979 and 1989 had been similarly reviewed and updated to reflect the changes and evolving progress of the profession. The reviewers found that the UT-III, though considered a valuable tool for occupational therapists, was lacking in clarity for both consumers and professionals regarding what occupational therapists do and how they do it. Furthermore, they found that the UT-III did not adequately describe or emphasize OT's focus on occupation, the foundation of the profession.

Given the feedback from the review, the COP determined the need for a new document that would preserve the intent of the UT-III (outlining and naming the constructs of the profession) while providing increased clarity about what occupational therapists and occupational therapy assistants do and how they do it. Additionally, it was determined that this new document would refocus attention to the primacy of occupation as the cornerstone of the profession and desired intervention outcome as well as show the process occupational therapists use to help their clients achieve their occupational goals.

NEED FOR THE OTPF

The OTPF makes it clear that the profession's central focus and actions are grounded in the concept of occupation. While some of what occupational therapists do could be construed by clients and other healthcare professionals as similar to or even duplication of the treatment efforts of other disciplines, formally delineating occupation as the overarching goal of all that OT does, and clearly documenting such goals, establishes the profession's unique contribution to client intervention.

This is not to say that prior to the OTPF, OT practitioners did not recognize or focus on occupation or occupational goals with their clients—most did; but in the physical disabilities practice setting, with the reductionistic, bottom-up approach and pervasive influence of the medical model, occupation was seldom mentioned or linked to what was being done in OT. A premium seemed to be placed on "medical speak" and it was difficult, if not impossible, to document occupational performance or occupational goals in the types of documentation that were characteristic of physical disabilities practice settings. Kent, the therapist from the case study, still occasionally experiences the medical team members' heightened interest as he reports muscle grades and sensory status, contrasted with their quizzical, glazed over looks when he describes his clients' difficulties with resuming homemaking, leisure, or other home and community skills. The OTPF provides a vehicle to communicate with others besides occupational therapists that engagement in occupation should be the primary outcome of all intervention.

The OTPF provides a language and structure that communicates occupation more meaningfully. It empowers occupational therapists to restructure evaluation, progress, and other documentation forms to reflect the primacy of occupation to what OT does, and shows the interaction of all the aspects that contribute to supporting or constraining the client's participation. Thus, by clearly showing and articulating the comprehensive nature of OT's domain of practice to clients, healthcare professionals, and other interested parties, occupational therapists enlist support and demand for their services and, most importantly, ensure that clients will receive the unique and important services that only OT provides. Of equal importance is that the Framework positions the client as a collaborator with the occupational therapist at every step of the process, thus empowering the individual as a change agent and reframing the image of the client as a passive recipient of services.

FIT BETWEEN THE OTPF AND THE ICF

There appears to be an excellent fit between the OTPF and the ICF. At about the same time the UT-III was being studied for continued suitability regarding contemporary language and practice, the WHO was also revising its language and classification model. The resulting WHO **International Classification of Functioning, Disability and Health** (ICF) contributes to the understanding of the complexity of having a physical disability.[16] The ICF "moved away from being a 'consequences of disease' classification to become a 'components of health' classification" (p. 4),[16] progressing from impairment, disability, and handicap to body functions and structures, activities, and participation. In the ICF, the term *body structures* refers to the anatomical parts of the body and *body functions* refers to a person's physiological and psychological functions. Also considered in this model is the impact of environmental and personal factors as they relate to functioning. The ICF adopted a universal model that considers health along a continuum where there is a potential for everyone to have a disability.

The ICF also provides support and reinforcement for OT to specifically address activity and activity limitations encountered by persons with disabilities.[16] This document describes, as well, the importance of participation in life situations, or domains, including (1) learning and applying knowledge, (2) general tasks and task demands, (3) communication, (4) movement, (5) self-care, (6) domestic life areas, (7) interpersonal interactions, (8) major life areas associated with work, school, and family life, and (9) community, social, and civic life. All of these domains are historically familiar areas of concern and intervention to the profession of OT. Although a physical disability may compromise a person's ability to reach up to brush his or her hair, the ICF redirects the service provider to also consider activity limitations that may result in restricted participation in desired life situations such as sports or parenting. A problem with a person's bodily structure, such as paralysis or a missing limb, is recognized as a potentially limiting factor, but that is not the focus of intervention.

Occupational therapy practitioners believe that intervention provided for people with physical disabilities should extend beyond a focus on recovery of physical skills and address the person's engagement, or active participation, in occupations. This viewpoint is the cornerstone of the Framework. Such active participation in occupation is interdependent upon the client's psychological and social well-being, which must be simultaneously addressed through the occupational therapy intervention. This orientation is congruent with the emphasis of the WHO ICF.

The language of the UT-III was, in many instances, different from that used and understood by the external audience of other healthcare professionals. Similarly, the terminology of the previous WHO classification was frequently different from that used by the audience with whom they were trying to communicate (e.g., healthcare professionals and other service providers). The goals of the new WHO classifications, the ICF, are to increase communication and understanding about the experience of having a disability and unify services. In a similar manner, the OTPF is designed to increase the knowledge and understanding of the OT profession to others and, where appropriate, incorporates the language of the ICF, as will be seen in the following discussion of the OT domain and process. Detailed information on the ICF can be found in the document referenced in this chapter[16] or an overview of

the document can be downloaded from *www3.who.int/icf/cfm*. (See Chapter 17 for further discussion of the integration of the ICF and the OTPF.)

THE OTPF: DESCRIPTION

The OTPF is composed of two interrelated parts, the domain and the process. The domain comprises the focus and factors addressed by the profession and the process describes how occupational therapy does what it does (evaluation, intervention, and outcomes), in other words, putting the domain into practice. Central to both parts is the essential concept of **occupation.** The definition of occupation used by the developers of the Framework is as follows:

Activities ... of everyday life, named, organized, and given value and meaning by individuals and a culture. Occupation is everything people do to occupy themselves, including looking after themselves, ... enjoying life, ... and contributing to the social and economic fabric of their communities ... (p. 32)[11]

Adopting this definition, the developers of the OTPF represented or characterized the profession's focus on occupation in a dynamic and action-oriented form, which they articulated as engagement in occupation to support participation in life (or context[s]). This phrase links both parts of the Framework, providing the unifying theme or focus of the occupational therapy domain, as well as the overarching outcome of the occupational therapy process.

THE OCCUPATIONAL THERAPY DOMAIN

The domain of occupational therapy encompasses the gamut of what occupational therapists do, along with the primary concern and focus of the profession's efforts. Everything that the OT does or is concerned about, as depicted in the domain of the OTPF, is directed at supporting the client's engagement in meaningful occupation that ultimately affects the health, well-being, and life satisfaction of that individual.

The six broad areas or categories of concern that comprise the occupational therapy domain include[1] performance in areas of occupation, performance skills, performance patterns, context, activity demands, and client factors (Figure 1-1). The developers of the Framework point out that there is a complex interplay among all of these areas or aspects of the domain, that no single part is more critical than another, and that all aspects are viewed as influencing engagement in occupations. Furthermore, the success of the occupational therapy process (evaluation, intervention, and outcomes) is incumbent upon the occupational therapist's expert knowledge of all aspects of the domain.

Performance in Areas of Occupation

Occupational therapists frequently use the terms *occupation* and *activity* interchangeably. The OTPF distinguishes between

ENGAGEMENT IN OCCUPATION TO SUPPORT PARTICIPATION IN CONTEXT OR CONTEXTS

Performance in Areas of Occupation

Activities of daily living (ADL)*
Instrumental activities of daily living (IADL)
Education
Work
Play
Leisure
Social participation

Performance Skills	**Performance Patterns**
Motor skills	Habits
Process skills	Routines
Communication/interaction skills	Roles

Context	**Activity Demands**	**Client Factors**
Cultural	Objects used and their properties	Body functions
Physical	Space demands	Body structures
Social	Social demands	
Personal	Sequencing and timing	
Spiritual	Required actions	
Temporal	Required body functions	
Virtual	Required body structures	

*Also referred to as basic activities of daily living (BADL) or personal activities of daily living (PADL)

Figure 1-1   Occupational therapy domain. (From American Occupational Therapy Association: Occupational therapy practice framework: domain and process, *Am J Occup Ther* 56(6):609, 2002.)

activities and occupations but confirms that both have similarities and are within the domain of occupational therapy. Activities are characterized as being meaningful and goal-directed but not considered by the individual to be of central importance to her or his life. Similarly, occupations are viewed as (1) activities in which the client engages, (2) activities that have the added qualitative criteria of giving meaning to the person's life and contributing to one's identity, and (3) activities in which the individual looks forward to engaging. For example, Karen, Kent's client with quadriplegia, regards herself as an excellent and dedicated clothes and accessories shopper; holidays and celebrations always include her engagement in her treasured occupation of shopping. Kent, on the other hand, regards the activity of shopping for clothes as important only to keep himself clothed and maintain social acceptance. Kent avoids the activity whenever possible. Each engages in this activity to support participation in life but with a qualitatively different attitude and level of enthusiasm. Within the OTPF, both of these closely related terms are used, recognizing that individual clients will determine which they regard as occupations and which are simply necessary activities that support their participation in life; for Kent shopping is an activity but for Karen it is a favorite occupation.

Included in the **areas of occupation** category of the domain are seven comprehensive types of human activities or occupations. Each is outlined below, with a listing of typical

activities that are included in each, and examples from the physical disability perspective as provided by Karen's circumstances.

Activities of daily living (ADLs) (also referred to as *personal activities of daily living* [PADLs] or *basic activities of daily living* [BADLs]) are those activities that have to do with accomplishing one's own personal body care. The body care activities included in this category are bathing/showering, bowel and bladder management, dressing, eating, feeding, functional mobility, personal device care, personal hygiene and grooming, sexual activity, sleep/rest, and toilet hygiene.

Instrumental activities of daily living (IADLs) are those "activities that are oriented toward interacting with the

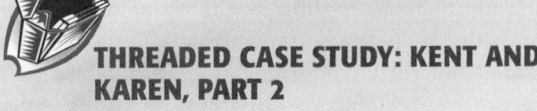

THREADED CASE STUDY: KENT AND KAREN, PART 2

As Kent perused the list of ADLs, he noted that virtually every category, with the exception of eating (which involves the ability to keep and manipulate food in the mouth and the ability to swallow), would be of concern to his client Karen because of the nature and extent of her SCI disability. When Kent discussed this list with Karen, she viewed practically all as necessary activities

THREADED CASE STUDY: KENT AND KAREN, PART 2—cont'd

but personally valued feeding, sexual activity, sleep/rest, and personal hygiene and grooming as being extremely important to her satisfactory participation in life. Karen was a little surprised to learn that sexual activity was included; "So this is occupational therapy? Maybe I'll wait awhile before I talk about this topic... but it's good to know I'm expected to be interested though," she thought.

For the present, Karen turned her attention to and took particular interest in the activities included in the personal hygiene and grooming category and its detailed description (found in Table 1 in the Appendix of the OTPF): "Obtaining and using supplies, removing body hair (use of razors, tweezers, lotions, etc.), applying and removing cosmetics, washing, drying, combing, styling, brushing and trimming hair; caring for nails (hands and feet), caring for skin, ears, eyes, and nose, applying deodorant, cleaning mouth, brushing and flossing teeth; or removing, cleaning, and reinserting dental orthotics and prosthetics" (p. 620).[1] The numerous details reminded her of how important all of these grooming activities were to her and were suggestive of the scope of the daily activities she would like to address in OT. Of particular concern to Karen were the grooming activities of plucking her eyebrows and styling her hair; these were bodily care activities she regarded as very personal. In fact, she was reluctant to let anyone do these for her. Though under similar circumstances these two ADLs might be gladly deferred by Kent, it was clear that Karen would prioritize them as personally meaningful occupational goals.

In studying the list of ADLs, Kent noted that each ADL item listed, just like personal hygiene and grooming, had a similarly helpful definition and detailed list of examples located in the Tables of the Appendix of the OTPF. He remembered reading that these lists were there to give a few examples, were not to be considered exhaustive, and in fact, there was an expectation that the lists would be modified and expanded upon as the OTPF became more familiar and integrated into practice.

environment and that are often complex. IADLs are generally optional in nature, that is, may be delegated to another" (p. 620).[1] The specific IADLs included in the domain are care of others (including selecting and supervising caregivers), care of pets, child rearing, communication device use, community mobility, financial management, health management and maintenance, home establishment and management, meal preparation and cleanup, safety procedures and emergency responses, and shopping. Knowing that the IADL of shopping was certain to be a priority occupation for Karen, Kent made a note of the full description of shopping from the corresponding lists of IADLs in Table 1 of the OTPF document. Shopping is described there as "Preparing shopping lists (grocery and other); selecting and purchasing items; selecting method of

payment; and completing money transactions" (p. 620).[1] This is not as detailed as some descriptions, but it is a good start for looking at the related activities that would have to be addressed if Kent and Karen were to collaborate on Karen's resumption of engagement in shopping. Kent noted too that community mobility included driving and using public transportation, another IADL that would be important to explore with Karen as she contemplates returning to paid work. In fact, the entire list of IADLs held numerous concerns to be addressed in OT.

Education is an area of occupation that includes "activities needed for being a student and participating in a learning environment" (p. 620).[1] Specific education activity subcategories include formal education participation, exploration of informal personal educational needs or interests (beyond formal education), and informal personal education participation. Table 1 of the OTPF similarly includes more details regarding what specific activities each of these subcategories could entail.

Work includes activities associated with both paid work and volunteer efforts. Specific categories of activities and concerns related to work include employment interests and pursuits, employment seeking and acquisition, job performance, retirement preparation and adjustment, volunteer exploration, and volunteer participation.

Activities associated with play are described as "Any spontaneous or organized activity that provides enjoyment, entertainment, amusement, or diversion" (p. 252).[12] Considered under this area of occupation are play exploration and play participation.

Leisure is defined as "...nonobligatory activity that is intrinsically motivated and engaged in during discretionary time, that is, time not committed to obligatory occupations such as work, self-care or sleep" (p. 250).[12] Leisure exploration and leisure participation are the major categories of activity in the leisure area of occupation. Karen shared with Kent her interests in spending leisure time listening to music, traveling, antiquing, swimming, playing bridge, and reading books. When looking at the description of leisure, it occurred to Kent that for Karen, shopping might also be characterized as a leisure activity as well as an IADL. It would probably depend upon the circumstances or context in which it was engaged, he thought, another parameter of the OTPF domain he would be learning.

Social participation is an area of occupation that encompasses the activities, occupations, and behaviors that support or constrain engagement in human relationships that are associated with participation in social interaction in the categories of community, family, peer, or friend. Just as in previously discussed areas of occupation, Table 1 of the OTPF provides definitions and more detailed information regarding the breadth of activities that comprise OT's involvement in work, play, leisure, and social participation. Like Kent, readers who are currently learning the OTPF could benefit from studying these expanded lists to broaden their understanding of occupational therapy's domain. As Kent studied these sections of Table 1, he found it helpful to make note of the content of each as illustrated by activities that were relevant to Karen in these areas of occupation. For example, Kent considered the range of job skills and work routines necessary for Karen to return to her paid work as an administrative assistant as well as similar concerns involved with resumption of her preferred play and leisure occupations including swimming, reading, and board games. Kent was also reminded of the importance of considering the activities that can support or constrain Karen's continued social participation in her community as a Girl Scout leader, in her family as the oldest daughter, and with her treasured circle of friends.

Performance Skills and Performance Patterns

The next main areas of the domain to consider are performance skills and performance patterns. Both are related to the client's capabilities in performance in the areas of occupation previously described and can be viewed as the actions and behaviors that are observed by the OT as the client engages in occupations.

The category of **performance skills** includes three components of concern: motor skills, process skills, and communication/interaction skills. The client's successful engagement in occupation or occupational performance is dependent upon having or achieving adequate ability in performance skills. Problems in any of the three areas of performance skills are the focus for formulating short-term goals or objectives to reach the long-term goal of addressing participation in occupation.

Motor skills consist of the movement and interactions observed while the individual is interacting with task objects and the environment while engaging in a particular activity or occupation including such aspects as posture, coordination, effort seemingly being exerted, and manipulation of objects. Kent observed Karen as she played a game of bridge with friends one afternoon in the OT clinic. Observing for performance skills, and in particular motor skills, Kent noted that Karen *looped* one elbow around the upright of her wheelchair, *leaned* her trunk towards the table, *reached* her other arm towards the card holder, and successfully *grasped* a card after three unsuccessful attempts (which Kent perceived as indicating *effort* and difficulty with the task).

Process skills include those observable actions taken to manage and modify the occupational task such as using knowledge, attending to, discerning solutions to problems with, and organizing the task including choosing appropriate tools and methods for performing the task. While Karen played cards, Kent also observed her process skills as she set up her card holder so that her cards were not visible to her opponents (selecting proper equipment and arranging the space), perused her cards, paused, rearranged them using her tenodesis hand splint (attending to the task, using both knowledge of bridge and selection of proper equipment), and then stated her bid (demonstrating discernment and problem solving).

Communication/interaction skills, the third category of performance skills, involve those observable actions and behaviors that indicate how the client "conveys his or her intentions and needs and coordinates social behavior to act together with people" (p. 612)[1] while engaging in activities or occupations. Such skills could include asking for information, expressing affect, and interacting or relating in a manner with others that supports engagement in the activity. While playing cards, Karen was observed to be furrowing her brow, squinting her eyes shut in a thoughtful cogitating manner, pursing her lips, and showing neither happiness nor despair on her face as she studied her cards in the card holder (expressing affect consistent with the activity of card playing). As she reached for the cards the holder moved out of her reach; she asked the friend next to her to push it back, cautioning her in a smiling and light manner "Don't dare look!" (demonstrating her ability to ask for assistance and using socially acceptable teasing behavior that enlists an opponent's cooperation in preserving the secrecy of her cards, thus conveying the image indicative of a savvy card player). Her observable communication/interaction behaviors support Karen's continued inclusion with friends in a favorite leisure occupation.

Each of these particular motor skills, process skills, and communication/interaction skills categories has detailed lists of representative skills annotated with definitions, descriptions, and examples outlined in Table 2: Performance Skills, in the OTPF document. (See Chapter 17 for additional and more detailed information regarding performance skills.)

Performance patterns are those observable patterns of behavior that support or constrain the client's engagement in occupation. Types or categories of patterns include habits, routines, and roles.

Habits are described as small patterns of behavior or small parts of occupations that with repetition become an automatic part of the individual's behavior. Routines reflect how the individual configures or sequences occupations throughout his or her daily life. Habits typically contribute (positively or negatively) to one's occupational routines and both are established with repetition over time. The role category of performance patterns is regarded as being composed of "sets of behaviors that have some socially agreed upon function and for which there is an accepted code of norms" (p. 603).[5]

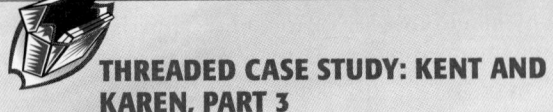

THREADED CASE STUDY: KENT AND KAREN, PART 3

Some might view Karen's engagement in the occupation of paid work as an example of the role of worker. Inherent in this role are accepted norms that customarily include regular attendance, timely adherence to schedules, and acceptance of responsibility for completing assignments. Karen's work role is consistent with the sets of behaviors that would be expected of an administrative assistant at a busy law firm including arriving at work on time, handling e-mail and other correspondence in a professional

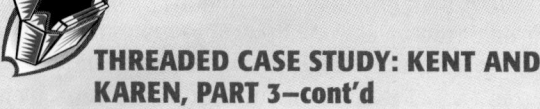

THREADED CASE STUDY: KENT AND KAREN, PART 3—cont'd

manner, managing the office budget and payroll according to accepted audit practices, and interacting with her supervisors, co-workers, and supervisees in a fair and respectful manner, to name just a few.

Karen's workday routine involves waking at 6:30 am, showering, grooming, and dressing, driving to work with a stop for breakfast on the way, and early arrival at work at 7:45 for an 8:00 am expected work start. For Karen, a habit she regards as beneficial to her workday routine is her prompt use of her day planner to record appointments, phone numbers, and additions to her things-to-do list. Another habit she believes contributes to the success of her workday routine is selecting her clothing the night before to save time in the morning, thus ensuring a punctual arrival at work. A habit that negatively affects her daily work routine is hitting the snooze button on her alarm clock. Both Kent and Karen recognize that though Karen may resume her work occupation or worker role, her ability to carry out the expected behaviors and her customary habits and routines will be substantially altered as the result of her SCI.

Karen's occupational performance, performance skills, and patterns will be significantly influenced by the next three main areas of the domain to be discussed, namely, contexts, activity demands, and client factors.

Contexts

In the OTPF, **contexts** are regarded as the circumstances or events that influence the client's occupational performance and form the environment within which engagement in occupation takes place. Contexts can either support or constrain engagement in occupation to support participation. In the OTPF domain, contexts are composed of seven categories or types including cultural, physical, social, personal, spiritual, temporal, and virtual. Several of the categories of context are regarded as external to the individual such as physical, social, and virtual contexts; some are viewed as internal to the client, such as personal and spiritual. Some contexts, such as culture, provide an external expectation of behavior that is often converted into an internal belief. Table 4 in the OTPF document provides detailed definitions and examples of each of these categories. For example, the category *physical* encompasses the "nonhuman aspects of contexts. Includes the accessibility to and performance within environments having natural terrain, plants, animals, buildings, furniture, objects, tools or devices" (p. 623).[1] Personal context describes "Features of the individual that are not part of the health status" (p. 17).[16] Personal context includes age, gender, socioeconomic status, and educational status.

Each of these contexts, as they pertain to Karen's specific circumstances, will significantly affect her future engagement in occupation. Karen's *physical context* includes aspects that will support her engagement in occupation including an accessible work site and a reliable and accessible system of public transportation in her neighborhood as well as a well-appointed downtown area of stores, shops, and restaurants within wheelchair distance. Those aspects of her physical context that may interfere with resumption of occupation include Karen's inaccessible 2nd floor apartment and small inaccessible bathroom. Supportive aspects of Karen's *personal context* are her college education in business and the fact that she has unemployment insurance that will supplement her sick leave and continue her health coverage. From a *social context* perspective, Karen is supported by both her family and friends; additionally, her employer and co-workers are anxious to have her come back to the law firm. Karen's *spiritual context* provides her the reassurance that her spinal cord injury (SCI) was part of a higher power's plan for her and that she will be given the strength to cope and succeed. The mainstream American *cultural context* in which Karen was reared, which values and supports the concepts of hard work overcoming adversity (doing rather than being) and the importance of independence (individualism), seemingly motivates Karen to resume engagement in previous levels of occupation for full participation in all contexts of her life.[7]

Given the difficulty that resuming Karen's shopping occupation may present, Kent suggested the possibility of using online shopping for some items. Although interested, Karen indicated that her preference was to shop "in the real world" instead of using the *virtual context* of computers and airways. Her ultimate decisions will no doubt be influenced by the changes she experiences in her *temporal contexts* as Karen experiences and adjusts to the increased amounts of time, and scheduling of and around the time of others, required to accomplish basic daily routines that, in turn, support her engagement in preferred occupations.

Activity Demands

Activity demands are focused on the activity and what is required to engage in the activity. Included in this section are several aspects that must be addressed for a client to perform that specific activity, including the following: objects and their properties, space demands, social demands, sequencing and timing, required actions, required body functions, and required body structures. Table 5 of the OTPF document provides a comprehensive list of definitions and examples for a clearer understanding of each of these categories.[1] Consider Karen's interest in shopping in the "real world" instead of making clothing purchases online using a virtual context. The *materials or tools needed* would be a purse or credit card holder. The *space demands* would be the accessibility of the store or shopping mall and the dressing room for Karen to try the clothes on before making a purchase. The *social demands* include paying for the items before leaving the store. The *sequence and timing* process includes being able to make a selection, go to the register, potentially wait in line, place the clothing on the counter, pay for the item, and then leave the store. The *required actions* refers to the necessary performance skills to engage in this activity such as the coordination needed to try on clothing, the process skills needed to select one sweater or blouse from a large array of possible choices, and the communication skills needed to ask for assistance or directions if needed.

These performance skills are not viewed in isolation but are seen as Karen engages in the activity of clothes shopping. The *required body functions and structures* refer to the basic client factors needed to perform the activity of shopping. The act of shopping requires a level of consciousness because inherent in the activity of shopping is having the opportunity to make a choice between available items. Karen's ability to engage in the activity demand of making a choice of purchases is indicative of her adequate level of consciousness for shopping.

Client Factors

The OTPF describes **client factors** in a manner similar to the ICF.[1,16] There are two categories in this portion of the OTPF: body functions and body structures. The body structure category refers to the integrity of the actual body part such as the integrity of the eye for vision (see Chapter 23) or the integrity of a limb (see Chapter 43). When the integrity of the body structure is compromised, it can impact function or require alternative approaches to engagement in activities, such as enlarged print for persons with macular degeneration or the use of a prosthetic device for a person who sustained a below elbow amputation. It is unlikely that this category of the domain would have application to Karen, because the integrity of her body structures is not necessarily compromised by her diagnosis. Should she develop a pressure sore, a possible complication of SCI, where the integrity of the body structure (i.e., skin) is compromised, her ability to engage in occupation could become significantly limited requiring alternative approaches such as positioning devices and adaptive equipment to compensate for the need to stay off the pressure sore.

The body function category of client factors refers to the physiological and psychological functions of the body and includes a variety of systems including for example the neuromusculoskeletal and movement-related functions. This category of body functions includes muscle function, which in turn includes muscle strength. A distinction is made between body functions and performance skills. Performance skills, as was described earlier, are observed as the client engages in an occupation or activity. The category of body function refers to the available ability of the client's body to function. A client may have the available neuromuscular function (client factor of body function; specifically, muscle strength) to hold a comb, bring the comb to the top of the head, and strength to pull the comb through the hair, but when you ask the client to comb his or her hair (an activity) you observe that the client has difficulties manipulating the comb in the hand

(motor skill of manipulation) and smoothly using the comb to comb hair (motor skill of flow). These motor skills are included as performance skills in the OTPF.

In Karen's case, absence of functioning muscles in her hands necessitates the use of a functional hand splint or adaptive writing device to enable her to sign the credit card receipt, a required action in her shopping occupation. In order to use a wrist-driven flexor hinge (i.e., tenodesis) hand splint to hold the pen, she must have adequate body function; in this case, Fair+ or better muscle strength in her radial wrist extensors. However, Karen must have adequate performance skills including the motor skills to exert enough force to adequately write her name, the process skills to select a type of pen that requires minimum effort to operate, and the communication/interaction skills to ask sales personnel for a firm writing surface (clip board) for her lap to compensate for the inaccessibility of the checkout counter.

The mental functions group includes affective, cognitive, and perceptual abilities. This group also includes the experience of self and body image (see Chapters 6, 24, and 25). A client, such as Karen, who has sustained a physically disabling injury, frequently may have an altered self-concept, lowered self-esteem, depression, anxiety, decreased coping skills, and other problems with emotional functions following the injury[14] (see Chapter 6). Sensory functions and pain are also included in the body functions category (see Chapters 22 and 27). Neuromuscular and movement-related functions refer to the available strength range of motion and movement (see Chapters 18-21), but do not refer to the client's application of these factors to activities or occupations as was seen in the example of Karen signing a credit card receipt as part of engaging in the occupation of shopping. The body functions category also refers to the ability of the cardiovascular, respiratory, digestive, metabolic, and genitourinary systems to function to support client participation. These are further described in both the OTPF and the ICF. The reader is referred to the OTPF Table 6 for a more detailed description of each function included in this category.

THE OCCUPATIONAL THERAPY PROCESS

As was described at the beginning of this chapter, the OTPF consists of two parts: the domain and the process (Fig. 1-2). From a very general perspective, the domain describes the scope of practice or answers the question: "What does an occupational therapist do?" The process describes the methods of providing occupational therapy services or answers the question: "How does an occupational therapist provide occupational therapy services?"

The process is briefly outlined here for continuity but the reader is referred to Chapter 3 for a more in-depth discussion. The primary focus of OTPF process is **evaluation** of the client's occupational abilities and needs to determine and provide services (intervention) that foster and support occupational performance (outcomes). Throughout the process the focus is on occupation; the evaluation begins with

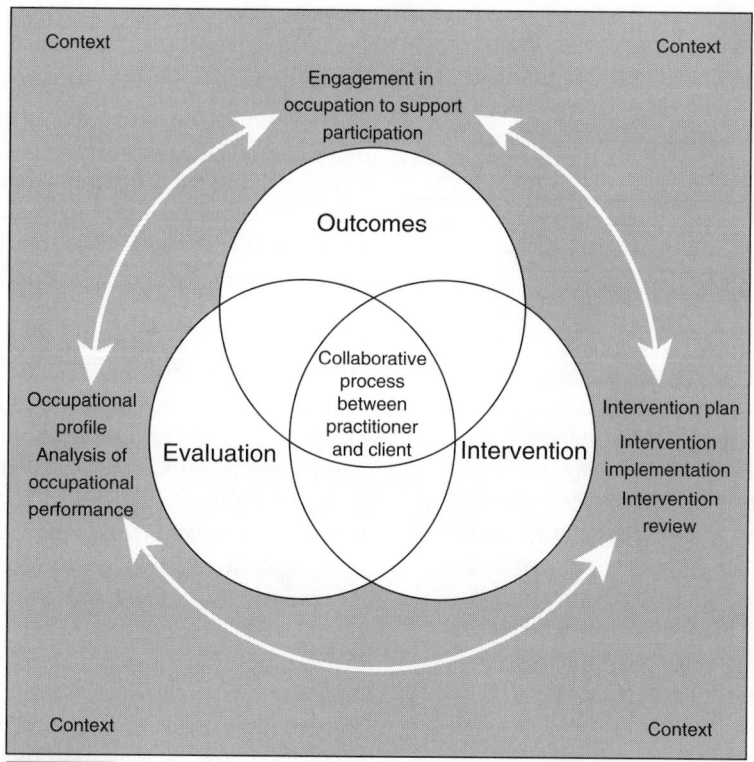

Figure 1-2   Occupational therapy process. (From American Occupational Therapy Association: Occupational therapy practice framework: domain and process, *Am J Occup Ther* 56(6):609, 2002.)

TABLE **1-1** **Types of Intervention**

Type of Intervention	Description
Therapeutic use of self	OT uses own self and all that entails (knowledge, personality, and experience), conveying empathy, active listening, and establishing trust
Therapeutic use of occupations and activities:	Client engages in the occupation
Occupation-based activity	Client learns and practices parts or portions of occupations
Purposeful activity	Methods that prepare client for
Preparatory methods	purposeful or occupation-based activity
Consultation process	OT uses knowledge and expertise in collaborating with client to ID problem and develop and try solutions; it is up to client to implement final recommendation
Education process	OT shares knowledge and expertise about engaging in occupation with the client but client does not actually engage in the occupation during the intervention

determining the client's occupational profile and occupational history. Preferred intervention methods are occupation-based and the overall outcome of the process is the client's engagement in occupation for participation in context(s).

Types of Occupational Therapy Intervention

Table 1-1 shows the types of occupational therapy intervention typically used in physical disability practice and their relationship to the domain of occupational therapy. Four general categories of intervention are presented in the OTPF: (1) therapeutic use of self, (2) therapeutic use of occupations and activities, a category composed of preparatory methods, purposeful activity, and occupation-based activity, (3) consultation process, and (4) education process. Because the OTPF has occupation as its primary focus, it is deceptive to think of the types of interventions as being selected or provided in any type of linear or stepwise order on a continuum. Rather, the occupational therapist reflects upon the client's goal of engagement in his or her preferred self-selected occupations and collaborates with the client in selecting the type, or types, of intervention the occupational therapist deems will most successfully facilitate achievement of the occupational goal. Since the inception of the OTPF, the previous concept of intervention levels has been dismissed in favor of viewing them as types of intervention in which no one type is considered of less or more importance than another, but rather each has a potential contribution in facilitating the ultimate goal of engagement in occupation to support participation in contexts.

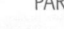

OT PRACTICE NOTE

Throughout the OT process, the therapist should convey to the client that *together* they will select the outcomes based upon the client's choice and collaborate in planning the intervention, thus establishing the beginnings of an atmosphere of caring and trust.

THREADED CASE STUDY: KENT AND KAREN, PART 4

Though Kent did not previously regard therapeutic use of self as an OT intervention, he has valued it highly and uses it in his practice. Clients respond well to Kent's caring and gentle approach. He enjoys the personal and interactive aspects of the therapeutic relationship, shows genuine interest in his clients' histories, actively listens to their responses, and makes it a practice to introduce himself and his role to his clients as the first step in the process. This practice allows Kent to assert the primacy of the client and associate and integrate the new information he is learning about the client with the image of the person he has just met.

Kent used therapeutic use of self as a type of intervention throughout the occupational therapy process with Karen. He brought to the process his 25 years of experience and knowledge of SCI as well as his experiential lessons of providing successful and not so successful OT intervention with numerous clients. Kent's college roommate and subsequent best friend has a physical disability, an experience that served to increase Kent's understanding and inform his attitudes and beliefs toward the experience of having a disability. His close and loving relationships with his sisters, wife, and teenage daughters provide him with an increased awareness of women's concerns and issues and cause him to consider how disability might be experienced differently by his women clients than by his men clients. All of these aspects of Kent's personal and professional repertoire support his ability to employ therapeutic use of self as an effective intervention in Karen's OT process.

Therapeutic use of self

The OTPF describes the therapeutic use of self as "A practitioner's planned use of his or her personality, insights, perceptions, and judgments as part of the therapeutic process" (p. 628).[1] Occupational therapy literature describes an OT who successfully uses therapeutic use of self for intervention as having the qualities or attributes of showing empathy (including sensitivity to the client's disability, age, gender, religion, socioeconomic status, education, and cultural background), being self-reflective and self-aware, and being able to communicate effectively using active listening and consistently keeping a client-centered perspective that in turn engenders an atmosphere of trust.[4,8,13]

The very focus of the occupational therapy process provides a favorable context to support the OT's use of therapeutic use of self as intervention. By using a client-centered approach and beginning the process with an evaluation that seeks information about the client's occupational history and occupational preferences, the therapist's initial interactions with the client are characterized to the client as being interested in what the client does (occupational performance), who the client is (contexts), and what occupations give meaning to the client's life.

Therapeutic use of occupations and activities

This category of occupational therapy intervention in the OTPF was adapted from the section "Treatment Continuum in the Context of Occupational Performance" (Chapter 1, p. 7) in the 5th edition of this book. The category is defined in the OTPF as "Occupations and activities selected for specific clients that meet therapeutic goals. To use occupations/activities therapeutically, context or contexts, activity demands, and client factors all should be considered in relation to the client's therapeutic goals" (p. 628).[1] Specific activities considered to be representative of the category, therapeutic use of occupations and activities, are further separated into three types including occupation-based activity, purposeful activity, and preparatory methods that will each be discussed below.

Occupation-based activity

In the OTPF, the purpose of occupation-based activity is described as allowing "clients to engage in actual occupations that are part of their own context and that match their goals" (p. 628).[1] Reading this description, Kent considers that occupation-based activity as intervention would include providing intervention to promote engagement in all areas of occupation including ADL, IADL, education, work, play, leisure, and social participation. The vast majority of occupational therapy intervention for Karen was occupation-based activity. To reach her targeted goal of resuming her favorite leisure occupation of clothes shopping, Kent and Karen took a trip to a nearby department store where Karen looked for a blouse with three-quarter-inch sleeves and a button-front closure. Karen perused the carousels inspecting the available blouses, asked for help from a sales person, tried on blouses in the dressing room, made her selection, and paid for her purchase, all parts of a typical shopping excursion in a natural shopping environment. Kent demonstrated and gave suggestions when necessary for how Karen could perform some of the more difficult shopping activities, such as accessing the crowded carousels, negotiating her wheelchair into the dressing room from a narrow hallway, and transporting the hangers with blouses on her lap without having them slide to the ground.

Purposeful activity

This type of intervention "allows the client to engage in goal-directed behaviors or activities within a therapeutically designed context that lead to an occupation or occupations"

(p. 628).[1] A few examples offered in the OTPF document include "practice vegetable slicing" and "role play to learn ways to manage anger" (p. 628).[1] The description of the purpose and the examples offered caused Kent to reframe or slightly reconfigure his view of what purposeful activity entailed. Given the OTPF categorization, he considered that he was providing purposeful activity intervention when he had Karen practicing activities that she would encounter as part of the occupation-based activity of clothes shopping. In the OT clinic, prior to the shopping trip, Karen and Kent collaborated on her being able to perform the purposeful activities of tearing checks out of her check book, accessing her credit card from her wallet, using a button hook to button her sweater, and lifting clothes on hangers out of a closet. Some of the shopping activities she encountered while buying her blouse were learned as part of other occupation-based interventions such as wheelchair mobility, writing, and dressing. When using purposeful activity, the OT practitioner is concerned primarily with assessing and remediating deficits in performance skills and performance patterns.

Preparatory methods

Intervention that is in nature preparatory "prepares the client for occupational performance. It is used in preparation for purposeful and occupation-based activities" (p. 628).[1] Preparatory methods used by occupational therapy may include exercise, facilitation and inhibition techniques, positioning, sensory stimulation, selected physical agent modalities, and provision of orthotic devices such as braces and splints. Occupational therapy services for persons with physical disabilities often introduce these methods and devices during the acute stages of illness or injury. When using these methods, the occupational therapist is likely to be most concerned with assessing and remediating problems with client factors such as body structures and body functions. It is important for occupational therapists to plan the progression of this type of intervention so that the selected methods are used as preparation for purposeful or occupation-based activity and are directed toward the overarching goal of engagement in the areas of occupation to support participation in contexts.

Kent reflected that in preparation for Karen's occupation-based intervention of clothes shopping he used several interventions that would be considered as preparatory methods. For example, he and Karen looked at her options for grasping items and decided upon a tenodesis hand splint, using orthotics as an intervention. To use the splint more effectively she had to have stronger wrist extensors and, to push her wheelchair or to reach for and lift hangers with clothes, she needed stronger shoulder muscles; thus, the preparatory intervention of exercise was chosen to facilitate ultimate engagement in purposeful and occupation-based activities.

Consultation process

Consultation is not a new activity or service provided by OT but is now viewed or labeled as an intervention and situated or integrated into what is considered part of the occupational therapy process. It is defined as "A type of intervention in which practitioners use their knowledge and expertise to collaborate with the client. The collaborative process involves identifying the problem, creating possible solutions, trying solutions, and altering them as necessary for greater effectiveness. When providing consultation, the practitioner is not directly responsible for the outcome of the intervention" (p. 113).[10]

As Kent studied this description, he considered that throughout his career he has provided occupational therapy services that he would now regard as consultative in nature as described in the OTPF. For example, Kent provided consultation with a small chain of grocery stores where he assessed the accessibility and made recommendations to help them reach compliance with the guidelines of the Americans with Disability Act (ADA) (see Chapter 14). Based upon his extensive knowledge of the ADA and his expertise in the activity demands for grocery shopping, his recommendations included suggestions for accessible parking and store layout, arrangement of shelves, adaptive equipment to enhance the shopping activity for people with a variety of disabilities, employee training to increase awareness of the shopping needs of people with disabilities, and many other ideas for streamlining the shopping experience for this population. After Kent completed the report of his recommendations and shared them with his client (the owners of the grocery store chain) he had completed his OT intervention and it was up to the client to implement his suggestions. Many of Kent's clients with SCI could potentially benefit from the implemented suggestions he had made, but this is not part of the consultation process intervention.

Education process

The OTPF describes education process as a "type of intervention process that involves the imparting of knowledge and information about occupation and activity and that does not result in the actual performance of the occupation/activity" (p. 628).[1] Kent also considered this definition, thinking of instances when he provided this type of intervention. Most recently, with Karen, he responded to her concerns about returning to her job as an administrative assistant. She was having misgivings about the amount of physical work and energy involved; the modest amount of salary she received, which barely covered her pre-injury expenses; and the additional expenses she would have for personal and household assistance. Using his years of knowledge and experience, Kent provided intervention in the form of educating Karen about her options by informing her about the services offered by vocational rehabilitation, educating her about the possibilities and opportunities for further education to support her work goal of becoming an attorney, a job position, he pointed out, that held potential for higher pay and one that could be less physically demanding than her administrative assistant position. He informed her about the similar circumstances of some of his former clients, describing the various scenarios and outcomes of each (being mindful to preserve the former clients' anonymity and privacy), as well as using his wealth of experience to discuss the many resources available to facilitate such options. Karen was already preparing to resume her job (an occupational goal she prioritized) and was actively participating in OT by engaging in occupation-based activity that involved her actual work occupations and supporting activities. The education process intervention described, however, provided her knowledge of options but did not involve any actual performance of an activity during the intervention.

Having studied the OTPF domain, process, and types of interventions and reinforcing his learning through application of his new knowledge to his own circumstances and those of his client Karen, Kent still felt the need for some additional suggestions or strategies for learning the OTPF more thoroughly. Such strategies are explored in the next section.

STRATEGIES FOR LEARNING THE OTPF

The most effective first step in learning the OTPF may be to obtain and thoroughly read the original document, making notations as points arise, drawing diagrams for increased understanding, writing questions or observations in the margins, and consulting tables, figures, and the glossary when directed, to reinforce or explicate new learning. The OTPF is a comprehensive conceptualization of the profession that requires a substantial investment of time and commitment to study and apply to practice before one feels comfortable in its use. Box 1-1 provides an abbreviated list of some of the core terminology and concepts of the framework to serve as a quick reference or to jog the reader's memory when first learning and using the OTPF.

More experienced occupational therapists who are accustomed to using the UT-III will find it helpful to consult the comparison of terms section at the end of the *AJOT* article on the OTPF,[2] where terminology used in the Framework is compared to that of the rescinded UT-III and the current ICF. Another, lengthier article entitled "From UT-III to the Framework: Making the Language Work,"[9] similarly compares the three documents. Both articles provide helpful tables showing the language of the UT-III, the OTPF counterpart, and that of the ICF. For example, one section of this table shows Performance Area (UT-III), Performance in Areas of Occupation (OTPF), and Activities and Participation (ICF), giving indications of the specific language used by each to name similar constructs. The occupational therapist can easily find the previous or older designation in one column, consider the new replacement terminology of the OTPF in another column, and locate the corresponding term from the ICF in yet another column.

BOX **1-1**	OCCUPATIONAL THERAPY PRACTICE FRAMEWORK QUICK GUIDE

I. Engagement in occupation to support participation in life: OT's unique contribution to health
   A. Overarching theme of the domain
   B. Overarching outcome of the process
II. Framework composed of two interrelated parts: domain and process
III. Domain = What OTs do; no single aspect considered more critical than another
   A. Performance in areas of occupation (ADL, IADL, education, work, play, leisure, social participation)
   B. Performance skills (motor skills, process skills, communication/interaction skills)
   C. Performance patterns (habits, routines, roles)
   D. Context (cultural, physical, social, personal, spiritual, temporal, virtual)
   E. Activity demands (space demands, social demands, sequencing and timing, required actions, required body functions, required body structures)
   F. Client factors (body functions, body structures)
IV. Process = How OTs provide their services; collaborative process between client and OT
   A. Evaluation (occupational profile, analysis of occupational performance)
   B. Intervention (preferred term over *treatment*; includes intervention plan, intervention implementation, intervention review)
   C. Outcomes: all goals aimed at overarching goal of engagement in occupation to support participation in life
V. Client: recipient of OT services (preferred term but actual term varies by practice setting; could be patient, student, consumer, employees, employer)
   A. Individual (broad view of client; could be actual person with a disability or individual providing support for the client such as caregiver)
   B. Groups (individuals within the context of a group)
   C. Populations/organizations/communities (individuals within)
VI. Client-centered approach or top-down approach to the evaluation and provision of the intervention: emphasis on the client and his or her goals
VII. Occupation vs. activity: activities are characterized as being meaningful and goal-directed but not of central importance to the life of the individual whereas occupations are viewed as activities that give meaning to the person's life, contribute to one's identity, and those to which the individual looks forward to engaging
VIII. Engagement: includes both the subjective (emotional or psychological) and objective (physically observable) aspects of performance

Several pioneering authors wrote helpful articles demonstrating application of the OTPF for the various AOTA Special Interest Sections. Siebert, writing for the Home and Community Health SIS, encouraged that it is "not as important to learn the OTPF as to use it as a tool to communicate practice, to support practice patterns that facilitate engagement in occupation, and to reflect on and refine our practice" (p. 4).[15] She also points out the dominant role that context plays in home and community practice by providing continuity to the client, noting how firmly the OTPF supports this concept. She expresses her belief that the focus of the framework on occupation and the beginning of the process with the client's occupational profile assures that the results of OT intervention will matter to the client.[15]

Coppola, writing for the *Gerontology SIS*, describes how the framework can be applied to geriatric practice and explains that the evaluation is one of OT's most powerful ways of informing others (including clients and colleagues) what OT is and what OT does. She provides a working draft of an Occupational Therapy Evaluation Summary Form that was developed to incorporate the OTPF and highlight occupation in a very visual way into her practice in a geriatric clinic. The draft is unconstrained by the more traditional documentation forms that seem to bury occupation under diagnostic and clinical terminology.[6]

Similarly, Boss offered readers of the *Technology SIS* his reflection upon how the framework can be operationalized in an assistive technology setting. Addressing each of the categories of the domain, he offers examples of how assistive technology both supports engagement in occupation (allowing completion of an activity or occupation) and use of assistive technology (personal device care and device use) can be an occupation in, and of, itself. He concludes his article by pointing out that "assistive technologies are all about supporting the client's participation in the contexts of their choice and are therefore part of the core of occupational therapy" (p. 2).[3]

Another strategy intended to facilitate the reader's education in the OTPF is the format of the chapters in this book as described below.

THE OTPF: ITS USE IN THIS BOOK

In keeping with the OTPF's central focus on the client and the importance of contexts and participation in occupation, each chapter begins with a case study and then integrates the information presented with consideration of that client and circumstances, similar to the use of Kent and Karen's experiences as described throughout this chapter. As the particular content information is presented, the reader is frequently asked to reflect back to the case scenario and consider how the information applies to the specifics of the client portrayed. The probative questions asked at the conclusion of the case study are also answered throughout the text or addressed at the end of the chapter.

SUMMARY

The Occupational Therapy Practice Framework was developed by the profession to reassert its focus on occupation and clearly articulate and enhance the understanding of the domain of occupational therapy (what OT practitioners do) and the occupational therapy process (how they do it) to both internal audiences (members of the profession) and external audiences (clients, healthcare professionals and interested others). The overarching goal of the Framework is engagement in occupation to support participation in context or contexts, which emphasizes the primacy of occupation, regarding it both as the theme of the domain and the outcome of the process.

The domain includes six categories that comprise the scope of occupational therapy, including performance in areas of occupation, performance skills and performance patterns, contexts, activity demands, and client factors. The OT process involves three interactive phases of occupational therapy services including evaluation, intervention, and outcomes, which occur in a collaborative and nonlinear manner. The types of occupational therapy intervention included in the Framework and typically employed in physical disabilities practice settings include therapeutic use of self, therapeutic use of occupations and activities (including occupation-based activity, purposeful activity, and preparatory methods), consultation process, and education process. In addition to studying the chapter, readers are encouraged to explore the AOTA's OTPF document in its entirety and reinforce their learning by applying the framework to their own life experiences and those of the clients they encounter in the case studies presented throughout the chapters of the book as well as those they experience in the clinic.

Review Questions

1. Briefly describe the history of the evolution of the Occupational Therapy Practice Framework.
2. Describe the need for the OTPF in the practice of occupational therapy for persons with physical disabilities.
3. Describe the fit between the OTPF and the ICF and how they inform and enhance the occupational therapist's understanding of physical disability.
4. List and describe the components that comprise the occupational therapy domain and give examples of each.
5. List and describe the components that comprise the occupational therapy process and give examples of each.
7. Briefly describe the occupational therapy intervention levels and give an example of each as it might be used in a physical disability practice setting.

REFERENCES

1. American Occupational Therapy Association: Occupational therapy practice framework: domain and process, *Am J Occup Ther* 56(6):609, 2002.
2. American Occupational Therapy Association: Uniform terminology for occupational therapy, ed 3, *Am J Occup Ther* 48:1047, 1994.

3. Boss J: The occupational therapy practice framework and assistive technology: an introduction, *Technol Special Interest Section Quarterly* 13(2), 2003.

4. Cara E: Methods and interpersonal strategies. In Cara E, MacRae A, editors: *Psychosocial occupational therapy: a clinical practice*, p. 359, Clifton Park, NY, 2005, Thomson/Delmar Learning.

5. Christiansen CH, Baum CM, editors: *Occupational therapy: enabling function and well-being*, Thorofare, NJ, 1997, Slack Publishers.

6. Coppola S: An introduction to practice with older adults using the occupational therapy practice framework: domain and process, *Gerontol Special Interest Section Quarterly* 26(1), 2003.

7. Crabtree JL, et al: Cultural proficiency in rehabilitation: an introduction. In Royeen M, Crabtree JL, editors: *Culture in rehabilitation: from competency to proficiency*, p. 1, Upper Saddle River, NJ, 2006, Pearson/Prentice Hall.

8. Crawford K, et al: *Therapeutic use of self in occupational therapy*, Unpublished Master's project, San Jose State University, San Jose, CA, 2004.

9. Delany JV, Squires E: From UT-III to the Framework: making the language work, *OT Practice* May 10, 20, 2004.

10. Dunn W: *Best practice in occupational therapy in community service with children and families*, Thorofare, NJ, 2000, Slack Publishers.

11. Law M, et al: Core concepts of occupational therapy. In Townsend E, editor: *Enabling occupation: an occupational therapy perspective*, p. 29, Ottawa, ONT, 1997, CAOT.

12. Parham LD, Fazio LS, editors: *Play in occupational therapy for children*, St Louis, 1997, Mosby.

13. Peloquin S: The therapeutic relationship: manifestations and challenges in occupational therapy. In Crepeau EB, Cohn ES, Schell BAB, editors: *Willard and Spackman's occupational therapy*, ed 10, p. 157, Philadelphia, 2003, Lippincott Williams & Wilkins.

14. Pendleton HMH, Schultz-Krohn W: Psychosocial issues in physical disability. In Cara E, MacRae A, editors: *Psychosocial occupational therapy: a clinical practice*, p. 359, Clifton Park, NY, 2005, Thomson/Delmar Learning.

15. Siebert C: Communicating home and community expertise: the occupational therapy practice framework, *Home Community Special Interest Section Quarterly* 10(2), 2003.

16. World Health Organization: *International classification of functioning, disability, and health (ICF)*, Geneva, 2001, WHO.

17. Youngstrom MJ: The occupational therapy practice framework: the evolution of our professional language, *Am J Occup Ther* 56(6):607, 2002.

SUGGESTED READING

Law M, et al: *Occupation-based practice: fostering performance and participation*, Thorofare, NJ, 2002, Slack Publishers.

Law M: *Evidence-based rehabilitation: a guide to practice*, Thorofare, NJ, 2002, Slack Publishers.

Youngstrom MJ: *Introduction to the occupational therapy practice framework: domain and process*, AOTA Continuing Education Article, OT Practice, Bethesda, MD, September, CE-1-7, 2002,

2

HISTORY AND PRACTICE TRENDS IN PHYSICAL DYSFUNCTION INTERVENTION

KATHLEEN BARKER SCHWARTZ

KEY TERMS

Moral treatment
Arts and crafts movement
Scientific management

Rehabilitation model
Medical model
Disability rights movement

Social model
Independent living movement

LEARNING OBJECTIVES

After studying this chapter the student or practitioner will be able to do the following:

1. Trace the ideas, values, and beliefs that have influenced the development of occupational therapy as a profession.
2. Analyze the development of occupational therapy within the larger context of cultural, social, political, and legislative forces.

3. Explain how some of the opportunities and challenges that physical disabilities practitioners face today are a result of the way the history of occupational therapy has evolved.

CHAPTER OUTLINE

Roots of occupational therapy
  Moral treatment
  Arts and crafts
  Scientific management
Expansion and specialization
  The rehabilitation model
  Physical dysfunction as a specialty

A new paradigm of disability: disability rights/independent living movements
A clash of paradigms: the medical model vs. moral treatment and the social model
Present practice: a unifying paradigm
Using history to understand today's practice

ROOTS OF OCCUPATIONAL THERAPY

Even into the early 20th century individuals with physical disabilities "were kept at home, out of sight, in back bedrooms, by families who felt a mixture of embarrassment and shame about their presence"[16] (p. 29). This detrimental and pervasive reaction to physical disability began to change with the introduction of the medical model. From a medical perspective, disability was seen as a biological deficit that could be ameliorated with professional treatment. In fact, in the early 20th century "progressive reformers" were looking to medical professionals to assist individuals with disability to reclaim their place in the community and the workplace.[43] It was against this backdrop that the profession of occupational therapy was founded in 1917.

The founders of occupational therapy believed that they could help to rehabilitate individuals with disability through engagement in occupation. They chose the term occupational therapy to reflect this goal, because in 1917 occupation was commonly used to mean "being occupied or employed with, or engaged in something"[29] (p. 682). At the time the founders were aware that such broad terminology could be confusing.[13] However, they valued the breadth of the term for the freedom it would give occupational therapists to use a wide range of modalities and approaches, individually tailored to meet each person's desires and needs.

The founders included William Rush Dunton, a psychiatrist; Herbert J. Hall, a physician; Eleanor Clarke Slagle, a social welfare worker; Susan Johnson, a former arts and crafts teacher; Thomas Kidner and George Barton, both former architects; and Susan Tracey, who was a nurse. They were influenced in their views of occupational therapy by ideas and beliefs prevalent during the latter part of the 19th century and the early years of the 20th. The ideas that seemed to have most shaped the profession's early development were reflected in three movements: moral treatment, arts and crafts, and scientific management.

MORAL TREATMENT

Moral treatment originated in 19th century Europe and was promoted by physicians such as Philippe Pinel of France and Samuel Tuke of England. It represented a shift in thinking from a pessimistic viewpoint that labeled the mentally ill as subhuman and incurable to an optimistic one that viewed the mentally ill as capable of reason and able to respond to humane treatment. The main features of moral treatment included a respect for human individuality, acceptance of the unity of mind and body, and belief that a humane approach using daily routine and occupation could lead to recovery.[7] Occupations included music, physical exercise, and art[33] and agriculture, carpentry, painting, and manual crafts.[12]

Building on these ideas half a century later, the famous neuropsychiatrist Adolf Meyer proposed that many illnesses were "problems of adaptation" that could be remedied through involvement in curative occupations.[26] Dunton and Slagle enthusiastically supported this view, and Meyer's philosophy of "occupation therapy" was published in the first issue of the profession's journal. Slagle, who worked with Meyer at Phipps Clinics, developed habit training programs in mental hospitals to re-establish healthy habits of self-care and social behavior.[37]

ARTS AND CRAFTS

The rise of the **arts and crafts movement** in the 1890s was in reaction to the perceived social ills created by the Industrial Revolution.[9] The economy was changing from an agrarian to a manufacturing society, so that what had previously been made by hand was now produced in factories. Proponents of the arts and crafts movement asserted that this resulted in a society of dissatisfied workers who were bored by monotonous and repetitive working conditions.

The use of arts and crafts as a therapeutic medium in occupational therapy (OT) arose from this trend. The arts and crafts approach was based on the belief that craftwork improved physical and mental health through exercise and the satisfaction gained from creating a useful or decorative article with one's own hands. According to Johnson, the therapeutic value of handicrafts lay in their ability to provide occupation that stimulated "mental activity and muscular exercise at the same time."[21] Different handicrafts could also be graded for the desired physical and mental effects. Crafts were successfully used by OT reconstruction aides during World War I for the physical and mental restoration of disabled servicemen.[35] For treating tuberculosis, Kidner advocated a graduated approach that began with bedside crafts and habit training and proceeded to occupations related to shop work and ultimately actual work within the institution.[23]

Thus, the ideas from the moral treatment and arts and crafts movements became intertwined as a definition of OT evolved to include treatment of individuals with physical and mental disabilities. In its early years, occupational therapists worked with patients throughout three stages of recovery.[23] During convalescence, patients would engage in bedside occupations that primarily consisted of handicrafts such as embroidery and basket weaving. Once patients were able to get out of bed, they would engage in occupations designed to strengthen both body and mind, such as weaving or gardening, and occupations designed to re-establish basic habits of self-care and communication. When they were almost ready to return to the community, patients would engage in occupations that would prepare them for vocational success, such as carpentry, painting, or manual crafts.

SCIENTIFIC MANAGEMENT

Frederick Taylor, a prominent engineer, introduced his theory of **scientific management** in 1911.[40] He proposed that rationality, efficiency, and systematic observation could be applied to industrial management and to all other areas of life, including teaching, preaching, and medicine. Progressive reformers of the period advocated that the ideology of scientific management address societal problems such as poverty and illness. These reformers criticized the noisy, dirty asylum of the 19th century and urged that the image of medical care be transformed into the clean, efficient hospital.[20] The idea that knowledge could be developed through research and observation and applied to patient care became an underlying tenet of the science of medicine and ultimately resulted in the development of reliable protocols for surgical and medical interventions.[43]

The founders of OT were attracted to the idea of a scientific approach to treatment. Barton was particularly taken with Taylor's time and motion studies and thought they might provide a model for OT research.[6] Dunton advocated that those who entered the profession be capable of engaging in systematic inquiry in order to further the profession's goals.[14] Similarly, Slagle urged research in OT to validate its efficacy.[37] By 1920 the profession was promoting the notion of the "science" of occupation by calling for "the advancement of occupation as a therapeutic measure, the study of the effects of occupation upon the human being, and the dissemination of scientific knowledge on this subject."[10]

However, there is little in the OT literature of the early 20th century to suggest that OT practice was informed by systematic observation. One exception was the Department of Occupational Therapy at Walter Reed Hospital in Washington, D.C., under the direction of psychologist Bird T. Baldwin.[5] OT reconstruction aides were assigned to the orthopedic ward, where methods of systematically recording range of motion and muscle strength were established. Activities were selected based on an analysis of the motions involved, including joint position, muscle action, and muscle strengthening. Methods of adapting tools were suggested, and splints were fabricated to provide support during the recovery process. Treatment with this systematic approach was more narrowly focused at times but was applied within the context of what Baldwin called "functional restoration," in which OT's purpose was to "help each patient find himself and function again as a complete man [sic] physically, socially, educationally, and economically."[4]

Besides advocating a scientific approach to practice, the scientific management ideology emphasized efficiency and a mechanistic approach to medical care. Using the factory analogy, patients were the product, and nurses and therapists were the factory workers. It was assumed that doctors had the most scientific knowledge and therefore should be positioned at the top of the medical hierarchy. Dunton, a physician himself, seemed to support this arrangement: "The occupational therapist, therefore, has the same relation to the physician as the nurse, that is, she is a technical assistant."[11] As the profession evolved, an emphasis on efficiency and deference to medical authority became problematic for the profession. The focus on science and the resulting growth of the medical model were both beneficial and detrimental to OT practice.

EXPANSION AND SPECIALIZATION

THE REHABILITATION MODEL

The growth of the **rehabilitation model** began after World War II and peaked with the health care industry boom in the 1970s, following the passage of bills establishing Medicare and Medicaid. Although this growth was initially driven by the need to treat the country's wounded soldiers, care of injured and chronically ill civilians also became a concern.

World War II revived the need for the United States to provide medical care for its wounded soldiers. Many more soldiers survived than in World War I because of recent scientific discoveries such as sulfa and penicillin. The Second World War also served to highlight the value of OT services: "Although occupational therapy started during the last World War, it developed slowly [until] now when doctors are finding this aid to the sick and wounded invaluable."[27] A major effort was launched to reorganize and revitalize the Veterans Administration (VA) hospital system. Departments of physical medicine and rehabilitation were created to bring together all the services needed to care for the large number of war injured. "The theory that handicapped persons can be aided by persons who understand their special needs originated during World War II. The armed services established such hospitals for disabled veterans such as the one for paraplegics in Birmingham, California. They helped the morale and physical condition of the patients so much that others were built for civilians."[28]

The interdisciplinary approach to care was emulated in the private sector. Demand for medical services increased in the civilian population as the treatment of chronic disability became a priority. Howard Rusk, a prominent voice in the development of rehabilitation medicine, asserted that the critical shortage of trained personnel would impede the country's ability to deliver services to the "5,300,000 persons in the nation who suffer from chronic disability."[22] He cited OT as one of the essential rehabilitation services. In response to the growing demand for rehabilitation services, Congress passed the Hill-Burton Act in 1946 to provide federal aid for the construction of rehabilitation centers. A proviso of the legislation was that rehabilitation centers must "offer integrated services in four areas: medical, including occupational and physical therapy, psychological, social, and vocational."[44] The passage of legislation establishing Medicare and Medicaid in 1965 put further demands on rehabilitation services to serve the chronically ill and elderly within healthcare institutions, as well as the community.

PHYSICAL DYSFUNCTION AS A SPECIALTY

The creation of a specialty in physical dysfunction within occupational therapy came about as a response to the changing demands of the marketplace and its requirement that specialists possess particular kinds of medical knowledge and technological skills.[18] This new specialty began with an increasing focus on occupations that would promote physical strength and endurance: "The Army is death on the old-time invalid occupations of basket weaving, chair caning, pottery and weaving. These are 'not believed to be interesting occupation for the present condition of men in military service,' says an officer from the Surgeon General's office. The stress now is on carpentry, repair work at the hospital, war-related jobs like knitting camouflage nets, and printing."[41]

The scientific approach of joint measurement and muscle strengthening that Baldwin pioneered at the end of World War I was adopted and improved upon. Claire Spackman, who along with Helen Willard wrote the profession's first textbook on occupational therapy, argued that therapists must become skilled in carrying out new treatments based on improved techniques. According to Spackman, the occupational therapists serving people with physical disability needed to be skilled in teaching activities of daily living (ADL), work simplification, and training in the use of upper extremity prostheses. But first and foremost, she asserted, "Occupational therapy treats the patient by the use of constructive activity in a simulated, normal living and/or working situation.... Constructive activity is the keynote of occupational therapy."[38]

As the rehabilitation movement helped to establish the importance of OT, it further positioned the profession within the **medical model**. OT was urged to specialize and separate into two distinct fields, physical dysfunction and mental illness. The head orthopedist at Rancho Los Amigos Hospital in Downey, California argued that the separation would result in "strengthened treatment techniques" and thus more credibility among the medical profession who "does not recognize your field as an established necessary specialty."[19] The American Occupational Therapy Association sought closer ties with the American Medical Association in order to increase occupational therapy's visibility and reputation as a profession dedicated to rehabilitation of the individual through engagement in occupation.

The closer relationship with medicine probably helped the profession gain credibility, at least within the medical model. The positive aspect of the medical model is that it emphasized the importance of the rehabilitation of those with disabilities, and it helped stimulate the development of new scientific techniques. The negative aspect of the medical model is that it presumed that the individual is a passive participant in the process. In response to this view, a new social model was proposed that placed the individual at the center of the rehabilitation process.

A NEW PARADIGM OF DISABILITY: DISABILITY RIGHTS/INDEPENDENT LIVING MOVEMENTS

The advocacy for disability rights that took hold in the 1970s had its roots in the social and political activism of the 1960s.

During the sixties, disabled people were profoundly influenced by the social and political upheaval that they witnessed. They identified with the struggles of other disenfranchised groups to achieve integration and meaningful equality of opportunity. They learned the tactics of litigation and the art of civil disobedience from other civil rights activists. They absorbed reform ideas from many sources—consumerism, demedicalization, and de-institutionalization[15] (pp. 15-16).

Like the civil rights and women's movements, the **disability rights movement** was rooted in self-advocacy. That is, it was the individuals with disability themselves who were promoting their own cause. Their activism took many forms including lawsuits, demonstrations, founding of a plethora of organizations dedicated to achieving disability rights, and political lobbying for legislation to address inequality and protect rights.

The ideas underlying the disability rights movement were based on a social rather than a medical model. The medical model had provided the predominant view of individuals with disability for much of the 20th century. It placed the medical professional at the center of the rehabilitation process and the patient on the periphery as the person who was being helped by the experts. It categorized individuals according to their medical disability, i.e., the paraplegic or quadriplegic, and it saw the remediation of that medical condition as the way to eradicate disability. Disability rights advocates rejected this view as too paternalistic, passive, and reductionistic. Instead they advocated a paradigm that put the individual with disability at the center of the model as the expert in knowing what it was like to have a disability.

The **social model** proposed that disability was created because of environmental factors that prevented individuals from being fully functioning members of society. Physical boundaries prevented individuals from having access to schools, workplace, and home. Social views of individuals as pathetic cripples blocked full participation in life activities. Political and legal interpretations advocated "separate but equal" participation rather than inclusion. The social model argued that disability must be viewed from a cultural, political, and social lens rather than a biomedical one:

This model makes us aware that a complex system of mutually supporting beliefs and practices can impact those with disability by: stigmatizing them as less than full humans, isolating them by policies of confinement or the built environment, making them overly dependent on professionals rather than helping them develop responsible behaviors, robbing them of independent decision making that others enjoy, undermining their self-confidence in their many capabilities, over-generalizing the significance of some impairment, and defining them as tax-eaters rather than tax-contributors[39] (p. 22).

Aligning itself with the social model, the **independent living movement** got its start when Edward Roberts was admitted to the University of California, Berkeley in fall 1963.[39] The polio that Roberts had contracted at the age of 14 left him paralyzed from the neck down and in need of a respirator during the day and an iron lung at night. It was arranged that Roberts would stay in Cowell Hospital on the Berkeley campus with his brother Ron providing him personal assistance. Although Roberts was the first, in the following years Berkeley admitted other students with severe disabilities. They formed the "Rolling Quads," and were dedicated to making the campus and environs physically accessible.

Having completed his master's degree, Roberts, and his fellow Rolling Quads, were invited in 1969 to Washington to help develop a program aimed at retention of students with disability on college campuses. They created the Physically Disabled Students' Program (PDSP), which included provision for personal assistants, wheelchair repair, and financial aid. In 1972 Roberts became the first executive director of the first Center for Independent Living (CIL), located in Berkeley. Roberts based the CIL on the principles underlying the PDSP:[1] "that the experts on disability are the people with the disabilities;[2] that the needs of the people with disabilities can best be met by a comprehensive, or holistic program, rather than by fragmented programs at different agencies and offices;[3] that people with disabilities should be integrated into the community"[31] (p. 61). Since the founding of the first CIL, hundreds of other centers have been developed throughout the country.

A CLASH OF PARADIGMS: THE MEDICAL MODEL VS. MORAL TREATMENT AND THE SOCIAL MODEL

The clash of paradigms within occupational therapy was expressed in terms of moral treatment vs. the medical model. A cry arose in the late 1960s and 1970s from some of the profession's leaders to return to its roots in moral treatment and to forego what Shannon referred to as the "technique philosophy."[36] In his article on what he called "the derailment of occupational therapy," Shannon described two philosophies at odds with each other. One, he asserted, viewed the individual "as a mechanistic creature susceptible to manipulation and control via the application of techniques"; the other, based on the profession's early philosophy of moral treatment, emphasized a holistic and humanistic view of the individual.

Kielhofner and Burke described the situation as a conflict between two paradigms.[24] Early OT practice, they asserted, was based on the paradigm of occupation that had moral treatment as its foundation. This paradigm provided a "holistic orientation to Man [sic] and health in the context of the culture of daily living and its activities." Post-World War II practice, they asserted, was based on the paradigm of reductionism, a mode of thinking characteristic of the medical model. This view emphasized the individual's "internal states" and represented a shift in focus to "internal muscular, intrapsychic balance and sensorimotor problems." The authors acknowledged that practice based on the reductionist paradigm "would pave the way for the development of more exact technologies for the treatment of internal deficits"; however, they were concerned it "necessitates[d] a narrowing of the conceptual scope of occupational therapy."[24]

The claim that early OT practice was based on the humanistic and holistic philosophy of moral treatment is accurate, but does not tell the full story. As this chapter describes, the founders also valued the medical model and the importance that "science" could play in establishing the profession's credibility. For example, the Committee on Installations and Advice, directed by Dunton, was formed to scientifically analyze the most commonly used crafts and to match the therapeutic value of each craft to a particular disability.[34]

How could the founders have supported what came to be viewed in the 1970s as the two opposing views of moral treatment and the medical model? The answer may be that in 1917 when the profession was founded, the models were not considered to be incompatible because the scientific medical model had not fully taken hold. It appears that in the founding years, OT primarily *practiced* moral treatment and *talked about* how practice should also be medical and scientific. When early practitioners were asked to treat patients in order to "restore the functions of nerves and muscles" or to make use of "the affected arm or leg,"[38] they based their treatment on their belief in the importance of occupation, habit training, and their knowledge of crafts. Once knowledge and technologic advances were sufficient and occupational therapists could actually practice using a scientific, medical perspective, it became apparent that the ideas underlying these two paradigms were in conflict.

The physical dysfunction therapist was faced with the problem of how to give treatment that was, on the one hand, holistic and humanistic and, on the other, medical and scientific. Baldwin's answer in 1919 was to see activities such as muscle strengthening and splint fabrication as techniques that contributed to the larger goal of "functional restoration" of the individual's social, physical, and economic well-being.[5] Spackman's answer in 1968 was that the occupational therapist should use "constructive activity in a simulated, normal living and/or working situation. This is and always has been our function."[38] She emphasized the teaching of ADL and work simplification, and was critical of treatment that consisted of having patients sand or use a bicycle saw with no "constructive activity" involved.

Another answer to the question of differing paradigms was to move outside the medical model. Bockoven urged OT practitioners to set up services in the community based on moral treatment. He said, "It is the occupational therapist's inborn respect for the realities of life, for the real tasks of living, and for the time it takes the individual to develop his modes of coping with his tasks, that leads me to urge haste on the profession . . . to assert its leadership in fashioning the design of human service programs. . . . Don't drop dead, take over instead!"[8] Yerxa urged therapists not to rely solely on doctor's orders: "The written prescription is no longer seen by many of us as necessary, holy or healthy. . . . The pseudo-security of the prescription required that we pay a high price. That price was the reduction of our potential to help clients because we often stagnated at the level of applying technical skills."[46]

However, as practice moved into the 1980s, there was much concern that if occupational therapists did as their critics suggested, they would jeopardize reimbursement as well as referrals. They argued that they were being asked to exclude skills and knowledge they believed were valuable in patient treatment, such as exercise, splinting, and facilitation techniques. They further argued that many patients receiving OT services were initially not at the level of motor capability that would enable them to engage in satisfying occupations. It was proposed that adjunctive techniques such as exercise and biofeedback should be considered legitimate when used to prepare the patient for further engagement in occupation.[42] A study conducted in 1984 by Pasquinelli[30] showed that although therapists valued occupation, they used a wide variety of treatment techniques and approaches, including facilitation and nonactivity-oriented techniques. Both Ayres and Trombly argued that instead of attempting to redirect the focus of OT, the profession should include current clinical practices that had proved effective on an empirical and practical basis.[3,42]

Others, such as Gill,[17] brought the perspective of the disability rights/independent living movements to the discussion of what constituted ideal occupational therapy practice.

A conceptualization of disability that differs significantly from the medical model and that is rapidly gaining adherents among disability experts is the interactional or sociopolitical model. From this perspective, disability is defined not only by the physical qualities of the individual but also by the corresponding response of the social environment. Disability, in this view, does not reside solely in the individual; rather it derives from the interaction between the individual and society. Furthermore, the correction of disability-related problems is no longer solely the province of health professionals but may also be affected by peer support, political activism, and self-help[17] (p. 50).

Gill argued that the medical model exempted society from taking any responsibility for its role in creating the climate that restricted the rights and opportunities of the disabled. She urged occupational therapists to examine their practice and make sure that their treatment did not focus solely on the individual's physical condition.

For rehabilitation to be helpful, it must address the reality of what life is like for disabled persons. If rehabilitation professionals fail to fit their services to the patient's needs, values, and interests, they fail both the patient and their own professional aspirations.....Without a proper balance of physical treatment and realistic social information, rehabilitation cannot enable patients....What good are increased range of motion and finger dexterity when a patient's morale can be crushed by job discrimination or social rejection?[17] (p. 54)

Indeed a study conducted by Pendleton in 1990 found that occupational therapists were much less likely to provide training in independent living skills than physical remediation.[32] She defined independent living skills as "those specific abilities broadly associated with home management and social/community problem solving." She argued that "Mastering such skills could contribute to the achievement of control over one's life based on the choice of acceptable options that minimize reliance on others...The result of achieving such control is that the person can actively participate in the day-to-day life of the community"[32] (pp. 94-95). She recommended that if occupational therapists are not able to provide sufficient independent living skills training in inpatient rehabilitation centers, they should shift their treatment to community-based programs. Pendleton saw independent living skills as the essence of occupational therapy, and urged therapists to make it one of their priorities.

Longmore, a well-known historian and disability rights activist, emphasized the importance of the issues raised by Gill and Pendleton. Although he acknowledged that disability rights activism has been responsible for numerous pieces of legislation since the 1970s aimed at giving those with disability equal access to all parts of society including schools, work, public places, and transportation, he warned that there is still much to be done. The most important legislation passed during this period included the Rehabilitation Act of 1973, the Individuals with Disabilities Education Act of 1973 (IDEA), and the Americans with Disabilities Act of 1990 (ADA). However, Longmore argued, despite this legislation, people with disabilities continue to experience marginalization and financial deprivation. "Depending on age and definition of disability, poverty rates among disabled people range anywhere from 50 percent to 300 percent higher than in the population at large..."[25] (p. 19). He worries that most people assume that the ADA has eradicated the major problems for those with disabilities, when in fact "to a surprising extent U.S. society continues to restrict or exclude people with disabilities"[25] (p. 21).

PRESENT PRACTICE: A UNIFYING PARADIGM

Early treatment in occupational therapy was based on belief in the importance of occupation, habit training, and knowledge of crafts. As scientific knowledge and technology advanced, OT defined a role for itself within the rehabilitation model. This resulted in the emergence of physical dysfunction as a specialty within OT. The closer relationship with medicine helped the profession gain credibility; however, it became apparent by the late 1960s that the scientific reductionism of the medical model was at odds with the holistic humanism of moral treatment. It was also at odds with the social model advocated by disability rights activists.

In an attempt to bridge the medical and social models, the World Health Organization published in 2001 the International Classification of Functioning, Disability and Health (ICF).[45] The ICF provides a classification model that considers physical and mental impairments as well as environmental and personal factors, any or all of which may result in activity limitations and participation restrictions.

Based on the conceptual scheme of the World Health Organization, The American Occupational Therapy Association issued the Occupational Therapy Practice Framework (OTPF) in 2002.[1] It provides a construct that promotes client-centered engagement in occupation as the central focus of practice. This construct addresses issues raised by proponents of moral treatment, as well as the social and medical models. It reclaims the values of moral treatment by its focus on occupation-based treatment that is both holistic and humanistic. It integrates aspects of the medical model by advocating the reduction of functional impairments caused by physical and psychological limitations. Finally, it supports the social model of the disability rights movement by emphasizing the need for client-centered treatment within the context of the social, cultural, and political environment.

Having reviewed the history of occupational therapy practice in the United States, one can conclude that although treatment techniques have changed throughout the 20th century, the values and beliefs established in the formative years continue to influence practice. The most enduring belief is this: That occupation as prescribed by OT practitioners promotes health, prevents and remedies dysfunction, and elicits adaptation to the environment. As new treatment techniques and technologies are developed in the future, OT intervention that promotes occupational function will remain consistent with the philosophical base of the profession.

USING HISTORY TO UNDERSTAND TODAY'S PRACTICE

In lieu of a case study, we will demonstrate how we can use our knowledge about occupational therapy's history to answer a question that is prevalent among students and therapists today: **Why do occupational therapists continually have to define "occupational therapy" to others?**

First we should acknowledge that more people than ever do understand occupational therapy. Most of these people are individuals who have received treatment or have had personal contact with someone who received occupational therapy. So each time an occupational therapist successfully engages a client in treatment he or she is providing a positive definition of occupational therapy. That being said, it can feel as though occupational therapists spend quite a bit of time educating others as to what we do. We can look back to the founding years to understand why this is so. The answer is complex and includes several factors.

The first relates to the profession's purpose: As this chapter describes, in naming the profession, the founders were looking for a term that was broad enough to encompass all of the things that occupational therapists did. The AOTA in 1923 described occupational therapy in this way: "Occupational Therapy is a method for training the sick or injured by means of instruction and employment in productive occupation. The objects sought are to arouse interest, courage, and confidence: to exercise mind and body in healthy activity;

to overcome disability; and to re-establish capacity for industrial and social usefulness."[2] This definition reflects a holistic, humanistic, and all-encompassing view of the individual, the rehabilitative process, and the role of occupational therapy within it. It addresses the mind as well as the body, and social as well as medical goals. The founders ultimately decided that "occupational therapy" was the term that best reflected the profession's goals. This is not to say that the founders did not consider the possible negative aspects of the term. It is clear from their writings that they were aware that such a broad term might cause some misunderstanding. However, in the end, they felt that this negative would be offset by the positive of providing occupational therapists with a wide range of freedom to treat each individual in the best way possible.

Secondly, we must consider that the name was chosen in 1917, and meanings of terms do change over time. For example, children with disabilities were placed in "asylums for the crippled" in the early 1900s. We would never use that terminology today. Fortunately, occupation does not carry such a negative connotation in today's lexicon, but the term has shifted in meaning. In 1917 "occupation" was most commonly used to mean an important activity in which one engages. For example, in a novel, one might read about a woman who was searching for an occupation that would satisfy her free time. As the century progressed, the term occupation came to be more closely aligned with the kind of paid work you do, as in "what is your occupation?" When looked at in this light, it is easier to understand any confusion someone today may have about the term, and the continual need for the occupational therapist to educate people about the term's meaning within today's context.

Thirdly, we must also consider that the professions that exist today did not exist at the time of occupational therapy's founding. That is one reason the definition of OT was so broad. At the time of the founding of occupational therapy, society was looking for a profession that could help remediate the wounds and illnesses of returning soldiers and enable them to become productive members of society. Occupational therapy offered that promise. Professions such as social work and physical therapy were still in their fledgling stage and it was unclear which profession would ultimately be involved in the soldiers' rehabilitation. In addition, art, music, recreation, and vocational therapy had yet to be introduced.

Finally, as has been discussed throughout this chapter, the ideas underlying occupational therapy do not fit neatly into just one theoretical paradigm. Occupational therapy uses an occupation-based, client-centered approach that bridges both the medical and social models, as is evidenced in the Occupational Therapy Performance Framework. While this sounds good in theory, in practice it means that if occupational therapists are working with people who use a strict medical model (including third parties), there will be misunderstandings about OT's proper role. This is where occupational therapists must be proactive in describing what we do.

History tells us that occupational therapy has always had a humanistic, holistic approach to viewing its clients and its role, and it cannot be neatly confined to the medical or social paradigms. The blending of these paradigms by the ICF and OTPF finally offers occupational therapy a suitable home. However, these are new ideas and it will take time for them to be accepted. This is one more reason why occupational therapists will not be finished defining what we do any time soon. But is it not a worthy challenge? History would suggest that it is. So the next time you have to define occupational therapy, think of yourself as the latest generation to carry on the proud tradition of defining your goals by what is good for the client rather than what "fits" into the prevailing theoretical model.

Review Questions

1. Name the seven founders of occupational therapy, and list the professional background of each.
2. What ideologies shaped the development of occupational therapy in the late 19th and early 20th centuries?
3. What were the main features of the philosophy of moral treatment?
4. Describe the ideas that were the foundations of occupation as a remedy for mental and physical illness.
5. What provoked the rise of the arts and crafts movement?
6. How did the arts and crafts movement influence occupational therapy?
7. Describe scientific management. How did it influence the development of occupational therapy?
8. When did the rehabilitation model evolve? How did the world wars influence the development of the rehabilitation model?
9. How did physical dysfunction become a specialty?
10. What factors influenced occupational therapy to adopt the medical model?
11. What was the apparent conflict between moral treatment and the medical model?
12. What impact has the disability rights and independent living movement had on occupational therapy?
13. How is the apparent conflict between the medical model and the social model being resolved in occupational therapy practice?

REFERENCES

1. American Occupational Therapy Association: Occupational therapy practice framework: domain and process, *Am J Occup Ther* 56:69-639, 2002.
2. American Occupational Therapy Association: *Principles of occupational therapy*, Bulletin 4, Bethesda, MD, 1923, Wilma West Archives.
3. Ayres AJ: Basic concepts of clinical practice in physical disabilities, *Am J Occup Ther* 12:300, 1958.
4. Baldwin BT: Occupational therapy, *Am J Care Cripples* 8:447, 1919.
5. Baldwin BT: *Occupational therapy applied to restoration of function of disabled joints*, Washington, DC, 1919, Walter Reed General Hospital.
6. Barton GE: *The movies and the microscope*, Bethesda, MD, 1920, Wilma West Archives.
7. Bing R: Occupational therapy revisited: a paraphrastic journey: 1981 Eleanor Clark Slagle lecture, *Am J Occup Ther* 35:499, 1981.
8. Bockoven JS: Legacy of moral treatment: 1800s to 1910, *Am J Occup Ther* 25:224, 1971.
9. Boris E: *Art and labor: Ruskin, Morris and the craftsman ideal in America*, Philadelphia, 1986, Temple University.
10. *Constitution of the National Society for the Promotion of Occupational Therapy*, Baltimore, MD,1917, Sheppard Pratt Hospital Press.
11. Dunton WR: *Prescribing occupational therapy*, Springfield Ill, 1928, Charles C Thomas.
12. Dunton WR: History of occupational therapy, *Modern Hospital* 8:60-382, 1917.
13. Dunton WR: *The growing necessity for occupational therapy. An address delivered before the class of nursing and health, Columbia University*, Bethesda MD, 1917, Wilma West Archives.
14. Dunton WR: The three "r's" of occupational therapy, *Occup Ther Rehab* 7:345-348, 1928.
15. Funk R: *Challenges of emerging leadership: community-based independent living programs and the disability rights movement*, Washington DC, 1984, Institute for Educational Leadership.
16. Gallagher H: *FDR's splendid deception*, Arlington, VA, 1999, Vandamere Press.
17. Gill C: A new social perspective on disability and its implications for rehabilitation, *Occup Ther Health Care* 4:49-55, 1987.
18. Gritzer G, Arluke A: *The making of rehabilitation*, Berkeley, 1985, University of California Press.
19. *Higher status near, doctor tells therapists: department scrapbooks, 1955-63*, Archives of the Department of Occupational Therapy, San José State University, San José, CA.
20. Hofstadter R: *The age of reform*, New York, 1969, Knopf.
21. Johnson SC: Instruction in handcrafts and design for hospital patients, *Modern Hosp* 15:1, 69-72, 1920.
22. Lack of trained personnel felt in rehabilitation field, *The New York Times*, Jan 25, 1954.
23. Kidner TB: Planning for occupational therapy, *Modern Hosp* 21:414-428, 1923.
24. Kielhofner G, Burke JP: Occupational therapy after 60 years, *Am J Occup Ther* 31:15-689, 1977.
25. Longmore P: *Why I burned my book and other essays on disability*, Philadelphia, 2003, Temple University Press.
26. Meyer A: The philosophy of occupation therapy, *Arch Occup Ther* 1:1-10, 1922.
27. *Occupational therapy classes have outstanding guest speakers from various army and civilian hospitals: department scrapbook, 1943-54*, Archives of the Department of Occupational Therapy, San José State University, San José, CA.
28. OT instructor says San José needs rehabilitation center, *Spartan Daily*, San José, Calif, Feb 9, 1953, San José State College, San José, CA.
29. *Oxford English Dictionary*, ed. 2, 10:681-683, 1989.

30. Pasquinelli S: *The relationship of physical disabilities treatment methodologies to the philosophical base of occupational therapy,* unpublished thesis, 1984, San José State University, San José, CA.

31. Pelka F: *The ABC-CLIO Companion to the disability rights movement,* Santa Barbara, 1997, ABC-CLIO.

32. Pendleton H: Occupational therapists current use of independent living skills training for adult inpatients who are physically disabled, *Occup Ther Health Care* 93-108, 1990.

33. Pinel P: *Traite medico-philosophique sur l'alienation mentale,* Paris, 1809, JA Brosson.

34. Putnam ML: Report of the committee on installations and advice, *Occup Ther Rehab* 4:57-60, 1924.

35. Quiroga V: *Occupational therapy: the first 30 years, 1900-1930,* Bethesda, MD, 1995, American Occupational Therapy Association.

36. Shannon PD: The derailment of occupational therapy, *Am J Occup Ther* 31:229, 1977.

37. Slagle EC: A year's development of occupational therapy in New York State hospitals, *Modern Hosp* 22:98-104, 1924.

38. Spackman CS: A history of the practice of occupational therapy for restoration of physical function: 1917-1967, *Am J Occup Ther* 22:67-71, 1968.

39. Stroman D: *The disability rights movement,* Lanham, MD, 2003, University Press of America.

40. Taylor F: *The principles of scientific management,* New York, 1911, Harper.

41. *The gift of healing,* 1943, Occupational Therapy Department Archives: San José State University, San José, CA.

42. Trombly CA: Include exercise in purposeful activity, *Am J Occup Ther* 36:467, 1982 (letter).

43. Weibe R: *The search for order, 1877-1920,* New York, 1967, Farrar, Straus & Giroux.

44. *Workshop on rehabilitation facilities, 1955: department scrapbooks 1955-63,* Archives of the Department of Occupational Therapy, San José State University, San José, CA.

45. World Health Organization: *International classification of functioning, disability and health (ICF),* Geneva, Switzerland, 2001, WHO.

46. Yerxa EJ: 1966 Eleanor Clarke Slagle Lecture: Authentic occupational therapy, *Am J Occup Ther* 21:1-9, 1967.

SUGGESTED READING

Kielhofner G: *Conceptual foundations of occupational therapy,* ed. 3, Philadelphia, 2004, FA Davis.

Occupational Therapy Process and Practice

3

Application of the Occupational Therapy Practice Framework to Physical Dysfunction

WINIFRED SCHULTZ-KROHN
HEIDI McHUGH PENDLETON

KEY TERMS

Occupational therapy practitioners	Intervention plan	Frame of reference	Acute rehabilitation
Referral	Clinical reasoning	Occupational therapy aide	Subacute rehabilitation
Occupational therapist	Procedural reasoning	Ethics	Skilled nursing facility
Screening	Interactive reasoning	Ethical dilemmas	Community-based settings
Evaluation	Conditional reasoning	Practice setting	
Occupational therapy assistant	Narrative reasoning	Inpatient settings	
	Pragmatic reasoning	Acute care	

LEARNING OBJECTIVES

After studying this chapter the student or practitioner will be able to do the following:

1. Identify and describe the major functions of the occupational therapy (OT) process.
2. Describe how clinical reasoning adjusts to consider various factors that may be present in the intervention context.
3. Identify how theories, models of practice, and frames of reference can inform and support OT intervention.
4. Identify appropriate delegation of responsibility among the various levels of OT practitioners.
5. Discuss ways in which OT practitioners may effectively collaborate with members of other professions involved in client care.
6. Recognize ethical dilemmas that may occur frequently in OT practice, and identify ways in which these may be addressed and managed.

7. Describe the various practice settings for OT practice in the arena of physical disabilities.
8. Discuss the type of services typically provided in these settings.
9. Identify ways in which different practice settings affect the occupational performance of persons receiving occupational therapy services.
10. Identify the environmental attributes that afford the most realistic projections of how the client will perform in the absence of the therapist.
11. Identify environmental and temporal aspects of at least three practice settings.
12. Describe ways in which the therapist can alter environmental and temporal features to obtain more accurate measures of performance.

CHAPTER OUTLINE

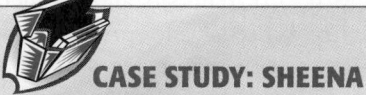

CASE STUDY: SHEENA

Sheena is an occupational therapy student who began her first fieldwork internship 2 weeks ago. She felt very fortunate to be assigned a site that provides a wide array of services. Sheena's site is a community hospital providing a continuum of care from emergency services and critical care (intensive care unit–ICU) to outpatient rehabilitation services. Her internship includes providing OT intervention in a variety of settings. Her clinical instructor (CI) requested that she review the process of developing an intervention plan and be prepared to differentiate the role of occupational therapy in the various settings.

Critical Thinking Questions

1. What process should be used when developing an intervention plan?
2. How do theories, models of practice, and frames of reference serve to guide an intervention plan?
3. What forms of clinical reasoning are employed when providing occupational therapy services?

This chapter is divided into two sections. The first section introduces the *occupational therapy* (OT) process, summarizing the function of evaluation, intervention, and outcomes described in the *Occupational Therapy Practice Framework* (OTPF).[6] The chapter will acquaint the reader with the complexity and creativity of clinical reasoning within the context of the contemporary clinical environment. The complementary roles of different **occupational therapy practitioners**, as well as relationships between OT and the other professional disciplines involved in the care of the client with physical dysfunction, are described. Common ethical dilemmas are introduced and ways to analyze these are presented.

The second section describes various practice settings where occupational therapy services are provided for individuals who have physical disabilities with a discussion of typical services in each setting.

SECTION 1: THE OCCUPATIONAL THERAPY PROCESS

Winifred Schultz-Krohn
Heidi McHugh Pendleton

THE OCCUPATIONAL THERAPY PROCESS

The OTPF discusses both the domain and the process of the profession.[6,77] The domain is described in Chapter 1 and the reader should be familiar with the domain prior to reading about the process of occupational therapy.

The occupational therapy process should be conceptualized as a circular process initiated by a **referral** (Fig. 3-1). Following the referral, an evaluation is conducted to identify the client's occupational needs. The intervention is developed based on the evaluation results. The targeted outcome of intervention is the client's engagement in occupations that support participation in context. The steps of evaluation, intervention, and outcome should not be viewed in a linear fashion but instead should be seen as a circular or spiraling process where the parts are mutually influential.

REFERRAL

The physician or other legally qualified professional requests occupational therapy services for the client. The referral may

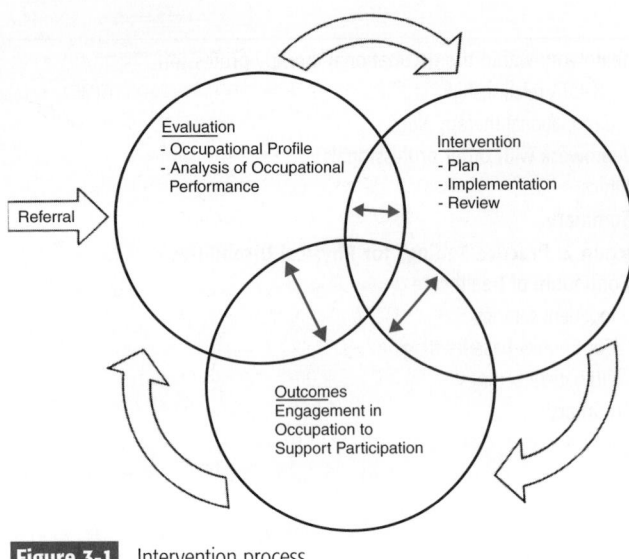

Figure 3-1 Intervention process.

be oral, but a written record is also necessary. Guidelines for referral vary and in some situations occupational therapy services may require a physician's referral. The **occupational therapist** (OT) is responsible for responding to the referral. Although clients may seek occupational therapy services without first obtaining a referral, the occupational therapist may need a referral prior to the initiation of intervention services. State regulatory boards and licensing requirements should be reviewed prior to initiation of services to determine if a referral for service is necessary.

SCREENING

The OT determines whether further evaluation is warranted and if occupational therapy services would be helpful to this client. The therapist may perform a **screening** independently or as a member of the healthcare team. Screening procedures are generally brief and do not cover all areas of occupation. A formal screen is not always conducted with the client but, during the review of the client's record prior to the evaluation, the OT considers the diagnosis, physical condition, referral, and information from other professionals. This information is then synthesized by the therapist prior to initiating an evaluation. In some settings the screening process flows directly into the evaluation of the client in a seamless manner.

EVALUATION

Evaluation refers to "the process of obtaining and interpreting data necessary for intervention. This includes planning for and documenting the evaluation process and results." Assessment refers "to specific tools or instruments that are used during the evaluation process."[1] Two parts of the evaluation process have been identified: the generation of an occupational profile and then the analysis of occupational performance. The assessments chosen help in developing the

occupational profile. The OT then analyzes the client's occupational performance through synthesis of data collected using a variety of means.

The evaluation portion begins with the OT and client developing an occupational profile that reviews the client's occupational history and describes the client's current needs and priorities.[6] This portion of the evaluation process includes the client's previous roles and the contexts for occupational performance. For example, Sheena has been assigned to develop an occupational profile for a 56-year-old man who recently had a tumor removed from his right cerebral hemisphere, resulting in dense left hemiplegia. He has been married to his wife for 27 years and reports that he never cooks. On further exploration during the development of the occupational profile, the man reports that one of his most treasured occupations is being able to grill, and discusses the importance of grilling over charcoal versus using a gas grill. Although Sheena may have initially ignored the need to work on cooking skills with this man, she now understands the occupational significance of grilling and, from the client's perspective, the difference between grilling and cooking! The occupational profile allows the OT to understand the client's occupational history, current needs, and priorities, and identifies which occupations or activities are successfully completed and those that are problematic for the client.

The occupational profile is most often initiated with an interview with the client, and significant others in the client's life, and by a thorough review of available records.[6] Interviews may be completed using a formal instrument or informal tools. Although the occupational profile is used to focus subsequent intervention, this profile is often revised throughout the course of intervention to meet a client's needs. The purpose of the occupational profile is to answer the following questions as articulated in the AOTA document:[6]

1. *Who is the client?* This requires consideration of not only the individual but includes the significant others in the client's life. In some settings the client may be identified as a group and not as an individual. For example, a 28-year-old woman, Nora, who sustained a traumatic brain injury resulting in memory deficits and slight difficulties with coordination, is a wife and a mother to two young children. During the evaluation process, Sheena considers not only Nora's occupational needs but also the needs of her family and her roles as a family member.

2. *Why is the client seeking service?* This relates to the occupational needs identified by the individual and significant others. The needs of not only Nora but also the needs of her husband and children should be included in answering this question.

3. *Which specific occupations are problematic for the client?* This would also include understanding which occupations are successfully completed by the client. Nora may have the physical ability to drive and yet has severe memory problems and has difficulties remembering the route to drive her children to school and various activities.

4. *How does context influence engagement in occupations?* Some contexts may be supportive where others present challenges or prohibit occupational performance. Nora's parents expect her to be the primary caregiver for her children and when her husband attempts to support Nora, her parents interfere.

5. *What is the client's occupational history?* This includes the level of engagement in various occupations and activities along with the value attributed to those occupations by the client. Although prior to her traumatic brain injury Nora was responsible for the majority of the housecleaning tasks, these were not highly valued by Nora. She was also responsible for meal preparation and reports that she enjoys cooking. She places a much higher value on being able to drive her children to school and various after-school activities.

6. *What are the client's priorities and desired outcomes?* These may be identified as occupational performance, role competence, adaptation to the circumstance, health and wellness, prevention, or quality of life issues. For Nora, the need to safely drive and resume responsibility for fostering community participation for her children was a primary outcome. This reflects her interest in occupational performance. She was not interested in having her parents or her husband assume these roles.

After the occupational profile is developed, the OT identifies the necessary additional information to be collected, including areas to be evaluated and what assessment instruments should be used prior to the analysis of occupational performance. The OT may delegate some parts of the evaluation, such as the administration of selected assessment tools, to the **occupational therapy assistant** (OTA). The interpretation of data is the responsibility of the OT. This requires the OT to direct the evaluation by completing an occupational profile, interpreting the data collected from the profile, and then analyzing the client's occupational performance prior to proceeding to assessment of client factors. The selection of additional information beyond the occupational profile should answer the following questions:

1. What additional data are needed to understand the client's occupational needs including contextual supports and challenges?

2. What is the best way (most efficient and accurate) to collect these data?

3. How will this information support the intervention plan?

The ability of the client to successfully plan, initiate, and complete various occupations is then evaluated. The occupations chosen are based on the occupational profile. The data are then analyzed by the OT to determine the client's specific strengths and weaknesses that impact occupational performance. The impact of contextual factors on occupational performance is included in the analysis of data. This can easily be seen when a client who is dependent upon a wheelchair for all mobility is faced with several stairs to enter an office building to conduct business. The client has functional mobility skills but is prohibited from participating due to an environmental factor that restricts access. The analysis includes integrating data regarding the activity demands, the client's previous and current occupational patterns, and the client factors that support or prohibit occupational performance. Data about specific client factors may be helpful in developing an intervention plan but should be performed after the occupational profile is completed and an analysis of occupational performance has been initiated. The information generated from the profile and analysis will allow more careful selection of necessary assessment tools to collect further data. The OT also considers if the client would benefit from a referral to other professionals.

Now consider the case presentation from the beginning of the chapter. Although Sheena is able to competently perform a manual muscle test and range of motion assessment, these assessments would not be necessary for all clients. Sheena must first develop the client's occupational profile as a guide to then select the most appropriate assessment instruments to complete her evaluation of the client's occupational performance. After she has completed these steps, Sheena is able to more clearly identify what additional information is needed to plan and implement intervention services.

INTERVENTION PLANNING

Working with the client, the occupational therapy practitioners (OT and OTA) develop a plan using the following approaches or strategies to enhance the client's ability to participate in occupational performance.[6] Although the OT is responsible for the plan, the OTA contributes to the plan and must be "knowledgeable about the evaluation results" (p. 665).[3] The strategies selected should be linked to the intended outcomes of service.[6] These approaches or strategies answer the question: "What type (approach/strategy) of intervention will be provided to meet the client's goals?" Examples of each form of intervention approach or strategy are provided with selected literature to support this form of occupational therapy intervention:

1. *Prevention of disability:* This approach is focused on developing the performance skills and patterns that support continued occupational performance and provides intervention that anticipates potential hazards or challenges to occupational performance. Contextual issues are also addressed using this approach and environmental barriers would be similarly considered. An example of services representing a preventative approach would be instructing a client who has compromised standing balance in fall prevention techniques and asking the family to remove loose throw rugs from the home to avoid falls.[22] The beneficial effects of preventative occupational therapy services were demonstrated by Clark et al.[19] in the investigation of well, elderly adults. Adults who received preventative occupational therapy displayed far fewer health and functional problems when compared to adults who did not receive these services.

2. *Health promotion*: A disabling condition is not assumed, but instead occupational therapy services are provided to enhance and enrich occupational pursuits. This approach may be used to help clients who are transitioning in roles or used to foster occupational performance across contexts. An example would be using narratives to promote a healthy transition from the role of a worker to retirement.[38] As workers described what they anticipated in retirement they linked "past, present, and future" (p. 49). This process of anticipating changes and making choices was considered to be an important factor in "understanding how people adapt to life changes" (p. 49).

3. *Establish or restore a skill or ability*: This strategy is aimed at improving a client's skills or abilities thus allowing greater participation in occupations. Evidence of the effectiveness of occupational therapy services provides this form of intervention as demonstrated by several investigators. Walker et al.[74] investigated the effectiveness of occupational therapy services in restoring *activities of daily living* (ADL) and *instrumental activities of daily living* (IADL) skills in clients who had sustained a *cerebrovascular accident* (CVA) but had not received inpatient rehabilitation services. They used a randomized controlled trial and demonstrated that clients receiving occupational therapy services had significantly better ADL and IADL performance when compared to clients who had not received these services. Rogers et al.[63] also demonstrated that performance of ADLs can be significantly improved when provided with systematic training.

4. *Adapt or compensate*: This approach is focused on modifying the environment, the activity demands, or the client's performance patterns to facilitate engagement in occupations. Instruction and use of energy conservation techniques for clients who have dyspnea (shortness of breath or difficulty breathing) as a result of chronic obstructive pulmonary disease is an example of this approach.[48] The use of *electronic aids to daily living* (EADL) is another example of how the activity can be modified to promote participation.[26] When clients who had acquired brain damage were provided with training in the use of EADL, they reported a sense of mastery. Even if a client's previous abilities cannot be restored, employing this adaptive or compensatory approach can promote participation in occupations.

5. *Maintain current functional abilities*: This approach recognizes that many clients are faced with degenerative disorders, and occupational therapy services should actively address the need to maintain occupational engagement.[17,28] Intervention may focus on the activity demands, performance patterns, or context for occupational performance. As an example, an individual in the early stage of Parkinson's disease is still able to complete many self-care activities but should develop the habits that will maintain these skills as motor function continues to deteriorate. Maintenance also includes clients who have a chronic, non-progressive disorder; in this situation there is a need

for maintaining physical conditioning to meet activity and environmental demands.

Through collaboration with the client and significant others, the intervention plan identifies not only the specific focus of the goal but also the explicit content of the goal. For example, Nora, who sustained a traumatic brain injury, indicated that she wanted to be able to return to driving her children to various community-based activities. Services would focus on two approaches: restoring the skills needed to engage in this occupation of driving her children to community activities and adapting the performance by avoiding community activities that necessitate driving during heavy traffic periods in the morning and late afternoon.

Specific driving skills would be improved using strategies to enhance reaction time, problem solving, and attention to potential safety risks. Due to Nora's diminished memory and difficulties with processing complex information, the occupation of driving her children to community activities should be modified. Nora could select community activities that are close to her children's school and home thereby decreasing the length of time she is driving her children. If these intervention approaches are unsuccessful, the OT may explore alternatives to driving with Nora, such as bicycling or walking with her children to nearby community activities or carpooling with another parent where the other parent assumes the actual driving role and Nora contributes by providing snacks or gas money. Such alternatives could provide a safer solution and still meet the need for Nora to be involved in the occupation of driving or transporting her children to their community activities.

The OT is responsible for the plan and for any parts delegated to the OTA. The plan includes client-centered goals and methods for reaching them using the above-mentioned approaches or strategies. The values and goals of the client are primary; those of the therapist are secondary.[6] Cultural, social, and environmental factors are incorporated into the plan. The plan must identify the scope and frequency of the intervention and the anticipated date of completion. The outcomes of the intervention must be written at the time the intervention plan is developed. Discharge planning is initiated during the intervention planning process. This is accomplished by developing clear outcomes and targeted time frames for completion of goals.

The generation of clear and measurable goals is a very important step in the planning process. Long-term goals or terminal behaviors must reflect a change in occupational performance. For a client to receive authentic occupational therapy services, there must be "engagement in occupation to support participation in context" (p. 611).[6] This may be achieved through several means including improved occupational performance, role competence, adaptation, prevention, or quality of life. To meet this outcome, short-term goals or behavioral objectives reflect the incremental steps that must occur to reach this target. An example would be Nora returning to driving. Several short-term steps would be

TABLE **3-1**   **Format for Writing Goals**

A. Actor	Begin the goal with a statement such as "Nora will ..." Name the client as the performer of the action for the goal.
B. Behavior	The occupation, activity, task, or skill to be performed by the client. If this is an outcome or terminal goal, the behavior must reflect occupational performance. Short-term goals or behavioral objectives are often steps to reaching a long-term goal or outcome. A short-term goal or objective may identify a client factor or performance skill as the targeted behavior. An outcome behavior for Nora would be the ability to drive a car where a short-term behavior would be to enter the car and fasten a seatbelt.
C. Condition	The situations for the performance of the stated behavior include social and physical environmental situations for the behavior. Examples of conditions included in a goal are the equipment used, social setting, and training necessary for the stated behavior. In the situation of Nora, driving a car with an automatic transmission is a far different condition than driving a car with a manual transmission.
D. Degree	The measure applied to the behavior and the criteria for how well the behavior is performed. These may include repetitions, duration, or the amount of the activity completed. A client may only be expected to complete a small portion of an activity as a short-term goal but the long-term goal would address the targeted occupation. The amount of support provided serves as a measure of degree of behavioral performance. This would include whether the client required minimal assistance, verbal prompts, or performed the task independently. The criteria must be appropriate for the behavior. Safely driving 50% of the time is an inappropriate criterion but using a percentage to indicate that Nora will independently fasten her seat belt 100% of the time provides an appropriate criterion for the behavior.
E: Expected timeframe	When is the goal to be met, the time period that is anticipated to meet the goal as stated.

Adapted from Kettenbach G: *Writing SOAP notes,* ed 2, Philadelphia, 2004, FA Davis.

necessary prior to meeting this terminal behavior or long-term goal. An intervention plan may address bilateral coordination and speed of reaction prior to having Nora return to driving. Several authors have provided detailed descriptions of the critical parts of a well-written goal.[39] Table 3-1 serves as a brief guide for the development of goals and objectives. (For additional details regarding goals and documentation see Chapter 8.)

INTERVENTION IMPLEMENTATION

The **intervention plan** is implemented by the OT practitioners. The OT may assign to the OTA specific responsibilities in delivery of the intervention plan. Nonetheless, the OT retains the responsibility to direct, monitor, and supervise the intervention and must ensure that relevant and necessary interventions are provided in an appropriate and safe manner and that documentation is accurate and complete.[3] The method used to provide interventions could include therapeutic use of self, therapeutic use of occupations and activities, consultation, and/or education.[6] (See Chapter 1 for a more detailed description of these methods of providing intervention.) These methods answer the question "How will intervention strategies be provided?" The intervention plan would identify which approach or strategy would be used in combination with the method of intervention. During the actual implementation of intervention services a clinician may seamlessly shift between different methods, depending on the needs of the client.

OT PRACTICE NOTES

The implementation of the intervention plan does not occur in isolation but requires the clinician to continuously review the effectiveness of the services delivered by monitoring the client's response to intervention. At the beginning of each intervention session the OT should answer the following questions:
* What is the primary focus of intervention for this session?
* How will this service meet the client's goals and needs?

Implementation of services should also include helping the client anticipate needs and solutions. A method developed by Schultz-Krohn[68] provides a structure to this process and was labeled anticipatory problem solving. This process was developed from client-centered models such as the Model of Human Occupation[40] and the Person-Environment-Occupation[44,45] model described later in this chapter. This process was designed to empower the client to anticipate potential challenges and develop solutions prior to encountering the challenges. The key elements of the anticipatory problem-solving process are as follows:

1. The client and clinician identify the occupation or activity to be performed.
2. The specific features of the environment that are required for occupational/activity performance are identified. This includes contextual factors and the necessary equipment to engage in the occupation/activity.

3. The OT and client identify potential safety risks or challenges to engagement in the occupation/activity that are located in the environment or with the objects required.
4. The OT and client develop a solution for these risks or challenges.

An example would be Nora, who would like to be able to drive her children to after-school activities. As she regains her abilities to drive, anticipatory problem-solving strategies are employed to prepare her for potential environmental challenges. The process follows these steps:

1. Nora and the OT identified the occupation of driving her children to after-school music lessons as the focus for intervention.
2. The car has an automatic transmission. The route typically used to drive her children from school to the lessons includes a busy street with four lanes but no highway driving is required. She does need to make one left-hand turn on this street but there is a left turn light. The travel time typically takes 10 minutes.
3. Nora reports that traveling on the one busy street can be a challenge because many drivers exceed the speed limit on this road and drive erratically. This is the quickest route to the music lessons and since she is very familiar with the route, it provides less challenge to her memory. Nora's husband also reports that this road often has construction, presenting an additional challenge.
4. Instead of changing the route, Nora develops a solution whereby she allocates an additional five minutes to transport her children to lessons, allowing her to feel less pressure when drivers are exceeding the speed limit. Strategies to address the erratic drivers encountered on this road included frequent checks of her side mirrors and moving to the left lane two intersections before the left-hand turn light. An alternate route is also mapped out to be used when road construction presents a challenge.

This process provides a brief illustration of how anticipatory problem-solving methods can be used during the intervention implementation. This process can be equally applied to bathing, where a client anticipates the potential hazard of a slippery surface and makes appropriate plans before bathing. The foundation of this process is to engage the client in developing solutions for everyday challenges encountered as he or she engages in occupations/activities. The client is actively involved in identifying not only the occupation/activity but also potential challenges or risks encountered and generating solutions for the identified challenges or risks.

INTERVENTION REVIEW

The occupational therapy practitioners evaluate the intervention plan on a regular basis to determine if the client's goals are being met.[6] The OT is "responsible for determining the need for continuing, modifying, or discontinuing occupational therapy services" (p. 665) but the OTA contributes to this process.[3] The review may include a re-evaluation of the client's status to determine what changes have occurred since the previous evaluation. This measurement of the outcomes of intervention is critical in showing the effectiveness of the intervention. The intervention plan may be changed, continued, or discontinued, based on the results of the re-evaluation. This re-evaluation also offers an opportunity to determine if the intervention provided is focused on the outcomes articulated in the plan.

OUTCOMES

Working in collaboration with the client, the client's family, and the intervention team, the OT and OTA identify the intended outcome of the intervention. Although the OTPF clearly states that the outcome of occupational therapy services is focused on the client's ability to engage in occupations to support participation in context, this outcome can be measured in several ways. Outcomes may be written to reflect a client's improved occupational performance; a change in the client's response to an occupational challenge; effective role performance; habits and routines that foster health, wellness and/or the prevention or lessening of further disability; and client satisfaction in the services provided. Client satisfaction can also include overall quality of life outcomes that often incorporate several of the previously mentioned outcomes.

Although the overarching outcome of occupational therapy intervention is to promote "engagement in occupation to support participation in context or contexts" (p. 611), this goal can be achieved through several types of outcomes.[6] The decision of whether the selected outcomes are successfully met is made collaboratively with the members of the intervention team including the client. The outcomes may require periodic revisions due to changes in the client's status. When the client has reached the established goals or achieved the maximum benefit from occupational therapy services, the OT formally discontinues service and creates a discontinuation plan that documents follow-up recommendations and arrangements. Final documentation includes a record of any change in the client's status from first evaluation through the end of services.

Figure 3-1 shows the relationship between the various parts of the intervention process. This process is not completed in a linear fashion but instead requires constant monitoring, and each section informs the other parts of the process. The outcome generated during the planning step should direct an OT to select intervention methods best suited to reach the desired client goals. During the intervention process, it may become apparent that the desired outcome is not realistic, necessitating revision of the client's goals and outcome of services.

CLINICAL REASONING IN THE INTERVENTION PROCESS

Since 1986, the *American Occupational Therapy Association* (AOTA) has funded a series of studies to examine how occupational therapists think and reason in their work with clients.[32]

Clinical reasoning can be defined informally as the process used by OT practitioners to understand the client's occupational needs, make decisions about intervention services, and as a means to think about what we do. There are several forms of clinical reasoning and authors do not consistently use the same term for specific forms of clinical reasoning. Fleming[30] identified three "tracks" of clinical reasoning used by the expert clinician to organize and process data: *procedural, interactive,* and *conditional.* Yet another dimension of clinical reasoning, identified as *narrative reasoning,* has been discussed in the literature by Mattingly.[47] The fifth form of clinical reasoning, *pragmatic reasoning,* describes the practical issues and contextual factors that must be addressed.[50,66] This section will describe how the five basic forms of clinical reasoning, discussed in current literature, can be applied to practice.

Procedural reasoning is concerned with getting things done, with what "has to happen next." This reasoning process is closely related to the medical form of problem solving. The emphasis is often placed on client factors and body functions and structures when this form of reasoning is employed. A connection between the problems identified and the interventions provided is sought using this form of reasoning, and can be seen in critical pathways developed in some hospitals. A *critical pathway* is a form of a decision-making tree based on a series of yes/no questions that can direct client intervention. For example, a client who had a total hip replacement would receive intervention that follows a predicted or anticipated trajectory of recovery. Critical pathways are often developed to support best practice when there is substantial information about a client's course of recovery from a surgical procedure or medical treatment. Procedural reasoning would be used to develop critical pathways and is driven by the client's diagnosis and potential outcomes anticipated for individuals with this diagnosis.

Interactive reasoning is concerned with the interchanges between the client and therapist. The therapist uses this form of reasoning to engage with, to understand, and to motivate the client. Understanding the disability from the client's point of view is fundamental to this type of reasoning. This form of reasoning is used during the evaluation to detect the important information provided by the client and to further explore the client's occupational needs. During intervention, this form of reasoning is used to assess the effectiveness of the intervention selected in meeting the client's goals. The therapeutic use of self fits well with this form of clinical reasoning as a therapist employs personal skills and attributes to engage the client in the intervention process.

Conditional reasoning is concerned with the contexts in which interventions occur, the contexts in which the client performs occupations, and the ways in which various factors might affect the outcomes and direction of therapy. Using a "what if?" or conditional approach, the therapist imagines possible scenarios for the client. The therapist engages in conditional reasoning to integrate the client's current status

with the hoped-for future. Intervention is often revised on a moment-to-moment basis to proceed to an outcome that will allow the client to participate in various contexts. Although an intervention is designed and implemented to foster occupational pursuits, conditional reasoning is not singularly focused on reaching the outcome. Conditional reasoning recognizes that the process of intervention often necessitates a re-appraisal of outcomes. This re-appraisal should be encouraged to help the client refine goals and outcomes.

Narrative reasoning uses story making or story telling as a way to understand the client's experience. The client's explanation or description of life and the disability experience reveal themes that permeate the client's understanding and that will affect the enactment and outcomes of therapeutic intervention. In this sense, narrative reasoning is phenomenological. Narrative reasoning is also used by therapists to plan the intervention session, to create a story line of what will happen for the client as a result of therapy. Here the therapist draws on both interactive and conditional reasoning using the client's words and metaphors to project possible futures for the client. The therapeutic use of self is critical when employing this form of clinical reasoning. Providing an opportunity for the client to share the meaning of the disability experience helps with formulating plans and projecting future occupational performance. This is where the context and occupational performance intersects. A person may be able to engage in an activity with modifications, but those modifications may be unacceptable within the client's cultural and social context. For example, an individual who, prior to a stroke, was an avid motorcyclist is now unable to control the clutch and hand controls necessary to safely drive a motorcycle and also has impaired balance. Although automatic motorcycles are now available with three wheels, this client refuses the option, considering this to be not part of the motorcycle culture.

Pragmatic reasoning extends beyond the interaction of the client and therapist. This form of reasoning integrates several variables including the demands of the intervention setting, the therapist's competence, the client's social and financial resources, and the client's potential discharge environment. Pragmatic reasoning recognizes the constraints faced by the practicing therapist by forces beyond the client-therapist relationship. For example, a hospital that provides inpatient services may not have the resources for a therapist to make a home visit prior to a client being discharged. A therapist, working solely through a home health agency, will not have full access to clinic equipment when working in the client's home. These challenges to providing intervention would be considered when developing an intervention plan using pragmatic reasoning.

Experienced master clinicians engage in all forms of reasoning to develop and modify their plans and actions during all phases of the occupational therapy process. Some of the questions a therapist might consider related to each form of clinical reasoning are listed in Box 3-1.

Box **3-1**   QUESTIONS TO ENGAGE IN CLINICAL REASONING

PROCEDURAL QUESTIONS

What is the diagnosis?

What prognosis, complications, and other factors are associated with this diagnosis?

What is the general protocol for assessment and intervention with this diagnosis?

What interventions (adjunctive methods, enabling activities, purposeful activities) might be employed?

INTERACTIVE QUESTIONS

Who is the client?

What are the client's goals, concerns, interests, and values?

How does the client view his or her occupational performance status?

How does the illness or disability fit into the client's performance patterns?

How might I engage this client?

How can we communicate?

CONDITIONAL QUESTIONS

What contexts has the client identified as important in his or her life?

What future(s) can be imagined for the client?

What events could or would shape the future?

How can I engage the client to imagine, believe in, and work toward a future?

NARRATIVE REASONING

What does the change in occupational performance mean to this client?

How is this change positioned within the client's life history?

How does the client experience the disabling condition?

What vision does the therapist hold for the client in the future?

What "unfolding story" will bring this vision to fruition?

PRAGMATIC REASONING

What organizational supports and constraints must be incorporated into the provision of services?

What physical environmental factors must be considered when designing an intervention plan?

What is the therapist's knowledge and skill level?

CLINICAL REASONING IN CONTEXT

Pressures for cost containment and reduction of unnecessary services require therapists to balance the needs of the client and the practical realities of healthcare reimbursement and documentation. Thus, on first meeting the client, the therapist will want to know the anticipated or required date of discharge, as well as the scope of services that will be reimbursed and those that are likely to be denied. Simultaneously, the therapist is formulating an occupational profile with the client, evaluating the client's occupational performance, engaging the client in identifying outcomes and goals, and determining which interventions would best meet the desired outcomes. The OT also considers the contextual factors that will influence occupational performance. Further, the therapist is alert to requirements for documentation and the particular *current procedural terminology* (CPT) codes that may apply. The OT must document service accurately and effectively so that reimbursement will not be challenged and the client's needs may be adequately addressed. (For a more detailed discussion of documentation see Chapter 8.)

From first meeting the client, the therapist is guided by the client's goals and preferences. Client-centered service delivery requires client (or family) involvement and collaboration at all stages of the intervention process.[6] To effectively engage the client and the family demands, cultural sensitivity and an ability to communicate with people of diverse backgrounds is required.[15,70,73,75] In some cultures, the idea of participating equally in decision making with a health professional may be unknown. Being asked by a therapist to

make decisions may feel quite unfamiliar and uncomfortable to the client. Thus, the therapist must support the client's ability to collaborate, adjust to the client's point of view, and find other ways to ensure that the intervention plan, including intended outcomes, is acceptable to the client and significant others in the client's life. Understanding the influence of culture on the client's occupational performance and performance patterns is fundamental to the provision of services.[15] The OT should pose the following questions to foster cultural competence in the provision of services:

1. *What do I know about the client's culture and beliefs about health?* This represents the basic knowledge of cultural health practices and beliefs. Conclusions or judgments should not be formed about why these practices are present.

2. *Does the client agree with these beliefs?* Although a client may affiliate with a specific cultural group, the OT must investigate if the cultural beliefs of health and the client's beliefs of health are similar.

3. *How will these beliefs influence the intervention and outcomes of services provided?* The OT must acknowledge and respond to the influences of cultural beliefs and practices within the intervention plan. To design a plan that conflicts with cultural beliefs would not only be counter productive to client-centered services but would be disrespectful of the client's belief system. If a client, in deference to the authority of the OT, follows an intervention that conflicts with cultural practices, the client may risk receiving support and affiliation with that cultural group.

4. *How can the intervention plan support culturally endorsed occupations, roles, and responsibilities to promote the client's engagement in occupation?* The OT must consider the important occupations from a cultural perspective. Evening meals may include specific behaviors that possess strong cultural symbols for one client but another client may view an evening meal as merely taking in food with no prescribed rituals.

CLIENT-CENTERED PRACTICE

Involving clients in identifying their own goals and in making decisions about their own care and intervention is highly valued by leaders in the OT profession[29,56,67] and is endorsed by the AOTA in its policy and practice guidelines.[8] Client-centered practice begins when the therapist first meets the client. Therapists using an occupation-based assessment model, such as the *Canadian Occupational Performance Measure* (COPM),[43] initiate assessment by asking clients to identify and choose goals early in the evaluation process. This process can be fostered when the therapist is aware of potential biases that could influence the development of goals.[65] Regardless of disability status or perceived limitations in cognitive functioning, every client should be invited to participate in evaluation and intervention decisions. Client-centered practice is guided by the following concepts:[10]

- Language used reflects the client as a person first and the condition second.
- The client is offered choices and is supported in directing the occupational therapy process.
- Intervention is provided in a flexible and accessible manner to meet the client's needs.
- Intervention is contextually appropriate and relevant.
- There is clear respect for differences and diversity in the occupational therapy process.

THEORIES, MODELS OF PRACTICE, AND FRAMES OF REFERENCE

The profession of occupational therapy acknowledges the need for theories, models of practice, and frames of reference to advance the profession, demonstrate evidence-based intervention, and more clearly view occupation.[40] Theories, models of practice, and frames of reference offer the clinician a means to understand and interpret information to develop an effective intervention plan. These terms require definition and understanding prior to application to practice.

THEORY

This term refers to the process of understanding phenomena including articulating concepts that describe and define phenomena and the relationships between observed events across situations or settings. A theory is tested across settings for confirmation of concepts and relationships. Although a theory may be generated from one profession, it is often applied across professions when the theory is an accepted method of understanding phenomena. According to Reed,[60] "theory attempts to:

- Define and explain relationships between concepts or ideas related to the phenomenon of interest (for example: occupational performance and occupation)
- Explain how these relationships can predict behavior or events
- Suggest ways that the phenomenon can be changed or controlled."[60]

A clear example of a theory that meets these expectations and is well known is germ theory.[13] Widely accepted and tested, germ theory states that microorganisms produce infections. Prior to understanding the relationship between these microorganisms and infections, physicians would perform an autopsy and then go to an adjacent room to deliver a baby without washing hands between the two events. The number and severity of infections occurring after childbirth dramatically decreased when germ theory was accepted and then functionally applied to practice (a frame of reference) through the use of proper hand washing procedures. From an occupational therapy perspective, theories provide the profession with a means to examine occupation and occupational performance and understand the relationship between engagement in occupations and participation in context.[40] The main purpose of a theory is to understand the specific phenomena. Mary Reilly's theory of occupational behavior was designed to explain the importance of occupation and the relationship between occupation and health.[61,62] Her theory served as a foundation for several models of practice within the profession of occupational therapy.

MODEL OF PRACTICE

Model of practice refers the application of theory to occupational therapy practice. This process is achieved through several means such as the development of specific assessments and articulation of principles to guide intervention. Models of practice are not intervention protocols but instead serve as a means to view occupation through the lens of theory with the focus on the client's occupational performance. Models of practice often serve as a mechanism to engage in further testing of the theory.[40] Some authors refer to models of practice as conceptual models[16] whereas other authors include models of practice in the discussion of professional theories.[21] In the profession of occupational therapy, several models of practice exist but the commonality seen in each is the focus on occupation. The main purpose of a model of practice is to facilitate the analysis of the occupational profile and consider potential outcomes with selected interventions. Models should be applicable across settings and client groups instead of designed primarily for a specific diagnostic group. From a very colloquial expression, a model of practice is where the clinician "puts on the OT eye glasses" to bring into focus the client's needs and abilities, various contextual issues, and engagement in occupation. Three of these models of practice will be briefly described. The reader is encouraged to seek additional information from the materials used in this brief description.

Model of Human Occupation

In the **model of human occupation** (MOHO),[40] the engagement in occupation is understood as the product of three interrelated subsystems that cannot be reduced to a linear process. These three subsystems are linked to produce occupational performance. The *volitional* subsystem refers to the client's values, interests, and personal causation. A client may clearly identify values and interests to a clinician but then express a sense of incompetence to engage in a desired occupation. Volition is the client's thoughts and feelings. The *habituation* subsystem refers to the habits and roles that are often critical to a sense of self. Colloquial phrases such as "I don't feel myself" often speak of a distortion of habit or role experienced in life. A client, faced with a disabling condition, often experiences a severe disruption in roles and habits. The sense of self can deteriorate when roles such as driving to work, driving to go shopping, or driving friends to enjoy a picnic are eliminated due to a disabling condition. The *performance capacity* subsystem reflects the client's lived experience of the body. This is not the strength or range of motion available but refers to the client's previous experience, changes, and expectations of performance capacity. Again using a colloquial phrase, "once you've ridden a bicycle you never forget" captures a portion of this concept and requires the therapist to consider the client's experience of successes or failures in using the body to engage in occupations.

Ecology of Human Performance

Ecology of human performance (EHP)[24] was not designed to be used exclusively within the profession of occupational therapy but was intended to serve as a mechanism to understand human performance across professions. An important concept expressed in the EHP is the interaction of the person, the task (activity demands), and the context. Occupational performance is intertwined with, and the product of, the interaction of these three variables. EHP is a client-centered model in which each person is viewed as unique and complex and includes past experiences, skills, needs, and attributes. The task is understood as the objective and observable behaviors to accomplish a goal. The context includes the person's age, life cycle, and health status from a perspective of the cultural and societal meanings of each. Context also addresses the physical, social, and cultural factors that influence performance. EHP recognizes that these three factors influence each other and that the person and task are inextricably linked with the context. Performance is the product of the person engaged in a task within a context. A significant contribution of this model is the equal importance placed on each variable in producing occupational performance. Instead of focusing only on improving skills in the person, intervention using

this model can assume several forms. Five intervention strategies are described and a close similarity to the OTPF can be seen. The five strategies include the following:[25]

1. Establish/restore: Although focused on improving the person's abilities and skills, the intervention includes the context for performance.
2. Alter: Intervention is designed to alter the contextual factors to foster occupational performance; an example would be home modifications to allow wheelchair access.
3. Adapt/modify: The task or context is adapted or modified to support performance such as use of a reacher to obtain objects or using elastic shoelaces to eliminate the need to tie shoes.
4. Prevent: Intervention may address the person, the context, or the task to prevent potential problems from occurring; examples would be back-safety techniques taught to prevent back injuries in a person, removing rugs in an environment to reduce the risk of falls as a contextual prevention method, and turning down the water temperature for a client with sensory problems to reduce the risk of burns when bathing.
5. Create: Intervention addresses all three variables of the person, task, and context and is designed to develop or create opportunities for occupational performance.

Person-Environment-Occupation Model

The person-environment-occupation model (PEO)[44,45] shares characteristics with EHP where occupational performance is seen at the intersection of the person, environment, and occupation. It is a client-centered approach but equal emphasis is placed on the environment and the occupation when designing intervention. PEO defines the person as a dynamic and changing being with skills and abilities to meet roles over the course of time. The environment includes the physical, social, cultural, and institutional factors that influence occupational performance. Occupations include self-care, and productive and leisure pursuits. PEO further differentiates the progression from an activity, a small portion of a task, a task that is a clear step towards an occupation, and the occupation itself, which often evolves over time. An example would be the activity of safely handling a knife. This is a very small portion of the task of making a peanut butter and jelly sandwich and the task of making a sandwich is seen as a part of the occupation of meal preparation. Occupational performance is the result of the person, environment, and occupation interacting in a dynamic manner.

FRAME OF REFERENCE

The purpose of a **frame of reference** (FOR) is to help the clinician link theory to intervention strategies and to apply clinical reasoning to the chosen intervention methods.[41,49] A FOR tends to have a more narrow view of how to approach occupational performance when compared to models of practice. The intervention strategies described within various FORs are not meant to be used as a protocol but offer the practitioner a way to structure intervention and think about intervention progressions. The clinician must always engage in the various forms of clinical reasoning to question the efficacy of the intervention in meeting the client's goals and outcomes.

A frame of reference should be well fitted to meet the client's goals and hoped-for outcomes. The colloquial concept of "one size fits all" definitely does not apply to the use of a FOR to guide intervention. That is why there is a need for multiple FORs to meet varied client goals and outcomes. A clinician may blend intervention strategies from several FORs to effectively meet the client's needs. As an example, a client may be able to recover control of both arms following a *traumatic brain injury* (TBI) by using a biomechanical and sensorimotor FOR, but have persistent memory deficits requiring the use strategies following a rehabilitative FOR. The following brief descriptions are not meant to be an exhaustive review of all possible FORs that can be used in occupational therapy. Examples are provided to illustrate how an FOR can be used to guide the intervention process.

Biomechanical

The understanding of kinematics and kinesiology serves as the foundation for the biomechanical FOR.[69] The clinician views the limitations in occupational performance from a biomechanical perspective, analyzing the movement required to engage in the occupation. Based on principles of physics, the force, leverage, and torque required to perform a task or activity are assessed. These also serve as the basis for intervention. A client may be unable to open a jar of peanut butter or jelly due to limitations in grip strength or the available range of motion required of the hands to hold the jar. A biomechanical approach would focus intervention on addressing these basic client factors to improve occupational performance. Although intervention may take the form of exercises, splinting, or other orthopedic approaches, the outcome must reflect engagement in occupation.[37]

Rehabilitation

The rehabilitation FOR is focused on the client's ability to return to the fullest physical, mental, social, vocational, and economic functioning as is possible. The emphasis is placed on the client's abilities and using the current abilities coupled with technology or equipment to accomplish occupational performance. Compensatory intervention strategies are often employed and examples include teaching one-handed dressing techniques to an individual who, following a CVA, no longer has functional use of one hand. The focus of intervention is often engagement in occupation through alternative means. (For additional examples of intervention strategies supported by the rehabilitation FOR, see Chapters 10, 11, and 16.) Returning to the same example of making a peanut butter and jelly sandwich, instead of having the client work on strengthening the hands to finally open the jar, the clinician would suggest using a device to stabilize the jar and use a gripper to

help accomplish the task with current abilities. Regardless of the technology or equipment available, the clinician must always link the intervention to the client's occupational performance.

Sensorimotor

Several FORs are included in this grouping, such as Rood techniques, *proprioceptive neuromuscular facilitation* (PNF), and *neurodevelopmental treatment* (NDT) (see Chapters 30 and 31 for additional information). These approaches share a common foundation of viewing a client who has sustained a central nervous system insult to the upper motor neurons, as having poorly regulated control of the lower motor neurons. To recapture the control of the lower motor neurons, various techniques are employed to promote reorganization of the sensory and motor cortices of the brain. The specific techniques vary but the basic premise is that by providing systematic sensory information to the client, the brain will reorganize and the return of motor function will be obtained.

MEETING THE CLIENT'S NEEDS

The OT relies on theories, models of practice, and FORs to interpret and integrate evaluation data to meet the client's identified outcomes. These are used in conjunction with clinical reasoning to develop an intervention plan and critically review the successfulness of the plan. For example, the OT would use procedural reasoning to select a theory, model, or FOR that has proven successful with clients who have a similar diagnosis. Interactive reasoning is used to assess if the chosen model or FOR is meeting the client's needs. As a therapist applies theories, models, or FORs to meet the client's needs, a series of professional questions should be posed:

1. Does the theory, model of practice, or frame of reference help with understanding and interpreting the evaluation data while considering the client's expressed needs?
2. Does the theory, model of practice, or frame of reference provide a good fit for the type of intervention that will meet the client's needs?
3. What evidence is available that the theory, model of practice, or frame of reference can efficiently produce the results requested by the client?

The above questions should be posed throughout the intervention process as a review of the effectiveness of services provided. Although the OT is responsible for interpreting and integrating evaluation data, collaborating with the client to develop the intervention plan, and engaging in ongoing review of the effectiveness of intervention, the OTA contributes to the evaluation and intervention process.

TEAMWORK WITHIN THE OCCUPATIONAL THERAPY PROFESSION

The OT profession recognizes and certifies two levels of practitioners, the OT and the OTA. The AOTA has provided many documents to guide practice and to clarify the relationship between the two levels of practitioner.[3,8] The OT operates as an autonomous practitioner with the ability to provide occupational therapy services independently, whereas the OTA "must receive supervision from an occupational therapist to deliver occupational therapy services" (p. 663).[3] Even though OTs are considered able to independently provide occupational therapy services, they should seek supervision and mentoring to foster professional growth. The OT who is managing a case or providing services to clients should use the following as a guide:

- Services are to be provided by personnel who have demonstrated service competency. Some states require advanced training and proficiency in specified arenas of practice. For example, an advanced certification in dysphagia (difficulty swallowing) and physical agent modalities is required in the state of California for an OT to provide those services.
- In the interests of rendering the best care at the least cost, the OT may delegate tasks to OTAs and, in some specific instances, to aides or other personnel, provided these providers have the competencies to render such services. This requires the OT to establish the level of competence required, and assess the ability of the OTA, aides, or other personnel to perform those duties.
- The OT retains final responsibility for all aspects of care, including documentation.

OT-OTA RELATIONSHIPS

To work effectively with OTAs, the OT must understand the role of the practitioner trained at the technical level.[3] It is common for OTs to alternately overestimate and underestimate the capabilities of OTAs. In overestimating the training and abilities of OTAs, OTs might assume that the OTA is trained to provide services identical to those of the OT but perhaps at a lesser pace and level and with a smaller caseload. In underestimating the OTA, the OT might assume that the OTA is capable of performing only concrete and repetitive tasks under the strictest supervision.

The appropriate role of the OTA is complementary to that of the OT. Employed effectively, the OTA can provide occupational therapy services under supervision that ranges from close to general. AOTA has identified critical factors to consider in the delegation of delivery of occupational therapy services.[3] These factors include the severity and complexity of the client's condition and needs, the competency of the OT practitioner, the type of intervention selected to meet the identified outcomes, and the requirements of the practice setting. Working together with several OTAs, the OT will be able to manage a larger caseload and will have the option of introducing more advanced and specialized services, since the role of the OTAs is often to provide routine services. Many variations in the use of OTAs exist across settings. Some services the supervising OT may delegate to the service-competent OTA include the following:

1. Administering selected screening instruments or assessments such as *range of motion* (ROM) tests, interviews and questionnaires, ADL evaluations, and other assessments that follow a defined protocol.[8]
2. Collaborating with the OT and client to develop portions of the intervention plan (e.g., planning for dressing training and planning for kitchen safety training).[8]
3. Implementing interventions supervised by the OT in the areas of ADL, work, leisure, and play. With appropriate training and supervision, the OTA can implement interventions related to other areas of occupational performance.[8] As determined by the OT, an OTA can also implement interventions where competence has been demonstrated. An example would be intervention related to the client factors of strength or range of motion.
4. As assigned by the OT, assisting with the transition to the next service setting by, for example, making arrangements with or educating family members or contacting community providers to address the client needs.
5. Contributing to documentation, record keeping, resource management, quality assurance, selection and procurement of supplies and equipment, and other aspects of service management.
6. Under the supervision of the OT, educating the client, family, or community about OT services.

OCCUPATIONAL THERAPY AIDES

The OT may also extend the reach of services by employing aides. AOTA guidelines stipulate that the **occupational therapy aide** works only under direction and close supervision of an OT practitioner (OT or OTA) and provides supportive services; "Aides do not provide skilled occupational therapy services" (p. 666).[3] Aides may perform only specific, selected, delegated tasks. While the OTA may direct and supervise the aide, the OT is ultimately responsible for the actions of the aide. Tasks that might be delegated to an aide include transporting clients, setting up equipment, preparing supplies, and performing simple and routine client services for which the aide has been trained. Individual jurisdictions and healthcare regulatory bodies may restrict aides from providing client care services; reimbursement may also be denied for some services provided by aides. Where permitted, the OT may delegate routine tasks to aides to increase productivity.[7]

TEAMWORK WITH OTHER PROFESSIONALS

Many healthcare workers collaborate in the care of persons with physical disabilities. Depending on the setting, the OT may work together with *physical therapists* (PT), *speech and language pathologists* (SLP), activity therapists, recreational therapists, nurses, vocational counselors, psychologists, social workers, pastoral care specialists, orthotists, prosthetists, rehabilitation engineers, vendors of durable medical equipment, and physicians from many different specialties.

Relationships among and expectations of various healthcare providers are often determined by the context of care or setting. For example, in some situations, home care services are coordinated by a nurse. In a hospital or rehabilitation setting using a medical model, the physician most often directs the client care program. Some rehabilitation facilities employ a team approach to assessment and intervention, which reduces duplication of services and increases communication and collaboration. Several individuals from different professions may together perform a single evaluation. For example, the OT may be the lead member of the team in some settings, or may be the director of rehabilitation services. In a team, members adjust scheduling and expectations to collaborate with one another to promote effective client care.

Many factors affect relationships among professionals across disciplines: the intervention setting, reimbursement restrictions, licensure laws and other jurisdictional elements, and the training and experience of the individuals involved. Relationships develop over time, based on experience and interaction and sometimes on personality. Even where formal jurisdictional boundaries may appear to limit roles for OT, informal patterns often develop at variance with the prescribed rules. For example, while in some states a physician's referral may be required to initiate OT service, the physicians may expect the OT to initiate the referral and actually perform a cursory screening before the physician becomes involved. Some physicians rely on OT staff to identify those clients who are most likely to benefit from occupational therapy service, and then generate referrals upon the recommendation of the OT.

Another example in which interdisciplinary boundaries may be at variance with actual practice is in the relationships among the rehabilitation specialists of OT, PT, and SLP. By formal definition, each discipline has a designated scope of practice, with some areas of overlap and occasional dispute. The scope of occupational therapy practice is described in the Domain of the Occupational Therapy Practice Framework.[6] Nonetheless, it is common for practitioners to share skills and caseloads across disciplines and to train each other to provide less complex aspects of each discipline's care. Two terms used to describe this are *cross training* and *multiskilling.*

Cross training is the training of a single rehabilitation worker to provide services that would ordinarily be rendered by several different professions. Multiskilling is sometimes used synonymously with cross training, but may also mean the acquisition by a single healthcare worker of many different skills. Arguments have been made for and against cross training and multiskilling.[20,31,55,76] The consumer may benefit by having fewer healthcare providers and better integration of services. Involving fewer providers may reduce costs.

The disadvantages cited include the prospect of erosion of professional identity, possible risk to consumers of harm at the hands of less skilled providers, and ceding the control of individual professions to outside parties such as insurers and advocates of competing professions.

ETHICS

Although the study of **ethics** within an OT curriculum may be addressed as a separate course or topic, clinicians encounter **ethical dilemmas** with surprising frequency. In an ethics survey conducted by Penny Kyler for the AOTA in 1997 and 1998,[42] clinician respondents ranked the following as the five most frequently occurring ethics issues confronting them in practice:

1. Cost-containment policies that jeopardize client care
2. Inaccurate or inappropriate documentation
3. Improper or inadequate supervision
4. Provision of treatment to those not needing it
5. Colleagues violating client confidentiality[42]

Additional concerns were related to conflict with colleagues, lack of access to OT for some consumers, and discriminatory practice. Further, 21% of clinicians reported they faced ethical dilemmas daily, 31% weekly, and 32% at least monthly.[42]

The AOTA has provided several documents to assist OT practitioners in analyzing and resolving ethical questions: the Occupational Therapy Code of Ethics,[5] the Guidelines to the Occupational Therapy Code of Ethics,[4] and Core Values and Attitudes of Occupational Therapy Practice.[2] While these documents provide a basis for resolving ethical issues, practitioners may find additional resources and support if they also approach institutional ethics committees and review boards for guidance. Kyler[42] also suggests that OT practitioners act to formalize resolutions for recurring questions by engaging with peers and others to analyze and consider courses of action.

ETHICAL CONSIDERATIONS

One process of ethical decision making within clinical practice includes the following:[58]

1. Gather sufficient data about the problem.
2. Clearly articulate the problem including the action and consequences.
3. Analyze the problem using theoretical constructs and principles.
4. Explore practical options.
5. Select and implement an action plan to address the problem.
6. Evaluate the effectiveness of the process and outcome.

Lohman et al.[46] expand the discussion of ethical practice to include the public policy arena. Instead of occupational therapy only considering ethical practice from a perspective of service delivery to an individual, they recommend the OT practitioner consider the need to influence public policy to better serve all clients.

To reiterate, OT practitioners should anticipate that they will frequently encounter ethical distress (defined as the subjective experience of discomfort originating in a conflict between ethical principles) in clinical practice. Many approaches may be useful. A plan of action for addressing ethical distress and resolving ethical dilemmas may involve the following:

1. Reviewing AOTA guidelines[2,4,5]
2. Seeking guidance from institutional ethics and review boards
3. Approaching and engaging colleagues, peers, and the community to identify and debate ethical questions and formalize resolutions

SUMMARY

The occupational therapy process begins with referral and ends with discontinuation of service. While discrete stages can be named and described as evaluation, intervention, and outcomes, the process is more spiraling and circular than stepwise. The processes of evaluation, intervention, and outcomes influence and interact with one another. This may look confusing to the novice, but it is actually a hallmark of clinical reasoning.

Different types of clinical reasoning are simultaneously employed to make decisions about the form and type of service provided. While logically analyzing how to proceed through the steps of therapy using procedural reasoning, the therapist also considers how best to interact with the client. Further, the therapist creates scenarios of possible future situations. The expert clinician seeks to uncover how the client understands the disability and uses a narrative or story making approach to capture the client's imagination of how therapy will benefit him or her. This process is also influenced by the pragmatic reasoning that draws attention to the demands of the current healthcare arena.

The OT profession endorses client-centered practice, engaging the client in all stages of decision making, beginning with assessment. To make this ideal a clinical reality requires that the OT approach every client as a co-participant and assist the client in identifying and prioritizing goals and in considering and selecting intervention approaches.

The occupational therapist and occupational therapy assistant have specific responsibilities and areas of emphasis within the OT process. The OT is the manager and director of the process and delegates specific tasks and steps to the qualified OTA. Aides may also be employed to extend the reach of OT services.

Effective practice typically involves interactions with members of other professions. This requires that the OT practitioner consider the intervention setting, the scope of practice of other professions, the applicable jurisdictions and healthcare regulations, and other factors (e.g., culture, personality, and history) that affect the individual situation.

Ethical questions arise with increasing frequency in modern healthcare. The AOTA provides guidelines and other resources; practitioners are urged to consider institutional and local resources as well, and to take an active role in identifying and resolving ethical concerns.

SECTION 2: PRACTICE SETTINGS FOR PHYSICAL DISABILITIES

Winifred Schultz-Krohn
Heidi McHugh Pendleton
with contributions from:
Maureen Michele Matthews
Michelle Tipton-Burton

Individuals who have a physical disability receive occupational therapy services in a variety of settings. These may include acute care hospitals, acute inpatient rehabilitation, subacute rehabilitation, outpatient clinics, skilled nursing facilities, assistive living units, home health, day treatment, community care programs, and work sites. Regardless of the physical setting in which services are delivered, the OT should always focus on enhancing occupational performance to support participation across contexts. The OT practitioner needs to be mindful of the supports and constraints encountered in the various practice settings.

A **practice setting** refers to the environment in which OT intervention occurs, an environment that includes the physical facility or structure along with the social, economic, cultural, and political situation that surrounds it. Several factors influence the delivery of OT service within a specific practice setting including the following: (1) government regulations, (2) the economic realities of reimbursement rules, (3) the workplace pressures of critical pathways and other clinical protocols, (4) the range of services that are considered customary and reasonable, and (5) the traditions and culture that the staff have developed over time.

In addition, there are physical aspects such as the building itself, the temperature and humidity of the air, the colors and materials that are used, the layout of the space, and the furnishings and lighting. Practitioners must always be aware that context influences client performance in evaluation and intervention. The practice setting also influences the type of intervention available.[53] *Length of stay* (LOS) and limitations on the numbers of visits require the OT practitioner to carefully examine intervention that can produce outcomes within the allotted time. Each practice setting has unique physical, social, and cultural circumstances that influence the individual's ability to engage in occupations or activities. These environmental features are important to consider when projecting how the client will perform in another setting. For example, individuals who are in control in their home environment may abdicate control for even simple decisions in an acute care hospital, giving the erroneous impression of being passive and indecisive.[14] The following section describes the typical practice settings in which OT services are provided for persons with physical disabilities. Table 3-2 provides a comparison of the approaches used at the various settings, length of time services are provided, and the frequency of services. Notice that although the typical client conditions do not substantially change across settings, the approaches change to

TABLE **3-2** **Comparison of Practice Settings**

Practice Setting	Length of Time Services Are Provided	Examples of Client Conditions Needing OT Services	Examples of Typical OT Approaches Used in Setting	Frequency of Services
Acute care hospitalization	Days to 1 or 2 weeks	Acute injuries and illnesses, exacerbations of chronic conditions	Restore ability or skill, modify the activity or context, prevention of further disability with an emphasis on discharge setting	Daily
Acute rehabilitation	Weeks	Neurological, orthopedic, cardiac, and general medical conditions	Restore ability or skill, modify the activity or context, prevention of further disability with emphasis on occupational performance	Daily, 3 hours a day
Subacute rehabilitation	Weeks to months	Neurological, orthopedic, cardiac, and general medical conditions	Restore ability or skill, modify the activity or context, prevention of further disability with emphasis on occupational performance	Daily to weekly
Skilled nursing facilities	Months to years	Neurological, orthopedic, cardiac, and general medical conditions	Restore ability or skill, modify the activity or context, prevention of further disability, preserve current skills	Daily, weekly, monthly consultation
Home- and community-based settings	Weeks to months	Neurological, orthopedic, cardiac, and general medical conditions	Restore ability or skill, modify the activity or context, prevention of further disability with emphasis on occupational performance	Daily to weekly
Residential care and ALUs	Months to years	Neurological, orthopedic, cardiac, and general medical conditions	Restore ability or skill, modify the activity or context, prevention of further disability, preserve current skills, health promotion	Weekly, monthly consultation
Home health care	Weeks to months	Neurological, orthopedic, cardiac, and general medical conditions	Restore ability or skill, modify the activity or context, prevention of further disability	Weekly
Outpatient	Weeks to months	Neurological, orthopedic, cardiac, and general medical conditions	Restore ability or skill, modify the activity or context, prevention of further disability with emphasis on occupational performance	Weekly
Day treatment	Months to years	Neurological, orthopedic, cardiac, and general medical conditions	Restore ability or skill, modify the activity or context, prevention of further disability, preserve current skills, health promotion	Daily, weekly
Work site	Weeks to months	Neurological, orthopedic, cardiac, and general medical conditions	Restore ability or skill, modify the activity or context, prevention of further disability with emphasis on occupational performance	Weekly, monthly consultation

meet the client's needs. Suggestions for modifications of the therapeutic environment and clinical approach are given.

CONTINUUM OF HEALTHCARE

The variety of settings forms a continuum of care, albeit not always in a sequential fashion, for the client who has a physical disability. Persons with physical disabilities who are referred to occupational therapy services may enter the healthcare system at any point on the continuum and do not necessarily follow a direct progression through the various settings described below. A client in an acute hospital might be referred for bed mobility, transfers, and self-care retraining. Depending on the severity of the condition and the potential to improve, the client may be seen in a rehabilitation or day treatment program. A home health or outpatient therapist may see the same individual to address unresolved problems and modify the home environment to maximize occupational performance.

Should the client return to the workforce, he or she may benefit from occupational therapy services, such as an assessment and recommendations about modifications to the work environment or job tasks (see Chapter 13). Some hospitals offer a range of healthcare services from an emergency room and acute care or *intensive care unit* (ICU), to inpatient and outpatient rehabilitation services. Other settings may offer only outpatient rehabilitation services.

INPATIENT SETTINGS

Settings in which the client receives nursing and other healthcare services while staying overnight are classified as **inpatient settings**.

Acute Care Inpatient Setting

Clients in an **acute care** inpatient setting typically have a new medical condition, such as a heart attack, burn, or a traumatic brain injury (TBI), that led to hospitalization or an exacerbation of a chronic condition, for example multiple sclerosis. An acute decline in a chronically progressive condition abruptly confronts the client with a long-term prognosis of increasing disability. The client may require life support due to the severity of the condition. Terminally ill clients, who have managed in their own home with support from a hospice program, may require acute hospitalization for pain management, placement, or imminent death; in such cases, a client's hospice goals should be clearly stated and respected by the hospital staff. (For additional information on hospice care see the section on skilled nursing facilities later in this chapter and Chapter 45).

Acute hospitalization, especially when unplanned, results in a sudden change in the client's context(s). Previous social roles may be abandoned when the person becomes hospitalized. External stressors such as financial issues or disruption of career and educational pursuits must be considered when providing services in an acute care setting. An individual who felt in control of his or her life becomes controlled by the circumstances requiring the hospitalization. Nora had a sudden change in her ability to control her environment and exercise her role as a wife and mother. When she sustained her TBI, she was admitted through the emergency room, hospitalized in an ICU to stabilize her condition, and had both a *naso-gastric* (NG) tube and a catheter inserted. On the second day in the ICU, the occupational therapist evaluated Nora's ability to manage oral secretions and swallow her own saliva. She would continue to receive the majority of her nutrition through the NG tube but was cleared to begin to eat thick liquids such as nectar. When her vital signs stabilized on day three, she was transferred to an acute rehabilitation setting for continued therapy services.

Three general roles have been identified for the occupational therapist working in the acute care setting: education, initiation of the rehabilitation process, and consultation.[12] Education may address safety precautions and activity analysis. Rehabilitation services may be initiated for clients who will be transferred to a rehabilitation facility. Consultation is focused on the discharge environment and client needs after leaving the acute care hospital. An experienced occupational therapist, equipped with knowledge of available resources in the hospital and community, can offer a better coordinated and efficient intervention plan to promote client progress and anticipate outcomes. For example, a therapist who determines that a client living alone at discharge would be unable to prepare meals should contact the social worker who would help arrange for the delivery of meals to the home. Another example is a therapist who evaluates a client scheduled for imminent discharge and finds that the client is impulsive, lacks insight into the consequences of his or her actions, and is confused when performing self-care tasks. In this instance, the therapist expresses these concerns to the discharge coordinator or the physician. The social worker might be consulted about family support available, or discharge may be delayed to determine if appropriate environmental supports are available for the client.

Acute hospitalizations are frequently stressful and frustrating for clients. Away from home while ill, subjected to multiple tests and examinations with sleep interrupted, clients are in a socially compromised environment. They may experience sleep deprivation and over-stimulation due to the frequency of procedures or interventions. Some clients, after 2 or 3 days in the ICU, may display marked difficulties with orientation, appearing confused, agitated, and disorganized.[54] This has been referred to as ICU psychosis and clients may experience hallucinations in addition to anxiety and confusion. The client's history should be reviewed to determine if previous episodes of disorientation and confusion were present, or if they are produced by the disorienting effects of being hospitalized in an intensive care unit (ICU). Concerns as to whether they might be able to return home after the hospitalization, who will help with care, or who is helping care for dependent loved ones may add to the client's feelings of stress.

The acute hospitalization has many physical environmental factors that present a challenge to clients. Often clients have several monitors in place and/or tubes inserted such as oxygen saturation monitors, cardiac monitors, arterial lines, and catheters that may compromise engagement in occupations.[36] The arrangement of the hospital rooms and extra equipment can further impact the client's occupational performance. The absence of carpeting and the presence of a slippery floor surface may prove challenging for clients during a transfer and when walking. The incidence of falls in the geriatric population is higher in acute hospitals than in either the community or skilled nursing facilities.[18]

Providing OT intervention services in an acute care setting may be challenging for therapists, because it is often necessary to perform assessments in client rooms rather than in more natural environments designed for ADLs. Performance of various activities may be influenced by catheters, feeding tubes, or monitors. Likewise, client performance in some self-care activities may be artificially enhanced by a lack of the extraneous stimuli found in the home and by the physical attributes of hospital equipment. For example, a client whose home includes three very active cats, several throw rugs on a slippery floor, a very soft bed several feet from the bathroom, and a tiny bathroom faces far more challenges to get up in the middle of the night to use the toilet when compared to the same activity performed in the hospital. The hospital has no throw rugs or active cats as obstacles and often the bathroom is adapted to support safety and performance in toileting. To partially replicate the home environment during the intervention session, the therapist might position the client's bed flat, eliminate the bed rails, and lower the bed to better simulate the client's home. Most hospitals would not allow further challenges such as bringing a cat into the room or scattering throw rugs on the floor as an obstacle for the client. Using clinical experience and judgment, along with information provided by the client regarding the home environment, the therapist must be able to anticipate the client's performance at home. However, referral to a home health therapist is also advisable to assess occupational performance and accessibility in the client's home.

The acute care hospital also presents unique economic, social, and physical challenges to the occupational therapist. Medical intervention is directed toward promoting medical stability and providing for safe, expedient discharge. It is not unusual for the individual in acute care to receive OT services for the first time on the day of discharge. During this single visit, the therapist must communicate the role of OT, establish an occupational profile, and assist the client in identifying problems and assets in the discharge environment. The client and the family frequently look to the therapist to identify what the client will need at home. The therapist, in collaboration with the client and family, must develop intervention priorities by identifying issues and concerns after discharge from the acute care setting. The intervention plan may include purchase of durable medical equipment and referral for further intervention to inpatient rehabilitation, a skilled nursing facility, an outpatient clinic, or home health therapy providers. By contacting other members of the healthcare team and communicating concerns, the therapist can facilitate implementation of the recommendations.

Inpatient Rehabilitation Setting

Clients may be admitted to an **inpatient rehabilitation** unit when they are able to tolerate several (usually 3) hours of therapy per day and are deemed capable of benefiting from rehabilitation. Rehabilitation settings may be classified as acute or subacute (see below). Clients are generally medically stable in this setting and require less acute medical care when compared to services provided in an acute care hospital. Pain, which may be present and affecting client performance, should be addressed in this setting. Performance in ADLs will reflect the client's adaptation to pain, and the energy expended to perform self-care tasks should be considered (see Chapter 27 for a further discussion of pain).

During Nora's acute rehabilitation hospitalization she received occupational therapy services twice a day along with

daily services from a speech and language pathologist and a physical therapist. These services were coordinated to support client outcomes. As is common during acute rehabilitation hospitalization, Nora was expected to dress in her typical street clothing and eat meals at a table in a dining area. This environmental feature of the acute rehabilitation setting provides a social element that is not present in the acute care hospital.

Acute Rehabilitation

When clients are medically stable and able to tolerate 3 hours of combined therapy services for 5 to 6 days a week, they may be transferred to an acute inpatient rehabilitation setting. Clients may still require some level of acute medical care in this setting. The *length of stay* (LOS) in **acute rehabilitation** settings generally ranges from 2 to 3 weeks, but varies according to the client's needs. The usual discharge plan from acute rehabilitation is to a lesser level of care (e.g., residential care or client's home with assistance such as a home health aide or personal care attendant).

The process of adjustment to disability has begun by the time the client has entered acute rehabilitation. As the client begins to participate in areas of occupation, deficits and strengths become more defined. An improvement in the client's function from the onset of the disabling condition may have occurred. Within a rehabilitation center, many clients form new social relationships with individuals who have similar disabilities. The advantages of these relationships are emotional support and encouragement from the progress of others. In rehabilitation, interventions are focused on resuming those roles and occupations deemed important to the client's life. For example, an adolescent will re-establish social roles with peers; a parent will resume child-care responsibilities.

Although bedrooms in acute inpatient rehabilitation settings are similar to those found in acute care hospitals, clients are often encouraged to personalize their room by having family and friends bring in pictures, comforters, and other items from home. In this setting, clients are expected to wear street clothes rather than pajamas. Most clothing selected by clients is easy-to-don leisure wear. The OT practitioner must consider the range of clothing the client will be expected to wear for resumption of his or her occupational roles upon discharge and include training with appropriate clothes such as neckties, button-front shirts, and panty hose if necessary.

Simulated living environments, family rooms, kitchens, bathrooms, and laundry facilities can be found at most rehabilitation centers. These environments may be inaccurate replicas of the client's home. For example, laundry machines may be side-by-side and top loading rather than coin operated and front loading. Kitchens may be wheelchair accessible in the facility but inaccessible in the home. Clutter, noise, and types of appliances encountered in the rehabilitation setting often vary from the client's natural environment.

Access to the community is not generally evaluated during the acute rehabilitation hospitalization. Some urban facilities are able to integrate community training more smoothly because stores, restaurants, and theaters are located near the hospital. Although the community surrounding the hospital may differ from the client's neighborhood, this offers an opportunity to experience a more natural environment.

The culture of rehabilitation facilities is focused on client performance and goal attainment. The client's own culture may be compromised in the process of rehabilitation unless the team is sensitive to and incorporates client's perspective into the intervention plan.[15] For example, some cultures view hospital settings as a place for respite and passive client involvement. Engaging clients in ADL performance can be in direct conflict with client and family expectations. When cultural perspectives clash, unrealistic goals may result. As is the case in any setting, meeting the established outcomes is dependent upon clear communication and identification of goals that are relevant and meaningful to the client.[65]

Upon completion of the acute inpatient rehabilitation program, some clients return home and receive home health services. Unfortunately, not all clients eligible to receive home health services are referred for these services.[51] The occupational therapist should actively participate in discharge planning for clients to ensure they receive the necessary services when discharged from the acute rehabilitation setting. Clients are also referred to a subacute rehabilitation setting upon discharge from the acute rehabilitation hospitalization for continued services. There are several similarities between the acute and subacute rehabilitation settings. The primary differences found in subacute settings are discussed in the following section.

Subacute Rehabilitation

Subacute rehabilitation facilities are found in skilled nursing facilities and other facilities that do not provide acute medical care. The equipment available to the occupational therapist for intervention and evaluation in the subacute setting may be comparable to that found in the acute rehabilitation facility. The focus of intervention continues to address restoring functional abilities but with the slower rate of change the occupational therapist must also consider the need to adapt or modify the environment to promote occupational performance. Lengths of stay in the subacute setting varies and may last from a week to several months. This setting is also known as a short-term skilled nursing facility admission. Clients are usually discharged to a lesser level of care when they leave a subacute rehabilitation setting.

The pace of intervention services varies, and engaging in 3 hours of therapy per day is not mandatory. Client endurance will influence the frequency and duration of therapies. A client may continue to make steady gains but at a slower pace than was seen during the acute inpatient rehabilitation stay.

Because many subacute rehabilitation programs are located in skilled nursing facilities, the client may have roommates who are convalescing rather than actively participating in rehabilitation services. This presents as an additional variable to be considered in the intervention plan since the social context does not always support participation in the rehabilitation services provided at the setting. Staff may be more oriented to the skilled nursing care services and not allocate similar efforts toward the rehabilitation goals of independence.

Skilled Nursing Facilities

A **skilled nursing facility** (SNF) is an institution that meets Medicare or Medicaid criteria for skilled nursing care, including rehabilitation services. Although subacute and short-term rehabilitation programs may be housed in SNFs, occupational therapy services are also provided to individuals who are not in a subacute rehabilitation program. They are known as long-term skilled programs. Many residents (the preferred consumer label for persons who live in long-term care settings) will remain in SNFs for the remainder of their lives; others will be discharged home.[11] Goals should be directed toward independence and meaningful occupational pursuits and may include fostering engagement in occupations through environmental modifications and adaptations. An example would be reading materials and playing cards with enlarged print to foster leisure pursuits for clients with macular degeneration. Hospice services may be included in this setting if appropriate.[72] Hospice care requires the physician to document that the client "probably has 6 months or fewer to live" (p. 8).[72] The services provided do not focus on rehabilitation but instead address palliative care and environmental modifications. Occupational therapy services for hospice clients should address access to the environment and participation in occupation through support and modifications. For example, occupational therapy services could address participation in leisure pursuits as a hospice client creates a memory book for significant others.

The physical and social environment in skilled nursing facilities may impede the natural performance of ADLs. Clients often receive additional assistance with self-care tasks to expedite task completion but this assistance is not focused on fostering engagement in occupational performance.[64] An investigation within SNFs demonstrated that even clients who were severely cognitively impaired benefited from intervention that was focused on fostering client participation in ADLs. Not only did clients increase participation in self-care tasks but there was also a reduction in disruptive behavior.

Extreme variations in disability status are present in SNFs. Observing residents who are severely and permanently disabled may lead newly disabled individuals to form negative expectations of their own prognosis and performance. Younger adults placed in SNFs (where most residents are older adults) may feel isolated and abandoned, which can adversely affect performance. Friends are less likely to visit in this environment. Family and friends may expect less of the individual than they would in other settings. Maintaining connections with friends from the community may require the client to actively pursue these relations. A therapist who facilitates identification of realistic and meaningful expectations and goals with the resident can promote a more positive outlook and outcome. A strong family commitment can support outside relationships by providing transportation to various community gatherings.

COMMUNITY-BASED SETTINGS

These settings often afford the therapist access to the client's natural physical, social, and cultural environments. Services provided in community settings can foster not only skill acquisition and habit formation but also engagement in occupations in context(s). **Community-based settings** may include a residential aspect but the client is not hospitalized. Clients also reside in their home when receiving community-based services.

Home- and Community-Based Settings

An alternative to an acute inpatient rehabilitation program for clients with traumatic injuries such as head or spinal cord injuries is a home- and community-based therapy program. This type of program provides intensive rehabilitation in the client's own home and community. The client receives comprehensive rehabilitation services and acquires functional skills in daily activities in the normal environments of home, school, work site, and community. This enhances the likelihood of a successful and functional outcome.

For example, Nora may benefit more from working on tasks in her home and community than in a clinic or acute rehabilitation setting. The client is performing in her natural physical, social, and cultural environment. Scheduling is within control of the client, and intervention sessions vary in length and frequency depending on the goals. An all-morning session to work with the client as she moves through her daily routine (e.g., bathing and dressing her child, going grocery shopping, and performing various household chores) would be possible.

OT PRACTICE NOTE

The therapist must be able to adapt the intervention to the natural social and cultural aspects present in the home. Attempts to alter the natural social and cultural order are ill advised, since things are likely to return to their natural state when the session ends and the therapist leaves.

When practice is necessary for goal attainment, a rehabilitation technician or therapy aide may be charged with carrying out specific and limited programs established by the therapist. The technician who spends many hours with the client can provide insight when the program is not succeeding because it interferes with the natural context of the client's lifestyle. Adjusting intervention strategies to adapt to these lifestyle differences will ensure better clinical outcomes.

Intermediate Care Facilities (Residential Care)

Generally, **residential facilities** more closely resemble home situations; persons may reside there on a permanent or transitional basis, depending on prognosis.[57] Similarities in the age of residents, their disability status, and even diagnoses are commonly present. Although clients do not require ongoing intensive medical care, the facilities are staffed with care providers 24 hours a day due to clients' need for safety and supervision. OT services may not be available on a daily basis and rehabilitation technicians may implement the unskilled portions of the intervention plans addressing ADLs, select IADLs, and leisure. Often clients require ongoing assistance for portions of these tasks, and personal care attendants or technicians complete portions of the activity or task. The therapist can identify key performance issues in this context. Difficulties with evening self-care, follow-through with safety guidelines, problem solving, schedules, and client performance are reviewed and discussed with the OT. Modifications in the intervention plan can be more easily tailored to promote independence under such close supervision.

Assisted Living Units or Residence

An **assisted living unit** (ALU) provides health services in a cooperative living setting. A client may live in an apartment or cottage where one or more meals are provided on a daily basis, medication management is provided as needed, and 24-hour support is available. These settings usually have age restrictions and residents must be over the age of 55 years old, or if a couple, one person must be over the age of 55. The client generally does not plan or anticipate a move to another type of setting and is often expected to own or rent the living space in the ALU. Since there is an age restriction for most ALUs, the social and environmental support is present to preserve living in one's own space. For example, apartments or cottages may be equipped with safety railings in the bathroom and walk-in closets for ease of accessibility.

In this setting, occupational therapy services are provided to foster and enhance the habits and routines necessary to remain housed in this environment, which often includes personal care skills such as dressing, grooming, hygiene, and simple home care tasks. Some household tasks may be partially assumed by the services provided in the assisted living setting. For example, an ALU may provide a service of laundering towels and bed linen but the individual is responsible for the care of his or her own clothing items. Some ALU settings provide all meals whereas other settings provide only one meal and the individual will need simple meal preparation skills to remain living in that setting. It is important for the OT to determine what services are available at the ALU prior to designing an intervention plan with the client. An important occupational pursuit for those in this setting would be leisure activities. Environmental supports such as magnifiers for reading, enlarged print playing cards, and a universal remote to access the television may provide opportunities for leisure activities in this setting.

Home Health

Home health care provides services within the client's home and affords the most natural context for intervention. Blue Cross of California defines a meaningful therapeutic outcome as "one in which the activity level achieved by the patient . . . is . . . necessary for the patient to function most effectively at home or work."[71] The client, returning home from the hospital, begins to resume life roles at home. The focus of occupational therapy intervention would be to support participation in those roles.

A visiting therapist is a guest in the client's home and is subject to certain social rules associated with guests. For example, the family may practice the custom of removing street shoes within the home and the therapist should respect and comply with this practice. Daily schedules for meals, waking, and sleeping are established by the client and family. Appointments should support the family's routines and not interfere with daily schedules. For example, if the client is accustomed to eating a larger meal during the middle of the day and a very small evening meal, an intervention to address meal preparation skills should be scheduled to support this routine.

Self-care, homemaking, and cooking tasks evaluated in the context of the home clearly identify the challenges that the client meets daily. The familiar clothing, furniture, appliances, and utensils used in everyday life are present and promote orientation and task performance. However, moving of furniture to make things more accessible and safe for the client, or modifying equipment to be used within the home may challenge orientation skills and increase confusion. Caring for and feeding pets, answering the door safely, and determining a grocery list for the week are potential issues to be addressed within the home setting. Self-care tasks such as bathing can be addressed within the natural environment and when appropriate modifications to the home are made, the client's dependence on others may decrease.[27]

Social and family support, or lack thereof, is readily evident to the home health therapist. Individuals who appeared alone and unsupported while hospitalized may have a network of friends and family members who lend support at home. Conversely, other individuals who had frequent visitors in the hospital may be abandoned when the realities of disability reach the home setting.

The client who receives home health services typically requires assistance for some aspects of his or her ADLs. Nearly 20% of all family caregivers are employed full-time outside the home.[9] These caregivers are available for only part of the client's day and will be concerned primarily with the safety of the client during their absence.

Stress is common among caregivers. Respite care, which temporarily places the client under the care and supervision of an alternative caregiver for a few hours and up to several days, can provide necessary relief for a caregiver.[9] Caring for a person with a disability in one's home is not an easy task.

Box **3-2**   Concerns in Caring for a Person with Disability in One's Home

AMOUNT AND TYPE OF CARE NEEDED

Long-term versus temporary, intensive supervision or assistance versus minimal, help available to the caregiver, presence of alternative solutions, and personal feelings about the client and the type of care required (intimate assistance versus household tasks).

IMPACT ON THE HOUSEHOLD

Effect on spouses, children, and others living in the home; possible involvement of family in making decisions.

ENVIRONMENTAL CONCERNS

Need and possibility of adapting the home, expenses of adaptations.

WORK AND FINANCE

Options for family medical leave; ability and need to quit work; benefits available.

Adapted from Visiting Nurses Association of America: *Caregiver's handbook: a complete guide to home medical care,* New York, 1997, DK Publishing.

Box 3-2 identifies practical concerns surrounding the presence of a client in the home. By providing individualized occupational therapy recommendations for home modifications, caregiver approaches, and community-based resources for clients who had Alzheimer's disease, caregivers reported a decrease in a sense of burden and improved quality of life.[23]

When viewing the client's home environment, the therapist can make recommendations for environmental adaptations, see them implemented, and modify those changes as needed to best meet the client's needs.[35] Physical changes to the home, including moving furniture, dishes, or bathing supplies, should not be undertaken without the permission of the client and are best considered through a team approach to support the collaboration between professionals and client.[59] If the client is in the home of a family member or friend, the permission of the homeowner must also be sought.

The client and family are in control of the home environment. Clinicians who fail to ask permission before adapting the environment will rapidly alienate their clients. A throw rug, viewed by the therapist as a tripping hazard, may be a precious memoir from the client's childhood home. In seeking permission of the client and family and providing options, the therapist opens communication. An adhesive mat placed beneath the throw rug will provide a safer surface on which to walk. Another possible solution is to hang the rug as a wall tapestry, where it will be more visually prominent and less prone to damage.

Healthcare workers in the home occasionally encounter ethical dilemmas, typically involving safety.[52] The therapist must determine the best method for resolving issues of safety hazards. Fire and health hazards must be discussed and corrected when the safety of the client or adjacent households is in jeopardy. By broaching the subject diplomatically and directly, the therapist can address most hazards and provide acceptable solutions. Inclusion of the client, family, and other team members in the process of problem identification and solution generation is strongly recommended.

When Nora returned home after her acute rehabilitation hospitalization, Sheena arranged for her to receive OT services through a home health agency. Nora, Sheena, and the home health OT identified concerns with meal preparation, laundry, and playing with her children as important occupations to be addressed. Sheena was not able to make a home visit prior to Nora's discharge from the acute rehabilitation program but was able to coordinate continued services through the home health agency. The home health OT worked with Nora on strategies to improve her safety in meal preparation, helped her to simplify her laundry and cleaning routines, and provided suggestions for leisure activities in which Nora could engage with her children in the home.

OUTPATIENT SETTINGS

Outpatient OT service is provided in hospitals and freestanding clinics to clients who reside elsewhere. Clients receiving services in this setting are medically stable and able to tolerate a few hours of therapy and travel to an outpatient clinic. Although many clients are adjusting to a new disability, some persons with long-standing disability may be referred for re-evaluations of functional status and equipment-related issues. The frequency of services provided in this setting varies substantially, with some clients receiving services several times a week and other clients seen once every few months. The frequency of service is determined by the client's needs and the services offered at the outpatient clinic.

Clients exert more control over outpatient therapy schedules when compared to inpatient therapy schedules. Transportation issues and pressing family matters necessitate that clinics offer a variety of times from which a client may choose. Otherwise, the client may select a different clinic or choose to forego therapy.

To evaluate a client's performance of ADLs or IADLs in an outpatient setting, the therapist must extrapolate how task performance would occur at home.[64] Engaging in self-care tasks in an outpatient clinic may be awkward for the client. Individuals who have been assisted with bathing and dressing before coming to the clinic may resist working on these same tasks during therapy. The more contrived and inappropriate a task and context seems to clients, the less likely they will perform well and benefit from services addressing those needs.

The physical design and equipment seen in outpatient clinics vary to meet the intervention needs of specific disabilities. Hand therapy programs, for example, will have treatment tables for exercise and activities and areas for splint fabrication. A clinic designed to address industrial work is often equipped with special exercise equipment such as Baltimore Therapeutic Equipment (BTE), which mimics work tasks. Less commonly found in the outpatient setting are complete kitchens with cooking equipment and therapeutic apartments with bathing facilities, living rooms, and bedrooms.

The social context found in outpatient programs is quite distinctive. The client has begun to resume life in the home and community and may be newly aware of problems not previously foreseen or acknowledged. If the therapist is viewed as an ally in resolving problems and promoting a smooth transition to home, the client or family members may easily disclose concerns. However, if the client and family fear that the client will be removed from the home because of an inability to manage there, they may actively hide concerns from the therapist. In the former instance the client and family view themselves as being in control of the situation. In the latter, control and power are assumed to belong to the healthcare professional. An outpatient therapist must be skilled in empowering the client. Soliciting client opinion and listening for unspoken needs are two methods for increasing the client's sense of control.[35] Providing choices for intervention does much to motivate clients and improve performance in desired tasks.

Day Treatment

Day treatment programs are becoming more popular as a community-based intervention setting. Programs vary, but the underlying philosophy is to provide an intensive interdisciplinary intervention for clients who do not need to be hospitalized.[33] Clients receiving day treatment typically live at home but frequently require support and assistance for ADLs or IADLs. Most programs offer a team approach. Professionals from all disciplines are engaged cooperatively, sharing their expertise to meet the client's individual goals. Clients may seek services from a day treatment program to further recover functional skills following an acute injury or illness such as a TBI or CVA, or clients with a progressively deteriorating disorder, such as Parkinson's disease or Alzheimer's disease, may benefit from a day treatment program to foster continued participation in occupations through environmental modifications and adaptations.

Many day treatment programs are designed without the time constraints seen in many outpatient programs. Lengthy community outings and home and work site intervention sessions may be used as a method of attaining goals. In a day treatment setting, the occupational therapist may have the best opportunity to evaluate and provide intervention for clients in all of their natural environments.

Work Site Therapy Settings

Industrial rehabilitation can be conducted in the context of the employee's place of work. Work site therapy programs are designed to address an employee's therapy needs related to work injury. The injured worker receives intervention to foster the occupational performance necessary in the work place, which may include work hardening, back safety, energy conservation, and work simplification techniques. This approach places the client back into the work role. Prevention of further injury occurs in a more natural context when employees are treated at the work site.

Providing OT services to individuals at their place of work helps them make the transition from the patient role to the role of worker. The therapist providing service at the work site must avoid compromising the worker's status.[34] The employer and peers view the employee as a worker rather than as a client. Maintaining confidentiality can be challenging because the co-workers' curiosity is often aroused by the unfamiliar face of the therapist in the work place. The therapist should remember never to answer queries that would compromise client-therapist confidentiality. Unsolicited requests from co-workers for medical advice and work site modifications are best referred to that employee's doctor or manager.

In the work setting, the therapist interacts not only with the client, but also the employer and often the insurance company. By encouraging the injured employee to communicate his or her needs for work modification and how productivity might be maintained, the therapist will pave the way for a successful transition to work. The therapist strives to balance the needs of both the employee and employer while promoting resolution of work-related issues that would interfere with a smooth transition to productive work. Scheduling of therapy visits to the workplace should meet the needs of both the employee and employer. Work site visits should be scheduled in a manner that minimizes interfering with the natural flow of work.

The financial impact of work modifications will concern the employer. Employers do not have unlimited resources for modifying work environments. Only reasonable and necessary work modifications should be considered. Suggestions for work modifications that have an associated cost should be discussed with the employer. The therapist can suggest work modifications, but must also consider the impact of these modifications on co-workers using the same equipment. As a general rule, modifications that affect workers other than the employee must be discussed with management before they are presented to the employee as possible options.

In a traditional clinic setting, a secretary who sustained a repetitive motion injury of her wrist may receive various modalities to control her symptoms of pain and edema and may be educated on joint and tendon protection techniques while performing various movements. When the secretary receives occupational therapy services in her work environment, additional benefits often occur. Joint and tendon protection techniques are applied at work while performing day-to-day work tasks. Since the client's injury occurred at work, it could be exacerbated or prevented at work. See also Chapters 13 and 14 with regard to the role of the occupational therapist in relation to workers and work settings.

SUMMARY

Practice settings, the environment in which intervention occurs, have temporal, social, cultural, and physical contextual dimensions that affect both the therapist and the person receiving therapy services. Knowing the features of each practice setting and anticipating how the context will affect occupational performance prepares the therapist to best meet client needs. The continuum of care must be considered as the occupational therapist develops the intervention plan with the client in a specific intervention setting. A skilled therapist collaborates with the client to develop meaningful and attainable goals and then clearly communicates those goals from one setting to the next to foster meaningful outcomes. Sensitivity to the unique needs of each individual in each practice setting is critical.

Review Questions

1. What are the major functions of the OT process?
2. How are the various forms of clinical reasoning used to guide the OT process?
3. How do theories, models of practice, and frames of reference inform and support OT intervention?
4. What is the appropriate delegation of responsibility among the various levels of OT practitioners (OT and OTA)?
5. What services may be assigned to the OT aide? What are the limits, and why?
6. How should OT practitioners effectively collaborate with members of other professions involved in client care?
7. What are some of the ethical dilemmas that occur frequently in OT practice, and how can these be addressed and managed?
8. What are the various practice settings for OT services in the arena of physical disabilities?
9. What types of services are typically provided in these settings?

REFERENCES

1. American Occupational Therapy Association: Clarification of the use of terms assessment and evaluation, *Am J Occup Ther* 49:1072, 1995.
2. American Occupational Therapy Association: Core values and attitudes of occupational therapy practice, *Am J Occup Ther* 47:1083, 1993.
3. American Occupational Therapy Association: Guide for supervision, roles, and responsibilities during the delivery of occupational therapy services, *Am J Occup Ther* 58:663, 2004.
4. American Occupational Therapy Association: Guidelines to the occupational therapy code of ethics, *Am J Occup Ther* 52:881, 1998.
5. American Occupational Therapy Association: Occupational therapy code of ethics, *Am J Occup Ther* 54:614, 2000.
6. American Occupational Therapy Association: Occupational therapy practice framework: domain and process, *Am J Occup Ther* 56:609, 2002.
7. American Occupational Therapy Association: Position paper: use of occupational therapy aides in occupational therapy practice, *Am J Occup Ther* 49:1023, 1995.

8. American Occupational Therapy Association: Standards of practice for occupational therapy, *Am J Occup Ther* 52:866, 1998.

9. Atchison B: Occupational therapy in home health: rapid changes need proactive planning, *Am J Occup Ther* 51(6):406, 1997.

10. Baptiste SE: Client-centered practice: implications for our professional approach, behaviors, and lexicon. In Kramer P, Hinojosa J, Royeen CB, editors: *Perspectives in human occupation,* Baltimore, MD, 2003, Lippincott, Williams & Wilkins.

11. Bausell RK, et al: *How to evaluate and select a nursing home,* Beverly, MA, 1988, Addison-Wesley.

12. Belice PJ, McGovern-Denk M: Reframing occupational therapy in acute care, *OT Practice,* April 29, 2002, 21.

13. Black JG: *Microbiology. Principles and applications,* ed 3, pp. 9-25, Upper Saddle River, NJ, 1996, Prentice Hall.

14. Blau SP, Shimberg EF: *How to get out of the hospital alive: a guide to patient power,* New York, 1997, Macmillan.

15. Bonder BR, et al: *Culture in clinical care,* Thorofare, NJ, 2002, Slack Publishers.

16. Burke JP: Philosophical basis of human occupation. In Kramer P, Hinojosa J, Royeen CB, editors: *Perspectives in human occupation,* Baltimore, MD, 2003, Lippincott, Williams & Wilkins.

17. Chan SCC: Chronic obstructive pulmonary disease and engagement in occupation, *Am J Occup Ther* 58:408, 2004.

18. Chu LW, et al: Risk factors for falls in hospitalized older medical patients, *J Gerontol A Biol Sci Med Sci* 54(1):M38, 1999.

19. Clark F, et al: Occupational therapy for independent-living older adults: a randomized controlled trial, *JAMA* 278:1321, 1999.

20. Collins AL: Multiskilling: a survey of occupational therapy practitioners' attitudes, *Am J Occup Ther* 51:749, 1997.

21. Crepeau EB, Schell BAB: Theory and practice in occupational therapy. In Crepeau EB, Cohn ES, Schell BAB, editors: *Willard and Spackman's occupational therapy,* ed 10, Baltimore, MD, 2003, Lippincott, Williams & Wilkins.

22. Cumming RG, et al: Home visits by an occupational therapist for assessment and modification of environmental hazards: a randomized trial of falls prevention, *J Am Geriatr Soc* 47:1397, 1999.

23. Dooley NR, Hinojosa J: Improving quality of life for persons with Alzheimer's disease and their family caregivers: brief occupational therapy intervention, *Am J Occup Ther* 58:561, 2004.

24. Dunn W, et al: The ecology of human performance: a framework for considering the effect of context, *Am J Occup Ther* 48:595, 1994.

25. Dunn W, et al: Ecological model of occupation. In Kramer P, Hinojosa J, Royeen CB, editors: *Perspectives in human occupation,* Baltimore, MD, 2003, Lippincott, Williams & Wilkins.

26. Erikson A, et al: A training apartment with electronic aids to daily living: lived experiences of persons with brain damage, *Am J Occup Ther* 58:261, 2004.

27. Fange A, Iwarsson S: Changes in ADL dependence and aspects of usability following housing adaptation: a longitudinal perspective, *Am J Occup Ther* 59:296, 2005.

28. Finlayson M: Concerns about the future among older adults with multiple sclerosis, *Am J Occup Ther* 58:54, 2004.

29. Fisher AG: Uniting practice and theory in an occupational framework: 1998 Eleanor Clarke Slagle Lecture, *Am J Occup Ther* 52:509, 1998.

30. Fleming MH: The therapist with the three-track mind, *Am J Occup Ther* 45:1007, 1991.

31. Foto M: Multiskilling: who, how, when, and why? *Am J Occup Ther* 50:7, 1996.

32. Gillette NP, Mattingly C: Clinical reasoning in occupational therapy, *Am J Occup Ther* 41:399, 1987.

33. Gilliand E: The day treatment program: meeting rehabilitation needs for SCI in the changing climate of health care reform, *SCI Nurs* 13(1):6, 1996.

34. Haffey WJ, Abrams DL: Employment outcomes for participants in a brain injury reentry program: preliminary findings, *J Head Trauma Rehabil* 6(3):24, 1991.

35. Head J, Patterson V: Performance context and its role in treatment planning, *Am J Occup Ther* 51(6):453, 1997.

36. Hogan-Kelley D: Occupational therapy frames of reference for treatment in the ICU, *OT Practice,* Feb. 7, 2005, 15.

37. James AB: Biomechanical frame of reference. In Crepeau EB, Cohn ES, Schell BAB, editors: *Willard and Spackman's occupational therapy,* ed 10, Baltimore, MD, 2003, Lippincott, Williams & Wilkins.

38. Jonsson H, et al: Anticipating retirement: the formation of narratives concerning an occupational transition, *Am J Occup Ther* 51:49, 1997.

39. Kettenbach G: *Writing SOAP notes,* ed 2, Philadelphia, 2004, FA Davis.

40. Kielhofner G: Motives, patterns, and performance of occupation: basic concepts. In Kielhofner G, editor: *Model of human occupation,* ed 3, Baltimore, MD, 2002, Lippincott, Williams & Wilkins.

41. Kramer P, Hinojosa J: Developmental perspective: fundamentals of developmental theory. In Kramer P, Hinojosa J, editors: *Frames of reference for pediatric occupational therapy,* ed 2, Baltimore, MD, 1999, Lippincott, Williams & Wilkins.

42. Kyler P: Issues in ethics for occupational therapy, *OT Practice* 3(8):37, 1998.

43. Law M, et al: *Canadian occupational performance measure,* ed 2, Toronto, 1994, Canadian Association of Occupational Therapists.

44. Law M, et al: Theoretical contexts for the practice of occupational therapy. In Christensen C, Baum C, editors: *Enabling function and well being,* ed 2, Thorofare, NJ, 1997, Slack Publ.

45. Law M, et al: The person-environment-occupation model: a transactive approach to occupational performance, *Canad J Occup Ther* 63:9, 1996.

46. Lohman H, et al: Bridge from ethics to public policy: implications for occupational therapy practitioners, *Am J Occup Ther* 58:109, 2004.

47. Mattingly C: The narrative nature of clinical reasoning, *Am J Occup Ther* 45:998, 1991.

48. Migliore A: Case report: improving dyspnea management in three adults with chronic obstructive pulmonary disease, *Am J Occup Ther* 58:639, 2004.

49. Mosey AC: *Three frames of reference for mental health,* Thorofare, NJ, 1970, Slack Publishers.

50. Neistadt ME: Teaching clinical reasoning as a thinking frame, *Am J Occup Ther* 52:221, 1998.

51. Neufeld S, Lysack C: Allocation of rehabilitation services: who gets a home evaluation, *Am J Occup Ther* 58:630, 2004.

52. Opachich KJ: Moral tensions and obligations of occupational therapy practitioners providing home care, *Am J Occup Ther* 51(6):430, 1997.

53. Park S, et al: Using the assessment of motor and process skills to compare occupational performance between clinics and home setting, *Am J Occup Ther* 48:697, 1994.

54. Paz JC, West MP: *Acute care handbook for physical therapists,* ed 2, Boston, 2002, Butterworth Heinemann.

55. Pew Health Professions Commission: *Health professions education for the future: schools in service to the nation,* San Francisco, 1993, The Commission.

56. Pollock N: Client-centered assessment, *Am J Occup Ther* 47:298, 1993.

57. Proctor D, Kaplan SH: The occupational therapist's role in a transitional living program for head injured clients, *Occup Ther Health Care* 9(1):17, 1995.

58. Purtillo R: *Ethical dimensions in the health professions,* ed 3, Philadelphia, 1999, WB Saunders.

59. Pynoos J, et al: A team approach for home modifications, *OT Practice,* April 8, 2002, p. 15.

60. Reed KL: Theory and frame of reference. In Neistadt ME, Crepeau EB, editors: *Willard and Spackman's occupational therapy,* ed 9, Philadelphia, 1998, JB Lippincott.

61. Reilly M: Occupational therapy can be one of the great ideas of 20th century medicine, *Am J Occup Ther* 16:1, 1962.

62. Reilly M: The educational process, *Am J Occup Ther* 23:299, 1969.

63. Rogers JC, et al: Improving morning care routines of nursing home residents with dementia, *J Am Geriatr Soc* 47:1049, 1999.

64. Rogers JC, et al: Evaluation of daily living tasks: the home care advantage, *Am J Occup Ther* 51(6):410, 1997.

65. Rosa SA, Hasselkus BR: Finding common ground with patients: the centrality of compatibility, *Am J Occup Ther* 59:198, 2005.

66. Schell BA, Cervero RM: Clinical reasoning in occupational therapy: an integrative review, *Am J Occup Ther* 47:605, 1993.

67. Schlaff C: From dependency to self-advocacy: redefining disability, *Am J Occup Ther* 47:943, 1993.

68. Schultz-Krohn WA: ADLs and IADLs within school-based practice. In Swinth Y, editor: *Occupational therapy in school-based practice,* 2004. Online course: Elective Sessions (Lesson 10). *www.aota.org.*

69. Smith LK, et al: *Brunnstrom's clinical kinesiology,* ed 5, Philadelphia, 1996, FA Davis.

70. Spector RE: *Cultural diversity in health and illness,* ed 6, Upper Saddle River, NJ, 2004, Prentice Hall.

71. Stewart DL, Albin SH: *Documenting function in physical therapy,* St Louis, 1993, Mosby.

72. Trump SM: Occupational therapy and hospice: a natural fit, *OT Practice,* Nov. 5, 2001, p. 7.

73. Velde BP, Wittman PP: Helping occupational therapy students and faculty develop cultural competence, *Occup Ther Health Care* 13:23, 2001.

74. Walker MF, et al: Occupational therapy for stroke patients not admitted to hospital: a randomized controlled trial, *Lancet* 354:278, 1999.

75. Well SA, Black RM: *Cultural competency for health professionals,* Bethesda, MD, 2000, American Occupational Therapy Association.

76. Yerxa EJ: Who is the keeper of occupational therapy's practice and knowledge? *Am J Occup Ther* 49:295, 1995.

77. Youngstrom MJ: From the Guest Editor: The Occupational Therapy Practice Framework: The revolution of our professional language, *Am J Occup Ther* 56:607, 2002.

SUGGESTED READING

Heron E: *Tending lives—nurses on the medical front pulse,* New York, 1998, Ballantine.

Visiting Nurses Association of America: *Caregiver's handbook: a complete guide to home medical care,* New York, 1997, DK Publ.

4

Evidence-Based Practice for Occupational Therapy

LYNN GITLOW
ELIZABETH DEPOY

KEY TERMS

Evidence-based practice
Systematic OT practice
Thinking processes
Action processes

Evidence
Inductive reasoning
Deductive reasoning
Problem statement

Problem mapping
Need statement
Goals
Objectives

Process objectives
Outcome objectives
Specificity

LEARNING OBJECTIVES

After studying this chapter the student or practitioner will be able to do the following:

1. Distinguish among diverse models of evidence-based practice.
2. Define systematic occupational therapy practice (SOTP).
3. List, in sequence, the five steps of systematic occupational therapy practice (SOTP) and detail the content and processes of each step.

4. Compare SOTP with the OT process as articulated in the occupational therapy practice framework.

CHAPTER OUTLINE

Models of EBP
The SOTP model
  Theoretical and logical foundations of SOTP

Complementarity with contemporary practice models
Summary

In this chapter, we present, discuss, and apply systematic occupational therapy practice (SOTP), a model that synthesizes and builds on evidence-based approaches, to professional practice. The importance of systematically grounded practice is now an established concept within OT and the broader health care arena. The need for empirical analysis of the problems and needs that occupational therapy (OT) practitioners address continues to be emphasized at local, national, and international levels as reflected by initiatives from the American Occupational Therapy Association (AOTA) and the American Occupational Therapy Foundation (AOTF). These include, but are not limited to, the Center for Outcomes Research and Education (CORE), an evidence-based practice forum addition to the *American Journal of Occupational Therapy*,[27] the Evidence Based Literature Project,[20] and the Evidence-Based Practice (EBP) Resource Directory on AOTA's website. Educators, scholars, and practitioners increasingly discuss and encourage the use of theoretically grounded and supported OT interventions and the development of solid evidence of successful outcomes of interventions. We assert that current and ongoing systematic OT practice is needed in all professional domains (individual, group, community, agency, and government) if OT is to remain a viable and valued field that will continue to flourish in the competitive environment of managed care and fiscal scarcity.

Systematic OT practice involves the integration of research-based techniques into all elements of OT practice. This chapter provides a framework through which readers will understand and learn the research-based thinking and action processes necessary to conduct all or part of the sequence of SOTP. The chapter begins with a discussion and analysis of current models of **evidence-based practice (EBP)**. We then define systematic OT practice and proceed through the presentation and application of our model. As you will see below, SOTP is valuable in all arenas of OT concern.

In this chapter, we present our model as a set of practice guidelines for clinical practice.

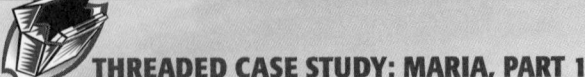

THREADED CASE STUDY: MARIA, PART 1

Maria is an occupational therapist who receives a referral to treat a client who has been diagnosed with carpal tunnel syndrome. The referral states "improve hand strength to increase independence in ADLs."

Critical Thinking Questions

Think about how to answer the following questions as you proceed through this chapter.

1. How do you clarify the OT problem and what is needed to resolve it? What evidence do you need to support your decision?

2. What factors do you need to consider in examining your professional activity and interventions, and what evidence do you need to consider?

3. How do you determine the extent to which you have determined the need and resolved the problem? What evidence do you need?

MODELS OF EBP

There are many models of evidence-based practice that have been presented in the literature. Practice models that integrate multiple methods of inquiry into all domains of professional practice have been called evidence-based medicine,[6,22,24] evidence-based practice,[5] evidence-based rehabilitation,[16] outcomes research,[15] etc. Because of the expansive literature on EBP approaches, it is beyond the scope of a single chapter to review all of the work in its entirety. Therefore, we have selected to present important definitions that have been advanced in the literature and to discuss their variations. This discussion then provides a rationale for systematic OT practice, our model for the application and use of evidence-based approaches relevant to and consistent with OT practice. At this point, you may be asking, "Why create another model if there are so many"? Our approach is not entirely new. However, we developed it as a comprehensive organizational framework that sees systematic OT practice and inquiry as one in the same. In other words, following the steps of SOTP in all professional activity leads not only to sound practice but also to the creation of OT knowledge.

Table 4-1 presents diverse approaches to evidence and inquiry-based practice. As you look at these descriptions, you will notice that each approach identifies different sources as credible evidence in three categories: client-generated, professionally generated, and/or scientifically grounded. By client-generated we mean that information put forth by the client is considered as part of the evidence base for professional interaction. Professionally generated refers to provider education and experience as a valued source of knowledge for use. Scientific evidence is that which is developed by rigorous methods of inquiry. Not all models may value all three sources as we depict in Table 4-1.

ETHICAL CONSIDERATIONS

Consistent with OT ethics, philosophy, values, and theory, we subscribe to the principle that it is our ethical obligation as professionals[1,2,21] to collaborate with clients regarding all aspects of their service need, provision, risk, and outcome. Therefore, we not only support the value of evidence generated by client, practitioner, and science, but encourage critical use of diverse sets of evidence as viable and purposive.

TABLE **4-1** **Approaches to Evidence- and Inquiry-Based Practice**

Author/s	Description	Client	Science	Profession
Sackett[23]	Evidence-based medicine is the conscientious, explicit, and judicious use of current best evidence in making decisions about the care of individual patients. The practice of evidence-based medicine means integrating individual clinical expertise with the best available clinical evidence from systematic research.		X	X
IOM[13]	Evidence-based practice is the integration of best research evidence with clinical expertise and patient values.	X	X	X
Law[16] (pp. 10-11)	Evidence-based rehabilitation is a subset of EBP that consists of four concepts: (1) *awareness*—being aware of the existence of and strength of evidence in one's field, (2) *consultation*—collaboration between the client and clinician in determining relevant problems and their clinical solutions, (3) *judgment*—being able to apply best evidence to the individual with whom you are working, and (4) *creativity*—which emphasizes that evidence based practice is not a "cookie cutter approach" practice but the combination of art and science.	X	X	X
Lee and Miller[19]	Process of evidence-based clinical decision making encourages us to include client and clinician "values, knowledge and experience."			
Kielhofner, Hammel, Helfrich, et al.[15] (p. 16)	Investigation that provides evidence about the effects of services. Identifying client need. Creating the best possible services to address those needs. Generating evidence about the nature of specific services and their impact. Accumulating and evaluating a body of evidence about specific OT services.			

THE SOTP MODEL

Building on and synthesizing the excellent work in evidence-based practice, we define **systematic OT practice** as the integration of critical, analytic, scientific thinking, and action processes throughout all phases and domains of OT practice. Let us look at this definition more closely. First, we distinguish thought and action from each other. In systematic inquiry, it is essential for the thinking sequence and its rationale to be presented clearly. Thinking processes are composed of the reasoning sequence and logic that OT practitioners use to conceptualize intervention and specify desired outcomes. **Thinking processes** involve the selection of a theoretical framework in which the OT practitioner plans the steps necessary to assess problems, evaluate intervention, specify desired outcomes, and plan a strategy to determine and systematically demonstrate the degree to which client-centered outcomes were met for an individual receiving OT services. Sometimes we are not fully aware of our thought processes, but they are there nonetheless and are the foundation of systematic OT practice, as we will see later in this chapter.

Action processes are the specific behaviors involved in implementing thinking processes.[8] Action processes are behavioral steps. In systematic OT practice, these steps are founded on logical inquiry such that any claim is supported with empirically derived information from a variety of sources.

Although SOTP is not research in itself, it is the organized application of research to the conceptualization, enactment, and investigation of the process and outcome of intervention.

OT and healthcare researchers, educators, and practitioners have identified many arenas in which EBP is valuable. Consistent with our chapter focus on clinical practice, Tickle-Degnan[26] states, "Evidence based practice (EBP) is like a toolbox of methods available to the occupational therapy practitioner to aid clinical reasoning. The toolbox consists primarily of methods designed to integrate current and best evidence from research studies into the clinical reasoning process" (p. 102). We add to this the integration of the client's perspective throughout the entire process.[2]

What is meant by **evidence**? This question is not easily answered. Synonyms for evidence include terms such as data, documentation, indication, sign, proof, authentication, and confirmation. In some models of evidence-based practice, the highest evidence in the hierarchy of credibility is considered to be data that are generated by positivist, experimental-type inquiry. This perspective is reflected in the AOTA'S Evidence-Based Literature Review Project.[20] However, other OTs and authors suggest that a full range of methods can generate useful evidence.[7,18]

In this chapter and in SOTP, we define evidence as information that is used to support a claim. This expansive definition allows for the identification and acceptance of a broad scope of evidence as the basis for decision making in practice as long as the evidence is identified and used within the systematic thinking and action processes that we discuss in detail below.

Within the profession, OT practitioners can use the information obtained from SOTP not only to improve the processes

ETHICAL CONSIDERATIONS

Unsubstantiated beliefs or claims are insufficient in themselves to support professional activity in an increasingly competitive, quality, safety and cost conscious, and accountability-demanding healthcare context.

and outcomes of their practices, but also to engage in informed thinking when choosing among possible interventions and to contribute to the overall knowledge base of our profession. Studies of practitioners' perceptions[9] of evidence-based practice suggest that OT practitioners view scientific literature as a valuable resource to share with other professionals when supporting the effectiveness of OT interventions. However, for informing intervention choice, practitioners tended to consult and depend on trusted personal sources.[9] SOTP systematically guides practitioners in determining which interventions are effective to produce desired outcomes, which interventions need to be improved, and what kinds of new knowledge need development. Additionally, having credible evidence to demonstrate that the interventions OT practitioners use produce desirable outcomes provides concrete feedback to the consumer.[12,27] Finally, by systematically evaluating interventions, OT practitioners can provide evidence for advancing clinical practices in the profession.

Pressures and demands on health practitioners from external sources render SOTP even more critical for three reasons. First, the location of service delivery and the time allowed for service delivery are in flux. Long-term hospital stays and treatments in acute care settings have been replaced by community-based treatment, and the length of time for delivery of treatment is shortening as third-party payers demand more efficient and cost-effective healthcare. SOTP guides the practitioner in balancing the multiple factors involved in practicing within a quality-focused fiscally driven healthcare environment. Second, by systematically examining the processes and outcomes of current practice, OT practitioners can provide an evidentiary basis for clinical thinking and action, which then can be presented to consumers, other professionals, insurers, and policy makers. Third, systematic inquiry transcends professional boundaries through shared language and theory. Within the context of physical rehabilitation, for example, the systematic foundation of the International Classification of Functioning, Disability and Health[28] is consistent with the Occupational Therapy Practice Framework (OTPF) and provides a common forum and language for cross-disciplinary communication.

As we proceed through SOTP, we will draw your attention to the skills and knowledge you already possess that are relevant to this conceptual approach. Let us now turn to the philosophical foundation and steps of the model.

OT PRACTICE NOTE

It is no secret that OT practitioners have always had difficulty in clearly describing what they do to those outside the profession. Moreover, OT practitioners have typically placed more emphasis on providing direct services than on publishing studies that document the results or that attribute successful outcomes to OT intervention. In today's increasingly complex and competitive healthcare environment, OT practitioners must clearly demonstrate their contribution to achieving clinical outcomes. It is particularly critical to do this if referral sources are to understand the benefits of OT to diverse client groups.

THEORETICAL AND LOGICAL FOUNDATIONS OF SOTP

SOTP is grounded in logic and the systematic thinking that undergirds all research thinking processes. Inductive and deductive reasoning form the basis for these thinking processes. Moreover, the two major research design traditions, naturalistic and experimental-type inquiry, are based on these logic structures.[8] Therefore, OT practitioners must understand them and use them to guide thinking and action and to support claims regarding the process and outcomes of OT intervention.

Inductive reasoning is a thinking process whereby one begins with seemingly unrelated data and links these data together by discovering relationships and principles within the data set. In inductive systematic approaches, the data may take many forms. Inductive reasoning leads us to select naturalistic strategies, those in which theory is derived from gathered evidence rather than tested by scientific experimentation. Among the methods used in naturalistic design are interview, observation, and textual analysis.[8] Data are collected and themes that emerge from repeated examination of the data are named, defined, and placed in a theoretical context.

Deductive reasoning begins with a theory and reduces the theory to its parts, which are then verified or discounted through examination. Deductive reasoning provides the foundation for experimental-type research, in which theories or parts are stated in measurable terms and standardized measurement forms the basis of all inquiry. Strategies used in deductive traditions include sampling, measurement, and statistical analysis. Because the rules of logic guide thinking, one can easily follow thinking processes and identify the basis on which guesses, claims, decisions, and pronouncements are made and verified.

COMPLEMENTARITY WITH CONTEMPORARY PRACTICE MODELS

Although it may seem difficult at first to engage in the formal, logical thinking processes that undergird research, we do it every day. Look at how the decision-making skills used in

OT practice mirror the logical thinking processes that form the foundation of SOTP. Box 4-1 presents the steps of SOTP and Table 4-2 illustrates the relationship between the occupational therapy process/clinical decision-making and systematic thinking processes.

Sequence of SOTP

Our model of SOTP has five steps, as listed in Box 4-1. The process begins with a conceptualization of the problem to be addressed. This leads to the question, "What exactly is a problem?"

Statement of the Problem

Although we often see problems as entities existing outside ourselves, problems are contextually embedded in personal and cultural values. A problem is value judgment about what is undesirable or in need of modification. Therefore, a **problem statement** is defined as a specific claim of what is not desired or of what should be changed. Although it seems simple to specify a problem, we often see problems stated in terms of a preferred solution; this error limits our options in analyzing problem components and solutions. Moreover, in systematic OT practice, problem statements must be derived from credible, systematically generated knowledge, including scholarly literature and inquiry, client report and data, and other sources that we discuss below.

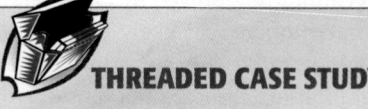

THREADED CASE STUDY: MARIA, PART 2

Remember that Maria received a referral that specifies the client's problem as "client needs to improve hand strength in order to increase independence in ADLs." This problem as stated suggests only one solution—to increase hand strength. Through systematic thinking together with the client, Maria however, expands her analysis of the problem to "limited hand strength does not allow the client to participate in work or self-care occupations," which allows Maria to generate additional potential solutions. For example, the client may take the following measures: look for alternative work, increase hand strength, work with adaptive equipment, adapt the environment, and so forth. By expanding a problem statement,

the OT practitioner moves beyond the obvious primary difficulty or impairment and a singular solution and can capture the breadth of focus of the problem as revealed by systematically derived evidence from literature, the client, or others.

TABLE **4-2** **Relationship Between the OT Process and SOTP**

SOTP	The OT Process/Clinical Decision Making
Initial problem statement	Referral to OT
Need statement	Systematic assessment of client/occupational profile and analysis of occupational performance
Goals and objectives	Intervention goals and objectives
Reflexive intervention	Regular progress monitoring and revision of intervention in response
Outcome assessment	Final assessment of client progress

If proceeding from the initial problem statement in the referral, the therapist may have missed the essence of the client's problem and thus may have selected inappropriate interventions and outcomes. The OTPF[2] guides us to define problems for OT by using a client centered approach. Thus in SOTP, it is critical to include the client and other diverse sources of knowledge beyond practitioner guessing in formulating the problem statement.

There are many ways to identify problems. Problem mapping is a method in which one expands a problem statement beyond its initial conceptualization by asking two questions repeatedly:[1] What caused the problem? and What are the consequences of the problem?[2] Similar to other professionals, OTs do not address all aspects of the problem statement. **Problem mapping** helps us operationalize the OTPF in that it provides a thinking process to locate impairment and individual function within seven broad contexts: cultural, physical, social, personal, spiritual, temporal, and virtual.[2] As we see in our example below, the problem areas for OT intervention are defined by the scope of our professional activity.

Apply the problem mapping method to the statement, "Jane has impaired short-term memory resulting from traumatic brain injury sustained in an automobile accident caused by a drunk driver." To conduct problem mapping, we first need to conceptualize the problem as a river. Articulating the original statement of the problem is analogous to stepping into the river and picking up one rock. As we look upstream, we see causes of the problem, and as we look downstream, we see the problem's consequences. How does this mapping technique work? See Figure 4-1 to look at the problem map. Each box above the initial problem contains a possible answer to the question of what caused the problem. Once we determine first-level causes of the problem, we ask, "What caused the cause of the problem?" and so on, until we reach cultural

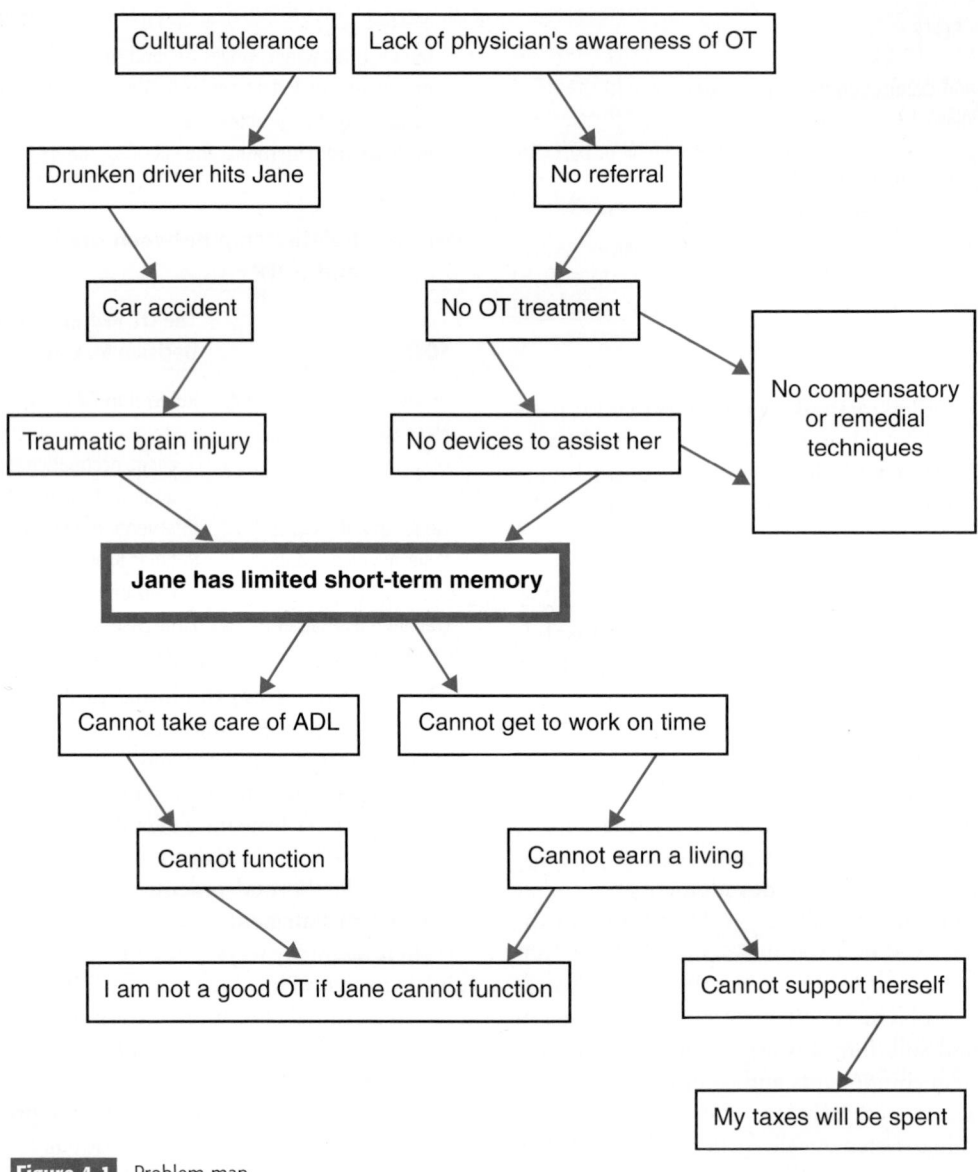

Figure 4-1 Problem map.

and social value statements, both of which are specified as contexts for OT practice in the OTPF. Keep in mind that the evidence that is used to identify causes and consequences must be generated from credible, identifiable sources, including client, professional, and scientific sources.

Below the initial problem statement, we repeatedly ask the question, "What is the consequence of the problem?" As with the upstream map, this question about the consequences of consequences is repeated until we reach the effect of the problem on ourselves. At this point, you may be asking "why?" It is because problems are values, and thus are in the eye of the beholder. The problem map expands the problem statement from documented cultural, social, and environmental causes to personal effect and suggests many different sites or targets for intervention.

As you might imagine from this example of Jane, many causes and consequences of problems are not within the scope of OT practice and thus cannot be resolved by OT intervention. While many OT practitioners will likely expand their efforts into political action or other areas at some point in their careers, others will look for clinical interventions that can improve the occupational performance of individuals. Given the focus of this text, we will concentrate this chapter on clinical interventions rather than the other roles that OTs might assume. Jane's problem map suggests numerous points of intervention for clinical OT in cognitive remediation, compensatory training, and provision of assistive devices and services such as assistive technology (AT). Within our chapter the focus on clinical practice, an area of occupational performance will be considered: developing vocationally related strategies that will enable Jane return to work. The OT practitioner could also make a referral to a social service agency for Jane, who might be eligible for social security disability income; thus the OT practitioner would intervene, through referral to another professional on the team, at the level of Jane's inability to support herself financially. In addition, as we look at the expanded problem, the OT practitioner may also want to intervene on the macro level by promoting stricter legislation and cultural "zero tolerance" of drunk driving, perhaps by educating adolescents and young adults. These areas of practice are beyond the scope of this chapter.

Consider the initial problem statement focusing on Jane's impaired short-term memory. This is not a problem that can be resolved by an OT practitioner as it is stated. Therefore, the OT in collaboration with the client must reconceptualize and restate the problem so that he or she can intervene using meaningful and systematic methods within OT's professional scope of practice.[3] Problem mapping or other logical, evidence-based problem identification techniques help in examining and analyzing problems beyond their initial presentation and identifying the strength of the evidence on which problems are analyzed. In SOTP, problem analysis and a careful statement of the part of the problem to be addressed are critical if the rest of the steps are to be implemented. Including evidence from the client's perspective in the process is essential in our model. Furthermore, clarifying the problem will help the therapist ascertain what is needed to resolve the part of the problem that will be addressed.

Now let us move to the next step of SOTP, determining need.

Ascertaining Need

After problem mapping, the next step is ascertaining need. In this step, one must clarify exactly what is needed to resolve the part of the problem that has been targeted for change. Let us examine the distinction between *problem* and *need*. As discussed earlier, a *problem* is a value statement about what is not desired. For a problem to be relevant to OT practitioners, it must concern improvement or maintenance of occupational performance. Thus, the problem area on the map that the OT practitioner would target for resolution would be delimited and guided by the professional and theoretical domains of OT concern. A **need statement** is a systematic, evidence-based claim, linked to all or part of a problem that specifies what conditions and actions are necessary to resolve the part of the problem to be addressed. Thus, the identification of need involves collecting and analyzing diverse sets of information such as assessment data and the information from the client interview, thus forming an occupational profile to ascertain what is necessary to resolve a problem.

At this needs assessment stage of the SOTP sequence, the OT may already have information on which to formulate need or may collect data in a systematic fashion to clearly delimit and identify need. A need statement should specify who is the target of the problem, what changes are desired, what degree of change is desired, and how one will recognize that the change has occurred. The need statement must be based on systematically derived data already contained in credible resources such as the relevant practice and research literature or documentation, professional education, knowledge, and experience, or revealed by the client in a needs assessment inquiry. Can you see that the need statement uses systematic research-based processes to define the next steps of specifying goals and objectives, determining the intervention, and specifying the evaluative criteria to find out if the desired outcomes of an intervention have been met?

Let us advance an example from our problem statement again. As already mentioned, the problem as stated (impaired short-term memory) is not a problem that can be resolved by an OT practitioner. Yet it is common for referrals for OT intervention to identify problems such as this one. Thus, the use of a problem map or similar problem analysis strategy is not only a reasonable thinking tool, but also is essential if we are to define the nature of our interventions more clearly and thereby document the unique contributions and outcomes of OT both within and outside of our field. We thus choose to reason about the causes and consequences of the problem to identify whether an area exists in which Jane would require OT intervention. As we mapped the problem, we found that OT did indeed have a critical role to play in Jane's treatment. Her ability to engage in meaningful occupational performance is impaired in that she is unable to manage her time and arrive at work on time as a result of her impaired short-term memory.

Given the problem statement, the therapist chooses to conduct a research-based needs assessment to determine what is necessary to resolve the targeted part of the problem, to set goals and objectives to guide the selection of an intervention, and to determine what processes and outcome should be expected.

Using a systematic approach to data collection, the OT practitioner uses naturalistic techniques including an interview and systematic observation of Jane to ascertain Jane's desires and skills. The OT practitioner also administers a standardized cognitive assessment and an occupational performance assessment. In this instance the OT practitioner is integrating qualitative and quantitative inquiry strategies to document a complete understanding of need and to provide the empirical basis for clinical decisions, as well as expected outcomes. One of the tools that the OT practitioner may use to collect data is the Canadian Occupational Performance Measure (COPM). This criterion-referenced measure is used to identify client-perceived problems in daily functioning in the areas of self-care, productivity, and leisure. By means of a semi-structured interview format, the COPM may be used to assess the performance skills and patterns the client identifies as interfering with the client's ability to function in a particular area. The data from the COPM are credible, outcome-based, and accepted as evidence in the research world.[17]

Systematic assessment reveals that Jane identifies returning to her job as a saleswoman in a boutique as her most important goal. Additionally, the results of the COPM interview reveal that Jane is not satisfied with her ability to manage her time or her ability to be punctual and that she perceives these two issues as the greatest barriers to achieving her desired goal of returning to work. She recognizes that her difficulties with short-term memory will affect her ability to do other work-related tasks, but she reports being most concerned about time management and promptness.

Standardized testing indicates that Jane's short-term memory is impaired but that her capacity to respond well to external cues remains intact. Additionally, Jane's performance on the Wisconsin Card Sorting Test (WCST) reveals that she is able to solve problems and that she demonstrates abstract reasoning. The WCST is a standardized cognitive assessment of executive function that was developed to assess problem solving, abstract reasoning, and the ability to shift cognitive strategies.[11] The results of standardized testing also suggest that Jane is able to learn new behaviors with specific, well-structured practice in the environment in which she will function. The WCST provides an assessment of cognitive flexibility and those data can be extrapolated to imply that she will be able to learn new skills in a structured environment, but the number of variables and complexity of her work setting should also be considered. Based on this empirically generated information, the therapist and Jane have a sound and credible basis for deciding that the intervention will be directed to the need to find and teach Jane compensatory strategies for time management and promptness. Further, Jane indicated in her occupational profile that she is married and that her husband would be supportive in helping her get to work.

Based on this information generated from naturalistic inquiry, the therapist and Jane decide to include Jane's husband in the intervention and to work first in Jane's home environment and then transfer her treatment to the work environment. Can you see from this example how SOTP both provides the guidance and the documentation for clinical decisions and suggests future steps in the intervention and outcome assessment processes? Anyone who observes the intervention process can easily see the rationale for decisions and actions. Credible, evidence-based knowledge is structured in a manner that provides a clear reasoning trail.

The desired outcomes are implicit in the need statement, which provides a basis for formulating measurable outcomes of intervention. According to the literature on closed head injury and professional wisdom,[14] what is needed is contextually based OT intervention in the home and in the workplace to assist Jane with time management and promptness, as a skill to facilitate her return to work. The evidence for targeting this intervention and for the goals and objectives to follow is clear and specified, as is the desired outcome.

The case example of the OT practitioner, George, considers a different type of need statement that illustrates why OT practice requires systematic inquiry.

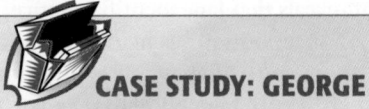

CASE STUDY: GEORGE

George, an OT practitioner, is asked by an employer to address a problem involving several computer operators whose ability to

perform their jobs has been impaired or lost as a result of neck pain. After constructing a problem map, based on literature about causes and consequences of neck pain, George formulates a need statement based on two areas that he believes will address the problem: instruction in proper body mechanics and instruction in a regularly scheduled upper body stretching routine. A literature review provided him with empirical evidence on which to base his intervention. He begins his intervention by teaching proper body mechanics and upper body stretching techniques to the computer operators, but the problem is not resolved. The computer operators continue to be unable to do their jobs and their complaints of neck pain continue. George's intervention is not successful in resolving the problem for which he was hired.

What was missing from George's reasoning? He based his problem map on empirical literature and educated but preconceived guesses without fully assessing the situation. Had he conducted a systematic needs assessment that included interview, testing, and observation of the workers in the process, he might have found that the monitors were too high for the operators and the chair heights were not adjustable. Thus, the intervention of body mechanics instruction and upper body stretching that may have been viable in another situation did not address the specific needs that George failed to identify. Had he used systematic thinking and action to ascertain need rather than guessing and then jumping from the problem to the intervention, George would quickly have identified the appropriate target areas.

In needs assessment, many systematic approaches can be useful in identifying and documenting needs, including but not limited to formal research strategies, well-conducted *a priori* studies, or mixed methods of information gathering and analysis. For individual clinical problems, strategies such as single case design are extremely useful for guiding and testing the efficacy of intervention decisions with a client. For program development, the therapist may want to use "group" (also called nomothetic) approaches, such as survey, interview, or standardized testing strategies, to yield needed information on which to support a needs claim. Naturalistic inquiry or integrated thinking and action strategies may be valuable to ascertain the perspectives of client groups about whose problems and needs the therapist knows little. Many excellent research texts exist from which to build research knowledge. (See the Suggested Reading at the end of this chapter.)

The next step in the process of systematic OT practice is translating the needs into goals and objectives.

Goals and Objectives

Goals and *objectives* are two words with which OT practitioners are familiar, since these concepts are used to structure treatment. In SOTP, goals and objectives emerge from the need statement and are essential not only for structuring intervention, but also for specifying how the process and outcome of intervention will be examined and supported.

A definition of the two terms is helpful. According to Bloom and Orme,[4] **goals** "are statements about what clients and relevant others would like to happen or do or to be." In other words, a goal is a vision statement about future desires that is delimited by the need that it addresses. **Objectives** are statements about both how to reach a goal and how to determine if all or part of the goal has been reached. The objective sets up the systematic approach to attaining the goal as well as the empirical measurement or assessment thereof.[10]

There are two basic types of objectives: process and outcome. **Process objectives** define concrete steps necessary to attain a goal. Process objectives are those interventions or services that will be provided or structured by the OT practitioner.[7] **Outcome objectives** define the criteria that must occur or exist to determine that all or part of the goal has been reached; outcome objectives further specify how these criteria will be demonstrated. Ultimately, assessing the attainment of outcome objectives is focused on ascertaining if the desired change has taken place as a result of participation in the OT process.

To develop goal and objective statements in our model, the therapist examines the need carefully, including the evidence to support the need statement. Then, the therapist and the client formulate conceptual goal and objective statements that guide and imply how the process and outcomes of intervention will be assessed. Goals are overall conceptual statements about what is desired; objectives are statements that are operationalized (i.e., stated in terms of how they will be measured or known). Both are based on systematically generated knowledge from the needs assessment.[7]

Let us now return to Jane to illustrate goals and objectives. From the problem and need statements, we have determined that an overall goal for Jane's intervention is to develop, teach, and have Jane learn compensatory strategies for promptness and time management so she can improve her performance in these areas and return to work. Based on the evidence given in the needs assessment, the OT intervention will be carried out at first in Jane's home with her husband participating, and then a transition will be made to the workplace.

One critical element of goal setting in SOTP is **specificity**. The following example uses the treatment goal that we discussed above as the basis for writing specific goal and objective statements:

GOAL: JANE WILL IMPROVE HER PROMPTNESS TO BE ABLE TO GET TO WORK ON TIME (PERFORMANCE) AND TO HER SATISFACTION

The process (P) and outcome (O) objectives we will use to attain this goal include the following:

1. Jane will be presented with assistive technology supports and services and catalogues of assistive devices from which she can select those she thinks will be most useful for her to achieve the goal. (P)
2. Given a choice of a variety of assistive devices (e.g., alarm watches, paging devices, and clocks), Jane will choose one or more devices to use as an external cue provider for promptness. (P)

3. Jane will select one daily activity at home for which she needs an external promptness cue. (P)
4. With assistance from the OT practitioner, Jane and her husband will configure the device to cue Jane to attend to this daily event. (P)
5. Jane's husband will monitor her promptness and provide feedback to Jane and the therapist regarding the effectiveness of the assistive device in meeting the goal. (P)
6. Once Jane has demonstrated that she can promptly attend to her schedule at home, she will begin to use the promptness cue to arrive at work. (O)
7. Once Jane has demonstrated that she can arrive at work on time, the therapist will work with Jane at the work site so that she can use the device to attend promptly to her work schedule to her and her employer's satisfaction. (P)
8. Using the most effective strategy and devices, Jane will improve her promptness and satisfaction with her performance at work. (O)

As you can see by reading this goal and its related objectives, in SOTP, objectives are very directive conceptual statements designed to achieve broad goal statements based on an empirical understanding of need. As we will see in the sections on reflexive intervention and outcome assessment, stating the goals and objectives as demonstrated above determines what will be formatively monitored and examined to ascertain treatment success.

Reflexive Intervention

Extrapolated from naturalistic methods of inquiry,[25] DePoy and Gilson[7] advanced the term reflexive intervention to highlight that systematic thinking does not cease during the implementation of interventions. We therefore have integrated this term into our model to remind us that as practice proceeds, the OT makes decisions based on feedback from the actual intervention itself, as well as from examination of therapeutic use of self and other influences on the intervention process. By reflexive intervention, we refer to the thinking and action strategies during the intervention phase of OT practice. In reflexive intervention, the OT systematically monitors the client, the collaboration, professional practice, setting-based resources, and therapeutic use of self and other internal and external influences that impact practice process and outcome. That is not to say that practice wisdom and intuition do not occur or are not used as evidence. Not only do they occur, but in SOTP, the OT makes it a point to be well aware of the pluralistic evidentiary basis from which he or she is making decisions, to carefully look at all practice to obtain clarity about what was done, and to consider feedback from engaging in practice.

Process assessment, the systematic monitoring of process objectives (denoted in the objective list above with a P) occurs throughout the reflexive intervention phase in order to provide the evidence on which to describe intervention and the context in which the intervention occurs, and to yield the evidence on which decisions are made regarding the need for intervention or programmatic change. Knowing what outcomes occurred without knowing what was done to cause them limits our knowledge base and our ability to communicate the benefits of OT practice to those outside of the profession. Thus, reflexive intervention is critical to the growth of OT knowledge, theory, and practice strategies. Let us return to Jane to illustrate.

As we mentioned previously, the COPM is an excellent measure to document performance that is meaningful to the client. In process assessment, the COPM can be used to document changes in occupational performance and illustrate the benefits of OT to Jane and other diverse audiences. Using this tool to collect data at multiple points during intervention can support the intervention "as is" or reconceptualize it. The OT might also track and document Jane's promptness over the course of her treatment to determine if revisions in the intervention are necessary or not. Moreover, documentation is an excellent way to show Jane and others that Jane has improved through OT. Similar strategies could be used to examine and document time management and other areas that Jane and the OT are addressing. It is useful to refer to the OTPF to guide reflexive intervention.

Outcome Assessment

Outcome assessment is a set of thinking and action processes conducted to ascertain and document what occurs as a result of being voluntarily or involuntarily exposed to a purposive intervention process, and to assess the worth of an intervention. In the objective list above, outcome objectives are identified with an "O." These objectives can be assessed by using both quantitative and naturalistic techniques and by applying systematic inquiry to examine whether objectives have been attained. To brush up on inquiry, we suggest that you consult one of the many excellent research method texts, some of which we list at the end of this chapter.

To carry out outcome assessment of Jane's intervention, a pre-post test design is selected using the COPM and the other documentation that we discussed in reflexive intervention. Although Jane's performance will be measured multiple times, only the change from beginning to end will be used for outcome assessment. As you can see, all OTs already do outcome assessment. The trick is to realize that you do it and to purposefully select methods that are credible and useful. We suggest that you choose strategies that are multi-method. Look at Box 4-2 to see how each objective will be assessed.

Box **4-2**   GOALS, OBJECTIVES, EVIDENCE, AND SUCCESS CRITERIA

Goal No. 1: Jane will Improve Her Promptness to be Able to Get to Work on Time (Performance) and to Her Satisfaction

1. **(P)** Jane will be supplied with catalogues and assistive devices from which to select those that she thinks will be most useful for her to achieve the goal.
   Criterion for success: completion of activity
   Evidence: notes of each session documenting progress toward goal
2. **(P)** Given a variety of assistive devices (e.g., alarm watches, paging devices, and clocks), Jane will choose a device to use as an external cue provider for promptness.
   Criterion for success: selection of device
   Evidence: notes of each session documenting progress toward goal
3. **(P)** Jane will select one activity at home for which she needs an external promptness cue.
   Criterion for success: selection of activity
   Evidence: notes of each session documenting progress toward goal
4. **(P)** With assistance from the OT, Jane and her husband will configure the device to cue Jane to attend to this daily event.
   Criterion for success: demonstration of completion of objective by Jane and her husband
   Evidence: progress notes indicating mastery of task
5. **(P)** Jane's husband will monitor her promptness and provide feedback to Jane and the therapist regarding the effectiveness of the assistive device in meeting the goal.
   Criterion for success: daily record of Jane's promptness supplied to her each evening after dinner
   Evidence: husband's written time charts

6. **(O)** Jane will demonstrate that she can promptly attend to her schedule at home.
   Criterion for success: daily record of Jane's promptness at home
   Evidence: husband's written time charts
7. **(P)** Once Jane has demonstrated that she can promptly attend to her schedule at home, she will begin to use the promptness cue to arrive at work.
   Criterion for success: daily record of Jane's use of cues
   Evidence: client self-report
8. **(O)** Jane will regularly arrive at work on time.
   Criterion for success: daily record of Jane's promptness at work
   Evidence: client's documented arrival time
9. **(P)** Once Jane has demonstrated that she can arrive at work on time, the therapist will work with Jane at the work site so that she can use the device to attend promptly to her work schedule to her and her employer's satisfaction.
   Criterion for success: OT will meet Jane at work daily for one week to support use of device
   Evidence: OT notes
10. **(O)** Using the most effective strategy and devices, Jane will improve her promptness sufficient to work and sufficient for her satisfaction.
    Criterion for success: significant improvement in Jane's promptness
    Evidence: COPM score on this item, compared with COPM score on pretest on this item

OT PRACTICE NOTE

SOTP IN PROFESSIONAL PRACTICE

An OT should deliberately perform each of the steps of SOTP and find a personal style for using evidence in professional practice. SOTP is not only a valuable approach in direct intervention, but provides the foundation for knowledge building and intervention development in all professional domains.

SUMMARY

In this chapter we presented SOTP, a practice approach in which systematic thinking and action are not only valued but are essential tools in OT practice. Our model begins with a clear problem statement that guides all of the remaining steps. Naturalistic and experimental research traditions are applied to clinical decision making to guide the subsequent steps of identifying and documenting need, positing goals and objectives, reflexive intervention, and outcome assessment. Reexamine Table 4-2 now in light of the need statement. The links among problem, needs, goals and objectives, process, and outcome have been clearly illustrated. Each step of SOTP emerges from and is anchored in the previous step. Moreover, systematic thinking and action provide the specificity and credible evidence supporting the extent to which the intervention resolved the part of the problem that was identified as falling within the OT domain.

Review Questions

1. List three reasons why OT practitioners need to use SOTP to demonstrate the efficacy of OT to external audiences.
2. Name and describe each of the steps of SOTP.
3. Compare the steps of SOTP to the steps of the OT process.
4. Using a potential OT client as a case study, select a problem and develop a problem map.
5. Pose strategies to ascertain the need based on your problem statement.
6. Identify the need for your client based on your problem statement.
7. What is the difference between a goal and an objective, and what is their relationship?
8. How do goals and objectives relate to need?
9. How do goals and objectives relate to a problem?
10. Identify goals for your client.
11. What are the two types of objectives described in this chapter, and what are the differences between them?
12. Based on your goals for your client, identify at least two process objectives and two outcome objectives.
13. Identify how you will know that your objectives have been met.
14. Chose at least two interventions to achieve the goals and objectives you have established in question 12.
15. Identify what questions you will ask and how you will answer them in reflexive intervention.
16. Discuss how you will use reflexive intervention and outcome assessment data to contribute to OT knowledge.

REFERENCES

1. American Occupational Therapy Association: occupational therapy code of ethics, *Am J Occup Ther* 53:614-616, 2000.
2. American Occupational Therapy Association: occupational therapy practice framework: domain and process, *Am J Occup Ther* 56:609-639, 2002.
3. American Occupational Therapy Association: *Scope of practice*, 2004. Retrieved June 29, 2004, from *http://www.aota.org/members/area2/docs/scope.pdf*.
4. Bloom M, Fischer J, Orme JG: *Evaluating practice: guidelines for the accountable professional*, ed 2, Boston, MA, 1998, Allyn & Bacon.
5. Brownson RC, Baker EA, Left TL, et al.: *Evidence-based public health*, Oxford, 2003, Oxford University Press.
6. *Cochrane Collaboration.* Retrieved June 29, 2004, from *http://www.cochrane.org/*.
7. Depoy E, Gilson S: *Evaluation practice: thinking and action principles for social work practice*, Belmont, CA, 2003, Wadsworth.
8. DePoy E, Gitlin L: *Introduction to research: understanding and applying multiple strategies*, ed 3. St. Louis, 2005, Mosby.
9. Dubouloz C, Egan M, Vallerand J: Occupational therapists' perceptions of evidence-based practice, *Am J Occup Ther* 53:445-453, 1999.
10. Fitzpatric JL, Sanders JR, Worthen BR: *Program evaluation: alternative approaches and practical guidelines*, ed. 3, Boston, 2003, Allyn & Bacon.
11. Haase B: Cognition. In Van Dusen J, Brunt D, editors: *Assessment in occupational therapy and physical therapy*, Philadelphia, 1997, WB Saunders.
12. Holm M: Our mandate for the new millennium: evidence based practice, 2000 Eleanor Clarke Slagle lecture, *Am J Occup Ther* 54:575-585, 2000.
13. Institute of Medicine: *Crossing the quality chasm: a new health system for the 21st century*. Committee on Quality of Health Care in America, Washington, DC, 2001, National Academies Press.
14. Johnstone B, Stonnington H, Stonnington HH, editors: *Rehabilitation of neuropsychological disorders: a practical guide for rehabilitation professionals and family members*. Brighton, NY, 2001, Psychology Press.
15. Kielhofner G, Hammel J, Helfrich C, et al.: Studying practice and its outcomes: a conceptual approach, *Am J Occup Ther* 58:15-23, 2004.
16. Law MC, editor: *Evidence-based rehabilitation: a guide to practice*, Thorofare, NJ, 2002, Slack Publishers.
17. Law MC, Baptiste S, Carswell A, et al.: *The Canadian Occupational Performance Measure*, Ottawa, Ontario, 1998, CAOT Publications.
18. Law MC, Philp I: Evaluating the evidence. In Law MC, editor: *Evidence-based rehabilitation: a guide to practice*, Thorofare, NJ, 2002, Slack Publishers.
19. Lee C, Miller L: The process of evidence-based clinical decision making in occupational therapy, *Am J Occup Ther* 57:473-477, 2001.
20. Lieberman D, Scheer J: AOTA's evidence-based literature review project: an overview, *Am J Occup Ther* 56:344-346, 2002.

21. Moyers P: Continuing competence & competency: what you need to know, *OT Practice* 7:178-22, 2002.

22. *OTseeker*. Retreived June, 20, 2004 from *www.OTseeker.com.*

23. Sackett DL, Rosenberg WM, Gray JA, et al.: Evidence based medicine: what it is and what it isn't, *BMJ* 312:70231-70272, 1996.

24. Sackett DL, Straus SE, Richardson WS, et al.: *Evidence-based medicine: how to practice and teach EBM,* ed 2, New York, 2000, Churchill Livingstone.

25. Steier F: *Research and reflexivity,* Newbury Park, CA, 1991, Sage.

26. Tickle-Degnan L: Gathering current research evidence to enhance clinical reasoning, *Am J Occup Ther* 54:102-105, 2000.

27. Tickle-Degnan L: Organizing, evaluating, and using evidence in occupational therapy practice, *Am J Occup Ther* 53:537-539, 1999.

28. World Health Organization: *International classification of functioning, disability and health (ICF),* Geneva, Switzerland, 2001, WHO.

SUGGESTED READING

Atkinson P, Coffey A, Delamont S, editors: *Handbook of ethnography,* Thousand Oaks, CA, 2001, Sage.

Babbie E: *The practice of social research,* ed 9, Belmont, CA, 2001, Wadsworth.

Coley SM, Scheinberg CA: *Proposal writing,* Thousand Oaks, CA, 2000, Sage.

Denzin NK, Lincoln YS: *Handbook of qualitative research,* ed 2, Thousand Oaks, CA, 2000, Sage.

Gambrill E: Authority-based profession, *Res Social Work Practice* 11:166-175, 2001.

Grinell RM: *Social work research and evaluation,* ed. 6, Itasca, IL, 2001, Peacock.

Mullen E: *Evidence-based knowledge: designs for enhancing practitioner use of research findings (a bottom up approach),* 4th International Conference on Evaluation for Practice, University of Tampere, July 4-6, 2002, Tampere, Finland.

Patton MQ: *Qualitative research and evaluation methods,* Thousand Oaks, CA, 2001, Sage.

Rosen A: Evidence-Based Social Work Practice: Challenges and Promises, Address at the Society for Social Work and Research, San Diego, CA, 2002.

Royse D, Thyer B, Padgett DK, et al.: *Program evaluation: an introduction,* Belmont, CA, 2000, Wadsworth.

Sonnert G: *Ivory bridges: connecting science and society,* Cambridge, 2002, MIT Press.

Stringer E: *Action research in health,* Englewood, NJ, 2003, Prentice Hall.

Sullivan T: *Methods of social research,* Fort Worth, FL, 2001, Harcourt College.

Tripodi T: A primer on single-subject design for clinical social workers, Washington, DC, 2000, NASW.

Thyer B: *The handbook of social work research methods,* Thousand Oaks, CA, 2001, Sage.

Unrau YA, Gabor PA, Grinnell RM: *Evaluation in the human services,* Itasca, IL, 2001, Peacock.

Yin R: *Case study research: design and methods,* ed 2, Thousand Oaks: CA, 2003, Sage.

5

HEALTH PROMOTION AND WELLNESS FOR PEOPLE WITH PHYSICAL DISABILITIES

MICHAEL A. PIZZI

MARJORIE E. SCAFFA

S. MAGGIE REITZ

KEY TERMS

Moral treatment	Primary prevention	PRECEDE-PROCEED model	Enablement
Occupational justice	Secondary prevention	Disability prevention	Expert-centered
Health promotion	Tertiary prevention	Wellness	Secondary conditions
Health protection	Risk factors	Client-centered care	Quality of life
Prevention	Transtheoretical model	Empowerment	

LEARNING OBJECTIVES

After studying this chapter the student or practitioner will be able to do the following:

1. Discuss historical influences on occupational therapy's role in health promotion and wellness
2. Define key health promotion and prevention concepts and terminology
3. Describe the potential impact of *Healthy People 2010* on occupational therapy practice
4. Identify strategies for integrating health promotion into physical disability practice
5. Develop a holistic, client- and occupation-centered health promotion perspective for physical disability practice

CHAPTER OUTLINE

Historical influences and considerations
  Early history and symbolism
  The development of a profession
  The AOTA's milestones in health promotion
  USC well-elderly program and study
  International trend
Health promotion principles and practice
Models of health promotion practice
  Transtheoretical model
  PRECEDE-PROCEED model
OT involvement in health promotion and prevention
Health promotion and occupational participation
Secondary conditions and people with disabilities
Evaluation: emphasizing the promotion of health and well-being
Intervention
Summary

The AOTA supports and promotes involvement of occupational therapy practitioners in the development and provision of health promotion and disease/disability prevention programs and services. These health promotion programs and services may target individuals, groups, organizations, communities, and policymakers. Their focus is to (a) prevent or reduce the incidence of illness, accidents, and injuries in the population; (b) improve the overall health and well-being of persons with chronic conditions or disabilities and their caregivers; and (c) promote healthy living practices, social opportunities, and healthy communities, with respect for cross-cultural issues and concerns (p. 1).[9]

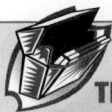

THREADED CASE STUDY: JEAN, PART 1

Jean is a 49-year-old with three grown children, two of whom live away from home. She has been married for 27 years. Jean developed gestational diabetes with her first-born child and has been insulin dependent for most of her married life. Jean is knowledgeable about diet, the need for exercise and activity, and insulin regulation. She is active in her community, works part-time to supplement her husband's income, and enjoys bowling, playing cards with friends every Friday night, crocheting, and maintaining her home.

Jean developed symptoms later confirmed to be a minor stroke. She lost sensation in her fingertips and in both lower extremities. As a result, she developed altered dynamic balance and grasp in both hands. She has coped with beginning glaucoma and diabetic neuropathies for several years. She has had a weakened cardiac status secondary to her diabetes despite her being active much of her life. Jean is overweight and has smoked a pack of cigarettes per day since she was 18 years old. Her husband also smokes regularly.

Critical Thinking Questions

1. How would you evaluate this client from a health promotion perspective?
2. In addition to standard occupational therapy services, what health promotion interventions might you use with this client and/or her family?

The value a society places on the health and welfare of its people can be measured by its level of commitment to policies and funding for healthcare. The wisdom of a society can also be measured by its commitment to prevention and health promotion. This chapter will begin with a description of how the profession of occupational therapy has been involved in health promotion and prevention activities as well as with policy development. A new direction, which may come to be identified as a historical shift back to occupational therapy's concern with societal level problems, will also be described.

This historical overview is followed by a review of health promotion principles and a description of health promotion-focused evaluation and intervention for individuals with physical disabilities. A case study assists readers in the integration of principles and practice of health promotion and prevention for people with physical disabilities and impairments.

HISTORICAL INFLUENCES AND CONSIDERATIONS

EARLY HISTORY AND SYMBOLISM

Humans have long appreciated the health-promoting and healing qualities of engagement in occupation.[43,46] History and anthropology,[17] as well as archaeology,[67] provide rich examples of how people through time from cultures around the world have used occupations not only for survival, but also as a means of healing and expressing identity and spirituality.[7,18,67] In the U.S., *petroglyphs* (cliff carvings) are as important to the living as those who fabricated them in the past, as Herman Agoyoyo, All-Indian Pueblo Council Chairman (1988) points out:

To us, these petroglyphs are not the remnants of some long lost civilization that has been dead for many years ... they are part of our living culture. What is stored in the petroglyphs is not written in any book or to be found in any library. We need to return to them to remind us of who we are and where we came from, and to teach our sons and daughters of it.[61]

When searching for supporting pictorial evidence of this history, often what is found are pictorial representations of humans engaged in hunting or other subsistence activities through the use of symbols or representations of the human hand or animals.[22,61] When living conditions allowed time for occupations other than for subsistence (i.e., activities of daily living and instrumental activities of daily living), humans turned their energy to identify these very occupations and the animals they shared their world with though symbols and artwork. These symbols convey feelings, identity, beliefs, and knowledge of these important occupations. Humans currently use symbols, often subconsciously, for these same purposes.[19] The production of petroglyphs is early evidence of the importance of symbols and their influence on health. Through these symbols early humans could communicate their essence to future generations and demonstrate that "through the use of his hands, as they are energized by mind and will, [man] can influence the state of his own health" (p. 2).[45]

The meanings or relevance of specific symbols can change through time in a society or within an individual. The symbolism of a handprint made during the Paleolithic period on the wall of the Cave of Chauvet-Pont-d'Arc[22] could carry both similar and different symbolism than that of a handprint of a small child to a parent of today. For individuals with disabilities, the familiar stick person in a wheelchair symbol used to denote accessibility might have held little or no meaning prior to sustaining a physical disability. However, after an

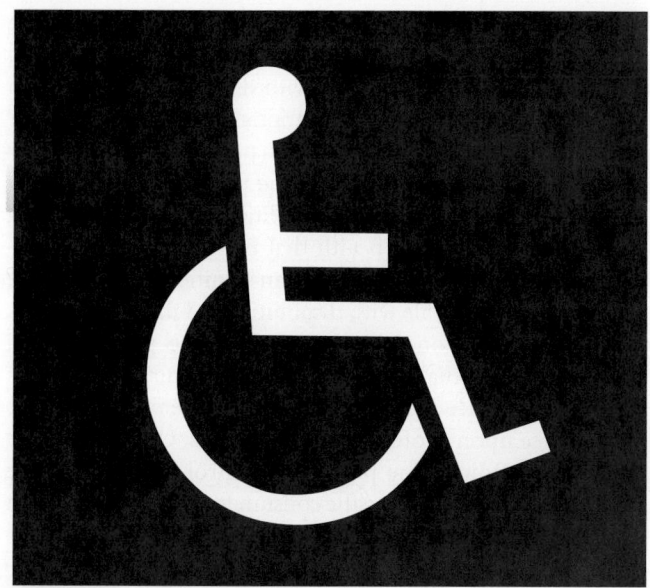

Figure 5-1 International symbol for access.

individual is diagnosed with or sustains a physical disability, this symbol (Figure 5-1), the *International Symbol for Access* (ISA), may take on new meaning and relevance for both that person and his or her family.

THE DEVELOPMENT OF A PROFESSION

Many descriptions of the development of occupational therapy as a profession either start with or include a discussion of moral treatment.[30,43,44] *Moral treatment* was defined as a "humane approach to the insane" that included occupation-based intervention that emphasized self-discipline, hard work, and learning self-control while developing "good habits."[67] (Chapter 2 provides a rich description of this time period and those who influenced the practice of occupational therapy with people with disabilities in the U.S.) The values and beliefs of the founders of occupational therapy in the U.S. were consistent with and influenced by the values and beliefs of the mental hygiene movement, the arts and crafts movement, the settlement house movement, and the actions of other social activists and reformers in the U.S. at that time.[8,32] These idealistic individuals and groups influenced the social injustice of their time. The backgrounds and contributions of the founders of occupational therapy in the U.S. are well documented.[5,8,30,34,43,44,51] Therefore, the rest of this discussion will focus on (1) a summary of key events for involvement in health promotion and policy development in the U.S. and (2) recent international developments that may influence practice in the U.S. in the coming decades.

AOTA'S MILESTONES IN HEALTH PROMOTION

Leaders within the field of occupational therapy and the *American Occupational Therapy Association* (AOTA) have

been encouraging the profession's increased attention to health promotion for many decades. As early as the 1960s, leaders[10,62,63,65,66] articulated their vision of the role of occupational therapy in prevention and health promotion. Themes included (1) concerns of emphasis on cure or the saving of life versus the provision of services to maximize the quality of a saved life or better yet the prevention of the illness or injury, (2) the match of occupational therapy values and principles with those of public health, (3) the untapped potential and responsibility for occupational therapy to contribute to the well-being of society, (4) the need to build and re-define the knowledge base of the profession, and (5) the responsibility to conduct research to determine effectiveness of community-based health promotion and prevention initiatives. Finn continued to encourage this involvement through an Eleanor Clarke Slagle Lecture[20] and subsequent work.[21]

Through the years the AOTA has developed a series of statements, as well as used other means to focus attention on health promotion. In 1979, "Role of the Occupational Therapist in the Promotion of Health and the Prevention of Disabilities," the first official document related to health promotion and prevention, was published.[1] In 1986, the AOTA supported this role by devoting an entire issue of its journal, the *American Journal of Occupational Therapy* (*AJOT*), to health promotion.[64]

In 1989, the AOTA's Representative Assembly rescinded the original statement and adopted the position paper "Occupational Therapy in the Promotion of Health and the Prevention of Disability."[2] This position paper remained in place until it was replaced with "Occupational Therapy in the Promotion of Health and the Prevention of Disease and Disability Statement" by the 2000 AOTA Representative Assembly.[9] In 1992, an article on the history of occupational therapy's role in preventive health appeared in the Special 75th Anniversary issue of the *American Journal of Occupational Therapy*.[46]

Besides promoting occupational therapy's role in health promotion within the profession, the AOTA has also promoted it to external audiences. The AOTA was a participant in the Healthy People 2000 Consortium.[4] The consortium, together with 22 expert groups and numerous state and national governmental agencies and services, worked cooperatively to set the Nation's health agenda for the next decade.[59] Both this document and its current version *Healthy People 2010*[60] include targeted health goals for individuals with physical disabilities. A review of the current version can encourage occupational therapists to develop new intervention strategies to address the documented unmet health needs of U.S. citizens, both with and without disabilities.

USC WELL-ELDERLY PROGRAM AND STUDY

The development of the Well-Elderly Program by faculty at the University of Southern California (USC) Department of Occupational Science and Occupational Therapy was a significant event in health promotion occupational therapy practice. The outcome of this program was published in a landmark article in the *Journal of the American Medical Association.*[14] The intervention protocol that evolved for the Well Elderly Study was eventually named "lifestyle redesign."[36] Results of this lifestyle redesign program indicated that "preventive occupational therapy greatly enhances the health and quality of life of independent-living adults" (p. xi).[36]

INTERNATIONAL TREND

An international discussion started by Wilcock and Townsend has the potential to shape the future history of occupational therapy's involvement in health promotion and prevention worldwide. Wilcock and Townsend have called attention to the potential for occupational therapists and occupational therapy assistants to combat social and occupational injustice.[57,67,68] The idea of occupational justice first emerged in Australia and Canada. *Occupational justice* is "the promotion of social and economic change to increase individual, community, and political awareness, resources, and equitable opportunities for diverse occupational opportunities which enable people to meet their potential and experience well-being" (p. 257).[67]

The World Federation of Occupational Therapists is also active in the call for the profession's involvement in promoting occupational justice by supporting the potential for occupational therapists to make significant contributions to the eradication of occupational deprivation.[53] The discussion is slowly emerging in the U.S.[47,49,58]

 ETHICAL CONSIDERATIONS

The profession of occupational therapy has the potential to be able to conduct an assessment of societal issues that impact the daily occupational rights and function of marginalized individuals, groups, and communities. Through education, political advocacy, and activism, occupational therapists can draw attention to the inequities that exist.

As occupational therapy practitioners further gain a working knowledge of the political process, they can advocate for both the prevention of disability as well as the promotion of health and prevention of secondary conditions for individuals with disabilities who have been marginalized. In preparation for this advocacy, occupational therapy practitioners should familiarize themselves with the goals, especially "Goal 2: Eliminate Health Disparities" (p. 11), and other data available in *Healthy People 2010*[60] concerning reducing disparities and improving quality of life for individuals with disabilities.

One possible action occupational therapists and occupational therapy assistants can take is increasing their awareness of what history-making efforts are currently underway

that can be joined and supported. The Independent Living Movement, which is working to combat these disparities and social injustice for individuals with disabilities, is one such example. However, if an occupational therapy practitioner singularly embraces the rehabilitation paradigm, he or she may not feel comfortable with either the principles of the independent living movement or its political agenda. Integrating a proactive approach to health that includes health promotion, wellness, and rehabilitation can significantly impact the quality of life of people with disabilities and their loved ones.

The rehabilitation paradigm defines the problem with disability as the actual physical or mental impairment whereas the independent living paradigm defines the problem as the dependence upon professionals and others. Under the rehabilitation paradigm, the person in control of service is the person with a disability, i.e., the consumer. In the rehabilitation model, the desired outcome of service delivery is maximum physical or mental functioning (or, as in vocational rehabilitation, gainful employment). Desired outcomes in independent living are tied to having control over one's daily life. Control does not necessarily mean having the physical or mental capacity to do everyday tasks for one's self. For some disability groups, complete control may not be possible, but the independent living movement continues to work toward complete consumer control wherever and whenever possible.[52]

Occupational therapists and occupational therapy assistants dedicated to enabling individuals with physical disabilities to participate in occupations need to look beyond the immediate rehabilitation goals to be truly client-centered in their practice.[57] Time must also be found to advocate for equal access and rights for all people, marginalized or not, with or without physical disabilities. In a sense this discussion has come full circle, with the opportunity to emulate the original founders of the profession by becoming social activists.

HEALTH PROMOTION PRINCIPLES AND PRACTICE

The vision of *Healthy People 2010: Understanding and Improving Health* challenges individuals to make healthy lifestyle choices and challenges healthcare practitioners to incorporate health promotion and prevention strategies in their practice. The overall comprehensive goals of *Healthy People 2010* are to (1) increase quality and years of healthy life for people of all ages and (2) eliminate health disparities among different groups within the population.[60]

Healthy People 2010 recognizes that the health of individuals and families is inseparable from and dependent upon the health of the communities in which they live, go to school, work, and play. Community health is affected not only by the physical environment, but also by the cultural, social, spiritual, temporal, and virtual contexts. Health is a constant interplay of a variety of factors and therefore is not static but always changing. Health and illness/disease, like functional ability/disability, are not mutually exclusive categories, but rather a finely graded continuum.[16] Important determinants of health status include individual biology and behavior, social and physical environments, policies and interventions, and access to health care (Figure 5-2).[60]

Examining birth and death rates, incidence and prevalence of disease, injury and disability, use of healthcare services, life expectancy, quality of life, and other factors can evaluate the health status of a population. Leading health indicators were established during the development of *Healthy People 2010* in an effort to focus the national health promotion agenda. The leading health indicators that serve as the foundation for the strategic planning process include "physical activity, overweight and obesity, tobacco use, substance abuse, responsible sexual behavior, mental health, injury and violence, environmental quality, immunization and access to health care" (p. 24).[60]

Health promotion can be defined as "any planned combination of educational, political, regulatory, environmental, and organizational supports for actions and conditions of living conducive to the health of individuals, groups or communities" (p. 656).[9] Health promotion encompasses both **health protection** and prevention of disease and disability. Health protection strategies are targeted at populations and include control of infectious diseases, immunizations, protection from occupational hazards, and governmental standards for the regulation of clean air and water, sanitation, and food and drug safety among other things.[16] **Prevention** refers to "anticipatory action taken to reduce the possibility of an event or condition from occurring or developing, or to minimize the damage that may result from the event or condition if it does occur" (p. 81).[38] Prevention strategies can be categorized on three levels: primary, secondary, and tertiary.

Primary prevention focuses on healthy individuals in order to decrease vulnerability or susceptibility to disease, disability, or dysfunction. Primary prevention strategies include good nutrition, regular physical activity, adequate housing, recreation and working conditions, genetic screening, periodic physical examinations, and seatbelt laws. **Secondary prevention** focuses on persons at risk or in the early stages of disease with the goal of arresting the disease progression and preventing complications and disability. Secondary prevention strategies include early detection and intervention, as well as screening for chronic diseases such as cancer, coronary artery disease, and diabetes. **Tertiary prevention** focuses on persons with disease or disability and attempts to prevent further complications, minimize the effects of the condition, and promote social opportunity. Tertiary prevention strategies include rehabilitation services and the removal of architectural and attitudinal barriers to social participation.[16,26,50]

Health promotion and prevention approaches attempt to reduce risk factors and enhance protective or resiliency factors. **Risk factors** are human characteristics or behaviors, circumstances, or conditions that increase the likelihood or predispose an individual or community to manifest certain health problems. Risk factors include not only physical conditions such as hypertension and behaviors such as smoking but also social, economic, and environmental conditions such as poverty, homelessness, exposure to radiation, and pollution.[16,50] Research indicates that "it is usually the accumulation of risk rather than the presence of any single risk factor that affects outcomes, and that multiple risks usually have multiplicative rather than merely additive effects" (p. 512).[15] Protective or resiliency factors are human characteristics or behaviors, circumstances, or conditions that decrease susceptibility or increase an individual's or community's resistance to illness, disability, dysfunction, or injury. Protective factors include not only an individual's genetic profile, personality, and health behaviors, but also peer and family relationships, social norms, and social support.[15,50]

MODELS OF HEALTH PROMOTION PRACTICE

In the health promotion field there are a number of individual, interpersonal, and community models and theories of health behavior change. Two models will be presented here briefly in order to help the practitioner better conceptualize health promotion interventions. One model, the Transtheoretical Model and Stages of Change, was designed to facilitate individual health behavior change and is therefore extremely relevant to occupational therapy practitioners. The second model, PRECEDE-PROCEED, is an approach to planning that facilitates the design, implementation, and evaluation of health promotion interventions.[23]

TRANSTHEORETICAL MODEL

The **Transtheoretical Model** (TTM) is based on the premise that change occurs in stages. The model consists of six stages: precontemplation, contemplation, preparation, action, maintenance, and termination. Precontemplation is the stage in which the person has no intention of taking action to modify health behaviors. This may be due to lack of knowledge, previous failed attempts at health behavior change, or simply a lack

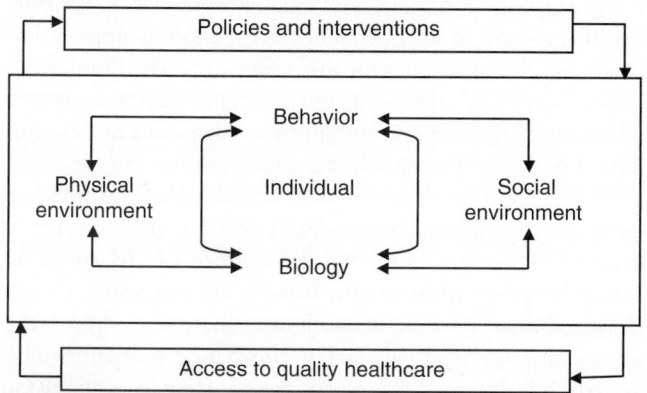

Figure 5-2   Determinants of health. (From U.S. Department of Health and Human Services: *Healthy people 2010: understanding and improving health,* ed 2, Washington, DC, 2000, U.S. Government Printing Office.)

of motivation. The contemplation stage is characterized by intention to modify behaviors within the next six months, but with some ambivalence regarding the costs and benefits of doing so. The preparation stage is an indication that the person is ready to take action in the very near future (30 days or less) and has demonstrated some initiative to plan their change strategies such as reading a self-help book, joining a health club, or talking to their physician. Action refers to specific overt manifestations of lifestyle modification. The duration of this stage is a minimum of six months. After six months of sustained health behavior change, a person is considered to be in the maintenance stage. The goal of this stage is to prevent relapse into previous unhealthy behaviors. Termination is the stage at which a person is no longer tempted and has a sense of self-efficacy that permits them to maintain their healthy behaviors even in stressful, high-risk situations. True termination may be unrealistic for most behavioral changes, and lifelong maintenance may be the appropriate goal for the majority of people.[42]

According to the TTM, change occurs through "covert and overt activities that people use to progress through the stages" (p. 103).[42] These activities or processes of change include consciousness raising, dramatic relief, self–re-evaluation, environmental re-evaluation, self-liberation, helping relationships, counter-conditioning, contingency or reinforcement management, stimulus control, and social liberation. The developers of the TTM discovered that each of these processes is more or less effective during different stages of change. For example, consciousness raising is critical in the precontemplation stage in order for the person to progress to the contemplation stage. Contingency management and stimulus control strategies are most useful in the maintenance stage to prevent relapse.[42]

PRECEDE-PROCEED MODEL

The **PRECEDE-PROCEED Model** is used for planning interventions and consists of 9 steps (Box 5-1). The PRECEDE portion of the model is based on the assumption that health

---

Box 5-1 STEPS OF THE PRECEDE-PROCEED MODEL

Step 1: Social Assessment
Step 2: Epidemiological Assessment
Step 3: Behavioral and Environmental Assessment
Step 4: Educational and Ecological Assessment
Step 5: Administrative and Policy Assessment
Step 6: Implementation
Step 7: Process Evaluation
Step 8: Impact Evaluation
Step 9: Outcome evaluation

From Green LW, Kreuter MW: *Health promotion planning: an educational and ecological approach,* ed 3, Mountain View, CA, 1999, Mayfield.

---

behaviors are the result of a complex interaction of multiple factors. In the PRECEDE framework, these factors are identified and specific objectives are developed for a population. The PROCEED portion of the model consists of policy development, intervention implementation, and evaluation. The first 5 steps represent a comprehensive needs assessment that evaluates a number of social, epidemiological, behavioral, environmental, educational, ecological, administrative, and policy issues that might affect the development, implementation, and ultimate success of a health promotion intervention. After all of these factors are considered, the intervention is developed and implemented. The final 3 steps represent a comprehensive evaluation of the intervention, including process, impact, and outcome measures.[25]

PRECEDE-PROCEED has been used to plan, implement, and evaluate health promotion interventions in school, work, healthcare, and community settings. It has been used to address a number of health issues including smoking cessation, HIV prevention, seat belt use, driving under the influence of alcohol, nutrition, exercise and fitness, blood pressure control, and stress management.[25] Typically interventions designed using the PRECEDE-PROCEED model address multiple risk factors and health behaviors and use multiple intervention strategies.

OT INVOLVEMENT IN HEALTH PROMOTION AND PREVENTION

The *Healthy People 2010* goal in the area of disability and secondary conditions is to "promote the health of people with disabilities, prevent secondary conditions, and eliminate disparities between people with and without disabilities in the U.S. population" (p. 6-3).[60] Several objectives in this area are appropriate for occupational therapy intervention (see Box 5-1). The objectives in *Healthy People 2010* address both individuals with disabilities and the environments in which they function, as it is recognized that disability is the result of the interaction between individual limitations and barriers in the environment.[60]

The Occupational Therapy Practice Framework describes health promotion and disability prevention as appropriate intervention approaches for the profession.[3] The Framework defines health promotion from an occupational therapy perspective as "an intervention approach that does not assume a disability is present or that any factors would interfere with performance. This approach is designed to provide enriched contextual and activity experiences that will enhance performance for all persons in the natural contexts of life" (p. 627).[3] **Disability prevention** is defined as "an intervention approach designed to address clients with or without a disability who are at risk for occupational performance problems. This approach is designed to prevent the occurrence or evolution of barriers to performance in context. Interventions may be directed at client, context, or activity variables" (p. 627).[3] **Wellness** is the outcome of health promotion programming.

It is defined in the Framework as "the condition of being in good health, including the appreciation and the enjoyment of health. Wellness is more than a lack of disease symptoms; it is a state of mental and physical balance and fitness" (p. 628).[3] Occupational therapy practitioners facilitate wellness through their holistic and client-centered practice.

Three potential roles for occupational therapy in health promotion include (1) promoting healthy lifestyles for patients, clients, and their caregivers and families; (2) complementing existing health promotion programs offered by public health professionals through inclusion of occupation-based interventions; and (3) designing and implementing occupation-focused health promotion programs at individual, group, organizational, community, and governmental levels.[9]

Occupational therapy involvement in prevention can assume a variety of forms. For example, primary prevention could include providing education to workers regarding their personal risk factors for injury on the job (such as poor body mechanics) or altering the environment to reduce the incidence of workplace accidents. Secondary prevention strategies in occupational therapy practice include joint protection, energy conservation, and work simplification techniques. Fall prevention programs and home safety evaluations for frail elderly clients are other examples of secondary prevention. Occupational therapists and occupational therapy assistants are experts in tertiary prevention, as they provide services to maximize function and minimize barriers to occupational performance.[26,50]

Occupational therapists and occupational therapy assistants who develop occupation-based health promotion and prevention programs should be cognizant of the literature in public health and use existing evidence on best practice. The American Public Health Association (APHA) developed standards for the design and implementation of health promotion programs that can guide occupational therapy health promotion efforts. These five principles include the following:[35]

- Addressing multiple risk factors that are measurable and clearly defined
- Focusing on the identified and expressed needs and preferences of the client or target population
- Including evidence-based interventions with demonstrated effectiveness
- Effectively using client and community strengths and available resources
- Designing programs that can be sustained and evaluated

Within the context of being a person with a disabling condition, health and well-being issues are often minimized, as people with disabilities are medicalized, rehabilitated, and looked upon as in need of long-term care financing.[60]

Four main misconceptions emerge from this contextual approach: (1) all people with disabilities automatically have poor health, (2) public health should focus only on preventing disabling conditions, (3) a standard definition of disability or people with disabilities is not needed for public health purposes, and (4) the environment plays no role in the disabling process[60] (p. 6-3).

A health promotion framework is needed that focuses on client needs (and those of caregivers) and one that explores the holistic needs of people with disabilities and their caregivers. The health and wellness approach to care would still include the functional needs of people, but will help occupational therapy practitioners to focus on health needs, issues of well-being, quality of life, and participation in society. This approach will also help the profession to examine more closely the role of occupational therapy in the prevention of secondary disabilities in order to promote healthy and meaningful participation.

HEALTH PROMOTION AND OCCUPATIONAL PARTICIPATION

A health promotion perspective will assist in enabling people with disabilities to more fully engage and participate in society. According to Hills,[27] there are three "pillars and related assumptions" of health promotion: (1) the primacy of people, (2) empowerment, and (3) enablement.

All three of the concepts listed above, especially the primacy of people, focus on what the profession of occupational therapy calls **client-centered care**. The Canadian Association of Occupational Therapy (CAOT) defines client-centered practice as the following:[11]

Collaborative approaches aimed at enabling occupation with clients who may be individuals, groups, agencies, governments, corporations or others. Occupational therapists demonstrate respect for clients, involve clients in decision making, advocate with and for clients in meeting clients' needs, and otherwise recognize clients' experience and knowledge (p. 49).

It is this client-centered approach that is health promoting for individuals with physical disabilities. The respect for and involvement in decision making, particularly in occupational participation, is a foundational similarity in both health promotion and occupational therapy. Occupational therapists facilitate meaning and assist people in seeing a hopeful future through occupational engagement and enablement of participation. This focus will help foster optimal health and wellness for people with disabilities.

Empowerment speaks to the development of autonomy and self-control. Occupational therapists are skilled at creating contexts and occupation-based interventions that support and facilitate the feeling of being empowered. "To increase control over and to improve one's health, one must not only be *empowered* to do so but also *able* to do so. To be able, one must possess the requisite skills, resources and knowledge" (p. 232).[27] People with impairments and disabilities and those at risk for impairment and disability can be knowledgeable about the need to change health behaviors that undermine the promotion of healthy living (e.g. smoking); however, they may be lacking skills and resources to achieve optimal well-being. "The fundamental assumption underlying the notion of **enablement** is that people have capacity to identify their own needs, to solve their own problems and to generally know what is best for them" (p. 232).[27]

In order to effectively promote health and well-being, occupational therapists should embrace the belief that people are capable of identifying needs and being able to problem-solve life challenges. Implementing client-centered approaches versus **expert-centered** approaches (those approaches that come from therapists without inclusion of clients or their caregivers) will empower people with disabilities to view themselves as valued and contributing members of society.

OT PRACTICE NOTE

It behooves occupational therapists and occupational therapy assistants to begin to make that paradigm shift and transition from defining oneself as a rehabilitation specialist to a specialist in occupation, health promotion, and well-being using occupation to facilitate healthy living. Through listening to the narratives of people with disabilities, and engaging in client-centered evaluation and interventions, occupational therapists and occupational therapy assistants can assist people with disabilities and chronic illnesses to maximize QOL and participation in society.[39]

Powers[41] provides a glimpse into the lived experiences of people with disabilities and their perceptions of health and well-being. She believes there is need to develop more models of health and wellness that specifically address the needs of people with disabilities. However, the models currently used, some of which are discussed earlier, do enhance the knowledge of health professionals regarding people with disabilities. Health and illness can and do coexist on a daily basis for people with physical impairments and disabilities:

...living healthy and well is not something new for people with disabilities. Currently, a stereotype exists that suggests people with disabilities are "sick" or are "perpetual patients" who cannot be considered "healthy" or "well." However, for years people with disabilities have used strategies to maintain health and wellness, created supportive relationships, and accessed needed resources from various service systems. It is from these resourceful people that health professionals need to be willing to continue learning about issues related to health, wellness and long-term disability[41] (p. 73).

SECONDARY CONDITIONS AND PEOPLE WITH DISABILITIES

Secondary conditions can be defined as "those physical, medical, cognitive, emotional, or psychosocial consequences to which persons with disabilities are more susceptible by virtue of an underlying impairment, including adverse outcomes in health, wellness, participation and quality of life" (p. 162).[28] The term secondary conditions expanded the term co-morbidity, which is a term often used in medical settings.

However, [the term] secondary condition adds three dimensions not fully captured by the term co-morbidity. It includes: (1) nonmedical events, e.g. isolation; (2) conditions that affect the general population, e.g. obesity, with higher prevalence among people with disabilities; and (3) problems that arise any time during the lifespan, e.g. inaccessible mammography. Children and adults with disabilities can experience secondary conditions any time during their lifespan.[12]

Occupational therapists can aid in the prevention of secondary conditions through increasing client awareness and patient education about health, healthy habits and routines, and strategies to offset increasing secondary conditions or other disability. *Healthy People 2010* set clear objectives for the reduction of secondary conditions (Box 5-2).

In view of the increased rates of disability among youth, it is particularly important to target activities and services

---

Box 5-2 Healthy People 2010 Disability and Secondary Conditions Objectives

- Reduce the proportion of children and adolescents with disabilities who are reported to be sad, unhappy, or depressed
- Reduce the proportion of adults with disabilities who report feelings such as sadness, unhappiness, or depression that prevent them from being active
- Increase the proportion of adults with disabilities who participate in social activities
- Increase the proportion of adults with disabilities reporting sufficient emotional support
- Increase the proportion of adults with disabilities reporting satisfaction with life
- Reduce the number of people with disabilities in congregate care facilities, consistent with permanency planning principles
- Eliminate disparities in employment rates between working-aged adults with and without disabilities
- Increase the proportion of children and youth with disabilities who spend at least 80% of their time in regular education programs
- Increase the proportion of health and wellness treatment programs and facilities that provide full access for people with disabilities
- Reduce the proportion of people with disabilities who report not having the assistive devices and technology that they need
- Reduce the proportion of people with disabilities reporting environmental barriers to participation in home, school, work, or community activities

Adapted from U.S. Department of Health and Human Services: *Healthy people 2010: understanding and improving health*, ed 2, Washington, DC, 2000, U.S. Government Printing Office.

that address all aspects of health and well-being, including promoting health, preventing secondary conditions, and removing environmental barriers, as well as providing access to medical care. For an older person with a disability, it is important to target worsening coexisting conditions that may intensify and thus threaten general well-being. For example, declining vision combined with declining hearing can greatly impair mobility, nutrition, and fitness, conditions that may intensify and thus threaten general well-being[60] (pp. 6-4, 6-5).

Hough[28] believes that a paradigm shift from disability prevention to prevention of secondary conditions is needed. After the inability to prevent primary disability, "it is within the environment that the negative effects of secondary conditions could be ameliorated and even prevented" (pp. 187-188). Public health agencies often focus efforts towards primary prevention; and secondary conditions need to be of equal concern. The emphasis on policy change and education of health professionals on health promotion for people with disabilities can help foster interventions towards self-management of one's disability.

Stuifbergen, Gordon, and Clark[54] emphasize the need for health practitioners to integrate health promotion strategies in neurorehabilitation for people with stroke. Krahn[31] emphasizes the need to encourage self-responsibility for health to promote health and well-being while living with a disability, while Rimmer[48] views health promotion as a means to maintain functional independence by preventing secondary conditions. "People with disabilities have increased health concerns and susceptibility to secondary conditions. Having a long-term condition increases the need for health promotion that can be medical, physical, social, emotional, or societal" (p. 6-4).[60]

The development of secondary conditions and occupational impairments can be directly related to one's mental health. Psychosocial aspects of physical disabilities are as important to identify and help ameliorate as the physical barriers to occupational participation.

People who have activity limitations report having had more days of pain, depression, anxiety, and sleeplessness and fewer days of vitality during the previous month than people not reporting activity limitations. Increased emotional distress, however, does not arise directly from the person's limitations. The distress is likely to stem from encounters with environmental barriers that reduce the individual's ability to participate in life activities and that undermine physical and emotional health[60] (pp. 6-4, 6-5).

Exploration of a person's disability, in the context of one's life situations, and the physical and emotional impacts of that disability on participation exemplifies occupational therapy practice committed to optimizing **quality of life** (QOL). QOL is an outcome of occupational therapy as defined by the Framework. QOL is "a person's dynamic appraisal of his or her life satisfactions (perceptions of progress toward one's goals), self-concept (the composite of beliefs and feelings about oneself), health and functioning (including health status,

self-care capabilities, role competence), and socioeconomic factors (e.g., vocation, education, income)"[3] (p. 628).

Stuifbergen and Rogers[55] interviewed 20 individuals with MS who shared their stories about health promotion, QOL, and factors that affected these areas of health. They identified six life domains related to QOL including family (most frequently identified domain), functioning to maintain independence, spirituality, work, socioeconomic security, and self-actualization. Six broad themes also emerged related to health-promoting behaviors. These included exercise or physical activity, nutritional strategies, lifestyle adjustment, maintaining a positive attitude, health responsibility behaviors, and seeking and receiving interpersonal support.[39] Occupational therapy practitioners play a key role in helping people actualize QOL through interventions that include the themes above. Physical disability does not translate to being unable to participate and experience a good QOL. The paradigm shift to promoting health and wellness is necessary to optimize QOL.

EVALUATION: EMPHASIZING THE PROMOTION OF HEALTH AND WELL-BEING

Evaluation of people with disabilities must include the life story or narrative of the person as elicited through careful occupational history taking. This occupational profile is coupled with physical, sensorimotor, social, psychological, and emotional assessments to create a holistic view of the person. The most important element in evaluation is incorporating the client's perspectives of health and well-being, as well as his or her values, beliefs, and contexts of living experiences. Client-centered care promotes healthy views of living for the client and the family system, from the beginning of occupational therapy intervention through discharge.

The *Pizzi Holistic Wellness Assessment* (PHWA)[40] was created for adults and is a subjective, occupation-focused, and client-centered assessment tool. It measures, both qualitatively and quantitatively, self-perceptions of a person's health and wellness in eight different categories. It is an assessment that is not focused on the disability, but instead emphasizes one's abilities and current levels of well-being. Collaboratively, the client and therapist work on strategies that the client identifies as health promoting for each area, as well as using the clinical reasoning of the therapist to problem-solve health issues related to occupational performance. A systems perspective was used during its development. Thus, it is a useful assessment and research tool for clients as well as caregivers of people with disabilities. For example, a caregiver may report additional burden achieving occupational balance of roles and occupations, as well as the caregiving responsibilities. The caregiver could benefit from occupational therapy intervention to address identified needs, based on responses from the PHWA.

Table 5-1 shows a number of assessments from a variety of disciplines that may be helpful to occupational therapists as they consider how to enhance their health promotion

THREADED CASE STUDY: JEAN, PART 2

For Jean, the PHWA could be used to evaluate the following:

- Occupational habits, routines, and patterns that may be barriers to general health (e.g., smoking, eating habits)
- Balance in daily life activity and barriers to fuller participation in occupation
- Stress and psychosocial areas that may exacerbate cardiac insufficiency, increase smoking and eating problems, and create insulin imbalance (use stress and depression scales to help assess these areas)
- Physical versus sedentary activity levels and reasons for these activity patterns
- Risk factors for development of secondary conditions related to her physical function and past medical history
- Contexts for occupation including current support system. Caregiver assessment, especially level of support for Jean, can be crucial for health promotion programming

interventions with people with disabilities.[29] The purpose of this table is to encourage practitioners to seek resources outside of the discipline that may increase options to facilitate the end goal of enhanced participation in occupations. Inclusion of a tool in this table should not be considered an endorsement of the tool. Readers are encouraged to critically examine assessment tools in terms of reliability, validity, sensitivity, and practicability, as well as possible training or certification required prior to use. Similar tables and lists of assessments that are more commonly used and known by occupational therapy practitioners exist that include assessments developed both within and external to the field.[6,13] These compilations include numerous additional assessments, which along with other resources, should be reviewed and considered prior to an assessment being selected for a specific client or client group. Assessments, when chosen appropriately and used competently, can be an important tool in implementing client-centered care.[33,37] Table 5-2 offers additional guidance and considerations for the selection of an assessment.[56]

INTERVENTION

For people with disabilities, health promotion interventions are designed to optimize health status. One focus is to help prevent secondary conditions from occurring and thus help people with disabilities to maintain a level of well-being in order to occupationally engage in meaningful life roles. The Framework identifies six areas of focus for intervention: (1) areas of occupation, (2) performance skills, (3) performance patterns, (4) context or contexts, (5) activity demands, and (6) client factors.[3] All of these areas affect each other, which, in turn, affect occupational performance and participation.

TABLE 5-1   A Selection of Assessments for Use in Health Promotion Physical Disabilities Practice

Assessment Type	Examples
Adjustment Scales	Profile of Adaptation to Live
	Social Support Questionnaire
Other Well-being Scales	Perceived Well-being Scale
Arthritis	Arthritis McMaster-Toronto Arthritis Patient Reference Disability Questionnaire (MACTAR)
	Health Assessment Questionnaire (HAQ)
	Arthritis Impact Measurement Scales (AIMS)
Back Pain	Disability Questionnaire
Cancer	Karnofsky Performance Status Measure (KPS)
	Functional Living Index: Cancer
COPD	American Thoracic Society Respiratory Questionnaire and Grade of Breathlessness Scale
Depression	Beck Depression Inventory
Diabetes	DCCT Questionnaire
Family Scales	Caregiver Time-Tradeoff Scale
	Family Hardiness Inventory
Hardiness Scales	Hardiness Scale
Health Risks Appraisals	The Healthier People Network Risk Appraisal
	1999 Youth Risk Behavior Survey
HIV/AIDS	AIDS Health Assessment Questionnaire
Heart	New York Heart Association Functional Classification (NYHA)
Life Satisfaction Scales	Kansas Family Life Satisfaction Index
	Index of Life Satisfaction
Multiple Sclerosis	Expanded Disability Status Scale
Neurologic Head Injury	Modified Sickness Impact Profile
Orthopedic	Musuloskeletal Outcomes Data Evaluation and Management System (MO-DEMS)
Pain	MOS Pain Measures
Quality of life	Overall Life Status

Data from Hyner GC, Peterson KW, Travis JW, et al, editors: *Society of prospective medicine handbook of health assessment tools,* Stoughton, WI, 1999, Wellness Associates Publications.

Interventions to promote health and well-being are implemented with consideration of all of these areas. Five approaches to intervention are listed in the Framework. While all of them can relate to health promotion, the Framework specifically cites the area of "create, promote" (p. 627)[3] as the intervention approach that is more focused on health promotion. Even though the Framework states that this approach is not one that "assumes a disability is present" (p. 627),[3] it relates to people with occupational impairments and disability. "This approach is designed to provide enriched contextual and activity experiences that will enhance performance for all

TABLE **5-2** **Organizing the Search for Assessment Evidence to Discuss with Different Decision Makers**

Decision Maker	Decision Maker's Use of Evidence	Question that Guides the Search for Evidence
Client and family members	To make informed decisions related to choosing assessment procedures	Is goal attainment scaling a reliable and valid method for assessing personally meaningful goal achievement among 75-year-old men with Parkinson's disease?
Manager	To decide which assessment procedures should be supported and provided by the organization	What are the most reliable and valid methods for assessing personally meaningful goal achievement among persons with Parkinson's disease?
Funder	To determine whether or not assessment procedures will effectively document important attributes of clients and their responses to rehabilitation	Same question as for manager

From Tickle-Degnen L: Communicating evidence to clients, managers, and funders. In Law M, editor: *Evidence-based rehabilitation: a guide to practice,* p. 225, Thorofare, NJ, 2002, Slack Publishers.

persons in the natural contexts of life" (p. 627).[3] Stated earlier, a paradigm shift for therapists' therapeutic reasoning is needed to understand that health, wellness, *and* disability can be co-mingled and interventions to promote healthy living *while* living with a disability is quintessentially vital for a person with disability.

Although the intervention approach of create/promote is identified as the one most closely related to health promotion, the other four (establish/restore, maintain, modify, and prevent)[3] are all related to the creation of healthy lifestyles and well-being. They can be considered factors for occupational health restoration within the context of health promotion.

THREADED CASE STUDY: JEAN, PART 3

The case example of Jean illustrates how a health promotion approach for a person with disability can be implemented. In addition to standard occupational therapy services, a health promotion approach might be appropriate with this client and/or her family. Potential health promotion interventions are described below.

If Jean's occupational habits, routines, and patterns are maladaptive and are barriers to healthy living, then patient education around developing healthy habits (including how her habits can result in further medical complications) should be implemented.

An imbalance in occupations and occupational performance can contribute to the exacerbation of stress, cardiac issues, and affect insulin production. Increasing awareness of the need for balance in daily life, including balance of work, play, rest, sleep, and leisure, can assist Jean in creating a new structure for her occupational living and optimize quality of life

Stress, depression, and other psychosocial factors can exacerbate pre-existing conditions and lead to inactivity, poor self-esteem, and eventually poorer health. Client-centered care that incorporates meaningful and interesting occupation relevant to the person in your care can help offset psychosocial conditions. Areas of concern could be feeling worthless or ineffective because one cannot occupationally engage in meaningful life activity. Jean may experience these issues due to her limited (and potentially limiting) medical condition. Exploring the impacts of stress, depression, and other factors on occupational performance and creating new occupational strategies for Jean can improve occupational performance and lead to Jean developing a future that includes "preventive occupations,"

in this case, preventing further or future depression and managing her stress.

After assessing activity levels, occupational interventions that promote a healthy heart, decrease smoking and overeating, and improve general mental and physical fitness are primary in Jean's case. Once Jean is aware of her abilities and develops a knowledge based on her real and perceived levels of activity, the occupational therapy practitioner can help her modify and adapt her lifestyle to incorporate activity that optimizes mental and physical health. It is important for Jean to optimize health for both present and future occupational performance in multiple contexts.

Interventions must include measures to prevent the development of secondary conditions. For example, Jean has developed the warning sign (transient ischemic attack, TIA) of potential future stroke. Preventive occupations can include increasing walks outdoors by 5 minutes each week to reach a daily target of 30 minutes maximum, working with an occupational therapy practitioner to help decrease smoking and overeating habits, or developing a stress management program. These health promotion program ideas can be habituated in the acute care and home care settings and followed through by Jean and her loved ones.

The caregiver support is critically important to implement and follow-through with a health promotion program. In Jean's case, she requires strong support to help her recognize and prevent future health problems (e.g., reminders, environmental and verbal cues, ongoing education). She also will need support with smoking cessation, developing healthy eating (and cooking) habits, and increasing optimism for a healthy and bright future.

SUMMARY

This chapter has introduced readers to health promotion and wellness concepts within the context of physical disability practice. An introduction to the power of symbols, important concepts such as occupational justice, and principles and practice of health promotion help to expand the reader's knowledge base for best practice. While practitioners have long promoted optimal health for their clients of all ages, there has been little discussion about theoretical foundations for evaluation and intervention in health promotion and wellness. This chapter addresses these issues and supports the Framework as a guide to helping practitioners integrate health promotion and wellness into their everyday practice.

The Framework emphasizes occupational engagement and participation in life as the means to health, wellness, and optimizing quality of life. Occupational therapy practitioners create and promote healthy living via careful attention to the physical, psychosocial, spiritual, social, and emotional abilities and challenges that support, or are barriers to, occupational performance. Holistic evaluation and goal planning utilizing a client-centered approach are implemented with health promotion goals being co-developed between client and practitioner.

Engagement in occupation to support participation in context is a key focus of the Framework. A health promotion approach enhances awareness of barriers to health and wellness, and strategies are developed to optimize health, as well as prevent future health problems. Risk factors are considered and interventions are implemented to support participation while creating a new lifestyle structure that is meaningful to the client. Client factors, while important to address to optimize occupational performance, are integrated into a top-down approach to care when providing a health promotion program. In the case example, Jean can engage in a physical activity program designed to improve her cardiac status while she develops strategies to control the pain and discomfort, which are the secondary complications of her diabetes.

As practitioners learn more about health promotion, prevention, and wellness, they will be better equipped to promote healthy living within the context of a person's lifestyle. Client-centered and occupation-centered care that includes health promotion and focuses on the whole person living with disability can be our unique contribution to humanity.

Review Questions

1. Consider the importance of symbols. Do you think the current international symbol for accessibility is inclusive of all individuals with physical disabilities? Why or why not? Sketch an alternative symbol.
2. Describe the historical relationship between social activism and occupational justice for individuals with disabilities.
3. Identify an objective from *Healthy People 2010* to support a new health promotion program you want to develop for your client group.
4. Describe the determinants of health as identified in *Healthy People 2010* and discuss how occupational therapy can address these determinants.
5. Identify the levels of prevention and give examples of potential occupational therapy interventions at each level.
6. Choose a health behavior of interest and describe the stages of change associated with that health behavior using the Transtheoretical Model.
7. Discuss how occupational therapists can facilitate resiliency for their clients with disabilities.
8. How would health promotion approaches fit within the Occupational Therapy Practice Framework?

REFERENCES

1. American Occupational Therapy Association: Association official position paper: role of the occupational therapist in the promotion of health and the prevention of disabilities, *Am J Occup Ther* 26(2): 59, 1979.
2. American Occupational Therapy Association: Occupational therapy in the promotion of health and the prevention of disease and disability (position paper), *Am J Occup Ther* 43:1206, 1989.
3. American Occupational Therapy Association: Occupational therapy practice framework: domain and process, *Am J Occup Ther* 56(6): 609, 2002.
4. American Occupational Therapy Association: Year 2000 health consortium meets, *OT Week*, December 7, p. 9, 1989.
5. Bing RK: Point of departure (a play about founding the profession), *Am J Occup Ther* 46(1): 27, 1992.
6. Boop C: Appendix A: Assessments: listed alphabetically by title. In Crepeau EB, Cohn ES, Schell BA, editors: *Willard & Spackman's occupational therapy*, ed 10, p. 981, Philadelphia, 2003, Lippincott, Williams & Wilkins.
7. Breines EB: *From clay to computers*, Philadelphia, 1995, FA Davis.
8. Breines EB: *Origins and adaptations*, Preface, pp. ix-xii; ch. 2 & 8, Lebanon, NJ, 1986, Geri-Rehab.
9. Brownson CA, Scaffa ME: Occupational therapy in the promotion of health and the prevention of disease and disability statement, *Am J Occup Ther* 55(6):656, 2001.
10. Brunyate RW: After fifty years, what stature do we hold? *Am J Occup Ther* 21(5):262, 1967.
11. Canadian Association of Occupational Therapists: *Enabling occupation: an occupational therapy perspective*, Ottawa, ON, 1997, CAOT Publications ACE.
12. Centers for Disease Control: *Secondary conditions: children and adults with disabilities*, 2003. Retrieved July 26, 2004, from *http://www.cdc.gov/ncbddd/factsheets/secondary_cond.pdf*.
13. Christiansen C, Baum C: Index of assessments. In Christiansen C, Baum C, editors: *Occupational therapy: enabling function and well-being*, ed 2, p. 607, Thorofare, NJ, 1997, Slack Publishers.
14. Clark F, Azen SP, Zemke R, et al: Occupational therapy for independent-living older adults: a randomized controlled trial, *J Am Med Assoc* 278(16): 1312, 1997.
15. Durlak JA: Common risk and protective factors in successful prevention programs, *Am J Orthopsychiatry* 68(4): 512, 1998.
16. Edelman CL, Mandle CL: *Health promotion throughout the lifespan*, ed 5, St. Louis, 2002, Mosby.
17. Fidler G: Introductory overview. In Fidler G, Velde B, editors: *Activities: reality and symbols*, p. 1, Thorofare, NJ, 1999, Slack Publishers.

18. Fidler G, Velde B, editors: *Activities: reality and symbols,* Thorofare, NJ, 1999, Slack Publishers.

19. Fine S: Symbolization: making meaning for self and society. In Fidler G, Velde B, editors: *Activities: reality and symbols,* p. 11, Thorofare, NJ, 1999, Slack Publishers.

20. Finn G: The occupational therapist in prevention programs, *Am J Occup Ther* 26(2):59, 1972.

21. Finn G: Update of Eleanor Clarke Slagle Lecture: the occupational therapist in prevention programs, *Am J Occup Ther* 31(10):658, 1977.

22. French Ministry of Culture and Communication, Great Archeological Sites: *The Cave of Chauvet-Pont-d'Arc,* 2000. Retrieved August 4, 2004, from *http://www.culture.gouv.fr/ culture/arcnat/chauvet/en/index.html.*

23. Glanz K, Rimer BK, Lewis FM: *Health behavior and health education: theory, research and practice,* ed 3, San Francisco, 2002, Jossey-Bass.

24. Green LW, Kreuter MW: *Health promotion planning: an educational and ecological approach,* ed 2, Mountain View, CA, 1999, Mayfield.

25. Green LW, Kreuter MW: *Health promotion planning: an educational and ecological approach,* ed 3, Mountain View, CA, 1999, Mayfield.

26. Harlowe D: Occupational therapy for prevention of injury and physical dysfunction. In Pedretti LW, Early MB, editors: *Occupational therapy practice skills for physical dysfunction,* ed 5, St. Louis, 2001, Mosby.

27. Hills MD: Perspectives on learning and practicing health promotion in hospitals: nursing students' stories. In Young L, Hayes V, editors: *Transforming health promotion practice: concepts, issues and applications,* p. 229, Philadelphia, 2002, F.A. Davis.

28. Hough J: Disability and health: a national public health agenda. In Simeonsson RJ, Bailey DB, editors: *Issues in disability and health: the role of secondary conditions and quality of life,* p. 161, Chapel Hill, 1999, North Carolina Office on Disability and Health.

29. Hyner GC, Peterson KW, Travis JW, et al., editors: *Society of prospective medicine handbook of health assessment tools,* Stoughton, WI, 1999, Wellness Associates Publications.

30. Kielhofner G: The development of occupational therapy knowledge. In Kielhofner G, editor: *Conceptual foundations of occupational therapy,* ed 3, p. 27, Philadelphia, 2004, FA Davis.

31. Krahn G: *Keynote: changing concepts in health, wellness, and disability.* Paper presented at the Changing Concepts of Health & Disability State of the Science Conference & Policy Forum, Bethesda, MD, 2003. Retrieved December 10, 2003, from *http://healthwellness.org/WIP/training/sciconf/sciconf_proceedings/ Proceedings03.pdf.*

32. Larson E, Wood W, Clark F: Occupational science: building the science and the practice of occupation through an academic discipline. In Crepeau EB, Cohn ES, Schell BA, editors: *Willard & Spackman's occupational therapy,* ed 10, p. 15, Philadelphia, 2003, Lippincott, Williams & Wilkins.

33. Law M: *Evidence-based rehabilitation,* Thorofare, NJ, 2002, Slack Publishers.

34. Licht S: The founding and the founders of the American Occupational Therapy Association, *Am J Occup Ther* 21(5): 269, 1967.

35. Lissi PE: Setting goals in health promotion: a conceptual and ethical platform, *Med Healthcare Philosophy* 3(20):169, 2000.

36. Mandel DR, Jackson JM, Nelson L, et al: *Lifestyle redesign: implementing the well-elderly program,* Bethesda, MD, 1999, American Occupational Therapy Association.

37. Ottenbacher KJ, Christiansen C: Occupational performance assessment. In Christiansen C, Baum C, editors: *Occupational therapy: enabling function and well-being,* ed 2, p. 104, Thorofare, NJ, 1997, Slack Publishers.

38. Pickett G, Hanlon JJ: *Public health: administration and practice,* St. Louis, 1990, Mosby.

39. Pizzi M: Health promotion for people with disabilities. In Scaffa M, Reitz SM, Pizzi M, editors: *Occupational therapy in the promotion of health and wellness,* Philadelphia, in press, FA Davis.

40. Pizzi M: The Pizzi Holistic Wellness Assessment, *Occup Ther Health Care* 13(3/4):51, 2001.

41. Powers L: *Health and wellness among persons with disabilities.* Paper presented at the Changing Concepts of Health & Disability State of the Science Conference & Policy Forum, Bethesda, MD, 2003. Retrieved December 10, 2003, from *http://healthwellness.org/ WIP/training/sciconf/sciconf_proceedings/Proceedings03.pdf,* pp. 73-77.

42. Prochaska JO, Redding CA, Evers KE: The transtheoretical model and stages of change. In Glanz K, Rimer BK, Lewis FM, editors: *Health behavior and health education: theory, research and practice,* ed 3, p. 99, San Francisco, 2002, Jossey-Bass.

43. Punwar AJ: The development of occupational therapy. In Punwar AJ, Peloquin SM, editors: *Occupational therapy: principles and practice,* p. 21, Baltimore, 2000, Lippincott, Williams & Wilkins.

44. Reed K: The beginnings of occupational therapy. In Hopkins H, Smith H, editors: *Willard & Spackman's occupational therapy,* ed 8, p. 26, Philadelphia, 1993, Lippincott, Williams & Wilkins.

45. Reilly M: Occupational therapy can be one of the great ideas of the 20th century medicine, *Am J Occup Ther* 16(1): 1, 1962.

46. Reitz SM: A historical review of occupational therapy's role in preventive health and wellness, *Am J Occup Ther* 46:50, 1992.

47. Reitz SM: Functional ethics. In Sladyk K, Ryan SE, editors: *Ryan's occupational therapy assistant: principles, practice issues, and techniques,* ed 4, Thorofare, NJ, 2005, Slack Publishers.

48. Rimmer JH: Health promotion for people with disabilities: the emerging paradigm shift from disability prevention to prevention of secondary conditions, *Phys Ther* 79:495, 1999.

49. Rybski D, Arnold MJ: *Broadening the concepts of community and occupation: perspectives in a global society.* Paper presented at the Society for the Study of Occupation: USA Second Annual Research Conference, Park City, Utah, October 17, 2003.

50. Scaffa ME: *Occupational therapy in community-based practice settings,* Philadelphia, 2001, FA Davis.

51. Schwartz KB: The history of occupational therapy. In Crepeau EB, Cohn ES, Schell BA, editors: *Willard & Spackman's occupational*

therapy, ed 10, p. 5, Philadelphia, 2003, Lippincott, Williams & Wilkins.

52. Shreve M: *The movement for independent living: a brief history*, 1982. Retrieved August 4, 2004, from *http://www.ilusa.com/articles/mshreve_article_ilc.htm*.

53. Sinclair K: Message to the AOTA Representative Assembly from the WFOT President, Department of Rehabilitation Sciences, Hong Kong Polytechnic University, May 2004.

54. Stuifbergen AK, Gordon D, Clark AP: Health promotion: a complementary strategy for stroke rehabilitation, *Topics Stroke Rehabil* 52(2):11, 1998.

55. Stuifbergen AK, Rogers S: Health promotion: an essential component of rehabilitation for persons with chronic disabling conditions, *ANS Adv Nurs Sci* 19(4):1, 1997.

56. Tickle-Degnen L: Communication evidence to clients, managers, and funders. In Law M, editor: *Evidence-based rehabilitation*, p. 221, Thorofare, NJ, 2002, Slack Publishers.

57. Townsend E: Invited comment: enabling occupation in the 21st century: making good intentions a reality, *Austr Occup Ther J* 46:147, 1999.

58. University of Southern California, Department of Occupational Science and Occupational Therapy: 14th Annual Occupational Science Symposium, Occupational Science and the Making of Community. Davidson Center, Los Angeles, January 26, 2002.

59. U.S. Department of Health and Human Services, U.S. Public Health Service: *Healthy people 2000: national health promotion and disease prevention objectives*, conference edition, Washington, DC, 1990, U.S. Government Printing Office.

60. U.S. Department of Health and Human Services: *Healthy people 2010: understanding and improving health*, ed 2, Washington, DC, 2000, U.S. Government Printing Office.

61. U.S. Department of the Interior, National Park Service: *Petroglyph national monument photos*. Retrieved August 4, 2004 from *http://www.nps.gov/petr/Images/Petroglyphs/PMdeerhunt.JPG*.

62. West WL: The growing importance of prevention, *Am J Occup Ther* 23(3):226, 1969.

63. West WL: The occupational therapist's changing responsibility to the community, *Am J Occup Ther* 21(5):312, 1967.

64. White V, editor: Special issue on health promotion, *Am J Occup Ther* 40(10), 1986.

65. Wiemer R: Some concepts of prevention as an aspect of community health, *Am J Occup Ther* 26(1):1, 1972.

66. Wiemer R, West W: Occupational therapy in community health care, *Am J Occup Ther* 24(5):323, 1970.

67. Wilcock AA: *An occupational perspective of health*, Thorofare, NJ, 1998, Slack Publishers.

68. Wilcock AA, Townsend E: Occupational terminology interactive dialogue: occupational justice, *J Occup Sci* 7(2):84, 2000.

6

PERSONAL AND SOCIAL CONTEXTS OF DISABILITY: IMPLICATIONS FOR OCCUPATIONAL THERAPISTS

SANDRA E. BURNETT*

KEY TERMS

Independent living movement	Social model	Liminality
Devaluation	Stigma	Spread
Medical model	Stereotype	Person-first language

LEARNING OBJECTIVES

After studying this chapter the student or practitioner will be able to do the following:

1. Describe the philosophy of the independent living movement and compare and contrast its view of the medical model and the social model of disability. Discuss implications of the philosophy of the independent living movement with occupational therapy practice.
2. Describe the personal context of the disability experience, noting the effect of individual differences, gender, type of disability, interests, beliefs, stage of life, and the usefulness of the stage models of disability adaptation.

3. Describe the social context of disability using the concepts of stigma, stereotypes, liminality, and spread. Discuss the effect on social context of person-first language, the culture of disability, and universal design principles.
4. Describe the ways the International Classification of Functioning, Disability, and Health (ICF) challenges mainstream ideas of health and disability.
5. Discuss various relationship issues between the occupational therapist and the person with a disability.

CHAPTER OUTLINE

---

*Dr. Elizabeth J. Yerxa's personal encouragement and foundation work were essential to the creation of this revised chapter.

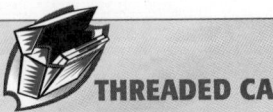

THREADED CASE STUDY: NANCY, PART 1

I was never a beautiful woman, and for that reason I've spent most of my life (together with 95% of the female population of the United States) suffering from the shame of falling short of an unattainable standard. The ideal woman of my generation was ... perky, I think you'd say, rather than gorgeous. Blond hair pulled into a bouncing ponytail. Wide blue eyes, a turned-up nose with a maybe a scattering of golden freckles across it, a small mouth with full lips over straight white teeth. Her breasts were large but well harnessed high on her chest; her tiny waist flared to hips just wide enough to give the crinolines under her skirt a starting push. In terms of personality, she was outgoing, even bubbly, not pensive or mysterious. Her milieu was the front fender of a white Corvette convertible, surrounded by teasing crew-cuts, and dressed in black flats, a sissy blouse, and the letter sweater of the Corvette owner. Needless to say, she never missed a prom.

Ten years or so later, when I first noticed the symptoms that would be diagnosed as MS, I was probably looking my best. Not beautiful still, but the ideal had shifted enough so that my flat chest and narrow hips gave me an elegantly attenuated shape, set off by a thick mass of long, straight, shining hair. I had terrific legs, long and shapely, revealed nearly to the pudendum by the fashionable miniskirts and hot pants I adopted with more enthusiasm than delicacy to taste. Not surprisingly, I suppose, during this time I involved myself in several torrid love affairs.

The beginning of MS wasn't too bad. The first symptom, besides the pernicious fatigue that had begun to devour me, was "foot drop," the inability to raise my left foot at the ankle. As a consequence, I'd started to limp, but I could still wear high heels, and a bit of a limp might seem more intriguing than repulsive. After a few months, when the doctor suggested a cane, a crippled friend gave me quite an elegant wood-and-silver one, which I carried with a fair amount of panache.

The real blow to my self-image came when I had to get a brace. As braces go, it's not bad: lightweight plastic molded to my foot and leg, fitting down into an ordinary shoe, and secured around my calf by a Velcro strap. It reduces my limp and, more importantly, the danger of tripping and falling. But it meant the end of high heels. And it's ugly. Not as ugly as I think it is, I gather, but still pretty ugly. It signified to me, and perhaps still does, the permanence and irreversibility of my condition. The brace makes my MS concrete and forces me to wear it on the outside. As soon as I strapped the brace on, I climbed into trousers and stayed there (though not in the same trousers, of course). The idea of going around with my bare brace hanging out seemed almost as indecent as exposing my breasts. Not until 1984, soon after I won a Western States Book Award for poetry, did I put on

a skirt short enough to reveal my plasticized leg. The connection between winning a writing award and baring my brace is not merely fortuitous; being affirmed as a writer did really embolden me. Since then, I've grown so accustomed to wearing skirts that I don't think about my brace any more than I think about my cane. I've incorporated them, I suppose: made them, in their necessity, insensate but fundamental parts of my body.

Meanwhile, I had to adjust to the most outward and visible sign of all, a three-wheeled electric scooter called an Amigo. This lessens my fatigue and increases my range terrifically, but it also shouts out to the world, "Here is a woman who can't stand on her own two feet." At the same time, paradoxically, it renders me invisible, reducing me to the height of a 7-year-old, with a child's attendant low status. "Would she like smoking or nonsmoking?" the gate agent assigning a seat asks the friend traveling with me. In crowds I see nothing but buttocks. I can tell you the name of every type of designer jeans ever sold. The wearers, eyes front, trip over me and fall across my handlebars into my lap. "Hey!" I want to shout to the lofty world, "Down here! There's a person down here!" But I'm not by their standards, quite a person anymore.

My self-esteem diminishes further as age and illness strip from me the features that made me, for a brief while anyway, a good-looking, even sexy, young woman. No more long, bounding strides; I shuffle along with the timid gait I remember observing with pity and impatience, in the little old ladies at Boston's Symphony Hall on Friday afternoons. No more lithe girlish figure: my belly sags from the loss of muscle tone, which also creates all kinds of interesting disruptions, hopelessly humiliating in a society in which excretory functions remain strictly unspeakable. No more sex, either, if society had its way. The sexuality of the disabled so repulses most people that you can hardly get a doctor, let alone a member of the general population, to consider the issues it raises. Cripples simply aren't supposed to "Want It," much less "Do It." Fortunately, I've got a husband with a strong libido and a weak sense of social propriety, or else I'd find myself perforce, practicing a vow of chastity I never cared to take.*

Critical Thinking Questions

1. How does Nancy's view of herself as a "good-looking, even sexy, young woman" change as the MS progresses?
2. What are the impairment-based difficulties and the participation restrictions described?
3. How do you explain her use of language referring to disability, particularly her use of the word "cripples"?

*This excerpt was originally published in *Staring Back: The Disability Experience from the Inside* Out,[45] and is Nancy Mairs' autobiographical account of living with multiple sclerosis.

Occupational therapy (OT) has the overarching goal to promote independence and self-direction with those whose lives include the experience of disability. Over the past 30 years the independent living movement has gained both scholarly and public support to promote the same end goal and has transformed models of disability, as well as the ways we think about disability. How the occupational therapy practitioners, as members of the healthcare and rehabilitation team, and independent living movement activists, comprised primarily of leaders with disabilities, interact can lead to a marriage of commonly held goals or produce a battleground of cross purposes. This chapter describes the ways that *occupational therapists* (OTs) may approach a call for an accord with activists.

Social scientists, such as Irving Zola, who had both high academic, scholarly credentials and personal experience with physical disability, began an infusion of their work into the rehabilitation and social program literature in the early 1980s. *Missing Pieces: A Chronicle of Living with a Disability*[76] and *Ordinary Lives: Voices of Disability and Disease*[77] provide an insider's discovery of the then unspoken social experience of disability that had been concealed in plain view. Zola's field notes chronicle a discovery self-framed within the social status of the researcher having a physical disability that was easily seen by others. For many also drawn to the independent living movement, it was the proverbial elephant in the room, finally acknowledged in their professional lives.

The **independent living movement**, which achieved public recognition in the early 1970s, is a political social justice, civil rights challenge to prior disability policy, practice, and research.[21] It is aligned with other minority groups (e.g., race, gender, ethnicity) in a call for equality in the dominant society, a civil rights movement, founded upon the idea that the difficulties of having a disability are primarily based on the myths, fears, and stereotypes established in society today.[59] This movement seeks to modify the convention of habilitating the isolated individual with disability through social and environmental changes.[59] A major political achievement was passage of the Americans with Disabilities Act signed into federal law in 1990 (see Chapter 2).

Occupational therapy proclaims the necessity and power of occupation in the everyday lives of all human beings. The disruption and return of occupation for those with disability is our therapeutic focus. Health is supported and maintained when individuals are able to engage in their valued occupations. Occupation always occurs within the context of interrelated conditions that will affect client performance.[3] The social and personal context of disability is inextricably linked when considering the lived experience of those with disability and ways to facilitate engagement in occupation. This chapter seeks to illuminate these contexts so that valued goals are achieved.

CLIENT-CENTERED SELF-REPORT

A justified complaint by those who have found their voice within the independent living movement is that medical and rehabilitation professionals focus on the attempt to classify an individual and do not listen to the personal account of the individual with the disability.[35,49] The medical rehabilitation tradition of case presentation seeks to frame the individual with the disability in the professional's point of view. There can be numerous goals for a "case" description: treatment justification, entitlement to support services, legal testimony as an expert witness, reimbursement of costs, social science research, educational process, etc. The role of the occupational therapist is to work *with* the client to achieve an individual desired outcome.[66] Occupational therapists are called to create a client-centered description of the individual's occupational self, one that must include the interrelated conditions of the social and personal context both surrounding and within the client. We must include the personal view of his or her own context in order to frame an accurate occupational picture that is responsive to individual values and goals.

PERSONAL CONTEXT

DISABILITY EXPERIENCE

People who acquire disability share the common experience of feelings of shame and inferiority along with avoidance of being identified as a person with disability.[74]

Neuroscience research, using state-of-the-art brain imaging, confirms what biological, psychological, and sociological studies and theory have posed; chiefly, that humans are social beings and a neurological response at the most basic physiological level is evident when conditions of social interaction are varied.[2] In short, we are drawn toward interaction with "our kind," and isolation from others may be deemed socially abnormal.

Community psychologists note that the individual forms an identity in relation to the social environment. In discussing those who deviate from societal-based norms, problems arise when individuals are assigned an identity and status that is demeaning and lacks elements of personal choice and human rights.[53]

A commonly experienced effect of having a disability is the social stigma associated with all individuals with a disability regardless of the condition.[69] The psychological effects of being labeled a "disabled individual" is considered to be the process of **devaluation**. To be continuously perceived as an individual "blemished" in form or function is psychologically demeaning, regardless of the nature of the individual condition.[69] The broadness of the term "disabled" imbues each individual with a disability with characteristics that are outside the norm.[69]

The individual with a disability must attend to an array of stimuli perceived as abnormal: some biological, such as being paralyzed; some environmental, such as inaccessible entrances; and some social, such as the patronizing behavior of others or preferential access to an event. It is a continuous flow of perceptions, which are not experienced by those who are not disabled. In short, many of the experiences of an individual with a disability are not shared by the normative society. Isolation and a lack of accord with one's thoughts and feelings compound the list of non-normative situations.[69]

In defining the experience of disability, social scientists[69] and psychologists have constructed what can only be described as the psychology of disability. Of interest, however, is that by exploring the differences inherent in the social experience of the individual with a disability, the gap in perceived differences from the social norm may be widened by exaggerations. Thus, the devaluation of the individual with a disability may be perpetuated by those seeking to understand and even modify the conventional social perceptions. The fact is, human beings are more alike than different, regardless of variances in their physical bodies, sensory capacities, or intellectual abilities.[13]

It has been suggested that individuals with a disability shape their personal identities and social conception from their personal experiences through the modes of non-conformity and the outcomes of interactions with others in society. Specifically, if the individual considers his or her situation as non-conformative, it is due to the imposition of external societal factors and not a symptom of a condition.[62] What is actually known about the similarities and differences between people with and people without disability? Siller reported that as soon as one departs from the direct fact of disability, evidence can be provided to demonstrate that persons with disabilities do or do not have different developmental tracks, social skills and precepts, defensive orientations, empathetic potential, etc. The data suggest that if the disabled do present themselves as different, it is often a secondary consequence of the social climate rather than inherent disability-specific phenomena.[62]

Another study[70] reported that a group of people with disability showed no differences in life satisfaction, frustration, or happiness, compared with a group without disability. The only difference found was on ratings of the difficulty of life. People with disability judged their lives to be more difficult and more likely to remain so. For example, people with chronic, but not fatal, health problems may not only seem to be quite happy, but also may derive some happiness from their ability to cope with their difficulty. We may question the assumption that physical limitations are directly related to happiness. Instead, many people with disabilities may find happiness despite their disabilities, even though the able-bodied public may expect otherwise.

INDIVIDUAL DIFFERENCES

Social scientists observe that an individual's reactions to having disability are influenced not only by the time of onset, type of onset, functions impaired, severity and stability, visibility of disability, and the experiences of pain, but also by the person's gender, activities affected, interests, values and goals, inner resources, personality and temperament, self-image, and environmental factors.[69]

Vash and Crewe[69] believed that different disabilities (such as blindness or paralysis) generate different reactions because each creates different problems or challenges. However, the insider-outsider perspective also applies to people with disability. Thus, the person with disability may feel that his or her condition is not as difficult as that of others. For example, a person who is blind may feel that it would be worse to be deaf. This idea has also proven to hold for the severity of the individual condition. A person with the inability to walk may have the view that this disability is not nearly as difficult as someone without legs. Reactions are also tempered by the impact of the disability on the valued skills and capacities the person has lost. For example, a person who loves music more than the visual arts may have a stronger reaction to loss of hearing than a visual person with the opposite pattern. Similarly, the severity of disability may not have a direct, one-to-one relationship with the person's reaction to it. (Note the use of the word *may* throughout this paragraph, indicating that reactions are individualized and unpredictable.)

The visibility or invisibility of impairment may influence a person's response to his or her disability because of social reactions. For example, invisible disabilities such as pain may create difficulties because other people expect the person to perform in impossible ways. One woman with arthritis indicated that it was easier for her to go grocery shopping when she wore her hand splints because then her disability was visible and people would carry her packages for her without her having to ask.[69]

The stability of the disability or the extent to which it changes over time may influence reactions both for the individual with a disability and for those surrounding him or her. In some progressive disabilities the individual faces uncertainty as to the degree of limitations, as well as (in some cases) a hastened death. Reactions to such disabilities are shaped by these realities and by what the affected people tell themselves about their projected futures.[69] When hope for neither containment nor cure is substantiated, the person may experience a new round of disappointment, fear, or anger. The prospect of a terminal condition can affect each person in individual ways. Even the experience of pain, which tends to overtake consciousness, may be ignored by some individuals. Reactions to pain are highly influenced by culture. Particularly important for occupational therapists is the issue of finding and implementing resources to assist the client in developing effective and gratifying lifestyles. The activities and behavior patterns affected by an impairment become the focus of the OT. Core issues addressed by the OT must include the individual client's spiritual or philosophical base (i.e., what makes the individual fulfilled).

Gender has also been found to elicit some of the most problematic issues for clients in their relationships with others. Gendered societal expectations dictate that individuals strive toward achieving, often idyllic, sexual roles. For example, the ideal for women to be physically perfect specimens or to carry the major responsibility for managing the home and caring for children may be of more concern for a female client than a male client.

Temporal elements of activity are part of the impact of disablement. The ways it interferes with what one is doing, with the interruption of ongoing activities, will influence the person's reactions. Additionally, activities never done but imagined as future goals also may be equally powerful influences in the person's reactions.

Interests, values, and goals influence a person's reaction to his or her disablement. The individual with a limited range of interests may react more negatively to a disability that prevents their expression, whereas an individual with a wide range of interests and goals may adapt more readily. Many people may not even be aware of their own interests, values, and goals and, therefore, may not be conscious of the ones that have the potential to lead to satisfaction after acquiring a disability. Thus, the client with multiple interests, activities, and goals has a greater probability of attaining engagement in satisfying activities. The resources that the individual possesses for coping with and enjoying life are assets that may counterbalance the devastation of loss of function. Some of these, such as social skills and persistence, may be developed to a level enabling paid employment, whereas others, such as artistic talent or leisure skills, may contribute to a more satisfying life.[69]

An often overlooked aspect of the individual with a disability is the importance of spiritual and philosophical beliefs toward that person's disablement. People who acknowledge a spiritual dimension of life and who have a philosophy of life into which disablement can be integrated in a meaningful, nondestructive way may be better able to deal with having a disability.[69] Specific religious beliefs may or may not be helpful. The person who views having a disability as punishment for past sins will respond differently from one who views the disability as a test or opportunity for spiritual development.

Lastly, the OT must acknowledge the importance of the person's environment in influencing his or her reactions to having disability. Immediate environmental qualities such as family support and acceptance, income, community resources, and loyal friends are powerful contributors. The institutional environment if one is hospitalized also has a profound effect, especially the attitudes and behaviors of the staff members. The culture and its support (or lack thereof) for resolving functional problems or protecting the civil rights of people with disability is another significant influence.

STAGE MODELS OF ADJUSTMENT TO DISABILITY

The **medical model** generally provides the medical rehabilitation team with a four-stage process of adjustment or adaptation to the experience of disability (Box 6-1).[46]

Box **6-1** FOUR-STAGE PROCESS OF ADJUSTMENT TO EXPERIENCE OF DISABILITY

STAGE 1: VIGILANCE

Becoming engulfed at the initial point of injury or acute illness. Within the intense, immediate crisis of the event, many individuals report a separation of the subjective and objective body. They experience an internal state of calmness contrasted with outward behavior of extreme distress and screaming, in response to severe pain. The stage ends when the person surrenders to care of others, often emergency medical personnel.

STAGE 2: DISRUPTION

Taking time out, a disruption of reality, often described as feeling as if in a fog. Significant others do not merely provide emotional support but serve as an orienting force in an otherwise confusing, chaotic environment; they are an emotional anchor in a disordered world of the acute care medical environment.

STAGE 3: ENDURING THE SELF

Confronting and regrouping, improvement in reality orientation with the implications of the injury recognized. This is the stage at which the severity of the physical limitations is faced. Support from others is needed to control a sense of panic and fear of the diminished physical ability. At this stage even small gains witnessed in therapy sessions are interpreted as evidence that a full recovery is possible. This preserved sense of hope to reclaim previous abilities may help endure the initial healing process from burns, amputations, and spinal cord injuries, by holding onto the faith in medical miracles, and return to prior physical ability.

STAGE 4: STRIVING TO REGAIN SELF

Merging the old and the new reality is marked with frustration in attempting to regain previously taken-for-granted tasks such as walking and feeding oneself by the use of compensatory methods. There is a feeling of exhaustion in developing new routines, frustration with the limited physical capacity to participate in a range of activities, and a need to reformulate goals.

Adapted from Morse JM, O'Brien B: Preserving self: from victim, to patient, to disabled person, *J Adv Nurs* 21:886, 1995.

Evidence only exists for emotional distress, commonly experienced as an initial response, and that it tends to diminish over time, but even that is not universal. Rehabilitation researchers are turning to a far more complex process of involving changes in the body, body image, self-concept, and the interactions between the person and the environment. For example, little attention has been given to individual personality differences (i.e., personal context), well recognized as contributors to all human endeavors (e.g., work, marriage, play, education, and occupations) expressed in an environment.

Rather, the disability has been seen as the sole determinant of the individual personal experience.

The terms adaptation, adjustment, and acceptance are commonly applied to the process of resolving the negative experiences of having a disability. In recent years the usefulness of such terms has been questioned by the social scientists aligned with the **social model** of disability. They point out the preoccupation by service professionals with the psychological loss, or stages of bereavement, process to describe appropriate adjustment by those with an impairment. The studies usually cited, which contain a four-stage process of psychological adjustment and rehabilitation applied to those with spinal cord injury, are troublesome for the social model scientists.[6] That process is usually thus: the initial reaction of shock and horror is followed by denial of the situation, leading to anger at others, bargaining, and finally to depression as a necessity for coming to terms with the acquired impairment. The acceptance, or adjustment, process takes one to two years to resolve.[6] The process draws from Kubler-Ross's seminal work describing the grief process, stages of loss, of those who are dying, with an implicit assumption that the former, non-disabled, self is dead and must be mourned.[37]

The social model views the notion of adaptation, adjustment, or acceptance with an unjust society as abhorrent at the most basic level of human rights and social justice. Other minority groups have not tolerated such treatment within democratic societies, and disability rights activists believe that those with disabilities should not either. They point to a major flaw in these stage models: what about the physical condition that is progressive in nature (such as multiple sclerosis, rheumatoid arthritis, etc.) or limiting, physical changes as the body ages associated with life-long disorders, such as spina bifida, or early in life trauma, such as spinal cord injury, or post-polio? The stages of loss concept common with the medical model, gives little to community-based occupational therapy in which the issues of chronic and/or progressive disability-related problems are more typically addressed. One might speculate that the stages of loss concept, at best, suits the emotional needs of clinicians, to have a sense of closure and resolution, as patients move out of acute medical rehabilitation.

STAGES OF LIFE AND SELF-CONCEPT

Many views of the individual and groups of people divide the human life cycle into three categories: childhood, adulthood, and the elderly. Its stages, statuses, and transitions are constructed in large by social institutions (i.e., the family, economic demands, and education) and the dominant culture. One might expect that by identifying the onset of a physical impairment in the life cycle, one may know the trajectory of many factors including self-concept. The stage of life at which disability occurs is thought to influence the person because it affects the way he or she is perceived by others and the developmental tasks that might be interrupted. In that vein, the three main trajectories commonly identified are as follows: (1) people whose impairment is diagnosed at birth or in early childhood, (2) those who acquire an impairment during the adolescent or early adult years, usually through illness or injury, and (3) older people whose impairment is most often attributed to the aging process.[6]

The person who is born with disability or acquires disability in infancy or childhood may experience isolation or separation from the mainstream in family life, play, and education. The trajectory of an early onset disability is thought to include socialization with pervasively abnormal low expectations, and lifestyle, with few positive role models to exhibit alternative models. Children with congenital impairments may be hidden by families and special-needs schools to protect them from discrimination and rejection from bullying peers. A "disabled identity" results from the child with a disability, growing up in a household and community with no other disabled person, lengthy periods of hospitalization, segregated special education, or a largely inaccessible physical environment.[6]

A recent study of self-image of a group of Swedish young persons with cerebral palsy revealed that most respondents viewed themselves in a very positive manner and rated markedly higher self-image than norm groups.[1] The influence of a generally positive or negative attitude toward oneself formed early in life and the sparse interaction with others outside of the family are posed as explanations of the research findings. Future studies must focus on the relationship between self-image and the social interaction with persons outside the immediate family as the individual with an impairment begins to interact with a wider social group.

Barnes and Mercer have concluded that many youth with disabilities do not experience the full impact of disablement until participation in more peer-directed leisure pursuits or joining the workforce is expected. When young people with disabilities are compared with non-disabled, they report lower job aspirations, poor or nonexistent career advice, employer discrimination, and a feeling of marginalization in the job market. There is evidence that the age of key major life transition indicators, such as leaving home, getting married, becoming a parent, and entry into the job market, occurs later among those with disabilities compared with those without disabilities.[6]

One cannot assume there will be continuing negative effects on self-esteem if there is an early onset disability. A longitudinal study found that, although adolescent girls with cerebral palsy scored significantly lower on physical, social, and personal self-esteem evaluations, as adults the same individuals no longer scored significantly different from able-bodied groups.[44] The authors speculated that factors in their subjects' changed self-esteem may have been due to an expanded range of environments in which to interact, better social relationships, or a wider variety of experiences in education, work, and commerce (than in earlier years).

It has been suggested that self-evaluations of global self-worth in adolescents with disability (e.g., cerebral palsy, oro-facial clefts, and spina bifida) found that the participants did not differ from those of an able-bodied comparison group. The assumption that self-esteem is necessarily reduced by a disability effect needs to be reassessed in light of recent studies.[36]

A person who acquires disability later in life may face different issues, such as the need to change vocations, find a marital partner, or remain a part of his or her culture via the routines of daily life.[9,69] Some are forced into a sudden and substantial re-evaluation of their identities, perhaps reinforced within a short time period by downward economic and social mobility. A distinction can be made between those who experience discontinuity with a sharp shift into unemployment, contrasted with the drift of a more gradual process of downward mobility. Generally, a chronic illness is less drastic than an accident resulting in disability, affording the individual the opportunity to plan and adjust to threats to self-identity.[6]

It has been posed that individuals who acquire an impairment in middle age may, more often than those who are aged, view the onset of a disability as an unexpected, personal tragedy. In comparison, those who are aged, and those who surround them, both family and service providers, may interpret the disability experience as an inevitable fact of life and, therefore, more of a normal course of events.[6]

Social scientists are calling for research on those with disabilities that includes much more descriptive factors such as the visibility of the impairment, the distinct type of impairment, whether the impairment was preventable, the age of onset, the influence of public perception on the individual, and social interactions. Increasingly, many persons who have disabilities from various backgrounds are learning to think about disability as a social justice issue rather than as a category of individual deficiency. Some surveys indicated that disabled Americans who are young enough to have been influenced by the disability rights movement are more likely than older counterparts to identify themselves as members of a minority group, namely, the disability community.[28]

Gill[28] calls for "deindividualizing the problem of disability," contrasting this view with seeing disability as a personal tragedy. In understanding the social determinants of the devalued status by challenging the disabling society, one reinforces the valid and whole feelings held by those who are disabled. Plainly stated, if the individual with a disability views personal experience as a problem highly influenced by factors outside of oneself, this perspective provides a way to effectively challenge societal perceptions of a devalued status.

Individuals with disabilities often demonstrate remarkable strength and achievement in the face of environmental obstacles and social exclusion. Those that seek to truly understand the disability experience should consider the aspects of the disability identity that engender creativity and an enhanced awareness of many commonly unappreciated aspects of human experience.[28]

UNDERSTANDING INDIVIDUAL EXPERIENCE

To avoid turning a category such as disability into an inflexible framework for identity, occupational therapists must develop methods that elicit the personal experiences and opinions of those who are disabled.[1] The narrative process for discovery of the individual is a recommended method. The process relies less on observable behavior and more on how people use their own stories to gain an understanding of everyday experience and emotion. It allows us to analyze the ways that personal identity is shaped by social interaction while maintaining the individual studied as an active agent.[6]

Part of a therapy program for clients with a disability should include client-centered exploration into the individual perspective. Initially, to help better define the client perspective, research has shown that discussing the *meaning* of core categories can lead to insight about the feelings and attitudes of the client.[22] Examples of core meaning categories have included (but are not restricted to): illness, independence, activity, altruism, self-caring, and self-respect. Researchers demonstrated that the independence, activity, and altruism categories actively directed behavior before and during treatment, and that the last two meanings emerged as treatment produced as a transformation process. Explanation of the categories identified should be a part of the rehabilitation intervention, with both therapists and clients benefiting from the increased awareness and self-reflection of the individual clients.

One study[49] employed this phenomenological approach to describe the lived experience of disability of a woman who sustained a head injury 21 years ago. The woman identified themes of nostalgia, abandonment, and hope and what the core categories meant to her. More importantly than simply defining these terms, she reflected upon how these meanings had shaped her life experiences for those 21 years. The outcome for this individual focused on changing her perspective from that of a passive victim to an active constructor of her own identity.[6] Revaluating these themes with the individual may allow both the therapist and the client discovery of the unique disability experience.

SOCIAL CONTEXT

SOCIAL STATUS AND DISABILITY

The historical Chicago city ordinance recorded in Box 6-2 is an example of the segregation and discrimination society has openly communicated to those with disabilities. A more extreme example, the extermination of 200,000 people with disabilities in the death camps of the Nazi regime in World War II, is yet another. Our 21st century perspective may scoff and feel distanced from such obvious prejudice. These may seem to be events consigned to another place, another time. To see our own present-day society behaving somewhere

---

BOX **6-2** CHICAGO CITY ORDINANCE, 1911, REPEALED IN 1974

No person who is diseased, maimed, mutilated, or in any way deformed so as to be unsightly or disgusting object or improper person to be allowed in or on the public ways or other public places in this city, shall therein or thereon expose himself to public view.

---

along the continuum that still includes discrimination and injustice is difficult. This is an inquiry we must not shy away from; the cost to our professional integrity would be too high without it; and, our ability to provide a useful service would be compromised without such an understanding.

Goffman's classic work[29] used the term **stigma** to describe the social discrediting process in strained relations between disabled and non-disabled people[28] that reduces the life chances of people with disability or other differences. In the process, an obvious impairment or knowledge of a hidden one signifies a moral deficiency. The individual with stigma is seen as not quite human. Society tends to impute a wide range of imperfections on the basis of the impairment.

As with individuals from other minority groups, those with disabilities are categorized with stereotypes. The standard definition of a **stereotype** is an unvarying form or pattern, a fixed notion, having no individuality, as though cast from a mold.[71] Stereotyping is part of the stigmatization process, applied to those perceived to exhibit certain qualities. Stigma may be

expressed as a societal reaction to fear of the unknown. One explanation for stereotypes applied to those with disabilities is that little direct experience, despite recent mainstreaming in education and the removal of some environmental barriers, produces little real knowledge of what to expect in daily life.

Individuals with visible disabilities may be discredited in social situations, without regard for their actual abilities. "The exclusion of persons with physical disabilities from educational settings and work situations regardless of their ability to participate in and perform all required activities is well recorded in the literature."[58]

Several researchers have noted the popular media portrayals of those with disabilities, forming and reinforcing the basis of our common stereotypes, even for those of us in health professions[49] (Box 6-3). For example, "Films present people with disabilities either condescendingly as 'inspirational,' endeavoring to be as 'normal' as possible by 'overcoming' their limitations, or as disfigured monsters 'slashing and hacking their way to box office success.'"[24] Cahill and Norden,[16] in their discussion of such stereotypic characterization of women with disabilities in the media, found the two most frequent categories of portrayal: the disabled ingénue-victim and the awe-inspiring overachiever. The disabled ingénue is young and pretty but significantly helpless because of her disability. The ingénue may be victimized or terrorized by others. Usually she is cured of her malady and able to return to the mainstream by the end of the story. Her return, or "reabsorption," often produces an ability to have a new perspective on life. Similarly, the awe-inspiring overachiever is

---

BOX **6-3** SEVEN MEDIA DEPICTION IMAGES OF "HANDICAPIST STEREOTYPES"

1. *The disabled person as pitiable and pathetic.* Found in charity telethons, perpetuating the image of people with disabilities as objects of pity. Their stories are often told in terms of people who are victims of a tragic fate.

2. *The disabled person as Supercrip.* Heartwarming stories that depict great courage, wherein someone likeable either succeeds in triumphing or succumbs heroically; these are usually considered "inspirational" stories. This image leaves a lot of ordinary people with disabilities feeling like failures if they haven't done something extraordinary.

3. *The disabled person as sinister, evil, and criminal.* This stereotype plays on deeply held fears and prejudices; the disabled villain (especially one with a psychiatric illness) is almost always someone who is dangerous, unpredictable, and evil.

4. *The disabled person as better off dead.* The "better dead than disabled syndrome" is one way in which the media imply that with medical costs soaring and resources limited, a disabled person would seek suicide because life is unbearable. Society, especially the family, is thereby relieved of caring for the disabled individual, who is not whole or useful.

5. *The disabled person as maladjusted—his or her own worst enemy.* "If only disabled persons were not so bitter and would accept themselves, they would have better lives" is the general statement of this stereotype. Usually it involves a non-disabled person who helps someone with a disability see the "bright side" of his or her impairment. It contains the mythology that persons with disabilities need guidance because they are unable to make sound judgments.

6. *The disabled person as a burden.* Family responsibilities and duty form the core of this stereotype, which is built on the assumption that persons with disabilities need someone else to take care of them. Like the stereotype of disabled persons as better off dead, it engenders the belief that the burden, whether financial or emotional, is so compelling that it ruins families and their lives.

7. *The disabled person as unable to live a successful life.* The media have distorted society's view of people with disabilities by limiting their presence in the portrayal of day-to-day life. Although more disabled people are beginning to appear in cameo-like scenes, or as a walk-on extra, they are seldom seen in ordinary workplace situations or as happy, healthy family members.

From Switzer JV: Disability rights: *American disability policy and the fight for equality,* Washington DC, 2003, Georgetown University Press.

attractive and succeeds in reaching extraordinary levels of competitive acclaim only to be taken down by an incurable disability. She eventually "overcomes" her disability with unrelenting personal fortitude, and often unexplained economic resources.[16]

The traditional approach used in telethons or other fundraising ventures, in which people with disabilities may be portrayed as victims, serves to reinforce our negative attitudes, stereotypes, and stigma. More recently, with pressure from disability advocacy groups, some network television programs and commercials include people with disabilities as regular participants in daily life, as workers or family members.

DISABILITY AS A COLLECTIVE EXPERIENCE

Vash and Crewe[69] recounted a rehabilitation conference a number of years ago when an address by a psychiatrist included the speaker alternatively standing up and then sitting back down in a wheelchair several times. The speaker challenged the audience to deny that their sense of his competence changed as he stood before them or sat in the wheelchair. Vash reported that when discussion followed, most acknowledged that their perception of his competence fluctuated; the speaker was more credible and worth attention when he was standing. The demonstration forced them to acknowledge their own, previously denied, prejudice and was emotionally charged for much of the audience. A wheelchair can be a powerful social symbol, conveying devaluation of the person in it.

Zola[76] observed that, at its worst, society denigrates, stigmatizes, and distances itself from people with chronic conditions. He experienced little encouragement to integrate his disability identity into his life because this would be interpreted as foregoing the fight to be normal. In letting his disability surface as a real and not necessarily bad part of himself, he was able to shed his super strong, "I can do it myself" attitudes and be more demanding for what he needed. Only later did he come to believe that he had the right to ask for or demand certain accommodations. He began to refuse invitations for speaking engagements unless they were held in a fully accessible facility (not only for him as the speaker, but also for the audience).

Another insider's view of disability is provided by Robert Murphy,[47] an anthropologist who developed a progressive spinal cord tumor that ultimately led to quadriplegia. His account particularly captures the medical and rehabilitation setting from the perspective of the client. He described his initial reaction: "But what depressed me above all else was the realization that I had lost my freedom, that I was to be an occasional prisoner of hospitals for some time to come, that my future was under the control of the medical establishment."[47] He reported the feeling as like falling into a vast web, a trap from which he might never escape.

The hospitalized individual must conform to the routine imposed by the medical establishment. For example, Murphy spent 5 weeks on one ward where he was bathed at 5:30 every morning because the day shift nurses were too busy to do it. The chain of authority from physicians on down creates a bureaucratic structure that breeds and feeds on impersonality.[47] The totality (of social isolation) of such institutions is greater in long-term care facilities, such as mental health and rehabilitation centers. A closed-off, total institution generally attempts to erase prior identity and make the person assume a new one, imposed by authority. The hospital requires that the "inmates" think of themselves primarily as patients, a condition of conformity and subservience.

Murphy[47] highlighted the experience of an increased social isolation as some of his friends avoided him. He often encountered physical barriers in his environment, which restricted opportunities for social contact. He applied a term from anthropology, **liminality**, to the observation that people with disability have the social experience of pervasive exclusion from ordinary life, the denial of full humanity, an indeterminate limbo-like state of being in the world, in other words, the marginal status of individuals who have not yet passed a test of full societal membership. Those with such social status have a kind of invisibility; as their bodies are impaired, so is their social standing. "Caught in a transitional state between isolation and social emergence" people with disabilities 'do not count as proven citizens of the culture.'"[28] This limbo-like state affects all social interaction. "Their persons are regarded as contaminated; eyes are averted and people take care not to approach wheelchairs too closely."[28] One of his colleagues viewed wheelchairs as portable seclusion huts or isolation chambers.

Murphy[47] was surprised to discover that in attending meetings of organizations formed by people with disability, often more attention was paid to the opinions of experts who were able bodied than to his views, in spite of his having disability and being a professor of anthropology. Those with disabilities may hold the same social attitudes from the culture about disability and behave in ways consistent with those negative views.

A major aspect of Murphy's life was his work as a professor, which he continued as long as possible. But even with his status as an internationally recognized anthropologist and researcher, hospital personnel often saw him as an anomaly. A hospital social worker asked him, "What *was* your occupation?" even though he was working full-time and doing research in areas related to medical expertise. With their mindset, hospital workers seemed unable to place him in the mainstream of society. Murphy[47] concluded that people with disability must make extra efforts to establish themselves as autonomous, worthy individuals.

Gill stated that, "In certain ways, many disabled persons are forced to lead dual lives. First, they are repeatedly mistaken for something they are not: tragic, heroic, pathetic, not full humans. Persons with a wide range of impairments report extensive experience with such identity misattributions. Second, disabled people must submerge their spontaneous reactions and authentic feelings to smooth over relations with others, from strangers to family members to the personal assistants they rely on to maneuver through each day."[28]

Murphy's book ended with this observation: "But the essence of the well-lived life is the defiance of negativity, inertia and death. Life has a liturgy which must be constantly celebrated and renewed; it is a feast whose sacrament is consummated in the paralytic's breaking out from his prison of flesh and bone, and in his quest for autonomy."[47]

Wright,[74] a social psychologist, studied and wrote about society's reactions to people with disability for many years. She used the term **spread** to describe how the presence of disability or an atypical physique serves as a stimulus to inferences, assumptions, or expectations about the person who has disability. For example, a person who is blind may be shouted at, as though lack of vision indicates impaired hearing as well, or a person with cerebral palsy and a speech impairment may be assumed to be mentally retarded. One extreme manifestation of spread is the belief that an individual's life must be a tragedy because of having a disability. This attitude may be expressed in such statements as, "I would rather be dead than have multiple sclerosis." The assumption that the presence of a disabling condition is a life sentence to a tragic existence denies that satisfaction and happiness may ever be achieved. This attitude is of particular ethical concern today, when genetic counseling and euthanasia may provide a socially acceptable means of exterminating people with disability.[67] If life is seen as tragic or not worth living, it is a fairly easy step to argue that it would be better for everyone if people with disability ceased to exist.[52]

Wright's work describing efforts to integrate disability with a positive sense of self has explicit recognition that the devalued status of those with disability is imposed on such persons *collectively*.[28] Gill points out that individuals with disabilities make assessments (of asset values in comparison with comparative-status values) in terms of contributions to one's life. She uses the example of the skill in using adaptive equipment; although others may judge the use of such devices as inferior (compared with "normal" functioning), persons with disabilities regard them as assets because they have learned to appreciate the benefit derived from their use.[28]

OCCUPATIONAL THERAPY PRACTICE AND THE INDEPENDENT LIVING PHILOSOPHY

Until recently, much of the emphasis in rehabilitation has been on modifying the individual to adapt to the existing environment. Individuals have been modified by machines, surgery, physical therapy, occupational therapy, psychotherapy, vocational counseling, social work, prosthetic and orthotic devices, education, training and so on.[69] This emphasis on modification of the person is termed the *medical model* (or biomedical model) of intervention. It is based on the thought that there must be intervention, treatment, repair or correction of pathology, of that which is a deviation from the norm. The norm may be physiological, anatomical, behavioral, or functional.

The cause of problem, in this model, is intrinsic to the person; normalization is the goal. In contrast, these normalization models are considered erroneous and dangerous by those aligned with the independent living philosophy, the *social model* of disability. Of particular concern is the tendency to isolate specific differences and then use those differences to determine and explain the consequences at a societal level.[25] This tendency creates a kind of logical fallacy, in which the evidence for what is normal is then used to explain the resultant problems that prevent participation in society.

In his landmark article in 1979, DeJong described the differences between the medical rehabilitation model and the independent living model, and its sister, the social model of disability.[21] In the medical model, the physician is the primary decision maker, and healthcare professionals are considered the experts. The problem is defined as the patient's impairment or disease; the solution lies in the services delivered by the healthcare professionals. Oftentimes, the goal of rehabilitation is for the patient to be independent in *activities of daily living* (ADL) performance. The client is expected to participate willingly in the program established by the healthcare professionals, and success is determined by the patient's compliance with the prescribed program and attainment of goals established by the medical rehabilitation team.[13]

Fleischer and Zames[24] point out that with the emergence of those with severe disabilities from secluded institutions in combination with independent living, strategies that produced participation in the community, a critical force gained momentum, creating the disability rights movement. Previously, many who became prime movers in the fledgling civil rights struggle for people with disabilities might have been hidden away in segregated institutions or become homebound. Edward Roberts, father of the worldwide Independent Living Movement, had to sleep in an iron lung. Both Judith E. Heumann, the former Assistant Secretary of Education and founder of Disabled in Action, and Roberts of the World Institute on Disability, require attendant care for activities of daily living. In the 1990s, it was reported that Fred Fay, cofounder of the Center for Independent Living and the American Coalition of Citizens with Disabilities, would lie on his back all day, every day, managing not only his home, but also state and national political campaigns and international disability advocacy programs using a combination of personal assistance and three computers.[13]

Bowen pointed out that occupational therapy practitioners should not deceive themselves into believing they are using an independent living, or social, model because the professional role is to help people live independently. This is merely a simple shift of words, not the core of the model. The independent living movement and the associated model are quite different and separate approaches to practice from the traditional medical model used by most practitioners.[13]

When the independent living model is used, the person receiving services is considered a consumer, not a patient, is the expert who knows his or her own needs, and is the one who should be the primary decision maker. In this model, the healthcare service provider describes what they can do with the consumer, and the consumer then decides what aspects of the service he or she wants to use. The foremost issues addressed are: the inaccessible environment, negative attitudes held by others about disabilities, and the medical rehabilitation process, which tends to produce dependence upon others. These problems are best resolved through self-help and consumer control of decision making, self advocacy, peer counseling, and removal of attitudinal and architectural barriers. The goal of independent living is full participation and integration into the entire society.[13]

Consumer-controlled and consumer-directed independent living programs offering a broad spectrum of services, including some that occupational therapy practitioners have considered hallmarks of the profession, such as assistive device recommendation and daily living skills training, are funded through federal, state, local, and private resources. In 1993, the *American Occupational Therapy Association* (AOTA) published a position paper outlining the role of occupational therapy in such programs. The general practice of the professional per se does not differ from other settings. The major difference is that the consumer selects which services to use, rather than receiving those chosen by the therapist. With the community-based nature of the settings, as contrasted with healthcare facility-based settings, the services are directly related to the consumer's ability to function within his or her roles in the local community. The practitioner may need a higher level of creativity to address the diverse role-related functional activities.

 OT PRACTICE NOTE

The independent living philosophy requires that the therapist play a supporting role in helping the consumer be the principal player as problems with the environment are solved. This role contrasts with the therapist's more common approach in which therapeutic activities are directed to restore abilities.[13]

Bowen stated that practitioners often fall short in implementation of a independent living philosophy, namely, striving to make others aware of the handicapping nature of the environment. The focused goal, using the independent living philosophy, is on problems that reside in the physical and social environment, not on a deficit within the person with a disability. Research noted that practitioners write therapeutic goals that seek to change the client 12 times more often than goals that focus on altering the environment.[13] Other occupational therapy researchers reported an extreme lack of practitioners' knowledge related to architectural accessibility regulations that, thereby, compromised their ability to promote integration into the community and empower consumers who use wheelchairs.[54]

PERSON-FIRST LANGUAGE

The language used to communicate ideas about people with disability is important because it conveys images about the people that may diminish their status as human beings. Kailes, a disability policy consultant who has a life-long disability, wrote "Language is powerful. It structures our reality and influences our attitudes and behavior. Words can empower, encourage, confuse, discriminate, patronize, denigrate, inflame, start wars and bring about peace. Words can elicit love and manifest hate, and words can paint vivid and long lasting pictures."[31] For example, in the jargon of the medical environment, disabled people may be called "quads," "paras," "CPs" or "that stroke down the hall." Such categorization leads to viewing individuals as stereotypic examples, engulfed by their impairments.[10] Some individuals are of the opinion that referring to people as "the disabled" or "a disabled person" makes the disability swallow up their entire identity, leaving them outside the mainstream of humanity. How, then, might occupational therapy practitioners use language in a spirit of dignity?

Switzer noted in her discussion of the complexities of disability policy that there is "virtually universal agreement that pejorative terms that objectify disabled persons (such as deformed or wheel-chair bound) diminish the importance of the individual and create the perception of people only in terms of their disability. Similarly, attempts to develop euphemisms (physically challenged, height-impaired) generally are thought to be misguided attempts that still identify persons by their disability alone."[64]

For PWDs (*persons with disabilities*) to develop a sense of pride, culture, and community, past negative attitudes must be changed. The use of language that recognizes that the person comes first, namely, a person with a disability, is yet again another acknowledgment that the individual is a human being before being someone with a disability.[64] This shift in use of language is widely known as **person-first language**.[40]

All struggles for basic human rights have included the significant issue of what labels will be used by and about a particular people. With other minority groups, examples include the following: "Negro" was replaced by "Black" and then changed to "African-American"; "Indian" changed to "Native American" or "People of First Nations"; and "ladies" or "girls" are now more commonly called "women". Kailes reminds us that terms such as "crippled", "disabled", and "handicapped" are labels imposed from outside the community of people with disabilities, from definitions constructed by social services, medical institutions, governments, and employers. The preferred terms continue to evolve and change. Negative attitudes, values, biases, and stereotypes can be amended by using disability-related language that is precise, objective, and neutral. Disability-related terms are often subjective and indirectly carry a feeling or bias through innuendo and tone. But the effect of these terms on those with disabilities can be very direct and disturbing with a sharp cringe, a flash of anger, or shutting down the interaction when confronted with "ablest" and "handicapist" language. Use of such language creates social distance, establishes an inequality in the interaction, and produces demeaning expectations.[31]

What should we call the recipient of occupational therapy—*patient, client,* or *patient-client* (Box 6-4)? *Patient* conveys both a sense of ethical responsibility[56] by practitioners, as well as passivity and dependence[47] for those people receiving care. *Client,* on the other hand, conveys merely an economic relationship,[60] as does *consumer.* One might sell a product or service to a client with the buyer beware ethic of a free market economy, whereas our professional ethics demand the provision of service based entirely on the benefits it affords its recipients. Perhaps a sensitive inquiry by the therapist is needed, asking what term that particular individual prefers might give the answer.

CULTURE OF DISABILITY

Shapiro, a highly regarded journalist, wrote about the new group consciousness emerging through a powerful coalition of literally millions of people with disabilities, their families, and those that work with them. He noted the start of a disability culture, which did not exist nationally even as recently as the late 1970s.[59] Barnes and Mercer,[7] British social scientists, more recently stated that the disability culture is a sense of common identity and interests that unites disabled people and separates them from those who are non-disabled.

Steven Brown, cofounder of the Institute on Disability Culture in Las Cruces, New Mexico, said, "People with disabilities have forged a group identity. We share a common history of oppression and a common bond of resilience. We generate art, music, literature, and other expressions of our lives and our culture, infused from our experience of disability. Most importantly, we are proud of ourselves as people with disabilities. We claim our disabilities with pride as part of our identity. We are who we are: we are people with disabilities."[24]

The notion of "disability pride," as an echo of "Black pride" or "gay pride," was dismissed as unachievable even within independent living movement circles during the mid-1970s. In the summer of 2004, however, was the first Disability Pride Parade in Chicago. Sarah Triano, Disabilities Pride Parade Planning Co-Chair, said, "It takes a lot for people with disabilities, particularly non-apparent disabilities, to get to a place where they openly and proudly identify themselves as disabled. Just as in other social/human rights movements, the first arena of acceptance comes from the internalized feelings of pride and power." She goes on to say, "It's time that we reclaim the definition of Disability and take control over the naming of our own experience ... disability is a natural and beautiful part of human diversity ... The barrier to be overcome is not my disability; it is societal oppression and discrimination based on biological differences (such as disability, gender, race, age, or sexuality)" (*www.disabledandproud.com/selfdefinition.htm*).

The emergence of the disability arts movement marks a significant stage in the transition to positive portrayal of disabled people building on the social model of disability. From the mid-1980s, there has been a substantial increase in work by disabled poets, musicians, artists, and entertainers that articulates the experience and value of the "disabled" lifestyle.[7] Art, literature, and performance, from the time of Shakespeare to the present day Axis Dance Company, aspire to convey the universality of human experience that we all share. For over 10 years, John Callahan, an irreverent cartoonist and self-stated "quadriplegic in a wheelchair" has depicted a point of view of life, including the experience of disability, which is published in newspapers across the nation. Callahan's autobiography, *Don't Worry He Won't Get Far on Foot,* made it to the New York Times best seller list.

"Disdainful of pity, disability culture celebrates its heritage and sense of community, using various forms of expression common to other cultures such as, for example, film, literature, dance, and painting."[24] The UCLA National Arts and Disability Center is dedicated to promoting the full inclusion of children and adults with disabilities into the visual-, performing-, media-, and literary-arts communities.

Sports and games, heralds of cultural pursuit, are also evident in the culture of disability. The term, "disabled athlete" has been reclaimed from sports medicine and orthopedics to mean competitive athletes with disabilities. Every major city marathon includes "runners" with wheels. The international Paralympics occur every four years in tandem with the Olympic games, with 4000 entrants from 130 countries (*www.paralympic.org*).

Charlton's *Nothing About Us Without Us: Disability Oppression and Empowerment* details the worldwide "grassroots disability activism" of those with disabilities. He states, "A consciousness of empowerment is growing among people with disabilities. ... it has to do with being proud of self and having a culture that fortifies and spreads the feeling."[17]

The well-known journalist and author of *Moving Violations, A Memoir, War Zones, Wheelchairs and Declarations of Independence,*[30] John Hockenberry, who had a spinal cord injury and uses a wheelchair, sees disability in a novel way, as a cultural resource, and is quoted as follows: "Why is it that a person would not be considered educated or privileged if he went to school and never learned there was a France or a French language? But if a person went through school and knew nothing about disability, never met a disabled person, never heard of American Sign Language, he might be considered not only educated, but also lucky? Maybe we in the disability community need to get out of the clinical realm, even out of the equity realm, into the cultural realm, and show that a strategy that leads to inclusion makes a better community for everyone."[30]

Murphy, in *The Body Silent,*[47] describes how his degenerative disability impelled him to examine the society of people with disabilities with the same analytical tools he used to study esoteric cultures in remote geographical areas, the classic field study location of his discipline. He stated: "Just

BOX **6-4**   USE OF LANGUAGE

DISABLED VS. HANDICAPPED

Handicapped connotes the negative image of a person on the street corner with a "handicap" in hand, begging for money. The word *disability* is not perfect, as it still implies a negative–what a person cannot do–but it has become the most widely used and accepted among people with disabilities. A disability is a condition, and a handicap is a barrier or obstacle that a person with a disability may encounter in the environment. People are not handicapped by their disability all the time. A wheelchair user is not handicapped in an environment where there are no steps. A disability can mean that a person may do something differently as compared to a person without a disability, but with equal participation and equal results. The phrase *disabled people* is a shortcut to the more involved and sometimes more awkward, but preferred expression, *people with disabilities*. It depicts people with disabilities as people, with multi-dimensional characteristics in addition to their disability.

For example, a woman who has a disability as a result of polio and uses a wheelchair may also be a mother, a wife, an executive, a student, a citizen, a board member, a gifted public speaker, etc. A man who has quadriplegia as a result of an auto accident is not a "vegetable." Although he has a significant physical disability, he may also be an active, contributing, productive member of society. *Disabled people* can represent differentness and separateness, and reduce a person's identity to only their disability; we don't refer to people with broken legs as "broken-leg people." An exception to this guideline is for people who are deaf who refer to themselves as the "Deaf with a capital D." Many people who are deaf consider themselves members of a culture that has its own language. There is also emerging discussion within the disability community that supports the phrase *disabled people* as representing a sense of pride, culture, common history, and experience.

WHEELCHAIR USER VS. WHEELCHAIR-BOUND OR CONFINED TO A WHEELCHAIR

People are not bound to wheelchairs. "Wheelchair-bound" or "confined to a wheelchair" conveys a stereotype that sets people with disabilities apart from others, and portrays people who use wheelchairs as devalued, impotent, slow, and passive. People use wheelchairs to increase their mobility, similar to the way people use cars. Many people who use wheelchairs can walk but choose to use a wheelchair or a scooter because of such functional limitations as reduced endurance, decreased balance, or slow walking speed. Often, ability, productivity, independence, ease, and speed of movement are increased by wheelchair use. For many, a wheelchair means increased mobility and freedom, it does not mean imprisonment! People who use wheelchairs can transfer to cars and chairs. Thus, they are neither confined nor bound to their wheelchairs.

PATIENT

Most people are patients at some point, but this does not mean that people are constant patients and always should be called patients. Patient is an adjective that frequently gets paired with people with disabilities. It is common to hear expressions like "a multiple sclerosis patient is in my class," "he is an Alzheimer's patient," or "stroke patients walk in the mall every day." The words conjure up a vision of a people walking in the mall, with IVs and EKG wires attached to their chests and accompanied by their doctors. Pairing people with disabilities with "patient" "over-medicalizes" people. It gives them a permanent status of "eternal and chronic patients" and reinforces a common misconception that people with disabilities are all sick. People with disabilities are not constant patients and most people with disabilities are not sick.

CRIPPLED

"Crippled" is derived from an old English word meaning "to creep." *Webster's New World Dictionary* gives a second meaning to the word "cripple," which is "inferior." These are derogatory images that perpetuate negative stereotypes!

OVERCOME

People cope with, adjust to, and live with a disability. Disability is a characteristic and just as one does not overcome being Black, one does not overcome having a disability. People overcome social, economic, psychological, attitudinal, architectural, transportation, educational, and employment barriers.

SPECIAL

People with disabilities should not be labeled as being "special." Although the term is often used in descriptions such as "special education," it is patronizing, inappropriate, and distancing. It is not necessary. "Special" is often viewed by the disability community as a euphemism for segregated, as it implies "differentness" and apartness.

SUFFER

An individual who has a disability does not necessarily suffer. "Suffer" conveys a stereotypical attitude of never-ending mourning. If one wants to say a particular person is suffering, this point should be developed explicitly. Mourning is one of the stages involved in adjusting to disability. It is not a chronic state.

VICTIM

The word "victim" is appropriate to use immediately after a diagnosis, an injury, or having experienced some form of abuse (victim of a violent crime, accident victim, or rape victim). It is inappropriate to use the word to describe an ongoing status. A person is not a lifetime multiple sclerosis victim, cerebral palsy victim, or stroke victim. Being constantly referred to as a victim reinforces the helplessness and degradation of the initial experience.

From Kailes JI: *Language is more than a trivial concern!* 1999, Author (available from www.jik.com).

as an anthropologist gets a better perspective on his own culture through the long and deep study of a radically different one, my extended sojourn in disability has given me, like it or not, a measure of estrangement far beyond the yield of any trip. I now stand somewhat apart from American culture, making me in many ways a stranger. And with this estrangement has come a greater urge to penetrate the veneer of cultural differences and reach an understanding of the underlying unity of all human experience."[47]

Why should an occupational therapist know about this evolving social phenomenon—disability culture? Is our contribution so bound to a medical model that we cannot acknowledge this cultural expression? What value is our relationship with those that have disabilities if not to support participation in all aspects of occupation, including those expressing a disability cultural perspective?

DESIGN AND DISABILITY

Bickenbach, a disability rights law and policy maker, draws on Irving Zola's work,[11] reminding us that the "special needs" approach to disability is inevitably short-sighted. If we see the mismatch between impairments and the social, attitudinal, architectural, medical, economic, and political environment as merely a problem facing the individual with a disability, then we are ignoring that disability is an essential feature of the human condition. It is not whether a disability will occur, but when; not so much which one, but how many and in what combination. The entire population is at risk for the impairments associated with chronic illness and disability. As people live longer lives, the incidence of disability increases. Viewing disability as an abnormality does not provide a realistic picture of the human experience. Bickenback, in his discussion of disability as a human rights issue, underlines the fact that disability is a constant and fundamental part of human experience, and that no individual has a perfect set of abilities for all contexts; there are no fixed boundaries dividing all the variations in human abilities. Our usual description of contrast between ability and disability is, in fact, a continuum of functionality in various settings.[11]

This perspective impacts the occupational therapy role in the realm of assistive technology and modification of the environment to enhance individual performance of occupational behavior. Our literature is overflowing with discussions about assistive technology (see Chapter 16) and environmental modifications: applications with various diagnostic classifications, methods for training the use of assistive technology, the usefulness of providing a specialized device to enhance performance, and home modifications. The concept of universal design (the way the environment may be designed to support individual differences) is not as prominent in our professional literature. This idea includes the built environment, information technology, and consumer products, as well as a host of commercial and social transactions, usable by all people, to the greatest extent possible, without the need for adaptation or specialized design. The concept is thus: if devices (buildings, computers, educational services, etc.) are designed with the needs of people with disabilities in mind, they will be more usable for all users, with or without disabilities.

Disability is just one of many characteristics that an individual might possess that should influence the design of our environments. An example of universal design is ramped entries, which are required by federal law (ADAAG regulations) in public buildings (including transportation services such as airports and train stations), and designed for those who use wheelchairs. As that design requirement has become increasingly implemented, the pervasive use of wheeled luggage by all travelers, as well as parents pushing children in strollers and delivery staff with rolling carts, has become commonplace. Just imagine the impact on home modification if new housing construction design included the requirement for one entrance easily adaptable and a bathroom door wide enough for wheelchair access.

Activists from the independent living movement influenced the fledgling personal computer revolution to integrate a multitude of individual preferences from the size and type of the font to the ease with which adaptive technologies such as speech recognition and alternative keyboards interact with operating systems. Universal design of instruction is evident as educators are increasingly trained to include multiple modalities of visual, auditory, and tactile systems to address the needs of people with wide differences in their abilities to see, hear, speak, move, read, write, understand English, attend, organize, engage, and remember.[14]

It is argued that universal design principles could make assistive technology unnecessary in many situations involving an impairment. A can opener that has been designed for one-handed use by anyone busy preparing multiple steps in a recipe also will also be usable by the cook who has a CVA-caused hemiparesis impairment.

Universally designed devices and aids may be one remedy for the stigmatization attached to special equipment. We know from research with older persons that "potential usefulness of a device is often offset in the minds of clients by concerns about social acceptability and aesthetics."[20] There will always be a need for individually prescribed equipment because impairments and individual needs are associated with so many variations of disability.

INTERACTIONAL PROCESS: PERSON WITH A DISABILITY AND THE ENVIRONMENT

INTERNATIONAL CLASSIFICATION OF FUNCTIONING, DISABILITY, AND HEALTH

In 2001, the World Health Organization restructured its classification (the *International Classification of Functioning, Disability and Health,* known as ICF) of health and health-related domains that describe body functions and structures, activities, and participation. The domains are classified from body, individual, and societal perspectives. The ICF also includes a list of environmental factors, since the individual performs within a context. The ICF classification's aim is to provide a unified and standard language and framework to describe changes in body function and structure, what a person with a health condition can do in a standard environment (their level of capacity), as well as what they actually do in their usual environment (their level of performance). The text produced with the language will depend on the users, their creativity, and their scientific orientation. This document is a companion to WHO's *International Classification of Disease, Tenth Revision* (ICD-10).[72] For health practitioners, including occupational therapists, the ICF challenges mainstream ideas on how health and disability are understood.

The ICF stresses health and functioning, rather than disability. Abandoned is the notion that disability begins at the point where health ends. The ICF is a tool for measuring the act of functioning, without regard for the etiology of the impairment. This radical shift emphasizes the person's level of health, not the individual disability.[73]

Fougeyrollas and Beauregard point out that the revision of the ICF is more aligned with social ecology's theoretical description of disability and is distanced from reductionist social theory by emphasizing the role of environmental factors. It is also more in accord with the disability rights movement.[25] Disciplines such as ergonomics and occupational therapy consider the environment to be an essential component of human behavior. To illustrate this shift in thinking, social ecologists point particularly to models of human occupation used in occupational therapy, such as the ecology of human performance,[23] the human occupation model,[33] and the person-environment-occupational model.[39] Occupational therapy theory development has had significant influence in changing the paradigm used in rehabilitation by applying holistic and ecological principles to an understanding of the human condition.[25]

Historically, occupational therapy has been associated with the field of medicine and its emphasis on etiology, or causation, to explain function and disability. In contrast, our profession is presently building an understanding of occupation as a social construction. In keeping consistent with a social model of disability, our focus on occupation produces an "understanding of people for who they are, have come to be, and are in the process of becoming."[49]

Health, as defined by the WHO, is a state of physical, mental, and social well-being. It is the capacity of the individual to function optimally within his or her environment or the adaptation of the person to his or her environment or setting.[25] The ICF moved away from being "a consequences of disease" classification in 1980 to become instead a "components of health" classification. Components of health identify the constituents of health (Table 6-1), whereas consequences of health focused on what may follow as a result of disease. This shifted from an exclusive view of disability from the medical model,

TABLE **6-1**   **ICF Parts and Components**

Part	Component
Functioning and disability	Body functions and structures
	Activities and participation
Contextual factors	Environmental factors
	Personal factors

Box **6-5**   **ICF DEFINITION OF ENVIRONMENTAL FACTORS**

Products and technology
Natural environment and human-made changes to environment
Support and relationships
Attitudes
Services, systems, and policies

directly caused by disease, trauma, or other health conditions that require individual treatment by professionals, to a paradigm that allows for integration of a social model, where disability is not an attribute of an individual but rather a complex collection of conditions, many of which are created by the social environment (Box 6-5). The social model requires social action and is the collective responsibility of society at large to make the environmental modifications necessary for the full participation of people with disabilities in all areas of social life.[72]

According to WHO, neither the medical model nor the social model provides a complete picture of disability, although both are partially useful. The complex phenomenon called disability can be viewed at the level of a person's body, as well as primarily viewed at the social level. It is always a dynamic exchange between characteristics of the person and the overall context within which the person is operating, but some aspects of disability reside within the person (e.g., the cellular changes associated with a disease process), while other aspects are essentially external (e.g., fears and prejudice of others about the disease). Thus, both application of the medical and social model are appropriate. The best model of disability is one that synthesizes what is accurate in each model, without the exclusion of the other viewpoint. WHO proposes calling such a model the *biopsychosocial model* and has based the ICF on such a synthesis. The aim is an integration of the medical and the social to produce a coherent view of health, incorporating biological, individual, and social perspectives.[73]

The ICF allows for the real world observation that two persons with the same disease can have different levels of functioning, and two persons with the same level of functioning do not necessarily have the same health problem (Table 6-2). Two individuals will generally have different environmental and personal factors interacting with distinct body function.

The shift from the medical model, namely, away from fixing a problem residing within the individual, to an integration

TABLE 6-2 **Example of ICF Terminology Usage**

Health Condition	Impairment	Activity Limitation	Participation Restriction
Spinal injury	Paralysis	Incapable of using public transportation	Lack of accommodations in public transportation leads to no participation in religious activities
Bipolar illness	Cognitive and emotional dysfunction	Incapable of managing finances	Lack of credit leads to homelessness

in occupational therapy practice of the social model, that accounts for the interaction of the person and the environment, has led to evolving theoretical constructs.[19,34] For example, the therapeutic notion of adaptation to environment, whereby individuals are expected to transform themselves through therapy, has been questioned by occupational science theorists. Rather, an interactional, dynamic, reciprocal adaptation of both the person and the environment emphasizes more the social model approach. Cutchin proposes the concept of place integration instead of adaptation to environment, whereby "people are more a part of their environment, and environments more a part of people,"[19] with the person's "motivations and processes never fully independent from the physical, social, and cultural realms that shape the self and desires."[19] In Cutchin's conclusion, he underlined that client and practitioner are reflexive social selves, with the potential for "the therapeutic moment, one in which the client and therapist are united by place and social ties and by the collaborative effort to coordinate occupation so that person and place become once again integrated and whole."[19]

A Canadian study of women wheelchair users underscored these evolving theoretical constructs. The researchers concluded that the barriers they experienced were a lack of space, stairs, difficult to reach spaces, poor transportation, and limited community access. The study recognized the importance of the many strategies used by the women to regain control over their environment and to attain autonomy and participation in the community. The researchers call on clinicians to have sensitivity to the meaning of home by including the relationship between body and environmental features that surround that meaning.[55]

RELATIONSHIP BETWEEN THE OT AND PERSON WITH A DISABILITY

Nancy Mairs' account of her experience with multiple sclerosis in the case study at the beginning of the chapter does not describe her relationships with medical or rehabilitation specialists. One might assume that, at times, there were reasons for her to seek advice, treatment, or consultation with such professionals. The determination of a diagnosis with multiple sclerosis can be a long and arduous journey fought with miscalculations, multiple speculations of cause, and little of the support one might expect in other aspects of medical rehabilitation, when there is a distinct, sudden onset or trauma.

 ETHICAL CONSIDERATIONS

The need for professional healthcare consultation is generally not a choice; rather, the need arises from trauma or a more insidious dysfunction impacting an individual's well-being. Healthcare providers must honor the vulnerability of those who engage us in their quest for restored well-being. Care and thoughtfulness must prevail to ensure respect, dignity, and ethical responsibility with those who engage occupational therapy.

Occupational therapy values center on a humanistic concern for the individual,[49] particularly individuals who have a chronic, severe, and lifelong disability and who will never be cured.[75] Some occupational therapy practitioners may be engaged by a person with a temporary disability (e.g., an injury to the hand that gains most or even all of its former function) or work in prevention programs designed to reduce work injuries and without contact with those who are considered disabled. However, the majority of people served by occupational therapists have lifelong conditions that cannot be "cured"[4] and, therefore, most of those served do not escape the potential for devaluation, stigma, liminality, stereotyping, and the experience of a world designed primarily for those without their differences. Some will have differences that are not observable in casual contact, for example, those with autoimmune deficiencies, seizure disorders, pain, or heart and pulmonary dysfunctions, and yet, once discovered or disclosed by others, produce similar personal and social results.

Rather than eradicating disease, occupational therapists identify and strengthen the healthy aspects or potential of the person. Self-directedness and self-responsibility of the person are emphasized rather than compliance or adherence to orders. A generalist, integrated view of the person as one who interacts with his or her environment guides OT practice rather than a specialist, reductive perspective. This integration requires emphasis on daily life activities and engagement in the occupations expected by the culture. The therapeutic relationships of occupational therapists should be based upon mutual cooperation[61] rather than an active therapist and passive patient approach. The recipient of our service should be viewed as an agent or actor with goals, interests, and motives and not as one whose behavior is determined by merely physical laws;[42] rather, we possess faith in potential ability, actualized by engagement in activity. The recipient's productivity and participation, rather than relief from responsibility, are emphasized.

OT PRACTICE NOTE

Occupational therapists seek to facilitate a balance among performance in areas of occupation[3] such as work, rest, play, sleep, ADLs, and a restored sense of well-being. To accomplish this goal, the occupational therapist must understand the experience and point of view, instead of relying on observation as the only credible source of information.

Although many occupational therapists provide services in a medical model milieu, we view the client different in a way from the traditional medical perspective of diagnosis, cure, and recovery, and should follow a different thought process. Our concern with the capacity to engage in daily life activities means that our scope of practice must include not only the hospital setting, but also home and community. Thus, occupational therapy may practice both within and outside of the medical milieu, often helping clients to become agents in their own return to health and well-being. In this sense, OT practice bridges the sometimes alien world of acute medical care with engagement in the world of home, family, and culture.

THERAPIST AS AN ENVIRONMENTAL FACTOR

OTs and other rehabilitation professionals are a distinct part of the social context for those with disabilities; OTs are an environmental factor for an individual as he or she seeks a sense of well-being. Behaviors, beliefs, and demonstrated attitudes have a bearing on the lived experience of the person OTs seek to serve. OTs bring to the environment cultural biases (e.g., woman as homemaker, man as breadwinner), religious beliefs (e.g., illness as a manifestation of sin or divine intervention), and attitudes towards disability and disablement (e.g., the mass media stereotypes). Personal mindset may be in conflict with the desire for an authentic understanding of each individual; for example, Asch, discussing bioethics, reported that "Rehabilitation specialists...dramatically underestimate life satisfaction of people with disabilities, regardless of the length of time they had been in the field or the number of people they had worked with."[5] It is reasonable to conclude that such an underestimate impacts the quality of the interaction between the person served and the specialist, and that it must influence the social context of the relationship.

Basnett,[8] a physician with a cervical spinal cord injury, argued that the predominant influences on healthcare professionals and their attitudes are the norms of society. Often reinforced by training and practice and biased predominantly by seeing disabled people when they are sick, health professionals can develop a view of disability that is at substantial variance from its reality for many disabled people. This can affect vital decisions involving health professionals that affect disabled people. His research results included (1) general health professionals' attitudes, in which attitudes become more negative as professional education proceeds, (2) a power imbalance in the relationship between professional and patient, and (3) functional limitations and the differences of disabled people are highlighted, rather than contacts emphasizing the strengths and similarities. He noted that other professionals, such as occupational therapists who specialize more in disability and varying functional limitations, may develop a different view than physicians.

Wright[74] observed that the goals of rehabilitation, independence, and self-directedness must be nurtured during rehabilitation. She proposed that co-management could result in improved outcomes. She observed that helping relationships might get in the way by conveying subservience and less power for the person being helped, and reinforcing the view that the expert has or should have the answers. The client might expect and want the professional to take complete charge. In some circumstances, such as acute medical care, this approach is necessary and commendable. However, shifting responsibility and power to the therapist can interfere substantially with the goals of rehabilitation and OT, especially the goal of independent living. Wright, therefore, asserted that, "It is essential that the client be brought into a directorship role as soon as [is] feasible."[74]

Wright[74] also acknowledged that rehabilitation specialists may have needs that interfere with co-management. They might need to assert themselves, display their knowledge, gain power, or achieve satisfaction in an authoritative role. Wright also cited the increasing pressure for efficiency and cost containment in the system as a stumbling block because co-management may require more time and effort than would professional prescriptions. Her advice was, "Don't get stuck with the problem; move on to the solution" to prod constructive thinking.

Research supported the findings about long-term effects of co-management.[74] A group of 100 patients with severe disability underwent rehabilitation in a hospital that encouraged their maximum involvement and participation. One year after discharge, their status was compared with that of a control group who had completed a conventional rehabilitation program at the same hospital. The experimental group showed a greater degree of sustained improvement in self-care and ambulation and a lower mortality rate.

Wright[74] concluded with the conviction that, whenever feasible, co-management on the part of the client should be promoted. The therapist should support this belief by showing that he or she respects the patient, by being friendly and caring, and by showing concern about the patient's overall welfare. Basic social civilities such as knocking at the door of the hospital room, introducing oneself, and addressing the recipient of services by name are important. The professional person needs "to question at all times whether the client is at the helm" or whether the person is being "paternalistically directed." This last test is especially important for occupational therapists who may work in an environment in which professional authoritarianism is the norm.

THERAPEUTIC USE OF SELF

Gill[28] stated that even though there are negative depictions in the literature, many people with disabilities have commendable relationships with non-disabled family members, friends, intimate partners, health professionals, and employers, relationships that, in fact, promote health. She reports that many individuals with disabilities have descriptive narratives of their lives in which key non-disabled persons are themselves without disability prejudice, are aware of prejudice when it appears, and are allied in despising it. These allies appear to learn who their disabled associates are in their "full glory and their full ordinariness."[28]

Neville-Jan,[48] an occupational therapist and professor with spina bifida, in her autoethnography of the "world of pain," described how an authentic and respectful relationship may be created. She refers back to Yerxa's 1967 Eleanor Clarke Slagle lecture, and reminds us that "authentic occupational therapy implies a commitment to a patient's meaning system and a relationship that is best described as "being there" with our patients."[48] Quoting Clark, Ennevor, and Richardson, she states, "'Techniques of collaboration, building empathy, inclusion of the ordinary, listening, and reflection'[18] are important for understanding patients' stories of their world of occupation, and, thereby, developing trust and hope." Neville-Jan stated, "In my story there were two professionals who engendered trust and hope consistently whether treatment worked or not. We were partners; they listened and shared stories from their lives, their families, and their interests. They were empathetic listeners. ... They were not rushed or impatient as I told them about my daily struggles with pain. They didn't try to change the topic to one that was not pain-related."[48] Darragh et al., from their research with participants with brain injury, described similar qualities and traits necessary for the positive perception of treatment.[20]

Neville-Jan's account of the authentic practitioner's behavior contrasts discernibly with Vash and Crewe's description of devaluation: distain for a lesser, inferior being, seen as incapable, not useful, probably a burden, unattractive, and of a lower status.[69] The call for the authentic practitioner is for one who does not devalue the individual with a disability.

Another professor, Smith, in the field of education, who also has a disability, calls for a relationship of ally, joined with another for a common purpose; a person who respects, values, and supports in a collaborative manner, the goals and aspirations of another, with knowledge that that person may speak and act on his or her own behalf. It's not the same as the advocate who speaks for another, or presumes to know what the other wants or needs.[63]

CLIENT-CENTERED PRACTICE: A SHIFT FROM THE MEDICAL TO SOCIAL MODEL

Client-centered practice has gained importance over the past 20 years. Occupational therapists consider it necessary to have a partnership with the client, one in which the client identifies issues to be addressed and collaborates in the selection and implementation of interventions. Adoption of this approach coincides with more therapists working in settings that expect a client-centered practice: schools, independent living centers, community settings, and health promotion centers.[41]

Chuck Close, a highly regarded visual artist, was interviewed several years after his successful return to the competitive world of art, after extensive rehabilitation for a collapsed spinal artery which left him almost completely paralyzed. A brace device on his partially mobile hand, a sophisticated wheelchair, and other aids allow him to paint. He rightfully criticized the attempts by therapists to engage him in housekeeping tasks when engagement in art and art creation was the defining occupation of his being and continues to be, despite his physical limitations. Finding a few paints and a way to make marks with paint in the basement of the rehabilitation center was the turning point of his "recovery."[26]

Occupational therapists working in rehabilitation centers frequently place much more emphasis on technical goals (such as range of motion and muscle strengthening) than on the skills needed for independent living.[50] Independent living skills require the OT to include a client's participation in preferred occupations, which involves not only the environment in which these occupations take place but the socialization that supports engagement in these occupations. Occupational therapists should devote more time and energy to preparing patients for the capacity to function in their own communities.[50]

Lyons, Phipps, and Berro,[43] occupational therapy practitioners in a major rehabilitation center, noted that the "shift from the medical model which encourages the client to take responsibility for making decisions" about the course of treatment, presents a unique opportunity for OTs to return to a more authentic, occupation-based approach to practice and to rediscover their roots in client-centered practice. They extol the virtue of their re-invention of practice to a truly client-centered and occupation-based approach within a medical model setting, thereby declaring occupational therapy's unique approach to client care, and positioning their leadership in client-centered care on the rehabilitation team. Their methods for achieving such a focus include use of a semi-structured occupational performance questionnaire, the *Canadian Occupational Performance Measure (COPM)*,[38] an occupational story-telling and story-making narrative designed to better know the client, and occupational kits to engage clients in *occupations of their choice*, such as gardening, letter writing, pet care, fishing, scrapbooking, and car care. The re-invention of practice, to return to an authentic, occupation-based approach is a win for the profession and a win for those we hope to serve.

Occupational therapists can help redefine disability.[57] This redefinition would include working for changes in social attitudes and practices so that society would recognize the dignity and worth of people with disability, granting their rights to self-definition and self-direction. The occupational therapist would strive to work in (social model) as a consultant, helper, and advocate, rather than as a diagnostician or a prescriber and manager of treatment. "The consumer is or becomes self-directed, and both the consumer and occupational therapist work to remove community barriers and disincentives"[57] for economic independence.

LIFE SATISFACTION AND QUALITY OF LIFE

The concepts of life satisfaction and quality of life are very important when discussing personal and social context of physical disabilities.[51] Life satisfaction is considered to be the subjective component of an individual's overall quality of life.[68] How satisfied an individual is with his or her life may include such factors as satisfaction with family life, engagement in leisure activities, vocational pursuits, self-care, and sexual expression. Satisfaction does not require the same level of participation from each individual, but instead reflects the person's value regarding his or her level of participation in various life situations. A preponderance of the literature regarding psychosocial issues of physical disability for those with a variety of chronic disabling conditions (whether acute,

progressive, or congenital onset) describes using an individual's perceived quality of life or life satisfaction as a measure of the person's success in adapting to or overcoming the emotional consequences of these diagnoses. Self-reported absence of depression, anxiety, and suicidal ideation are deemed evidence of mental health, which is frequently equated with high quality of life and life satisfaction.[32,65]

Of particular relevance to occupational therapy is what clients report as contributing to their quality of life and life satisfaction. Over 20 years ago, Burnett and Yerxa[15] found that individuals with disability, while satisfied with their performance of personal ADLs after discharge from rehabilitation, felt ill-prepared for functioning in the home and community. More recent studies indicate that those individuals with disability who report high quality of life and life satisfaction regarded socialization (friendship), leisure, and productive occupations as most responsible for their reported high quality of life and life satisfaction. In fact, for the four participants in Pendleton's qualitative study of the friendships of successful women with physical disability, friendship supported participation in occupation, and participation in occupation, in turn, facilitated their friendship.[51]

Studies in Sweden showed that among community-based people who had had strokes, life satisfaction was not correlated with the degree of physical impairment. Rather, it was related to people's ability to achieve their own valued goals.[10]

THREADED CASE STUDY: NANCY, PART 2

Nancy's account of the experience of living with MS was not written to form a relationship with an occupational therapy practitioner, or for that matter, any other professional. Rather, this insider's reflection was written, in the editor Fries' words, to "affirm our lives by putting the world on notice that we are staring back."[26] Fries quotes the question: "Who should have the power to define the identities of people with disabilities and to determine what it is they *really* need?" With that admonition, one should not be drawn into speculation based on her account about what Nancy may or may not find useful from a practitioner. We may, however, glimpse into a description of a type of cross-cultural identity, one with and without disability.

How does Nancy's view of herself as a "good-looking, even sexy, young woman" change as the MS progresses?

One might consider that being a "good looking, even sexy, young woman" is an area of occupation that includes social participation, leisure, play, IADLs, and ADLs. The performance skills needed to engage in the occupation are numerous and, from Nancy's account, changed as the MS progressed. Mainstream cultural expectations regarding the correct expression of the occupation are elegantly described by Nancy. Luckily, her social environment includes "a husband with a strong libido and a weak sense of social propriety."

What are the impairment-based difficulties and the participation restrictions described?

Nancy describes several impairment-based difficulties: "pernicious fatigue that had begun to devour me, 'foot drop,' limp, timid gait, loss of muscle tone, as well as 'disruptions...excretory functions.'" The participation restrictions described include social reactions to a cane, leg brace, a three-wheeled scooter. "I'm not by their standards, quite a person anymore," and with reference to sexuality, "you can hardly get a doctor, let alone a member of the general population, to consider the issues it raises."

How do you explain her use of language in referring to disability, particularly her use of the word "cripples"?

As with others who identify with a minority group, especially a group historically referred to by a pejorative, such as "cripples," Nancy may be evoking her right to use the word from an insider's point of view. This turning of tables through the use of highly charged language can be viewed as a rite of passage as a minority group member develops a sense of pride and cultural identity. Switzer[64] points out that "just as the civil rights movements for people of color raised questions about the propriety of terms such as 'Chicano' and 'Afro-American,' those in disability activism are not in agreement among themselves about terminology...The more militant activists have called for a return to the stereotypical terminology of prior centuries [such as] 'cripple.'"

SUMMARY

This chapter explores the personal and social contexts of physical disability and implications for occupational therapists. The individual experiences of people with disabilities are necessary resources for practitioners to create a meaningful and useful approach to the problems of living with disability.

Distinctions between the medical model and the social model and its sister, the independent living philosophy, as applied to the experience of disability, give us important lessons for creating useful relationships with those who may benefit from our professional knowledge and skills. As we explore engagement in a unique pattern of occupations, in unique environments with individuals who have specific interests, we seek to improve the potential satisfaction of that experience for that individual. Our attention must include the removal of barriers to that engagement in occupations.

Using our professional expertise, we practitioners, become an integral part of a client's environment through our direct contact and construction of a rehabilitation (or health promotion) environment along with other professionals. We are held by the ethical standards and the mission of our profession, to foster relationships that promote quality of life and personal autonomy. The language we use conveys a powerful affective message and must reflect our values. As members of the larger society exposed to mass media images of disability, we may need to examine our own biases, namely, "handicapist" stereotypes, that create attitudinal barriers for those with disabilities.

Our commitment to improving the life opportunities of people with disabilities directs us to always strive for improvement in our practice and knowledge base. Our thoughtful desire for, and value of, positive change in the human condition must lead us to continual self-examination, throughout our individual careers.

Review Questions

1. How would a therapist approach a clinical situation if employing an independent living movement philosophy? In what ways does the approach differ from traditional treatment?
2. What are some of the individual elements that affect the personal context of the disability experience?
3. What do we know about stage models of disability adaptation? In what ways are they useful?
4. How do stigma, stereotypes, liminality, and spread influence the social context of disability?
5. What are innovative ways of conceptualizing disability, culture, and the environment?
6. In what ways does the WHO ICF promote a biopsychosocial model of disability? How has this model gained support from occupational therapy theorists?
7. In what ways does the occupational therapist become an environmental factor with the person who has a disability?
8. What is therapeutic use of self and why is it important?
9. How can practice become occupation-centered and client-centered?
10. What do we know about quality of life and life satisfaction with those who have disabilities?

REFERENCES

1. Adamson L: Self-image, adolescence, and disability, *Am J Occup Ther* 57(5):578, 2003.
2. Amen DG: *Healing the hardware of the soul: how making the brain-soul connection can optimize your life, love, and spiritual growth*, New York, 2002, The Free Press.
3. American Occupational Therapy Association: Occupational therapy practice framework: domain and process, *Am J Occup Ther* 56(6):609, 2002.
4. American Occupational Therapy Association: *Summary report: 1990 member data survey*, Rockville MD, 1990, AOTA.
5. Asch A: Disability, bioethics, and human rights. In Albrecht GL, Seelman KD, Bury M, editors: *Disability handbook*, Thousand Oaks, CA, 2001, Sage Publishers.
6. Barnes C, Mercer G: *Disability*, Malden MA, 2003, Blackwell Publishers.
7. Barnes C, Mercer G: Disability culture: assimilation or inclusion? In Albrecht GL, Seelman KD, Bury M, editors: *Handbook of disability studies*, Thousand Oaks, CA, 2001, Sage Publishers.
8. Basnett I: Health care professionals and their attitudes toward and decision affecting disabled people. In Albrecht GL, Seelman KD, Bury M, editors: *Disability studies handbook*, Thousand Oaks, CA, 2001, Sage Publishers.
8. Beisser A: *Flying without wings: personal reflections on being disabled*, New York, 1989, Doubleday.
9. Bernspang B: *Consequences of stroke: aspects of impairments, disabilities and life satisfaction with special emphasis on perception and occupational therapy*, Umea, Sweden, 1987, Umea University Printing Office.
11. Bickenbach JE: Disability human rights, law, and policy. In Albrecht GL, Seelman KD, Bury M, editors: *Handbook of disability studies*, Thousand Oaks, CA, 2001, Sage Publishers.
12. Bickenbach JE: *Physical disability and social policy*, Toronto, Canada, 1993, University of Toronto Press.
13. Bowen R: *Practice what we preach*, OT Practice, Bethesda MD, May 1996, American Occupational Therapy Association.
14. Burgstahler S: Universal design of instruction. In Cory R, Taylor S, Walker P, et al, editors: *Beyond compliance: an information package on the inclusion of people with disabilities in postsecondary education*, Syracuse, NY, Center on Human Policy, September 2003, Syracuse University.
15. Burnett SE, Yerxa EJ: Community based and college based needs assessment of physically disabled persons, *Am J Occup Ther* 34(3):201, 1980.
16. Cahill MA, Norden MF: Hollywood's portrayals of disabled women. In Hans A, Patri A, editors: *Women, disability and identity*, Thousand Oaks, CA, 2003, Sage Publications.
17. Charlton JI: *Nothing about us without us: disability oppression and empowerment*, Berkeley, CA, 1998, University of California Press.
18. Clark F, et al: A grounded theory of techniques for occupational storytelling and occupational story making. In Zemke R, Clarke F, editors: *Occupational science: the evolving discipline*, Philadelphia, 1996, FA Davis.

19. Cutchin MP: Using Deweyan philosophy to rename and reframe adaptation-to-environment, *Am J Occup Ther* 58(3):303, 2004.

20. Darragh AR, et al: "Tears in my Eyes 'cause somebody finally understood": client perceptions of practitioners following brain injury, *Am J Occup Ther* 55(2):191, 2001.

21. DeJong G: Defining and implementing the independent living concept. In Crewe NM, Zola IK, editors: *Independent living for physically disabled people*, San Francisco, 1983, Jossey-Bass.

22. Dubouloz CJ, et al: Transformation of meaning perspectives in clients with rheumatoid arthritis, *Am J Occup Ther* 58(4):399, 2004.

23. Dunn W, et al: The ecology of human performance: a framework for considering the effects of context, *Am J Occup Ther* 48(7):595, 1994.

24. Fleischer DZ, Zames F: *The disability rights movement: from charity to confrontation*, Philadelphia, 2001, Temple University Press.

25. Fougeyrollas P, Beauregard L: An interactive person-environment social creation. In Albrecht GL, Seelman KD, Bury M, editors: *Handbook of disability studies*, Thousand Oaks, CA, 2001, Sage Publishers.

26. Fresh Air (National Public Radio): Interview with Chuck Close by Terry Gross, Philadelphia, April 14, 1998.

27. Fries K: Introduction. In Fries K, editor: *Staring back: the disability experience from the inside out*, New York, 1997, Plume.

28. Gill CJ: Divided understandings: the social experience of disability. In Albrecht GL, Seelman KD, Bury M: *Handbook of disability studies*, Thousand Oaks, CA, 2001, Sage Publishers.

29. Goffman E: *Stigma, notes on the management of spoiled identity*, Englewood Cliffs, NJ, 1963, Prentice-Hall.

30. Hockenberry J: *Moving violations, a memoir, war zones, wheelchairs and declarations of independence*, New York, 1995, Hyperion.

31. Kailes JI: *Language is more than a trivial concern!* rev ed, 1999, Author. Available at www.jik.com

32. Kemp BJ, Kraus JS: Depression and life-satisfaction among people ageing with post-polio and spinal cord injury, *Disabil Rehabil* 21(5/6):241, 1999.

33. Kielhofner G: Functional assessment: toward a dialectical view of person-environment relations, *Am J Occup Ther* 47(3):248, 1993.

34. Kielhofner G, Forsyth K: Commentary on Cutchin's using Deweyan philosophy to rename and reframe adaptation-to-environment, *Am J Occup Ther* 58(3):313, 2004.

35. Kielhofner G, et al: Documenting outcomes of occupational therapy: the center for outcomes research and education, *Am J Occup Ther* 58(1):15, 2004.

36. King GA, et al: Self-evaluation and self-concept of adolescents with physical disabilities, *Am J Occup Ther* 47(2):132, 1993.

37. Kubler-Ross E: *On death and dying*, New York, 1969, Macmillan.

38. Law M, et al: *Canadian Occupational Performance Measure Manual*, ed 3, Ottawa, Ontario, 1998, CAOT Publ.

39. Law M, et al: The person-environment-occupation model: a transactive approach to occupational performance, *Can J Occup Ther* 63(1):9, 1996.

40. Lehrer S: *The language of disability*, OT Practice, Bethesda MD, American Occupational Therapy Association, January 26, 2004.

41. Letts L: Occupational therapy and participatory research: a partnership worth pursuing, *Am J Occup Ther* 57(1):77, 2003.

42. Lewontin RC: *Biology as ideology*, New York, 1991, Harper Collins.

43. Lyons A, et al: Using occupation in the clinic, *OT Practice*, Bethesda MD, AOTA, July 26, 2004.

44. Magill-Evans JE, Restall G: Self-esteem of persons with cerebral palsy: from adolescence to adulthood, *Am J Occup Ther* 45 (9):819, 1991.

45. Mairs N: Carnal acts. In Fries K, editor: *Staring back: the disability experience from the inside out*, New York, 1997, Plume.

46. Morse JM, O'Brien B: Preserving self: from victim, to patient, to disabled person, *J Adv Nurs* 21:886, 1995.

47. Murphy RF: *The body silent*, New York, 1990, WW Norton.

48. Neville-Jan A: Encounters in a world of pain: an autoethnography, *Am J Occup Ther* 57(1):88, 2003.

49. Padilla R: Clara: A phenomenology of disability, *Am J Occup Ther* 57(4):413, 2003.

50. Pendleton HM: Occupational therapists' current use of independent living skills training for adult inpatients who are physically disabled, *Occup Ther Health Care* 6:93, 1989.

51. Pendleton H. McH (1998) Establishment and sustainment of friendship of women with physical disability: The role of participation in occupation. Doctoral dissertation, University of Southern California, Los Angeles. Available through UMI.

52. Proctor RN: *Racial hygiene: medicine under the Nazis*, Cambridge, MA, 1988, Harvard University Press.

53. Rappaport J: *Community psychology: values, research, action*, New York, 1977, Holt, Rinehart & Winston.

54. Redick AG, et al: Consumer empowerment through occupational therapy: the Americans with Disabilities Act Title III, *Am J Occup Ther* 54(2):207, 2000.

55. Reid D, et al: Home is where their wheels are: experiences of women wheelchair users, *Am J Occup Ther* 57(2):186, 2003.

56. Reilly M: The importance of the client versus patient issue for occupational therapy, *Am J Occup Ther* 38(6):404, 1984.

57. Schlaff C: Health policy from dependency to self-advocacy: redefining disability, *Am J Occup Ther* 47(10):943, 1993.

58. Segal R, et al: Stigma and its management: a pilot study of parental perceptions of the experience of children with developmental coordination disorder, *Am J Occup Ther* 56(4):422, 2002.

59. Shapiro JP: *No pity: people with disabilities forging a new civil rights movement*, New York, 1993, Times Books.

60. Sharrott GW, Yerxa EJ: Promises to keep: implications of the referent "patient" versus "client" for those served by occupational therapy, *Am J Occup Ther* 39(6):401, 1985.

61. Shortell SM: Occupational prestige differences within the medical and allied health professions, *Soc Sci Med* 8(1):1, 1974.

62. Siller J: The measurement of attitudes toward physically disabled persons. In Herman CP, Zanna MP, Higgins ET, editors: *Ontario symposium on personality and social psychology*, vol. 3, Hillsdale, NJ, 1986, Lawrence Erlbaum.

63. Smith V: Why being an ally is important. In Cory R, Taylor S, Walker P, et al, editors: *Beyond compliance: an information package on the inclusion of people with disabilities in postsecondary education*, Syracuse NY, National Resource Center on Supported Living and Choice, Center on Human Policy, September 2003, Syracuse University.

64. Switzer JV: *Disability rights: American disability policy and the fight for equality*, Washington DC, 2003, Georgetown University Press.

65. Tate DG, Forchheimer M: Health-related quality of life and life satisfaction for women with spinal cord injury, *Topics Spinal Cord Inj Rehabil* 7(1):1, 2001.

66. Townsend E, et al: Professional tensions in client-centered practice: using institutional ethnography to generate understanding and transformation, *Am J Occup Ther* 57(1):17, 2003.

67. Turner C: Death of Canada "right to die" advocates triggers new debate, *Los Angeles Times*, p. A5, April 8, 1994.

68. Tzonichaki I, Kleftaras G: Paraplegia from spinal cord injury: self-esteem, loneliness, and life satisfaction, *Occup Ther J Res* 22:96, 2002.

69. Vash CL, Crewe NM: *Psychology of disability*, New York, 2004, Springer.

70. Weinberg N: Another perspective: attitudes of people with disabilities. In Yuker E, editor: *Attitudes toward persons with disabilities*, New York, 1988, Springer.

71. *Webster's New World Dictionary*, college ed, Cleveland/New York, 1966, New World Publishing.

72. World Health Organization: *ICF introduction*, Geneva, 2001, WHO. Available from *http://www3.who.int/icf/icftemplate.cfm*.

73. World Health Organization: *ICF towards a common language for functioning, disability and health*, Geneva, 2002, WHO. Available from *http://www3.who.int/icf/beginners/bg.pdf*.

74. Wright B: *Physical disability: a psychological approach*, ed 2, New York, 1983, Harper & Row.

75. Yerxa EJ: Audacious values: the energy source for occupational therapy practice. In Kielhofner G, editor: *Health through occupation*, Philadelphia, 1983, FA Davis.

76. Zola IK: *Missing pieces: a chronicle of living with a disability*, Philadelphia, 1982, Temple University Press.

77. Zola IK, editor: *Ordinary lives: voices of disability and disease*, Cambridge/Watertown, 1982, Apple-wood Books.

7

TEACHING ACTIVITIES IN OCCUPATIONAL THERAPY

PAMELA RICHARDSON

KEY TERMS

Transfer of learning	Visual instruction	Contextual interference	Strategies
Procedural learning	Somatosensory instruction	Blocked practice	
Declarative learning	Intrinsic feedback	Random practice	
Verbal instruction	Extrinsic feedback	Metacognition	

LEARNING OBJECTIVES

After studying this chapter the student or practitioner will be able to do the following:

1. Discuss specific outcome goals for which occupational therapists teach activities.
2. Analyze how therapeutic interventions will differ, depending on the types of learning processes a client needs to develop.
3. Apply current knowledge about factors that influence motivation and active participation to occupational therapy interventions.
4. Provide appropriate instruction, feedback, and practice tailored to individual tasks and client goals.
5. Promote transfer of learning to real-life situations through effective approaches to teaching activity.
6. Implement occupational therapy intervention designed to promote active strategy development.

CHAPTER OUTLINE

Why occupational therapists teach activities
Phases of learning
Learning capacities
Procedural and declarative learning
Principles of teaching and learning in OT
  Identify a meaningful activity
  Choose instructional mode compatible with client's cognition

Structure the learning environment
Provide reinforcement and grading of activities
Structure feedback and practice
Help client develop self-awareness and self-monitoring skills
Factors that influence the learning process
Summary

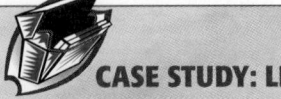

CASE STUDY: LI

Li is a 67-year-old retired high school science teacher who was hit by a car as he walked across a city street. Prior to his accident, he was active in a variety of volunteer activities that included teaching English as a second language at the local adult education program, working as a docent at the local botanical gardens, and leading nature hikes in a nearby county park. He also was an amateur watercolor artist who had recently begun to receive recognition for his landscape paintings.

Upon referral to occupational therapy, he was nonambulatory due to a fracture of the pelvis and right femur. He also had fractures of his right clavicle, humerus, and multiple fractures of his dominant right forearm and hand. He had a severe concussion and experienced dizziness and impaired balance, memory loss and confusion, and episodes of agitation.

Critical Thinking Questions

1. What types of activities should Li learn how to do? Should the activities/tasks be related to an occupation?
2. What strategies should Li's therapist use to facilitate his learning?

Teaching is a fundamental skill for occupational therapists. Therapists spend much of their time with clients teaching a variety of activities. Effectiveness as a teacher depends on the therapist's ability to organize the environment and the instructional methods to meet the learning needs of the individual client. This chapter discusses the process of teaching for occupational therapists working with clients who have physical disabilities, and presents the reasons occupational therapists teach activities, the phases and types of learning, and principles of teaching and learning with this population.

WHY OCCUPATIONAL THERAPISTS TEACH ACTIVITIES

Occupational therapists use a variety of teaching techniques in their interventions. Occupational therapists engage in teaching activities for the following reasons:

1. *To help clients relearn skills that have been lost as a result of illness or injury.* Clients may need to relearn how to perform daily tasks such as eating and dressing. They may also need to relearn basic performance skills such as the ability to maintain sitting or standing balance, reaching, or grasping. In the case of Li, his head injury affected both short- and long-term memory, affecting his ability to perform self-care skills. One of the first goals for his OT program was to relearn hygiene and grooming skills so that he could regain independence in this aspect of self-care.

2. *To develop alternative or compensatory strategies for performing valued activities or occupations.* Clients may need to be taught new ways to perform familiar activities. Alternative or compensatory strategies can also be taught to prevent injury and increase safety. These strategies may be either temporary, as in the case of an individual who needs to learn hip precautions after hip replacement surgery, or permanent, as in the case of an individual who needs to learn to use a tenodesis grasp after a complete spinal cord injury at the C6 level. In some cases, adaptive equipment may be necessary to achieve independence, and instruction in the use of adaptive equipment must be included in the teaching of compensatory strategies. Li's occupational therapist instructed him in adaptive dressing and bathing techniques so that he could maintain independence in these activities while his fractures healed.

3. *To develop new performance skills to support role performance in the context of a disabling condition.* In some cases, clients will need to learn new skills to enable participation in daily occupations. Driving a wheelchair, operating a prosthetic device, and managing a bowel and bladder program are examples of new skills that clients with specific disabilities must learn. Li's therapist worked with him to develop a reminder system to compensate for his memory loss. He learned to record and keep important information with him in a small notebook so that he could easily access phone numbers, appointments, and other needed information.

4. *To provide therapeutic challenges that will help to improve performance skills to support participation in areas of occupation.* Therapists may teach clients activities that provide physical and/or cognitive challenges to facilitate the rehabilitation process. Activities such as board games and crafts can be used to improve strength, dexterity, postural control, and problem-solving and sequencing skills, among others. Clients may need to be instructed in the rules or procedures of the activity, as well as how to position or organize themselves in order to engage in the activity. To improve dexterity in Li's injured right arm after the cast was removed as well as to increase his attention and task orientation, his therapist instructed him in paint by number activities. This activity addressed his deficits in both motor and process skills, and supported his return to participation in his valued occupation of watercolor painting.

5. *To instruct family members or caregivers in activities that will enhance the client's independence and/or safety in daily occupations.* If the client is not able to learn to perform an activity using compensatory and/or adaptive strategies, it is necessary to teach family members or caregivers how to assist or supervise the client in the activity. Many self-care and home activities may require assistance or supervision to ensure safety. Environmental modifications may also need to be made in order to ensure the safety of the client and caregiver and facilitate maximal independence for

the client. Li's wife was instructed in how to help him with wheelchair transfers. She was also instructed on how to cue him to use his reminder notebook at home.

PHASES OF LEARNING

Learning generally proceeds through three phases. These phases include the *acquisition phase*, the *retention phase,* and the *generalization,* or *transfer, phase.* The acquisition, or learning, phase that occurs during initial instruction and practice is often characterized by numerous errors of performance, as the learner develops strategies and schema for how to successfully complete the task. The retention phase is demonstrated during subsequent sessions, when the learner demonstrates recall or retention of the task in a similar situation. **Transfer of learning**, or generalization of skill, is seen when the learner is able to spontaneously perform the task in different environments, such as a client who is able to correctly apply hip precautions at home after learning the precautions in the therapy clinic.

LEARNING CAPACITIES

Not all clients are able to transfer skills learned in one environment into other contexts. Clients who cannot transfer learning will need environmental modifications, supervision, and/or cueing to engage successfully in the activity being taught. Therefore, the therapist needs to determine each client's capacity for retaining and transferring knowledge so that therapist and client can establish appropriate goals and use appropriate teaching methods.

Transfer of knowledge can be evaluated by changing one or more attributes of the task and observing whether the client is still able to perform the task. For instance, a therapist who has been teaching upper body dressing can change the type of garment used in the task, the location or orientation of the garment relative to the client, or the client's positioning. A client who is not able to perform the task with one or more attributes changed may not be capable of transferring new skills.

OT PRACTICE NOTE

Learning capacities can change dramatically in some clients due to spontaneous recovery from neurological insults, so therapists should frequently reassess clients to determine if teaching methods and goals need to be adjusted.

PROCEDURAL AND DECLARATIVE LEARNING

Therapists teach tasks in which learning occurs both consciously and unconsciously. Knowledge is demonstrated in different ways for the two types of tasks. **Procedural learning** occurs for tasks that are typically performed automatically,

without attention or conscious thought, such as many motor and perceptual skills. Procedural knowledge is developed through repeated practice in varying contexts. An individual learns to maneuver a wheelchair through a process of procedural learning, gradually developing a movement schema for the activity.[19] Verbal instruction alone is of little value. Rather, the procedures for performing this activity are learned through opportunities to experiment with different combinations of arm or arm and leg movements to achieve propulsion in a variety of directions and speeds. Learning is expressed through performance; therefore, individuals who have limitations in cognition or language can still demonstrate procedural knowledge.

Declarative learning creates knowledge that can be cognitively recalled. Learning a multi-step activity such as tying a shoelace or performing a transfer is often facilitated if the client can verbalize the steps of the task while completing it. Learning can also be demonstrated by verbally describing (declaring) the steps involved in completing the activity. Through repetition of an activity, declarative knowledge can become procedural, as the movement becomes more automatic and requires less cognitive attention. Mental rehearsal is an effective technique for enhancing declarative learning. During mental rehearsal the individual practices the activity sequence by reviewing it mentally or by verbalizing the process. This method can be used effectively with clients who are limited in their ability to physically practice an activity to due to weakness or fatigue. However, due to the cognitive requirements, clients with significant cognitive or language deficits may not be able to express declarative knowledge.

PRINCIPLES OF TEACHING AND LEARNING IN OT

The process of teaching activities involves a sequence of clinical reasoning decisions. Regardless of the characteristics of the client and the activity, basic learning principles can be applied to any teaching and learning situation. These principles are presented in Box 7-1.

The principles presented in Box 7-1 illustrate that prior to initiating a teaching activity, the occupational therapist must

---

Box **7-1**   PRINCIPLES OF TEACHING AND LEARNING IN
OCCUPATIONAL THERAPY

- Identify an activity that has meaning or value to the client and/or family
- Choose an instructional mode that is compatible with the client's cognition and the characteristics of the task to be taught
- Organize the learning environment
- Provide reinforcement and grading of activities
- Structure feedback and practice schedules
- Help client develop self-awareness and self-monitoring skills

be aware of the client's cognitive capacity, occupations that have value to the client and family, the attributes of the task being taught, and the context in which the client will be expected to perform the activity after discharge from therapy. The therapist needs to gather this information during the initial assessment, in order to have an accurate knowledge base from which to develop the intervention plan, the choice of activities, and the method of teaching. The principles of teaching and learning in occupational therapy are further discussed below.

IDENTIFY A MEANINGFUL ACTIVITY

When conducting a client-centered assessment, the therapist explores which occupations have the greatest value and importance to the client. Engagement in these occupations can serve both as outcomes of intervention and as activities used in the intervention process. The client will be motivated to be an active partner in the therapy process if the activities are perceived to be meaningful.[22] If the client does not have the capability to engage in the occupation itself, performance skills and activities that contribute to participation in the occupation are often addressed in the intervention. The client needs to be informed of how developing or improving these skills will contribute to the ability to engage in the valued occupation. Doing so helps the client to ascribe meaning to the activities and facilitates optimal participation.

Li's occupational therapist learned of his skill as a painter during the initial interview with Li and his wife. The therapist was able to use Li's motivation to return to this valued occupation to guide the choice of drawing and painting activities to increase function in his injured arm. The therapist also was able to explain to Li how his participation in other therapeutic activities to improve strength, range of motion, and endurance would contribute to his ability to resume his occupation of painting, as well as independence in daily living skills. The therapist's attention to Li's interests and values created trust that led to a productive learning partnership.[5]

CHOOSE INSTRUCTIONAL MODE COMPATIBLE WITH CLIENT'S COGNITION

When many people think about the act of teaching, verbal instruction is what comes to mind. **Verbal instruction** is an effective means of conveying information in many situations. It is an efficient method for instructing groups, such as in back safety classes, training in hip precautions after hip replacement surgery, and instruction in body mechanics and ergonomic principles for employee groups. Verbal instruction can also be used effectively when instructing individual clients. Verbal cues can be used to provide reinforcement, or to give information about the next step in the sequence or of the quality of performance. Verbal cues can be an effective way to provide feedback in the early and middle stages of learning, but if possible, should be phased out as soon as

possible so that the client does not become dependent on the verbal cues to complete the task. Family members and caregivers can also be instructed in how to provide appropriate verbal cues, if the client is unable to recall a task sequence independently.

Visual instruction is effective for clients who have cognitive and/or attention deficits and difficulty processing verbal language, as well as for tasks that are too complex to describe verbally. The therapist demonstrates the activity and the client observes the therapist and follows the therapist's example. The therapist can repeat the demonstration as many times as is necessary for the client to accurately reproduce the task. The therapist can also break the task into steps, demonstrating one step at a time and continuing to the next step as the client completes the previous step. Other forms of visual instruction include drawings or photographs that can be used to remind a client and/or caregiver about the task sequence or desired performance outcome. Visual instruction can effectively be paired with verbal instruction, but therapists must avoid overwhelming the client with combined verbal and visual input.

Somatosensory instruction is a third mode of instruction. This involves the use of tactile, proprioceptive, and kinesthetic cues to help guide the speed and direction of a movement. Manual guidance is a form of somatosensory instruction that is especially effective for procedural learning, such as the process of weight-shifting and postural adjustment involved in coming from sit to stand. Hand-over-hand assistance is also effective when teaching activities to clients who have cognitive and/or sensory processing deficits; the therapist guides the client's hands in completion of a task.

Li's therapist used all three instructional modes. Verbal instruction was most effective for reteaching self-care skills; verbal cueing was also used to orient Li to the task sequence during the acquisition phase of learning. Visual instruction was used to teach many of the therapeutic activities the therapist used to increase upper extremity function. Somatosensory instruction was effective for balance retraining.

STRUCTURE THE LEARNING ENVIRONMENT

Choosing the appropriate environment in which to instruct a client is critical to teaching success. If a client is confused or easily distracted, a quiet environment with minimal visual distractions is often needed when initiating teaching of a task. As the client becomes more proficient in the skill being taught, visual and auditory distractions need to be introduced so that the environment more closely resembles the one in which the client will eventually engage in the activity. For instance, a therapist working with a client on self-feeding may initially conduct the intervention in the client's room. As the client becomes more proficient and confident, the therapist may move the intervention to the facility dining room, where multiple distractions are present. While providing more challenges to the client's attention, the dining room also provides opportunities for social interaction, which may act as a motivator for the client to further improve self-feeding skills. Similarly, clients need opportunities to practice new skills in a variety of environments so that they are proficient in meeting environmental challenges. A client learning how to control a wheelchair needs to practice both outdoors and indoors on a variety of surfaces. A client who is working on refining grasp and dexterity needs experience manipulating objects of a variety of sizes, shapes, and weights while engaging in functional tasks with a variety of demands similar to those that will be encountered in the client's daily activities.

Li's therapist determined that his initial confusion and agitation necessitated the use of a quiet, minimally stimulating environment to initiate teaching in self-care skills. As Li's confusion cleared he was able to work in the therapy clinic on activities to improve balance and upper extremity skills and later to work in the kitchen and garden areas on more demanding and varied home skills.

PROVIDE REINFORCEMENT AND GRADING OF ACTIVITIES

The concept of reinforcement comes from operant conditioning theory, which states that behaviors that are rewarded or reinforced tend to be repeated.[9] There are many types of reinforcement. For some clients, social reinforcement such as a smile or verbal encouragement creates motivation to continue. Some clients may require more tangible rewards, such as rest periods, snacks, favorite activities, etc. Other clients are motivated by visible indications of their progress. Use of a graph or chart to demonstrate daily improvement in performance skills or client factors such as grip strength, sitting tolerance, or range of motion can help a client to engage more actively in the therapy process. These are examples of extrinsic reinforcement.

Many clients are motivated by completion of a task, for instance preparing a snack and then eating it, or dressing themselves independently so they can visit with friends. The task completion provides intrinsic reinforcement, or the individual's satisfaction in the ability to participate in desirable activities as a result of completing the task. An activity that is motivating and meaningful to the client can increase active participation and improve intervention outcomes.

Several studies have shown that adding purposeful or imagery-based occupations to rote exercise results in more repetitions than for rote exercise alone,[6] that clients select occupationally embedded activities over rote exercise tasks,[25] and that added purpose occupations result in greater retention and transfer of motor learning than rote exercise.[4] Sietsema and colleagues found that better scapular abduction and efficiency of forward reach were achieved when clients with traumatic brain injury focused on reaching to control a game panel than when they focused on how far they could reach an arm forward.[20] Similarly, Nelson and colleagues[14] showed

that intervention to improve coordinated forearm pronation-supination was more effective in stroke rehabilitation when clients focused on turning an adapted dice-thrower in the context of a game than when they focused on the movement itself. Wu and colleagues[24] found that intervention to improve symmetrical posture in adults with hemiplegia had significantly better outcomes when the subjects focused on wood sanding and bean bag toss games.

In addition to structuring the type of reinforcement, the therapist also needs to carefully grade the challenges of the activity so that the client can experience success and mastery during the process of learning the activity. If the client has too much difficulty completing a task, social reinforcement or inherent meaningfulness of the activity will not be enough to override frustration or fatigue. Therefore, therapists must analyze the activity and determine how to grade the activity to meet the learning and reinforcement needs of the individual client. This includes deciding on the most appropriate mode of instruction as described in the previous section, what type of reinforcement will facilitate intrinsic motivation, and structure of feedback and practice schedules, which are described in the next section.

Li's therapist knew that his strong desire to return to his occupation of leading nature hikes would motivate him to improve his balance and standing tolerance. The therapist explained how a variety of activities involving challenges to Li's sitting and standing balance would help him regain his postural stability. Li participated actively in these tasks and generated ideas for additional tasks that could be incorporated into his OT program as well as practiced outside of the therapy environment. His intrinsic motivation to perform these tasks in varied contexts was instrumental in his improved balance skills.

STRUCTURE FEEDBACK AND PRACTICE

Feedback is information about a response[15] that can provide knowledge about the quality of the learner's performance or the results of the performance. **Intrinsic feedback** is generated by an individual's sensory systems. An individual learning to hit a golf ball uses visual and somatosensory feedback to evaluate performance. The visual system is used to align the head of the golf club and the golfer's body in correct orientation to the ball. Kinesthetic and proprioceptive inputs inform the golfer about joint position and location of body segments in space, which allow the golfer to make the necessary postural adjustments and upper extremity movements to bring the club head into contact with the ball using appropriate speed and force.

Extrinsic feedback is information from an outside source. The trajectory of the golf ball, the distance of the drive, and location of the ball on the fairway all provide extrinsic feedback about the results of the golfer's actions. An observer can provide extrinsic feedback about task performance by giving the golfer information such as, "Your stance was too open,"

"You did not follow through far enough on the swing," or "Your head position was good." For clients whose sensory recognition or processing abilities have been impaired, extrinsic feedback from a therapist or technological device can provide useful supplementary information to facilitate learning during the acquisition phase. Technological feedback mechanisms include biofeedback systems, as well as digital displays of kinetic or cardiovascular data on exercise equipment. These feedback systems provide more immediate and consistent feedback than from a therapist.

Although extrinsic feedback may be helpful early in the learning process, clients will achieve greater independence and efficiency in activities by developing the ability to continue learning through intrinsic rather than extrinsic feedback. In fact, extrinsic feedback may not produce optimal learning, and may create dependency, with deterioration in performance if the feedback is removed.[12] Therefore, extrinsic feedback must be gradually decreased if the client's goal is independent performance in a variety of performance contexts.

Practice is a powerful component of the occupational therapy process. The ways in which a therapist structures the practice conditions can influence a client's success in retention and transfer of learning. Several aspects of practice are discussed below.

Li experienced mild sensory loss in his right arm as part of his injury. When his cast was removed and active rehabilitation commenced, he benefited from extrinsic verbal and somatosensory feedback from his therapist about the quality of his movement. As his upper extremity function improved, the therapist gradually decreased the amount of extrinsic feedback provided. Li learned to use intrinsic feedback to adjust the timing, speed, and direction of his movements while engaged in a variety of functional activities designed to improve strength, range of motion, and dexterity. Participation in practice sessions that included varied task challenges helped him to learn strategies that could be transferred to many activities.

Contextual Interference

Contextual interference refers to factors in the learning environment that increase the difficulty of initial learning. Limiting the extrinsic feedback provided about the results of performance is one example of contextual interference. A therapist who is attempting to limit extrinsic feedback will minimize the amount of verbal feedback about performance and/or the amount of manual guidance provided during the task. While performance during the acquisition phase may be poorer with high contextual interference, retention and generalization are more effective. This may be because a high level of contextual interference forces the learner to rely on intrinsic feedback and to adapt motor and cognitive strategies in order to complete the task, resulting in more effective learning.[7]

Blocked and Random Practice Schedules

Blocked and random practice schedules are examples of low and high contextual interference, respectively. During **blocked practice**, clients practice one task until they master it. This is followed by practice of a second task until it is also mastered. In **random practice**, clients attempt multiple tasks or variations of a task before they have mastered any one of the tasks. A random practice schedule may be used to teach wheelchair transfer skills. The client practices each of several transfers during the course of a single session. For example, the client will practice moving between the wheelchair and a therapy mat, between wheelchair and chair, and between a toilet and the wheelchair. A random practice schedule for improving postural stability might include having the client stand on a variety of unstable surfaces such as an equilibrium board, balance beam, or foam cushion while playing a game of catch. These types of practice schedules may slow the initial acquisition of skills, but are better for long-term retention of these skills.[18]

Whole Versus Part Practice

Breaking a task into its component parts for teaching purposes is useful only if the task can naturally be divided into discrete, recognizable units.[23] This is because *continuous skills* (or whole task performance) are easier to remember than discrete responses.[18] For example, once a person has learned to ride a bicycle, this motor skill will be retained even without practicing for many years. Continuous skills should be taught in their entirety rather than in segments. For example, the activity of making vegetable soup includes several discrete tasks, including chopping vegetables, measuring ingredients, assembling the ingredients in the soup pot, and cooking the ingredients. A therapist could teach a client to chop the vegetables during one session and teach other components of the task in subsequent sessions. However, for the activity of making a pot of coffee, the task components (measuring the water, pouring it into the coffeemaker, measuring the coffee, putting the coffee into the coffeemaker, turning on the coffeemaker) need to be completed in a specific order. Teaching any of these task components in isolation would not result in meaningful learning or independent activity performance. For best retention and generalization, it is better to teach making coffee as a complete task than to practice a different portion of the task during each therapy session.

To facilitate the learning process, the therapist may provide demonstration, verbal cueing, or manual guidance as needed for selected aspects of the task. This way, the client experiences completion of the task on each trial and the therapist gradually gives less assistance as practice sessions continue.

Practice Contexts

Practice under variable contexts enhances transfer of learning. Optimal retention and transfer of motor skills occur when the practice context is natural, rather than simulated.[11,13] This may be because the enriched, natural environment provides more sources of feedback and information about performance than the more impoverished simulated environment.

However, transfer of learning is better when the demands of the practice environment more closely resemble the demands of the environment in which the client will eventually be expected to perform.[23] Therefore, teaching kitchen skills in a client's own home or in a kitchen environment that is very similar to the client's kitchen will result in better task performance when the client engages in the task at home.

Client factors may also influence outcomes related to the practice context. A meta-analysis of the effects of context found that treatment effects were much larger for populations with neurological impairments than for those without neurological impairment.[10] One aspect of the practice context that has received little research attention is the role of the social environment in task learning. The importance of the social context of occupational performance and of the occupation of social participation is endorsed by the Occupational Therapy Practice Framework.[1] Working with other clients in a group promotes socialization, cooperation, and competition, which can increase clients' motivation. Acquisition of skills is enhanced through observation of others learning a task. Additionally, group intervention can facilitate development of problem-solving skills and create a bridge between the supervised therapy environment and the unsupervised home environment.[3]

HELP CLIENT DEVELOP SELF-AWARENESS AND SELF-MONITORING SKILLS

To maximize the retention and transfer of learning, clients must develop the ability to self-monitor, so that they are not dependent on extrinsic feedback and reinforcement. The knowledge and regulation of personal cognitive processes and capacities is known as **metacognition**.[8] It includes an awareness of personal strengths and limitations and the ability to evaluate task difficulty, plan ahead, choose appropriate strategies, and shift strategies in response to environmental cues. Although metacognition is typically discussed in relation to improving cognitive skills, self-awareness and monitoring of relevant performance skills may be equally important prerequisites to developing effective motor, interpersonal, and coping strategies. Specifically, intervention directed toward helping clients develop enhanced awareness of body kinematics and alignment may be an important component of motor learning.[2] Self-review of performance and guided planning for tackling the challenges of future tasks are key factors in the therapeutic process and are critical prerequisites to a person's ability to generate and apply appropriate strategies.

Strategies are organized plans or sets of rules that guide action in a variety of situations.[16] *Motor strategies* include the repertoire of kinematic linkages and schema that underlie performance of skilled, efficient movement. The process of stepping to the side when one is abruptly jostled is a motor strategy for the maintenance of standing balance.[19] *Cognitive strategies* include the variety of tactics used to facilitate processing, storage, retrieval, and manipulation of information.

Using a mnemonic device to remember a phone number is a cognitive strategy. *Interpersonal strategies* help in social interactions with other individuals. A person who uses direct eye contact and greets another by name when being introduced is using an interpersonal strategy. *Coping strategies* allow people to adapt constructively to stress. Coping strategies can include deep breathing, exercise, or relaxation activities.

Strategies provide individuals with foundational skills that can be adapted to the changing demands of occupational tasks within a variety of contexts. Thus, learning is more likely to be transferred to new situations when opportunities exist to develop foundational strategies.[21] Individuals develop strategies through a process of encountering problems, implementing solutions, and monitoring the effects of these solutions. Occupational therapists use activities to help clients develop useful strategies by presenting task challenges within a safe environment that provide opportunities to try out different solutions.[16]

As Li was nearing discharge from occupational therapy services, the therapist worked with him to develop strategies to facilitate his occupational performance. Although his memory was improved, recall of names and numbers was still poor, so the cognitive strategy of using a notebook for recording important information was continued. In addition, to cope with persistent mild deficits in balance, Li and his therapist developed a motor strategy of keeping a sturdy table nearby when he stood to talk to visitors at the botanical gardens. This provided a support that he could lean on or hold on to if needed, and was a strategy that could be used in other situations as well.

FACTORS THAT INFLUENCE THE LEARNING PROCESS

The ultimate goal of learning is to create strategies and skills that individuals can apply flexibly in a variety of contexts and occupations. As this chapter has presented, occupational therapists have many methods available to them to help their clients achieve this goal. The concepts discussed in this chapter that facilitate transfer of learning to other environments are listed in Box 7-2.

Box **7-2** FACTORS THAT SUPPORT TRANSFER OF LEARNING

- Active participation
- Occupationally embedded instruction
- Intrinsic feedback
- Contextual interference
- Random practice schedules
- Naturalistic contexts
- Whole-task practice
- Strategy development

SUMMARY

Occupational therapists teach activities for a variety of reasons. They re-teach familiar activities, teach alternate or compensatory strategies of performing valued activities, teach new performance skills to support role performance, teach therapeutic challenges to improve performance skills to support occupational participation, and teach caregivers and/or family members to facilitate client independence and safety in the home environment.

Occupational therapists use a variety of teaching strategies to promote skill acquisition, skill retention, and transfer of learning. Procedural and declarative learning represent unconscious and conscious learning processes, respectively.

Occupational therapists maximize the learning process by (1) identifying activities that have meaning or value to the client/family, (2) providing instruction tailored to the needs of the individual and the task, (3) structuring the environment to facilitate learning, (4) providing reinforcement and grading of activities to establish intrinsic motivation, (5) structuring feedback and practice to facilitate acquisition, retention, and transfer of learning, and (6) helping clients develop self-awareness and self-monitoring skills.

Review Questions

1. What is the difference between acquisition, retention, and transfer of learning? Apply these terms to describe the learning stages in a client you have observed.
2. When are declarative learning and procedural learning processes used? How will teaching methods differ when declarative or procedural processes are required?
3. What are the reasons therapists teach activities? Give an example of desired teaching outcomes for each of the reasons presented in the chapter.
4. In which situations is extrinsic feedback valuable to the therapeutic process? What are some advantages and disadvantages to providing extrinsic feedback to clients?
5. Why does contextual interference contribute to transfer of learning? Think of an example of how contextual interference can be incorporated into an OT session.
6. Differentiate between random and blocked practice schedules. In which situations would each of these practice schedules be chosen?
7. Provide examples of how a therapist might structure whole practice versus part practice. In which situations might each of these types of practice be appropriate?
8. In which ways can occupational therapists enhance the variability of practice contexts? Give practical examples of how occupational therapists working in inpatient settings can provide treatment in natural contexts.
9. How can occupational therapists help clients develop metacognitive skills? Why are these skills important in the learning process?

REFERENCES

1. American Occupational Therapy Association: Occupational therapy practice framework: domain and process, *Am J Occup Ther* 56(6):609, 2002.
2. Carr JH, Shepherd RB: *Neurological rehabilitation: optimizing motor performance*, Oxford, England, 1998, Butterworth Heinemann.
3. Carr JH, Shepherd RB: *Stroke rehabilitation: guidelines for exercise and training to optimize motor skill*, London, 2003, Butterworth-Heinemann.
4. Ferguson JM, Trombly CA: The effect of added-purpose and meaningful occupation on motor learning, *Am J Occup Ther* 51:508, 1997.
5. Guidetti S, Tham K: Therapeutic strategies used by occupational therapists in self-care training: a qualitative study, *Occup Ther Internat* 9(4):257, 2002.
6. Hsieh C, Nelson DL, Smith DA, et al: A comparison of performance in added-purpose occupations and rote exercise for dynamic standing balance in persons with hemiplegia, *Am J Occup Ther* 50:10, 1997.
7. Jarus T: Motor learning and occupational therapy: the organization of practice, *Am J Occup Ther* 48(9):810, 1994.
8. Katz N, Hartman-Maier A: Metacognition: the relationships of awareness and executive functions to occupational performance. In Katz N, editor: *Cognition and occupation in rehabilitation: cognitive models for intervention in occupational therapy*, Bethesda, MD, 1998, American Occupational Therapy Association.
9. Kupferman I: Learning and memory. In Kandel ER, Schwartz JH, Jessell TM, editors: *Principles of neuroscience*, ed 3, New York, 1991, Elsevier.
10. Lin K-C, Wu C-Y, Tickle-Degnan L, et al: Enhancing occupational performance through occupationally embedded exercise: a meta-analytic review, *Occup Ther J Res* 17:25, 1997.
11. Ma H, Trombly CA, Robinson-Podolski C: The effect of context on skill acquisition and transfer, *Am J Occup Ther* 53:138, 1999.
12. Magill RA: *Motor learning: concepts and applications*, ed 6, New York, 2001, McGraw-Hill.
13. Mathiowetz V, Haugen JB: Motor behavior research: implications for therapeutic approaches to central nervous system dysfunction, *Am J Occup Ther* 48:733, 1994.
14. Nelson DL, Konosky K, Fleharty K, et al: The effects of an occupationally embedded exercise on bilaterally assisted supination in persons with hemiplegia, *Am J Occup Ther* 50(8):639, 1996.
15. Poole J: Application of motor learning principles in occupational therapy, *Am J Occup Ther* 45(6):530, 1991.
16. Sabari J: Activity-based intervention in stroke rehabilitation. In Gillen G, Burkhardt A, editors: *Stroke rehabilitation: a function-based approach*, ed 2, St Louis, 2004, Mosby.
17. Sabari J: Using activities as challenges to facilitate development of functional skills. In Hinojosa J, Blount ML, editors: *Activities, the texture of life: describing purposeful activities*, Bethesda, MD, 2000, American Occupational Therapy Association.
18. Schmidt RA: *Motor performance and learning: principles for practitioners*, Champaign, IL, 1992, Human Kinetics.
19. Shumway-Cook A, Woollacott M: *Motor control: theory and practical applications*, ed 2, Baltimore, MD, 2001, Williams & Wilkins.

20. Sietsema JM, Nelson DL, Mulder RM, et al: The use of a game to promote arm reach in persons with traumatic brain injury, *Am J Occup Ther* 47(1):19, 1993.

21. Singer RN, Cauraugh JHL: The generalizability effect of learning strategies for categories of psychomotor skills, *Quest* 37:103, 1985.

22. Trombly CA: Occupation: purposefulness and meaningfulness as therapeutic mechanisms. 1995 Eleanor Clark Slagle Lecture, *Am J Occup Ther* 49:960, 1995.

23. Winstein CJ: Designing practice for motor learning clinical implications. In Lister MJ, editor: *Contemporary management of motor control problems: proceedings of the II STEP conference,* Alexandria, VA, 1991, Foundation for Physical Therapy.

24. Wu SH, Huang HT, Lin CF, et al: Effects of a program on symmetrical posture in patients with hemiplegia: a single-subject design, *Am J Occup Ther* 50(1):17, 1996.

25. Zimmerer-Branum S, Nelson DL: Occupationally embedded exercise versus rote exercise: a choice between occupational forms by elderly nursing home residents, *Am J Occup Ther* 49:397, 1995.

8

Documentation of Occupational Therapy Services

JERILYN (GIGI) SMITH

KEY TERMS

Documentation
Clinical reasoning
Scientific reasoning
Narrative reasoning
Pragmatic reasoning
Ethical reasoning

Evaluation
Assessments
Objective
Discharge goal
Client-centered goals
Progress report

Skilled interventions
SOAP note
Problem-oriented medical record (POMR)
Narrative note
Descriptive note

RUMBA
Discharge reports
Health Insurance Portability and Accountability Act (HIPAA)

LEARNING OBJECTIVES

After studying this chapter the student or practitioner will be able to do the following:

1. Identify five purposes of documentation.
2. Describe the basic technical points that should be adhered to when writing in the medical record.
3. Explain why only approved abbreviations should be used in occupational therapy documentation.
4. Describe the acceptable method of correcting an error in the medical record.
5. Explain why occupational therapy documentation should reflect the terminology outlined in the Occupational Therapy Practice Framework.
6. Describe the components of a well written progress note.
7. Identify the different places where documentation is required.
8. Briefly summarize the content of the initial evaluation.
9. Define assessments as they apply to the occupational therapy process.
10. Describe the purpose of the intervention plan.
11. Explain why the establishment of goals should be a collaborative effort between the client and therapist.
12. Explain the meaning of client-centered goal.
13. Describe the purpose of progress reports.
14. Explain what a skilled intervention is.
15. List the components of a SOAP note and give an example of each component of the note.
16. Identify the purpose of the discharge report.
17. List the primary reimbursement systems of occupational therapy services in the physical disabilities setting.
18. Describe two ways that ensure that confidentiality in documentation is maintained (refer to AOTA Code of Ethics and HIPAA regulations).

CHAPTER OUTLINE

Purposes of documentation
Best practices
Clinical reasoning skills
Legal liability
Initial evaluation
Intervention plan
Progress reports
  SOAP notes

Narrative notes
Descriptive notes
RUMBA
Discharge reports
Types of reporting formats
Confidentiality
Summary

THREADED CASE STUDY: JANE, PART 1

Jane just started her first job as an occupational therapist at a skilled nursing facility. This week she had to complete two initial evaluations and has seen four clients for therapy each day. Jane knows the importance of accurate documentation and she wants to make sure that she includes data that will communicate the necessary information for reimbursement. She also knows that documentation is essential to demonstrate the value of occupational therapy. However, she has never worked in this practice setting and is worried about what terminology to use and how to effectively document to guarantee reimbursement.

Critical Thinking Questions

As you read this chapter, reflect upon the following questions as they pertain to the case study:

1. What specific skills must Jane employ as she decides upon how she will document the evaluation process?
2. What information is important to include in the SOAP note for reimbursement? Will the practice setting have an influence on what is included in the note?
3. How might the federal regulations (HIPAA) and the principles put forth in the Occupational Therapy Code of Ethics influence how Jane communicates the results of the occupational therapy evaluation and intervention program?

OT PRACTICE NOTE

EXAMPLES OF DOCUMENTATION

Documentation is an ongoing process that continues throughout the client's therapy program. Screening reports, initial evaluation reports, reevaluation reports, progress notes, discharge summaries, other medical record entries (e.g., interdisciplinary care plans, MD telephone orders), intervention and equipment authorization requests, letters and reports to families and other healthcare professionals, and data collection of outcomes are examples of documentation completed by occupational therapists.

Box **8-1**   THE PURPOSE OF DOCUMENTATION

- Articulates the rationale for provision of occupational therapy services and the relationship of this service to the client's outcome
- Reflects the therapist's clinical reasoning and professional judgment
- Communicates information about the client from the occupational therapy perspective
- Creates a chronological record of client status, occupational therapy services provided to the client, and client outcomes

---

PURPOSES OF DOCUMENTATION

Documentation is a permanent record of what occurred with the client. It is also a legal document and as such must follow the guidelines that will withstand a legal investigation. Reimbursement depends upon accurate, well-written documentation that provides the necessary information to justify the need for occupational therapy services. The American Occupational Therapy Association (AOTA) has identified four main points that articulate the purpose of documentation (Box 8-1).

Clear, concise, and objective information is essential to communicate the occupational therapy process to others. The expectations of documentation are so important that our professional survival may be dependent on accurate, consistent, and relevant documentation.[9]

Documentation is required whenever occupational therapy services are performed. This includes recording what occurred during direct client care as well as supportive documentation required to justify the need for occupational therapy intervention.

Documentation is an essential component of occupational therapy practice. It is the primary method of communication that is used to convey what was done with the client. It demonstrates to others the value of occupational therapy intervention.

BEST PRACTICES

Regardless of where documentation takes place, there are basic technical points that are important to adhere to when writing in a medical record. Proper grammar and correct spelling are essential components in any professional correspondence. Keeping lists of commonly used terms or using a handheld spell-check device are two strategies that may assist with spelling difficulties. Poor grammar or inaccurate spelling can lead the reader to question the skills of the therapist. Legibility is important to ensure that misinterpretations do not occur. Only approved abbreviations are to be used in the medical record. Each clinical site should have a printed list of acceptable abbreviations that can be used at their site. It is important to obtain this list and use it as a reference when documenting. Examples of common abbreviations used in clinical practice are listed in Box 8-2. Misinterpretation of intended meaning can occur when unfamiliar abbreviations or casual language unsuitable for therapeutic context are used. Language particular to a profession (slang or jargon) should never be used in the client record.

All entries made into the medical record must be signed with the therapist's legal name. Your professional initials (OTR/L, OTL) should follow your signature. Do not leave blank spaces at the end of an intervention note. Instead, draw a single line that extends from the last word to the signature. This prevents additional information from being added after the entry has been completed.

ETHICAL CONSIDERATIONS

Documentation must be written by the therapist providing the intervention. It is never acceptable to write a note for another therapist, and in fact it is considered fraudulent to do so.

The best practice is to complete documentation as soon after the therapy session as possible. The longer the time interval between the evaluation or intervention and the completion of the written record of the event, the greater the chance of forgetting details or other important information.

Altering, substituting, or removing information from the client record should never take place. Changes made to the original documentation could be used to support allegations of tampering with the medical record,[14] even when this was not the intent of the writer. However, there are times when corrections must be made. There are several principles that should be followed to avoid questioning of the validity of

Box **8-2**	ABBREVIATIONS FOR CLINICAL DOCUMENTATION		
A	assessment	P.M.H.	past medical history
Add	adduction	post	posterior
ADL	activities of daily living	PTA	prior to admission
adm	admission, admitted	PWB	partial weight bearing
AE	above elbow	q	every
AFO	ankle-foot orthosis	qd	every day
AK	above knee	qh	every hour
a.m.	morning	qid	four times a day
ant	anterior	qn	every night
AP	anterior-posterior	R	right
AROM	active range of motion	re	regarding
Assist.	assistance, assistive	rehab	rehabilitation
B/S	bedside	reps	repetitions
BE	below elbow	R/O	rule out
BM	bowel movement	ROM	range of motion
BOS	base of support	RR	respiratory rate
BR	bedrest	RROM	resistive range of motion
c/o	complains of	Rx	intervention plan, therapy
cal	calories	sec	seconds
cont.	continue	SLR	straight leg raise
D/C	discontinued or discharged	SNF	skilled nursing facility
dept.	department	SOB	short of breath
DNR	do not resuscitate	S/P	status post
DOB	date of birth	stat	immediately
DOE	dyspnea on exertion	sup	superior
Dx	diagnosis	Sx	symptoms
ECF	extended care facility	ther ex	therapeutic exercise
eval.	evaluation	tid	three times daily
ext.	extension	t.o.	telephone order
FH	family history	Tx	treatment
flex	flexion	UE	upper extremity
FWB	full weight bearing	VC	vital capacity
fx	fracture	v.o.	verbal orders
h, hr	hour	v.s.	vital signs
p.o.	by mouth	w/c	wheelchair
P.H.	past history	WNL	within normal limits
p.m.	afternoon		

Data from Kettenbach G: *Writing SOAP notes,* ed 3, Philadelphia, 2004, FA Davis.

OT PRACTICE NOTE

While documenting at the time of service delivery is ideal, it is not always possible. At these times it may be beneficial for the therapist to carry a notepad or clipboard and record data that can later be included in the official write up.

the information. Never use correction fluid when correcting an entry in the client's record. An acceptable method of correcting an error in the documentation is to draw a single line through the word or words, initial and date the entry, and indicate that this was an error. Do not try to obliterate the sentence or word as this may appear to be an attempt to prevent others from knowing what was originally written. Late entries to the medical record cannot be back-dated. If it is necessary to enter information that is out of sequence (i.e., a note that the therapist forgot to write), it must be entered into the medical record as a late entry and must be identified as such. Words or sentences cannot be squeezed into existing text after the fact. Attempts to do this may be interpreted as adding missing information to support something that occurred after the original documentation was completed.

ETHICAL CONSIDERATIONS

Although no fraudulent intent may be present, it could be interpreted as such if the content is ever called into question.

Do not leave blank spaces on evaluation and preprinted forms. If it is not appropriate to complete a section, "N/A" can be inserted to indicate that the particular area was not addressed. If sections are left blank, others reading the chart may think these areas were overlooked.

Documentation should reflect the terminology outlined in the *Occupational Therapy Practice Framework* (OTPF).[4] One of the purposes of the OTPF is to assist therapists in communicating occupational therapy's unique focus on occupation and daily life activities to other professionals, consumers of services, and third-party payers. Documentation focuses on occupational therapy's emphasis on supporting function and performance in daily life activities and those factors that influence performance (performance skills, performance patterns, context, activity demands, and client factors) during the evaluation and intervention process.[4] Many practice settings that follow the medical model, such as hospitals, use the term *patient* to describe the recipient of services. Other settings may prefer the term *resident*. Although these are acceptable, the OTPF advocates use of the term *client*.

Client encompasses not only the individual receiving therapy, but also others who are involved in the person's life such as spouse, parent, child, caregiver, employer, or larger groups such as organizations or communities. The OTPF provides terminology that can be used at each stage of the therapy process. This will be explained in further detail when the various parts of the therapy evaluation, intervention, and discharge processes are described.

CLINICAL REASONING SKILLS

Occupational therapists must use **clinical reasoning** throughout the occupational therapy process. This includes determining how to appropriately document information obtained during the evaluation, intervention, and discharge process. Clinical reasoning is used to plan, direct, perform, and reflect upon client care.[16] Documentation must demonstrate that clinical reasoning was used in the decision-making process during all aspects of the client's therapy program.

Clinical reasoning is comprised of many different aspects of reasoning: scientific, narrative, pragmatic, and ethical. **Scientific reasoning** is used to help the therapist understand the client's impairments, disabilities, and performance contexts and to determine how these might influence occupational performance. **Narrative reasoning** guides the therapist to evaluate the meaning that occupational performance limitations might have on the client. **Pragmatic reasoning** is used when addressing the practical realities associated with the delivery of therapy services. **Ethical reasoning** is the process by which the therapist determines the most appropriate therapy intervention to address the client's occupational performance needs.[16] Keeping these points in mind and using clinical reasoning skills when determining what to document will facilitate client care and reimbursement for therapy services.

One of the greatest challenges for students and new therapists is developing skill for writing notes that are concise yet comprehensive, including all of the relevant information necessary to meet the purposes of documentation as described earlier. Most third-party payers do not reimburse for the time spent in documentation, so efficiency becomes essential. Although it is very important to accurately describe what occurred in the therapy session, care must be taken to keep this information to the point and relevant to the established goals identified in the intervention plan. A common error is to describe each event that occurred in the intervention session in a step-by-step format. This is far too time consuming and in fact does not meet the objectives of good documentation. Rather, short statements should be used that clearly and objectively convey necessary information to the reader. Acceptable abbreviations can be used to save time and space. Customized forms and checklists that include information relevant to the practice setting help streamline documentation and reduce time spent on narrative writing.

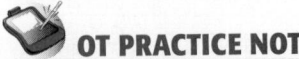
OT PRACTICE NOTE

Concise, clear, accurate documentation that keeps the target audience in mind will ensure that appropriate information is conveyed to other healthcare professionals and will meet the criteria for reimbursement.

LEGAL LIABILITY

The medical record is a legal document. All written or computerized therapy documentation must be able to endure a legal review. The medical record may be the most important document in a malpractice suit because it outlines the type and amount of patient care or services that were given.[7] The therapist must know what information is necessary to include in the client record to reduce the risk of malpractice in a legal proceeding. All information must be accurate and based on firsthand knowledge of care. Deductions and assumptions are to be avoided; judgmental statements do not belong in the therapy notes. The therapist should instead describe the action, behavior, or signs and symptoms that are observed. As described earlier, it is considered fraudulent to alter the medical record in any way.

INITIAL EVALUATION

The initial evaluation is a very important document in the occupational therapy process. It is the foundation upon which all other components of the client's program (including long- and short-term goals, the intervention plan, progress notes, and therapy recommendations) are based. **Evaluation** is the process of obtaining and interpreting data necessary for understanding the individual, system, or situation. It includes planning for and documenting the evaluation process, results, and recommendations, including the need for intervention.[5] The Occupational Therapy Practice Framework[4] stresses that the evaluation process should focus on identifying what the client wants and needs to do, as well as on identifying those factors that act as supports or barriers to performance. The client's participation in this process is key in guiding the therapist in choosing appropriate tools to assess these areas. The occupational therapist takes into account the performance skills, performance patterns, context, activity demands, and client factors that are required for the client to successfully engage in occupation.

A clear, accurately written accounting of the client's current status as well as a description of his or her prior status is essential to justify the need for occupational therapy services. It is also provides necessary information to establish a baseline from which re-evaluation data and progress notes can be compared, in order to demonstrate the efficacy of therapy intervention. The evaluation must clearly paint a clinical picture of the client's current functional status, strengths, impairments, and need for occupational therapy.

The evaluation should include an occupational profile of the client. The occupational profile includes information about the client's occupational history and experiences, patterns of daily living, interests, values, and needs.[4] Information obtained from the occupational profile is essential in guiding the therapist to make clinically sound decisions about appropriate assessments, interventions, and goals.

Assessments are the tools, instruments, or interactions used during the evaluation process.[5] These include standardized and nonstandardized tests. They can be written tests or performance checklists. Interviews and skilled observations are examples of assessments frequently used in the evaluation process. The specific assessments used are determined by the needs of the client and the practice setting in which the client is being seen. Assessments should be chosen that will evaluate the client's occupational needs, problems, and concerns. Clinical judgment skills are used to decide which assessments are appropriate and which areas should be evaluated. It is not necessary to evaluate every area of occupation and all performance skills for every individual. For example, it is not appropriate to assess a client's ability to cook a meal if he or she lives in a setting where meals are provided. The results of the assessment should be clearly identifiable and stated in measurable terminology that is standardized to the practice setting. Table 8-1 shows an example of terminology that can be used to describe the level of assistance required during the performance of a functional task.

AOTA has outlined the recommended components of professional documentation used in occupational therapy in Guidelines for Documentation of Occupational Therapy.[1] Suggestions for what information should be included in the recording of information for the evaluation and re-evaluation reports, intervention plan, progress reports, transition plan, and discharge report are described.

The evaluation report should contain the following content:
1. Client information: name/agency; date of birth; gender; applicable medical, educational, and developmental diagnosis; precautions; and contraindications
2. Referral information: date and source of referral, services requested, reason for referral, funding source, and anticipated length of service
3. Occupational profile: client's reason for seeking occupational therapy services; current areas of occupation that are successful and areas that are problematic; contexts that support or hinder occupations; medical, educational, and work history; occupational history; client's priorities; and targeted outcomes
4. Assessments: types of assessments used and results (e.g., interviews, record reviews, observations, and standardized or nonstandardized assessments), description of the client factors, contextual aspects or features of the activities that facilitate or inhibit performance, and confidence in test results

TABLE **8-1**   **Levels of Assistance**

Level	Description
Independent	Client is completely independent.
	No physical or verbal assistance is required to complete the task.
	Task is completed safely.
Supervised	Client requires supervision to safely complete task.
	May require a verbal cue for safety.
Contact guard/standby assistance	Hands-on, contact guard assistance is necessary for the client to safely complete the task or caregiver must be within arm's length for safety.
Minimum assistance	Client requires 25% physical or verbal assistance of one person to safely complete the task.
Moderate assistance	Client requires 50% physical or verbal assistance of one person to safely complete the task.
Maximal assistance	Client requires 75% physical or verbal assistance of one person to safely complete the task.
Dependent	Client requires 100% assistance to complete the task.

Note: It is important to state whether assistance provided is physical or verbal assistance.

5. Summary and analysis: interpretation and summary of data as they are related to occupational profile and referring concern
6. Recommendation: judgment regarding appropriateness of occupational therapy services or other services

INTERVENTION PLAN

Upon completion of the assessment, the intervention plan is established. Information obtained from the occupational profile and the various assessments is analyzed and a problem list is generated. The therapist must use theoretical knowledge and clinical reasoning skills to develop long- and short-term goals, intervention approaches, and the types of interventions to be used to achieve the goals. The intervention plan also includes recommendations or referrals to other professionals or agencies.[1] The intervention plan is based on selected theories, frames of reference, and evidence-based practice.[4] It is directed by the client's goals, values, and beliefs.

The establishment of goals should be a collaborative effort between the client and the therapist or, if the client is unable, the client's caregiver or guardian.[3,4] Goals must be measurable and directly related to the client's ability to engage in desired occupations. The overarching goal of occupational therapy intervention is "engagement in occupation to support participation."[4] This must be kept in mind at all times when developing the long- and short-term goals. The Occupational Therapy Practice Framework further identifies the outcome of occupational therapy intervention to be improvement in the following areas: occupational performance, client satisfaction, role competence, adaptation, health and wellness, prevention, and quality of life.[4] Documentation that incorporates this terminology will support the unique focus that occupational therapy contributes to the client care plan.

The client intervention plan contains both short- and long-term goals. Some therapists prefer to use the term *objective*

in place of short-term goal. Short-term goals or objectives are written for specific time periods (e.g., one or two weeks) within the overall course of the client's therapy program. They are periodically updated as the client progresses or in accordance with the guidelines of the practice setting. Short-term goal achievement leads to attainment of the established long-term goal, which usually encompasses the entire therapy stay. Short-term goals are the steps that lead to the accomplishment of the long-term goal, which is also called the **discharge goal** in some settings. The long-term goal is generally considered to be the overall functional goal of the intervention plan and is broader in nature than the short-term goal. For example, the client's long-term goal may be to become independent with dressing. One short-term goal to accomplish this might be that the client is to be able to dress in a simple pullover shirt without fasteners. When this short-term goal is achieved, a subsequent goal might be for the client to be able to dress independently in a shirt with buttons. Eventually lower extremity dressing would be added as an objective, then outerwear, until the long-term goal of independent dressing is achieved.

Establishing functional, client-centered goals that focus on engagement in occupations and activities to support participation in life is central to the philosophy of occupational therapy. **Client-centered goals** are written to reflect what the client will accomplish or do, not what the therapist will do, and are written in collaboration with the client. Goals must be objective, measurable, and include a time frame. The expected behavior is clearly stated (the client will don pants), a measurable expectation of performance is identified (independently), with conditions or circumstances that support the outcome listed (using a dressing stick). An indication of the time frame in which the outcome will be achieved (within one week) may also be included, although this may be written in a separate section of the evaluation form. Well-written goals contain all of the components listed above (Table 8-2).

TABLE 8-2 **Examples of Short- and Long-Term Goals**

Area	Short-Term Goal (to be completed in 2 weeks)	Long-Term Goal (to be completed in 4 weeks)
Cooking	Client will prepare a cup of tea with minimal verbal assistance for safety and technique	Client will independently adhere to safety precautions during simple cooking tasks 100% of the time
Hygiene	Client will brush teeth with moderate physical and verbal assistance while seated at the sink	Client will complete morning hygiene and grooming independently after task set up while seated at the sink
Dressing	Client will don socks with minimal assistance using a sock aid while seated in a wheelchair	Client will independently complete lower body dressing without assistive devices while seated at the edge of the bed

Once goals are established, the therapist chooses the appropriate interventions that will lead to goal attainment. This plan is comprised of the skilled interventions that the therapist will provide throughout the intervention program. Interventions that involve the therapeutic use of self, therapeutic use of occupations or activities (i.e., occupation-based activity, purposeful activity, preparatory methods), and consultation and client/caregiver education are chosen. Examples of occupational therapy interventions include ADL training; IADL training; therapeutic activities; therapeutic exercises; splint/orthotic fabrication, modification, and application; neuromuscular retraining; cognitive-perceptual training; and discharge planning. The OTPF outlines the various approaches that are used to guide the intervention process (Table 8-3). These approaches are based on theory and evidence. It is expected that the intervention plan will be modified based upon client needs and priorities. Modifications to the intervention plan must be documented in the client record.

PROGRESS REPORTS

Progress towards goal attainment is an expected criterion for reimbursement of occupational therapy services. Documentation that demonstrates the progression towards

goal achievement is critical to support the need for ongoing therapy. The purpose of the **progress report** is to document the client's improvement, to demonstrate the skilled therapy provided, and to update goals. Progress reports can be written daily or weekly depending upon the requirements of the work site and the payer source. There are various reporting formats that are used to document client progress. The most prevalent formats used in physical disabilities settings include SOAP notes, checklist notes, and narrative notes.

Regardless of the format used, progress reports should identify these key elements of the intervention session: (1) what was the client outcome (using measurable terminology from the OTPF), (2) what skilled interventions were provided by the occupational therapist, and (3) what progress resulted as a result of occupational therapy intervention. **Skilled interventions** are those that require the unique skills of an occupational therapist. Skilled therapy services have a level of inherent complexity such that they can only be performed safely and/or effectively by or under the general supervision of a qualified therapist. Skilled services include (1) evaluation, (2) determination of effective goals and services with the patient and the patient's caregivers and other medical professionals, (3) analysis and modification of functional tasks, (4) determination that the modified task obtains optimum performance through

TABLE 8-3 **Occupational Therapy Intervention Approaches**

Approach	Description
Create, promote (health promotion)	An intervention approach designed to provide enriched contextual and activity experiences to enhance performance for persons in the contexts of life.
Establish, restore (remediation, restoration)	An intervention approach designed to change client variables to develop a skill or ability that has not yet been developed or to restore a skill or ability that has been impaired.
Maintain	An intervention approach designed to provide the supports that will allow the client to maintain their performance capabilities. Without continued maintenance intervention, client performance would decline and/or occupational needs would not be met, thereby affecting health and quality of life.
Modify (compensation, adaptation)	An intervention approach designed to find ways to revise the current context or activity demands to support performance. This includes using compensatory techniques, enhancing some features to provide cues, or reducing features to reduce distractibility.
Prevent (disability prevention)	An intervention approach designed to prevent the occurrence or development of barriers to performance in context. This approach is directed towards clients with or without a disability who are at risk for occupational performance problems.

Adapted from American Occupational Therapy Association: Occupational therapy practice framework: domain and process, *Am J Occup Ther* 56(6):609, 2002.

tests and measurements, (5) providing instructions for the task(s) to the patient, family, caregivers, and (6) periodically re-evaluating the client's status with corresponding readjustment of the occupational therapy program.[11] Box 8-3 shows examples of terminology that can be used to demonstrate skilled service provision.

Documentation of skilled services includes a description of the type and complexity of the therapeutic activity and must reflect the therapeutic rationale underlying the task. Reimbursement for clinical services provided is dependent upon documentation that demonstrates the clinical reasoning that underlies the intervention. The progress note must also reflect progress made towards the established goals. Comparison statements are an excellent way to convey this information. Current status information is compared to baseline evaluation findings to clearly identify progress: *client now requires minimal assistance to regain sitting posture during lower body dressing (last week required moderate assistance)*. A statement explaining why further therapy services are needed provides justification for ongoing therapy: *occupational therapy services are required for facilitation of balance and postural corrections during lower body dressing training*. Goals are modified and updated based upon the client's progress: *client will don pants independently, without loss of balance, while seated at the edge of the bed*. This is an ongoing process and meticulous documentation is necessary to demonstrate the need for continued occupational therapy services.

Box **8-3**   SERVICE PROVISION TERMINOLOGY

SKILLED TERMINOLOGY

- Assess
- Analyze
- Interpret
- Modify
- Facilitate
- Inhibit
- Instruct in compensatory strategies, hemiplegic dressing, techniques, safety, and adaptive equipment
- Fabricate
- Design
- Adapt
- Environmental modifications
- Determine
- Establish

UNSKILLED TERMINOLOGY

- Maintain
- Help
- Watch
- Observe
- Practice
- Monitor

SOAP NOTES

The **SOAP note** format was first introduced by Dr. Lawrence Weed in 1970 as a method for charting in the **problem-oriented medical record (POMR)**.[17] In the POMR, which focuses on a client's problems instead of his diagnosis, a numbered problem list is developed and becomes an important part of the medical record. Each member of the healthcare team writes a SOAP note to address the problems in the list that are specific to their area of expertise. The POMR is constantly modified and updated throughout the client's stay. The SOAP note is one of the most frequently used formats used by therapy for documenting patient status in this system. SOAP is an acronym, with each letter standing for the name of a section of the note.

S = Subjective
O = Objective
A = Assessment
P = Plan

The *Subjective* (S) part of the note is the section where the therapist includes information reported by the client. This can also include information provided by the family or caregivers. There are many different types of statements that can be included in the subjective section of the SOAP note. Any information that the client tells the therapist about his or her current condition, functional performance, limitations, general health status, social habits, medical history, or client goals can be appropriate to include in this section.[10] A client's subjective response to treatment is recorded in this section. Direct quotes can be used when appropriate. Family, caregivers, and others involved in the client's care can also provide valuable information. For example, nursing may report that the client was unable to feed him or herself at breakfast or a family member may supply information on the client's normal routine prior to hospitalization. If the client is nonverbal, gestures, facial expressions, and other types of nonverbal responses are appropriate to include. This information can be used to demonstrate improvement, support the benefit of chosen interventions, document the client's response, and show client compliance. However, discretion must be used when deciding what information to include.

The Subjective section should only include relevant information that will support the therapist's decision on which assessments to use and which goals are appropriate for this client. The therapist should avoid statements that can be misinterpreted or jeopardize reimbursement. Subjective statements that do not relate to information in the other parts of the note are not useful. Negative quotes from the client that do not relate to the intervention session are also not necessary or beneficial to include. If there is nothing relevant to report in the Subjective section, it is permissible to not include a statement. In this case, write a circle with a line through it, (O) indicating that you have intentionally left the section blank.[15]

The *Objective* (O) section of the SOAP note is where the therapist documents the results of assessments performed and objective observations.[10] Data that are recorded in the Objective section are measurable or observable. Only factual information may be included. Results of standardized and nonstandardized tests are documented in this part of the note. Measurable performance of functional tasks (*basic activities of daily living* [BADLs], *instrumental activities of daily living* [IADLs]), ROM measurements, muscle grades, results of sensory evaluations, and tone assessments are examples of appropriate information for this section of the SOAP note. It is important that the therapist not interpret or analyze data in the Objective section. Rather, statements should only include objective recordings of the client's performance. Simply listing the activities that the client engaged in is not sufficient.[15] The emphasis is on the results of the interventions, not on the interventions themselves.[6]

In the *Assessment* (A) section of the SOAP note, the therapist draws from the subjective and objective findings and interprets the data in order to establish the most appropriate therapy program. In this section, impairments and functional deficits are analyzed and prioritized to determine what impact they have on the client's occupational performance. Clinical reasoning is required to analyze the information and develop the intervention plan. The Assessment portion of the SOAP note is where the therapist demonstrates his or her ability to summarize relevant assessment findings, synthesize the information, analyze its impact on occupational performance, and use it to formulate the intervention plan. It requires keen clinical reasoning and judgment skills, as well as an ability to identify relevant factors that inhibit or facilitate performance. Insight and skill in completing the assessment section improve with clinical experience.

The intervention plan is outlined in the *Plan* (P) section. As the client achieves the short-term goals, the plan is revised and new short-term goals are established. Documentation reflects the client's updated goals as well as any modifications to the frequency of therapy. Suggestions for additional interventions are also included in this section. This information will guide subsequent treatment sessions. Figure 8-1 is an example of a progress note using the SOAP format.

NARRATIVE NOTES

The **narrative note** is another format used to document daily client performance. One way to organize the narrative note is to categorize the information into the following subsections: problem, program, results/progress, and plan. The *problem* being addressed in the treatment intervention should be clearly identified. The impairment as well as the functional impact is stated. The intervention or intervention modality is identified in the *program* section. The *results*, including progress, are documented in measurable, objective terminology. Barriers to progress are included in this section. The plan for future intervention is outlined in the *plan* section. The need to modify goals and the rationale for this would be included here. Figure 8-2 is an example of a narrative note using this format.

S: Client states that "it takes too much energy to dress each day and my hands are too stiff to manage buttons and ties anyways." Client's family reports that client no longer seems interested in self-care activities.

O: Client became SOB with seated self-care task (dressing) after 5 minutes of activity. Client required minimal assistance for upper body dressing, moderate assistance to don pants and maximal assistance to don shoes (last week she required maximal assistance with all tasks). Client had moderate difficulty with buttons (last week she was unable to button blouse). Client was unable to tie shoes. BUE shoulder strength is 3+/5 (was 3/5).

A: Client is improving in her ability to complete her self-care tasks. COPD still interferes with ADL independence. She may benefit from adaptive equipment for lower body dressing.

P: Continue ADL training: assess for independence with adaptive equipment (dressing stick, long-handled shoe horn, and elastic shoe laces). Instruct client in energy-conservation techniques during ADL task completion. Instruct client in AROM exercises before beginning morning ADL tasks.

Figure 8-1 SOAP note.

Problem: Client was seen for 60 minutes. IADL task: light meal preparation

Results: Client was able to assemble necessary items to prepare a simple sandwich with minimal verbal cues, which were necessary because of unfamiliarity with clinic kitchen. Minimal verbal assistance was necessary for task initiation and progression from one step to the next. Although physical assistance was not required, client demonstrated mild coordination deficits resulting in difficulty opening jars, manipulating knife, and opening packages. Endurance was good for this activity — client was able to stand for 30 minutes without rest.

Plan: Therapeutic exercise and activities will be performed to improve coordination.
Instruct client in strategies for improving task initiation.
Progressive IADL assessment — hot meal preparation

Figure 8-2 Narrative progress note.

DESCRIPTIVE NOTES

At times, a short **descriptive note** is useful to relay important information about the client. Although it is preferable to keep notes as objective as possible, there are times when subjective information is appropriate to include. Judgmental comments, negative statements, comments about other staff members, and information not directly related to the client's intervention program do not belong in the official medical record.

RUMBA

According to Perinchief,[13] using a tool such as the RUMBA test can be beneficial in organizing the therapist's thought process for effective documentation. **RUMBA** is an acronym with each letter identifying something that the therapist should keep in mind when documenting the therapeutic process.

- Is the information Relevant (the outcome must be relevant)?
- Is the information Understandable?
- Is the information Measurable?
- Is the information Behavioral (describes behaviors)?
- Is the outcome Achievable (realistic)?

Therapists can review their documentation to determine if these questions are answered, all the while keeping the target audience in mind.

DISCHARGE REPORTS

Discharge reports are written at the conclusion of the therapy program. A comparison statement of functional performance from the initial evaluation to the discharge is documented to demonstrate progress. Emphasis should be placed on the progress the client has made in engagement in occupations. A summary of the skilled interventions provided to the client is also included. Discharge recommendations (e.g., home programs, therapy follow-up, referral to other programs) are made to assist in a smooth transition from therapy. Clients are discharged from therapy when they have achieved the established goals, received maximal benefit from occupational therapy services, refused to participate in further therapy, or exceeded reimbursement allowances. The discharge summary should clearly demonstrate the efficacy of occupational therapy services and is often used to obtain information for outcome studies.

TYPES OF REPORTING FORMATS

Documentation can either be paper-based (written record) or computer-generated. The written medical record is still the most widely used method for recording information; however, computer-based documentation is becoming more common, especially in large hospital settings. Computerized documentation can be used to record all aspects of the occupational therapy process from the evaluation report to the discharge report. Reporting forms can be input into the computer and results of the initial evaluation and discharge report can be typed directly onto the forms. This guarantees legibility and ensures that no areas are left uncompleted.

Computerized evaluation forms and progress notes are formatted to meet the needs of the facility and include information required for reimbursement (Figure 8-3).

Therapists are often able to choose responses from a pull down menu, reducing time spent in deciding upon the appropriate terminology to use. There is usually space to include narrative information as well. Since all healthcare providers enter information on a common database, members of the team are able to quickly access information about the patient by reviewing relevant sections on the computerized medical chart.

One of the problems or inconveniences that may occur with using computerized documentation involves the accessibility of computers. Therapists must allow time to locate a computer that is not in use so that they can enter their data. Since notes must be entered in chronological order, this sometimes becomes an issue if a computer is not available, as the therapist may not be able to wait until the next day to enter information. Some forms that are on the computer are very restrictive in what information the therapist may enter. This may make it difficult for the therapist to adequately document the session. There is often a long time lapse between updates of the computer programs. In general, however, computerized documentation and billing can be an asset in the therapy setting. It can allow for greater therapist productivity by reducing the amount of time spent writing and will assist in guiding the new therapist in choosing appropriate responses and terminology to document what occurred with the client.

There are many different written formats for documenting occupational therapy services. The content of the form used is usually determined by the requirements of the third-party payer reimbursing the service, and the unique needs of the practice setting. As stated before, documentation must contain the information necessary to justify the need for occupational therapy services, demonstrate the provision of skilled therapeutic interventions, and show client progress towards identified goals. Occupational therapy documentation should address all of these components to assure reimbursement as well as to convey accurate information about client performance.

The primary reimbursement systems of occupational therapy services in the physical disabilities setting include Medicare, Medicaid, various health maintenance organizations (HMOs), and preferred provider organizations (PPOs) and worker's compensation. Each of these organizations requires specific information that must be included in the documentation for reimbursement to occur. Individual facilities (e.g., hospitals, clinics, home health agencies, and skilled nursing facilities) will design documentation forms to meet their specific needs and ensure that the information necessary for reimbursement is included. Billing systems may also influence the type of documentation format that is used in a particular setting.

Medicare is a major payer source in the geriatric physical disability setting. This government agency has set forth detailed guidelines stating their expectations for what information must be included in the medical record to justify the need for occupational therapy services. Intermediaries will reimburse occupational therapy services only if they meet all of the requirements established by the Medicare guidelines and regulations. The Medicare Program Integrity Manual

DATE:		PAGE 1
TIME:	NURSING ASSESSMENT	
	O.T. PROGRESS REPORT	

Client :	Age/Sex :
Account :	Unit # :
Admit Date :	Location :
Status : ADM IN	Room/Bed :
Attending :	

Diagnosis :
Precautions :
Onset Date :   Equipment :

	INITIAL STATUS	STATUS WEEK
FUNCTIONAL SKILLS	Date :	From : To :
Eating :	.	:
Grooming :	.	:
Sponge Bathing UB/LB :	.	:
Showering :	.	:
Toileting :	.	:
Dressing UB :	.	:
Dressing LB :	.	:
Kitchen/Homemaking :	.	:
Bed/Chair Transfers :	.	:
Toilet Transfer :	.	:
Tub/Shower Transfer :	.	:

Pain :   Pain Scale : (1-10)   /10
Pain Location :   Quality of Pain:
Effects of pain on ADLs :
 Pain Comment :

CURRENT SHORT-TERM GOALS
1 :   MET :
2 :   :
3 :   :

Current Problems :
1 :   4 :
2 :   5 :
3 :   6 :

NEW SHORT-TERM GOALS
1 :
2 :
3 :

COMMENTS :   Conferred with OT for Treatment Plan Adjustment:
 :
 :
 :
 :
 :

EDUCATED
Client Instructed :   Parent/Significant Other Instructed :   Translator Used :
Instruction Given On :
 :

Figure 8-3 Computerized documentation form.

```
DATE:                                                              PAGE 2
TIME:                        NURSING ASSESSMENT
                             O.T. PROGRESS REPORT

Client :                                                Age/Sex :
Account :                                               Unit  # :
Admit Date :                                            Location :
Status : ADM IN                                         Room/Bed :
Attending :

                      :

     Mode of Instruction :

        Fact Sheet/Handout Title :

     Instruction comment :
Understanding Validated By :
MD aware of current status via conference notes (SNU)


Occurred Date :                                         Occurred Time :
Monogram :          Initials :           Name :         Nurse Type :
```

Figure 8-3, cont'd

(*www.hcfa.gov/pubforms/83*) describes the key words and phrases medical reviewers are looking for when they review a claim for payment. Each part of the therapy process has specific information that Medicare requires be clearly documented in order for therapy to be reimbursed. Understanding these requirements is critical to assure reimbursement for the services provided. The therapist working with Medicare clients must become familiar with these guidelines and regulations. Detailed information can be found at the Medicare website.

Although Medicare no longer requires its exclusive use, it has designed a specific form for outpatient evaluations called the Medicare 700 form, the "Plan of Treatment for Outpatient Rehabilitation." This form specifies the information required by Medicare. Figure 8-4 shows this form and directions for completing it. Documentation on the initial evaluation must demonstrate that it is reasonable and necessary for the therapist to complete the evaluation to determine if there is an expectation that either restorative or maintenance services are appropriate.[11] It is important to fill in all spaces on the 700 form. Failure to complete a section on the form could result in a technical denial. It is important to include a statement of the client's prior level of function and the change in function that precipitated the occupational therapy referral. Results from assessments that support the need for therapy intervention are recorded in this section. Objective tests and measurements are used to establish baseline data. This information will serve as the basis for the short- and long-term goals.

Many rehabilitation companies and hospitals have modified the 700 form with headings and checklists to assist the therapist in providing the type of information that will support the need for therapy services (Figure 8-5). Space on the 700 form is limited, and the therapist must be able to concisely present data that will clearly demonstrate the need for occupational therapy. A recent change in function (either a decline or an improvement) is required to justify therapy. The plan of treatment (section 12) includes functional, measurable goals based upon assessment results described in section 18. Goals cannot address issues that do not have supporting baseline data in the assessment section. The plan of treatment is the skilled intervention that the therapist will provide. The 700 form also functions as the end of month progress report and/or the discharge form. Section 20 is completed at the end of the billing period. Progress, current functional status, and the skilled interventions that were provided during the previous month are included here.

Figure 8-6 is an example of an initial evaluation form used in a rehabilitation center. It has been modified to meet the specific needs of the practice setting. Figure 8-7 shows an example of an occupational therapy evaluation report and initial intervention plan that incorporates the OTPF language and process. As facilities develop updated evaluation forms, the OTPF language should be incorporated.

CONFIDENTIALITY

Maintaining confidentiality in documentation is the responsibility of the occupational therapist. Principle 3E of the AOTA Code of Ethics addresses the issue of privacy and confidentiality in all forms of communication, including documentation. "Occupational therapy personnel shall protect all privileged confidential forms of written, verbal, and electronic communication gained from educational, practice, research, and investigational activities unless otherwise mandated by local, state, or federal regulations."[3]

ETHICAL CONSIDERATIONS

The AOTA *Guidelines to the Code of Ethics*[2] speaks directly to confidentiality issues: "Information that is confidential must remain confidential. This information cannot be shared verbally, electronically, or in writing without appropriate consent. Information must be shared on a need-to-know basis only with those having primary responsibilities for decision making."

5.1 All occupational therapy personnel shall respect the confidential nature of information gained in any occupational therapy interaction.

5.2 Occupational therapy personnel shall respect the individual's right to privacy.

5.3 Occupational therapy personnel shall take all due precautions to maintain the confidentiality of all verbal, written, and electronic communications that are confidential.

5.4 Occupational therapy personnel shall maintain as confidential, information derived from working relationships with other occupational therapy practitioners.

Ethical practice demands that the therapist understand what is meant by confidential information and is knowledgeable about how to maintain client confidentiality. Information about clients including their names, diagnoses, and intervention programs cannot be discussed outside of the treatment environment. Client charts should not be removed from the facility. Reports containing personal information (name, social security number, medical diagnosis) cannot be left out in plain view where others can read the information. Therapists, students, and staff cannot discuss clients in public areas where others may overhear the conversation.

There are now federal laws to protect the consumer against breaches of confidentiality. The privacy sections of the **Health Insurance Portability and Accountability Act (HIPAA)** clearly outline the expectations of healthcare professionals in issues of confidentiality. HIPAA was initially enacted in 1996 and consisted of a series of provisions that required the Department of Health and Human Services to adhere to national standards for electronic transmission of healthcare information. The law also required that healthcare providers adopt privacy and security standards to protect confidential medical information of patients. Beginning in April 2003, healthcare providers were required to adhere to the privacy standards mandated by HIPAA. Individually identifiable health information, also known as **protected health information** (PHI), is federally protected under HIPAA regulations. PHI is health information that relates to a past, present, or future physical or mental health condition. This rule limits the use and disclosure of PHI to the minimum necessary to carry out the intended purpose. It also gives the patient the right to access their medical records. This regulation protects medical records of clients, whether the information is written, electronic (computer), or verbally communicated. Violations of the HIPAA rulings are subject to criminal or civil sanctions.[8]

The law requires that all staff be trained in HIPAA policies and procedures and understand the implications specific to the work setting. In addition to client confidentiality procedures explained earlier, additional safeguards must now be adhered to in order to be compliant with HIPAA regulations. The therapist has a responsibility to protect confidential information from unauthorized access, use, or disclosure. This includes information documented in the medical record. Papers, reports, and forms containing PHI should not be disposed in the regular trash. Instead, they must be shredded. Never leave medical records or portions of the record (i.e., therapy notes) unattended in public view. Information (written, verbal, or electronic) cannot be shared with the family members unless permission has been provided in writing by the client.

If documentation is done electronically, special care must be taken to prevent unauthorized persons from accessing client information. Login pass codes cannot be shared among staff. Therapists must take care to assure privacy when entering information.

ETHICAL CONSIDERATIONS

Special safety measures such as personal identification and user verification codes for access to records should be established to prevent unauthorized persons from accessing client records.[7,12]

Text continued on p. 129

DEPARTMENT OF HEALTH AND HUMAN SERVICES
CENTERS FOR MEDICARE & MEDICAID SERVICES

PLAN OF TREATMENT FOR OUTPATIENT REHABILITATION
(COMPLETE FOR INITIAL CLAIMS ONLY)

1. PATIENT'S LAST NAME	FIRST NAME	M.I.	2. PROVIDER NO.	3. HICN

4. PROVIDER NAME	5. MEDICAL RECORD NO. *(Optional)*	6. ONSET DATE	7. SOC. DATE

8. TYPE □PT □OT □SLP □CR □RT □PS □SN □SW	9. PRIMARY DIAGNOSIS *(Pertinent Medical D.X.)*	10. TREATMENT DIAGNOSIS	11. VISITS FROM SOC.

12. PLAN OF TREATMENT FUNCTIONAL GOALS

GOALS *(Short Term)*

OUTCOME *(Long Term)*

PLAN

13. SIGNATURE *(professional establishing POC including prof. designation)*	14. FREQ/DURATION *(e.g., 3/Wk. x 4 Wk.)*

I CERTIFY THE NEED FOR THESE SERVICES FURNISHED UNDER THIS PLAN OF TREATMENT AND WHILE UNDER MY CARE □ N/A

15. PHYSICIAN SIGNATURE | 16. DATE

17. CERTIFICATION
FROM   THROUGH   N/A

18. ON FILE *(Print/type physician's name)*
□

20. INITIAL ASSESSMENT *(History, medical complications, level of function at start of care. Reason for referral.)*

19. PRIOR HOSPITALIZATION
FROM   TO   N/A

21. FUNCTIONAL LEVEL *(End of billing period)* PROGRESS REPORT   □ CONTINUE SERVICES **OR**   □ DC SERVICES

22. SERVICE DATES
FROM   THROUGH

Form CMS-700-(11-91)

Figure 8-4 Medicare evaluation form and instructions. (Courtesy Medicare, *www.medicare.org.*)

Continued

INSTRUCTIONS FOR COMPLETION OF FORM CMS-700

(Enter dates as 6 digits, month, day, year).

1. **Patient's Name** - Enter the patient's last name, first name and middle initial as shown on the health insurance Medicare card.

2. **Provider Number** - Enter the number issued by Medicare to the billing provider *(i.e., 00–7000)*.

3. **HICN** - Enter the patient's health insurance number as shown on the health insurance Medicare card, certification award, utilization notice, temporary eligibility notice, or as reported by SSO.

4. **Provider Name** - Enter the name of the Medicare billing provider.

5. **Medical Record No.** - *(optional)* Enter the patient's medical/clinical record number used by the billing provider.

6. **Onset Date** - Enter the date of onset for the patient's primary medical diagnosis, if it is a new diagnosis, or the date of the most recent exacerbation of a previous diagnosis. If the exact date is not known enter 01 for the day *(i.e., 120191)*. The date matches occurrence code 11 on the UB-92.

7. **SOC** *(start of care)* **Date** - Enter the date services began at the billing provider (the date of the first Medicare billable visit which **remains the same on subsequent claims** until discharge or denial corresponds to occurrence code 35 for PT, 44 for OT, 45 for SLP and 46 for CR on the UB-92).

8. **Type** - Check the type therapy billed; i.e., physical therapy (PT), occupational therapy (OT), speech-language pathology (SLP), cardiac rehabilitation (CR), respiratory therapy (RT), psychological services (PS), skilled nursing services (SN), or social services (SW).

9. **Primary Diagnosis** - Enter the pertinent written medical diagnosis resulting in the therapy disorder and relating to 50% or more of effort in the plan of treatment.

10. **Treatment Diagnosis** - Enter the written treatment diagnosis for which services are rendered. For example, for PT the primary medical diagnosis might be Degeneration of Cervical Intervertebral Disc while the PT treatment DX might be Frozen R Shoulder or, for SLP, while CVA might be the primary medical DX, the treatment DX might be Aphasia. If the same as the primary DX enter SAME.

11. **Visits From Start of Care** - Enter the **cumulative total** visits *(sessions)* completed since services were started at the billing provider for the diagnosis treated, through the last visit on this bill. *(Corresponds to UB-92 value code 50 for PT, 51 for SLP, 52 for SLP, or 53 for cardiac rehab.)*

12. **Plan of Treatment/Functional Goals** - Enter brief current plan of treatment goals for the patient for this billing period. Enter the major short-term goals to reach overall long-term outcome. Enter the major plan of treatment to reach stated goals and outcome. Estimate time-frames to reach goals, when possible.

13. **Signature** - Enter the signature *(or name)* and the professional designation of the professional establishing the plan of treatment.

14. **Frequency/Duration** - Enter the current frequency and duration of your treatment; e.g., 3 times per week for 4 weeks is entered 3/Wk x 4Wk.

15. **Physician's Signature** - If the form CMS-700 is used for certification, the physician enters his/her signature. **If certification is required and the form is not being used for certification, check the ON FILE box in item 18.** If the certification is not required for the type service rendered, check the N/A box.

16. **Date** - Enter the date of the physician's signature only if the form is used for certification.

17. **Certification** - Enter the inclusive dates of the certification, **even if the ON FILE box is checked in item 18.** Check the N/A box if certification is not required.

18. **ON FILE** (Means certification signature and date) - Enter the **typed/printed name of the physician** who certified the plan of treatment that is on file at the billing provider. If certification is not required for the type of service checked in item 8, type/print the name of the physician who referred or ordered the service, **but do not check the ON FILE box.**

19. **Prior Hospitalization** - Enter the inclusive dates of recent hospitalization *(1st to DC day)* **pertinent** to the patient's current plan of treatment. Enter N/A if the hospital stay does not relate to the rehabilitation being rendered.

20. **Initial Assessment** - Enter only **current relevant history** from records or patient interview. Enter the major functional limitations stated, if possible, in objective measurable terms. Include only relevant surgical procedures, prior hospitalization and/or therapy for the same condition. Include only pertinent baseline tests and measurements from which to judge future progress or lack of progress.

21. **Functional Level** (end of billing period) - Enter the pertinent progress made and functional levels obtained at the end of the billing period compared to levels shown on initial assessment. Use objective terminology. Date progress when function can be consistently performed. When only a few visits have been made, enter a note indicating the training/treatment rendered and the patient's response if there is no change in function.

22. **Service Dates** - Enter the From and Through dates which represent this billing period *(should be monthly)*. Match the From and Through dates in field 6 on the UB-92. DO NOT use 00 in the date. Example: 01 08 91 for January 8, 1991.

Figure 8-4, cont'd

☐ Part A   ☐ Part B   ☐ Other _____   Room No. _____   ☐ F.F.S.   ☐ Direct Bill   Facility: _____

700 FORM OCCUPATIONAL THERAPY PLAN OF TREATMENT
(Complete For Initial Claims Only)   ☐ E.O.M.   ☐ D/C Sum

1. Patient's Last Name	First Name M.I. ☐ M ☐ F	2. Provider No.	3. Provider Name
4. HIC#	5. Medical Record No.	6. Onset Date	7. SOC Date

8. DOB	9. Primary Diagnosis (Pertinent Medical DX) (ICD-9)	10. Treatment Diagnosis (ICD-9)	11. Visits From SOC

12. Functional Goals (Short Term) - In ___ weeks, patient will:

1.

2.

3.

4.

I have reviewed this Plan of Treatment and certify the need for service.
13. PHYSICIAN SIGNATURE   DATE   ☐ N/A

18. INITIAL ASSESSMENT :
Reason for Referral:

Prior Level of Function:

History/Medical Complications:

Precautions/Contraindications:

Check and document with skilled objective data, on the areas that impact function.
☐ Cognition/Safety Judgment:

☐ Visual Motor/Perception:

☐ Neuromotor:

☐ Sensorimotor:

☐ Balance: Sitting Static: Dynamic:

☐ Balance: Standing Static: Dynamic:

19. SIGNATURE (professional establishing POT, including credentials)   DATE

20. FUNCTIONAL LEVEL (End of Billing Period)
Skilled Interventions:

☐ Evaluation

PLAN OF TREATMENT
☐ Self Care/Home Management Training   ☐ Cognitive Retraining
☐ Therapeutic Activities   ☐ Orthotics Fitting Training/UE Splinting
☐ Neuromuscular Re-education   ☐ Other _____
☐ Therapeutic Exercise   ☐ Other _____
☐ *In Individual and/or Group Treatment*

OUTCOME (Long Term Goal) - In ___ weeks, patient will:

14. Frequency/Duration
(e.g., 5x/wk x 4 wks)

15. Certification
From   Through   ☐ N/A

16. Physician's Name

17. Prior Hospitalization
From   Through   ☐ N/A

Scoring Key: **MDS ADL Self Performance:** *0=Independent 1=Supervision→Supervision(SBA)*
2=Limited→C.G.A.   3=Extensive→ **Min, Mod, Max Assist** *4=Total→***Dependent**
Support (SUP): *0=No Set-up   1=Set-up help only   2=1 person assist   3=2 person assist*

☐ ROM:

ADL Status	0 Ind	1 Sup	2 CGA	3 Min	3 Mod	3 Max	4 Total	SUP
Self Feeding								
Hygiene / Grooming								
Dressing-Upper Body								
Dressing-Lower Body								
Toileting								
Toilet Transfers								
Bathing-Upper Body								
Bathing-Lower Body								
Functional Mobility								

☐ Strength:

☐ Activity Tolerance:

☐ Other/Comments

Clinical Impressions:

Positive Prognostic Indicators:

Rehab Potential: ☐ Good   ☐ Excellent   Patient aware of prognosis: ☐ Yes ☐ No
Admit Cond: ☐ Mild ☐ Mod ☐ Sev ☐ Dep   Patient aware of diagnosis: ☐ Yes ☐ No

Document Impairments and Reason to:
☐ Continue Services   *or*   ☐ D/C Services

Resident/Caregiver Training:

Recommendations:

D/C Prognosis to Maintain Function: ☐ Good   ☐ Fair   ☐ N/A
D/C Condition: ☐ Goals Met   ☐ Improved   ☐ Declined   ☐ No Change
D/C Location: ☐ Home ☐ ALF ☐ LTC ☐ SNF ☐ Hospital ☐ Other ☐ Expired

21. THERAPIST SIGNATURE:
Service Dates: From: Through:

ADL Status	0 Ind	1 Sup	2 CGA	3 Min	3 Mod	3 Max	4 Total	SUP
Self Feeding								
Hygiene / Grooming								
Dressing-Upper Body								
Dressing-Lower Body								
Toileting								
Toilet Transfer								
Bathing-Upper Body								
Bathing-Lower Body								
Functional Mobility								

REHABWORKS
A Division of Symphony Health Services   Modified OT 700 Form   **RW5904** OT Plan of Treatment 11/2004

Figure 8-5   Modified Mediare700 form—occupational therapy plan of treatment. (Courtesy Rehabworks, a Division of Symphony Rehabilitation, Hunt Valley, MD.)

County of Los Angeles   **RANCHO LOS AMIGOS NATIONAL REHABILITATION CENTER**   **Department of Health Services**

DIAGNOSIS: | ONSET DATE: | ADMIT DATE:

LIVING SITUATION / LIFE ROLES:

DISCHARGE PLAN:

MAJOR PROBLEMS / INTERFERING FACTORS:

BEHAVIOR / COGNITION / COMMUNICATION:

ADL STATUS	INITIAL	GOAL	CURRENT	KEY (Status): 7 = Complete independence/no helper, 6 = Modified independence/device, 5 = Supervision or set up, 4 = Minimum assist (patient does 75-100%), 3 = Moderate assist (patient does 50-74%), 2 = Maximum assist (patient does 25-49%), 1 = Total assist (patient does <25%), 0 = Not tested
SELF FEEDING				**Precautions:**
HYGIENE GROOMING				**Self-care:**
BATHING				
WET TUB / SHOWER TRANSFER				**Upper Extremity Status:**
UPPER BODY DRESSING				**Motor Control:**
LOWER BODY DRESSING				**RUE:**
				LUE:
TOILET ACTIVITIES				
WRITING / TYPING				**Sensation:**
TELEPHONE				**RUE:**
DIRECTING (OWN) CARE				**LUE:**
MEAL PREPARATION				**Occupational History:**
SHOPPING				
LAUNDRY				
DRIVING				
PUBLIC TRANSPORTATION				
LIGHT HOUSEKEEPING				
HEAVY HOUSEKEEPING				
AVOCATIONAL				
VOCATIONAL				
OTHER				

PATIENT / FAMILY GOALS:

O.T. PROGRAM:

ANTICIPATED FREQUENCY AND DURATION:

FOLLOW UP PLAN:

760193E (R 11/97)

☐ ADMISSION

☐ INTERIM

☐ DISCHARGE

THERAPIST'S SIGNATURE _____ Date

PHYSICIAN'S SIGNATURE _____ Date

NAME

RLANRC #

B.D. SEX

UNIT

OCCUPATIONAL THERAPY NOTE

Figure 8-6   OT initial evaluation form. (Courtesy Rancho Los Amigos National Rehabilitation Center, Downey, CA.)

Occupational Therapy Initial Assessment

Name: _____ DOB: _____ Start of Service Date: _____

HICN: _____ Onset: _____

Medical Dx/ICD-9 # _____Treatment Dx/ICD-9# _____

Past Medical History:_____

Occupational Profile:

Areas of Occupation:

ADL Status	dep	max	mod	min	sup	indep	comments:
Self-feeding							
Hygiene/grooming							
UB bathing							
UB dressing							
LB dressing							
Wet tub/shower							
Toilet transfer							
Toileting skills							
Functional mobility:							
Personal device care							

IADL Status							
Kitchen survival skills							
Meal preparation							
Shopping							
Laundry							
Light housekeeping							
Community mobility							
Financial mgmt							
Care of others							

Work/Leisure/social participation

Figure 8-7 Occupational therapy initial assessment.

Continued

Vocational:	
Avocational:	
Leisure participation:	
Social participation:	

Client Factors:

Functional cognition	
Perceptual status	
Memory	
Vision/hearing	
Pain	

ROM:
  RUE:
  LUE:	

Motor control:
  RUE:
  LUE:	

Strength:
  RUE:
  LUE:	

Muscle tone	
Coordination/bilateral integration	
Body system function	

Performance Skills: Patient/family goals:

Posture
  Sit:
  Stand:	

Mobility	
Endurance/effort	

| Short-term goals: | Long-term goals: |
| OT intervention plan: | Frequency/duration: |

Therapist's Signature   Date

Figure 8-7, cont'd

THREADED CASE STUDY: JANE, PART 2

Reflect upon the questions posed earlier regarding the case presented at the beginning of this chapter. Jane, the new occupational therapist beginning her first job at the skilled nursing facility, must use clinical reasoning skills at all stages of the therapy process, including the documentation of services delivered. The evaluation, intervention plan, and short- and long-term goals are written based upon sound clinical reasoning. Evidence of this must be reflected in the documentation provided by Jane. It is essential that occupational therapy notes also indicate the skilled service or skilled intervention that was provided for reimbursement purposes. The format used for recording this information, as well as the terminology used, may be specific to the practice setting. Federal privacy mandates (HIPAA) as well as the Occupational Therapy Code of Ethics must be adhered to at all times during all methods of documentation, whether written, verbal, or computer-generated.

SUMMARY

Documentation is a necessary part of the occupational therapy process. The occupational therapist has a responsibility to the client, the employer, and to the profession to develop the skills that will allow him or her to accurately document the therapy process. Well-written documentation promotes the profession by providing proof of the value of occupational therapy intervention. It can provide valuable information for outcome research and evidence-based practice. It is a professional expectation that the occupational therapist will keep current on documentation requirements for his or her practice area and will acquire the skills necessary to accurately document the occupational therapy process.

Review Questions

1. Why is documentation an essential component of occupational therapy practice?
2. How is language found in the OTPF incorporated into occupational therapy documentation?
3. How does the occupational therapy profile influence what is included in the client evaluation?
4. How is clinical reasoning used during the intervention planning process?
5. What should client-centered goals focus on?
6. Give an example of each of the following occupational therapy intervention approaches:
   Create, promote (health promotion)
   Remediation, restoration
   Compensation, adaptation
   Prevention
7. Name three criteria that would make an intervention skilled.

8. What information is appropriate to include in the "S" section of a SOAP note?
9. How is the information included in the "A" section of the SOAP note different than that in the "O" section?
10. What is the RUMBA test used for in documentation?
11. How does the clinician decide which forms are appropriate to use during documentation?
12. What ethical issues must be considered during the documentation process?

REFERENCES

1. American Occupational Therapy Association: *Guidelines for documentation of occupational therapy*, Bethesda, MD, 2003, AOTA.
2. American Occupational Therapy Association: Guidelines to the occupational therapy code of ethics, *Am J Occup Ther* 52:881, 1998.
3. American Occupational Therapy Association: Occupational therapy code of ethics, *Am J Occup Ther* 54:614, 2000.
4. American Occupational Therapy Association: Occupational therapy practice framework: domain and process, *Am J Occup Ther* 56(6):609, 2002.
5. American Occupational Therapy Association: Standards of practice for occupational therapy, *Am J Occup Ther* 52:866, 1998.
6. Borcherding S, Kappel C: *The OTA's guide to writing SOAP notes*, Thorofare, 2002, Slack Publishers.
7. Fremgen B: *Medical law and ethics*, Upper Saddle River, NJ, 2002, Prentice-Hall.
8. Health Resources and Services Administration: *Plain language principles and thesaurus for making HIPAA privacy notices more readable*, 2003. Retrieved from *http://hrsa.gov/language.htm*.
9. Hinojosa J, Kramer P: *Occupational therapy evaluation: obtaining and interpreting data*, Bethesda, MD, 1998, AOTA.
10. Kettenbach G: *Writing SOAP notes*, ed 3, Philadelphia, 2004, FA Davis.
11. *Medicare Program Integrity Manual*, 2001. Retrieved from *http://www.hcfa.gov/pubforms/83*.
12. Meyer MJ, Schiff M: *HIPAA: the questions you didn't know to ask*, Upper Saddle River, NJ, 2004, Pearson/Prentice-Hall.
13. Perinchief JM: Documentation and management of occupational therapy services. In Crepeau EB, Cohn ES, Schell BAB, editors: *Willard and Spackman's occupational therapy*, ed 10, p. 897, Philadelphia, 2003, Lippincott Williams & Wilkins.
14. Ranke BAE: Documentation in the age of litigation, *OT Practice* 3(3):20, 1998.
15. Sames KM: *Documenting occupational therapy practice*, Upper Saddle River, NJ, 2005, Pearson/Prentice-Hall.
16. Schell BAB: Clinical reasoning: the basis of practice. In Crepeau EB, Cohn ES, Schell BAB, editors: *Willard and Spackman's occupational therapy*, ed 10, p. 131, Philadelphia, 2003, Lippincott Williams & Wilkins.
17. Weed LL: *Medical records, medical education and patient care*, Chicago, 1971, Year Book Medical Publishers.

9

INFECTION CONTROL AND SAFETY ISSUES IN THE CLINIC

ALISON HEWITT GEORGE

KEY TERMS

Fowler's position
Endotracheal tube
Arterial monitoring line
Nasogastric (NG) tube
Intravenous (IV) feeding
Total parenteral nutrition
Hyperalimentation

Feeding pump
Intravenous lines
Catheter
Universal precautions
Centers for disease control
and prevention
Pathogens

Standard precautions
Occupational safety and health
administration
Autoclave
Isolation systems
Transmission-based
precautions

Nosocomial infection
Cardiopulmonary resuscitation
Antiseptic
Dyspnea control postures

LEARNING OBJECTIVES

After studying this chapter the student or practitioner will be able to do the following:

1. Recognize the role of occupational therapy personnel in preventing accidents.
2. Identify recommendations for safety in the clinic.
3. Describe the purposes of special equipment.
4. Identify precautions when treating clients who require special equipment.
5. Identify universal precautions and explain the importance of following them with all clients.
6. Describe proper techniques of hand washing.
7. Recognize the importance for all healthcare workers to understand and follow isolation procedures used in client care.
8. Identify procedures for handling client injuries.
9. Describe guidelines for handling various emergency situations.

CHAPTER OUTLINE

Safety recommendations for the clinic
Precautions with special equipment
  Hospital beds
  Ventilators
  Monitors
  Feeding devices
  Catheters
Infection control
  Isolation systems
Incidents and emergencies

Falls
Burns
Bleeding
Shock
Seizures
Insulin-related illnesses
Respiratory distress
Choking and cardiac arrest
Summary

THREADED CASE STUDY: DONNA, PART 1

Donna is a registered occupational therapist hired as Director of occupational therapy (OT) services in a recently opened community hospital. This 300-bed general acute care hospital provides inpatient and outpatient services for individuals with a wide range of medical needs including cardiac problems, brain injury, neurological and orthopedic problems, oncology, obstetrics, and gynecology. Occupational therapy services are provided in acute care, skilled nursing, acute rehabilitation, and outpatient units.

As Director of OT Services, Donna must establish policies and procedures pertaining to client safety, infection control, medical emergencies, and precautions with special equipment. Donna must develop written guidelines and identify and/or develop training requirements to ensure adequate orientation and preparation of the occupational therapy personnel.

Critical Thinking Questions

In preparing these policies and procedures, D.F. must consider the following:

1. What general safety procedures and infection control standards should be followed to maintain a safe clinic environment?
2. What specialized medical equipment are occupational therapy personnel likely to encounter in their intervention with clients, and what precautions should be taken when treating a client who requires special equipment?
3. What are the basic guidelines and/or procedures to be used in emergency situations?
4. What resources are available to healthcare providers that offer the most current information pertaining to safety procedures and infection control?

As you read through the chapter keep in mind these questions as well as any other concerns confronting Donna in developing protocols, policies, and procedures for the safety of the clients and occupational therapy personnel.

The *Occupational Therapy Practice Framework* (OTPF) describes occupational therapy service delivery as a collaborative process between the client and occupational therapy practitioner.[2] This collaboration can occur in a variety of settings (hospitals, schools, community settings, home). An important concept of the OTPF is context, which is "the variety of interrelated conditions within and surrounding the client that influence performance" (p. 613).[2] Contexts can be "cultural, physical, social, personal, spiritual, temporal and virtual" (p. 613).[2] Therefore, the setting, or physical context, in which occupational therapy intervention occurs plays a significant role in the delivery of services in either supporting or inhibiting the client's performance.

ETHICAL CONSIDERATIONS

Occupational therapists have an ethical obligation to take the necessary precautions to avoid harming the recipients of OT services.[1] In order to meet the ethical obligation to clients, and provide a physical context that supports the clients' engagement in meaningful occupations, occupational therapists need to be educated in proper safety procedures, infection control standards, and emergency interventions.

Medical technology and cost control pressures have made it necessary for rehabilitation professionals to treat seriously ill clients early in their illness and for shorter periods. In the hospital setting, it is not unusual for occupational therapists to work with clients using interventions that include specialized medical equipment such as catheters, IV lines, monitoring devices, and ventilators. These circumstances increase the potential for injuries to the clients. In addition to ethical obligations to provide safe and proper intervention, *occupational therapy* (OT) personnel can be held legally liable for negligence if a client is injured because staff failed to follow proper procedures or standards of care.[6]

This chapter reviews specific safety precautions for use with a variety of clients. It identifies precautions to consider when encountering equipment commonly used with clients. Guidelines for handling various emergency situations are reviewed. It is important to note that the chapter is only an overview and cannot substitute for training in specific procedures used in many facilities. In addition to following these procedures, it is incumbent upon the occupational therapist to teach clients and their families applicable techniques that can be followed at home.

SAFETY RECOMMENDATIONS FOR THE CLINIC

Prevention of accidents and subsequent injuries begins with consistent application of basic safety precautions for the clinic:

1. Wash your hands for at least 15 seconds before and after treating each client to reduce cross-contamination.[4]
2. Make sure space is adequate to maneuver equipment. Avoid placing clients where they may be bumped by equipment or passing personnel. Keep the area free from clutter.[11]
3. Do not attempt to transfer clients in congested areas or in areas where your view or movement is blocked.[11]
4. Routinely check equipment to be sure it is working properly.
5. Make sure the furniture and equipment in the clinic are stable. When not using items, store them out of the way of the treatment area.

6. Keep the floor free of cords, scatter rugs, litter, and spills. Ensure that the floors are not highly polished, because polished floors may be very slippery.[11]

7. Do not leave clients unattended. Use restraint belts properly to protect clients when they are not closely observed.

8. Have the treatment area and supplies ready before the client arrives.

9. Allow only properly trained personnel to provide client care.

10. Follow the manufacturer's and facility's procedures for handling and storing potentially hazardous material. Be sure such materials are marked and stored in a place that is in clear view. Do not store such items above shoulder height.

11. Clearly label emergency exits and evacuation routes.

12. Have emergency equipment, such as fire extinguishers and first aid kits, readily available.

PRECAUTIONS WITH SPECIAL EQUIPMENT

Newly hired OT personnel need orientation and education regarding the types of medical equipment they are likely to encounter when treating clients. Before providing any intervention to a client at bedside, the OT should carefully review the medical chart to determine whether there are any specific instructions regarding movement precautions, positioning, or handling. For example, a client may need to follow a turning schedule and may be limited in the length of time allowed to remain in one position. There may be certain joint movements that are contraindicated, or special bed and wheelchair positioning requirements, such as with clients recovering from burn injury, spinal cord injury, stroke, hip replacement surgery, or others. Special handling techniques may be required when working with clients who have catheters, feeding tubes, IV lines, or special monitors. The various chapters throughout this book that address specific diagnoses will identify necessary precaution and handling recommendations.

HOSPITAL BEDS

OT personnel must be educated in the proper use of hospital beds to ensure client safety. Two of the beds most commonly used in hospitals are the standard manually operated and standard electrically operated beds. Both beds are designed to make it easier to support the client and to change a client's position. Other, more specialized beds are needed for management of more complicated or more traumatic cases. Whatever type is used, the bed should be positioned so that the client is easily accessed and the therapist can use good body mechanics (see Chapter 11).

Most *standard electrically adjustable beds* are adjusted by means of electrical controls attached to the head or the foot of the bed or to a special cord that allows the client to operate the controls. The controls are marked according to their function and can be operated with the hand or foot. The entire bed can be raised and lowered, or upper and lower sections of the bed can be elevated or lowered to meet client needs. When the upper portion is raised 45-60°, the client's position is referred to as **Fowler's position**.[10] This commonly used position facilitates lung expansion, improves breathing, and decreases cardiac workload (as compared to supine lying). However, an important precaution for the OT to observe and address is that, in this position, the client may slide down in the bed, which increases shearing forces on the back tissues.[5]

Side rails are attached to most beds as a protective measure. Some rails are lifted upward to engage the locking mechanism, whereas others are moved toward the upper portion of the bed until the locking mechanism is engaged. If a side rail is used for client security, the OT should be sure the rail is locked securely before leaving the client. The rail should be checked to ensure it does not compress, stretch, or otherwise interfere with any IV or other tubing.

A rotating *kinetic bed* allows for re-alignment and stabilization of the client and also places him/her in perpetual slow motion from side to side, which provides pressure relief and mobilization of respiratory secretions. The bed is constructed with hinged sections that can be removed to allow access to all areas of the body so that healthcare providers can perform necessary care and treatment.[5] This bed is used most frequently with clients who have spinal cord injuries requiring immobilization. Another option is a *turning frame* (e.g., Stryker wedge frame), which has front and back frames that are covered with canvas. The support base allows elevation of the head or foot ends of the frames or of the entire bed. One person can easily turn the client horizontally from prone to supine or from supine to prone. The turning frame allows access to the client and permits the client to be repositioned without being removed from the frame.[5] Because of the limited number of possible positions, the skin of clients using this type of bed should be monitored frequently.

The *circular turning frame* (CircOlectric bed) has a front and a back frame attached to two circular supports. The frames on which the client is positioned move the client vertically from supine to prone or from prone to supine. The circular support frames are moved by an electric motor and can be stopped at any point within a 210° range.[10] The client or other persons can use a control switch to adjust the position. The circular turning bed is used with clients in traction, and to facilitate turning clients with severe burn injury. It provides the benefit of frequent position changes to relieve skin pressure. However, a client is still at risk for skin problems because of the pressure forces that may occur when the bed is turned or rotated vertically. The bed can also serve as a standing frame when stopped in the vertical position, which is helpful for clients who can benefit from increased weight bearing and stress to the bones and muscles of the lower extremity.[5] However, clients may experience symptoms of motion sickness such as vertigo, nausea, or hypotension when being turned. Devices that turn the client, such as the CircOlectric bed, are potentially dangerous. Personnel should be fully trained in correct operation, and patients need to be carefully monitored for signs of discomfort, dizziness, respiratory changes, or faintness following repositioning. This bed is contraindicated for use with clients with unstable spinal fractures or certain other pathological conditions.[5]

The *air-fluidized* support bed (e.g. Clinitron) rests the client on an air-permeable mattress that contains millions of silicon-coated beads called microspheres.[10] Heated, pressurized air flows through the beads to suspend a polyester cover that supports the client. When set in motion, the microspheres develop the properties associated with fluids. Clients feel as if they are floating on a warm waterbed. The risk for skin problems is reduced because of the minimal contact pressure between the client's body and the polyester sheet, which allows for even weight distribution and improved capillary blood flow to the skin. Friction and shearing of the skin are minimal. This bed is used with clients who have several infected lesions, or who require skin protection and whose position cannot be altered easily.[5] Care should be taken to prevent puncturing the polyester cover (which would allow the microspheres to be expelled).

VENTILATORS

Ventilators (respirators) move gas or air into the client's lungs and are used to maintain adequate air exchange when normal respiration is decreased.[10] Two frequently used types of ventilators are the *volume-cycled ventilators* and the *pressure-cycled ventilators*. Both ventilators deliver a predetermined volume of gas (air) during inspiration and allow for passive expiration.[8] The gas delivered by the ventilator usually will be induced into the client through an **endotracheal tube** (ET), which is a catheter inserted through the nose or mouth into the trachea.[10] When the tube is in place, the client is *intubated*. Insertion of the ET will prevent the client from talking. When the ET is removed, the client may complain of a sore throat and may have a distorted voice for a short period. It is important to avoid disturbing, bending, kinking, or occluding the tubing or accidentally disconnecting the ventilator tube from the ET. The client who uses a ventilator may participate in various bedside activities, including sitting and ambulation. Make sure the tubing is sufficiently long to allow the activity to be performed. Because the client will have difficulty talking, ask questions that can be answered with head nods or other nonverbal means. A client using a ventilator may have a lower tolerance for activities and should be monitored for signs of respiratory distress such as a change in the respiration pattern, fainting, or blue lips.

MONITORS

Various monitors are used to observe the physiologic state of clients who need special care. Therapeutic activities can be performed by clients who are being monitored, provided

that care is taken to prevent disruption of the equipment. Many of the units have an auditory and a visual signal that are activated by a change in the client's condition or position or by a change in the function of the equipment. It may be necessary for a nurse to evaluate and correct the cause of the alarm unless the OT has received special instruction.

The *cardiac monitor* provides a continuous check on the function of the client's heart including electrical activity (electrocardiogram or EKG), heart rate, blood pressure, and respiration rate.[10] Acceptable or safe ranges for the three physiologic indicators can be set in the unit. An alarm is activated when the upper or lower limits of the ranges are exceeded or if the unit malfunctions. A monitoring screen provides a graphic and digital display of the values so that healthcare staff can observe the client's responses to treatment.

The *pulmonary artery catheter* (PAC) (e.g., Swan-Ganz catheter) is a long, plastic IV tube that is inserted into a thoracic vein, through the right side of the heart and terminated in the pulmonary artery. It provides accurate and continuous measurements of pulmonary artery pressures and will detect subtle changes in the client's cardiovascular system, including responses to medications, stress, and activity.[3] Activities, including OT intervention, can be performed with the PAC in place, providing they do not interfere with the location of the catheter's insertion. For example, if the catheter is inserted into the subclavian vein, elbow flexion should be avoided and shoulder motions restricted.

The *intracranial pressure (ICP) monitor* measures the pressure exerted against the skull by brain tissue, blood, or cerebrospinal fluid (CSF).[10] It is used to monitor ICP in clients with a closed head injury, cerebral hemorrhage, brain tumor, or overproduction of CSF. Some of the complications associated with this device are infection, hemorrhage, and seizures. Two of the more commonly used ICP monitoring devices are the ventricular catheter and the subarachnoid screw. Both are inserted in a hole drilled in the skull. Physical activities should be limited when these devices are in place. Activities that would cause a rapid increase in ICP, such as isometric exercises, should be avoided. Positions to avoid include neck flexion, hip flexion greater than 90°, and the prone position. The client's head should not be lowered more than 15° below horizontal. Care must be taken to avoid disturbing the plastic tube.

The **arterial monitoring line** (A line) is a catheter that is inserted into an artery to continuously and accurately measure blood pressure or to obtain blood samples without repeated needle punctures.[3] OT intervention can be provided with an A line in place, but care should be taken to avoid disturbing the catheter and inserted needle.

FEEDING DEVICES

Special feeding devices may be necessary to provide nutrition for clients who are unable to ingest, chew, or swallow food. Some of the more commonly seen devices are the nasogastric tube, the gastric tube, and IV feedings.

The **nasogastric** (NG) *tube* is a plastic tube inserted through a nostril, terminating in the client's stomach. The tube may cause the client to have a sore throat or an increased gag reflex. Feeding training can be initiated while the NG tube is in place. However, care should be taken as the tube may desensitize the swallow mechanism.[3] Caution should be used when moving the client's head and neck, especially forward flexion, to prevent dislodging of the tube.

The *gastric tube* (G tube) is a plastic tube inserted through an incision in the client's abdomen directly into the stomach.[3] The tube should not be disturbed or removed during intervention.

Intravenous feeding, total parenteral nutrition (TPN), or **hyperalimentation** devices permit infusion of large amounts of nutrients needed to promote tissue growth. A hyperalimentation device is used when a client is unable to eat or absorb nutrients through the gastrointestinal tract.[3] A catheter is passed into a large vein (typically the subclavian vein) that empties directly into the heart. The catheter may be connected to a semi-permanently fixed cannula, or sutured at the point of insertion. The OT should carefully observe the various connections to be certain they are secure before and after intervention. A disrupted or loose connection may result in the development of an air embolus, which could be life threatening.[3]

The system usually includes a specialized **feeding pump**, which will administer fluids and nutrients at a preselected, constant flow rate. An audible alarm will be activated if the system becomes imbalanced or when the fluid source is empty.[3] Intervention activities can be performed as long as the tubing is not disrupted, disconnected, or occluded and as long as undue stress to the infusion site is prevented. Motions of the shoulder on the side of the infusion site may be restricted, especially abduction and flexion.

Most **intravenous** (IV) **lines** are inserted into superficial veins. Various sizes and types of needles or catheters are used, depending on the purpose of the IV therapy, the infusion site, the need for prolonged therapy, and site availability. Care should be taken during intervention to prevent any disruption, disconnection, or occlusion of the tubing. The infusion site should remain dry, the needle should remain secure and immobile in the vein, and no restraint should be placed above the infusion site.[3] For example, a blood pressure cuff should not be applied above the infusion site. The total system should be observed, to be certain it is functioning properly when intervention begins and ends. If the infusion site is in the antecubital area, the elbow should not be flexed. The client who ambulates with an IV line in place should be instructed to grasp the IV support pole so that the infusion site will be at heart level.[3] If the infusion site is allowed to hang lower, blood flow may be affected. Similar procedures to maintain the infusion site in proper position should be followed when the client is treated while in bed or at a treatment table. Activities involving elevation of the infusion site above the level of the heart for a prolonged period should be avoided.

Problems related to the IV system should be reported to nursing personnel. Simple procedures such as straightening the tubing or removing an object that is occluding the tubing may be performed by the properly trained therapist.

CATHETERS

A urinary **catheter** is used to remove urine from the bladder when the client is unable to satisfactorily control retention or release.[10] The urine is drained through plastic tubing into a collection bag, bottle, or urinal. Any form of trauma, disease, condition, or disorder affecting the neuromuscular control of the bladder sphincter may necessitate the use of a urinary catheter. The catheter may be used temporarily or for the remainder of the client's life.

A urinary catheter can be applied internally (*indwelling catheter*) or externally. Female clients require an indwelling catheter inserted through the urethra and into the bladder. Males may use an *external* catheter. A condom catheter is applied over the shaft of the penis and is held in place by an adhesive applied to the skin or by a padded strap or tape encircling the proximal shaft of the penis. The condom is connected to a drainage tube and urine collection bag.[3]

When clients with urinary catheters are receiving OT intervention, several precautions are important. Disruption or stretching of the drainage tube should be prevented and no tension should be placed on the tubing or the catheter. The urine collection bag must not be placed above the level of the bladder for more than a few minutes to avoid back flow of the urine into the bladder or kidneys (if indwelling catheter) or soiling the client (if external catheter). The bag should not be placed in the client's lap when the client is being transported. The production, color, and odor of the urine should be observed. The following observations should be reported to a physician or nurse: foul-smelling, cloudy, dark, or bloody urine, or a reduction in the flow or production of urine. The collection bag must be emptied when it is full.[3]

Infection is a major complication for persons using catheters, especially for those using indwelling catheters. Everyone involved with the client should maintain cleanliness during treatment. The tubing should be replaced or reconnected only by those properly trained. Treatment settings in which clients with catheters are routinely treated have specific protocols for catheter care.[3]

Two types of internal catheters that are frequently used are the *Foley catheter* and *suprapubic catheter*. The Foley catheter is a type of indwelling catheter that is held in place in the bladder by a small balloon inflated with air, water, or sterile saline solution. For removal of the catheter, the balloon is deflated and the catheter is withdrawn. The suprapubic catheter is inserted directly into the bladder through incisions in the lower abdomen and the bladder. The catheter may be held in place by adhesive tape, but care should be used to avoid its removal, especially during self-care activities.[3] Catheter application and bladder management are *activities of daily living* (ADLs) that are frequently taught to clients as part of a comprehensive OT intervention program (see Chapters 10 and 36 for examples).

INFECTION CONTROL

Infection control procedures are used to prevent the spread of disease and infection among clients, healthcare workers, and others. They are designed to interrupt or establish barriers to the infection cycle. **Universal precautions** (UP) were first established by the **Centers for Disease Control and Prevention (CDC)** to protect the health care worker from infectious agents such as the human immunodeficiency virus (HIV) and diseases such as acquired immunodeficiency syndrome (AIDS), hepatitis B, and hepatitis C. UP place an emphasis on preventing the transmission of **pathogens** (infectious microorganisms) through contact with blood and bodily fluids. The CDC has developed further guidelines for a new system of isolation, called *body substance isolation* (BSI), which focuses on "the isolation of all moist and potentially infectious body substances (blood, feces, urine, sputum, saliva, wound drainage and other body fluids) from all patients."[8] The CDC's most recent guidelines for isolation precautions in hospitals recommends the use of **standard precautions**, which synthesize the primary features of BSI and UP. Standard precautions apply to blood, all bodily secretions and fluids, mucous membranes, and nonintact skin, and are used with all clients, not just those identified as infected (Box 9-1 and Figure 9-1).[8]

The **Occupational Safety and Health Administration** (OSHA) issues regulations to protect the employees of healthcare facilities. All healthcare settings must do the following to comply with federal regulations:

1. Educate employees on the methods of transmission and the prevention of hepatitis B, HIV, and other infections.
2. Provide safe and adequate protective equipment and teach employees where the equipment is located and how to use it.
3. Teach employees about work practices used to prevent occupational transmission of disease, including, but not limited to, universal precautions, proper handling of client specimens and linens, proper cleaning of body fluid spills (Figure 9-2), and proper waste disposal.
4. Provide proper containers for the disposal of waste and sharp items, and teach employees the color coding system used to distinguish infectious waste.
5. Post warning labels and biohazard signs (Figure 9-3).
6. Offer the hepatitis B vaccine to employees who are at substantial risk of occupational exposure to the hepatitis B virus.
7. Provide education and follow-up care to employees who are exposed to communicable disease.

OSHA has also outlined the responsibilities of healthcare employees. These responsibilities include the following:

1. Using protective equipment and clothing provided by the facility whenever the employee contacts, or anticipates contact, with body fluids

Box **9-1**   SUMMARY OF STANDARD PRECAUTIONS
1. Use extreme care to prevent injuries caused by sharp instruments. 2. Cover minor, nondraining, noninfected skin lesions with an adhesive bandage. 3. Report infected or draining lesions and weeping dermatitis to your supervisor. 4. Avoid personal habits (e.g., nail biting) that increase the potential for oral mucous membrane contact with body surfaces. 5. Perform procedures involving body substances carefully to minimize splatters. 6. Cover environmental surfaces with moisture-proof barriers whenever splattering with body substances is possible. 7. Wash hands regularly, whether or not gloves are worn. 8. Avoid unnecessary use of protective clothing. Use alternate barriers whenever possible. 9. Wear gloves to touch the mucous membrane or nonintact skin of any client, and whenever direct contact with body substances is anticipated. 10. Wear protective clothing (e.g., gown, mask, and goggles) when splashing of body substances is anticipated. 11. Ensure that the hospital has procedures for care, cleaning, and disinfection of environmental surfaces and equipment. 12. Handle and process soiled linens in a manner to minimize the transfer of microorganisms to other patients and environments. 13. Handle used patient-care equipment appropriately to prevent transfer of infectious microorganisms. Ensure that reusable equipment is thoroughly and appropriately cleaned.

2. Disposing of waste in proper containers, applying knowledge and understanding of the handling of infectious waste, and using color-coded bags or containers
3. Disposing of sharp instruments and needles into proper containers without attempting to recap, bend, break, or otherwise manipulate them before disposal
4. Keeping the work environment and client care area clean
5. Washing hands immediately after removing gloves and at any other times mandated by hospital or agency policy
6. Immediately reporting any exposures such as needle sticks or blood splashes or any personal illnesses to immediate supervisor and receiving instruction about any further follow-up action

Although it is impossible to eliminate all pathogens from an area or object, the likelihood of infection can be greatly reduced. The largest source of preventable client infection is contamination from the hands of healthcare workers. Hand washing (Box 9-2 and Figure 9-4) and the use of gloves are the most effective barriers to the infection cycle.[4] The use of gloves does not eliminate the need for hand washing, and vice versa. Latex gloves provide the best protection from infectious materials. However, many individuals have latex allergies so

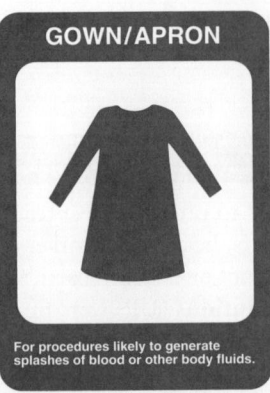

GLOVE

Before touching blood, body fluids, mucous membranes, non-intact skin or performing venipuncture. Change gloves after contact with each patient.

WASH

Wash hands immediately after gloves are removed. Wash hands and other skin surfaces immediately if contaminated with blood or other body fluids.

GOWN/APRON

For procedures likely to generate splashes of blood or other body fluids.

MASK/EYEWEAR

Masks and protective eyewear or face shields for procedures likely to generate splashes of blood or other body fluids.

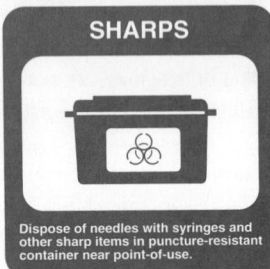
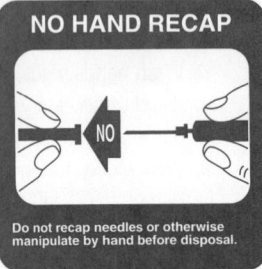
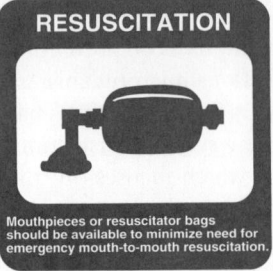
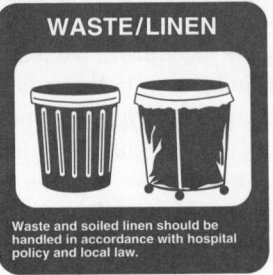

SHARPS

Dispose of needles with syringes and other sharp items in puncture-resistant container near point-of-use.

NO HAND RECAP

Do not recap needles or otherwise manipulate by hand before disposal.

RESUSCITATION

Mouthpieces or resuscitator bags should be available to minimize need for emergency mouth-to-mouth resuscitation.

WASTE/LINEN

Waste and soiled linen should be handled in accordance with hospital policy and local law.

Universal Precautions apply to blood, visibly bloody fluid, semen, vaginal secretions, tissues and to cerebrospinal, synovial, pleural, peritoneal, pericardial and amniotic fluids.

Figure 9-1 Universal blood and body fluid precautions. (Courtesy Brevis Corp., Salt Lake City, UT.)

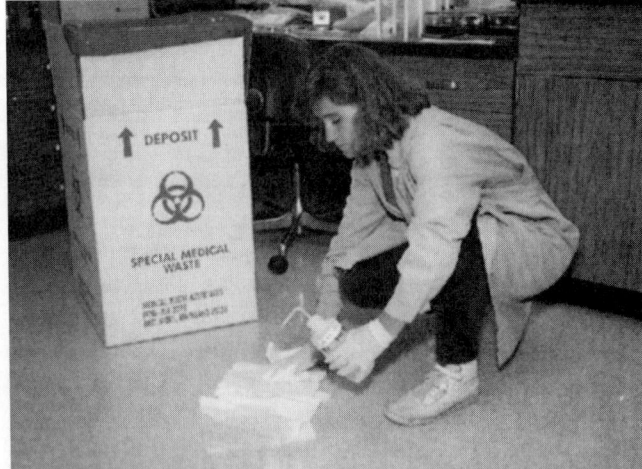
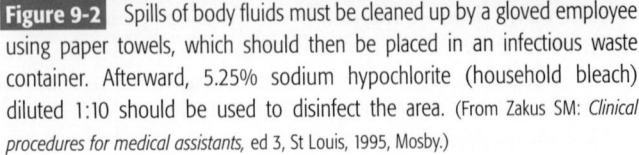

Figure 9-2 Spills of body fluids must be cleaned up by a gloved employee using paper towels, which should then be placed in an infectious waste container. Afterward, 5.25% sodium hypochlorite (household bleach) diluted 1:10 should be used to disinfect the area. (From Zakus SM: *Clinical procedures for medical assistants,* ed 3, St Louis, 1995, Mosby.)

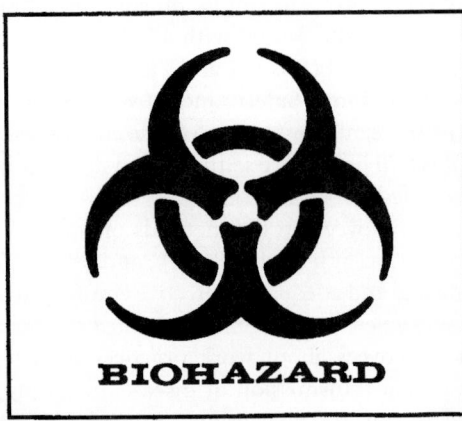

BIOHAZARD

Figure 9-3 Biohazard label. (From Zakus SM: *Clinical procedures for medical assistants,* ed 3, St Louis, 1995, Mosby.)

non-latex gloves should be used for activities that are not likely to involve contact with infectious materials (food preparation, routine housekeeping, general maintenance, etc.).[5] The CDC also recommends the use of alcohol-based hand rubs as an acceptable alternative to hand washing. Alcohol-based hand rubs are fast acting, cause minimal skin irritation, and significantly reduce the presence of microorganisms on the skin.[4]

In the clinic, general cleanliness and proper control of heat, light, and air are also important for infection control. Spills should be cleaned up promptly. Work areas and equipment should be kept free from contamination.

To *decontaminate* is to "remove, inactivate, or destroy blood-borne pathogens on a surface or item to the point where they are no longer capable of transmitting infectious particles and the surface or item is rendered safe for handling, use, or disposal."[13] Items to be sterilized or decontaminated should first be cleaned thoroughly to remove any residual matter. Sterilization is used to destroy all forms of microbial life, including highly resistant bacterial spores. An **autoclave** is used

Box **9-2**	TECHNIQUE FOR EFFECTIVE HAND WASHING

1. Remove all jewelry, except plain band-type ring. Remove watch or move it up. Provide complete access to area to be washed.
2. Approach the sink and avoid touching the sink or nearby objects.
3. Turn on the water and adjust it to a lukewarm temperature and a moderate flow to prevent splashing.
4. Wet your wrists and hands with your fingers directed downward and apply approximately 1 teaspoon of liquid soap or granules.
5. Begin to wash all areas of your hands (palms, sides, and backs), fingers, knuckles, and between each finger, using vigorous rubbing and circular motions (Figure 9-4, **A**). If wearing a band, slide it down the finger a bit and scrub skin underneath it. Interlace fingers and scrub between each finger.
6. Wash for at least 15 seconds, keeping the hands and forearms at elbow level or below, with hands pointed down. Wash longer if you have treated a client known to have an infection.
7. Rinse hands well under running water.
8. Wash wrists and forearms, as high as contamination is likely.
9. Rinse hands, wrists, and forearms under running water (Figure 9-4, **B**).
10. Use an orangewood stick or nail brush to clean under each fingernail at least once a day when starting work and each time hands are highly contaminated. Rinse nails well under running water (Figure 9-4, **C**).
11. Dry your hands, wrists, and forearms thoroughly with paper towels. Use a dry towel for each hand. The water should continue to flow from the tap as you dry your hands.
12. Use another dry paper towel to turn water faucet off (Figure 9-4, **D**). Discard all towels in an appropriate container.
13. Use hand lotion as necessary.

Modified from Zakus SM *Clinical procedures for medical assistants,* ed 3, St Louis, 1995, Mosby.

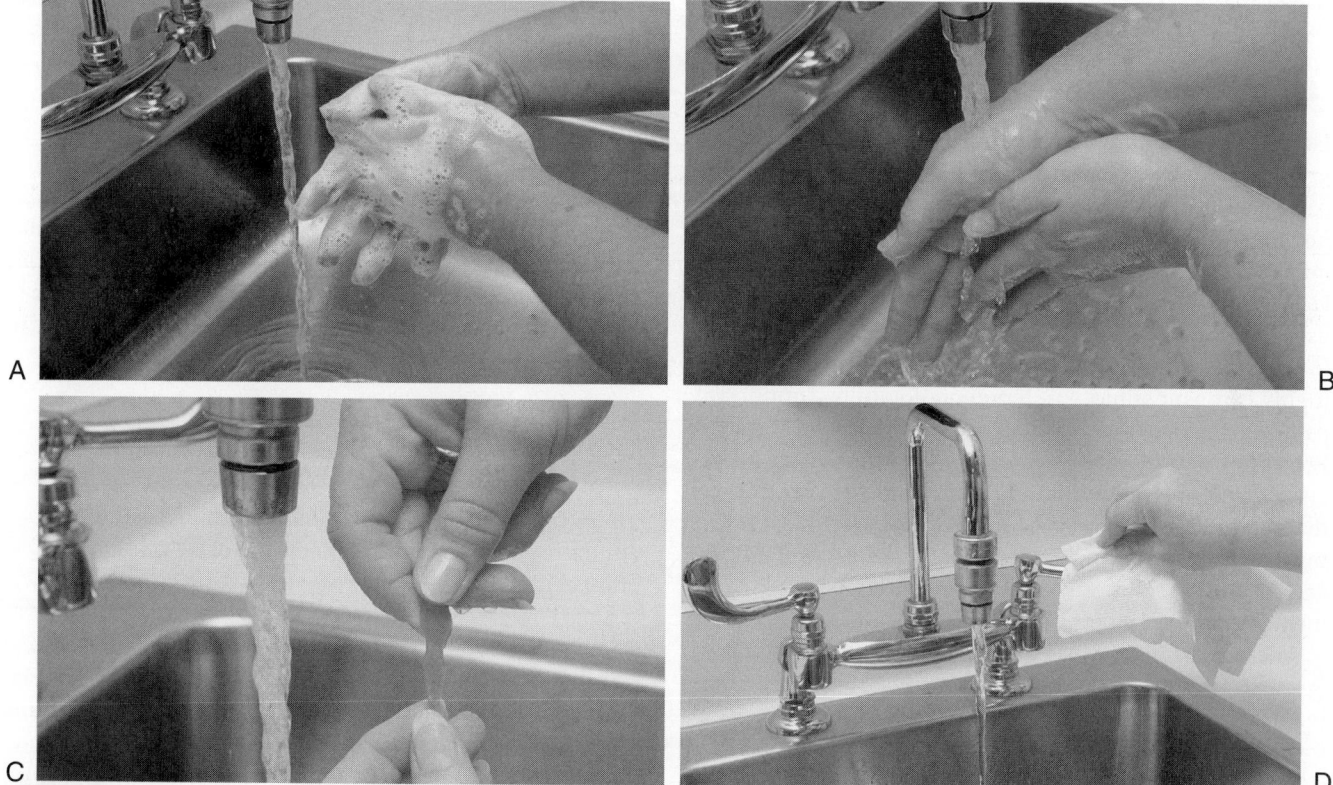

Figure 9-4   **A,** Handwashing technique. Interlace fingers to wash between them. Create a lather with soap. Keep hands pointed down. **B,** Rinse hands well, keeping fingers pointed down. **C,** Use blunt edge of an orangewood stick to clean under the fingernails. **D,** After drying your hands, turn water faucet off, using a dry paper towel. (From Zakus SM: *Clinical procedures for medical assistants,* ed 3, St Louis, 1995, Mosby.)

to sterilize items by steam under pressure. Ethylene oxide, dry heat, and immersion in chemical disinfectants are other methods of sterilization.[3]

A variety of disinfectants may be used to clean environmental surfaces and reusable instruments. When liquid disinfectants and cleaning agents are used, gloves should be worn to protect the skin from repeated or prolonged contact. The CDC, local health department, or hospital infection control department can provide information about the best product and method to use.

Instruments and equipment used to treat a client should be cleaned or disposed of according to institutional or agency policies and procedures. Contaminated reusable equipment should be placed carefully in a container, labeled, and returned to the appropriate department for sterilization. Contaminated disposable items should be placed carefully in a container, labeled, and disposed of.

Contaminated or soiled linen should be disposed of with minimal handling, sorting, and movement. It can be bagged in an appropriate bag and labeled before transport to the laundry, or the bag can be color coded to indicate the type or condition of linen it contains. Other contaminated items such as toys, magazines, personal hygiene articles, dishes, and eating utensils should be disposed of or disinfected. They should not be used by others until they have been disinfected.

OT PRACTICE NOTE

Therapists should routinely clean and disinfect personal items such as pens, keys, and clipboards because these objects are touched frequently and may become contaminated.

ISOLATION SYSTEMS

Isolation systems are designed to protect a person or object from becoming contaminated or infected by transmissible pathogens. Various isolation procedures are used in different institutions. It is important for all healthcare workers to understand and follow the isolation approach used in their facilities so protection can be ensured. The CDC has established **transmission-based precautions**, which are "designed for patients documented or suspected to be infected with highly transmissible or epidemiologically important pathogens for which additional precautions beyond Standard Precautions are needed to interrupt transmission in hospitals."[8] There are three types of transmission-based precautions that may be used singly or in combination to control infectious transmission: contact precautions, droplet precautions, and airborne precautions. The CDC provides specific recommendations for each infection control measure.

When transmission-based precautions are needed, a client is usually isolated from other clients and the hospital environment when he or she has a transmissible disease. Isolation involves placing the client in a room either alone or with one or more clients with the same disease to reduce the possibility of transmitting the disease to others. Specific infection control techniques must be followed by all who enter the client's room. These requirements are based upon the type of infectious organism and common routes of transmission (i.e., airborne, direct or indirect physical contact, and droplets). Specific instructions are listed on a color-coded card and placed on or next to the door of the client's room. Strict isolation and respiratory isolation procedures are shown in Figure 9-5. Protective clothing, including gown, mask, cap, and gloves, may be needed. When leaving the client, the caregiver must dispose of protective clothing before leaving the room and dispose of it in an appropriately designated area or container for storage, washing, decontamination, or disposal. Examples of diseases that require transmission-based precautions include tuberculosis, SARS, chicken pox, measles, and meningitis.[8]

Occasionally, a client's condition (e.g., burns or a systemic infection) makes him or her more susceptible to infection. This client may be placed in *protective isolation*. In this approach, persons entering the client's room may have to wear protective clothing to prevent the transmission of pathogens to the client. The sequence and method of donning the protective garments are more important than the sequence used to remove them.

Nosocomial infections, or hospital-acquired infections, are a significant problem in hospital environments. Approximately 5% of American hospital clients acquire a clinically significant nosocomial infection.[8] It is critical that OT personnel be given proper education and training in infection control standards to prevent the spread of unnecessary infections.

INCIDENTS AND EMERGENCIES

Occupational therapists should be able to respond to a variety of medical emergencies and to recognize when it is better to get assistance from the most qualified individual available, such as a doctor, emergency medical technician, or nurse. Securing such assistance should be relatively easy in a hospital but may require an extended period before response if the OT intervention is conducted in a client's home or outpatient clinic. It is a good idea to keep emergency telephone numbers readily available. The therapist will need to determine at the time of the incident whether it is wiser to ask for assistance before or after beginning emergency care.

ETHICAL CONSIDERATIONS

In most cases, it is best to call for assistance before initiating emergency care, unless the delay is life threatening to the client.

All OTs should be certified in **cardiopulmonary resuscitation** (CPR) and have basic first aid training. Training and certification can be obtained through organizations such as the American Heart Association (www.americanheart.org) and the American Red Cross (www.redcross.org).

Consistently following safety measures will prevent many accidents. However, the therapist should always be alert to the possibility of an injury and expect the unexpected to happen. Most institutions have specific policies and procedures to follow. In general, the therapist should do the following when there is an injury to a client:

1. Ask for help. Do not leave the client alone. Prevent further injury to the client and provide emergency care.
2. When the emergency is over, document the incident according to the institution's policy. Do not discuss the

STRICT ISOLATION

VISITORS: REPORT TO NURSES' STATION BEFORE ENTERING ROOM

1. Masks are indicated for all persons entering the room.
2. Gowns are indicated for all persons entering the room.
3. Gloves are indicated for all persons entering the room.
4. HANDS MUST BE WASHED AFTER TOUCHING THE PATIENT OR POTENTIALLY CONTAMINATED ARTICLES AND BEFORE TAKING CARE OF ANOTHER PATIENT.
5. Articles contaminated with infective material should be discarded or bagged and labeled before being sent for decontamination and reprocessing.

A

RESPIRATORY ISOLATION

VISITORS: REPORT TO NURSES' STATION BEFORE ENTERING ROOM

1. Masks are indicated for those who come close to the patient.
2. Gowns are not indicated.
3. Gloves are not indicated.
4. HANDS MUST BE WASHED AFTER TOUCHING THE PATIENT OR POTENTIALLY CONTAMINATED ARTICLES AND BEFORE TAKING CARE OF ANOTHER PATIENT.
5. Articles contaminated with infective material should be discarded or bagged and labeled before being sent for decontamination and reprocessing.

B

Figure 9-5   **A,** Strict isolation procedures sign. Card will be color-coded yellow and placed on or next to the door of the client's room. **B,** Respiratory isolation procedures sign. Card will be color-coded blue and placed on or next to the door of the client's room.

incident with the client or significant others or express information to anyone that might indicate negligence.[13]

3. Notify the supervisor of the incident and file the incident report with the appropriate person within the organization.

FALLS

There is always the risk of falling when addressing functional mobility with clients. The OT can reduce the risk of falling by carefully preparing the environment prior to initiating intervention. This includes use of a gait belt during mobility activities, clearing the environment of potential hazards, and having a wheelchair or chair nearby to pull into position for clients who might be prone to falling. The therapist can prevent injuries from falls by remaining alert and reacting quickly when clients lose their balance. Proper guarding techniques must be practiced. In many instances it is wise to resist the natural impulse to keep the client upright. Instead, the therapist can carefully assist the client to the floor or onto a firm object.

If a client begins to fall forward, the following procedure should be used: Restrain the client by firmly holding the gait belt. Push forward against the pelvis and pull back on the shoulder or anterior chest. Help the client stand erect once it is determined there is no injury. The client may briefly lean against you for support. If the client is falling too far forward to be kept upright, guide the client to reach for the floor slowly. Slow the momentum by gently pulling back on the gait belt and the client's shoulder. Step forward as the client moves toward the floor. Tell the client to bend the elbows when the hands contact the floor to help cushion the fall. The client's head should be turned to one side to avoid injury to the face.

If the client begins to fall backward, the following procedure should be used: Rotate your body so one side is turned toward the client's back, and widen your stance. Push forward on the client's pelvis and allow the client to lean against your body. Then, assist the client to stand erect. If the client falls too far backward, to stay upright, continue to rotate your body until it is turned toward the client's back, and widen your stance. Instruct the client to briefly lean against your body or to sit on your thigh. You may need to lower the client into a sitting position on the floor using the gait belt and good body mechanics.

BURNS

Generally, only minor, first-degree burns are likely to accidentally occur in occupational therapy. These can be treated with basic first aid procedures. Skilled personnel should be contacted for immediate care if the burn has any charred or missing skin or shows blistering. The following steps should be taken for first-degree burns in which the skin is only reddened:[7]

1. Rinse or soak the burned area in cold (not iced) water.
2. Cover with a clean or sterile dressing.
3. Do not apply any cream, ointment, or butter to the burn because this will mask the appearance and may lead to infection or a delay in healing.
4. Report the incident so that the injury can be evaluated by a physician.

BLEEDING

A laceration may result in minor or serious bleeding. The objectives of first aid treatment are to prevent contamination of the wound and to control the bleeding. The following steps should be taken to stop the bleeding:

1. Wash your hands and apply protective gloves. Continue to wear protective gloves while treating the wound.
2. Place a clean towel or sterile dressing over the wound and apply direct pressure to the wound. If no dressing is available, use your gloved hand.
3. Elevate the wound above the level of the client's heart to reduce blood flow to the area.
4. In some instances the wound can be cleansed with an **antiseptic** or by rinsing it with water.
5. Encourage the client to remain quiet and avoid using the extremity.
6. If there is arterial bleeding (demonstrated by spurting blood), it may be necessary to apply intermittent, direct pressure to the artery, above the level of the wound. The pressure point for the brachial artery is on the inside of the upper arm, midway between the elbow and armpit. The pressure point for the femoral artery is in the crease of the hip joint, just to the side of the pubic bone.
7. Do not apply a tourniquet unless you have been trained to do so.

SHOCK

Clients may experience shock as a result of excessive bleeding, sepsis, and respiratory distress; as a reaction to the change from a supine to an upright position; or as a response to excessive heat or *anaphylaxis* (severe allergic reaction). Shock causes a drop in blood pressure and inefficient cardiac output, resulting in inadequate perfusion of organs and tissues. Signs and symptoms of shock include pale, moist, and cool skin; shallow and irregular breathing; dilated pupils; a weak or rapid pulse; dizziness or nausea; and altered level of consciousness.[7] Shock should not be confused with fainting, which would result in

a slower pulse, paleness, and perspiration. Clients who faint will generally recover promptly if allowed to lie flat. If a client exhibits symptoms of shock, the following actions should be taken:[7]

1. Get medical assistance as soon as possible, as shock can be life-threatening.
2. Try to determine the cause of shock and correct it if possible. Monitor the client's blood pressure, breathing, and pulse rate.
3. Place the person in a supine position, head slightly lower than the legs. If there are head and chest injuries or if respiration is impaired, it may be necessary to keep the head and chest slightly elevated.
4. Do not add heat, but prevent loss of body heat if necessary, by applying a cool compress to the client's forehead and covering the client with a light blanket.
5. Do not allow exertion. Keep the client quiet until emergency medical help arrives.

SEIZURES

Seizures may be caused by a specific disorder, brain injury, or medication. The OT should be able to recognize a seizure and take appropriate action to keep the client from getting hurt. A client having a seizure will usually become rigid for a few seconds and then begin to convulse with an all-over jerking motion. The client may turn blue and may stop breathing for up to 50 to 70 seconds. A client's sphincter control may be lost during or at the conclusion of the seizure, so the client may void urine or feces involuntarily.[7] When a client shows signs of entering a seizure, the following steps should be taken:[7]

1. Place the person in a safe location and position away from anything that might cause injury. *Do not* attempt to restrain or restrict the convulsions.
2. Loosen clothing around the person's neck to assist in keeping the client's airway open.
3. *Do not* insert any objects in the person's mouth; this can cause injury.
4. Remove sharp objects (glasses, furniture and other objects) from around the person to prevent injury.
5. When the convulsions subside, lay the person on his or her side to maintain an open airway and prevent the person from aspirating any secretions.
6. After the convulsions cease, have the client rest. He or she may experience confusion for a period of time. It may be helpful to cover the client with a blanket or screen to provide privacy.
7. Get medical help.

INSULIN-RELATED ILLNESSES

Many clients seen in OT have insulin-related episodes. These episodes can occur due to severely inadequate insulin levels (*hyperglycemia*) or from excessive insulin (*hypoglycemia*).[7] It is

TABLE **9-1** **Warning Signs and Symptoms of Insulin-Related Illnesses**

	Insulin Reaction (Insulin Shock)	Ketoacidosis (Diabetic Coma)
Onset	Sudden	Gradual
Skin	Moist, pale	Dry, flushed
Behavior	Excited, agitated	Drowsy
Breath odor	Normal	Fruity
Breathing	Normal to shallow	Deep, labored
Tongue	Moist	Dry
Vomiting	Absent	Present
Hunger	Present	Absent
Thirst	Absent	Present

very important for the OT to be able to differentiate between the conditions of hypoglycemia (insulin reaction) and hyperglycemia (ketoacidosis), which can lead to diabetic coma as shown in Table 9-1. Both conditions can result in a loss of consciousness, but medical intervention for each condition is very different.

An *insulin reaction* (also called insulin shock) can be caused by too much systemic insulin, the intake of too little food or sugar, or too much physical activity.[7] If the client is conscious, some form of sugar (e.g., candy or orange juice) should be provided. If the client is unconscious, glucose may have to be provided intravenously. The client should rest, and all physical activity should be stopped. This condition is not as serious as ketoacidosis, but the client should be given the opportunity to return to a normal state as soon as possible.

Hyperglycemia can develop when a person with diabetes fails to take enough insulin or deviates significantly from a prescribed diet. Ketoacidosis and dehydration occur, and can lead to a diabetic coma and eventual death if not treated.[7] It should be considered a medical emergency requiring prompt action, including assistance from qualified personnel. The client should not be given any form of sugar. Usually, an injection of insulin is needed, followed by IV fluids and salt. A nurse or physician should provide care as quickly as possible.

RESPIRATORY DISTRESS

Dyspnea control postures may be used to reduce breathlessness in clients in respiratory distress.[9] The client must be responsive and have an unobstructed airway. The *high-Fowler's* position (Figure 9-6, *A*) may be used for clients in bed. The head of the bed should be in an upright position at a 90° angle. If available, a footboard should be used to support the client's feet. The *orthopneic* position (Figure 9-6, *B*) may be used for clients who are sitting or standing. In either case, the client bends forward slightly at the waist and supports the upper body by leaning the forearms on a table or counter. Pursed-lip breathing, which is a breathing pattern of inhaling through the nose and slowly exhaling through pursed lips, can also help decrease dyspnea and respiratory rate[9] (see Chapter 44 for additional suggestions).

CHOKING AND CARDIAC ARREST

All healthcare practitioners should be trained to treat clients who are choking or suffering from a cardiac arrest. Specific training courses are offered by both the American Heart Association and the American Red Cross. *The following information is presented as a reminder of the basic techniques and is not meant to be substituted for training.*

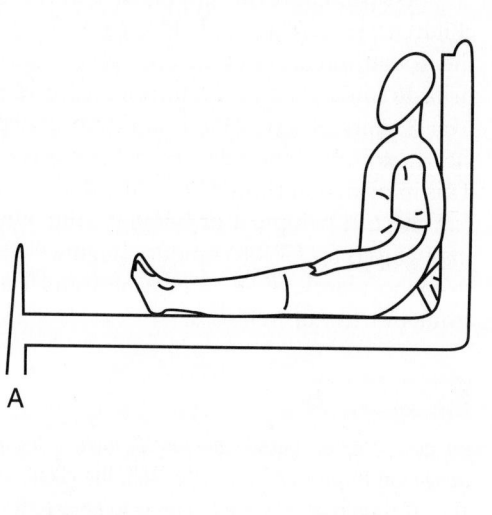

A

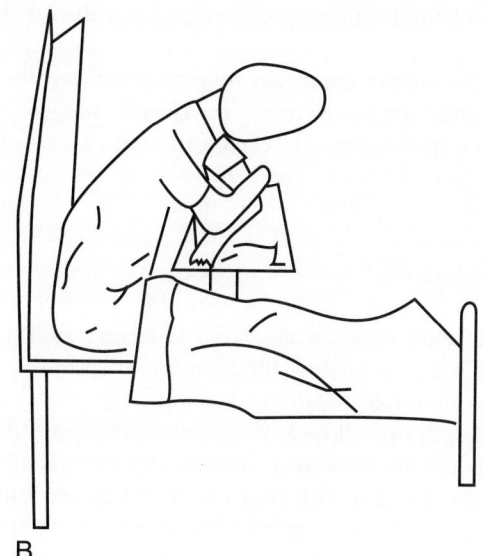

B

Figure 9-6 **A,** Orthopneic position. **B,** High-Fowler's position.

The urgency of choking cannot be overemphasized. Immediate recognition and proper action are essential. When assisting a conscious adult or a child who is more than 1 year old, the following steps should be taken:

1. Ask the client, "Are you choking?" If the client can speak, or cough effectively, *do not* interfere with the client's own attempts to expel the object.
2. If the client is unable to speak, cough, or breathe, check the mouth and remove any visible foreign object.
3. If the client is unable to speak or cough, position yourself behind the client. Clasp your hands over the client's abdomen, slightly above the umbilicus but below the diaphragm.
4. Use the closed fist of one hand, covered by your other hand, to give three or four abrupt thrusts against the person's abdomen by compressing the abdomen in and up forcefully (Heimlich maneuver). Continue to apply the thrusts until the obstruction becomes dislodged or is relieved, or the person becomes unconscious.
5. Seek medical assistance.

When assisting an unconscious adult or child who is more than 1 year old, the following steps should be taken:

1. Place the person in a supine position and call for medical help.
2. Open the person's mouth and use your finger to attempt to locate and remove the foreign object (finger sweep).
3. Open the airway by tilting the head back and lifting the chin forward. Attempt to ventilate using the mouth-to-mouth technique. If unsuccessful, kneel behind or over the person and deliver up to five abdominal thrusts (Heimlich maneuver), repeat the finger sweep, and attempt to ventilate. It may be necessary to repeat these steps. Be persistent and continue these procedures until the object is removed or medical assistance arrives.

It may be necessary to initiate CPR techniques to stabilize the person's cardiopulmonary functions after the object has been removed. The following procedures are recommended for CPR:[12]

1. Determine the client's condition by gently shaking the client and asking, "Are you all right?" or, "How do you feel?"
2. If there is no response, place the client in a supine position on a firm surface. Open the client's airway by lifting up on the chin and pushing down on the forehead to tilt the head back.
3. Check for respiration by observing the chest or abdomen for movement, listen for sounds of breathing, and feel for breath by placing your cheek close to the person's mouth. If no sign of breath is present, the client is not breathing, and you should initiate breathing techniques.
4. Pinch the client's nose closed and maintain the head tilt to open the airway. Place your mouth over the client's mouth and form a seal with your lips. Perform two full breaths, then evaluate the circulation. Some persons prefer to place a clean cloth over the client's lips before initiating mouth-to-mouth respirations. If available, a plastic intubation device can be used to decrease the contact between the caregiver's mouth and the client's mouth and any saliva or vomitus.
5. Palpate the carotid artery for a pulse. Sometimes it can be difficult to locate a pulse, so also observe the client for signs of life—breathing, movement, consciousness. If there is no pulse or signs of consciousness, you must begin external chest compressions.
6. To initiate chest compressions, kneel next to the client, place the heel of one hand on the inferior portion of the sternum just proximal to the xiphoid process, and place your other hand on top of the first hand. Position your shoulders directly over the client's sternum, keep your elbows extended, and press down firmly, depressing the sternum approximately 1 1/2 to 2 inches with each compression. Relax after each compression, but do not remove your hands from the sternum. The relaxation and compression phases should be equal in duration. This can be accomplished by mentally counting "one thousand one," "one thousand two," "one thousand three," and so on for each phase.
7. If you perform all CPR procedures without assistance, you should perform 30 chest compressions and then perform two breaths. You must compress at the rate of approximately 100 times per minute. Continue these procedures until qualified assistance arrives or the client is able to sustain independent respiration and circulation. If you are alone, attempt to gain assistance from other persons by calling loudly for help. If a second person is present, the person should contact an advanced medical assistance unit before beginning to assist with CPR. In most instances the client will require hospitalization and evaluation by a physician.

(*Note:* Extreme care must be used to open the airway of a person who may have experienced a cervical spine injury. In such cases, use the chin lift, but avoid the head tilt. If the technique does not open the airway, the head should be tilted slowly and gently until the airway is open.)

These procedures are appropriate to use for adults and for children 8 years of age and older. New CPR guidelines recommend that rescuers initiate emergency assistance (911, etc.) prior to initiating CPR on unresponsive adults and children over 8 years of age. CPR is contraindicated if clients have clearly expressed their desire for "do not resuscitate" (DNR). This information should be clearly documented in the medical chart. A pamphlet or booklet containing diagrams and instructions for CPR techniques (Figure 9-7) can be obtained from most local offices of the American Heart Association or from a variety of web sites.

SUMMARY

All occupational therapy personnel have a legal and professional obligation to promote safety for self, the client, visitors, and others. The OT should be prepared to react to emergency situations quickly, decisively, and calmly. The consistent use of safe practices helps reduce accidents for both clients and workers and reduces the length and cost of treatment.

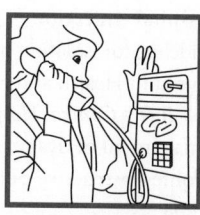

STEP 1

Call 911

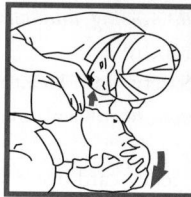

STEP 2

Tilt head,
lift chin,
check
breathing

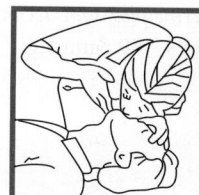

STEP 3

Give two
breaths

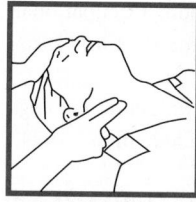

STEP 4

Check
pulse

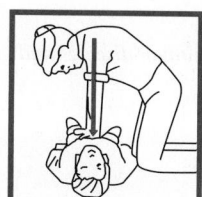

STEP 5

Position
hands in the
center of
the chest

STEP 6

Firmly
push down
2 inches
on the chest
30 times

**Continue with two breaths
and 30 pumps until help arrives**

Figure 9-7 Standard CPR. (From *www.learncpr.org/pocket.html.*)

THREADED CASE STUDY: DONNA, PART 2

To adequately prepare the OT clinic as a safe environment for clients and staff, clear policies and procedures pertaining to client safety, medical emergencies, client safety, infection control, and precautions with special equipment need to be developed and implemented. In the case study presented at the beginning of this chapter, Donna, the Director of OT Services, was responsible for developing such policies and procedures. It should be mandatory for all OT personnel to become certified in CPR and first aid. Employee manuals can be produced that orient staff to general safety procedures and infection control standards. Furthermore, inservice education should be developed for newly hired personnel that familiarizes them with the types of specialized medical equipment that occupational therapy personnel are likely to encounter in their interventions with clients.

There are many resources available that can assist Donna in establishing these policies and procedures. The Centers for Disease Control and Prevention (*www.cdc.gov*), the Occupational Safety and Health Administration (*www.OSHA.gov*), and the National Institutes of Health (*www.NIH.gov*) are government organizations that provide the most current information pertaining to health standards, infection control, medical research, and workplace safety. Information on first aid, choking, and CPR can be obtained from most local offices of the American Heart Association and from the American National Red Cross. In addition, information on emergency procedures may be found at a variety of web sites.

Review Questions

1. Why is it important to teach the client and significant others guidelines for handling various emergency situations?
2. Describe at least four behaviors you can adopt to improve client safety.
3. Why is it important to review a client's chart prior to initiating intervention?
4. What types of activities are appropriate when providing intervention to a client that is ventilator dependent? What precautions must be taken during such activities?
5. Define the following: IV line, A line, NG tube, TPN or hyperalimentation, and catheter.
6. Describe standard precautions.
7. Why is it important to follow standard precautions with all clients?
8. Demonstrate the proper technique for hand washing.
9. How should you respond to a client emergency?
10. Distinguish between an insulin reaction and ketoacidosis (diabetic coma). What is the appropriate medical intervention for each condition?
11. Describe how you would help a client who is falling forward and one who is falling backward?
12. Which emergency situations might require getting advanced medical assistance and which situations could a therapist handle alone?

REFERENCES

1. American Occupational Therapy Association: Occupational therapy code of ethics, *Am J Occup Ther* 54:614, 2000.

2. American Occupational Therapy Association: Occupational therapy practice framework: domain and process, *Am J Occup Ther* 56(6):609, 2002.

3. Bolander VB, editor: *Sorensen and Luckmann's basic nursing: a psychophysiologic approach*, ed 3, Philadelphia, 1994, WB Saunders.

4. Centers for Disease Control and Prevention: Guideline for hand hygiene in health-care settings, *MMWR* 51(RR-16):1, 2002.

5. Dubois R: Preventing complications of immobility. In Bolander, VB, editor: *Sorensen and Luckmann's basic nursing: a psychophysiologic approach*, ed 3, Philadelphia, 1994, WB Saunders.

6. Ekelman Ranke BA, Moriarty MP: An overview of professional liability in occupational therapy, *Am J Occup Ther* 51(8):671, 1996.

7. Frazier MS, Drzymkowski JW: *Essentials of human diseases and conditions*, ed 3, St Louis, 2004, Elsevier.

8. Garner JS, Hospital Infection Control Practices Advisory Committee: Guideline for isolation precautions in hospitals: from the US Department of Health and Human Services, Centers for Disease Control, *Infect Control Hosp Epidemiol* 17:53, 1996.

9. Migliore A: Management of dyspnea: guidelines for practice for adults with chronic obstructive pulmonary disease, *OT Health Care* 18(3):1, 2004.

10. *Mosby's medical, nursing and allied health dictionary*, ed 6, St Louis, 2002, Mosby.

11. Occupational Safety and Health Administration: *Hospital etool: ergonomics*, http:www.osha,gov/SLTC, etools/hospital/index.html.

12. Ornato J: Emergency cardiovascular care: new guidelines for basic life support, *J Critical Illness* 16(9):416, 2001.

13. Pierson FM: *Principles and techniques of client care*, ed 2, Philadelphia, 1999, WB Saunders.

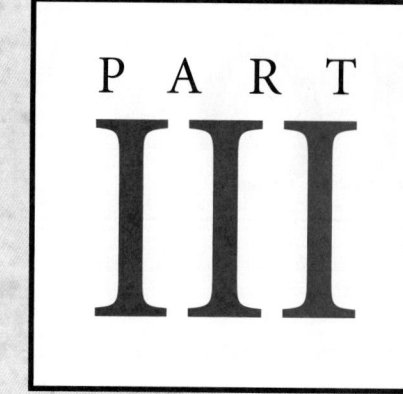

OCCUPATIONAL PERFORMANCE AND THE PERFORMANCE AREAS: EVALUATION AND INTERVENTION

10 ACTIVITIES OF DAILY LIVING

DIANE FOTI
LISA M. KANAZAWA

KEY TERMS

Activities of daily living
Instrumental activities of daily
  living

Client-centered approach
Levels of independence
Home assessment

Accessibility
Backward chaining

LEARNING OBJECTIVES

After studying this chapter the student or practitioner will be able to do the following:

1. Define activities of daily living (ADL) and instrumental activities of daily living (IADL).
2. Name two standardized tests of ADLs.
3. Describe a client-centered approach to evaluation.
4. Define levels of independence.
5. Explain the usual procedures for ADL and IADL assessments.
6. Explain the benefits of a home evaluation.

7. Explain how to record and summarize results of the ADL assessment and training program.
8. Discuss various methods of teaching ADLs.
9. Discuss considerations for selecting adaptive equipment.
10. Describe, perform, and teach ADL techniques for individuals with limited range of motion (ROM) and strength, incoordination, paraplegia, quadriplegia, and low vision.

CHAPTER OUTLINE

Definitions of ADLs and IADLs
Evaluation of areas of occupation
Considerations in ADL and IADL occupational analysis and training
ADL and IADL performance analysis
  General procedure
  Recording results of ADL assessment
Instrumental activities of daily living
  Home management assessment
  Home assessment
  Financial management
  Community mobility
  Health management and maintenance

ADL and IADL training
  Methods of teaching ADLs
  Recording progress in ADL performance
  Assistive technology and adaptive equipment
Specific ADL techniques
  ADLs for the person with limited ROM or strength
  ADLs for the person with incoordination
  ADLs for the person with hemiplegia or use of only one upper extremity
  ADLs for the person with paraplegia
  ADLs for the person with quadriplegia
  ADLs for the person with low vision
Summary

Anna is a 24-year-old woman who incurred a C7 *spinal cord injury* (SCI) from a car accident. She is currently in an inpatient rehabilitation program. Prior to her injury, Anna lived in a house with two bedrooms and one bathroom with her husband and two-year-old daughter. Anna's mother has been caring for her granddaughter since Anna's accident. Anna worked part-time as a bookkeeper and was active in her church.

Previously, Anna's typical weekday included driving her daughter to daycare in the morning while she worked. After lunch, she picked her daughter up from daycare and returned home to prepare meals, perform chores, tend to household money management, and shop. Anna's husband returned home before dinner, helped with their daughter's bedtime routine, and performed yard work around the home.

Anna and her husband are concerned about the amount of assistance they may require when Anna is discharged from the rehabilitation program. She expresses concern that she may need assistance with her personal care but really wants to be as independent as possible in that area. Ideally, she would like to be able to participate in her previous household duties, especially providing her daughter's care. Anna says she misses driving her daughter home from daycare and hearing her daughter tell about her day.

Critical Thinking Questions

1. What are the occupational areas Anna has identified as a priority for engagement?
2. What specific activities within those areas of occupation has Anna expressed a want or need to maximize her independence?
3. In addition to ADL training, what other assessments or intervention recommendations will be required?

Activities of daily living (ADLs) and **instrumental activities of daily living** (IADLs) are areas of occupation that include routine tasks of personal care, functional mobility, communication, home management, and community mobility.[2,8,27] Evaluation and training in the performance of these important life tasks have long been important aspects of *occupational therapy* (OT) programs in virtually every type of healthcare service. Loss of ability to care for personal needs and to manage the environment can result in loss of self-esteem and a deep sense of dependence. Family roles are also disrupted, requiring partners to assume the function of caregiver when one loses the ability to perform ADLs or IADLs independently.[23]

According to the Occupational Therapy Practice Framework, service delivery in the areas of occupation begins with the OT practitioner collecting information from the client, caregivers, and family members as appropriate to create an occupational profile. The OT practitioner and client collaborate to identify which areas of occupation, such as ADLs and IADLs, the client wants or needs to participate in and the specific activities that are important. The OT practitioner may also be involved in removing or reducing physical, cognitive, social, and emotional barriers that are interfering with performance of those occupations. The need to learn new methods or use assistive devices to perform daily tasks may be temporary or permanent, depending upon the particular dysfunction and the prognosis for recovery.

DEFINITIONS OF ADLs AND IADLs

Daily living activities can be separated into two areas: **activities of daily living** (ADLs) [also called *personal activities of daily living* (PADLs) and *basic activities of daily living* (BADLs)] and **instrumental activities of daily living** (IADLs). ADLs require basic skills, whereas IADLs require more advanced problem-solving skills, social skills, and more complex environmental interactions. ADL tasks include self-care, functional mobility, sexual activity, and sleep/rest.[2] IADL tasks include communication device use, health management and maintenance, financial management, meal preparation and cleanup, and community mobility (Box 10-1).

EVALUATION OF AREAS OF OCCUPATION

A comprehensive evaluation of occupational performance involves collaborating with the client to determine what he or she wants and needs to do and the barriers or supports to participation.[2] Areas of occupation include ADLs, IADLs, education, work, play, leisure, and social participation. The role of occupational therapy is to facilitate engagement in occupation to support participation in context(s).[2] It is important to help the individual with a disability to balance activity in each of these areas of occupation according to his or her personality, skills, limitations, needs, cultural values, and lifestyle.

The process of occupational therapy outlined by the Framework is described in three broad areas: evaluation, intervention, and outcomes. The client in this process may be defined as an individual, those in a group (family), or those in a population (community). The process is dynamic and interactive, client-centered, with the outcome comprising engagement in occupation.[2] In a **client-centered approach** the therapist collaborates with the client and/or the family/caregivers, centering the occupational therapy process on the client's priorities and fostering an active participation towards the outcome. Evaluation consists of creating an occupational profile and a performance analysis of skills and patterns and the factors that influence performance.

Box **10-1** Activities in ADL and IADL

ACTIVITIES OF DAILY LIVING (ADLs)

Bathing/showering
Bowel and bladder management
Dressing
Eating
Feeding
Functional mobility
Personal device care
Personal hygiene and grooming
Sexual activity
Sleep/rest
Toilet hygiene

INSTRUMENTAL ACTIVITIES OF DAILY LIVING (IADLs)

Care of others
Care of pets
Child rearing
Communication device use
Community mobility
Financial management
Health management and maintenance
Home establishment and management
Meal preparation and cleanup
Safety procedures and emergency responses
Shopping

Data from American Occupational Therapy Association: Occupational therapy practice framework: domain and process, *Am J Occup Ther* 56(6):620, 2002.

Using a top-down approach to the evaluation process, the therapist will begin to understand the client's occupational history and interests. The evaluation may include the charting of a daily or weekly schedule, an activities configuration, an interest checklist, or an occupational role history.[9,13,23,25,33] The activities configuration protocol can be used to gather data about the client's values, education, work history, and vocational interests and plans. The interest checklist can be used to determine the degree of interest in five categories of activities: manual skills, physical sports, social recreation, ADLs, and cultural and educational activities.[23] The occupational role history is used to indicate the balance between work and leisure roles.[13] Although the interest checklist and the occupational role history were developed for a psychiatric population, they can be adapted for application to clients with a physical dysfunction.

A bottom-up approach to the evaluation process focuses on identifying problems in specific performance skills or client factors. This approach may fail to identify how a deficit in a specific skill or client factor affects the client's ability to engage in a chosen occupation.[14] For example, a therapist determines

that a client has impaired fine motor control. A general evaluation may indicate that the client has difficulty with simple tasks such as tying shoes and buttoning clothes. After completing an interest checklist and occupational role history, the occupational therapist also determines that the fine motor control deficit will affect the client's job as a computer operator and limit her ability to continue with a hobby of jewelry making. Although these two approaches to evaluation are discussed separately, a skilled clinician blends the two in practice. Once a performance skill deficit is identified, the body function deficit that causes the performance skill deficit is identified. The therapist can then determine if it is possible to restore or provide remediation for the body function factor or if a compensatory method will be needed to improve occupational performance.

An interview and performance analysis can yield a well-rounded picture of the client's occupational performance. Deficits and imbalances in occupational performance will be apparent. The performance analysis is fundamental to the development of a comprehensive intervention plan. The assessments to be addressed in this chapter are for ADLs and IADLs. Work evaluation is assessment of specific work skills using real or simulated work situations[11] and is discussed in Chapter 13. Leisure activities are discussed in Chapter 15.

CONSIDERATIONS IN ADL AND IADL OCCUPATIONAL ANALYSIS AND TRAINING

The analysis of occupational performance in ADLs/IADLs includes observing the client's performance and noting skills and patterns and the factors that support them.[2] Performance skills such as strength, range of motion (ROM), coordination, sensation, and balance should be assessed to determine the potential for remediation and possible need for adaptive equipment. Perceptual and cognitive functions should be assessed to determine the potential for learning ADL skills. Specific assessments to identify and measure activity demands and client factors contribute information influencing ADL and IADL performance. General mobility in bed or wheelchair or ambulation should also be assessed and is discussed in more detail in Chapter 11.

OT PRACTICE NOTE

In addition to these relatively concrete and objective assessments, the occupational therapist should be familiar with the context of the occupation including the client's culture and the culture's values in relation to self-care, the sick role, family assistance, and independence. The values of the client and the client's peer group and culture should be important considerations in selecting objectives and initial activities in the ADL program. The demands of time and energy for the balance of activities in the client's day may influence how many ADLs can be performed independently.

The environment to which the client will return is an important consideration. Will the client live alone or with his or her family or a roommate? Will the client go to a skilled nursing facility or to a board and care home, and will the client go permanently or temporarily? Will the client return to work and community activities? The type and amount of assistance available in the home environment must be considered if the caregiver is to receive training to provide assistance and supervision.

The finances available for assistant care, special equipment, and home modifications are important considerations. For example, a client who must use a wheelchair for mobility and who has the financial resources necessary, may be willing and able to make major modifications in the home, such as installing an elevator, lowering kitchen counters, widening doorways, and replacing carpeting to accommodate a wheelchair lifestyle. A client with fewer financial resources may need the assistance of an occupational therapist in making less costly modifications, such as removing scatter rugs and door sills, installing a ramp at the entrance, and attaching a handheld shower head to the bathtub faucet.

The ultimate goal of any ADL and IADL training program is for the client and family to learn to adapt to the life changes that necessitated a referral to the occupational therapist. For the individual who values independence, the goal may be to achieve the maximal level of independence. It is important to note that this level is different for each client. For the client with mild muscle weakness in one arm, complete independence in ADLs may be the maximal. In contrast, for the individual with a high-level quadriplegia, self-feeding, oral hygiene, and communication activities with devices and assistance may be the maximal level of independence that can be expected.

For the individual whose culture does not value independence as highly as does Western culture, the occupational therapist may focus primarily on teaching the client and family to adapt. The focus would be on family training and identifying the activities of highest value to the client. The potential for independence depends upon each client's unique personal needs, values, capabilities, limitations, and social and environmental resources.

ADL AND IADL PERFORMANCE ANALYSIS

Performance analysis of ADLs and IADLs may include using a checklist as a guide for questioning and selection of performance activities as identified during the interview for the occupational profile. Several types of ADL and IADL checklists and standardized tests are available. They all cover similar categories and performance tasks.[5] The use of a standardized test will ensure a more objective assessment and provide a standard means of measurement. A standardized assessment tool can be used at a later time for reevaluation, and some assessments allow for comparison to a norm group. Asher[5] has developed an annotated index of assessment tools that can be used as a resource for selecting appropriate tools

TABLE **10-1** **Examples of Standardized Assessments for ADLs and IADLs**

ADL Assessments	IADL Assessments	Measures of ADLs and IADLs
Klein-Bell ADL Scale[16]	Assessment of Motor and Process Skills (AMPS)[12]	Canadian Occupational Performance Measure (COPM)[19]
Functional Independence Measure (FIM)[32]	Kitchen Task Assessment (KTA)[6]	Kohlman Evaluation of Living Skills (KELS)[18]

for evaluation. Some examples of standardized ADL and IADL assessments are listed in Table 10-1. The occupational therapist should review the literature periodically to learn about new assessments developed by occupational therapists and about those that have been developed as interdisciplinary assessments, such as the Assessment of Motor and Process Skills[12] and the Functional Independence Measure (FIM).[32]

GENERAL PROCEDURE

When data have been gathered about the client's physical, psychosocial, and environmental resources, the feasibility of ADL assessment or ADL training should be determined by the occupational therapist in concert with the client, supervising physician, and other members of the rehabilitation team. In some instances, ADL training should be delayed because of limitations of the client or in favor of more immediate intervention objectives that require the client's energy and participation.

The interview may serve as a screening device to help determine the need for further assessment by observation of performance. This need is determined by the therapist based on knowledge of the client, the dysfunction, and previous assessments. A partial or complete performance analysis is invaluable in assessing ADL performance. The interview alone can lead to inaccurate assumptions. The client may recall performance before the onset of the dysfunction, may have some confusion or memory loss, and may overestimate or underestimate individual abilities because there has been little opportunity to perform routine ADLs since the onset of the physical dysfunction.

Ideally, the occupational therapist assesses the performance of activities in the environment and context where they usually take place.[3] For example, a dressing assessment could be arranged early in the morning in the treatment facility when the client is dressed by nursing personnel, or in the client's home. Self-feeding assessment should occur at regular meal hours. If this timing is not possible, the assessment may be conducted during regular treatment sessions in the OT clinic under simulated conditions. Requiring the client to perform routine self-maintenance tasks at irregular times in an artificial environment may contribute to a lack of carry-over, especially for clients who have difficulty generalizing learning.

The therapist should select relatively simple and safe tasks from the ADL and IADL checklist and should progress to more difficult and complex items, including some that involve safety measures. The ADL assessment should not be completed at one time because this approach would cause fatigue and create an artificial situation. Tasks that would be unsafe or that obviously cannot be performed should be omitted and the appropriate notation made on the assessment form.

During the performance analysis, the therapist should observe the methods the client is using or attempting to use to accomplish the task and try to determine causes of performance problems. Common causes include weakness, spasticity, involuntary motion, perceptual deficits, cognitive deficits, and low endurance. If problems and their causes can be identified, the therapist has a good foundation for establishing training objectives, priorities, methods, and the need for assistive devices.

Other important aspects of this analysis that should not be overlooked are the client's need for respect and privacy and the ongoing interaction between the client and the therapist. The client's feelings about having his or her body viewed and touched should be respected. Privacy should be maintained for toileting, grooming, bathing, and dressing tasks. The therapist with whom the client is most familiar and comfortable may be the appropriate person to conduct ADL assessment and training. As the therapist interacts with the client during performance of daily living tasks, it may be possible to elicit the client's attitudes and feelings about the particular tasks, priorities in training, dependence and independence, and cultural, family, and personal values and customs regarding performance of ADLs.

RECORDING RESULTS OF ADL ASSESSMENT

During the interview and performance analysis, the therapist makes appropriate notations on the checklists. If a standardized assessment is used, the standard terminology identified for that assessment is used to describe or measure performance. Nonstandardized tests may include separate checklists for self-care, home management, mobility, and home environment assessments. When describing **levels of independence,**

occupational therapists often use terms like *maximum, moderate,* and *minimal assistance*. These quantitative terms have little meaning to healthcare professionals unless they are defined, or unless supporting statements are included in progress summaries to give specific meanings for each. It also should be specified whether the level of independence refers to a single activity, a category of activities such as dressing, or all ADLs. In designating levels of independence, an agreed-upon performance scale should be used to mark the ADL checklist. The following general categories and their definitions are suggested:

1. *Independent:* can perform the activity or activities without cueing, supervision, or assistance, with or without assistive devices, at normal or near normal speeds. If the client requires assistive devices or an adaptive environment to perform the activity but no other assistance, the term *modified independence* may be used.

2. *Supervised:* can perform the activity alone but needs someone available for safety. In many settings, the terms *standby assist* (verbal cue) and *contact guard* (physical cue) may also be used to indicate a safety concern in the client's performance of an activity.

3. *Minimal assistance:* supervision, cueing, or less than 20% physical assistance.

4. *Moderate assistance:* supervision, cueing, and 20% to 50% physical assistance.

5. *Maximal assistance:* supervision, cueing, and 50% to 80% physical assistance.

6. *Dependent:* can perform only one or two steps of the activity or very few activities independently, may fatigue easily and perform very slowly, may require elaborate equipment and devices to perform basic skills such as feeding, needs more than 80% physical assistance.

These definitions are broad and general. They can be modified to suit the approach of the particular treatment facility.

Information from the ADL assessment is summarized succinctly for inclusion in the client's permanent record so that it can be referred to by interested professional co-workers. A sample case study (Loretta), with resulting ADL and home management checklists, and summaries of an initial assessment and progress report are included in Figures 10-1 and 10-2. When reviewing these, the reader should keep in mind that the assessment and progress summaries relate only to the ADL and IADL portions of the intervention program.

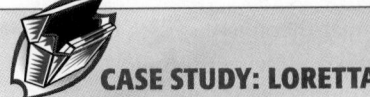 **CASE STUDY: LORETTA**

Loretta is a 72-year-old married woman who incurred a cerebral thrombosis resulting in a *cerebrovascular accident* (CVA) 3 months ago. She lives in a modest home with her husband. Loretta was active before her CVA, volunteering 10 hours a week at a local charity thrift store, walking a mile a day with friends, and caring for her husband, who is diabetic and has poor vision. She was independent with all of the indoor home management activities. She and her husband have a gardener, but Loretta enjoyed gardening with potted plants.

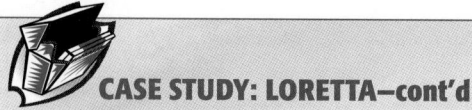

CASE STUDY: LORETTA—cont'd

The CVA resulted in an ataxic gait, mild *dysarthria* (slurred speech), *dysphagia* (swallowing deficit), and slight hand incoordination. Loretta is easily frustrated and concerned about how she and her husband will manage, since her adult children live 5 hours away. She was referred to OT for evaluation and training in ADLs and IADLs and for treatment of dysphagia.

The initial evaluation process involved an interview with the client and her husband to create an occupational profile. Based on the priorities and problems identified by the client and her husband, the occupational performance analysis included the use of the Kitchen Task Assessment and an ADL performance evaluation. The evaluation was completed in a 1-hour session. Loretta became restless after 15 minutes, but with redirection continued to attend to the tasks. Loretta is independent with eating, upper body dressing, and grooming while seated. Loretta is independent with toileting. She has been receiving maximum assistance for lower body dressing and bathing. She has difficulty with handwriting, use of the telephone, and handling keys. She requires moderate assistance to walk, using a *front-wheeled walker* (FWW), but is independent with wheelchair mobility on flat surfaces. Her visual fields are intact. She has no visual-spatial deficit. Her upper extremity strength and range of motion are *within normal limits* (WNL). Hand coordination is mildly impaired, as demonstrated with moderate difficulty pushing buttons on the phone and shoe tying. She is able to stand while holding on to a stable surface but cannot use her hands for a task while standing.

Results of the Kitchen Task Assessment[5] demonstrated deficits in organization of the task, at which point she required physical assistance. Loretta is highly motivated and has the potential to do simple, hot meal preparation and basic self-care independently, except for showering, for which she requires supervision.

A swallow assessment demonstrated moderately impaired tongue coordination and minimal delay with a swallow. Loretta has already modified her diet by selecting very soft foods and slightly thickened liquids.

Progress Report

Loretta has attended OT two times a week for 4 weeks. She is generally cooperative and motivated, although periodically she becomes discouraged as she continues to have an ataxic gait and requires the use of the wheelchair for independent mobility. Treatment has focused on lower extremity dressing, oral-motor exercises to improve swallowing, and simple meal preparation. Loretta has made significant progress in the treatment program. She has progressed from maximum assistance with lower extremity dressing to independent while seated. She has improved from chair-level grooming to standing with one-hand stabilization while using the other to brush her hair and teeth. Progress has been made from maximum assistance with bathing to supervised with transfer to a shower seat. From moderate difficulty with use of phone, she has progressed to independent, and from dependent with oral-motor exercises she has progressed to supervised. Loretta is now independent in cold meal preparation after initially requiring maximum assistance.

Loretta continues to require a soft diet and slightly thickened liquids because of swallowing difficulties. She is consistent with use of safety techniques for swallowing. She continues to have impaired hand coordination but is learning compensatory techniques to adapt her method of performing various ADL tasks as demonstrated with her progress in ADLs.

Occupational therapy has coordinated treatment and goals with the physical therapist and social worker. The therapist has recommended that the social worker refer the client's husband to a low vision center for evaluation, since he was dependent on his wife and never received instruction in low vision training. His independence will relieve some of Loretta's burden of care giving.

Occupational therapy will focus on hot meal preparation, bed making, and exploring leisure interests with gardening, along with continuing to work toward improvement of oral-motor and hand coordination.

INSTRUMENTAL ACTIVITIES OF DAILY LIVING

HOME MANAGEMENT ASSESSMENT

Home management tasks are assessed similarly to self-care tasks. First, the client should be interviewed to elicit a description of the home and of former and present home management responsibilities. Tasks the client needs to perform when returning home, as well as those that he or she would like to perform, should be ascertained during the interview. If the client has a communication disorder or a cognitive deficit, aid from friends or family members may be enlisted to get the information needed. The client may also be questioned about his or her ability to perform each task on the activities list. The assessment is much more meaningful and accurate if the interview is followed by a performance assessment in the

ADL kitchen or apartment of the treatment facility, or if possible, in the client's home.

The therapist should select tasks and exercise safety precautions consistent with the client's capabilities and limitations. The initial tasks should be simple one- or two-step procedures that are not hazardous, such as wiping a dish, sponging a table top, and turning the water on and off. As the assessment progresses, tasks graded in complexity and involving safety precautions should be performed, such as making a sandwich and a cup of coffee and vacuuming the carpet.

Home management skills apply to women, men, and sometimes adolescents and children. Individuals may live independently or share home management responsibilities with their partners. In some homes, it is necessary for a role

Text continued on p. 158

OCCUPATIONAL THERAPY DEPARTMENT
ACTIVITIES OF DAILY LIVING

Name _Loretta_   Age _72_   Diagnosis _CVA_

Disability _ataxia; dysarthria; dysphagia; hand incoordination_

Activity Precautions _none_

Mode of Ambulation _w/c; FWW with mod A_   Hand Dominance _R_

Previous Functional Level _Independent_

Social/Home environment _Pt. is caregiver to husband; lives in own home_

Grading Key:
- I = Independent
- S = Supervised
- Min A = Minimal Assistance
- Mod A = Moderate Assistance
- Max A = Maximum Assistance
- D = Dependent
- N/A = Not applicable
- N/T = Not tested

TRANSFERS AND AMBULATION

Date	1/29	2/24		Remarks
Tub or shower	Mod A	S		2° to slippery surfaces
Toilet	I	I		
Wheelchair	I	I		
Bed and chair	I	I		
Ambulation	Mod A	Min A		FWW
Wheelchair mgt.	I	I		On flat surfaces
Car	N/T	S		

FUNCTIONAL BALANCE

Date	1/29	2/24		Remarks
Sitting	I	I		
Standing	Mod A	S		Must use hands for balance
Walking	Mod A	Min A		FWW

EATING

Date	1/29	2/24		Remarks
Butter bread	I	I		
Cut meat	I	I		With effort and built-up handle
Eat with spoon	I	I		
Eat with fork	I	I		
Drink w/ straw	I	I		
Drink w/ glass	I	I		
Drink w/ mug	I	I		
Pour from pitcher	N/T	I		

UNDRESS

Date	1/29	2/24		Remarks
Underwear	Max A	I		
Slip/undershirt	I	I		
Dress	N/A	N/A		
Skirt	N/A	N/A		
Blouse/shirt	Min A	I		Difficulty with buttons
Slacks/jeans	Max A	I		
Necktie	N/A	N/A		

Figure 10-1 ADL evaluation form.

UNDRESS (continued)

Date	1/29	2/24		Remarks
Nylons	N/T	N/A		
Housecoat/robe	Min A	I		To pull robe up
Jacket	I	I		
Belt/suspenders	N/A	N/A		
Hat	N/T	I		
Coat	N/T	I		
Sweater	I	I		
Mittens/gloves	N/T	I		
Glasses	I	I		
Brace	N/A	N/A		
Shoes	Max A	I		
Socks	Max A	I		
Boots	Max A	N/T		

DRESS

Date	1/29	2/24		Remarks
Underwear	Max A	I		
Slip/undershirt	I	I		
Dress	N/A	N/A		
Skirt	N/A	N/A		
Blouse/shirt	Min A	I		Difficulty with buttons
Slacks/jeans	Max A	I		
Necktie	N/A	N/A		
Nylons	N/T	N/A		
Housecoat/robe	Max A	I		To pull robe down
Jacket	I	I		
Belt/suspenders	N/A	N/A		
Hat	N/T	I		
Coat	N/T	I		
Sweater	I	I		
Mittens/gloves	N/T	I		
Glasses	I	I		
Brace	N/A	N/A		
Shoes	Max A	I		
Socks	Max A	I		
Boots	Max A	N/T		

FASTENERS

Date	1/29	2/24		Remarks
Button	Min A	I		
Snap	Min A	I		
Zipper	I	I		
Hook and eye	N/A	N/A		
Untie shoes	Max A	I		
Velcro	N/A	N/A		

HYGIENE

Date	1/29	2/24		Remarks
Blow nose	I	I		
Wash face/hands	I	I		While seated
Wash upper body	I	I		While seated
Wash lower body	Max A	I		
Brush teeth	I	I standing		While seated
Brush dentures	N/A	N/A		

Figure 10-1, cont'd

Continued

HYGIENE (continued)

Date	1/29	2/24		Remarks
Brush/comb hair	/	/ standing		While seated
Curl hair	N/A	N/A		
Shave	N/A	N/A		
Apply makeup	N/T	/		
Clean fingernails	N/T	/		
Trim nails	N/T	S		
Apply deodorant	/	/		While seated
Shampoo hair	Min A	/		Needs items in reach
Use toilet paper	/	/		
Use tampons/napkins	N/A	N/A		

MEDICATION MANAGEMENT

Date	1/29	2/24		Remarks
Identify proper medication	N/T	/		
Open bottle	N/T	/		
Handle pills	N/T	/		Needs pill organizer
Manage syringe	N/T	Min A		Did this for husband before CVA
Draw medication	N/T	Min A		

COMMUNICATION

Date	1/29	2/24		Remarks
Verbal	/	/		Dysarthric
Read	/	/		
Hold book	/	/		
Turn page	/	/		
Write	Mod A	/		Poor legibility
Use telephone	Mod A	/		
Type/keyboard	N/T	N/T		
Handle mail	N/T	N/T		

COMBINED PERFORMANCE ACTIVITIES

Date	1/29	2/24		Remarks
Open/close door	Max A	/		
Remove/replace objects	/	/		
Carry objects while walking/wheeling	Max A	/		From wheelchair
Retrieve object from floor	Max A	/		With reacher

OPERATE

Date	1/29	2/24		Remarks
Light switches	/	/		
Doorbell	/	/		
Door locks/handles	/	/		From wheelchair
Faucets	/	/		From wheelchair
Shades/curtains	N/T	N/T		
Open/close window	N/T	N/T		
Hang up garment	N/T	/		From wheelchair

SUMMARY OF EVALUATION RESULTS

SENSORY STATUS

Date	1/29		2/24				Remarks
Intact (IN) or impaired (IM)	IN	IM	IN	IM	IN	IM	
Touch	✓		✓				

Figure 10-1, cont'd

SENSORY STATUS (continued)

Date	1/29		2/24				Remarks
Intact (IN) or impaired (IM)	IN	IM	IN	IM	IN	IM	
Pain	✓		✓				
Temperature	✓		✓				
Proprioception		✓		✓			
Stereognosis	✓		✓				
Visual fields	✓		✓				

PERCEPTUAL/COGNITIVE

Date	1/29		2/24				Remarks
Intact (IN) or impaired (IM)	IN	IM	IN	IM	IN	IM	
Follows directions	✓		✓				
Orientation	✓		✓				
Memory	✓		✓				
Attention span		✓	✓				*Needed redirection after 15 min*
Problem solving		✓	✓				*KTA—problems with organization*
Visual spatial	✓		✓				
Left/right discrimination	✓		✓				
Motor planning	✓		✓				

FUNCTIONAL RANGE OF MOTION

Date	1/29		2/24				Remarks
Intact (IN) or impaired (IM)	IN	IM	IN	IM	IN	IM	
Comb hair	✓		✓				
Feed self	✓		✓				
Fasten buttons	✓		✓				*Impaired coordination*
Pull up back of pants	✓		✓				
Zip zipper	✓		✓				
Tie shoes	✓		✓				*ROM WNL; impaired balance*
Reach self	✓		✓				*From wheelchair*
Stoop	✓		✓				*Balance impaired*

STRENGTH: indicate muscle grade

Date	1/29		2/24				Remarks
Left (L) or right (R)	L	R	L	R	L	R	
Head/neck	WNL	WNL	WNL	WNL			
Shoulder flexion	WNL	WNL	WNL	WNL			
Shoulder extension	WNL	WNL	WNL	WNL			
Elbow flexion	WNL	WNL	WNL	WNL			
Elbow extension	WNL	WNL	WNL	WNL			
Supination	WNL	WNL	WNL	WNL			
Pronation	WNL	WNL	WNL	WNL			
Wrist extension	WNL	WNL	WNL	WNL			
Wrist flexion	WNL	WNL	WNL	WNL			
Gross grasp	WNL	WNL	WNL	WNL			

COORDINATION

Date	1/29		2/24				Remarks
Left (L) or right (R)	L	R	L	R	L	R	
Fine motor	IM	IM	IM				*2/24 slightly improved; pt. is compensating for deficits*
Gross U.E.	IM	IM	IM				

Figure 10-1, cont'd

OCCUPATIONAL THERAPY DEPARTMENT
ACTIVITIES OF HOME MANAGEMENT

Name _Loretta_   Date _1/29 (Initial eval)_
Address _Anytown, USA_
Age _72_   Role in Family _Wife, caregiver_
Diagnosis _CVA_
Activity Precautions _None_

DESCRIPTION OF HOME
Owns home _X_   Apartment _____   Board & care _____
   No. of rooms _7_   Bathroom description _____
   No. of floors _1_   _Small 27" wide door_
   Stairs   _3 to enter_   _Tub - shower combination_
   Elevator   _N/A_   _Closed sink_

Will client be required to perform the following activities? If not, who will perform? x = yes

   Meal preparation   _X_
   Serving   _X_
   Wash dishes   _X_
   Shopping   ___   _Will need assist as she isn't driving_
   Child care   _N/A_
   Laundry   _X_
   Housecleaning   ___   _Will hire housekeeper_
   Pet care   _X_
   Sewing   _no_
   Hobbies   _X_   _Volunteer work_

Does the client really like housework?   _Yes_

Grading Key: I   =   Independent
                 S   =   Supervised
                 Min A = Minimal Assistance
                 Mod A = Moderate Assistance
                 Max A = Maximum Assistance
                 D   =   Dependent
                 N/A =   Not applicable
                 N/T =   Not tested

MEAL PREPARATION

Date	1/29	2/24		Remarks
Manage faucets	S	I		To stand
Handle stove controls	S	S		
Open packages	S	I		
Carry items	Max A	I		From wheelchair
Open cans	N/T	I		
Open jars	N/T	I		
Handle milk carton	I	I		
Empty garbage	N/T	N/T		
Retrieve refrigerator items	S	I		
Reach cupboards	S	I		
Peel vegetables	N/T	I		
Cut safely	N/T	I		

Figure 10-2   Activities of home management.

MEAL PREPARATION (continued)

Date	1/29	2/24		Remarks
Break eggs	N/T	N/T		
Use electric mixer	N/T	N/T		
Use toaster	N/T	I		
Use coffee maker	N/T	I		
Use microwave	N/T	I		
Manage oven	N/T	S to Min A		
Pour hot water	N/T	S		

SET UP/CLEAN UP FOR MEAL PREPARATION

Date	1/29	2/24		Remarks
Set table	S	I		From wheelchair
Carry items to table	Max A	I		With wheelchair
Load/empty dishwasher	N/T	I		
Wash dishes	Mod A	I		
Wash pots and pans	Mod A	I		Fatigued rapidly
Wipe counters/stove	S	I		To stand
Wring out dishcloth	S	I		

CLEANING ACTIVITIES

Date	1/29	2/24		Remarks
Pick up object from floor	N/T	I		
Wipe spills	N/T	S		
Make bed	N/T	N/T		
Use dust mop	N/T	N/T		
Dust high surfaces	N/T	N/T		
Dust low surfaces	N/T	N/T		
Mop floor	N/T	N/T		
Sweep	N/T	N/T		
Use dust pan	N/T	N/T		
Vacuum	N/T	N/T		
Clean tub and toilet	N/T	N/T		
Change sheets	N/T	N/T		
Carry pail of water	N/T	N/T		
Carry cleaning tools	N/T	N/T		

LAUNDRY/CLEANING ACTIVITIES

Date	1/29	2/24		Remarks
Do hand washing	N/T	I		
Wring out clothes	N/T	I		
Hang clothing	N/T	S		
Carry laundry to and from washer and dryer	N/T	N/T		
Manage controls on appliances	N/T	I		
Use washing machine	N/T	I		
Retrieve clothes from dryer	N/T	S		
Iron	N/T	N/T		

HEAVY HOUSEHOLD ACTIVITIES, WHO WILL DO THESE?

Date	1/29	2/24		Remarks
Clean stove and oven	N/T	D		
Clean refrigerator	N/T	Mod A		
Shopping	N/T	Mod A		

Figure 10-2 Cont'd

Continued

HEAVY HOUSEHOLD ACTIVITIES, WHO WILL DO THESE?
LAUNDRY/CLEANING ACTIVITIES (continued)

Date	1/29	2/24		Remarks
Put away groceries	N/T	Mod A		
Wash windows	N/T	D		
Change light bulbs	N/T	D		
Wash bathtub	N/T	D		
Maintain smoke alarms	N/T	D		
Recycle/compost	N/T	Mod A		

MISCELLANEOUS LAUNDRY/CLEANING ACTIVITIES

Date	1/29	2/24		Remarks
Retrieve newspaper	N/T	I		Needs reacher
Retrieve mail	N/T	N/T		
Feed pet	N/T	I		With reacher
Manage pet waste	N/T	D		
Let pet in and out	N/T	I		
Reach thermostat	N/T	I		
Thread needle/knot	N/T	N/T		
Sew on button	N/T	N/T		
Use scissors	N/T	N/T		
Water houseplants	N/T	N/T		

WORK HEIGHTS (Indicate best height)   *1/29 - evaluation*

Ironing	N/A
Cutting	Wheelchair level approx 31"
Dish washing	Standard sink adequate
General work	31"
Maximal depth of counter (reach)	16" (for side reach)
Maximal height of work surface	31"
Maximal reach for high cupboards	43"
Maximal reach for low cupboards	9"
Best height for chair	20-23"

SUGGESTIONS FOR HOME MODIFICATION:

- Transfer tub bench / bathtub mat / grab bar in shower
- Shower hose
- 3 in 1 commode for use at night beside bed & over toilet during day
- Widen bathroom door to 32"

Figure 10-2, Cont'd

reversal to occur after the onset of a physical disability, and the partner who usually stays at home may seek employment outside the home, while the disabled individual remains at home. In Anna's case, she has stated she would like to participate in previous home management activities. Anna's occupational therapist will collaborate with her on prioritizing tasks to be addressed during intervention. Meanwhile, Anna's mother is available to perform these tasks with direction from Anna.

If a client will be home alone, there are several basic ADL and IADL skills needed for safety and independence. Minimal ADL skills include independence with toileting and transfers, allowance for rest periods, and use of the telephone or special call system in case of emergency. Minimal IADL skills required to stay at home alone include the ability to[1] prepare or retrieve a simple meal,[2] employ safety precautions and exhibit good judgment,[3] take medication, and get emergency aid[4] if needed. The occupational therapist can assess potential for remaining at home alone through the activities of home management assessment. A child with a permanent disability also needs to be considered for assessment and training for IADL skills as he or she develops and matures with a growing need for independence.

HOME ASSESSMENT

When discharge from the treatment facility is anticipated, a **home assessment** should be carried out to facilitate the client's maximal independence in the living environment. Ideally, the occupational and physical therapists should perform the home assessment together. During the home visit, the client and family members or housemates must be present. Budget and time factors may not allow two professional workers to go to the client's home or may prohibit a home visit altogether. Therefore, the rehabilitation team along with the client and family members should identify the most serious concerns and develop a plan to address them. Figure 10-3 shows a home safety checklist. Family members or housemates could take pictures and measurements of the home and/or draw floor plans. The home assessment may also be referred to the home health agency that will provide home care services to the client.

The client and a family member should be interviewed to determine the client and family's expectations and the roles the client will assume in the home and community. The cultural or family values regarding a disabled member may influence role expectations and whether independence will be encouraged. Willingness and financial ability to make modifications in the home can also be determined.[31]

Sufficient time should be scheduled for the home visit so that the client can demonstrate the required functional mobility skills. The therapist may also wish to ask the client to demonstrate selected self-care and home management tasks in the home environment. During the assessment, the client should use the ambulation aids and any assistive devices that he or she is accustomed to using. The therapist should bring a tape measure to measure the width of doorways, the height of stairs, the height of the bed, and other dimensions. A digital camera can be useful to record arrangement of furniture, placement of bathroom fixtures, and other architectural structures/possible barriers for later reference when problem solving solutions.

 ETHICAL CONSIDERATIONS

Informed consent for photographing in the home should be obtained from the client prior to the home visit.

The therapist can begin by explaining the purposes and procedure of the home assessment to the client and others present, if this has not been done before the visit. The therapist can proceed to take the required measurements while surveying the general arrangement of rooms, furniture, and appliances. It may be helpful to sketch the size and arrangement of rooms for later reference and attach these sketches to the home assessment checklist (Figure 10-4). For more information on a variety of checklists, see Letts and associates.[20] Next, the client demonstrates functional mobility skills and essential self-care and home management tasks. The client's ability to use the entrance to the home and to transfer to and from an automobile, if it is to be used, should be included in the home assessment.

During the performance assessment the therapist should observe safety factors, ease of mobility and performance, and limitations imposed by the environment. If the client needs assistance for transfers and other activities, the caregiver should be instructed in the methods that are appropriate. The client may also be instructed in methods to improve maneuverability and simplify performance of tasks in a small space.

At the end of the assessment, the therapist can make a list of problems, recommended modifications, and additional safety equipment and assistive devices that are needed. The most common changes are the following:[31]

1. Installation of a ramp or railings at the entrance to the home
2. Removal of scatter rugs, extra furniture, and bric-a-brac
3. Removal of door sills
4. Addition of safety grab bars around the toilet and bathtub
5. Rearrangement of furniture to accommodate a wheelchair
6. Rearrangement of kitchen storage
7. Lowering of the clothes rod in the closet

Access into the bathroom and maneuvering with a wheelchair or walker are common problems. Frequently, a bedside commode is recommended until a bathroom can be made accessible or modified to allow independence with toileting (Figure 10-5). Shower seats can be used in the tub if a client can transfer over the edge of the tub, and also may be used in a shower. A transfer tub bench (Figure 10-6) is recommended for individuals who cannot safely or independently step over the edge of the tub. Installation of a hand-held shower hose increases access to the water and also eliminates risky turns and standing while bathing. The ADA Accessibility Guidelines for Buildings and Facilities are available at *www.access-board.gov/ adaag/html/adaag.htm*. When the home assessment is completed, the therapist should write a report summarizing the information on the form and describing the client's performance in the home. The report should conclude with a summary of the environmental barriers and the client's functional limitations that were encountered. Recommendations should include equipment or alterations needed with specific details about size, building specifications, costs, and sources. Recommendations may also include further functional goals to improve independence in the individual's home environment.

The therapist should carefully review all recommendations with the client and family. This review should be done with

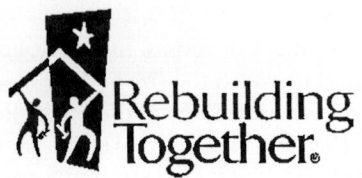

Home Safety Checklist

Created in partnership with the Administration on Aging

Rebuilding Together
1536 16th Street NW
Washington, DC 20036
800-4-REHAB-9
www.rebuildingtogether.org

Use this list to identify fall hazards and accessibility issues of the homeowner and family members. Home modification strategies on the reverse side of this page can help prioritize your work. Underline or use a highlighter to note problems and add comments.

1. EXTERIOR ENTRANCES AND EXITS
- ☐ Note condition of walk and drive surface; existence of curb cuts
- ☐ Note handrail condition, right and left sides
- ☐ Note light level for driveway, walk, porch
- ☐ Check door threshold height
- ☐ Note ability to use knob, lock, key, mailbox, peephole, and package shelf
- ☐ Do door and window locks work?

2. INTERIOR DOORS, STAIRS, HALLS
- ☐ Note height of door threshold, knob and hinge types; clear width door opening; determine direction that door swings
- ☐ Note presence of floor level changes
- ☐ Note hall width, adequate for walker/wheelchair
- ☐ Determine stair flight run: straight or curved
- ☐ Note stair rails: condition, right and left side
- ☐ Examine light level, clutter hazards
- ☐ Note floor surface texture and contrast

3. BATHROOM
- ☐ Are basin and tub faucets, shower control and drain plugs manageable?
- ☐ Are hot water pipes covered?
- ☐ Is mirror height appropriate, sit and stand?
- ☐ Note ability reach shelf above, below basin
- ☐ Note ability to step in and out of the bath and shower
- ☐ Can resident use bath bench in tub or shower?
- ☐ Note toilet height; ability to reach paper; flush; come from sit to stand posture
- ☐ Is space available for caregiver to assist?

4. KITCHEN
- ☐ Note overall light level, task lighting
- ☐ Note sink and counter heights
- ☐ Note wall and floor storage shelf heights
- ☐ Are undersink hot water pipes covered?
- ☐ Is there under counter knee space?
- ☐ Is there a nearby surface to rest hot foods on when removed from oven?
- ☐ Note stove control location (rear or front)

5. LIVING, DINING, BEDROOM
- ☐ Chair, sofa, bed heights allow sitting or standing?
- ☐ Do rugs have non-slip pad or rug tape?
- ☐ Chair available with arm rests?
- ☐ Able to turn on light, radio, TV, place a phone call from bed, chair, and sofa?

6. LAUNDRY
- ☐ Able to hand-wash and hang clothes to dry?
- ☐ Able to access automatic washer/dryer?

7. TELEPHONE AND DOOR
- ☐ Phone jack location near bed, sofa, chair?
- ☐ Able to get phone, dial, hear caller?
- ☐ Able to identify visitors, hear doorbell?
- ☐ Able to reach and empty mailbox?
- ☐ Wears neck/wrist device to obtain emergency help?

8. STORAGE SPACE
- ☐ Able to reach closet rods and hooks, open bureau drawers?
- ☐ Is there a light inside the closet?

9. WINDOWS
- ☐ Opening mechanism at 42 inches from floor?
- ☐ Lock accessible, easy to operate?
- ☐ Sill height above floor level?

10. ELECTRIC OUTLETS AND CONTROLS
- ☐ Sufficient outlets?
- ☐ Outlet height, wall locations
- ☐ Low vision/sound warnings available?
- ☐ Extension cord hazard?

11. HEAT, LIGHT, VENTILATION, SECURITY, CARBON MONOXIDE, WATER TEMP CONTROL
- ☐ Are there smoke/CO detectors and a fire extinguisher?
- ☐ Thermometer displays easily readable?
- ☐ Accessible environmental controls?
- ☐ Pressure balance valve available?
- ☐ Note rooms where poor light level exists
- ☐ Able to open windows; slide patio doors?
- ☐ Able to open drapes or curtains?

COMMENTS:

_____

_____

_____

_____

_____

_____

_____

Figure 10-3 Home safety checklist. (Courtesy Rebuilding Together, Washington, DC; *www.rebuildingtogether.org/downloads/home_safety_checklist.pdf*)

HELP PREVENT FALLS: Use this list to prioritize work tasks. Leave a copy of this list with the family so they can make further improvements.

I. EXTERIOR ENTRANCES AND EXITS

- ☐ Increase lighting at entry area
- ☐ Install stair rails on both sides
- ☐ Install door lever handles; double-bolt lock
- ☐ Install beveled, no step, no trip threshold
- ☐ Remove screen or storm door if needed
- ☐ Create surface to place packages when opening door
- ☐ Install peephole on exterior door
- ☐ Repair holes, uneven joints on walkway
- ☐ Provide non-slip finish to walkway surface
- ☐ Add ramp

2. INTERIOR DOORS, HALLS, STAIRS

- ☐ Create clear pathways between rooms
- ☐ Apply color contrast or texture change at top and bottom stair edges
- ☐ Install door lever handle
- ☐ Install swing-clear hinges to widen doorway. Minimum width: 32 inches
- ☐ Install beveled thresholds (max 1/2 inch)
- ☐ Replace or add non-slip surface on steps
- ☐ Repair or install stair handrails on both sides

3. BATHROOM

- ☐ Install swing-clear hinges to widen doorway. Minimum width: 32 inches
- ☐ Install secure wall reinforcement and place grab bars at toilet, bath and shower
- ☐ Install adjustable-height shower head
- ☐ Install non-slip strips in bath/shower
- ☐ Secure floor bathmat with non-slip, double-sided rug tape
- ☐ Elevate toilet height by adding portable seat or raising toilet base on a pedestal
- ☐ Adapt flush handle or install flush sensor
- ☐ Adapt or relocate toilet paper dispenser
- ☐ Round counter corners to provide safety
- ☐ Insulate hot water pipes if exposed
- ☐ Create sitting knee clearance at basin by removing vanity door and shelves underneath
- ☐ Install mirror for sitting or standing view
- ☐ Install good-quality non-glare lighting
- ☐ Install shower with no threshold if bathing abilities are severely limited

4. KITCHEN

- ☐ Increase task lighting at sink, stove, etc.
- ☐ Install D-type cupboard door handles
- ☐ Install adjustable shelving to increase access to upper cabinets
- ☐ Increase access to under counter storage space by installing pull-out units
- ☐ Insulate hot water pipes if exposed
- ☐ Install hot-proof surface near oven
- ☐ Install switches and outlets at front of counter
- ☐ Install pressure-balanced, temperature-regulated, lever faucets
- ☐ Create sitting knee clearance under work sites by removing doors or shelves
- ☐ Improve color contrast of cabinet and counters surface edges for those with low vision
- ☐ Add tactile and color-contrasted controls for those with low vision

5. LIVING, DINING, BEDROOM

- ☐ Widen or clear pathways within each room by rear- ranging furniture
- ☐ Secure throw and area rug edges with double-sided tape
- ☐ Improve access to and from chairs and beds by inserting risers under furniture legs
- ☐ Use side bed rail or chairs with armrests
- ☐ Install telephone jack near chair or bed
- ☐ Enlarge lamp switch or install touch-control lamp at bedside
- ☐ Install adjustable closet rods, shelving and light source for better storage access
- ☐ Install vertical pole adjacent to chair and sofa
- ☐ Raise furniture to appropriate height using leg extender products
- ☐ Install uniform level floor surfaces using wood, tile or low-pile rugs

6. LAUNDRY

- ☐ Build a counter for sorting and folding clothes
- ☐ Adjust clothesline to convenient height
- ☐ Relocate laundry appliances

7. TELEPHONE AND DOOR

- ☐ Install phone jacks near bed, sofa, and chair
- ☐ Install peephole at convenient height
- ☐ Install flashing light or sound amplifier to indicate ringing doorbell for those with visual or hearing problems
- ☐ Install mailbox at accessible height

8. STORAGE SPACE

- ☐ Install lights inside closet
- ☐ Install adjustable closet rods and shelves
- ☐ Install bi-fold or pocket doors

9. WINDOWS

- ☐ Install handles and locks that are easy to grip, placed at appropriate heights

10. ELECTRICAL OUTLETS AND CONTROLS

- ☐ Install light fixtures or outlet for lamps
- ☐ Install switches at top and bottom of stairs

II. HEAT, AIR, LIGHT, SECURITY, WATER TEMP, CARBON MONOXIDE CONTROLS

- ☐ Install smoke/CO detectors, fire extinguishers
- ☐ Increase residents' access to environmental control systems

Figure 10-3, Cont'd

HOME EVALUATION CHECKLIST

Name_____ Date_____
Address_____
Diagnosis_____

Mobility status
- ☐ ambulatory, no device   ☐ walker
- ☐ cane   ☐ wheelchair

Exterior

Home located on
- ☐ level surface
- ☐ hill

Type of house
- ☐ owns house   ☐ mobile home
- ☐ apartment   ☐ board and care

Number of floors
- ☐ one story   ☐ split level
- ☐ two story

Driveway surface
- ☐ inclined   ☐ smooth
- ☐ level   ☐ rough

Is the DRIVEWAY negotiable?   ☐ yes   ☐ no
Is the GARAGE accessible?   ☐ yes   ☐ no

Entrance

Accessible entrances
- ☐ front   ☐ side
- ☐ back

Steps
- number   _____
- height of each   _____
- width   _____
- depth   _____

Are there HANDRAILS?   ☐ yes   ☐ no
If yes, where are they located?   ☐ left   ☐ right
HANDRAIL height from step surface?   _____
If no, how much room is available for HANDRAILS?   _____

Are landings negotiable?   ☐ yes   ☐ no

Briefly describe any problems with LANDINGS:_____

Ramps ☐ yes   ☐ no
- ☐ front   ☐ back
- height   _____
- width   _____
- length   _____

Are there HANDRAILS?   ☐ yes   ☐ no
If yes, where are they located?   ☐ left   ☐ right   height_____
If no ramp, how much room is available for one? _____

Porch
- width   _____
- length   _____
- level at threshold?   ☐ yes   ☐ no

Door
- width   _____
- threshold height   _____   Negotiable?   ☐ yes   ☐ no
- ☐ swing in
- ☐ swing out
- ☐ sliding

Interior

Living Room
Is furniture arranged for easy maneuverability?   ☐ yes   ☐ no
Is frequently used furniture accessible?   ☐ yes   ☐ no
Type of floor covering: _____
Comments _____

Hallways
Can wheelchair or walking aide be maneuvered in hallway?   ☐ yes   ☐ no
- hall width   _____
- door width   _____
- sharp turns?   ☐ yes   ☐ no
- Steps?   ☐ yes   ☐ no
- number   _____
Are there HANDRAILS?   ☐ yes   ☐ no
If yes, where are they located?   ☐ left   ☐ right   height_____

Bedroom
- ☐ single
- ☐ shared
Is there room for a W/C?   ☐ yes   ☐ no

Door
- width   _____
- threshold height   _____   Negotiable?   ☐ yes   ☐ no
- ☐ swing in
- ☐ swing out

Bed:
- ☐ twin
- ☐ double
- ☐ queen
- ☐ king
- ☐ hospital bed

overall height _____   Accessible?   ☐ yes   ☐ no
Would hospital bed fit into room if needed?   ☐ yes   ☐ no

Clothing:
Are drawers accessible?   ☐ yes   ☐ no
    ☐ on right   ☐ on left
Is closet accessible?   ☐ yes   ☐ no
    ☐ on right   ☐ on left
Comments: _____

Bathroom

Door:
- width   _____
- threshold height   _____   Negotiable?   ☐ yes   ☐ no

Tub:
- height, floor-rim   _____
- height, tub bottom rim   _____
- tub width inside   _____
- glass doors?   ☐ yes   ☐ no
- width of tub doors   _____
- overhead shower?   ☐ yes   ☐ no
- Is tub accessible?   ☐ yes   ☐ no

Stall Shower: ☐ yes   ☐ no
- door width   _____
- height of bottom rim   _____
- Accessible?   ☐ yes   ☐ no

Sink:
- height   _____
- faucet type   _____
- ☐ open
- ☐ closed
- Accessible?   ☐ yes   ☐ no

Toilet:
- height from floor   _____
- location of toilet paper   _____
- distance from toilet to side wall L   _____
-     R   _____

Grab bars: ☐ yes   ☐ no
- Location   _____
Comments: _____

Kitchen

Door:
- width   _____
- threshold height   _____   Negotiable?   ☐ yes   ☐ no

Stove:
- height   _____
- location of controls   ☐ front   ☐ back
- Is stove accessible for use?   ☐ yes   ☐ no

Oven:
- height from floor to door hinge & door handle   _____
- location of oven   _____

Sink:
- Will w/c fit underneath?   ☐ yes   ☐ no
- type of faucets   _____

Cupboards:
- Accessible from w/c?   ☐ yes   ☐ no

Refrigerator:
- hinges on   ☐ left   ☐ right
- Accessible from w/c?   ☐ yes   ☐ no

Switches / outlets:
- Accessible?   ☐ yes   ☐ no

Kitchen table:
- height from floor   _____
- Accessible?   ☐ yes   ☐ no

Comments: _____

Laundry

Door: width   _____
- threshold height   _____   Negotiable?   ☐ yes   ☐ no

Steps: ☐ yes   ☐ no
- number   _____
- height   _____
- width   _____

Are there HANDRAILS?   ☐ yes   ☐ no
If yes, where are they located?   ☐ left   ☐ right   height_____

Figure 10-4   Home visit checklist. (Adapted from *Occupational/physical therapy home evaluation form,* San Francisco, 1993, Ralph K. Davies Medical Center; and *Occupational therapy home evaluation form,* Albany, CA, 1993, Alta Bates Hospital.)

Washer:
☐ Topload
☐ Front load
Accessible?   ☐ yes   ☐ no

Dryer:
☐ Topload
☐ Front load
Accessible?   ☐ yes   ☐ no

Safety

Throw rugs
☐ yes   ☐ no
Location _____

Phone
Accessible?   ☐ yes   ☐ no
Location _____

Emergency phone numbers
☐ yes   ☐ no
Location _____

Mailbox
Accessible?   ☐ yes   ☐ no
Location _____

Thermostat
Accessible?   ☐ yes   ☐ no
Location _____

Electric Outlets / switches
Accessible?   ☐ yes   ☐ no

Imperfect floor?
☐ yes   ☐ no
Location _____

Sharp-edged furniture?
☐ yes   ☐ no
Location _____

Insulated hot water pipes: ☐ yes   ☐ no
Location _____

Cluttered areas?
☐ yes   ☐ no
Location _____

Fire extinguisher?
☐ yes   ☐ no
Location _____

Equipment present: _____
_____

Problem list: _____
_____
_____

Recommendations for modifications: _____
_____
_____
_____

Equipment recommendations: _____
_____
_____

Figure 10-4, Cont'd

tact and diplomacy in a way that gives the client and family options and the freedom to refuse them or consider alternative possibilities. Family finances may limit implementation of needed changes. The social worker may be involved in working out funding for needed equipment and alterations, and the client should be made aware of this service when cost is discussed.[31]

The therapist should include recommendations regarding the feasibility of the client's discharge to the home environment or remaining in or managing the home alone, if applicable. If there is a question regarding the client's ability to return home safely and independently, the home assessment summary should include the functional skills the client needs to return home.

If a home visit is not possible, much of the information can be gained by interviewing the client and family member(s) following a trial home visit. The family member or caregiver may be instructed to complete the home visit checklist and provide photographs or sketches of the rooms and their arrangements. Problems encountered by the client during the home visit should be discussed and the necessary recommendations for their solution made, as described earlier.[31]

FINANCIAL MANAGEMENT

If the client is to resume management of money and financial matters independently, a cognitive and perceptual assessment that accurately tests these skills should be implemented. Because some persons with physical disabilities also have concurrent involvement of cognition and perception, the level of impairment should be determined. Caregivers may require training if the role of financial manager is new and must be assumed. The client may be capable of handling only small amounts of money or may need retraining in activities that require money management, such as shopping, balancing a checkbook, or making a budget. If a physical limitation is involved, the therapist may introduce adaptive writing devices to allow the client to handle the paperwork aspects of money management.

COMMUNITY MOBILITY

Some clients are fortunate enough to be able to drive and to adapt their own vehicle or purchase an adapted van (see Chapter 11). The client who does not meet these criteria must learn to use public transportation or to get around the community on foot or in a wheelchair. In this case, the occupational therapist must assess the client's physical, perceptual, cognitive, and social capabilities to be independent and safe with community mobility.

Physical capabilities to be considered are (1) whether the client has the endurance to be mobile in the community without fatigue and (2) whether the client is sufficiently independent with the walker, cane, crutch, or wheelchair skills and transfers needed to go beyond the home environment. These skills include managing uneven pavement, curbs, and inclines and crossing the street. Other skills to be evaluated before considering community mobility are how to (1) handle money, (2) carry objects in a wheelchair or with a walker, and (3) manage toileting in a public rest room.

Cognitive skills include the ability to be geographically oriented; if taking a bus, to know how to read a schedule and map or know how to get directions; and to have good problem-solving skills if a problem should occur in the community. If the disability is new, the client may be developing new social skills. At first, these skills will be stretched to the limit

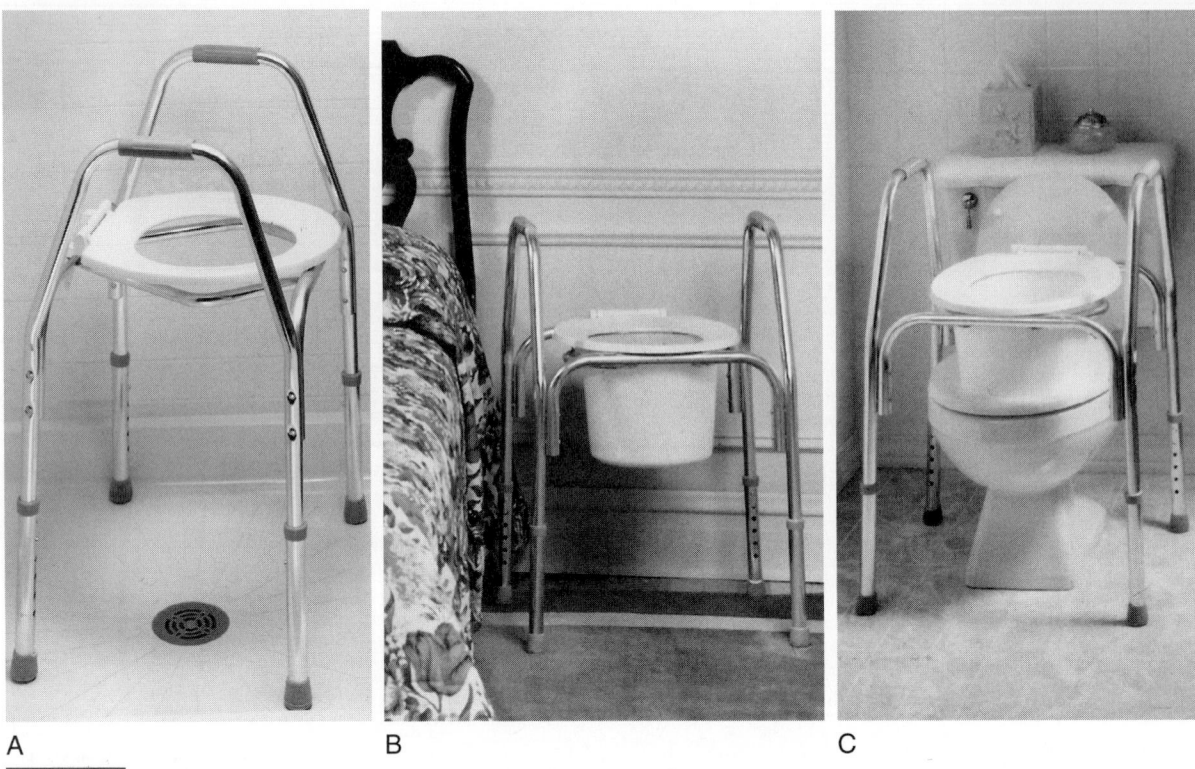

A   B   C

Figure 10-5   All-purpose commode. **A,** In shower. **B,** At bedside. **C,** Over toilet. (Courtesy Sammons Preston.)

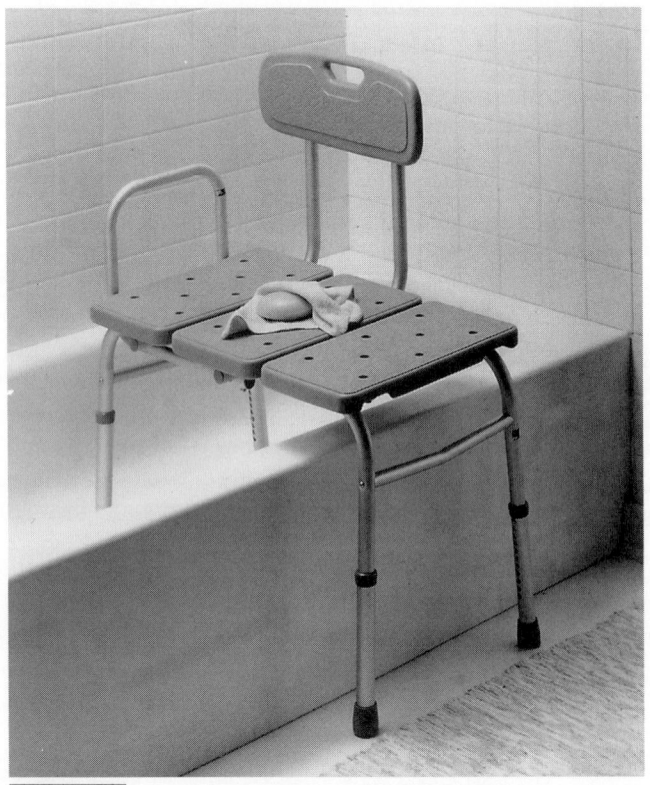

Figure 10-6   Transfer tub bench. (Courtesy Sammons Preston.)

once the client is out in the community—for example, learning how to be assertive to get an accessible table at a restaurant, obtaining assistance with unreachable items in the grocery store, and becoming comfortable with a new body image within the able-bodied community.

The therapist should also assess the client's community environment. For example, is the neighborhood safe enough for an individual who might be vulnerable because of physical limitations? What is the terrain like? Are there curb cut-outs? Are the sidewalks smooth and even? How far away are the closest store and bus stop? Are the traffic lights long enough for the client to negotiate safely given mobility limitations?

Accessibility of community transportation should also be considered. Some communities have door-to-door cab and van service, which have certain restrictions. Some of these restrictions include the need to arrange transportation one week in advance, the ability to get out the front door and to the curb independently, and the ability to transfer independently into the vehicle. If a public bus is to be used by the client, he or she must learn how to use the electric lifts and how to lock a wheelchair into place. Because not all bus stops are wheelchair accessible, the neighboring bus stops should be surveyed.

Community mobility requires preplanning by the occupational therapist and the client; accurate assessment of the client's abilities; and knowledge of potential physical, cognitive, and social barriers that may be encountered. A valuable resource by Armstrong and Lauzen, *Community Integration Program*,[4] provides practical treatment protocols to establish a community-living skills program. Attaining independence in community mobility is worth the investment because it allows the client to expand life tasks beyond those in the home and interact with the community.

HEALTH MANAGEMENT AND MAINTENANCE

Health management and maintenance include the client's ability to understand the medical condition and make decisions to maintain good health. The client's ability to handle medications, know when to call a physician, and know how to make a medical appointment is a practical aspect of health management. The evaluation of the client's ability to perform these activities may be completed solely by the occupational therapist but will probably include other team members such as the nurse and the physician.

Performance skills and patterns must be assessed in light of the skills required for each task. The OT assessment can be helpful in determining which aspects of the task need to be modified for the client to be independent. For example, the occupational therapist can work jointly with a nurse to ensure that a client with hemiplegia and diabetes can manage insulin shots. The OT evaluation considers the client's cognitive and perceptual abilities to make judgments about drawing the insulin out of the bottle, measuring the insulin, and injecting the insulin. Physical concerns include how to stabilize the insulin bottle, accurately see the measurement, and handle the syringe with one hand. Other medication management may involve how the client is able to open the medication and measure it, if the medication is a liquid. The occupational therapist may also evaluate and train the client in other skills that affect health management. Examples include using the phone, finding the appropriate phone numbers, and providing the needed information to make a medical appointment.

Health maintenance is an issue for the client and entire healthcare team. The occupational therapist plays an important role because of the scope of the ADL and IADL assessments, which may identify and help resolve problems related to health maintenance.

ADL AND IADL TRAINING

If it is determined after an assessment that ADL and IADL training are to be initiated, it is important to establish appropriate short- and long-term goals, based on the assessment and on the client's priorities and potential for independence. The following sequence of training for self-care activities is suggested: feeding, grooming, continence, transfer skills, toileting, undressing, dressing, and bathing. This sequence is based on the normal development of self-care independence in children.[31] It provides a good guide but may have to

be modified to accommodate the specific dysfunction and the capabilities, limitations, and personal priorities of the client.

The occupational therapist should estimate which ADL and IADL tasks are possible and which are impossible for the client to achieve. The therapist should explore with the client the use of alternative methods of performing the activities and the use of any assistive devices that may be helpful. He or she should determine for which tasks the client requires assistance and how much should be given. It may not be possible to estimate these factors until training is under way.

The ADL and IADL training program may be graded by beginning the intervention with a few simple tasks and gradually increasing the number and complexity of tasks taught. Training should progress from dependent to assisted to supervised to independent, with or without assistive devices.[31] The rate at which grading can occur depends on the client's potential for recovery, endurance, skills, and motivation.

METHODS OF TEACHING ADLs

The therapist must tailor methods of teaching the client to perform daily living tasks to suit each client's learning style and ability. The client who is alert and grasps instructions quickly may be able to perform an entire process after a brief demonstration and oral instruction. Clients who have perceptual problems, poor memory, and difficulty following instructions of any kind need a more concrete, step-by-step approach, reducing the amount of assistance gradually as success is achieved. For these clients it is important to break down the activity into small steps and progress through them slowly, one at a time. A slow demonstration of the task or step by the therapist in the same plane and in the same manner in which the client is expected to perform is helpful. Oral instructions to accompany the demonstration may or may not be helpful, depending on the client's receptive language skills and ability to process and integrate two modes of sensory information simultaneously.

Touching body parts to be moved, dressed, bathed, or positioned; passive movement of the part through the desired pattern to achieve a step or a task; and gentle manual guidance through the task are helpful tactile and kinesthetic modes of instruction (see Chapter 7). These techniques can augment or replace demonstration and oral instruction, depending on the client's best avenues of learning. It is necessary to perform a step or complete a task repeatedly to achieve skill, speed, and retention of learning. Tasks may be repeated several times during the same training session if time and the client's physical and emotional tolerance allow, or they may be repeated daily until the desired retention or level of skill is achieved.

The process of **backward chaining** can be used in teaching ADL skills. In this method, the therapist assists the client until the last step of the process is reached. The client then performs this step independently, which affords a sense of success and completion. When the last step is mastered, the therapist assists until the last two steps are reached and the client then completes these two steps. The process continues, with the therapist offering less and less assistance and the client performing successive steps of the task, from last to first, independently. This method is particularly useful in training clients with brain damage.[31]

Before beginning training in any ADL, the therapist must prepare by providing adequate space and arranging equipment, materials, and furniture for maximal convenience and safety. The therapist should be thoroughly familiar with the task to be performed and any special methods or assistive devices that will be used in its performance. The therapist should be able to perform the task skillfully, as he or she expects the client to perform it. After preparation, the activity is presented to the client, usually in one or more of the modes of guidance, demonstration, and oral instruction described earlier. The client then performs the activity either along with the therapist or immediately after being shown, with the required amount of supervision and assistance. Performance is modified and corrected as needed, and the process is repeated to ensure learning.

Because other staff or family members are frequently the individuals reinforcing the newly learned skills, family training is critical to reinforce learning and ensure that the client carries over the skills from previous treatment sessions. In the final phase of instruction, when the client has mastered one or more tasks, he or she is asked to perform them independently. The therapist should check performance in progress and later arrange to check on the adequacy of performance and carryover of learning with the client, nursing personnel, the caregiver, or the supervising family members.

RECORDING PROGRESS IN ADL PERFORMANCE

The ADL checklists used to record performance on the initial assessment usually have one or more spaces for recording changes in abilities and the results of reassessment during the training process. The sample checklist given earlier in this chapter is so designed and filled in (Figure 10-1). If a standardized assessment is used during the initial evaluation, it should be used in the reevaluation process to determine the level of progress the client has made.

Progress is usually summarized for inclusion in the medical record. The progress record should summarize changes in the client's abilities and current level of independence and should also estimate the client's potential for further independence, attitude, motivation for ADL training, and future goals for the ADL program. The information about the client's level of assistance needed for ADLs and IADLs will help with the discharge planning. For example, if a client continues to require moderate assistance with self-care, he or she may need to hire an attendant, or the occupational therapist may justify ongoing treatment when the client has potential for further independence.

ASSISTIVE TECHNOLOGY AND ADAPTIVE EQUIPMENT

Assistive technology is defined as any item, piece of equipment, or product system, whether acquired commercially, off the shelf, modified, or customized, that is used to increase or improve functional capabilities of individuals with disabilities. This is a definition provided in Public Law (PL) 100-47, the Technical Assistance to the States Act, in the United States (*www.resna.org/taproject/library/laws/techact94.htm*). The terms *assistive technology, adaptive equipment,* and *assistive devices* are generally used interchangeably throughout the profession. Adaptive equipment is used to compensate for a physical limitation, to promote safety, and to prevent joint injury. *Electronic aids to daily living* (EADLs) provide a bridge between an individual with limited function and an electrical device such as a telephone or door operator.[30] Physical limitations may include a loss of muscle strength, loss of *range of motion* (ROM), incoordination, or sensory loss. An example of using adaptive equipment to improve safety is the use of a bed or door alarm to alert a caregiver that a patient with impaired cognition is wandering. The use of adaptive equipment to prevent joint injury is indicated for the person with rheumatoid arthritis.

Before recommending a piece of adaptive equipment, the OT practitioner must complete a thorough assessment to determine the client's functional problems and causes of the problems. The OT practitioner may also consider practical solutions first, before settling on adaptive equipment as the solution. Some practical solutions would be to avoid the cause of the problem, use a compensatory technique or alternative method, get assistance from another person, or modify the environment. Typical of these considerations is the case example of Sadie.

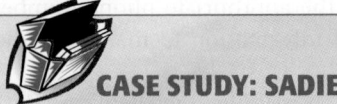

CASE STUDY: SADIE

Sadie is 75 years old and living in a nursing home. The occupational therapist received a referral for a self-feeding assessment because Sadie has recently lost weight and the nursing aides have reported that she needs assistance with eating. The nurse mentioned that she thought Sadie needed a built-up handle utensil to eat.

The OT assessment included an interview with Sadie, observation of Sadie eating lunch in her usual location (in her room with the use of an over-bed table), physical assessment (including strength, ROM, sensation, coordination), and gross cognitive and perceptual assessments. The results indicated that Sadie had problems with sitting properly in her wheelchair. The over-bed table was too high and limited her ability to reach the plate. Her strength, ROM, coordination, and sensation were within normal limits, except that bilateral shoulder flexors and abductors were F- (3-). Sadie's cognition and perception were adequate to relearn simple self-care tasks.

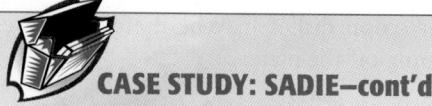

CASE STUDY: SADIE–cont'd

Treatment involved working on wheelchair positioning, lowering the over-bed table, and then teaching the client how to use a compensatory technique of elbow propping to bring her hand to her mouth during eating. The OT assessment did not indicate a need for adaptive equipment at this time; instead, the environment was adapted, wheelchair positioning modified, and a compensatory method taught.

If the results of the assessment had indicated that Sadie had a weak grasp and/or hand incoordination, a built-up handle utensil and plate guard might have been used to promote independence with self-feeding.

Other factors to consider when selecting adaptive equipment are whether the disability is short or long term, the client's tolerance for gadgets, the client's feelings about the device, and the cost and upkeep of the equipment.

SPECIFIC ADL TECHNIQUES

In many instances, specific techniques to solve specific ADL problems are not possible. Sometimes the occupational therapist has to explore a variety of methods or assistive devices to reach a solution. It is occasionally necessary for the therapist to design a special device, method, splint, or piece of equipment to make a particular activity possible for the client to perform. Many of the assistive devices available today through rehabilitation equipment companies were first conceived and made by occupational therapists and clients. Many of the special methods used to perform specific activities also evolved through the trial-and-error approaches of therapists and their clients. Clients often have good suggestions for therapists, because they live with the limitation and are confronted regularly with the need to adapt the performance of daily tasks.

The purpose of the following summary of techniques is to give the reader some general ideas about how to solve ADL problems for specific classifications of dysfunction. The focus is on compensatory strategies involving changing the method in which an activity is performed, changing the environment, or using an assistive device. If the client has the potential for improvement of specific deficits, treatment that includes remediation should be considered. The references at the end of this chapter provide more specific instruction in ADL methods. The following categories of physical deficits are addressed in this chapter:

- ADLs for the person with limited ROM or strength
- ADLs for the person with incoordination
- ADLs for the person with hemiplegia or use of only one upper extremity
- ADLs for the person with paraplegia
- ADLs for the person with quadriplegia
- ADLs for the person with low vision

The following ADLs and IADLs are addressed with each of the physical deficits listed above:

- Dressing activities
- Feeding activities
- Personal hygiene and grooming activities
- Communication and environmental adaptations
- Functional mobility
- Home management, meal preparation, and cleanup activities

ADLs FOR THE PERSON WITH LIMITED ROM OR STRENGTH

The major problem for persons with limited joint ROM is compensating for the lack of reach and joint excursion through such means as environmental adaptation and assistive devices. Individuals who lack muscle strength may require some of the same devices or techniques to compensate and to conserve energy. Some adaptations and devices are outlined here.[22,31,36]

Lower Extremity Dressing Activities

1. Use dressing sticks with a neoprene-covered coat hook on one end and a small hook on the other (Figure 10-7) for pushing and pulling garments off and on feet and legs.
2. For socks, use a commercially available sock aid (Figure 10-8).
3. Eliminate the need to bend to tie shoelaces or to use finger joints in this fine motor activity by using elastic shoelaces or other adapted shoe fasteners. Use Velcro-fastened shoes.

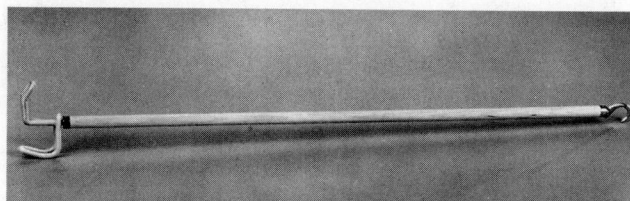

Figure 10-7   Dressing stick or reacher. (Courtesy Sammons Preston.)

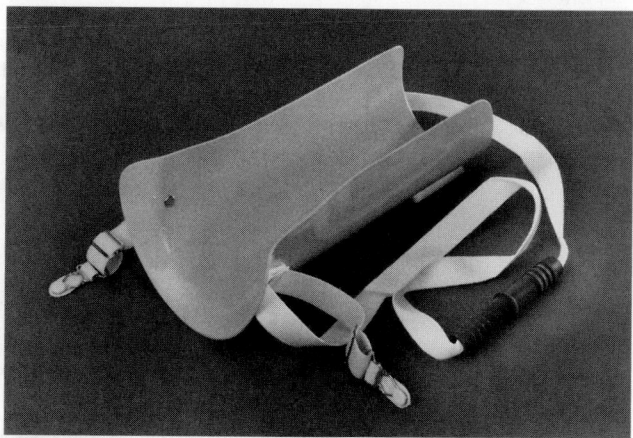

Figure 10-8   Sock aid. (Courtesy Sammons Preston.)

4. Use reachers (Figure 10-9) for picking up socks and shoes, arranging clothes, removing clothes from hangers, picking up objects on the floor, and donning pants.

Upper Extremity Dressing Activities

1. Use front-opening garments that are one size larger than needed and made of fabrics that have some stretch.
2. Use dressing sticks (Figure 10-7) to push a shirt or blouse over the head.
3. Use larger buttons or zippers with a loop on the pull tab.
4. Replace buttons, snaps, hooks, and eyes with Velcro or zippers (for those clients who cannot manage traditional fastenings).
5. Use one of several types of commercially available buttonhooks (Figure 10-10) if finger ROM is limited.

Feeding Activities

1. Use built-up handles on eating utensils that can accommodate limited grasp or prehension (grip or pinch pattern) (Figure 10-11).
2. Elongated or specially curved handles on spoons and forks may be needed to reach the mouth. A swivel spoon or spoon-fork combination can compensate for limited supination (Figure 10-12).
3. Long plastic straws and straw clips on glasses or cups can be used if neck, elbow, or shoulder ROM limits hand-to-mouth motion or if grasp is inadequate to hold the cup or glass.
4. Universal cuffs or utensil holders can be used if grasp is very limited and built-up handles do not work (Figure 10-13).

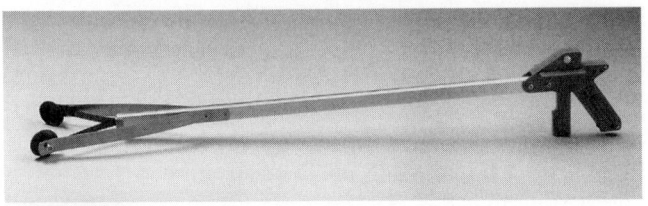

Figure 10-9 Extended-handle reacher.

5. Plate guards or scoop dishes may be useful to prevent food from slipping off the plate.

Personal Hygiene and Grooming Activities

1. A hand-held flexible shower hose for bathing and shampooing hair can eliminate the need to stand in the shower and offers the user control of the direction of the spray. The handle can be built up or adapted for limited grasp.
2. A long-handled bath brush or sponge with a soap holder (Figure 10-14) or long cloth scrubber can allow the user to reach legs, feet, and back. A wash mitt (Figure 10-15) and soap on a rope can aid limited grasp.
3. A wall-mounted hair dryer may be helpful. This device is useful for clients with limited ROM, upper extremity weakness, incoordination, or use of just one upper extremity. The dryer is mounted to allow the user to manage his or her hair with one arm or position himself or herself to compensate for limited ROM.[10]
4. Long handles on a comb, brush, toothbrush, lipstick, mascara brush, and safety or electric razor may be useful for clients with limited hand-to-head or hand-to-face movements. Extensions may be constructed from inexpensive wooden dowels or pieces of PVC pipe found in hardware stores.
5. Spray deodorant, hair spray, and spray powder or perfume can extend the reach by the distance the material sprays. Special adaptations may be required by some persons to operate the spray mechanism (Figure 10-16).
6. Electric toothbrushes and a Water-Pik may be easier to manage than a standard toothbrush.
7. A short reacher can extend reach for using toilet paper. Several types of toilet aids are available in catalogs that sell assistive devices.
8. Dressing sticks can be used to pull garments up after using the toilet. An alternative is the use of a long piece of elastic or webbing with clips on each end that can be hung around the neck and fastened to pants or panties, preventing them from slipping to the floor during use of the toilet.

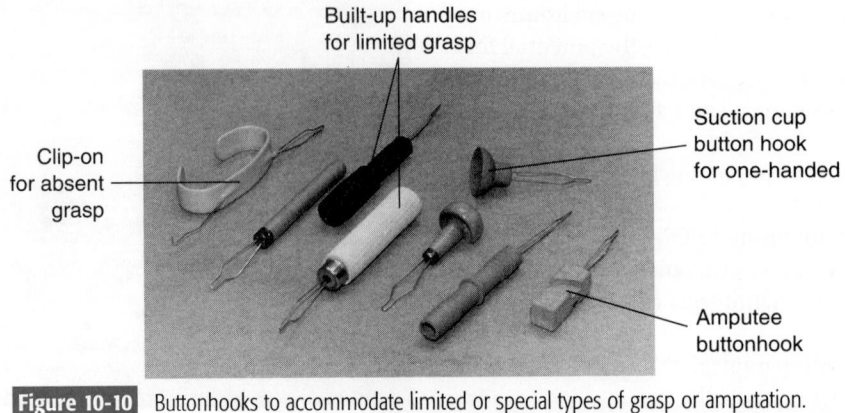

Built-up handles for limited grasp

Clip-on for absent grasp

Suction cup button hook for one-handed

Amputee buttonhook

Figure 10-10 Buttonhooks to accommodate limited or special types of grasp or amputation.

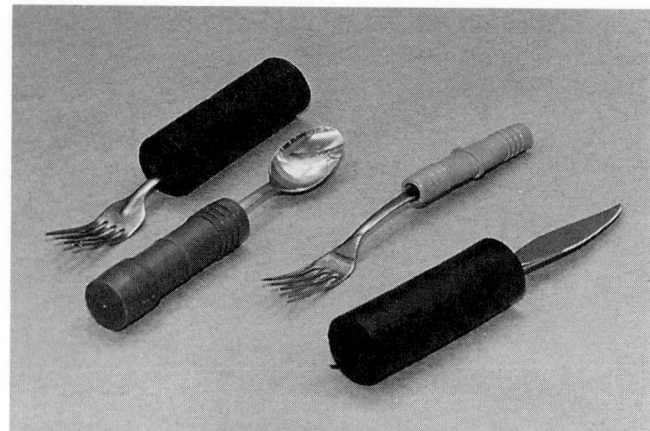

Figure 10-11   Eating utensils with built-up handles.

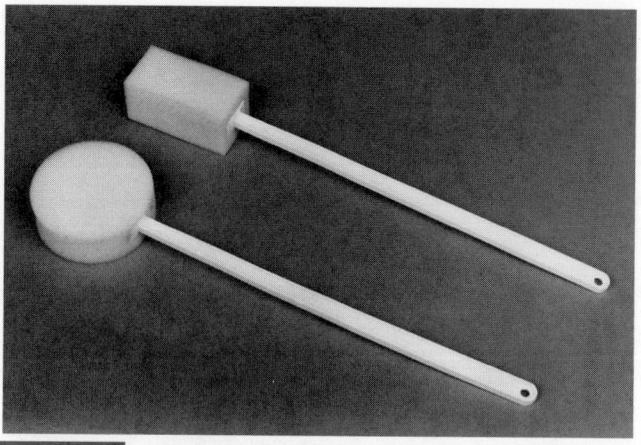

Figure 10-14   Long-handled bath sponges. (Courtesy Sammons Preston.)

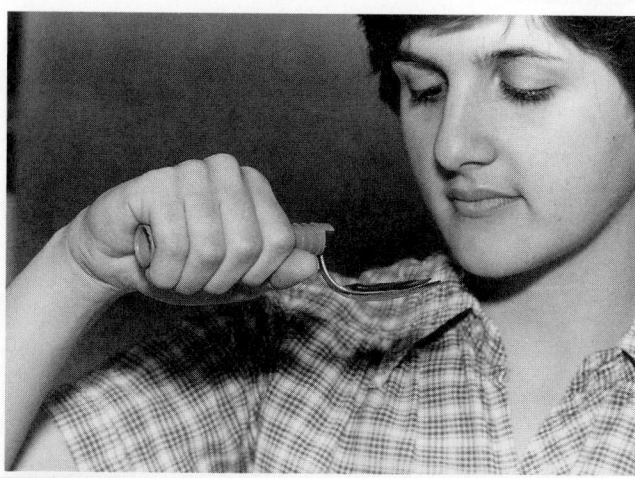

Figure 10-12   Swivel spoon compensates for limited supination or incoordination.

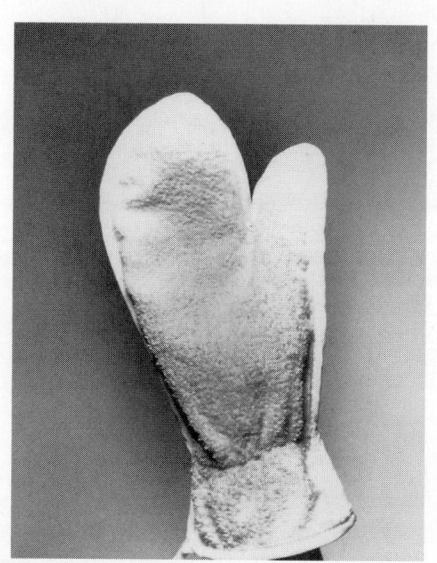

Figure 10-15   Terry cloth bath mitt. (Courtesy Sammons Preston.)

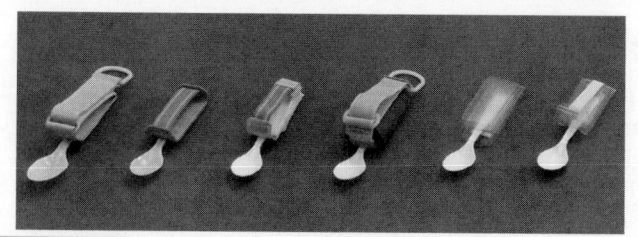

Figure 10-13   Utensil holders and universal cuffs. (Courtesy Sammons Preston.)

9. Safety rails (Figure 10-17) can be used for bathtub transfers, and safety mats or strips can be placed in the bathtub bottom to prevent slipping.
10. A transfer tub bench (Figure 10-6), shower stool, or regular chair set in the bathtub or shower stall can eliminate the need to sit on the bathtub bottom or stand to shower, thus increasing safety.

11. Grab bars can be installed to prevent falls and ease transfers.

Communication and Environmental Hardware Adaptations

1. Extended or built-up handles on faucets can accommodate limited grasp.
2. Telephones should be placed within easy reach, or portable phones can be used and kept with the client. A speakerphone may be necessary. A dialing stick is helpful if individual finger movements are not possible.
3. Built-up pens and pencils can be used to accommodate limited grasp and prehension. A Wanchik writer and several other commercially available or custom-fabricated writing aids are available (Figure 10-18).

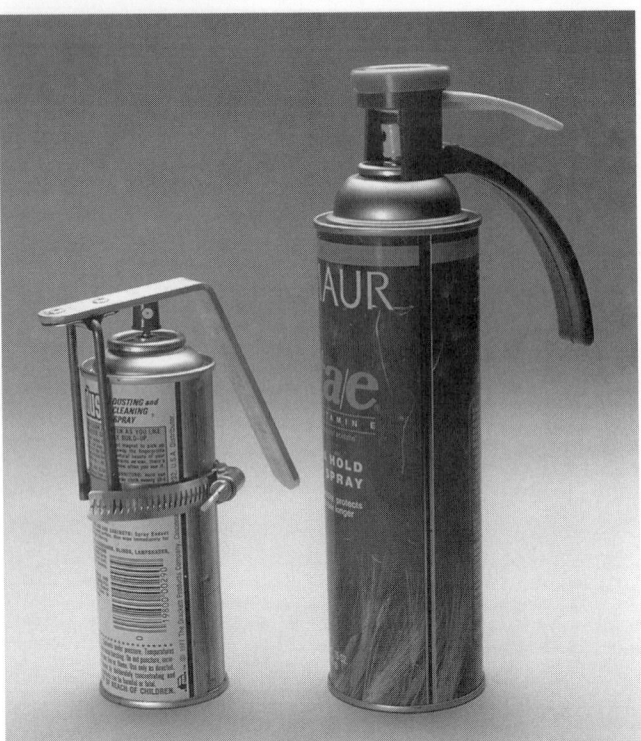

Figure 10-16 Spray can adapters. (Courtesy Sammons Preston.)

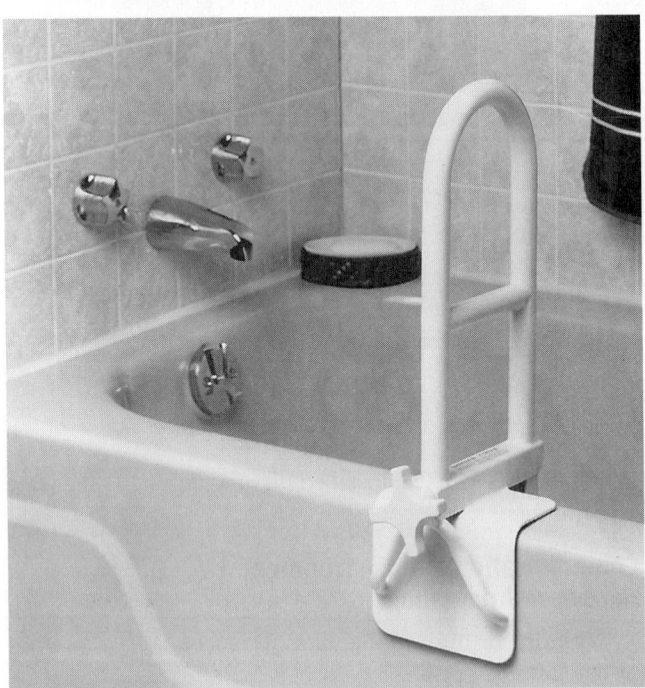

Figure 10-17 Bathtub safety rail. (Courtesy Sammons Preston.)

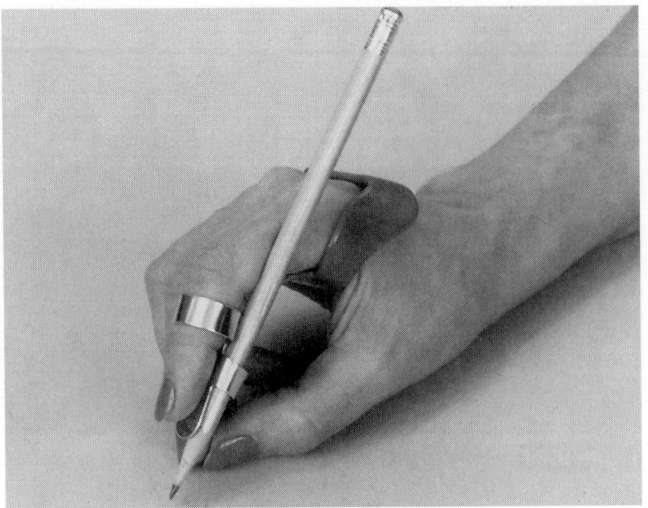

Figure 10-18 Wanchik writing aid. (Courtesy Sammons Preston.)

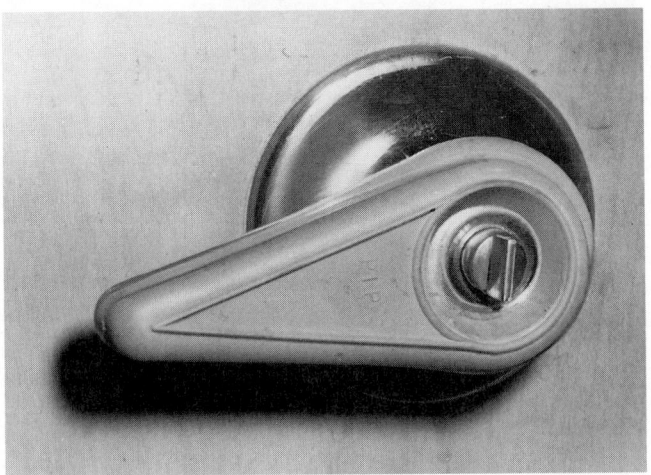

Figure 10-19 Rubber doorknob extension. (Courtesy Sammons Preston.)

Functional Mobility

The individual who has limited ROM without significant muscle weakness may benefit from the following assistive devices:

1. A glider chair that is operated by the feet can facilitate transportation if hip, hand, and arm motion is limited.
2. Platform crutches can prevent stress on hand or finger joints and can accommodate limited grasp.
3. Enlarged grips on crutches, canes, and walkers can accommodate limited grasp.
4. A raised toilet seat can be used if hip and knee motion is limited.
5. A walker with padded grips and forearm troughs can be used if marked hand, forearm, or elbow joint limitations are present.
6. A walker or crutch bag or basket can facilitate the carrying of objects.

4. Personal computers, word processors, and book holders can facilitate communication for those with limited or painful joints.
5. Lever-type doorknob extensions (Figure 10-19), car door openers, and adapted key holders can compensate for hand limitations.

Home Management, Meal Preparation, and Cleanup Activities

Home management activities can be facilitated by a wide variety of environmental adaptations, assistive devices, energy conservation methods, and work simplification techniques.[8,36] The principles of joint protection are essential for those with rheumatoid arthritis. These principles are discussed in Chapter 38. The following are suggestions to facilitate home management for persons with limited ROM:

1. Store frequently used items on the first shelves of cabinets, just above and below counters or on counters where possible.
2. Use a high stable stool to work comfortably at counter height, or attach a dropleaf table to the wall for planning and meal preparation area if a wheelchair is used.
3. Use a utility cart of comfortable height to transport several items at once.
4. Use reachers to get lightweight items (e.g., a cereal box) from high shelves.
5. Stabilize mixing bowls and dishes with nonslip mats.
6. Use lightweight utensils, such as plastic or aluminum bowls and aluminum pots.
7. Use an electric can opener and an electric mixer.
8. Use electric scissors or adapted loop scissors to open packages (Figure 10-20).
9. Eliminate bending by using extended and flexible plastic handles on dust mops, brooms, and dustpans.
10. Use adapted knives for cutting (Figure 10-21).
11. Use pull-out shelves to organize cupboards and eliminate bending.
12. Eliminate bending by using a wall oven, countertop broiler, microwave oven, and convection oven.
13. Eliminate leaning and bending by using a top-loading automatic washer and elevated dryer. Wheelchair users can benefit from front-loading appliances.
14. Use an adjustable ironing board to make it possible to sit while ironing, or eliminate ironing with the use of permanent press clothing.
15. Elevate the playpen and diaper table and use a bathinette or a plastic tub on the kitchen counter for bathing to reduce the amount of bending and reaching by the ambulatory parent during child care. The crib mattress can be in a raised position until the child is 3 or 4 months of age.
16. Use larger and looser fitting garments with Velcro fastenings on children.
17. Use a reacher to pick up clothing and children's toys.
18. Use a comforter instead of a top sheet and blanket to increase the ease of making the bed.

ADLs FOR THE PERSON WITH INCOORDINATION

Incoordination in the form of tremors, ataxia, or athetoid or choreiform movements can be caused by a variety of *central nervous system* (CNS) disorders, such as Parkinson's disease,

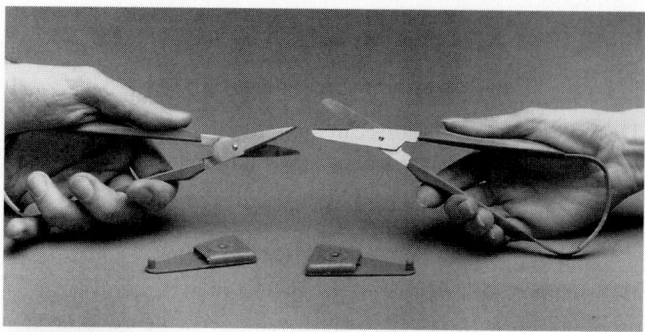

Figure 10-20   Loop scissors. (Courtesy Sammons Preston.)

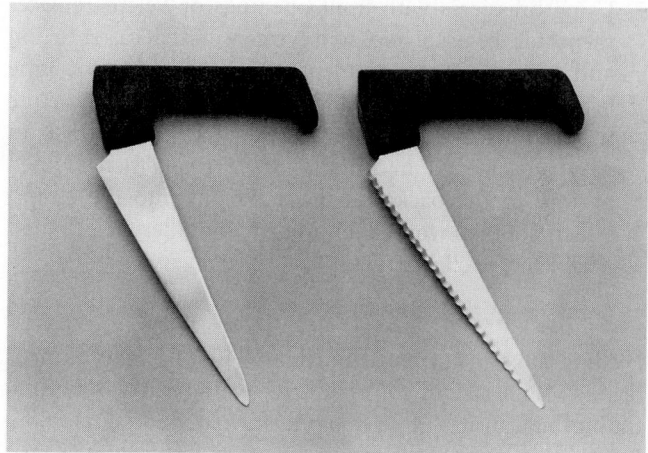

Figure 10-21   Right-angle knife. (Courtesy Sammons Preston.)

multiple sclerosis, cerebral palsy, and head injuries. The major problems encountered in ADL performance are safety and adequate stability of gait, body parts, and objects to complete the tasks.[22,31]

Fatigue, emotional factors, and fear may influence the severity of incoordinated movement.[22] The client must be taught appropriate energy conservation and work simplification techniques along with appropriate work pacing and safety methods to prevent the fatigue and apprehension that could increase incoordination and affect performance.

Stabilizing the arm reduces some of the incoordination and may allow the individual to accomplish gross and fine motor movements without assistive devices. A technique that can be used throughout all ADL tasks is the stabilization of the involved upper extremity. This technique is accomplished by propping the elbow on a counter or table top, pivoting from the elbow, and only moving the forearm, wrist, and hand in the activity. When muscle weakness is not a major deficit for the individual with incoordination, the use of weighted devices can help with stabilization of objects. A Velcro-fastened weight can be attached to the client's arm to decrease ataxia, or the device being used (e.g., eating utensils, pens, and cups) can be weighted.[31]

Dressing Activities

To avoid balance problems, the client should attempt to dress while sitting on or in bed or in a wheelchair or chair with arms. The following adaptations can reduce dressing difficulties:

1. Use of front-opening garments that fit loosely can facilitate their donning and removal.
2. Use of large buttons, Velcro, or zippers with loops on the tab can facilitate opening and closing fasteners. A button-hook with a large, weighted handle may be helpful.
3. Elastic shoelaces, Velcro closures, other adapted shoe closures, and slip-on shoes eliminate the need for bow tying.
4. Trousers with elastic tops for women or Velcro closures for men are easier to manage than trousers with hooks, buttons, and zippers.
5. Using brassieres with front openings or Velcro replacements for the usual hook and eye may make it easier to don and remove these garments. A slipover elastic-type brassiere or bra-slip combination also may eliminate the need to manage brassiere fastenings. Regular brassieres may be fastened in front at waist level, then slipped around to the back and the arms put into the straps, which are then worked up over the shoulders.
6. Men can use clip-on ties.[1,31]

Feeding Activities

Feeding can be a challenge for clients with problems of incoordination. A lack of control during eating is not only frustrating, but can also cause embarrassment and social rejection. It is important to make eating safe, pleasurable, and as neat as possible. The following are some suggestions for achieving this goal:

1. Use plate stabilizers, such as nonskid mats (Dycem), suction bases, or even damp dishtowels.
2. Use a plate guard or scoop dish to prevent pushing food off the plate. The plate guard can be carried away from home and clipped to any ordinary dinner plate (Figure 10-22).
3. Prevent spills during the plate-to-mouth excursion by using weighted or swivel utensils to offer stability. Weighted cuffs may be placed on the forearm to decrease involuntary movement (Figure 10-23).

4. Use long plastic straws with a straw clip on a glass, or use a cup with a weighted bottom to eliminate the need to carry the glass or cup to the mouth, thus avoiding spills. Plastic cups with covers and spouts may be used for the same purpose.[22,31]
5. Use a resistance or friction feeder similar to a mobile arm support to help control patterns of involuntary movement during feeding activities of adults with cerebral palsy and athetosis. These devices may help many clients with severe incoordination to achieve some degree of independence in feeding. The device is available in adaptive equipment catalogs and is listed as a Friction Feeder MAS (Mobile Arm Support) Kit.

Personal Hygiene and Grooming Activities

Stabilization and handling of toilet articles may be achieved by the following suggestions:

1. Articles such as a razor, lipstick, and a toothbrush may be attached to a cord if frequent dropping is a problem. An electric toothbrush may be more easily managed than a regular one.
2. Weighted wrist cuffs may be helpful during the finer hygiene activities, such as hair care, shaving, and applying make-up.[31]
3. A wall-mounted hair dryer described earlier for clients with limited ROM can also be useful for clients with incoordination.
4. An electric razor, rather than a blade razor, offers stability and safety.[31] A strap around the razor and hand can prevent dropping.
5. A suction brush attached to the sink or counter can be used for nail or denture care (Figure 10-24).
6. Soap should be on a rope. It can be worn around the neck or hung over a bathtub or shower fixture during bathing to keep it within easy reach. A bath mitt with a pocket to hold

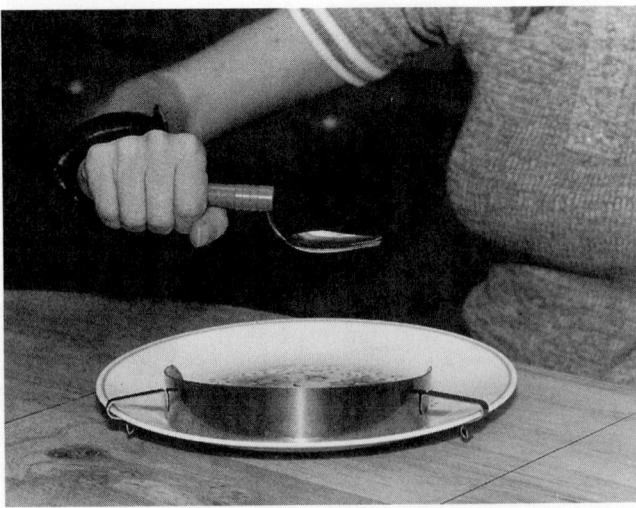

Figure 10-23 Weighted wrist cuff and swivel utensil can sometimes compensate for incoordination or involuntary motion and limited supination.

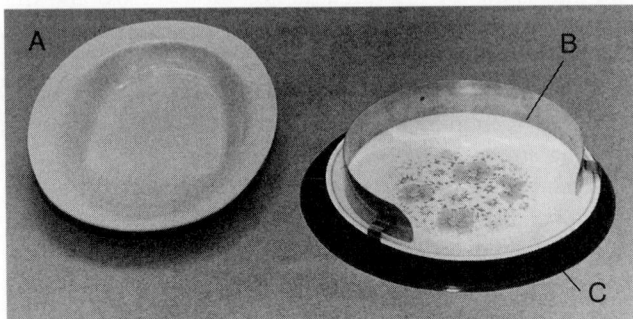

Figure 10-22 **A,** Scoop dish. **B,** Plate with plate guard. **C,** Nonskid mat.

the soap can be used for washing to eliminate the need for frequent soaping and rinsing and wringing a washcloth. A leg from a pair of pantyhose with a bar of soap in the toe may be tied over a faucet to keep soap within reach and will stretch for use. Liquid soap with a soft nylon scrubber may be used to minimize the handling of soap. Bath gloves can be worn and liquid soap applied to eliminate the dropping of the soap and washcloth.[31]

7. An emery board or small piece of wood with fine sandpaper glued to it can be fastened to the table top for filing nails.[31] A nail clipper can be stabilized in the same manner.

8. Large roll-on deodorants are preferable to sprays or creams.[31]

9. Sanitary pads that stick to undergarments may be easier to manage than tampons.[31]

10. Nonskid mats should be used inside and outside the bathtub during bathing. Their suction bases should be fastened securely to the floor and bathtub before use. Safety grab bars should be installed on the wall next to the bathtub or fastened to the edge of the bathtub. A bathtub seat or shower chair provides more safety than standing, while the individual is showering or transferring to a bathtub bottom.[31] Many clients with incoordination require supervisory assistance during this hazardous activity. Sponge bathing while seated at a bathroom sink may be substituted for bathing or showering several times a week.

Communication and Environmental Hardware Adaptations

1. Doorknobs may be managed more easily if adapted with lever-type handles or covered with rubber or friction tape (Figure 10-19).

2. Large button phones, speakerphones, or a holder for a telephone receiver may be helpful.

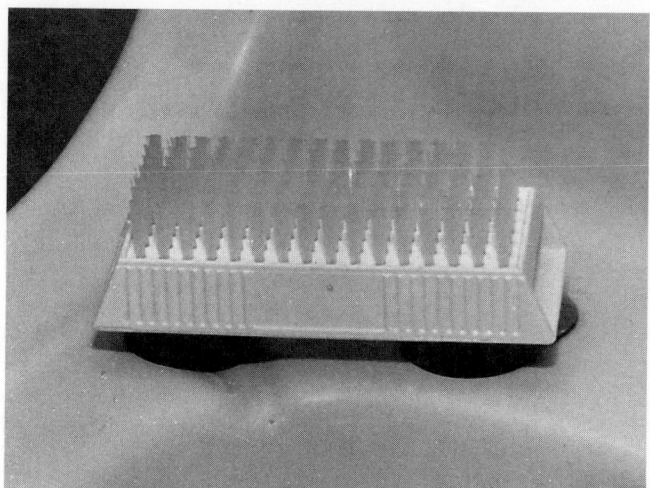

Figure 10-24   Suction brush attached to bathroom sink for dentures or fingernails. Can also be used in kitchen to wash vegetables and fruit.

3. Writing may be managed by using a weighted, enlarged pencil or pen. A personal computer with a keyboard guard is a helpful aid to communication. A computer mouse may frequently be substituted for the keyboard.[31] A voice-recognition program may be used with a personal computer to minimize use of the keyboard or mouse.

4. Keys may be managed by placing them on an adapted key holder that is rigid and offers more leverage for turning the key. Inserting the key in the keyhole may be difficult, however, unless the incoordination is relatively mild.

5. Extended lever-type faucets are easier to manage than knobs that turn and push-pull spigots. In order to prevent burns during bathing and kitchen activities, the person with incoordination should turn cold water on first and add hot water gradually.

6. Lamps that can be turned on and off with a wall switch, a light, or a signal-type device can eliminate the need to turn a small switch.

Functional Mobility

Clients with problems of incoordination may use a variety of ambulation aids, depending on the type and severity of incoordination. Clients with degenerative diseases sometimes need help to recognize the need for and to accept ambulation aids. This problem may mean moving gradually from a cane to crutches to a walker, and finally to a wheelchair for some persons. The following suggestions can improve stability and mobility for clients with incoordination:

1. Instead of lifting objects, slide them on floors or counters.

2. Use suitable ambulation aids.

3. Use a utility cart, preferably a heavy, custom-made cart that has some friction on the wheels.

4. Remove door sills, throw rugs, and thick carpeting.

5. Install banisters on indoor and outdoor staircases.

6. Substitute ramps for stairs wherever possible.

Home Management, Meal Preparation, and Cleanup Activities

It is important for the occupational therapist to carefully assess performance of homemaking activities to determine (1) which activities can be done safely, (2) which activities can be done safely if modified or adapted, and (3) which activities cannot be done adequately or safely and should be assigned to someone else. The major problems are stabilization of foods and equipment to prevent spilling and accidents, and the safe handling of appliances, pots, pans, and household tools to prevent cuts, burns, bruises, electric shock, and falls. The following are suggestions for the facilitation of home management tasks.[17,22,31]

1. Use a wheelchair and wheelchair lapboard, even if ambulation is possible with devices. The wheelchair saves energy and increases stability if balance and gait are unsteady.

2. If possible, use convenience and prepared foods to eliminate as many processes (e.g., peeling, chopping, slicing, and mixing) as possible.

3. Use easy-opening containers or store foods in plastic containers once opened. A jar opener is also useful.

4. Use heavy utensils, mixing bowls, and pots and pans to increase stability.

5. Use nonskid mats on work surfaces.

6. Use electrical appliances such as crock pots, electric fry pans, toaster ovens, and microwave or convection ovens because they are safer than using a range-top stove.

7. Use a blender and countertop mixer because they are safer than handheld mixers and easier than mixing with a spoon or whisk.

8. If possible, adjust work heights of counters, sink, and range to minimize leaning, bending, reaching, and lifting, whether the client is standing or using a wheelchair.

9. Use long oven mitts, which are safer than potholders.

10. Use pots, pans, casserole dishes, and appliances with bilateral handles because they may be easier to manage than those with one handle.

11. Use a cutting board with stainless steel nails (Figure 10-25) to stabilize meats and vegetables while cutting. When the board is not in use, the nails should be covered with a large cork. The bottom of the board should have suction cups or should be covered with stair tread, or the board should be placed on a nonskid mat to prevent slippage when in use.

12. Use heavy dinnerware, which may be easier to handle because it offers stability and control to the distal part of the upper extremity. (On the other hand, unbreakable dinnerware may be more practical if dropping and breakage are problems.)

13. Cover the sink, utility cart, and countertops with protective rubber mats or mesh matting to stabilize items.

14. Use a serrated knife for cutting and chopping because it is easier to control.

15. Use a steamer basket or deep-fry basket for preparing boiled foods to eliminate the need to carry and drain pots containing hot liquids.

16. Use tongs to turn foods during cooking and to serve foods because tongs may offer more control and stability than a fork, spatula, or serving spoon.

17. Use blunt-ended loop scissors to open packages.

18. Vacuum with a heavy upright cleaner, which may be easier for the ambulatory client. The wheelchair user may be able to manage a lightweight tank-type vacuum cleaner or electric broom.

19. Use dust mitts for dusting.

20. Eliminate fragile knickknacks, unstable lamps, and dainty doilies.

21. Eliminate ironing by using no-iron fabrics or a timed dryer or by assigning this task to other members of the household.

22. Use a front-loading washer, a laundry cart on wheels, and premeasured detergents, bleaches, and fabric softeners.

23. Sit when working with an infant and use foam-rubber bath aids, an infant bath seat, and a wide, padded dressing table with Velcro safety straps to offer enough stability for bathing, dressing, and diapering an infant. (Child care tasks may not be possible unless the incoordination is mild.)

24. Use disposable diapers with tape or Velcro fasteners, because they are easier to manage than cloth diapers and pins.

25. Do not feed the infant with a spoon or fork unless the incoordination is very mild or does not affect the upper extremities. This task may need to be performed by another household member.

26. Children's clothing should be large, loose, and made of nonslippery stretch fabrics, and should have Velcro fastenings.

27. Use front infant carriers or strollers for carrying.

ADLs FOR THE PERSON WITH HEMIPLEGIA OR USE OF ONLY ONE UPPER EXTREMITY

Suggestions for performing daily living skills apply to persons with hemiplegia, unilateral upper extremity amputations, and temporary disorders such as fractures, burns, and peripheral neuropathic conditions that can result in the dysfunction of one upper extremity.

The client with hemiplegia needs specialized methods of teaching, and many such clients have greater difficulty learning and performing one-handed skills than do those with orthopedic or lower motor neuron dysfunction. Because the trunk and leg are involved, as well as the arm, ambulation and balance difficulties may exist. Sensory, perceptual, cognitive, and speech disorders may be present in a mild to severe degree. These disorders affect the ability to learn and retain learning and performance. Finally, the presence of apraxia (or difficulty with motor planning) sometimes seen in this group of clients can have a profound effect on the potential for learning new motor skills and remembering old ones. Therefore, the client with normal perception and cognition and the use of only one upper extremity may learn the techniques quickly and easily.[31] The client with hemiplegia needs

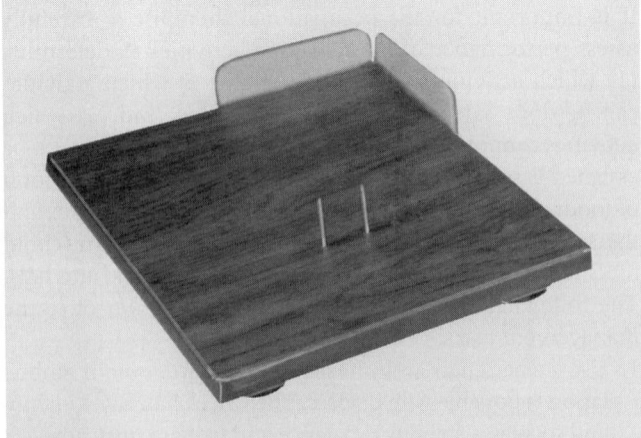

Figure 10-25   Cutting board with stainless steel nails, suction cup feet, and corner for stabilizing bread is useful for patients with incoordination or use of one hand. (Courtesy Sammons Preston.)

to be assessed for sensory, perceptual, and cognitive deficits to determine the potential for ADL performance and to establish appropriate teaching methods to facilitate learning.

The major problems for the one-handed worker are reduction of work speed and dexterity and stabilization to substitute for the role normally assumed by the nondominant arm.[22,31] The major problems for the individual with hemiplegia are balance and precautions relative to sensory, perceptual, and cognitive losses.

Dressing Activities

If balance is a problem, the client should dress while seated in a locked wheelchair or sturdy armchair. Clothing should be within easy reach. A reacher may be helpful for securing articles and assisting in some dressing activities. Assistive devices should be used minimally for dressing and other ADLs. Compensatory techniques are preferable. For the client with hemiplegia, dressing techniques that employ *neurodevelopmental treatment* (NDT or Bobath) principles are discussed in Chapter 31. The following one-handed dressing techniques* can facilitate dressing for persons with use of only

---

*Summarized from Activities of daily living for clients with incoordination, limited range of motion, paraplegia, quadriplegia, and hemiplegia, Cleveland, 1989, Metro Health Center for Rehabilitation, Metro Health Medical Center, unpublished.

one upper extremity. A general rule is to begin with the affected arm or leg first when donning clothing. Start with the unaffected extremity when removing clothing.

Shirts

One of the three following methods can be used to manage front-opening shirts. The first method can also be used for jackets, robes, and front-opening dresses.

Method I

Donning Shirt

1. Grasp the shirt collar with normal hand and shake out twists (Figure 10-26, *A*).
2. Position shirt on lap with inside up and collar toward chest (Figure 10-26, *B*).
3. Position sleeve opening on affected side so opening is as large as possible and close to affected hand, which is resting on lap (Figure 10-26, *C*).
4. Using normal hand, place affected hand in sleeve opening and work sleeve over elbow by pulling on garment (Figure 10-26, *D1, D2*).
5. Put normal arm into its sleeve and raise arm to slide or shake sleeve into position past elbow (Figure 10-26, *E*).
6. With normal hand, gather shirt up middle of back from hem to collar and raise shirt over head (Figure 10-26, *F*).
7. Lean forward, duck head, and pass shirt over head (Figure 10-26, *G*).

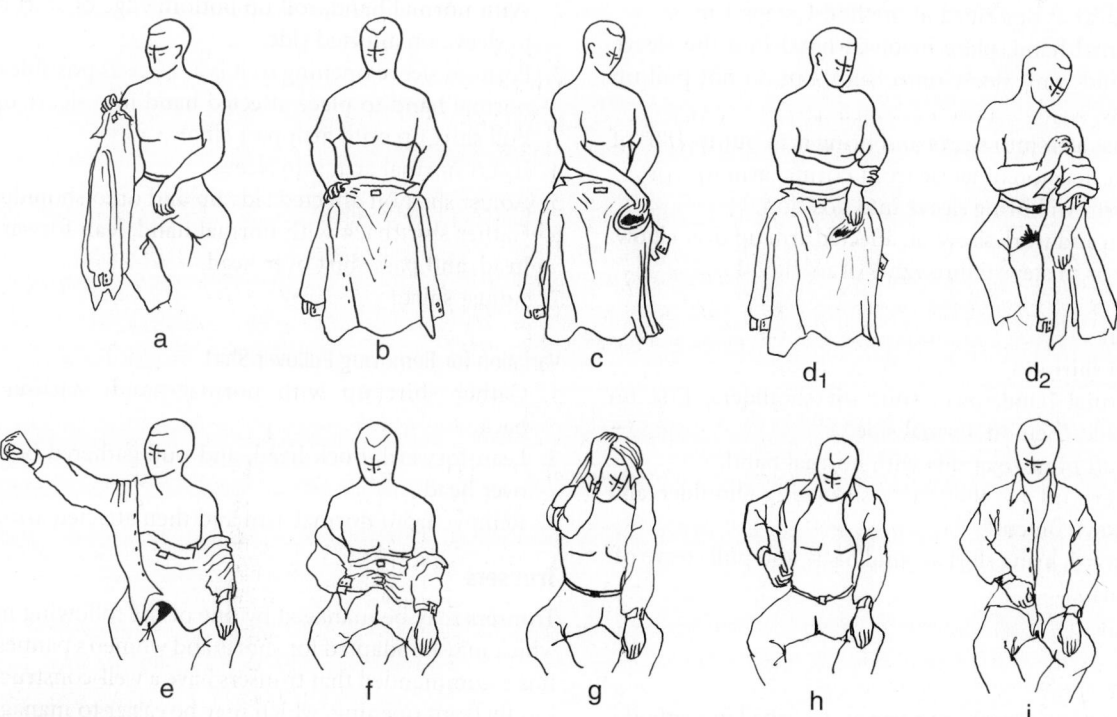

a   b   c   d₁   d₂

e   f   g   h   i

Figure 10-26   Steps in donning a shirt: method I. (Courtesy Christine Shaw, Metro Health Center for Rehabilitation, Metro Health Medical Center, Cleveland, Ohio.)

8. With normal hand, adjust shirt by leaning forward and working shirt down past both shoulders. Reach in back and pull shirt tail down (Figure 10-26, *H*).

9. Line up shirt fronts for buttoning and begin with bottom button (Figure 10-26, *I*). Button sleeve cuff of affected arm. Sleeve cuff of unaffected arm may be pre-buttoned if cuff opening is large. Button may be sewn on with elastic thread or sewn onto a small tab of elastic and fastened inside shirt cuff. A small button attached to crocheted loop of elastic thread is another option. Slip button on loop through buttonhole in garment so that elastic loop is inside. Stretch elastic loop to fit around original cuff button. This simple device can be transferred to each garment and positioned before shirt is put on. Loop stretches to accommodate width of hand as it is pushed through end of sleeve.[29]

Removing Shirt
1. Unbutton shirt.
2. Lean forward.
3. With normal hand, grasp collar or gather material up in back from collar to hem.
4. Lean forward, duck head, and pull shirt over head.
5. Remove sleeve from normal arm and then from affected arm.

Method II

Donning Shirt
Clients who get their shirts twisted or have trouble sliding the sleeve down onto the normal arm can use method II.
1. Position shirt as described in method I, steps 1 to 3.
2. With normal hand, place involved hand into the sleeve opening and work sleeve onto hand, but do not pull up over elbow.
3. Put normal arm into sleeve and bring arm out to 180° of abduction. Tension of fabric from normal arm to wrist of affected arm will bring sleeve into position.
4. Lower arm and work sleeve on affected arm up over elbow.
5. Continue as in steps 6 through 9 of method I.

Removing Shirt
1. Unbutton shirt.
2. With normal hand, push shirt off shoulders, first on affected side, then on normal side.
3. Pull on cuff of normal side with normal hand.
4. Work sleeve off by alternately shrugging shoulder and pulling down on cuff.
5. Lean forward, bring shirt around back, and pull sleeve off affected arm.

Method III

Donning Shirt
1. Position shirt and work onto arm as described in method I, steps 1 to 4.
2. Pull sleeve on affected arm up to shoulder (Figure 10-27, *A*).

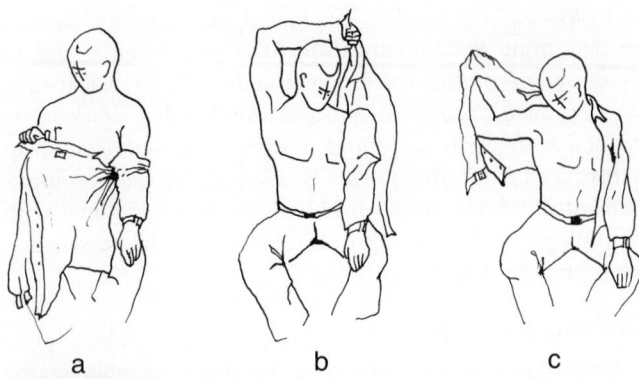

Figure 10-27 Steps in donning a shirt: method III. (Courtesy Christine Shaw, Metro Health Center for Rehabilitation, Metro Health Medical Center, Cleveland, Ohio.)

3. With normal hand, grasp tip of collar that is on normal side, lean forward, and bring arm over and behind head to carry shirt around to normal side (Figure 10-27, *B*).
4. Put normal arm into sleeve opening, directing it up and out (Figure 10-27, *C*).
5. Adjust and button as described in method I, steps 8 and 9.

Removing Shirt
The shirt may be removed using the procedure described previously for method II.

Variation for Donning Pullover Shirt
1. Position shirt on lap, bottom toward chest and label facing down.
2. With normal hand, roll up bottom edge of shirt back up to sleeve on affected side.
3. Position sleeve opening so it is as large as possible and use normal hand to place affected hand into sleeve opening. Pull shirt up onto arm past elbow.
4. Insert normal arm into sleeve.
5. Adjust shirt on affected side up and onto shoulder.
6. Gather shirt back with normal hand, lean forward, duck head, and pass shirt over head.
7. Adjust shirt.

Variation for Removing Pullover Shirt
1. Gather shirt up with normal hand, starting at top back.
2. Lean forward, duck head, and pull gathered back fabric over head.
3. Remove from normal arm and then affected arm.

Trousers

Trousers may be managed by one of the following methods, which may be adapted for shorts and women's panties as well. It is recommended that trousers have a well-constructed button fly front opening, which may be easier to manage than a zipper. Velcro may be used to replace buttons and zippers. Trousers should be worn in a size slightly larger than worn previously and should have a wide opening at the ankles. They should be put on after the socks have been put on but before the shoes are put on. If the client is dressing in a wheelchair, feet should be placed flat on the floor, not on the footrests of the wheelchair.

Method I

Donning Trousers

1. Sit in sturdy armchair or in locked wheelchair (Figure 10-28, *A*).
2. Position normal leg in front of midline of body with knee flexed to 90°. Using normal hand, reach forward and grasp ankle of affected leg or sock around ankle (Figure 10-28, B_1). Lift affected leg over normal leg to crossed position (Figure 10-28, *B2*).
3. Slip trousers onto affected leg up to position where foot is completely inside trouser leg (Figure 10-28, *C*). Do not pull up above knee or difficulty will be encountered in inserting normal leg.
4. Uncross affected leg by grasping ankle or portion of sock around ankle (Figure 10-28, *D*).
5. Insert normal leg and work trousers up onto hips as far as possible (Figure 10-18, E_1 and E_2).

6. To prevent trousers from dropping when pulling pants over hips, place affected hand in pocket or place one finger of affected hand into belt loop. If able to do so safely, stand and pull trousers over hips (Figure 10-28, F_1 and F_2).
7. If standing balance is good, remain standing to pull up zipper or button (Figure 10-28, F_3). Sit down to button front (Figure 10-28, *G*).

Removing Trousers

1. Unfasten trousers and work down on hips as far as possible while seated.
2. Stand, letting trousers drop past hips, or work trousers down past hips.
3. Remove trousers from normal leg.
4. Sit and cross affected leg over normal leg, remove trousers, and uncross leg.

Method II

Donning Trousers

Method II is used for clients who are in wheelchairs with brakes locked and footrests swung away; who are in sturdy, straight armchairs positioned with the back against the wall; and for clients who cannot stand independently.

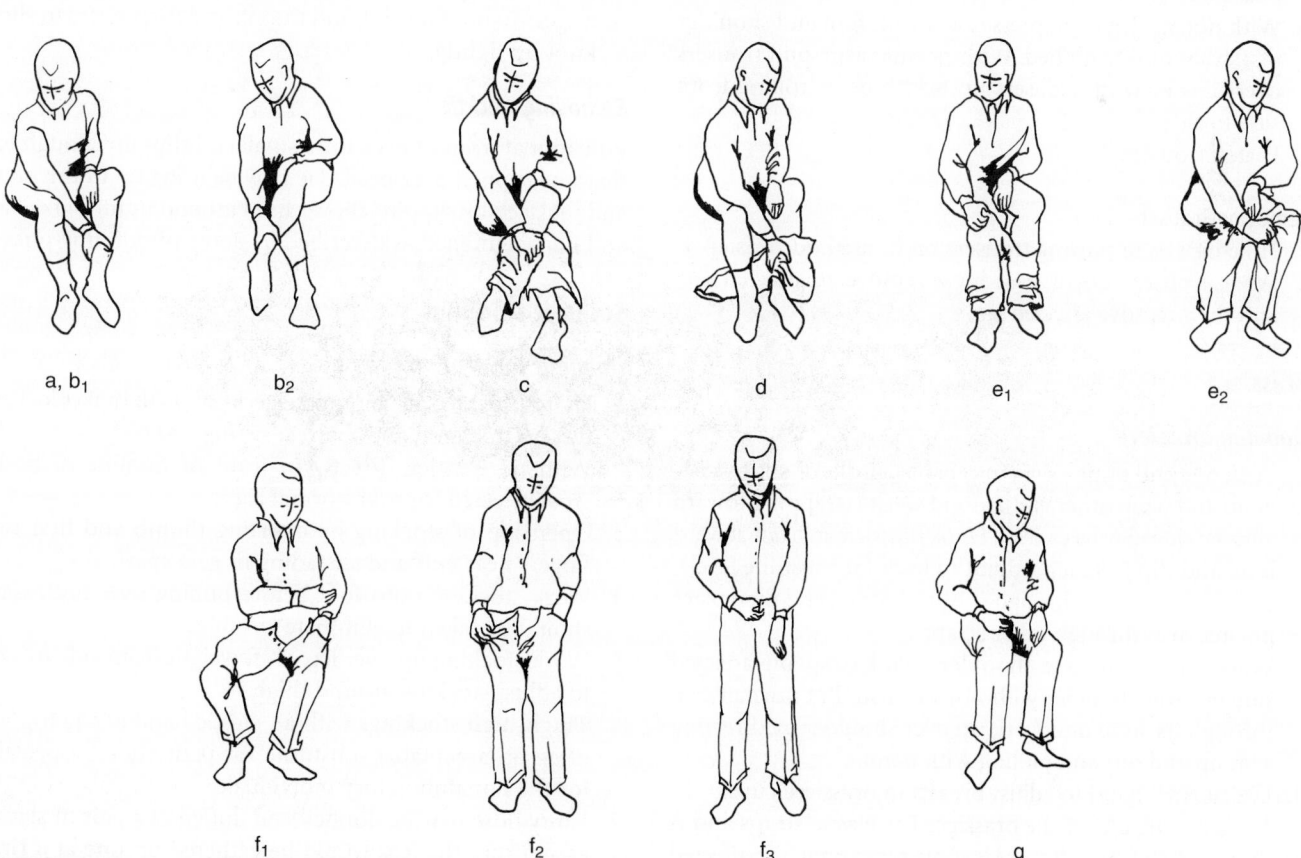

a, b₁   b₂   c   d   e₁   e₂

f₁   f₂   f₃   g

Figure 10-28 Steps in donning trousers: method I. (Courtesy Christine Shaw, Metro Health Center for Rehabilitation, Metro Health Medical Center, Cleveland, Ohio.)

1. Position trousers on legs as in method I, steps 1 through 5.
2. Elevate hips by leaning back against chair and pushing down against the floor with normal leg. As hips are raised, work trousers over hips with normal hand.
3. Lower hips back into chair and fasten trousers.

Removing Trousers

1. Unfasten trousers and work down on hips as far as possible while sitting.
2. Lean back against chair, push down against floor with normal leg to elevate hips, and with normal arm work trousers down past hips.
3. Proceed as in method I, steps 3 and 4.

Method III

Donning Trousers

Method III is for clients who are in a recumbent position. It is more difficult to perform than those methods done sitting. If possible, the bed should be raised to a semi-reclining position for partial sitting.

1. Using normal hand, place affected leg in bent position and cross over normal leg, which may be partially bent to prevent affected leg from slipping.
2. Position trousers and work onto affected leg first, up to the knee. Then uncross leg.
3. Insert normal leg and work trousers up onto hips as far as possible.
4. With normal leg bent, press down with foot and shoulder to elevate hips from bed. With normal arm, pull trousers over hips or work trousers up over hips by rolling from side to side.
5. Fasten trousers.

Removing Trousers

1. Hike hips as in putting trousers on in method III, step 4.
2. Work trousers down past hips, remove unaffected leg, and then remove affected leg.

Brassiere

Donning brassiere

1. Tuck one end of brassiere into pants, girdle, or skirt waistband and wrap other end around waist (wrapping toward affected side may be easiest). Hook brassiere in front at waist level and slip fastener around to back (at waistline level).
2. Place affected arm through shoulder strap, and then place normal arm through other strap.
3. Work straps up over shoulders. Pull strap on affected side up over shoulder with normal arm. Put normal arm through its strap and work up over shoulder by directing arm up and out and pulling with hand.
4. Use normal hand to adjust breasts in brassiere cups.
   Note: It is helpful if the brassiere has elastic straps and is made of stretch fabric. If there is some function in the affected hand, a fabric loop may be sewn to the back of the brassiere

near the fastener. The affected thumb may be slipped through the loop to stabilize the brassiere while the normal hand fastens it. All elastic brassieres, prefastened or without fasteners, may be put on by adapting method I for pullover shirts described previously. Front-opening bras may also be adapted with a loop for the affected hand with some gross arm function.

Removing brassiere

1. Slip straps down off shoulders, normal side first.
2. Work straps down over arms and off hands.
3. Slip brassiere around to front with normal arm.
4. Unfasten and remove.

Necktie

Donning necktie

Clip-on neckties are attractive and convenient. If a conventional tie is used, the following method is recommended:

1. Place collar of shirt in "up" position and bring necktie around neck and adjust so that smaller end is at desired length when tie is completed.
2. Fasten small end to shirt front with tie clasp or spring clip clothespin.
3. Loop long end around short end (one complete loop) and bring up between "V" at neck. Then bring tip down through loop at front and adjust tie, using ring and little fingers to hold tie end, and thumb and forefingers to slide knot up tightly.

Removing necktie

Pull knot at front of neck until small end slips up enough for tie to be slipped over head. Tie may be hung up in this state and replaced by slipping it over head around upturned collar, and knot tightened as described in step 3 of donning phase.

Socks or stockings

Donning socks or stockings

1. Sit in straight armchair or in wheelchair with brakes locked, feet on the floor, and footrest swung away.
2. With normal leg directly in front of midline of body, cross affected leg over normal leg.
3. Open top of stocking by inserting thumb and first two fingers near cuff and spreading fingers apart.
4. Work stocking onto foot before pulling over heel. Care should be taken to eliminate wrinkles.
5. Work stocking up over leg. Shift weight from side to side to adjust stocking around thigh.
6. Thigh-high stockings with an elastic band at the top are often an acceptable substitute for panty hose, especially for the nonambulatory individual.
7. Panty hose may be donned and doffed as a pair of slacks, except that the legs would be gathered up one at a time before placing feet into the leg holes.

Removing socks or stockings

1. Work socks or stockings down as far as possible with normal arm.
2. Cross affected leg over normal one as described in step 2 of process of putting on socks or stockings.
3. Remove sock or stocking from affected leg. Dressing stick may be required by some clients to push sock or stocking off heel and off foot.
4. Lift normal leg to comfortable height or to seat level and remove sock or stocking from foot.

Shoes

If possible, select slip-on shoes to eliminate lacing and tying. If an individual uses an *ankle-foot orthosis* (AFO) or short leg brace, shoes with fasteners are usually needed.

1. Use elastic laces and leave shoes tied.
2. Use adapted shoe fasteners.
3. Use one-handed shoe-tying techniques (Figure 10-29).
4. It is possible to learn to tie a standard bow with one hand, but this requires excellent visual, perceptual, and motor planning skills along with much repetition.

Ankle-foot orthosis

The individual with hemiplegia who lacks adequate ankle dorsiflexion to walk safely and efficiently frequently uses an AFO. It can be donned in the following manner.

Donning an AFO

Method I

1. Sit in straight armchair or wheelchair with brakes locked and feet on the floor (Figure 10-30, *A*). The fasteners are loosened and the tongue of the shoe is pulled back to allow the AFO to fit into the shoe (Figure 10-30, *B*).
2. AFO and shoe are placed on the floor between the legs but closer to the affected leg, facing up (Figure 10-30, *C*).

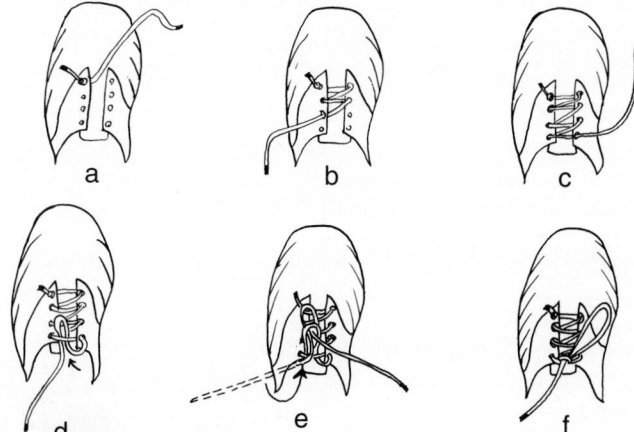

Figure 10-29 One-hand shoe-tying method. (Courtesy Christine Shaw, Metro Health Center for Rehabilitation, Metro Health Medical Center, Cleveland, Ohio.)

3. With the unaffected hand, lift the affected leg behind the knee and place toes into the shoe (Figure 10-30, *D*).
4. Reach down with unaffected hand and lift AFO by the upright. Simultaneously use the unaffected foot against the affected heel to keep the shoe and AFO together (Figure 10-30, *E*).
5. The heel will not be pushed into the shoe at this point. With the unaffected hand, apply pressure directly downward on the affected knee to force the heel into the shoe, if leg strength is not sufficient (Figure 10-30, *F*).
6. Fasten Velcro calf strap and fasten shoes (Figure 10-30, *G*). The affected leg may be placed on a footstool to assist with reaching shoe fasteners.
7. To fasten shoes, one-handed bow-tying may be used; elastic shoelaces, Velcro-fastened shoes, or other commercially available shoe fasteners may be required if the client is unable to tie shoes.

Method II

Steps 1 and 2 are the same as the positioning required for donning pants.

1. Sit in sturdy armchair or in locked wheelchair.
2. Position normal leg in front of midline of body with knee flexed to 90°. Using normal hand, reach forward and grasp ankle of affected leg or sock around ankle. Lift affected leg over normal leg to crossed position.
3. The fasteners are loosened and the tongue of the shoe is pulled back to allow the AFO to fit into the shoe; Velcro fastener on upright is unfastened.
4. Using normal hand, hold heel of shoe and work over toes of affected foot and leg. Once toes are in shoe, work top part of AFO around the calf.
5. Pull heel of shoe onto foot with hand or place foot on floor, place pressure on knee, and push heel down into shoe.
6. Fasten Velcro calf strap and fasten shoes.

Removing an AFO

Variation I

1. While seated as for donning an AFO, cross affected leg over normal leg.
2. Unfasten straps and laces with normal hand.
3. Push down on AFO upright until shoe is off foot.

Variation II

1. Unfasten straps and laces.
2. Straighten affected leg by putting normal foot behind heel of shoe and pushing affected leg forward.
3. Push down on AFO upright with hand and at same time push forward on heel of AFO shoe with normal foot.

Feeding Activities

The main problem encountered by the one-handed individual is managing a knife and fork simultaneously for cutting meat. This problem can be solved by the use of a rocker knife for cutting meat and other foods (Figure 10-31). This knife

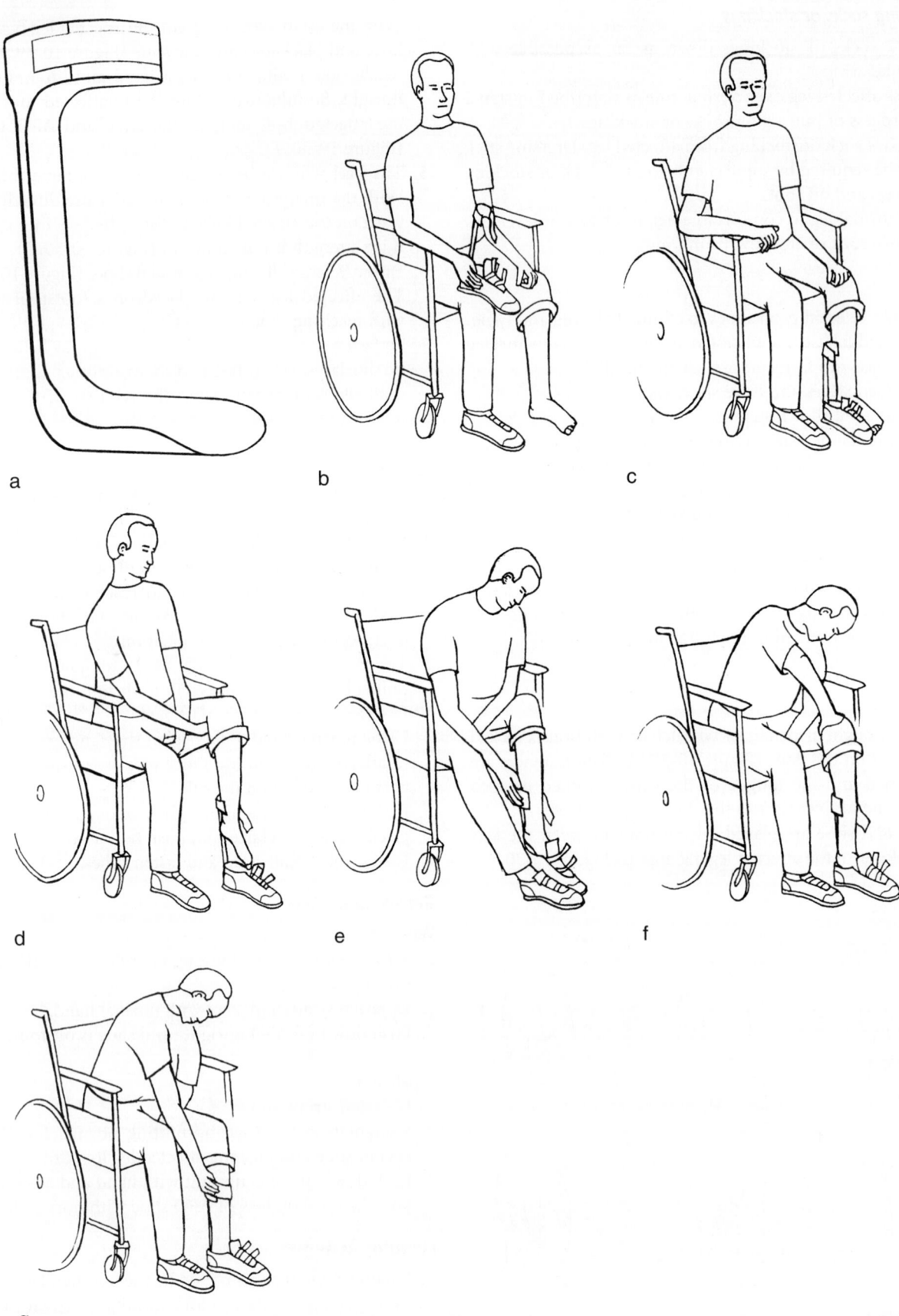

a

b

c

d

e

f

g

Figure 10-30   Steps in donning ankle-foot orthosis (AFO).

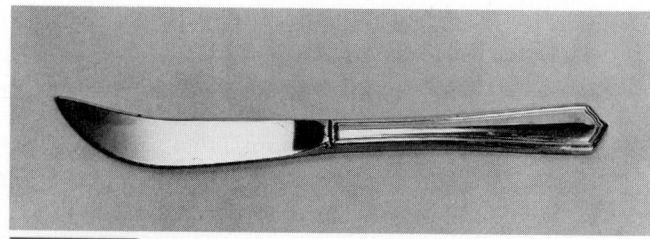

Figure 10-31 One-handed rocker knife. (Courtesy Sammons Preston.)

cuts with a rocking motion rather than a back-and-forth slicing action. Use of a rocking motion with a standard table knife or a sharp paring knife may be adequate to cut tender meats and soft foods. If such a knife is used, the client is taught to hold the knife handle between the thumb and the third, fourth, and fifth fingers, and the index finger is extended along the top of the knife blade. The knife point is placed in the food in a vertical position, and then the blade is brought down to cut the food. The rocking motion, using wrist flexion and extension, is continued until the food is cut.

 OT PRACTICE NOTE

The occupational therapist should keep in mind that one-handed meat cutting involves learning a new motor pattern. This skill may be difficult for clients with hemiplegia and apraxia.

Personal Hygiene and Grooming Activities

Clients with the use of one hand or one side of the body can accomplish personal hygiene and grooming activities by using assistive devices and alternative methods. The following are suggestions for achieving hygiene and grooming with one hand:

1. Use an electric razor rather than a safety razor.
2. Use a shower seat in the shower stall or a transfer tub bench in a bathtub-shower combination. Also use a bath mat, wash mitt, long-handled bath sponge, safety rails on the bathtub or wall, soap on a rope or suction soap holder, and suction brush for fingernail care.
3. Sponge bathe while sitting at the lavatory using the wash mitt, suction brush, and suction soap holder. The uninvolved forearm and hand may be washed by placing a soaped washcloth on the thigh and rubbing the hand and forearm on the cloth.
4. Use a wall-mounted hair dryer. Such a device frees the unaffected upper extremity to hold a brush or comb to style the hair during blow-drying.[12]
5. Care for fingernails as described previously for clients with incoordination.
6. Use a suction denture brush for care of dentures. The suction fingernail brush may also serve this purpose (Figure 10-22).

Communication and Environmental Hardware Adaptations

1. The primary problem with writing is stabilization of the paper or tablet. This problem can be overcome by using a clipboard, paperweight, or nonskid surface such as Dycem, or by taping the paper to the writing surface. In some instances, the affected arm may be positioned on the table top to passively stabilize the paper.
2. If dominance must be shifted to the nondominant extremity, writing practice may be necessary to improve speed and coordination. One-handed writing and keyboarding instruction manuals are available.
3. Book holders may be used to stabilize a book while reading or holding copy for typing and writing practice. A soft pillow will easily stabilize a book while the person is seated in an easy chair.
4. The telephone is managed by lifting the receiver to listen for the dial tone, setting it down, pressing the keys, and lifting the receiver to the ear. To write while using the telephone, a stand or shoulder telephone receiver holder must be used. A speakerphone can also leave hands free to take messages. One-touch dialing using preprogrammed phone numbers eliminates pressing as many keys, simplifies sequencing, and may help compensate for memory deficits.

Functional Mobility

Principles of transfer techniques for clients with hemiplegia are described in Chapter 11.

Home Management, Meal Preparation, and Cleanup Activities

Many assistive devices are available to facilitate home management and meal activities. Various factors determine how many home management and meal activities can realistically be performed, which methods can be used, and how many assistive devices can be managed. These factors include (1) whether the client is disabled by the loss of function of one arm and hand, as in amputation or a peripheral neuropathic condition, or (2) whether both arm and leg are affected along with possible visual, perceptual, and cognitive dysfunctions, as in hemiplegia. The references listed at the end of this chapter provide details of homemaking with one hand. The following are some suggestions for home management and meal activities for the client with use of one hand.[17]

1. Stabilizing items is a major problem for the one-handed homemaker. Stabilize foods for cutting and peeling by using a cutting board with two stainless steel or aluminum nails in it. A raised corner on the board stabilizes bread for making sandwiches or spreading butter. Suction cups or a rubber mat under the board will keep it from slipping. A nonskid surface or rubber feet may be glued to the bottom of the board (Figure 10-25).
2. Use sponge cloths, nonskid mats or pads, wet dishcloths, or suction devices to keep pots, bowls, and dishes from turning or sliding during food preparation.

3. To open a jar, stabilize it between the knees or in a partially opened drawer while leaning against the drawer. Break the air seal by sliding a pop bottle opener under the lid until the air is released, then use a Zim jar opener (Figure 10-32).

4. Open boxes, sealed paper, and plastic bags by stabilizing between the knees or in a drawer as just described, and cut open with household shears. Special box and bag openers are also available from ADL equipment vendors.

5. Crack an egg by holding it firmly in the palm of the hand. Hit it in the center against the edge of the bowl. Then using the thumb and index finger, push the top half of the shell up and use the ring and little finger to push the lower half down. Separate whites from yolks by using an egg separator, funnel, or large slotted spoon.

6. Eliminate the need to stabilize the standard grater by using a grater with suction feet, or use an electric countertop food processor instead.

7. Stabilize pots on the counter or range for mixing or stirring by using a pan holder with suction feet (Figure 10-33).

8. Eliminate the need to use hand-cranked or electric can openers, which necessitate the use of two hands, by using a one-handed electric can opener.

9. Use a utility cart to carry items from one place to another. For some clients a cart that is weighted or constructed of wood may be used as a minimal support during ambulation.

10. Transfer clothes to and from the washer or dryer by using a clothes carrier on wheels.

11. Use electrical appliances, such as a lightweight electrical hand mixer, blender, and food processor, that can be managed with one hand and save time and energy.

Safety factors and judgment need to be evaluated carefully when electrical appliances are considered.

12. Floor care becomes a greater problem if, in addition to one arm, ambulation and balance are affected. For clients with involvement of only one arm, a standard dust mop, carpet sweeper, or upright vacuum cleaner should present no problem. A self-wringing mop may be used if the mop handle is stabilized under the arm and the wringing lever operated with the normal arm. Clients with balance and ambulation problems may manage some floor care from a sitting position. Dust mopping or using a carpet sweeper may be possible if gait and balance are fairly good without the aid of a cane.

These are just a few of the possibilities for solving homemaking problems for one-handed individuals. The occupational therapist must evaluate each client to determine how the dysfunction affects performance of homemaking activities. One-handed techniques take more time and may be difficult for some clients to master. Activities should be paced to accommodate the client's physical endurance and tolerance for one-handed performance and use of special devices. Work simplification and energy conservation techniques should be employed. New techniques and devices should be introduced on a graded basis as the client masters first one technique and device and then another. Family members need to be oriented to the client's skills, special methods used, and work schedule. The therapist, with the family and client, may facilitate the planning of homemaking responsibilities to be shared by other family members and the supervision of the client, if that is needed. If special equipment and assistive devices are needed for ADL, it is advisable to acquire these through the health agency, if possible. The therapist can then train the client and demonstrate use of the equipment to a family member before these items are used at home. After training, the occupational therapist should provide the client with sources to replace items independently, such as a consumer catalog of adaptive equipment.

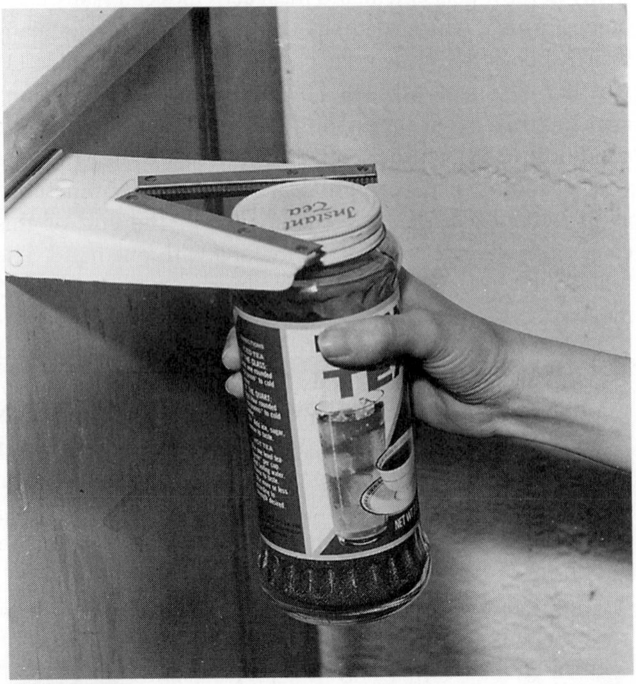

Figure 10-32   Zim jar opener.

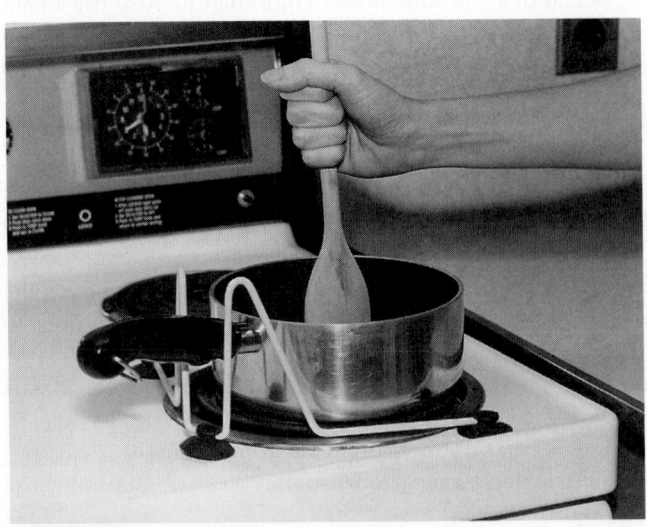

Figure 10-33   Pan stabilizer.

ADLs FOR THE PERSON WITH PARAPLEGIA

Clients who must use a wheelchair for mobility need to find ways to perform ADLs from a seated position, to transport objects, and to adapt to an environment designed for standing and walking. Given normal function in the upper extremities, the wheelchair ambulator can probably perform independently. The client should have a stable spine, and mobility precautions should be clearly identified.

Dressing Activities*

It is recommended that clients who must use wheelchairs put on clothing in this order: stockings, undergarments, braces (if worn), trousers or slacks, shoes, shirt, or dress.

Trousers

Donning trousers

Trousers and slacks are easier to fasten if they button or zip in front. If braces are worn, zippers in side seams may be helpful. Wide-bottom slacks of stretch fabric are recommended. The procedure for putting on trousers, shorts, slacks, and underwear is as follows:

1. Use side rails or a trapeze to pull up to sitting position, back supported with pillows or headboard of the bed.
2. Sit on bed and reach forward to feet, or sit on bed and pull knees into flexed position.
3. Holding top of trousers, flip pants down to feet.
4. Work pant legs over feet and pull up to hips. Crossing ankles may help get pants on over heels.
5. In semi-reclining position, roll from hip to hip and pull up garment.
6. A long-handled reacher may be helpful for pulling garment up or positioning garment on feet if there is impaired balance or range of motion in the lower extremities or trunk.

Removing trousers

Remove pants or underwear by reversing procedure for putting on. Dressing sticks may be helpful for pushing pants off feet.

Socks or stockings

Soft stretch socks or stockings are recommended. Panty hose that are slightly large may be useful. Elastic garters or stockings with elastic tops should be avoided because of potential skin breakdown. Dressing sticks or a stocking device may be helpful to some clients.

Donning socks or stockings

1. Put on socks or stockings while seated on bed.
2. Pull one leg into flexion with one hand and cross over the other leg.

*Summarized from Activities of daily living for clients with incoordination, limited range of motion, paraplegia, quadriplegia, and hemiplegia, Cleveland, 1989, Metro Health Center for Rehabilitation, Metro Health Medical Center, unpublished.

3. Use other hand to slip sock or stocking over foot and pull sock or stocking on.

Removing socks or stockings

Remove socks or stockings by flexing leg as described for donning, pushing sock or stocking down over heel. Dressing sticks may be needed to push sock or stocking off heel and toe and to retrieve sock.

Slips and skirts

Slips and skirts slightly larger than usually worn are recommended. A-line, wraparound, and full skirts are easier to manage and look better on a person seated in a wheelchair than narrow skirts.

Donning slips and skirts

1. Sit on bed, slip garment over head, and let it drop to waist.
2. In semi-reclining position, roll from hip to hip and pull garment down over hips and thighs.

Removing slips and skirts

1. In sitting or semi-reclining position, unfasten garment.
2. Roll from hip to hip, pulling garment up to waist level.
3. Pull garment off over head.

Shirts

Fabrics should be wrinkle-resistant, smooth, and durable. Roomy sleeves and backs and full shirts are more suitable styles than closely fitted garments.

Donning shirts

Shirts, pajama jackets, robes, and dresses that open completely down the front may be put on while the client is seated in a wheelchair. If it is necessary to dress while in bed, the following procedure can be used:

1. Balance body by putting palms of hands on mattress on either side of body. If balance is poor, assistance may be needed or bed backrest may be elevated. (If backrest cannot be elevated, one or two pillows may be used to support back.) With backrest elevated, both hands are available.
2. If difficulty is encountered in customary methods of applying garment, open garment on lap with collar toward chest. Put arms into sleeves and pull up over elbows. Then hold on to shirt tail or back of dress, pull garment over head, adjust, and button.

Removing shirts

1. Sitting in wheelchair or bed, open fastener.
2. Remove garment in usual manner.
3. If usual manner is not feasible, grasp collar with one hand while balancing with other hand. Gather material up from collar to hem.
4. Lean forward, duck head, and pull shirt over head.

5. Remove sleeves, first from supporting arm and then from working arm.

Shoes

Donning shoes

If an individual has sensory loss and is at risk for bruising during transfers, shoes should be donned in bed.

Variation I

1. In sitting position on bed, pull one knee at a time into flexed position with hands.
2. While supporting leg in flexed position with one hand, use free hand to put on shoe.

Variation II

1. Sit on edge of bed or in wheelchair for back support.
2. Bend one knee up to flexed position, while supporting leg with arm, and slip shoe onto foot with free hand.

Variation III

1. Sit on edge of bed or in wheelchair for back support.
2. Cross one leg over other and slip shoe onto foot.
3. Put foot on footrest and push down on knee to push foot into shoe.

Removing shoes

1. Flex or cross leg as described for appropriate variation.
2. For variations I and II, remove shoe with one hand while supporting flexed leg with other hand.
3. For variation III, remove shoe from crossed leg with one hand while maintaining balance with other hand, if necessary.

Feeding Activities

Eating activities should present no special problem for the person who uses a wheelchair but has good to normal arm function. Wheelchairs with desk arms and swing-away footrests are recommended so that it is possible to sit close to the table.

Personal Hygiene and Grooming

Facial and oral hygiene and arm and upper body care should present no problem. Reachers may be helpful for securing towels, washcloths, make-up, deodorant, and shaving supplies from storage areas, if necessary. Special equipment is needed for using tub baths or showers. Transfer techniques for toilet and bathtub are discussed in Chapter 11. The following are suggestions for facilitating bathing activities:

1. Use a hand-held shower hose and keep a finger over the spray to determine sudden temperature changes in water.
2. Use long-handled bath brushes with soap insert for ease in reaching all parts of the body.
3. Use soap bars attached to a cord around the neck, or use liquid soap.

4. Use shower chairs or bathtub seats.
5. Increase safety during transfers by installing grab bars on wall near bathtub or shower and on bathtub.
6. Fit bathtub or shower bottom with nonskid mat or adhesive material.
7. Remove doors on the bathtub and replace with a shower curtain to increase safety and ease of transfers.

Communication and Environmental Hardware Adaptations

With the exception of reaching difficulties in some situations, use of the telephone should present no problem. Short-handled reachers may be used to grasp the receiver from the cradle. A cordless telephone can eliminate reaching, except when the phone needs recharging. The use of writing implements, tape recorder, and personal computer should be possible. Managing doors may present some difficulties. If the door opens toward the person, it can be opened by the following procedure:

1. If doorknob is on the right, approach door from right and turn doorknob with left hand.
2. Open door as far as possible and move wheelchair close enough so that it helps keep door open.
3. Holding door open with left hand, turn wheelchair with right hand and wheel through door.
4. Start closing door when halfway through.

If the door is very heavy and opens out or away from the person, the following procedure is recommended:

1. Back up to door so knob can be turned with right hand.
2. Open door and back through so that big wheels keep it open.
3. Also use left elbow to keep door open.
4. Wheel backward with right hand.

Functional Mobility

Principles of transfer techniques are discussed in Chapter 11.

Home Management, Meal Preparation, and Cleanup Activities

When homemaking activities are performed from a wheelchair, the major problems are work heights, adequate space for maneuverability, access to storage areas, and transfer of supplies, equipment, and materials from place to place. If funds are available for kitchen remodeling, lowering counters and range to a comfortable height for wheelchair use is recommended. Such extensive adaptation is often not feasible, however. The following are some suggestions for homemaking activities.[17]

1. Remove cabinet doors to eliminate the need to maneuver around them for opening and closing. Frequently used items should be stored toward the front of easy-to-reach cabinets above and below the counter surfaces.
2. If entrance and inside doors are not wide enough, use a device to reduce wheelchair width or make doors slightly wider by removing strips along the door jambs. Offset hinges can replace standard door hinges and increase the door jamb width by 2 inches (Figure 10-34).

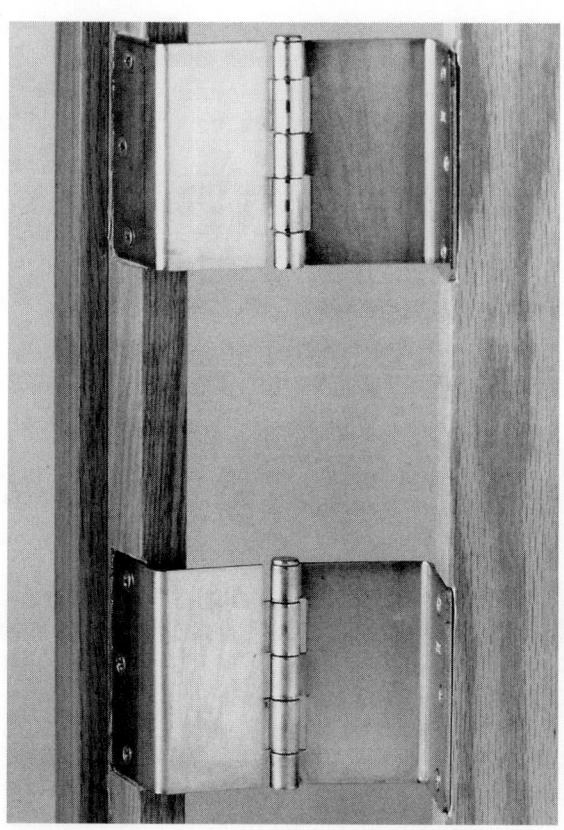
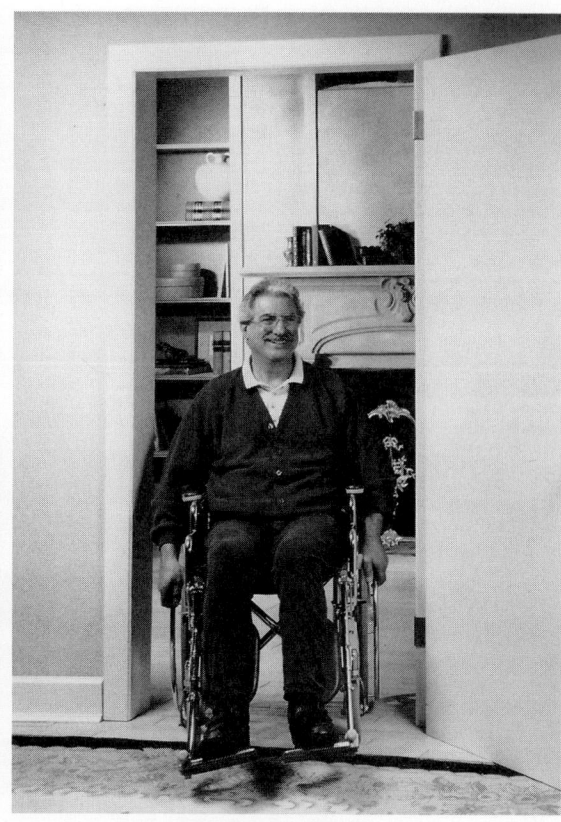

A   B

Figure 10-34   **A,** Offset door hinges. **B,** Offset hinges widen doorway for wheelchair user. (Courtesy Sammons Preston.)

3. Use a wheelchair cushion to increase the user's height so that standard height counters may be used.

4. Use detachable desk arms and swing-away detachable footrests to allow the wheelchair user to get as close as possible to counters and tables and also to stand at counters, if that is possible.

5. Transport items safely and easily with a wheelchair lap board. The lap board may also serve as a work surface for preparing food and drying dishes. It also protects the lap from injury from hot pans and prevents utensils from falling into the lap (Figure 10-35).

6. Fasten a dropleaf board to a bare wall, or install a slide-out board under a counter to provide a work surface that is a comfortable height in a kitchen that is otherwise standard.

7. Fit cabinets with custom- or ready-made lazy Susans or pull-out shelves to eliminate the need to reach to rear space (Figure 10-36).

8. Ideally, ranges should be at a lower level than standard height. If this arrangement is not possible, place the controls at the front of the range, and hang a mirror angled at the proper degree over the range so that the homemaker can see contents of pots.

9. Substitute small electric cooking units and microwave ovens for the range if the range is not safely manageable.

10. Use front-loading washers and dryers.

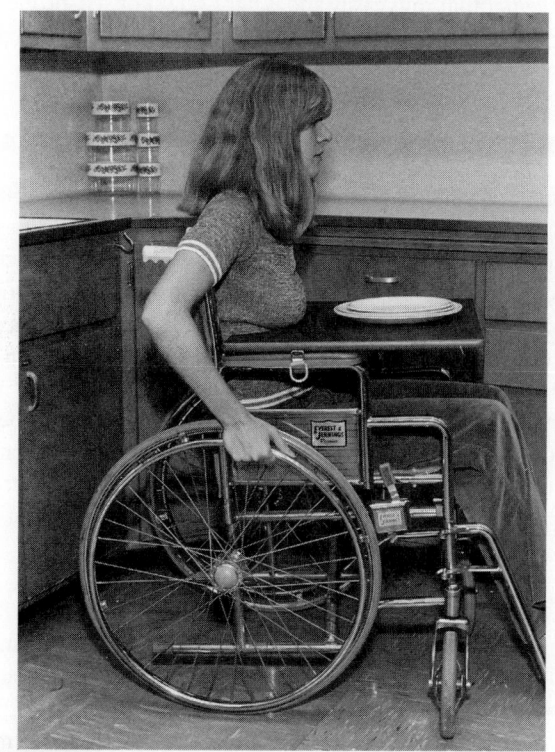

Figure 10-35   Wheelchair lapboard is used to transport items.

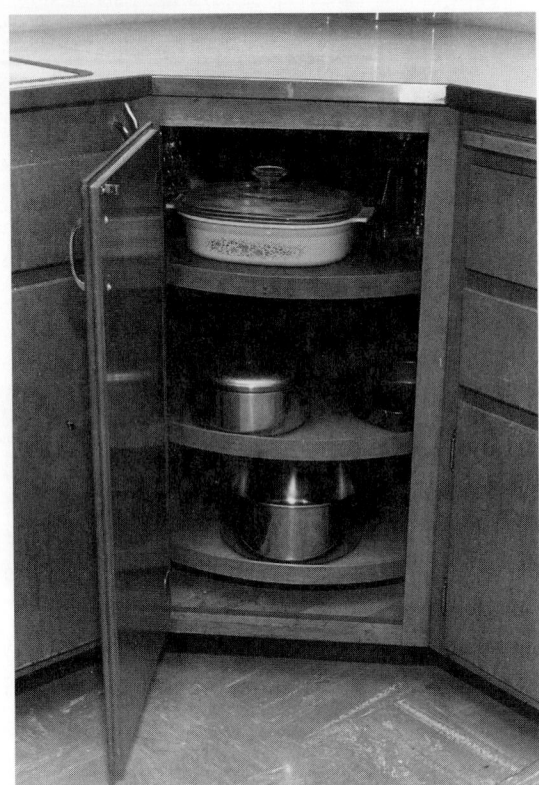

Figure 10-36 Lazy Susan in kitchen storage cabinet.

11. Vacuum carpets with a carpet sweeper or tank-type cleaner that rolls easily and is lightweight or self-propelled. A retractable cord may be helpful for preventing tangling of cord in wheels.

ADLs FOR THE PERSON WITH QUADRIPLEGIA

In general, persons with muscle function from spinal cord levels C7 and C8 can follow many of the methods just described for paraplegia, except for fine motor tasks such as buttoning or typing. Individuals with muscle function from C6 can be relatively independent with adaptations and assistive devices, whereas those with muscle function from C4 and C5 will require considerable special equipment and assistance. Clients with muscle function from C6 may benefit from the use of a wrist-driven flexor hinge splint. Externally powered splints and arm braces or mobile arm supports are recommended for C3, C4, and C5 levels of muscle function[1] and are discussed in Chapters 29 and 36.

Dressing Activities

Training in dressing can be commenced when the spine is stable.[7,28] *Minimum criteria* for upper extremity dressing are as follows:

1. Fair to good muscle strength in deltoids, upper and middle trapezii, shoulder rotators, rhomboids, biceps, supinators, and radial wrist extensors.

2. ROM of 0° to 90° in shoulder flexion and abduction, 0° to 80° in shoulder internal rotation, 0° to 30° in external rotation, and 15° to 140° in elbow flexion.

3. Sitting balance in bed or wheelchair, which may be achieved with the assistance of bed rails, electric hospital bed, or wheelchair safety belt.

4. Finger prehension achieved with adequate tenodesis grasp or wrist-driven flexor-hinge splint.

Additional criteria for dressing the lower extremities are as follows:[28]

1. Fair to good muscle strength in pectoralis major and minor, serratus anterior, and rhomboid major and minor.

2. ROM of 0° to 120° in knee flexion, 0° to 110° in hip flexion, and 0° to 80° in hip external rotation.

3. Body control for transfer from bed to wheelchair with minimal assistance.

4. Ability to roll from side to side, turn from supine position to prone position and back, and balance in side-lying.

5. Vital capacity of 50% or better.

Dressing is *contraindicated* if any of the following factors are present:[7,28]

1. Unstable spine at site of injury.

2. Pressure sores or tendency for skin breakdown during rolling, scooting, and transferring.

3. Uncontrollable muscle spasms in legs.

4. Less than 50% vital capacity.

Sequence of dressing

The recommended sequence for training to dress is to put on underwear and trousers while still in bed, then transfer to a wheelchair and put on shirts, socks, and shoes.[28] Some clients may wish to put the socks on before the trousers because socks may help the feet slip through the trouser legs more easily.

Expected proficiency

Clients with spinal cord lesions at C7 and below can achieve *total dressing*, which includes dressing skills for both the upper and lower extremities. Clients with lesions at C6 can also achieve total dressing, but lower extremity dressing may be difficult or impractical in terms of time and energy for these clients. Clients with lesions at C5 to C6 can achieve upper extremity dressing, with some exceptions. It is difficult or impossible for these clients to put on a brassiere, tuck a shirt or blouse into a waistband, or fasten buttons on shirt fronts and cuffs. Factors such as age, physical proportions, coordination, concomitant medical problems, and motivation will affect the degree of proficiency in dressing skills that can be achieved by any client.[7]

Types of clothing

Clothing should be loose and have front openings. Trousers need to be a size larger than usually worn to accommodate the urine collection device or leg braces if worn. Wraparound skirts and incontinence pads are helpful for women. The fasteners that are easiest to manage are zippers and Velcro closures. Because the client with quadriplegia often uses the thumb as a hook to manage clothing, loops attached to zipper pulls, undershorts, and even the back of the shoes can be helpful. Belt loops on trousers are used for pulling and should be reinforced. Brassieres should have stretch straps and no wires in them. Front-opening brassiere styles can be adapted by fastening loops and adding Velcro closures; back-opening styles can have loops added at each side of the fastening.

Shoes can be one-half size to one size larger than normally worn to accommodate edema and spasticity and to avoid pressure sores. Shoe fasteners can be adapted with Velcro, elastic shoelaces, large buckles, or flip-back tongue closures. Loose woolen or cotton socks without elastic cuffs should be used initially. Nylon socks, which tend to stick to the skin, may be used as skill is gained. If neckties are used, the clip-on type or a regular tie that has been preknotted and can be slipped over the head may be manageable for some clients.[7,28]

Trousers and undershorts

Donning Trousers and Undershorts

1. Sit on bed with bed rails up. Trousers are positioned at foot of bed with trouser legs over end of bed and front side up.[28]
2. Sit up and lift one knee at a time by hooking right hand under right knee to pull leg into flexion, then put trousers over right foot. Return right leg to extension or semi-extended position while repeating procedure with left hand and left knee.[7] If unable to maintain leg in flexion by holding with one arm or through advantageous use of spasticity, use a dressing band. This device is a piece of elasticized webbing that has been sewn into a figure-eight pattern, with one small loop and one large loop. The small loop is hooked around the foot and the large hoop is anchored over the knee. The band is measured for individual client so that its length is appropriate to maintain desired amount of knee flexion. Once the trousers are in place, knee loop is pushed off knee and dressing band is removed from foot with dressing stick.
3. Work trousers up legs, using patting and sliding motions with palms of hands.
4. While still sitting, with pants to midcalf height, insert dressing stick in front belt loop. Dressing stick is gripped by slipping its loop over wrist. Pull on dressing stick while extending trunk, returning to supine position. Return to sitting position and repeat this procedure, pulling on dressing sticks and maneuvering trousers up to thigh level.[28] If balance is adequate, an alternative is for client to remain sitting and lean on left elbow and pull trousers over right buttock, then reverse process for other side. Another alternative is for client to remain in supine position and roll to one side; throw opposite arm behind back; hook thumb in waistband, belt loop, or pocket; and pull trousers up over hips. These maneuvers can be repeated as often as necessary to get trousers over buttocks.[7]
5. Using palms of hands in pushing and smoothing motions, straighten the trouser legs.

6. In supine position, fasten trouser placket by hooking thumb in loop on zipper pull, patting Velcro closed, or using hand splints and buttonhooks if there are buttons or a zipper pull for zippers.[7,28]

Variation

Substitute the following for step 2: Sit up and lift one knee at a time by hooking right hand under right knee to pull leg into flexion, then cross the foot over the opposite leg above the knee. This position frees the foot to place the trousers more easily and requires less trunk balance. Continue with all other steps.

Removing Trousers and Undershorts

1. Lying supine in bed with bed rails up, unfasten belt and placket fasteners.
2. Placing thumbs in belt loops, waistband, or pockets, work trousers past hips by stabilizing arms in shoulder extension and scooting body toward head of bed.
3. Use arms as described in step 2 and roll from side to side to get trousers past buttocks.
4. Coming to sitting position and alternately pulling legs into flexion, push trousers down legs.[28]
5. Trousers can be pushed off over feet with dressing stick or by hooking thumbs in waistband.

Cardigans or pullover garments

Cardigan and pullover garments include blouses, vests, sweaters, skirts, and front-opening dresses.[7,28] Upper extremity dressing is frequently performed in the wheelchair for greater trunk stability. The procedure for putting on these garments is as follows:

Donning cardigans or pullover garments

1. Position the garment across thighs with back facing up and neck toward knees.
2. Place both arms under back of garment and in armholes.
3. Push sleeves up onto arms, past elbows.
4. Using a wrist extension grip, hook thumbs under garment back and gather material up from neck to hem.
5. To pass garment over head, adduct and externally rotate shoulders and flex elbows while flexing head forward.
6. When garment is over head, relax shoulders and wrists and remove hands from back of garment. Most of material will be gathered up at neck, across shoulders, and under arms.
7. To work garment down over body, shrug shoulders, lean forward, and use elbow flexion and wrist extension. Use wheelchair arms for balance, if necessary. Additional maneuvers to accomplish task are to hook wrists into sleeves and pull material free from underarms, or lean forward, reach back, and slide hand against material to aid in pulling garment down.
8. Garment can be buttoned from bottom to top with aid of button hook and wrist-driven flexor hinge splint if hand function is inadequate.

Removing cardigans or pullover garments

1. Sit in wheelchair and wear wrist-driven flexor hinge splints. Unfasten buttons (if any) while wearing splints and using buttonhook. Remove splints for remaining steps.
2. For pullover garments, hook thumb in back of neckline, extend wrist, and pull garment over head while turning head toward side of raised arm. Maintain balance by resting against opposite wheelchair armrest or pushing on thigh with extended arm.
3. For cardigan garments, hook thumb in opposite armhole and push sleeve down arm. Elevation and depression of shoulders with trunk rotation can be used to get garment to slip down arms as far as possible.
4. Hold one cuff with opposite thumb while elbow is flexed to pull arm out of sleeve.

Brassiere (Back-opening)

Donning brassiere

1. Place brassiere across lap with straps toward knees and inside facing up.
2. Using a right-to-left procedure, hold end of brassiere closest to right side with hand or reacher and pass brassiere around back from right to left side. Lean against brassiere at back to hold it in place, while hooking thumb of left hand in a loop that has been attached near brassiere fastener. Hook right thumb in a similar loop on right side, and fasten brassiere in front at waist level.
3. Hook right thumb in edge of brassiere. Using wrist extension, elbow flexion, shoulder adduction, and internal rotation, rotate brassiere around body so that front of brassiere is in front of body.
4. While leaning on one forearm, hook opposite thumb in front end of strap and pull strap over shoulder, then repeat procedure on other side.[7,28]

Removing brassiere

1. Hook thumb under opposite brassiere strap and push down over shoulder while elevating shoulder.
2. Pull arm out of strap and repeat procedure for other arm.
3. Push brassiere down to waist level and turn around as described previously to bring fasteners to front.
4. Unfasten brassiere by hooking thumbs into the adapted loops near the fasteners.

    Alternatives for a back-opening bra are (1) a front-opening bra with loops for using a wrist extension grip or (2) a fully elastic bra that has no fasteners and can be donned like a pullover sweater.

Socks

Donning socks

1. Sit in wheelchair, or on bed if balance is adequate, in cross-legged position with one ankle crossed over opposite knee.
2. Pull sock over foot with wrist extension grip and patting movements with palm of hand.[7,28]
3. If trunk balance is inadequate and cross-legged position cannot be maintained, balance by propping foot on stool, chair, or open drawer, while opposite arm is around upright of wheelchair. Using a wheelchair safety belt or leaning against wheelchair armrest on one side are options to maintain balance.
4. Use stocking aid or sock cone (Figure 10-8) to assist in putting on socks while in this position. Powder sock cone (to reduce friction) and apply sock to cone by using thumbs and palms of hands to smooth sock out on cone.
5. With the cord loops of sock cone around the wrist or thumb, throw cone beyond foot.
6. Maneuver cone over toes by pulling cords using elbow flexion. Insert foot as far as possible into cone.
7. To remove cone from sock after foot has been inserted, move heel forward off wheelchair footrest. Use wrist extension (of hand not operating sock cone) behind knee and continue pulling cords of cone until it is removed and sock is in place on foot. Use palms to smooth sock with patting and stroking motion.[28]
8. Two loops can also be sewn on either side of the top of the sock so that thumbs can be hooked into the loops and the socks pulled on.

Removing socks

1. While sitting in wheelchair or lying in bed, use a dressing stick or long-handled shoehorn to push sock down over heel. Cross the legs if possible.
2. Use dressing stick with cup hook on end to pull sock off toes.

Shoes

Donning shoes

1. Use same position for donning socks as for putting on shoes.
2. Use long-handled dressing aid and insert aid into tongue of shoe. Place shoe opening over toes. Remove dressing aid from shoe and dangle shoe on toes.
3. Using palm of hand on sole of shoe, pull shoe toward heel of foot. One hand is used to stabilize leg while other hand pushes against sole of shoe to work shoe onto foot. Use thenar eminence and sides of hand for this pushing motion.
4. With feet flat on floor or on wheelchair footrest and knees flexed 90°, place a long-handled shoehorn in heel of shoe and press down on flexed knee.
5. Fasten shoes.[28]

Removing shoes

1. Sitting in wheelchair with legs crossed as described previously, unfasten shoes.
2. Use shoehorn or dressing stick to push on heel counter of shoe, dislodging it from heel. Shoe will drop or can be pushed to floor with dressing stick.[28]

Feeding Activities

Feeding may be assisted by a variety of devices, depending on the level of muscle function.[1] An injury at C5 or above necessitates mobile arm supports or externally powered splints and braces. A wrist splint and universal cuff may be used together if a wrist-driven flexor hinge splint is not used. The universal cuff holds the eating utensil, and the splint stabilizes the wrist. A nonskid mat and a plate with plate guard may provide adequate stability of the plate for pushing and picking up food (Figure 10-37).

The spoon plate is an option for independent feeding for clients with high spinal cord injuries. The plate is a portable device that can be adjusted in height to the level of the client's mouth. The plate is made of a high-temperature thermoplastic and is formed over a mold that has a rim bowled to the approximate depth and length of a spoon. The client rotates the device with mouth and neck control. Food is removed from the rim of the plate with the mouth. Successful use of the device depends on adequate oral control, head and trunk control, and motivation. The reader is referred to the original source for information on making or obtaining this device.[34] Also available for clients who have no use of their upper extremities, is the electric self-feeder, which requires only slight head motion and is activated by a chin switch (Figure 10-38).

A regular or swivel spoon-fork combination can be used when there is minimal muscle function (C4 to C5). A long plastic straw with a straw clip to stabilize it in the cup or glass eliminates the need for picking up these drinking vessels. A bilateral or unilateral clip-type holder on a glass or cup makes it possible for many persons with hand and arm weakness to manage liquids without a straw.

Built-up utensils may be useful for those with some functional grasp or tenodesis grasp. Food may be cut with a quad-quip knife if arm strength is adequate to manage the device (Figure 10-39).

Personal Hygiene and Grooming

1. Use a shower or bathtub seat and transfer board for transfers.
2. Extend reach by using long-handled bath sponges with loop handle or built-up handle.
3. Eliminate need to grasp washcloth by using bath mitts or bath gloves.
4. Hold comb and toothbrush with a universal cuff.[1]
5. Use a wall-mounted hair dryer. Use a universal cuff to hold brush or comb for hair styling while using this mounted hair dryer.[10]
6. Use a clip-type holder for electric razor.
7. Persons with quadriplegia can use suppository inserters to manage bowel care independently.
8. Use skin inspection mirror with long stem and looped handle for independent skin inspection (Figure 10-40). Devices and methods selected must be adapted according to the degree of weakness of each client.

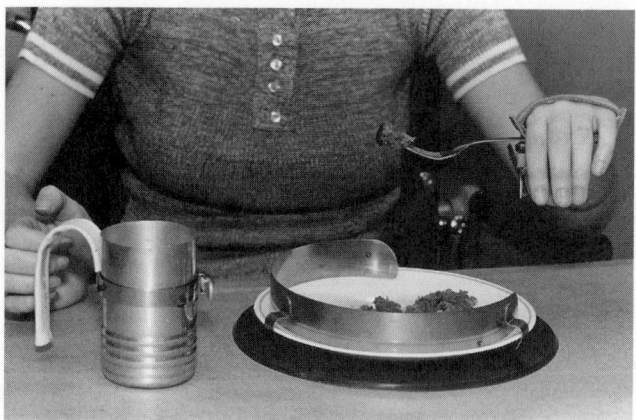

Figure 10-37 Self-feeding with aid of universal cuff, plate guard, nonskid mat, and clip-type cup holder to compensate for absent grasp.

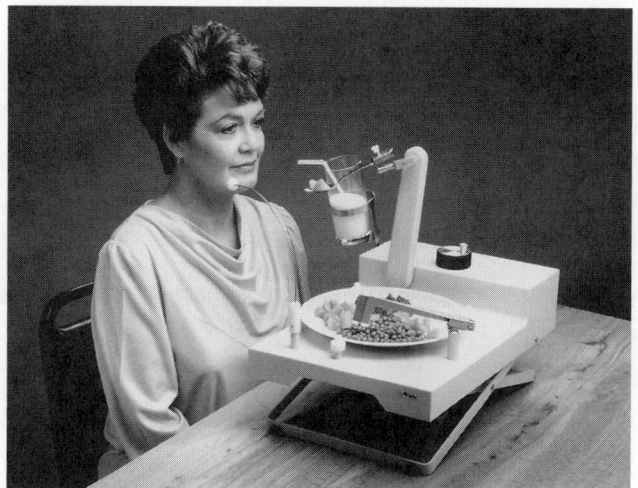

Figure 10-38 Electric self-feeder. (Courtesy Sammons Preston.)

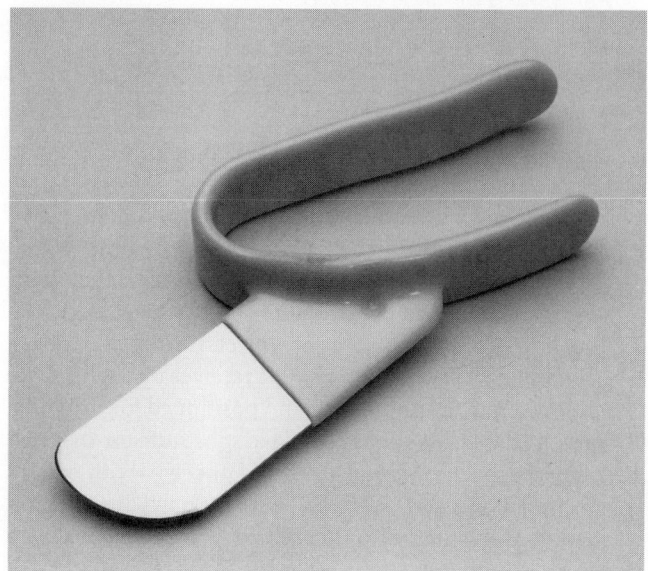

Figure 10-39 Quad-quip knife.

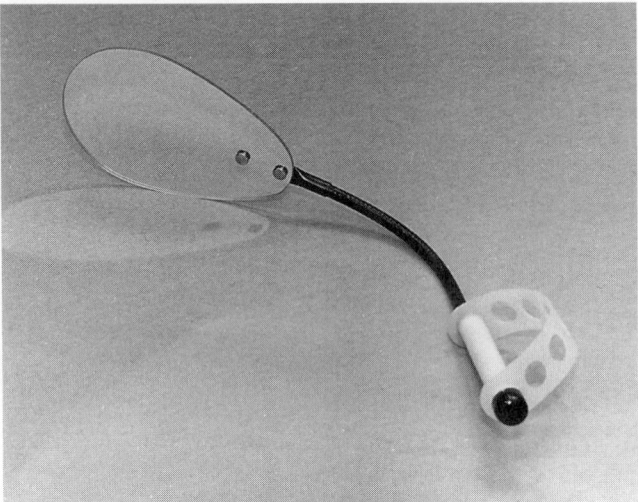

Figure 10-40 Skin inspection mirror.

Figure 10-41 Wand mouth stick is provided by Sammons Preston, An AbilityOne Company.

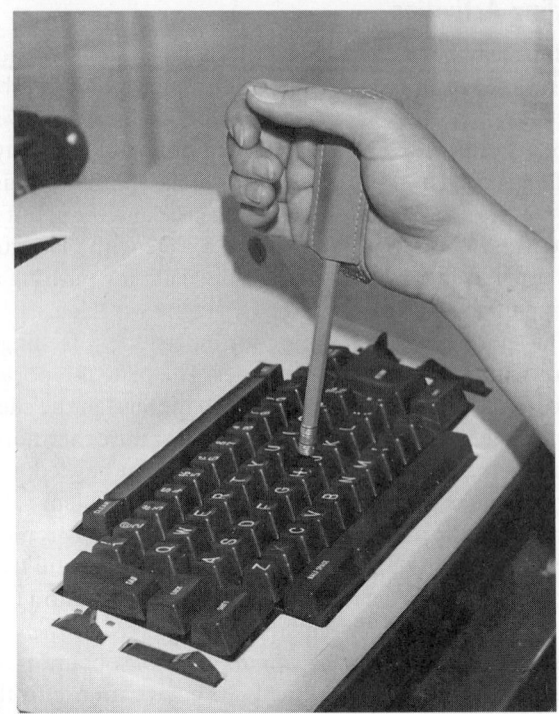

Figure 10-42 Typing with aid of utensil holder and typing stick

9. Adapted leg-bag clamps to empty catheter leg-bags are also available for individuals with limited hand function. Elastic leg-bag straps may also be replaced with Velcro straps.

Communication and Environmental Hardware Adaptations

1. Turn pages with an electric page-turner, mouth stick, or head wand if hand and arm function are inadequate (Figure 10-41).
2. For keyboarding, writing, operating a tape recorder, and painting, insert pen, pencil, typing stick, or paintbrush in a universal cuff that has been positioned with the opening on the ulnar side of the palm (Figure 10-42).
3. Touch telephone keys with the universal cuff and a pencil positioned with eraser down. The receiver may need to be stationed in a telephone arm and positioned for listening. Special adaptations are available to substitute for the need to replace the receiver in the cradle. For clients with no arm function, a speakerphone can be used along with a mouth stick to push the button to initiate a call. The operator assists with dialing.

4. Use personal computers or word processors. A computer mouse may be substituted for use of the keyboard. A variety of different mouse designs and sizes are available. Speech recognition programs are available for individuals with little or no arm movement.
5. Built-up pencils and pens or special pencil holders are needed for clients with hand weakness. The Wanchik writer is an effective adaptive writing device (Figure 10-18).
6. Sophisticated electronic communications devices operated by mouth, pneumatic controls, and head controls are available for clients with no function in the upper extremities.[31]
7. Kelly[15] describes a cassette tape holder and two mouth sticks that allow C3, C4, or C5 quadriplegic clients to operate a tape recorder or radio independently. The first mouth stick, with a friction tip, is used to depress the operating buttons and adjust the volume and selector dials of the radio. The second mouth stick is used to move the cassettes from the cassette holder to the tape recorder and to remove the cassettes from the recorder. The cassette tape stand has eight levels and is designed to hold eight tapes. The reader is referred to the original source for specifications on construction of these devices and to develop methods for a client to be able to manage a CD player.[15]
8. Environmental controls allow for easy operation from a panel designed to run multiple devices such as televisions,

radios, lights, telephones, intercoms, and hospital beds (see Chapter 16).

Functional Mobility

Principles of wheelchair transfer techniques for the individual with quadriplegia are discussed in Chapter 11. Mobility depends on degree of weakness. Electric wheelchairs operated by hand, chin, or pneumatic controls have greatly increased the mobility of persons with severe upper and lower extremity weakness. Vans fitted with wheelchair lifts and stabilizing devices permit such clients to be transported to pursue community, vocational, educational, and leisure activities with an assistant. In addition, adaptations for hand controls have made it possible for many clients with function of at least C6 level to drive independently.

Home Management, Meal Preparation, and Cleanup Activities

Clients with muscle function of C6 or better may be independent for light homemaking with appropriate devices, adaptations, and safety awareness. Many of the suggestions for wheelchair maneuverability and environmental adaptation outlined for the paraplegic apply here as well. In addition, clients with upper extremity weakness need to use lightweight equipment and special devices. The *Mealtime Manual for People with Disability and the Aging* compiled by Klinger[17] contains many excellent specific suggestions that apply to homemakers with weak upper extremities.

ADLs FOR THE PERSON WITH LOW VISION

The environmental modifications described in the following section are appropriate when performing ADLs for all persons with low vision.

Lighting and Magnifiers

1. Improve lighting by aiming light at the work area, not into the eyes.
2. Reduce glare by having adjustable blinds, sheer curtains, or tinted windows. Wearing dark glasses indoors may also reduce glare.
3. Maximize contrast by providing a work surface that is in contrast to the task. For example, serve a meal on a white plate if the table is dark. Paint a white edge on a dark step. Replace white wall switches with black to contrast with the wall.
4. Simplify figure-ground perception by clearing pathways and eliminating clutter.
5. Work in natural light by placing a chair by a window.[26,35]
6. Use magnifiers with lights. These come in a variety of sizes and degrees of magnification. Specialists in low vision can determine the appropriate degree of magnification needed. Some magnifiers are portable, others are attached to stands to do needle work or fine work, and others are sheets of plastic to magnify an entire page of print.[21]

Dressing Activities

1. Light closet to improve acuity. Hang matching clothes together.
2. Pin socks together when placing them in the washer and dryer so they will stay matched.

Feeding Activities

1. Provide high contrast. Ensure that plates contrast with table surface or place mats. Avoid patterned tablecloths.
2. Arrange food on the plate in a clockwise fashion and orient the person with low vision to the arrangement.

Personal Hygiene and Grooming Activities

1. Reduce clutter in bathroom drawers and cabinets.
2. Use electric razor.
3. Use magnified mirrors.
4. Use high-contrast bath mat in bathtub.
5. Install high-contrast grab bars in shower.

Communication and Environmental Hardware Adaptations

1. Use talking watches or clocks to tell time.
2. Use talking scale to determine weight.
3. Use large-print magnification screen on computer.
4. Technology for reading print is changing rapidly. Become familiar with the various types of adaptations for reading print.[21]
5. Use high-contrast door knobs. Paint the door frame a color that contrasts highly with the door to improve ease of identifying the door.[26]
6. Use speakerphones, preprogrammed phone numbers, or a phone with large print and high-contrast numbers. Identify phone buttons with contrasting tape or a Velcro dot to teach client how to turn phone on and the correct buttons to push.
7. Use writing guides to write letters, checks, or signatures.[21]
8. To read, use books on tape or "talking books."

Functional Mobility

Mobility is eased with the clearing of pathways and the minimizing of clutter and furniture. Lighting in hallways and entryways is also needed. The person with low vision needs to optimize visual scanning abilities by learning to turn and position the head frequently when mobile or participating in an activity.[35] The OT practitioner may need to refer a client to a specialist in low vision who is specifically trained in teaching mobility to persons with low vision or legal blindness.

Home Management, Meal Preparation, and Cleanup Activities

A variety of devices are available to compensate for low vision while managing the home. Organization and consistency are critical to the safe and efficient performance of home management tasks. Family members need to remember to replace items where they were found and not reorganize items without assistance from the person with low vision.

1. For safety, cleaning supplies should be placed separately from food supplies.
2. Eliminate extra hazardous cleaning supplies and replace with one multipurpose cleanser. Place this cleaning agent in a uniquely shaped bottle or in a specific location.
3. Mark appliance controls with high-contrast tape or paint to identify start and stop buttons or positions. Place Velcro tabs to mark frequently used positions on dials (e.g., on the 350° position for stove or for the wash and wear cycle on the washer or dryer).
4. Label cans by using rubber bands to attach index cards with bold, dark print to each can. When the can is used, the card may be placed into a stack to create a shopping list.
5. Indicate number of minutes needed for microwave cooking by placing rubber bands on the items. Two rubber bands would indicate that the item should be cooked for 2 minutes. Assistance will be needed for initial setup.
6. Use liquid level indicator to determine when hot liquid reaches 1 inch from top of cup or container.[26]
7. Use cutting guides or specially designed knives to cut meat or bread.[21]
8. Use a tape recorder to make reminder lists or grocery lists.

MEDICATION MANAGEMENT

1. Use medication organizer to organize pills.
2. For diabetic management, there are many different products available for individualized evaluation of the client (e.g., syringe magnifiers, talking or large-print glucometers, and a device to count the insulin dosages).
3. Use talking scales to evaluate weight.[24]

MONEY MANAGEMENT

1. Use a consistent method of folding money to identify denominations, as in the following example:

$1.00	Keep flat
$5.00	Fold in square half
$10.00	Fold lengthwise
$20.00	Fold in half and then lengthwise

2. Keep different denominations in different sections of the wallet. Learn to recognize coins by size and type of edge (smooth or rough).[35]

SUMMARY

ADLs and IADLs are areas of occupation that include activities of self-maintenance, mobility, communication, homemaking, and community living skills that enable a person to function independently and assume important occupational roles.

Occupational therapists routinely assess performance in ADLs to determine clients' levels of functional independence. Interviews and performance analysis are used to carry out the assessment. Results of the assessment and ongoing progress are recorded on one of many available ADL checklists or with a standardized assessment, the content of which is summarized for the permanent medical record (please refer to Chapter 8 for further information on documentation).

Intervention is client-centered and directed at training in independent living skills with activities such as feeding, dressing, mobility, homemaking, communication, and community living skills. The occupational therapist can include in the intervention plan special equipment and many methods of performing ADLs for clients with specific functional problems.

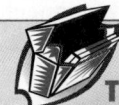

THREADED CASE STUDY: ANNA, PART 2

At the beginning of this chapter, Anna's case introduced questions regarding ADL and IADL participation. She prioritized ADLs and IADLs as the areas of occupation needing intervention. Anna identified self-care, child rearing, community mobility, financial management, home management, meal preparation and cleanup, and shopping as important activities that she wanted to engage in again and especially desired a high level of independence in self-care and child rearing. Both Anna and her husband were concerned about the level of assistance that might be required upon her discharge. A home assessment is recommended to ascertain needs that might require home modification or special equipment that would foster Anna's independence.

Review Questions

1. Define ADLs and IADLs. List three classifications of tasks that may be considered in each category.
2. What is the role of OT in restoring ADL and IADL independence?
3. List at least three activities that are considered self-care skills, three functional mobility skills, three functional communication skills, and three home management and/or meal preparation and cleanup skills.
4. List three factors that the occupational therapist must consider before commencing ADL performance assessment and training. Describe how each could limit or affect ADL performance.
5. What is the ultimate goal of the ADL and IADL training program?
6. Discuss the concept of maximal independence, as defined in the text.

7. List the general steps in the procedure for ADL assessment.
8. Describe how the occupational therapist can use the ADL checklist.
9. List the steps in the activities of home management assessment.
10. What is the purpose of the home assessment?
11. List the steps in the home assessment.
12. Who should be involved in a comprehensive home assessment?
13. What kinds of things are observed in a home assessment?
14. How does the therapist record and report results of the home assessment and make the necessary recommendations?
15. How does the occupational therapist, with the client, select ADL and IADL training objectives after an assessment?
16. Describe three approaches to teaching ADL skills to a client with perception or memory deficits.
17. List the important factors to include in an ADL progress report.
18. Describe the levels of independence, as defined in the text.
19. Give an example of a health management and maintenance issue.
20. Give three examples of adaptations that may be helpful for the person with low vision.

Exercises

1. Demonstrate the use of at least three assistive devices mentioned in the text.
2. Teach another person to don a shirt, using one hand.
3. Teach another person how to don and remove trousers, as if he or she had hemiplegia.
4. Teach another person how to don and remove trousers, as if the legs were paralyzed.
5. Prepare a meal using only one hand and write about your experience.

REFERENCES

1. Activities of daily living for patients with incoordination, *limited range of motion, paraplegia, quadriplegia, and hemiplegia,* Cleveland, 1968 (rev 1989), Metro Health Center for Rehabilitation, Metro Health Medical Center for Rehabilitation.
2. American Occupational Therapy Association: Occupational therapy practice framework: domain and process, *Am J Occup Ther* 56, 609, 2002.
3. Arilotta C: Performance in areas of occupation: the impact of the environment, *Phys Disabil Special Interest Section Quarterly* 26, 1, 2003.
4. Armstrong M, Lauzen S: *Community integration program,* ed 2, Enumclaw, WA, 1994, Idyll Arbor.
5. Asher IE: *Occupational therapy assessment tools: an annotated index,* ed 2, Bethesda, MD, 1996, American Occupational Therapy Association.
6. Baum C, Edwards D: Cognitive performance in senile dementia of the Alzheimer's type: the kitchen task assessment, *Am J Occup Ther* 47:431, 1993.
7. Bromley I: *Tetraplegia and paraplegia: a guide for physiotherapists,* ed 2, London, 1981, Churchill Livingstone.

8. Christiansen CH, Matuska KM, editors: *Ways of living: adaptive strategies for special needs,* ed 3, Bethesda, MD, 2004, American Occupational Therapy Association.
9. Cynkin S, Robinson AM: *Occupational therapy and activities health: toward health through activities,* Boston, 1990, Little, Brown.
10. Feldmeier DM, Poole JL: The position-adjustable hair dryer, *Am J Occup Ther* 41:246, 1987.
11. Fenton S, Gagnon P: Work activities. In Crepeau E, Cohn E, Schell B, editors: *Willard and Spackman's occupational therapy,* ed 10, Philadelphia, 2003, Lipponcott, Williams & Wilkins.
12. Fisher AG: *Assessment of motor and process skills (AMPS),* Fort Collins, CO, 1999, Three Star Press.
13. Florey LL, Michelman SM: Occupational role history: a screening tool for psychiatric occupational therapy, *Am J Occup Ther* 36:301, 1982.
14. Gray JM: Putting occupation into practice: occupation as ends, occupation as means, *Am J Occup Ther* 52:354, 1998.
15. Kelly SN: Adaptations for independent use of cassette tape recorder/radio by high-level quadriplegic patients, *Am J Occup Ther* 37:766, 1983.
16. Klein RM, Bell B: Self care skills: behavioral measurement with Klein-Bell ADL Scale, *Arch Phys Med Rehabil* 63(7):335, 1982.
17. Klinger JL: *Mealtime manual for people with disabilities and the aging,* Thorofare, NJ, 1997, Slack Publishers.
18. Kohlman-Thomson L: *The Kohlman evaluation of living skills (KELS),* ed 3, Bethesda, MD, 1993, American Occupational Therapy Association.
19. Law ML, Baptiste S, Carswell A, et al: *Canadian occupational performance measure (COPM),* ed 3, Ottawa, 1998, CAOT Publications.
20. Letts L, Law M, Rigby P, et al: Person-environment assessments in occupational therapy, *Am J Occup Ther* 48:608, 1994.
21. *The Lighthouse catalog,* New York, The Lighthouse Press.
22. Malick MH, Almasy BS: Activities of daily living and homemaking. In Hopkins HL, Smith HD, editors: *Willard and Spackman's occupational therapy,* ed 7, Philadelphia, 1988, JB Lippincott.
23. Matsusuyu J: The interest checklist, *Am J Occup Ther* 23:323, 1969.
24. *Maxi aids and appliances for independent living,* Farmingdale, NY, Maxi Aids.
25. Moorhead L: The occupational history, *Am J Occup Ther* 23:329, 1969.
26. Orr AL: *Issues in aging and vision: a curriculum for university programs and in-service training,* New York, 1998, American Foundation for the Blind Press.
27. Rogers JC, Holm MB: Activities of daily living and instrumental activities of daily living. In Crepeau E, Cohn E, Schell B, editors: *Willard and Spackman's occupational therapy,* ed 10, Philadelphia, 2003, Lippincott, Williams &Wilkins.
28. Runge M: Self-dressing techniques for clients with spinal cord injury, *Am J Occup Ther* 21:367, 1967.
29. Sokaler R: A buttoning aid, *Am J Occup Ther* 35:737, 1981.
30. Steggles E, Leslis J: Electronic aids to daily living, *Home & Community Health Special Interest Quarterly,* 8, 1, 2001.

31. Trombly CA: Activities of daily living. In Trombly CA, editor: *Occupational therapy for physical dysfunction,* ed 2, Baltimore, 1983, Williams & Wilkins.

32. Uniform Data System for Medical Rehabilitation: *Functional independence measure (FIM),* Buffalo, NY, 1993, State University of New York at Buffalo.

33. Watanabe S: *Activities configuration: regional institute on the evaluation process,* Final report. RSA-123-T-68, New York, 1968, American Occupational Therapy Association.

34. Wykoff E, Mitani M: The spoon plate: a self-feeding device, *Am J Occup Ther* 36:333, 1982.

35. Yano E: *Working with the older adult with low vision: home health OT interventions,* Presentation at Kaiser Permanente Medical Center Home Health Department, Hayward, CA, 1998.

36. Yasuda YL, Leiberman D: *Adults with rheumatoid arthritis: practice guidelines series,* Bethesda, 2001, American Occupational Therapy Association.

11 MOBILITY

DEBORAH BOLDING
CAROLE ADLER
MICHELLE TIPTON-BURTON
SUSAN M. LILLIE

KEY TERMS

Functional ambulation
Gait training
Ambulation aids
Rehabilitation technology
  supplier
Durable medical equipment
Skin breakdown

Vital capacity
Medical necessity
Body mechanics
Positioning mass
Pelvic tilt
Community mobility
Fixed route

Paratransit
Americans with Disabilities Act
Private transportation
Driving
Driver training
Driver competence
On-road evaluation

Older drivers
Clinical assessment
Primary controls
Secondary controls
Follow-up services
Driving retirement

LEARNING OBJECTIVES

After studying this chapter the student or practitioner will be able to do the following:

1. Define functional ambulation.
2. Discuss the roles of the physical and occupational therapists and other caregivers in functional ambulation.
3. Identify safety issues in functional ambulation.
4. Recognize basic lower extremity orthotics and ambulation aids.
5. Develop goals and plans that can help ambulatory clients resume occupational roles.
6. Identify the components necessary to perform a wheelchair evaluation.
7. Understand the process of wheelchair measurement and prescription completion.
8. Identify wheelchair safety considerations.
9. Follow guidelines for proper body mechanics.
10. Apply principles of proper body positioning.
11. Identify the steps necessary in performing various transfer techniques.
12. Identify considerations necessary to determine the appropriate transfer method based on the client's clinical presentation.
13. Identify different transportation systems and contexts and the treatment implications each system presents.
14. Understand the multi-level role of the therapist in the occupation of community mobility.
15. List performance skills and client factors needing assessment in a comprehensive driver evaluation.
16. Discuss the value of driving within this society and how loss of license or mobility affects participation in occupation.
17. Develop awareness of the complexities involved in a driver referral and evaluation.
18. Define primary and secondary controls.
19. Recognize that driver competency assessment is a specialty practice area requiring advanced training.

CHAPTER OUTLINE

Section 1: Functional ambulation
  Basics of ambulation
    Orthotics
    Walking aids
  Functional ambulation
    Kitchen ambulation
    Bathroom ambulation
    Home management ambulation
  Summary

Section 2: Wheelchair assessment and transfers
  Wheelchairs
  Wheelchair assessment
  Wheelchair ordering considerations
    Propelling the wheelchair
  Rental versus purchase
    Frame style
  Wheelchair selection
    Manual versus electric/power wheelchairs

Walking, climbing stairs, traveling within one's neighborhood, and driving a car are so universal and customary that most people would not consider these to be complex activities. The basic capacities to move within the environment, to reach objects of interest, to explore one's surroundings, and to come and go at will appear natural and easy. For persons with disabilities, however, mobility is rarely taken for granted or thought of as automatic. A disability may prevent a person from using the legs to walk or using the hands to operate controls of motor vehicles. Cardiopulmonary and medical conditions may limit aerobic capacity or endurance, which requires the person to take frequent rests and to curtail walking to cover only the most basic of needs, such as toileting. Deficits in motor coordination, flexibility, and strength may seriously compromise movement and may make difficult any activities that require a combination of mobility (e.g., walking or moving in the environment) and stability (e.g., holding the hands steady when carrying a cup of coffee or a watering can).

Occupational therapy (OT) practitioners assist persons with mobility restrictions to achieve maximum access to environments and objects of interest to them. Typically, OT practitioners provide remediation and compensatory training. In so doing, therapists must analyze the activities most valued and environments most often used by their clients and must consider any future changes that can be predicted from an individual's medical history, prognosis, and developmental status.

This chapter guides the practitioner in evaluation and intervention of persons with mobility restrictions. Three main topics are explored. The first section addresses functional ambulation, which combines the act of walking within one's immediate environment (e.g., home or workplace) with other activities chosen by the individual. Feeding pets, preparing a meal and carrying it to a table, and doing simple housework are tasks that may involve functional ambulation. Functional ambulation may be conducted with aids such as walkers, canes, or crutches.

The second section concerns wheelchairs, their selection, measurement, fitting, and use. For many persons with disabilities, mobility becomes possible only with a wheelchair and specific positioning devices. Consequently, individual evaluation is needed to select and fit this essential piece of personal medical equipment. Proper training in ergonomic use allows the person who is dependent on the use of a wheelchair many years of safe and comfortable mobility. Safe and efficient transfer techniques based on the individual's clinical status are introduced in this chapter. Attention also is given to the body mechanics required to safely assist an individual.

The third section covers community mobility, which for many in the United States is synonymous with driving. Increased advocacy by and for persons with disabilities has improved access and has yielded an increasing range of options for adapting motor vehicles for individual needs. Public transportation also has become increasingly accessible.

Driving is a complex activity that requires multiple cognitive and perceptual skills. Evaluation of individuals with medical conditions and physical limitations is thus important for the safety of the disabled person and the public at large.

Mobility is an area of OT practice that requires close coordination with other healthcare providers, particularly PTs (PTs) and providers of durable medical equipment. Improving and maintaining the functional and community mobility of persons with disabilities can be one of the most gratifying practice areas. Clients experience tremendous energy and empowerment when they are able to access and explore wider and more interesting environments.

SECTION 1: FUNCTIONAL AMBULATION

Deborah Bolding

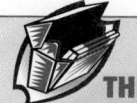

THREADED CASE STUDY: PYIA, PART 1

Pyia is a 75-year-old woman who was treated for breast cancer 8 years earlier. She developed spinal metastases, with an onset of acute, bilateral lower extremity weakness and loss of sensation. For 2 days she felt "unsteady" when she was walking and had one fall. By the time she was admitted to the hospital, she was unable to walk. She underwent a laminectomy and decompression of the spinal cord, with debulking of the tumor, followed by cyberknife treatment.

Pyia was hospitalized for 1 day before her surgery and for 4 days after the surgery. Postoperatively she learned to ambulate 50 feet with a front-wheeled walker and minimal assistance and to get on and off a commode chair. She required an ankle-foot orthosis (AFO) for her left foot. Pyia was discharged from the hospital to stay with her daughter and had a rental wheelchair for community mobility. A referral for home-based occupational and physical therapy was made through a home care agency.

An occupational profile provided the following information about Pyia. Pyia was widowed and lived alone in a three-bedroom house with three steps to enter the home. She retired from retail sales when she was 62. She was independent in driving and was active in her church and attended occasional programs at the local senior citizen's center. She volunteered 3 hours per week at a thrift shop that benefits the local children's hospital. Pyia has two close friends that she went to lunch with each Tuesday. Pyia has three children, two sons living in other states, and a daughter who lives in the same town. She has two grandchildren who live nearby, ages 10 and 13. Two to three times per year she would fly to visit her sons.

An important part of Pyia's life for the past few years was to go to her daughter's home one to two afternoons per week. She would help watch the grandchildren after school or drive them to activities

Continued

THREADED CASE STUDY: PYIA, PART 1—cont'd

while their parents worked. She would also help her daughter with laundry and dinner preparation.

After 3 weeks at her daughter's home, Pyia was asked to identify what areas of occupational performance were still problematic for her, what she could do well, and what her goals were. She replied that she was happy to be walking better but felt endurance was still a problem. She used the walker independently in the home but still needed assistance to get up and down stairs. The PT felt that she would soon be independent with stairs and may be able to transition to a cane, as her lower extremity strength, especially in her right leg, had improved. Pyia was able to walk to the bathroom and use a toilet independently and was independent in dressing. Her daughter helped her in and out of the tub for safety reasons, and she used a stool in the tub for bathing. She was able to prepare a simple breakfast and lunch but needed a rest period each morning and afternoon.

Pyia felt like a burden to her daughter and son-in-law. She felt guilty that her daughter had taken a week off work after her hospitalization to be with her at home and that her son had to visit to help her for the second week. She was happy that she could now take care of herself during the day but would like to be able to help with household chores. She had to rely on her family and friends to drive her to doctors' appointments and will need to drive her to therapy appointments the following week as she transitions to outpatient care. Pyia wished that she could return to her home but recognized that she was not yet ready. Her old friends brought lunch to her daughter's home the previous Tuesday, and she was grateful for their support, and the support from her pastor and church.

Critical Thinking Questions

1. How did Pyia's needs, goals, and occupational roles change during the course of her illness and recuperation?
2. Where would you start your intervention plan considering her current goals?
3. What are safety issues and how would you address them?

Occupational therapists (OTs) work with many types of clients who may have impaired ambulation because of disease or trauma. These impairments may be temporary or long term. For example, an elderly person with a hip fracture may require the use of a walker for several weeks or months until the bone is healed and strength is regained. Persons with a spinal cord injury may have permanent motor and sensory losses that require lower extremity bracing and the use of crutches for walking. They may be ambulatory only part of the time and use a wheelchair part of the time. This depends on several factors, including the level of injury, the amount of energy required for ambulation, and their occupational roles.

Functional ambulation, a component of functional mobility, is a term used to describe how a person walks while achieving a goal, such as carrying a plate to the table or carrying groceries from the car to the house. Functional ambulation training is applicable for all individuals with safety or functional impairments and for a variety of diagnoses, such as lower extremity amputation, cerebrovascular accident, brain trauma or tumors, neurological diseases, spinal cord injury, orthopedic injuries, and total hip or knee replacement.

Ambulation evaluation, gait training (treatments used to improve walking and ameliorate deviations from normal gait), and recommendations for bracing and ambulation aids are the professional role of the PT. The PT makes recommendations that can be followed by the client, families, hospital staff, or other caregivers. The OT works closely with colleagues in physical therapy to determine when clients may be ready to advance to the next levels of functional performance. For example, the OT may begin having a client walk to the bathroom for toileting instead of using a bedside commode when the PT reports that the client is safe to walk the distance from the bed to the bathroom. The PT may recommend certain techniques or cueing to improve safety. Mutual respect and good communication between all team members help coordinate the care for clients. For example, a client with Parkinson's disease may walk well with the PT immediately after taking his medication in the morning but may have difficulty preparing lunch a few hours later when the effects of medication are waning.

The following section is meant to provide an introduction to the OT about the basics of ambulation and aids such as crutches, canes, walkers, and braces to assist with the teaching of activities of daily living (ADL). It is not meant as a substitute for close collaboration with a physical therapist (PT).

BASICS OF AMBULATION

Normal walking is a method of using two legs, alternately, to provide support and propulsion. Gait and walking are often used interchangeably, but gait more accurately describes the style of walking. The "normal" pattern of walking includes the components of body support on each leg alternately (stance phase), advancement of the swinging leg to allow it to take over a supporting role (swing phase), balance, and power to move the legs and trunk. Normal walking is achieved without difficulty and with minimal energy consumption.

Descriptors of the events of walking include loading response, mid-stance, terminal stance and pre-swing, and mid-swing and terminal swing, with the duration of the complete cycle called *cycle time*. Cadence is the average step rate. Stride length is the distance between two placements of the same foot. It may be shortened in people with a variety of diseases. Walking base is the distance between the line of the two feet. It may be wider than normal for people with balance deficits.[62]

Abnormal gait is caused by disorders of the complex interaction between neuromuscular and structural elements of the body. It may result from problems with the brain, spinal cord, nerves, muscles, joints, and skeleton or from pain. Problems may include weakness, paralysis, ataxia, spasticity, loss of sensation, and inability to bear weight through the limb or pelvis. Deficits may include decreased velocity, decreased weight bearing, increased swing time of the affected leg, an abnormal base of support, and balance problems. Functional deficits may include loss of mobility, decreased safety (increased fall risk), and insufficient endurance. The OT should reinforce **gait training** by following recommendations of the PT.

ORTHOTICS

As the PT evaluates the causes of gait problems, orthotics and ambulatory aids may be recommended. The OT should be familiar with basic lower extremity (LE) orthotics, including the reason for bracing. The OT may teach clients to put on the orthotics as part of dressing training.

Orthotics, or braces, are used to provide support and stability for a joint, to prevent deformity, or to replace lost function. They should be comfortable, easy to apply, and lightweight, if possible. The more joints of the lower extremity that require bracing, the higher the energy cost of ambulation.

Orthotics are named by the part of the body that is supported. A supramalleolar orthosis (SMO or SMAFO) is made of plastic and fits into a shoe. It provides medial-lateral stability at the ankle, provides rear foot alignment during gait, supports midfoot laxity, and can control pronation/supination positions of the forefoot. It is not useful in cases of high tone or limited dorsiflexion. An ankle-foot orthosis (AFO) is usually made of plastic and inserts into a shoe and extends up the back of the lower leg. It is sometimes called a *"foot drop" splint*, because it is used in cases of central or peripheral nerve lesions, which cause weakness of ankle dorsiflexors. An AFO may be one piece or hinged to permit ankle dorsiflexion. A knee-ankle-foot orthosis (KAFO) may be recommended for clients with knee weakness or hyperextension or for foot problems. The KAFO might be used with diagnoses such as paraplegia, cerebral palsy, or spina bifida. For clients with spinal cord lesions or spina bifida involving the hip muscles, a hip-knee-ankle-foot orthosis (HKAFO) might be used. A reciprocating gait orthosis (RGO) is a type of HKAFO that may be used to help advance the hip in the presence of hip flexor weakness. High energy costs are associated with use of HKAFOs, and the clients' upper extremities are used for support on walkers and crutches. This makes functional ambulation tasks extremely challenging for these clients, and it may be more energy efficient and safer to perform some tasks while seated in a chair or wheelchair.

WALKING AIDS

Ambulation aids may be used to compensate for deficits in balance and strength, to decrease pain, to decrease weight bearing on involved joints and help with fracture healing, or in the absence of a lower extremity. Walking aids are generally classified as canes, crutches, and walkers. All three help support part of the body weight through the arm or arms during gait. They may also provide sensory cues for balance and enhance stability by increasing the size of the base of support.

A single point cane may be used with clients who have minor balance problems, by widening the base of support or providing sensory feedback through the upper extremity about position. For clients with a painful hip or knee, a cane is most commonly used on the contralateral side to reduce loading on the painful joint. The cane is advanced during the swing phase of the leg it is protecting. Variations of cane designs include quad canes and hemi-walkers that are heavier and bulkier than single-point canes but provide greater stability.

Crutches are able to transmit forces in a horizontal plane, because two points of attachment exist, one at the hand and one higher on the arm. Clients should be cautioned not to lean on the crutches at the axilla, because this may cause damage to blood vessels or nerves. The lever between the axilla and hand is long, and enough horizontal force can be generated to permit walking when one leg has restricted weight-bearing capacity, or when both legs are straight and have limited or no weight-bearing capacity. They are suitable for short-term use, such as for a fractured leg.

Forearm crutches may also be called *Lofstrand* or *Canadian crutches*. The points of contact are on the hand and forearm. The lever arm is shorter than with axillary crutches, and they are lighter. Mobility is easier for most people using the Lofstrand or forearm crutches than when using the axillary crutches, and they are useful for active people with severe leg weakness. All crutches require good upper body strength.

Walkers are more stable than canes or crutches. With a "pick-up" style walker, the walker is moved first, the client takes a short step with each foot and then moves the walker again. This type of walking can be slow. Most clients who need a walker are able to use a "front-wheeled walker," which has two wheels on the front, which makes it lighter and easier to advance. Another variation is to have four wheels, with a braking system. Some walkers have seats so that clients can rest when they become fatigued. Walkers require the use of both arms but do not require as much upper body strength or balance as crutches. Forearm platforms can be added to forearm crutches or walkers when clients are unable to bear weight through their hands or wrists, perhaps because of fractures or arthritis. For example, Pyia is currently using a walker that supplies substantial support during ambulation but also requires additional energy to use compared with a cane. The PT may recommend a cane as Pyia progresses, but a walker may still be necessary in some situations within the home environment.

Ambulation Techniques

Basic ambulation techniques recommended by the PT vary from client to client, depending on the individual's goals, strengths, and weaknesses and may be more complex than the descriptions provided above. The OT reinforces the PT's recommendations and incorporates them into functional ambulation activities.

During functional ambulation on a level surface, the OT is positioned slightly behind and to one side of the client. The therapist may be on the client's stronger or weaker side, based on the recommendations and preference of the PT or the goals of the activity. The therapist moves in tandem with the client when providing support during ambulation. The therapist's outermost lower extremity moves with the ambulation aid, and the therapist's inside foot moves forward with the client's lower extremity. Of course, some clients may be independent with basic ambulation and need guarding or assistance only when practicing new activities, such as transporting hot foods, mopping a floor, or reaching into a dryer.

Safety

OT PRACTICE NOTES

SAFETY FOR FUNCTIONAL AMBULATION

1. Know the client (e.g., status, orthotics and aids, and precautions).
2. Use appropriate footwear.
3. Monitor physiological responses.
4. Use a gait belt to guide the client. Do not use the client's clothes or upper extremity to guide the client.
5. Think ahead for the unexpected.
6. Do not leave the client unattended.
7. Clear potential hazards.

Safety is the number-one priority for clients during functional ambulation. Before beginning an evaluation of ADLs, the OT should know basic client information. The therapist reviews the medical record, especially the current status and precautions. Does the client use oxygen? Does it need to be increased during activity? In the hospital setting, it may be useful to be aware of hematocrit level, if available, to help predict how much activity the client may be able to tolerate. The therapist should review physical therapy reports and confer with the PT as needed about gait techniques, aids, orthotics, and ambulatory status. To prepare the client for functional ambulation, the therapist and client should have safe and appropriate footwear. Soft-soled shoes or shoes with a slippery sole should be avoided, and slippers or shoes without a heel support can compromise safety and stability for the client.

Another key to safe and successful ADLs is awareness of the client's endurance level, including distance the client is able to ambulate. It is very important to plan ahead for the activity. The therapist should have a wheelchair, chair, or stool readily available for use at the appropriate intervals or in case of need because of client fatigue. The area should be free of potential safety hazards, such as throw rugs or other objects on the floor. In certain cases, however, such as with a client with unilateral neglect, hemianopsia, or visual or perceptual deficits, the therapist may want to challenge the client to be able to manage in a complex environment.

The client's physiological responses should be monitored during the activity. The therapist should be aware of the client's precautions and respond appropriately. Physiological responses may include a change in breathing patterns, perspiration, reddened or pale skin, a change in mental status, and decreased responsiveness. These changes may require the termination of the activity to allow the client a period of rest. Recall that Pyia continues to experience limited endurance and easily fatigues. Activities that require sustained standing or walking may be too challenging at this time.

Elderly clients who use assistive devices for ambulation before hospitalization are particularly at risk for loss of ADL and IADL function after hospitalization. The history of use of assistive devices may be markers for decreased ability to recover.[36] It may be important to target these elderly for intensive therapy to maintain function.

Falls represent a major problem in the elderly. Studies suggest that one fourth of persons aged 65 to 79 and half of those older than 80 will fall every year.[21] Falls result from many factors, both intrinsic (e.g., health, existence of balance disorders) and external, or environmental, factors. Home hazards include poor lighting, inadequate bathroom grab rails, inadequate stair rails, exposed electrical cords, items on the floors, and throw rugs. Elderly people with health problems such as cardiac disease, stroke, and degenerative neurological conditions have an even greater risk of falling.[32,53] OTs may visit the client's home while the client is hospitalized or may work through home health agencies, fall prevention programs, or senior citizen centers to help evaluate homes for potential hazards.[47] All reasonable efforts should be made to decrease the risk of falls.

If a client loses his or her balance or stumbles, the therapist will have better control of the client if he or she is holding onto the client's trunk. Therapists may be less prone to injure their own backs if they are using their legs to support or lower the client to the floor instead of pulling or twisting with the upper body. For a client who feels faint or develops sudden leg weakness, the therapist lowers the client onto the therapist's flexed leg, like onto a chair, then down to the floor.

 OT PRACTICE NOTE

> All clients who are at risk for falling and who are alone for significant periods of time should be connected to a lifeline-type phone system, where help can be summoned in the event of a fall or other emergency. Local hospitals or senior citizen centers will have further information about lifeline services.

FUNCTIONAL AMBULATION

Functional ambulation integrates ambulation into ADLs and instrumental activities of daily living (IADL). Using an occupational-based approach, the OT assesses the client's abilities within the performance context and with an understanding of client habits, routines, and roles. What role(s) does the client have or want to have? What tasks does this role require? The OT plans for functional mobility activities with the goal of helping the client achieve valued roles and activities. Several typical functional ambulation activities follow. The activities must be individualized for clients. Functional ambulation may be incorporated during ADLs, IADLs, work, play, or leisure activities.

KITCHEN AMBULATION

Meal preparation and cleanup involve many different tasks, such as opening and reaching into a refrigerator, dishwasher, stove, microwave, and cupboards. It often involves transporting items within the kitchen and to a table. If something is dropped, the item will need to be retrieved from the floor. The task may be relatively quick and easy, such as heating food in a microwave, or require someone to stand while chopping, stirring, or cooking food. The OT can help the client engage in problem-solving strategies on how to safely accomplish these tasks. For example, clients with left hemiplegia who ambulate with a quad cane may be guided to the left of the oven so that they can open the oven door with use of the unaffected right upper extremity. The same concept should be kept in mind for opening cabinet doors or drawers or refrigerator doors. The therapist can help assess the client's safety during these tasks and recommend alternatives as needed. If the client is unable to successfully balance and reach into the oven, a toaster oven on the counter may be a safer alternative. Clients can place frequently needed items in convenient locations, or equipment such as a reacher may be needed. If the reacher is applied to a walker with Velcro, it is usually available when the client needs it. Clients may be able to pick up items from the floor by kicking or pushing the item close to a counter, where they can hold onto the counter while bending to pick up the item. If they have had a total hip replacement and have hip flexion precautions, they can position the affected leg behind them, being careful to not internally rotate the hip, while they reach down to the floor.

Transporting items such as food, plates, and eating utensils during functional ambulation invites creative problem solving on the part of the OT, particularly when the client is using an ambulation aid (Figures 11-1 and 11-2). The use of baskets attached to a walker, rolling carts, or the use of countertops to slide the item may be appropriate in these situations. Clients must clearly desire the equipment or adaptations, and care should be taken not to provide unwanted or unnecessary equipment. A client who does not live alone may prefer to share jobs with other family members; that is, the client may do the cooking while a family member sets and clears the table. Although Pyia was able to prepare a simple meal, she still experiences fatigue after doing so and is unable to assist her daughter in meal preparation. Suggestions regarding adaptations and energy conservation techniques may support Pyia's goal of being able to help with this activity while still living with her daughter.

BATHROOM AMBULATION

Functional ambulation to the sink, toilet, bathtub, or shower is an important concern for the client. Care should be taken during activities in the bathroom because of the many risks associated with water and hard surfaces. Spills on the floor are slipping hazards, and loose bath mats are tripping hazards. Clients must be educated about these dangers. Non-slip surfaces or mats should be used on tub and shower floors.

Functional ambulation to the sink, using a walker may be performed by having the client approach the sink as close as possible. If the walker has a walker basket, the client can position the walker at the side of the sink, then holding onto the walker with one hand and the sink or countertop with the other, turn to face the sink.

The importance of helping the client become as independent as possible in toileting cannot be overemphasized. People who are unsure about their abilities to safely use a toilet in friends' or families' homes, in restaurants, in the mall, or at gas stations may become homebound as a result. When safe to do so, practice toileting in a variety of settings and with and without equipment such as commodes or elevating toilet seats and grab bars. One limiting factor may be postoperative precautions: a tall client who has had a total hip replacement may not be able to sit safely on a regular toilet while observing their post-surgical precaution of no hip flexion greater than 90 degrees. A shorter client may be able to sit successfully on a regular-height toilet without difficulty. If a client is unable to get up and down from the toilet without assistance, or with difficulty, consult the PT, who can provide the client with lower extremity strengthening exercises.

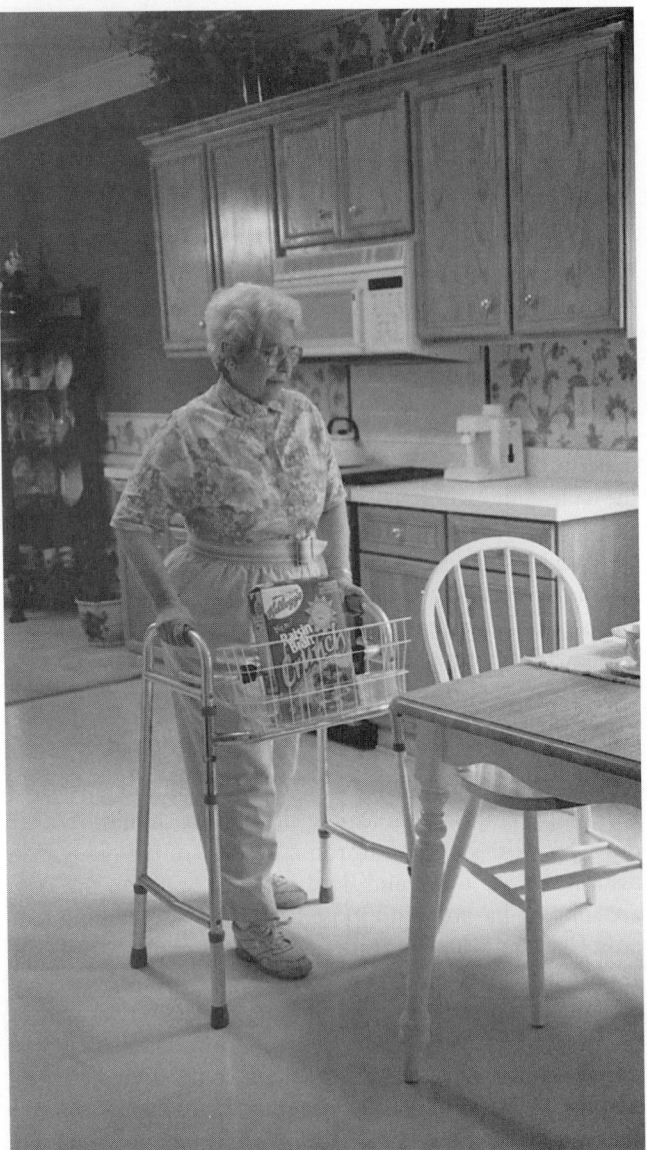

Figure 11-1   Functional ambulation with a walker and walker basket.

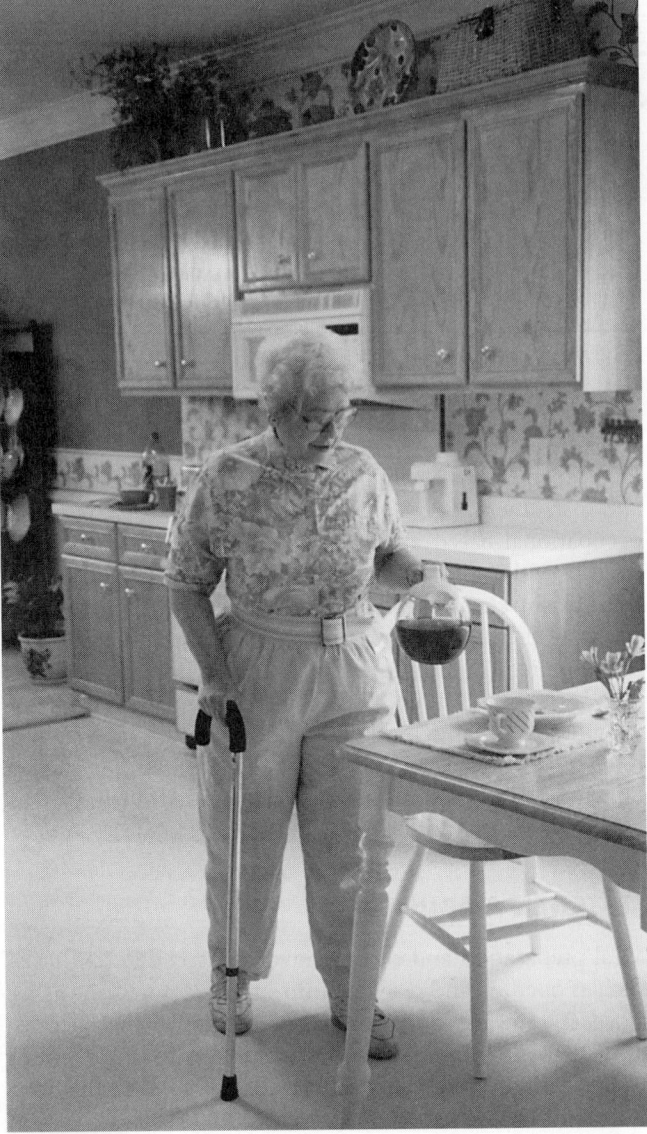

Figure 11-2   Functional ambulation with a straight cane.

When the client is ambulating to a tub or shower, make sure the equipment and supplies are in position for the client to use. While stepping into a shower stall with a low rim, clients use the same technique that they would use to go up a curb or step, using their walking aid if it fits into the door of the shower. If the walking aid does not fit, the therapist can evaluate the client's ability to safely step in without the equipment. A client who has non–weight-bearing precautions on a leg will not be able to step into a shower without walking aids or step into a tub. A tub bench must be used for non–weight-bearing clients who have access only to tubs. Pyia is able to negotiate her daughter's home and use the toilet but still requires assistance to transfer in and out of the tub. These skills will need to be addressed before Pyia can return to her own home.

Grab bars are important safety items for clients in the shower and tub. The therapist may want to practice shower or tub transfers under trial conditions before practicing an actual shower or bath. Some older persons have become accustomed to taking sponge baths because of a fear of falling in the bathroom. The therapist should determine whether the client is satisfied with this system or would like to work toward independent showering.

HOME MANAGEMENT AMBULATION

The ability to live alone is closely tied to the ability to perform IADLs.[35] Home management activities include cleaning, laundry, and household maintenance. Cleaning includes tidying, vacuuming, sweeping and mopping floors, dusting, and making beds. Clients may balance with one hand and hold onto a counter or sturdy piece of furniture while cleaning floors if they are not stable independently or with a walking aid. Lightweight duster-style sweepers, which come with dry or wet replaceable pads, are easy to handle and use. When making the bed, the client can stabilize himself or herself on the bed or walking aid while straightening and pulling up sheets and bedcovers. The client then moves around the bed to the other side to repeat the process. Some clients find that carrying items in a small fanny pack or shoulder bag slung over the neck is an easy way to transport small items such as cordless phones, bottled water, and books. Moving clothes to or from a laundry room may present a challenge for people with mobility impairments, particularly if they use a walking aid. Rolling carts may be useful to transport items to the laundry and in the kitchen. Some clients carry items over the front of their walkers, in a bag attached to the walker, or in a bag that they hold while walking with crutches or a cane. Whichever method that is safe for the client is acceptable. Watch to make sure that the clothes do not shift while clients carry them, which may throw them off balance.

Other home management activities may include maintenance of the yard, garden, appliances, and vehicles. The client should be consulted to determine the home management activity most valued by the client before the functional activity is begun. Sometimes the client has goals that the therapist does not feel are safe for the client to perform. For example, the client who has had a mild stroke who wants to climb a ladder and trim tree branches with his power saw may need to be persuaded to wait until his balance and strength are improved. Although this is a valued activity, it may be incompatible with the client's functional abilities at the time. Gardening is an area in which the PT and OT may want to collaborate. The PT helps the client learn to maneuver over uneven surfaces and get up and down from the ground, whereas the OT helps the client learn how to carry tools and other equipment and how to dispose of clippings and weeds.

In case of falls, clients should learn how to get up and down from the floor or ground during physical therapy sessions. It may be a functional activity with the OT when clients want to be able to get to the bottom of a tub, reach objects stored under a bed, or sit on the floor to play with their grandchildren.

Therapists should listen to clients about the techniques the clients have developed to be independent and safe. Some clients with fall risks manage to walk to the bathroom from their bed every night without putting on braces and/or using equipment. They will say things such as, "I lean against the wall as I walk," or "There is a couch there, and I brace myself on the back." If the technique is safe, and if the client has not had falls, the routine may not need modification.

SUMMARY

Functional ambulation may be incorporated during ADLs, IADLs, work and productive activities, and play or leisure.

OTs and PTs have an opportunity to collaborate, with the PT providing gait training, exercises, and ambulation aid recommendations, and the OT to reinforce training and integrate it during purposeful activities.

THREADED CASE STUDY: PYIA, PART 2

In regard to our case study, Pyia's roles as homemaker, caregiver, grandmother, mother, and volunteer changed with her illness. Her role became more passive as others became her caregivers. She was initially very concerned about her disease, whether and how long she would live, and if she would ever be able to walk again. After her surgery, her goals were to be able to walk, and to go to her daughter's home. Once this was achieved, she began to experience loss about her change in roles and to plan for the future: taking care of herself during the day, resuming homemaking activities, planning a return to her own home, visiting with her friends, and becoming more independent in the community.

Pyia is home alone during the day. She would like to be more active with homemaking, both to help her daughter and in preparation for the return to her own home. The therapist could begin practice on laundry and cleaning. She is already able to do basic meal preparation. The therapist could help assess safety in Pyia's home and make recommendations for equipment or modifications and refer the family for lifeline services. Pyia might arrange transportation services for the disabled through her county, or she could have a driver's evaluation to determine if she could start to drive again. She would need to be able to get in and out of the car safely, and to put her walker and other items in the car.

SECTION 2: WHEELCHAIR ASSESSMENT AND TRANSFERS

Carole Adler
Michelle Tipton-Burton

WHEELCHAIRS

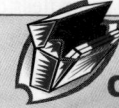

CASE STUDY: CHEN

Chen is a 17-year-old male who sustained a C6 spinal cord injury after a diving accident approximately 2 weeks ago. Sensation and motor function are absent below the level of the lesion. He is now medically stable, is receiving rehabilitation services, and is referred for a wheelchair assessment. Chen has a halo vest for

Continued

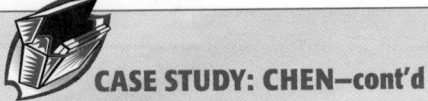

CASE STUDY: CHEN—cont'd

stabilization and is able to tolerate sitting upright for 1 hour before he complains of getting dizzy. He still asks the rehabilitation therapists, nurses, and his physician when he will be able to move his legs. He has been told that because he has had no return of function during the past 2 weeks it is unlikely that he will have significant changes in his current level of motor and sensory function.

Upon discharge from the inpatient rehabilitation unit, Chen will be returning to his home where he lives with his parents and younger brother. The home is two stories, and Chen's bedroom is located on the second floor. There is a bathroom located on the first floor.

Before his injury, Chen was very physically active and was on the track and field team of his high school. He was also an avid hiker and would often go camping with his family and friends. Chen is a high school senior and received early acceptance to a university located within 2 hours of his home. He was very excited about attending this university because of the track and field program in addition to his interest in becoming a marine biologist. Although Chen's friends have come to visit him, his girlfriend of 2 years has not visited.

Critical Thinking Questions

1. How would you anticipate Chen responding to being fitted for a wheelchair? What emotional responses may be evoked in Chen by this experience and how could you minimize his potential distress?
2. What decisions could Chen make regarding the selection of the wheelchair?
3. Considering Chen's needs across several contexts, what type of wheelchair would you recommend?
4. What client factors must be considered when selecting a wheelchair for Chen?

A wheelchair can be the primary means of mobility for someone with a permanent or progressive disability, such as cerebral palsy, brain injury, spinal cord injury, multiple sclerosis, or muscular dystrophy. Someone with a short-term illness or orthopedic problem may need it as a temporary means of mobility. In addition to mobility, the wheelchair can substantially influence the total body positioning, skin integrity, overall function, and general well-being of the client. Regardless of the diagnosis of the client's condition, the OT must understand the complexity of wheelchair technology, available options and modifications, the evaluation and measuring process, the use, care, and cost of the wheelchair and, importantly, the process by which this equipment is funded.

Wheelchairs have evolved considerably in recent years, with significant advances made in powered and manual wheelchair technology by manufacturers and service providers. Products are constantly changing. Many of the improvements result from user and therapist recommendations.

OTs and PTs, depending on their respective roles at their treatment facilities, are usually responsible for evaluation, measurement, and selection of a wheelchair and seating system for the client. They also teach wheelchair safety and mobility skills to clients and their caregivers. The constant evolution of technology and variety of manufacturers' products make it advisable to include an experienced, knowledgeable, and certified **rehabilitation technology supplier** (RTS) on the ordering team. The RTS is a supplier of **durable medical equipment** (DME) who is proficient in ordering custom items and can offer an objective and broad mechanical perspective on the availability and appropriateness of the options being considered. The RTS will be the client's resource for insurance billing, repairs, and reordering when returning to the community.

Whether the client requires a non-custom rental wheelchair for temporary use or a custom wheelchair for use over many years, an individualized prescription clearly outlining the specific features of the wheelchair is needed to ensure optimal performance, mobility, and enhancement of function. A wheelchair that has been prescribed by an inexperienced or non-clinical person is potentially hazardous and costly to the client. An ill-fitting wheelchair can, in fact, contribute to unnecessary fatigue, **skin breakdown,** and trunk or extremity deformity, and it can inhibit function.[49] A wheelchair is an extension of the client's body and should facilitate rather than inhibit good alignment, mobility, and function.

WHEELCHAIR ASSESSMENT

The therapist has considerable responsibility in recommending the wheelchair appropriate to meet immediate needs and long-term needs. When evaluating for a wheelchair, the therapist must know the client and have a broad perspective of the client's clinical, functional, and environmental needs. Careful assessment of physical status must include the following: the specific diagnosis, prognosis, and current and future problems (e.g., age, spasticity, loss of range of motion [ROM], muscle weakness, and reduced endurance) that may affect wheelchair use. Additional client factors that are also considered in assessment of wheelchair use are sensation, cognitive function, and perceptual skills. Functional use of the wheelchair in a variety of environments must be considered. Box 11-1 lists questions to consider before making specific recommendations.

Before the final prescription is prepared, collected information must be analyzed for an understanding of advantages and disadvantages of recommendations based on the client's condition and how all specifics will integrate to provide an optimally effective mobility system.

To ensure that payment for the wheelchair is authorized, the therapist should have an in-depth awareness of the client's insurance benefits and provide documentation with thorough justification of the **medical necessity** of the wheelchair and

OT PRACTICE NOTE

The therapist must develop a good working relationship with the equipment supplier (RTS) and the reimbursement sources to facilitate payment of the most appropriate mobility system for the client. The therapist must have the oral and written documentation skills to clearly communicate the medical necessity, appropriateness, and cost-effectiveness of each item throughout the assessment and recommendation process.

any additional modifications. Therapists must explain clearly why particular features of a wheelchair are being recommended. They must be aware of standard versus "up charge" items, the cost of each item, and the effect of these items on the end product.

WHEELCHAIR ORDERING CONSIDERATIONS

Before selecting a specific manufacturer and the wheelchair's specifications, the therapist should carefully analyze the following sequence of evaluation considerations.[2,49,60]

PROPELLING THE WHEELCHAIR

The wheelchair may be propelled in a variety of ways, depending on the physical capacities of the user. If the client is capable of self-propulsion by use of his or her arms on the rear wheels of the wheelchair, sufficient and symmetrical grasp,

arm strength, and physical endurance may be assumed present to maneuver the chair independently over varied terrain throughout the day.[60] An assortment of push rims are available to facilitate self-propelling, depending on the user's arm and grip strength. A client with hemiplegia may propel a wheelchair using the extremities on the unaffected side to maneuver the wheelchair. A client with tetraplegia may have functional use of only one arm and may be able to propel a one-arm drive wheelchair, or a power chair may be more appropriate. Although Chen, the 17-year-old who has a C6 spinal cord injury, has functional strength in both biceps, the energy expenditure must be considered if he is to use only a manual wheelchair.

If independence in mobility is desired, a power wheelchair should be considered for those who have minimal or no use of the upper extremities, limited endurance, or shoulder dysfunction. Power chairs are also preferred in situations involving inaccessible outdoor terrain.[60] Power wheelchairs have a wide variety of features and can be programmed; driven by foot, arm, head, or neck; or be pneumatically controlled. Given current sophisticated technology, assuming intact cognition and perception, even a person with the most severe physical limitations is capable of independently driving a power wheelchair.

If the chair is to be propelled by the caregiver, consideration must be given to ease of maneuverability and handling, in addition to the positioning and mobility needs of the client.

Regardless of the method of propulsion, serious consideration must be given to the effect the chair has on the client's current and future mobility and positioning needs. In addition, lifestyle and environment, available resources

---

Box 11-1   QUESTIONS TO ASK BEFORE MAKING SPECIFIC RECOMMENDATIONS FOR A WHEELCHAIR

Who will pay for the wheelchair?
Who will determine the preferred DME provider: the insurance company, the client, or the therapist?
What is the specific disability?
What is the prognosis?
Is range of motion limited?
Is strength or endurance limited?
How will the client propel the chair?
How old is the client?
How long is the client expected to use the wheelchair?
What was the client's lifestyle, and how has it changed?
Is the client active or sedentary?
How will the dimensions of the chair affect the client's ability to transfer to various surfaces?
What is the maneuverability of the wheelchair in the client's home or in the community (e.g., entrances and egress, door width, turning radius in bathroom and hallways, and floor surfaces)?

What is the ratio of indoor to outdoor activities?
Where will the wheelchair be primarily used—in the home, at school, at work, or in the community?
Which mode of transportation will be used? Will the client be driving a van from the wheelchair? How will it be loaded and unloaded from the car?
Which special needs (e.g., work heights, available assistance, accessibility of toilet facilities, and parking facilities) are recognized in the work or school environment?
Does the client participate in indoor or outdoor sports activities?
How will the wheelchair affect the client psychologically?
Can accessories and custom modifications be medically justified, or are they luxury items?
What resources does the client have for equipment maintenance (e.g., self, family, and caregivers)?

such as ability to maintain the chair, transportation options, and available reimbursement sources are major determining factors. Although Chen is physically fit, his upper body strength has been compromised by the spinal cord injury. If he is interested in engaging in outdoor activities, he may lack the physical strength to propel a manual wheelchair on varied terrains. A powered wheelchair seemed an appropriate option for Chen, but the therapist also considered his previous occupations of camping and hiking when selecting a wheelchair that could potentially be used in outdoor terrain.

RENTAL VERSUS PURCHASE

The therapist should estimate how long the client will need the chair and whether the chair should be rented or purchased, which will affect the type of chair being considered. This decision is based on several clinical and functional issues. A rental chair is appropriate for short-term or temporary use, such as when the client's clinical picture, functional status, or body size is changing. Rental chairs may be necessary when the permanent wheelchair is being repaired. A rental wheelchair also may be useful when prognosis and expected outcome are unclear or when the client has difficulty accepting the idea of using a wheelchair and needs to experience it initially as a temporary piece of equipment. Often the eventual functional outcome is unknown. In that case a chair can be rented for several months until a re-evaluation determines whether a permanent chair will be necessary.[2]

A permanent wheelchair is indicated for the full-time user and for the client with a progressive need for a wheelchair over a long period. It may be indicated when custom features are required and also when body size is changing, such as in the growing child.[2]

FRAME STYLE

Once the method of propulsion and the permanence of the chair have been determined, several wheelchair frame styles are available for consideration. The frame style must be selected before specific dimensions and brand names can be determined. The therapist needs to be aware of the various features, the advantages and disadvantages of each, and the effect of these features on the client in every aspect of his of her life, from a short-term and long-term perspective. Chen is still in emotional shock that he no longer has motor control of his legs and hands. These variables must be considered when approaching Chen about the wheelchair selection. Although a power wheelchair seemed the most appropriate choice for Chen, the therapist was concerned about the appearance of the wheelchair. The therapist actively engaged Chen in making choices regarding the type, model, and options available on various wheelchairs.

WHEELCHAIR SELECTION

The following questions regarding client needs should be considered carefully before the specific type of chair is determined.[2]

MANUAL VERSUS ELECTRIC/POWER WHEELCHAIRS

Manual Wheelchair

See Figure 11-3, *A*.

- Does the user have sufficient strength and endurance to propel the chair at home and in the community over varied terrain?
- Does manual mobility enhance functional independence and cardiovascular conditioning of the wheelchair user?
- Will the caregiver be propelling the chair at any time?
- What will be the long-term effects of the propulsion choice?

Power Wheelchair

See Figure 11-3, *B*.

- Does the user demonstrate insufficient endurance and functional ability to propel a manual wheelchair independently?
- Does the user demonstrate progressive functional loss, making powered mobility an energy-conserving option?
- Is powered mobility needed to increase independence at school, at work, and in the community?
- Does the user demonstrate cognitive and perceptual ability to operate a power-driven system safely?
- Does the user or caregiver demonstrate responsibility for care and maintenance of equipment?
- Is a van available for transportation?
- Is the user's home accessible for use of a power wheelchair?
- Has the user been educated regarding the rear, mid, and front wheel drive systems and been guided objectively in making the appropriate selection?

MANUAL RECLINE VERSUS POWER RECLINE VERSUS TILT WHEELCHAIRS

Manual Recline Wheelchair

See Figure 11-4, *A*.

- Is the client unable to sit upright because of hip contractures, poor balance, or fatigue?
- Is a caregiver available to assist with weight shifts and position changes?
- Is relative ease of maintenance a concern?
- Is cost a consideration?

Power Recline Versus Tilt

See Figure 11-4, *B* and *C*.

- Does the client have the potential to operate independently?
- Are independent weight shifts and position changes indicated for skin care and increased sitting tolerance?

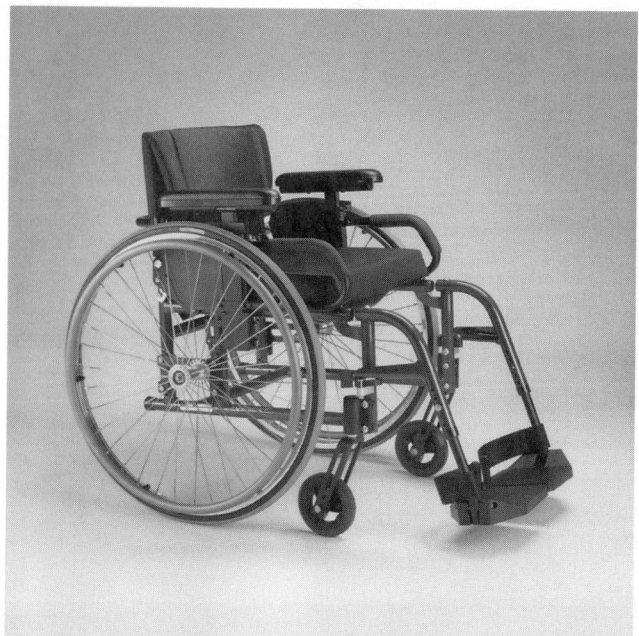

A

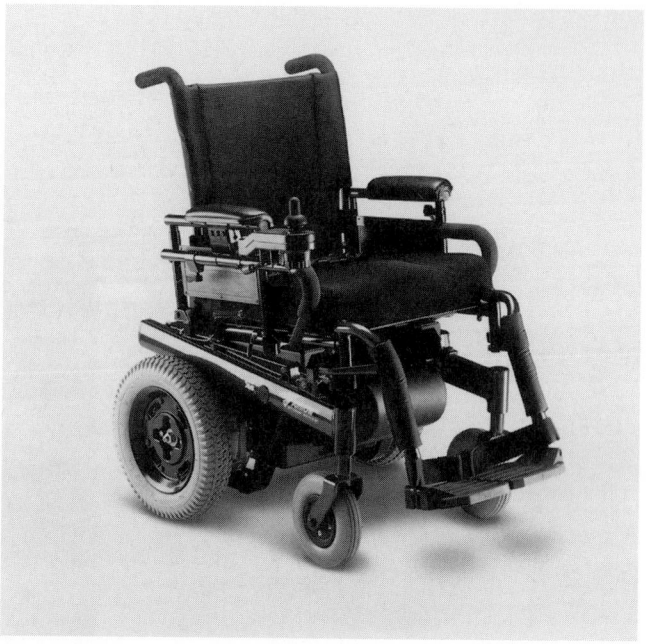

B

Figure 11-3 Manual versus electric wheelchair. **A,** Rigid frame chair with swing-away footrests. **B,** Power-driven wheelchair with hand control. (*A,* Courtesy Quickie Designs; *B,* courtesy Invacare Corporation.)

- Does the user demonstrate safe and independent use of controls?
- Are there resources for care and maintenance of the equipment?
- Does the user have significant spasticity that is facilitated by hip and knee extension during the recline phase?
- Does the user have hip or knee contractures that prohibit his or her ability to recline fully?
- Will a power recline or tilt decrease or make more efficient use of caregiver time?
- Will a power recline or tilt feature on the wheelchair reduce the need for transfers to the bed for catheterizations and rest periods throughout the day?
- Will the client require quick position changes in the event of hypotension and/or dysreflexia?
- Has a reimbursement source been identified for this add-on feature?

FOLDING VERSUS RIGID MANUAL WHEELCHAIRS

Folding Wheelchairs

See Figure 11-5, *A.*
- Is the folding frame needed for transport, storage, or home accessibility?
- Which footrest style is necessary for transfers, desk clearance, and other daily living skills? Elevating footrests are available only on folding frames.
- Is the client or caregiver able to load and fit the chair into necessary vehicles?

- Equipment suppliers should have knowledge and a variety of brands available. Frame weight can range approximately from 28 to 50 lb, depending on size and accessories. Frame adjustments and custom options depend on the model.

Rigid Wheelchairs

See Figure 11-5, *B.*
- Does the user or caregiver have the upper extremity function and balance to load and unload the nonfolding frame from a vehicle if driving independently?
- Will the user benefit from the improved energy efficiency and performance of a rigid frame?

Footrest options are limited and the frame is lighter (20 to 35 lb). Features include an adjustable seat angle, rear axle, caster mount, and back height. Efficient frame design maximizes performance. Options exist for frame material composition, frame colors, and aesthetics. These chairs are usually custom ordered; availability and expertise are usually limited to custom rehabilitation technology suppliers.

LIGHTWEIGHT (FOLDING OR NONFOLDING) VERSUS STANDARD-WEIGHT (FOLDING) WHEELCHAIRS

Lightweight Wheelchairs: Under 35 Pounds

See Figure 11-5, *A.*
- Does the user have the trunk balance and equilibrium necessary to handle a lighter frame weight?

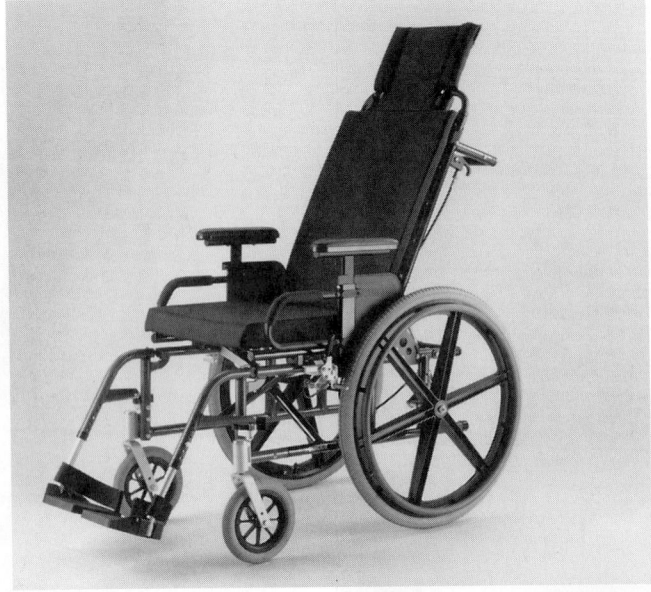

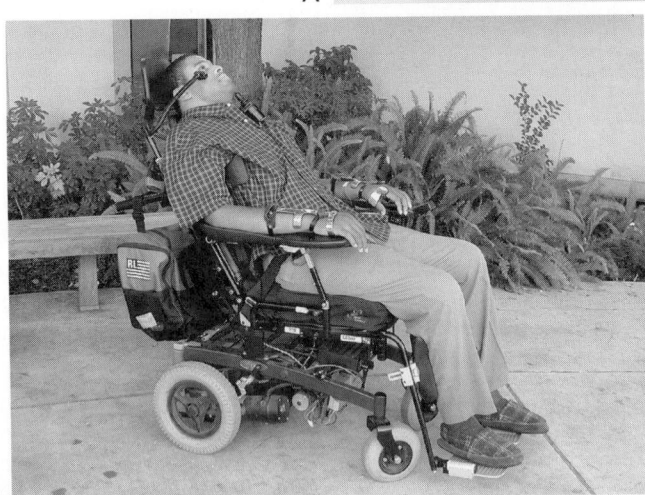

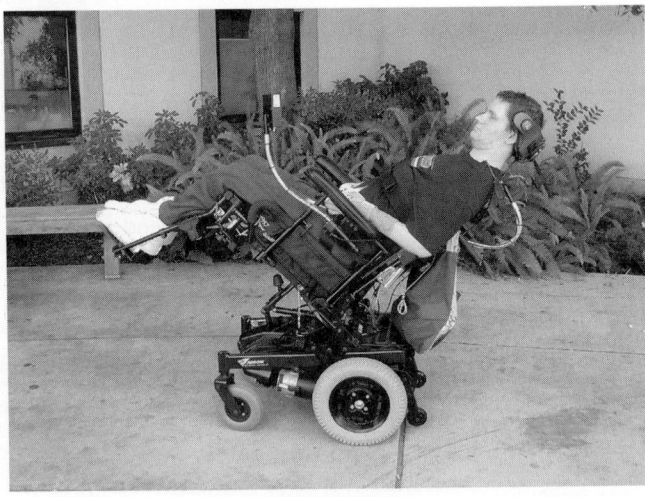

Figure 11-4   Manual recline versus power recline wheelchair. **A,** Reclining back on folding frame. **B,** Low-shear power recline with collar mount chin control on electric wheelchair. **C,** Tilt system with head control on electric wheelchair. (*A,* Courtesy Quickie Designs; *B* and *C,* courtesy Luis Gonzalez.)

- Does the lighter weight enhance mobility by reducing the user's fatigue?
- Will the user's ability to propel the chair or handle parts be enhanced by a lighter-weight frame?
- Are custom features (e.g., adjustable height back, seat angle, and axle mount) necessary?

Standard-Weight Wheelchairs: More Than 35 Pounds

See Figure 11-6.
- Does the user need the stability of a standard-weight chair?
- Does the user have the ability to propel a standard-weight chair?

- Can the caregiver manage the increased weight when loading the wheelchair and fitting into a vehicle?
- Will the increased weight of parts be unimportant during daily living skills?

Custom options are limited, and these wheelchairs are usually less expensive (except heavy-duty models required for users more than 250 lb).

STANDARD AVAILABLE FEATURES VERSUS CUSTOM, TOP-OF-THE-LINE MODELS

The price range, durability, and warranty within a specific manufacturer's model line must be considered.

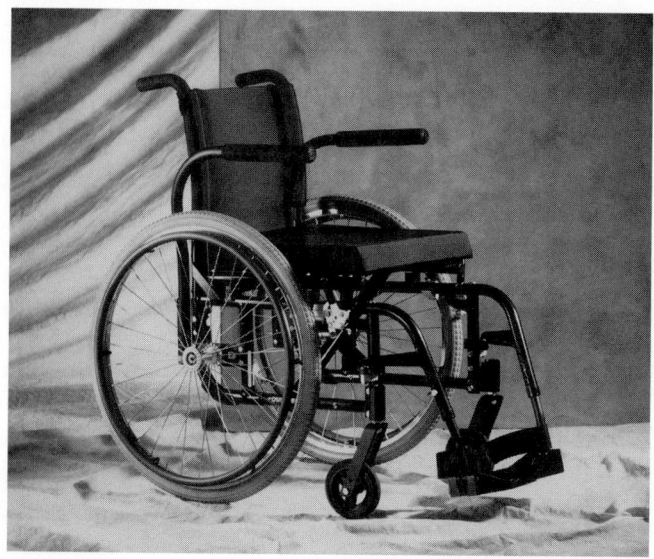
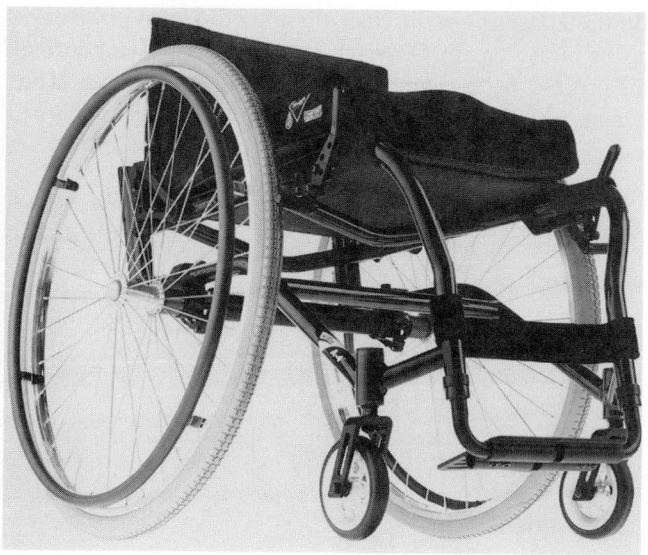

A

B

Figure 11-5   Folding versus rigid wheelchair. **A,** Lightweight folding frame with swing-away footrests. **B,** Rigid aluminum frame with tapered front end and solid foot cradle. (*A,* Courtesy Quickie Designs; *B,* courtesy Invacare Corporation.)

Standard Available Features

- Is the chair required only for part-time use?
- Does the user have a limited life expectancy?
- Is the chair needed as a second or transportation chair, used only 10% to 20% of the time?
- Will the chair be primarily for indoor or sedentary use?
- Is the user dependent on caregivers for propulsion?
- Will the chair be propelled only by the caregiver?
- Are custom features or specifications not necessary?
- Is substantial durability unimportant?

For standard wheelchairs, a limited warranty is available on the frame. These chairs may be indicated because of reimbursement limitations. Limited sizes and options and adjustability are available. These cost considerably less than custom wheelchairs.

Custom and Top-of-the-Line Models

- Will the client be a full-time user?
- Is there a likely prognosis for long-term use of the wheelchair?
- Will this be the primary wheelchair?
- Is the user active indoors and outdoors?
- Will this frame style improve prognosis for independent mobility?
- Is the user a growing adolescent, or does he or she have a progressive disorder requiring later modification of the chair?
- Are custom features, specifications, or positioning devices required?

Top-of-the-line wheelchair frames usually have a lifelong warranty on the frame. A variety of specifications, options, and adjustments are available. Many manufacturers will

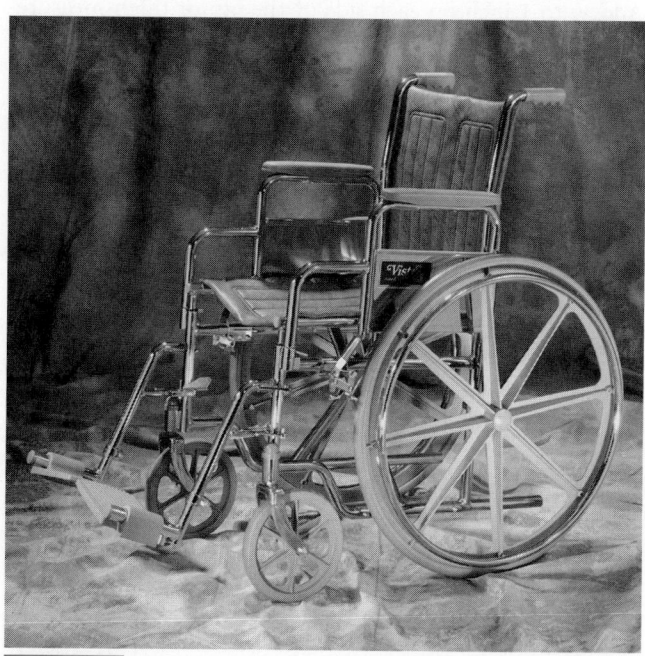

Figure 11-6   Standard folding frame (more than 35 lb) with swing-away footrests. (Courtesy Everest & Jennings, Inc.)

work with therapists and providers to solve a specific fitting problem. Experience is essential in ordering top-of-the-line and custom equipment.

WHEELCHAIR MEASUREMENT PROCEDURES

The client is measured in the style of chair and with the seat cushion that most closely resembles those being ordered. If the client will wear a brace or body jacket or need any additional devices in the chair, these should be in place during the measurement. Observation skills are important during this process. Measurements alone should not be used. The therapist should visually assess and monitor the client's entire body position throughout the measurement process.[2,59]

SEAT WIDTH

See Figure 11-7, *A*.

Objectives

1. Distributing the client's weight over the widest possible surface.
2. Keeping the overall width of the chair as narrow as possible.

Measurements

Measure the individual across the widest part of either the thighs or hips while the client is sitting in a chair comparable to the anticipated wheelchair.

Wheelchair Clearance

Add ½ to 1 inch on each side of the hip or thigh measurement taken. Consider how increasing the overall width of the chair will affect accessibility.

Checking

Place the flat palm of the hand between the client's hip or thigh and the wheelchair skirt and armrest. The wheelchair skirt is attached to the armrests in many models, and clearance should be sufficient between the user's thigh and the skirt to avoid rubbing or pressure.

Considerations

- User's potential weight gain or loss
- Accessibility of varied environments

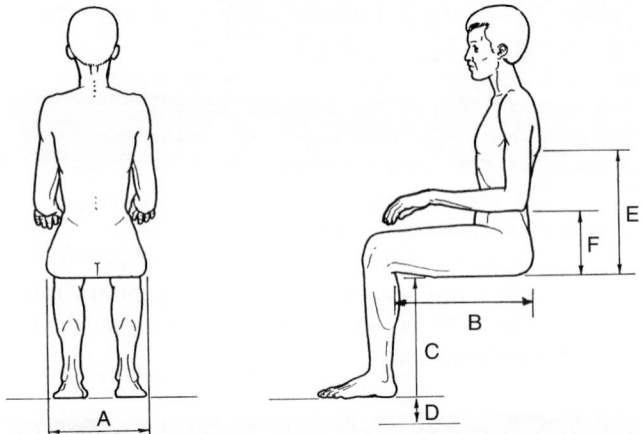

Figure 11-7 Measurements for wheelchairs. **A,** Seat width. **B,** Seat depth. **C,** Seat height from floor. **D,** Footrest clearance. **E,** Back height. **F,** Armrest height. (Adapted from Wilson A, McFarland SR: *Wheelchairs: a prescription guide,* Charlottesville, Va, 1986, Rehabilitation Press.)

- Overall width of wheelchair. Camber, axle mounting position, rim style, and wheel style can also affect overall wheelchair width.

SEAT DEPTH

See Figure 11-7, *B*.

Objective

The objective is to distribute the body weight along the sitting surface by bearing weight along the entire length of the thigh to just behind the knee. This approach is necessary to help prevent pressure sores on the buttocks and lower back and for optimal muscle tone normalization to assist in the prevention of pressure sores throughout the body.

Measurements

Measure from the base of the back (the posterior buttocks region touching the chair back) to the inside of the bent knee; the seat edge clearance needs to be 1 to 2 inches less than this measurement.

Checking

Check clearance behind the knees to prevent contact of the front edge of the seat upholstery with the popliteal space. (Consider front angle of leg-rest or foot cradle.)

Considerations

- Braces or back inserts may be pushing the client forward.
- Postural changes may occur throughout the day from fatigue or spasticity.
- Thigh length discrepancy; the depth of the seat may be different for each leg.
- If considering a power recliner, assume the client will slide forward slightly throughout the day and make depth adjustments accordingly.
- Seat depth may need to be shortened to allow independent propulsion with the lower extremities.

SEAT HEIGHT FROM FLOOR AND FOOT ADJUSTMENT

Objectives

1. Supporting the client's body while maintaining the thighs parallel to the floor (Figure 11-7, *C*)
2. Elevating the foot plates to provide ground clearance over varied surfaces and curb cuts (Figure 11-7, *D*)

Measurements

The seat height is determined by measuring from the top of the wheelchair frame supporting the seat (the post supporting the seat) to the floor and from the client's popliteal fossa to the bottom of the heel.

Wheelchair Clearance

The client's thighs are kept parallel to the floor so that the body weight is distributed evenly along the entire depth of the seat. The lowest point of the foot plates must clear the floor by at least 2 inches.

Checking

Slip fingers under the client's thighs at the front edge of the seat upholstery. Note: A custom seat height may be needed to obtain footrest clearance. An inch of increased seat height raises the foot plate 1 inch.

Considerations

If the knees are too high, increased pressure at the ischial tuberosities puts the client at risk for skin breakdown and pelvic deformity.

Sitting too high off the ground can impair the client's center of gravity, seat height for transfers, and visibility if driving a van from the wheelchair.

BACK HEIGHT

See Figure 11-7, *E*.

Objective

Back support consistent with physical and functional needs must be provided. The chair back should be low enough for maximal function and high enough for maximal support.

Measurements

For full trunk support for the client, the back must be of sufficient height. Full support height is obtained by measuring from the top of the seat frame on the wheelchair (seat post) to the top of the user's shoulders. For minimum trunk support, the top of the back upholstery is below the inferior angle of the client's scapulae and should permit free arm movement, not irritate the skin or scapulae, and provide good total body alignment.

Checking

Ensure that the client is not being pushed forward because the back of the chair is too high or leaning backward over the top of the upholstery because the back is too low.

Considerations

- Adjustable-height backs (usually offer a 4-inch range)
- Adjustable upholstery
- Lumbar support or another commercially available or custom back insert to prevent kyphosis, scoliosis, or other long-term trunk deformity

ARMREST HEIGHT

See Figure 11-7, *F*.

Objectives

1. Maintaining posture and balance
2. Providing support and alignment for upper extremities
3. Allowing change in position by pushing down on armrests

Measurements

With the client in a comfortable position, measure from the wheelchair seat frame (seat post) to the bottom of the user's bent elbow.

Wheelchair Clearance

The height of the top of the armrest should be 1 inch higher than the height from the seat post to the user's elbow.

Checking

The client's posture should look appropriately aligned. The shoulders should not slouch forward or be subluxed or forced into elevation when the client is in a relaxed sitting posture, with flexed elbows resting slightly forward on armrests.

Considerations

- Other uses of armrests exist, such as increasing functional reach or holding a cushion in place.
- Certain styles of armrests can increase the overall width of the chair.
- Are armrests necessary?
- Is the client able to remove and replace the armrest from the chair independently?
- Review all measurements against standards for a particular model of chair. Manufacturers have lists of the standard dimensions available and the cost for custom modifications.

PEDIATRICS

The goals of pediatric wheelchair ordering, as with all wheelchair ordering, should be obtaining a proper fit and facilitating optimal function. Rarely does a standard wheelchair meet the fitting requirements of a child. The selection of size is variable; therefore custom seating systems specific to the pediatric population are available. A secondary goal is to consider a chair that will accommodate the child's growth.

For children less than 5 years of age a decision must be made about whether to use a stroller base or a standard wheelchair base. Considerations are the child's ability to propel the chair relative to the developmental level and the parent's preference for a stroller or a wheelchair.

Many variables must be considered when customizing a wheelchair frame. An experienced RTS or the wheelchair manufacturer should be consulted to ensure that a custom request will be successful.

ADDITIONAL SEATING AND POSITIONING CONSIDERATIONS

A wheelchair evaluation is not complete until the seat cushion, back support, and any other positioning devices and the integration of those parts are carefully thought out, regardless of the diagnosis. The therapist must appreciate the effect that optimal body alignment has on skin integrity, tone normalization, overall functional ability, and general well-being (Figure 11-8).[2]

Consider Chen's potential need for a wheelchair seat cushion that will distribute weight evenly and avoid excessive pressure on his ischial tuberosities while sitting. He lacks sensory awareness in the buttocks region, and that places him at risk for developing decubitus ulcers. He should develop sitting tolerance that extends beyond the current 1-hour time period to help him pursue his educational goals of attending college. An appropriate seat cushion that distributes weight evenly will help Chen remain seated for a longer period of time. He will also need to develop the habit of shifting his weight while seated. This can be done by having Chen position his arm around the upright posts of the wheelchair back and pulling his body slightly to one side and then repeating the process on the other side. This shifting of the body from side to side reduces the risk of developing decubitus ulcers.

The following are the goals of a comprehensive seating and positioning assessment.

PREVENTION OF DEFORMITY

Providing a symmetrical base of support preserves proper skeletal alignment and discourages spinal curvature and other body deformities.

TONE NORMALIZATION

By providing proper body alignment, in addition to bilateral weight bearing and adaptive devices as needed, tone normalization can be maximized.

PRESSURE MANAGEMENT

Pressure sores can be caused by improper alignment and an inappropriate sitting surface. The proper seat cushion can provide comfort, assist in trunk and pelvic alignment, and create a surface that minimizes pressure, heat, moisture, and shearing, the primary causes of skin breakdown.

PROMOTION OF FUNCTION

Pelvic and trunk stability is necessary to free the upper extremity for participation in all functional activities, including wheelchair mobility and daily living skills.

MAXIMUM SITTING TOLERANCE

Wheelchair sitting tolerance will increase as support, comfort, and symmetrical weight bearing are provided.

OPTIMAL RESPIRATORY FUNCTION

Support in an erect, well-aligned position can decrease compression of the diaphragm and thus increase **vital capacity.**

PROVISION FOR PROPER BODY ALIGNMENT

Good body alignment is necessary for prevention of deformity, normalization of tone, and promotion of movement. The client should be able to propel the wheelchair and also to move around within the wheelchair.

A wide variety of seating and positioning equipment is available for all levels of disability. Custom modifications are continually being designed to meet a variety of client needs. In addition, technology in this area is ever growing, and interest in wheelchair technology as a professional specialty also is growing. However, the skill of clinicians in this field ranges from extensive to negligible. Although it is an integral aspect of any wheelchair evaluation, the scope of seating and positioning equipment is much greater than can be addressed in this chapter. The suggested reading list at the end of this chapter gives additional resources.

ACCESSORIES

Once the measurements and the need for additional positioning devices have been determined, a wide variety of accessories are available to meet a client's individual needs. It is extremely important to understand the function of each accessory and how an accessory interacts with the complete design and function of the chair and with seating and positioning equipment.[2,60]

Armrests come in fixed, flip-back, detachable, desk, standard, reclining, adjustable height, and tubular styles. The fixed armrest is a continuous part of the frame and is not detachable. It limits proximity to table, counter, and desk surfaces and prohibits side transfers. Flip-back, detachable desk, and standard length arms are removable and allow side-approach transfers. Reclining arms are attached to the back post and recline with the back of the chair. Tubular arms are available on lightweight frames.

Footrests may be fixed, swing-away detachable, solid cradle, and elevating. The fixed footrests are attached to the wheelchair frame and are not removable. These footrests prevent the person from getting close to counters and may make some types of transfers more difficult. The swing-away detachable footrests can be moved to the side of the chair or removed entirely. This allows a closer approach to bed, bathtub,

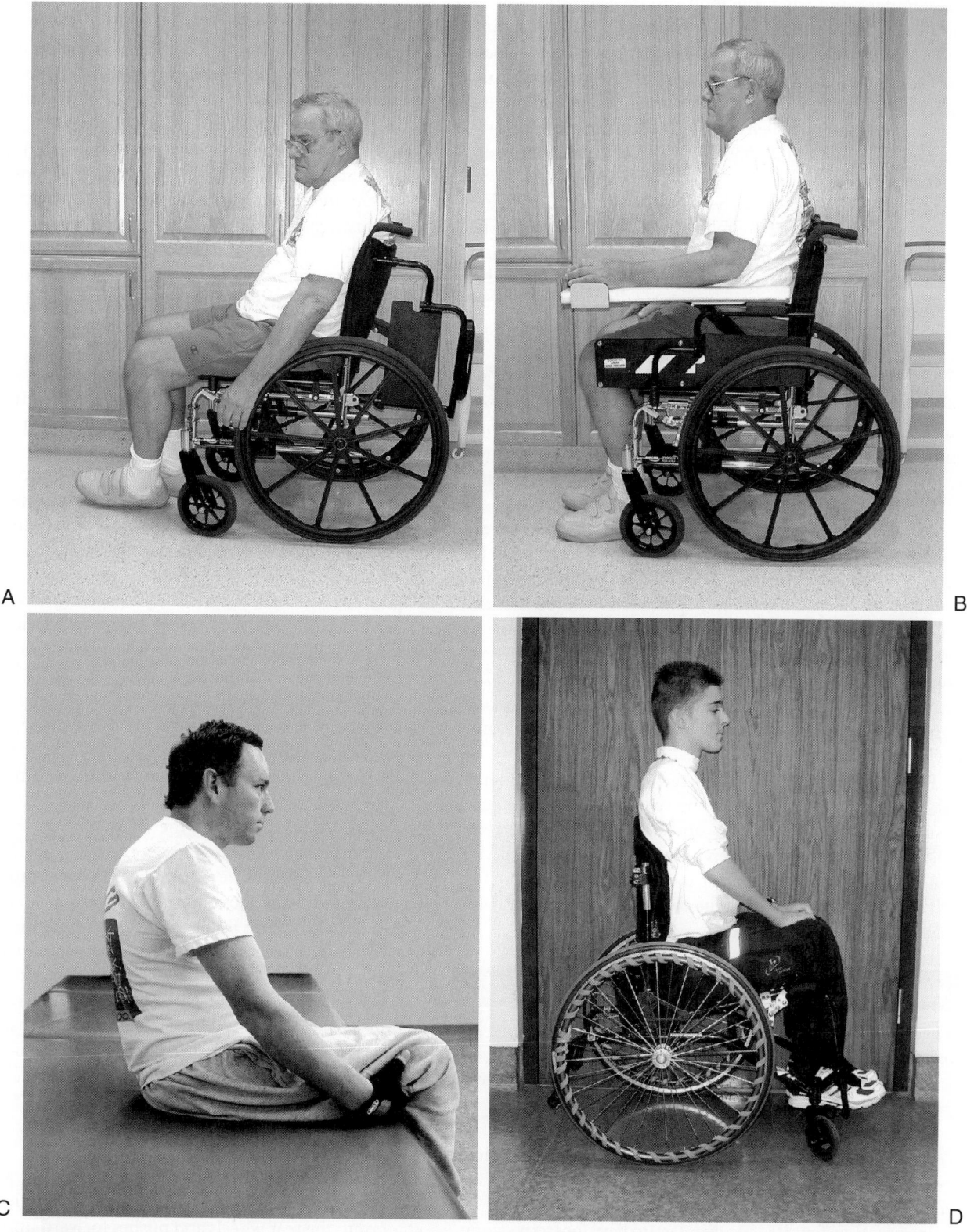

Figure 11-8   **A,** Client who had a stroke, seated in wheelchair. Poor positioning results in kyphotic thoracic spine, posterior pelvic tilt, and unsupported affected side. **B,** Same client now seated in wheelchair with appropriate positioning devices. Seat and back insert facilitate upright midline position with neutral pelvic tilt and equal weight bearing throughout. **C,** Client who sustained a spinal cord injury sitting with back poorly supported results in posterior pelvic tilt, kyphotic thoracic spine, and absence of lumbar curve. **D,** Same client seated with rigid back support and pressure-relief seat cushion, resulting in erect thoracic spine, lumbar curve, and anterior tilted pelvis.

and counters, and when the footrests are removed, reduces the overall wheelchair length and weight for easy loading into a car. Detachable footrests lock into place on the chair with a locking device.[60] A solid cradle footrest is found on rigid, lightweight chairs and is not removable. Elevating leg rests are available for clients with such conditions as lower-extremity edema, blood pressure changes, and orthopedic problems.

The foot plates may have heel loops and toe straps to aid in securing the foot on the foot plate.[60] A calf strap can be used on a solid cradle or when additional support behind the calf is necessary. Other accessories can include seat belts, various brake styles, brake extensions, anti-tip devices, caster locks, arm supports, and head supports.

PREPARING THE PRESCRIPTION

Once specific measurements and the need for modifications and accessories have been determined, the wheelchair prescription must be completed. It should be concise and specific so that everything requested can be accurately interpreted by the DME supplier, who will be submitting a sales contract for payment authorization. Before-and-after pictures can be helpful to illustrate medical necessity. The requirements for payment authorization from a particular reimbursement source must be known so that medical necessity can be demonstrated. The therapist must be aware of the cost of every item being requested and provide a reason and justification for each item. Payment may be denied if clear reasons are not given to substantiate the necessity of every item and any modification requested.

Before the wheelchair is delivered to the client, the therapist should check the chair to the specific prescription and ensure that all specifications and accessories are correct. When a custom chair has been ordered, the client should be fitted by the ordering therapist to ensure that the chair fits and that it provides all the elements that were expected when the prescription was generated.

WHEELCHAIR SAFETY

Wheelchair parts tend to loosen over time and should be inspected and tightened on a regular basis.

Elements of safety for the wheelchair user and the caregiver are as follows:

1. Brakes should be locked during all transfers.
2. The client should never stand on the foot plates, which are placed in the "up" position during most transfers.
3. In most transfers, it is an advantage to have footrests swung away if possible.
4. If a caregiver is pushing the chair, he or she should be sure that the client's elbows are not protruding from the armrests and that the client's hands are not on the hand rims. If approaching from behind to assist in moving the wheelchair, the caregiver should inform the client of this intent

and check the position of the client's feet and arms before proceeding.
5. To push the client up a ramp, he or she should move in a normal, forward direction. If the ramp is negotiated independently, the client should lean slightly forward while propelling the wheelchair up the incline.[61]
6. To push the client down a ramp, the caretaker should tilt the wheelchair backward by pushing the foot down on the tipping levers to its balance position, which is a tilt of approximately 30 degrees. Then the caregiver should ease the wheelchair down the ramp in a forward direction, while maintaining the chair in its balance position. The caregiver should keep his or her knees slightly bent and the back straight.[61] The caregiver may also move down the ramp backward while the client maintains some control of the large wheels to prevent rapid backward motion. This approach is useful if the grade is relatively steep. Ramps with only a slight grade can also be managed in a forward direction if the caregiver maintains grasp and pull on the hand grips and the client again maintains some control of the big wheels to prevent rapid forward motion. If the ramp is negotiated independently, the client should move down the ramp facing forward while leaning backward slightly and maintaining control of speed by grasping the hand rims. The client can descend a steep grade by traversing the ramp slightly back and forth to slow the chair. Gloves may be helpful to reduce the effect of friction.[61]
7. A caregiver can manage ascending curbs by approaching them forward, tipping the wheelchair back, and pushing the foot down on the tipping levers, thus lifting the front casters onto the curb and pushing forward. The large wheels then are in contact with the curb and roll on with ease as the chair is lifted slightly onto the curb.
8. The curb should be descended using a backward approach. A caregiver can move himself or herself and the chair around as the curb is approached and pull the wheelchair to the edge of the curb. Standing below the curb, the caregiver can guide the large wheels off the curb by slowly pulling the wheelchair backward until it begins to descend. After the large wheels are safely on the street surface, the assistant can tilt the chair back to clear the casters, move backward, lower the casters to the street surface, and then turn around.[61]

With good strength and coordination, many clients can be trained to manage curbs independently. To mount and descend a curb, the client must have a good bilateral grip, arm strength, and balance. To mount the curb, the client tilts the chair onto the rear wheels and pushes forward until the front wheels hang over the curb, then lowers them gently. The client then leans forward and forcefully pushes forward on the hand rims to bring the rear wheels up on the pavement. To descend a curb, the client should lean forward and push slowly backward until the rear and then the front wheels roll down the curb.[20]

The ability to lift the front casters off the ground and balance on the rear wheels ("pop a wheelie") is a beneficial skill and expands the client's independence in the community with curb management and in rural settings with movement over grassy, sandy, or rough terrain. Clients who have good grip, arm strength, and balance usually can master this skill and perform safely. The technique involves being able to tilt the chair on the rear wheels, balance the chair on the rear wheels, and move and turn the chair on the rear wheels. The client should not attempt to perform these maneuvers without instruction and training in the proper techniques, which are beyond the scope of this chapter. Specific instructions on teaching these skills can be found in the sources cited at the end of the chapter.[20]

TRANSFER TECHNIQUES

Transferring is the process of a client's moving from one surface to another. This process includes the sequence of events that must occur both before and after the move, such as the pre-transfer sequence of bed mobility and the post-transfer phase of wheelchair positioning. Assuming that a client has some physical or cognitive limitations, it will be necessary for the therapist to assist in or supervise a transfer. Many therapists are unsure of the transfer type and technique to employ or feel perplexed when a particular technique does not succeed with the client. Each client, therapist, and situation is different. This chapter does not include an outline of all techniques but presents the basic techniques with generalized principles. Each transfer must be adapted for the particular client and his or her needs. The discussion in this chapter includes directions for some transfer techniques that are most commonly employed in practice. These techniques are the stand pivot, bent pivot, and one-person and two-person dependent transfers.

PRELIMINARY CONCEPTS

The therapist must be aware of the following concepts when selecting and carrying out transfer techniques to ensure safety for the client and self:

1. The therapist should be aware of the client's status, especially the client's physical, cognitive, perceptual, and behavioral abilities and limitations.
2. The therapist should know his or her own physical abilities and limitations and whether he or she can communicate clear, sequential instructions to the client (and if necessary to the long-term caregiver of the client).
3. The therapist should be aware of and use correct moving and lifting techniques.

GUIDELINES FOR USING PROPER MECHANICS

The therapist should be aware of the following principles of basic **body mechanics**[3]:

1. Get close to the client or move the client close to you.
2. Position your body to face the client (face head on).
3. Bend knees; use your legs not your back.
4. Keep a neutral spine (not bent or arched back).
5. Keep a wide base of support.
6. Keep your heels down.
7. Don't tackle more than you can handle; ask for help.
8. Don't combine movements. Avoid rotating at the same time as bending forward or backward.

The therapist should consider the following questions before performing a transfer:

1. What medical precautions affect the client's mobility or method of transfer?
2. Can the transfer be performed safely by one person, or is assistance required?
3. Has enough time been allotted for safe execution of a transfer? Are you in a hurry?
4. Does the client understand what is going to happen? If not, does he or she demonstrate fear or confusion? Are you prepared for this limitation?
5. Is the equipment that the client is being transferred to and from in good working order and in a locked position?
6. What is the height of the bed (or surface) in relation to the wheelchair? Can the heights be adjusted so that they are similar?
7. Is all equipment placed in the correct position?
8. Is all unnecessary bedding and equipment moved out of the way so that you are working without obstructions?
9. Is the client dressed properly in case you need to use a waistband to assist? If not, do you need a transfer belt or other assistance?
10. What are the other components of the transfer, such as leg management and bed mobility?

The therapist should be familiar with as many types of transfers as possible so that each situation can be resolved as it arises.

Many classifications of transfers exist, based on the amount of therapist participation. Classifications range from *dependent*, in which the client is unable to participate and the therapist moves the client, to *independent*, in which the client moves independently while the therapist merely supervises, observes, or provides input for appropriate technique related to the client's disabling condition.

Before attempting to move a client, the therapist must understand the biomechanics of movement and the effect the client's center of **positioning mass** has on transfers.

PRINCIPLES OF BODY POSITIONING

Pelvic Tilt

Generally, after the acute onset of a disability or prolonged time spent in bed, clients assume a posterior **pelvic tilt** (i.e., a slouched position with lumbar flexion). In turn, this posture moves the center of mass back toward the buttocks. The therapist may need to verbally cue or assist the client into a neutral or slightly anterior pelvic tilt position to move the center of mass forward over the center of the client's body and over the feet in preparation for the transfer.[52]

Trunk Alignment

It may be observed that the client's trunk alignment is shifted to either the right or the left side. If the therapist assists in moving the client while the client's weight is shifted to one side, the movement could throw the client and the therapist off balance. The client may need verbal cues or physical assistance to come to and maintain a midline trunk position before and during the transfer.

Weight Shifting

The transfer is initiated by shifting the client's weight forward, removing weight from the buttocks. This movement allows the client to stand, partially stand, or be pivoted by the therapist. This step must be performed regardless of the type of transfer.

Lower Extremity Positioning

The client's feet must be placed firmly on the floor with ankles stabilized and with knees aligned at 90 degrees of flexion over the feet. This position allows the weight to be shifted easily onto and over the feet. Heels should be pointing toward the surface to which the client is transferring. The client should either be barefoot or have shoes on to prevent slipping out of position. The feet can easily pivot in this position, and the risk of twisting or injuring an ankle or knee is minimized.

Upper Extremity Positioning

The client's arms must be in a safe position or in a position in which he or she can assist in the transfer. If one or both of the upper extremities is nonfunctional, the arms should be placed in a safe position that will not be in the way during the transfer (e.g., in the client's lap). If the client has partial or full movement, motor control, or strength, he or she can assist in the transfer either by reaching toward the surface to be reached or by pushing off from the surface to be left. The decision to request the client to use the arms during the transfer is based on the therapist's prior knowledge of the client's motor function.

PREPARING EQUIPMENT AND CLIENT FOR TRANSFER

The transfer process includes setting up the environment, positioning the wheelchair, and helping the client into a pre-transfer position. The following is a general overview of these steps.

POSITIONING THE WHEELCHAIR

1. Place the wheelchair at approximately a 30-degree angle to the surface to which the client is transferring.
2. Lock the brakes on the wheelchair and the bed.
3. Place both of the client's feet firmly on the floor, hip width apart, with knees over the feet.

4. Remove the wheelchair armrest closer to the bed.
5. Remove the wheelchair pelvic seat belt.
6. Remove the wheelchair chest belt and trunk or lateral supports.

BED MOBILITY IN PREPARATION FOR TRANSFER

Rolling the Client Who Has Hemiplegia

1. Before rolling the client, you may need to put your hand under the client's scapula on the weak side and gently mobilize it forward to prevent the client from rolling onto the shoulder, potentially causing pain and injury.
2. Assist the client in clasping the strong hand around the wrist of the weak arm, and lift upper extremities toward the ceiling.
3. Flex the client's knees.
4. You may assist the client to roll onto his or her side by first moving the arms toward the side, then the legs, and finally by placing one of the therapist's hand at the scapula area and the other therapist's hand at the hip, guiding the roll.

Side-Lying to Sit Up at the Edge of Bed

1. Bring the client's feet off the edge of the bed.
2. Stabilize the client's lower extremities.
3. Shift the client's body to an upright sitting position.
4. Place the client's hands on the bed at the sides of his or her body to help maintain balance.

Scooting to the Edge of the Bed

When working with a client who has sustained a stroke or traumatic brain injury, walk the client's hips toward the edge of the bed. Shift the client's weight to the unaffected side, position your hand behind the opposite buttock, and guide the client forward. Then shift the client's weight to the affected side, and repeat the procedure if necessary. Move forward until the client's feet are flat on the floor.

In the case of an individual with spinal cord injury, grasp the client's legs from behind the knees and gently pull the client forward, placing the client's feet firmly on the floor and making sure that the ankles are in a neutral position.

STAND PIVOT TRANSFERS

The standing pivot transfer requires the client to be able to come to a standing position and pivot on one or both feet. It is most commonly used with clients who have hemiplegia, hemiparesis, or a general loss of strength or balance.

WHEELCHAIR TO BED OR MAT TRANSFER

1. Help the client scoot to the edge of the surface and put his or her feet flat on the floor. The client's heels should be pointed toward the surface to which the

client is transferring. The feet should not be perpendicular to the transfer surface but the heel should be angled towards the surface.

2. Stand on the client's affected side with your hands either on the client's scapulae or around the client's waist or hips. Stabilize the client's involved foot and knee with your own foot and knee. Provide assistance by guiding the client forward as the buttocks are lifted up from the present surface and toward the transfer surface (Figure 11-9, *A*).

3. The client either reaches toward the surface to which he or she is transferring or pushes off the surface from which he or she is transferring (Figure 11-9, *B*).

4. Guide the client toward the transfer surface and gently help him or her down to a sitting position (Figure 11-9, *C*).

VARIATIONS: STAND PIVOT AND/OR STAND/STEP TRANSFER

A stand pivot and/or stand/step transfer is generally used when a client can take small steps toward the surface goal and not just pivot toward the transfer surface. The therapist's intervention may range from physical assistance to accommodate for potential loss of balance to facilitation of near normal movement, equal weight bearing, and maintenance of appropriate posture for clients with hemiplegia or hemiparesis.

If a client demonstrates impaired cognition or a behavior deficit, including impulsiveness and poor safety judgment, the therapist may need to provide verbal cues or physical guidance.

SLIDING BOARD TRANSFERS

Sliding board transfers are best used with those who cannot bear weight on the lower extremities and who have paralysis, weakness, or poor endurance in their upper extremities. If the client is going to assist the caregiver in this transfer, the client should have good upper extremity strength. It is most often employed with persons who have lower extremity amputations or individuals with spinal cord injuries.

METHOD

See Figure 11-10.

1. Position and set up the wheelchair as previously outlined.

2. Lift the leg closer to the transfer surface and place the board under this leg, mid-thigh between the buttocks and knee, angled toward the opposite hip. The board must be firmly under the thigh and firmly on the surface to which the client is transferring.

3. Block the client's knees with your own knees.

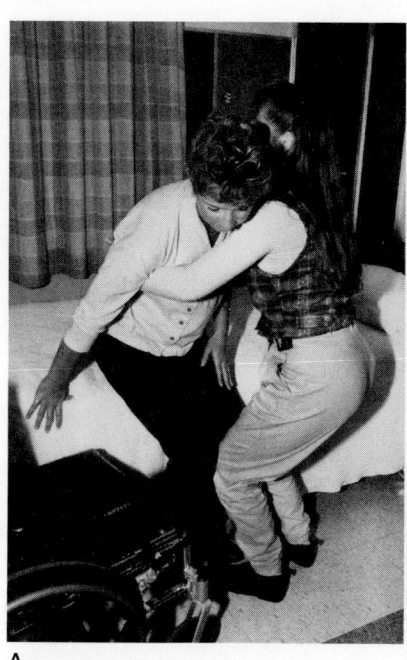 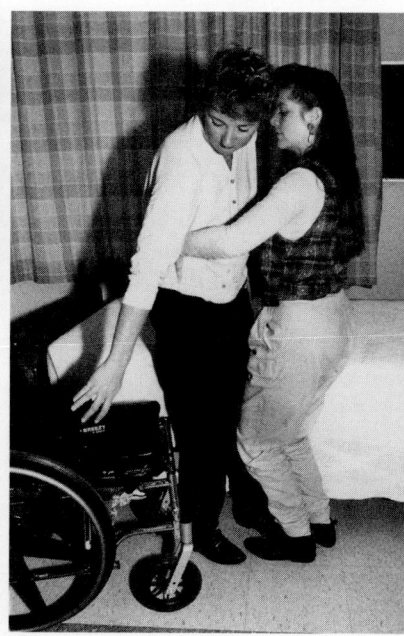 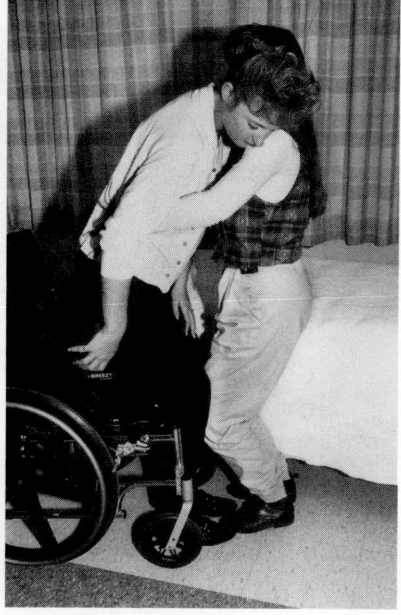

A B C

Figure 11-9 Standing pivot transfer; wheelchair to bed, assisted. **A,** Therapist stands on client's affected side and stabilizes client's foot and knee. She assists by guiding client forward and initiates lifting buttocks up. **B,** Client reaches toward transfer surface. **C,** Therapist guides the client toward transfer surface. (Courtesy Luis Gonzalez.)

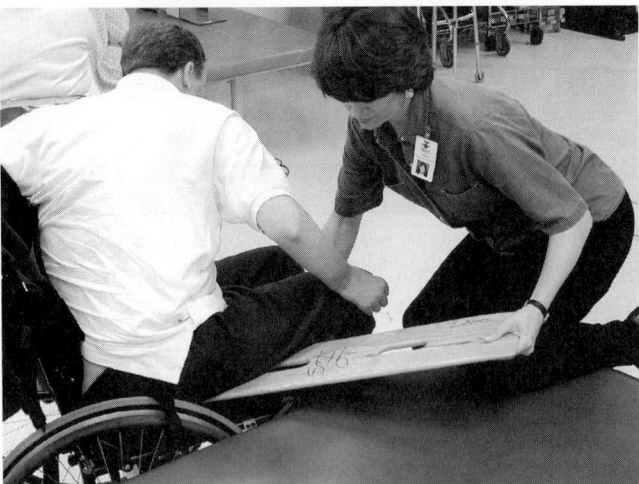

Figure 11-10 Positioning sliding board. Lift leg closest to transfer surface. Place board midthigh between buttocks and knee, angled toward opposite hip. (Courtesy Luis Gonzalez.)

4. Instruct the client to place one hand on the edge of the board and the other hand on the wheelchair seat.
5. Instruct the client to lean forward and slightly away from the transferring surface.
6. The client should transfer his or her upper body weight in the direction opposite to which he or she is going. The client should use both arms to lift or slide the buttocks along the board.
7. Assist the client where needed to shift weight and support the trunk while moving to the intended surface.

BENT PIVOT TRANSFER: BED TO WHEELCHAIR

The bent pivot transfer is used when the client cannot initiate or maintain a standing position. A therapist often prefers to keep a client in the bent knee position to maintain equal weight bearing, provide optimal trunk and lower extremity support, and perform a safer and easier therapist-assisted transfer.

PROCEDURE

1. Assist the client to scoot to the edge of the bed until both of the client's feet are flat on the floor. Grasp the client around the waist, hips, or even under the buttocks if a moderate or maximal amount of assistance is required.
2. Facilitate the client's trunk into a midline position.
3. Shift the weight forward from the buttocks toward and over the client's feet (Figure 11-11, *A*).
4. Have the client either reach toward the surface he or she is transferring to or push from the surface he or she is transferring from (Figure 11-11, *B*).
5. Assist the client by guiding and pivoting the client around toward the transfer surface (Figure 11-11, *C*).

Depending on the amount of assistance required, the pivoting portion can be done in two or three steps, with the therapist repositioning himself or herself and the client's lower extremities between steps. The therapist has a variety of choices of where to hold or grasp the client during the bent pivot transfer, depending on the weight and height of the

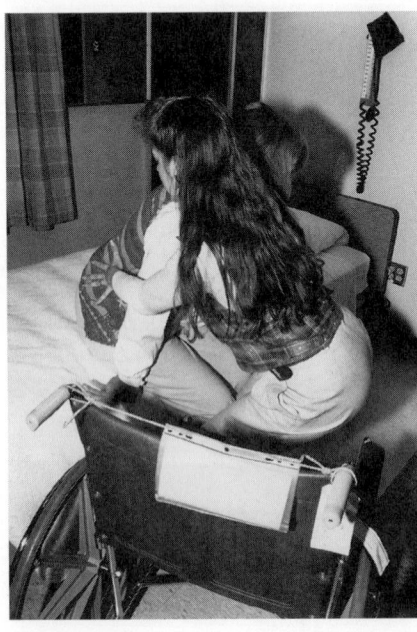 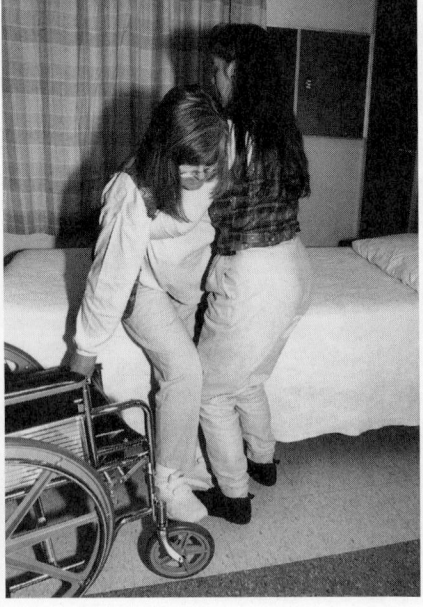 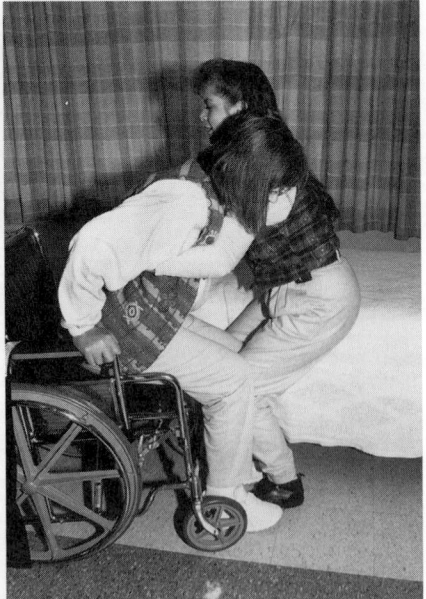

A   B   C

Figure 11-11 Bent pivot transfer; bed to wheelchair. **A,** Therapist grasps client around trunk and assists in shifting client's weight forward over feet. **B,** Client reaches toward wheelchair. **C,** Therapist assists client down toward sitting position. (Courtesy Luis Gonzalez.)

client in relation to the therapist and the client's ability to assist in the transfer. Variations include using both hands and arms at the waist, or trunk, or one or both hands under the buttocks. The therapist never grasps under the client's weak arm or grasps the weak arm, an action that could cause significant injury because of weak musculature and poor stability around the shoulder girdle. The choice is made with consideration to proper body mechanics. Trial and error of technique is advised to allow for optimal facilitation of client independence, safety, and the therapist's proper body mechanics.

DEPENDENT TRANSFERS

The dependent transfer is designed for use with the client who has minimal to no functional ability. If this transfer is performed incorrectly, it is potentially hazardous for therapist and client. This transfer should be practiced with able-bodied persons and initially used with the client only when another person is available to assist.[3]

The purpose of the dependent transfer is to move the client from surface to surface. The requirements are that the client be cooperative and willing to follow instructions. The therapist should be keenly aware of correct body mechanics and his or her own physical limitations. With heavy clients, it is always best to use the two-person transfer or at least to have a second person available to spot the transfer.

ONE-PERSON DEPENDENT SLIDING BOARD TRANSFER

See Figure 11-12.

The procedure for transferring the client from wheelchair to bed is as follows:

1. Set up the wheelchair and bed as described previously.
2. Position the client's feet together on the floor, directly under the knees, and swing the outside footrest away. Grasp the client's legs from behind the knees, and pull the client slightly forward in the wheelchair so that the buttocks will clear the large wheel when the transfer is made (Figure 11-12, A).
3. Place a sliding board under the client's inside thigh, midway between the buttocks and the knee, to form a bridge from the bed to the wheelchair. The sliding board is angled toward the client's opposite hip.
4. Stabilize the client's feet by placing your feet laterally around the client's feet.
5. Stabilize the client's knees by placing your own knees firmly against the anterolateral aspect of the client's knees (Figure 11-12, B).
6. Help the client lean over the knees by pulling him or her forward from the shoulders. The client's head and trunk should lean opposite the direction of the transfer. The client's hands can rest on the lap.
7. Reach under the client's outside arm and grasp the waistband of the trousers or under the buttock.

On the other side, reach over the client's back and grasp the waistband or under the buttock (Figure 11-12, C).
8. After your arms are positioned correctly, lock them to stabilize the client's trunk. Keep your knees slightly bent and brace them firmly against the client's knees.
9. Gently rock with the client to gain some momentum, and prepare to move after the count of three. Count to three aloud with the client. On three, holding your knees tightly against the client's knees, transfer the client's weight over his or her feet. You must keep your back straight and your knees bent to maintain good body mechanics (Figure 11-12, D).
10. Pivot with the client and move him or her onto the sliding board (Figure 11-12, E). Reposition yourself and the client's feet and repeat the pivot until the client is firmly seated on the bed surface, perpendicular to the edge of the mattress and as far back as possible. This step usually can be achieved in two or three stages (Figure 11-12, F).
11. You can secure the client on the bed by easing him or her against the back of an elevated bed or on the mattress in a side-lying position, then by lifting the legs onto the bed.

The one-person dependent sliding board transfer can be adapted to move the client to other surfaces. It should be attempted only when therapist and client feel secure with the wheelchair-to-bed transfer.

TWO-PERSON DEPENDENT TRANSFERS

Bent Pivot: With or Without a Sliding Board Bed to Wheelchair

A bent pivot transfer is used to allow increased therapist interaction and support. It allows the therapist greater control of the client's trunk and buttocks during the transfer. This technique can also be employed during a two-person dependent transfer. It is often used with neurologically involved clients because trunk flexion and equal weight bearing are often desirable with this diagnosis. The steps in this two-person procedure are as follows:

1. Set up the wheelchair and bed as described previously.
2. One therapist assumes a position in front of the client and the other in back.
3. The therapist in front assists in walking the client's hips forward until the feet are flat on the floor.
4. The same therapist stabilizes the client's knees and feet by placing his or her knees and feet lateral to each of the client's.
5. The therapist in back positions himself or herself squarely behind the client's buttocks, grasping either the client's waistband, grasping the sides of the client's pants, or placing his or her hands under the buttocks. Maintain proper body mechanics (Figure 11-13, A).

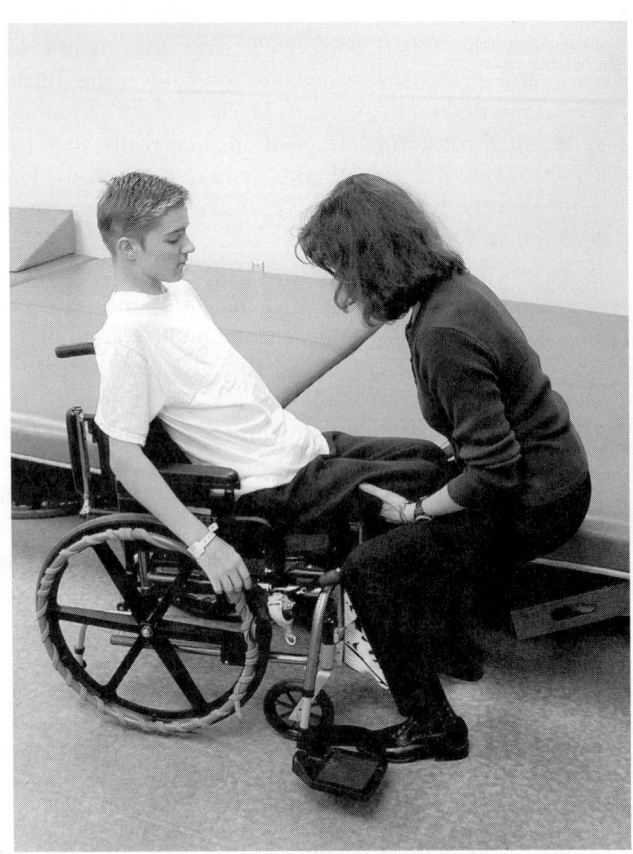
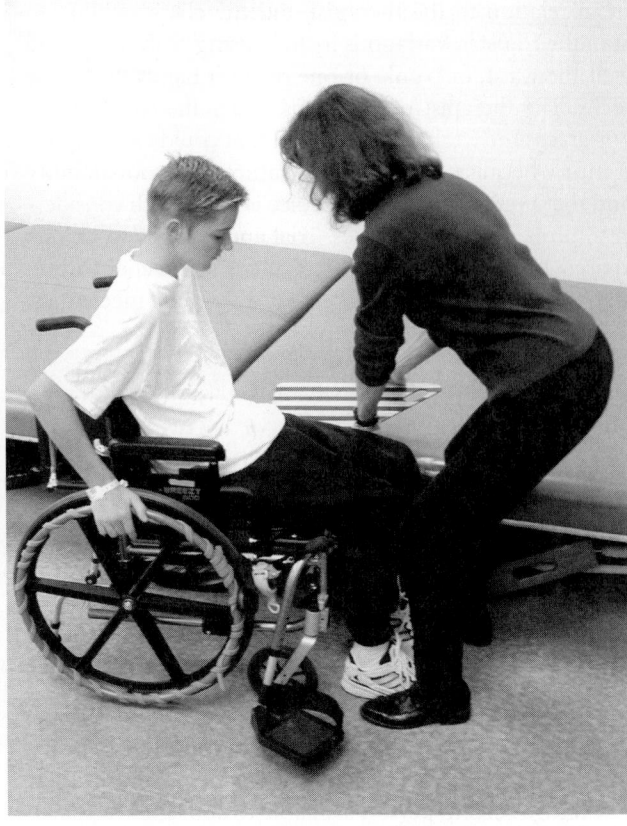
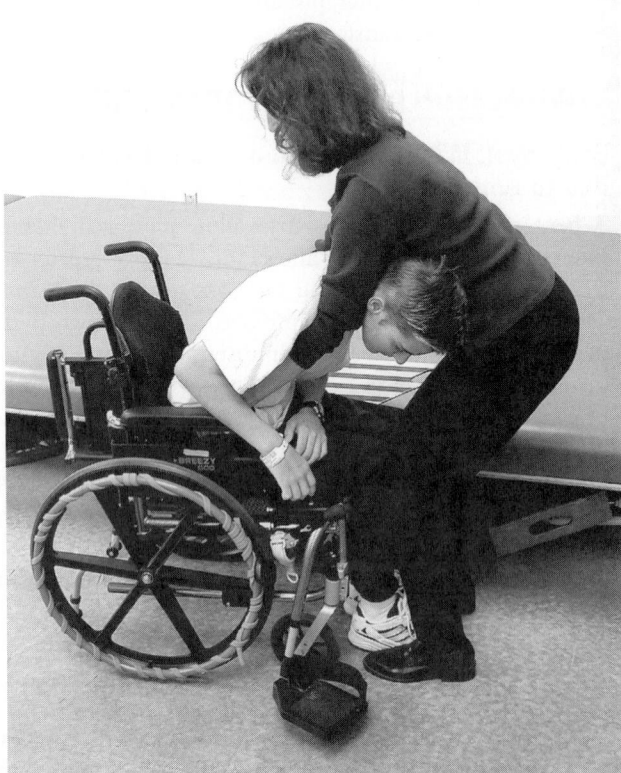
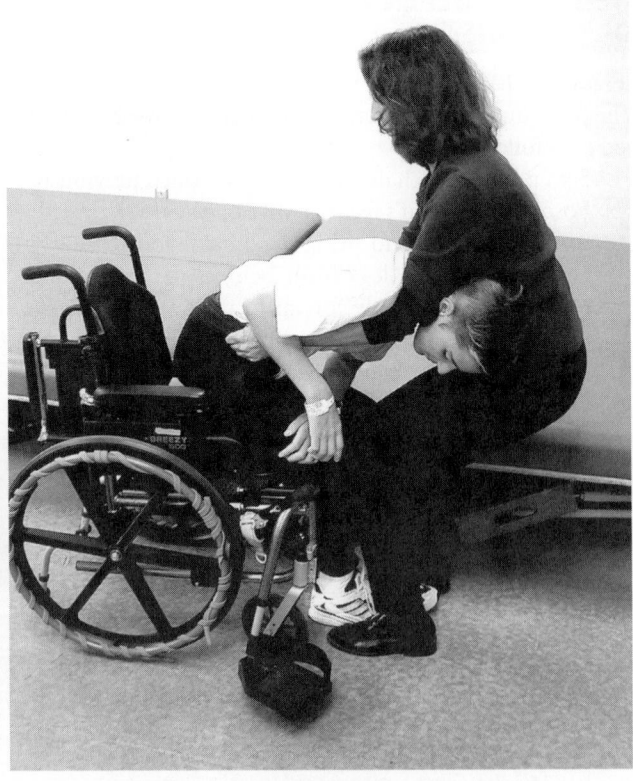

Figure 11-12 One-person dependent sliding board transfer. **A,** Therapist positions wheelchair and client, and pulls client forward in chair. **B,** Therapist stabilizes client's knees and feet after placing sliding board. **C,** Therapist grasps client's pants at lowest point of buttocks. **D,** Therapist rocks with client and shifts client's weight over client's feet, making sure client's back remains straight.

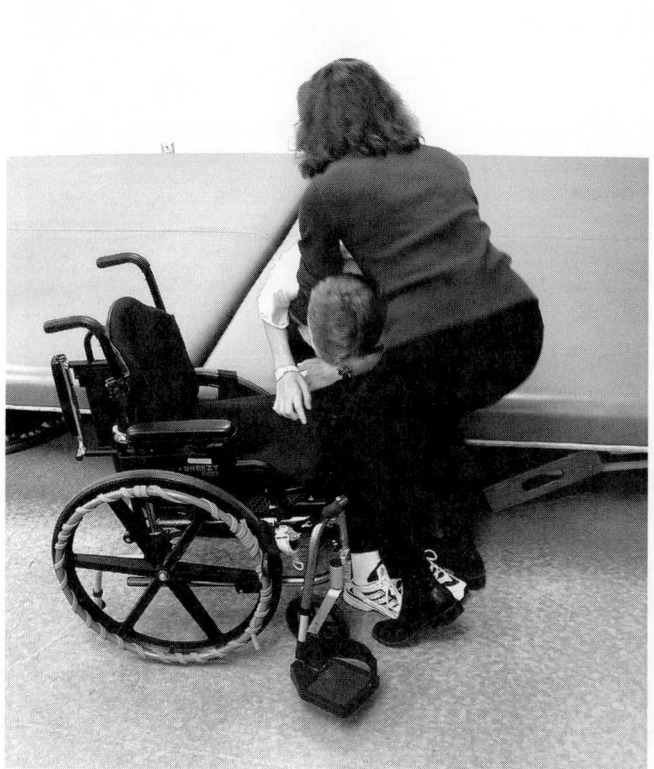
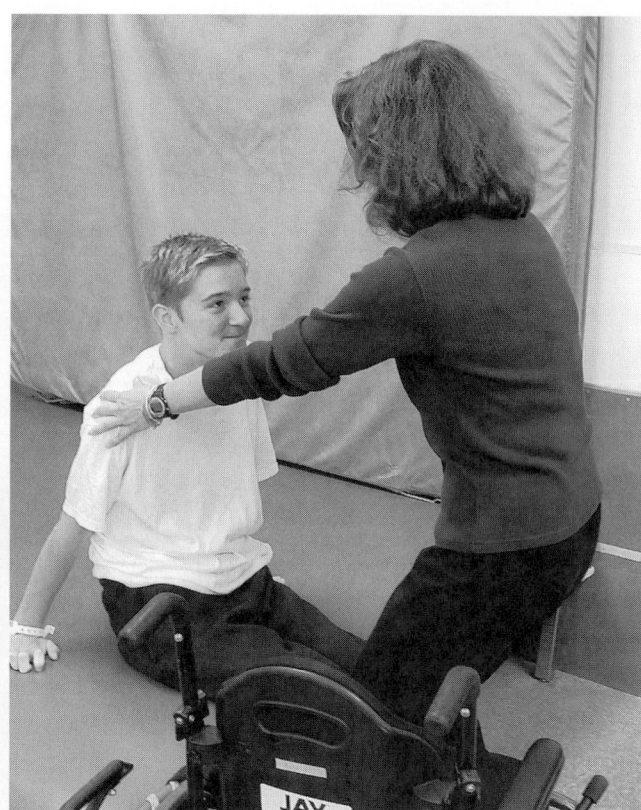

E   F

Figure 11-12, cont'd   **E,** Therapist pivots with client and moves client onto sliding board. **F,** Client is stabilized on bed. (Courtesy Luis Gonzales.)

6. The therapist in front moves the client's trunk into a midline position, grasps the client around the back of the shoulders, waist, or hips, and guides the client to lean forward and shift his or her weight forward, over the feet and off the buttocks. The client's head and trunk should lean in the direction opposite the transfer. The client's hands can rest on the lap (Figure 11-13, *B*).

7. As the therapist in front shifts the client's weight forward, the therapist in back shifts the client's buttocks in the direction of the transfer. This can be done in two or three steps, making sure the client's buttocks land on a safe, solid surface. The therapists reposition themselves and the client to maintain safe and proper body mechanics (Figure 11-13, *C*).

8. The therapists should be sure they coordinate the time of the transfer with the client and one another by counting to three aloud and instructing the team to initiate the transfer on three.

9. Transfer or gait belts may be employed to offer a place to grasp while assisting the client in a transfer. The belt is placed securely around the waist and often utilized instead of the client's waistband. The belt should not be allowed to slide up the client's trunk as leverage will be compromised.

MECHANICAL LIFT TRANSFERS

Some clients, because of body size, degree of disability, or the health and well-being of the caregiver, require the use of a mechanical lift. A variety of mechanical lifting devices can be used to transfer clients of any weight (Figure 11-14). A properly trained caregiver, even one who is considerably smaller than the client, can learn to use the mechanical lift safely and independently.[61] The client's physical size, the environment in which the lift will be used, and the uses to which the lift will be put must be considered to order the appropriate mechanical lift. The client and caregiver should demonstrate safe use of the lift to the therapist before the therapist prescribes it.

TRANSFERS TO HOUSEHOLD SURFACES

SOFA OR CHAIR

See Figure 11-15.

Wheelchair-to-sofa and wheelchair-to-chair transfers are similar to wheelchair-to-bed transfers; however, a few unique concerns should be assessed. The therapist and client need to be aware that the chair may be light and not as stable as a bed or wheelchair. When transferring to the chair, the client must

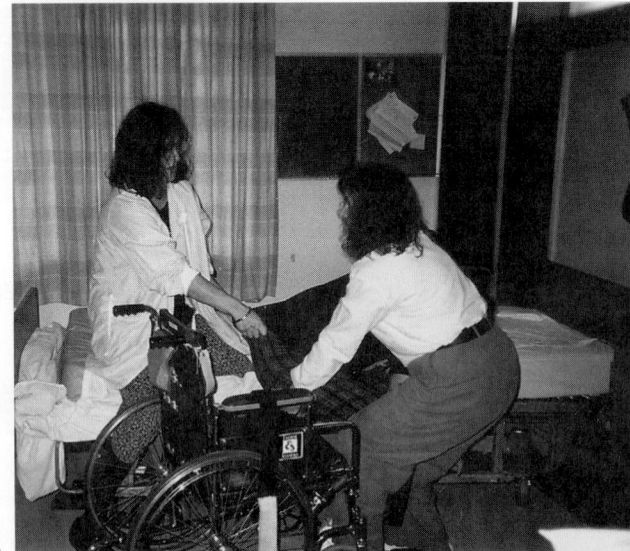
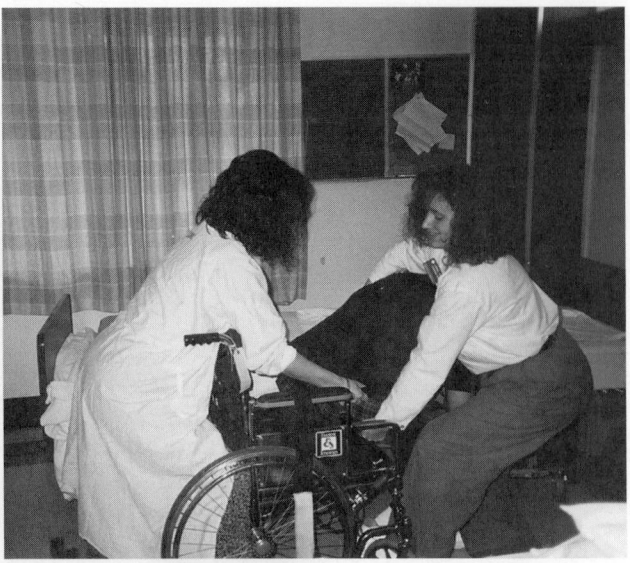
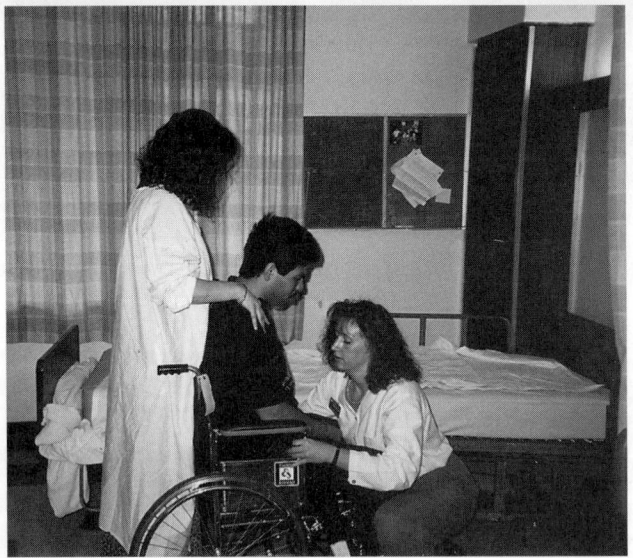

Figure 11-13   Two-person dependent transfer, bed to wheelchair. **A,** One therapist positions self in front of client, blocking feet and knees. The therapist in back positions self behind client's buttocks and assists by lifting. **B,** Person in front rocks client forward and unweights buttocks as the back therapist shifts buttocks toward wheelchair. **C,** Both therapists position client in upright, midline position in wheelchair. Seat belt is secured and positioning devices are added. (Courtesy Luis Gonzales.)

be instructed to reach for the seat of the chair. The client should not reach for the armrest or back of the chair because this action may cause the chair to tip over. When moving from a chair to the wheelchair, the client should use a hand to push off from the seat of the chair as he or she begins to stand. Standing from a chair is often more difficult if the chair is low or the seat cushions are soft. Dense cushions may be added to increase height and provide a firm surface to which to transfer.

TOILET

In general, wheelchair-to-toilet transfers are difficult because of the confined space in most bathrooms and the instability and lack of support of a toilet seat. The therapist and client should attempt to position the wheelchair next to or at an appropriate angle to the toilet. The therapist should analyze the space around the toilet and wheelchair to ensure no obstacles are present. Adaptive devices such as grab bars and raised toilet seats can be added to increase the client's independence during this transfer. (Raised toilet seats are poorly secured to toilets and may be unsafe for some clients.) The client can use these devices to support himself or herself during transfers and maintain a level surface to which to transfer.

BATHTUB

The OT should be cautious when assessing or teaching bathtub transfers because the bathtub is considered one of the

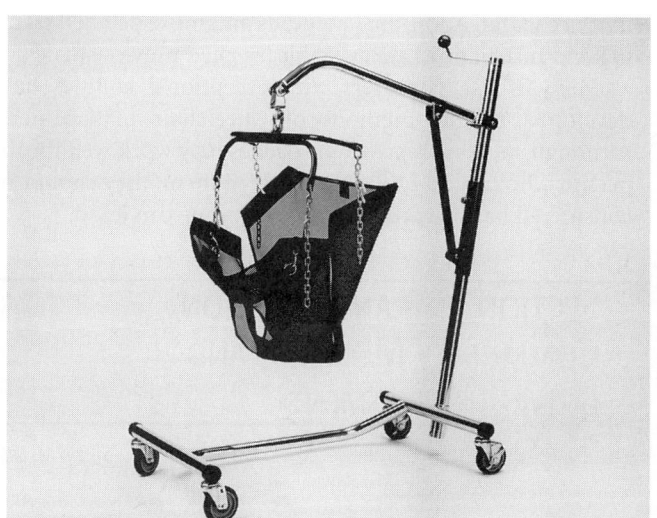

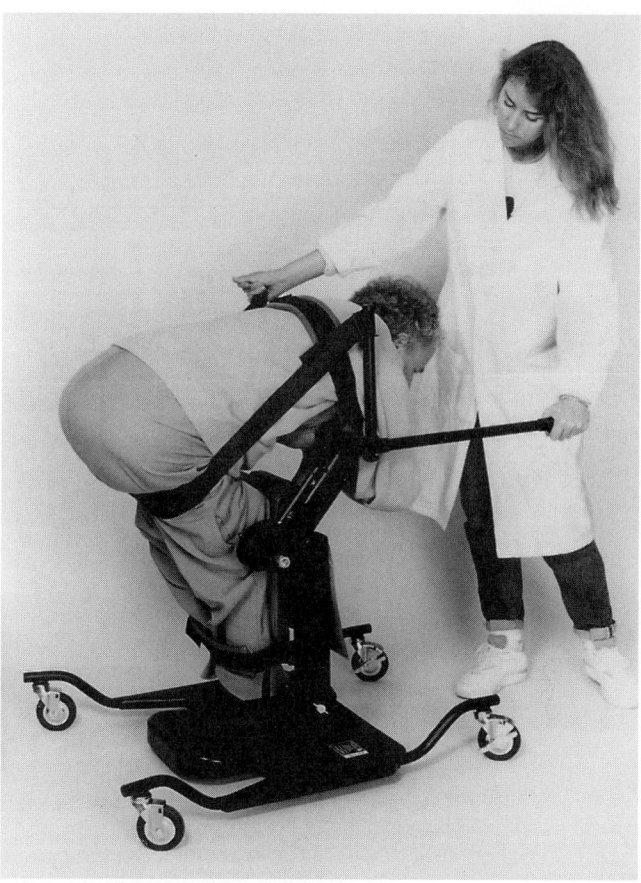

A   B

Figure 11-14   **A,** Traditional boom-style mechanical lift. **B,** Client lift useful in transferring individuals with spinal cord injury. (*A*, Courtesy Trans-Aid Lifts, Sunrise Medical; *B*, courtesy EZ-Pivot, Rand-Scott.)

most hazardous areas of the home. Transfers from the wheelchair to the bottom of the bathtub are extremely difficult and used with clients who have good bilateral strength and motor control of the upper extremities (e.g., clients with paraplegia and lower extremity amputation). A commercially produced bath bench or bath chair or a well-secured straight-back chair is commonly used by therapists for seated bathing. Therefore, whether a standing-pivot, bent-pivot, or sliding board transfer is performed, the technique is similar to a wheelchair-to-chair transfer. However, the transfer may be complicated by the confined space, the slick bathtub surfaces, and the bathtub wall between the wheelchair and the bathtub seat.

If a standing-pivot transfer is employed, it is recommended that the locked wheelchair be placed at a 45-degree angle to the bathtub if possible. The client should stand, pivot, sit on the bathtub chair, and then place the lower extremities into the bathtub.

If a bent-pivot or sliding board transfer is used, the wheelchair is placed next to the bathtub with the armrest removed. The transfer tub bench may be used, which removes the need for a sliding board. This approach allows the wheelchair to be placed right next to the bench, which allows a safe and easy transfer of the buttocks to the seat. Then the lower extremities can be assisted into the bathtub.

In general, the client may exit by first placing one foot securely outside the bathtub on a nonskid floor surface and then performing a standing or seated transfer back to the wheelchair.

CAR TRANSFERS

A car transfer is often the most challenging for therapists because it involves trial-and-error methods to develop a technique that is safe and easy for the client and caregiver to carry out. The therapist often uses the client's existing transfer technique. The client's size, degree of disability, and vehicle style (two-door versus four-door) must be considered. These factors will affect level of independence and may necessitate a change in the usual technique to allow a safe, easy transfer.

In general, it is difficult to get a wheelchair close enough to the car seat, especially with four-door vehicles. The following

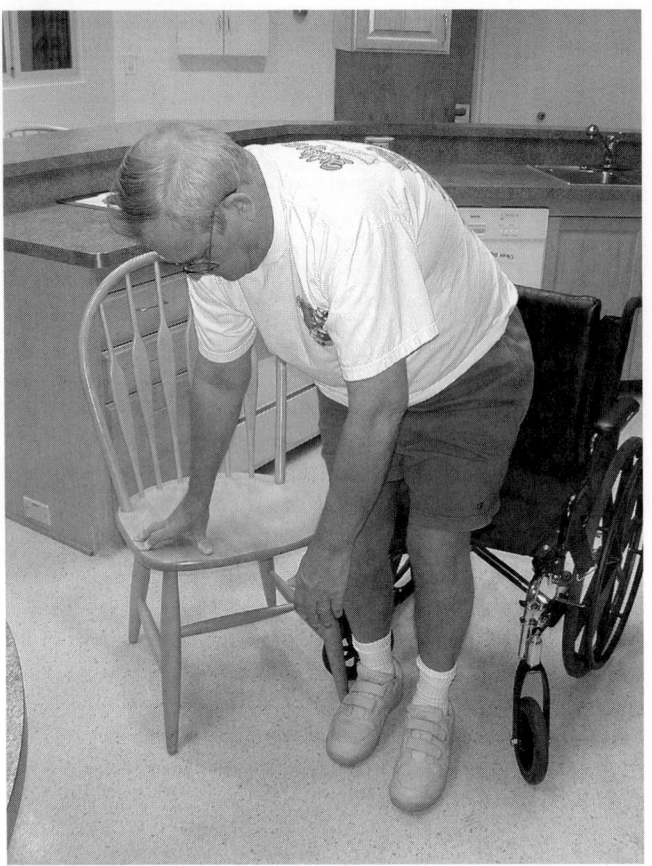

Figure 11-15 Client who sustained a stroke in midtransfer reaches for seat of chair, pivots, and lowers body to sitting. (Courtesy Luis Gonzales.)

are some additional considerations when making wheelchair-to-car transfers:

1. Car seats are often much lower than the standard wheelchair seat height, which makes the uneven transfer much more difficult, especially from the car seat to the wheelchair.

2. Occasionally, clients have orthopedic injuries that necessitate the use of a brace such as a halo body jacket or lower extremity cast or splint. The therapist often must alter technique to accommodate these devices.

3. The therapist may suggest use of an extra long sliding board for this transfer to compensate for the large gap between transfer surfaces.

4. Because uphill transfers are difficult and the level of assistance may increase for this transfer, the therapist may choose a two-person assist instead of a one-person assist transfer to ensure a safe and smooth technique.

SUMMARY

A wheelchair that fits well and can be managed safely and easily by its user and caregiver is one of the most important factors in the client's ability to perform ADLs with maximal

independence.[59] Each wheelchair user must learn the capabilities and limitations of the wheelchair and safe methods of performing all self-care and mobility skills. If a caregiver exists, he or she needs to be thoroughly familiar with safe and correct techniques of handling the wheelchair, positioning equipment, and the client.

Transfer skills are among the most important activities that must be mastered by the wheelchair user. The ability to transfer increases the possibility of mobility and travel. However, transfers can be hazardous. Safe methods must be learned and followed.[61] Several basic transfer techniques are outlined in this chapter. Additional methods and more detailed training and instructions are available, as cited previously.

Many wheelchair users with exceptional abilities have developed unique methods of wheelchair management. Although such innovative approaches may work well for the person who has devised and mastered them, they cannot be considered basic procedures that everyone can learn.[61]

SECTION 3: TRANSPORTATION, COMMUNITY MOBILITY, AND DRIVING ASSESSMENT

Susan M. Lillie

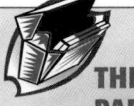

THREADED CASE STUDY: JACQUELINE, PART 1

Jacqueline is a 67-year-old retiree who has had increased difficulty in her ADLs because of painful arthritis in her neck, hands, back, hips, knees, and ankles. She is 5 feet, 6 inches tall and 138 lb and drives a 20-year-old sedan, meticulously maintained. Her husband has diabetes and no longer drives because of peripheral neuropathies in his legs. He is 6 feet tall and weighs 220 lb. Her role has dramatically changed; she was primarily the passenger and navigator until 1 year ago when her husband ceased driving upon the direction of his physician; she then assumed the primary role for transportation and driving, including assisting her husband with his wheelchair and car transfers.

Her doctor referred her to OT to increase independence with ADLs; she received four visits on an outpatient basis. The therapist worked with her in the kitchen and recommended larger grip kitchen utensils to facilitate performance in meal preparation. One day she escorted Jacqueline to her car to assess car transfers and noted difficulty in several areas: she had difficulty loading her husband's manual wheelchair, managing the key in the door, and opening the car door. She doesn't mind driving, "although it can be painful," she told her therapist, and on bad days, she doesn't drive at all.

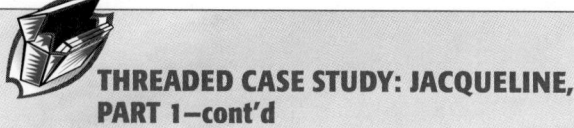

THREADED CASE STUDY: JACQUELINE, PART 1—cont'd

Jacqueline is in fine health, other than the limitations posed by her arthritis. During therapy sessions, she mentioned she feels fatigued from so much driving. She takes herself and her husband to all doctor appointments, the pharmacy for medicines, and to church, and she maintains their home and cares for her disabled husband. She stated she rarely participates in her hobby of scrapbooking anymore because of lack of time and fatigue. She is worried about what the future will bring because their two adult children both live out-of-state 500 miles away.

Critical Thinking Questions

1. What areas of Jacqueline's community mobility are appropriate for OT intervention?
2. Analyzing the task of driving relative to her diagnosis, what client factors can be predicted as needing assessment and intervention?
3. What adaptations or recommendations can Jacqueline and her therapist consider to improve mobility for her and her husband?

Mobility is a universal need at any age. Mobility allows one to participate in a desired occupation or activity throughout the lifespan, whether an infant lured to crawl by a shiny object or an adult moving about a kitchen to prepare a meal. Whatever the age and whether a passenger or driver, movement and transportation in the community are basic needs.

Community mobility is an area of occupation that affects all areas of practice. **Community mobility** is the action of moving oneself in the community; it also includes driving and the use of various forms of public and private transportation[18] and is considered an instrumental ADL under the OT Practice Framework.[8] Community mobility can be a means to an occupation (walking or driving to work) or an occupation in and of itself (a leisurely stroll or scenic drive).

Most adults in the United States consider community mobility, and the subset of driving in particular, to be the defining instrumental activity of daily living (IADL). In fact, this performance area is often viewed as synonymous with independence.[1,5,7,14,24] When transportation is unavailable for basic needs, such as visiting a grocery store, pharmacy, or physician, too often the result is social isolation, depression, and a diminishment or loss of life occupations.[14,16,24] Lack of transportation is cited as a significant factor in the unemployment of those who are disabled.[57] Competence in community mobility is essential to quality of life throughout the lifespan.[18] The OT is ideally suited to identify when community mobility occupations require assessment and intervention.

THE ROLE OF OCCUPATIONAL THERAPY

OTs are uniquely trained to address community mobility. Therapists address performance skills in the natural context or setting—in this case, the community itself—for therapeutic intervention.[39,58] The ability to analyze an activity from the client factors of performance, activity demands, performance skills, and contexts provides a framework for analyzing and developing treatment plans for all areas of community mobility (Figure 11-16).[8] This framework enables the OT to select an appropriate level of intervention and develop a plan to meet the client's needs.[7,18] All therapists have the skills and training necessary to ask basic questions about community mobility issues, such as are you comfortable with your transportation system or driving? The depth at which the individual therapist addresses the issue depends on the level of experience and specialized training received.[18,23,50] By returning to the case study at the beginning of this section, the therapist identified several areas that require intervention in Jacqueline's situation within her comfort zone of training; the driver assessment, however, is not within her purview and she referred the client to a driving program for that aspect of community mobility.

OTs have the ability to identify issues that may prevent safe mobility in the community.[23,50] Although driving may first come to mind, pedestrian safety, use of public transportation systems, passenger needs, and well adult programs are also aspects of community mobility within the OT's scope of practice.[23]

Advanced practice skills[23,50] and future specialty certification by AOTA (in progress) will formalize roles for different levels of intervention. Clients can derive benefit from therapeutic assistance in identifying a "next step" transportation plan if the client's primary transportation mode is no longer possible. This next step is sometimes better accepted as a back-up plan for IADL transportation needs. Early conversations regarding alternative transportation modes enable individuals and their families to initiate the process of considering appropriate resources and contingency planning before a transportation crisis occurs[5] and enable clients and their families to become familiar with and more readily participate in formal assessments, should the need arise in the future.[50]

In Jacqueline's case, she reported she is sometimes unable to drive because of arthritic flare-ups. This is a critical factor in development of intervention for personal transportation and alternative transportation. The therapist can follow this thread of conversation to elicit pertinent facts regarding needs and resources. As it turned out, Jacqueline qualified for alternate transportation systems, but she was unaware of them. The therapist was able to direct her to the appropriate resource and assist in developing a comprehensive transportation plan. After completing the application process and becoming an established member of the system, Jacqueline

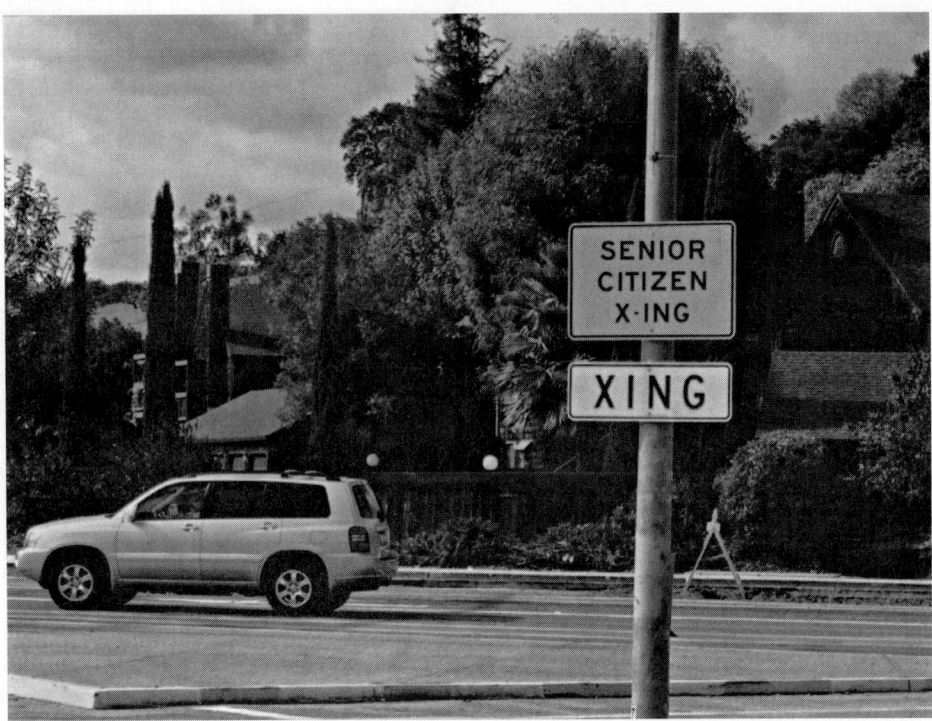

Figure 11-16   Community mobility in this context includes pedestrian and driver issues. The "Senior Citizen X-ing" sign reflects growing awareness of the needs of the aging population.

was relieved that a safety net was in place for her and her husband.

HISTORICAL CONTEXT

OTs have been involved from the infancy of this new specialty area of practice. The international association, ADED, The Association for Driver Rehabilitation Specialists (first known as the Association for Driver Educators for the Disabled) established a formal organization in 1977[11] with the mission of providing professional education and support in driver rehabilitation. OTs were a part of that founding movement.

As the field grew, safety issues were identified and addressed. A trade association, the National Mobility Equipment Dealers Association (NMEDA), founded a quality certification program for dealers that modified vehicles. The National Highway Traffic Safety Administration (NHTSA) became involved in the early 1990s and identified two areas of need: (1) a national safety plan for older drivers and (2) assurance that vehicle modifications for the disabled met with Federal Motor Vehicle Safety Standards, except where exempt. The American Occupational Therapy Association (AOTA) also became involved. These associations and agencies now work together to improve the quality and availability of service providers (Box 11-2).

It is interesting to note that Franklin Delano Roosevelt (FDR), former president of the United States, owned the first gas/brake hand control documented. The cultural contexts of the time caused FDR to conceal the impact of his polio from the public; he was seen walking and standing and was rarely photographed in a wheelchair, his primary method of mobility.[28] He enjoyed driving and while he was behind the wheel of a car he was not identified as someone with a disability.[51] For some clients, the social and cultural constraints and viewpoints on disability of the 1930s, such as those perceived by FDR, still exist within their own family and cultural contexts, and some clients may be hesitant to accept adaptations that look different. Many individuals take intrinsic pleasure from driving; they report that driving temporarily frees them from their disability because behind the wheel they look like everyone else.

PUBLIC TRANSPORTATION

Community mobility within public transportation includes the use and navigation of transportation systems offered by public and private entities. Public transportation "provides the general public with a general or special service on a regular and continuing basis."[12] Public transportation includes two key systems: **fixed route** and **paratransit.**

Fixed route systems use defined routes with predetermined stops; they run on a published schedule. Trains, city buses, and shuttles are types of fixed route transportation. The paratransit system provides demand-response service within a prescribed geographical area; vehicle dispatch occurs

Box **11-2** ADDITIONAL RESOURCES

American Medical Association
Physician's guide to assessment, older driver information
http://www.ama-assn.org (search for "older driver")

American Association of Retired Persons
Information and publications on older driver issues
http://www.aarp.org (search for "older drivers")

American Occupational Therapy Association
Physical Disability Special Interest Section–Driving Network Listserv
Listserv driving network for members, professional development tool,
older driver driving and older driver on-line courses, as offered
http://www.aota.org (click on AOTA Listserv, then on Driving/Driver
Rehabilitation)

Association for Driver Rehabilitation Specialists (ADED)
Best practices, standards of practice, models of practice, disability
fact sheets, bulletin board for members
http://www.aded.net

National Mobility Equipment Dealers Association
Trade association for manufacturers of equipment and vehicle
modifiers, QAP program
http://www.nmeda.org

National Highway Traffic Safety Administration
Consumer and disabled driver safety information
http://www.nhtsa.dot.gov
Older Driver Information

American Occupational Therapy Association
Numerous topics on older drivers and community mobility
http://www.aota.org/olderdriver/

---

only in response to a qualified rider's request. Jacqueline was able to qualify herself and her husband for their local paratransit system.

Inconvenience and fear for personal safety are frequently cited as a barrier to the use of fixed and demand-response public transportation and must be addressed to increase its use among the disabled and aging populations.[1,16]

AMERICANS WITH DISABILITIES ACT

The Americans with Disabilities Act (ADA) of 1990 was a landmark bill, which bans discrimination against the disabled; the act includes public transportation jurisdiction. One major purpose of the ADA was to provide disabled individuals equal access to transportation. The ADA regulates buses, trains, ships, and other means of transportation that use fixed and demand-response systems. The ADA does not regulate air travel, public school transportation at the K-12 level, or privately owned over-the-road buses, similar to full-size touring and for-profit travel buses.[26]

Disabled access to buses, trains, and light-rail systems occurs through the use of a wheelchair lift. The ADA specified lift dimensions (30-inch-wide by 48-inch-long platform lift), securements for mobility aid devices, priority seating, and a host of other features intended to facilitate navigation of the transportation system by those who are disabled.[26] The ADA also regulates paratransit, designated for persons who are disabled and unable to access or navigate a fixed route system.

The American Public Transportation Association estimated that nearly 30 million one-way rides were provided in the United States in the first quarter of 2004 alone; paratransit is an increasingly important tool for retaining community mobility.[9] The ADA specifies curb-to-curb service for paratransit, although door-to-door service is frequently still provided. An associate or attendant is able to accompany or assist a person with a disability on the paratransit vehicle.

The first 10 years of the ADA focused on the removal of physical barriers and providing accessible transport. The Federal Transit Administration is now focusing on improving paratransit service standards, reliability, and cost effectiveness; the paratransit system was so successful that actual use exceeded anticipated ridership and budgetary expectations. More stringent criteria will be used to determine who is paratransit-qualified as efforts to mainstream appropriate riders to fixed transit systems continue.[25] OTs have a leading role in matching task demands of local transit contexts to an individual's performance skills and client factors and recommending alternatives or intervention methods to meet desired outcomes. Transportation for those with impaired sensory performance areas, such as vision or hearing, is an increasing need.

INTERVENTION IMPLICATIONS FOR FIXED TRANSIT

The activity demands for fixed-route transportation include multiple steps required for ridership and also require the client to possess motor skills commensurate with the physical context of the community environment, process skills for route planning and navigation, and high-level cognitive functions sufficient to spontaneously problem solve during the activity. These activity demands also apply to pedestrians.

The OT determines barriers to successful outcomes; a focused intervention plan may be required to remediate or compensate for limited subskills. Mobility to and from the bus stop, to and from the destination, boarding and exiting the bus, dealing with the fare box and money handling, interpersonal skills, and contingency planning are common areas in which intervention is required. Several styles of lifts and locations of the lifts on buses exist, each with unique characteristics that must be considered; a repertoire of boarding techniques may be required depending on how a community's or region's fleet of vehicles is equipped.

Similarly, when making recommendations for a wheelchair or scooter, the therapist should consider the implications of using a fixed-route system; it cannot be assumed that mobility devices fit on fixed transit platform lifts; many, in fact, do not. Accessibility on an ADA-compliant lift is a function of the height of the lift end flap (ranging from 3 inches to 8 inches) and the footrest clearance of a given wheelchair. Lower footrests tend to make a wheelchair functionally longer and potentially incompatible with transit lifts.

Testing a proposed mobility device on an actual lift is recommended because the natural environment poses limitations that cannot be duplicated or foreseen in the clinic setting. A scooter may fit on the lift, for example, but have a turning radius that exceeds the physical environment of a bus or light rail system. Assessment in the community's physical context is an important step toward ensuring that an individual's mobility device will actually be able to provide the mobility needed for participation in occupations.

INTERVENTION IMPLICATIONS FOR PARATRANSIT

Paratransit requires ability to use the reservation system, and to function within the service limitations, and contingency plan. Intervention may include orientation to the local system, assessing ability to identify and locate access channels, planning a trip, preparing back-up safety plans, and accompanying an individual on an actual trip to a destination and back. The activity demands of curb-to-curb service are much greater than those of door-to-door service. For example, a client must navigate from a drop-off point to the final destination using a curb-to-curb service, whereas door-to-door service eliminates this demand.

Paratransit combines rider trips of several individuals to meet the capacity of the vehicles, and often travel takes longer than private transportation and can exceed fixed-route timelines. Extended travel can pose hardship to those whose medical conditions or symptoms include urinary urgency and frequency, pain with prolonged immobility, or decreased endurance. When no other transportation options are available, intervention may be required, such as additional positioning devices to decrease pain and fatigue.

Food, water, shelter, and public telephones may not be available at drop-off points. On some occasions, miscommunications or errors delay or outright cancel a ride. As with fixed transit, the unaccompanied rider needs a certain degree of resourcefulness and problem-solving skill to navigate the system safely and efficiently. Jacqueline became a paratransit rider to provide herself with transportation and accompany her husband to appointments. One concern she had was the long ride; Jacqueline's doctor was an hour away. Factoring in travel time, waiting, and the doctor visit, they could be away from home for 3 to 5 hours. The therapist recommended that Jacqueline pack appropriate diabetic snacks to properly maintain her husband's blood sugar level and avoid low blood sugar problems during their journey.

PRIVATE TRANSPORTATION

Private transportation relies on consumer vehicles that are privately owned. These vehicles can be owned individually or by an entity collectively. The primary advantage of private transportation is the on-demand, 24-hour availability with immediate origin-to-destination travel, flexibility to modify travel plans, and the strong sense of control over one's life. The primary disadvantage is cost: the individual is responsible for access needs, fuel, and keeping the adaptations and vehicle mechanically sound. Nondrivers who own vehicles face the additional costs of hiring drivers, which limits on-demand transportation.

Individuals preferring the convenience of private transportation must also plan for replacement costs of the vehicle to retain independence. Factors of aging or long-term disability may result in a higher level of compensatory adaptations being required in the future at greater cost.[14,33] A new trend results in further costs, as mobility equipment dealers are starting to require a driver assessment before adapting a vehicle. Costs and vehicle responsibilities prohibit many from private transportation options. Some clients will request consultations to identify the process and cost for private transportation, based on their diagnosis and function.

In one such case, a client with a C5 spinal cord injury discovered that the level of technology he was likely to need was expensive; should he be a successful driver candidate, the vehicle and adaptations alone would cost more than $100,000. This figure does not include the cost of the comprehensive evaluation or extensive driver's training. The client appreciated learning the assistive technology required for his injury, because it provided pivotal information for his transportation planning. Some clients value driving so highly that they would gladly pay the cost out of settlement or other funds. However, this client decided not to drive, stating, "That sure would buy a lot of taxi rides!" By providing a "mini" evaluation or consultation, the client obtained critical information he required to best plan his future. The client knew he could drive but chose to use his resources in a different transportation plan.

COLLABORATIVE OPTIONS

The aging of America has resulted in a focused effort on development of alternative transportation systems to accommodate nondrivers. The Beverly Foundation in Pasadena, California, joined with the AA Foundation for Traffic Safety in 1998[15] to support and promote collaborations and cooperatives within communities. Frequently churches, synagogues, and community centers serve as new sources for private transportation systems. Senior-friendly transportation must incorporate the 5 As: availability, accessibility, acceptability, affordability, and adaptability.[1] Charitable and non-profit agencies are beginning to create a unique resource for community mobility; such systems pair requests for transportation with a fleet of volunteer drivers. An added dimension is the social interaction and communication available within such a program.[1,16] By being involved in senior mobility issues in the community, therapists can learn of or even help develop appropriate alternatives to driving, adding their unique expertise to the process.

INTERVENTION IMPLICATIONS

Driving is but one aspect of private transportation within the practice area of community mobility. Other services that OTs provide include passenger evaluations. Passenger issues are too often overlooked as a focus of intervention, yet a trained therapist can significantly improve the safety of the caregiver and the rider. Supplemental trunk and head supports may be needed when an individual has inadequate motor and postural control to overcome dynamic forces of a vehicle in motion.[9] OTs can identify and recommend such devices, in addition to appropriate occupant restraint systems that match the performance of skills of the caregiver. In fact, caregivers should be screened to match adaptive devices to any limitations in the caregiver's physical performance or capacity. Education and training of body mechanics and joint protection are part of the caregiver training that is essential for

safety and injury prevention during the physical management of a person because the tight confines of a car or van can be challenging.[14]

SPECIALIZED NEEDS

When life support devices are required, safety dictates provision of a backup energy source in the vehicle through a device known as an *inverter*. An inverter converts a 12-volt DC battery source to common 110-volt AC power found in household power outlets, thereby providing an instantaneous plug-in source of power for life support equipment, should the device's battery supply fail.

Safe transport of infants and children with medical needs or disabilities is another area of practice that should not be overlooked. Car seats should not be modified unless the person performing the modification is certified to do so because of the life-threatening implications of inappropriate car seat adaptations that are recommended or made with good intentions.[13]

Assessment for children and teenagers must integrate future physical growth; a 6-year-old riding in a van seated in a wheelchair may no longer fit in the vehicle by age 12, for example, because of increased height. Also, activity demands associated with caregiving will be greater for a 12-year-old than a 6-year-old. Alternate mechanical or power lifts or adaptations may become necessary for children or adults when their body size becomes unmanageable (and therefore unsafe) for their caregiver. Jacqueline may need to consider specialized passenger seats designed for the elderly. These motorized seats move outside the car and rotate, easing the activity demand of car transfers through compensatory mechanical movement and power (Figure 11-17).

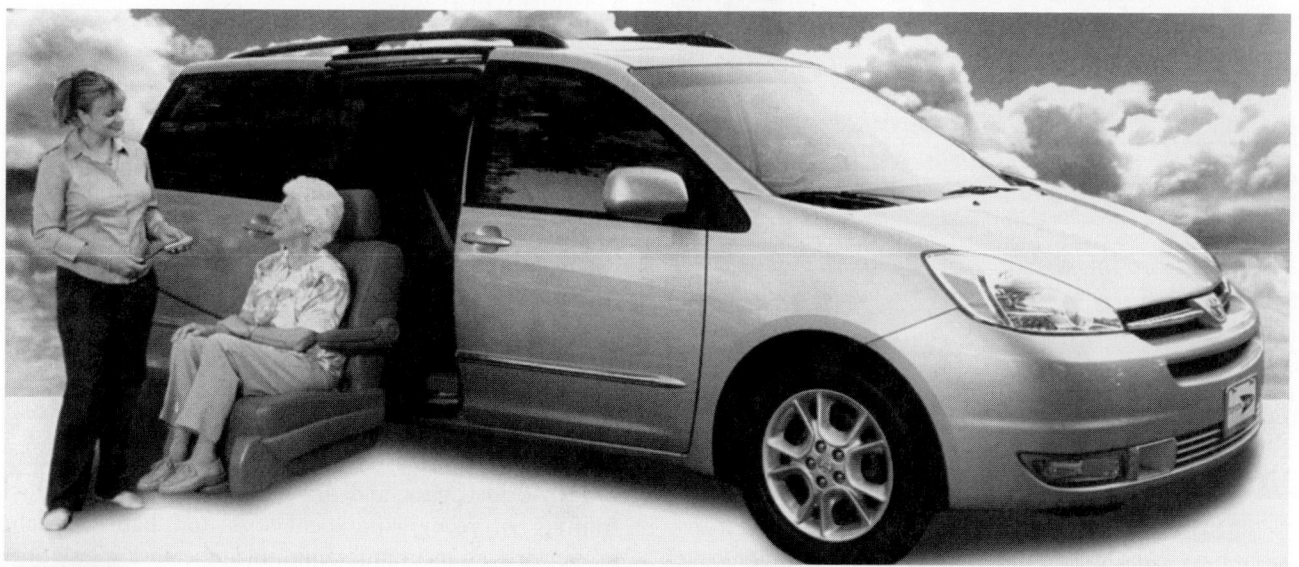

Figure 11-17 Bruno's Lift-Up power mobility seat for Toyota Sienna minivans aids vehicle entry by modifying activity demands for the caregiver and client. (Courtesy Bruno Independent Living Aids.)

DRIVING

Driving is cited again and again as the basis for personal independence, employment, and aging in place.[5,23,24,39] A driver's license has deep social and cultural contexts: a rite of passage for the teenager, ability to pursue employment and recreational opportunities for the adult, and competence and wellness for the aging population. Driving competence is regarded as instrumental in obtaining and maintaining an independent lifestyle and aging in place for the older adult (Figure 11-18).[1,16]

OCCUPATIONAL THERAPISTS AND DRIVING

OTs make up the overwhelming majority of professionals providing driver rehabilitation services for the physically disabled population.[30] Knowledge and training in implications of medical conditions and disease processes, ADLs and IADLs, adaptive devices, and occupation-based intervention make OT practitioners uniquely qualified. Even at the national level of government, therapists are recognized as having a unique skill set; the NHTSA is looking to the field of OT to provide services for older adult drivers. With nearly 27 million "baby boomers" turning 65 in the year 2010, the need to train additional therapists in this specialty practice area is tremendous.[11]

ADVANCED PRACTICE

As one of the top 10 emerging practice areas in the profession of occupational therapy, OTs offering driver evaluation services require advanced training.[23,39,50] Driving presents a greater possibility of personal and public harm than does any other ADL or IADL and therefore necessitates specialized skills. Conversely, the inadequately trained therapist can unnecessarily curtail driving and related independence by lacking the knowledge that would have provided a successful outcome. Therapists must receive specialized training[23,50] and educate themselves on the numerous guidelines, regulations, and ethics associated with this specialty practice area.[31,34]

 ETHICAL CONSIDERATIONS

Driver rehabilitation specialists have a responsibility to their clients and the larger community as well. Public safety is an important concern.

SPECIALTY TRAINING

A therapist's entry-level curriculum does not include driver education coursework. A comprehensive driving evaluation includes assessment of the client's skills in a specially equipped vehicle.

 ETHICAL CONSIDERATIONS

No therapist should proceed with driver evaluation on-road without first meeting the industry standard or equivalent for driver instructors within her or his own state. Proceeding without this basic driver instructor training is not recommended, having the potential to be unsafe as well as result in the therapist teaching techniques incorrectly that must later be unlearned.

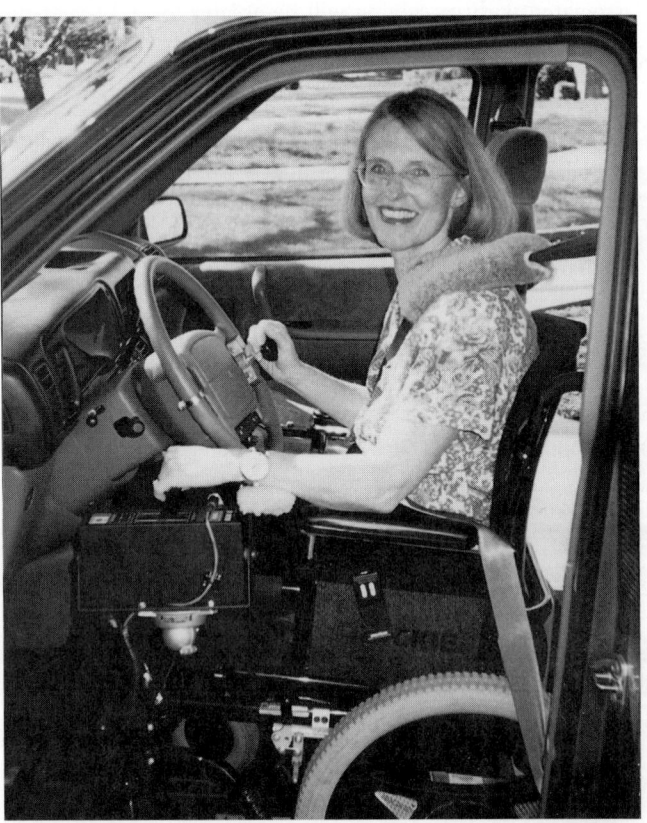

Figure 11-18 This client was experiencing difficulties driving and at work, as progression of her multiple sclerosis exceeded the activity demands of pushing a manual wheelchair. Driving from a power wheelchair and using electronic gas-brake hand control decreased the activity demands on her upper extremities, enabling her to drive safely and work full-time as a teacher.

Driver instructor and driver education courses provide training in recognizing behaviors and habits, teaching proper driving techniques, minimizing collision risk during the evaluation, recognizing specific driving pattern characteristics of novice and older drivers, and implementing training exercises and programs to improve outcomes.

⚖ ETHICAL CONSIDERATIONS

Principle C-46 of the Association for Driver Rehabilitation Specialists' (ADED) Code of Ethics, "Driver rehabilitation specialists use only assessment techniques that they are qualified and competent to use. They do not misuse assessment results or interpretations."

MODELS OF PRACTICE

Practice models provide additional guidance for established and new driving programs and identify conceptual areas and detailing practices that should be considered. In 2002 the NMEDA and ADED released Model Practices for Driver Rehabilitation for Individuals with Disabilities, focusing on agency-sponsored evaluations and vehicle modifications, such as the Department of Rehabilitation (DR).[41] In 2004 the ADED published Best Practices, delineating frameworks for driver rehabilitation services.[11] And in some states, the DR has existing guidelines and role delineations, which provides further models and references.[54,55] Therapists seeking advanced skills in driver rehabilitation need to be aware of the resources and guidelines available within the field.

CERTIFICATION PROGRAMS

Currently, ADED, the Association for Driver Rehabilitation Specialists, is the only association to offer certification in driver rehabilitation (Box 11-3). The certified driver rehabilitation specialists (CDRS) credential allows individuals from allied health or **driver training** backgrounds meeting criteria for educational background, and years of experience to sit for an examination covering driver education, disabilities, and vehicle modifications. In some states, agencies such as the Department of Rehabilitation require the CDRS credential to provide services.

A certification program is under development by the AOTA to promote specialization in community mobility and driving.[6] The resulting role delineation will help identify therapists with appropriate advanced training to more effectively meet the transportation needs of the aging population.[39] The AOTA's certification will cover a broad range of services: community

---

Box **11-3** CERTIFICATION PROGRAMS

Association for Driver Rehabilitation Specialists (ADED)
Certification requirements, testing dates, sample tests
http://www.aded.net (click on certification link)
American Occupational Therapy Association
Community Mobility & Driving Certification
Professional development certification updates, requirements, and application process once available
http://www.aota.org

---

mobility and driving. In partnership, the AOTA and NHTSA hope to address the more basic and populous needs of the aging driver, matching the differentiated levels of therapist's skills with the level of complexity an individual requires.

For example, arthritis is a common diagnosis in the older driver. Awareness of simple devices, such as blind spot mirrors or adaptive key holders, can restore or maintain the well older driver's competence when problems related to motor skills and mobility impede blind spot checks and turning the key in the door or ignition of a vehicle.

DRIVING PROGRAM STRUCTURE

Therapists can be based in an agency, private practice, or hospital and offer different levels of services, ranging from referrals, consultations, and clinical screenings to comprehensive **driver competence** assessments. Most programs have just one driving program staff member in the vehicle during an **on-road evaluation,** which is usually the therapist fulfilling the evaluator and driving instructor roles. Further specialized level of expertise and skill is needed of the therapist when higher levels of driving technology are introduced.

Some programs choose to use staff or contracted driver instructors for the on-road portion, and the therapist makes observations from the back seat. A variation of this is for the instructor to conduct the on-road evaluation alone without the therapist and report to the therapist on performance level. This is not recommended, especially when the client has significant mobility or performance skill involvement, because the therapist's unique training may identify an issue otherwise overlooked. Programs with just one professional in the vehicle should consider outlining special criteria that would dictate the need for two staff members during the on-road assessment. Two professionals in the vehicle can offer better security and protection, for example, when witnesses are desired for all direct client contact.

OCCUPATIONAL THERAPY ASSISTANTS

The OT assistant (OTA) is a valuable asset to driver rehabilitation. Completion of standardized testing, vehicle entry/exit and lift safety training, transfer training, and functioning in the role of driver instructor are just some of the ways the OTA can complement a driving program. The OTA must work under the supervision of the OT and restrict practice to OTA guidelines when billing under OT therapy services.[27]

Expanded roles are possible when documented intervention protocols are developed and followed, again under the OT's supervision. For example, training and establishment of criteria for observational skills and treatment progressions for driver training can be defined and formalized, thereby providing clear supervisory communication and an additional method to use the OTA. Because cost containment is an ongoing issue with driving programs, appropriate use of the OTA can greatly benefit a program.

Driving Program Goals

Driving competence can be disrupted by a single disability, multiple medical conditions, or factors of aging.[14] Driving programs seek to provide safe and independent transportation for individuals; transportation may be as a passenger or as a driver. Driver program services provide assessment in a natural environment under real-time conditions; an important aspect because outcomes in general can be overestimated in clinical settings.[10] The client's performance skills, activity demands, and client factors are assessed in efforts to determine what restorative, compensatory, or preventive interventions may be needed for safe transportation or driving.

Goals must include the specific driving occupations in which an individual wishes to engage. Although independent driving is the general goal, subset occupations exist within the task of driving. Some drivers only want to drive to the store, doctor, and church; others want to return to a job in which driving is an essential function of employment. A divorced or single mother with severe chronic pain may wish to regain the ability to transport her child for parental visitations. Driving needs and associated activity demands are personal and specific; identification of each client's occupational needs is paramount to a meaningful assessment and successful outcome. When identified early, the occupation of driving and required subskills can be interwoven into the fabric of intervention.

DRIVER EVALUATION

BEST PRACTICES IDENTIFIED

Driver evaluation is a process, dynamic and fluid (Figure 11-19). An individual's readiness, performance skills, and rate of learning can affect the ease and speed of completing the driver evaluation process. Recommended and best practices provide frameworks that accommodate any level of a client's performance skills.

Best practices from the ADED include a clinical evaluation followed by (1) an on-the-road evaluation in an actual driving environment, (2) subsequent vehicle modification recommendations and wheelchair measurements, (3) recommended driver training and education, (4) a final fitting, and (5) licensing assistance.[11,22,27] An on-road evaluation is indicated when program criteria are met; programs set varied criteria based on specialized training received, scope of program, comfort level, and safety issues. Recommendations for adaptive equipment are not advisable until a driver demonstrates competency to access or use the equipment or a similar device in a behind-the-wheel assessment.

PROGRAM CRITERIA

Driving programs must establish the necessary elements of an evaluation process and objective performance criteria for

 ETHICAL CONSIDERATIONS

Therapists in this practice area must be able to withstand significant pressure in their decision making. A novice driver with significant cognitive and perceptual impairments, for example, may press to curtail the assessment process prematurely because of time and financial considerations; pressure to sway the therapist's opinion before completion of an assessment may occur from biased third-party payers; even family members may strongly attempt to influence the outcomes of the assessment in a direction that is not supported by performance observations. This behavior may be due to pressures or dysfunctional dynamics within the family system.

decision making to provide consistent and accurate decision making. This also provides an objective means against which progress (or lack of it) can be measured. Use of best practices also provides a measure of liability protection. The American Medical Association recently published the *Physician's Guide to Assessing and Counseling Older Drivers*, in which different levels of assessment, from interviewing to a formal driver assessment, are presented.[5] Factors that are listed prompting a physician to be concerned about a client's driving skills include acute events, chronic medical conditions, questioning of safety by an individual or their family members, conditions that are unpredictable or episodic, and use of specific medications. These factors may also serve as a basis to construct program criteria.

REFERRAL PROCESS

Physicians, allied healthcare professionals, family members, and individuals are appropriate referral sources for community mobility and driving assessments. The referral process may be simple or complex and cannot always be completed in a seamless fashion. Verification of an individual's insurance coverage can be time consuming. Most private insurance sources do not pay for evaluations, and government insurance, such as Medicaid and Medicare, generally follows the private insurance industry. Although some therapists are able to obtain Medicare coverage, the reimbursement rate rarely covers the full costs of the assessment process.

Each program must set criteria for accepting a referral for driver evaluation. A physician's referral, recent medical records, confirmed payment source, and valid driver's license or permit (for on-road segment) are frequently required. Most programs also create an intake form to obtain background information on the client that is relevant to the process. During the referral process, it is important to communicate the program's intent to enable and assist the client's driving skills. Jacqueline was worried until the therapist

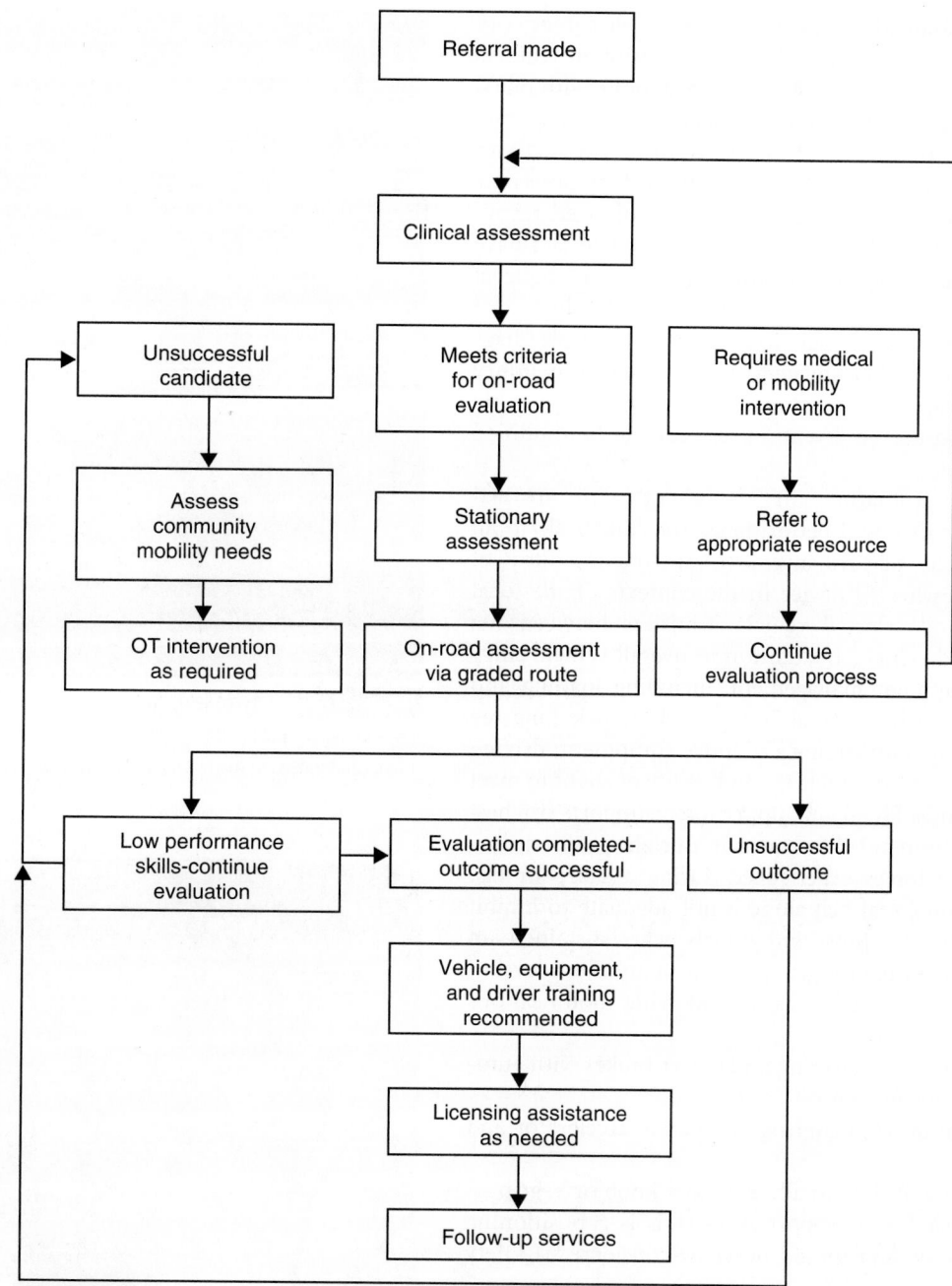

Figure 11-19   The flow chart illustrates the complexities and dynamics of the driving evaluation process.

from the driving program called and spoke with her. She was relieved to hear that an array of options was available to meet her needs. She had considered canceling the evaluation because of the devastating impact a loss of license would have but chose not to after reviewing goals with her therapist. As a result, she arrived for her evaluation optimistic and ready for productive changes in her driving system.

DRIVING EVALUATIONS AND DISABILITIES

SPINAL CORD INJURIES

Spinal cord injury (SCI) research has resulted in improved medical outcomes and resulted in 31.2% of quadriplegics and 28.2% of paraplegics sustaining incomplete spinal cord injuries.[42] Individuals who have an incomplete injury can be challenging in driver rehabilitation. Intervention requires the OT to engage in critical thinking, collaborate with physical therapy, and determine if the client can demonstrate the necessary performance skills to meet the activity demands of driving without undue fatigue. Adaptations may be temporarily needed for driving while prolonged recovery occurs. Clients who have sustained complete SCI have more prescribed intervention protocols based on the level of injury. All individuals who have sustained spinal cord injuries, however, have high frequency of multiple diagnoses, including mild or undiagnosed traumatic brain injury (TBI).[42] Therapists need to remain alert to possible signs of TBI so that intervention services can be modified accordingly.

A driving evaluation for the client with an SCI focuses on occupational performance subskills basic to all evaluations. The performance areas include mobility of wheelchair or wheeled device in the contexts of the local community and selected vehicle; transfers between the wheelchair and vehicle, in addition to overall vehicle entry and exit; equipment management, including loading and unloading wheelchairs or ability to lock/unlock long leg braces; need for compensatory adaptive equipment; driving competence in a natural setting; and ability of client to meet activity demands. Frequently upper torso supports or chest straps are recommended to maintain upright position during centrifugal forces experienced during a sharp or fast turn[12]; a diagonal seat belt alone is not adequate to inhibit lateral movements. Most individuals who sustained an SCI with resultant paraplegia and some at an injury level of C7-8 can drive a car that has the following modifications (Figure 11-20):

1. Standard power steering and power brakes with automatic transmission
2. Mechanical hand controls to operate accelerator and brake
3. A steering device, usually a spinner knob or V-grip
4. An upper torso support strap (this is a positioning device only and should never be considered a safety device.)
5. Accessible or remote switch for horn, dimmer, and wipers
6. A parking brake extension

An extensively modified van may be needed when transfers are overly exerting or when assistance is required for a transfer.[12] Structural modifications to the van (e.g., a raised door, raised roof, or lowered floor) may be necessary to accommodate the wheelchair and driver. With current technologies, and after extensive evaluation and training, some clients with C4-5 SCI can safely drive systems with high-technology modifications (Figure 11-21). As in all SCIs, presence of significant spasticity, especially in the upper extremities, can preclude a client from being able to drive.

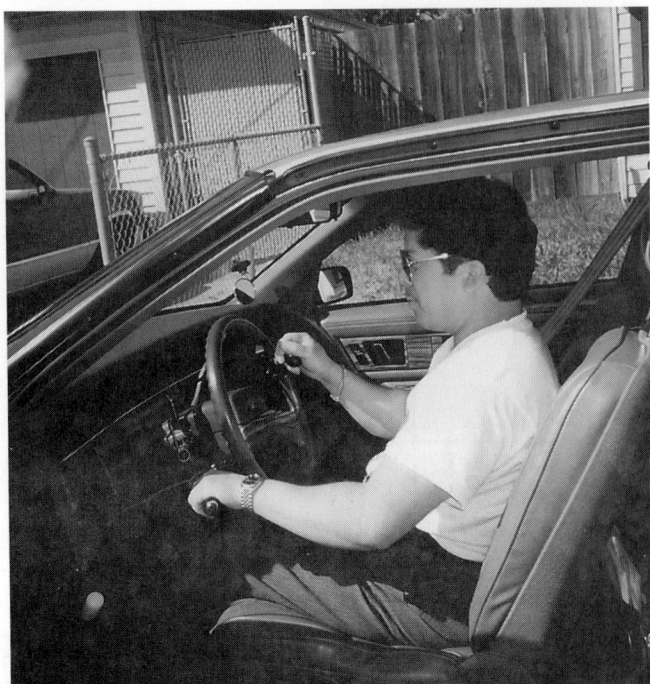

Figure 11-20 A basic setup for paraplegics includes spinner knob for steering and mechanical hand controls to operate accelerator and brake. This equipment can be used in many cars, vans, trucks, and sport utility vehicles.

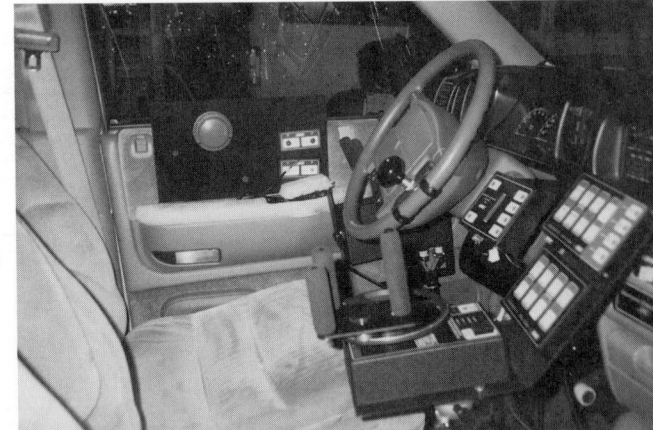

Figure 11-21 High-tech equipment compensates for limited motor skills. The evaluation van equipped with Electronic Mobility Controls (EMC) has a left-side electronic gas-brake, remote left elbow secondary control button, 7-inch remote steering wheel *(on right)* with tripin steering device, and membrane switch console for functions including gear shift, windows, and headlights.

DRIVING FROM A WHEELCHAIR

When a person needs to drive from the wheelchair, client education and informed choice are necessary to address increased safety risk. It is generally accepted that the hierarchy of safe seating for a driver is first to drive from the original equipment manufacturer's (OEM) driver seat, followed by an aftermarket powered seat base (which moves up/down, forward/back, and even rotates to facilitate transfers), a power wheelchair, and last, a manual wheelchair. It is not possible to drive from a scooter. Driving from a manual wheelchair should be approached very cautiously for three reasons: a lack of driver protection; the required wheelchair securement device to the wheelchair and van floor, because this device adds 10 to 15 lb to the wheelchair; and an inability for a folding manual wheelchair to fold after placement of the permanent securement device.

When the client is driving from a wheelchair, a wheelchair assessment is required to ensure appropriate positioning and stability and overall compatibility with driving.[12] For example, wheelchairs in which the seat rests on a single post are not advisable because of the ability of the post to shear on impact. Some wheelchair models have independent suspension, the motion of which can have a tremendous impact on driver stability; sometimes only thorough on-road assessments designed to test dynamic forces will reveal problems in this area. Last, wheelchairs must be secured to the floor of the van with an automatic lockdown mechanism. The powered devices are not available for all models of power wheelchairs.

NEUROLOGICAL CONDITIONS

Individuals who have acquired or traumatic brain injuries, cerebral palsy, and other neurological conditions may present with obvious or subtle disturbances in their performance and process skills needed for driving. The therapist is recommended to look for and analyze patterns in performance. Applying theoretical skills, knowledge of body functions, and diagnoses can lead the therapist to improve outcomes in specific client factors required during driving: vision, attention, judgment, and motor planning.[11] Clients with various neurological conditions or even aging can narrow the attentional window of visual information, which results in incomplete information being considered for decision making (Figure 11-22).[14,46]

The timing of consultations, pre-driving assessments, and referrals to on-road driving programs is an important aspect of intervention. A referral made too early in the client's recovery process uses up valuable resources, such as limited therapy visits from an insurance provider or financial resources of the individual or family. Consultation with the driving specialist can identify performance skill needs that can be integrated into inpatient, outpatient, day treatment, or community intervention programs. When evidence exists of functional performance in client factors such as new learning, divided attention, higher-level cognitive functions, and insight, it is appropriate to continue exploring driving potential. As driving is such a highly valued occupation, integration of driving into an intervention planning can enhance

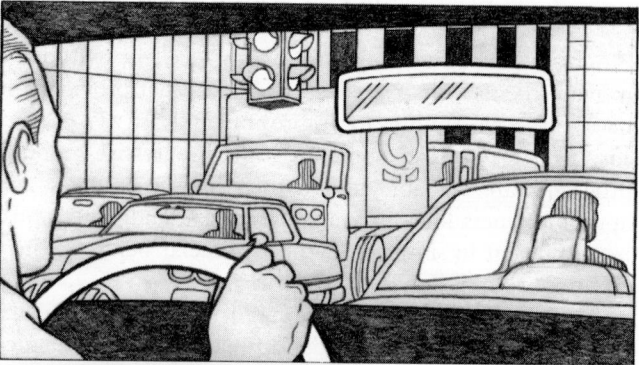

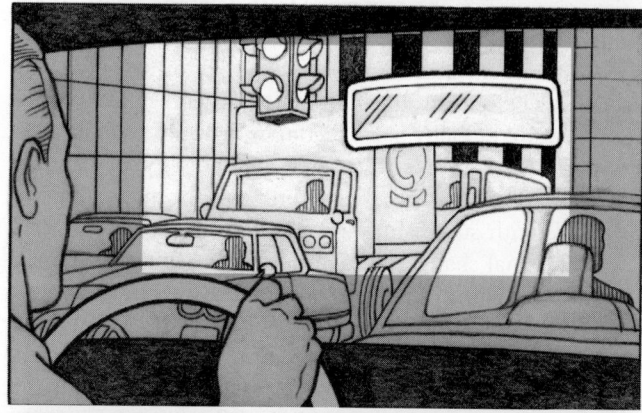

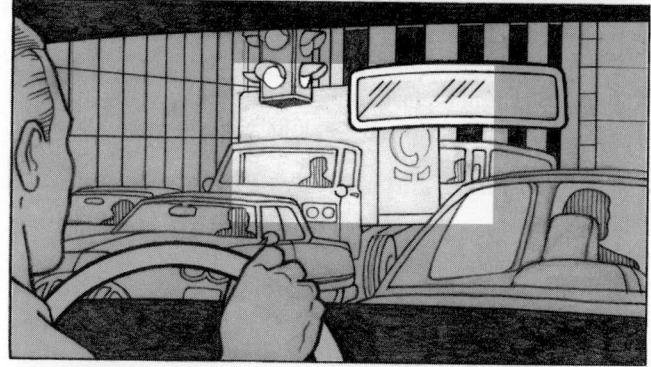

Figure 11-22   The attentional window or white area appears normal in the first slide and continues to shrink as visual processing speed and divided attention are increasingly impaired.

an individual's participation by motivating him or her to continue therapy.

Therapeutic Intervention: Facilitating Progress

More than any other diagnostic group, clients with neurological impairments can work slowly toward driving goals during therapy sessions or home programs. Baseline data can be established by a therapist or involved family member, and the client is able to work toward resuming the desired occupation: driving. Programs must be graded and need to be done with an involved family member or friend who can provide feedback to the therapist. Continual feedback and modification of the program are key to facilitating progress.

Progressive Mobility Programs

Progressive mobility programs are an excellent method to provide clients with a graded experience that provides the necessary opportunities for improvement. Used as a precursor to driving or as a home program, progressive mobility programs are valuable in identification of progress and appropriateness for a driving referral. The individual must be competent in simple, low-speed contexts before mastering more complex ones.

The concept is to increase the speed at which an individual is moving to provide the body opportunities to integrate appropriate responses to the contextual features of the environment. Collaboration or co-treatment with physical therapy is necessary to verify an individual's ability to perform the separate motor task before introducing additional therapeutic demands. A progressive mobility plan's hierarchy may look as follows:

- Low-speed ambulation or wheeled mobility graded from light to crowded indoor environments (hospital, shopping mall) with successful outcome indicated by appropriate directional changes, recognition and use of communication, and safe motor skills in a smooth, integrated pattern
- Moderate to fast-speed ambulation or wheeled mobility indoors and in natural community contexts with same parameters as above, with greater emphasis on dynamic and flexible responses to real-time changes in a situation
- Graded bicycling or wheeled mobility in light to congested outdoor areas (quiet park or residential street, surface streets) with emphasis on integration of visual/perceptual systems with performance skills and patterns

Active Passenger and Narrative Driving

This therapy program is performed in a moving vehicle, and the client can participate only as a passenger for safety reasons. Tasks of visual scanning and coordination within this program are performed with the client ideally in the front passenger seat of the vehicle. However, it has also successfully been assigned to those using paratransit, secured in the back while sitting in their wheelchair. The activity is designed to establish new behaviors and habits for novice drivers and to improve, speed up, or reinforce patterns and behaviors in experienced drivers. The goal of the "active passenger" is to visually scan and then verbally narrate the salient contextual changes in the environment such as road signs, road markings, traffic signals, hazards, or developing situations that require attention. This should only be done for a brief period, 10 to 15 minutes, until endurance is built up. For example, a client with a head injury may travel with a parent, and as they travel down the road, call out, "Pedestrian on the right, red light, 35 mph sign, car turning left," etc. Several variations of the activity exist:

- The driver and "active passenger" can play together and see who sees the situation or directional signs first.
- The "active passenger" performs all motions of driving—head turning, steering, gas/brake, turn signal indicators—in addition to narrating the route.

- The "active passenger" acts as navigator with written directions to a destination. The driver should know the route ahead of time.

Therapists using this program need to carefully match home program demands with the client's performance skill and other client factors. All variations of the program should start in low speed residential areas and increase to faster speed zones as visual scanning improves.

NEUROMUSCULAR CONDITIONS

The neuromuscular diseases (polio, muscular dystrophy, and multiple sclerosis) impair motor skills, endurance, and joint stability. Multiple sclerosis and some forms of muscular dystrophy can affect cognition, perception, and vision. Each diagnosis has a strikingly different pattern of symptoms and progression, and only specific parts of the body may be affected. To the extent possible, the recommended equipment must meet current and anticipated future needs. Drivers may ambulate with or without devices, push a wheelchair, or use a scooter or even a power wheelchair. Driving equipment is just as varied.

CHRONIC LONG-TERM DISABILITY AND ACCELERATED AGING

Long-term disability can cause significant symptoms or medical conditions in clients. Awareness of these issues can result in a more appropriate assessment that encompasses special needs of accelerated aging process associated with long-term disabilities. Accelerated aging is the premature physiological changes associated with aging; these effects will affect respiratory, cardiovascular, musculoskeletal, and connective tissue systems. Years of pushing a manual wheelchair, for example, can result in carpal tunnel syndrome, rotator cuff tears, and general overuse of the arms, which then affect all areas of living.[14] Overuse syndromes occur when the activity demands over time are too close to the maximum attainable exertion or capacity, which in turn affects mobility. Over time, personal mobility is on a continuum for some clients: walking with braces, manual wheelchairs, and then scooter or power wheelchairs. Depression and obesity are often common results with a long-term disability.[14] The key concept is that small or subtle physical changes can have a disproportionate functional effect for those who have chronic disabilities. Joint protection, energy conservation, and margins of function are all required to maximize and extend functional independence for those clients with chronic conditions.

OLDER DRIVERS: A GROWING POPULATION

The driving ability of older adults changes as they age, but most remain safe drivers. **Older drivers** adapt by gradually limiting their driving, such as omitting travel during rush hour and the evening.[24,43] Others experience an abrupt change in driver status because of a medical event such as a stroke.

The AMA is encouraging and supporting physicians to address community mobility needs and has provided many tools for appropriate intervention.[5]

To date, research has not identified the skills or qualities that make an older driver, or any driver for that matter, competent, which makes large-scale epidemiological screening difficult.[24,29,43,44,56] Older adults with multiple medical conditions are probably most at risk and in need of driver evaluation and intervention.[5,24] Many adult drivers benefit from simple devices or interventions that compensate for the physical changes of aging.

THREADED CASE STUDY: JACQUELINE, PART 2

Jacqueline has impaired neck and hand ROM because of arthritic changes. Jacqueline was issued an adaptive key holder to open the car door and recommended to purchase a steering wheel wrap to build up the grip on the steering wheel; the knobby wrap provided a larger diameter wheel to grip. When neck rotation for blind spot checks was discussed, she reported that she has had "near misses" while changing lanes, nearly colliding with cars she didn't see. It is important to note that many older drivers never received formal driver training and are unaware a blind spot check is required. In Jacqueline's case, it is a skill that was requires mobility she doesn't have, such as turning the head enough to look behind one's shoulder.

Introduction of a wide-angle interior rearview mirror and blind spot mirrors on her exterior mirrors greatly improved her safety and confidence of seeing what she needed to see. She also assisted in properly adjusting her driver seat to the appropriate position behind the wheel; in her current car the old seats caused her to sit too low. Sitting lower than was optimal resulted in poor field-of-view out the windshield in addition to poor mechanical advantage to turn the steering wheel. An additional cushion was required to raise her so that her eye level was 2 to 3 inches above the top of the steering wheel.

Her performance on road was greatly improved by these changes. Jacqueline's driving was now at a safer and more competent level. However, when the older adult has limited driving competence even with adaptations or interventions, the therapist should consider graded licensing, which permits driving under certain limitations (e.g., dawn to dusk or no freeway). A recommendation for a graded license extends the older adult's ability to function independently.[4,24]

Wellness Programs

In contrast to assessment and remediation programs, development of wellness programs provides opportunities for older drivers to extend their driving competence by focusing on habits and routines. Reinforcing or improving performance patterns commensurate with age and performance skills is thought to extend the years in which one can safely drive.[24] These already competent licensed drivers seek to fine-tune their driving performance with appropriate knowledge and subsequent voluntary changes in habits and routines. Programs may be developed and taught by a therapist or, in the case of the 55 Alive classroom program, taught by peers 55 years of age or older. Agencies and therapists are enhancing issues of safety and mobility for older drivers through development of wellness programs.

Early intervention through wellness programs is thought to be a viable method for prolonging independence and driving competence; this area of intervention may or may not include on-road assessments and is an area of practice expecting significant growth parallel to the aging of America. Referral processes are considerably less involved, because this is a voluntary improvement program.

THEORETICAL CONSTRUCTS

Activity analysis using the Occupational Therapy Practice Framework provides a strong foundation for a thorough driver evaluation. The therapist assesses an individual's performance skills and client factors first in the clinic. During the on-road test, the therapist then evaluates the client's ability to integrate performance skills and client factors within the physical context of actual driving conditions.

Occupational role theory is also helpful in driver assessment, which enables a therapist to match activity demands with desired roles. Occupational roles may carry specific needs related to transportation equipment and parking environments. A construction site inspector may enter or exit a vehicle more than 10 times daily and thus may need to consider a transfer seat or driving from a wheelchair in a van. A certified public accountant audits businesses that may have parking structures or covered parking, which therefore necessitates that the accountant's minivan not exceed certain height restrictions. The older driver is often satisfied with the freedom to drive to church, medical appointments, and the grocery store. In each example, the selection of the vehicle and its modifications are based largely on the occupational roles chosen by the client.

DRIVING ASSESSMENT

CLINICAL ASSESSMENT

The **clinical assessment** is also referred to as a *screening* or *pre-driving evaluation*. The clinical assessment can be performed solely by the OT or by many members of the rehabilitation team together.[19,30,50] Used to build rapport and identify strengths and weaknesses in potential performance skills and client factors related to driving, the clinical assessment begins with a review of medical information, medication and side effects, episodes of seizure or loss of consciousness, mobility status, social history, vocational history, driving history, and purpose of the evaluation. An interview process with open-ended questions often yields greater results and more readily unveils unexpected, pertinent, and critical information to pursue further. Open-ended questioning with Jacqueline revealed the lack of a back-up transportation plan; this identification enabled the therapist to provide appropriate intervention through a referral to paratransit services.

Before proceeding with an evaluation, the OT should determine whether a client's condition is stable, improving, or progressively deteriorating. In progressive conditions, a mobility history should be taken to determine and document the rate of progression; without this information, it is difficult to establish adequate safety margins. The clinical assessment will then independently assess the individual's performance skills and client factors required for safe driving.

VISUAL FUNCTIONING

A comprehensive vision screening is important because vision is the primary sense used to gather information needed for driving-related decision making. Vision testing is completed before other testing to eliminate impaired acuity as a factor. A comprehensive vision screening includes near and far acuity, phoria or alignment, saccades, occulomotor pursuits, range of motion, convergence, and field of vision.[11,17] Glare recovery is relevant to assess for the older adult evaluation and is a recommended best practice.[11]

MOTOR SKILLS

Muscle strength, active ROM, grip, and reaction time are frequently cited as the basic abilities that must be measured.[11,17,30,33] Ability to stabilize and align posture and position oneself (dynamic and static posture) is also important. Quality of performance skill elements, such as coordination, manipulation, and flow of movement, also should be included.[12] Force readings with a torque wrench or Chatillon scale provide data that aid appropriate matching of strength and effort performance with the activity demands of steering or braking, particularly in more complex modifications for driving.

COGNITIVE AND VISUAL-PERCEPTUAL SKILLS

The driver must have adequate mental functions commensurate with a rapidly changing environment, blending cognitive and visual-perceptual skills. Mental functions requiring assessment include sustained and selective attention, initiation, decision making, safety judgment, problem solving and planning, insight, and the mental flexibility to shift focus at will. The ability to multitask or divide attention is also a critical driving skill.[46] Multitasking is the simultaneous performance and monitoring of two or more equally important activities, such as maintaining lane positioning while turning one's head for a visual traffic check.

Visual-perceptual skills required for driving include visual organization, visual searching and scanning, spatial relations, directionality, and visual processing speed.[11,33,56] Visual memory is also important in driving. Older drivers and those who require additional concentration to engage in driving frequently have a decreased visual attention window.

Recommendations for driver's license status should not be made on the basis of clinical test scores alone. Still no clear evidence exists that any one test identifies at-risk drivers or accurately predicts driving competence.[24,29,37,45,56] Properly used and selected, however, cognitive and visual-perceptual testing helps the driver evaluator identify impairments, improve behind-the-wheel risk management, and plan appropriate treatment for driver rehabilitation interventions.

VEHICLE OPTIONS

Car Considerations

A basic level of service for the majority of driving programs is the car evaluation. A car is generally appropriate if a person can enter and exit the vehicle and load mobility equipment devices independently. The standard car recommendation is a midsize vehicle with power steering, power brakes, and an automatic transmission. Two-door cars can be advantageous for wheelchair loading by the driver, although some find the larger and heavier vehicle door difficult to manage; fewer two-door models continue to be manufactured, which results in the more frequent use of four-door vehicles.

When loading a manual wheelchair into a car is not feasible, sometimes the use of a mechanical device such as a car top loader can provide the driver with some independence. Clients with limited ambulation and using wheeled mobility devices for long distances may be able to continue using their standard minivan, sport utility vehicle, or truck with the assistance of a power hoist (Figure 11-23).

Van Considerations

Drivers who depend predominantly on a wheelchair most often choose between full-size vans and minivans. Providing information on the differences between minivans and full-size vans, including accessibility, ground clearance, load capacity, durability, and cost, enables clients to make educated choices that suit their needs, budget, and lifestyle. In any van, the interface of the needs of the driver who is dependent on use of a wheelchair with the vehicle are more complex, and a more highly skilled evaluation is required because of increased variables that affect driving performance and equipment selection.

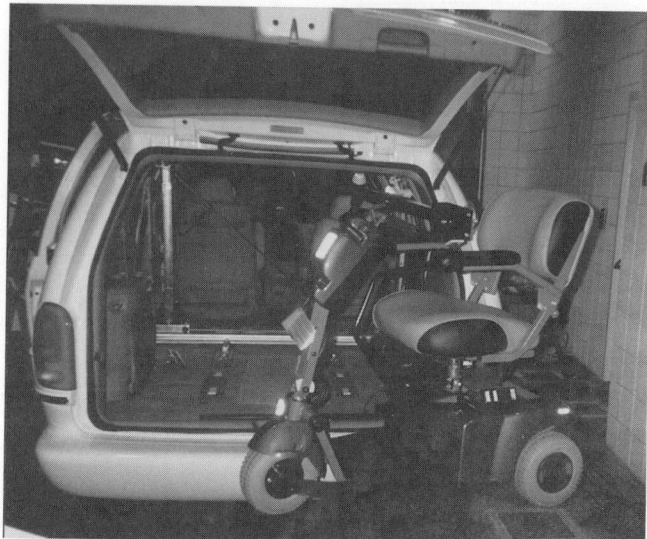

Figure 11-23 The Curbsider, by Bruno, hoists a scooter or fully assembled power wheelchair, up to 250 lb, from the sidewalk and lifts it into the back of a standard minivan.

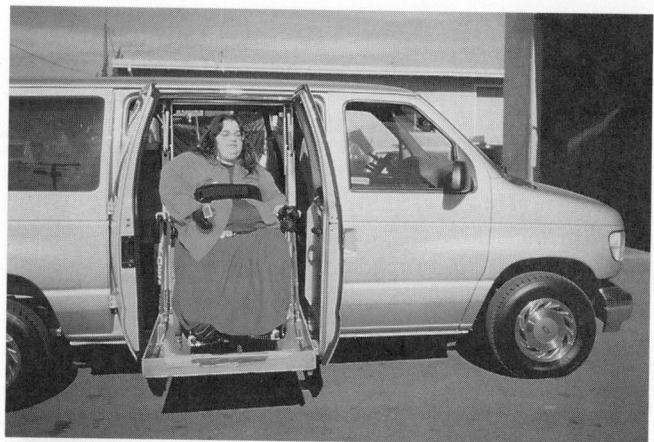

Figure 11-24 A platform-style lift can be located at the side or rear of a van. Additional entry headroom, obtained through a lowered floor, provides client with appropriate visibility when driving from a power wheelchair.

Full-size vans require an automatic mechanical lift for independent entry with a wheelchair or scooter. Mechanical lifts can be mounted on the rear or side of a full-size van or the side of a minivan. Lifts fall into two basic styles: platform-style lifts and rotary or swing in-style lifts (Figure 11-24). Each lift has unique characteristics that must be considered.[48]

Minivans have fully automatic mechanical side ramps for independent exit and entry (Figure 11-25). Minivans have limited interior space but much appeal because they drive like a car, are easier to park, and get better gas mileage.

Other Vehicles

Sport utility vehicles (SUVs) and trucks, both midsize and full size, are also options for individuals who require limited adaptive equipment to be able to successfully drive. Four-wheel drive is another area that can be included in a modified vehicle at great cost. In all these areas that go outside the typically modified vehicle, care should be taken to factor in all considerations that affect equipment compatibility and installation, function, and occupations desired by the client.

STATIONARY ASSESSMENT

The stationary component of the assessment involves an assessment of the pre-driving habits and routines in addition to the adaptive equipment setup with the vehicle parked, and, as needed, the engine on to assess performance skills in steering, acceleration, and braking. Stationary performance alone is inadequate to predict either on-road performance or final equipment needs. The stationary assessment process enables proposed equipment to be verified, modified, or discarded; the process continues until adequate results are obtained. If subsequent on-road performance indicates that the activity demands exceed performance skills, the stationary process is repeated with the next level of equipment. This trial-and-error approach is an expected and necessary step in assistive technology evaluation.[14,22]

PRE-DRIVING HABITS AND ROUTINES

Pre-driving tasks include mobility to the vehicle, inserting and turning a key (or keyless entry operation), opening and closing the door, entering and exiting the vehicle, loading and unloading mobility devices (e.g., cane, walker, and wheelchair), adjusting the driver seat, adjusting the mirrors, fastening the seat belt (and chest strap when needed), and having adequate visibility to scan dashboard light indicators. Adaptive devices to facilitate independence in pre-driving tasks include special key holders, loops for lower extremity management, a strap to extend reach for wheelchair loading, and modifications for independent retrieval of the seat belt.

PRIMARY CONTROLS

Steering Control Assessment

The first step in the primary control assessment phase is to position the driver to obtain optimal motor skill performance, including positioning for adequate field of view. Poor trunk stability may necessitate special positioning devices. The upper torso support or chest strap is a commonly used positioning device.[5,6] Once postural issues are resolved, equipment setups begins with the **primary controls**—those devices that control the steering, accelerator, and braking of a vehicle.

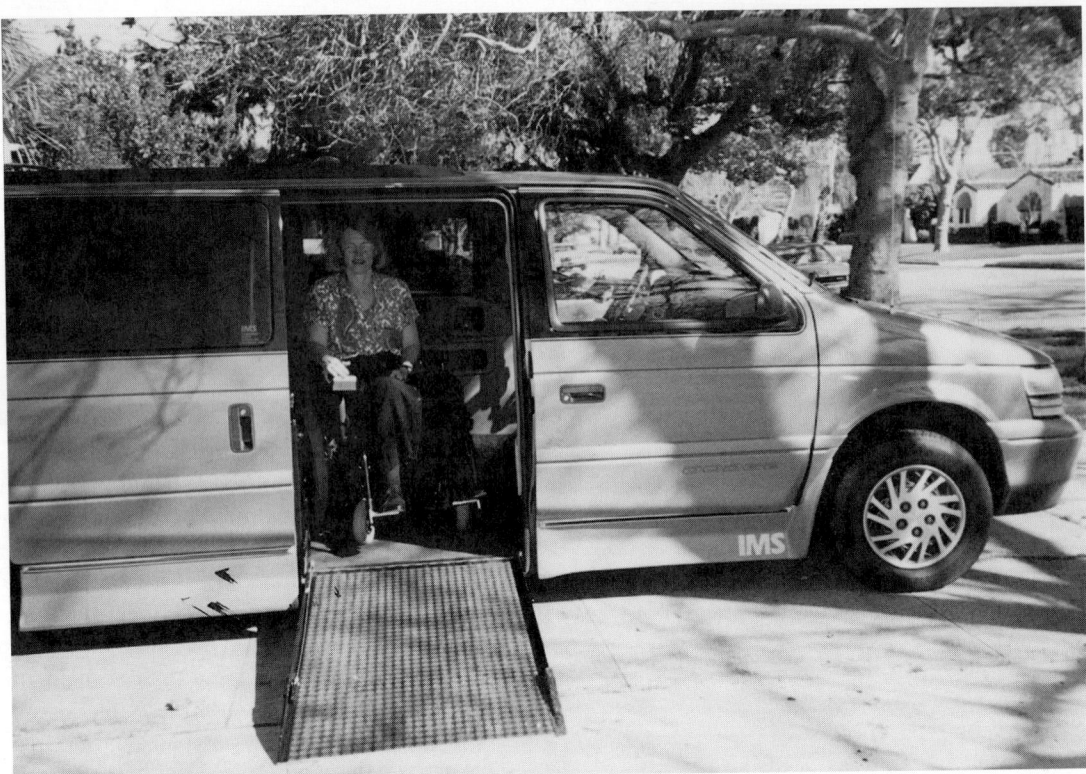

Figure 11-25   Minivan conversion with side ramp access and lowered 10-inch floor. The ramp angle can be decreased for easier entry and exit.

Steering systems all include an element of resistance and no universal standards exist for steering resistance labeling by automotive manufacturers. As a result, one car manufacturer's power steering can be as difficult or as easy to turn as another vehicle's manual steering. The first step in steering control is to assess whether a client's motor skills are adequate to turn the steering wheel on the intended vehicle. Therapists need to acquire knowledge of trends and patterns in steering system resistance for popular vehicle models for accurate outcomes and recommendations. In general, only after the stationary steering process is complete does the evaluation move to the accelerator and brake controls.

A client needs to demonstrate steering competence by slowly turning a steering wheel to lock in both directions without undue effort or pain to proceed. Rapid turning can cover substitution patterns or decreased strength and does not address performance skills adequately or allow motor performance to be analyzed. In foot steering, a specialized wheel is mounted on the floor of the vehicle.

When a driver cannot use two hands to steer, a steering device is frequently recommended as an initial step to improve mechanical advantage. One-handed steering by palming the wheel can result in inadequate control, especially in sharp, fast turns and evasive maneuvers. The use of adaptive steering devices—the spinner knob, V-grip, tri-pin, palmar cuff, or amputee ring—improves control and speed when turning the steering wheel (Figure 11-26).[22] Once the performance

skills are well matched to the activity demands of the steering setup in the stationary position, verification of competence through a dynamic on-road evaluation can begin.

Steering systems

Steering systems are divided into those that use a standard steering or OEM column and those higher-technology systems in which the OEM steering column is modified or absent. Steering modifications such as extended steering columns, smaller diameter steering wheels, and reduced levels of steering resistance are compatible with OEM columns. High-technology options include a 7-inch remote steering wheel that can be placed anywhere. Driving technology also enables a driver to combine steering, acceleration, and brake operations on a single lever operated by a single limb, such as the unilever and joystick systems. Van modifications, especially at these levels, require longer evaluations and extensive driver training for the client.

Airbag issues

A critical final step in steering assessment developed as a result of airbags.[40] Airbags are integrated in the steering wheel system; additional side and knee impact bags are being introduced in vehicles for additional safety. The impact of supplemental airbags on adaptive equipment is just beginning to be realized, and agencies and manufacturers of adaptive equipment are working on solutions. The NHTSA

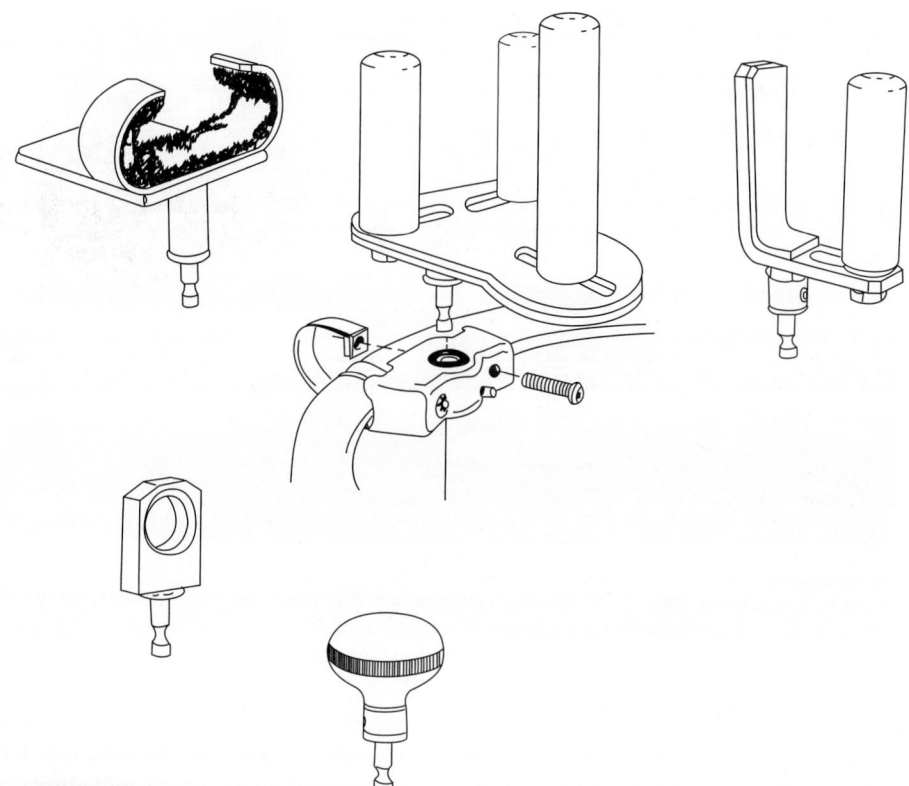

Figure 11-26 These steering devices accommodate a variety of hand and upper extremity impairments. (Courtesy Mobility Products and Design.)

established guidelines on airbag distance, which every therapist must address and document in an evaluation. The distance from a driver's sternum to the center of the steering wheel must be a minimum of 10 inches, as recommended by the NHTSA, to prevent serious injury or death from airbag inflation.[18] In certain cases, turning the airbag off is a necessary safety step but should be recommended only by an experienced therapist who has considered other alternatives.[38,40]

Accelerator and Brake Controls

Modified accelerator and brake controls can be installed in most vehicles. Simple modifications such as pedal extensions can be installed on the accelerator and brake pedals to compensate for limited reach. More drivers need extended pedals with airbags because maintaining proper distance from the airbag prevents fully reaching the accelerator and brake pedals.

With a significant right hemiplegia, the right foot is unable to operate the standard pedals. Intuitively, some clients try to use the left foot to cross over to the gas pedal, which is unsafe and can cause undue physical strain on the joints over time. A left-sided accelerator pedal can be placed to the left of the standard gas pedal to compensate for this condition.

When the driver lacks adequate performance skills in the lower extremities, a device called a "hand control" allows the driver to operate the accelerator and brake pedals by pushing and pulling with an upper extremity. Hand controls use rotary, push-pull, push-pull down, or push-rocker motions to activate the accelerator and the brake. High-technology accelerator and brake controls have servomotors activated by vacuum, hydraulic, or electronic means and require motor skills. Postural control is even more critical if such controls are used (Figure 11-27).

SECONDARY CONTROLS

All other controls are **secondary controls.** A driver must be able to activate four secondary controls at will when the vehicle is in motion: turn signal indicators, horn, dimmer, and windshield wipers.[27] These can be activated through a variety of adaptive switches that either can be placed on the hand control or can be controlled through elbow motion.

ON-ROAD ASSESSMENT

THE STANDARD OF COMPETENCE

Once the driver has been set up with primary controls (and secondary controls, when able) through the stationary assessment, the ability to use these controls must be observed during the process of actual driving. This assessment is commonly referred to as the behind-the-wheel or on-road portion of

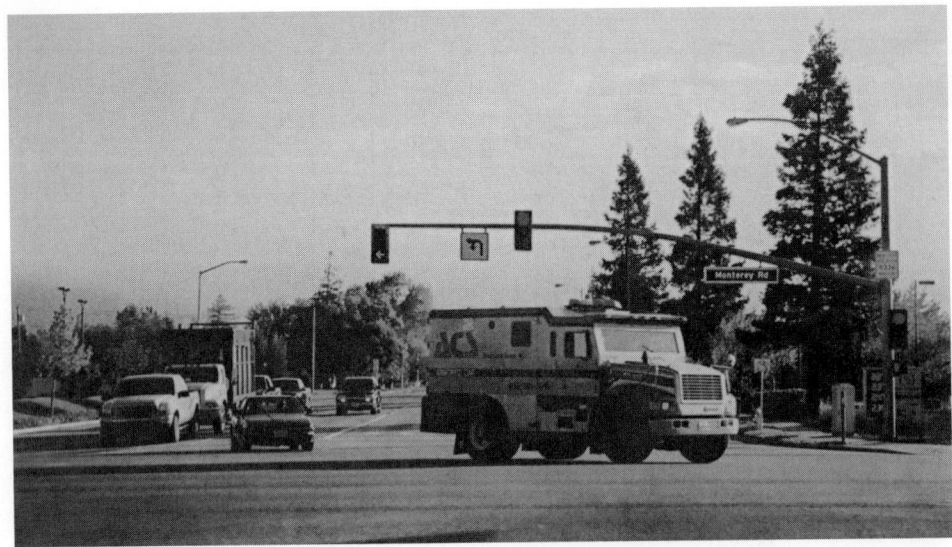

Figure 11-27 Assessment of visual processing, divided attention, coordination, and judgment must be made in the natural driving environment. Performance in complex and faster traffic situations is essential, because activity demands increase with speed and visual clutter.

the assessment. The current industry standard is to accept the on-road driving test as the optimal measure of driving competence.[17,29,37,44] The on-road assessment should be a minimum of 45 minutes long and no longer than 2 hours of actual driving time. A shorter period is inadequate for obtaining required information, particularly the assessment of the energy component of motor and process skills enabling adequate sustained effort throughout the task.

The driving instructor orients a driver in the use of adaptive driving equipment, maintains vehicle control by intervening for safety when necessary, and directs the route. A score sheet is recommended. Driving performance scores should reflect physical management of the vehicle, ability to use the adaptive equipment,[1] interaction with other traffic, adherence to rules of the road, and safety judgment.[29,56]

DRIVING ROUTE

Driving routes used in assessment should incorporate a sampling of road conditions, traffic patterns, and unusual settings common to the local region. The driving route initially should allow the driver time to become familiar with the vehicle and adaptive equipment in a low-stimulation environment. This period of learning and accommodation will be longer for the novice or apprehensive driver. The assessment route should progress through faster and more congested traffic and various dynamic traffic conditions to elicit information on the driver's performance in a wide variety of conditions (Figure 11-28). Competence implies that a client can repeat a performance skill consistently, that success was not based on encountering a lack of environmental or traffic challenges. Therefore repeat success is needed in maneuvers and judgment situations before competence is determined. As drivers' skills will

greatly vary, "bailout" points are needed along the route to provide the therapist the option of terminating the on-road assessment; therapists should always work within a window of comfort and only take clients in situations in which they are able to provide override control.

DRIVER RECOMMENDATIONS AND INTERVENTIONS

POSSIBLE OUTCOMES

Results of the driver evaluation require a decision on driver competency, need for adaptive equipment and vehicle, and when appropriate, the number of recommended driver training hours required to raise performance skill to a safe and independent level. New driver evaluators need to be cautious not to misconstrue new driver or older driver patterns as uncorrectable errors incompatible with driving. Conversely, less-experienced driver evaluators need to weigh errors, especially with neurologically involved clients, in whom consistency of performance can be an issue. The possible outcomes for a driver evaluation are as follows:

1. The client demonstrates driving competence: no adaptive equipment or driver training is required.
2. The client requires changes to achieve driving competence: adaptive driving equipment and/or training is required.
3. The client's performance skills are borderline: an extended evaluation and/or driver's training is required.
4. The client is not safe to drive at this time: continued therapy and time for additional recovery of function may change outcome. Re-evaluation in 6 to 12 months is recommended.

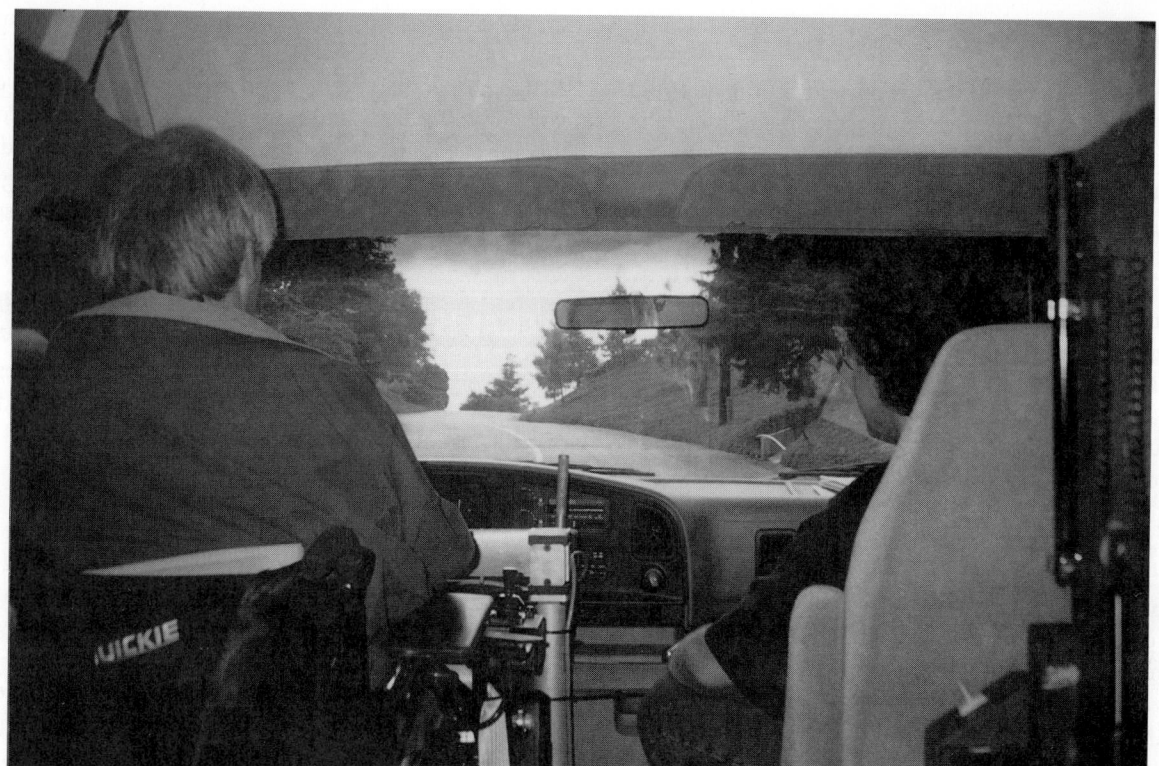

Figure 11-28   This client drives a steep mountain pass near his home. During the follow-up evaluation in his new Driving Systems, Inc. (DSI) unilever van, a test drive was performed in nearby foothills to ensure the adjustments were adequate for steep inclines. This essential step identified additional adjustments needed before delivery.

5. The client is unsafe to drive and no potential for improvement exists.

After the driving test is completed, the driving team reviews the results with the driver. Asking the client for feedback before reviewing results provides a valuable perspective on the driver's insight. Results cannot be shared with family without permission from the client; a verbal agreement from the client to share results should be documented.

Jacqueline was very nervous in freeway situations and made some non-critical errors; overall, she thought she did well, especially as the better positioning in the car seat decreased her shoulder pain. The therapist agreed. The therapist did recommend 4 hours of driver training to focus on defensive driving skills, compensatory strategies for older drivers, use of expanded mirrors, and freeway maneuvers. Involvement with professional organizations helps the therapist obtain knowledge to develop criteria for recommendations.

WRITTEN REPORT

The comprehensive driving report should contain a summary of the clinical assessment and a statement of the client's potential to be a safe and independent driver. The report should specify the type of vehicle necessary, the modifications needed, information about mobility equipment, dealer sources for providing the modifications, and other pertinent information. The report should include recommendations on the type of follow-up services required, explanation of what is needed, and who is best suited to provide the follow-up services. The report should also estimate the amount (duration, frequency, and total length) of driver training needed, indicate what specific areas of training should be emphasized, and provide resources where the training is available.[11,54,55]

DRIVER TRAINING

In the delivery of any assistive technology equipment, including adaptive driving equipment, training is a key part of the comprehensive intervention process.[22] Individuals who have cognitive and perceptual impairments will often need to relearn driving behaviors or implement compensatory skills to obtain consistent driving performance, even though adaptive equipment may not be needed. The use of high-technology equipment also necessitates extensive training, with a greater focus on the vehicle control and recovery, especially in unexpected situations and at high speeds. Depending on each state's requirements, the driver training may occur before or after the vehicle is modified.

FOLLOW-UP SERVICES

Follow-up services are also an important aspect of equipment delivery. When adaptive equipment is recommended, a follow-up evaluation ensures that the equipment is located and adjusted to meet the client's functional needs.[11,54] Follow-up services include midfit and final fitting sessions for quality assurance and safety measures. When an adapted vehicle is delivered, it will work as envisioned only if everything is modified correctly; it is the first time that the client, adaptations, and selected vehicle have interfaced and some adjustment is almost always needed to meet functional goals.[10] An on-road session is recommended to make sure adjustments are adequate for function when dynamic forces of driving come into play (Figure 11-29).

LICENSING ASSISTANCE

Dealing with licensing situations relative to a disability or medical condition can be daunting and intimidating to a client. The therapist must be knowledgeable of the licensing practices and protocols in his or her state; this knowledge enables the therapist to provide education and steps to follow to complete the licensing process. At times, the therapist may need to assist in licensing issues with the local agency to obtain or extend a learner's or special permit. Contact with such agencies requires the written authorization of the client, and only minimal information pertinent to the issue at hand should be revealed. Best practices include maintaining common agency forms or driver handbook materials in the clinic for distribution to the client as appropriate.[11]

DRIVING RETIREMENT

One of the most difficult tasks facing a driver evaluator is notifying a client that he or she is unable to achieve or no longer retains the performance skills required for safe and independent driving. Such decisions need to be carefully thought through and then communicated to the driver with compassion and understanding. The AMA has named this transition from driver to nondriver as **driving retirement**.[5] Referring the client to the motor vehicle department to exchange the driver's license for a photo identification card, which looks like a license, is essential for legal identification and psychosocial reasons. The therapist can work on community mobility goals when appropriate to maximize independence and well-being.

Educating individuals in alternative means of transportation and immediately providing materials regarding local options can prove helpful at a difficult time. Furthermore, when driving retirement is considered and planned for in advance, as recommended by many agencies, the transition is eased. However, early discussion is a new model and is just being implemented by the AMA and others. Occupational therapists will play a significant role in promoting long-term planning through community mobility interventions with their clients.[50]

Jacqueline isn't ready to retire from driving; she had competency verified and is receiving intervention for freeway situations. She feels confident and able to address any driving concerns raised by family members. She told her therapist that she shared the good news regarding her driving skills with her family, although not all were convinced. Her therapist encouraged her to rely on the outcome demonstrated by her performance skills and perhaps begin discussing her future transportation needs that will arise when she transitions into driving retirement.

LEGAL ISSUES AND PUBLIC POLICY

Therapists and physicians need to be aware of their states' laws concerning medical conditions and driving. Most states do not require the reporting of medical conditions, seizures, or loss of consciousness to the motor vehicle department.[27] Instead, most states rely on voluntary reporting of medical conditions by the driver who has the condition.[5,44,56] Although some states advocate reporting by the family, physician, or law enforcement officials, not all states provide immunity for such reporting. Once identified to the motor vehicle department, the client undergoes a license review process that varies from state to state; therapists should know their states' policies on graded licensing.[1,4,6]

SUMMARY

Community mobility, whether achieved by using public transportation or by driving one's own vehicle, is a pivotal IADL. Individual evaluation, with consideration of valued occupational roles and local transportation systems, provides a foundation for determining the necessary level of intervention. The implementation of ADA-mandated services and advances in assistive technology provide significant means to assist mobility-restricted individuals to move freely within their communities.

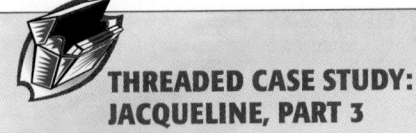

**THREADED CASE STUDY:
JACQUELINE, PART 3**

Jacqueline received intervention in private and public transportation arenas: She was referred for a driver evaluation by her primary therapist and is now participating in a paratransit program for respite and a supplemental transportation plan. She was anticipated to require adaptations because of her arthritis in her neck, shoulders, hands, and lower extremities: an adaptive key holder, door opener, blind spot mirror, and steering wheel cover improved function by modifying the physical context of her occupations. Jacqueline received training in adaptive techniques for vehicle entry/exit, car transfers, wheelchair loading, and driving performance. She could still use a wheelchair carrier but has chosen to wait because of the cost. Jacqueline's quality of life has been greatly improved through therapeutic intervention in many aspects of her community mobility. She is quite pleased with the driving outcomes achieved with her therapist.

Review Questions

1. Define functional ambulation. List three activities of daily living or instrumental activities of daily living in which functional ambulation may occur.
2. Who provides gait training?
3. What is the role of the OT practitioner in functional ambulation?
4. How do the OT and PT practitioners collaborate in functional ambulation?
5. List and describe safety issues for functional ambulation.
6. Name five basic ambulation aids in order of most supportive to least supportive.
7. Discuss why great care should be taken during functional ambulation within the bathroom.
8. List at least three diagnoses for which functional ambulation may be appropriate as part of OT services.
9. What purpose does a task analysis serve in preparation for functional ambulation?
10. What suggestions could be made regarding carrying items during functional ambulation when an ambulation aid is used?
11. What is the objective in measuring seat width?
12. What is the danger of having a wheelchair seat that is too deep?
13. What is the minimal distance for safety from the floor to the bottom of the wheelchair step plate?
14. List three types of wheelchair frames and the general uses of each.
15. Describe three types of wheelchair propulsion systems and tell when each would be used.
16. What are the advantages of detachable desk arms and swing-away footrests?
17. Discuss the factors for consideration before wheelchair selection.
18. Name and discuss the rationale for at least three general wheelchair safety principles.
19. Describe or demonstrate how to descend a curb in a wheelchair with the help of an assistant.
20. Describe or demonstrate how to descend a ramp in a wheelchair with the help of an assistant.
21. List four safety principles for correct moving and lifting technique during wheelchair transfers.
22. Describe or demonstrate the basic standing-pivot transfer from a bed to a wheelchair.
23. Describe or demonstrate the wheelchair-to-bed transfer, using a sliding board.
24. Describe the correct placement of a sliding board before a transfer.
25. In what circumstances would you use a sliding board transfer technique?
26. List the requirements for client and therapist to perform the dependent transfer safely and correctly.
27. List two potential problems and solutions that can occur with the wheelchair-to-car transfer.
28. When is the mechanical lift transfer most appropriate?
29. How is community mobility defined?
30. What are the primary advantages and disadvantages of public and private transportation?
31. What unique qualifications do therapists have, enabling them to address community mobility issues?
32. What basic element of community mobility can be addressed by the therapist?
33. Why are specialized skills needed for driver evaluations?
34. Describe the driving evaluation process and dynamics.
35. Name four ways the OTA may be used in a driver evaluation program.
36. What is the difference between a driver evaluation and wellness program?
37. What are the five Best Practices components in the driver evaluation process?
38. What is the best method to determine driver competency?
39. How long should the on-road evaluation session be?
40. Why are older driver issues of particular interest?
41. What additional credentials can therapists obtain in the field of driver rehabilitation?
42. What is the function of driver training?
43. Why is a follow-up evaluation necessary with adaptive equipment?
44. What legal issues must be considered by a driver rehabilitation therapist?
45. Where can the interested therapist go for additional information on this area of practice?

REFERENCES

1. AA Foundation for Traffic Safety, Beverly Foundation: Transportation alternatives for seniors: high cost problems low cost solutions. Retrieved September 11, 2004, from http://www.seniordrivers.org/STPs/whitepaper6.cfm
2. Adler C: Wheelchairs and seat cushions: a comprehensive guide for evaluation and ordering, San Jose, Calif, 1987, Santa Clara Valley Medical Center, Occupational Therapy Department.
3. Adler C, Musik D, Tipton-Burton M: Body mechanics and transfers: multidisciplinary cross training manual, San Jose, Calif, 1994, Santa Clara Valley Medical Center.
4. American Association of Retired Persons: Graduated driver licensing creating mobility choices, Pub No D15109, Washington, DC, 1993, AARP.
5. American Medical Association: Physician's guide to assessing and counseling older drivers, Chicago, 2003, The Association.
6. American Occupational Therapy Association: Commission on Continuing Competence and Professional Development (CCCPD): 2004. Retrieved Oct. 1, 2004 from *http://www.aota.org/members/area16/index.asp*
7. American Occupational Therapy Association: *Driving and transportation alternative for older adults (fact sheet)*, 2003, The Association.
8. American Occupational Therapy Association: Occupational therapy practice framework: domain and process, *Am J Occup Ther* 56(6):609, 2002.
9. American Public Transportation Association: *Transit ridership report first quarter 2004*. Retrieved Oct. 1, 2004 from *http://www.apta.com/research/stats/ridership/riderep/documents/04q1cvr.pdf*
10. Arilotta C: Performance in areas of occupation: the impact of the environment, *Physical Disabilities Special Interest Quarterly* 26(1):1, 2003.
11. Association of Driver Rehabilitation Specialists (ADED): *ADED documents & resources*, 2004, CD-ROM, Ruston, LA, ADED.

12. Blanc C: *Seating and positioning behind the wheel: special considerations when driving a vehicle from a wheelchair,* Presentation to the ADED annual conference, Dearborn, Mich, 1995.

13. Berres S: Keeping kids safe passenger restraint systems, *OT Practice* Oct 20, 2003, p 13.

14. Berlly M, Lillie SM: *Long term disability: the physical and functional impact on driving.* Presented at annual ADED conference, San Jose, 2000.

15. Beverly Foundation: About us. Retrieved October 11, 2004 from *http://www.seniordrivers.org/STPs/about_us.cfm*

16. Beverly Foundation: Community effectiveness in safeguarding at-risk senior drivers, Interim Report, Pasadena, Calif, February 1998, Beverly Foundation.

17. Bouska MJ, Gallaway M: Primary visual deficits in adults with brain damage: management in occupational therapy, *Occup Ther Pract* 3(1):1, 1991.

18. Brachtesende A: Ready to go? *OT Practice,* Oct 6, 2003, p 14.

19. Breske S: The drive for independence, *Adv Rehabil* 8(3):10, 1994.

20. Bromley I: *Tetraplegia and paraplegia: a guide for physiotherapists,* ed 3, London, 1985, Churchill Livingstone.

21. Cesari M: Prevalence and risk factors for falling in an older community-dwelling population, *Journal of Gerontology,* 57:722, 2002.

22. Cook AM, Hussey SM: *Assistive technologies: principles and practice,* St Louis, 1995, Mosby.

23. Davis ES: Defining OT roles in driving, *OT Practice,* Jan 13, 2004, p 15.

24. Eberhard J: A national perspective on older adult transportation: safe mobility for life. Presentation at Older Adults and Transportation: The New Millennium Regional Forum, Los Angeles, July 22, 1999.

25. Federal Transit Administration: Access for persons with disabilities. Retrieved Oct 5, 2004, from *http://www.fta.dot.gov/transit_data_info/transit_info_for/riders_with_disabilities/1631_4918_ENG_HTML.htm*

26. Golden M, et al: Explanation of the contents of the Americans With Disabilities Act of 1990, Washington, DC, 1990, Disability Rights Education and Defense Fund.

27. Green L: Keys to starting a driver rehabilitation program, *OT Practice,* Oct 6, 2003, p 18.

28. Howard Hughes Medical Institute: FDR and polio: public life, private pain. Retrieved September 13, 2004, from *http://www.hhmi.org/biointeractive/disease/polio/polio2.html*

29. Janke MK: Age related disabilities that may impair drivers and their assessment, Sacramento, 1994, State of California, Department of Motor Vehicles.

30. Kalina T: Starting a driver rehabilitation program, *Work* 8:229, 1997.

31. Kaplan W: The occupation of driving: legal and ethical issues, *Physical Disabilities Special Interest Quarterly* 22:1, 1999.

32. Lamb SE, et al: Risk factors for falling in home-dwelling older women with stroke. The women's health and aging study, *Stroke* 34:494, 2003.

33. Latson LF: Overview of disabled drivers' evaluation process, *Physical Disabilities Special Interest Quarterly* 10(4), 1987.

34. Lohman H, et al: The bridge from ethics to public policy: implications for occupational therapy practitioners, *Am J Occup Ther* 58(1):109, 2004.

35. Lysack CL, et al: After rehabilitation: an 18-month follow-up of elderly inner-city women, *Am J Occup Ther* 57:298, 2003.

36. Mahoney JE: Use of an ambulation assistive device predicts functional decline associated with hospitalization, *J Gerontol* 54:83, 1999.

37. Mallon K, Wood JM: Occupational therapy assessment of open-road driving performance: validity of directed and self-directed navigational instructional components, *Am J Occup Ther* 58(3):279, 2004.

38. National Highway Traffic Safety Administration: Air bags and on-off switches: information for an informed decision, Pub No DOT HS 808 629, Washington, DC, 1999, US Department of Transportation.

39. National Highway Traffic Safety Administration: Driver rehabilitation: a growing niche, *OT Practice,* May 10, 2004, p 13.

40. National Highway Traffic Safety Administration: Supplemental questions and answers regarding air bags, Retrieved October 11, 2004, from *http://www.nhtsa.dot.gov/people/injury/airbags/supplbag.qa.html.*

41. National Mobility Equipment Dealers Association, Association for Driver Rehabilitation Specialists (ADED): Model practices for driver rehabilitation for individuals with disabilities, Tampa, 2002, The Association.

42. National Spinal Cord Injury Association: More about spinal cord injury, Retrieved October 8, 2004, from *http://www.spinalcord.org/html/factsheets/spinstat.php*

43. Odenheimer GL: Cognitive dysfunction and driving abilities, Presentation to the annual meeting of the American Geriatric Society, Atlanta, May 18, 1990.

44. Odenheimer GL, et al: Performance based driving evaluation of the elderly driver: safety, reliability, and validity, *Gerontol Med Sci* 49(4):153, 1994.

45. Owen MM, Stressel DI: Motor-free visual perception test as a screening tool for driver evaluation and rehabilitation readiness, *Physical Disab Special Interest Q* 22:3, 1999.

46. Owsley C, et al: Visual processing impairment and risk of motor vehicle crash among older adults, *J Am Med Assoc* 279(14): 1083, 1998.

47. Pardessus V: Benefits of home visits for falls and autonomy in the elderly, *Am J Phys Med Rehabil* 81:247, 2002.

48. Perr A, Barnicle K: Van lifts: the ups and downs and ins and outs, *Team Rehabil Rep* 49, 1993.

49. Pezenik D, Itoh M, Lee M: Wheelchair prescription. In Ruskin AP, editor: *Current therapy in physiatry,* Philadelphia, 1984, WB Saunders.

50. Pierce S: The occupational therapist's roadmap to safety for seniors, *Gerontol Special Interest Q* 26(3):1, 2003.

51. Public Broadcasting System: Freedom: a history of us. Retrieved September 13, 2004, from *http://www.pbs.org/wnet/ historyofus/web12/segment3b.html*

52. Santa Clara Valley Medical Center, Physical Therapy Department: Lifting and moving techniques, San Jose, Calif, 1985, Santa Clara Valley Medical Center.

53. Schaafsma JD, et al: Gait dynamics in Parkinson's disease: relationship to Parkinsonian features, falls and response to levodopa, *J Neuro Sci* 212:47, 2003.

54. State of California Department of Rehabilitation, Mobility Evaluation Program: Interpretive guidelines for vehicle modification participants, Downey, 1998.

55. State of California Department of Rehabilitation, Mobility Evaluation Program: Statement of assurances for providers of driver evaluation services, Downey, 1990.

56. Summary of proceedings of the Conference on Driver Competency Assessment, CAL-DMV-RSS-91-132, Sacramento, 1993, State of California Department of Motor Vehicles, Program and Policy Administration, Research and Development Section.

57. Taylor H, Harris L: N.O.D. survey of Americans with disabilities: the new competitive advantage: expanding the participation of people with disabilities in the American work force. Reprinted from *Business Week,* May 20, 1994, Washington, DC, National Organization on Disability.

58. Wheatley C, et al: Report on community mobility/driver safety intervention as an area for specialty certification. Retrieved June 17, 2004, from *http://www.aota.org/members/area16/docs/ dri.pdf*

59. Wheelchair prescription: measuring the client (Booklet no. 1), Camarillo, Calif, 1979, Everest & Jennings.

60. Wheelchair prescription: wheelchair selection, (Booklet no. 2), Camarillo, Calif, 1979, Everest & Jennings.

61. Wheelchair prescription: safety and handling (Booklet no. 3), Camarillo, Calif, 1983, Everest & Jennings.

62. Whittle MW: Gait analysis: an introduction, Oxford, 2002, Mosby.

SUGGESTED READINGS

Adler C: Equipment considerations. In Whiteneck, et al, editor: *Treatment of high quadriplegia,* New York, 1988, Demos Publications.

Bergen A, Presperin J, Tallman T: *Positioning for function,* Valhalla, NY, 1990, Valhalla Rehabilitation Publications.

Davies PM: *Steps to follow: a guide to the treatment of adult hemiplegia,* New York, 1985, Springer-Verlag.

Ford JR, Duckworth B: *Physical management for the quadriplegic client,* Philadelphia, 1974, FA Davis.

Gee ZL, Passarella PM: *Nursing care of the stroke client: a therapeutic approach,* Pittsburgh, 1985, A.R.E.N. Publications.

Hill JP, editor: *Spinal cord injury: a guide to functional outcomes in occupational therapy,* Rockville, Md, 1986, Aspen.

Outcomes following traumatic spinal cord injury: clinical practice guidelines for health-care professionals, consortium for spinal cord medicine, 1999, Paralyzed Veterans of America.

12 SEXUALITY AND PHYSICAL DYSFUNCTION

GORDON UMPHRED BURTON

KEY TERMS

Sensuality
Sexuality
Self-perception
Emasculation

Sexual harassment
Sexual values
Sexual history
New body

Sexual abuse
Erogenous
Vaginal atrophy
Reflexogenic erection

Sexually transmitted diseases
Autonomic dysreflexia
PLISSIT

LEARNING OBJECTIVES

After studying this chapter the student or practitioner will be able to do the following:

1. Justify sexuality as a concern of the occupational therapist.
2. List at least five possible reactions of the person with physical disability to her or his sexuality.
3. List some attitudes and assumptions that the able-bodied population may make about the sexuality of people with physical disability.
4. Discuss how sexuality and sensuality are related to self-esteem and a sense of attractiveness.
5. Define sexual harassment and describe how to handle a situation in which clients harass staff members.
6. Describe the effects that such items as mobility aids and splints can have on sexuality.
7. List signs of potential sexual abuse of adults.
8. List at least two intervention goals designed to improve sexual functioning.
9. Discuss ways in which the occupational therapist can provide a safe environment for discussing sexual issues.
10. Describe how sexual values can be communicated.
11. List at least five effects that physical dysfunction can have on sexual functioning and possible solutions for each.
12. Discuss the potential hazards of birth control.
13. List the potential complications of pregnancy and childbirth for a woman with disability.
14. Discuss methods of sex education.
15. Define PLISSIT.

CHAPTER OUTLINE

Reactions to sexuality and disability
  Therapeutic communication
Values clarification
Sexual history
Sexual abuse
Effects of physical dysfunction
  Hypertonia
  Hypotonia
  Low endurance
  Loss of mobility and contractures
  Joint degeneration
  Pain
  Loss of sensation
  Aging and sexuality
  Isolation
  Medication

Performance anxiety
Skin care
Lubrication
Erection
Birth control
Adaptive aids
Safe sex
Hygiene
Pregnancy, delivery, and child care
Methods of education
  Repeat information
  Discovery of the "new" body
  PLISSIT
  Activity analysis
  Basic sex education
Summary

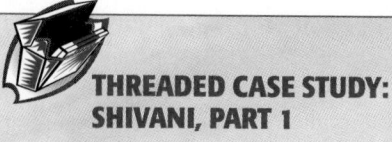

THREADED CASE STUDY: SHIVANI, PART 1

Shivani is a person with cerebral palsy. She is 29 years old and has been married for 2 years. She would like to have a child but has some barriers to overcome with this occupation of reproduction. To start with, as she was growing up she was never taught by her therapists, or anyone else, to enjoy her body and never had a role model with cerebral palsy to know if she could have and raise a child. Now she is trying to relax and enjoy sexual activities with her spouse. This has been further complicated by the fact that several people sexually molested her as she grew up (her doctor and a caretaker). Shivani has also found that sex is uncomfortable in the missionary position where she is lying on her back and her husband is positioned on top of her (the only position she is aware of); she feels like a failure as a partner and as a woman. In her culture she feels that she should not discuss this topic with anyone.

Critical Thinking Questions

Shivani has been referred to your agency.

1. Can she enjoy having sex, get pregnant, and raise a child?
2. Do issues such as sexual positioning, enjoyment of the body, and abuse have anything to do with OT?
3. How would you approach this situation with Shivani and her partner?

Sensuality and **sexuality** are important aspects of everyone's activities of daily living (ADLs) and directly relate to the quality of each person's life. As an ADL, sexual activity is in the domain of occupational therapy (OT). Occupational therapists work with clients in all areas related to sensuality and sexuality (Box 12-1).

Box **12-1**   FACTORS RELATED TO SEXUALITY AND SENSUALITY
Quality of life
Role delineation
Cultural aspects
Impulse control
Energy conservation
Muscle weakness
Hypertonicity and hypotonicity
Appreciation of body
Psychosocial issues
Range of motion
Joint protection
Motor control
Cognition
Increased or decreased sensation

Physical limitations may cause the client to question his or her ability to experience sexual pleasure. With the onset of physical disability, the client undergoes a significant change in the commonly held roles and practices of the able-bodied population.[8,46,55] The individual with a disability may be regarded by able-bodied persons as asexual, an object of pity, and unattractive.[3,31,35] Being perceived as unattractive and possibly unlovable can cause the client to believe that he or she can never be intimate with anyone. Holding this belief can lead the client and related others to a sense of despair. McCabe and Taleporos[37] found that "people with more severe physical impairments experienced significantly lower levels of sexual esteem and sexual satisfaction and significantly higher levels of sexual depression than people who had mild impairments or who did not report having a physical impairment."

Low and Zubir[35] and Kettl, Zarefoss, Jacoby, et al[29] found that females with acquired spinal cord injuries reported feeling less than half as attractive after they had acquired the disability, even though spinal cord injury is a disability with little observable physical change in body appearance. These studies showed a major decrease in the **self-perception** of attractiveness.[35] Another study found that with the advent of a disability, males felt a loss of their sense of masculinity and sensed a threat to the male role.[45]

These are just a few examples of the feelings and perceptions that affect the sensuality and sexuality of the person who has a physical disability. To accomplish comprehensive rehabilitation with the client, the OT and other health professionals must address self-perception, beliefs, and needs related to sexuality. This chapter examines issues related to sexuality and sensuality with physical disability.

REACTIONS TO SEXUALITY AND DISABILITY

The many obstacles encountered by people with disability should not interfere with the expression of sensuous and sexual needs. As an informed professional, each therapist can help the adult client eliminate unnecessary obstacles, overcome anxieties, and appreciate personal uniqueness. The expression of sexuality or sensuality is a sign of self-confidence, self-validation, and a sense of being lovable. When a person acquires a disability or is born with a disability, he or she can feel less positive about self and less lovable.[17,44,45]

Sexuality can symbolize how a person is dealing with the world. If a person feels inadequate as a sexual, sensual, and lovable human being, the motivation to pursue other avenues of life can be affected. When an individual has a negative self-image, coping with life's problems is difficult. Because sexuality is often used as a barometer of how one feels about oneself, it is productive for the therapist to help the client feel as positive as possible about her or his physical and personal qualities. A healthy attitude toward one's sexuality enhances motivation for all aspects of therapy. The therapist must try to help the client adjust self-perceptions enough to function positively in life.

Sexuality has been found to be a predictor of marital satisfaction, adjustment to physical disability, and success of vocational training. In society, people are often judged by physical attractiveness.[46] In Western civilization, physical intimacy is closely associated with love. Therefore, if a person perceives himself or herself as incapable of expressing sensuality or sexuality, it is possible that he or she feels incapable of loving and being loved. In the majority of people who have had a stroke they "reported a marked decline in all measured sexual functions."[20,30] Without the capability of loving and being loved, a sense of isolation and of being valueless may ensue.[6,35,41,44] Adaptive devices such as braces, wheelchairs, and communication aids can be a detriment to one's perceived attractiveness and sexuality. For example, it may be hard to perceive oneself as sexual when an indwelling catheter is present or when braces are worn. By discussing the effects of these devices on social interaction, the client can get some ideas about how to handle difficult situations when they arise.[1,34,41,58]

OT intervention should include goals that facilitate an increase in self-esteem and enable the client to feel lovable. The therapist's role is to foster feelings of self-worth and help the client engage in occupation and to help minimize feelings of worthlessness and hopelessness.[6,18,35,44,46] Feeling lovable engenders a sense of self-worth, attractiveness, sensuality, sexuality, and being capable of intimacy. Achieving this goal enhances the development of a healthy and realistic life balance (Figure 12-1) in which the client engages in occupations.

Whether sex is still possible is a concern that arises after the onset of physical disability. This concern is often set aside in the immediacy of coping with the adjustment to hospital life and activities that make up the daily routine. However, the concern is not forgotten. A common complaint made about medical staff by people with disabilities is that the staff members never deal with or let people with disability deal with the topic of their sexuality.[5,35,57] People with disabilities feel that if their sensuality and sexuality are negated, a significant facet of their personhood is negated. This lack of acceptance causes the person with a disability to lose the feeling that he or she is treated as a whole person.

Often men and women with disabilities have an increased dependence on an able-bodied partner, which results in a decrease in sex life.[15] One possible explanation is that the able-bodied partner is less inclined to be aroused when he or she has just bathed the partner or assisted the partner with toileting. The therapist must be sensitive to the possibility of these perceptions and help the client deal appropriately with the feelings they evoke.

The client's sense of masculinity or femininity may be threatened by the disability.[36,45,48] Men who have recently acquired a disability report that they feel emasculated.[45,48] Feelings of **emasculation** can be reinforced by physical limitations. For example, lifting weights may no longer be possible, sports participation may not be possible without adaptations, and attendance at sporting events may be limited by lack of access. The necessity to look up at others from a wheelchair and ask for assistance can engender feelings of dependency.

A man with a disability may react to feelings of dependency and emasculation[45] by flirting to prove his masculinity. The client may attempt to flirt or make passes at a therapist. Because it is estimated that up to 10% of the population is homosexual,[27] the therapist can expect that at some time clients of the same sex may make sexual advances.

Women experience many of the same feelings but probably interpret and react to them in a different way. Women with disabilities report feeling unattractive and undesirable. This can lead to despair if a woman feels that she cannot achieve some of her major goals in life. Thus, the female client may flirt to see if she is still attractive to others.

The therapist must realize that the client is seeking confirmation of her or his sexuality. The therapist should not be surprised by flirtations or sexual advances and should deal with them in a positive and professional manner, but the therapist should not be harassed. All of the therapist's interactions should be directed toward creating an environment that promotes the client's self-esteem, positive and appropriate sexuality, and adjustment to disability.

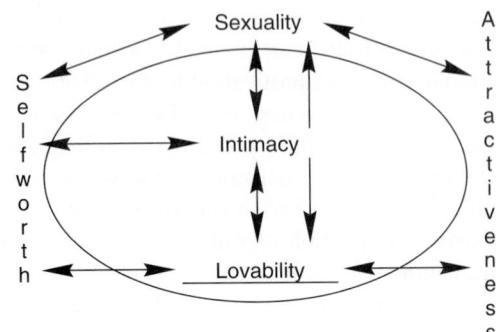

Sexuality and disability

Figure 12-1 Sexuality and disability.

ETHICAL CONSIDERATIONS

When responding to the client, the therapist should be alert to the client's current sexuality issues to prevent doing further damage to the client's sense of self. If the therapist rejects or ridicules the client, the client may hesitate to attempt such confirmation of personal attractiveness in future situations in which these behaviors are more socially appropriate. If the therapist rejects the client, the client may assume that if someone who is familiar with persons who have disabilities is rejecting, then one who is unfamiliar with them would not be likely to be accepting either.

Inappropriate sexual advances, **sexual harassment,** or exploitation of either the therapist or the client cannot be permitted.[38,51] Behavior is considered harassment when it causes the therapist to feel threatened, intimidated, or treated as a sexual object. If sexual harassment is allowed, it can be damaging to the client and to staff morale.[23] The therapist should provide direct feedback explaining that he or she feels offended and that the behavior is inappropriate and must cease. All of the staff members should be informed and develop and implement a plan to modify the client's behavior if it persists.

THERAPEUTIC COMMUNICATION

Conversations regarding sexuality can be opportunities for discussing personal feelings and perceptions. One way to approach discussion of intimate matters is by asking the female client how she will perform breast self-examination with her disability. A male client can be asked how he will perform self-examination of the testicles. If the treatment facility does not have information about these examinations, the client can obtain them from the American Cancer Society or the local Planned Parenthood Association. Each of these activities falls into the domain of health maintenance and may not have been discussed by other health team members. This interaction will set the stage for discussion of other personal matters, impress upon the client the necessity for concern about personal health, and reaffirm the client's sexual identity.

Clients often feel safe asking the OT about sexual matters related to their disabilities, because the therapist deals with other intimate activities such as bathing, dressing, and toileting. It is also important to discuss sexual hygiene as an ADL. The trust built up in the relationship encourages this communication. The therapist should be prepared with information and resources. The therapist does not need to know everything or be a sex counselor but should see that the client gets the necessary information or referral.

The OT is the most appropriate professional to solve some problems, such as motor performance needed for sexual activity.[9] For example, discussing positioning to reduce pain or hypertonicity or to enable the client to more comfortably engage in sexual relations will help the client deal with problems before they occur.[12,32,41]

Shivani, who has hypertonicity, particularly in hip adductors, experiences discomfort in a sexual position in which she abducts her legs during intercourse with her husband. She and her husband have not explored other positions but instead have decreased the number of times they have intercourse during the month. Shivani's sense of failure and feelings of diminished worth as a wife have further affected the intimacy of her marriage.

During all aspects of the rehabilitation process, the client needs to work on communication with the therapist, staff, and his or her sexual partner. The therapist can facilitate this process simply by giving the client permission to discuss feelings and potential problems, especially sexual problems. The client needs to learn how to accurately communicate sexual needs, desires, and position options to a partner, either verbally or nonverbally, to have a mutually satisfactory sexual relationship.[16,29] Each client will have unique problems or issues that are related to the nature of the disability. An example is a client with Parkinson's disease in whom the lack of facial expression impedes the nonverbal communication of intimacy. The client can be taught to communicate feelings verbally that were previously conveyed with facial expressions.

OT PRACTICE NOTE

Discussion of sexuality is a way to explore feelings of dependency, identity, attractiveness, and unattractiveness.[35,39] Communication must be established regarding the feelings of sexual role changes. If a client's perceived roles are threatened, this situation should be dealt with as early as possible during intervention. If it is not, the effects could persist throughout the client's life and impinge upon occupations important to the client.

VALUES CLARIFICATION

Sexual values of the client, the partner, and the therapist must be examined for the therapist to interact with the client in the most effective and positive manner.[3,14,36,41,46] Many professional schools do not train healthcare workers on the subject of sexuality and disability.[3,22,48,52] In-service training can be arranged to help the staff be aware of the sexual needs of people with disability.[19,29] Books, articles, videotapes, and training packets are available for professional education.[7,13,14,48]

Unless the staff is educated about the significance of sexuality and related issues, they could have negative feelings about dealing with these matters.[3,7,52,56] If the therapist is not aware of the thoughts and feelings of all of the individuals involved, the therapist could make incorrect assumptions that have negative results.[12] One of the most direct ways of gaining information is by taking a **sexual history.**[12,48,49] The purpose of a sexual history is to learn how a person thinks and feels about sex and bodily functions and to discover the needs of those concerned.[12,33,48] According to some researchers, many individuals with a disability had a sexual dysfunction before they acquired the physical disability. Taking the sexual history can help to identify such a problem.[34]

SEXUAL HISTORY

When taking a sexual history, the therapist should create an environment that will allow for confidentiality, comfort, and self-expression. In early intervention, the therapist should ask about the client's concerns regarding contraception, safe sex, homosexuality, masturbation, sexual health, aging, menopause, and physical changes.

Box 12-2 lists some questions that could be asked. All questions should not be asked at the same time, nor would all questions be asked of every client.

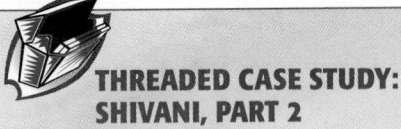

THREADED CASE STUDY: SHIVANI, PART 2

The following questions may have elicited important responses from Shivani.

1. How important is sexuality at this time in your life?

From her answer we would find out that Shivani does not feel that it is important to her but that it is for her spouse and to have a child.

2. How would you describe your sexual activities at this time?

We would find out that sex is uncomfortable for her and that she views sex as more of a necessary evil for her.

3. If you could change aspects of your current sexual situation, what would you change and how would you change it?

Shivani may say that she is uncomfortable during sex because she had been molested previously and that sex is physically uncomfortable for her now, which makes her feel like a failure. The therapist may not want to pursue the discussion regarding the sexual molestation and the psychological counseling aspects but may ask for a referral to a psychiatric professional. The physical discomfort may be then addressed. Positions could be found to make intercourse more comfortable and let Shivani feel less like a failure as a partner.

After taking the sexual history, the therapist can often ascertain whether guilt is connected with the sex act, body parts, or sexual alternatives (such as masturbation, oral sex, sexual positions, or sexual devices). For example, some clients report feelings of guilt or fear in relation to having sex after a heart attack or a stroke—fear that sex can cause a stroke or guilt that it may have caused the first episode. Another fear is that the partner will not accept the presence of catheters, adaptive equipment, or scars. Performance is often an issue. Able-bodied persons and those with disabilities ask questions regarding the sexual ability of the person with disabilities.

The therapist can furnish the necessary information by (1) directing the client to other professionals, (2) providing magazines and books that discuss the subject, (3) showing movies, or (4) suggesting role models. The therapist must be tactful and remember that the client is probably questioning her or his own values and previous notions about sexuality. Personal care such as toileting, personal hygiene, menstrual hygiene, bathing, and birth control are issues that can evoke reflection on values regarding sex and body image.

Self-care issues, particularly personal hygiene and sexuality, usually are not emphasized enough during acute illness

Box 12-2	QUESTIONS TO ASK IN A SEXUAL HISTORY

How did you first find out about sexuality?

When and how did you first learn about heterosexuality and homosexuality?

Who furnished you with information about sexuality when you were young?

Were you ready for the information when you first heard about sexuality?

How important is sexuality at this time in your life?

How would you describe your sexual activities at this time?

How do you feel sexuality expresses your feelings and meets your needs and those of others?

If you could change aspects of your current sexual situation, what would you change and how would you change it?

What concerns do you have about birth control, disease control, and sexual safety?

What physical, medical, or drug-related concerns do you have relating to your sexuality?

Have you ever been pressured, threatened, or forced into a sexual situation?

Which sexual practices have you engaged in, in the past (e.g., oral, anal, and genital)?

Do you consider certain sexual activities "kinky"? How do you feel about participating in such activities?

How important do you think sexuality will be in your future?

What concerns do you have about your sexuality?

Are there questions or concerns that you have regarding this interview?

and rehabilitation. Discussing such issues once or twice is not sufficient. The circumstances and environment in which these issues are discussed should also be considered. The therapist must create an environment that will allow personal discussions to occur. A personal conversation cannot take place in a crowded therapy room, during a rushed and impersonal treatment session, or with a therapist with whom a good personal rapport does not exist. Building rapport is a problem in healthcare facilities in which therapists are frequently rotated or work on a per-diem basis.

A discussion of feelings will also help the client explore her or his **new body** or adapt to ongoing degeneration of the body if there is a progressive disability. These conversations may take place while other therapeutic activities are in progress, so that billing insurers for time is not a barrier.

SEXUAL ABUSE

The **sexual abuse** of adults with disabilities is a considerable problem.[1,50,52,56] Some people who have disabilities have reported being approached by pimps representing prostitution rings that specialize in providing people with disabilities for their customers. Clients should be made aware of the possibility of this type of exploitation. Others have reported that medical staff members took inappropriate liberties with them and that personal care attendants, on whom they depended, demanded sexual favors. Clients can and should report such abuse to Adult Protective Services. The therapist also must report cases of suspected sexual abuse. The client may be reluctant to report abuse because of a concern that it will not be possible to get another aide or that, during the time it takes to hire another aide, essential assistance will not be available. These are major problems for a person who is dependent on others for care.

Therapists usually do not suspect caregivers, medical staff, aides, transportation assistants, or volunteers of sexual abuse, but the therapist should be alert to signs of possible abuse even from these sources.[47] Some individuals prey on adults and children with disabilities and are drawn to the health fields with this motive.[1] The therapist should watch for signs of potential abuse, such as clients usually being upset after interacting with a specific person, caregivers taking clients off alone for no apparent reason, excessive touching in a sensual manner by caregivers, the client being agitated when around a particular individual, and the client being overly compliant with a specific individual.

 ETHICAL CONSIDERATIONS

Therapists must increase their awareness of what constitutes sexual abuse. Children with disabilities have long been expected to undress and be examined or treated as part of their medical care. This treatment is sometimes necessary, but the preferences and dignity of the client should be respected at all times. A person of any age should not be forced to endure humiliation.

The therapy session should help the client develop a sense of personal ownership of her or his body. This goal may be neglected when working with adults and is often neglected in working with children. For example, a child who believes that he or she does not have the right to say no to being touched, who cannot physically resist unwanted advances, and who may not be able to communicate that abuse has taken place is in jeopardy for being a victim.[1]

The therapist should ask permission before touching the client and should touch with respect and maintain the client's sense of dignity. If the therapist does not ask permission to touch a client, the client can lose the sense of control over being touched by others. The therapist should guard against communicating this notion to the client.

Naming body parts and body processes is a good way of helping clients take charge of their bodies. Once the body parts and processes are named, using correct terminology rather than slang, the possibility exists for the client to communicate and to relate in an appropriate manner.[1,11,40,49] The use of the proper terms has the effect of helping the client

view the body in a more positive way, whereas slang tends to communicate negative images.[49]

EFFECTS OF PHYSICAL DYSFUNCTION

Specific physical problems that may create difficulties in sexual performance for people with disabilities and their partners and suggestions for management of the problems are outlined below and summarized in Table 12-1.

HYPERTONIA

Hypertonia can increase when muscles are stretched. To prevent quick stretching of muscles involved in a movement pattern, motion should be performed slowly. It is advisable to incorporate rotation into the movement to break up the tone. Slow rocking can be used to inhibit hypertonic musculature. Gentle shaking or slow stroking (massage) can also be inhibitory. Heat or cold can also be used to inhibit tone. Clients with hypertonia should review options for different positions in which to have sexual intercourse. Alternative ways of dealing with personal hygiene (e.g., toileting, inserting tampons, gynecological examinations, and birth control) may also need to be explored in relation to hypertonicity.

Shivani's OT discussed strategies that could be used to relax the hypertonicity in her legs, such as gently rocking her legs side to side while she was seated. Although initially presented as a means to decrease the hypertonicity affecting Shivani's sitting balance when toileting and for personal hygiene during menstruation, this technique also was suggested as a means to relax her legs before intercourse.

HYPOTONIA

Clients with low muscle tone (hypotonia) need physical support during sexual activity. Pillows, towels, or bolsters may be used to support body parts, allowing for endurance and protecting the body from overstretching and fatigue. Sexual positions that allow support of the joints involved should be explored. The client and her or his partner should also explore their attitudes about the positions.

LOW ENDURANCE

Prolonged sexual activity can be intolerable because of low physical endurance. Some techniques for dealing with low endurance are employing principles of work simplification to sexual activity, using timing to engage in sex when the client has the most energy, and assuming positions in which sexual performance uses less energy.

LOSS OF MOBILITY AND CONTRACTURES

Limited mobility and contractures prohibit many movement patterns and limit the number of positions for sex. Activity analysis must be done to find positions that will

TABLE 12-1   **Conditions and Possible Effects on Sexual Functioning**

Symptom

DIAGNOSIS	Anxiety/ Fear	Contractures	Cultural Barriers	Decreased Libido	Depression	Impotence	Incontinence	Limited ROM	Loss of Mobility	Loss of Sensation	Low Endurance	Medication	Paralysis/ Spasticity	Poor Body Image	Tremor	Catheter/ Ostomy
Amputations	X	X	X		X				X	X				X		
Arthritis	X	X	X	X	X			X	X		X	X		X		
Burns	X	X	X		X			X	X	X	X	X	X	X		
Cardiac disease	X		X	X	X	X			X		X			X		
Cerebral palsy	X	X	X		X		X	X	X	X	X	X	X	X	X	X
CVA	X	X	X	X	X	X	X	X	X	X	X	X	X	X	X	X
Diabetes	X	X	X	X	X	X		X	X	X	X		X	X	X	
Hand injury	X	X	X		X			X	X	X	X	X		X		
Head injury	X	X	X	X	X*	X	X	X	X	X	X	X	X	X	X	X
Musculo-skeletal	X	X	X		X		X	X	X	X	X	X	X	X	X	
Spinal cord injury	X	X	X		X	X	X	X	X	X	X	X	X	X	X	X

X, possible involvement. CVA, cerebrovascular accident. ROM, range of motion.

*Fear of medication as possible causes.

allow sexual activity. This system often requires creative problem solving on the part of the client, the partner, and the responsible professional counselor.

JOINT DEGENERATION

Conditions such as arthritis can cause pain, damage to the joints, and contractures. Avoiding stress and repetitive weight bearing on the joints can decrease joint damage. Activity analysis is needed to reduce joint stress and excessive weight bearing on the joints. It is necessary to find a position, such as that shown in Figure 12-2, that takes weight and stress off the knees or hips. This position is sometimes referred to as the missionary position. A position with substantial hip abduction may not be acceptable for the client, in which case a side-lying position may be more acceptable. If hip abduction is limited, the woman should avoid positions such as those shown in Figures 12-2, 12-5, and 12-9. After Shivani's OT introduced the technique of slow rocking, Shivani asked about other positions that would be more comfortable during intercourse. The OT discussed the possibility of using the side-lying position to decrease the stress on the hip joints and discomfort Shivani experiences during intercourse.

PAIN

Pain limits the enjoyment of sexual activities.[26] Usually at some time of day pain is diminished and energy is at its highest. Sexual activities can be scheduled for such times. After pain medication has taken effect, many people find that sexual activity is possible. Communication between partners is especially important when pain is involved. An unaffected partner who does not understand the negative effects of pain may believe that the affected partner is not considering her or his personal needs. A referral to a counselor who understands the effects of pain or to a pain specialist can help work out emotional and physical aspects of this problem. The OT can help the client think of acceptable ways of meeting the partner's sexual needs without causing pain. Masturbation and mutual masturbation with sexual fantasy are possible ways of meeting sexual needs in these circumstances. In this way the partners are interacting and neither person feels isolated.

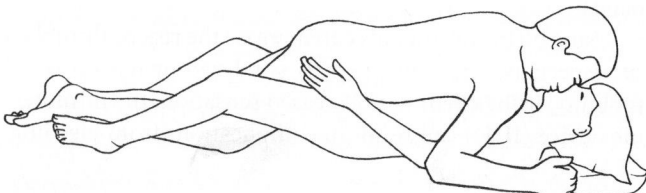

Figure 12-2 This position places pressure on a female's bladder and requires hip abduction but little energy expenditure for her.

LOSS OF SENSATION

The loss of sensation can affect the sexual relationship in several ways. The lack of **erogenous** sensation in the affected area can block proper warning that an area is being abraded (e.g., the vagina not being sufficiently lubricated) or damaged (e.g., bladder or even bones if the partner is on top and being too forceful). A lack of sensation may be a sign of disruption of the reflex loop responsible for sensation and erections in the male and sensation and lubrication in the female.

AGING AND SEXUALITY

With aging, changes take place that can affect sexuality. Menopause and the resulting hormonal changes cause **vaginal atrophy** in women and slower reactions to sexual stimulation. In the male, greater stimulation may be needed to develop and maintain an erection, and reaction time between erections may be greater. Partners can be informed of ways to increase stimulation and can be helped to understand that it is the quality, not the quantity, of sexual activity that is important in the relationship. The client should be made aware of the maturation process and its normal effect on sexuality so that the disability is not blamed for all of the problems.

ISOLATION

The environment is composed of objects, persons, and events. In all activities is an interaction between the person and environment. Some of the objects with which people with disabilities interact are wheelchairs, braces, canes, crutches, and splints. These objects are all hard, cold, and angular. They can communicate a hard exterior and a fragile interior and can convey the notion that no softness exists, that it is not safe to hug, and that a person in a wheelchair or in braces or on crutches can get hurt or toppled if touched. As a result of these ideas, the individual with a disability may feel isolated by the appliances.

Some people tend to withdraw from the objects around the client. This may reinforce the client's notion of a lack of sensuousness and increase the client's sense of isolation. Clients often feel isolated and different from the "normal" population.[14] This phenomenon is more common among clients who have been out of the healthcare facility for a period of time. In the early phases of the disability, the therapist and the client can role play about how to deal with a new partner or how to explain equipment used, such as a catheter. This approach may help ease the client's fears and increase the client's comfort with such issues. At the same time the therapist is communicating that sex may be a possibility in the future. It should be pointed out to clients that at no time in human history have people with disabilities not existed in society, that they are a part of society, and that it is not "abnormal" to have disability. All people who live long enough will acquire a disability to a greater or lesser extent at some time.

MEDICATION

Potential side effects of medication are impotence, delayed sexual response, or other problems. Diuretics and antihypertensives can cause impotence, decreased libido, and loss of orgasm. Tranquilizers and antidepressants can contribute to decreased libido and even impotence in some individuals.[48] Side effects of medication should be discussed with the physician and the pharmacist to see whether medications can be altered or changed. If they cannot, acknowledging that the problem is organic can be helpful to the client.

PERFORMANCE ANXIETY

At times of great emotional stress, a male client may find that the erection is inhibited. This problem can lead to increased anxiety in relation to sexuality and create a cycle of dysfunctional inhibition. It can be helpful for the client and his partner to take the focus off erection and genital intercourse and focus on sensuality and making each other feel good. A massage is one possibility that will allow for more normal physiological reactions. If this approach does not work, a trained counselor may be needed to help deal with the problem, if it has been determined that the problem is not organic in nature.

SKIN CARE

The person with a disability should be informed that positioning modifications might be needed to protect the skin, prevent skin breakdown, and increase pleasure. If a sexual position causes repeated rubbing on the skin, this friction can cause abrasions and result in skin damage. The therapist and client can discuss methods to prevent the friction—through an alternative position, for example. Pressure on bony prominences or pressure exerted in a specific area by a partner can also cause problems with skin irritation and must be avoided.

LUBRICATION

Stimulating natural lubrication in female clients is important. It may be overlooked in a woman with paralysis because she may not be able to feel the stimulation or lack of natural lubrication. Stimulation to cause reflexive lubrication should occur even when the woman does not feel it. Without proper lubrication, damage may occur without awareness of the problem. If needed, artificial water-based lubricants (such as K-Y Jelly) should be introduced. The individual should be warned that only water-based lubricants are appropriate because petroleum-based lubricants can cause irritation and can attack latex condoms, causing condom failure. This is a major concern because the female partner is more likely than the male to become infected with the human immunodeficiency virus (HIV) in any given heterosexual encounter.

ERECTION

Many men regard the ability to achieve an erection as one of the most significant signs of masculinity.[33] If awareness of sensory stimulation to the penis is blocked by the sensory loss associated with paralysis and if the male client does not try to stimulate a reflexogenic erection, he may believe that he is impotent. This is not necessarily true, and the client may go through much needless anguish. The client should be encouraged to explore his body. Rubbing the penis, the thighs, or the anus can be effective ways to evoke a **reflexogenic erection**. Even rubbing the big toe has been reported by some men with quadriplegia to stimulate an erection. If the normal reflex arc is interrupted, it is usually not possible to achieve an erection, and alternative methods must be explored.

Alternative methods can be forms of sex that do not require an erect penis, such as using a vibrator or trying oral or digital sex. If the client feels that penile intercourse is the only acceptable method, other possibilities do exist.* Injections of hormones that stimulate erections can be used, but this practice may have adverse reactions or lead to problems if the client does not have good judgment or lacks hand dexterity. The use of a vacuum tube is sometimes effective and is one of the less invasive techniques.[49] Surgical implants can be used but have disadvantages, such as the possibility of infection and skin breakdown. With a physician's prescription Viagra, Levitra, and Cialis are among the stimulants that are being developed and may be a possibility for some clients but have some major side effects.

BIRTH CONTROL

The client should consult with her or his physician in weighing the pros and cons of various methods of birth control. People with disabilities must consider a number of factors when planning birth control.[9,10,24,32,40] Because most disabling conditions do not impair fertility (especially for women), it is important for the client to be aware of birth control and potential complications of the use of birth control.

Condoms require good use of the hands. An applicator can be adapted in some cases, but someone with good hand dexterity must assemble the device beforehand. Diaphragms are not very feasible for people who have poor hand function, unless the partner does have hand function and both parties feel comfortable about inserting the diaphragm as part of foreplay. The contraceptive sponge also requires good use of hands.

Using birth control pills can increase the risk of thrombosis, especially when the client is paralyzed or has impaired mobility. If the client has decreased sensation, the intrauterine device (IUD) can result in complications from bleeding,

---

*An excellent discussion of these alternatives can be found in *Sexuality and Disability* 12:1, 1994.

cramping, puncturing of the uterus, or infection. The use of spermicides requires good control of the hands or the assistance of the partner who has normal hand function. The use of nonoxynol 9 has been suspected to increase the risk of HIV transmission and should be avoided.[42] The injectable type of birth control may allow for easy use but has many of the same side effects as the pill. In using any method of birth control, the client must always be concerned with decreasing the chance of infection and with practicing safe sex.

ADAPTIVE AIDS

Adaptive aids may be necessary, especially if the client lacks hand function. One aid is a vibrator for foreplay or masturbation.[21] Special devices have been adapted for men and women.[12,32,40] Pillows may be used for positioning, and other equipment may be used for clients who have special needs. The therapist must prepare the client for the concept of using sexual aids before suggesting the option to the client. For example, the therapist can suggest that the client privately explore the sensation that the vibrator produces in the lower extremities. The client might discover the possible use of the vibrator for sexual stimulation or at least, when told how it can be used, may be more open to the idea of using a vibrator as a sexual aid.

SAFE SEX

The issue of safe sex has increased considerably since the advent of the acquired immune deficiency syndrome (AIDS). Safe sex is important to protect against all forms of **sexually transmitted diseases** (STDs).[24] Clients need to be advised that this is an important issue. If there is a sensory impairment in and around the genital area, the person might not be aware of an abrasion or infection. Having any genital irritation or infection allows easy entrance for STDs. The person with disability must be informed of the increased risk for HIV and STDs so that extra caution can be taken.

HYGIENE

Catheter care is a concern, especially when hand function is impaired. Questions may be raised regarding how or if a person with an indwelling catheter can have sex. Sex is possible for both men and women, but some precautions should be taken. If the catheter becomes kinked or closed off (which will definitely happen in the case of a catheterized man having vaginal intercourse), pressure should not be placed on the bladder. The bladder should be fully voided before sexual activity. Urine flow should be restricted for as short a time as possible and no more than 30 minutes. Damage to the bladder and kidneys could result if these precautions are not followed. The client should not drink fluids for at least 2 hours before sex to prevent the bladder filling during

this time. Sexual positions that avoid placing pressure on the bladder should be used (Figures 12-3 to 12-10). Many of the same positions can be used if the client uses a stoma appliance.

Women who have various disabling conditions have reported irregular menstrual periods and deterioration of their neurological condition during menstruation.[57] Hygiene issues may occur for several reasons. Lack of education, poor hand function, and poor sensation are conditions that may contribute to menses complications. Information regarding toxic shock syndrome should be given to clients that may not feel or be aware of infection. A sanitary napkin or pad requires less fine motor skill and is less dependent upon intact sensation than a tampon. Although the client's preferences must be considered, the therapist is responsible for educating a woman regarding the pros and cons of using either a sanitary pad or a tampon during menstruation. Menopause complications may be increased but this area may need further research.

A person with an impairment of bowel or bladder function may have an occasional episode of incontinence during sexual activities. If the client and the therapist discuss this possibility and how to deal with it, some embarrassment can be averted when it occurs. The client and therapist can roleplay to explore various scenarios such as, "You are planning intimacy with a new partner. How will you explain your catheter and appliances to the person?" These may be awkward conversations for the therapist and the client, but dealing with these issues beforehand is usually easier than waiting for the situation to arise. Such topics must be approached with caution and discretion.

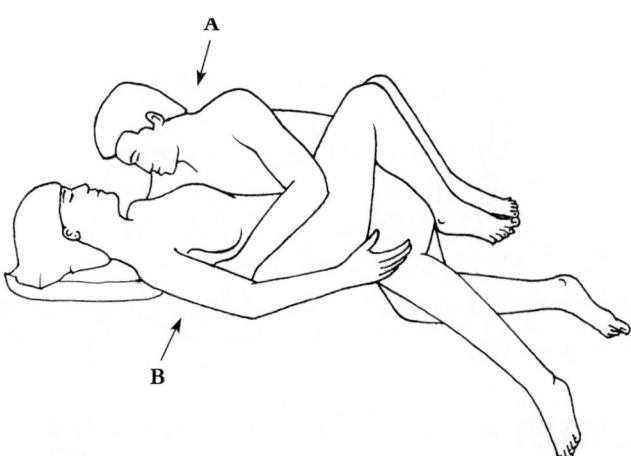

Figure 12-3 Vaginal entry of *B* requires no hip abduction, and hip flexion tightness would not impede performance. Energy requirements for both parties are minimal. Bladder pressure, catheter safety, and stoma appliance safety should not be an issue in this position for *B*. This position may be recommended if *B* has back pain or is paralyzed, especially if roll is used to support lumbar spine.

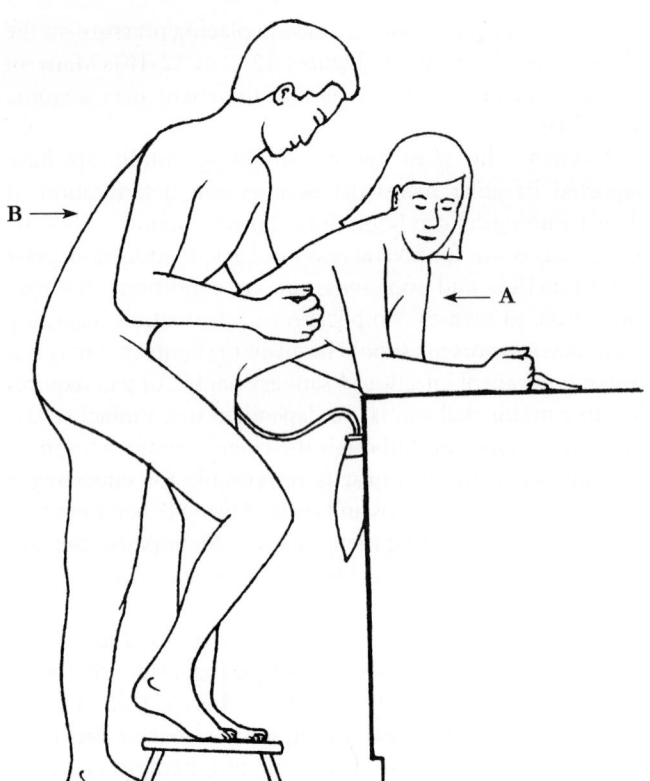

Figure 12-4   Partner *A* needs little hip abduction but good strength. Partner *B* may find decreased strain on his back. Hip, knee, or ankle joint degeneration would preclude this position for either partner.

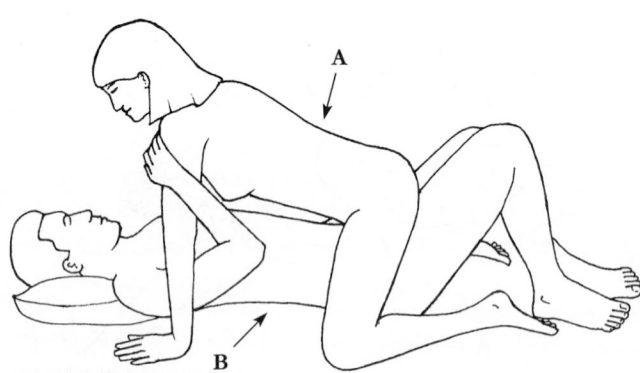

Figure 12-5   Person *A* must have hip abduction, balance, and endurance but pressure is off of bladder and stoma. If catheter is used it would be unrestricted. Back pain may be avoided by keeping trunk vertical. Person *B*'s hip flexors could be contracted. If low back pain is a problem, legs should be flexed and roll placed under low back. If stoma appliance is used, this position would prevent interference. If low endurance is a problem, this position can be used effectively for *B*.

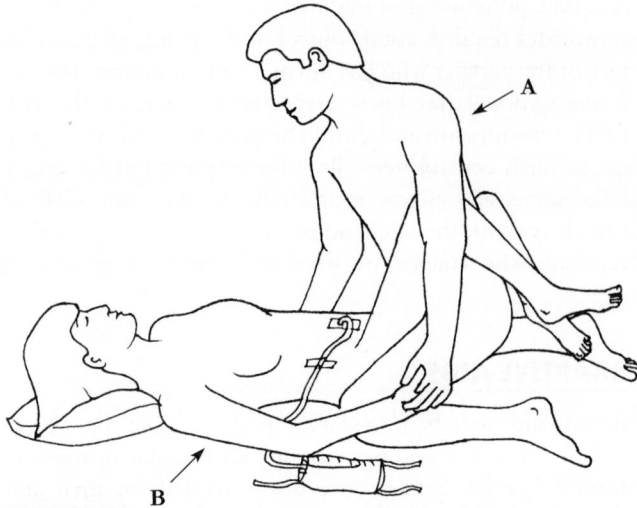

Figure 12-6   This position keeps pressure off bladder, lessens chance of tubing becoming bent, reduces pressure on back (especially if small roll is used under low back), and does not require *B* to use much energy. Legs do not need to be as high as is shown, but if hip flexors are contracted, this position may be comfortable.

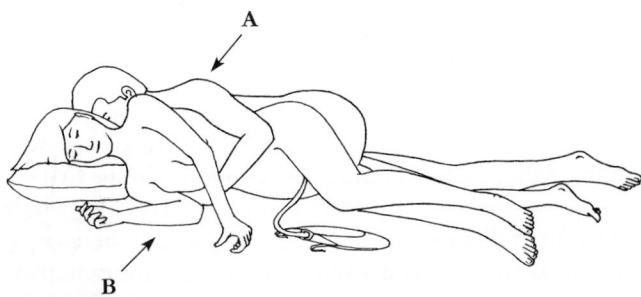

Figure 12-7   Partner *B* need not expend much energy in this position. Both partners may avoid swayback in this position. Either person may have hemiparesis. Person *B* will not need hip abduction, and pressure on stoma bag may be avoided.

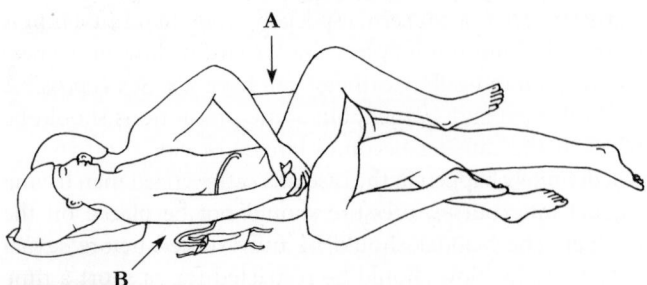

Figure 12-8   This position can be used if either partner has hemiparesis. If low endurance is a problem, this position can be used. Person *A* may avoid swayback in this position.

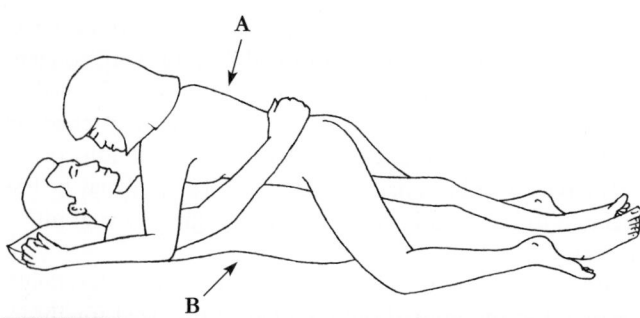

Figure 12-9   Partner *B* can be paralyzed or have limited range of motion. His back may need roll for support, and he must be concerned with pressure on his bladder.

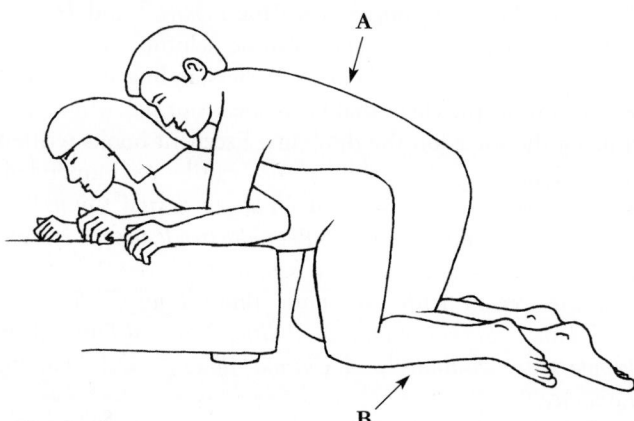

Figure 12-10   Rear vaginal entry of *B*, who does not need much energy because of support and little or no abduction of hips. Flexion tightness of hips does not affect performance. Because of weight on *B*'s knees, hips, and back, as well as inevitable repetitive movement at hips, this would not be a good position for individuals with back, hip, or knee joint degeneration.

PREGNANCY, DELIVERY, AND CHILD CARE

Before becoming pregnant, women must weigh the risks and benefits of pregnancy, childbirth, and child care. Complications of pregnancy may affect the client's function and mobility. These include the potential for respiratory or kidney problems. The effect of the increased body weight on transfers, an increased possibility of **autonomic dysreflexia,** and the need for increased bladder and bowel care should all be considered when pregnancy is contemplated.[54] Labor and delivery can present some special problems, such as a lack of awareness of the beginning of labor contractions. Induction of labor may be contraindicated if a person has a spinal cord injury at T6 or above and the medical staff members are not trained to deal with the respiratory problems or dysreflexia that can result. After delivery, the parent with disability will need to have modifications made to the wheelchair. The client may need consultations to achieve an optimal level of function in the parenting role.[24]

Using Shivani as an example, the therapist may help her with where to find information. Introducing her to sites appropriate for an online search, or encouraging her to contact Planned Parenthood and/or United Cerebral Palsy to gain the information to make informed decisions would help her locate necessary information. She could also ask these agencies for a list of doctors who have experience with women who were pregnant and have cerebral palsy.

The therapist may then simulate situations during the first year after birth. This may include how to transport an infant, change diapers and dress the child at different stages, play with the child, bathe the child, and/or deal with parenting when one has mobility impairments, just to name a few possible scenarios.

METHODS OF EDUCATION

The following techniques or approaches have been used effectively to deal with the emotional aspects of sex education of people with disability.

REPEAT INFORMATION

Mentioning sexual issues just once is not enough. Whether they have a disability or not, most people need to hear information more than once. This fact is especially true for people who are in crisis or who are in the process of adjustment to a disabling condition. Too much information, or more than is asked for, should not be offered at one time. Whenever possible, the therapist should try to say something positive in every conversation. Holding out hope for the restoration of function or alternative function is important. The therapist should not assume that the client understands all of the information. To verify that the information is understood, the therapist should invite the client to ask questions and to paraphrase what has been said.

DISCOVERY OF THE "NEW" BODY

With any disability, the client's body image and perception of the body are altered. In effect, the client has a new body and must find altered ways of moving, interpreting sensations, and performing ADLs. A large part of the therapeutic experience is directed toward helping the client discover how to use this new body as effectively as possible. The therapist can facilitate this discovery of the new body by creating situations that encourage awareness of the body through the input of sensation and function.[34] The client alone or with her or his sexual partner can accomplish this awareness through exercises that encourage exploration of the body. Exercises such as the gentle tapping or rubbing of a specific area can be developed to see if sensation exists or if the stimulation causes a change in muscle tone. Many people with a disability such as paralysis report that they have experienced non-genital orgasms[9] by stimulating other new erogenous areas, often in the area just above where sensation starts to appear. The therapist may suggest ways to use this sensation or change in tone in ADLs or may ask the client to think of ways this change in tone could be used, such as triggering reflex leg extension to help putting on pants. This discussion stimulates problem solving by the client.

PLISSIT

The acronym **PLISSIT** stands for *permission, limited information, specific suggestions, and intensive therapy.* PLISSIT is a progressive approach to guide the therapist in helping the client deal with sexual information.[2] *Permission* refers to allowing the client to feel new feelings and experiment with new thoughts or ideas regarding sexual functioning. *Limited information* refers to explaining what effect the disability can have on sexual functioning. An explanation with great detail is not usually necessary early in the counseling process. The next level of information is providing *specific suggestions.* It may be in the therapist's domain to give specific suggestions on dealing with specific problems that relate to the disability, such as positioning. This is the highest level of input the average occupational therapist should attempt without advanced education and training in sexual counseling. *Intensive therapy* should be reserved for the rare client who has an abnormal coping pattern in dealing with sexuality. An extensive counseling background is needed to provide intensive therapy.

ACTIVITY ANALYSIS

To assess the client's positioning needs, the therapist must analyze the demands of the particular activity. This analysis entails looking at the physical, psychological, social, cultural, and cognitive aspects of the client's functioning. Activity analysis should be implemented using an objective and professional perspective. The therapist must realize that the sex act itself, if one exists, is only a small part of the act of making love and should be treated as just one more ADL that must be analyzed and with which the client needs professional assistance. The therapist must also remember that not all partners had sex on a daily, weekly, or even yearly basis before the onset of the disability. The therapist's values and biases should not be imposed on the client. Same-sex partners, multiple partners, masturbation, or a preference for no sexual activities are some of the client's practices that could evoke bias.

BASIC SEX EDUCATION

Some clients need basic sex education if they didn't have the information before the onset of disability. Some clients may not have been informed because of the disability, or they may be misinformed about sexual practices.[1,9,35] Research has shown that people with hearing impairments have substantially less information regarding sex than do those without hearing impairments.[53] In one study of adolescents with congenital disabilities, it was found that they were misinformed or not informed about sexual issues and that they relied on health professionals and parents to keep them informed.[4] Women who had not had sex before age 18 years may be less inclined to have sex later if they are not given sexual information.[16,21,35]

If the OT is not the one to educate the client or the client's partner, the therapist should anticipate the need for information and have resources available for the client to acquire the information. It is not advisable to recommend only books about sexuality and people with disabilities. Such books are useful, but their focus on the disability may be discouraging to some. Books written for the able-bodied, such as *The Hite Report on Male Sexuality,*[28] *The Hite Report,*[27] and *How to Satisfy a Woman Every Time,*[25] can be helpful. These books will not only give the client an understanding of sex, but will also show the client that he or she is normal, while minimizing the focus on the disability. Excellent books written for individuals with disabilities also can be recommended. Some of these are *Choices: A Guide to Sexual Counseling with the Physically Disabled,*[40] *Reproductive Issues for Persons with Physical Disabilities,*[24] *The Sensuous Wheeler,*[43] *Sexuality and the Person with Traumatic Brain Injury,*[23] *Sex and Back Pain,*[26] *Sexuality and Disabilities,*[36] *Sexual Function in People with Disability and Chronic Illness,*[48] and *Enabling Romance.*[32]

SUMMARY

This chapter began with the case of Shivani and examined some of the possible needs of people with disabilities that affect the ADLs of sexuality. This topic is a very powerful one that must be dealt with in a professional and sensitive manor by the OT. We have seen that Shivani can engage in sexual activity, become pregnant, and be a good parent. She may need assistance with finding the better positions to have sex, and she may learn to enjoy her body and sex even though she was abused. All of these issues may be within the role of the OT and should be dealt with to improve the quality of life for the client.

OTs are concerned with the sexuality of their clients because sexuality is related to self-esteem and influences the adjustment to disability and because sexual activity is an activity of daily living. As with other ADLs, a physical dysfunction can necessitate some change in performance of sexual activities. Education, counseling, and activity analysis can be used to solve many common sexual problems confronted by persons with physical dysfunction.

OTs can provide information and referrals to clients who are concerned with sexual issues. Trained therapists can provide counseling. Issues of sexual function, sexual abuse, and values need to be considered in providing sex education and counseling. Through activity analysis and problem solving, physical limitations that affect sexual functioning can usually be managed. A wide variety of sexual practices, modes of sexual expression, and expressions of sensuality are possible. The client needs the opportunity to explore her or his needs and acceptable options to meet those needs. The OT is one of the members of the rehabilitation team who has something to offer the client in the area of rehabilitation and sexuality and sensuality.

Review Questions

1. List at least five areas related to sensuality or sexuality that are usually the concerns of the OT.
2. What are some common attitudes of the able-bodied population about the sexuality of persons with physical dysfunction?
3. How do these attitudes affect the disabled person's perception of self and attitudes toward his or her own sexuality?
4. How is sexuality related to self-esteem and a sense of attractiveness?
5. Describe some typical questions for taking a sexual history. How can these questions be used to clarify values about sexuality?
6. How do mobility aids and assistive devices affect sexual functioning? How can this concern be managed?
7. What are some signs of potential sexual abuse of adults?
8. What are some suggestions for dealing with the following physical symptoms during sexual activity: hypertonia, low endurance, joint degeneration, and loss of sensation?
9. List some medications that may cause sexual dysfunction.
10. Discuss some issues and precautions relative to birth control for the woman with a physical disability.
11. How is a catheter managed during sexual activity?
12. What are some potential problems in pregnancy, delivery, and child care?
13. Discuss some techniques for educating a person about sexual issues.
14. How should sexual harassment of staff members by clients be handled?

REFERENCES

1. Andrews AB, Veronen LJ: Sexual assault and people with disabilities, *J Soc Work Human Sexuality* 8(2):137, 1993.
2. Annon JS: *The behavioral treatment of sexual problems,* vol 1-2, Honolulu, 1974, Enabling Systems.
3. Becker H, Stuifbergen A, Tinkile M: Reproductive health care experiences of women with physical disabilities: a qualitative study, *Arch Phys Med Rehabil* 78(12 Suppl 5):S26, 1997.
4. Berman H, Harris D, Enright R, et al: Sexuality and the adolescent with a physical disability: understandings and misunderstandings, *Issues Compr Pediatr Nurs* 22(4):183, 1999.
5. Black K, Sipski ML, Strauss SS: Sexual satisfaction and sexual drive in spinal cord injured women, *J Spinal Cord Med* 21(3):240, 1998.
6. Blum RW: Sexual health contraceptive needs of adolescents with chronic conditions, *Arch Pediatr Adolesc Med* 151(3):330-337, 1997.
7. Boyle PS: Training in sexuality and disability: preparing social workers to provide services to individuals with disabilities, *J Soc Work Human Sexuality* 8(2):45, 1993.
8. Braithwaite DO: From majority to minority: an analysis of cultural change from able-bodied to disabled, *Int J Intercultural Relations* 14:465, 1990.
9. Choquet M, Du Pasquier Fediaevsky L, Manfredi R: National Institute of Health and Medical Research (INSERM), Unit 169, Villejuif, France: Sexual behavior among adolescents reporting chronic conditions: a French national survey, *J Adolesc Health* 20(1):62, 1997.
10. Cole SS, Cole TM: Sexuality, disability, and reproductive issues for persons with disabilities. In Haseltine FP, Cole SS, Gray DB, editors: *Reproductive issues for persons with physical disabilities,* Baltimore, 1993, Paul H Brooks.
11. Cole SS, Cole TM: Sexuality, disability, and reproductive issues through the life span, *Sexuality and Disability* 11(3):189, 1993.
12. Cole TM: Gathering a sex history from a physically disabled adult, *Sexuality and Disability* 9(1):29, 1991.
13. Cornelius DA, Chipouras S, Makas E, et al: *Who cares? A handbook on sex education and counseling services for disabled people,* Baltimore, 1982, University Park Press.
14. Ducharme S, Gill KM: Sexual values, training, and professional roles, *J Head Trauma Rehabil* 5(2):38, 1991.
15. Edwards DF, Baum CM: Caregivers' burden across stages of dementia, *Occup Ther Practice* 2(1):13, 1990.
16. Ferreiro-Velasco ME, Barca-Buyo A, Salvador De La Barrera S, et al: Sexual issues in a sample of women with spinal cord injury, *Spinal Cord* Aug. 10, 2004.
17. Fisher TL, Laud PW, Byfield MG, et al: Sexual health after spinal cord injury: a longitudinal study, *Arch Phys Med Rehabil* 83(8):1043, 2002.
18. Froehlich J: Occupational therapy interventions with survivors of sexual abuse, *Occup Ther in Health Care* 8(2-3):1, 1992.
19. Gender AR: An overview of the nurse's role in dealing with sexuality, *Sexuality Disability* 10(2):71, 1992.
20. Giaquinto S, Buzzelli S, Di Francessco L, et al: Evaluation of sexual changes after stroke, *J Clin Psychiatry* 64(3):302, 2003.
21. Goldstein H, Runyon C: An occupational therapy education module to increase sensitivity about geriatric sexuality, *Phys Occup Ther Geriatrics* 11(2):57, 1993.
22. Greydanus DE, Rimsza ME, Newhouse PA: Adolescent sexuality and disability, *Adolescent Med* 13(2):223, 2002.
23. Griffith ER, Lemberg S: *Sexuality and the person with traumatic brain injury: a guide for families,* Philadelphia, 1993, FA Davis.
24. Haseltine FP, Cole SS, Gray DB: *Reproductive issues for persons with physical disabilities,* Baltimore, 1993, Paul H Brooks.
25. Hayden N: *How to satisfy a woman every time,* New York, 1982, Bibli O'Phile.
26. Hebert L: *Sex and back pain,* Bloomington, Minn, 1987, Educational Opportunities.
27. Hite S: *The Hite report,* New York, 1976, Macmillan.
28. Hite S: *The Hite report on male sexuality,* New York, 1981, Knopf.
29. Kettl P, Zarefoss S, Jacoby K, et al: Female sexuality after spinal cord injury, *Sexuality Disability* 9(4):287, 1991.

30. Korpelainen JT, Nieminen P, Myllyla VV: Sexual functioning among stroke patients and their spouses, *Stroke* 30(4):715, 1999.

31. Krause JS, Crewe NM: Chronological age, time since injury, and time of measurement: effect on adjustment after spinal cord injury, *Arch Phys Med Rehabil* 72:91, 1991.

32. Kroll K, Klein EL: *Enabling romance,* New York, 1992, Harmony Books.

33. Lefebvre KA: Sexual assessment planning, *J Head Trauma Rehabil* 5(2):25, 1990.

34. Lemon MA: Sexual counseling and spinal cord injury, *Sexuality Disability* 11(1):73, 1993.

35. Low WY, Zubir TN: Sexual issues of the disabled: implications for public health education, *Asia Pac J Public Health* 12 Suppl:S78, 2000.

36. Mackelprang R, Valentine D: *Sexuality and disabilities: a guide for human service practitioners,* Binghamton, NY, 1993, Haworth Press.

37. McCabe MP, Taleporos G: Sexual esteem, sexual satisfaction, and sexual behavior among people with physical disability, *Arch Sexual Behavior* 32(4):359, 2003.

38. McComas J, Hebert C, Giacomin C, et al: Experiences of students and practicing physical therapists with inappropriate patient sexual behavior, *Phys Ther* 73(11):762-769, 1993.

39. Neufeld JA, Klingbeil F, Bryen DN, et al: Adolescent sexuality and disability, *Phys Med Rehabil Clin N Am* 13(4):857, 2002.

40. Neistadt ME, Freda M: *Choices: a guide to sexual counseling with physically disabled adults,* Malabar, Fla, 1987, Krieger.

41. Nosek M, Rintala D, Young M, et al: Psychological and psychosocial disorders: sexuality issues for women with physical disabilities, *Rehabil Res Development Progress Reports* 34:244, 1997.

42. Phillips DM, Sudol KM, Taylor CL, et al: Lubricants containing N-9 may enhance rectal transmission of HIV and other STI's, *Contraception* 70(2):1007, 2004.

43. Rabin BJ: *The sensuous wheeler,* Long Beach, Calif, 1980, Barry J Rabin.

44. Rintala D, Howland C, Nosek M, et al: Dating issues for women with physical disabilities, *Sexuality Disability* 15(4):219, 1997.

45. Romeo AJ, Wanlass R, Arenas S: A profile of psychosexual functioning in males following spinal cord injury, *Sexuality Disability* 11(4):269, 1993.

46. Sandowski C: Responding to the sexual concerns of persons with disabilities, *J Soc Work Human Sexuality* 8(2):29, 1993.

47. Scott R: Sexual misconduct, *PT Magazine Phys Ther* 1(10):78, 1993.

48. Sipski M, Alexander C: *Sexual function in people with disability and chronic illness,* Gaithersburg, Md, 1997, Aspen Publishing.

49. Smith M: Pediatric sexuality: promoting normal sexual development in children, *Nurse Pract* 18(8):37, 1993.

50. Sobsey D, Randall W, Parrila RK: Gender differences in abused children with and without disabilities, *Child Abuse Negl* 21(8):707, 1997.

51. Stockard S: Caring for the sexually aggressive patient: you don't have to blush and bear it, *Nursing* 21(11):72, 1991.

52. Suris JC, Resnick MD, Cassuto N, et al: Sexual behavior of adolescents with chronic disease and disability, *Adolesc Health* 19(2):124, 1996.

53. Swartz DB: A comparative study of sex knowledge among hearing and deaf college freshmen, *Sexuality Disability* 11(2):129, 1993.

54. Verduyn WH: Spinal cord injured women, pregnancy, and delivery, *Sexuality Disability* 11(3):29, 1993.

55. Yim SY, Lee IY, Yoon SH, et al: Quality of marital life in Korean spinal cord injured patients, *Spinal Cord* 36(12):826, 1998.

56. Young ME, Nosek MA, Howland C, et al: Prevalence of abuse of women with physical disabilities, *Arch Phys Med Rehabil* 78(12 suppl 5):S34, 1997.

57. Weppner DM, Brownscheidle CM: The evaluation of the health care needs of women with disabilities, *Prim Care Update Ob Gyns* 5(4):210, 1998.

58. Zani B: Male and female patterns in the discovery of sexuality during adolescence, *J Adolesc* 14:163, 1991.

SUGGESTED READINGS

Gregory MF: *Sexual adjustment: a guide for the spinal cord injured,* Bloomington, Ill, 1993, Accent On Living.

Greydanus DE: *Caring for your adolescent: the complete and authoritative guide,* New York, 2003, Bantam Books.

Kempton W, Caparulo F: *Sex education for persons with disabilities that hinder learning: a teacher's guide,* Santa Barbara, Calif, 1989, James Stanfield.

Leyson JF: *Sexual rehabilitation of the spinal-cord-injured patient,* Totowa, NJ, 1991, Humana Press.

Mackelprang R, Valentine D: *Sexuality and disabilities: a guide for human service practitioners,* Binghamton, NY, 1993, Haworth Press.

Sandowski C: Sexual concern when illness or disability strikes, Springfield, Ill, 1989, Charles C Thomas. In *Resources for people with disabilities and chronic conditions,* ed 2, Lexington, Ky, 1993, Resources for Rehabilitation.

Shortridge J, Steele-Clapp L, Lamin J: Sexuality and disability: a SIECUS annotated bibliography of available print materials, *Sexuality Disability* 11(2):159, 1993.

Sipski M, Alexander C: *Sexual function in people with disability and chronic illness,* Gaithersburg, Md, 1997, Aspen.

Sobsey D, Gray S, editors: *Disability, sexuality, and abuse,* Baltimore, 1991, Paul H Brooks.

RESOURCES

American Association of Sex Education Counselors and Therapists
435 N. Michigan Avenue, Suite 1717, Chicago, IL 60611
(312) 644-0828

Association for Sexual Adjustment in Disability
PO Box 3579, Downey, CA 90292

Coalition on Sexuality and Disability
122 East Twenty-third Street, New York, NY 10010
(212) 242-3900

Sex Information and Education Council of the United States
    (SIECUS)
130 West Forty-second Street, Suite 2500, New York, NY 10036
(212) 819-9770

Sexuality and Disability Training Center
University of Michigan Medical Center
Department of Physical Medicine and Rehabilitation
1500 E. Medical Center Drive, Ann Arbor, MI 48109
(313) 936-7067

The Task Force on Sexuality and Disability of the American
    Congress of Rehabilitation Medicine
5700 Old Orchard Road, Skokie, IL 60077
(708) 966-0095

http://www.lookingglass.org

http://www.sexualhealth.org

13 WORK EVALUATION AND WORK PROGRAMS

DENISE HARUKO HA

JILL J. PAGE

CHRISTINE M. WIETLISBACH

KEY TERMS

Vocational evaluation
Industrial rehabilitation
Functional capacity evaluation
General vocational evaluation
Specific vocational evaluation

Job demands analysis
Essential tasks
Work hardening
Work conditioning
Worksite evaluations

Ergonomics
System theory
Ergonomic evaluation
Primary prevention
Secondary prevention

Tertiary prevention
Work-related musculoskeletal disorders
Work readiness program

LEARNING OBJECTIVES

After studying this chapter the student or practitioner will be able to do the following:

1. Understand the role of occupational therapy in the development of work programs.
2. Describe the different types of work evaluation and work programs that are currently being practiced.
3. Identify the components of an industrial rehabilitation program.
4. Understand the difference between work hardening and work conditioning.
5. Identify the aspects of a well-designed functional capacity evaluation.
6. Explain the importance of reliability and validity in the context of evaluation.

7. Understand the differences between a job demands analysis, ergonomic evaluation/hazard identification, and a worksite evaluation.
8. Discuss the application of job demands analysis.
9. Discuss basic ergonomic interventions.
10. Describe the components of injury prevention programs.
11. Describe school-to-work transition services.
12. Describe the purpose of a work readiness program.
13. Identify various community-based work programs.

CHAPTER OUTLINE

THREADED CASE STUDY: JOE, LORNA, AND HENRY, PART 1

Joe is a 26-year-old male who worked two jobs to support himself and his daughter who lived with his ex-wife. He worked as a janitor during the day at a hotel and spa, and cleaned offices at night. Due to a motor vehicle accident, he sustained a T-11 spinal cord injury, which resulted in complete paralysis of his legs. Since this injury affected his mobility, strength, and effort, he could not return to janitorial work because he would not be able to effectively carry out the essential functions of the job from a wheelchair. Fortunately one of Joe's employers, the hotel and spa, liked him because he was a good worker and was willing to offer him an alternative job as a laundry attendant if he could meet the physical demands of the job. Joe was referred to occupational therapy by his physician.

Lorna is a 39-year-old single mother who has been doing the same job at a St. Louis upholstery factory for the past 20 years. Lorna's job is to pull heavy fabric tightly over a padded wooden frame, and then staple the fabric to the frame. Once she is finished stapling, she pushes the piece of furniture over to a co-worker who checks her work and then wraps the piece of furniture in thick plastic. It is hard work and her hands and back often ache at the end of the day from pulling the fabric tightly, using the heavy staple gun, and handling the awkward furniture. With the holidays approaching, Lorna and co-workers decide to put in extra hours to make some extra money to buy presents for their children. Lorna is now experiencing significant pain, numbness, and tingling in her hands. She no longer can just shake her hands out to make this go away. She is having trouble holding onto the fabric and often drops the staple gun. She has had to take a few days off work due to the pain in her back and hands.

Henry is a 42-year-old father and husband who has been supporting his family by working as a roofer for the past 15 years. On one of his work assignments, he fell off the roof and sustained a traumatic brain injury and a couple of lower extremity fractures. As the result, his motor, process, and communication/interaction skills have been affected. He has been receiving worker's compensation for two years; now Henry feels ready to return to some type of work but does not know what he can do. He has enough insight to know that he cannot return to roofing, but would like to do something with his life.

Critical Thinking Questions

As you read through the following information on occupational therapy work evaluation and intervention keep in mind the circumstances of Joe, Lorna, and Henry to determine which services they may benefit from most.

1. What type of evaluation and services could occupational therapy offer to assist Jose, his physician, and the employer?
2. What occupational therapy interventions can help Lorna and her work environment?
3. What work-related occupational therapy services can help Henry discover what type of work he can do at this point?

One of the most significant occupations in which adults engage is work. A stable job provides the means to acquire the most basic physiological and safety requirements that humans need to survive and thrive: food and water, a safe place to sleep, and the security of knowing these resources will continue to be available. For many, belonging and esteem needs are also met at the workplace. Anything that prevents an adult from participating in the occupation of work will have significant consequences for that individual's health and well being. Occupational therapy practitioners play a key role in helping workers maintain their employment despite symptoms they experience as well as facilitating one's entry or re-entry into the workforce.

HISTORY OF OCCUPATIONAL THERAPY INVOLVEMENT IN WORK PROGRAMS

The therapeutic use of work has always been a core tenet of occupational therapy since the inception of the profession.[31] Work programs have their roots for those with mental illness during the Moral Treatment movement, which started in Europe in the late 18th and early 19th centuries.[74] In 1801, Philippe Pinel, one of the founders of Moral Treatment, first introduced work treatment in the Bicentre Asylum for the Insane. He suggested that "prescribed physical exercises and manual occupations should be employed in all mental hospitals... Rigorously executed manual labor is the best method of securing good morale...The return of convalescent patients to their previous interests, to industriousness and perseverance have always been for me the best omen of a final recovery."[77] Later in the 1800s, several psychiatric settings instituted productive activity programs.

In 1914, George Barton, one of the founding fathers of the occupational therapy profession, who was disabled by tuberculosis and a foot amputation, established the Consolation House in New York.[85] This program enabled convalescents to use occupations to return to productive living.[85] Barton stated, "the purpose of work was to divert the mind, exercise the body, and relieve the monotony and boredom of illness."[80]

In 1915, Eleanor Clarke Slagle, another founder of the occupational therapy profession, was hired to create a program for persons with mental or physical disabilities to work and become self-sufficient.[85] The program was located at Hull House, a settlement house in Chicago, and was funded by philanthropic contributions. The participants involved in the program produced goods such as baskets, needlework, toys, rugs, and cabinets, while developing manual skills and receiving wages for their work.

The early leaders of occupational therapy identified the importance of work when defining the profession's focus and purpose. Adolph Meyer, a psychiatrist who emigrated from Germany at the time and who was an early proponent of moral treatment, observed that healthy living involved a "blending of work and pleasure."[59] Dr. Herbert Hall helped establish a medical workshop at Massachusetts General Hospital in Boston, where clients were involved in "work cure."[30] In this workshop, clients produced marketable goods and received a share of the profits. The focus of treatment in these curative workshops was to restore the impaired body part to as normal function as possible, with the goal of returning the client to work.

While this curative workshop movement was transpiring on the East Coast, similar programs were developing elsewhere in the United States. For example, at the Los Angeles County Poor Farm, now recognized as Rancho Los Amigos National Rehabilitation Center in Downey, California, "all inmates were requested to do an amount of work that was commensurate with their physical strength and mental capacity, which was determined by the admitting doctor."[28] Inmates built a large amount of the furniture that was used at the farm with woodworking machinery. Commodes, bedside tables, wheelchair tables, park benches, cabinets, etc. were built in the shops. In later years when there was a true occupational therapy department, patients made Navajo-type rugs, rag or braided rugs, brushes, shawls, pottery, pictures, baskets, and leatherwork (Figure 13-1, A). Patients took special occupational therapy classes, "which were designed to enable those who are crippled, blinded or otherwise handicapped to make themselves useful" by producing articles that could be used at the County Farm, or sold to employees or the California Crafts and Industries Society in Los Angeles (Figure 13-1, B).[28]

In the early 1900s, the medical profession did not seem to consider vocational readiness programs to be important. The focus of care for persons with physical illnesses was primarily palliative, involving immobilization and bed rest. This attitude shifted after World War I with the need to rehabilitate the large numbers of injured soldiers to help them become functional and gain employment.

The U.S. Federal Board for Vocational Education (FBVE) was created after the adoption of the Vocational Education Act of 1917.[40] In 1918, the Division of Orthopaedic Surgery in the Medical Department of the Army organized a reconstruction program for disabled soldiers.[74] One of the founders of occupational therapy, Thomas Kidner, served as an advisor. This program led to the development of reconstruction aides, who were the precursors to occupational and physical therapists. Treatment involved both handicrafts and vocational education. The reconstruction aides used work activities to

return the injured soldiers to military duty or civilian life to the highest degree possible.

In 1920, Congress passed the Civilian Rehabilitation Act of 1920 (Smith-Fess Act, Public Law 66-236). This law provided funds for vocational guidance and training, work adjustment, prostheses, and placement services.[40] If therapy was part of a medical treatment program, the law provided payment for occupational therapy services; however, it did not provide payment for physician services. Physicians either provided free services or received payment through state or volunteer contributions. This limited the use of occupational therapy services in vocational rehabilitation to the states that supplemented federal program funds to support services such as the curative workshops.

The Social Security Act of 1935 defined rehabilitation as "the rendering of a person disabled fit to engage in a remunerative occupation."[52] This was the first attempt to provide vocational rehabilitation to the physically handicapped in the community.

In 1937 industrial therapy, called employment therapy, was born.[56] The occupational therapist used activities as treatment modalities. It was common for patients to have work assignments in the hospital that matched their experience, aptitude, and interest. Sheltered work environments within the hospital were used, including the hospital laundry, barber shop, and carpenter shop.

The term *prevocational* started appearing in the literature by the late 1930s. It referred to the use of crafts to develop skills readily transferable to industry.[97] Prevocational therapy prepared patients for the work role. Occupational therapists worked as directors, work evaluators, and prevocational therapists of work programs. In the 1940s, prevocational programs and work evaluation were accepted as part of the occupational therapy practice. Patients in acute care facilities who were physically disabled were transferred to outpatient or rehabilitation prevocational and vocational programs.

World War II brought more opportunities for occupational therapists to become involved in work programs. With the advancement of medicine and pharmacology, many injured soldiers survived their wounds. Federal funding for rehabilitating the disabled veterans increased as the government discharged the disabled soldiers. This led to an increase in the development of work programs designed to evaluate and rehabilitate injured veterans.[17]

In 1943, the Barden-LaFollette Act (Public Law 78-113) modified the original provisions of the Civilian Rehabilitation Act of 1920.[40] This new law, called the Vocational Rehabilitation Act, covered many medical services, including occupational therapy and vocational guidance. Services were expanded to those with physical and mental limitations. This law also created the Office of Vocational Rehabilitation, a state and federally funded agency, which is still in existence today providing job training and placement services to people with disabilities. Industrial therapy continued in various settings as a form of vocational rehabilitation.

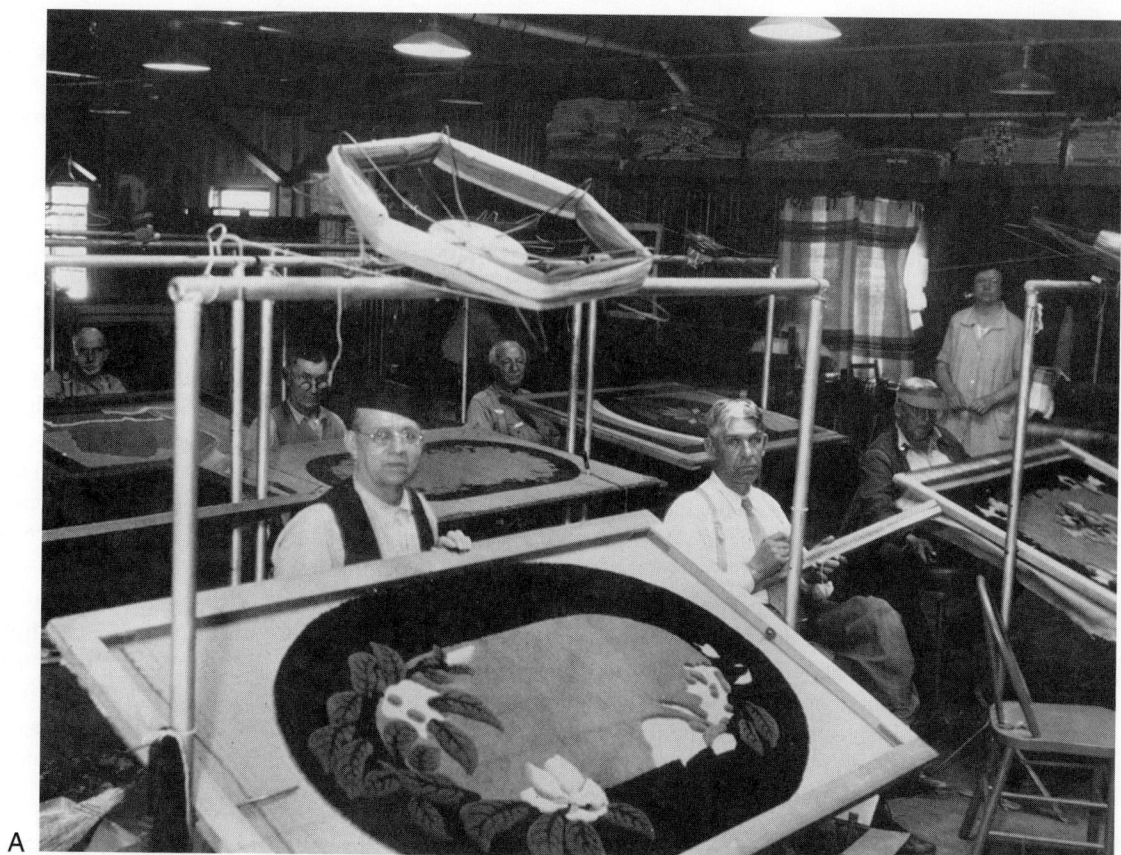

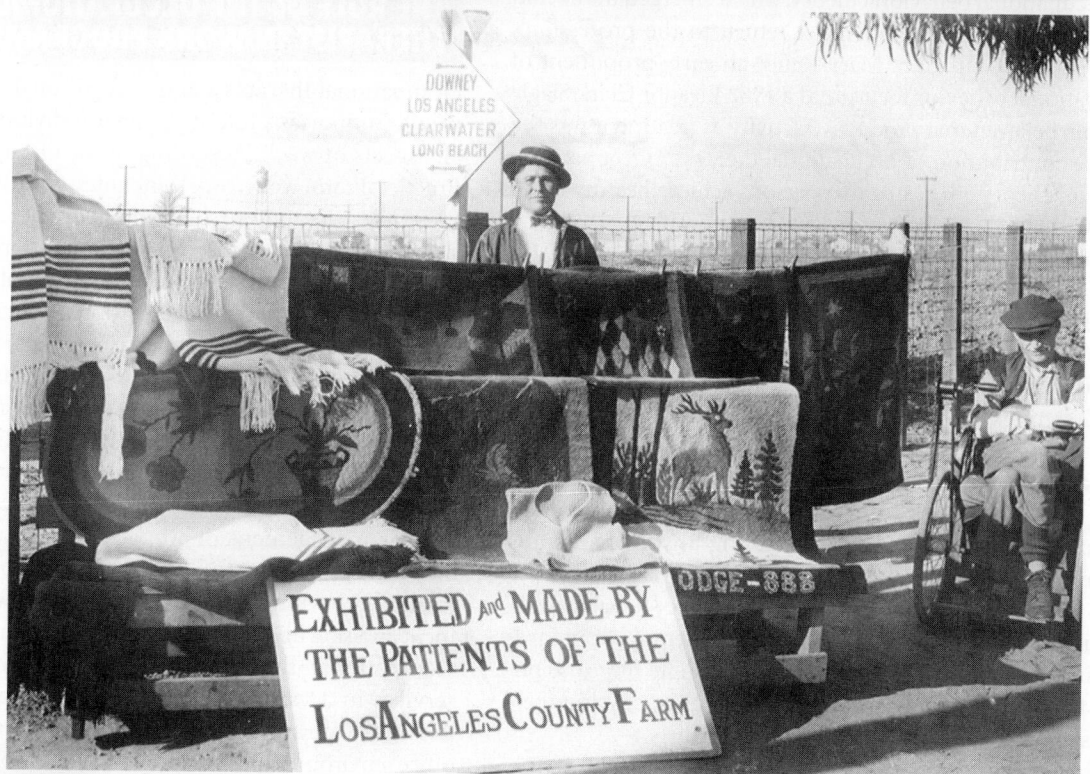

Figure 13-1 **A**, Patients at work weaving rugs in the OT shop at the LA County Poor Farm. **B**, Patients with a display of their products made at the LA County Poor Farm. (From Fliedner CA: Occupational therapy: for the body and the mind. In Rodgers GM, editor: *Centennial Rancho Los Amigos Medical Center 1888-1988*, Downey, CA 1990, Rancho Los Amigos Medical Center.)

During the 1950s, many occupational therapists believed that work evaluation belonged to a newly established profession of vocational rehabilitation rather than to occupational therapy.[56] Occupational therapy involvement declined and vocational counselors, vocational evaluators, and work adjusters were primarily the leaders in this field. There were, however, still a few occupational therapists that remained active in work programming.

A high point in the development of prevocational exploration and training techniques in the field of occupational therapy occurred in 1960.[40] Rosenberg and Wellerson published an article on the development of the TOWER (Testing, Orientation, and Work Evaluation in Rehabilitation) System in New York.[81] The TOWER system was one of the first work sample programs to use real job samples in a simulated work environment.[81] In 1959, Lilian S. Wegg gave the Eleanor Clarke Slagle Lecture on "Essentials of Work Evaluation" based on her experiences at the May T. Morrison Center for Rehabilitation in San Francisco. Wegg promoted the need for both sound testing procedures and training programs.[96] Florence S. Cromwell, a president of the American Occupational Therapy Association (AOTA), established norms for disabled populations on certain prevocational tests while evaluating the performance of adults with cerebral palsy at the United Cerebral Palsy Organization.[40] Cromwell continued to be an important work-related therapy advocate for the coming decades.

Occupational behavioral theory, which emerged in the mid 1960s and early 1970s, offered a return to the profession's concern for occupation. Mary Reilly, an early proponent of occupational behavior theory and a 1962 Eleanor Clark Slagle lecturer, believed that productive activity as treatment was the unique contribution of occupational therapy.[40] Occupational behavior theory advocated that persons achieve healthy living only with a balance between work, rest, and play.

The increasing numbers of industries in the late 1970s and early 1980s opened up a whole new arena for occupational therapists: industrial rehabilitation and work hardening.[40] **Work hardening** used actual work tasks in a simulated structured work environment, generally in community-based settings.[4] Occupational therapists used their knowledge of neuromuscular characteristics, including **range of motion** (ROM) and endurance, along with task analysis skills and knowledge of the psychosocial aspects of work in evaluating, planning, and implementing a work hardening program.

In 1989, the Commission on Accreditation of Rehabilitation Facilities (CARF) developed work hardening standards requiring an interdisciplinary approach.[15] The interdisciplinary team consisted of occupational therapists, physical therapists, psychologists, and vocational specialists.

The Americans with Disabilities Act of 1990 (ADA; Public Law 101-336) was important legislation that opened major markets for occupational therapists.[40] Occupational therapists were involved with providing work training for persons with disabilities and assistance to employers with meeting the requirements of the ADA. This legislation continues to have important implications for work practice.[23] (See Chapter 14 for more information.)

In 1992, the AOTA defined work as "all productive activities and included life roles such as homemaker, employee, volunteer, student, or hobbyist."[3] This document was replaced in 2000 by the "Occupational Therapy Services In Facilitating Work Performance (Statement)." This statement asserts that "occupational therapists and occupational therapy assistants contribute to the delivery of services for the promotion and management of productive occupations as well as the prevention and treatment of work-related disability."[2]

In 2002, the Occupational Safety and Health Administration (OSHA) unveiled a comprehensive approach to ergonomics to reduce musculoskeletal disorders (MSDs) in the workplace. Their four-pronged, comprehensive approach includes guidelines, enforcement, outreach and assistance, and a national advisory committee on ergonomics.

Occupational therapists have traditionally consulted and continue to consult with employers and employees on making recommendations about equipment, posture, and body mechanics to prevent injuries. Ergonomic intervention continues to be an area of many opportunities for occupational therapists who have received additional training and education in the area of ergonomics.

THE ROLE OF THE OCCUPATIONAL THERAPIST IN WORK PROGRAMS

Occupational therapists and occupational therapy assistants play an important role in helping individuals participate in all aspects of work. According to the Occupational Therapy Practice Framework, work includes the following: employment interests and pursuits, employment seeking and acquisition, job performance, retirement preparation and adjustment, volunteer exploration, and volunteer participation.[1] The statement: Occupational Therapy Services in Facilitating Work Performance, documents that occupational therapists provide "consultative, preventive, evaluative, restorative, and compensatory services that are designed to improve the functional work status of individuals in all age groups."[2] It further contends that occupational therapists are able to make a unique contribution to society for the prevention or management of work-related disability due to the occupational therapist's educational background in the biological and behavioral sciences, including knowledge of development and skill in evaluating all aspects of human performance. Occupational therapy practitioners provide work-related services in a variety of settings, including, but not limited to, "acute care and rehabilitation facilities; industrial sites and office environments; work-evaluation, work tolerance, and work-hardening programs, sheltered work programs, school-to-work transition programs, psychiatric treatment centers, programs for elderly persons, educational systems, community programs; and home environments."[2]

Occupational therapy practitioners are involved in assessment, direct intervention, consultation, and making recommendations for the worker, work, and workplace.[25]

Baseline information is gathered about the worker through a functional capacity evaluation. This is an objective one- to two-day assessment to determine present physical abilities to determine whether a person is able to return to any job or a specific job. A more comprehensive assessment of the worker, a **vocational evaluation**, can also be conducted by an occupational therapist when it is questionable whether a person can return to a specific job or to explore other work options. A vocational evaluation assesses work habits, work behaviors, physical and cognitive abilities, psychosocial skills, and work skills in relation to the client's interests, motivation, age, and educational level to determine a reasonable occupation for the client to pursue. These types of evaluations are being done less frequently because they are less cost efficient than a functional capacity evaluation. A vocational evaluation is typically conducted over a three- to ten-day period whereas a functional capacity evaluation is generally only a one- to two-day assessment.

After an assessment is conducted, therapy may be indicated to remediate a worker's performance deficits, or improve work behaviors or work tolerance. An occupational therapist may develop a work hardening or work conditioning program to address these deficits and build important skills and tolerances to prepare for returning to work. Other interventions may also be indicated for the worker such as providing reasonable accommodations to enable a person to work effectively.

The second component that the occupational therapist evaluates is the work that the worker performs. The occupational therapist can perform a job analysis (as well as a worksite evaluation when necessary) to look at the skills and abilities the job requires. This information about the job is used to look at the relationship between the worker and the work to determine whether the worker can perform the job despite performance deficits.[45] Therapeutic intervention may be indicated to modify how one performs the job or to modify tools and equipment. This may involve teaching an individual strategies to enable him or her to perform the job to compensate for specific deficits.

The third component that the occupational therapist evaluates is the workplace. The occupational therapist analyzes the need for modification of the equipment the worker is using or the workplace to help the person perform with greater efficiency, effectiveness, and safety.[4] The occupational therapist assesses the workplace environment to identify factors in the work environment that may be contributing to performance deficits. Recommendations for ergonomic changes to prevent work injury or fatigue may be given, as well as reasonable accommodations for the employer to enable worker performance may be indicated.

The occupational therapist practitioner thus evaluates the worker, the work, the workplace, and the relationship among them. Therapeutic intervention is employed when performance deficits are found. The occupational therapist can modify the way the worker performs the work or modify the work environment to allow the worker to perform optimally.

INDUSTRIAL REHABILITATION

The range of services provided to injured workers and industry is often encompassed by the terms "industrial" or "occupational rehabilitation." The terms will be used interchangeably in this chapter. **Industrial rehabilitation** includes functional capacity evaluation, vocational evaluation, job demands analysis, worksite evaluation, pre-employment screening, work hardening/conditioning, on-site rehabilitation, modified/transitional employment, education, ergonomics, wellness, and preventative services. Occupational therapists are integral in providing these services, and this area of practice provides a tangible way for therapists to experience the tremendous reward of seeing lives changed through their efforts. AOTA has developed a work special interest section (SIS) for those who are involved with or wish to know more about this area of specialization.

FUNCTIONAL CAPACITY EVALUATION

A **functional capacity evaluation** (FCE) is an objective assessment of an individual's ability to perform work-related activity.[51] These functionally based tests have been used since the early 1970s to assist in making return-to-work decisions and were primarily performed by occupational and physical therapists.[36] Today, however, the results of such an evaluation can be used in many different ways and are performed by a multitude of disciplines. An FCE can be used to set goals for rehabilitation and readiness for returning to work, assess residual work capacity, determine disability status, and screen for physical compatibility prior to hiring a new employee and case closure.[72]

An FCE usually consists of a review of medical records, an interview, musculoskeletal screening, evaluation of physical performance, formation of recommendations, and report generation.[43] The evaluation of physical performance usually takes the form of assessing the client's physiology, both cardiovascular and muscular endurance, over the course of strength, static, and dynamic tasks. The report usually contains information regarding the overall level of work, tolerance for work over the course of a day, individual task scores, job match information, level of client participation (cooperative or self-limiting), and interventions for consideration.[43,48]

There are a wide variety of FCEs currently used in practice today, both commercially available systems and evaluations developed by individual therapists or clinics (Box 13-1, Figure 13-2).

FCEs can be (1) all-inclusive when looking at case closure or settlement, (2) job-specific when making a match between a person's abilities and their job description, such as "cashier at XYZ store" or a broader occupational title like "cashier," or

OT PRACTICE NOTE

The referral source for an FCE can and does vary. Physicians, attorneys, case managers, insurance carriers, and other therapists are the primary sources for FCE referrals. Some states, institutions, and insurance carriers require a physician's prescription for an FCE; therefore, it is important to be aware of each state's practice act, employer, and insurance carrier guidelines for accepting referrals. Reimbursement also varies with geographical location.

(3) injury-specific, such as an upper extremity evaluation post bilateral carpal tunnel release. Joe, the 26-year-old man with T11 paraplegia, could benefit from a job-specific FCE to determine whether he can meet the physical demands of the alternative job as a laundry attendant.

A well-designed FCE is comprehensive, standardized, practical, objective, reliable, and valid.[43,48,83]

A comprehensive FCE will include all of the physical demands of work as defined by the *Dictionary of Occupational Titles*, published by the U.S. Department of Labor, last revised in 1991 (Box 13-2).[93] The main focus of Joe's FCE will be on the physical demands of work that he can still reasonably do from the wheelchair, such as lifting, sitting, carrying, pushing, pulling, balancing, reaching, handling, fingering, feeling, talking, hearing, and seeing.

It is also important for the individual being tested to understand the correlation between the test items and the functions of their job. The application of meaningful activity can improve their cooperation during testing and encourage maximum effort. For example, an individual who performs secretarial duties may have difficulty understanding the need

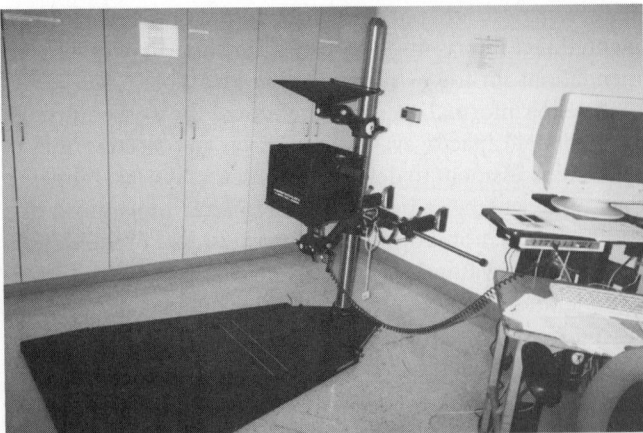

Figure 13-2 An example of a functional capacity evaluation system.

to test her ability to climb ladders if she doesn't actually perform this function during the course of her job.[72]

An FCE needs to be practical in terms of length of testing, cost, space, and report generation.[48,72]

ETHICAL CONSIDERATIONS

The tasks need to take clients' safety into account and not jeopardize their health or put them at risk for injury by allowing them to perform in an unsafe manner or push beyond their maximum level of performance.[48]

Standardization in FCEs means having a procedure manual, task definitions and instructions, a scoring methodology, and equipment requirements and set-up.[48,51,73] This type of structure helps to ensure that individuals are being assessed in a fair and consistent manner and demonstrates the effort

---

Box **13-1** VARIOUS FCE SYSTEMS
Blankenship
Key
Isernhagen
Arcon
Ergos
BTE Technologies
ErgoScience
Saunders
West/Epic
Valpar Joule
Smith
Assessworks
Assessability
Worksteps
Intertek
ISO-Machines
Company Developed Rehabilities
HealthSouth

Box **13-2** TWENTY PHYSICAL DEMANDS OF WORK	
Lifting	Kneeling
Standing	Crouching
Walking	Crawling
Sitting	Reaching
Carrying	Handling
Pushing	Fingering
Pulling	Feeling
Climbing	Talking
Balancing	Hearing
Stooping	Seeing

Data from US Department of Labor, Employment and Training Administration: *Revised dictionary of occupational titles*, Vols. I & II, ed 4, Washington, DC, 1991, US Government Printing Office.

to minimize observer bias. Verbal instructions are critical in establishing rapport between the evaluator and the individual being tested. During the initial interview, the tone is set for the course of the evaluation, and the individual's trust in the evaluator is implicit in maximizing cooperation and effort during the evaluation.[48] Objectivity is not limited to weights, distances, heights, or some other numeric quantity; subjective measures can be made objective with operational definitions. Objectivity during the course of the FCE does not exclude clinical judgment and decision making but it does require the measure to be as free as possible of examiner bias.[83] This includes physical performance as well as client cooperation during testing. This is accomplished through standardization of the testing protocol and a structured scoring methodology.

The most important aspects of an FCE are reliability and validity of the testing protocol. There are two types of reliability that are deemed to be important in an FCE: inter-rater and test-retest.[51] Inter-rater reliability in an FCE means consistency; if two therapists administer the same test to the same client will they get the same results?[43] King et al. state that, "Test-retest reliability or intra-rater reliability refers to the stability of a score derived from one administration of an FCE to another when administered by the same rater."[43] Being able to establish reliability is the first step in determining validity or accuracy of the results.[83] If there is not agreement between evaluators, then it is difficult to determine whose results are correct.[43] Once reliability has been proven, then validity can be assessed. The term validity is used in many ways, often with significance placed upon issues surrounding sincerity of effort. In scientific terms, validity means accuracy; in other words, does the FCE provide results that truly describe how the client can perform at work?[48,83]

There are several types of validity, with content, criterion (both concurrent and predictive), and construct validity having the most impact on FCE results.[43,48] *Content validity* is the easiest to establish in an FCE, as this measure refers to whether or not the evaluation tests the physical demands of work, as defined by a panel of experts, by job analysis, or by a recognized document, such as the *Dictionary of Occupational Titles* (DOT).[48,51,72,93]

Criterion validity refers to whether or not conclusions can be drawn from the measures taken and, in an FCE, this refers to whether or not a person can actually perform at the level that they demonstrated during testing.[43,48,51] This is often determined by comparing the methodology in question against a "gold standard"—another instrument that has been proven reliable and valid.[43,48,51] This is difficult to do in an FCE, as there are a limited number of available assessments with proven reliability and validity to compare against, and other methods, such as comparing the person's tested ability with their actual work level, can be seriously flawed.[54,48,51] Criterion validity includes concurrent and predictive validity.

Concurrent validity refers to the ability of a test to measure existing abilities and in an FCE this would be demonstrated by the test's ability to determine which clients can perform

at a given level and which clients cannot perform at a given level.[43,48,51]

Predictive validity is indicated by the test's capacity to predict future ability and has great value in an FCE by determining who can safely return to work and remain without injury.[43,48,57] The first FCE to be studied for validity and published in peer-reviewed literature was developed by Susan Smith, OT, and has served as an important contribution to the knowledge base.[88] Without reliability and validity, a referral source cannot know that the results of the evaluation would not vary if the individual were tested by another therapist, or if the results are accurate.[43,48,51]

VOCATIONAL EVALUATIONS

Work evaluations or vocational evaluations are "a comprehensive process that systematically uses work, real or simulated, as the focal point for vocational assessment and exploration to

ETHICAL CONSIDERATIONS

The FCE is a tremendous tool in the course of rehabilitation, allowing a therapist to have objective findings in order to make thoughtful and appropriate recommendations regarding beginning, continuation, or cessation of treatment or referring the client along to another service. Great care must be taken to ensure that the results are not derived lightly due to the enormous impact such results can have on a person's life.[43,48]

assist individuals in their vocational development."[25] According to CARF, the following factors are addressed in the traditional vocational evaluation model: physical and psychomotor capacities; intellectual capacities; emotional stability; interests, attitudes, and knowledge of occupational information; aptitudes and achievements (vocational and educational); work skills and work tolerances; work habits; work-related capabilities; and job-seeking skills.[34] These assessments can last from three to ten consecutive days depending on the goals of the assessment. Vocational evaluators generally conduct these types of assessments in private vocational agencies; however, some occupational therapists have been involved in conducting these evaluations as well in public and private medical or nonmedical settings. Vocational Rehabilitation (VR), worker's compensation, and long-term disability carriers pay for these services but most medical plans do not.

Standardized work samples such as the Valpar Component Work Sample System or the Jewish Employment Vocational Services are used to assess specific skills in the areas of data or things (Figure 13-3). Dexterity tests such as the Bennett Hand Tool, Crawford Small Parts, and the Purdue Pegboard are used to evaluate motor skills (Figure 13-4).[34] When there are no standardized work samples available to assess specific

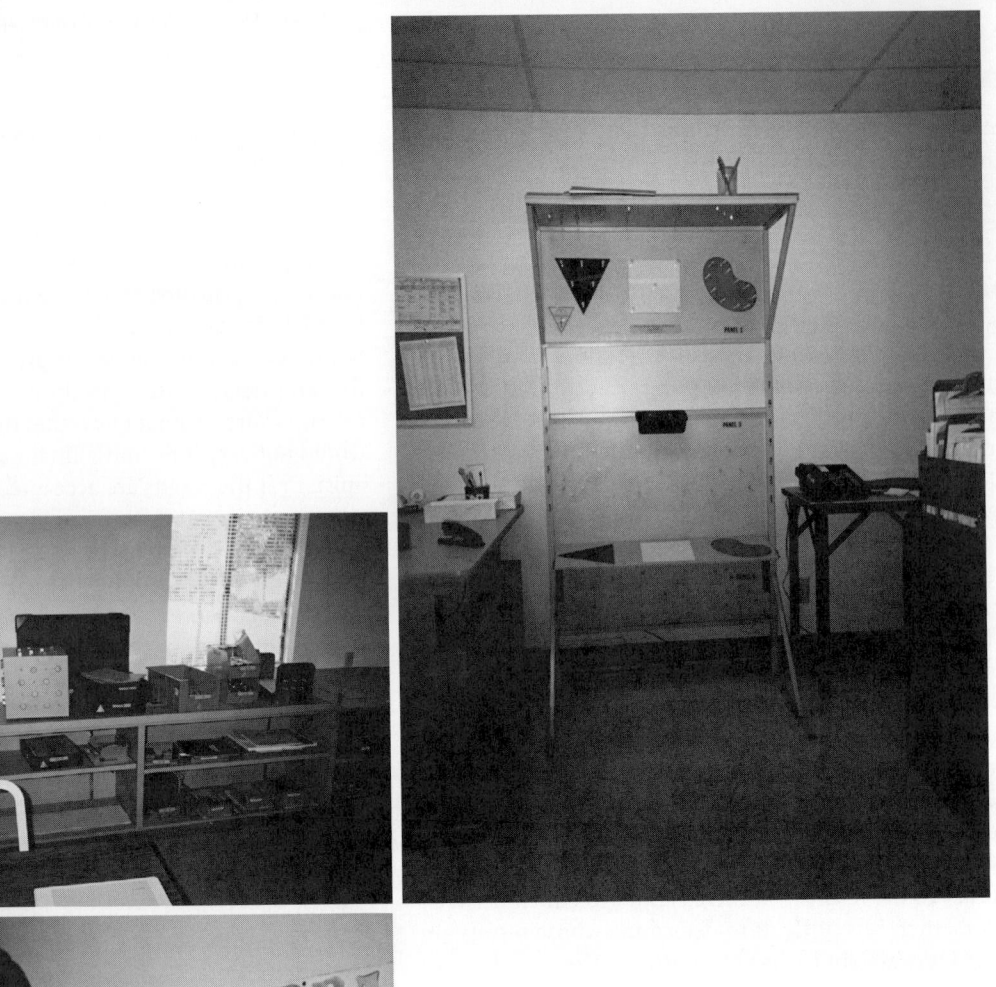

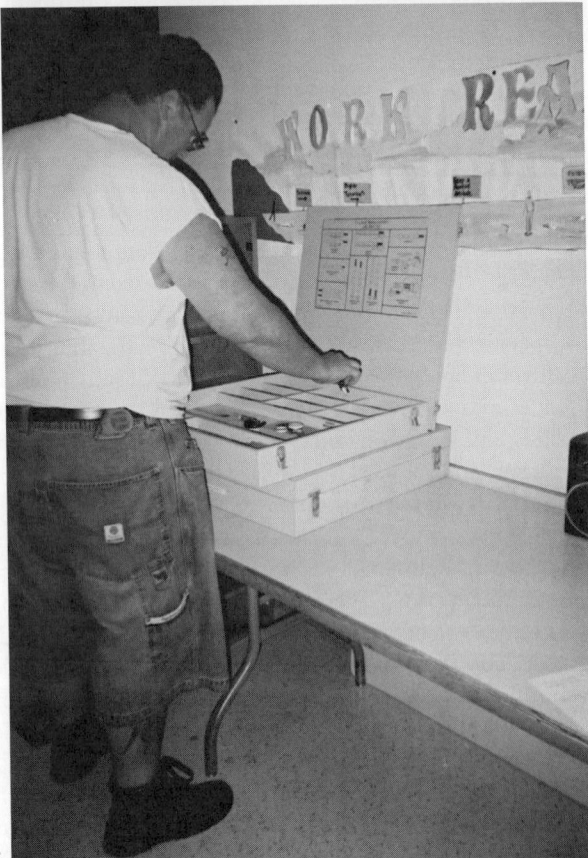

Figure 13-3 **A**, Valpar and JEVS work samples. **B**, Valpar 9 Total Body Range of Motion work sample, which is used to evaluate functional abilities such as standing, bending, crouching, reaching, and gross manipulation and handling. **C**, The Valpar 10 Tri-Level Measurement is used to evaluate a person's ability to follow a multi-step sequence to inspect metal parts using various jigs and tools.

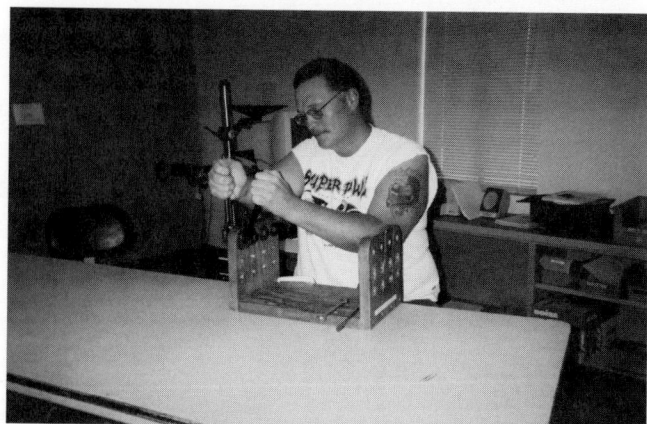

Figure 13-4 The Bennett Hand Tool is a dexterity test to assess a person's ability to use hand tools.

skills needed for a particular occupation, specially designed situational assessments are also used to create real life work situations that are related to actual work tasks that would be conducted on particular jobs. For example, a person who is interested in working as a floral arranger could be evaluated on her motor skills to see if she has the coordination, energy, and strength and effort to grip and manipulate tools to cut the stems of flowers and plants and arrange them in floral containers. Individuals can also be evaluated in real work-sites and perform actual job tasks that one would perform on the job.

There are generally two different types of vocational evaluations: a general vocational evaluation and a specific vocational evaluation. A **general vocational evaluation** is a comprehensive assessment to evaluate a person's potential to do any type of work. For an individual who has never worked, does not have a job to return to, or cannot return to the previous job because of their disability, this type of evaluation is beneficial in determining one's aptitudes, abilities, and interests to explore all reasonable options for work. For example, Henry, the roofer who experienced a traumatic brain injury due to a fall while working, could benefit most from a general vocational evaluation to explore other options for employment. A general vocational evaluation could help identify other vocational interests and abilities by exploring this person's cognitive and motor skills and physical and mental tolerances that could be applied to a different occupation. A **specific vocational evaluation** assesses a person's readiness to return to a particular occupation. For a person who had a stroke and wants to return to work as a general office clerk, a specifically tailored vocational evaluation to assess the person's ability to return to this particular type of work can be done. Clerical work samples and specially designed situational assessments that gauge the person's ability to multi-task, pay attention to detail, file, answer a telephone, and take messages can be incorporated as an integral component of the vocational evaluation.

JOB DEMANDS ANALYSIS

Assessing the physical demands of a job is often beneficial in the rehabilitation process, as recommendations for initial or return to work require objective information about both the client's abilities and the job itself. A well-written job description, which includes the essential tasks of the job, physical requirements, cognitive aptitudes, educational requirements, equipment operated, and environmental exposures, assists in selecting suitable candidates for employment, setting compensation packages, and making appropriate return-to-work decisions after an injury.[8]

A **job demands analysis** (JDA) does not need to be confused with ergonomic evaluations or hazard identification and abatement. A JDA looks to define the actual demands of the job, while ergonomic evaluations and hazard assessment focus more on the work practice and the risk for injury secondary to postural or manual material-handling extremes or excesses.[8] Certainly, these areas can overlap, but it is important to be clear on the differences and the reasons behind the request for information and to use suitable methods for each.[8]

Approaches to a JDA include questionnaires, interviews, observations, and formal measurement.[8] It is common to interview incumbents or supervisors about the job requirements.[72] Such an informal approach often leads to narrative descriptions with little functional information and questionable accuracy of demand estimates.[72] As with other types of assessment, it is important to have an objective process for analyzing the demands of the job. In the context of attempting to make return-to-work decisions based upon matching the results of an FCE with the job description, many FCEs include a JDA component.[48] However, these are often subjective interviews with the client and can lack accuracy regarding the physical demands.

The occupational therapist who was working with Joe contacted the employer and conducted a JDA to obtain a complete picture of the job demands and requirements of the laundry attendant position. The occupational therapist spoke to the supervisor as well as other employees while they were performing the actual job at the worksite. Being able to actually observe the job being done in the real work environment allowed the occupational therapist to gather the information needed to adequately assess Joe's ability to carry out the essential functions of this job.

It is crucial to have a standardized classification system in order to have consistency among terminology and professionals. The *Dictionary of Occupational Titles* (DOT) defines the physical demands of work and defines occupations in the United States (Tables 13-1 through 13-3).[93] It provides definitions for the overall level of work, strength demands, and frequencies for the physical demands.[93,94] Many countries around the world also refer to the DOT as their primary reference for generic occupational descriptions.

The DOT was last revised in 1991, and in the early 1990s, the US government made the decision not to revise the DOT

TABLE 13-1 **Definitions for Overall Level of Work**

Level of Work	Definition
Sedentary	Exerting up to 10 pounds of force occasionally or a negligible amount of force frequently to lift, carry, push, pull, or otherwise move objects, including the human body. Sedentary work involves sitting most of the time, but may involve walking or standing for brief periods of time. Jobs are Sedentary if walking and standing are required only occasionally, but all other Sedentary criteria are met.
Light	Exerting up to 20 pounds of force occasionally, or up to 10 pounds of force frequently, or a negligible amount of force constantly to move objects. Physical demand requirements are in excess of those for Sedentary Work. Even though the weight lifted may be only a negligible amount, a job should be rated Light Work: (1) when it requires walking or standing to a significant degree; or (2) when it requires sitting most of the time, but entails pushing or pulling of arm or leg controls; or (3) when the job requires working at a production rate pace entailing the constant pushing or pulling of materials even though the weight of those materials is negligible. NOTE: The constant stress and strain of maintaining a production rate pace, especially in an industrial setting, can be and is physically demanding of a worker even though the amount of force exerted is negligible.
Medium	Exerting 20-50 pounds of force occasionally, or 10-25 pounds of force frequently, or greater than negligible up to 10 pounds of force constantly to move objects. Physical demand requirements are in excess of those for Light Work.
Heavy	Exerting 50-100 pounds of force occasionally, or 25-50 pounds of force frequently, or 10-20 pounds of force constantly to move objects. Physical demand requirements are in excess of those for Medium Work.
Very Heavy	Exerting force in excess of 100 pounds of force occasionally, or in excess of 50 pounds of force frequently, or in excess of 20 pounds of force constantly to move objects. Physical demand requirements are in excess of those for Heavy work.

Data compiled from US Department of Labor, Employment and Training Administration: *Revised Dictionary of Occupational Titles*, Vol. I & II, ed 4, Washington, DC, 1991, US Government Printing Office; US Department of Labor, Employment and Training Administration: *The Revised Handbook for Analyzing Jobs*, Indianapolis, IN, 1991, JIST Works.

TABLE 13-2 **Definitions for Physical Demand Frequencies**

Physical Demand Frequency	Definition
Never	Activity or condition does not exist
Occasionally	Up to 1/3 of the day
Frequently	1/3 to 2/3 of the day
Constantly	2/3 to full day

Data compiled from US Department of Labor, Employment and Training Administration: *Revised Dictionary of Occupational Titles*, Vol. I & II, ed 4, Washington, DC, 1991, US Government Printing Office; US Department of Labor, Employment and Training Administration: *The Revised Handbook for Analyzing Jobs*, Indianapolis, IN, 1991, JIST Works.

TABLE 13-3 **Strength Demands of Work**

	Frequency of force exertion or weight carried		
Strength Rating	**Occasional (up to 1/3 of the day)**	**Frequent (1/3 to 2/3 of the day)**	**Constant (over 2/3 of the day)**
Sedentary	10 lb	Negligible	Negligible
Light	20 lb	10 lb	Negligible
Medium	20-50 lb	10-25 lb	10 lb
Heavy	50-100 lb	25-50 lb	10-20 lb
Very Heavy	Over 100 lb	50-100 lb	20-50 lb.

Data from US Department of Labor, Employment and Training Administration: *Revised Dictionary of Occupational Titles*, Vol. I & II, ed 4, Washington, DC, 1991, US Government Printing Office.

again, but instead to create a new format for classifying occupations.[27] The intent was to create a more generic classification system or framework for defining work. The American Institutes of Research (AIR) was awarded a contract by the Utah Department of Employment Security on behalf of the US. Department of Labor and they developed the O*NET 98 Database. While the new format includes an enormous amount of data, its design makes it very difficult for rehabilitation professionals to use in a qualitative fashion. Based upon feedback from professional organizations and the rehab community, the design is being revisited before any final adoptions are made. It is recommended that both the DOT and O*NET be consulted when obtaining occupational information.[27]

In terms of recent legislation that impacts employment law, both the Americans With Disabilities Act (ADA) and the Equal Employment Opportunities Commission (EEOC) define **essential tasks** as being the reason that the job exists.[5,8] The ADA further defines essential tasks as being those that are highly specialized, i.e., the reason the incumbent was hired to perform the job, and that there are a limited number of people available at the job site to perform the tasks.[5] During the course of JDA, it is important to distinguish between tasks that are essential and those that are not. This can be challenging because it is a nontraditional way to look at the job for both the employee and the employer. It is important that both hiring and *return-to-work* (RTW), decisions be based upon job descriptions that define the essential tasks to be congruent with both ADA and the EEOC language.

OT PRACTICE NOTE

In preparation for an observational JDA, an interview can be conducted on the telephone to glean initial information about the job to allow for adequate research on the job title and equipment. Advance preparation also aids in selecting personal protective equipment that needs to be worn while performing the analysis.

Jobs are composed of the tasks that are performed, the physical demands that make up the tasks, and the frequency with which the physical demands are performed, including weights handled, forces exerted, and distances both ambulated and reached.[8] The frequency of each physical demand must be weighted appropriately for the given duration of each task, as there is often significant difference in the amount of time spent on each task during the workday. For example, the job of "loader" in ABC warehouse is composed of two tasks: (1) loading crates with boxes and (2) wrapping the crate with packing tape when loaded. The loader completes 48 cycles of loading and taping in an eight-hour shift, with loading the crate taking approximately 80% of the work-shift. The boxes weigh 10 lb. each. To correctly assess the overall level of work, the amount of weight lifted must be determined, as well as the frequency of the manual materials handling.

Task 1 is composed of the physical demands of lifting, carrying, stooping, walking, reaching, handling, and standing. Task 2 is composed of walking, reaching, handling, fingering, and standing. To correctly sum the amount of the physical demands for the job of loader, one must determine how much time is spent in each physical demand within each task and then account for the proportion of the time that the task is performed during the workday. This type of assessment can be performed manually, as well as with the application of various software protocols available in the marketplace, such as the ErgoScience Quantitative Job Demands Analysis.[49]

ETHICAL CONSIDERATIONS

Whatever methods are selected, clinicians should strive towards providing an accurate picture of the job and its requirements, with an emphasis on functional demands for easier application in the rehabilitation continuum.

WORK HARDENING/WORK CONDITIONING

The idea of using work for rehabilitation is at the very core of occupational therapy. In the 1970s, the idea of occupational rehabilitation developed from the necessity of improving strategies to control work-related injuries.[19,42,50,71] Work hardening was first illustrated conceptually by Leonard Matheson, a psychologist at Rancho Los Amigos, who worked very closely with Linda Dempster, an OT, in developing his materials.[42,50,71] The goal was then, and remains now, to rehabilitate injured workers, maximize their function, and return them to work as quickly and safely as possible. The delivery system for this type of rehabilitation has evolved over time from a lengthy hospital-based program, to structured interdisciplinary programs in outpatient settings, to the more progressive partnership between outpatient intervention and transitional work, as well as rehabilitation occurring at the workplace in company-sponsored clinics. In the 1980s, the Commission on Accreditation of Rehabilitation Facilities (CARF) developed guidelines for work hardening programs and offered certification for a fee through adherence to their guidelines and periodic survey.[19,42,50,71] In 1991, a committee from the American Physical Therapy Association (APTA) developed another set of principles for clinics that wanted to follow recognized standards, but did not want to undertake the accreditation process of the CARF.[19,42,50]

Work hardening refers to formal, multidisciplinary programs for rehabilitating the injured worker.[19,42,50,71] The disciplines represented on the team can often include occupational and physical therapists and assistants, psychologists, vocational evaluators and counselors, licensed professional counselors, addiction counselors, exercise physiologists, and dieticians.[19,42,50] The programs typically range from 4-8 weeks, with entry and exit evaluation (usually an FCE or a derivative thereof), a job site evaluation, graded activity, both work simulation and strength and cardiovascular conditioning, education, and individualized goal setting and program modification, with a goal of return to work at either full or modified duty.[19,42,50] Actual equipment from the job is preferred during the work simulation, to maximize the cooperation of the worker and more closely replicate the actual demands of the job.[42] **Work conditioning** is more often defined as physical conditioning alone, which covers strength, aerobic fitness, flexibility, coordination, and endurance and generally involves a single discipline.[19,42,40] Both approaches involve evaluation of the worker to establish a baseline from which to plan treatment and measure progress.

Motivational issues are a constant concern and are often thought to be at the forefront of unsuccessful return to work.[87] The injured worker can develop maladaptive behaviors regarding return to work influenced by depression, financial issues, family pressures, and feeling manipulated by the "system."[87] This can lead to employer mistrust, interest in litigation, and the need to exaggerate symptoms. Fraud on the part of the injured worker is also a concern.[87] Employer indifference is a concern and can have remarkable impact on a worker's attitude toward returning to their job.[87] Surveys of attitudes among employers have indicated that activity on the part of the employer can affect costs; as many as 90% of respondents indicated that how well the employee perceived that he or she was treated at the time of injury was associated with decreased injury costs.[87]

OT PRACTICE NOTE

It is essential for the therapist to encourage the employer to be involved with the employee after the injury, investigating injury claims that are worthy of investigation, calling to inquire about how the employee is feeling, and considering modified duty and transitional work options to promote a successful return to work.

Think about Lorna, the upholsterer who is experiencing hand problems, and the difficulties she is experiencing at work. An occupational therapist could evaluate her symptoms and her job description and make suggestions to the employer about modifying her job demands to allow her to continue to work during treatment. This demonstrates to Lorna that her well-being matters and can help her to have a positive outcome with treatment.

Ensuring positive outcome for the injured worker requires early intervention and a customized plan of treatment to address the various areas impacted by the injury, which includes both physical and psychosocial.[87] The incorporation of a multidisciplinary team allows the patient to have the benefit of many areas of expertise working toward his or her common good. Intervening and initiating the rehabilitation program as soon as possible following the injury dramatically increases the chances for a successful return to work. Based upon a study of 5620 worker's compensation beneficiaries, there was a 47% return-to-work rate for workers referred to rehabilitation within the first three months post injury with a cost savings of 71%. When referred during months 4 through 6, the rates dropped to 33% for return to work and 61% for cost savings. For those referred beyond 12 months after injury, only 18% returned to work, with cost savings dropping to 51%.[87]

Transitional work and modified duty programs involve a combination or a progression of acute rehabilitation and return to work at a level consistent with the individual's current ability, with a goal of returning to work full duty, or to maximize the individual's work capacity. An example of transitional duty would have a worker performing work conditioning activities under supervision in an outpatient clinic from 8-10 AM and then going to the worksite and performing the less physically demanding portions of his job from 11 AM to 1 PM, breaking for lunch, and then returning to the "lighter" duties of his job for the duration of the shift. More regular duty activities are added under supervision as his skill and strength improve, eventually returning to full duty. This type of structure provides a much better environment for the worker to be involved in the work culture and allows the co-workers and supervisors to participate in job modification and the overall recovery of the injured worker.[87] Modified duty follows a similar path but typically does not include the clinical portion of the day. There are challenges with return to work at less than full duty, however, as some employers do not want a worker to return to the site unless they are at "100%." It is imperative to demonstrate the benefit to the company and the employee, both economically and psychologically, of the early transitional return to the long-term success of returning the employee to the work force.

Industrial rehabilitation programs will continue to change as the tides of economy, industry needs, and legislation move forward. Occupational therapists are key in directing the changes that lie ahead.

WORKSITE EVALUATIONS

Worksite evaluations are on-the-job assessments to determine if an individual can return to work after onset of a disability or whether a person can benefit from reasonable accommodations to maintain employment.[39,91] For example, a man who worked at a manufacturing company as a machine operator incurs a stroke and the employer is willing to take him back as long as he can meet the physical and cognitive demands of the job. An occupational therapist can go to the worksite to evaluate the person's ability to safely and adequately operate the machinery and carry out the essential functions of the job. Consider another example. A person who previously worked as an office clerk without any difficulties is now experiencing extreme fatigue, pain, and muscle weakness with repetitive tasks due to post polio syndrome. This person could benefit from a worksite evaluation to identify reasonable accommodations to allow her to continue working at this job while minimizing her symptoms. Several factors are assessed at the worksite with the worker present: the essential functions of the job, the functional assets and limitations of the worker, and the physical environment of the workplace.[53]

A worksite evaluation is usually conducted after a job analysis has been done. Larger companies may already have information on job analyses done on specific jobs. If a job analysis has not been done then the occupational therapist can conduct a job analysis if the employer is willing, or a job description could be obtained from the employer before going out to the worksite. If there is no written job description, then a phone call to the supervisor/manager of the worker should be made to obtain verbal information regarding the essential functions of the job and the physical and cognitive requirements of the job. After this information is obtained, then the occupational therapist schedules a time with the employer and the worker to meet at the worksite. This is exactly what happened with Joe as he prepared to switch from the job of janitor to laundry attendant at the hotel and spa. After the occupational therapist conducted the job analysis, Joe met with both the occupational therapist and the employer at the worksite for the worksite evaluation.

When the occupational therapist meets the employer and worker at the worksite, the occupational therapist assesses the work, the worker, and the workplace. The evaluation begins with the analysis of the essential functions that may require accommodation.[91] The occupational therapist should have an idea of what these are based on the information obtained prior to going out to the worksite. The desired outcome of the work tasks should be emphasized, not just the process of performing the essential function.[91] The occupational therapist should find out certain details, such as how the outcome will be affected if a particular task is done incorrectly, in a different sequence, or omitted; whether there are quotas, standards, or time constraints that must be met;[76] and whether the frequency with which a task is done will affect the outcome.

Activity analysis is a useful tool in evaluating a person at their worksite.[10] It can be used to address all areas including the following: motor, sensory, cognitive, perceptual, emotional and behavioral, cultural, and social. When assessing the person's ability to carry out the essential functions of the job, the occupational therapist has expertise in breaking down the tasks and determining with which parts of the task the worker is having difficulty or may have difficulty over the course of a workday. The occupational therapist can suggest accommodations to allow the worker to carry out the essential functions of the job.

The final step in the worksite evaluation is to assess the work environment. The environment outside the immediate work area should be assessed (parking if driving or access to public transportation; access into the building, break room, and restroom), as well as the workstation itself. All work areas that the worker may use need to be investigated to identify obstacles and solutions to increase accessibility. The location and placement of machines, supplies, and equipment that the worker needs to access should be assessed as well as other environmental factors, such as lighting, temperature, and noise level.

Taking photographs or video recordings at the worksite can be very useful; however, permission must be obtained from the employer as well as the worker to do so. The occupational therapist should also bring a tape measure to measure heights of work surfaces, widths of doorways, etc. depending on the person's needs. Drawing a layout of the work area using graph paper to draw the room to scale is also very helpful, especially when the worker is in a wheelchair. Critical measurements can be recorded on the diagram.

The outcome of the worksite evaluation is to determine whether the person can safely and adequately carry out the essential functions of the job with or without any reasonable accommodations. Ergonomic principles (addressed in the following section) should be considered and applied when recommending reasonable accommodations. The process of identifying reasonable accommodations requires cooperation between the person with the disability, the employer, and the occupational therapist.[76] Each person has valuable insights and information to contribute to the process of identifying the best accommodations. The Job Accommodation Network (JAN), a product of the President's Committee for the Employment of People with Disabilities, is the best resource for assisting employers and disabled workers with reasonable accommodations (*http://janweb.icdi.wvu.edu/*).[84] Their website points out that most job accommodations are not usually expensive. According to the JAN, over half of all accommodations cost under $500. They can involve any of the following: altering the job duties or work schedule, modifying the facility, purchasing adaptive equipment or assistive technology, or modifying or designing a new product (Table 13-4).

After the worksite evaluation is completed, a report is prepared and sent to the qualified employee, the referring party, and the employer. The problem areas that relate to the essential

TABLE **13-4** **Examples of Accommodations**

Job	Functional Problem	Accommodation	Approximate Cost
Forklift driver	Difficulty gripping steering wheel due to arthritis	Steering ball	$100
CAD/CAM drafting specialist	Limited use of upper extremities due to tetraplegia	Speech-activated software	$500
Factory worker	Difficulty standing 10 hours a day due to back impairment	Sit-lean stool and anti-fatigue matting	$250
Retail salesperson	Fatigue from diabetes and needed extra breaks to administer medication	Schedule was altered to allow for a longer meal break and periods during the day to administer medication	$0
Elementary school teacher	Having difficulty hearing students due to the noise of screeching chairs moving against the floor	Teacher was permitted to cut holes in donated tennis balls and place them on the legs of the chairs	$0

Data from Job Accommodation Network website, *www.jan.wvu.edu.*

job functions should be clearly listed as well as the accommodations necessary to solve them. If training is necessary to use a recommended accommodation, those sources for the training should be identified. If commercially available equipment is recommended, exact model numbers, local sources, and approximate expenses should be provided.[91] If custom equipment needs to be fabricated, then sources, cost estimates, and the amount of time required to fabricate the equipment should be included as well. The report should summarize the evaluation findings and the accommodations that were recommended.

After Joe's worksite evaluation, it was determined that he could safely and dependably carry out the essential functions of the job from his wheelchair. Just one accommodation was recommended and implemented. Since it got very hot in the laundry room and Joe was sensitive to the heat, the employer agreed to purchase additional fans to ventilate the room better as well as allow the door to the laundry room to be propped open. The employer agreed to schedule Joe's shift in the evening or early morning when it was cooler to avoid having to work in the heat of the day.

ERGONOMICS

All aspects of the domain of occupational therapy must be in harmony in order for people to fully engage in the occupation of work. The activity demands of the job and context in which the job is performed must fit with the employee's abilities and physical/psychosocial makeup. Any mismatch between the activity demands of the job and context, individual client factors, and performance patterns will interfere with successful execution of appropriate performance skills required to do the job.

Occupational therapists use the science of ergonomics to assist clients in fully engaging in the occupation of work. **Ergonomics** addresses human performance and well-being in relation to one's job, equipment, tools, and environment. The goal of ergonomics is to improve the health, safety, and efficiency of both the worker and the workplace.[65] The term *ergonomics* comes from the Greek words *ergos*, meaning "work," and *nomos*, meaning "laws"—hence, the laws of work.[20] A Polish educator and scientist, Wojciech Jastrzebowski (1799-1882), introduced the term *ergonomics* in the literature about 150 years ago.[18] However, the concept of ergonomics—that there is some connection between physical well-being and type of work performed—is as old as humanity: "From the very first tool of the Stone Age, humans have tried to find better ways of working, taking advantage of human talents and making up for human shortcomings."[54]

The idea behind ergonomics is that every worker brings his or her own unique set of performance skills, performance patterns, and client factors to the workplace. Many times work settings and work processes are designed to satisfy space and budget limitations and the demands of productivity and aesthetics. When these designs fail to take into account the *people* who will be using the work setting and process, injury and inefficiency can result. Finding a way to match individual employees' strengths and limitations with the context and activity demands of a job can improve both worker safety and workplace productivity.

The principles of ergonomics help to address a variety of work-related issues. Common issues include workplace and work process design, work-related stress, the disabled and aging workforces, tool and equipment design, and architectural design and accessibility. Ergonomic intervention can be applied proactively, preventing problems before they occur, or reactively, adjusting the worker-job-context "fit" when problems do occur. Many occupational therapists use ergonomic principles as part of their comprehensive rehabilitation or wellness and prevention client-centered programs. A few occupational therapists specialize in ergonomics and become professional ergonomists.

With regard to ergonomic services, the occupational therapist's client base may include the individual worker, workers in the context of employee groups, and/or the employer itself. The environment for the occupational therapist providing ergonomic services is generally at the client's place of work. These occupational therapists must become skilled in navigating what can be an unfamiliar business world with its unique lingo, social norms, and traditions. However, the occupational therapist providing ergonomic services shares a similar focus with occupational therapists in all areas of practice, that is, a focus on marketing and sale of the product (in ergonomics-wellness), cost effectiveness, definable outcomes, and client satisfaction.

Occupational therapists are not the only professionals suited to specialize in the field of ergonomics. Ergonomics professionals come from a variety of backgrounds. It is not unusual to see ergonomists who have been academically trained in industrial hygiene, engineering, safety, business administration, human resources, medicine, physical/occupational rehabilitation, psychology, architecture, epidemiology, or computer science.[18] For the occupational therapist, the road to becoming a professional ergonomist can take many paths. Box 13-3 outlines a variety of methods for acquiring advanced knowledge and certification in the field of ergonomics.

For the occupational therapist interested in the field of ergonomics, the holistic nature of occupational therapy training is an asset. The occupational therapist immediately understands that the goal of ergonomic intervention, achieving the perfect fit between an individual worker and his or her job and context, is never simplistic. In the domain of occupational therapy, the worker component is composed of performance skills, performance patterns, and client factors. The job component is composed of activity demands, both of the job tasks and tools/equipment. Engaging in the occupation of work occurs in a variety of contexts, including the environment and organization, as well as the worker's personal, cultural, social, and spiritual contexts.

Box **13-3**   EDUCATION AND TRAINING OPPORTUNITIES IN ERGONOMICS

Education and training beyond occupational therapy entry-level practice is necessary for achieving advanced competence in ergonomics.

- University-sponsored graduate certificate programs in ergonomics are available through Texas Women's University, Cleveland State University, University of Central Florida, and the University of Massachusetts. These graduate-level courses typically require four to five courses for a total of 12-16 credit hours.
- Continuing education providers offer several-day courses that, upon completion, allow the occupational therapist eligibility for certifications such as the Ergonomics Evaluation Specialist available through Roy Matheson and Associates, Inc. (*www.roymatheson.com*) and the Certified Ergonomics

Assessment Specialist available through the Back School of Atlanta (*www.backschoolofatlanta.com*).

- The Oxford Research Institute (*www.oxfordresearch.org*) offers the following advanced-level certifications: Certified Industrial Ergonomist, Certified Associate Ergonomist, and Certified Human Factors Engineering Professional.
- The Board of Certification in Professional Ergonomics (BCPE) (*www.bcpe.org*) offers the highest level of certification in the field of ergonomics—the Certified Professional Ergonomist. Other advanced-level certifications available through the BCPE include Associate Ergonomics Professional, Certified Ergonomics Associate, Certified Human Factors Professional, and Associate Human Factors Professional.

Data from Snodgrass J: Getting comfortable: developing a clinical specialty in ergonomics has its own challenges and rewards, *Rehab Management* p. 24, July 2004.

Observing independent aspects of the domain offers the observer limited insight. Rather, it is the interactions between the various aspects of the domain that reveal the whole picture. This way of looking at worker performance via the interactions of all aspects of the domain of occupational therapy is known as **system theory**. Rannell Dahl, MS, OTR, explains that the "components of work systems are workers, job tasks, tools and equipment, work environments, and organizational structure, and the interactions among these components."[18] Dahl offers an excellent schematic of this concept of the ergonomics work system (Figure 13-5).

In his groundbreaking text, *Conceptual Aspects of Human Factors*, David Meister explained that in human factors (ergonomics), the system concept is the belief that human performance in work can only be meaningfully conceptualized in terms of organized wholes. He emphasized the fundamental Gestalt ideas that "the whole is more than the sum of its parts, that the parts cannot be understood if isolated from the whole, and that the parts are dynamically interrelated or interdependent."[57] Occupational therapists understand that one can conceive of worker performance only in terms of the interaction between performance skills, performance patterns, context, activity demands, and client factors. The Occupational Therapy Practice Framework supports this concept:

Engagement in occupation includes both the subjective (emotional or psychological) aspects of performance and the objective (physically observable) aspects of performance. Occupational therapists and occupational therapy assistants understand engagement from this duel and holistic perspective and address all aspects of the performance (physical, cognitive, psychological and contextual).[1]

Jeffrey Crabtree, OTD, OTR, FAOTA, adds that it is "the subjective meaning of the interactions in the human-work-machine-environment model (that) is central to occupational therapy and ergonomics."[16]

The system theory does not discount the importance of adequacy of the independent aspects of the domain of occupational therapy. The quality of the work system can suffer if there are deficiencies or deviations in performance skills, performance patterns, context, activity demands, or individual client factors. Dahl explains that each component of the ergonomics work system (see Figure 13-5) "has its own set of characteristics that affect the performance of the work system"[18] as a whole. It is here that ergonomic assessment and intervention seek to make a difference in the quality of our clients' engagement in the occupation of work. The ergonomic practitioner modifies and strengthens certain aspects of the system with the goal of enhancing the overall quality of the work system interactions (i.e., improving the fit between the worker and his or her job).

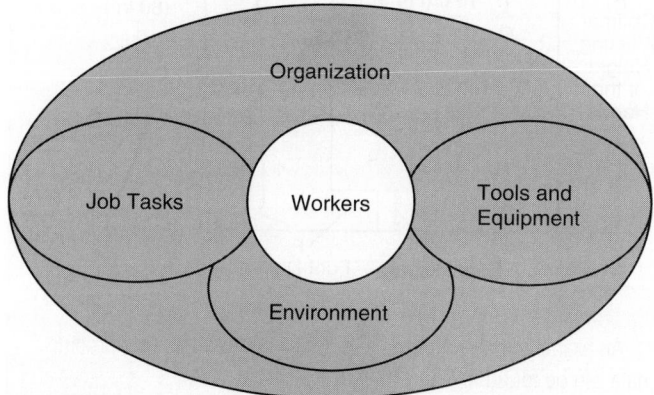

Figure 13-5   Dahl's ergonomics work system. (From Dahl R: Ergonomics. In Kornblau B, Jacobs K, editors: *Work: principles and practice*, Bethesda, MD, 2000, AOTA.)

Improving the fit between workers and their jobs requires a good understanding of human anatomy and *kinesiology* as well as expertise in occupational performance analysis and environmental modification. Ergonomics practitioners must also familiarize themselves with architectural and engineering codes, as well as local, state, and federal regulations.[18] Employers often call upon the ergonomics practitioner to consult with in-house safety and engineering professionals. The ergonomist provides the human understanding link in workplace design or redesign to reduce injury and improve efficiency. Ergonomic design principles are based on current knowledge of anatomy, kinesiology, biomechanics, *anthropometry* (comparative measurements of the human body; Box 13-4), cognitive-perceptual processing and integration, management theories, mechanical work-capacity models, psychology, and social/legal considerations.[12,18]

Though it is beyond the scope of this chapter to comprehensively review the complete array of ergonomic design considerations, the following is a discussion of selected ergonomic design principles. There are, however, a multitude of resources for the occupational therapist interested in learning more about the science of ergonomics. The authors of this chapter direct you to the references listed at the end of the chapter. Additionally, readers may be interested in the ergonomics information available through the Occupational Safety and Health Administration (*www.osha.gov*) and the National Institute for Occupational Safety and Health (*www.cdc.gov/niosh/homepage.html*).

When discussing ergonomic design it is important to understand that it is the relationship between the worker and work equipment, tools, or processes that is the problem, not any particular characteristic on either side. This can be confusing to an employer who orders expensive ergonomic tools and equipment for his or her workers and is disappointed when the workers continue to suffer work-related injuries and illnesses. The specialists in ergonomics must explain to their clients that a tool or piece of equipment is never in itself ergonomic; rather, it is the *fit* between a particular piece of equipment, tool, or process and the intended user of that equipment, tool, or process that creates a proper ergonomic situation.

WORKSTATIONS

There are three major types of workstations: seated, standing, and combination sit/stand. The type of task being performed dictates the best choice. Seated workstations are best for fine assembly and writing tasks and when all required task items can be supplied and handled within comfortable arm's

---

BOX 13-4 ANTHROPOMETRY

Anthropometry is the study of people in terms of their physical dimensions. It includes the measurement of human body characteristics, such as size, breadth, girth, and distance between anatomical points. It also includes segment masses, the centers of gravity of body segments, and the ranges of motion, which are used in biomechanical analysis of work and postures. Standard anthropometric tables exist to assist designers of work areas, work surfaces, chairs, and equipment. The tables outline the average dimensions of adult males and females in the 5th, 50th, and 95th percentile of the population. Ideally, designs should "fit" a wide range of persons between the 5th percentile (smallest people) and the 95th percentile (largest people). Retail merchandise labeled "ergonomic" is based on these anthropometric dimensions. In practice, however, few designs meet the needs of such a wide range of people. This explains why expensive equipment labeled "ergonomic" does not always produce the desired results. Professional ergonomic intervention seeks to create a better "fit" for the individual user.

Following is an example of ergonomic design recommendations based on anthropometric data:

WORKSTATION DESIGN

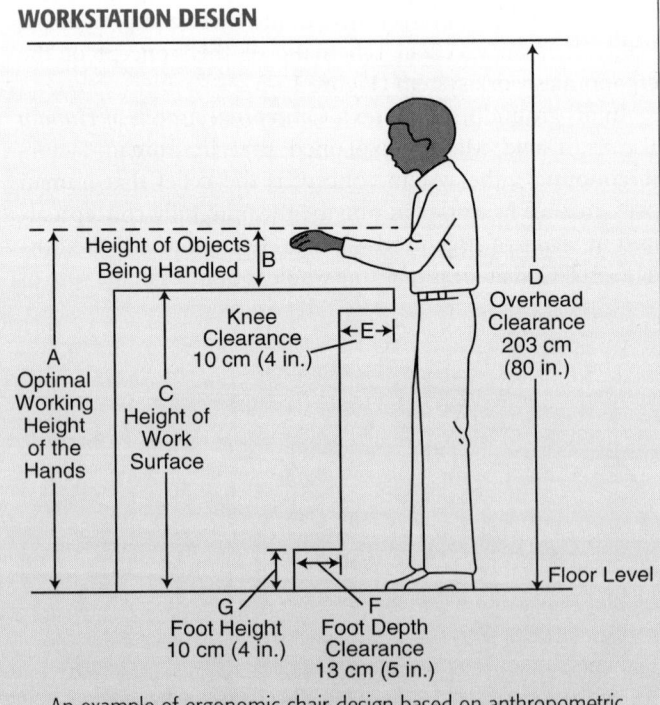

An example of ergonomic chair design based on anthropometric data can be found in Figure 13-7, *A*.

From Eggleton E, editor: *Ergonomic design for people at work*, Vol 1, New York, 1983, Van Nostrand Reinhold.

reach in the seated work space. Items handled in a seated workstation should not require hands to work more than 6 inches (15 cm) above the work space, and items handled should not weigh more than 10 lb (4.5 kg). For this reason, the work surface height should be above elbow height for precision work. Standing workstations are appropriate for all kinds of work tasks, but are preferred when downward forces must be exerted (i.e., packaging and wrapping tasks) and frequent movement and when or multi-level reaching is required around the work area. Items weighing more than 10 lb (4.5 kg) should be handled in a standing workstation. Work surface heights for heavy work should be 4-6 inches (10-15 cm) below elbow height for heavy work. The combination sit/stand workstation is best for jobs consisting of multiple tasks, some best done sitting and some best done standing.[22] Figure 13-6 shows the recommended dimensions of both a seated workstation and a standing workstation.

SEATING

If seating is required, the design of the chair is of paramount importance for worker comfort and support. Poor seating leads to poor working posture. The result can be fatigue, musculoskeletal injury, and/or poor work performance. Although chair preference is highly variable among the population, there are some basic characteristics to consider. Chairs should be easily adjustable for height, backrest position, and seat pan tilt. Appropriate lumbar support is important. Seats upholstered in woven fabric are cooler and more comfortable in warmer work environments.[22] Chair casters should match the flooring (i.e., hard floor versus carpet casters). A seat pan that is too deep will cut into the back of the leg and compromise lower extremity circulation. Sitting in a chair without the feet supported will also cause pressure on the back of the legs. When the worker is seated at the workstation and performing a task, both feet should be supported on the floor or a footrest. Choosing a seat pan with a front-edge "waterfall" design will also decrease pressure on the back of the legs. Armrests are an area of controversy but generally should be provided when the work task requires the arms to be held away from the body.[35] Figure 13-7, *A* illustrates recommended chair characteristics for generalized seated workstations. Figure 13-7, *B* illustrates a seated position for computer users.

VISUALIZING THE JOB TASK

Visual factors to consider are location of task items and lighting. Again, recommendations depend on the type of task being performed. The goal is clear and direct viewing without straining the eyes or neck. Tasks should be located as directly in front of the worker as possible. Tasks requiring close range viewing should be positioned 6-10 inches (15-25 cm) above the work surface. Minimum and maximum viewing distances depend on the size of the object being viewed.

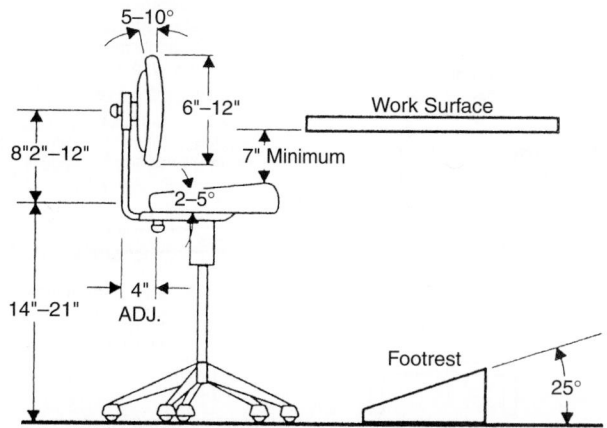

Seated Work

Optimal work surface height varies with perrformed:
Precision work = 31–37 inches
Reading/writing = 28–31 inches
Typing/light assembly = 21–28 inches
Seat and back rest heights should be adjustable
as noted in chair requirements.

A

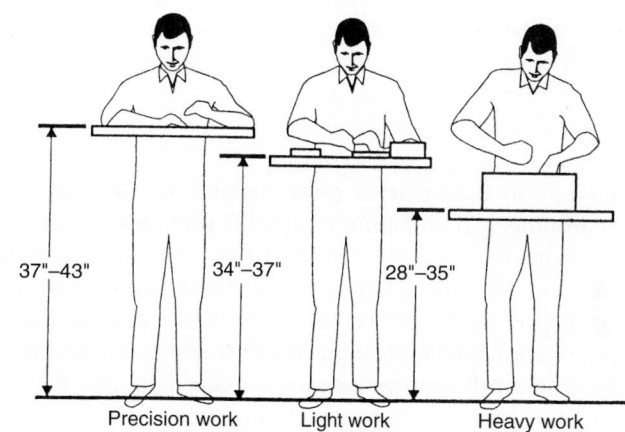

Standing Work

Precision work   Light work   Heavy work

Workbench heights should be:
Above elbow height for precision work
Just below elbow height for light work
4-6 inches below elbow height for heavy work

B

Figure 13-6 Recommended dimensions of workstations. **A,** Seated work. **B,** Standing work. (From Cohen AL, et al: *Elements of ergonomics programs: a primer based on workplace evaluations of musculoskeletal disorders*, Washington DC, 1997, US Government Printing Office.)

Bifocal eyeglass wearers have difficulty observing any object closer than 7 inches (18 cm) in front of the body that is above eye level or near the floor. Additionally, bifocal wearers have difficulty focusing on signs or dials located from 24 to 36 inches (61-91 cm) in front of them.[20]

There are three basic lighting factors to consider for performance of work: quantity, contrast, and glare. Lighting should be adequate for the worker to perform the job task,

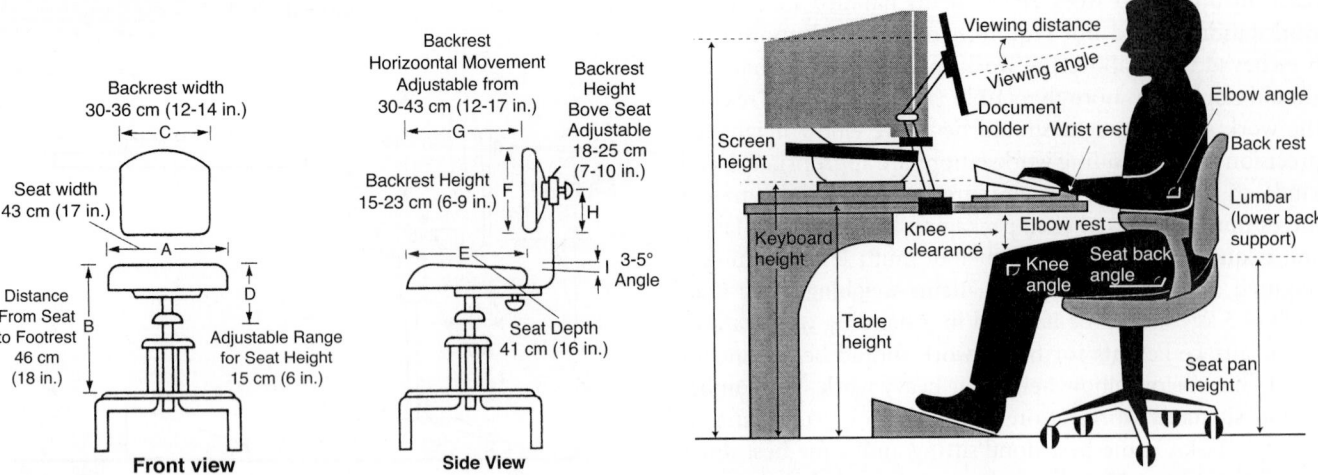

Figure 13-7 **A,** Recommended chair characteristics. Dimensions are given using both front and side views for width (A), depth (E), vertical adjustability (D), and angle (I) and for backrest width (C), height (F), and vertical (H) and horizontal (G) adjustability relative to the chair seat. The angle of the backrest should be adjustable horizontally from 12-17 inches (30-43 cm), by either a slide-adjust or a spring, and vertically from 7-10 inches (18-25 cm). The adjustability is needed to provide back support during different types of seated work. The seat should be adjustable within at least a 6-inch (15-cm) range. The height above the floor of the chair seat with this adjustment range will be determined by the workplace, with or without a footrest. (From Eggleton E, editor: *Ergonomic design for people at work*, Vol 1, New York, 1983, Van Nostrand Reinhold.) **B,** Proper seated position for computer user. (From Occupational Safety and Health Administration: *Working safely with video display terminals*, Washington DC, 1997, US Government Printing Office, *www.osha.gov/Publications/osha3092.pdf.*)

but not so bright as to cause discomfort. General work environment illumination is typically provided by sunlight and light fixtures at 50 to100 foot-candles (ft-c). Computer users may find that this amount of illumination washes out the display screen and causes eyestrain. The recommended illumination level for computer-user workstations is 28 to 50 ft-c. Too much contrast between the task items and the surrounding areas can also stress the eyes. Therefore the illuminance between the task items, equipment, horizontal work surface, and surrounding areas should be minimized. Finally, the color and finish of the workstation walls and equipment, as well as the arrangement of the lighting sources, should all be designed to avoid reflective glare on the job task (Figure 13-8).[70]

TOOLS

Tools should be designed to protect the worker from hand vibration, extreme temperatures, and soft tissue compression. Therefore, handles on tools are essential. "A properly designed tool handle should isolate the hand from contact with the tool surface, enhance tool control and stability, and serve to increase the mechanical advantage while reducing the amount of required exertion."[78] Since the average worker's hand is 4 inches (10 cm) across, the length of the tool handle must be at least 4 inches to avoid unnecessary pressure in the palm of the hand.

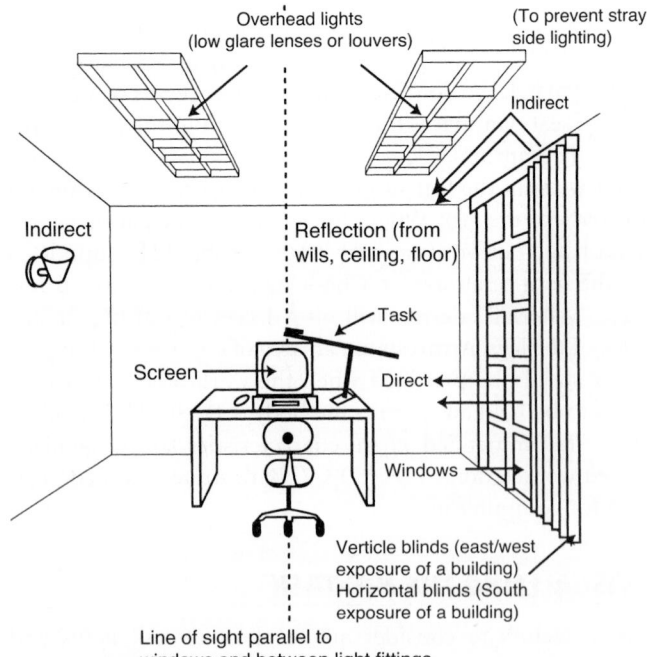

Figure 13-8 Lighting position considerations for computer-user workstations. Most of these lighting position principles can be applied to workstations in general. (From Occupational Safety and Health Administration: *Working safely with video display terminals*, Washington DC, 1997, US Government Printing Office, *www.osha.gov/ Publications/osha3092.pdf.*)

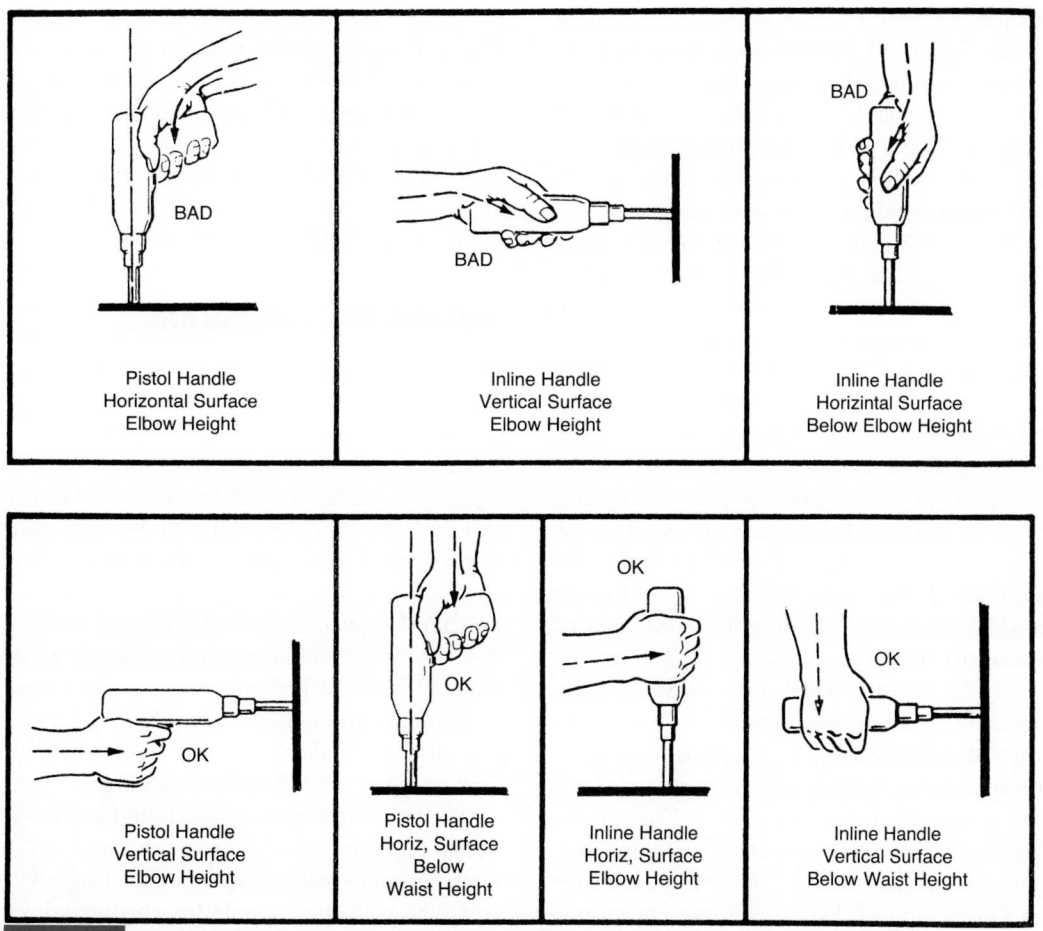

Figure 13-9   Hand tool design and wrist posture. (From Armstrong T: *An ergonomic guide to carpal tunnel syndrome,* Akron, Ohio, 1983, American Industrial Hygiene Association.)

Handles of scissors and pliers should be spring-loaded to avoid trauma to the back and sides of hands.[78]

Tool design should minimize muscular effort and awkward posturing of the upper extremity. Whenever possible, opt for power tools to minimize the human effort required. Choose tool shapes that allow the wrist to stay straight and the elbow to stay bent and close to the body during use. The shape of the tool will depend on the job task and work surface (Figure 13-9). Tools that weigh between 10 and 15 lb (4-6.5 kg) cannot be held in a horizontal position more than a couple of minutes without the worker experiencing pain and fatigue. Suspension systems and counterweights should be designed for use with heavy hand tools.[78]

Whole-body vibration can cause back pain and performance problems when the workstation vibrates, as in the case of long-distance truck drivers and in production industries using high-powered drills or saws in the work area.[14] Hand-arm vibration has been linked to vascular compromise, peripheral nerve damage, muscular fatigue, bone cysts, and central nervous system disturbances.[29] The effects of hand tool vibration should be minimized as much as possible.

Use anti-vibration tools at low speeds when available. Ensure that tool handles and gloves fit the workers' hands. Train workers to grip tool handles as lightly as possible and allow the tool to do all the work instead of the worker adding force behind the tool. Encourage frequent rest breaks and educate workers that smoking increases the risk for vibration-related hand problems.[18,29]

MATERIALS HANDLING

Concerns regarding handling materials center on back injury and include lifting, pushing, pulling, bending, and twisting. The heavier the materials, the more risk for injury. Low back injuries are seldom the result of a single traumatic episode but rather the result of repeated micro-traumas that ultimately lead to injury.[32] Therefore, workstation and work process design become integral for materials handling worker safety.

Design considerations for heavy lifting include use of mechanical assist devices whenever feasible (e.g., use of a Hoyer Lift for moving immobile patients in the hospital).

Where mechanical assist devices are not available, training in proper lifting technique and proper body mechanics is important to promote worker safety. Providing workers with back supports is controversial but many believe that use of an elastic back support "has a preventative function, protecting the tissues...thus making injury less common."[44] Training workers and providing them with back supports is only effective, however, when "supervisors and managers encourage the use of safe procedures and write policies that enforce them."[82]

The following suggestions are useful for addressing safe handling of materials. Design workstations to keep large items that require lifting off the floor. Provide platforms that will keep items at mid-thigh height to allow workers to stand nearly erect for lifting. Provide foot clearance so that workers can get as close to the item as possible when lifting and face the load head-on. Adjustable lift tables are excellent for this purpose. Objects should be against the torso during the lift to minimize force on the spine. Workers should never be forced to twist their torsos to lift an object. Use carts or conveyors to transport heavy materials instead of carrying them. Orient packages for easy pick-up and provide adequate handles or handhold cutouts on packages.[18]

As stated earlier, these ergonomic design principles can be applied proactively to work situations, preventing problems before they even occur. For many occupational therapists, however, introduction to ergonomic considerations comes secondarily as part of a comprehensive rehabilitation program for injured workers. Following a work-related injury, ergonomic intervention is essential to the client's successful re-engagement in the occupation of work. Without the ergonomic intervention aspect, the rehabilitation process cannot be considered complete.

A significant amount of effort goes into the rehabilitation of an injured worker. Physical injuries require the attention of a medical doctor to prescribe rest, medications, and rehabilitative therapies. The occupational therapist will provide acute care to the injuries by fabricating splints, instructing in stretching and strengthening exercise, and using physical agent modalities such as heat and ice to calm the soft tissues in preparation for functional rehabilitative activities. Other aspects of the occupational therapy treatment plan include educating the injured worker about the nature of the injury and training in general body mechanics and personal injury management strategies to help prevent injury recurrence upon return to work. In some cases, the injured worker will require specialized conditioning prior to return to work and will be referred to a work hardening program. When the client is ready to return to work, it is important to remember that an injured worker cannot safely be returned to the same job without ergonomic intervention.

It seems obvious that returning an injured worker to the same conditions that caused the injury will certainly result in re-injury if not eliminated prior to the employee's return to work. However, ergonomic intervention is sometimes overlooked as an integral part of the rehabilitation program. The goal of ergonomic evaluation and intervention in the injured employee's work environment is to eliminate those factors that contributed to the injury in the first place. If we don't eliminate the major cause of the original injury, it won't be long before the worker suffers a recurrence. If that happens, we have failed as occupational therapists to provide a successful rehabilitation process.

ERGONOMIC EVALUATION

The **ergonomic evaluation** is an important assessment and intervention tool when used as part of a comprehensive rehabilitation or injury prevention program. This tool can be used along the entire continuum of prevention services. Ergonomic evaluation can be performed during workstation and work methods planning to assist in efforts to prevent worker injury. Ergonomic evaluation can also be performed for workers who develop symptoms of a **work-related** *musculoskeletal disorder* (WMSD) and workers who come to therapy for rehabilitation and are ready to return to work, the goal being to prevent re-injury. And finally, ergonomic assessment can be useful in modifying a job in preparation for a disabled worker's return to work with the goal to prevent further injury related to the disability.

The ergonomic evaluation should begin with the occupational therapist scheduling a time to meet with both the worker(s) to be assessed and the direct supervisor of the work area. The evaluation should be scheduled during the normal work hours of the worker(s). The goal is to get the best understanding of what actually occurs during a typical work shift, so the conditions should be closely approximated. It is extremely important that the actual worker(s) be present. The purpose of the evaluation is to look at the fit between the specific worker(s) and the specific job methods, equipment, and set-up. If any element is missing, the evaluation is of little, or even no, value.

Ideally, the occupational therapist evaluator will arrive at the worksite and meet first with the direct supervisor of the work area to be evaluated. The supervisor will be asked to give an overview of the circumstances leading up to the request for ergonomic evaluation. The occupational therapist will want to know what kinds of injuries are occurring in the work area, when the problem started, and how many employees have been affected. The supervisor will be able to review how the organization has dealt with the problem to date. Often, the supervisor will also describe what sorts of psychosocial and environmental influences may be affecting the situation. Occasionally, an ergonomic assessment is requested before any problems occur at all. The supervisor may explain that the employer is just trying to be proactive. Either way, this brief encounter with the supervisor will give the observant occupational therapist evaluator a very good feel for the organization's management culture and organizational priorities.

Following the supervisor interview, the occupational therapist evaluator will want to see the work area and meet the employees. The supervisor may give the evaluator a brief tour of the work area, describing the job tasks and methods that occur there. If the supervisor has identified any problem areas (areas the supervisor thinks are contributing to injury), the supervisor should be encouraged to point those out. This part of the evaluation will give the evaluator an understanding of how management views the situation. Next, the evaluator will ask to meet with the workers.

Once alone with the worker(s) it is important to establish some level of trust. The evaluator will explain to the workers(s) why the organization has asked for an ergonomic evaluation. It should be explained that the purpose of the evaluation is to make the job safer and more comfortable for the worker(s). The worker(s) should be encouraged to give the evaluator a tour of the work area and to explain their job tasks. If there are any discrepancies between management's understanding of the job situation and the workers' understanding of the same, the evaluator must seek definitive clarification.

Finally, the worker(s) should be asked to begin performing the job as normally as possible. The evaluator will explain that he/she will be watching and perhaps videotaping or taking notes. The evaluator should assure the worker(s) that the information that is being recording will be used to develop strategies to make the job tasks safer and more comfortable to perform. The evaluator must stress that he or she wants the workers(s) to do the job just like any other day. The evaluator will not begin analysis of the work methods until at least 10 minutes have passed. This will allow workers time to fall into a more normal work pattern.

The ergonomic workstation and work methods assessment should focus on identifying known risk factors for MSD. It is often very useful to videotape the work area and work methods performed. Recording the worker(s) performing their job tasks will allow the evaluator to return to his or her office and further analyze the data. If the evaluator plans to videotape any work areas or work methods, he or she should ask permission from the company before taping. It is becoming increasingly more difficult to gain permission for in-house videotaping due to confidentiality and trade secrets concerns. However, some companies are still willing to allow videotaping for the purpose of ergonomic evaluation. Always obtain prior written permission allowing you to videotape in-house. Box 13-5 suggests a protocol for videotaping jobs for the purpose of ergonomic evaluation.

In light of these concerns, it may be helpful to develop an ergonomic checklist to assist in performing the on-site evaluation. The checklist should include the most common ergonomic risk factors and be tailored to the specific needs and conditions of the workplace the occupational therapist intends to evaluate. Figure 13-10 is an example of a typical ergonomic risk factor identification checklist. Figure 13-11 is an example of a checklist for computer-user workstation evaluation. Figure 13-12 is a typical hand tool risk factor checklist.

The risk factors to look for include the following:
1. *Forceful exertions*: Heavy lifting, pushing, pulling, twisting, gripping, or pinching. Handling heavy tools, equipment, or product. Difficulty maintaining control of equipment or tools, or lifting and moving an object of asymmetrical size. Also using inappropriate or inadequate tools.
2. *Repetition*: Performing the same motion or series of motions continually or frequently for an extended period of time (Table 13-5).
3. *Awkward or static posturing, either repetitively or for prolonged periods*: Assuming positions that place stress on the body such as reaching above shoulder height, kneeling, squatting, leaning over a work surface, using a knife or keyboard with wrists bent, twisting the torso while lifting, or looking at a computer monitor off to one side causing the neck to twist all day. Also, sitting all day at a desk with poor posture.
4. *Contact stress*: Pressing the body or part of the body (such as a hand or forearm) against hard or sharp surfaces and edges (e.g., using the hand as a hammer, resting the forearms on a sharp desk edge while typing, and using pliers with the handle pressing into the palm).
5. *Excessive vibration*: For example, from power tools or sitting in a truck cab all day while driving.
6. *Cold temperatures*: Either working in cold temperature or handling cold tools or products (e.g., construction workers outside during winter handling metal tools and equipment, or meat packers or butchers handling frozen meat).

Once the workstation and work methods risk factors have been identified and the worker(s) have had a chance to familiarize themselves with the occupational therapist, focus should turn to the psychosocial aspects of the job. Often, these factors will surface during the evaluation process without any prompting whatsoever. Factors such as workload and productivity stressors, relationship quality between the worker(s) and other coworkers and the supervisor, genuine job task enjoyment, and overall health and fitness cannot be overlooked. Work-related musculoskeletal injury is never the result of any one factor; rather, it is the accumulation of a variety of risk factors and situations that ultimately result in injury. Occupational therapists look at the entire occupational profile to determine what is occurring.

Finally, it is important to ask the workers for their perspective on problem areas or risk factors in their work area. If their perspective matches what has been identified in the ergonomic evaluation of the work area and work methods, the workers should be encouraged to share their ideas for correcting the problem. Although the occupational therapist is the expert in workstation and work methods analysis, the on-site workers know their job better than anyone. The workers have likely spent hours formulating and discussing how they would change things if ever given the chance. Ask them. Often, one will find a wealth of knowledge and many useful ideas for reducing or eliminating risk factors among the people who perform the job. It is important to use caution before using

---

BOX **13-5** PROTOCOL FOR VIDEOTAPING JOBS FOR ERGONOMIC EVALUATION

The following is a guide to preparing a videotape and related task information for facilitating job analyses and assessments of risk factors for WMSDs.

MATERIALS NEEDED

- Video camera and blank tapes.
- Spare batteries (at least 2) and battery charger.
- Clipboard, pens, paper, blank checklists.
- Stopwatch, strain gauge (optional) for weighing objects.

VIDEOTAPING PROCEDURES

1. To verify the accuracy of the video camera to record in real time, videotape a worker or job with a stopwatch running in the field of view for at least 1 min. The play back of the tape should correspond to the lapsed time on the stopwatch.
2. Announce the name of the job on the voice channel of the video camera before the taping of any job. Restrict running time comments to the facts. Make no editorial comments.
3. Tape each job long enough to observe all aspects of the task. Tape 5 to 10 minutes for all jobs, including at least 10 complete cycles. Fewer cycles may be needed if all aspects of the job are recorded at least 3 to 4 times.
4. Hold the camera still, using a tripod if available. Don't walk unless absolutely necessary.
5. Begin taping each task with a whole-body shot of the worker. Include the seat/chair and the surface the worker is standing on. Hold this for 2 to 3 cycles, then zoom in on the hands/arms or other body parts which may be under stress due to the job task.
6. It is best to tape several workers to determine if workers of varying body size adopt different postures or are affected in

other ways. If possible, try to tape the best and worst case situations in terms of worker fit to the job.

The following suspected upper body problems suggest focusing on the parts indicated:

Wrist problems/complaints
Hands/wrists/forearms
Elbow problems/complaints
Arms/elbows
Shoulder problems/complaints
Arms/shoulders

For back and lower limb problems, the focus would be on movements of the trunk of the body and leg, knee, and foot areas under stress due to task loads or other requirements.

7. Tape from whatever angles are needed to capture the body part(s) under stress.
8. Briefly tape the jobs performed before and after the one under actual study to see how the targeted job fits into the total department process.
9. For each taped task, obtain the following information to the maximum extent possible:

- If the task is continuous or sporadic
- If the worker performs the work for the entire shift, or if there is rotation with other workers
- Measures of work surface heights and chair heights and whether adjustable
- Weight, size, and shape of handles and textures for tools in use; indications of vibration in power tool usage
- Use of handwear
- Weight of objects lifted, pushed, pulled, or carried
- Nature of environment in which work is performed (too cold or too hot?)

From Cohen AL, et al: *Elements of ergonomics programs: a primer based on workplace evaluations of musculoskeletal disorders,* Washington DC, 1997, US Government Printing Office.

---

each suggestion. As the expert, it is the occupational therapist's responsibility to assure that the changes implemented will serve to reduce and prevent injury. Sometimes, worker-driven suggestions inadvertently cause new problems if not assessed appropriately by the ergonomic consultant.

Following the on-site evaluation, the occupational therapist returns to his or her office to analyze the data and prepare a report. The report will be shared with whomever requested the ergonomic evaluation. The report should contain an introduction explaining the background and purpose of the ergonomic evaluation, a description of the actual work area and work methods assessment, and finally the evaluator's findings and recommendations with clear and comprehensive information regarding how to implement the recommendations and resources for securing and purchasing any equipment or services. Job tasks found to contain several

risk factors for development of WSMD contain the greatest risk for injury and should be addressed first by the company. Recommendations will focus on ways to eliminate or reduce risk factors (Table 13-6).

Lorna benefited from a worksite evaluation. The occupational therapist went to her worksite to observe her and the other workers perform some of the essential functions of the job in their actual work environment. Risk factors were identified such as excessive force from pinching and pulling the fabric tightly over the padded wooden frame and from using the heavy staple gun. A significant amount of force is required to push the heavy furniture to the next workstation. Her work tasks are repetitive, for example, pulling the trigger of the staple gun and pushing and pulling the fabric and furniture all day long. Lorna and the other workers were observed to have awkward posturing with frequent bending, twisting,

General Ergonomic Risk Analysis Checklist

Check the box if your answer is "yes" to the question. A "yes" response indicates that an ergonomic risk factor that requires further analysis may be present.

Manual Material Handling
- ❑   Is there lifting of loads, tools, or parts?
- ❑   Is there lowering of loads, tools, or parts?
- ❑   Is there overhead reaching for loads, tools, or parts?
- ❑   Is there bending at the waist to handle loads, tools, or parts?
- ❑   Is there twisting at the waist to handle loads, tools, or parts?

Physical Energy Demands
- ❑   Do tools and parts weigh more than 10 lbs?
- ❑   Is reaching greater than 20 inches?
- ❑   Is bending, stooping, or squatting a primary task activity?
- ❑   Is lifting or lowering loads a primary task activity?
- ❑   Is walking or carrying loads a primary task activity?
- ❑   Is stair or ladder climbing with loads a primary task activity?
- ❑   Is pushing or pulling loads a primary task activity?
- ❑   Is reaching overhead a primary task activity?
- ❑   Do any of the above tasks require five or more complete work cycles to be done within a minute?
- ❑   Do workers complain that rest breaks and fatigue allowances are insufficient?

Other Musculoskeletal Demands
- ❑   Do manual jobs require frequent, repetitive motions?
- ❑   Do work postures require frequent bending of the neck, shoulder, elbow, wrist, or finger joints?
- ❑   For seated work, do reaches for tools and materials exceed 15 inches from the worker's position?
- ❑   Is the worker unable to change his or her position often?
- ❑   Does the work involve forceful, quick, or sudden motions?
- ❑   Does the work involve shock or rapid buildup of forces?
- ❑   Is finger-pinch gripping used?
- ❑   Do job postures involve sustained muscle contraction of any limb?

Computer Workstation
- ❑   Do operators use computer workstations for more than 4 hours a day?
- ❑   Are there complaints of discomfort from those working at these stations?
- ❑   Is the chair or desk nonadjustable?
- ❑   Is the display monitor, keyboard, or document holder nonadjustable?
- ❑   Does lighting cause glare or make the monitor screen hard to read?
- ❑   Is the room temperature too hot or too cold?
- ❑   Is there irritating vibration or noise?

Environment
- ❑   Is the temperature too hot or too cold?
- ❑   Are the worker's hands exposed to temperatures less than 70° F?
- ❑   Is the workplace poorly lit?
- ❑   Is there glare?
- ❑   Is there excessive noise that is annoying, distracting, or producing hearing loss?
- ❑   Is there upper extremity or whole body vibration?
- ❑   Is air circulation too high or too low?

General Workplace
- ❑   Are walkways uneven, slippery, or obstructed?
- ❑   Is housekeeping poor?
- ❑   Is there inadequate clearance or accessibility for performing tasks?
- ❑   Are stairs cluttered or lacking railings?
- ❑   Is proper footwear worn?

Figure 13-10   General ergonomic risk analysis checklist. (From Cohen AL, et al: *Elements of ergonomics programs: a primer based on workplace evaluations of musculoskeletal disorders*, Washington DC, 1997, US Government Printing Office.)

Tools

❏ Is the handle too small or too large?
❏ Does the handle shape cause the operator to bend the wrist in order to use the tool?
❏ Is the tool hard to access?
❏ Does the tool weigh more than 9 pounds?
❏ Does the tool vibrate excessively?
❏ Does the tool cause excessive kickback to the operator?
❏ Does the tool become too hot or too cold?

Gloves

❏ Do the gloves require the worker to use more force when performing job tasks?
❏ Do the gloves provide inadequate protection?
❏ Do the gloves present a hazard of catch points on the tool or in the workplace?

Administration

❏ Is there little worker control over the work process?
❏ Is the task highly repetitive and monotonous?
❏ Does the job involve critical tasks with high accountability and little or no tolerance for error?
❏ Are work hours and breaks poorly organized?

Figure 13-10, cont'd

and squatting to move the bulky furniture around to staple the fabric down.

Lorna's employer was open to the suggestions that the occupational therapist made and was willing to make the appropriate accommodations. A special tool with a padded and curved handle to fit the shape of most hands was purchased to allow the workers to use a grasp-release motion to activate a material clamp, rather than using the fingers so forcefully to pinch and pull the fabric. To lessen the amount of bending, twisting, and squatting required, it was recommended that the company purchase commercially available platforms on wheels to easily move the wooden furniture frames around. Additionally, the platforms contain a simple hydraulic lift that elevates the frame to whatever height was needed for easy stapling. The occupational therapist researched and located a resource for purchase of this helpful equipment, which facilitated the employer's timely implementation of the worksite recommendations. Worksite evaluations and ergonomic interventions can also comprise important aspects of a comprehensive injury prevention program as will be discussed in the next section.

INJURY PREVENTION PROGRAMS

For decades, the majority of occupational therapy practice has been in the area of rehabilitation. Occupational therapists are unquestionably skilled in facilitating client independence during and/or following an injury, illness, or disease. Although not an entirely new concept, we are now recognizing occupational therapy's potential to facilitate and perpetuate independence prior to or even in avoidance of these events. As we move into the 21st century, increasing numbers of occupational therapists are broadening their practices to include wellness and prevention.

Support for this movement is ubiquitous. The 1994-1996 landmark University of Southern California's *Well Elderly Study* supports occupational therapy's preventative intervention role in enhancing physical and mental health, occupational functioning, and life satisfaction.[38] The adoption of the Occupational Therapy Practice Framework in 2002 provides further support, listing health promotion and prevention as occupational therapy intervention approaches that "facilitate engagement in occupation to support participation in life."[1] Finally, in 2004, AOTA President, Carolyn Baum, PhD, OTR/L, FAOTA, identified several prevention-related businesses as "hot" occupational therapy emerging practice areas.[55]

With regard to occupational therapy and work, prevention can take on three forms: primary prevention, secondary prevention, and tertiary prevention. **Primary prevention** efforts help protect healthy workers against a targeted condition before the condition occurs. Interventions are directed to an entire workforce to prevent a specific work-related medical problem. **Secondary prevention** emphasizes early identification and intervention of asymptomatic workers who have risk factors for developing work-related medical problems, as well as identification and treatment of workers with mild medical symptoms in the early reversible stages of injury. The goal is to identify risk factors so that they can be minimized or eliminated and to reverse any medical problems that might be developing. **Tertiary prevention** occurs after a worker suffers nonreversible injury, illness, or disease. Interventions include treatment of the medical problem, attempts to restore maximum function in the workplace, and prevention of injury, illness, or disease-related complications. The goal is to return the affected worker to gainful employment within the confines of the medical problem *and* to prevent further injury. Once a permanent work-related injury occurs, primary and secondary prevention measures

Risk Analysis Checklist for Computer-User Workstations

"No" responses indicate potential problem areas which should receive further investigation.

1. Does the workstation ensure proper worker posture, such as

   - horizontal thighs? ☐ Yes ☐ No
   - vertical lower legs? ☐ Yes ☐ No
   - feet flat on floor or footrest? ☐ Yes ☐ No
   - neutral wrists? ☐ Yes ☐ No

2. Does the chair

   - adjust easily? ☐ Yes ☐ No
   - have a padded seat with a rounded front? ☐ Yes ☐ No
   - have an adjustable backrest? ☐ Yes ☐ No
   - provide lumbar support? ☐ Yes ☐ No
   - have casters? ☐ Yes ☐ No

3. Are the height and tilt of the work surface on which the keyboard is located adjustable? ☐ Yes ☐ No

4. Is the keyboard detachable? ☐ Yes ☐ No

5. Do keying actions require minimal force? ☐ Yes ☐ No

6. Is there an adjustable document holder? ☐ Yes ☐ No

7. Are arm rests provided where needed? ☐ Yes ☐ No

8. Are glare and reflections avoided? ☐ Yes ☐ No

9. Does the monitor have brightness and contrast controls? ☐ Yes ☐ No

10. Do the operators judge the distance between eyes and work to be satisfactory for their viewing needs? ☐ Yes ☐ No

11. Is there sufficient space for knees and feet? ☐ Yes ☐ No

12. Can the workstation be used for either right- or left-handed activity? ☐ Ye ☐ No

13. Are adequate rest breaks provided for task demands? ☐ Yes ☐ No

14. Are high stroke rates avoided by

    - job rotation? ☐ Yes ☐ No
    - self-pacing? ☐ Yes ☐ No
    - adjusting the job to the skill of the worker? ☐ Yes ☐ No

15. Are employees trained in

    - proper postures? ☐ Yes ☐ No
    - proper work methods? ☐ Yes ☐ No
    - when and how to adjust their workstations? ☐ Yes ☐ No
    - how to seek assistance for their concerns? ☐ Yes ☐ No

Figure 13-11 Risk analysis checklist for computer-user workstations. (From Cohen AL, et al: *Elements of ergonomics programs: a primer based on workplace evaluations of musculoskeletal disorders*, Washington DC, 1997, US Government Printing Office.)

Handtool Risk Factor Checklist

"No" responses indicate potential problem areas which should receive further investigation.

1. Are tools selected to limit or minimize

   - exposure to excessive vibration?   ☐ Yes   ☐ No
   - use of excessive force?   ☐ Yes   ☐ No
   - bending or twisting the wrist?   ☐ Yes   ☐ No
   - finger pinch grip?   ☐ Yes   ☐ No
   - problems associated with trigger finger?   ☐ Yes   ☐ No

2. Are tools powered where necessary and feasible?   ☐ Yes   ☐ No

3. Are tools evenly balanced?   ☐ Yes   ☐ No

4. Are heavy tools suspended or counterbalanced in ways to facilitate use?   ☐ Yes   ☐ No

5. Does the tool allow adequate visibility of the work?   ☐ Yes   ☐ No

6. Does the tool grip/handle prevent slipping during use?   ☐ Yes   ☐ No

7. Are tools equipped with handles of textured, non-conductive material?   ☐ Yes   ☐ No

8. Are different handle sizes available to fit a wide range of hand sizes?   ☐ Yes   ☐ No

9. Is the tool handle designed not to dig in the palm of the hand?   ☐ Yes   ☐ No

10. Can the tool be used safely with gloves?   ☐ Yes   ☐ No

11. Can the tool be used by either hand?   ☐ Yes   ☐ No

12. Is there a preventative maintenance program to keep tools operating as designed?   ☐ Yes   ☐ No

13. Have employees been trained

    - in the proper use of tools?   ☐ Yes   ☐ No
    - when and how to report problems with tools?   ☐ Yes   ☐ No
    - in proper tool maintenance?   ☐ Yes   ☐ No

Figure 13-12   Hand tool risk factor checklist. (From Cohen AL, et al: *Elements of ergonomics programs: a primer based on workplace evaluations of musculoskeletal disorders*, Washington DC, 1997, US Government Printing Office.)

TABLE **13-5** **High Risk Repetition Rates for the Upper Extremity**

Body Part	Repetitions Per Minute
Shoulder	More than 2½
Upper arm/elbow	More than 10
Forearm/wrist	More than 10
Finger	More than 200

From Kilbom A: Repetitive work of the upper extremity; Part II: The scientific basis for the guide, *Int J Ind Erg* 14:59, 1994.

have failed. However, early risk factor detection and intervention through secondary prevention may have minimized the severity of the permanent injury.[82,95]

Most occupational therapists are familiar with the process of tertiary prevention of work-related medical problems. Typically, the OT becomes involved after a worker suffers an injury and it becomes OT's job to help the client regain maximum function in the workplace and prevent further injury. Occupational therapists are also commonly involved with secondary prevention efforts. Workers are referred with mild work-related medical conditions and intervention is planned to reverse the symptoms. When these clients get ready to return to work, the OT may assist the client in risk-factor identification and modification to reduce the risk for re-injury. Worksite evaluation and ergonomic intervention are generally part of the process for successfully re-engaging these workers.

TABLE **13-6** **Combating Ergonomic Risk Factors**

Risk Factor	Suggestions for Improvement
Using excessive force	***Reduce force required to perform activity***
OT lifts/transfers heavy clients several times daily	Use Hoyer lift or get help from co-worker
Employee uses heavy drill in a manufacturing plant	Suspend tools from ceiling with tension wire
Chef has difficulty cutting chicken in restaurant kitchen	Provide equipment to sharpen knives after every shift
Repetition	***Reduce prolonged exposure to repetitive activity***
Multiple scans required to activate grocery scanner	Implement program for regular preventative maintenance on scanners
Executive secretary required to do five hours typing in an 8-hour work day	Alternate typing task every 30 minutes with other office tasks like making phone calls and filing
Awkward/static posturing	***Reduce or eliminate awkward/static posturing***
Medical transcriptionist types with her head turned to the right in order to see computer screen	Move computer monitor on desk so that it is directly in line with the computer keyboard and worker's face as she looks straight ahead
Same medical transcriptionist sits in same position all day to type	Require worker to stand and gently march in place for 60 seconds after every 30 minutes of typing; provide timer to remind worker
Grocery store checkout clerk bends at waist and grabs case of soda from bottom of cart with right hand several times daily	Teach body mechanics for proper lift technique and use of two-hand power grip
Contact stress	***Reduce or eliminate contact stress***
Typist rests her forearms on sharp desk edge to type	Provide soft wrist rest until budget allows for purchase of new desk with rounded edges
Jewelry maker uses pliers with short handle to twist wires; end of handle rests in palm of hand	Provide pliers with longer handle that is gently curved to fit hand
Teacher uses side of fist to punch stapler several times daily	Provide electric stapler
Excessive vibration	***Reduce vibration***
Drill vibrates in hand of assembly-line worker in manufacturing plant	Wrap handle of power tool in vibration dampening tape and have the worker wear anti-vibration gloves that fit correctly (to avoid grasping tighter than necessary to handle tool)
Cold temperature	***Reduce exposure to cold***
Construction workers outside in winter handle cold metal equipment and tools	Wrap tool and equipment handles with neoprene and provide workers with thermal gloves to wear, making sure gloves fit the workers correctly to avoid grasping objects tighter than necessary
Meat and deli team at grocery store handle frozen foods frequently	Provide well-fitting thermal gloves to wear when handling frozen items and provide grasping tool to use to handle smaller frozen packages

Worksite evaluation and ergonomic intervention can also be part of a comprehensive primary prevention program designed to prevent work-related injury, illness, and disease.

Helping employers improve worker fitness, job comfort, and workplace safety reduces work-related medical problems. It can also lead to improved employee morale and increased productivity.[37] Occupational therapists, acting as consultants, can assist corporate clients in establishing injury prevention programs. This is one way occupational therapists can incorporate the concepts of wellness and health promotion into their daily practices.

Melnick writes that "the success or failure of a prevention program has less to do with specific activities implemented and more to do with the methods of implementation."[58] Melnick outlines the four characteristics that are common among successful injury prevention programs: ongoing management support, supervisor "buy in," employee participation, and ongoing support and reinforcement.[58] Melnick explains that successful prevention programs are grounded in the consultant's ability to instill in the corporate client a culture of safety and wellness. The focus should be on the process of implementing safety and wellness activities and not on the activities themselves.

One common reason that an occupational therapist might be asked to consult with an industrial client is to control the severity and incidence of work-related musculoskeletal disorders (WMSDs). WMSDs are a class of soft injuries affecting the muscles, tendons, and nerves. Other names for WMSDs are cumulative trauma disorders, over-use syndromes, and repetitive strain disorders. WMSDs come on slowly and develop over time. They are thought to be the result of repeated micro-traumas to a body and occur when the body is denied the opportunity to adequately rest and repair itself. Common diagnoses within the class of WMSDs include carpal tunnel syndrome, de Quervain's tendinitis, lateral epicondylitis, and some types of back injuries.[78]

WSMDs account for approximately one third of all occupational injuries and illnesses reported to the United States Bureau of Labor Statistics; employers pay more than $45 billion annually in workers' compensation and other expenses associated with these disorders.[3] In 1999, carpal tunnel syndrome itself accounted for an average of 27 days missed work compared to an average of 6 lost work days for all other types of work-related injuries and illnesses.[26] These statistics indicate that WMSDs are at crisis level in the workplace. However, the financial losses to industry and the economy pale in comparison to the physical and emotional pain and suffering endured by today's injured workers.

Lorna and several of her co-workers were experiencing WMSDs. Their employer agreed to implement an in-house ergonomics program and injury prevention program at the recommendation of the occupational therapy consultant. An ergonomic team was developed consisting of the company's chief financial officer, the stapling station supervisor, the employee health nurse, the safety manager, the occupational therapist consultant, and three employees who worked in the stapling station, including Lorna.

There are a multitude of resources available for prevention consultants interested in helping corporate clients develop effective programs for evaluating and addressing musculoskeletal concerns in the workplace. OSHA and the National Institute for Occupational Safety and Health (NIOSH) are excellent starting points. Box 13-6 offers information on these two government entities, and provides a partial listing of their ergonomic and injury prevention resource materials.

It is important to remember that every corporate client is unique and the consultant's recommendations must work with the corporate culture, goals, and budget constraints. Melnick also reminds us that we must help our corporate clients recognize that "injury prevention consultants do not reduce injuries. This would occur only if the consultant stepped in and performed each worker's job. Rather, prevention consultants help companies reduce their losses by guiding them through various activities."[58]

As a guiding framework, however, the injury prevention consultant will want to incorporate the following elements into the corporate plan:

- A process for the organization to initially identify the potential risk for musculoskeletal problems or other risk factors in the workplace.
- A strategy for showcasing management's commitment to addressing problems and encouraging open worker involvement in problem-solving activities.
- Skill training to assure that management and worker can assess work areas and work methods for risk factors that could lead to musculoskeletal problems.
- Protocols for gathering data to identify jobs or work conditions that are most problematic and at-risk, using strategies such as ergonomic evaluation.
- A strategy for developing effective controls for identified risk factors that, left untouched, could lead to musculoskeletal injury.
- Protocols for outcomes assessment to see if the musculoskeletal injury risk factor controls have actually reduced or eliminated the problem.
- A plan for establishing a healthcare management program that emphasizes the importance of early detection and treatment of musculoskeletal disorders, recognizing that early identification and treatment of these disorders almost always reduces the severity of injury and disability and their associated costs.
- A plan for minimizing future musculoskeletal injury risk factors when new work processes and work areas are in development, recognizing that it is less costly to build good design into the workplace than it is to redesign or retrofit later.

The essential elements of musculoskeletal injury prevention programs listed above are based on recommendations from both the United States Occupational Safety and Health

Box **13-6** OSHA AND NIOSH

The Occupational Safety and Health Act of 1970 created both the National Institute for Occupational Safety and Health (NIOSH) and the Occupational Safety and Health Administration (OSHA). Although NIOSH and OSHA were created by the same act of Congress, they are two distinct agencies with separate responsibilities.

OSHA is in the U.S. Department of Labor and is responsible for developing and enforcing workplace safety and health regulations. Since its inception in 1971, OSHA has helped to cut workplace fatalities by more than 60% and occupational injury and illness rates by 40%. At the same time, U.S. employment has doubled from 56 million workers at 3.5 million worksites to more than 115 million workers at 7.1 million sites. In fiscal year 2004, OSHA had an authorized staff of 2220, including 1123 inspectors. OSHA is headquartered in Washington DC, and has offices in 26 states.

OSHA developed the following publication guidelines to assist industries in developing in-house ergonomic programs:

- *Ergonomic Program Management Guidelines for Meatpacking Plants (OSHA Publication 3123)*
- *Guidelines for Nursing Homes: Ergonomics for the Prevention of Musculoskeletal Disorders* (OSHA Publication 3182)
- *Guidelines for Retail Grocery Stores: Ergonomics for the Prevention of Musculoskeletal Disorders* (OSHA Publication 3192)
- *Guidelines for Poultry Processing: Ergonomics for the Prevention of Musculoskeletal Disorders* (OSHA Publication 3213-09N)

These publications can be ordered at *www.osha.gov* or by calling 1-800-321-OSHA.

NIOSH is in the U.S. Department of Health and Human Services and is an agency established to help assure safe and healthful conditions for working men and women by providing research, information, education, and training in the field of occupational safety and health. NIOSH and OSHA often work together toward the common goal of protecting worker safety and health. NIOSH is headquartered in Washington, DC, with research laboratories and offices in Cincinnati, Ohio; Morgantown, West Virginia; Pittsburgh, Pennsylvania; Spokane, Washington; and Atlanta, Georgia. NIOSH is a professionally diverse organization with a staff of over 1400 people representing a wide range of disciplines including epidemiology, medicine, industrial hygiene, safety, psychology, engineering, chemistry, and statistics.

NIOSH developed the following publication to assist organizations in developing in-house ergonomic programs:

- *Elements of Ergonomic Programs: A Primer Based on Workplace Evaluations of Musculoskeletal Disorders* (NIOSH Publication 97-117)

This publication can be ordered from the National Technical Information Service (NTIS) by calling 703-487-4650. Ask for PB97 144901. It can also be found at the NIOSH website: *http://www.cdc.gov/niosh/homepage.html*; NIOSH 1-800-356-4674.

Administration (OSHA) and the National Institute of Occupational Safety and Health (NIOSH).[14,66-69] In the 1990s and early 2000s, these two entities developed guidelines and recommendations for public and private sector organizations seeking to establish in-house musculoskeletal injury prevention programs. These informational documents are available through OSHA and NIOSH and are an invaluable resource for occupational therapists wanting to offer prevention consulting services to address work-related MSDs.

EMPOWERING CORPORATE CLIENTS: THE INJURY PREVENTION TEAM

Corporate clients initially realize they may have a problem with WMSDs in a variety of ways. Signs of potential problems include worker reports of frequent aches and pains via employee health visits or organized symptom surveys, injury and illness trends among workers performing the same job tasks, and identification of injury risk factors as a result of preventative ergonomic job analysis.[14] Figure 13-13 gives an example of a typical symptom survey used by companies to screen for potential work-related musculoskeletal problems.

Once an organization recognizes it has a problem with work-related musculoskeletal disorders, it must develop a strategy to address the problem. At this point, corporate clients frequently seek an injury prevention consultant to "make the problem go away."

Corporate clients frequently seek injury prevention specialists with the hope for a quick and definitive fix. However, controlling WMSDs needs to be an ongoing process of control and management. The injury prevention consultant must work toward empowering the corporate client to maintain a successful injury prevention program consistently over time. The consultant must assure that the client company has the knowledge and skills to follow through with the program. The role of the injury prevention consultant is to help the organization put together a team and a strategy for ongoing implementation of musculoskeletal injury risk factor identification and control.

In the same way that occupational therapists teach individuals to be self-sufficient in performing activities of daily living, they can also teach their corporate clients to be self-sufficient in controlling musculoskeletal injury risk factors in the work environment. This client-centered approach has

Symptoms Survey: *Ergonomics Program*

Date _____/_____/_____/

_____   _____   Job Name _____
Plant   Dept #

_____   _____   _____ years _____ months
Shift   Hours worked/week   Time on THIS Job

Other jobs you have done in the last year (for more than 2 weeks)

_____   _____   _____   _____ months _____ weeks
Plant   Dept #   Job Name   Time on THIS Job

_____   _____   _____   _____ months _____ weeks
Plant   Dept #   Job Name   Time on THIS Job

(If more than 2 jobs, include those you worked on the most)

Have you had any pain or discomfort during the last year?

☐ Yes   ☐ No (If NO, stop here)

If YES, carefully shade in area of the drawing which bothers you the MOST.

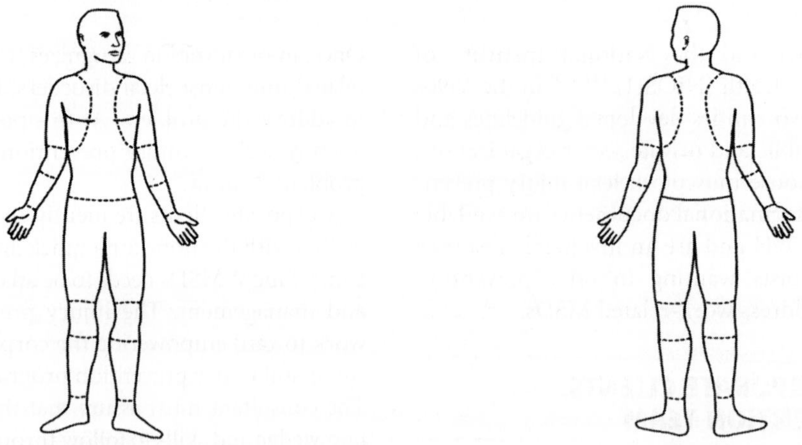

Front   Back

(Continued)

Figure 13-13 Symptom surveys are sometimes used as screening tools in companies that suspect problems with work-related musculoskeletal disorders. Workers are asked to voluntarily fill out the survey. The surveys are analyzed for trends indicating similar musculoskeletal symptoms within certain work groups. If workers from a specific work group tend to have similar complaints, the job tasks and workstations should be further analyzed. (From Cohen AL, et al: *Elements of ergonomics programs: a primer based on workplace evaluations of musculoskeletal disorders*, Washington DC, 1997, US Government Printing Office.)

Continued

(Complete a separate page for each area that bothers you)

Check Area: ☐ Neck ☐ Shoulder ☐ Elbow/Forearm ☐ Hand/Wrist ☐ Fingers
☐ Upper Back ☐ Low Back ☐ Thigh/Knee ☐ Low Leg ☐ Ankle/Foot

1. Please put a check by the words(s) that best describe your problem

☐ Aching ☐ Numbness (asleep) ☐ Tingling

☐ Burning ☐ Pain ☐ Weakness

☐ Cramping ☐ Swelling ☐ Other

☐ Loss of Color ☐ Stiffness

2. When did you first notice the problem?_____ (month)_____ (year)

3. How long does each episode last? (Mark an X along the line)

_____/_____/_____/_____/_____/
 1 hour   1 day   1 week   1 month   6 months

4. How many separate episodes have you had in the last year?_____

5. What do you think caused the problem?_____

_____

6. Have you had this problem in the last 7 days? ☐ Yes ☐ No

7. How would you rate this problem? (mark an X on the line)
   NOW

   None   Unbearable
   When it is the WORST

   None   Unbearable

8. Have you had medical treatment for this problem? ☐ Yes ☐ No

   8a. If NO, why not?_____

   8a. If YES, where did you receive treatment?

   ☐ 1. Company Medical   Times in past year _____

   ☐ 2. Personal doctor   Times in past year _____

   ☐ 3. Other   Times in past year _____

   Did treatment help? ☐ Yes ☐ No _____

9. How much time have you lost in the last year because of this problem?____ days

10. How many days in the last year were you on restricted or light duty because of this problem?
    ____ days

11. Please comment on what you think would improve your symptoms

_____

_____

_____

_____

Figure 13-13 cont'd

occupational therapy intervention focused on the corporate client's priority of controlling work-related injuries and their associated costs. The occupational therapy intervention plan is the development of a corporate in-house injury prevention team. Another name for this team is the *ergonomics team*.

Usually, the injury prevention consultant will decide with corporate management who will be a part of the ergonomics team. Ideally, the team will be composed of representatives from management, front-line supervisors, production workers, labor unions, employee health, safety and/or industrial hygiene, engineering, and the injury prevention/ergonomic consultant. The exact makeup of the team will vary depending on the nature of the organization and corporate structure. The team meets and formulates a strategy for developing and implementing the injury prevention program.

Initial meetings will typically focus on the nature and scope of reported injuries and the effects these injuries have had on production, worker's compensation and associated costs, employee retention, and employee morale. An analysis of existing medical, safety, and insurance records can be conducted for the purpose of identifying injuries associated with MSDs. Healthcare team members should be encouraged to present medical record and injury information in a way that protects the confidentiality of individual workers. The team can then determine incidence rates of MSDs and look at trends that indicate problem work areas or job tasks.

Once the scope of the problem has been analyzed, the team will decide on a plan of attack for injury prevention. In general, the magnitude and location of existing problems will suggest the magnitude and direction of initial team efforts. The consultant will want to direct the corporate client to address the most grievous and resource-draining problems first. If, upon analysis of the data, the problems seem widespread and involve a large percentage of the workforce, then the plan of attack will likely be an aggressive company-wide program. On the other hand, if the problems seem isolated to just a few work areas or employees, the initial plan would likely be more focused and direct.[14]

MANAGEMENT COMMITMENT

Industrial safety and health literature stresses that management support for injury prevention efforts is crucial for successful implementation and outcomes.[14] The consultant will want to assure that management commitment to the process is genuine. If there is a lack of sincere top-level support for the injury prevention program, a consultant would be wise to pass on his or her involvement. Consultants are judged on their record of success. Prevention efforts without management support are destined to fail.

A good injury prevention consultant knows that employees want to see evidence of management support for all new programs. One of several ways to assist the corporate client in demonstrating support to the workforce is to encourage management to issue policy statements that give injury prevention efforts equal priority with productivity standards and cost control. Management should also meet with employee or union representatives (who should ideally be part of the ergonomics team) to discuss new policy and injury prevention program plans and show evidence of committing resources to implement the injury prevention program. Goals should be set and timelines established for meeting these goals, with specific people assigned responsibility and held accountable for overseeing various aspects of the program. Finally, information about the program should be disseminated to the entire workforce, from planning, to implementation, to evaluation. Employees want and need to feel they are a part of the organization's commitment to safety.[9,14]

TRAINING IN RISK FACTOR IDENTIFICATION/ERGONOMIC EVALUATION AND PROBLEM SOLVING

Research has identified specific physical activity demands that place people at risk for developing WMSDs: repetition, force, awkward or static posturing, prolonged direct pressure on soft tissue, vibration, exposure to cold, and inappropriate or inadequate hand tools.[14,66-69,78] Additionally, psychosocial stressors at work can contribute to development of WMSDs.[14] Although this is an area in need of further study, these types of stressors can include excessive volume or productivity expectations, work that is "too difficult" or beyond the intellectual or emotional capacity of the employee, or a superior who does not express appreciation for a job well done. It is the combination of physical and psychosocial risk factors that the ergonomics team must address as part of an injury prevention program for WMSDs.

The ergonomics team will likely have the injury prevention consultant perform the first ergonomic evaluations at the workplace and present the first suggestions for improvement. However, key members of the injury prevention team should receive training in performing these evaluations themselves and training in how to formulate solutions. In this way, the evaluation part of the process is not reliant on an outside source. The goal, eventually, is to have the injury prevention consultant step out of the picture and leave behind a self-sufficient team of in-house experts to implement an on-going process of risk factor identification MSD control.

Figure 13-10 is an example of a general ergonomic injury risk analysis checklist. Members of the injury prevention team could be trained to use this tool to screen a variety of jobs for musculoskeletal injury risk factors. Similarly, Figure 13-11 is an example of a job-specific screening tool. This checklist helps evaluators identify musculoskeletal injury risk factors for computer users. Figure 13-12 is a hand tool analysis checklist. The injury prevention consultant or ergonomics team members could choose to modify any of these screening tools to match jobs specific to the organization.

The NIOSH publication *Elements for Ergonomics Programs* 12 lists several objectives for team member training. The successfully trained team member will be able to do the following:

- Recognize musculoskeletal injury risk factors and understand basic methods for their control
- Identify signs and symptoms of musculoskeletal injury in workers
- Understand the company's injury prevention program thoroughly and everyone's role and responsibility from top-level management to front-line worker
- Know the company's procedure for reporting identified risk factors and signs and symptoms of musculoskeletal injury
- Demonstrate the ability to do a basic ergonomic evaluation for identifying musculoskeletal injury risk factors
- Recommend ways to control injury risk factors based on collaboration with employees, management, and other members of the ergonomics team
- Select ways to implement and evaluate the control measures
- Demonstrate skill in team building, consensus development, and problem solving

Some companies will decide to extend training to other members of the workforce. General employee training can be provided to employees who may potentially be exposed to musculoskeletal injury hazards. Training can include how to recognize and report early signs and symptoms of musculoskeletal injury, information on identifying musculoskeletal injury risk factors both at work and outside of work, and strategies for workers to protect themselves from developing musculoskeletal injury. Supervisors should receive the same training as workers, as well as training in techniques to reinforce proper body mechanics and other important aspects of the injury prevention program.[69]

Training the ergonomics team in skills required to sustain the injury prevention program is a substantial aspect of the consultant's role. The consultant selects or designs the training and training materials to be understandable to the lay person, considering the participants' educational levels and literacy abilities. Language skill consideration is also important and attempts should be made to provide the materials in the primary language of the employee.[14] Outside training courses are also valuable in bringing perspective to the organization's situation. Interaction with other companies' course attendees provides opportunities for company-to-company networking. Many resources exist for locating appropriate training courses, including NIOSH and OSHA.

DEVELOPING RISK FACTOR CONTROLS

The ergonomic evaluations will identify known risk factors for development of MSDs. Risk factors might include forceful exertions, awkward or static posturing, repetition, contact stressors, vibration, exposure to cold, and/or psychosocial stressors. These identified risk factors will be brought back to the ergonomics team for discussion. Once high-risk areas or tasks have been identified, the task of the team then becomes formulating ways to reduce or eliminate the musculoskeletal injury risk factors.

At this point, it is important to use as many front-line production workers in the problem-solving process as possible. Workers know their jobs better than anyone and may have already formulated some ideas about improving the work area or work methods. Promoting worker involvement at this point has several benefits: enhanced worker motivation and job satisfaction, added team problem-solving capabilities, greater acceptance of workplace change, and greater knowledge of the work and organization.[11,14,46,47,64]

When workers present ideas for risk factor modification, it is essential that the injury prevention consultant and the in-house ergonomics team assure that these potential solutions are appropriate and do not carry with them potential for creating new problems. Union representatives should ensure that the suggested solutions do not violate employee-management understandings and contracts. Engineering's role is to evaluate suggested solutions for practical and physical feasibility. Management's role is to provide input regarding the organizational and financial appropriateness of the suggested solutions.

There are a variety of ways to reduce or eliminate musculoskeletal injury risk factors. The 1991 OSHA publication, *Ergonomics Program Management Guidelines for Meatpacking Plants*, outlines a variety of risk factor control strategies applicable to most any workplace situation. These strategies can be categorized as either engineering controls, work practice controls, administrative controls, or use of personal protective equipment.[69]

Engineering controls include strategies for designing or modifying the workstation, work methods, and/or tools. The goal is to eliminate or reduce excessive exertion, awkward postures, and repetition. Workstations should be designed or modified to accommodate the actual worker at that workstation. If more than one person uses a workstation, then elements of the workstation should be adjustable to fit each worker and be comfortable for the workers to use. Work methods should be designed or modified to minimize static and awkward posturing, repetitive motions, and excessive force. Tools and handles should be designed for a specific job and minimize contact stress, vibration, and forceful motions/gripping by the workers' hands.[69]

Work practice controls include policy and procedures for safe and proper task performance that are understood by all and enforced by supervisors. Workers should receive training in proper body mechanics, tool maintenance, and use of workstation adjustability features. New workers and those workers who have been away for awhile should be allowed adequate break-in periods in order to condition and recondition their bodies for the physical demands of the job. Supervisors and management should constantly monitor the use and effectiveness of work practice controls, and make adjustments to techniques, line speeds, and staffing as needed to maintain a safe and healthy work environment.[69]

Selection and use of personal protective equipment should be in-line with the overall injury prevention program. Equipment should be available in a variety of sizes to accommodate the size differences among workers. Proper fit is especially important for gloves because improperly fitting gloves can reduce blood flow and sensory feedback, leading to slippage and use of excessive grip and pinch forces. Protection against extreme cold (< 40° F) is required to protect joints and soft tissues. Back braces and upper extremity splints should not be considered personal protective equipment. These devices are part of the medical management aspect of the program, and should only be used with the advice and under the supervision of the healthcare team.[69]

Finally, administrative controls must be an option in situations in which musculoskeletal risk factors cannot be adequately reduced or eliminated via engineering controls, work practice controls, and use of personal protective equipment. Administrative controls reduce the duration, frequency, and severity of exposure to risk factors. Methods include decreasing production rates, limiting overtime work, providing periodic rest breaks throughout the day, increasing staffing levels, and using job rotation/job enlargement to other jobs and tasks that use different muscle-tendon groups.[69]

When the team comes to a consensus on which methods to employ to reduce or eliminate the musculoskeletal injury risk factors, it is time to formulate a plan and implement the proposed solutions. However, before any changes are made, it is important to again solicit employee feedback regarding these plans, especially from employees who are not involved with the ergonomics team. Most people are resistant to change; it is human nature. Soliciting and sincerely listening to feedback improves employee buy-in for the proposed changes. Additionally, this feedback might identify implementation problems that the ergonomics team overlooked. Even the best idea for improving the comfort and safety of a job cannot be successfully implemented without employee support. Performing this step in the process is well worth the time and effort.

MEDICAL MANAGEMENT STRATEGIES

In addition to identifying musculoskeletal injury risk factors and implementing plans to reduce or eliminate these risk factors, it is important for the ergonomics team to develop a medical management plan. Initiating early conservative medical treatment is key to minimizing serious disorder and dysfunction.[60] Workers should be trained to identify early symptoms of developing MSDs so that they can seek medical care. The employee health staff should formulate guidelines for management of employees with early symptoms of MSDs. This plan might include oral anti-inflammatories, splinting, rotation to light duty or time off from work, and occupational therapy. The physician and/or employee health nurse will usually lead the effort in developing medical management guidelines for the organization.

As occupational therapists, it is important to understand the role and implications for upper extremity splinting of work-related injuries. The healthcare team should think about the possible ramifications of prescribing an upper extremity splint to the worker who plans to remain on the job. It is true that splinting helps rest the injured body part and this can be helpful for recovery from a musculoskeletal injury. However, when a worker is restricted from moving, for example, the wrist during work, the result is often that the elbow or shoulder will compensate by positioning itself awkwardly to get the task accomplished. Splinting during work may protect the wrist, but the result could be injury to the elbow, shoulder, neck, or back. Therefore, splints should not be used at work unless the healthcare team understands the worker's job tasks and can assure that using the splint will not place stress on other parts of the body.

OUTCOMES ASSESSMENT AND PREVENTING FUTURE PROBLEMS

Finally, once the ergonomics team has implemented both the musculoskeletal injury risk factor control efforts and the medical management process, the entire injury prevention program must be evaluated for effectiveness. Outcomes measures are useful in determining if the program is working and to what extent. If the program does not seem to be working to any significant degree, the team will continue to modify their efforts until the incidence of WMSDs has declined to acceptable levels. The injury prevention program should be considered an ongoing process rather than a short-term solution to an identified incident or problem work area. Most ergonomics teams find that as soon as one problem work area is under control, another problem is identified that requires the focus of the team's efforts.

The occupational therapist is an invaluable resource for helping organizations develop in-house injury prevention programs to control risk factors related to musculoskeletal injury development. The occupational therapist's basic training in occupational performance analysis, problem identification, intervention planning and implementation, and outcomes assessment make the fields of ergonomics and injury prevention ideally suited for practitioners of our profession. The National Institute of Occupational Safety and Health and the United States Occupational Safety and Health Administration are valuable resources for the occupational therapist interested in working in ergonomics and injury prevention.

PRE-EMPLOYMENT TESTING

A frequent use of functional testing includes assessing a person's ability to meet certain physical requirements before they are hired for a job.[75] Some pre-employment testing may consist of isometric strength testing, ROM testing, or actual measurement of a person's ability to perform selected tasks from the job description. Pre-employment screening can be an integral part of a company's comprehensive injury prevention and management strategy.[75]

When a company is looking at the overall impact of an employee injury on their bottom line, it goes much further than simply the cost of the injury itself. It extends beyond the medical costs to include the employee's compensation, benefit package payments, training of replacement personnel, replacement personnel's wages, and overtime payment for existing personnel if they are needed for coverage. This does not include the indirect costs of diminished productivity during the period of time when coverage is being arranged. The total impact can be quite staggering. The cost of developing an employment screening process is significant; however, the cost savings to the company can be dramatic.[75]

OT PRACTICE NOTE

Due to task analysis training and a holistic approach, occupational therapists are excellent candidates for assisting companies with the expansion of plans to more effectively manage employee injuries.

The EEOC's Uniform Guidelines on Employee Selection Procedures sets forth guidelines for the structure and function of human resource departments within companies and businesses. The guidelines also address how an organization can select and manage employees, and places strong emphasis on the necessity of policies and procedures being job related.[24,75] The EEOC also mandates that an employer's selection process not have adverse impact on any group of people and must not discriminate on the basis of race, color, religion, sex, or national origin, as established by Title VII of the Civil Rights Act of 1964.[24,75] Meeting these criteria requires that the selection procedures demonstrate validation, be of business necessity, and be a bona fide occupational requirement.[24,75] To be ADA compliant, pre-employment screening must be based upon an accurate job description, test only the essential functions (although not every function need be assessed), and have high face validity (often referred to as content validity—tests what you really

want to know), or closely mirror the aspects of the job that is being tested.[5,75] Dynamic testing (actually replicating physical tasks from the job) is recommended and can be conducted on-site at the company, or off-site and needs to use equipment from the job, as it is available.[75] It is vital that a company take the time to thoroughly develop their screening process to be able to defend why the screening was considered necessary, maintain awareness and vigilance in the development phase of good test design, and be prepared to explain and demonstrate the applicability of the screen to the job in question.[75]

Pre-employment testing can also occur at several points in the hiring process; however, many healthcare providers and legal experts recommend conducting such testing after an offer of employment has been extended. With post-offer screening (POS), the most advantageous progression is to interview the applicant and determine if the person is an acceptable candidate for employment.[75] A conditional offer is extended to the applicant, based upon the applicant's ability to meet a variety of conditions, such as passing a drug screen, acceptable background check, and physical testing. A problem with pre-offer testing is that Title 29 of the Code of Federal Regulations specifically states that medical examination is permissible "after making an offer of employment to a job applicant."[13] Monitoring blood pressure or heart rate or inquiring about past medical history are all considered to be part of a medical examination and are precluded in pre-offer testing.[75]

Anything that a therapist does in the way of evaluating an applicant might be deemed medical, simply because an occupational therapist is a medical professional. It is also important to look critically at any testing that is considered to be general strength testing as it has been found to be a poor predictor of potential for injury.[21,63,75] Normative databases are of little use in making hiring decisions, too, as according to both the ADA and the EEOC, it doesn't matter if the applicant falls into the 5th percentile or the 95th percentile; the only thing of importance is whether the applicant can perform the tasks of the job.[5,24]

If the applicant passes the screening, then he or she is hired and begins working. If the applicant does not pass, then the employer must assess whether or not the applicant has a disability, as defined under the ADA (see Chapter 14).[5] If the applicant does, then the employer must determine if they are able to offer reasonable accommodation to the applicant in order that that the individual may be able to perform the job. Reasonable accommodation means providing accommodation in such a way that the employer is not placed under undue financial strain in order for the accommodation to be implemented. If the company can and does offer accommodation to the applicant, the hiring process is completed and their employment begins. If the company cannot offer reasonable accommodation, or if the applicant does not have a disability, yet fails the screening, then the employer can choose to rescind the offer of employment, examine opportunities for alternative placement elsewhere in the company, or offer remediation of some type and allow the applicant to re-test if certain criteria are met.[75] For example, if a non-disabled applicant does not pass the lifting portion of a POS and otherwise meets the employment criteria, the company might elect to allow the applicant two weeks to improve their strength with the goal of returning to re-test the screen in an attempt to pass the lifting portion.

Suppose Henry had difficulty balancing on one leg as a result of an early childhood accident, but that this balance problem was not something that readily presented itself. If a POS was conducted with Henry prior to his being hired at the roofing company and balance was a component of testing for working as a roofer, his difficulty could have been detected and Henry could have been declined the job or offered alternative placement. Either way Henry would have been protected from a fall that would radically change his life.

A company does not have to test applicants for every job. Typically, it is suggested that a company survey all of its injuries and determine where the majority of injuries are occurring and determine if injuries are occurring within the first six months of hiring. If so, this company is a good candidate for implementing a physical screen as part of their hiring process. Once it is determined which jobs are going to be selected for testing, then the physical demands of the job must be evaluated. This can be done by survey, questionnaire, or observation (either direct or video).[8] The job description must include information that is functional in terms of physical demands, describe the essential tasks of the job, and be presented in such language that one can test for an individual's ability to perform them.[8] In the case of a company requesting that existing job descriptions be used for the development of the screen, it is extremely important to document that the company provided the job descriptions and that the therapist does not assume any liability for errors in their accuracy.

Physical demand items can then be selected for testing during screening, either based on the difficulty or the frequency of the item. It is not necessary to test all of the physical demands for each job. For instance, a job might include carrying 10 lb a distance of 10 feet twice a day and lifting 40 lb from pallet height to waist height 200 times per day. Testing the ability to lift 40 lb would be a better selection for testing, for if the applicant is able to lift 40 lb from pallet height to waist height, it is likely that he or she will also be able to carry 10 lb a distance of 10 feet. It is important to select a method of testing the tasks that is reliable and valid and demonstrates job applicability, whether choosing from a standardized battery of physical demand tests or developing job-specific tasks to improve applicant understanding of the relevance of the task and defensibility of hiring decisions.[24,75]

 ETHICAL CONSIDERATIONS

It is imperative for the clinician to encourage companies to have written policies regarding the screening process, including how to handle screening failures.[75] It is also important to extricate the therapist from the hiring process, in that all communications come from the employer, so the therapist is allowed to maintain objectivity and third-party distance to the course of action.[75] Continuing documentation and follow-up help to establish a definitive paper trail demonstrating the business necessity for implementing a pre-employment screening process, the steps taken to select and analyze the job and tasks to be tested, the implementation phase, ongoing quality assurance to monitor any changes in the job and reflect subsequent changes in the screen and the actions taken to handle screening failures, reasonable accommodation, and avoiding adverse impact.[75]

After tasks are selected, then implementation can begin. It is suggested that a statistically significant sample of incumbents be tested to assure that the correct demands have been selected and that the minimum requirements for each demand have been set appropriately. Once pilot testing is complete, the screening can be administered consistently to all applicants for a given job. It is also recommended that the screening process be monitored to ensure that fair and nondiscriminatory selection of applicants is occurring and that modifications to the screening process can occur as needed.[75]

TRANSITION SERVICES FROM SCHOOL TO WORK

Occupational therapy practitioners can make a valuable contribution to students with disabilities transitioning from school to the community. The 1997 amendments to the Individuals with Disabilities Education Act (IDEA) of 1990 specified that transition planning is to be part of the Individualized Education Program (IEP). Representatives from community agencies that provide post-school services, such as state-sponsored vocational rehabilitation, must join the education team. Related services such as occupational therapy are formal contributors to the transition planning for students who need these type of services.[90] Transition services are defined by IDEA as "a coordinated set of activities for a student designed within an outcome-oriented process, which promotes movement from school to post-school activities, includes postsecondary education, vocational training, integrated employment (including supported employment), continuing and adult education, adult services, independent living, or community participation."[89] Occupational therapy's unique focus on occupational performance can be a strong asset to the transition team.

The three main roles that an occupational therapist will participate in are transition-related evaluation, service planning, and service implementation. The occupational therapist contributes vital information about students' performance abilities and needs in any of the transition domains: domestic, vocational, school, recreational, and community.

TRANSITION-RELATED EVALUATION

Effective transition-related evaluation primarily uses nonstandardized interviews, situational observation, and activity analysis approaches. These approaches are top-down, meaning that they first consider what the student wants or needs to do and secondarily they identify the occupational performance issues that are causing difficulties.[6] The transition team helps the student identify a positive, shared vision for the future. This can include living alone or with others in the community, attending postsecondary schools or training programs, working in a paid or volunteer job, using community services, and participating in activities of interest. The occupational therapist and other members on the team work together to identify the student's present interests and abilities within the context in which performance is expected or needed. The evaluation process also allows the team to identify areas in which the student is likely to need ongoing support and resources to achieve his or her vision and goals for the future.

SERVICE PLANNING

In a collaborative transition team, the team members collectively share information and write the student's goals.[90] The team members do not write discipline-specific goals that focus on remediating the student's underlying deficits. The occupational therapist, for example, does not need to write specific goals addressing cognitive, motor, or psychosocial skills. Instead, two or more group members gather together to write the goals and work collaboratively together with the student to accomplish the goals. A student with limited movement in her arms and hands may have the goal of being able to complete written assignments. The occupational therapist may take the lead in evaluating the effectiveness of using alternative writing methods such as assistive technology. Recommendations are made to the student and the team. If the team supports the recommendations, then the team would assign responsibility for obtaining the equipment as well as providing training to the student and other team members. Rainforth and York-Barr define collaboration as "an interactive process in which persons with varied life perspectives and experiences join together in a spirit of willingness to share resources, responsibility, and regards in creating inclusive and effective educational programs and environments for students with unique learning needs."[79]

PROGRAM IMPLEMENTATION

The occupational therapist provides services in collaboration with the student and his or her teachers, parents, employers, co-workers, and others as necessary to address the student's goals in the areas of domestic, vocational, school, recreation, and community. Occupational therapy personnel (including the occupational therapist and the occupational therapy assistant) deliver transition services in the student's natural environments. Therefore, occupational therapy may provide intervention in the student's school, workplace, home, or any other relevant setting in the community. Collaborative problem solving with others involved in the student's environment is essential to help the student use alternative methods to complete necessary activities. For example, an occupational therapist may introduce and train the teacher on using assistive technology to help a student be able to access the computer at school to do written assignments. The occupational therapy practitioner may provide direct or consultative services to help minimize discrepancies in the student's abilities and the demands of any environment. Evaluating whether the student reaches his or her goals should be the outcome measure to evaluate the effectiveness of occupational therapy services.

WORK READINESS PROGRAMS

Many times, people who have survived a major accident or illness cannot return to their prior employment and need to explore other options for employment. For example, Henry can no longer carry out the job demands of a roofer. Henry may really want to return to some type of meaningful work, but needs guidance and direction to explore what his present abilities and work skills are so that he can set some realistic vocational goals.

A **work readiness program** is designed to help individuals who desire to work identify vocational options that match their interests, skills, and abilities. At Rancho Los Amigos National Rehabilitation Center in Downey, California, an occupational therapist leads a work readiness program along with a vocational evaluator. This is a six-week program that meets three times a week for two hours. It consists primarily of group sessions with a few individual sessions. Topics addressed include the following: work habits, values, goals, interests, work skills, vocational exploration, job hunting strategies, and community resources. Instruction, group discussion, and hands-on exploration of work skills using standardized work samples and situational assessments are used to help people explore their readiness to work and discover their potential for pursuing training for a different occupation. Each person's program is individualized to address specific goals and interests. For example, Henry may be interested in working with a computer. He would be given the opportunity to do different work-related tasks using a computer so Henry could see if he has an aptitude for this type of work. If Henry was not familiar with the types of jobs a person could do using a computer, then he would learn how to do vocational research by using various reference books in the library or on the Internet.

A work readiness program can help people identify specific goals to pursue, and develop a plan to help them work toward their goals. This program can help a person prepare for returning to work, but it does not provide a job for the participant. At the completion of the program, if a person demonstrates readiness to work, then he or she can be referred to the state department of rehabilitation for assistance with job training and job placement. After completing a work readiness program, the occupational therapist can provide valuable information on a person's skills, aptitudes, and interests to assist the rehabilitation counselor with developing a feasible plan for the worker. While Henry was attending the work readiness program, he identified the goal to become a computer support technician. Based on the vocational testing and research that he did during the program, this was determined to be a reasonable goal for him to pursue. He was referred to the state department of rehabilitation for job training and job placement in his new career.

COMMUNITY-BASED SERVICES

Historically, work-related programs took place within medical model clinics, such as rehabilitation programs or settings designed for work intervention as opposed to the site where the worker actually performed his or her role.[86] Today, work programs are increasingly located in the community in which the participant resides or within the work setting itself.[86] This trend toward increased community practice is probably due to changes within the field of occupational therapy and external forces influencing the practice. Current thinking in occupational therapy recognizes that "occupational dysfunction is multidimensional, resulting from the interplay of biological, psychological, and ecological factors."[86] Decreasing reimbursement in medical model settings has resulted in occupational therapists exploring other options for reimbursement in the community.

Funding for most community-based programs is from grants or contracts through local, state, or federal governments, as well as foundations. Grants are funds that are awarded for a specific purpose and a specific time period, usually for research or a service project, "based on a submission of a creative original proposal."[86] Contracts also provide funding for research or service projects; however, the funding agency defines the scope of the project and requests bids from competing organizations in the community. The majority of funding for community-based programs comes from foundations; "Foundations are operated by philanthropic families, corporations, or community agencies that have reserved significant amounts of money for the purpose of supporting charitable organizations and programs to address specific community needs."[86] Many associations and civic groups, such as the United Way, American Head Injury Foundation, Kiwanis Club, etc. provide funding for community projects related to

specific interest areas. It is important to note that community-based programs should develop a broad financial base with multiple funding sources in order for programs to "survive and thrive" in the long run.

COMMUNITY REHABILITATION PROGRAMS

There are almost 600 community rehabilitation programs (CRPs) with federal contracts under the Javits-Wagner-O'Day (JWOD) Program according to NISH, formerly the National Industries for the Severely Handicapped. These community-based non-profit organizations train and employ individuals with severe disabilities (primarily developmental disabilities and blindness) and provide quality goods and services to the federal government. The CRPs subcontract work with various industries to allow individuals with severe disabilities the opportunity to be productive, earn a competitive wage, and contribute to society. See the NISH website (*www.NISH.org*) for more details. These programs receive most of their funding from regional centers or the Office of Vocational Rehabilitation (OVR). Although most of these programs are run by non-occupational therapy personnel, this is an area some occupational therapists may want to explore for future involvement. There is a great need for these types of programs for those with other severe, chronic disabilities (such as brain and spinal cord injuries), but creative funding needs to be obtained to support them.

HOMELESS SHELTER PROGRAMS

An emerging practice area for occupational therapists is working with persons who are homeless. Due to the increasing number of persons experiencing homelessness, Congress enacted the Stewart McKinney Homeless Assistance Act of 1987 (Public Law 100-77).[33] This act was designed to meet the needs of those who are homeless by providing funds for emergency shelters, food, healthcare, housing, education, job training, and other community services. The act funded a Department of Labor (DOL) project to plan, implement, and evaluate the effectiveness of a comprehensive spectrum of employment, training, and other support services to help persons who are homeless to locate and sustain employment. Based on the Job Training for the Homeless Demonstration Program (JTHDP), which consisted of 63 organizations across the United States that provided comprehensive services for persons who were homeless from September 1988 to November 1995, the DOL created a best practices guide.[86] Box 13-7 lists the findings of the JTHDP, which recommended that a sponsoring agency provide the core services or that the agency develop linkages with other local human service providers to assist persons who are homeless in obtaining and sustaining employment.

Occupational therapists have the skills to design and implement programs that incorporate the JTHDP recommendations for best practices. Client-centered job readiness and job training programs can be developed for community service

Box **13-7**   CORE SERVICES NECESSARY ACCORDING TO THE JTHDP

- Case management and counseling
- Evaluation and employability development planning
- Job training services (e.g., remedial education, basic skills training, literacy instruction, job-search assistance, job counseling, vocational and occupational skills training, and on-the-job training
- Job development and placement services
- Post-placement follow-up and support services (e.g., additional job placement services, training after placement, self-help support groups, mentoring)
- Housing services (e.g., emergency housing assistance, evaluation of housing needs, referrals to appropriate housing alternatives)
- Other support services (e.g., child care, transportation, chemical dependence evaluation, counseling, and referral to outpatient or inpatient treatment as appropriate)
- Mental health evaluation, counseling, and referral to treatment
- Other healthcare services
- Clothing
- Life skills training

From Herzberg GL, et al: Work and the underserved: homelessness and work. In Kornblau BL, Jacobs K, editors: *Work: principles and practice*, Bethesda, 2000, AOTA.

agencies to address the concerns of persons who are homeless. This population desires intervention services that are "sensitive, respectful, and responsive to their self-identified needs."[9]

Occupational therapy practitioners work with those who are homeless as well as the agencies providing services for people who are homeless to build skills for accessing resources, solving problems by identifying strengths and assets, and learning to critically analyze situations for win-win situations for employers and the persons who are homeless.

WELFARE-TO-WORK PROGRAMS

Congress passed the Personal Responsibility and Work Opportunity Reconciliation Act (Public Law 104-193) in 1996, to move people from welfare to work.[9] It required welfare recipients to find work after receiving two years of public assistance. The Balanced Budget Act of 1997 (BBA; Public Law 105-33) provided funds for welfare-to-work grants. These grants are for training long-term recipients of welfare or public assistance to enter the job market in unsubsidized jobs. People who are most difficult to place because of multiple barriers to work, such as low academic skills, poor work history, or those who need substance abuse treatment, are the target of these grants. A substantial percentage of welfare recipients have learning problems, mental health and substance use disorders, and issues of domestic violence interfering with their sustained employability.[86]

Welfare-to-work programs are another innovative practice area for occupational therapists. Therapists who are interested in entering this area of practice must find out which agencies within the local or state communities control the welfare-to-work funds. Occupational therapists can subcontract with these agencies and collaborate with them. This information can be accessed from the National Governors Association (NGA) Center for Best Practices welfare reform website.[61] Private foundations that are involved with the welfare-to-work programs may also be a source of entry for occupational therapists.

There are many barriers that a person receiving welfare must face in order to enter into competitive employment. Lack of transportation, lack of childcare, problems with domestic violence, illiteracy, lack of housing, substance abuse, and medical needs can interfere with a welfare recipient's ability to obtain and retain a job.[9] Successful welfare-to-work programs attempt to break down these barriers. For example, programs combine basic education and job development, provide refurbished cars for transportation to work, and provide one-on-one mentoring for improving self-sufficiency.[62] Transitioning welfare recipients to the workplace presents a challenging practice area for occupational therapists to use their creativity to design and deliver effective services to help clients set goals, explore vocational options, and introduce them to different community resources to achieve successful and continued employment.[41]

TICKET TO WORK

The Ticket to Work and Work Incentives Improvement Act was enacted in December 1999. This law created a voluntary program for Supplemental Security Income (SSI) and Social Security Disability Insurance (SSDI) recipients to receive job-related support services and encourage beneficiaries to return to work and pursue their employment goals.[92] Those who have tickets can go to any employment network such as a local office of vocational rehabilitation (OVR) to receive services. Interested individuals can contact MAXIMUS Toll free at 1-866-968-7842 or visit the website *www.yourticket-towork.com* or *www.ssa.gov/work*. The Ticket to Work program creates opportunities for occupational therapists to serve on advisory panels, work as program managers, or provide employment support services.[41]

SUMMARY

This chapter gives an overview of the varying types of work programs in which occupational therapists are currently practicing. There are tremendous opportunities for occupational therapists and certified occupational therapy assistants to expand their role and involvement in hospitals, schools, industrial settings, and in the community in general in the area of work practice. Occupational therapy practitioners involved in work programs need to take a proactive approach in advocating the need and benefit of these types of programs in all communities to help restore the worker role in many people's lives.

THREADED CASE STUDY: JOE, LORNA, AND HENRY, PART 2

Reflecting back upon the introductory case scenarios, the reader sees opportunities for the application of these comprehensive work-related occupational therapy interventions. For example, Joe's occupational therapist could conduct a job demands analysis of the laundry attendant position and a worksite evaluation at the hotel and spa where he worked prior to his spinal cord injury. Then the occupational therapist could determine if Joe could successfully carry out the essential functions of that alternate job. The occupational therapist could recommend any modifications that needed to be done to make the work area wheelchair accessible. A functional capacity evaluation may be helpful to determine whether Joe could carry out any of the specific physical demands of the job on an occasional or frequent basis. Based upon the results, the occupational therapist could then make recommendations to the physician and the employer on any reasonable accommodations that may be necessary for Joe to successfully return to work as well as inform them of any concerns of Joe's ability to safely meet the physical demands of the job.

After Lorna, the upholsterer with the repetitive stress hand injury, obtains a general occupational therapy evaluation and intervention for her acute injuries in the clinic, she could similarly benefit from an ergonomic assessment and intervention at her workplace.

The goal of an ergonomic assessment and intervention would be to eliminate the risk factors that contributed to her original injury and to avoid recurrence of future problems. The occupational therapist could communicate with Lorna's employer about developing an in-house ergonomic and injury prevention program at the company to reduce the number of work-related musculoskeletal disorders occurring at the workplace.

Finally, contemplate the third scenario which involves Henry. Henry needs the assistance of an occupational therapy practitioner to help him discover what type of work he would be best suited for while taking into consideration his present physical and cognitive abilities and limitations. He could also benefit from a comprehensive vocational evaluation to assess his cognitive and physical abilities, work habits, work skills, and work tolerances, as well as interests and attitudes to determine if he could return to any other type of work. Another alternative would be for Henry to participate in a work readiness program. The same areas assessed during a vocational evaluation would also be addressed in the work readiness program; however, Henry could also benefit from a discussion on work-related topics as well as receive peer interaction and feedback on his work performance, work habits, and attitudes.

Review Questions

1. How has occupational therapy involvement in work programs evolved over the years?
2. What is the role of occupational therapy in work programs?
3. Describe the difference between a functional capacity evaluation and a vocational evaluation.
4. What components are usually included in an FCE report?
5. Describe the difference between work hardening and work conditioning.
6. Name the common applications of the results of a job demands analysis.
7. What interventions are used to determine if someone is capable of returning to a specific occupation after an injury?
8. Discuss the ergonomic design considerations for workstations, seating, visualizing job tasks, tools, and materials handling.
9. List and discuss the eight important elements of corporate injury prevention plans.
10. Why are occupational therapists good candidates for assisting companies in the development of injury management programs?
11. Name and describe some innovative types of work programs in which occupational therapists can be involved in the community.

REFERENCES

1. American Occupational Therapy Association: Occupational therapy practice framework: domain and process, Am J Occup Ther 56(6):609, 2002.
2. American Occupational Therapy Association: Statement: Occupational therapy services in facilitating work performance, Am J Occup Ther 54(6):626, 2000.
3. American Occupational Therapy Association: Occupational therapy services in work practice, Am J Occup Ther 46(12):1086, 1992.
4. American Occupational Therapy Association: Work hardening guidelines, Am J Occup Ther 40(12):841, 1986.
5. Americans with Disabilities Act: Technical Assistance Manual, Washington, DC, 1992, Equal Employment Opportunity Commission.
6. Baum CM, Law M: Occupational therapy practice: focusing on occupational performance, Am J Occup Ther 51(4):277, 1997.
7. Biddle J, Roberts K: More evidence of the need for an ergonomic standard, Am J Ind Med 45(4):329, 2004.
8. Bohr PC: Work analysis. In King PM, editor: Sourcebook of occupational rehabilitation, New York, 1998, Plenum Press.
9. Callahan SR: Understanding health-status barriers that hinder the transition from welfare to work, Washington, DC, 1999, National Governors Association Center for Best Practices, Health Policy Status Division.
10. Canelon MF: An on-site job evaluation performed via activity analysis, Am J Occup Ther 51(2):144, 1997.
11. Cascio WF: Applied psychology in personnel management, Englewood Cliffs, NJ, 1991, Prentice-Hall.

12. Chaffin DB, Andersson GB: *Occupational biomechanics*, ed 2, New York, 1991, John Wiley & Sons.

13. Code of Federal Regulations, Title 29, Vol 4. Revised as of July 1, 2003. Part 1630: *Regulations to implement the equal employment provisions of the Americans with Disabilities Act*. Section 1630.14, Washington DC.

14. Cohen AL, et al: *Elements of ergonomics programs: a primer based on workplace evaluations of musculoskeletal disorders*, Washington DC, 1997, US Government Printing Office.

15. Commission on Accreditation of Rehabilitation Facilities: *Standards manual for organizations serving people with disabilities*, Tucson, AZ, 1989, CARF.

16. Crabtree J: The end of occupational therapy, *Am J Occup Ther* 52(3):205, 1998.

17. Cromwell FS: Work-related programming in occupational therapy: its roots course and prognosis, *Occup Ther in Healthcare* 2(4):9, 1985.

18. Dahl R: Ergonomics. In Kornblau B, Jacobs K, editors: *Work: principles and practice*, Bethesda, MD, 2000, AOTA.

19. Darphin LE: Work-hardening and work-conditioning perspectives. In Isernhagen SJ, ed: *The comprehensive guide to work injury management*, Gaithersburg, FL, 1995, Aspen Publishers.

20. Davis H, Rodgers S: Using this book for ergonomics in industry: introduction. In Eggleton E, editor, Rodgers S, technical editor: *Ergonomic design for people at work*, Vol 1, New York, 1983, Van Nostrand Reinhold.

21. Deuker JA, et al: Isokinetic trunk testing and employment, *J Occup Med* 36(1):42, 1994.

22. Eggleton E, ed; Rodgers S, technical ed: *Ergonomic design for people at work*, Vol 1, New York, 1983, Van Nostrand Reinhold.

23. Ellexon M: *What every rehab professional in the U.S.A. should know about the ADA*, Miami, 1992, ADA Consultants.

24. Equal Employment Opportunity Commission: *Uniform guidelines on employee selection procedures*, Washington, DC, 1978, EEOC.

25. Eser G: *Overview of vocational evaluation*, Las Vegas, 1983, Stout Univ. Training Workshop.

26. Falkiner S, Myers S: When exactly can carpal tunnel syndrome be considered work-related? *ANZ J Surg* 72(3):204, 2002.

27. Field JE, Field TF: *COJ 2000 with an O*NET™ 98 Crosswalk*, Athens, GA, 1999, Elliot & Fitzpatrick, Inc.

28. Fliedner CA: Occupational therapy: for the body and the mind. In Rodgers GM, ed: *Centennial Rancho Los Amigos Medical Center 1888-1988*, Downey, CA, 1990, Rancho Los Amigos Medical Center.

29. Grubbs R, Hamilton A, eds: Criteria for a recommended standard: occupational exposure to hand-arm vibration, Washington DC, 1989, US Government Printing Office.

30. Hall H, Buck M: *The work of our hands*, New York, 1919, Moffat Yard & Co.

31. Harvey-Krefting L: The concept of work in occupational therapy: a historical review, *Am J Occup Ther* 39(5):301, 1985.

32. Hepper E, et al: Back school. In Kirkaldy-Willis WH, Burton CV, eds: *Managing low back pain*, ed 3, New York, 1992, Churchill Livingstone.

33. Herzberg GL, et al: Work and the underserved: homelessness and work. In Kornblau, BK, Jacobs K, eds: *Work: principles and practice*, Bethesda, MD, 2000, AOTA.

34. Holmes D: The role of the occupational therapist-work evaluator, *Am J Occup Ther* 39(5), 308, 1985.

35. *IBM ergonomics handbook*, New York, 2000, IBM Corp.

36. Isernhagen SJ: Advancements in functional capacity evaluation. In D'Orazio BP, ed: *Back pain rehabilitation*, Boston, 1993, Butterworth.

37. Isernhagen SJ: Corporate fitness and prevention of industrial injuries. In Rothman J, Levine R, eds: *Prevention practice: strategies for physical therapy and occupational therapy*, Philadelphia, 1992, WB Saunders.

38. Jackson J, et al: Occupation in lifestyle redesign: the well elderly study occupational therapy program, *Am J Occup Ther* 52(5):326, 1998.

39. Jacobs K: Preparing for return to work. In Trombly K, editor: *Occupational therapy for physical dysfunction*, ed 4, Baltimore, MD, 1995, Williams & Wilkins.

40. Jacobs K, Baker NA: The history of work-related therapy in occupational therapy. In Kornblau BL, Jacobs K, eds: *Work: principles and practice*, Bethesda, MD, 2000, AOTA.

41. Johannson C: Top 10 emerging practice areas to watch in the new millennium, *OT Pract*, Jan. 31, 2000.

42. King PM: Work hardening and work conditioning. In King PM, ed: *Sourcebook of Occupational Rehabilitation*, New York, 1998, Plenum Press.

43. King PM, Barrett T: A critical review of functional capacity evaluations, *Phys Ther* 78(8), 852, 1998.

44. Kirkaldy-Willis WH: Energy stored for action: the elastic support and bodysuit. In Kirkaldy-Willis WH, Burton CV, eds: *Managing low back pain*, ed 3, New York, 1992, Churchill Livingstone.

45. Kornblau B: *The occupational therapist and vocational evaluation*, Work Programs Special Interest Section Newsletter, 10:1, 1996.

46. LaBar G: Safety at Saturn: a team effort, *Occup Hazards* 56(3):41, 1994.

47. Lawler EE: *High involvement management*, San Francisco, 1991, Jossey-Bass.

48. Lechner DE: Functional capacity evaluation. In King PM, editor, *Sourcebook of occupational rehabilitation*, New York, 1998, Plenum Press.

49. Lechner DE: *Quantitative job demands analysis* (procedure manual), Birmingham, AL, 1999, ErgoScience, Inc.

50. Lechner DE: Work hardening and work conditioning interventions: do they affect disability? *Phys Ther*, 74(5):102, 1994.

51. Lechner D, et al: Functional capacity evaluation in work disability, *Work* 1:37, 1991.

52. Legislative Committee, National Rehabilitation Association: Meeting the nation's needs by the expansion of the program of vocational rehabilitation of physically handicapped persons, *Occup Ther Rehab* 16(3):186, 1937.

53. MacFarlane B: Job modification, *Work Special Interest Section Newsletter* 2(1):1, 1988.

54. MacLeod D, et al: *The ergonomics manual: guidebook for managers, supervisors, and ergonomic team members,* Minneapolis, MN, 1990, Comprehensive Loss Management, Inc.

55. Malugani M: Emerging areas in OT, Monster Worldwide (*http://content.monster.com*) on the AOTA website 12/24/04 (*http://www.otjoblink.org/links/link09.asp*), 2004.

56. Marshall EM: Looking back, *Am J Occup Ther* 39(5):297, 1985.

57. Meister D: *Conceptual aspects of human factors,* Baltimore, MD, 1989, John Hopkins Press.

58. Melnick M: Injury prevention. In Kornblau B, Jacobs K, eds: *Work: principles and practice,* Bethesda, MD, 2000, AOTA.

59. Meyer A: The philosophy of occupational therapy, *Am J Occup Ther,* 31(10):639, 1977.

60. Mosely LH, et al: Cumulative trauma disorders and compression neuropathies of the upper extremities. In Kasdan ML, editor: *Occupational hand and upper extremity injuries and diseases,* Philadelphia, 1991, Hanley & Belfus.

61. National Governors Association Center for Best Practices. *Welfare reform* (online) Available at *http://www.nga.org/cbp/activities/welfarereform.asp,*1999.

62. Network WI; *Promising practices* (online) Available at *http://www.welfareinform.org/promising.htm,* 2000.

63. Newton M, Waddell G: Trunk strength testing with iso-machines: Part I. Review of a decade of scientific evidence, *Spine* 18(7):801, 1993.

64. Noro K, Imada AS: *Participatory ergonomics,* Bristol, PA, 1991, Taylor and Francis.

65. O'Callaghan J: Primary prevention and ergonomics: the role of rehabilitation specialists in preventing occupational injury. In Rothman J, Levine R, eds: *Prevention practice: strategies for physical therapy and occupational therapy,* Philadelphia, 1992, WB Saunders.

66. Occupational Safety and Health Administration: *Ergonomics for the prevention of musculoskeletal disorders: guidelines for nursing homes,* Washington, DC, 2003, US Government Printing Office.

67. Occupational Safety and Health Administration: *Ergonomics for the prevention of musculoskeletal disorders: guidelines for poultry processing,* Washington, DC, 2004, US Government Printing Office.

68. Occupational Safety and Health Administration: *Ergonomics for the prevention of musculoskeletal disorders: guidelines for retail grocery stores,* Washington, DC, 2004, US Government Printing Office.

69. Occupational Safety and Health Administration: *Ergonomics program management guidelines for meatpacking plants,* Washington, DC, 1990, US Government Printing Office.

70. Occupational Safety and Health Administration: *Working safely with video display terminals,* Washington, DC, 1997, US Government Printing Office.

71. Ogden-Niemeyer L, Jacobs K: Definition and history of work hardening. In Ogden-Niemeyer L, Jacobs K, editors: *Work hardening state of the art,* Thorofare, NJ, 1989, Slack Publ.

72. Owens LA, Buchholz RL: Functional capacity assessment, worker evaluation strategies, and the disability management process. In Shrey DE, Lacerte M, eds, *Principals and practices of disability management in industry,* Winter Park, FL, 1995, GR Press, Inc.

73. Page J: Functional capacity evaluation—making the right decision, *RehabPro* 9(4), 2001.

74. Patterson C: A historical perspective of work practice services. In Pratt J, Jacobs K, eds, *Work practice: international perspectives,* Boston, 1997, Butterworth.

75. Perry L: Preemployment and preplacement testing. In King PM, ed: *Sourcebook of Occupational Rehabilitation,* New York, 1998, Plenum Press.

76. Peterson W, Perr A: Home and worksite accommodations. In Galvin JC, Scherer J, eds, *Evaluating, selecting and using appropriate assistive technology,* Gaithersburg, 1996, Aspen Publ.

77. Pinel P: *A treatise on insanity,* New York, 1962, Hafner Publ.

78. Putz-Anderson V, editor: *Cumulative trauma disorders: a manual for musculoskeletal diseases of the upper limbs,* Bristol, PA, 1988, Taylor & Francis.

79. Rainforth B, York-Barr J: *Collaborative teams for students with severe disabilities: integrating therapy and educational services,* ed 2, Baltimore, MD, 1997, Brookes.

80. Reed K: The beginnings of occupational therapy. In Hopkins HL, Smith, HD: *Willard and Spackman's occupational therapy,* Philadelphia, 1993, Lippincott.

81. Rosenberg B, Wellerson T: A structured pre-vocational program, *Am J Occup Ther* 14:57, 1960.

82. Rothman J, Levine R: *Prevention practice: strategies for physical therapy and occupational therapy,* Philadelphia, 1992, W.B. Saunders.

83. Rothstein J, Echternach J: *Primer on measurement: an introductory guide to measurement issues featuring the APTA's standards for tests and measurements in physical therapy practice,* Alexandria, VA, 1993, APTA.

84. Ryan DJ: *Job search handbook for people with disabilities,* Indianapolis, IN, 2000, JIST Publ.

85. Sabonis-Chafee B: *Occupational therapy: introductory concepts,* St. Louis, 1989, Mosby.

86. Scaffa ME, et al: Future directions in community-based practice. In Scaffa ME: *Occupational therapy in community-based practice settings,* Philadelphia, 2001, F.A. Davis.

87. Shrey DE: Worksite disability management and industrial rehabilitation: an overview. In Shrey DE, Lacerte M, eds: *Principals and practices of disability management in industry,* Winter Park, FL, 1995, GR Press.

88. Smith SL, et al: The predictive validity of the functional capacities evaluation, *Am J Occup Ther* 40:564, 1986.

89. Snodgrass JE: Getting comfortable: developing a clinical specialty in ergonomics has its own challenges and rewards, *Rehab Management* p.24, July 2004.

90. Spencer K: Transition from school to adult life. In Kornblau B, Jacobs K, eds: *Work: principles and practice,* Bethesda, MD, 2000, AOTA.

91. Symons J, Veran A: Conducting worksite evaluations to identify reasonable accommodations. In Hamil J, editor: *Integrating assistive technology into your practice,* AOTA on-line course, Bethesda, MD, 2000, AOTA.

92. The Work Site. Ticket to work fact sheet (online). Available at *www.ssa.gov.*

93. US Department of Labor, Employment and Training Administration: *Revised dictionary of occupational titles.* Vol I & II, ed 4, 1991, Washington, DC, US Government Printing Office.

94. US Department of Labor, Employment and Training Administration: *The revised handbook for analyzing jobs,* Indianapolis, IN, 1991, JIST Works.

95. US preventive services task force: *Guide to clinical preventive services,* ed 2, Washington DC, 1996, US Government Printing Office.

96. Wegg LS: The essentials of work evaluation, *Am J Occup Ther,* 14:65, 1960.

97. Young ES: Setting up an industrial program for the tuberculosis, *Occup Ther Rehab* 18(3):163, 1939.

14

AMERICANS WITH DISABILITIES ACT AND RELATED LAWS THAT PROMOTE PARTICIPATION IN WORK, LEISURE, AND ACTIVITIES OF DAILY LIVING

BARBARA L. KORNBLAU

KEY TERMS

Individual with a disability
Major life activities
Qualified person with a
   disability

Essential job functions
Reasonable accommodations
Undue hardship
Discrimination

Direct threat
Places of public accommodation
Auxiliary aids
Accessibility audit

LEARNING OBJECTIVES

After studying this chapter the student or practitioner will be able to do the following:

1. Explain how the Americans with Disabilities Act (ADA) defines disability and how that definition may apply to clients seen by occupational therapists.
2. Compare and contrast definitions of discrimination and discuss how they may apply to clients served by occupational therapy.
3. Recognize and define specific terms used in the ADA, Fair Housing Act, and Air Carrier Access Act.
4. Discuss the roles occupational therapy can play in advocating for clients under the ADA, Fair Housing Act, and Air Carrier Access Act.
5. Discuss the roles occupational therapy can play in consulting with employers, places of public accommodation, airline carriers, and landlords.

6. Explain the process used to determine essential job function.
7. Analyze reasonable accommodations as an intervention strategy in occupational therapy and explain the decision-making process involved in making reasonable accommodations.
8. Outline the process for removing physical and other barriers to access to places of public accommodation and the steps necessary to perform an accessibility audit.
9. Prepare and train employers, co-workers, supervisors, airline employees, and those who work with the public to treat individuals with disabilities with dignity and respect.

CHAPTER OUTLINE

Americans with Disabilities Act
   Title I: Employment
Reasonable accommodations
   Title II: State and local government services
   Title III: Public accommodations
Air Carrier Access Act

Discrimination prohibited under ACAA
Air carrier obligations
   The Role of the occupational therapist
Fair Housing Act
Advocacy as intervention
Summary

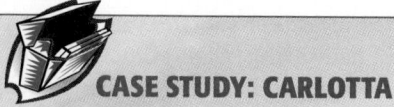

CASE STUDY: CARLOTTA

Carlotta is a 50-year-old woman with severe rheumatoid arthritis. Since her most recent exacerbation, she finds she must use a wheelchair for mobility. She has always prided herself in her independence and does not want to rely on her children or husband for assistance. She loves going to the movies, shopping, and traveling. Carlotta works as a Spanish teacher at the local high school.

She comes to OT concerned about several things. How will she be able to participate in her work and leisure occupations from her wheelchair when some places (and people) in the community, including her classroom, are not wheelchair friendly or accessible? How will she manage airplane travel from a wheelchair? How can she independently participate in activities of daily living from a wheelchair when her landlord of 12 years will not allow her to make needed changes in her apartment?

This chapter addresses Carlotta's concerns by expanding the concept of OT interventions to include advocacy as a key concept of intervention. As we address the occupations significant to Carlotta, we look at three laws for guidance and support in promoting occupational performance. We also look to these laws to support our intervention plan. These laws include the Americans with Disabilities Act,[60] the Air Carrier Access Act,[59] and the Fair Housing Act.[69] Each law provides an avenue for OT intervention that promotes the greater good for many individuals with disabilities. Each law also provides specific support for our efforts to promote our client's desire to increase and improve her participation at work, at home, and in the community.

Carlotta's evaluation shows that as a person with a chronic disability, she is a very sophisticated player. Over almost 25 years of living with arthritis, she has acquired many adaptive devices, such as reachers, jar openers, and bathtub benches to make her life easier, facilitate independent participation, and prevent further damage to the joints of her hands. She requires assistance of others for some tasks.

Her occupational profile shows that her job as a Spanish teacher at a large private school where she has worked for 18 years is very important to her. She believes she can do her job but will have some difficulty navigating the classroom from her wheelchair because of the presence of multiple levels. Her classroom is the former orchestra classroom. She also expresses concerns about continuing her weekly excursions to the movies. How can she navigate the old theater in town that turned the old upstairs balcony into a separate screen theater with a one flight walk up? Before she began to use a wheelchair herself, she saw wheelchair users at the local shopping mall struggling to get in the door and she believes this will present a barrier to her shopping or, as she puts it, "retail therapy." How will she manage at the airport and aboard airplanes in her quest to find the perfect bed and breakfast (another hobby)? Finally, from her experience as an individual with a disability, she knows she will need more adaptations in her bathroom to participate in activities of daily living. She is particularly concerned because her landlord has already told her that she cannot widen the bathroom door or install grab bars in the bathtub. She is interested in finding alternatives so that she can take care of herself and not have to move. She also expressed her concern about her difficulty with carrying out a home aquatics program from her previous occupational therapist. She now requires assistance to get into the pool at her apartment complex but the complex's rules do not allow guests on weekends.

Disability laws heavily influence the facilitation of participation in work, leisure, and the community. Ignoring disability laws can promote ineffective intervention plans. To move forward with an occupational therapy intervention plan, one must first understand the disability laws that affect the areas of concern to Carlotta and how these laws can provide a basis for intervention.

AMERICANS WITH DISABILITIES ACT

To understand the protection the ADA affords Carlotta and the roles the American with Disabilities Act (ADA) provides for occupational therapists (OTs) and occupational therapy assistants (OTAs), one must first have a basic understanding of the ADA, its definitions, and how the courts have interpreted the law. Congress passed the ADA in 1990 in an effort to decrease discrimination against individuals with disabilities and promote their inclusion in the mainstream of society. The law's anti-discrimination provisions cover employment, certain state and local government services, public accommodations, communications, and public transportation. This chapter explores Title I (employment), Title II (state and local government services), and Title III (public accommodations) and how they affect occupational therapy (OT) practice.

TITLE I: EMPLOYMENT

Before the ADA became law, the Rehabilitation Act of 1973 prohibited discrimination against qualified individuals with disabilities in employment by three categories of employers: (1) the federal government, (2) employers who contract with the federal government to provide goods and service, and (3) employers who were recipients or beneficiaries of federal funding.[74] Congress extended that protection by expanding it to private employers who are not dependent on federal funding by passing the ADA in 1990. Because one of Carlotta's concerns is her work and whether she can continue to participate in her work from a wheelchair, knowledge of Title I of the ADA can provide a foundation for OT intervention.

Title I of the ADA prohibits discrimination against individuals with disabilities in employment with private, non-government employers who have 15 or more employees. In a nutshell, the prohibition against discrimination in Title I states:

> No covered entity may discriminate against a qualified individual with a disability because of the individual's disability, in regard to job application procedures, the hiring, advancement or discharge of employees, employee compensation, job training, social and recreational programs sponsored by the employer, and other terms, conditions, and privileges of employment.[48]

To understand this statement, one must understand the terms used by answering the following questions:
- Who is considered "an individual with a disability" under the ADA?
- What is a "qualified individual with a disability" under the ADA?
- What is considered "discrimination" under the ADA?

An Individual with a Disability Defined

The ADA refers to *individuals with disabilities* as opposed to *disabled individuals* to give voice to politically correct terminology that stresses the individual first, not the disability. It defines the phrase **individual with a disability** broadly under the three umbrella categories.

The first definition states that an individual with a disability includes "one who has a *physical or mental impairment* that *substantially limits* one or more *major life activities.*"[28] A physical or mental impairment includes "any physiological disorder or condition, cosmetic disfigurement or anatomical loss affecting one or more of the following body systems: neurological, musculoskeletal, special sense organs, respiratory (including speech organs), cardiovascular, reproductive, digestive, genito-urinary, hemic and lymphatic, skin, and endocrine."[31] Physical or mental impairment as defined includes most of the traditional medical diagnoses OTs treat including, for example, multiple sclerosis, spinal cord injury, cerebral vascular accident, cerebral palsy, and Carlotta's arthritis, which affects the musculoskeletal system. Mental or psychological disorders include "mental retardation, organic brain syndrome, emotional or mental illness, and specific learning disabilities."[32]

Under the ADA the phrase *substantially limits* means "unable to perform a major life activity that the average person in the general population can perform" or "significantly restricted as to the condition, manner or duration under which an individual can perform a particular major life activity as compared to the condition, manner, or duration under which the average person in the general population can perform that same major life activity."[34] Determining whether one is substantially limited considers "the nature and severity of the impairment; the duration or expected duration of the impairment; and the permanent or long-term impact, or the expected permanent or long-term impact of or resulting from the impairment."[35]

Major life activities include many areas of occupation and related activities of daily living (ADLs) functions such as caring for oneself, performing manual tasks, talking, seeing, hearing, speaking, learning, and working.[33] In the work context, *substantially limited in the major life activity of work* means significant limitations in the ability to perform either a class of jobs or a broad range of jobs in various classes as compared with the average person having comparable training, skills, and abilities.[34]

Since the ADA became law, the U.S. Supreme Court took the opportunity to review what it means to be substantially limited in a major life activity in the case of *Williams v. Toyota Motor Mfg.*[78] Mrs. Williams had tendinitis and cumulative trauma syndrome. She claimed she was restricted in her ability to do her job and limited in the major life activity of manual tasks associated with her job. The evidence showed that she was able to perform her ADLs.

The U.S. Supreme Court said that looking only at manual tasks associated with one's job was not enough. The court said:

> When addressing the major life activity of performing manual tasks, the central inquiry must be whether the claimant is unable to perform the variety of tasks central to most people's lives, not whether the claimant is unable to perform the tasks associated with her specific job...Manual tasks unique to any particular job are not necessarily important parts of most people's lives. As a result, occupation [meaning "work"] specific tasks may have only limited relevance to the manual task inquiry.[78]

Reading between the lines almost makes it seem as though the U.S. Supreme Court is endorsing OT or, at the very least, acknowledges OT's potential role. The OT evaluation provides the information the Court believes necessary to make a determination as to whether an individual is substantially limited in major life activities. OTs may find themselves assisting employers, attorneys, and others by providing this information, if requested.

The OT evaluation of Carlotta shows that Carlotta has arthritis, which substantially limits the major life activity of walking. She also has difficulty participating in or is unable to participate in a variety of tasks central to everyday living. In light of these limitations, she probably falls under the first definition of disability.

The second definition of an individual with a disability under the ADA includes someone who has a record of having had such an impairment as described in the first definition.[29] This category includes persons with a history of a disabling condition, such as an individual who had multiple sclerosis that is now in remission, or someone cured of hepatitis C.

The third definition of an individual with a disability includes situations in which someone is regarded as having a substantially limiting impairment, which is a perception of a disability based on myths, misperceptions, fears, and stereotypes.[30] For example, suppose a morbidly obese individual, Sue, seeks a promotion to a position that requires frequent trips out of town. The person empowered to decide whether Sue gets that promotion assumes that Sue will have difficulty managing the traveling because of her size. The manager is concerned that Sue will struggle with walking through the airports, breathing, and other non-sedentary aspects of her job. Sue has had a perfect attendance record and has always received excellent performance appraisals. The manager bases his failure to hire Sue on his assumptions about her supposed difficulty walking, breathing, and completing non-sedentary tasks, and these assumptions are simply not true. The manager regards Sue as being an individual with a substantially limiting impairment.

Individuals Not Covered by the ADA

The ADA provides its protection against disability discrimination only for those who meet the criteria outlined above. This means that individuals with temporary impairments, such as a broken leg or after a knee replacement that is likely or expected to heal normally, will not find the ADA protects them. Individuals who have impairments that are not substantially limiting, such as a vision limitation correctable with eyeglasses, will not find benefits under the ADA.

Further, the ADA enumerates specific exclusions to its definition of disability. The ADA does not provide protection for individuals who fall into one of the following categories: transvestites, homosexuals, pedophiles, exhibitionists, voyeurs, and gender disorders not caused by physical impairments, and other sexual behavior disorders.[46] The ADA further excludes from its protection illegal drug users, compulsive gamblers, kleptomaniacs, pyromaniacs, and alcoholics whose alcohol use prevents them from performing their jobs.[47] The ADA does provide protection against discrimination based on disability for recovering illegal drug users, as long as they participate in a rehabilitation program.

Qualified Person with a Disability

Title I of the ADA does not protect all individuals with disabilities. It protects only qualified individuals with a disability. The ADA defines a **qualified person with a disability** as "an individual with a disability who satisfies the requisite skill, experience, education and other job related requirements of the employment position" he or she holds or desires, "and who, with or without reasonable accommodation, can perform the essential functions of the employment position that the individuals holds or desires."[36] The first inquiry in deciding whether an individual with a disability meets the basic job requirements looks at individuals' amount of experience, level of education, and skills necessary to perform the job. Carlotta meets these requirements since the school hired her as a qualified teacher more than 18 years ago, and thus, she meets the basic education, skills, and experience requirement. The next inquiry is whether the individual in question can perform the essential functions of the job.

Essential Job Functions

The ADA defines **essential job functions** as those job duties fundamental to the position the individual holds, or desires to hold, as opposed to functions that are marginal functions.[37] The essential functions are those functions that the individual who holds the position must be able to perform with or without the assistance of a reasonable accommodation. One may consider a function essential because the position exists to perform the particular function. These essential functions are usually obvious. For example, a typist must type and a proofreader must proofread.

A function is essential because of the limited number of employees available who can share the particular function. For example, because only three Spanish teachers are at Carlotta's school, Carlotta must collaborate with the other two Spanish teachers to write and direct the annual Spanish language pageant. If the school employed 20 Spanish teachers, responsibilities may be divided so that Carlotta did not have to participate in the annual Spanish language pageant.

An essential function also is one in which the function is so specialized that the employer hires the person in the position for his or her particular expertise or ability to perform that function. For example, a brain surgeon is a highly specialized position, and the person in this position is hired to perform highly technical surgery.

Whether a function is an essential function is determined on a case-by-case basis. Specific evidence will support whether a particular function is an essential function. The Equal Employment Opportunity Commission (EEOC), the federal agency that provides enforcement for Title I's provisions, and the Courts will look at seven factors[38] as evidence of whether a function is essential (Box 14-1).

In some situations essential functions are obvious. For example, the essential functions of a receptionist's position may include answering telephones, taking messages, and greeting and announcing visitors. Typing may be a marginal function for a receptionist in a very busy office where the receptionist has not had to type anything at all over the last 6 months. One determines essential job functions on a case-by-case basis looking at the facts of each situation. OTs can

Box **14-1**	SEVEN DETERMINING FACTORS OF ESSENTIAL FUNCTIONS

The employer's judgment of which functions are essential
Written job descriptions prepared before the hiring process begins
The amount of time spent performing the job function
The consequences of not requiring the performance of a particular function
The terms of the collective bargaining agreement
The work experience of previous employees who held the job
The current work experience of incumbents in similar positions

help determine essential job functions by looking at the job description, by conducting focus groups with employees, and by performing a job analysis as discussed in Chapter 13.

In determination of essential job functions, the focus must be on the outcome or job tasks employers expect employees to perform. The definition of essential job functions focuses on the concept of job duties, not the physical demands required to perform a job duty. In other words, the essential function is a task one must perform to perform the job, not a physical function. Essential functions are not bending, lifting, walking, climbing, or other physical demands. For example, a mail clerk for a large corporation includes delivering mail as one of his essential functions. The essential function is not *walking* and *carrying* the mail but rather the outcome of *delivering* the mail. If the mail clerk were not able to carry the mail, he could push the mail on a cart to accomplish the same result or outcome. Essential functions are *what* you do, not *how* you do it.

The job description, job analysis, and discussions with Carlotta about her job show that as a teacher Carlotta must perform several essential functions, including grading papers and tests and recording their results, discussing student progress with parents, preparing lesson plans, motivating students, and maintaining order in the classroom. (Note that these essential functions are all specific job tasks and not physical functions such as "hand manipulation skills for writing" or "walking around the classroom.") The OT evaluation shows that Carlotta is able to perform these functions for her position as a Spanish teacher. However, she may have difficulty maneuvering around the classroom to the desks of the individual students because of steps and multiple levels in the former band classroom in which she currently teaches Spanish. Carlotta will also have difficulty writing on the

blackboard from a wheelchair. The key to facilitating Carlotta's continued participation in the workplace lies with reasonable accommodations.

REASONABLE ACCOMMODATIONS

The ADA defines **reasonable accommodations** as any change in the work environment or in the way work is customarily performed that enables an individual with a disability to enjoy equal employment opportunity.[39] Not all employees are entitled to reasonable accommodation. Employers need make reasonable accommodations only for employees who are qualified individuals with disabilities (Box 14-2).

Reasonable accommodations include three subcategories. First, reasonable accommodations include modifications or adjustments to the job application process that enable consideration for employment of a qualified applicant with a disability.[40] This would include reading a job application to an individual with dyslexia or modifying the way a pre-placement screening is performed to accommodate an individual with one hand. If Carlotta were to apply for another position, her potential employer would need to provide her with an accessible entrance to the human resources department so that she could obtain a job application. The potential employer would also have to allow her to use a larger pen for filling out an application because she uses the larger pen to prevent joint changes in her hand. As an alternative, the potential employer can provide someone to assist her in filling out the application.

The modifications and adaptations that OT most typically provides fall under the umbrella of the second category of reasonable accommodations. The second category includes modifications or adjustments to the work environment or to

---

Box **14-2**   REASONABLE ACCOMMODATIONS DECISION PROGRESSION

STEP 1: IS THE WORKER AN INDIVIDUAL WITH A DISABILITY (IWD)?

Does the individual meet one or more of the following criteria?
- A physical or mental impairment that substantially limits one or more major life activities
- A history of having had such an impairment
- Regarded as having such an impairment

If the worker is *not* an IWD, the employer does *not* have to accommodate.

STEP 2: IS THE WORKER A QUALIFIED INDIVIDUAL WITH A DISABILITY (QIWD)?

Does the individual meet both of the following criteria?
- Individual satisfies the requisite skills, experience, education, and other job-related requirements of the job

- Individual can perform the essential functions of such position with or without reasonable accommodations

If the worker is *not* a QIWD, the employer does *not* have to accommodate.

STEP 3: IS THE ACCOMMODATION REASONABLE?

- How much does the accommodation cost in relationship to the size and budget of the business?
- Are there tax credits or deductions or outside funding sources to pay for the accommodation?
- Does the accommodation interfere with the operation of the business or the ability of other employees to perform their duties?

If it is *not* reasonable, the employer does *not* have to accommodate.

Courtesy Barbara L. Kornblau, ADA Consultants.

OT PRACTICE NOTE

OTs may assist human resources personnel in understanding how disabling conditions and the limitations in performance skills and client factors that accompany them can affect the hiring process. In addition, OTs can suggest appropriate reasonable accommodations available for the application and interview process that can prevent unintentional discrimination.

the manner or circumstances under which the position is customarily performed, which enable a qualified individual with a disability to perform the essential functions of that position.[41] OTs have traditionally been involved in this area by modifying job sites, including raising or lowering work heights, making a jig, or using a piece of equipment such as a cart to move objects rather than carrying them. Carlotta's continued participation in her work environment will require reasonable accommodations in her intervention plan in the form of changes to the way the work is performed. For example, Carlotta's employer could reasonably accommodate her by moving Carlotta to a different classroom—one that is all on one level and without steps or risers throughout the room to provide physical access to the students at their desks. Carlotta could also benefit from a laptop computer with an LCD projector, which will eliminate the need for her to write on the board—an impossible task from a wheelchair level. (See Chapter 13 for more detailed discussion of job modifications.)

OTs and OTAs working with development of reasonable accommodations should note that employers must provide an effective reasonable accommodation, meaning one that works, not the most expensive accommodation or the specific accommodation the employee wants. Although the employee suggests the specific type of accommodation, ultimately, the employer gets to select the accommodation used. If a shoebox with some rubber bands wrapped around it works as well as the high-tech computerized gadget the employee requests, the employer need only provide the shoebox.

The third category of reasonable accommodations includes modifications or adjustments that enable employees with a disability to enjoy equal benefits and privileges of employment as other similarly situated employees without disabilities enjoy.[42] For example, suppose the language department at Carlotta's school customarily holds an annual international fair for all of the students and their families at the school. The teachers compete by class for the best food, costumes, and projects. The teacher of the winning class wins prizes supplied by the PTA. Under the ADA, the school would be required to hold the fair at an accessible location so that Carlotta could participate. This also would apply to school's annual holiday party and all other school functions for employees. OTs can improve awareness for employers, assist them with making reasonable accommodations, and help

sensitize employers to the needs of individuals with disabilities in these situations.

According to the ADA, reasonable accommodations may include physical changes to make facilities accessible in addition to other non-environmental changes. Depending on the individual circumstances, reasonable accommodations can include job restructuring, part-time or modified work schedules, reassignment to a vacant position, acquisition or modification of equipment or devices (such as Carlotta's laptop computer and LCD projector), appropriate adjustment or modification of examinations, training materials or policies, the provision of qualified readers or interpreters, and other similar accommodations for individuals with disabilities.[40,41]

For example, an individual who needs to begin kidney dialysis may find leaving work early 3 days a week reasonably accommodates his needs. Allowing a cashier with fatigue from multiple sclerosis to sit instead of stand while working may reasonably accommodate her needs. Because of their knowledge of limitations of disabling conditions and adapting the work environment to the individual, OTs can suggest and/or design many of these accommodations working together with the client. Carlotta has a good understanding of much of what she needs to reasonably accommodate her work needs, and her intervention plan should incorporate her insights and suggestions.

The most efficient way for employers to identify the reasonable accommodations an individual employee may need is to initiate an informal, interactive process with the qualified individual with a disability in need of the accommodation.[61] Employers will find that the individual with a disability is often in the best position to determine which reasonable accommodations he or she may need to enable job performance. The OTs may participate in this effort in which the parties need additional expertise to make those accommodations. The EEOC, the federal government agency charged with enforcing the ADA, recognizes the expertise of OTs in assisting with making reasonable accommodations.[67]

The ADA provides an exception to the employer's requirement to provide reasonable accommodations for qualified individuals with disabilities. Employers need not provide reasonable accommodations where the provision of the accommodation would cause an **undue hardship** to the employer. Undue hardship refers to any accommodation that would be unduly costly, extensive, substantial, or disruptive, or that would fundamentally alter the nature or operation of the business.[43] For example, it would probably be an undue hardship for the school to fix Carlotta's classroom by ripping out the floor in the old band room to remove the risers and level the floor because it would eliminate the use of a very needed classroom for an extended period of time and might present a significant expense. The alternative, to swap classrooms with another teacher, would be more cost effective and less disruptive.

The determination of whether an accommodation presents an undue hardship to the employer looks at whether the proposed action requires significant difficulty or expense when the following factors are considered[44]:

- Nature and cost of accommodation needed in light of tax credits and deductions, and/or outside funding
- Overall financial resources of the facility, the number of persons employed at the facility, and the effect on the expenses and resources
- Overall financial resources, overall size of the business, and the number, type, and location of facilities
- Composition, structure, and functions of the workforce
- Impact of the accommodation upon the operation of the facility, including the impact on the ability of other employees to perform their duties, and the impact on the facilities' ability to conduct business

According to the Job Accommodations Network, a federally funded program that has provided technical assistance for making accommodations for more than 12 years, the data show that more than 50% of all accommodations cost less than $500. Further, its statistics also show that employers experience financial gains from the decreased costs of training new employees, a decrease in insurance costs, and an increase in worker productivity.[70]

Discrimination Under the ADA

The ADA does not give one specific definition of **discrimination**. Instead, it specifies at least nine categories of activities considered discriminatory.

Limiting, classifying, or segregating

The first prohibited activity includes limiting, classifying, or segregating the employee because of his or her disability.[49] For example, if Carlotta's school were to require all employees who use wheelchairs for mobility to work in one wing of the first floor, it would be segregating the employees with disabilities. This section also forbids employers from asking any questions about an applicant's worker's compensation history during the interview or on the employment application because employers can use this information to limit or classify individuals because of their disability.

Poor disability etiquette can lead to limiting, classifying, and segregating individuals with disabilities in the workplace. The way co-workers treat people with disabilities and the language they use to refer to individual with disabilities can also make people feel bad or left out of the workplace culture. One method employers may use to avoid limiting, classifying, or segregating employees because of their disabilities is to sensitize supervisors and other employees to working with individuals with disabilities. Non-disabled individuals who lack familiarity in socializing with individuals with disabilities may not know how to shake hands with a person who does not have a right hand. They may shout at a person who is deaf instead of speaking clearly and facing the person with the hearing impairment.

OTs can work with supervisors and co-workers on basic disability etiquette tips such as using politically correct

OT PRACTICE NOTE

OTs can assist employers with providing sensitivity training experiences similar to those used in some OT program classrooms to develop an understanding of the disability experience. Giving co-workers time in a wheelchair or with a blindfold during planned activities can help them experience functional limitations, if only for a brief time, that may encourage development of some sensitivity to how it feels to have limitations in performance and participation. Using lay language, free of confusing jargon, during this kind of training makes it easier to get the message across to co-workers unfamiliar with OT lingo.

terminology, in which, as mentioned above, the person comes before the disability. For example, using the phrase *a person who had a stroke* is better than calling someone a *stroke patient* or *stroke victim*, because the word *victim* has negative connotations. Using the phrase *wheelchair user* is more appropriate than *wheelchair-bound*, because no one is physically bound to the wheelchair as a book is bound to its binding. Box 14-3 gives more tips on disability etiquette. For tips with the interview process see Box 14-4.

Contractual relationships that discriminate

The second prohibited activity includes participating in a contractual or other relationship that results in discrimination against qualified applicants or employees because of their disability.[50] This provision applies to collective bargaining agreements, contracts with employment agencies, and other contracts. For example, suppose Carlotta's employer contracted with an outside company to provide continuing education courses at her school. The continuing education company would have to comply with the ADA by offering reasonable accommodations where needed, such as allowing Carlotta to tape sessions or providing her with a note-taker if she is unable to take notes during the classes. The OT could work with the continuing education provider to help develop other reasonable accommodations for Carlotta and other individuals with disabilities.

Using standards, criteria, and methods of administration that discriminate

The third prohibited activity includes use of standards, criteria, or methods of administration that are not job-related and consistent with business necessity and have the effect of discriminating based on the disability.[45] For example, an employer could not require that Carlotta possess a driver's license for promotion to Chair of the Spanish Department if driving is not an essential function of the position.

Employers may use a **direct threat** standard to exclude from employment individuals whose disabilities pose a direct threat to the health and safety of themselves or others in the workplace.[45] However, the direct threat must be a significant

Box **14-3**   DISABILITY ETIQUETTE DOS AND DON'TS

- Do try to treat an individual with disabilities as you would treat any other person.
- Don't raise your voice at someone because he or she is in a wheelchair or has a visual or hearing impairment.
- Do address the person, not the wheelchair, interpreter, or guide.
- Don't trap yourself into thinking, "If I were disabled how would I feel?"
- Do refer to an individual with a disability as "an individual with a disability."
- Don't refer to an individual with a disability as "the quadriplegic," or "Mary is diabetic or epileptic."
- Do cleanse your vocabulary of offensive, outdated terms such as wheelchair-bound or stroke "victim," or "afflicted with..." or "suffering from..."
- Don't refer to able-bodied persons as "normal."
- Do avoid generalizations such as, "People with epilepsy are unpredictable" or "People with learning disabilities are not very intelligent."
- Don't apologize for comments such as, "Let's take a walk" to an individual in a wheelchair or "Do you see my point?" to a person with a visual impairment.

- Do avoid statements such as, "I admire your courage" or "You've done so much for a person in a wheelchair."
- Don't use outdated terminology such as "handicapped," "crippled," "retarded," "lame," "*the* disabled," or "*the* handicapped."
- Do provide assistance only in the manner requested.
- Don't take hold of an individual's wheelchair or push his or her wheelchair unless asked to do so.
- Do put yourself on the same level as the individual in a wheelchair as soon as possible by sitting down during the conversation or interview.
- Don't turn away when conversing with an individual with a hearing impairment.
- Do speak directly to the person, not the interpreter.
- Don't complete the sentences of an individual with communication impairments.
- Do rid your thinking of stereotypes about disabilities.
- Don't perpetuate another person's insensitivity to an individual with a disability.

Courtesy Barbara L. Kornblau, ADA Consultants.

Box **14-4**   INTERVIEW DOS AND DON'TS

- Don't make notes about an individual's physical or mental condition.
- Do discuss reasonable accommodations where possible. The interviewee is an expert on accommodating his or her disability.
- Don't rely on body language as a measure during the interview process. Lack of eye contact or a mild grip handshake may be caused by an applicant's disability, not his or her lack of confidence.
- Do remember that individuals with disabilities may make poor interviewees if judged against many "traditional" interviewing standards.
- Don't try to put yourself in the applicant's place and ask yourself, "Could I do this job if I were disabled?"
- Do offer an applicant a job based on his or her abilities—not disabilities.
- Don't job stereotype.
- Do remember that communications skills are often an inaccurate measure of the intelligence, ability, or confidence of an individual with a speech or hearing problem.
- Don't patronize the applicant with a disability with your own body language.

Courtesy Barbara L. Kornblau, ADA Consultants.

risk of substantial harm to the health or safety of the individual or others that employers or others cannot eliminate or reduce to less a significant risk by reasonable accommodation. Employers must consider the duration of the risk, the nature and severity of the potential harm, the likelihood that the potential harm will occur, and the imminence of potential harm.[45]

For example, suppose Carlotta wanted to swap classrooms with a teacher whose classroom is on the second floor of the school, which has three stories and an elevator. The headmaster could not refuse to allow Carlotta to use this second-floor classroom because he fears Carlotta, as a wheelchair user, would pose a direct threat in the event of a fire. The chances of a fire occurring are small; therefore, little likelihood exists that any harm will occur. Moreover, the school could develop an emergency plan in advance that would further lower the risk.

Employers must base the determination that an individual poses a direct threat on an individualized assessment of the individual's present ability to safely perform the essential functions of the job. Employers must base the assessment on a reasonable medical judgment that relies on the most current medical knowledge and/or on the best available objective evidence.[45]

The regulations suggest that employers seek opinions from professionals who have expertise in the disability involved or direct knowledge of the individual with the disability. The EEOC recognizes that documentation of direct threat can come from OTs "who have expertise in the disability involved and/or direct knowledge of the individual with a disability."[67] Often a reasonable accommodation can reduce the risk. For example, a teenager with epilepsy has a seizure every time the buzzer goes off on the French-fryer while working at the local fast food restaurant. The OT suggests the employer could reasonably accommodate him by changing the buzzer to a bell.

Discrimination based upon association with an individual with a disability

The fourth prohibited activity includes excluding or otherwise denying equal job or benefits to a qualified individual because of the known disability of an individual with whom the qualified individual is known to have a family, business, social, or other relationship or association.[52] For example, an employer could not refuse to hire Carlotta's husband because Carlotta has arthritis and is in a wheelchair and the employer is worried that Carlotta's husband may have excessive absences because of Carlotta's condition. In fact, this principle prohibits the employer from asking any questions of him that may reveal information about his wife's disability.

Failing to make a reasonable accommodation

The fifth prohibited activity includes failing to make a reasonable accommodation after a request for a particular accommodation, for a known disability of a qualified individual, or denying someone employment to avoid providing a reasonable accommodation, unless the employer can show that the accommodation would impose undue hardship on the business operation.[53] As previously discussed, the OT can play a major role in assisting employers to determine reasonable accommodations. As previously mentioned, Carlotta's intervention plan includes her need for the following reasonable accommodations: a laptop computer and LCD computer and a one-level classroom. Carlotta must request the specific accommodations she wants. As part of the intervention plan, the OT may prepare a report as documentation to the school explaining Carlotta's need for the particular accommodations for submission with Carlotta's accommodation request. The OT may meet with the school to help staff members understand the needed accommodations. Should Carlotta's school fail to make the reasonable accommodations she requests, it would violate this provision of the ADA.

The employer must know that a prospective or actual employee is an individual with a disability before its obligation to make accommodation arises. Courts have found that an employer cannot discriminate based on disability if it does not know about the disability (*Morisky v. Broward County*).[72] Vague statements about one's limitations or past are not sufficient to put the employer on notice of a disability.[72] Disabilities such as multiple sclerosis, arthritis, learning disabilities, and mental health disorders may not be as obvious to an employer as seeing someone in a wheelchair. For employees to obtain reasonable accommodations for these hidden disabilities, employees or potential employees must disclose

their disability to the employer. OTs can work with clients as employees or potential employees on whether to disclose the disability, when to disclose, and how to disclose their disability.

Employment tests that screen out individuals with disabilities

The sixth prohibited activity involves using employment tests that tend to screen out individuals with disabilities on the basis of their disability, unless the test is shown to be job-related for the position in question and is consistent with business necessity.[54] The EEOC considers a test job-related if the test measures a legitimate qualification for the specific job in question.[67] A test is not consistent with business necessity if it excludes an individual with a disability because of the disability and is not related to the essential functions of the job.[67] For example, under this section of Title I, the private school where Carlotta works could not give a written, twelfth grade–level reading test to an individual with a known learning disability who applies for a janitorial position. The janitorial position requires reading labels, which are on a fourth-grade reading level. That test would screen out the applicant based upon her disability and is neither job-related nor consistent with business necessity.

Administering tests to measure physical attributes, not skills or aptitudes

The seventh prohibited activity involves failing to administer tests in a manner to ensure that when administered to a job applicant or employee with a disability—which impairs sensory, manual, or speaking skills—the test results accurately reflect the skill, aptitude, or whatever other factor of the applicant or employee that the test purports to measure, rather than the sensory, manual, or speaking skills, except where such skills are the factors that the test purports to measure.[55] For example, in *Stutts v. Freeman*,[76] an individual with dyslexia was denied a heavy equipment job because he could not pass a written test required to enter a training program. The standard that he pass a written test had the effect of discriminating against the plaintiff because of his disability because the test was not meant to test the applicant's ability to read and write but rather his knowledge of heavy equipment operation. Had the employer administered the test orally, the potential employer would have focused on evaluation of the applicant's qualifications for the job, not his ability to read the material.

Retaliating against individuals who file discrimination claims

The eighth prohibited activity prevents employers from retaliating against individuals who file claims for discrimination under Title I.[56] Before an applicant can file a lawsuit in court under Title I, he or she must file a complaint with the EEOC. This section prohibits an employer from firing, demoting, or otherwise retaliating against an employee who files a charge of discrimination with the EEOC or otherwise pursues his or her rights under this law.

Conducting pre-employment medical exams or inquiries

The final prohibited activity keeps employers from conducting pre-employment medical examinations of an applicant or employee or inquiring into whether the applicant is an individual with a disability or the nature and extent of the person's disability before the employer extends an offer of employment to the applicant.[57] Under the ADA, a medical examination means a "procedure or test that seeks information about an individual's physical or mental impairments or health."[68] The EEOC considers a variety of factors in deciding whether a test is a medical exam. These include, among others, whether the test is administered or the results interpreted by a healthcare professional or someone trained by a health professional, whether the test is designed to reveal an impairment, and whether the test measures the applicant's performance of a task or his or her physiological responses to performing the task.[68]

Pre-placement Screenings and Functional Capacities Assessments

This provision of Title I affects the way OTs do business. OTs are often involved in pre-placement screenings and functional capacity evaluations, which are sometimes considered under the category of fitness for duty exams. Employers often hire OTs to perform these tests, which are described more fully in Chapter 13. The ADA regulations outline the types of testing that employers (or those acting on their behalf) may perform and the stages at which they may perform them.

The hiring process includes two relevant stages. The first stage, the pre-offer, occurs during the interview process, before an employer extends an offer of employment to an applicant or candidate. The second stage, the post-offer, occurs after the employer has made a hiring decision and extends an offer of employment to the applicant or candidate. We often speak of this offer of employment as a conditional offer of employment because it is subject to withdrawal under certain circumstances, which this chapter addresses below.

During the pre-offer stage, an employer may conduct only a simple agility test. Employers and OTs acting on their behalf may not conduct medical examination or inquiries, pre-employment physical, pre-placement screening, or functional capacity assessments during the pre-offer stage. An agility test is a simple test that looks at one's physical agility. It is not a medical test. Agility tests do not involve medical examinations, physicians, or medical diagnoses. Employers may request clearance from the applicant's physician before administration of the agility test.[67] The classic agility test for police recruits shows them running through tires, scaling a wall, and climbing ropes. Another example of a permissible agility test would allow the employer to ask an applicant to carry a piece of wallboard from one end of the construction site to the other.

Although employers may perform these agility tests, ADA rules govern their use. If an employer chooses to use an agility test, it must give the test to all similarly situated applicants or employees. If the agility test screens out individuals with disabilities, the employer must show that the test is job-related, consistent with business necessity, and that the applicant could not perform the job with a reasonable accommodation.

During the post-offer stage, employers or those acting on their behalf may conduct agility tests, medical exams and inquiries, pre-employment physicals, pre-placement screenings, and functional capacity assessments. If the employer chooses to give medical exams once it makes a conditional offer of employment, it must give the exam to all employees entering the same job category. The ADA does not require that a medical exam satisfy the job-related and consistent with business necessity standards. However, if the employer withdraws a conditional offer of employment because of the medical exam results, the employer must be able to show the following: (1) the reasons for the exclusion are job-related and consistent necessity or the person is being excluded to avoid a direct threat to health or safety and (2) no reasonable accommodation was available that would enable this person to perform the essential functions without a significant risk to health or safety, or that the accommodation would cause an undue hardship.

As mentioned above, during the post-offer stage employers, and OTs acting on their behalf, may perform pre-placement screenings and functional capacity assessments. Both are subject to the same requirements as medical exams. In other words, although the tests need not comply with the job-related and business necessity requirements, should the tests screen out individuals with disabilities, job-related and business necessity becomes the required standard to meet. Reality dictates then that to comply with the ADA, the pre-placement screening must be job-related and test only the essential functions of the job. For example, assessing Carlotta's hand strength as a part of the interview process for hiring her as a Spanish teacher would violate this provision of the ADA because hand strength is not job-related and not related to an essential job function.

Employers and those acting on their behalf must keep results of all medical exams and inquiries confidential with some limited exceptions. These exceptions include work restrictions information, insurance purposes, government investigations of ADA complaints, and state worker's compensation and second injury funds, which are funds set up by some states to encourage employers to hire individuals with previous worker's compensation–related or other injuries.

This prohibition against inquiries into medical and disability-related information also extends to job applications and interviews. Employers cannot ask questions about someone's disability or questions that will lead to information about someone's disability during the job interview process. Box 14-5 shows examples of questions employers cannot ask during the interview process.

Box **14-5**	QUESTIONS NOT PERMITTED UNDER THE ADA

- How did you become disabled?
- Are you in good health?
- Have you recovered from your prior disability?
- How much can you lift?
- How far can you walk?
- Have you been in a wheelchair your whole life?
- Do you have a driver's license? (If the job doesn't require driving or if a reasonable accommodation can't eliminate the driving.)
- Does your wife, husband, child, or roommate have a disability?
- Who takes care of your disabled husband (or wife or child)?
- Have you ever been injured in an accident?
- Have you ever filed a claim for workers' compensation?
- How were you burned?
- Do you have any physical conditions that would prevent you from doing your job?
- Do you have a good back?
- Have you ever been hospitalized?

OTs can assist human resources professionals in the proper way to inquire into an individual's ability to perform the essential function of a position without asking prohibited questions. Employers must base their interview questions on specific job functions, information that OTs gather from the job analysis described in more detail in Chapter 13. Ideally, the interviewer should have a job description prepared from the OT's job analysis and ask interviewees questions about the match between their skills and abilities and the job's essential functions.

The Role of the Occupational Therapist

OTs can work together with individuals with disabilities as part of their intervention plans to identify needed accommodations that will enable participation in the workplace and plan a strategy to obtain those accommodations from the employer. OTs can help their clients understand their right to reasonable accommodations under Title I of the ADA. This includes the need to request the specific accommodations needed and to furnish documentation of the need, which the OT can prepare for the client's submission to the employer. OTs may find themselves advocating for the accommodations to their clients' employer.

For example, as described above, Carlotta's OT can play a major role in her employer's provision of the accommodations she needs. Carlotta and her OT identified the accommodations she needs as part of her occupational profile and intervention plan. If the employer refuses to provide the accommodations after Carlotta provides the OT's documentation and if Carlotta eventually files a lawsuit, the OT may find himself or herself testifying in court about Carlotta's need for the accommodations.

OTs can also provide consultation services for employers who want to avoid litigation and seek advice on making reasonable accommodations for its employees with disabilities. If Carlotta's employer were proactive, he may have contacted an OT for advice on how to accommodate Carlotta.

This kind of consultation, in which the client is the employer, not the individual with a disability, usually begins with a job analysis (described in detail in Chapter 13) to see what the job requires. The therapist takes this information, compares it to the individual's limitations, and tries to develop accommodations to enable performance. This accommodation development stage cannot proceed without input from the person with the disability.

For example, the author was hired by a hospital to look at whether a nurse affected by some post-polio weakness and arthritis could use a scooter (wheelchair-substitute type scooter) as her requested accommodation to cut down on the number of steps she took during the day. The nurse had filed a charge of discrimination with the EEOC and the hospital's attorney suggested hiring an OT to see if the requested accommodations were reasonable, so it could avoid a full-blown lawsuit. The head nurse could not imagine a nurse using a scooter. The author performed a job analysis and determined that the scooter was a reasonable accommodation. Convincing the head nurse that the scooter was reasonable took more work in the form of sensitivity training, which the OT also contributes.

TITLE II: STATE AND LOCAL GOVERNMENT SERVICES

Title II of the ADA prohibits state and local government entities and those with whom they contract from denying a qualified individual with a disability participation in or the benefits of services, programs, or activities that it provides to individuals without disabilities.[13] Title II's antidiscrimination protection in employment of individuals with disabilities by state governments has been limited by cases decided by the U.S. Supreme Court. Individual state employees can no longer bring lawsuits for money damages in federal court where a state discriminates in its employment practices based on the disability.[65]

Title II's other requirements look similar to those of Title III, described in detail for non-government entities below. However, Title II goes further in its requirement for state and local government services than for those privately owned entities in one particular concept.

Title II requires that government agencies give qualified individuals with disabilities equal opportunity to participate in or benefit from the state or local government aid, benefits, or services.[14] This requires providing more access than in Title III's requirements to provide what is readily achievable, as described later in this chapter. Providing equal opportunity to state and local government services requires taking measures such as making facilities physically accessible, making policy changes, providing reasonable accommodations in the form of auxiliary aids and services, providing accessibility in public transportation, and communication such as 911 services for the hearing impaired, and others described more fully under Title III below. OTs can help state and local governments make some of the needed changes as will be discussed further in this chapter.

TITLE III: PUBLIC ACCOMMODATIONS

Title III of the ADA prohibits discrimination against individuals with disabilities in **places of public accommodation**. One may find this description slightly misleading because in spite of its name, this section of the ADA covers *privately* owned entities that own or lease to others, places that affect commerce. In other words, **places of public accommodation** are privately owned entities where business of some kind is transacted or affected. *Places of public accommodation* covers 12 broad categories enumerated in the ADA (Table 14-1).[15] The U.S. Department of Justice, the federal government agencies charged with overseeing and enforcing Title III, reports that more than 5 million places of accommodations exist in the United States.[77]

The super rule, which forms the basis for Title III, prohibits discrimination as follows:

> No individual shall be discriminated against on the basis of disability in the full and equal enjoyment of the goods, services, facilities, privileges, advantages, or accommodations of any place of public accommodation by any private entity who owns, leases (or leases to), or operates a place of public accommodation.[16]

TABLE **14-1**   **Places of Public Accommodation Under Title III**

Category of Public Accommodation	Examples
Places of lodging	Hotels, motels
Establishments serving food or drink	Restaurants, bars
Places of exhibition or entertainment	Movie theaters, stadiums
Places of public gathering	Convention centers
Sales or rental establishments	Bakeries, shopping malls
Service establishments	Laundromats, funeral homes, doctors' offices
Public transportation terminals	Train stations
Places of public display or collection	Museums, libraries
Places of recreation	Parks, zoos, amusement parks
Places of education	Pre-schools, private schools, colleges
Social service establishments	Day care centers, senior centers
Places of exercise or recreation	Health clubs, bowling alleys, golf courses

Under Title III, places of public accommodation must remove barriers to access and if it cannot remove the barriers, the place of public accommodation (PPA) must provide an alternative or reasonable accommodation to provide access to the goods and services it provides. Many think of the barriers Title III addresses as architectural barriers or those barriers in the physical environment, such as steps and curbs, that limit physical access to a place one desires to go. Although many view the requirements of Title III as a quasi-building code, removing barriers to access as described in the ADA refers to more than mere access through removal of physical barriers. It also refers to access caused by attitudinal barriers and rules, and policies based on myths, misperceptions, and fears about individuals with disabilities that act as barriers to their access to places of public accommodations. For example, before the ADA became law, in some banks it was a common policy to not allow individuals who are blind to have safe deposit boxes. The rationale behind it asserts that because individuals who are blind cannot see what is in their safe deposit boxes, how can they remove things they need from the box? Only the safe deposit box holder can go into the viewing booth. Based upon misperceptions, banks believed themselves at risk for accusations of theft from the boxes and as a result, disallowed individuals who were blind from benefiting from the services they provided to individuals who were not blind. This practice discriminated against individuals with visual impairments. The ADA prohibits these practices and seeks to break down these kinds of barriers.

To further its mission of breaking down physical and attitudinal barriers, Title III specifies three broad principles that provide the foundation for its philosophy of inclusion of individuals with disabilities in society. First, PPA must provide individuals with disabilities with an equal opportunity to participate in or benefit from the goods and services offered.[17] Further, the PPA must give individuals with disabilities an equal opportunity to benefit from the goods and services it offers.[17] Finally, PPA must provide the benefits in the most integrated setting possible.[17,18]

The PPA can violate Title III's mandates against discrimination by the following, among other things.
- *Refusing to admit an individual with a disability merely because he or she has a disability.*[17] For example, a restaurant cannot refuse to admit and/or serve an individual with cerebral palsy because he or she drools.
- *Failing to provide goods and services to individuals with disabilities in the most integrated setting appropriate to the individual's needs.*[18] For example, a professional or college football team cannot segregate all wheelchair users in a "handicapped" section in the end zone. It must allow wheelchair users to sit with family members and disperse wheelchair seating throughout the stadium.
- *Using eligibility criteria that screen out or tend to screen out individuals with disabilities from full and equal enjoyment of goods and services.*[20] For example, retail stores located in a busy tourist area require that individuals using credit cards

show a driver's license as proof of identification as a way of cutting down on the use of stolen credit cards. However, this practice screens out individuals with visual impairments or other disabilities who do not qualify for driver's licenses. The retail stores would have to accept state identification cards in place of a driver's license from individuals with disabilities who do not qualify for driver's licenses.

- *Failing to make reasonable modifications in policies, practices, or procedures, when the modifications are necessary to afford goods, services, or facilities to individuals with disabilities.*[21] The example given above regarding bank policies for safe deposit boxes and individuals who are blind is a good illustration of a policy that discriminates on the basis of disability. Another example, Great Grocery Store has a policy whereby cashiers must place all checks in a specific column in the cash drawer. Carlotta's OT recommended that she use large print checks because she can write more legibly using larger print. She attempts to give the cashier a large print check. The cashier refuses to take the check because it does not fit in the cash drawer column for checks. She also tells Carlotta that their policy is to accept large print checks only from blind people. Great Grocery Store must modify its policies and accept Carlotta's check.

- *Failing to take steps to ensure that individuals with disabilities are not excluded or denied services, segregated, or otherwise treated differently from individuals without disabilities because of the absence of auxiliary aides and services.*[22] **Auxiliary aids** as used in the ADA include devices that OTs usually refer to as adaptive equipment or assistive technology. According to the regulations auxiliary aids and services includes, among other things, qualified interpreters, assistive listening devices, closed caption decoders on televisions, Braile materials, taped texts, and "acquisition or modification of equipment or devices."[22]

    For example, suppose Carlotta stays at restored historic hotel in her quest for the perfect bed and breakfast. She finds that she can use the bathing facilities in her room only if she has a tub bench. The hotel would have to provide her with a bathtub bench as an auxiliary aid so that it will not exclude or deny her bathing services.

    Two exceptions exist to the auxiliary aide provision requirement. The PPA need not provide an auxiliary aide that fundamentally alters the nature of the goods and services offered or causes an undue burden.[22] An undue burden means the provision of the auxiliary aide would cause significant difficulty or expense. The impact to the PPA varies, considering such elements as the size of the business and its budget. A major corporation should expect to spend more money on auxiliary aids and services than a neighborhood "mom and pop" operation. A fundamental alteration to the nature of the goods and services offered would occur, for example, if an individual with a visual impairment requested management to raise the lights in a bar, where the lights are customarily turned down low to create a particular ambiance or atmosphere.

    The PPA need not provide personal devices and services such as individually prescribed devices (e.g., eyeglasses) or services of a personal nature (e.g., eating, toileting, or dressing).[25] However, it would probably be a reasonable auxiliary service should Carlotta request the restaurant cut her meat in the kitchen before serving her steak should weakness in her hands prevent her from performing this task.

- *Failing to furnish auxiliary aids and services when necessary to ensure effective communication, unless an undue burden or fundamental alteration would result.*[22] For example, Bob is deaf. He needs a sign language interpreter to converse with others. He seeks counseling services at a private mental health clinic. He requests a sign language interpreter to enable him to communicate with the mental health therapist. The mental health clinic must provide the sign language interpreter unless it is an undue burden.

- *Refusing to remove architectural and structural communication barriers in existing facilities where readily achievable.*[23] *Readily achievable* means barrier removal that is easily accomplishable and can be carried out without much difficulty or expense.[23] The ADA regulations provide 21 examples of steps places of public accommodation can take to remove barriers (Box 14-6).

Box **14-6** EXAMPLES OF STEPS TO REMOVE BARRIERS

Installing ramps

Making curb cuts in sidewalks and entrances

Repositioning shelves

Rearranging tables, chairs, vending machines, display racks, and other furniture

Repositioning telephones

Adding raised markings on elevator control buttons

Installing flashing alarm lights

Widening doors

Installing offset hinges to widen doorways

Eliminating a turnstile or providing an alternative accessible path

Installing accessible door hardware

Installing grab bars in toilet stalls

Rearranging toilet partitions to increase maneuvering space

Insulating lavatory pipes under sinks to prevent burns

Installing a raised toilet seat

Installing a full-length bathroom mirror

Repositioning the paper towel dispenser in a bathroom

Creating designated accessible parking spaces

Installing an accessible paper cup dispenser at an existing inaccessible water fountain

Removing high pile, low density carpeting

Installing vehicle hand controls

PRIORITY ONE: ACCESS INTO THE PPA (PLACE OF PUBLIC ACCOMMODATION)

First, the PPA should try to provide access to and into the place of public accommodation from public sidewalks, parking, or public transportation. In other words, provide a way for individuals with disabilities to get into the building. For example, this includes, among other things as may prove necessary in individual circumstances, installing a ramp to the entrance, widening entrances, and providing accessible parking spaces.[23] Under this provision, the PPA would be responsible for making sure Carlotta can get from her parking space into the lobby of the movie theater.

PRIORITY TWO: ACCESS TO AREAS WHERE GOODS AND SERVICES ARE AVAILABLE

The second priority PPA should focus on is providing access to those areas of public accommodation where it makes goods and services available to the public. This step answers the following question: Now that individuals with disabilities can enter through our door, how do we get them to the actual part of the PPA where we provide the goods and services? This can include changes such as adjusting the layout of display racks, providing Braile and raised character signage, widening doorways, providing visual alarms, and installing ramps.[22] The movie theater, under this section, would want to make sure Carlotta could get

to the snack bar to purchase her popcorn and into the theater to watch the movie.

PRIORITY THREE: ACCESS TO RESTROOMS

The third priority for access is access to the restroom facilities. This may include modifications such as removing obstructing furniture or vending machines, widening doorways, installing ramps, providing accessible signage, widening toilet stalls, lowering paper towel dispensers and mirrors, and installing grab bars, usable faucet handles, and soap dispensers, to name a few. The movie theater would provide Carlotta access to the restrooms under this provision.[22]

PRIORITY FOUR: ACCESS TO THE GOODS & SERVICES

The fourth and final priority for access is access to the goods, services, facilities, privileges, advantages, or accommodations offered at the place of public accommodation. This includes access to the actual goods or services that the PPA provides.[23] For Carlotta, the PPA needs to consider whether a place exists for Carlotta to sit in the movie theater so that she can watch the movie she wishes to see. Can they remove seats to provide her a place to sit where she can sit with her family? Can they disperse the seats in the theater so that they do not have to segregate all of the wheelchair users in the back or front of the theater?

The ADA regulations recognize that not all changes are immediately readily achievable. In concert with input from members of the disability community, the Justice Department set forth four priorities in the ADA regulations that PPA should take to comply with the barrier removal requirements (Box 14-7).[22]

- *Refusing to provide access to goods and services through alternative readily achievable measures when removal of barriers is not readily achievable.*[24] The ADA regulations give three examples of alternatives to barrier removal. These include providing curb service or home delivery for an inaccessible restaurant, for example, retrieving merchandise from inaccessible shelves or racks in the grocery store, and relocating activities to accessible locations.[24] For example, in pursuit of her movie hobby, Carlotta wishes to see the latest popular art film. A multi-screen cinema is showing the film, but the particular theater requires climbing a flight of steps. The theater must rotate the films to provide Carlotta access to the film she wishes to see.[24]
- *Failing to provide equivalent transportation services and purchase accessible vehicles in certain circumstances.*[26] For example, Robby Rat's Fantasy Garden, a large amusement park, provides trams to take people to their cars in its enormous

parking lots. On one of her trips, Carlotta takes her grandchildren to the Fantasy Garden. The Fantasy Garden must provide an accessible transportation from the parking lot to the entry gates for Carlotta.

- *Failing to maintain accessible features of facilities and equipment.*[19] For example, a Streams Department Store must maintain its accessible ramped entrance into the store. This means shoveling snow in the winter and raking leaves in the fall so that Carlotta has access into the store on her trips to this city.
- *Failing to design and construct new facilities and, when undertaking alterations, alter existing facilities in accordance with the Americans with Disabilities Act Accessibility Guidelines issued by the Architectural and Transportation Barriers Compliance Board and incorporated in the final Department of Justice Title III regulations.*[27] This is where the "building code" flavor of the ADA comes in. Specific requirements dictate how builders should design and decorate buildings to provide access. Readers will find the specifics of these ADA Accessibility Guidelines for Buildings and Facilities (ADAAG) requirements online at *http://www.access-board.gov/adaag/html/adaag.htm*. The government agencies periodically update the accessibility guidelines. For example, the current

version of ADAAG now includes standards for play areas for children and recreational facilities which, though they are not enforceable at this time, provide guidelines for PPA to improve access and enable participation.[62,63] Readers should keep in mind that some state regulations differ from the ADAAG requirements. For example, Florida requires accessible parking spaces of a 12-foot width (144 inches) with a 5-foot access aisle,[73] whereas the ADAAG rules requires a width of 8 feet (96 inches) with a 5-foot access aisle.[58] ADA regulations advise PPA to follow the rule that provides the most access to individuals with disabilities.

The Role of the Occupational Therapist

Even though Congress passed the ADA more than 15 years ago, research shows that individuals with disabilities continue to feel their participation limited by access problems, and many do not even know what their rights are under the ADA.[71] OT is in a unique position to promote Title III's access and inclusion mandates. With our knowledge of performance in areas of occupation, performance skills, performance patterns, activity demands in context, and client factors, we have skills to look at how the physical environment can affect performance. We know how to make adaptations to the environment, the task, or the person to enable performance in spite of the limitations an individual may have in performance skills. This knowledge base equips OT to help PPA comply with Title III's access requirement as consultants by looking at accessibility limitations and making recommendations to the PPA to improve access, physical and non-physical (including attitudes, policies, and procedures).

OTs may find themselves working from two angles in providing access intervention. Their clients may include individuals with disabilities seeking to increase their participation in the community through increasing their access and inclusion, such as Carlotta is. Alternatively, OTs may find their clients include proactive PPA seeking to make their goods and services accessible to individuals with disabilities to avoid lawsuits and/or do the right thing.

In the case in which the individual with the disability serves as the client, the OT will want to do an occupational profile that will delve into the client's interests in the community as was done with Carlotta. The OT works with the client to determine what the barriers are to the client's participation in the community activities of his or her choice. In Carlotta's case, we know that movies and going to the mall are important to her. Part of our intervention plan will include problem solving the changes that Carlotta will need to be able to participate in these occupations, explaining her right to accommodations under Title III, and suggesting ways to advocate for those needed changes to the PPA. If the PPA fails to make changes to provide access to Carlotta, she can file an administrative complaint with the Department of Justice in Washington* or immediately file a lawsuit. The OT may serve as a witness in Title III litigation should it come to that.

Under circumstances in which the PPA is his or her client, the OT will look at the goods and services the PPA offers, the policies and procedures it uses (especially customer service–related policies), and the physical access offered in the ADA-delineated priority order. Just as the employment-related ADA consultation with an employer usually begins with a job analysis, the access consultation with a PPA begins with the accessibility audit. An **accessibility audit** is a review of the access and inclusion practices of a PPA from a physical and policy perspective. The accessibility audit looks at the ADAAG requirements, the kinds of modifications one can make to increase access, and readily achievable changes one can make according to the priorities set in Title III. Figure 14-1 contains an accessibility audit that includes examining physical as well as non-physical barriers to access according to ADAAG and follows the priorities specified in Title III.

OTs can also provide consultation services for employers.

OT PRACTICE NOTES

ADVOCATING FOR EMPLOYEES WITH DISABILITIES

Analyze physical functions to determine, for the employee, whether he or she can perform the essential functions of a given job with or without reasonable accommodations.

Suggest specific reasonable accommodations, such as adaptive equipment, auxiliary aids, or modifications to the worksite to enable the prospective or returning employee to perform the essential functions of his or her job.

Obtain adaptive devices or auxiliary aids to facilitate performance in the workplace and in the community.

Develop strategies to prepare the prospective employee to suggest reasonable accommodations to human resources personnel during the interview and hiring process.

Teach adolescents with disabilities entering the job market for the first time how to manage the application, hiring, and interview processes.

Expand access to public accommodations in the mainstream of independent living, such as theaters, conference centers, hotels, and restaurants through focusing on mobility in the community; identification of equipment, aids, and services; and advocacy to obtain them.

Provide information to clients so they can develop a basic understanding of what their rights are under the ADA.

*See *http://www.usdoj.gov/crt/ada/enforce.htm#anchor 218282.*

OT PRACTICE NOTES

CONSULTING WITH PLACES OF PUBLIC ACCOMODATION

Advise businesses that offer public accommodations, such as restaurants, movie theaters, hospitals, medical clinics, and hotels, how to make their facilities accessible to individuals with disabilities.

Ensure that places of public accommodations are accessible to individuals with disabilities and make recommendations to remove architectural and other barriers.

Assist with the acquisition of auxiliary aids to allow individuals with disabilities to have an equal opportunity to participate in or benefit from programs offered.

Prevent lawsuits by performing accessibility audits and making recommendations for increased access and barrier removal on a proactive basis.

Locate and/or acquire auxiliary aids and services for places of public accommodation.

Train employees in how to make people with disabilities feel welcome in their facilities, how to use the auxiliary aids, and how to provide auxiliary services to individuals with disabilities.

OT PRACTICE NOTES

CONSULTING WITH EMPLOYERS

Analyze jobs to determine essential job functions and possible accommodations that one can easily make to a specific job.

Develop or rewrite job descriptions based on job analysis that include specific descriptions of essential job functions.

Modify job sites to make reasonable accommodations for individual employees with disabilities.

Suggest specific devices and adaptive equipment that allows the employer to hire an individual with a disability who, with the assistance of the device, can now perform the essential functions of a given job.

Sensitize co-workers and supervisors to interacting, supervising, and working effectively with individuals with disabilities.

Train supervisors to develop reasonable accommodations for injured workers returning to the job, including worker's compensation claimants.

Ensure that job sites are accessible to individuals with disabilities and make recommendations to remove architectural barriers where inaccessible features are found.

Propose post-offer, job-related employee screenings and/or evaluations for high injury risk positions.

Perform an individualized assessment of a worker's present ability to safely perform the essential functions of the job to determine whether the worker with a disability poses a direct threat to the health and safety of himself, herself, or others.

Save businesses money by promoting cost-effective reasonable accommodations during the complaint or mediation process to avoid costly litigation.

AIR CARRIER ACCESS ACT

Carlotta's occupational profile shows that travel is a meaningful occupation for her. To pursue that occupation now that she uses a wheelchair for mobility, she will need to know what to expect while traveling and how she can advocate for herself. The key is the Air Carrier Access Act of 1986. The Air Carrier Access Act of 1986 (ACAA)[59] prohibits discrimination against qualified individuals with physical or mental impairments in air transportation by foreign and domestic air carriers. The ACAA applies only to air carriers that provide regularly scheduled services for hire to the public. As with the ADA and FHA, the ACAA lists specific actions it considers discriminatory.

DISCRIMINATION PROHIBITED UNDER ACAA

Airline carriers may not refuse to transport qualified individuals with disabilities on the basis of their disability.[3] The definitions of disability are similar to the definitions found in the ADA. A qualified individual with a disability in the airline travel context means he or she seeks to purchase or has a ticket to fly. The ACAA would protect Carlotta because she has arthritis and an airline ticket. By federal statute, carriers may exclude anyone from a flight if carrying the person would be "inimical to the safety of the flight."[3] This parallels the direct threat criteria under the ADA. If the airline carrier excludes persons with disabilities on safety grounds, the carrier must provide a written explanation of the decision within 10 days of the refusal.[3]

Airline carriers may not deny transportation to a qualified individual with a disability "because the person's disability results in appearance or involuntary behavior that may offend, annoy, or inconvenience crewmembers or other passengers."[3] Airline carriers cannot limit the number of people with disabilities it will allow on a flight as a means of refusing transportation based on disability.[3] The ACAA prohibits airlines from requiring a person with a disability to accept special services, such as pre-boarding, if the passenger does not request them.[1] Similarly, air carriers cannot segregate passengers with disabilities, even if separate or different services are available to them.[1]

Under the ACAA, airline carriers cannot require a qualified individual with a disability to provide advance notice of his or her intention to travel or of his or her disability as a condition of receiving transportation or of receiving services or required accommodations.[4] Carlotta would not have to notify the airline in advance that she planned to fly. A limited exception to this rule exists, however. An airline carrier may require up to 48 hours notice for certain specific accommodations that require advance preparation such as medical oxygen use, the transportation for an electric wheelchair in a plane with fewer than 60 seats, and the provision of an on-board wheelchair in an aircraft that lacks an accessible lavatory.[4]

How To Do An Accessibility Audit Under The ADA

A. Remember Title III, Public Accommodations, is not limited to the physical accessibility of a building. Title III includes meaningful access and equal participation in all programs and services offered by the public accommodation.

> 1. Making something accessible is worthless if you do not identify its location. For example, public accommodations must include accessible signage to assist individuals in locating accessible bathrooms and building entrances.

B. Title III sets forth the following priorities for accessibility:

> 1. **Access to and into the place of public accommodation** from public sidewalks, parking, or public transportation. This includes installing a ramp to the entrance, widening entrances, and providing accessible parking spaces.

> 2. **Access to those areas of public accommodation where goods and services are made available to the public.** This includes adjusting the layout of display racks, providing Brailed and raised character signage, widening doorways, providing visual alarms, and installing ramps.

> 3. **Access to restroom facilities.** This includes removing obstructing furniture or vending machines, widening doorways, installing ramps, providing accessible signage, widening toilet stalls, lowering paper towel dispensers and mirrors, and installing grab bars.

> 4. **Access to the goods, services, facilities, privileges, advantages, or accommodations offered at the place of public accommodation.** This includes access to the actual goods or services themselves.

C. **The Accessibility Audit should follow the priorities set forth in Title III.**

STEP ONE: According to the first priority, look at the access to and into the place of public accommodation from public sidewalks, parking, or public transportation:

		YES	NO
1.	Are parking spaces 96 inches wide with an adjacent access aisle of 60 inches?	_____	_____
2.	Is one in every eight parking spaces served by a 96-inch access aisle marked "van accessible?"	_____	_____
3.	How many parking spaces are designated for individuals with disabilities? _____ (_____% of spaces) (compare with chart at ADAAG § 4.1.2(5)(a); 10% of total number provided for outpatient units or facilities should be accessible.)	_____	_____
4.	If covered parking is provided, is the ceiling at least 114 inches high to allow access to high-top vans?	_____	_____
5.	Are all curb ramps (curb cuts) from the parking spaces at a gradient of 1:20 with a textured, non-slip surface?	_____	_____

Figure 14-1 How to do an accessibility audit under the ADA. (Courtesy Barbara L. Kornblau, ADA Consultants, Inc., 1992, 2002.)

6.   Are parking area and building separated by a street?   _____ _____

7.   Are the accessible parking spaces located on the shortest
       accessible route of travel from the parking to the
       accessible building entrance?   _____ _____

8.   Is the surface of the accessible route smooth (no sand,
       gravel, or utility hole covers)?   _____ _____

9.   Are all ramps along the accessible route at a gradient of at
       least 1:12 (1:16 - 1:20 preferred)?   _____ _____

10.   Do ramps have 5-foot level landings at the bottom and top
       that are as wide as the ramp itself?   _____ _____

11.   Do all ramps have handrails with top handrail, non-slip,
       gripping surfaces mounted between 34 inches and 38 inches above
       the ramp surface?   _____ _____

12.   Is the accessible route walkway at least 48 inches wide?   _____ _____

13.   Is the accessible route marked with appropriate signage?   _____ _____

14.   Is there a passenger loading and unloading zone?   _____ _____

15.   The accessible entrance is located _____
       _____   _____ _____

16.   Is the accessible door marked with appropriate signage?   _____ _____

17.   Is the entrance door a minimum of 32 inches wide?   _____ _____

18.   Is the door automatic?   _____ _____

19.   Is the door opening mechanism set to less _____ pounds
       of pressure (as measured by a push than pull scale, although no
       specific requirements are set for exterior doors at this time)?   _____ _____

20.   If there are two doors in series at the entrance, do the
       doors open in the same direction or away from the space
       between the two doors and is the space at least 48 inches plus
       the width of any door opening into the space?   _____ _____

21.   Is there an alternative to a revolving door?   _____ _____

22.   Is door hardware shaped so as to require one hand to
       open and not to require tight grasping, tight pinching, or
       twisting of the wrist to operate?   _____ _____

23.   Are thresholds less than ½ inch high?   _____ _____

24.   If the primary entrance has steps, is there a proper sign
       directing patrons to the accessible entrance?   _____ _____

Figure 14-1, cont'd

(Continued)

STEP TWO: Look at access to those areas of public accommodation where goods and services are made available to the public. This includes adjusting the layout of display racks, providing Brailed and raised character signage, widening doorways, providing visual alarms, and installing ramps.

A. List all areas in the facility where goods, services, and programs are provided to the public. (Remember, this includes areas in places that are not normally considered places of public accommodations, but parts of those facilities where members of the public would go, i.e., the showroom of a factory not open to the general public but where outside buyers and salespersons might go.)

B. Are all areas where goods, services, and programs are located accessible?
(This section should be repeated for all goods, services, and programs offered at the location.)

Goods/Service/Program and Location

Figure 14-1, cont'd

Airlines cannot exclude a passenger with disabilities from a particular seat or require him or her to sit in a certain seat, except to comply with FAA safety regulations, such as exit row seating, which requires passengers have specific abilities to open the exit door in case of an emergency.[6] Airlines must accommodate passenger seat assignments if required based on the person's disability and requested 24 hours in advance. For example, if Carlotta traveled with a service animal that assisted her with tasks such as pulling her wheelchair and picking up items from the floor, the carrier would have to assign them to a bulkhead seat or another seat that could accommodate the service animal.[7]

Airline carriers may not require a person with a disability to travel with an attendant, except in certain limited circumstances.[5] These limited circumstances include those in which a person with mobility impairment is unable to assist in his or her own evacuation and in which a person with a mental disability cannot understand or respond to the crew's safety instructions.[5] If the person with a disability and the carrier disagree about whether the individual's circumstances meet the ACAA's criteria, the carrier may require the attendant, but the carrier may not charge for the attendant's transportation cost.[5]

Text continued on p. 331

		YES	NO
1.	Is the width of the pathway to the area, including corridors and aisles, at least 32 inches of usable space?	_____	_____
2.	Is the pathway free of protruding telephones, water fountains, or other items?	_____	_____
3.	Is the pathway flooring covered with high-density, low-pile (½ inch) carpeting, non-slip tile, or vinyl?	_____	_____
4.	Are doorways at least 32 inches wide?	_____	_____
5.	If there are steps along the pathway, is the area also served by an elevator?	_____	_____
6.	Are steps covered with non-slip surfaces, provided with adequate lighting, and designed with curved nosers and sloped risers?	_____	_____
7.	Do all stairways have handrails positioned at both sides of the stairs with top handrail, non-slip, gripping surfaces mounted between 34 inches and 38 inches above the stair nosing?	_____	_____
8.	Do the handrails extend 12 inches beyond the top riser and 12 inches plus the width of one thread beyond the bottom riser?	_____	_____
9.	Are thresholds at ½ inch high or less for interior doors?	_____	_____
10.	Is the door-opening mechanism set to 5 pounds of pressure or less?	_____	_____
11.	Is door hardware shaped so as to require one hand to open and not to require tight grasping, tight pinching, or twisting of the wrist to operate?	_____	_____
12.	If doorways have two independently operated door leaves, is one leaf at least 32 inches wide?	_____	_____
13.	If there are two doors in series along the pathway, do the doors open in the same direction or away from the space between the two doors and is the space at least 48 inches plus the width of any door opening into the space?	_____	_____
14.	Are elevator call buttons centered at 42 inches above the floor and at least ¾ inch in diameter?	_____	_____
15.	Do objects mounted below the elevator call button protrude more than 4 inches into the elevator lobby?	_____	_____
16.	Are visible and audible signals provided at each elevator entrance to indicate which car is answering the call and the direction the car is going (once for up and twice for down)?	_____	_____

Figure 14-1, cont'd

(Continued)

17. Are raised and Braille characters at least 2 inches high, provided on both jams of the elevators, and centered 60 inches above the floor?   _____ _____

18. Are elevators provided with an automatic reopening device?   _____ _____

19. Is the minimum amount of time the elevators remain open in response to a call at least 3 seconds?   _____ _____

20. Are control buttons inside the elevator designated by Braille and raised letters?   _____ _____

21. Are floor buttons 54 inches or less above the floor for a side wheelchair approach and 48 inches or less for a front approach?   _____ _____

22. If public telephones are provided, are they on an accessible floor at an accessible location?   _____ _____

23. Is at least one telephone mounted so that its operable parts are no more than 54 inches or less above the floor for a side wheelchair approach and 48 inches or less for a front approach?   _____ _____

24. Is there a clear floor or ground space of at least 30 inches by 48 inches under the telephone absent bases, enclosures, fixed seats, and protruding objects of more than 4 inches?   _____ _____

25. Is at least one telephone equipped with an amplifier for individuals with hearing impairments and located near an electrical outlet for portable TTDs?   _____ _____

26. Is the telephone cord at least 29 inches long?   _____ _____

27. Is at least one text telephone provided?   _____ _____

28. Where are the accessible telephones located?   _____ _____

29. Are accessible telephones marked with appropriate signage?   _____ _____

30. Are water fountains mounted so that spouts are no higher than 36 inches from the floor?   _____ _____

31. Are fire alarms and other warning signals provided in both a visual and audible manner?   _____ _____

32. Are room numbers, directional signs, emergency directions, and other signs and markings indicated in large, block letters and numerals, using contrasting colors so they can be read by individuals with visual impairments?   _____ _____

33. Are signs provided in raised and Brailled letters and numbers?   _____ _____

Figure 14-1, cont'd

If the answer to any of the above questions is no, what reasonable accommodations may be made to allow access to the area where the goods, services, and programs are provided?

_____

_____

_____

STEP THREE : Look at access to restroom facilities.

	YES	NO
1. Where are the accessible restrooms located? _____		
_____	_____	_____
2. Is the accessible restroom designated with appropriate signage?	_____	_____
3. Is the restroom on an accessible pathway?	_____	_____
4. Can one use the restroom without going up or down steps?	_____	_____
5. Is the width of the pathway to the restrooms, including corridors, and aisles, at least 32 inches of usable space?	_____	_____
6. Is the pathway to the restrooms free of protruding telephones, water fountains, or other items?	_____	_____
7. Is the pathway flooring to the restrooms covered with high-density, low-pile (½ inch) carpeting, non-slip tile, or vinyl?	_____	_____
8. Are the doorways to the restrooms at least 32 inches wide?	_____	_____
9. Do doorways to the restroom require 5 pounds or less of pressure to open?	_____	_____
10. Is the entrance to the toilet stall at least 32 inches wide?	_____	_____
11. Is the top of the seat of the accessible toilet between 17 inches and 19 inches from the floor?	_____	_____
12. Does the toilet paper dispenser allow for the continuous flow of toilet paper without delivery control?	_____	_____
13. Does the toilet stall have a minimum depth of 56 inches where toilets are wall mounted and 59 inches where toilets are floor mounted?	_____	_____
14. Is at least one stall a minimum of 36 inches wide with an outwardly opening, self-closing door?	_____	_____

Figure 14-1, cont'd

(Continued)

15.   Are there a minimum of two grab bars at least 36 inches long in
       the accessible toilet stall with one grab bar mounted
       behind the toilet?   _____ _____

16.   Are grab bars between 33 inches and 36 inches from the floor?   _____ _____

17.   Are urinal rims at a maximum of 17 inches from the floor?   _____ _____

18.   Is there a clear space in front of the urinal of 30 inches by 48 inches to
       allow a front approach?   _____ _____

19.   Are soap dispensers, paper towel dispensers, hand dryer,
       and feminine product dispensers within 48 inches from the floor?   _____ _____

20.   Are mirrors mounted so that the bottom edge is within 40 inches
       from the floor?   _____ _____

21.   Are sinks mounted so that the rim or counter surface is
       within 34 inches of the floor and a 29-inch clearance space is
       provided from the floor to the bottom of the apron?   _____ _____

22.   Is there a clear space in front of the sink of 30 inches by 48 inches to
       allow a front approach?   _____ _____

23.   Are hot water pipes insulated or configured to avoid
       contact?   _____ _____

24.   Are sink faucets lever-operated, push-type, electronically
       controlled, or otherwise operable with one hand without
       requiring tight grasping, pinching, or twisting of the wrist?   _____ _____

25.   Do self-closing faucets remain open for at least 10
       seconds?   _____ _____

STEP FOUR: Look at access to the goods, services, facilities, privileges, advantages, or accommodations offered at the place of public accommodation.

This step answers the question, "Can people use or take advantage of the goods, services, facilities, or programs provided at the place of public accommodation?"

Look back at the goods, services, facilities, or programs identified in **STEP TWO** and determine whether they are usable. **For example**…

		YES	NO

1.   Are printed materials provided in alternative formats where
      needed?   _____ _____

2.   Are items in racks or on walls within reach?   _____ _____

3.   Are special listening devices provided for individuals with
      hearing impairments in theaters, conference centers, and
      concert halls?   _____ _____

Figure 14-1, cont'd

4.   Can individuals in wheelchairs reach the microfilm machines at the library?

_____   _____

5.   Is there an integrated location for individuals in wheelchairs to sit at the football stadium without having to transfer out of one's chair?

_____   _____

6.   Can individuals with disabilities reach the items on the grocery store shelves?

_____   _____

STEP FIVE: If STEPS ONE through STEP FOUR identify goods, services, facilities, or programs that are not usable by individuals with disabilities, can an accommodation be made to enable the individual to take advantage of the goods, services, facilities, or programs?

Are there policies that need to be changed to enable participation by individuals with disabilities?

Figure 14-1, cont'd

AIR CARRIERS' OBLIGATIONS

Airline carriers must provide assistance with boarding and deplaning by providing personnel, ground wheelchairs, boarding wheelchairs, and ramps or mechanical lifts.[8] If no jet bridge is available, airlines can use lifts and other devices not normally used for freight. Exceptions exist for certain small airplanes and low volume airports. OTs should review with Carlotta how to explain to the airline personnel the safest way to transfer her. Carlotta should also know that the carrier could not leave her unattended in a ground or boarding wheelchair for more than 30 minutes if she cannot independently operate that wheelchair.[8] The carrier must also accept her wheelchair as carry-on baggage if a place exists to store it on the plane or as gate-checked baggage, which the airline returns to her as soon as possible, and as close to the airplane door as possible if she wishes. She can also choose to have it delivered to her in the baggage claim area.[9]

The ACAA requires airlines to provide other assistance to individuals with disabilities as outlined in Box 14-8.[8] Carriers cannot charge for providing these services.[10]

Wide-bodied aircraft must have accessible lavatories and those with 100 seats or more must have priority space for storing wheelchairs in the cabins.[2] This information may help Carlotta select her flights based on the services the

Box 14-8	SERVICES AIRLINES MUST PROVIDE IF REQUESTED

Assistance moving to and from seats during boarding and deplaning

Assistance in preparation for eating, such as opening cartons (but not assistance in eating)

Assistance to and from the lavatory if the aircraft has an on-board wheelchair (but no assistance in the lavatory)

Assistance moving to and from the lavatory for a semi-ambulatory person, not involving lifting or carrying

Assistance loading and retrieving carry-on items, including mobility aids stored on board

plane provides. In addition to services and access on the airplanes themselves, airlines must make sure their terminals are accessible.

The ACAA requires airline carriers to train their employees in awareness and appropriate response to persons with a disability, "including persons with physical, sensory, mental, and emotional disabilities, including how to distinguish among the differing abilities of individuals with a disability."[11] This could provide opportunities for advocating for a particular client such as Carlotta or for consulting with the airline to provide sensitivity training and disability awareness.

Each airline must designate a complaints resolution official at each airport it serves to receive and make efforts to resolve complaints. If it cannot resolve the complaint, it must give the passenger a written summary of the problem and outline the steps the carrier will take to solve it. It must also notify the passenger of his or her right to pursue the complaint with the U.S. Department of Transportation.[12] Passengers may refer to *http://airconsumer.ost.dot.gov/ACAAcomplaint.htm* for information about filing a complaint with the U.S. Department of Transportation.

THE ROLE OF THE OCCUPATIONAL THERAPIST

OTs can work with their clients to understand what their needs will be in air travel and help them develop a strategy to follow to meet their needs. They can also play a key role in informing clients of the rights to which they are entitled in air travel and how to advocate for those rights for themselves.

 ## ETHICAL CONSIDERATIONS

As OTs we are in a unique position to facilitate an understanding of disabilities and the impact disabilities play on everyday activities and functions. OTs can use this knowledge to work directly with airlines as consultants, conducting the training mandated by the law to promote a culture of sensitivity and awareness.

FAIR HOUSING ACT

Congress passed the Fair Housing Amendments Act of 1988, to add "handicaps" (hereafter referred to as *individuals with disabilities*, a more politically correct term with the same legal meaning[66]) to the list of those protected against discrimination in housing. Before the passage of the Fair Housing Act Amendments, the Fair Housing Act prohibited discrimination based only upon race, color, religion, sex, handicap, familial status, or national origin.[69]

Generally, the Fair Housing Act (FHA) prohibits discrimination in the sale, rental, or advertising of housing dwellings, in the provision of brokerage services, or in other residential real estate–related transactions such as the provision of mortgage loans. The FHA covers private housing, housing that receives federal government assistance, and state and local government housing. Some exceptions exist to the FHA. For example, the FHA does not apply to owner-occupied apartment buildings with four or fewer units or private homes where the owner owns fewer than three single-family homes and is not in the business of selling or renting dwellings.

The FHA defines individuals with disabilities using the same definition as the one found in the ADA. Discrimination means denying or making a sale or rental unavailable because of the disability of buyer or renter, the disability of intended resident, or the disability of any person associated with a person with a disability. Landlords may not inquire as to whether the applicant for sale or rental is an individual with a disability, and they cannot charge a higher price or provide different services because a renter or purchaser of a dwelling unit is an individual with a disability.

The passage of the Fair Housing Act Amendments gave individuals with disabilities certain additional rights to use and enjoy their dwellings. These additional rights play a significant role in promoting independent living and participation for individuals with disabilities. Under the FHA it is illegal to refuse to permit reasonable modification of existing premises occupied or to be occupied by individuals with disabilities, if the proposed modification is necessary to allow the person with the disability full use and enjoyment of the dwelling. Unlike the ADA, where businesses have to pay for the modifications that provide access, the FHA does not require landlords to pay for the modifications. It only requires that the landlord allow the tenant to make modifications at the expense of the person with a disability who needs those modifications.

The landlord may, if reasonable, condition permission for modification on the renter agreeing to restore the interior to the condition before the modification. If the renter plans to make a modification to the dwelling, the landlord may not increase a security deposit. The landlord may, however, condition permission for modification on provision of a reasonable description of the proposed modification and assurances the work will be properly performed by licensed professional with permits, etc.

The FHA also makes it illegal for any person to refuse to make reasonable accommodations in rules, policies, practices, or services when needed to afford a person with a disability equal opportunity to use and enjoy a dwelling unit, including public and common use areas. For example, an apartment building management company would have to make an exception to a "no pets" policy so that an individual with a spinal cord injury could keep a service dog. Another often-disputed example involves parking. A person with a disability may need an assigned parking space close to his or her apartment in a development that prides itself on unassigned parking. It would be a reasonable accommodation to modify the parking policy to allow assignment of a parking space to the person with the disability.

Research shows that intervention based upon home assessments, such as providing bath benches and recommending grab bars, helps prevent falls in the home and encourages safe and independent participation in everyday home life.[64,75] Part of Carlotta's intervention plan would include a home assessment. Applying the provisions of the FHA to Carlotta affords her some assistance in her quest for independent participation. First, the landlord would have to allow Carlotta to install the grab bars her OT recommended for her bathtub, as long as this was done in a workman-like manner, with permits, etc. The landlord would probably have to allow Carlotta to widen her bathroom door as the OT recommended so that Carlotta could wheel her wheelchair into the bathroom. With these modifications and others developed by the OT in collaboration with Carlotta, Carlotta can independently participate in her ADLs.

The second issue for Carlotta involves her need for assistance to carry out her aquatics home program. To do this, she must be able to use the pool, an amenity to which she is entitled like all residents of the apartment complex. Carlotta has no access to the pool unless her friend can help her get in and out of the pool each day. The landlord would probably have to modify the "no guests in the pool on weekends" policy to allow Carlotta access to and use of the pool on weekends.

What if the landlord does not want to allow Carlotta to make these accommodations? Even the most wonderful accommodation suggestions the OT and/or OTA makes are worthless if the client cannot use them. Because the success of the OT intervention plan may rest on the provision of these accommodations, the OT and/or OTA will want to steer Carlotta to the website for the United States Department of Housing and Urban Development (HUD).* At this website, Carlotta can file an administrative complaint to encourage the landlord to allow her to make the needed accommodations. Remember, under the FHA, the landlord is not responsible for making the accommodations but must allow the tenant to make needed reasonable accommodations. HUD staff will contact the landlord and/or property management

company, mediate the situation by encouraging them to follow the law, and try to resolve the issues without the necessity of filing a lawsuit.

OTs and OTAs will also find the FHA helpful in other very commonly encountered situations. For example, OTs who make home visits to patients' and clients' homes before hospital discharge will appreciate the support of the FHA. During these home visits, OTs customarily evaluate the individual's ability to function in the home as independently as possible. This assessment includes making recommendations about adaptive equipment and other modifications to the home to promote independent participation. The FHA gives the therapist's recommendations clout should the landlord refuse to allow the modifications to the dwelling unit. Clients in need of grab bars and other accommodations in their homes have an alternative route to take should the landlord say "no" to the needed accommodations.

ADVOCACY AS INTERVENTION

OTs promote participation in work, leisure, and ADLs. As shown above, sometimes barriers to participation exist in spite of OT's efforts with its clients. For example, the client successfully transfers from wheelchair to toilet and bath bench in the clinic but cannot get into the bathroom at home if the landlord will not allow modifications to the apartment. Carlotta can do her job from a wheelchair, but the headmaster will not transfer her to an accessible classroom.

To promote participation in these instances, the OT may have to include advocacy as an intervention strategy. The OT may need to act as an advocate or he or she may have to guide the client through a self-advocacy process.

 ETHICAL CONSIDERATIONS

EIGHT RULES OF ADVOCACY

Know your laws.

Read the regulations.

Believe you or your client has a right to what you seek.

Organize yourself, document your efforts, get everything in writing, and keep copies of all correspondence.

Start with the source of the problem.

Be specific; tell them exactly what you want.

File a complaint with the administrative agency that oversees the matter.

Follow through.

SUMMARY

The ADA, ACAA, and FHA exist to provide individuals with disabilities certain rights. These laws, in concert with OT intervention, have the potential to open many avenues to participation for individuals

---

*http://www.hud.gov/complaints/housediscrim.cfm

with disabilities. By familiarizing themselves with these laws and sharing that information with clients, OTs can play a major role in ensuring that those whom they serve have more opportunities to participate in work, leisure, and ADLs.

With the assistance of the ADA, ACAA, and, FHA, Carlotta should be able to continue in her job as a teacher with the reasonable accommodations provided by her employer under Title I of the ADA. Carlotta can continue traveling by airplane to find the perfect bed and breakfast with accommodations provided to her under the ACAA. She can continue shopping and movie going with the protection afforded to her under Title III of the ADA. The FHA will provide the tools Carlotta needs to stay in her current apartment and care for herself independently and with cooperation from her landlord for the accommodations she needs.

Review Questions

1. What qualifies a person for protection under the ADA?
2. What is meant by "substantially limits a person"?
3. How can a person with a specific learning disability be tested for ability to perform the essential functions of a job?
4. What may and may not an employer do during the two stages of the hiring process?
5. How can OTs help employers develop employment application forms and interview questions that comply with the ADA?
6. What are some of the ways qualified persons with disabilities can be accommodated if they are unable to perform an essential function of a job?
7. Must all job applicants or only applicants with disabilities be required to pass a screening of physical ability before they begin a new job?
8. Does public access to buildings apply only to government facilities, or does it apply to buildings owned by private parties?
9. How should an OT plan an evaluation of a building for accessibility?

REFERENCES

1. 14 C.F.R. §§ 382.7(a)(2)-(3) (2003)
2. 14 C.F.R. § 382.21 (2003)
3. 14 C.F.R. § 382.31(a)–(e) (2003)
4. 14 C.F.R. §§ 382.33(a)-(b) (2003)
5. 14 C.F.R. §§ 382.35(a)-(c) (2003)
6. 14 C.F.R. § 382.37(a) (2003)
7. 14 C.F.R. § 382.38 (2003)
8. 14 C.F.R. § 382.39 (2003)
9. 14 C.F.R. § 382.41 (2003)
10. 14 C.F.R. § 382.57 (2003)
11. 14 C.F.R. § 382.61 (a)(2) (2003)
12. 14 C.F.R. § 382.65 (2003)
13. 28 C.F.R. § 35.130 (1991)
14. 28 C.F.R. § 35.130(b)(1)(ii) (1991)
15. 28 C.F.R. § 36.104 (1991)
16. 28 C.F.R. § 36.201(a) (1991)
17. 28 C.F.R. §§ 36.202(a)-(c) (1991)
18. 28 C.F.R. § 36.203(a)(b) (1991)
19. 28 C.F.R. § 36.211(a) (1991)
20. 28 C.F.R. § 36.301(a) (1991)
21. 28 C.F.R. § 36.302(a) (1991)
22. 28 C.F.R. §§ 36.303(a)(b)(c) (1991)
23. 28 C.F.R. §§ 36.304 (a)-(c) (1991)
24. 28 C.F.R. §§ 36.305 (a)-(c) (1991)
25. 28 C.F.R. § 36. 307 (1991)
26. 28 C.F.R. § 36.310 (1991)
27. 28 C.F.R. § 36.401 (1991)
28. 29 C.F.R. § 1630.2(g)(1) (1991)
29. 29 C.F.R. § 1630.2(g)(2) (1991)
30. 29 C.F.R. § 1630.2(g)(3) (1991)
31. 29 C.F.R. § 1630.2(h)(1) (1991)
32. 29 C.F.R. § 1630.2(h)(2) (1991)
33. 29 C.F.R. § 1630.2(i) (1991)
34. 29 C.F.R. § 1630.2(j) (1991)
35. 29 C.F.R. §§1630.2(j)(2)(i)—(iii) (1991)
36. 29 C.F.R. §1630.2(m) (1991)
37. 29 C.F.R. §1630.2(n)(1) (1991)
38. 29 C.F.R. § 1630.2(n)(3) (1991)
39. 29 C.F.R. § 1630.2(o) (1991)
40. 29 C.F.R. § 1630.2(o)(1)(i) (1991)
41. 29 C.F.R. § 1630.2(o)(1)(ii) (1991)
42. 29 C.F.R. § 1630.2(o)(1)(iii) (1991)
43. 29 C.F.R. § 1630.2(p) (1991)
44. 29 C.F.R. § 1630.2(p)(2)(i)-(v) (1991)
45. 29 C.F.R. § 1630.2(r) (1991)
46. 29 C.F.R. § 1630.3(d)(1) (1991)
47. 29 C.F.R. § § 1630.3(d)(2)(3) (1991)
48. 29 C.F.R. § 1630.4 (1991)
49. 29 C.F.R. § 1630.5 (1991)
50. 29 C.F.R. § 1630.6 (1991)
51. 29 C.F.R. § 1630.7 (1991)
52. 29 C.F.R. § 1630.8 (1991)
53. 29 C.F.R. § 1630.9 (1991)
54. 29 C.F.R.§ 1630.10 (1991)
55. 29 C.F.R. § 1630.11 (1991)
56. 29 C.F.R. § 1630.12 (1991)
57. 29 C.F.R. § 1630.14 (1991)
58. ADAAG § 4.6.3
59. Air Carrier Access Act, codified at 14 C.F.R. § 382.1 *et. seq.* (2003)
60. Americans With Disabilities Act, codified at 29 § 1630 *et. seq.* & 28 § 36.101 *et. seq.* (1991)
61. Appendix to Part 1630-Interpretive Guidance on Title I of the Americans With Disabilities Act 29 C.F.R. § 1630 (1992)
62. Architectural and Transportation Barriers Compliance Board: *About this edition of ADAAG*, amended September 2002. From *http://www.access-board.gov/adaag/html/intro.htm.*
63. Architectural and Transportation Barriers Compliance Board: *ADA Accessibility Guidelines for Buildings and Facilities (ADAAG) Appendix A to 36 C.F.R. 28 § 101 et. seq.* as amended September 2002. From *http://www.access-board.gov/adaag/html/adaag.htm.*

64. Baker R: Elder design: home modifications for enhanced safety and self-care, *Care Management J* 1(1):47, 1999.

65. *Board of Trustees of the University of Alabama v. Garrett* 531 U.S. 356, (2001)

66. *Bragdon v. Abbott*, 524 U.S. 624, 631 (1998)

67. EEOC: *A technical assistance manual on the employment provisions (Title I) of the Americans with Disabilities Act*, Washington, DC, 1992, U.S. Government Printing Office.

68. EEOC: *EEOC: enforcement guidance on disability-related inquiries and medical examinations of employees under the Americans with Disabilities Act (ADA)*, 2000. From *http://www.eeoc.gov/policy/docs/guidance-inquiries.html*.

69. Fair Housing Act 42 U.S.C. § 3601 *et. seq.* (1989)

70. Job Accommodation Network: *Frequently asked questions*, March 24, 2004. Retrieved January 18, 2005, from *http://www.jan.wvu.edu/portals/faqs.html#fund*.

71. McClain L, Medrano D, Marcum M, et al: A qualitative assessment of wheelchair users experience with ADA compliance, physical barriers and secondary health conditions, *Topics Spinal Cord Injury Rehabil* 6(1):99, 2000.

72. *Morisky v. Broward County*, 80 F.3d 445, 447 (11th Cir.1996)

73. Parking spaces for persons who have disabilities. Fl. Stat. § 553.5041

74. Rehabilitation Act of 1973, 29 USC 791 §§ 501, 503, 504.

75. Rogers J: The occupational therapy home assessment: the home as a therapeutic environment, *J Home Health Care Pract* 2(1):73, 1989.

76. *Stutts v. Freeman*, 694 F.2d 666, (11th Cir, 1983)

77. U.S. Department of Justice: *Title III highlights*, 1996. Retrieved January 18, 2005, from *http://www.usdoj.gov/crt/ada/t3hilght.htm*.

78. *Williams v. Toyota Motor Mfg.*, 534 U.S. 184 (2002)

15 LEISURE OCCUPATIONS

MARTI SOUTHAM

KEY TERMS

Leisure

Play

Humor

Modeling

Leisure exploration

Leisure participation

LEARNING OBJECTIVES

After studying this chapter the student or practitioner will be able to do the following:

1. Discuss the benefits of leisure for adults.
2. Describe the key areas in which humor can be used.
3. Understand the differing needs that people in different stages of life have.
4. Identify specific strategies to promote leisure activity for persons with disabilities.

CHAPTER OUTLINE

Leisure and life satisfaction for persons with physical disabilities

Benefits of play and laughter in leisure occupations

Meaningful leisure occupations: age, cultural issues, and gender

  Age and leisure

  Culture and leisure

Leisure occupations: evaluation and intervention

  Intervention: where there's a will, there's a way

  Level of functioning

Summary

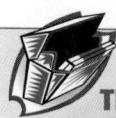

THREADED CASE STUDY: JERI, PART I

Prior to a traffic accident, Jeri, a 29-year-old newly married woman, lived a full and happy life. She was employed as an interior designer, spent time with her husband, friends, and family, and participated in leisure occupations. She particularly enjoyed scrapbooking, going to a nearby lake to boat and fish, playing with and caring for her dogs, and shopping. As Jeri was driving home from running errands one evening, a drunk driver hit her car. It rolled over and she was trapped inside. After being removed from the car and taken by paramedics to the local hospital, she was diagnosed with a traumatic head injury, a broken wrist, and a broken leg. Jeri was transported to the regional head trauma center for rehabilitation. She recovered over a period of months and returned home.

Jeri continues rehabilitation as an outpatient for the residual problems from her head injury as well as for continuing problems using her dominant hand due to the wrist fracture. She receives twice-weekly occupational therapy and is demonstrating significant improvement, progressing from needing maximum assistance for ADLs to minimum assistance. Jeri has no apparent cognitive deficits, uses a walker to ambulate, and still needs a family member or aide at home on a full-time basis due to poor balance that impairs her safety when moving around in her environment. The occupational therapist is ready to discharge Jeri, as her ADL goals have been met. During the intervention review prior to discharge, Jeri reports that she spends most of her days hanging out at home watching TV, feels lonely and disengaged from her friends, and will miss OT because it is her only activity outside of the home.

Critical Thinking Questions

1. Is Jeri ready to be discharged from occupational therapy?
2. Why is Jeri dissatisfied with her current lifestyle?
3. What intervention could the occupational therapist provide to improve Jeri's quality of life?

Participating in meaningful leisure occupations is vital to a healthy, balanced lifestyle. As an area of occupation, **leisure** is defined in the Occupational Therapy Practice Framework[44] as "a nonobligatory activity that is intrinsically motivated and engaged in during discretionary time, that is, time not committed to obligatory occupations such as work, self-care, or sleep"[46] (p. 621). Key phrases in the definition are that these activities are *intrinsically motivated* and that they are *not obligatory*. In other words, people participate in leisure occupations that they choose and that they enjoy. For instance, for some people cooking could be a chore while for others it is a joyful pleasure.

Leisure time may be spent in a variety of ways indicative of an individual's unique interests. Examples of leisure occupations are reading, playing games, participating in sports, doing arts and crafts, participating in outdoor activities (biking, hiking, fishing), cooking, taking a yoga class, exercising at the gym, going to concerts, watching movies, and so on. Due to the uniqueness of individuals, this list is as long as there are people who participate in leisure occupations.

LEISURE AND LIFE SATISFACTION FOR PERSONS WITH PHYSICAL DISABILITIES

When adults sustain injuries (e.g., traumatic head injury, stroke, spinal cord injury, carpal tunnel syndrome) or develop health conditions (e.g., multiple sclerosis, Parkinson's disease, arthritis) that disrupt normal habits and routines, they face devastating losses. Loss of work, social activities, and meaningful leisure activities may contribute to depression, and the self must be redefined.[56]

Occupational therapists (OTs) are skilled in collaborating with people with physical disabilities to assist them in resuming a full life. It has been suggested that one method of measuring whether or not a person is fully engaged in life is to consider the individual's participation in leisure activities.[47] This is especially important because research indicates that the perception of leisure satisfaction by adults with physical disabilities is the most significant predictor of life satisfaction.[26,32] Depressive symptoms have also been shown to decrease when the number and variety of pleasant activities increase.[20] Engaging in leisure activities provides a receptive environment for opportunities for socialization and friendship making, providing people with physical disabilities a chance to demonstrate their occupational skill to others who might not otherwise view the person with a disability as capable or as a friendship candidate.[48]

OT PRACTICE NOTES

BENEFITS OF LEISURE ACTIVITIES

Participation in leisure activities can offer many psychosocial and physical benefits, such as the following:

PSYCHOSOCIAL BENEFITS

- Increased sense of self-worth
- Release of hostility and aggression
- Shared control of self and environment
- Experience of choice
- Increased socialization
- Development of leadership
- Practice in adaptive behavior and coping skills
- Increased attention span
- Adjustment to living arrangements
- Increased tolerance of groups and other people
- Experience of intellectual stimulation

Continued

OT PRACTICE NOTES–cont'd

PHYSICAL BENEFITS

- Increased circulation
- Promotion of gross, fine, bilateral, and eye-hand coordination
- Provision of vestibular stimulation
- Provision of sensory stimulation
- Promotion of motor planning
- Improvement or maintenance of perceptual abilities
- Maintenance or improvement of adaptive and coping skills
- Increased strength, range of motion, and physical tolerance
- Improved balance
- Provision of opportunity to grade activities

OT PRACTICE NOTE

THE THERAPIST'S ROLE IN ENCOURAGING LEISURE ACTIVITIES

If therapists only provide interventions aimed at physical rehabilitation (e.g., strengthening, range of motion exercises) and improving performance in activities of daily living and instrumental activities of daily living, the recovering individual may never experience the opportunity of resuming old leisure interests or developing new ones.

Sadly, however, studies indicate that most leisure activities are abandoned after the onset of a physical disorder such as rheumatoid arthritis or stroke.[47,58] Adults with physical disabilities seem to relinquish activities that are purely for enjoyment, especially community-based social activities, and focus their effort and time on activities of daily living and work.[18,26,47] The emphasis on the physical model of recovery is most likely due to (1) the health professionals who deliver treatment with focus on mobility and independence in activities of daily living and (2) the fact that rehabilitation outcome measures are commonly based on these factors.[47] Occupational therapists need to recognize that people often experience difficulty in adapting their interests and activities by themselves after a physical or neurological disorder.

A randomized, controlled study of stroke survivors[20] supports the need for occupational therapists to address the leisure area of occupation in order for clients to engage in leisure interests and activities after therapy is discontinued. Sixty-five clients were randomly assigned to three groups: leisure rehabilitation, conventional occupational therapy treatment, and control. A baseline for the three groups for the number and frequency of leisure activities demonstrated no significant difference between the three groups upon admission to the hospital.

After hospital discharge, the leisure rehabilitation group and the conventional occupational therapy group were treated by the same occupational therapist one time a week for 30 minutes for 3 months, and then one 30-minute session every 2 weeks for 3 months. Each person in the leisure rehabilitation group was given an individualized program that included "advice and help ... in the following broad categories: treatment (e.g., practice of transfers needed for leisure pursuits); positioning; provision of equipment; adaptations; advice on obtaining financial assistance and transportation; liaison with specialist organization, and providing physical assistance (e.g., referral to voluntary agencies)."[20]

The occupational therapy group received individualized treatment by the same therapist for the same amount of time. Interventions included "transfers, washing and dressing practice, and, where appropriate, perceptual treatments ... No reference was made to the importance of continuing previous interests, and no help or advice was offered to encourage participation in leisure pursuits"[20] (p. 285). At 3 and 6 months post-discharge, an independent assessor re-administered the leisure questionnaire. Results showed that the leisure rehabilitation group had significantly higher leisure scores than the conventional occupational therapy group and the control group.[20]

Thus, adults with physical disabilities may give up leisure activities because they are not aware of ways to adapt valued activities so that they may participate in them again. Or they may not know about new hobbies or crafts that they might enjoy. Occupational therapists have an important role in helping people to both explore and to plan engagement in leisure occupations so that they may participate in activities that bring joy to life.[56]

BENEFITS OF PLAY AND LAUGHTER IN LEISURE OCCUPATIONS

When talking about participating in leisure occupations, people often use the word **play.** Some examples are to play golf, play the piano, play sports, play cards, play board games, and so on. Play suggests fun, and fun is often accompanied by laughter.

Many physical health benefits of laughter have been demonstrated through numerous research studies. For example, immune cells increase and stress hormones decrease thereby possibly preventing illness or helping in recovery.[3,11-13,49,55] Some people experience relief from pain and a sense of well being after hearty laughter.[14,17] Laughter also benefits people psychologically and psychosocially.[21,36,39,52,54,59] Laughing together facilitates bonding, reduces anxiety, and improves coping—all important factors in a therapeutic alliance between occupational therapist and client (Box 15-1).

Facilitating psychosocial and physical adaptations is integral to occupational therapy, and given the current health care climate of high productivity and short hospital and rehabilitation stays, it is imperative that occupational therapists be able to quickly form a therapeutic alliance with their clients. Humor and laughter are natural ways that therapists and clients connect. Recent studies have found that all of the occupational therapists who were interviewed or

Box **15-1** HEALTH BENEFITS OF LAUGHTER

PHYSICAL HEALTH BENEFITS OF LAUGHTER[17,21,52]

- Stress hormones (e.g., cortisol and noradrenaline) decrease[11,39,59]
- Immune functions increase (e.g., immunoglobulin A and natural killer cells)[11-13,55]
- Muscle tension relaxes
- Blood pressure drops and cardiovascular functions improve; increases blood flow to aid healing
- Respiratory airways are cleared (through laughing and coughing)
- Pain relief may be attained after hearty laughter and last for several hours due to release of opioids and endorphins[49]
- "Feel good" hormones (e.g., beta-endorphins and serotonin) are released

PSYCHOLOGICAL AND PSYCHOSOCIAL HEALTH BENEFITS OF LAUGHTER[3,36,52,54]

- Facilitates bonding—laughter occurs more often with others than when alone[14]
- Improves coping with problems
- Increases well-being and promotes hope and optimism
- Diverts negative thoughts—it is hard to maintain destructive thoughts when laughing
- "Saves face" in embarrassing situations
- Facilitates mental clarity, creativity, and brainstorming because the two hemispheres communicate better during humor and the limbic system is aroused
- Adds vibrancy to facial tone and sparkle to the eyes

surveyed agreed that humor has a place in occupational therapy.[38,54,57]

In a recent national cross-sectional randomized survey of 283 occupational therapists that examined their attitudes and uses of humor with adult clients with physical disabilities, humor was classified into four key areas: (1) building relationships, (2) helping clients cope with adversity, (3) promoting clients' physical health, and (4) facilitating compliance with treatment.[54] While therapists reported positive attitudes about humor in all four of these areas, most were actually only using humor to build relationships and to help clients cope. The majority of therapists felt comfortable using spontaneous humor with clients as a part of the therapeutic use of self, rather than using planned humor as a therapeutic intervention.

People who are disabled may need to learn ways to adapt to their new circumstances. **Humor** is a skill that can be learned that may provide the client with the ability to manage concerns related to his or her health and life situations. Within a larger relational context, humor may be modeled by occupational therapists to teach coping skills. Bandura[7] described four essential factors for **modeling** to be an effective intervention. First, the client must have adequate attention span to

focus on the modeled behavior. Second, he or she must be able to cognitively form and retain a mental image of the behavior. Third, the client must be able to recall the image and then to produce the behavior. Last, and perhaps most importantly, the client must have the motivation to engage in the behavior.

ETHICAL CONSIDERATIONS

The establishment of trust through the bond of a therapeutic relationship may provide the encouragement that clients need to try new behaviors such as humor and laughter.[28]

The intimacy that humor presumes may provide the client with a sense of connection with the therapist. This connection, which occurs on conscious and unconscious levels, has many positive benefits for clients. When the therapist is able to demonstrate professionalism and empathy with a touch of humor, a client may feel less alone and more cared for as an individual.[25,29,54] An improved sense of equality with the healthcare provider may occur that could increase the client's active involvement in her or his treatment.[1,21]

Although laughter has been shown to be beneficial, there are times when humor may not be a good choice, and laughter must be used with caution or avoided altogether. Seizures and cataleptic or narcoleptic attacks may follow a laughter episode in a small number of people.[24] Also, because laughing increases abdominal and thoracic pressure, people with recent abdominal surgery, upper body fractures, acute asthma, or "preexisting arterial hypertension and cerebral vascular fragility"[24] (p. 1857) should not be encouraged to laugh.

ETHICAL CONSIDERATIONS

Occupational therapists also need to be aware that humor possesses destructive elements, and may be used to intentionally or unintentionally hurt a person. Use of the "AT&T" principle[53] helps to determine the appropriateness of humor use. Klein describes this principle as Appropriate, Timely, and Tasteful, meaning that the therapist must be attuned to the patient's humor style, culture, and current status (physical, emotional, and cognitive) before introducing humor and facilitating laughter.

Leisure exploration is defined by the Occupational Therapy Practice Framework[44] as "identifying interests, skills, opportunities, and appropriate leisure activities" and **leisure participation** is "planning and participating in appropriate leisure activities; maintaining a balance of leisure activities with other areas of occupation; and obtaining, using, and maintaining equipment and supplies as appropriate" (p. 621). While exploring leisure with the client, the OT will be concerned with the appropriateness of such occupations as to age, gender, and cultural fit for the specific individual—concerns that will be addressed in the next section.

MEANINGFUL LEISURE OCCUPATIONS: AGE, CULTURAL ISSUES, AND GENDER

Clients choose the leisure occupations that they want to pursue.[44] Choices may be based on past experiences or on a desire to explore something new. As people move through the developmental stages of adulthood, the occupation of leisure may vary in intensity and time use. The continuity theory of aging suggests that personality plays a major role in adjustment to aging. As the personality does not radically change throughout life, one's preferences, lifestyle, and activities remain relatively the same in successful aging.[5,10]

AGE AND LEISURE

Knowledge of the typical progression through adulthood, common life stage choices of leisure activities, and the ways that physical disabilities may disrupt leisure participation is critical for occupational therapists. Armed with this information, therapists are able to discover gaps in developmental stages and to assist clients in the mastery of valued and meaningful occupations.[40]

Young Adulthood (20-40 Years)

Young adults are typically healthy, active, working, and engaged in relationships. Erikson's sixth stage of psychosocial development, intimacy versus isolation, describes young adulthood as a time in life when people know who they are and are ready to form intimate relationships with others.[45] Inability to make commitments on an intimate level may lead to isolation. Levinson views this age period as a time of becoming independent from parents, choosing and beginning an occupation, and imagining one's dream future.[45] Young adults typically settle down and choose interests that encompass family, work, and leisure activities.

Examples of leisure activities in which young adults engage may include: social and family group activities, sports (e.g., basketball, off-road biking), exercise, travel, computer games and Internet surfing, hobbies and crafts (e.g., scrapbooking), outdoor activities, dancing, dating, and sex.

Accidents or physical disorders affecting an individual's areas of occupation, performance skills, and body functions can severely impede progress through the normal activities of young adulthood and may delay the development of age-related roles such as spouse, parent, employer/employee, social participant, participator in leisure occupations, and sexual being. Persons who are at the beginning stage

of adulthood and who sustain an irreversible injury may need to redefine themselves to successfully navigate the aging process. Leisure problems may include social isolation and changes in relationships, lack of ability to perform favorite sports, difficulty in traveling, and decreased knowledge of how to creatively express the self.[56] A sense of incompetence may ensue that could lead to depression.

Middle Adulthood (40-65 Years)

People in this age group are typically immersed in work and family life. They usually have developed expertise in their chosen field of employment and may have risen to supervisory levels. Financial independence is attained as people purchase homes and cars and build a nest egg. Some adults in this age group experience midlife review of self and career, and may change careers or retire. This is the stage of generativity versus stagnation (Erikson's 7(th) stage of psychosocial development) in which the person enjoys developing the skills and talents of younger people (e.g., serving as sports coach or work mentor).[45] Lack of generativity may lead to stagnation in life, disappointment, and burnout.[40]

Examples of leisure activities typical of this age group are friend and family activities, sports (e.g., golf, bowling, coaching), card games, Internet surfing and shopping, travel, pet care, gardening, movies, attending plays and concerts, boating, fishing, reading, television, bike riding, and sexual activity with spouse or partner.

Disruption caused by a physical disability can impair the individual's ability to engage in cherished leisure occupations. Spouses or significant others are called upon to be caregivers and the relationship may undergo changes. Leisure occupations such as travel and fishing may be put aside for the more immediate concerns of learning to cope with self-care, rehabilitation exercises, and therapeutic equipment.[58] Friend relationships often change as well. For example, if two men had a friendship based on golfing every Saturday, and one of them suffers a stroke and needs to use a wheelchair, they will either have to be proactive and figure out a way to enjoy each other's company in a new way (such as playing golf with adapted equipment or trying out a new activity that they both enjoy), or they may drift apart.

Late Adulthood (65 Years and Older)

Occupational roles typically go through transformations during this age span. Some changes seen with older adults include a shift of emphasis from parent to grandparent and worker to retiree or volunteer. As time spent in work/career diminishes, free time increases, and leisure occupations come into full bloom. The interests and activities that were put aside during career attainment can now be given full rein.[40] Erikson's last stage of psychosocial development (Stage 8, ego integrity versus despair) is described as the time when people review their lives and hopefully accept the life cycle as complete and satisfying.[45] The "use it or lose it" principle is particularly important as people age. If activity levels are not maintained, strength, coordination, and skills may deteriorate rapidly.[45] Some aspects of aging that are considered fairly normal include diminishing hearing and eyesight, arthritis and decreased sensory abilities, as well as general aches and pains.

Examples of leisure activities in which older adults engage are dining with or cooking for friends and family, social activities, card games, bingo, travel, sports (e.g., golf, game attendance or viewing on TV), walking, exercise at the gym, swimming, boating, sexual activity with spouse or partner, reading, television, pet care, gardening, hobbies (e.g., crafts, collecting, scrapbooking).

If a physically disabling event or disease progression occurs, spouses or significant others may be called upon to assist their partners in performing daily living activities, including leisure. This can be problematic because the caregiver may also be advanced in age and may not be well suited to provide the needed care. Consequently, leisure activities may be forgotten except for sedentary activities such as television viewing.[58]

For some, isolation and depression could set in and diminish the person's quality of life. A longitudinal study of 66 people over 60 years of age who were at risk for needing assistive devices indicated that the leisure activities they missed the most were crafts, walking, gardening, and participating in sports.[41] In another study of 324 older Swedes living in the community, researchers discovered that people who increased participation in leisure activities reported being more satisfied with life. "The results suggest that maximizing activity participation is an adaptive strategy taken by older adults to compensate for social and physical deficits in later life"[53] (p. 528). Mental acuity may also be strengthened or preserved by engaging in novel activities. Engagement with life is vital to successful aging.

CULTURE AND LEISURE

Because of the increasing diversity of the United States populace, occupational therapists must have knowledge of how culture affects the choices and performance of leisure activities for clients. The U.S. Census Bureau (*www.census.gov*) reports that, while the white population is still the majority (70%), by the year 2050, whites and minority groups overall will be roughly equal in size. Ethnic groups are currently concentrated in various areas of the country (Table 15-1). Thus, depending upon where occupational therapy is delivered, therapists should make themselves familiar with leisure activities related to the culture of their clients (Table 15-2).

Leisure Occupations Related to Culture

Games and leisure occupations instruct, inspire, and reflect the values and beliefs of the parent cultures. For persons

TABLE **15-1**   **Ethnic Groups in the United States, 2000 Census**

Ethnic Group	Percent of Population	Population Centers
White	70%	Midwest and Northeast
Hispanic or Latino	13% (Of these, 67% are Mexican)	Southwest and California
Black or African American	12%	Southeast and Mid-Atlantic
Asian-American	4%	West and Northeast
American Indian and Alaskan Native	0.9%	Northwest, West, Southwest, and Midwest
Native Hawaiian and other Pacific Islanders	0.1%	Hawaii and West

Data from U.S. Bureau of the Census, Census 2000, *www.census.gov*.

TABLE **15-2**   **Examples of Leisure Interests and Occupations by Ethnicity**

Ethnic Group	Possible Leisure Interests and Occupations
Hispanic/Latino	Music, dancing, video games, sports (e.g., soccer, races, arena football), needlework, concerts, movies, TV, socializing, cooking, travel to Mexico and Central/South America (minimal domestic U.S. travel)
Black/African American	Socializing, sports (e.g., bowling, baseball, basketball), cooking, games (e.g., cards, gambling, board), TV, computers/Internet, running, weightlifting, woodworking, remodeling, sewing, quilting, gardening, music, dancing
Asian American	Board games (e.g., GO), tile games (e.g., Mah Jong), traditional cooking and arts, Asian language classes, gardening, sewing, t'ai chi, yoga, walking, computers, Internet surfing/shopping, travel to Asian destinations[4]
American Indian	Sports (e.g., running, lacrosse, longball), outdoor traditions (e.g., canoe, kayak, archery), recreational pastimes (e.g., cup and ball, dice or deer button game, snowsnake), powwow (dancing, arts)

Sources: *www.artsedge.kennedy_center.org; www.diversitylab.uiuc.edu/shinew; www.combose.com/Society/Ethnicity/The_American/Indigenous/Native_Americans/ Sports; www.goldsea.com/Features2/Essays/get;* Allison & Geiger (1993).

immigrating to a new country (e.g., Hispanics to the United States), leisure activities can be used to maintain connections with their heritage. Other possible uses of leisure that aid community integration are to (1) gain pleasure from the new environment and people and (2) learn language and customs.[31] Watching television and reading are two ways that newcomers use leisure to improve conversational skills and to understand cultural features.[4] Depending upon the interest of the client involved, occupational therapists may offer leisure occupations that (1) reflect the client's traditional background, thus fostering security in a new country or (2) provide leisure experiences of the new country to increase learning, comfort, and integration (Table 15-2). Keeping the leisure interventions client-centered is the critical element to a successful outcome. Table 15-3 gives ideas for leisure resources.

Leisure-Time Physical Activity by Gender, Age, and Racial/Ethnic Groups

Physical inactivity has been associated with various health risk factors such as obesity, cardiovascular disease including stroke, diabetes, some cancers, and premature mortality.[42]

Occupational therapists can aid clients to live a healthy lifestyle by encouraging them to participate in some type of leisure-time occupation that employs physical exercise at least several times a week. Some examples of leisure occupations that provide physical exercise but could be more attractive alternatives to some people are dancing, swimming, boating, bowling, golfing, gardening, and yoga.

In order to discover trends in physical activity levels, the Centers for Disease Control (CDC) researchers conducted a randomized telephone survey of 170,423 persons from 35 states and the District of Columbia asking, "During the past month, other than your regular job, did you participate in any physical activities or exercise such as running, calisthenics, golf, gardening, or walking for exercise?" Analysis of the data revealed that women, older adults, and the majority of racial/ethnic groups participated the least in leisure-time physical activities.[27] Blacks, Hispanics, and American Indians or Alaska Natives more often reported fair or poor health, obesity, diabetes, and lack of leisure-time physical activity than Whites, Asians, or Pacific Islanders. Women in all cultures surveyed engaged in the least amount of physical activity.[22]

TABLE 15-3   **Resources for Leisure Occupations**

Media	Titles
Examples of books	Adams/McCubbin:[2] *Games, Sports and Exercises for the Physically Disabled*, 4th edition
	Kenney:[30] *Have Crutch, Will Travel*
	Klinger:[34] *Meal Preparation and Training: The Health Care Professional's Guide*
	Willan: *The Good Cook* (step-by-step photographs)
Examples of journals	*Adapted Physical Activity Quarterly* (*www.humankinetics.com*): "The official journal of the International Federation of Adapted Physical Activity. This multidisciplinary journal provides the latest scholarly inquiry related to physical activity for special populations. Regular features include case studies; techniques for adapting equipment, facilities, methodology, and settings; editorial commentary; article abstracts; and books."
	Leisure Science (research journal)
	Journal of Leisure Science
Examples of magazines	*New Mobility Magazine* (*www.newmobility.com*): Serves people with disabilities by providing information, humor, and inspiration to unite the disabled community.
	Sports 'n Spokes (*www.sportsnspokes.com*): "A monthly magazine from the Paralyzed Veterans Association for wheelchair athletes and other people who use a wheelchair who pursue an active lifestyle. Check out their annual survey of lightweight wheelchairs in the Online Article Library."
Examples of Web sites	Animal Assisted Therapy (AAT) (*www.deltasociety.org*): "A goal-directed intervention in which an animal that meets specific criteria is an integral part of the treatment process. AAT is directed and/or delivered by a health/human service professional with specialized expertise, and within the scope of practice of his/her profession."
	Canine Companions for Independence (*www.caninecompanions.com*): "A national nonprofit that enhances the lives of people with disabilities by providing highly-trained *assistance dogs* and ongoing support to ensure quality partnerships."
	Gardening (*www.gonegardening.com*) and (*http://gardening.tamu.edu*): provides tips for tools, raised garden beds, garden design, planting, watering, etc.
	Video Games Accessibility
	(*http://www.igda.org/articles/twestin_access.php*): gives examples of Braille games, audio-only games, and ways to access games through specialized hardware, e.g., head movement or breath-controlled.

Some barriers to leisure-time physical activities have been identified. While many people of different cultures and ages believe that movement (e.g., exercise, gardening, walking) yields positive benefits such as improved health and appearance, they do not engage in physical activities because of "self-consciousness and lack of discipline, interest, company, enjoyment and knowledge."[19] Other barriers to activity were identified as lack of transportation, prohibitive cost, and perceived lack of safety. Social issues such as gender roles for activity and poor support from the family were also identified by minority women. As a barrier to activity, these women also reported problems with (1) language, (2) isolation in the community, and (3) child care due to lack of relatives in the area. While planning intervention, occupational therapists can collaborate with clients to address these problems, find community resources, and develop strategies to improve participation in leisure-time physical activities.

LEISURE OCCUPATIONS: EVALUATION AND INTERVENTION

The Occupational Therapy Practice Framework focuses on a client-centered approach and mandates that the first step in the process is for occupational therapists to develop an occupational profile collaboratively with clients and family/caregivers.[44] The profile includes the client's occupational history, past and current interests, performance, and values. Knowledge of the problems and goals that the client and family/caregivers consider important gives the therapist a basis for a meaningful intervention plan. Evaluation includes formal and informal assessments conducted initially and over the course of the therapy process to guide the therapist in providing an individualized intervention program that meets the client's expressed needs and desires. Examples of possible assessments that address the leisure area of occupation and a description of each are presented in Table 15-4.

TABLE 15-4 **Leisure Assessments and Descriptions Used by Occupational Therapists**

Assessments	Descriptions
Occupational Profile[44]	Interview with client (and family/caregivers, if appropriate) to gather information about demographics, language, health status, social and medical history. Questions addressing why client needs OT services, what his or her concerns are, occupational history (e.g., values, meanings associated with life experiences, etc.), and what client's priorities are.
Canadian Occupational Performance Measure[37]	Interview conducted pre- and post-intervention to describe problems, level of satisfaction with performing activities, and level of perceived performance abilities in areas of self-care, productivity, and leisure.
Role Checklist[43]	Interview to discover past, present, and future occupational roles (including leisure roles) and their value to client.
Activity Card Sort[8]	Picture cards of adults performing instrumental, social-cultural, and leisure activities. Client sorts them into piles depending upon interest level. Provides a "retained activity level" score indicating engagement levels of activity performance of past and current activities.
Modified Interest Checklist (available from Model of Human Occupation Clearinghouse)	Checklist of 68 activity items that assesses client's level of interest (casual, strong, or no interest). Includes many leisure-time activities.
Leisure Attitude Measurement Scale[50]	Scale of 36 items addressing attitudes towards leisure in three areas: cognitive, affective, and behavioral. Rated on a 5-point scale from "never true" to "always true."
Leisure Motivation Scale[9]	Scale of 48 items addressing motivation to participate in leisure in four areas: intellectual activities, social activities, mastery activities, and stimulus-avoidance activities. Rated on a 5-point scale from "never true" to "always true."
Quality of Life Scale[15,23,58]	Perceived quality of life on a scale of 16 items (e.g., material comforts, expressing yourself creatively, socializing, participating in active recreation) rated on a Likert scale of "very satisfied" to "very dissatisfied."
Play and Laughter Assessment[35]	Informal interview to determine client's attitude toward humor use, sense of humor, kinds of humor client has enjoyed, etc.
Performance Skills	Assessment of client's ability to perform leisure occupations includes motor skills, process skills, communication, and interaction skills. These may be assessed using formal tests and by observation and analysis of client's performance during activity engagement in the appropriate context (e.g., analyze the client's ability to hold and manipulate cards during a card game; analyze client's ability to put bait on a fish hook, manage the rod and reel, catch and remove fish from hook while seated by a lake).
Context	Assessment of cultural, physical, social, personal, spiritual, temporal, and virtual contexts that may influence participation in leisure occupations.
Client Factors	Assessment of bodily systems that support participation in leisure occupations (e.g., mental, sensory, neuromusculoskeletal, cardiovascular, respiratory and speech functions, pain, skin, etc.).

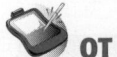

INTERVENTION: WHERE THERE'S A WILL, THERE'S A WAY

Using information gathered during the evaluation process, an intervention plan incorporating leisure occupations is developed that the client and family/caregivers view as important to improving quality of life. Clients (including family or caregivers, as necessary) and therapists develop goals and plan interventions together, thus assuring that the client is motivated to engage in therapy sessions to the best of his or her ability.[44] In occupational therapy, leisure occupations can be a *means* and an *end*. As a means of intervention, the client is provided with the therapeutic use of leisure that is motivating because it is chosen and fun. Leisure as an end is seen when the client voluntarily engages in leisure occupations after therapy intervention ceases.[44] When developing discharge plans that include leisure, the therapist should consider "attributes of novelty and challenge, meaningful use of time, and identity construction," which are imperative to the continued growth, adaptation, and quality of life for clients.[56] Occupational therapists may offer a variety of leisure activities delivered to individuals or groups, depending upon the relevance to the client's interests, abilities, and activity demands. In the case of Kris (see Case Study), individual activities need to be mastered before group activity can be considered.

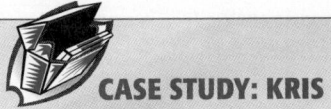

CASE STUDY: KRIS

For example, Kris, a 22-year-old man with a spinal cord injury (paraplegia), has an avid interest in playing wheelchair basketball.

In order to prepare him for this sport, the occupational therapist works with him individually to order the correct wheelchair, strengthen his upper extremities, and develop skill in dribbling, catching/throwing the ball, and making baskets from the wheelchair. A referral is then made to a recreational therapist who helps Kris incorporate these basic skills into an existing team of players. By developing his individual skills before entering the group activity, his potential to successfully participate in his leisure activity of choice is increased.

Balloon volleyball is a fun and social activity. For example, in a long-term care facility, residents with appropriate cognitive and motor skills can be organized into two teams, seated and facing each other. A real or simulated volleyball net is erected between the two teams and a balloon is hit back and forth. Music adds to the enjoyable atmosphere. This game can meet several occupational therapy goals such as improving eye pursuits, upper extremity range of motion, socialization, and cognition (keeping track of the score). Also, because joking and laughing often occur, physical, social, and psychological benefits may be gained (Box 15-1). The therapist must ensure that each person is safe, with wheelchairs locked, and if necessary, seat belts attached. Cardiac patients may not be appropriate to include because of the upper extremity workout and increased respiration, heart rate, and blood pressure that could occur.

Adapting the Activity for Success

Occupational therapists are uniquely qualified to adapt the activity, including the equipment or the environment, to make leisure occupations accessible to clients. By participating in leisure occupations that are meaningful, clients are able to continue to make positive adaptations that lead to greater life satisfaction. Table 15-5 describes some leisure occupations and possible adaptations.

LEVEL OF FUNCTIONING

Occupational therapists view the client as a whole person with a myriad of dimensions (e.g., physical, cognitive, spiritual, psychological). Leisure occupations are self-enhancers that add joy and pleasure to life. For effective implementation, activities need to be analyzed according to the individual's level of functioning (e.g., performance skills, performance patterns, client factors, activity demands, and context). Examples of clients by level of function, along with leisure occupations that are meaningful to the individual, are described in the Case Studies examining Tina, John, and Miguel.

TABLE 15-5 Examples of Adapted Leisure Occupations

Leisure Occupation	Possible Adaptations
Gardening	Raised flower or vegetable garden beds to be accessible from chair or wheelchair. Nonskid surface under pots to prevent sliding during potting.
Golf	Adapted golf clubs (e.g., constructed to be used from seated or wheelchair position, or to be used one-handed), lower extremity prosthetics specially made for golf.
Playing cards	Card shuffler, card holder (Figure 15-1), large print or Braille cards
Computer activities or Internet surfing	Large monitor screen, large print font, voice activated controls or software (e.g., Dragonspeak).
Cooking	Energy conservation techniques, sliding instead of lifting heavy pots, nonskid surface to prevent slippage, rocker knife, perching stool.
Pets	Canine Companions to manage daily tasks (e.g., open drawers and doors, acknowledge phone ringing, obtain objects) as well as provide love and licks. Therapy dogs to visit clients in hospitals, skilled nursing facilities, and homes to bring joy and opportunities for touch (Figure 15-2). Pets such as fish, cats, dogs, etc. provide companionship and may promote motivation for engagement in caring activities.
Bike riding	For persons with lower extremity weakness or paralysis, handcycles may be purchased. These bikes are propelled and controlled by arm strength and coordination (Figure 15-3).

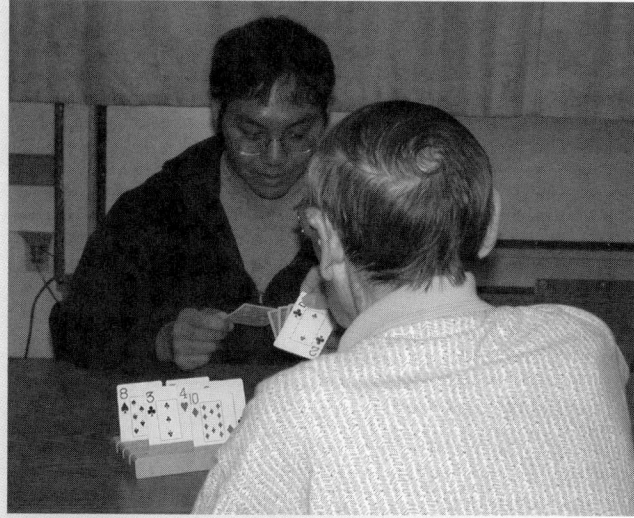

Figure 15-1 Use of an adapted card holder placed on the left side to encourage Ray to scan to that side while enjoying a game of cards with a friend.

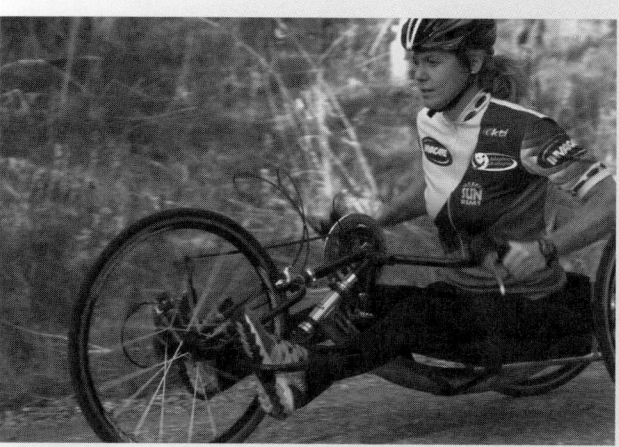

Figure 15-3 Monica, a vivacious woman with paraplegia, rides a hand-cycle racing bike.

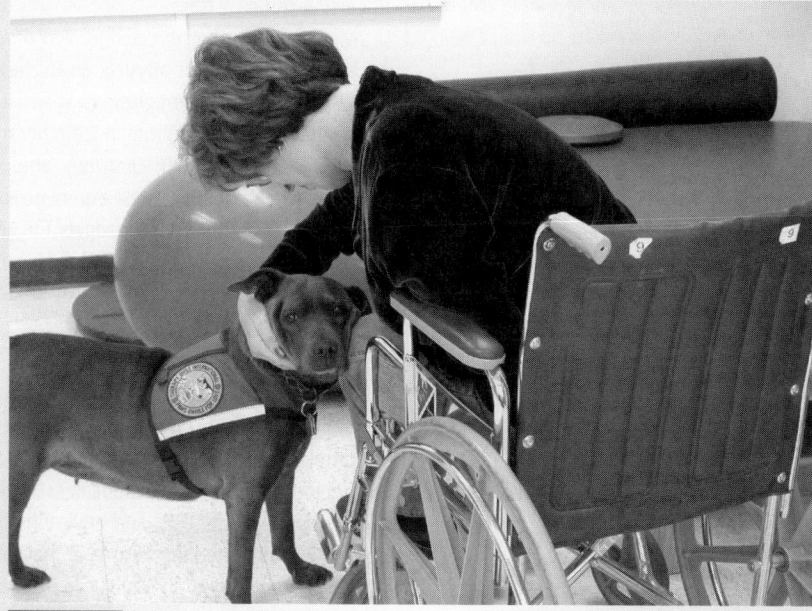

Figure 15-2 Certified Therapy Dog visiting an occupational therapy client.

CASE STUDIES: TINA, JOHN, AND MIGUEL

Level of Functioning: Clients and Leisure Occupations.

Tina

Level of Function: Maximum Assistance Needed

Tina, a 41-year-old mother of two, had a severe stroke which left her unable to smoothly coordinate movement. She enjoys listening to tapes of her son playing the guitar.

Leisure Occupation

Occupational therapy assessment revealed that when Tina was positioned correctly, her left hand could be guided to hit a large button switch. Stephanie, the occupational therapist, connected the button switch to a tape player, which held a tape of her son's recent musical accomplishments. Her family members were instructed in how to assist Tina so that they could all participate in a valued leisure activity together (Figure 15-4).

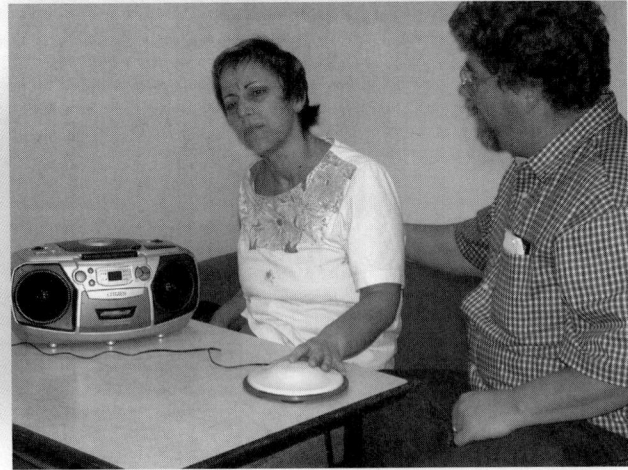

Figure 15-4   Tina, with husband, Scott, using a large button device to turn on a tape player to listen to her son playing guitar.

John

Level of Function: Moderate Assistance Needed

John, a 50-year-old man, had a traumatic head injury 3 years ago. He demonstrates poor dynamic balance, short-term memory deficits, and weakness on his right side. He uses a 3-wheeled walker for ambulation. John lives with his wife and is independent in the majority of activities of daily living. His passion is bowling.

Leisure Occupation

After assessing his interests and performance abilities, his occupational therapist, DeShawn, accompanied John, his wife, and his adult son to the bowling alley. DeShawn called ahead to make sure that the bowling alley was accessible and had accommodations for persons with disabilities. The lanes were set up with gutter bumpers and a bowling ball ramp. With a gait belt and moderate assistance, John was able to place a light-weight ball on the ramp, set up his shot, release the ball, and knock down some of the pins. When he, his wife, and his adult son saw that bowling was possible again, they set up a family night once a week to resume a cherished fun activity.

Miguel

Level of Function: Independent

Miguel, a 25-year old single man, was in a skiing accident 5 years ago and incurred a spinal cord injury (SCI) resulting in paraplegia. He progressed through rehabilitation and is independent in activities of daily living and instrumental activities of daily living. He uses a power wheelchair, drives, and has a job as a police dispatcher. Miguel has come in to occupational therapy to upgrade his wheelchair and discuss leisure occupations. He reports that his free time is boring and he wants to return to a sport.

Leisure Occupation

Wheelchair sports abound in variety. Miguel's occupational therapist, Eric, began by helping Miguel to explore the many options for persons wishing to participate as a wheelchair athlete, including basketball, mountaineering, hunting, rugby (the fastest growing wheelchair sport), weight lifting, racing (including hand-cycle racing), tennis, javelin throwing, and snow skiing. When Miguel indicated that he might be interested in resuming a previously loved leisure occupation of camping, Eric showed him how to locate helpful resources such as magazines, journals, Web sites, catalogs and other related publications. For example, Butler[16] wrote an article that reviews sports wheelchairs that might provide information on the chairs' suitability for traversing camping trails.

Miguel was further directed to *New Mobility*, a magazine written for and by people with physical disabilities, which had an excellent article on accessible campgrounds as well as suggestions for making a trip successful. Eric recommended other magazines as well, such as *Adapted Physical Activity Quarterly* and *Sports & Spokes* so that Miguel can read about others' experiences and stories and broaden his ideas of equipment and gadgets for wheelchair users. Eric was thrilled to hear back from Miguel a few months later that he had, indeed, gone camping and that it was a "super experience!"

SUMMARY

Occupational therapists assist clients in attaining life satisfaction through a variety of occupations that are meaningful to the individual. Engaging and re-engaging in leisure occupations, which may include social interactions, movement, playfulness, and pleasure, are important aspects of a balanced lifestyle. Realizing that lack of leisure activities may lead to isolation and depression and detrimentally affect an individual's recovery and joy of life, occupational therapists need to include leisure evaluation, intervention planning, and implementation for persons with physical disabilities. Consideration of the client's age, gender, culture, interests, and environment is paramount when investigating or implementing leisure so that intervention is client-centered. A skilled occupational therapist can facilitate participation in meaningful leisure occupations that may lead to improved psychological and physical well-being, social relationships, and quality of life.

THREADED CASE STUDY: JERI, PART 2

Reconsider the questions posed regarding Jeri, a 29-year old, newly married woman, whose case study opened the chapter:

Question 1: Is Jeri really ready to be discharged from occupational therapy?

Probably not. While the occupational therapist has done a thorough job of teaching Jeri how to be competent in activities of daily living, we now know there is more to life for occupational therapists to consider than instructing clients in personal care techniques. Occupational therapy assessments of leisure attitudes, interests, skills, and abilities need to be undertaken and a further intervention plan developed that addresses quality of life issues.

Question 2: Why is Jeri dissatisfied with her current lifestyle?

Jeri is leading a restricted life compared to her life prior to the accident. She has lost many of the activities that brought joy to her life. She is unable to do scrapbooking because she still lacks the fine motor coordination in her dominant hand to manipulate scissors and small decorative paper pieces. She wants to drive again and misses her work as in interior designer, shopping, meeting friends for lunch, and running errands. Her husband treats her like she will break and is unsure that she is capable of boating and fishing again. Jeri is no longer engaging in leisure activities that reaffirm her age-related competencies.

Question 3: What interventions could the occupational therapist provide to improve Jeri's quality of life?

To improve Jeri's ability to resume her cherished hobby of scrapbooking, the occupational therapist could provide fine motor activities that incorporate scrapbooking materials. Manipulation of materials can be improved by gluing small paper pieces onto sturdy cards to make them easier to hold and using adapted scissors to cut. A pre-driving assessment, and perhaps driver training, may help Jeri resume her outside activities, or the assessment may determine that driving is not advisable at this time. If Jeri is unable to drive, the occupational therapist may determine that an intervention aimed at accessing and using public transportation may be the first step in increasing community independence.

A collaborative session with Jeri's husband can be set up to talk through his concerns and to instruct him in the use of adaptive equipment, transfers, etc. to assist her in resuming former life roles such as fishing. Jeri, her husband, and the occupational therapist could discuss Jeri's missed social roles and need for emotional expression. They may set mutual goals that encourage Jeri and her husband to invite friends and family over for a few hours for socializing. She may also be interested in joining a head injury support group that the occupational therapy department runs to provide her with needed peer interaction; the husband may also wish to be included in a support group for families. Sexual and sensual expression may be brought up in this meeting and the occupational therapist could offer suggestions regarding communication of perceived changes, use of touch, and positions to enhance intimacy. The occupational therapist may also indicate referrals, as necessary. All of these leisure-related accomplishments will help reestablish 29-year-old Jeri's perception of herself as a whole human being.

Review Questions

1. Name five psychosocial benefits and five physical benefits of leisure activities.
2. What four factors are essential for modeling to be an effective intervention?
3. When should humor and laughter be used with caution?
4. What can the absence of meaningful leisure occupation lead to?
5. Why is the client's cultural background important?
6. Why is it important for the client to be involved in setting his or her own goals?

REFERENCES

1. Adams P (with Mylander M): *Gesundheit!* Rochester, VT, 1998, Healing Arts Press.
2. Adams RC, McCubbin JA: *Games, sports and exercises for the physically disabled*, ed 4, Philadelphia, 1990, Lea & Febiger.
3. Ader R: Historical perspectives on psychoneuroimmunology. In Friedman H, Klein TW, Friedman AL, editors: *Psychoneuroimmunology, stress, and infection*, Boca Raton, FL, 1995, CRC Press.
4. Allison MT, Geiger CW: Nature of leisure activities among Chinese-American elderly, *Leisure Sci* 15(4):309, 1993.
5. Atchley RC: *Social forces and aging: an introduction to social gerontology*, ed 10, Belmont, CA, 2004, Wadsworth.
6. Bachner S: *Picture this: an illustrated guide to complete dinners*, 1984, Special Additions.
7. Bandura A: *Social foundations of thought and action: a social cognitive theory*, Englewood Cliffs, NJ, 1986, Prentice-Hall.
8. Baum CM, Edwards D: *Activity card sort*, St. Louis, 2001, Washington University at St. Louis.
9. Beard JB, Ragheb MG: Measuring leisure motivation, *J Leisure Res* 15:219, 1983.
10. Bearon LB: Successful aging: what does the good life look like? Concepts in gerontology, *Forum Family Consumer Issues* 1(3), 1996.
11. Bennett MP, et al: The effect of mirthful laughter on stress and natural killer cell activity, *Altern Ther Health Med* 9(2):38, 45, Mar-Apr 2003.
12. Berk L: The laughter-immune connection: new discoveries, *Humor Health J* 5:1, 1996.
13. Berk L, Tan S, Fry W: Eustress of humor associated laughter modulates specific immune system components, *Annals of Behav Med* 15:111, 1993.
14. Black DW: Laughter, *JAMA* 252(21):2995, 1984.
15. Burckhardt C, et al: Measuring the quality of life of women with rheumatoid arthritis or systemic lupus erythematosus.

A Swedish version of the Quality of Life Scale (QoLS), *Scandinavian J Rheum* 21(4):190, 1992.

16. Butler B: Overview of sports wheelchairs, *Brit J Occup Ther* 4(2):66, 1997.

17. Cousins N: *Head first: the biology of hope and the healing power of the human spirit*, New York, 1989, Penguin Books.

18. Dekker R, et al: Functional status and dependency of stroke patients five years after clinical rehabilitation, *J Rehab Sciences* 8(4):99, 1995.

19. Dergance JM, et al: Barriers to and benefits of leisure-time physical activity in the elderly: differences across cultures, *J Am Geriatr Soc* 51(6):863, 2003.

20. Drummond AER, Walker MF: A randomized controlled trial of leisure rehabilitation after stroke, *Clin Rehab* 9:283, 1995.

21. Du Pre, A: *Humor and the healing arts: a multimethod analysis of humor use in health care.* Mahwah, NJ, 1998, Lawrence Erlbaum Associates.

22. Eyler AE, et al: Correlates of physical activity among women from diverse/racial groups, *J Womens Health Gender Based Med* 11(3):239, 2002.

23. Flanagan J: A research approach to improving our quality of life, *Amer Psychologist/J Amer Psychol Assoc* 33(2):138, 1978.

24. Fry W: The physiologic effects of humor, mirth, and laughter, *JAMA* 267(13):1857, 1992.

25. Gilfoyle EM: Caring: a philosophy for practice, *Am J Occup Ther* 34(8):517, 1980.

26. Giogino K, et al: Appraisal of and coping with arthritis-related problems in household activities, leisure activities, and pain management, *Arthritis Care Res* 7(1):20, 1994.

27. Ham SA, et al: *Centers for Disease Control Weekly: prevalence of no leisure-time physical activity—35 states and the District of Columbia*, 1988-2002, 2/6/04. Available online at *http://wwwcdc.gov/mmwr/preview/mmwrhtml/mm5304g4.htm.*

28. Hampes WP: The relationship between humor and trust, *Humor* 12(3):253, 1999.

29. Jordan JV: The meaning of mutuality. In Jordan JV, Kaplan AG, Miller JB, et al: *Women's growth in connection: writings from the Stone Center*, New York, 1991, The Guilford Press.

30. Kenney C: *Have crutch, will travel*, Denver, CO, 2002, Tell Tale Publ.

31. Kim E, et al: Leisure activity, ethnic preservation, and cultural integration of older Korean Americans, *J Gerontol Soc Work* 36(1/2):107, 2001.

32. Kinney WB, Coyle CP: Predicting life satisfaction among adults with physical disabilities, *Arch Phys Med Rehabil* 73(9):863, 1992.

33. Klein A: *The healing power of humor*, Los Angeles, CA, 1989, Jeremy P. Tarcher.

34. Klinger JL: *Meal preparation and training: the health care professional's guide*, Thorofare, NJ, 1997, Slack Publ.

35. Kolkmeier LG: Play and laughter: moving toward harmony. In Dossey BM, Keegan L, Kolkmeier LG, et al: *Holistic health promotion: a guide for practice*, Rockville, MD, 1989, Aspen Press.

36. Kuhlman TL: *Humor and psychotherapy*, Homewood, IL 1984, Dow Jones-Irwin,

37. Law M, et al: *Canadian occupational performance measure*, ed 3, Canadian Association of Occupational Therapy, 1999, Toronto.

38. Leber DA, Vanoli EG: Brief report: therapeutic use of humor: occupational therapy clinicians' perceptions and practices, *Am J Occup Ther* 50:221, 2000.

39. Lefcourt HM, Martin RA: *Humor and life stress: antidote to adversity*, New York, 1986, Springer-Verlag.

40. Llorens L: Performance tasks and roles throughout the life span. In Christiansen C, Baum C, editors: *Occupational therapy: overcoming human performance deficits*, Thorofare, NJ, 1991, Slack Publ.

41. Mann WC, et al: Assistive devices used by home-based elderly persons with arthritis, *Amer J Occup Ther* 49(8):810, 1995.

42. *Morbidity & Mortality Weekly Report*, Mar 24 49(SS-2):1, 2000.

43. Oakley F, et al: The Role Checklist: development and empirical assessment of reliability, *Occup Ther J Res* 6(3):157, 1986.

44. Occupational therapy practice framework: domain and process, *Amer J Occup Ther* 56(6):609, 2002.

45. Papalia DE, et al: *Human development*, ed 9, New York, 2004, McGraw-Hill.

46. Parham LD, Fazio LS: *Play in occupational therapy for children*, St. Louis, 1997, Mosby.

47. Parker CJ, et al: The role of leisure in stroke rehabilitation, *Disabil Rehabil* 19(1):1, 1997.

48. Pendleton HM: *Establishment and sustainment of friendship of women with physical disability: the role of participation in occupation*, Doctoral dissertation, 1998, University of Southern California, Los Angeles. Available through UMI.

49. Pert C: *Molecules of emotion: why you feel the way you feel*, New York, 1997, Scribner.

50. Ragheb MG, Beard JG: Measuring leisure attitude, *J Leisure Res* 14:155, 1982.

51. Rickards P: *Popular activities and games: for blind, visually impaired and disabled people* (large print), Association for the Blind, 1986.

52. Robinson VM: *Humor and the health professions: the therapeutic use of humor in health care*, ed 2, Thorofare, NJ, 1991, Slack Publ.

53. Silverstein M, Parker MG: Leisure activities and quality of life among the oldest old in Sweden, *Res Aging* 24(5):528, 2002.

54. Southam M: Therapeutic humor: attitudes and actions by occupational therapists in adult physical disabilities settings, *Occup Ther Health Care* 17(1):23, 2003.

55. Takahashi K, et al: The elevation of natural killer cell activity induced by laughter in a crossover designed study, *Int J Mol Med* 8(6):645, 2001.

56. Taylor LPS, McGruder JE: The meaning of sea kayaking for persons with spinal cord injuries, *Am J Occup Ther* 50(1):39, 1996.

57. Vergeer G, MacRae A: Therapeutic use of humor in occupational therapy, *Am J Occup Ther* 47:678, 1993.

58. Wikstrom I, et al: Leisure activities in rheumatoid arthritis: change after disease onset and associated factors, *Brit J Occup Ther* 64(2):87, 2001.

59. Wooten P: Humor: an antidote for stress, *Hol Nrs Prac* 10(2):49, 1996.

16 ASSISTIVE TECHNOLOGY

DENIS ANSON

KEY TERMS

Rehabilitation technology
Assistive technologies
Universal design
Human interface assessment
  (HIA) model
Electronic aids to daily living
Power switching
Augmentative and alternative
  communications
User control system
Message composition system
Message transmission system
Graphical communications
Pointing systems

LEARNING OBJECTIVES

After studying this chapter the student or practitioner will be able to do the following:

1. Describe the range of assistive technologies options currently available for persons with physical disabilities.
2. Explain the human interface assessment (HIA) model.
3. Identify common solutions for enabling control of daily living devices through technology.
4. Discuss options for augmentative and alternative communications
5. Analyze input and output options for assistive technologies and match these to the needs of consumers.

CHAPTER OUTLINE

THREADED CASE STUDY: GIANNA, PART 1

Gianna, a 26-year-old, has completed her undergraduate degree and applied to law school with the hopes of becoming a lawyer. Her path to the legal profession is obstructed by her C4 level complete spinal cord injury, which she sustained 12 years previously in an automobile accident that killed her parents. Gianna is bright, articulate, and exceptionally popular in her rural community. She recently received a new wheelchair with sip-and-puff controls, which allows her mobility in her home and community, and now she would like to attend law school. Ultimately, Gianna would like to specialize in disability rights, to support the civil rights of others with profound disabilities. She feels that her insider perspective on the issues might make her arguments more compelling when disabled workers are seeking reasonable accommodations.

The admissions office at the nearby university, which includes a law program, suggests that Gianna may have a difficult time completing the required work. As a law student, Gianna will have to research legal precedence in case law and write briefs. She can get into the library, which meets many of the requirements of the ADA, but will need to be able to navigate the legal records, take notes of her findings, and write formal responses to legal challenges. The counselor feels that Gianna, who has no movement below her neck, may find the challenge of the legal profession to exceed her capabilities.

Gianna does have full-time attendant care and the attendant would be allowed to sit with Gianna in the classroom, acting as a note-taker for her. (The school also provides lecture notes to disabled students within three days of a class session, if requested.)

However, since Gianna's attendant must constantly monitor Gianna's physical needs, the ability of the attendant to focus on the lecture may be impaired. Also, since the attendant does not have the interest or background to study law, the ability of the attendant to identify what is important within the lecture is limited. Finally, due to the required hours and hourly wage, Gianna generally changes attendants every 6 months or so. The new attendant would not have a complete background to help with interpretation of the material Gianna is studying. In her home life, Gianna would like to be able to adjust the lights in the room, the room temperature, and radio station (she prefers to study with music in the background) that is playing without interrupting her attendant. She knows that she will always be dependent on others for bathing, dressing, meal preparation, and many other aspects of her ADLs. However, she feels that if she were able to make fewer demands on her attendants, they might be able to remain in her employ longer.

Gianna is seeking an assistive technology consultation to explore technological aids to assist her in reaching her life goals.

Critical Thinking Questions

1. Which of Gianna's areas of occupation might be improved through the application of assistive technology?
2. What types of assistive technologies might assist Gianna in pursuing her activities and occupations?
3. What control strategies might be appropriate for Gianna?
4. Would Gianna benefit from output enhancement technologies?

WHAT IS ASSISTIVE TECHNOLOGY?

A discussion of **assistive technology** should begin with a description of the general limits of the topic. This is made difficult because the legal definitions of assistive technology are not uniform. Assistive technologies are sometimes included in the category of rehabilitation technology.[12] In other cases, rehabilitation technology is considered as an aspect of assistive technologies.[8] A third category of universal designed technologies doesn't seem to fit into either category.[11] For purposes of this discussion, the author will present a set of definitions that are within the current definitions, but not necessarily congruent with any particular statute.

REHABILITATIVE/ASSISTIVE/UNIVERSAL TECHNOLOGIES

The category into which an enabling technology falls depends largely on its application, not on the specific device. What is for some people a convenience, may be an assistive technology for another.

REHABILITATION TECHNOLOGY

To rehabilitate is to restore to a prior level of function. To be consistent with general usage, therefore, the term **rehabilitation technology** should be used to describe those technologies that are intended to restore an individual to a previous level of function following the onset of pathology. When an occupational therapist (OT) uses a technological device to establish, restore, or modify functioning in the client, he or she is using a rehabilitative technology. Physical agent modalities such as ultrasound, diathermy, paraffin, and functional electric stimulation are examples of rehabilitative technologies. When these technologies have done their job, the client will have improved intrinsic function, and the technology will be removed.

ASSISTIVE TECHNOLOGY

Central to occupational therapy is the belief that active engagement in meaningful activity supports the health and well being of the individual. When an individual has

ETHICAL CONSIDERATIONS

Rehabilitative technologies are generally intended to be used within a therapy setting by trained professionals, and over a short period of time. Because the technologies are intended to be used by trained professionals, they can have fairly complex or cryptic controls. The expectation is that the professional may have significant training before applying the technology. The professional guiding the use of such technologies is expected to assure the correct application of the technology, and to protect the safety of the individual using the device.

functional limitations secondary to some pathology, they may not have the cognitive, motor, or psychological skills necessary to engage in a meaningful activity, and may require assistance to participate in the desired task.

To assist is to help, aid, or support. There is no implication of restoration in assistance. **Assistive technologies**, therefore, are those technologies that assist a person with a disability in performing tasks. More specifically, assistive technologies are those technologies, whether designed for a person with a disability or designed for mass market and used by a person with a disability, that allow that person to perform tasks that an able-bodied person can do without technological assistance. It may be that an able-bodied person would prefer to use a technology to perform a task, using a television remote control, for example, but it does not rise to the level of assistive technology as long as it is possible to perform the task without the technology.

Assistive technologies replace or support an impaired function of the user without being expected to change the native functioning of the individual. A wheelchair, for example, replaces the function of walking, but is not expected to teach the user to walk. Similarly, forearm crutches support independent standing, but do not, of themselves, improve strength or bony integrity, so will not change the ability of the user to stand without them.

Because they are not expected to change the native ability of the user, assistive technologies have different design considerations. They are expected to be used over prolonged periods of time, by individuals with limited training, and possibly with limited cognitive skills. The technology, therefore, must be designed so that it will not inflict harm on the user through casual misuse. The controls of the device must be readily understood, so that, while some training may be required to use the device, constant retraining will not be. The device should not require deep understanding of its principles and functions to be useful.

One significant difference between rehabilitation technology and assistive technology occurs at the end of the rehabilitation process. At this point, the client no longer uses rehabilitation technologies, but may have just completed training in the use of assistive technologies. The assistive technologies go home with the client; the rehabilitation technologies generally remain in a clinic. Some technologies do not fit neatly into these categories since they may be used differently with different clients. Some clinicians use assisted communication as a tool to train unassisted speech for their clients. For other clients, assisted communication may be used to support or replace speech. In the first case, the technology is rehabilitative. In the second, the same technology may be assistive.

UNIVERSAL DESIGN

Universal design is a very new category of technology. The principles of universal design were published by the Center for Universal Design at North Carolina State University in 1997,[11] and their application is still very limited. The concept of universal design is very simple: if devices are designed with the needs of people with a wide range of abilities in mind, they will be more usable for all users, with and without disabilities.

This design philosophy could, in some cases, make assistive technology unnecessary. A can opener that has been designed for one-handed use by a busy housewife will also be usable by the cook who has had a cerebral vascular accident (CVA), and now only has use of one hand. Since both individuals are using the same product for the same purpose, it is just technology, not assistive technology. Electronic books will include features to allow them to be used as "talking books." The goal here is to provide a "hands-free, eyes-free" interface so that the books can be used by commuters while driving. However, the same interface will meet the needs of the individual who is blind and cannot see the screen, or who has mobility limitations and cannot operate the manual controls. No adaptation is necessary because the special needs of the person with a disability have already been designed into the product.

THE ROLE OF ASSISTIVE TECHNOLOGY IN OCCUPATIONAL PARTICIPATION

The Occupational Therapy Practice Framework[7] defines the appropriate domain of occupational therapy as including the analysis of the performance skills and patterns of the individual and the activity demands of the occupation the individual is attempting to perform.

HUMAN INTERFACE ASSESSMENT

Anson's **human interface assessment (HIA) model** provides a detailed look at the skills and abilities of the human in the skill areas of motor, process, and communication/interaction as well as the demands of an activity (Figure 16-1, *A*). The HIA model suggests that when the demands of a task do not exceed the skills and abilities of an individual, no assistive technology is required, even when a functional limitation

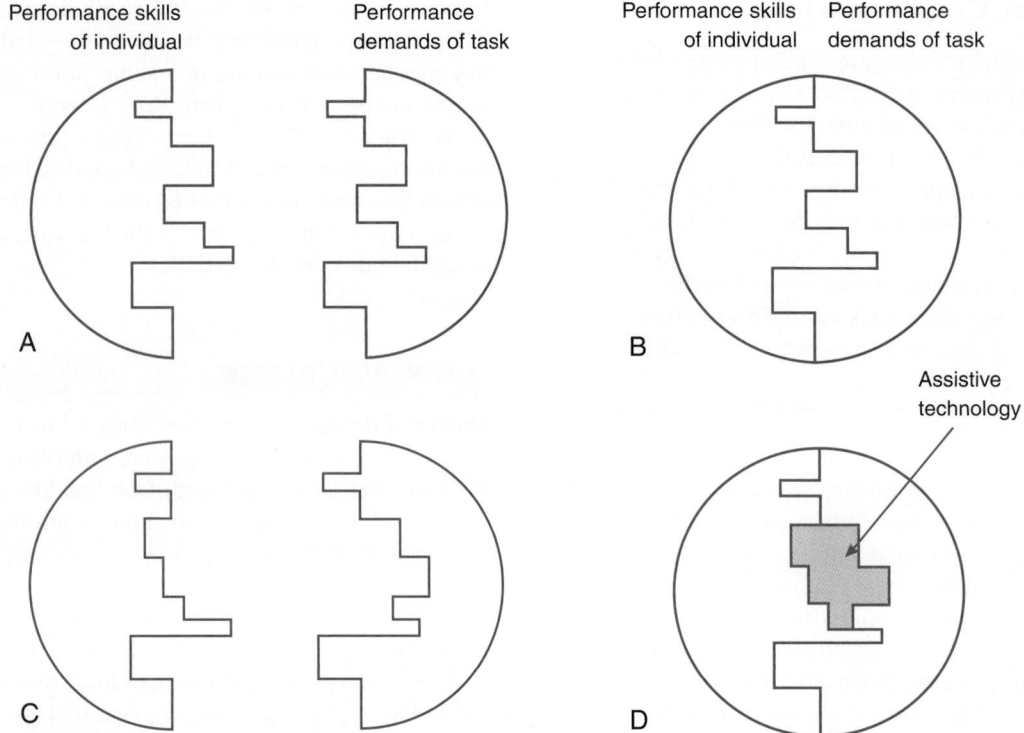

Figure 16-1 **A**, Skills of the individual and the demands of the task. **B**, Match of skills of the individual with the demands of the task. **C**, Skills of the individual and demands of the task mismatch. **D**, Assistive technology used to bridge gap between the skills of the individual and the demands of the task.

exists (Figure 16-1, *B*). On the other hand, when a task makes demands that exceed the native abilities of the individual, the individual will not be able to perform the task in the prescribed manner (Figure 16-1, *C*). In these cases, an assistive technology device may be used to bridge the gap between the demands and abilities (Figure 16-1, *D*).

While an assistive technology must be able to assist in performing the desired task, it also presents an interface to the individual, which must also match the needs of the client. A careful match between the abilities of the human for sensory perception, cognitive processing, and motor output and the input and output capabilities of assistive technologies is necessary for assistive technologies to provide effective interventions.

TYPES OF ELECTRONIC ENABLING TECHNOLOGIES

While modern technology can blur some of the distinctions presented below, it is useful to consider assistive technologies in categories by the application to which it is applied. This chapter deals only with electronic assistive technologies, which, in terms of their primary application, may be considered to fall into three categories: electronic aids to daily living (EADLs), alternative and augmentative communications (AAC), and general computer applications.

ELECTRONIC AIDS TO DAILY LIVING

Electronic aids to daily living (EADLs) are devices that can be used to control electrical devices in the client's environment. Prior to 1998,[31] this category of device was generally known as an environmental control unit (ECU), though technically, this terminology should be reserved for furnace thermostats and similar controls. The more generic EADL applies to control of lighting and temperature, but also applies to control of radios, televisions, telephones, and other electrical and electronic devices in the environment of the client (Figure 16-2).[9,13]

EADL systems may be thought of in terms of the degree and types of control that they provide to the user. These levels of control are simple *power switching, control of device features, and subsumed devices* (Figure 16-3).

Power Switching

The simplest EADLs provide simple switching of the electrical supply for devices in a room. Although not typically considered as EADLs, the switch adaptations for switch-adapted toys provided to severely disabled children would, formally, be included in this category of device. Primitive EADL systems consisted of little more than a set of electrical switches and outlets in a box that connected to devices within a room via extension cords. These devices are limited in their utility

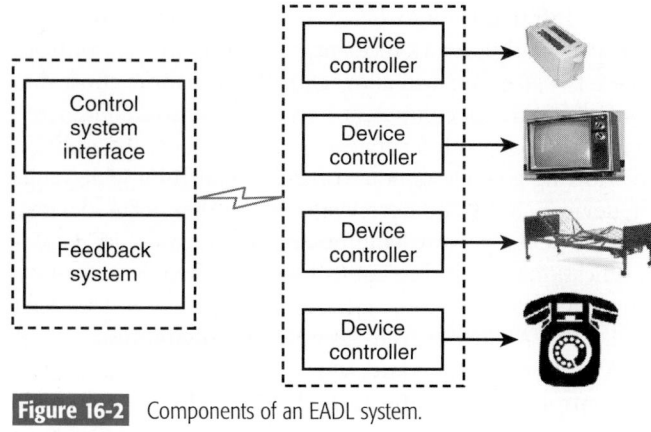

Figure 16-2 Components of an EADL system.

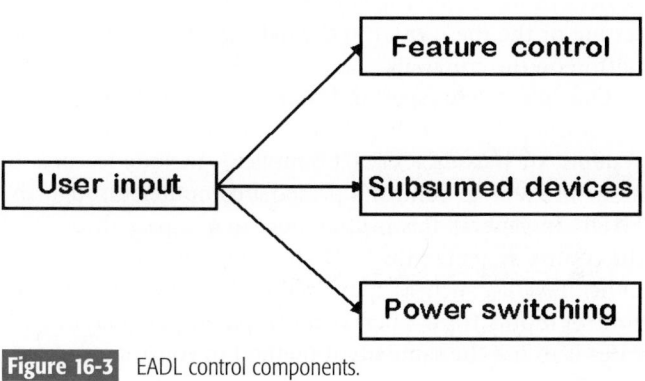

Figure 16-3 EADL control components.

and safety, since extension cords pose safety hazards to people in the environment through risks of both falls (tripping over the extension cords) and fires (overheated or worn cords). Because of the limitations posed by extension cords, EADL technology was driven to use remote switching technologies.

Second generation EADL systems used various remote control technologies to remotely switch power to electrical devices in the environment. These strategies include the use of ultrasonic pulses (e.g., TASH Ultra 4), infrared light (e.g., Infrared Remote Control), and electrical signals propagated through the electrical circuitry of the home (e.g., X-10). All of these switching technologies remain in use, and some are used for much more elaborate control systems. Here we are only considering power switching, however.

The most prevalent power-switching EADL control system is that produced by X-10 Corporation. The X-10 system uses electrical signals sent over the wiring of a home to control power modules that are plugged into wall sockets in series with the device to be controlled. (In a series connection, the power module is plugged into the wall, and the remotely controlled device is plugged into the power module.) X-10 supports up to 16 channels of control, with up to 16 modules on each, for a total of up to 256 devices controlled by a single system. The signals used to control X-10 modules will not travel through the home's power transformer so, in single family dwellings, there is no risk of interfering with devices in a neighbor's home.

This is not necessarily true, however, in an apartment setting, where it is possible for two X-10 users to inadvertently control each other's devices. The general set-up of early X-10 devices was to control up to 16 devices on an available channel, so that such interference would not occur. In some apartments, the power within a single unit may be on different "phases" of the power supplied to the building. (These phases are required to provide 220-volt power for some appliances.) If this is the case, the X-10 signals from a controller plugged into one phase will not cross to the second phase of the installation. A special "phase cross-over" is available from X-10 to correct this problem. X-10 modules, in addition to switching power on and off, can be used via special lighting modules, to dim and brighten room lighting. These modules work only with incandescent lighting, but add a degree of control beyond simple switching. For permanent installations, the wall switches and receptacles of the home may be replaced with X-10 controlled units. Because X-10 modules do not prevent local control, these receptacles and switches will work like standard units, with the added advantage of remote control.

When they were introduced in the late 1970s, X-10 modules revolutionized the field of EADLs. Prior to X-10, remote switching was a difficult and expensive endeavor, restricted largely to applications for people with disabilities and to industrial applications. The X-10 system, however, was intended as a convenience for able-bodied people who did not want to walk across a room to turn on a light. Because the target audience was able to perform the task without remote switching, the technology had to be inexpensive enough that it was easier to pay the cost than get out of a chair. X-10 made it possible for an able-bodied person to remotely control electrical devices for under $100, where most disability-related devices cost several thousand dollars. Interestingly, the almost universal adoption of X-10 protocols by disability related EADLs did not result in sudden price drops in the disability field, so many clinicians continue to adapt mass-market devices for individuals with disabilities.

Feature Control

As electronic systems became more pervasive in the home, simple switching of lights and coffee pots failed to meet the needs of the individual with a disability who wanted to control the immediate environment. With wall current control, a person with a disability might be able to turn radios and televisions on and off, but would have no control beyond that. A person with a disability might want to be able to surf cable channels as much as an able-bodied person with a television remote control. When advertisements are blaring from the speakers, a person with a disability might want to be able to turn down the sound or tune to another radio station. Nearly all home electronic devices are now delivered with a remote control, generally using infrared signals. Most of these remote controls are not usable by a person with a disability, however, due to dependence on fine motor control and good sensory discrimination.

EADL systems designed to provide access to the home environment of a person with a disability must provide more than on/off control of home electronics. They must also provide control of the features of home electronic devices. Because of this need, EADL systems frequently have hybrid capabilities. They will incorporate a means of directly switching power to remote devices, often using X-10 technology. This allows control of devices such as lights, fans, and coffee pots, as well as electrical door openers and other specialty devices.[37] They will also typically incorporate some form of infrared remote control, which will allow them to mimic the signals of standard remote control devices. This control will be provided either by programming in the standard sequences for all commercially available VCRs, televisions, and satellite decoders, or through teaching systems, where the EADL learns the codes beamed at it by the conventional remote. The advantage of this latter approach is that it can learn any codes, even those that have not yet been invented. The disadvantage is that the controls must be taught, requiring more set-up and configuration time for the user and caregivers.

Infrared remote control, as adopted by most entertainment systems controllers, is limited to approximate line of sight control. Unless the controller is aimed in the general direction of the device to be controlled (most have wide dispersion patterns), the signals will not be received. This means that an EADL cannot directly control, via infrared, any device not located in the same room. However, infrared repeaters such as the X-10 Powermid can overcome this limitation by using radio signals to send the control signals received in one room to a transmitter in the room of the device to be controlled. With a collection of repeaters, a person would be able to control any infrared device in the home from anywhere else in the home.

One problem that is shared by EADL users and able-bodied consumers is the proliferation of remote control devices. Many homes now are plagued with a remote control for the television, the cable/satellite receiver, the DVD player/VHS recorder (either one or two devices), the home stereo/multimedia center, and other devices, all in the same room. Universal remote controls allow switching from controlling one device to another, but are often cumbersome to control. Some hope is on the horizon for improved control of home audio-visual devices with less difficulty. In November of 1999, a consortium of eight home electronics manufacturers released a set of guidelines for home electronics called HAVi. The HAVi specification will allow compliant home electronics to communicate so that any HAVi device can control the operation of all of the HAVi devices sharing the standard. A single remote control can control all of the audio-visual devices in the home, through a single interface. (As of the summer of 2004, the HAVi site lists six products, from two manufacturers, that actually use the HAVi standard.)

The Infrared Data Association (IrDA) is performing similar specifications work focusing purely on infrared controls. The IrDA standard will allow an infrared remote control to control features of computers, home audio-visual equipment, and appliances with a single standard protocol. In addition to allowing a single remote control to control a wide range of devices, IrDA standards will allow other IrDA devices, such as PDAs, personal computers, and augmentative communications systems, to control home electronics. Having a single standard for home electronics will allow much easier design of EADL systems for people with disabilities.

A more recent standard, V2,[23] offers a much greater level of control. If fully implemented, V2 would allow a single EADL device to control all of the features of all electronic devices in its vicinity, such as the volume of the radio, the setting of the thermostat in the hall, or the "Push to Walk" button on the crosswalk.

One interesting aspect of feature control by EADLs, is the relationship between EADLs and computers. Some EADL systems, such as the Quartet Simplicity, include features to allow the user to control a personal computer through the EADL. In general, this is little more than a pass-through of the control system of the EADL to a computer access system. Other EADLs, such as the PROXi, are designed to accept control inputs from a personal computer. The goal in both cases is to use the same input method to control a personal computer as to control the EADL. In general, the control demands of an EADL system are much less stringent than those for a computer. An input method that is adequate for EADL control may be very tedious for general computer controls. On the other hand, a system that allows fluid control of a computer will not be strained by the need to also control an EADL. The "proper" source of control will probably have to be decided on a case-by-case basis, but the issue will appear again in dealing with augmentative communication systems.

Subsumed Devices

Finally, modern EADLs frequently incorporate some common devices that are more easily replicated than controlled remotely. Some devices, such as the telephone, are so pervasive that an EADL system can assume that a telephone will be required. Incorporating telephone electronics into the EADL is actually less expensive, due to the standardization of telephone electronics, than inventing special systems to control a conventional telephone. Other systems designed for individuals with disabilities are so difficult to control remotely that the EADL must generate an entire control system. Hospital bed controls, for example, have no provisions for remote control, but should be usable by a person with a disability.

Many EADL systems include a speakerphone, which will allow the user to originate and answer telephone calls using the electronics of the EADL as the telephone. Because of the existing standards, these systems are generally analog, single-line telephones, electronically similar to those found in the typical home. Many business settings now use multi-line sets, which are not compatible with home telephones. Some businesses are converting to digital interchanges, which are also not compatible with conventional telephones. Because of this, the telephone built into a standard EADL may not meet the needs of a disabled client in an office setting. Before recommending an EADL as an access solution for a client's office, therapists should check that the system is compatible with the telecommunications systems in place in that office.

Because the target consumer for an EADL will often have severe restrictions in mobility, the manufacturers of many of these systems consider that a significant portion of the customer's day will be spent in bed, and so include some sort of control system for standard hospital beds. These systems commonly allow the user to adjust head and foot height independently, extending the time the individual can be independent of assistance for positioning. As with telephone systems, different brands of hospital bed use different styles of control. It is essential that the clinician match the controls provided by the EADL with the inputs required by the bed to be controlled.

Controlling EADLs

EADL systems are designed to allow the individual with limited physical capability to control devices in the immediate environment. As such, the method used to control the EADL must be within the capability of the client. Since these controls share many features in common with other forms of electronic enablers, the control strategies will be discussed below.

AUGMENTATIVE AND ALTERNATIVE COMMUNICATIONS

The phrase **augmentative and alternative communications** (AAC) is used to describe systems that supplement (augment) or replace (alternative) communication by voice or gestures between people.[30] Formally, it incorporates all assisted communication, including tools such as pencils and typewriters as used to communicate either over time (as in leaving a message for someone who will arrive at a location after you leave) or over distance (sending a letter to Aunt May). However, as used in assistive technology, AAC is considered as the use of technology to allow communication in ways that an able-bodied individual would be able to accomplish without assistance. Thus, using a pencil to write a letter to Aunt May would not be an example of AAC for a person who is unable to speak, since an able-bodied correspondent would be using the same technology (pencil and paper) for the same purpose (social communication). However, when a person who is nonvocal uses the same pencil to explain to the doctor that she has sharp pains in her right leg, it becomes an AAC device, since an able-bodied person would communicate this by voice.

There are two very different reasons that an individual might have a communication disorder. Following a brain injury that affects Wernicke's area, an individual may exhibit a language disorder. In a language disorder, the individual has difficulty in understanding and/or formulating messages, regardless of means of production. A person with a language disorder, in most cases, will not benefit from AAC. On the other hand, an individual with difficulty in motor control or muscle tone may be perfectly able to understand and formulate messages, but not be able to speak intelligibly because of difficulty in controlling the oral musculature. Such a person has no difficulty with language composition, only with language transmission. (In cases of apraxia, the motor control of writing can be as impaired as that of speaking, without affecting language.) This person may well benefit from an AAC device.

AAC devices range from extremely low technology to extremely high technology. In hospital intensive care units, low-tech communication boards can allow a person on a respirator to communicate basic needs (Figure 16-4). A low-tech communication board can allow a client to deliver basic messages or spell out more involved messages in a fashion that can be learned quickly. For a person with only Yes/No response, the communication partner can indicate the rows of the aid one at a time, asking if the desired letter is in the row. When the correct row is selected, the partner can move across a row until the communicator indicates the correct letter. This type of communication is inexpensive, quick to teach, and very slow to use. In settings where there are limited communication needs, it is adequate, but will not serve for long-term or fluent communication needs.

To meet the communication needs of a person who will be nonvocal over a longer period of time, electronic AAC devices are frequently recommended by clinicians (Figure 16-5).

 OT PRACTICE NOTE

In selecting a communication device, the clinician must consider the type of communication the individual will employ as well as the settings in which communication will take place.

A	B	C	D	E	F	I hurt
G	H	I	J	K	L	I'm thirsty
M	N	O	P	Q	R	Head/neck
S	T	U	V	W	X	Trunk
Y	Z	1	2	3	4	Arms
5	6	7	8	9	0	Legs

Figure 16-4 Low-technology AAC system.

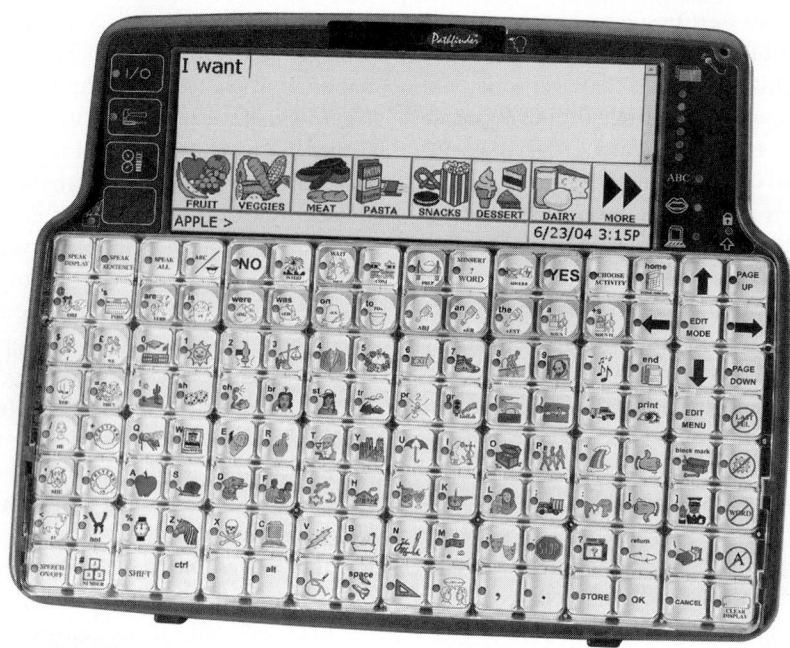

Figure 16-5 High-technology AAC system (Pathfinder Plus). (Courtesy of Prentke Romich Company, Wooster, Ohio.)

Light[29] describes four types of communication that we participate in: (1) expression of needs and wants, (2) information transfer, (3) social closeness, and (4) social etiquette. In the intensive care setting noted above, most communication will occur at the first two levels. The communicator will want to express their basic needs of hunger, thirst, and relief of pain. He or she will wish to communicate with the doctor providing care, convey information about where it hurts, and determine whether treatment seems to be working. In work or school settings, communication is often intended to convey information.

When participating in a classroom discussion, a student may want to be able to describe the troop movements in the Battle of Gettysburg, for example. In math class, the student may need to present a proof involving oblique angles and parallel lines. Such information exchange may be spontaneous, as when called on in class, or may be planned, as in a formal presentation.

In a social or interpersonal setting, communication has a markedly different flavor. Teenagers may spend hours on the telephone with very little "information" exchanged, but communicating shared feelings and concerns. At a faculty tea, much of the communication is very formulaic, such as "How are you today?" Such queries are not intended as questions into medical status, but simply recognition of your presence and an indication of wishing you well. The planning and fluency of communication in each domain are substantially different, and the demands on AAC systems in each type of communication are likewise very different.

An AAC system used solely for expression of needs and wants can be fairly basic. The vocabulary used in this type of communication is limited, and, because the expressions tend to be fairly short, the communication rate is not of paramount importance. In some cases, the entire communication system may be an alerting buzzer, indicating that the individual is in need, to summon a caregiver. Low-tech communication systems such as that described earlier can meet basic communication needs for individuals whose physical skills are limited to eye blinks or directed eye movement.

Low-tech devices may enable expression of more complex ideas. For example, a therapist became aware that his client with aphasia wished to communicate something. Since no AAC was available to this client, the therapist began attempting to guess what he wanted to communicate. After exhausting basic needs ("Do you need a drink? Do you need to use the bathroom?"), the therapist was floundering. Over the next 20 minutes, the client was able to communicate that his ears were the same shape as Cary Grant's! Even a basic communication aid, such as the ICU aid described above, would have allowed much faster transfer of this information.

Most development in AAC seems to be focused around the level of communicating basic needs and information transfer. Information transfer presents some of the most difficult technological problems, because the content of information to be communicated cannot be predicted. The designer of an AAC device would probably not be able to anticipate the need to discuss the shape of Cary Grant's ears during vocabulary selection. To meet such needs, AAC devices must have the ability to generate any concept possible in the language being used. Making these concepts available for fluent communication is the ongoing challenge of AAC development.

Social communication and social etiquette present significant challenges for users of AAC devices. While the information content of these messages tends to be low, since the communication is based on convention, the dialog should be both varied and spontaneous. AAC systems, such as the Dynavox, have provisions for pre-programmed messages that can be retrieved for social conversation, but providing both fluency and variability of social discourse through AAC remains a challenge. Current devices allow somewhat effective communication of wants. They are not nearly so effective in discussing dreams.

Parts of AAC Systems

In general, electronic AAC systems have three components (Figure 16-6): a **user control system**, which allows the user to generate messages and control the device; a **message composition system**, which allows the user to construct messages to be communicated to others; and a **message transmission system**, which allows the communication partner to receive the message from the user. The issues of user control of AAC devices are essentially the same as those for other electronic assistive technologies, and will be discussed with access systems in general.

Message composition

Most of the time, able-bodied people as well as individuals with disabilities plan their messages before speaking. (Many of us can remember the taste of foot when we have neglected this process.) An AAC device should allow the user to construct, preview, and edit communication utterances before they become apparent to the communication partner. This gives the user of an AAC device the ability to think before speaking. It also allows compensation for the rate difference between message composition via AAC and communication between able-bodied individuals.

Able-bodied individuals typically speak between 150 and 175 words per minute.[35] Augmentative communication rates are more typically on the order of 10 to 15 words per minute,

resulting in a severe disparity between the rate of communication construction and expected rate of reception. While input techniques (discussed below) offer some improvement in message construction rates, the rate of message assembly using AAC is such that many listeners will lose interest before an utterance can be delivered. If words are spaced too far apart, an able-bodied listener may not even be able to assemble them into a coherent message!

The message construction area of an AAC device allows the individual to assemble a complete thought, and then transmit it as a unit. A typical AAC device will include a display in which messages can be viewed prior to transmission. This area allows the communicator to review and edit the message that is being composed prior to transmitting it to the communication partner. This has two beneficial effects: the communicator can select words with care before communicating them, and it relieves the communication partner from the need for constant vigilance in conversation. The Atkinson-Shiffrin Model of human memory suggests that human sensory memory will retain spoken information for only 4 or 5 seconds before it fades.[1] Communication between able-bodied people generally happens quickly enough for a complete sentence to be held in sensory memory at once. When an able-bodied person is communicating with a person using an AAC device, the time between utterances may be too long to remain in memory. The able-bodied person loses focus, and may not be able to maintain attention to the conversation. If messages come as units, the communication partner can respond to a query, and then busy himself/herself in another activity while the communicator composes the next message. This is not unlike having a conversation via e-mail.

Message transmission

When the communicator has finished composing a message, it can be transmitted to the communication partner. The means of transmission varies with the device and the setting. Some AAC devices use exclusively printed transmission. One of the first true AAC devices, the Canon Communicator, was a small box, which included an alphanumeric keyboard. The box was strapped to the user's wrist, allowing the user to tap out messages that were printed on paper tape (message composition). When the message was completed, it was removed from the communicator, and passed to the communication partner (message transmission).[20] On devices like the Zygo LightWRITER, the message may be displayed on an electronic display that is made visible to the communication partner. Other systems use auditory communication, speaking the message out-loud using speech synthesis. There is a tendency to think of voice output as more appropriate than text, since able-bodied people generally communicate by voice.[20] In activities such as classroom discussion, voice communication may be the most appropriate method of communication. In other settings, such as a busy sidewalk or a noisy shop, voice output may be drowned out or unintelligible, and printed output may result in more effective communication.

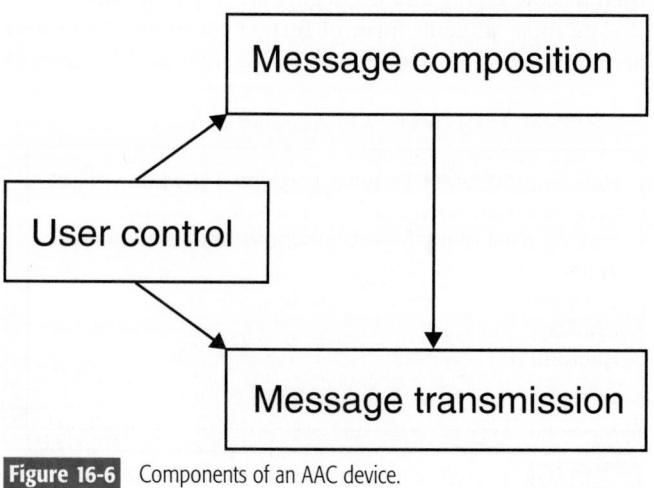

Figure 16-6 Components of an AAC device.

In a setting where verbalization may disturb others, printed output may, again, be the transmission method of choice.

In settings where voicing is the preferred method of communication, voice quality must be considered. Early AAC devices used voices that, to novice listeners, were only slightly more understandable than the communicator's unassisted voice. As speech synthesis technology has improved, AAC voices have become more generally intelligible. The high-quality voices of modern speech synthesizers have vastly improved intelligibility, but continue to provide only a narrow range of variation and vocal expression. Although the AAC user has the option of deciding what he or she would like to sound like, the choices are very few.

Communication Structure

Communications to be augmented may be categorized in terms of their intent, as well as in the content as Light[29] proposed. At the top level, communication may be divided, with the conditions discussed above, into primarily verbal and primarily written. In these cases, the categorization would be based on the mode of communication that would typically be used by an able-bodied person, not on the form that is being used by the augmented communicator.

Verbal communications

One category of verbal communication is conversation. Conversation implies a two-way exchange of information. This includes face-to-face communication with a friend, oral presentation when question and answer sessions are included, small group discussions, and a conversation over a telephone. In all of these cases, rapid communication is required and the user is expected to compose and respond immediately. If the composition rate is too slow, communication will break down, and the conversation will cease. The augmented communicator may use "telegraphic" speech styles, but this results in a primitive style of language ("want food") that may be taken to indicate poor cognition.

Another form of verbal communication is the oral presentation in which no question-and-answer component is included or in cases in which such a component is considered separately. In these cases, the augmented communicator has ample preparation time to generate communications before delivery, and an entire presentation may be stored in a communication device prior to the time of delivery. In such cases, while the time taken to prepare the message may be long, that does not inhibit the delivery of the message, as long as the device has adequate storage for the entire presentation. Stephen Hawking, through the use of an ACC device, is able to present formal papers at conferences orally, just as well as his colleagues. His ability to respond to questions, however, is severely constrained.

Graphical communications

The category of **graphical communications** includes all forms of communication that are mediated by graphic symbols.

This includes writing using paper and pencil, typewriter, computer/word processor, calculator, or drawing program. In this form of communication, the expectation is that there is a difference between the time to create the message and the time to receive it. Within the realm of graphical communications, there are a wide range of conditions and intents of communication that may influence the devices selected for the user.

One type of graphical communication is note taking. Note taking is a method of recording information as it is being transmitted from a speaker, so that the listener can recall it later. The intended recipient of this form of communication is the person who is recording the notes. It is a violation of social convention to ask the speaker to speak more slowly to accommodate the note-taker, so a note-taking system must allow rapid recording of information. However, since the listener is also the intended recipient, notes can be very cryptic, and may be meaningless to anyone other than the note taker.

Messaging is a form of graphical communication that shares many characteristics with note taking. Although the intended recipient is another person, shared abbreviations and non-grammatical language are common in messaging. The language that is common in adolescent e-mail today is very cryptic and only barely recognizable as English (Figure 16-7), but is a form of graphical messaging that communicates to its intended audience. In general, messaging does not demand the speed of input of note taking, since encoding and receiving are not linked in time. However, instant messaging, which has become nearly ubiquitous among teens, blurs the lines between messaging and conversation. The expectation is generally of an immediate response, as in conversation.

The most language-intensive form of graphical communication is formal writing. This includes writing essays for school, writing for publication, and writing business letters or contracts. Formal writing differs from the previously discussed forms of graphical communication in that it must follow the rules of written grammar. It is expected that the communicator will spend significant time and effort in preparing a formal written document, and the abbreviations used in note taking and messaging are not allowed.

The most difficult form of formal communication may be mathematical notation. The early target of AAC devices

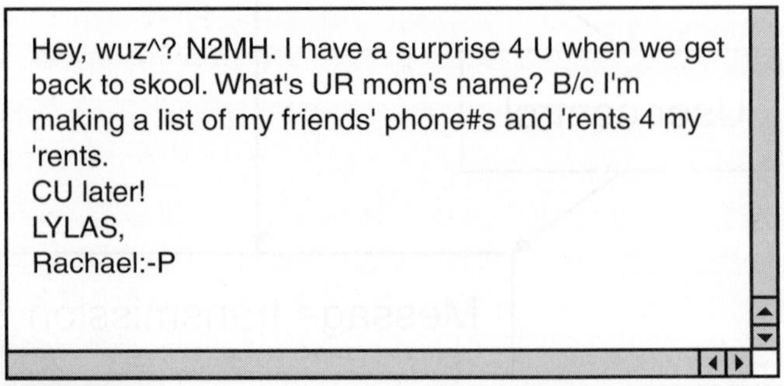

Hey, wuz^? N2MH. I have a surprise 4 U when we get back to skool. What's UR mom's name? B/c I'm making a list of my friends' phone#s and 'rents 4 my 'rents.
CU later!
LYLAS,
Rachael:-P

Figure 16-7 Example of message encryption in adolescent e-mail.

was narrative text as used in messaging and written prose. Such language is commonly linear, and can be composed in the same order it is to be read. Mathematical expressions, on the other hand, may be two dimensional and nonlinear. Simple arithmetic, such as $2 + 2 = 4$, is not excessively difficult. But algebraic expressions such as:

$$x = \frac{-b \pm \sqrt{b^2 - 4ac}}{2a}$$

can be much more difficult for an AAC device to create. A relatively basic calculus equation, such as:

$$\sum_{n=1}^{+\infty} \frac{(-1)^{n+1} \cdot 1 \cdot 3 \cdot 5 \cdots (2n-1)}{2 \cdot 4 \cdot 6 \cdots 2n} x^n$$

can be an impossible barrier to write, much less solve for the user of an AAC device. While current technology allows prose construction with some facility, an AAC user will have marked difficulty with higher mathematics. Because similar issues are experienced on the World Wide Web, new communication protocols such as MathML[17] are being developed that may, if incorporated into augmentative communication devices, provide improved access to higher mathematics for AAC users.

GENERAL COMPUTER ACCESS

The third category of electronic enabler is general computer access. While computer use is ubiquitous among able-bodied individuals, it is an assistive technology for individuals with a wide range of disabilities, because the computer allows them to perform tasks for which they have no alternative method. Computers can be used to write messages or to research school subjects. For the person with a print impairment, the computer can provide access to printed information either through electronic documents or through optical character recognition of printed documents, which can convert the printed page into an electronic document. Once a document is stored electronically, it can be presented as large text for the person with a visual acuity limitation, or read aloud for the person who is blind or profoundly learning disabled. Computers can allow the manipulation of "virtual objects" to teach mathematical concepts, form constancy, and develop spatial relations skills that are commonly learned by manipulation of physical objects.[22] *Personal digital assistants* (PDAs) may be useful for the busy executive, but may be the only means available for a person with *attention deficit hyperactivity disorder* (ADHD) to get to meetings on time.[39] For the executive, they are conveniences, but for the person with ADHD, they can be assistive technologies.

Individuals using computers can locate, organize, and present information at levels of complexity that are not possible without electronic aids. Through the emerging area of cognitive prosthetics, computers can be used to augment

attention and thinking skills in people with cognitive limitations. Computer-based biofeedback can monitor and enhance attention to task. Research in temporal processing deficits has led to the development of computer modified speech programs that can be used to enhance language learning and temporal processing skills.[33,38]

Beyond such rehabilitative applications, the performance-enhancing characteristics of the conventional computer can allow a person with physical or performance limitations to participate in activities that would be too demanding without the assistance of the computer. An able-bodied person would find having to retype a document to accommodate edits frustrating and annoying. A person with a disability may lack the physical stamina to complete the task without the cut-and-paste abilities of the computer. For the able-bodied person, the computer is a convenience. For the person with a disability, it is an assistive technology because the task is impossible without it. The applications of the computer for a person with a disability include all of the applications of the computer for an able-bodied person.

CONTROL TECHNOLOGIES

All of these electronic enabling technologies depend on the ability of the individual to control them. Although the functions of the various devices differ, the control strategies for all of them share common characteristics. Since the majority of electronic devices were designed for use by able-bodied persons, the controls of assistive technologies may be categorized in the ways that they are adapted from the standard controls. Electronic control may be divided into three broad categories: (1) input adaptations, (2) performance enhancements, and (3) output adaptations.

INPUT TO ASSISTIVE TECHNOLOGIES

Although there is a wide range of input strategies available to control electronic enablers, they can be more easily understood by considering them in subcategories. Different authors have created different taxonomies for the categorization of input strategies, and some techniques are classified differently in these taxonomies. The categorization presented here should not be considered as uniquely correct, but merely as a convenience. Input strategies may be classified as those using physical keyboards, those using virtual keyboards, and those using scanning techniques.

Physical Keyboards

Physical keyboards generally supply an array of switches, with each switch having a unique function. On more complex keyboards, modifier keys may change the base function of a key, usually to a related function.[2] Physical keyboards appear on a wide range of electronic technologies, including typewriters/computers, calculators, telephones, and microwave ovens. In these applications, sequences of keys are used to generate meaningful units such as words, checkbook balances, telephone numbers, and the cooking time for a baked potato. Other keyboards may have immediate action when a key is pressed. For example, the television remote control has keys that switch power, or raise volume when pressed.

Physical keyboards can be adapted to the needs of the individual with a disability in a number of ways (Figure 16-8). Most alphanumeric keyboards, for example, are arranged in the pattern of the conventional typewriter. This pattern was intentionally designed, for reasons relating to mechanical limitations, to slow down the user. Most individuals with disabilities do not require artificial restraints to slow them down, so this pattern of keys is seldom optimum for assistive technologies. Alternative keyboard patterns include the Dvorak Two Handed, Dvorak One Handed, and Chubon (Figure 16-9).[2] These patterns offer improvements in efficiency of typing that may allow a person with a disability to perform for functional periods of time.[4]

The standard keyboard is designed to respond immediately when a key is pressed, and, in the case of computer keyboards,

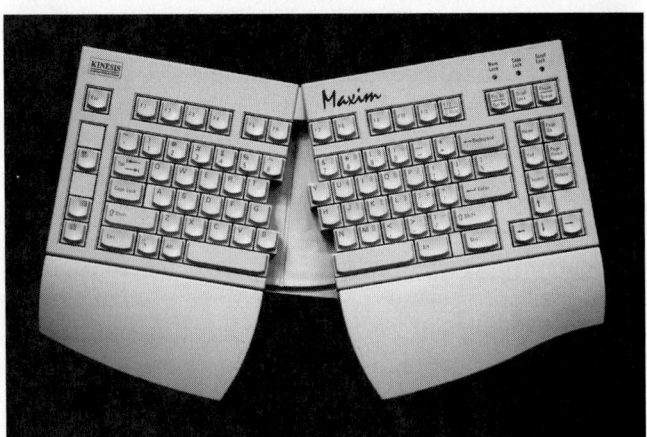

Figure 16-8   Physical keyboard with adaptive features.

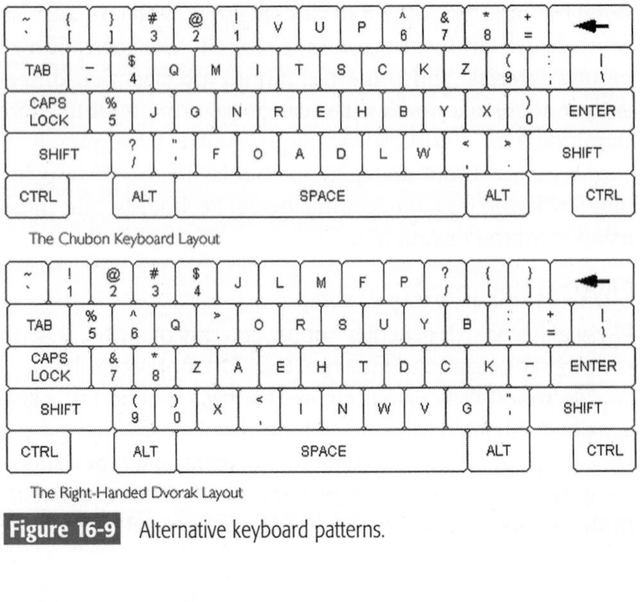

The Chubon Keyboard Layout

The Right-Handed Dvorak Layout

Figure 16-9   Alternative keyboard patterns.

to repeat when held depressed. This behavior benefits the individual with rapid fine motor control, but penalizes the individual with delayed motor response. Fortunately, on many devices, the response of the keyboard can be modified. Delayed acceptance provides a pause between the instant a key is pressed and when the key-press takes effect. Releasing the key during this pause will prevent the key from taking effect. This adaptation, if carefully calibrated, can allow a person to type with fewer mistakes, resulting in higher accuracy and, sometimes, higher productivity.

The scale of the standard keyboard provides a balance between the fine-motor control and range of motion (ROM) of an able-bodied individual. The client with limitations in either ROM or motor control may find the conventional keyboard to be difficult to use. If the client has limitations in motor control, a keyboard with larger keys and/or additional space between keys may allow independent control of the device. This adaptation may also assist the person with a visual limitation. However, to provide an equivalent number of options on larger keys increases the size of the keyboard, which may make it unusable for the person with limitations in ROM.

To accommodate limitations in ROM, the keyboard controls can be reduced in size. Smaller controls, placed closer together, will allow the selection of the full range of options with less demand for joint movement. However, the smaller controls will be more difficult to target for the person with limited motor control. A mini-keyboard is usable only by a person with good fine motor control, and may be the only scale of keyboard usable by a person with limited ROM.

To accommodate both limited ROM and limited fine motor control, a keyboard can be designed with fewer options. Many augmentative communication devices can be configured with 4, 8, 32, or 64 keys on a keyboard of a single size. Modifier or "paging" keys can allow access to the full range of options for the keyboard, but with an attendant reduction in efficiency. In this approach, the person uses one or more keys of the keyboard to shift the meanings of all of the other keys of the keyboard. Unless this approach is combined with a dynamic display, the user must remember the meanings of the keys.

Virtual Input Techniques

When an individual lacks the motor control to use an array of physical switches, a virtual keyboard may be used in its place. Virtual keyboards provide the functionality of a physical keyboard system, allowing the user to directly select from the array of options through a unique action, but may not have physical switches for the actions to be performed. Instead, the meaning of the "selection" action may be encoded spatially, via pointing, or temporally, via sequenced actions.

Pointing Systems

Pointing systems are analogous to using a physical keyboard with a physical pointer, such as a head or mouth stick.[15]

In these systems, a graphical representation of a keyboard is presented to the user, and the user is able to make selections from it by pointing to a region of the graphical keyboard and performing a selection action. The selection action is typically either the operation of a single switch (e.g., clicking the mouse) or the act of holding the pointer steady for a period of time.

The pointer used for these systems may range from a beam of light projected by the user through the reflection of a light source from the user, to sound waves received by a microphone that the user carries.[6] Changing the orientation or position of the sensor moves an indicator over the graphical image of the keyboard, informing the user of the current meaning of the selection action.

Several augmentative communication systems now use a dynamic display on which the graphical keyboard can be changed as the user makes selections, so that the meaning of each location of the keyboard changes as a message is composed. Dynamic displays free the user from having to either remember the current meaning of a key, or decode a key with multiple images on it.

Pointing systems behave very much like physical keyboard systems and many of the considerations of physical keyboards apply. The key size must balance the demands for fine-motor control with the ROM available to the client. The keyboard pattern should be selected to enhance, not hinder, function. The selection technique should facilitate intentional selections while minimizing accidental actions.

The ultimate pointing system to date is eye-tracking input. *Eye-tracking systems* generally are based on reflected infrared light from the surface of the eye. In general, these systems require extreme stability in the physical location of the eye and the camera observing the reflections.[28] Traditionally, this has meant that the user must hold his/her head extremely still in order for the system to be usable. Because of cost considerations, this input method has not been a reasonable option for a person who could produce head movement, so the requirement of head stabilization has not been a major issue. However, as eye-gaze moves into mainstream technologies, there may be changes in these requirements.

The first mainstream products that incorporated eye tracking were hand-held camcorders, which had eye tracking built into the viewfinder. By tracking the portion of the screen being focused on, this eye tracking allowed the camera to focus on the part of the display that was of special interest to the person taking the video.

The demonstrated utility of these products has led to two divergent approaches to eye tracking in mainstream products. In the first approach, personal computer developers are exploring eye tracking as a means of detecting the action that the user would like to perform.[34] This tracking will allow the computer to anticipate the needs of the user. To work as a mainstream product, the system must be able to track the user's gaze anywhere in front of the computer monitor. Challenges encountered developing adequate technology to

allow free movement while tracking eye-gaze is delaying introduction of such products.

The second approach to using eye-tracking devices is similar to video cameras with built-in eye tracking; these work because the camera is held to the eye, and moved with the eye. If an eye-tracking system were small enough to be head-mounted, it would be much easier to use, as the system would remain in fixed relationship to the eyes. Currently, systems that combine head-mounted displays with eye tracking are being made available for development of future products. A number of possibilities are opened by this combination. For example, a head-mounted display might project a control system that the user looked at to control devices, and looked through for other activities. With binocular eye tracking combined with head tracking, an EADL system might be constructed that would allow the user to control devices simply by looking at them. There is currently no affordable, easy-to-use, and effective eye-gaze input system. While eye-gaze is available for those who have no other option, it is currently competitive as an input method for those who do have other options to control their computer. However, now that mainstream engineers have discovered this technology, it will probably become less costly and more effective.

Switch Encoding Inputs

The individual who lacks the ROM or fine-motor control necessary to use a physical or graphical keyboard may be able to use a switch encoding input method. In *switch encoding*, a small set of switches (from one to nine) is used to directly access the functionality of the device. The meaning of the switch may depend on the length of time it is held closed, as in Morse code, or on the immediate history of the switch set, as in the Tongue Touch Keypad.

In Morse code, a very small set of switches is used to type. In single-switch Morse, a short switch closure produces an element called a "dit," which is typically written as an "*". A long switch closure produces the "dah" element, which is written as a "-". Formally, a "long switch closure" is three times longer than a short switch closure, which can be adjusted to the needs of the individual. Patterns of switch closures produce the letters of the alphabet, numbers, and punctuation. Pauses longer than five times the short switch closure indicate the end of a character. Two-switch Morse is similar, except two switches are used: one to produce the "dit" element, and a second to produce the "dah". Because the meaning of the switches is unambiguous, it is possible for the dit and dah to be the same length, potentially doubling typing speed. Three-switch Morse breaks the time dependence of Morse by using a third switch to indicate that the generated set of dits and dahs constitutes a single letter.

Morse code is a highly efficient method of typing for a person with severe motor control limitations and has the advantage over other virtual keyboard techniques of eventually becoming completely automatic.[5,32] Many Morse code users indicate that they do not "know" Morse code. They think in words, and the words appear on the screen, just as happens in touch-typing. Many Morse code users type at speeds approaching 25 words per minute, making this a means of functional writing. The historical weakness of Morse is that each company creating a Morse interface for assistive technology has used slightly different definitions of many of the characters. To address this issue, and to promote application of Morse code, the Morse 2000 organization has created a standard for Morse development.[36]

Another variety of switch encoding involves switches monitoring their immediate history for selection. The Tongue Touch Keypad (TTK), from newAbilities Systems, uses a set of nine switches on a keypad built into a mouthpiece and resembling a dental orthotic.

Early versions of the product used an "on-screen keyboard" called MiracleTyper (Figure 16-10). When using this input method, the first switch selection selected a group of nine possible characters, and the second switch action selected a specific character. This approach to typing is somewhat more efficient physically than Morse, but does require the user to observe the screen to know the current switch meaning. Later versions of the TTK used the keypad only as a mouse emulator, allowing the user to select any on-screen keyboard desired for text entry.

A different approach to switch encoding is provided by the T9 keyboard (Figure 16-11). In this novel interface, each key

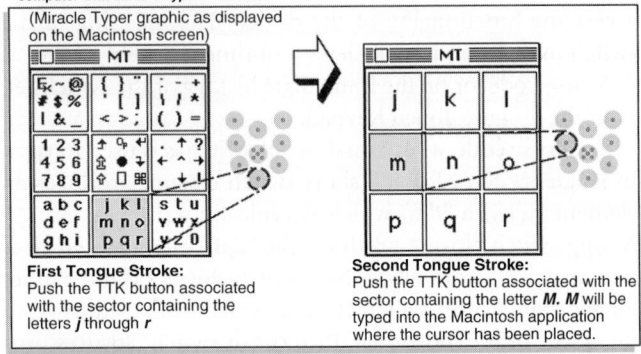

Figure 16-10 MiracleTyper enabling character selection, by selection history.

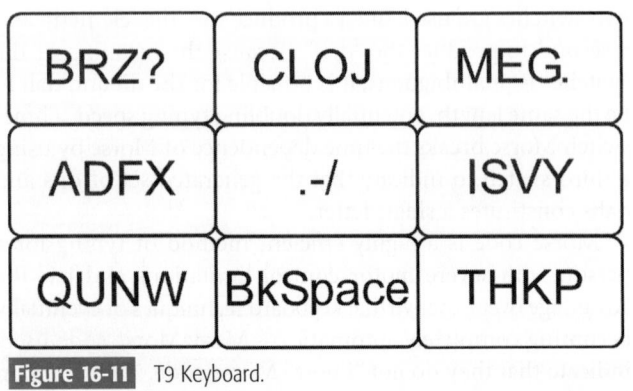

Figure 16-11 T9 Keyboard.

of the keyboard has several letters on it, but the user types as if only the desired character were present. The keyboard software determines from the user's input what word might have been intended. The disambiguation process used in the T9 keyboard allows a high degree of accuracy in determining which character the user intended, and also allows rapid learning of the keyboard. This input technology is potentially compatible with pointing systems, described above, providing an excellent balance of target size and available options.

Speech Input

For many, speech input has a magical allure. What could be more natural than to speak to an EADL or computer, and have one's wishes carried out. When first introduced by Dragon Systems in 1990, large vocabulary speech input systems were enormously expensive, and, for most, of limited utility. While highly dedicated users were able to type using voice in 1990, almost no one with the option of the keyboard would choose to use voice for their daily work. These early systems required the user to pause between each word, so that the input system could recognize the units of speech. Today,[24] the technology has evolved to allow continuous speech, with recognition accuracy greater than 90%.[26] (The companies producing speech products claim accuracy of greater than 95%.) While this advance in speech technology is remarkable, it does not mean that speech input is the control of choice for people with disabilities, for a number of reasons.

Speech recognition requires consistent speech. While it is not necessary that the speech be absolutely clear, the user must say words the same way each time for an input system to recognize them. Because of this, the majority of people with speech impairments cannot use a speech input system. Slurring and variability of pronunciation will result in a low recognition rate.

Speech input requires a high degree of vigilance during training and use. Before current speech technology can be used, it must be "trained" to understand the voice of the intended user. To do this, the system presents text to the potential user, which must be read into the microphone of the recognition system. If the user lacks the cognitive skills to respond appropriately to the presented cues, the training process will be very difficult. A few clinicians have reported success in training students with learning disabilities or other cognitive limitations to use speech input systems, but in general, the success rate is poor. Even after training, the user must watch carefully for misrecognized words, and correct them at the time the error is made. Modern speech recognition systems depend on context for their recognition. Each uncorrected error slightly changes the context, until the system can no longer recognize the words being spoken. Spell checking a document will not find misrecognized words, since each word on the screen is a correctly spelled word. It just may not be the word the user intended!

Speech input is intrusive. One person in a shared office space talking to a computer will reduce the productivity of every other person in the office. If everyone in the office were talking to their computers, the resulting noise levels would be chaotic. Speech input is effective for a person who works or lives alone, but is not a good input method for most office or classroom settings.[25]

The type of speech system used depends on the device being controlled. For EADL systems, discrete speech (short, specific phrases such as "light on") provides an acceptable level of control. The number of options is relatively small, and there is seldom a need for split-second control. Misrecognized words are unlikely to cause difficulty. Text generation for narrative description, however, places higher demands for input speed and transparency, and may call for a continuous input method. Other computer applications may work better with discrete than continuous input methods. Databases and spreadsheets typically have many small input areas, with limited information in each. These applications are much better suited to discrete speech than continuous.

The optimum speech recognition program would be a system that would recognize any speaker, with an accuracy of better than 99%. Developers of current speech systems say that, based on advances in processor speed and speech technologies, this level of usability should be possible within about 5 years. However, they have been making the same prediction (with 5 years) for the past 10 years! Modern speech recognition systems are vastly better than those available 10 years ago, and are also available at just over 1% of the cost of the early systems. However, even with these improvements, they are still not preferable to the conventional keyboard for most users.

Scanning Input Methods

For the individual with very limited cognition and/or motor control, a variation in row-column scanning is sometimes used.[2,14,20] In scanning input, the system to be controlled sequentially offers choices to the user and the user indicates affirmation when the correct choice is offered. Typically, such systems first offer groups of choices, and, when a group is selected, offer the items of the group sequentially. Because the items were, in early systems, presented as a grid being offered a row at a time, such systems are commonly referred to as "row-column" scanning, even when no rows or columns are present.

Scanning input allows selection of specific choices with very limited physical effort. Generally, the majority of the user's time is spent waiting for the desired choice to be offered, so the energy expenditure is relatively small. Unfortunately, the overall time expenditure is generally relatively large. When the system has only a few choices to select among, as in most EADL systems, scanning is a viable input method. The time spent waiting while the system scans may be a minor annoyance, but the difference between turning on a light now versus a few moments from now is relatively small. EADL systems are used intermittently throughout the day, rather than continuously, so the delays over the course of the day are acceptable in most cases. For AAC or computer systems, however,

the picture is very different. In either application, the process of composing thoughts may require making hundreds or thousands of selections in sequence. The cumulative effect of the pauses in row-column scanning will slow productivity to the point that functional communication is very difficult, and may be impossible. Certainly, when productivity levels are mandated, the communication rate available via scanning input will not be adequate.

Integrated Controls

One area of current development is the long advocated idea of integrated controls.[16] An individual with a profound disability is likely to require more than one type of control device. A person with severe motor involvement from cerebral palsy, for example, may require an augmentative communication system for interpersonal communication, an EADL for control of the local environment, a computer access system to complete job-related tasks, and a powered mobility device to navigate the community. Historically, each of these systems had their own control systems, with slightly different control strategies. The user of these multiple systems would have to move from control system to control system, and have to learn how to control each of the systems.

With an integrated control system, the user would have a single interface that could control each assistive technology device. Since both AAC and computer access commonly involve language, means of using an AAC device to control a computer was an early goal. The 1994 standard for General Input Device Emulating Interface (GIDEI)[18] defined characters to be sent from an AAC device to a supporting computer to provide control, equivalent to the keyboard and mouse. With GIDEI, an AAC user could use the same control interface to communicate with friends in the same room, or to write a business proposal.

Since many devices can be used with a moving pointer, the joystick control of a powered wheelchair may offer another avenue to integrated controls. The same joystick could be used to move a selection icon on the display of an EADL or AAC device, or the mouse pointer of a computer screen. Ideally, the communication between devices would be wireless, and the current Bluetooth standard for short range, wireless communications offers to make such controls possible. (Bluetooth is a consortium of electronics companies whose goal is to develop a flexible low-cost wireless platform capable of short-distance communication.)

The question, for the clinician, will be whether the advantages of a single, generic control that is not optimum for any particular device would outweigh the costs of learning individual, optimal control strategies for each device. Because the demands of controlling a powered wheelchair are significantly different than those for writing a formal proposal, changing channels on a television, or answering a question in a classroom, different control strategies might be necessary for each device. Whether a single control interface can support the optimal strategy for each device remains to be seen.

RATE ENHANCEMENT OPTIONS

For EADL systems, rate of control input is relatively unimportant. As noted above, the number of control options is relatively limited, and selections are rarely severely time constrained. However, for AAC and computer control systems, the number of selections to be made in sequence is high, and rate is frequently very important. Because a person with a disability can generally not make selections at the same rate as an able-bodied person, rate enhancement technologies may increase the information transmitted by each selection. In general, language can be expressed in one of three ways: letter-by-letter spelling, prediction, and compaction/expansion. The latter two options allow enhancement of language generation rates.

Letter-by-Letter Spelling

Typical typing is an example of letter-by-letter representation, and is relatively inefficient. In all languages and alphabets, there is a balance between the number of characters used to represent a language, and the number of elements in a message. English, using the conventional alphabet, averages about 6 letters (selections) per word (including the spaces between words). When represented in Morse code, the same text will require roughly 18 selections per word. By comparison, the basic Chinese vocabulary can be produced by selecting a single ideogram per word; however, thousands of ideograms exist. In general, having a larger number of characters in an alphabet allows each character to convey more meaning, but may make the selection of each specific character more difficult.

Many AAC systems use an expanded set of characters in the form of pictograms or icons to represent entire words that may be selected by the user. Such semantic compaction allows a large vocabulary to be stored within a device, but requires a system of selection that may add complexity to the device.[13] For example, a device may require the user to select a word group (e.g., food) prior to selecting a specific word (e.g., hamburger) from the group. Using subcategories, it is theoretically possible to represent a vocabulary of over two million words on a 128-key keypad with just three selections.

Prediction

Because messages in a language tend to follow similar patterns, it is possible to produce significant savings of effort using prediction technology. There are two types of prediction used in language: (1) word completion and (2) word/phrase prediction.

In word completion, a communication system (AAC or computer based) will, after each keystroke, present a number of options to the user representing words that might be typed. When the appropriate word is presented by the prediction system, the user may select that word directly rather than continuing to type out the entire word. Overall, this strategy may reduce the number of selections required to complete a message.[21] However, it may not improve typing speed.[27]

Anson[3] demonstrated that when typing from copy using the keyboard, typing speed was reduced in direct proportion to the frequency of using word prediction. The burden of constantly scanning the prediction list overwhelms the potential speed savings of word completion systems under these conditions. However, when typing using an on-screen keyboard or scanning system, where the user must scan the input array in any case, word completion does appear to increase typing speed as well as reduce the number of selections made.

Because most language is similar in structure, it is also possible, in some cases, to predict the word that will be used following a specific word. For example, after a person's first name is typed, they frequently will type their surname. When this prediction is possible, the next word may be generated with a single selection. When combined with word completion, next-word prediction has the potential to decrease the effort of typing substantially. However, in many cases, this potential is unrealized. Many users, even when provided with next-word prediction, become so involved in spelling words that they ignore the predictions even when they are accurate. The cognitive effort of switching between "typing mode" and "list scanning" mode may be greater than the cognitive benefit of not having to spell the word out.[19]

Compression/Expansion

Compression/expansion strategies allow limited sets of commonly used words to be stored in unambiguous abbreviations. When these abbreviations are selected, either letter-by-letter or through word completion, the abbreviation is dynamically replaced by the expanded form of the word or phrase.[2,14]

Because the expansion can be many selections long, this technology offers an enormous potential for energy and timesavings. However, the potential savings are available only when the user remembers to use the abbreviation rather than the expanded form of a word. Because of this limitation, abbreviations must be carefully selected. Many abbreviations are already in common use, and can be stored conveniently. Most people will refer to the television by the abbreviation TV, which requires just 20% of the selections to represent. With an expansion system, each use of TV can automatically be converted to "television" with no additional effort of the user. Similarly, TTFN might be used to store the social message, "Ta-ta for now."

Effective abbreviations will be unique to the user, rather than general. An example of an effective form of abbreviation would be the language shortcuts commonly used in note taking. These abbreviations form a shorthand generally unique to the individual, which allows complex thoughts to be represented on the page quickly in the course of a lecture. A clinician should work carefully with the client to develop abbreviations that will be useful and easily remembered.

Another form of "abbreviations" that is less demanding to create involves corrections of common spelling errors. For persons, either students or adult writers, who have cognitive deficits that influence spelling skills, expansions can be created to automatically correct misspelled words. In these cases, the "abbreviation" is the way that the client generally misspells the word, and the "expansion" is the correct spelling of the word. Once a library of misspelled words is created, the individual is relieved of the need to worry about the correct spelling. There are those who will maintain that this form of adaptation will prevent the individual from ever learning the correct spelling. In cases in which the client is still developing spelling skills, this is probably a valid concern, and the adaptation should not be used. But for the individual with a cognitive deficit, in which remediation is not possible, accommodation, through compression/expansion technology is a desirable choice.

None of these technologies will allow a person with a disability to produce messages at the same rate as an able-bodied person. However, individually and collectively, they can make generation of the message significantly more efficient than it would be without them. The techniques are not mutually exclusive. Icons can be predicted using "next word" techniques. Abbreviations can be used in conjunction with word completion and word prediction technologies.

OUTPUT OPTIONS

The control of assistive technologies involves a cycle of both human output and human input, matched to technology input and technology output. Individuals who have sensory limitations may have difficulty controlling assistive technologies (or common technologies) because they are unable to perceive the messages that are being sent to them by the technology. For these individuals, adaptations of the output of the technology may be required. These adaptations generally depend on one of three sensory modalities: (1) vision, (2) hearing, or (3) tactile sensation.

Visual Output

The default output of many types of electronic technology is visual. Computer screens are designed to resemble the printed page. AAC systems have input that looks like a keyboard and, generally, a graphical message composition area. EADLs use display panels and lighted icons to show current status of controlled devices. The perception of all of these controls depends on the user having visual acuity at nearly normal levels. When the client has some vision, but that vision is limited, some adaptations may be required.

Colors and contrast

Many types of visual impairment affect the ability to separate foreground and background colors. In addition, bright background colors can produce a visual glare that makes the foreground difficult to perceive. In accommodating visual deficits, the clinician should explore the colors that are easily perceived by the individual, and those that are difficult. Background colors, for most people, should be muted, soft colors that do not produce strong visual response. Icons and letters, on the other hand, may be represented in colors that provide visual contrast with the background. Very bright or strident colors should be avoided in both cases, and the specific colors and contrast levels required by the user must be selected on an individual basis.

Image size

Visual acuity and display size present difficulty in output displays that closely mirror the issues that ROM and fine motor skills present in keyboard design. A person with 20/20 vision can generally easily read text that is presented in letters about 1/6 of an inch high. (This is equivalent to a page printed in a 12-point font.) On a typical display, this allows the presentation of between 100 and 150 words of text at a time, or a similar number of icons for selection. If the user has lower visual acuity, the letter/icon size must be increased to accommodate that loss of acuity. Larger icons, however, require either fewer letters shown at a time, or increased display size. For people with severe visual limitations, as with individuals with severe fine motor limitations, it would be impractical to display all choices at once.

Screen enlargement programs[2] typically overcome this limitation by showing a part of the full screen at a time, and moving the portion that is expanded to the area most likely of interest to the user. The visual effect is similar to viewing the screen through a magnifying glass that the user moves over the display. Most programs can be configured to follow the text insertion point, the mouse pointer, or other changes on the display. Navigation is a serious problem with all such programs. When the user can see only a small portion of the screen at a time, the landmarks that are normally available to indicate the layout of the text on a page may be invisible because they are not in the field of view. Any screen enlargement program must provide a means of orienting to the location on the screen that is usable by the client.

AAC systems can accommodate the needs of a user with low visual acuity using precisely the same techniques that are used for the person with limited fine motor control. The keyboard of the device can be configured with fewer, larger keys, each of which has a larger symbol to represent its meaning. However, as with keyboards for those with physical limitations, the result is either fewer communication options or a more complex interface for the user. Also, these accommodations do not adapt the size of the message composition display, which may be inaccessible to the user with visual limitations.

Speech Output

It is very important to keep the difference between voice input and voice output clearly in mind. In voice input, the user speaks, and the spoken word is converted into commands within the assistive technology. In voice output, the device communicates with the user through auditory means, converting printed words or commands into voice. Voice output technology has been in existence for much longer than voice input, and is a more mature technology—not perfect, but more mature.

The demands of voice output are very different depending on the application and the intended listener. In general, this can be divided as systems where a second person is the listener, or the user is listener.

Second person as listener

When used in AAC applications, voice output is almost always intended to be understood by a person who may have little experience with synthetic voices. For example, if an AAC user is at the corner market, buying two pounds of hamburger for dinner, the butcher will have had very little experience with a synthetic voice. When asking for directions on the street corner, the listener will not only have little prior experience, but the AAC's voice will be competing with the sounds of trucks and buses.

To be understandable by novice listeners in real-world environments, a synthetic voice should be clear and as human sounding as possible. The voice will be easily understood to the extent that it sounds like what the listener expects to hear. Ideally, the voice should provide appropriate inflection in the spoken material, and should be able to convey emotional content. Current AAC systems do not convey emotional content well, but high-end voices do sound very much like a human speaker. Under adverse conditions, they will remain less understandable than a human speaker because facial and lip movements do not accompany synthetic voices and they provide additional cues as to the sounds being produced.

User as listener

When used for computer access or EADLs, voice quality need not be as human sounding. In either case, the user has the opportunity to learn to understand the voice during training. In EADL applications, there will be relatively few utterances that must be produced, and they can be designed to sound as different as possible, so that there is little chance of confusion. General voice output for an entire language is somewhat more difficult, however, because many words sound similar, and can be easily confused.

For general text reading, however, the primary issue is voicing speed. As noted earlier, humans generally talk between 150 and 175 words per minute. However, most humans also read between 300 and 400 words per minute. A person who depends on a human sounding voice for reading printed material will be limited to reading at less than half the speed of able-bodied readers. To be an effective text access method, synthetic voice must be understandable at speeds in excess of 400 words per minute. This will obviously require significant training, since untrained people without disabilities can't understand speech at such speeds. However, with training, speech output is a very useful way for a person with a visual limitation to access printed material.

Speech is a useful tool in two cases: (1) when it replaces voice for a person with a disability and (2) when the user is not able to use vision to access the technology. AAC devices using voice provide the most "normal" face-to-face communication available. Able-bodied people, in most conditions, communicate by voice. People with disabilities generally want to communicate in similar fashion. The other application of voice is "eyes-free" control. In the mass market for able-bodied consumers, these applications include presenting information over the telephone, while driving, or in other settings where a visual display might be difficult to use. All of these situations are important for people with disabilities as well. In addition, assistive technologies using voice output may be intended for use by people with print impairments. The category of print impairments includes conditions that result in very low vision and/or blindness, as well as conditions that result in the inability to translate visual stimuli to language and those that make manipulation of printed materials difficult.

The one weakness of voice output technologies lies in its use with people who are developing language skills. Because English is an irregular language, with many letter combinations making similar sounds, it is almost impossible to learn spelling by listening to the sound of words. As such, children who are blind from birth may not be good candidates for speech output as the primary language access method because the structure of words is lost when converted to speech. For these children, and for many others, tactile access is a better tool, and is, in fact, mandated under IDEA.[40]

Tactile Output

The oldest method for individuals with visual deficits to access printed material is Braille. In 1829, Louis Braille developed the idea of adapting a military system that allowed aiming artillery in darkness and writing secret messages, to provide a method of reading for students at the National Institute for the Young Blind in Paris.[9] Over time, this original system has been extended to allow communication of music, mathematics, and computer code to readers without vision. Basic Braille uses an array of six dots to represent letters and numbers. Traditional Braille, however, is only usable for static text, such as printed books. Dynamic information cannot be represented by raised dots on a sheet of paper.

Technology access requires the use of refreshable Braille. Refreshable Braille displays use a set of piezoelectric pins to represent Braille letters. Changing electrical signals to the display moves the pins up and down, allowing a single display to represent different portions of a longer document.

Braille is not widely used among individuals who are blind.[9] By some estimates, only 10% of the blind population know and use Braille. It is not usable by those who have limited tactile sensation as well as blindness. In spite of this, Braille is a skill that probably should be taught to a person who is blind. Most Braille readers are employed. Most people who are blind but do not read Braille are not employed. While Braille may not be an essential skill for employment, the ability to learn Braille certainly correlates with the ability to hold a job.[9]

SUMMARY

An occupational therapist should always keep in mind that disability makes few things impossible. It does make many things harder, and some sufficiently hard that they are "not worth it." Assistive technology can make many things easier for the person with a disability. Because they are easier, many things that were previously not worth the effort can become reasonable activities for a person with a disability. Assistive technology will never, in the terminology of the model of disability, remove the functional limitation. It can, however, prevent that functional limitation from resulting in a disability.

THREADED CASE STUDY: GIANNA, PART 2

Gianna has difficulty in her current areas of occupation of instrumental activities of daily living, education, and social participation, which might be addressed through assistive technology. She will continue to have deficits in her ADLs that will not be addressed through assistive technology. Through the use of an EADL, Gianna can gain control over her immediate environment. She will be able to control the temperature of her home, the radio, and/or television; control the lighting; and open doors as desired. Her verbal communication skills are excellent, but her ability to write letters to friends (graphical communications) would benefit from the same technologies (primarily mobility [not addressed in this chapter] and computer access) that will allow her to pursue her education. Although Gianna can write and print papers, she will not be able to hand them in without assistance, unless her professors allow electronic submission.

Considering Gianna's level of motor control, she might consider head pointing, Morse code, or speech recognition as a means of controlling her assistive technology. All of these technologies can be applied to computer control and to her EADL. A careful assessment by her therapist would determine which control strategy best meets her needs, and if the same control strategy would work for all of her AT applications.

Depending on the input method selected, Gianna might benefit from word prediction and abbreviation expansion for her text input. Since her vision and hearing are not affected, no changes to the output systems of her computer would be necessary.

Through the application of appropriate assistive technology, it becomes possible for Gianna to have more control over her life, both in terms of her immediate surroundings, and her future occupations. Gianna will be able to access online resources, write her papers for college, and ultimately, if she has the cognitive skills, become a successful lawyer. Her assistive technology does not guarantee that Gianna will succeed. It does give her the same opportunities to succeed or fail that her peers without functional limitations enjoy.

Review Questions

1. Compare and contrast rehabilitative and assistive technologies.
2. In what way do devices using universal design assist individuals with disabilities? Why aren't they considered to be assistive technologies?
3. According to the Human Interface Assessment model, why might a person with a disability not require any assistive technology in the completion of some tasks?
4. In pediatric applications, complex EADL devices might not be considered appropriate. What sort of EADL might be used with a very young child?
5. Some EADL devices allow control of the features of devices in the environment. Discuss the benefit of providing such control. What additional load does this place on the user?
6. AAC devices can be used to provide alternative or augmentative communication. Discuss the difference between these two strategies. Might an AAC device be a rehabilitation technology in some applications?
7. What is the value of having a message composition area that is independent from the message transmission feature of an AAC device? Discuss the value for the communicator and for the communication partner.
8. Discuss the difference between "conversation" and "formal presentation." How might each of these be important in an educational setting? What are the dominant demands of each type of communication?
9. How does a language disorder differ from a communication disorder? What sort of AAC device would help a person with a language disorder?
10. If an individual is able to use a physical keyboard, but is able to use only one hand, what keyboard options might help him or her with text production?
11. Consider the keypad providing control to a microwave oven. How might the keypad present difficulty to an individual who is blind? How might it be modified by an occupational therapist to improve its usability?
12. Word prediction and word completion are often touted as means to improve typing speed, yet the research suggests that it does not. What advantage might these technologies offer to improve productivity for a person with a disability?
13. Abbreviation expansion is generally considered as a means to type long words and phrases with only a few keystrokes, though this requires the user to remember the abbreviation. How else can this technology be used for individuals with learning disabilities, in ways that do not require memorization of keystroke sequences?
14. Refreshable Braille is expensive while text to speech is quite inexpensive. Yet Braille training is mandated by IDEA. What factors support the learning of this old technology for individuals who are blind?
15. Integrated control systems will allow a single control device to serve as the interface to a range of assistive technologies. What are the advantages of integrated control systems? Why might an integrated control system not be desirable for an individual user?

REFERENCES

1. Abbott B: *Human memory: Atkinson-Shiffrin model,* 2000. Retrieved July 29, 2004 from *http://users.ipfw.edu/abbott/120/ AtkinsonShifrin.html.*

2. Anson D: *Alternative computer access: a guide to selection,* Philadelphia, 1997, FA Davis.

3. Anson DK: The effect of word prediction on typing speed, *Am J Occup Ther* 47(11):1039, 1993.

4. Anson D, et al: Efficiency of the Chubon vs. the QWERTY keyboard, *Assistive Technol* 13:40, 2001.

5. Anson D, et al: *Long-term speed and accuracy of Morse code vs. head-pointer interface for text generation,* Paper presented at the RESNA 2004 Annual Conference, Orlando, FL, 2004.

6. Anson D, et al: Efficacy of three head-pointing devices for a mouse emulation task, *Assistive Technol* 14:140, 2002.

7. American Occupational Therapy Association Commission on Practice: Occupational therapy practice framework: domain and process, *Am J Occup Ther* 56:609, 2002.

8. Assistive Technology Act of 1998: 105-394, S.2432.

9. Canadian National Institute for the Blind: *Braille information center.* Retrieved July 29, 2004 from *http://www.cnib.ca/eng/braille_information/.*

10. Center for Assistive Technology: *Environmental control units.* Retrieved July 26, 2004 from *http://cat.buffalo.edu/newsletters/ecu.php.*

11. Center for Universal Design: *What is universal design?: principles of UD,* 1997. Retrieved July 29, 2004 from *http://www.design.ncsu.edu:8120/cud/univ_design/princ_overview.htm.*

12. Commission for the Blind and Visually Handicapped: *CBVH manual, rehabilitation technology - 8.20,* 3/31/2000, revised 2002. Retrieved July 29, 2004 from *http://www.nls.org/cbvh/8.20.htm.*

13. Conti B: *Semantic compaction systems — the home of Minspeak,* 2004. Retrieved July 30, 2004, from *http://www.minspeak.com/about1.html.*

14. Cook AM, Hussey SM: *Assistive technologies: principles and practice,* ed 2, St. Louis, 2002, Mosby.

15. DeVries RC, et al: A comparison of two computer access systems for functional text entry, *Am J Occup Ther* 52:656, 1998.

16. Ding D, et al: Integrated control and related technology of assistive devices, *Assistive Technol* 15:89, 2003.

17. Froumentin M: *W3C Math Home,* 2004. Retrieved July 30, 2004, from *http://www.w3.org/Math/.*

18. *General input device emulating interface (GIDEI) proposal,* 1994, revised 2002. Retrieved Aug. 1, 2004, from *http://trace.wisc.edu/docs/gidei/gidei.htm.*

19. Gibler CD, Childress DS: *Language anticipation with a computer-based scanning communication aid.* Paper presented at the IEEE Computer Society Workshop on Computing to the Handicapped, Charlottesville, VA, 1982.

20. Glennen SL, DeCoste DC: *The handbook of augmentative and alternative communication,* San Diego, 1997, Singular Publishers.

21. Hunnicutt S, Carlberger J: Improving word prediction using Markov models and heuristic methods, *Augmentative Alternative Communication* 17:255, 2001.

22. Intellitools: *Number Concepts 2,* 2004. Retrieved July 30, 2004, from *http://intellitools.com/.*

23. InterNational Committee for Information Technology Standards: *What exactly is V2 — and how does it work?* 2004. Retrieved July 30, 2004, from *http://www.myurc.com/whatis.htm.*

24. *International Morse Code basics,* 2001. Retrieved June 4, 2003, from *http://ac3l.com/morse.htm.*

25. Koester HH: *Abandonment of speech recognition by new users.* Paper presented at the RESNA 26th International Annual Conference, Atlanta, 2003.

26. Koester HH: *Performance of experienced speech recognition users.* Paper presented at the RESNA 26th International Annual Conference, Atlanta, 2003.

27. Koester HH, Levine SP: Effect of a word prediction feature on user performance, *Augmentative Alternative Communication* 12:155, 1996.

28. LC Technologies: *Detailed medical and technical information,* 2003. Retrieved July 30, 2004, from *http://www.eyegaze.com/2Products/Disability/Medicaldata.html.*

29. Light J: Interaction involving individuals using augmentative and alternative communication systems: state of the art and future directions, *Augmentative Alternative Communication* 4(2):66, 1988.

30. Lloyd LL, et al: *Augmentative and alternative communication: a handbook of principles and practices,* Boston, 1997, Allyn and Bacon.

31. MacNeil V: Electronic aids to daily living, *Team Rehabilitation Report* 9(3):53, 1998.

32. McDonald JB, et al: Advantages of Morse code as a computer input for school aged children with physical disabilities. In *Computers and the handicapped,* Ottawa, 1982, National Research Council of Canada.

33. Merzenich M, et al: Temporal processing deficits of language-learning impaired children ameliorated by training, *Science* 271:77, 1996.

34. Microsoft Research: *Machine learning and perception group: home & projects,* 2004. Retrieved July 30, 2004, from *http://research.microsoft.com/mlp/pages/home.htm.*

35. Miller GA: *Language and speech,* San Francisco, 1981, WH Freeman.

36. Morse 2000: *Development specification: Morse code input system for the Windows 2000 operating system,* 1999. Retrieved June 13, 1999, from *http://www.uwec.edu/academic/hss-or/Morse2000/MorseSpecification.doc.*

37. Quartet Technology: *Quartet Technology, Inc. — News,* 2004. Retrieved July 29, 2004, from *http://www.qtiusa.com/ProdOverview.asp?ProdTypeID=1.*

38. Tallal P, et al: Language comprehension in language-learning impaired children improved with acoustically modified speech, *Science* 271:81, 1996.

39. TechDis Accessibility Database Team: *TechDis PDA project — time management and organization,* 2002. Retrieved July 30, 2004, from *http://www.techdis.ac.uk/PDA/time.htm.*

40. Warger C: *New IDEA '97 requirements: factors to consider in developing an IEP,* 1999. Retrieved July 30, 2004, from *http://www.hoagiesgifted.org/eric/e578.html.*

RESOURCES

Tash Inc.
3512 Mayland Ct.
Richmond, VA 23233
http://www.tashinc.com

DU-IT Control Systems Group, Inc.
8765 Township Road #513
Shreve, OH 44676
216-567-2906
800-463-5685 or 905-686-4129

SmartHome, Inc.
16542 Millikan Avenue
Irvine, CA 92606-5027
221-9200 x109

asiHome
36 Gumbletown Rd. CS1
Paupack, PA 18451
800-263-8608
http://www.asihome.com/cgi-bin/ASIstore.pl?user_action=
detail&catalogno=X10PEX01

HAVi, Inc.
40994 Encyclopedia Circle Fremont, CA 94538
510-979-1394
Fax: 510-979-1390
www.havi.org

Infrared Data Association
http://www.irda.org/index.cfm

Quartet Technology, Inc.
87 Progress Avenue
Tyngsboro, MA 01879
978-649-4328

Madentec, Ltd.
4664 99 St.
Edmonton, Alberta
Canada T6E 5H5
877-623-3682
http://madentec.com

DynaVox Systems LLC
2100 Wharton Street, Suite 400
Pittsburgh, PA 15203
800-344-1778
http://www.dynavoxsys.com

ZYGO Industries, Inc.
P.O. Box 1008
Portland, OR 97207-1008
800-234-6006
http://www.zygo-usa.com/lighwrts.htm

newAbilities System Inc.
2938 Scott Blvd.
Santa Clara, CA 95054
http://www.newabilities.com/

Tegic Communications
2001 Western Avenue, Suite 250
Seattle, WA 98121
http://www.tegic.com

Dragon Systems, Inc.
320 Nevada Street
Newton, MA 02460
617-965-5200
FAX: 617-965-2374

PERFORMANCE SKILLS AND CLIENT FACTORS: EVALUATION AND INTERVENTION

17

OVERVIEW OF PERFORMANCE SKILLS AND CLIENT FACTORS

ANNE FISHER

KEY TERMS

Occupation
Task
Areas of occupation
Performance skills

Motor skills
Process skills
Communication/interaction
 skills

Body functions
Activities
Participation
Performance analysis

Client-centered assessment
Adaptive occupation
Restorative occupation

LEARNING OBJECTIVES

After studying this chapter the student or practitioner will be able to do the following:

1. Describe the relationship between performance skills and the Occupational Therapy Practice Framework areas of occupation and client factors (specifically, body functions).
2. Describe the relationship between performance skills and the International Classification of Functioning, Disability, and Health components of activities and participation, and body functions and body structures (specifically, body functions).
3. Explain why performance skills are parallel concepts to many of the International Classification of Functioning, Disability, and Health activity and participation domain subcategories.

4. Explain the difference between performance skills and body functions.
5. Understand how performance skills are observed and assessed, using both informal and standardized assessment methods.
6. Understand the differences among tasks, activities, and occupations.
7. Explain the differences between performance analyses and task analyses.
8. Discuss the difference between top-down and bottom-up reasoning and evaluation.

CHAPTER OUTLINE

Occupation and performance skills (vs. tasks)
 Areas of occupation
 Performance skills
International classification of functioning, disability, and health
 Body functions
 Activities and participation
 Differentiating among body functions, actions, and tasks
Comparing the ICF to the framework

Avoiding confusion between framework performance skills and ICF
 body functions
Evaluation of performance skills
 Nonstandardized performance analysis
 Standardized performance analysis
 Assessment of motor and process skills
 Performance analyses vs. task analyses
Summary

THREADED CASE STUDY: JOHN, PART 1

Kim and Maria (Kim's supervisor) both observed Kim's client John, a 72-year-old man who was 3 months post bilateral *cerebral vascular accident* (CVA). When Kim was asked to describe the results of her occupational therapy evaluation, she shared the following information with the team: John wants to return home to his own apartment. To be able to do this, he prioritized several daily life tasks he felt most important. One of them was to be able to prepare a pot of coffee independently.

When Kim observed John in the kitchen making a pot of coffee, he demonstrated markedly increased effort and moderate inefficiency. He needed frequent verbal and standby assistance with preparing coffee and was at risk for a fall when standing and reaching for task objects from overhead cupboards.

More specifically, John had marked increase in effort and moderate inefficiency when moving his wheelchair around the kitchen. As a result, he also had marked increase in effort and moderate inefficiency when positioning his wheelchair at the refrigerator or the counter, and transporting task objects from the refrigerator to the counter and back again. When he stood up to reach for the coffee cups from an overhead cupboard, he was very unstable and at risk of a fall. He was able to grasp and lift task objects, and to remove and replace the lid of the coffee can by stabilizing the can between his knees and using his right arm to remove and reapply the lid. Although he selected the task tools and materials he had said he would use,

he collected needed task objects (coffee, coffee cup, milk, sugar) into different workspaces. He paused frequently as he carried out the coffee-making task, and his overall performance was slow. Finally, John was unable to independently adapt his performance to overcome these problems, and his problems persisted throughout the task performance.

When Kim evaluated John, she used a true top-down reasoning and evaluation process. That is, after gathering background information about John, including his interests, goals, and priorities for intervention, she focused the next phase of her evaluation first on global occupation and then on performance skills, the smallest observable units of occupation. She reported the results of this evaluation process to the team. Her implementation of this top-down reasoning and evaluation process that included the evaluation of performance skills will enable Kim to implement true top-down, occupation-focused, and client-centered occupational therapy services to enable John to achieve his goal of returning to his own apartment.

Critical Thinking Questions

1. What are performance skills and how do occupational therapists evaluate them?
2. How do performance skills differ from body functions?
3. What are performance analyses and why are they critical to true top-down reasoning and evaluation?

The focus of this chapter is to provide background information needed for occupational therapists to understand and evaluate performance skills. Performance skills are the smallest observable units of occupation and this chapter will clarify how occupation and performance skills are virtually synonymous. To accomplish this, performance skills will first be introduced and defined, then placed in the context of both the Occupational Therapy Practice Framework (Framework)[1] and the World Health Organization's (WHO) *International Classification of Functioning, Disability, and Health* (ICF).[65] Performance skills will then be placed into the context of the Framework by first discussing areas of occupation and then relating performance skills to these areas of occupation. In that process, performance skills will be defined in more detail. From there, performance skills will be compared and contrasted to the body functions and the activities and participation domains categorized in the ICF. Then, after discussing the interrelationship among performance skills, the activities and participation domains, and occupation, a description will be provided of how we can evaluate performance skills in everyday practice using both informal and standardized performance analyses. As part of that discussion, the importance of an evaluation focused on occupational performance, also known as a top-down approach to evaluation, will be included, and

then contrast (1) performance evaluations and analyses with (2) evaluations of body functions, the environment, and task analysis. Finally, how the results of a standardized performance analysis, the *Assessment of Motor and Process Skills* (AMPS),[16,18] can be used to facilitate intervention planning and document intervention outcomes will be demonstrated.

OCCUPATION AND PERFORMANCE SKILLS (VS. TASKS)

Occupation is the action of seizing, taking possession of, or occupying space or time. It is also a series of actions in which one is engaged.[56] Occupation, therefore, clearly pertains to the carrying out of actions—doing something—not what is done. What is done is the task; a **task** is the unit of action that will be done once the person is finished performing.[50] To complete the circle, we can say that the *doing* of it— *performing* the task—is occupation.

As we continue to analyze our definition of occupation, we can begin with the idea that occupation is action or a series of actions. In the Framework,[1] these actions are called performance skills. If we think about a person's observable actions, we can also consider the idea that each action may be more or less skilled. If these actions are more or less skilled, then the occupation will be more or less skilled. That is, when we observe a person performing a task, we might observe skilled task performance; each individual action the person performs will be detectable as a skilled action. Likewise, if some or all of the actions the person performs reflect less skill, we will observe a task performance that reflects less skill. Therefore, we can view performance skill, skilled task performance, and skilled occupation as virtual synonyms (Box 17-1).

In looking further at the definition of occupation, we realize that the definition tells us that occupation is not just action or a series of actions, but a series of actions in which one is engaged. That we are engaged in the actions stresses the important relationship between the performance of daily life tasks and engagement in that performance. The Framework states that "occupational therapy's unique focus [is] on occupation and daily life activities and the application of an intervention process that facilitates engagement in occupation" (p. 609).[1] The task performances that we engage in are those that we experience as having meaning, purpose, and relevance to life. Thus, the Framework goes on to stress that occupations are activities that have "unique meaning and purpose in a person's life" (p. 610).[1] If we look more carefully at the terms *action*, *activity*, *doing*, and *occupation*, they all relate to the idea that something is happening or that something is moving.

Contrast these terms with the term task. Task does not convey a sense that something is happening or that there is movement. Rather, the task is more accurately viewed as the specified or defined piece of work to be done,[50] in other words, what will be (or was) done when the performance or series of actions comes to a termination point. For example, we might say that we read a chapter in a book, got dressed, went for a walk, or took a nap. It is only when we are reading the chapter, getting dressed, going for the walk, or taking a nap

that we have occupational or task performances. Now we can observe action or a series of actions.

What is unique about the term "occupation" as we use it in our profession, is that we emphasize the idea of one being engaged in what is happening or what one is doing. According to the Framework, this engagement in what is happening or what one is doing is the ultimate goal of occupational therapy.

AREAS OF OCCUPATION

As we use the Framework to think more about occupation, we begin by focusing on areas of occupation. **Areas of occupation** represent a taxonomy for categorizing daily life activities (occupations, not tasks) into groups (Box 17-2). For example, bathing, dressing, and feeding are included in the category of activities of daily living (ADLs).

In the Framework, most of the definitions of activities listed in each area of occupation are clearly defined in terms of action, doing, or occupation. Unfortunately, not all of the activities have been defined in this way. Instead, some are defined more like tasks or as a list of tasks. In Box 17-3, two

---

BOX 17-2   AREAS OF OCCUPATION CATEGORIZED IN THE FRAMEWORK

Activities of daily living (ADLs)
Instrumental activities of daily living (IADLs)
Education
Work
Play
Leisure
Social participation

BOX 17-1   WHY DON'T WE TALK ABOUT SKILLED OCCUPATION?

While we do not commonly talk about skilled occupation, the reason is not clear. We can speculate, however, about possible reasons. First, to talk of skilled occupation feels unfamiliar and, hence awkward, almost as if we are grammatically incorrect. The result may be that occupational therapy authors (including myself) instead tend to use the phrases *skilled occupational performance* and *skilled task performance* to convey skilled occupation—actually performing the task in a skilled manner. Second, many occupational therapy authors incorrectly use the terms *task* and *occupation* interchangeably, or they use the term *occupation* as a replacement for the term *task*. For example, such an author may incorrectly call the occupation of *dressing* a task. The task is to dress oneself or to get dressed. It becomes occupation when the person is dressing or getting dressed. Therefore, if we prefer not to talk about skilled occupation, we should refer instead to skilled task performance, not skilled occupational performance.

BOX 17-3   EXAMPLES OF ACTIVITIES CORRECTLY DEFINED IN THE FRAMEWORK AS OCCUPATIONS VS. EXAMPLES INCORRECTLY DEFINED IN TERMS OF TASKS PERFORMED

Occupations (something is happening, the person is doing something):
- Shopping: Preparing shopping lists (grocery and other), selecting and purchasing items, selecting method of payment, and completing money transactions
- Informal personal education participation: Participating in classes, programs, and activities that provide instruction/ training in identified areas of interest
Tasks (what the person will do or what will be done if the person does it):
- Sleep/rest: A period of inactivity in which one may or may not suspend consciousness
- Formal educational participation: Including the categories of nonacademic (e.g., recess, lunchroom, hallway), extracurricular (e.g., sports, band, cheerleading, dances, and vocational) participation

sets of activity definitions from the Framework are presented. The first set, labeled occupations, has been defined in terms of action, doing, or occupation. The second set, labeled tasks, has been defined in terms of tasks. If we compare the two sets of definitions in Box 17-3, we can see that in the first set there is a clear sense of something happening, typically conveyed by the use of the continuous or progressive verb tense, taking the form of "-ing" (e.g., preparing something, selecting something, participating in something). In the second set, we find definitions and names of what is done or what is to happen (e.g., a period of inactivity, recess, sports).

We might be tempted to think that sleep and rest are not associated with action or something happening. Yet even when we think of someone doing nothing (e.g., sleeping, listening to the radio, or sitting under a tree and watching the clouds pass overhead), we can observe an action or series of actions that unfolds over time (e.g., walking over to the bed, lying down, closing one's eyes, sleeping, snoring, waking up, rolling over, standing up, rubbing one's eyes).[21]

PERFORMANCE SKILLS

Performance skills pertain to the individual goal-directed actions of occupation. More specifically, **performance skills** are small units of observable action that are connected or linked together one-by-one in the process of building or executing a daily life task performance.[16,21,23] These small units of action are always goal-directed because they are enacted in the context of carrying out and completing a daily life task (Box 17-4). If we think of a task performance as a chain (which can vary in length just as task performances vary in complexity or duration), then the performance skills are the individual links (rings) that must be connected together to construct the more global, larger whole, i.e., the chain.[21] For example:

As Mark observed Sara, a 7-year-old student referred to him for an occupational therapy evaluation because of concerns

---

Box **17-4**   DEFINING GOAL DIRECTED WHEN CONSIDERED IN THE CONTEXT OF A DAILY LIFE TASK PERFORMANCE

Goal directed means that there is a specific purpose or outcome of the action and also that the action is performed in the natural context of the overall daily life task performance. The purpose of the action is always intrinsic to the execution of the task, whether or not the overall task performance has an intrinsic or extrinsic purpose.

While one can argue that (1) raising one's arm to 90° of flexion when directed to do so or (2) turning a door knob, out of the context of opening a door for purposes of going through the doorway, are goal directed, they do not meet the criterion of being a goal directed action performed within the context of a daily life task performance.

---

about her schoolwork task performance, he observed the following actions as she colored a picture of a cat:

Sara *reached* for, *chose*, *grasped*, and *lifted* a red crayon. She then *manipulated* the crayon to reposition it in her hand and alter her grasp of the crayon as she prepared to begin to color. After pausing, she *initiated* coloring the body of the cat. As she *continued* to color, she *moved* the crayon back and forth across the paper, *pressing* downward on the crayon with so much force that the crayon broke.

It does not matter what task performance we observe, we can always observe and then describe, action by action, what we observed. The smallest occupations (actions) we observe are the performance skills. The task was to color the cat. The more global occupation was *coloring* a picture of a cat. The smallest occupations included reaching for and grasping the crayon, and so forth. They were occupations because Sara was engaged in the task performance.

In Sara's case, we can note that some actions seemed to have been more skilled than were others. Of course, we do not know for sure, because the description above does not include any qualifiers that describe the quality of her performance. Adding those qualifiers will become part of the evaluation process discussed later in this chapter. Nevertheless, we can conclude that Sara pressed too hard on the crayon, a behavior that reflects less "pressing" skill.

In social contexts, we can also observe actions related to social interactions with others. For example:

When Stephan was sitting at a table with a group of his clients who were planning a group outing to a local restaurant, he focused his observations on José as he interacted with the other clients. This is a brief segment from what he observed (and heard):

When the other clients spoke to José, he often *looked* down toward his hands and did not *turn* or *look* at whoever was speaking to him. When Mike (another client) asked José what type of food he wanted to eat, Stephan could faintly hear José *mumbling*, "D'know."

Origin of Performance Skills

Performance skills have been divided into three taxonomies in the Framework: motor skills, process skills, and communication/interaction skills.[1] The first two taxonomies are derived from the AMPS.[16-18] The earliest work on the process skill definitions began as a collaborative effort between this author and Gary Kielhofner in 1987 and 1988. The first complete set of operational definitions of the motor and process skills was reported in 1989 in the first research edition of the AMPS.[15] Since that time, they have been incorporated into the Model of Human Occupation,[38,39] the Occupational Therapy Intervention Process Model,[21,23] and, most recently, the Framework.[1] The definitions in the Framework come from an earlier edition of the AMPS.[17] More recently, I have modified the definitions of the motor and process skills presented in the Framework.[16,18,25] They also can be used for informal

Box **17-5**	MOTOR SKILLS AND THEIR RELATED ICF CODES

MOTOR SKILLS: Observed actions that represent the quality of occupational performance as a person interacts with and moves task objects, and moves oneself around the task environment.

BODY POSITION

- Stabilizes: Maintains an upright sitting or standing position while moving through the task environment or interacting with task objects such that there is no evidence of *momentary* propping or loss of balance that affects task performance (**d4153**, **d4154**).
- Aligns: Sustains an upright sitting or standing position, as required during the task performance, such that there is no evidence of *persistent* propping, leaning, or loss of balance that affects the ongoing task performance (**d4153**, **d4154**).
- Positions: Positions body, arms, or wheelchair in relation to task objects (i.e., not too close or too far away) and as required for promoting the use of *efficient arm movements* during task performance (no parallel ICF code).

OBTAINING AND HOLDING OBJECTS

- Reaches: Extends the arm, *and when appropriate, bends the trunk*, to effectively grasp or place task objects that are out of reach; includes skillfully using a reacher to obtain task objects (**d4452**).
- Bends: Actively flexes, rotates, or twists the trunk in a manner and direction appropriate to the task, as when bending to pick up a task object from the floor or to sit down in a chair or on a bed (**d4105**, **d4104**).
- Grips: Pinches or grasps task objects such that the task object does not slip (e.g., from the person's fingers or hand, from between the teeth) (**d4400**, **d4401**).
- Manipulates: Uses dexterous grasp and release patterns, isolated finger movements, and coordinated *in-hand manipulation* patterns when interacting with small task objects (e.g., difficulty manipulating buttons when buttoning, difficulty using isolated finger movements to open and close scissors when cutting) (**d4402**).
- Coordinates: Uses two or more body parts together to stabilize and manipulate task objects during bilateral motor tasks, such as when holding paper in one hand when cutting with scissors held

in the other hand, or holding a jar between the knees when removing the lid (no parallel ICF code; do *not* confuse with Body Functions code **b7602**).

MOVING SELF AND OBJECTS

- Moves: Pushes or pulls task objects along a supporting surface, pulls to open or pushes to close doors and drawers, or pushes on wheels to propel a wheelchair (**d4450**, **d4451**).
- Lifts: Raises or lifts task objects; includes lifting an object from one place to another, but without ambulating or moving from one place to another (**d4300**).
- Walks: Ambulates on level surfaces and changes direction while walking without shuffling the feet, lurching, instability, propping, or using assistive devices (e.g., cane, walker, wheelchair) during the task performance (**d450**, especially **d4500**).
- Transports: Carries task objects from one place to another while walking, seated in a wheelchair, or using a walker (**d4301**, **d4302**, **d4303**, **d4304**).
- Calibrates: Regulates or grades the force, speed, and extent of movements when interacting with task objects (e.g., not too much or too little—not crushing task objects, not banging a task object when placing it on a table, pushing a door with enough force that it closes) (no parallel ICF code; do *not* confuse with Body Functions codes **b760** or **b765**).
- Flows: Uses smooth and fluid *arm and wrist* movements when interacting with task objects (no parallel ICF code; do *not* confuse with Body Functions codes **b7650** or **b7651**).

SUSTAINING PERFORMANCE

- Endures: Persists and completes the task without *obvious* evidence of physical fatigue, pausing to rest, or stopping to "catch ones breath" (no parallel ICF code; do not confuse with Body Functions code **b445**, as the focus of Endures is not on underlying respiratory or cardiovascular capacity).
- Paces: Maintains a consistent and effective rate or tempo of performance throughout the performance of actions and steps of the entire task (**d2100**, **d2101**, **d2200**, **d2201**, **d2302**). (Note: Paces is both a motor skill and a process skill, but we score it only once, based on the person's overall rate or tempo of performance.)

From Fisher AG: *Occupational therapy intervention process model: a model for planning and implementing top-down, client-centered, and occupation-based occupational therapy interventions,* manuscript in preparation, 2005.

evaluation of performance skills.[21] These modified definitions are shown in Boxes 17-5 and 17-6.

The communication/interaction skills were first operationalized and reported in *The Assessment of Communication and Interaction Skill.*[27] They also have been incorporated into the Model of Human Occupation[38,39] and the Framework.[1] In 1995, Fisher and Kielhofner[26] reported two social skill taxonomies, the communication/interaction skills and the social interaction skills. The latter were based on the Assessment of Social Interaction[14] but have recently been

updated to provide an even more comprehensive taxonomy.[21] These revised and expanded social interaction skills are listed in Box 17-7.

Motor skills

Motor skills are the observable, goal-directed actions that a person carries out one-by-one during naturalistic and relevant daily life task performances as the person interacts with and moves task objects, and moves oneself around the task environment (Box 17-8).

| Box **17-6** | PROCESS SKILLS AND THEIR RELATED ICF CODES |

PROCESS SKILLS: Observed actions that represent the quality of occupational performance as a person (1) selects, interacts with, and uses task tools and materials; (2) carries out individual actions and steps; and (3) modifies performance when problems are encountered.

SUSTAINING PERFORMANCE

- Paces: Maintains a consistent and effective rate or tempo of performance throughout the performance of actions and steps of the entire task (**d2100, d2101, d2200, d2201, d2302**). (Note: Paces is both a motor skill and a process skill, but we score it only once, based on the person's overall rate or tempo of performance.)
- Attends: Maintains focus on the task performance such that the person does not look away from what he or she is doing (e.g., toward extraneous auditory or visual stimuli), thus interrupting the ongoing task progression (**d160**).
- Heeds: Uses goal-directed task actions that are focused toward carrying out and completing a specified task (i.e., the outcome originally agreed on or specified by another), and using task materials that were specified (e.g., making brewed coffee, not instant coffee, if the client specified that he or she would make brewed coffee; writing sentences with a pencil, not a marker, if the students' teacher specified that they were to write with pencils) (possibly **d210**, but **d210** is more vague in that it only includes carrying out and completing a task).

APPLYING KNOWLEDGE

- Chooses: Selects necessary and appropriate type and number of tools and materials for the task; includes choosing the tools and materials that the person specified he or she would use prior to the initiation of the task (no parallel ICF code, but choosing needed task objects can be viewed as an undefined element of **d210**).
- Uses: Employs tools and materials (1) as they are intended (e.g., using a knife to cut or spread, but not to stir foods; using a pencil sharpener to sharpen a pencil, but not to sharpen a crayon), and (2) in a reasonable (including hygienic) fashion, given their intrinsic properties and the availability (or lack of availability) of other objects (no parallel ICF code, but using needed task objects appropriately can be viewed as an undefined element of **d210**).
- Handles: Supports, stabilizes, and holds tools and materials in an appropriate manner, protecting them from damage, slipping, moving, or falling (no parallel ICF code, but handling task objects appropriately can be viewed as an undefined element of **d210**).
- Inquires: (1) Seeks needed verbal or written information by asking questions or reading directions or labels and (2) does not ask for information in situations where the person has been fully oriented to the task and environment and had immediate prior awareness of the answer (e.g., asking where task tools or materials are located after having just placed them where he or

she wanted them) (**d166** [reading directions or labels]; asking questions has no parallel ICF code, but can be viewed as an undefined element of **d350**).

TEMPORAL ORGANIZATION

- Initiates: Starts or begins *the next* action or step without hesitation; does not include having to complete the action or step (**d210**, but **d210** places the emphasis on initiating the overall task, not the individual actions or steps that comprise the task).
- Continues: Performs single sustained actions or a series of step actions (e.g., cutting actions when slicing a carrot, erasing actions when erasing a mistake, letter writing actions when writing a word) without unnecessary interruptions or pauses such that once an action or task step is initiated, the individual continues on until the action or step is completed (no parallel ICF code, but continuing action without interruption can be viewed as a component of sustaining a task, **d210**, or as part of carrying out simple or complex and coordinated actions of integrated or complex tasks, **d220**).
- Sequences: Performs steps in an effective or logical order for efficient use of time and energy; and with an absence of (1) randomness or lack of logic in the ordering and/or (2) inappropriate repetition of steps (no parallel ICF code, but sequencing task steps appropriately can be viewed as a component of sustaining a task, **d210**, or as part of carrying out simple or complex and coordinated actions of integrated or complex tasks, **d220**).
- Terminates: Brings to completion *single actions* or *single steps* without inappropriate persistence (i.e., continues to perform the action or step beyond what is needed or required) or premature cessation (i.e., stops performing the action or step before it is completed) (no parallel ICF code, but terminating single actions and single steps can be viewed as a component of sustaining a task, **d210**, or as part of carrying out simple or complex and coordinated actions of integrated or complex tasks, **d220**).

ORGANIZING SPACE AND OBJECTS

- Searches/Locates: Looks for and locates *tools and materials* in a logical manner, both within and beyond the immediate environment; includes not asking where task objects are located before looking for them, provided the person was aware prior to beginning the task where tools and materials are located (no parallel ICF code, but searching for and finding task objects can be viewed as a component of preparing and organizing materials, **d210**).
- Gathers: Collects together needed or misplaced tools and materials, including (a) collecting related tools and materials into the same workspace; and (b) collecting and replacing materials that have spilled, fallen, or been misplaced (no parallel ICF code, but gathering task objects can be viewed as a component of preparing and organizing materials, **d210**).

Continued

BOX **17-6** PROCESS SKILLS AND THEIR RELATED ICF CODES—CONT'D

- Organizes: Logically positions or spatially arranges tools and materials in an orderly fashion (1) within a single workspace and (2) between multiple appropriate workspaces, in order to facilitate ease of task performance (e.g., the workspace is not too spread out or too crowded); includes spatially arranging clothing such as when getting dressed or ironing (no parallel ICF code, but organizing task objects within and between workspaces can be viewed as a component of organizing space and materials, **d210**).
- Restores: (1) Puts away tools and materials in appropriate places, (2) restores immediate workspace(s) to original condition (e.g., wiping work surface clean, putting tools and materials away in cupboards or drawers), (3) closes and seals containers and coverings when indicated, and (4) saves work on a computer before exiting the program (no parallel ICF code, but restoring task objects appropriately can be viewed as an undefined element of **d210**).
- Navigates: Modifies the movement pattern of the arm, body, or wheelchair to maneuver around obstacles that are encountered in the course of moving through space, such that undesirable contact with obstacles (e.g., knocking over, bumping into) is avoided; includes holding and maneuvering objects around obstacles (no parallel ICF code, but navigating the body or body parts around obstacles can be viewed as an undefined element of **d210**). (Note: Navigates should be viewed as a skill related to organizing oneself in space, not a skill related to mobility.)

ADAPTING PERFORMANCE

- Notices/Responds: Responds appropriately to (1) nonverbal task-related cues (e.g., task object rolling, appliance heating, liquid dripping) that provide feedback regarding task progression, (2) the spatial arrangement of objects to one another (e.g., alignment of objects during stacking, alignment of numbers on a page), and notices and responds to cupboard doors or drawers that have been left open during the task performance. Notices and, when indicated, makes an effective and efficient response (no parallel ICF code; noticing and responding to task-related cues is related to modification of one's task performance to prevent or correct errors, possibly an undefined adaptation element in **d2**).

- Adjusts: Changes working environments in anticipation of, or in response to, problems that arise; anticipates or responds to problems effectively by making some change (1) between workspaces by moving to a new workspace or bringing in or removing tools and materials from the present workspace or (2) in an environmental condition (e.g., turning on or off the tap, turning up or down the temperature) (no parallel ICF code; adjusting by changing the working environment is related to modification of one's task performance to prevent or correct errors, possibly an undefined adaptation element in **d2**).
- Accommodates: Modifies actions or the location of objects within the workspace, in anticipation of, or in response to, problems that might arise; anticipates or responds to problems effectively by (1) changing the method with which one is performing an action sequence, (2) changing the manner in which one interacts with or handles tools and materials already in the workspace, and (3) asking for assistance when appropriate or needed (no parallel ICF code; accommodating by changing how one interacts with task objects is related to modification of one's task performance to prevent or correct errors, possibly an undefined adaptation element in **d2**).
- Benefits: Anticipates and prevents undesirable circumstances or problems from recurring or persisting; includes responding appropriately to verbal cues intended to lead to correction of errors (no parallel ICF code; benefiting such that problems in performance do not recur or persist is related to modification of one's task performance to prevent or correct errors, possibly an undefined adaptation element in **d2**).

From Fisher AG: *Occupational therapy intervention process model: a model for planning and implementing top-down, client-centered, and occupation-based occupational therapy interventions,* manuscript in preparation, 2005.

Mark observed motor skills during a naturalistic and relevant daily life task performance when he saw Sara reach for, grasp (*grip*), and *lift* the crayon. He also observed motor skills when he observed her *manipulate* the crayon as she repositioned it in her hand and altered her grasp. Finally, he observed motor skills when he saw her *move* the crayon back and forth across the paper, and press downward (*calibrate*) on the crayon with so much force that the crayon broke (see Box 17-5).

Process skills

Process skills are the observable, goal-directed actions that a person carries out one-by-one during naturalistic and relevant daily life task performances as the person (1) selects, interacts with, and uses task tools and materials; (2) carries out individual actions and steps; and (3) modifies performance when problems are encountered.

Mark observed process skills during a naturalistic and relevant daily life task performance when he saw Sara *choose* the red crayon, and then pause before she *initiated* coloring the body of the cat. He also observed a process skill as he watched her *continue* to color (see Box 17-6).

Communication/interaction skills

Like motor and process skills, **communication/interaction skills** (and their social interaction skills counterpart) are observable, goal-directed actions that a person carries out one-by-one during naturalistic and relevant daily life task performances. The key difference is that, while motor and

Box **17-7** SOCIAL INTERACTION SKILLS AND THEIR RELATED ICF CODES

SOCIAL INTERACTION SKILLS: Observed actions that represent the quality of occupational performance as a person communicates and interacts with others in the social task environment.

INITIATING AND TERMINATING SOCIAL INTERACTION

- Approaches/Starts: Uses appropriate strategies to approach and initiate interaction with the social partner; includes catching the attention of the social partner through (a) asking a question or (b) sending a greeting or introductory phrase to start a social interaction (**d3500**).
- Greets: Uses appropriate words, phrases, gestures, and ceremonies to greet the social partner, as appropriate, given the social context and the degree of familiarity with the social partner; includes responding to the arrival of or greeting from the social partner by (1) turning toward and making eye contact with the social partner and/or (2) verbalizing a responsorial greeting to (e.g., saying, "Hi"), gesturing toward (e.g., waving, nodding), or touching (e.g., shaking hands, embracing) the social partner (no parallel ICF code).
- Concludes/Disengages: Terminates the conversation or social interaction using customary termination statements, brings to closure the topic under discussion, and disengages or says goodbye using appropriate phrases and ceremonies as appropriate to the context and degree of familiarity with the social partner; includes the ability to send verbal and nonverbal messages that termination is desired, and then using appropriate strategies to carry the termination of the conversation or social interaction through to an appropriate end (**d3502**).

PRODUCING SOCIAL INTERACTION

- Produces Speech: Produces spoken or signed messages with literal meaning; includes producing clearly articulated speech that is audible and expresses meaning, given the social context (**d330, d335**).
- Gesticulates: Uses socially appropriate gestures (e.g., shaking one's head, frowning, smiling, waving one's hand) to send signals to one's social partner (**d3350**).
- Speaks Fluently: Speaks in a fluent and continuous manner with an even flow (not too fast, not too slow) and appropriate intonation; includes speaking without too many pauses and awkward or long delays *during* the message (no parallel ICF code; do not confuse with Body Functions codes **b3300, b3301,** and **b3302** that focus on speech impairments).

PHYSICALLY SUPPORTING SOCIAL INTERACTION

- Turns Toward: Actively positions or turns the body and face toward the social partner or the person who is speaking (no parallel ICF code).
- Looks: Makes eye contact with the social partner in a manner that is relaxed; includes adjusting the frequency and duration of eye contact to match that of the social partner (no parallel ICF code).

- Places Self: Places oneself at an appropriate distance from the social partner, given the context and the degree of familiarity with the social partner; implies acting according to the social partner's cues about personal space, and adjusting one's distance to the type of social interaction and degree of familiarity with social partner (**d7204**).
- Touches: Responds to and uses touch or bodily contact in a manner that is socially appropriate (**d7105**).
- Regulates: Controls impulses and behaviors that are not appropriate to a social situation; includes assuming body positions that are appropriate to type of social interaction and degree of familiarity with the social partner (**d7202** and, possibly, **d3350**).

SHAPING CONTENT OF SOCIAL INTERACTION

- Questions: Requests facts and information or asks questions that are relevant to the social context and the degree of familiarity with the social partner (e.g., asking questions in order to seek socially relevant information about the partner's opinions, interests, or needs; asking questions needed to manage a task); includes asking and then waiting for the answer (possibly **d3503** as part of shaping a conversation).
- Answers: Gives relevant replies to questions; includes providing factual information and/or elaborating (i.e., by providing personal opinions, expressing feelings); also includes giving a relevant reply to an apology or feedback expressed by the social partner (no parallel ICF code).
- Discloses: Shares personal information, experiences, feelings, opinions, and thoughts in an appropriate manner, given the social context and degree of familiarity with the social partner; implies sharing at a level that corresponds to social partner's degree of openness, provided that level is also appropriate; includes revealing personal information in a gradual, step by step manner that matches the social partner's level of disclosure (**d710**).
- Expresses Emotions: Shares emotions in a way that is socially acceptable and appropriate to the context and the level of familiarity with the social partner; includes expressing emotion through one's facial expression or tone of voice in a manner that reflects the same emotion as the social partner's message (e.g., showing empathy, expressing concern); also includes expressing appropriate affect with words and/or corresponding nonverbal signals (e.g., facial expressions, hugs) (**d3350, d7202**).
- Critiques: Expresses differences of opinion in a socially appropriate manner and as appropriate to the social context and degree of familiarity with the social partner (**d7103**).
- Thanks: Uses appropriate words, phrases, gestures, and ceremonies to confirm receipt of services, offers, gifts, and/or compliments; includes expressing gratitude for the generosity or kindness shown by the social partner or showing conventional courtesy in the context of economical transactions involving goods and services (no parallel ICF code).

Continued

BOX **17-7**   SOCIAL INTERACTION SKILLS AND THEIR RELATED ICF CODES—CONT'D

MAINTAINING FLOW OF SOCIAL INTERACTION

- Extends/Sustains: Keeps the conversation going by adding ideas or elaborating on the topics being discussed, introducing new ideas, or returning to previously mentioned topics; includes sending messages that are more than one or two words (when more would be appropriate), are not circuitous, and that focus on the topic being discussed (**d3501**).
- Transitions: Smoothly transitions the conversation to a closely related topic, and/or changes the topic without disrupting the conversation (**d3505**).
- Completes: Sends a complete message with a clear end-point (possibly **d3503** as part of maintaining a conversation).

TIMING SOCIAL INTERACTION

- Times Response: Replies to social messages without delay or hesitation (no parallel ICF code).
- Times Duration: Speaks for reasonable time periods that are appropriate, given the social partner and the context; includes adjusting the length of one's turn, depending on the situation and the complexity of the message (possibly **d3503** as part of maintaining a conversation).
- Takes Turns: Awaits one's turn and gives social partner the freedom to take his or her turn; includes sending cues or messages that signal whose turn it is to send a message, as well as taking one's own turn at the appropriate time; also includes not allowing oneself to be dominated by others (**d3501**).

VERBALLY SUPPORTING SOCIAL INTERACTION

- Matches Language: Uses language and level of address that is appropriate to the situation and social partner's abilities and level of understanding; implies being able to control and vary one's level of language according to (1) the type of social interaction (e.g., formal speech vs. casual conversation), (2) the level of language used by the social partner (e.g., that of the child vs. that of an adult), and (3) the degree of familiarity with the social partner (no parallel ICF code).
- Clarifies: Ensures, in a manner appropriate to the social context and the degree of familiarity with the social partner, that the social partner "follows" the conversation or social interaction; includes recognizing when the social partner does not comprehend or understand a message and then responding appropriately by clarifying or giving an explanation (possibly **d3503** as part of maintaining a conversation).
- Confirms: Acknowledges that a social message has been received by nodding, changing facial expressions (e.g., smiling), or verbalizing (possibly **d3503** as part of maintaining a conversation).
- Encourages: Makes supportive, encouraging statements to the social partner; includes using gestures of encouragement (**d710**).
- Appreciates: Expresses a positive, benevolent attitude towards the social partner by agreeing with, empathizing with, or expressing satisfaction with the social partner; includes using gestures of concern or satisfaction (e.g., hugging, patting the social partner on the back, shaking hands) as appropriate, given the social context and degree of familiarity with the social partner (**d7101**, **d7104**).

From Fisher AG: *Occupational therapy intervention process model: a model for planning and implementing top-down, client-centered, and occupation-based occupational therapy interventions*, manuscript in preparation, 2005.

BOX **17-8**   DEFINING NATURALISTIC AND RELEVANT TASK PERFORMANCES

In using the term "naturalistic," I mean that the task performance occurs in an ecologically appropriate environment. That is, the environment is the person's usual environment and if not, is as much like his or her environment as possible. The environment includes the physical spaces, objects, and people who might usually be present. This means that a naturalistic task performance is one where the person performs the task in the type of space where it would usually be performed, using the types of tools and materials that would typically be used by the person, and in the presence of the people that usually would be present.

In using the term "relevant," I mean that the task is one that the person perceives as not only applicable to his or her life, but also as important. For example, a person may have a yard with grass that needs cutting. But if the person typically hires someone to cut the grass, cutting the grass may be applicable to his or her life, but not important for him or her to be able to do. Cutting the grass would therefore not be a relevant occupation for that client.

process skills can be observed during virtually any daily life task performance, communication/interaction skills are only observable in the context of a social task such as the one Stephan observed when he focused his observation on José. Communication/interaction skills are those we can observe (or hear) when a person conveys intentions and needs and coordinates social behavior.

> Stephan observed communication/interaction skills when he observed José look down (*gaze*) toward his hands and not turn or look (*orient, gaze*) at whoever was speaking to him. Stephan also observed communication/interaction when José mumbled a barely audible, "D'know" (*articulate, modulate*).
>
> If Stephan had used the social interaction taxonomy, he would have observed José *look, turn toward, produce speech*, and *extend/sustain* (see Box 17-7).

In each of the examples presented, the occupational therapist was able to observe and describe the actions he observed. Because these two therapists (Mark and Stephan) observed the client performing tasks, action by action, the therapists could also have evaluated the actions (performance skills) in terms of the degree of skill observed. But before we discuss the evaluation of performance skills, they should be placed into the context of the *International Classification of Functioning, Disability, and Health.*[65]

INTERNATIONAL CLASSIFICATION OF FUNCTIONING, DISABILITY, AND HEALTH

The *International Classification of Functioning, Disability, and Health* (ICF) has been developed by the World Health Organization to provide a language that could be used internationally to classify a person's functioning and related contextual factors that support or restrict functioning.[65] More specifically, as shown in Table 17-1, the ICF includes two parts: functioning and disability and contextual factors. Each of these is further divided into components. Three of the components (activities and participation, body functions and body structures, and environmental factors), in turn, comprise several coded domains. Finally, each domain is broken down into even more detailed categories and subcategories. The domains included in each component are shown in Table 17-2. Since the body structure domains have no immediate relevance to this chapter, they are not included in Table 17-2.

TABLE **17-1**   **Structural Organization of the ICF**

	Parts	*Functioning and Disability*			*Contextual Factors*	
More Broad	*Components*	*Activities and Participation*	*Body Functions*	*Body Structures*	*Environmental Factors*	*Personal Factors*
	Domains	Nine coded activity and Participation domains	Eight coded Body Functions domains	Eight coded Body Structures domains	Five coded Environmental Factors domains	List of internal influences from within the person (not coded)
More Detail	*Categories and subcategories*	Coded domains are further broken down into second level categories and third and fourth level subcategories				Not coded

Data from World Health Organization: *International classification of functioning, disability, and health: ICF*, p. 7, Geneva, 2001, WHO.

TABLE **17-2**   **Overview of the Domains (and Respective Codes) of the ICF**

Part	*Functioning and Disability*		*Contextual Factors*	
Components	*Activities and Participation*	*Body Functions*	*Environmental Factors*	*Personal Factors*
Domains	d1: Learning and applying knowledge d2: General tasks and demands d3: Communication d4: Mobility d5: Self-care d6: Domestic life d7: Interpersonal interactions and relationships d8: Major life areas d9: Community, social life, and civic life	b1: Mental functions b2: Sensory functions and pain b3: Voice and speech functions b4: Functions of the cardiovascular, hematological, immunological, and respiratory systems b5: Functions of the digestive, metabolic, and endocrine systems b6: Genitourinary functions b7: Neuromusculoskeletal and movement-related functions b8: Functions of the skin and related structures	e1: Products and technology e2: Natural environment and human-made changes to environment e3: Support and relationships e4: Attitudes e5: Services, systems, and policies	Gender Age Race Fitness Lifestyle Habits Upbringing Coping styles Socioeconomic status Education Profession Religion Social background Past and current life experiences Overall behavior patterns Character style Psychological assets Other personal characteristics

Data from World Health Organization: *International classification of functioning, disability, and health: ICF*, p. 7, Geneva, 2001, WHO.

When looking at Table 17-2, it is important to note that in the ICF coding system, single digit codes (e.g., d1) refer to domains, each of which is further described. The letter "d" refers to the activities and participation domain, the letter "b" refers to the body functions domain, and the letter "e" refers to the environment domain. The number of digits after the letter code denotes the level of the code, with smaller numbers being more global (e.g., d4) and larger numbers being more discrete (e.g., d4401).[65]

The WHO provides a single list of nine domains under the double rubric of activities and participation (see Table 17-2).[65] The user may make a distinction and divide these nine domains in such a way that activities and participation may contain (1) all nine domains in their entirety, (2) distinctly different domains, (3) some overlapping and some distinctly different domains, or (4) different categories from each domain.

BODY FUNCTIONS

Body functions are "the physiological functions of body systems (including psychological function" (p. 47).[65] Here, the focus is on the various functions of body systems, not the body structures themselves. The functions of the brain, for example, include mental functions (e.g., perception, cognition, emotion).[65] Some examples of the body function codes in the ICF are shown in Table 17-3. Note that they focus on what the person's body systems do, not what the person does. For example, Group A in Table 17-3 pertains to what the muscles do, which is generate force. Likewise, Group B has examples of what the brain does, which is perform mental functions related to attention, concentration, and executive functions. Finally, Group C shows the function of the larynx, surrounding muscles, and the respiratory system, which is to produce voice and speech.

ACTIVITIES AND PARTICIPATION

Activities are the "execution of a task or action by an individual" (p. 123)[65] and the perspective is more at the level of the individual. The key point here is that the definition conveys doing, and that doing can occur at two levels: small discrete actions and larger tasks. Note that WHO has chosen to use the term "task" in the same sense as action. This is just one of the many places where there is confusion between (1) words that connote activity or doing something and (2) words that connote or name something that was done. As we will see, WHO (like the Framework) frequently uses the continuous or progressive form of the verb "-ing" when defining both actions and tasks in the activities and participation domains, suggesting that indeed, they mean activity or occupation and not task.

Finally, **participation** has been defined in the ICF as "involvement in a life situation" (p. 123)[65] within the natural context of daily life; the point of view is more from a societal perspective. While the use of the term "involvement" within the ICF is acknowledged to convey the idea of engagement,

TABLE **17-3** **Body Functions: Three Groups of Examples from Selected Categories and Subcategories (with Respective Codes) within ICF Domains**

Group	Body Functions Domain	Category and Subcategories
A	b7: Neuromusculoskeletal and movement related functions	b730: Muscle power functions: Functions related to generating force by contracting muscles b7300: Power of isolated muscles and muscle groups: Functions related to generating force by contracting specific muscle groups (e.g., muscles of the hand) b7301: Power of muscles of one limb: Functions related to generating force by contracting the muscles of the arm or leg
B	b1: Mental functions	b140: Attention functions: Mental functions related to focusing on external stimuli for a given period of time b1400: Sustaining attention: Mental functions that produce concentration b1402: Dividing attention: Mental functions that allow one to focus on two or more stimuli simultaneously b164: Higher-level cognitive functions: Mental functions primarily related to frontal lobes; often referred to as executive functions b1641: Organization and planning: Mental functions related to organizing parts into a whole and developing a method for acting
C	b3: Voice and speech functions	b310: Voice functions b3100: Production of voice: Coordination of the larynx, surrounding muscles, and the respiratory system to produce sounds b330: Fluency and rhythm of speech functions b3300: Fluency of speech: Functions related to producing smooth, uninterrupted flow of speech

Data from World Health Organization: *International classification of functioning, disability, and health: ICF*, p. 47, Geneva, 2001, WHO.

WHO is clear to separate involvement and engagement from the idea of having a sense of belonging.[65]

Again, it is important to point out that there is only one list of categories and subcategories in the ICF activities and participation domains.[65] The ICF user must decide if the problem observed or the evaluation method used is more focused on the person and what he or she can do (activities) or if the problem or evaluation method is more focused on what the person actually does in the natural context, including his or her degree of involvement (participation).

The evaluation of mobility provides one such example. Mobility, as defined within the ICF, pertains to (1) changing body positions; (2) movement transitions from one position or place to another (e.g., standing, walking, transferring); and (3) carrying, moving, and manipulating task objects.[65] The actions listed do not need to be observed within the context of a larger daily life task performance. That is, one could evaluate d4500, walking short distances, by observing the person walking, upon command or direction from a therapist, up and down a hallway or across a room; the task is to walk from point A to point B. When walking is assessed in this manner, it is generally outside of the natural context of engagement in a more global and relevant daily life task. When this occurs, we are not assessing occupation. Occupation involves engagement in the performance of a task one perceives as having meaning, purpose, and relevance to daily life.

To get a clearer picture of this distinction, compare the evaluation of walking by asking a person to walk up and down a hallway (for the sole purpose of evaluating the person's ability to walk) to observing a person perform a chosen and valued task (e.g., vacuuming the living room, gardening, going for a walk in the nearby woods). In the latter case, we can evaluate walking in the natural context of the person engaged in the performance of a more global and relevant daily life task and evaluate the quality of walking and its impact on the overall task progression. In the former context, the evaluator asks, "Is the person able to walk without instability or need to support him or herself on external objects?" In the latter, more natural context, the evaluator asks, "Is there instability or a need to support oneself on external objects while walking that impacts the overall effectiveness of the chosen, life-relevant task performance in which the person was engaged?" The former more closely reflects the ICF definition for activities, while the latter more closely reflects the ICF definition for participation.[65]

DIFFERENTIATING AMONG BODY FUNCTIONS, ACTIONS, AND TASKS

Body functions pertain to what the person's body systems (e.g., muscles, brain) do, not what the person does (see Table 17-3). Table 17-4 has some examples of ICF activities and participation domain categories and subcategories that often become confused with their counterpart in the body functions domain categories. Compare the Group A examples in Table 17-3 with the Group A examples in Table 17-4.

TABLE **17-4**   **Actions: Three Groups of Examples from Selected Categories and Subcategories (with Respective Codes) within ICF Activities and Participation Domains**

Group	Activities and Participation Domain	Category and Subcategories
A	d4: Mobility	d440: Fine hand use: "Performing the coordinated actions of handling objects, picking up, manipulating and releasing them using one's hand, fingers and thumb, such as required to lift coins off a table or turn a dial or knob" (p. 142)[65]
		d4401: Grasping: Using the hand to hold or grasp something (e.g., tool, door knob)
		d430: Lifting and carrying: Raising up or taking an object from one place to another (e.g., lifting a plate, carrying a book from one room to another)
		d4300: Lifting: "Raising up an object in order to move it from a lower to a higher level, such as when lifting a glass from the table" (p. 141)[65]
B	d1: Learning and applying knowledge	d160: Focusing attention: Intentionally focusing on specific stimuli (e.g., by filtering out distracting sounds)
	d2: General tasks and demands	d210: Undertaking a single task: "Carrying out simple or complex and coordinated actions related to the mental and physical components of a single task, such as initiating a task, organizing time, space and materials for a task, pacing task performance, and carrying out, completing, and sustaining a task" (p. 129)[65]
C	d3: Communication	d330: Speaking: Producing spoken messages to express a fact or tell a story
		d350: Conversation: Starting, sustaining, and ending a conversation with others
		d3500: Starting a conversation
		d3501: Sustaining a conversation
		d3502: Ending a conversation

Data from World Health Organization: *International classification of functioning, disability, and health: ICF*, p. 123, Geneva, 2001, WHO.

Note again that body functions pertain to what the person's body systems do (e.g., muscle contract, fingers close), whereas actions pertain to what the person does as he or she interacts with task objects (e.g., grasp coins, lift a plate). As with mobility, we could tell a person to perform an action and then observe him or her grasp a tool or lift a glass from the table outside the context of engagement in a more global task performance (activity). We also have the opportunity to observe these same actions while the person is engaged in the performance of a daily life task that has greater meaning and purpose than simply grasping a tool or lifting a glass because we have directed them to do so (participation).

In a similar manner, we can compare the examples in Group B and Group C between Tables 17-3 and 17-4. Those related to attention in Group B are the most difficult to differentiate. Those in Table 17-3 have to do with what the person's brain is doing. The examples in Table 17-4 have to do with what the person does. For example, while cooking a meal, we might observe a woman to look away from the performance of a cooking task toward a radio that is playing in the next room. In this case, we observe that she looked away and we must judge if she inappropriately focused on something that was not related to the task of cooking (see Table 17-4). When we consider the examples in Table 17-3, we progress one step further in our reasoning process and interpret the person's behavior (i.e., why she looked away and focused on the radio). If we conclude that she looked away and focused on the radio because she is distractible and cannot concentrate, then we are actually referring to mental functions within the person's brain (see Table 17-3).

Consider another example. A young man is driving a car and briefly looks away from the road toward a bicyclist approaching from the right. When we consider what the person does, we see the exact same behavior, looking away and focusing on something else (see Table 17-4). Again, we must judge if it was appropriate for him to do so. In this circumstance, once we consider the behavior we observed and then progress to our interpretation of it at the level of Group B body functions (see Table 17-3), most of us would conclude that this man was not distractible. Instead, we would conclude that he is able to divide his attention in order to be able to take note of a potential danger on the road (see Table 17-3).

In summary, when it is an action in the activities and participation domains, we are referring to what we observe the person doing—looking toward specific stimuli (e.g., noises, movement). When it is body functions, we must infer what is happening in the brain to cause (or support) the person to do what he or she does. Of course, we need body systems that function reasonably well to be able to perform, but that does not mean that what we do is equivalent to what our brains or muscles do.

Table 17-5 provides examples of activities and participation domain tasks. Here the distinction should be clearer. Few would be tempted to confuse washing oneself with the functions of the muscles or the brain. The main difference between actions and tasks relates to the earlier analogy of the links and the chain. Actions are the links. Tasks are the chains that have been constructed once the links have been connected together. Constructing the chain is the task performance. The task codes in the ICF activities and participation domains have generally been described or defined more like activities through the use of the progressive or continuous verb tense.

COMPARING THE ICF TO THE FRAMEWORK

It should come as no surprise that the content and language of the ICF and the Framework are often very similar; the Framework was based largely upon the ICF. This is especially

TABLE **17-5**   **Tasks: Examples from Selected Categories and Subcategories (with Respective Codes) within ICF Activities and Participation Domains**

Group	Activities and Participation Domain	Category and Subcategories
A	d5: Self-care	d510: Washing oneself: Washing and drying one's body or body parts
		d540: Dressing: "Carrying out the coordinated actions and tasks of putting on and taking off clothes and footwear in sequence" (p. 151),[65] as appropriate to climatic and social context
		d5403: Putting on footwear: Carrying out putting on socks, shoes, and footwear
B	d6: Domestic life	d630: Preparing meals: Includes getting together ingredients, cooking, and serving simple and complex meals
		d6300: Preparing simple meals: "Organizing, cooking and serving meals with a small number of ingredients that require easy methods of preparation and serving" (p. 154)[65]
		d640: Doing housework: Performing tasks required to manage a household (e.g., cleaning the house, washing laundry, sweeping, ironing, and folding clothes)
C	d8: Major life areas	d820: School education: Includes engaging in school-related activities (e.g., working together with other students, taking directions from the teacher, and completing assigned schoolwork tasks)

Data from World Health Organization: *International classification of functioning, disability, and health: ICF*, p. 123, Geneva, 2001, WHO.

clear when one compares the categorization of body functions within the Framework with the classification system presented in the ICF. The relationship between areas of occupation in the Framework and the activities and participation domains of the ICF are less direct, but extensive overlap still exists. Moreover, the ICF includes actions in the activities and participation domains that can be likened to the performance skills listed in the Framework.

For example, the actions listed in Group A of Table 17-4 are examples that have parallels among the motor skills (see Box 17-5). Those actions listed in Group B of Table 17-4 have parallels among the process skills (see Box 17-6). Finally, those actions listed in Group C of Table 17-4 have parallels among the social interaction skills (see Box 17-7). Conversely, most of the performance skills included in the Framework have parallel codes in the ICF (see Boxes 17-5 through 17-7).

The majority of the parallel activities and participation ICF codes for motor skills come from the mobility domain (d4). In general, process skills provide a more detailed breakdown and operational definitions of the ICF codes included under the activities and participation domain general tasks and demands (d2). Finally, the majority of the parallel activities and participation ICF codes for the communication/interaction skills and the social interaction skills come from the communication domain (d3) and the interpersonal interactions and relationships domain (d7). Finally, while there are exceptions, general parallels between (1) the categorizations for areas of occupation and performance skills in the Framework and (2) the activities and participation domains of the ICF can be seen in Table 17-6.

Some of the performance skills listed in Boxes 17-5 to 17-7 have no parallel activities and participation ICF codes; where there is no parallel ICF code, one can question if the skill listed reflects a missing element in the ICF classification system. Likewise, there are some motor actions listed in the activities and participation domains of the ICF that are not included in the Framework. The motor and process skills listed in Boxes 17-5 and 17-6 represent universal actions that can be observed in virtually any daily life task performance. Some daily life task performances involve the performance of actions that are unique to the particular task. This means that we should not be limited to those listed in the Framework. Consider the following example:

When Brenda, the occupational therapist observed Kyle playing soccer, she observed him *squat* down, *pick up* the ball, *throw* it into play, and *run* onto the field. Later, she saw him *push* against an opponent and then *kick* the ball.

Each of the actions Brenda observed is included in the activities and participation mobility domain (d4) of the ICF, but not in the Framework. If Kyle was one of Brenda's clients, there is no reason that she could not evaluate the degree of skill Kyle demonstrated when performing these actions. Squatting, picking up, throwing, and so on are also performance skills.

TABLE **17-6** **Parallel Comparison of the OT Framework and ICF Categorization Schemes**

Framework	ICF Activities and Participation Domains
Areas of Occupation	
Activities of daily living	d5: Self-care
Instrumental activities of daily living	d6: Domestic life
Education	d8: Major life areas
Work	d8: Major life areas
Play	d9: Community, social, and civic life
Leisure	d9: Community, social, and civic life
Social participation	d7: Interpersonal interactions and relationships
Performance Skills	
Motor	d4: Mobility
Process	d2: General tasks and demands
Social interaction and communication/interaction skills	d3: Communication, and d7: Interpersonal interactions and relationships

Compiled from American Occupational Therapy Association: Occupational therapy practice framework: domain and process, *Am J Occup Ther* 56(6):609, 2002; World Health Organization: *International classification of functioning, disability, and health: ICF*, p. 123, Geneva, 2001, WHO.

AVOIDING CONFUSION BETWEEN FRAMEWORK PERFORMANCE SKILLS AND ICF BODY FUNCTIONS

Unfortunately, within the occupational therapy literature, there are numerous examples of performance skills being confused with body functions. Of concern here is that the Framework presents performance skills in a manner that, while accurately representing the original source,[17] can result in further misunderstanding. I believe this issue had its origin in the fact that in our early work together, Gary Kielhofner and I first grouped process skills into categories that we named *energy, knowledge, temporal organization, organizing space and objects*, and *adaptation*. These names had roots in earlier versions of the Model of Human Occupation.[40] When I determined a need to develop a set of motor skills, we again grouped them into categories—*posture, mobility, coordination, strength and effort*, and *energy*. Anyone (student, clinician, researcher, and scholar alike) who is not fully familiar with the Assessment of Motor and Skills[15-18] can easily think, "strength, that must be muscle strength" or "organizing space and objects, that sounds like planning." Indeed, even some of the performance skill names (e.g., *stabilizes, coordinates, attends*) tend to connote body functions.

Our original use of these terms might be why others have misunderstood the motor and process skills, viewing them as body functions. Therefore, in an attempt to reduce or prevent further confusion, I have recently reorganized the motor,

---

Box **17-9** CATEGORIES OF MOTOR SKILLS, PROCESS SKILLS,
AND SOCIAL INTERACTION SKILLS

MOTOR SKILLS

Body position
Obtaining and holding objects
Moving self and objects
Sustaining performance

PROCESS SKILLS

Sustaining performance
Applying knowledge
Temporal organization
Organizing space and objects
Adapting performance

SOCIAL INTERACTION SKILLS

Initiating and terminating social interaction
Producing social interaction
Physically supporting social interaction
Shaping content of social interaction
Maintaining flow of social interaction
Timing social interaction
Verbally supporting social interaction

---

process, and social interaction skills, grouping them into new categories[16,18,21,25] (Box 17-9). With hope that these new category labels will help us to avoid confusing performance skills with body functions, let us now turn to how we evaluate performance skills.

EVALUATION OF PERFORMANCE SKILLS

When the occupational therapist evaluates performance skills, he or she implements a performance analysis. A **performance analysis** is an evaluation of the quality of the smallest units of occupation that the occupational therapist can directly observe as a person engages in the performance of a daily life task. When we evaluate performance skills, therefore, we evaluate occupation. That is, to be able to obtain a richer and more detailed understanding of which of the smallest observable units of the daily life task performance were effective and which were not effective, we evaluate the quality of the learned, goal-directed actions that comprise the occupation: motor, process, and, when relevant, communication/interaction or social interaction skills. More specifically, the occupational therapist rates the quality (degree of skill observed) of the goal-directed actions (performance skills) that are carried out, one-by-one, in the context of naturalistic, relevant, and chosen daily life task performances.[21,23]

The concept of performance analysis is relatively new to our profession. Hagedorn[32,33] has also used the term "performance analysis" to refer to the evaluation of a person's ability to perform the daily life tasks one needs and wants

to perform. However, an important distinction between her application of the term and my own[21,23] is that she indicates that performance analyses were used to identify the performance skill deficits that are the underlying cause of the dysfunction. That is, Hagedorn used the term "performance skills" to refer to sensorimotor, cognitive, psychosocial, and other body functions. In contrast, as the term is used in the Framework, analyses of performance skills are what we do when we evaluate the quality of the smallest observable units of occupation, not the underlying body functions.

NONSTANDARDIZED PERFORMANCE ANALYSIS

The occupational therapist can implement an informal evaluation of performance skills based on the observation of performance of any daily life task. To do this, he or she must first have a clear idea of what the client plans or is directed to do. For example:

> When Mark observed Sara, he heard the teacher give directions to use crayons to color the picture of the cat. Moreover, the teacher told the students to color the cat so that it looked just like the cat in the picture in the book she had just read to them (orange).

Then, after observing the person's performance (in this case, observing Sara color), the occupational therapist must systematically consider the motor skills, process skills, and (when relevant) the communication/interaction or social interaction skills. For example, the occupational therapist might subjectively judge whether the observed actions were skilled, and if not, if the skills were mildly, moderately, or markedly ineffective.

> When Mark judged Sara's observed level of coloring skill, he concluded that she demonstrated effective skill as it pertained to *reaching* for, *grasping*, *lifting*, and *manipulating* the crayon. He judged her to have mildly ineffective *choosing* skill because the teacher had specifically stated that the students were to color the cat orange and Sara chose a red crayon. He also judged Sara to have very mildly ineffective *initiating* skill as she paused briefly before she began to color the cat. Mark's greatest concern, however, pertained to the skill, *calibrates*. Sara not only pressed so hard that she broke the red crayon, she also went on to break three more. In addition, her excessive pressure resulted in her tearing the paper as she moved the crayon back and forth. Hence, Mark judged Sara's calibration skill to be markedly ineffective.

STANDARDIZED PERFORMANCE ANALYSIS

When the occupational therapist wants to use a more objective and standardized method of documenting the quality of a person's occupation, he or she must use a standardized performance analysis. Standardized performance analyses have several advantages, but they also have disadvantages. Among the advantages, standardization allows the respective test developers to create possibilities for users to generate a client summary score or measure that can be used to document outcomes and implement evidence-based practice. Second, because the administration and scoring procedures are standardized, there is more consistent evaluation practice that can lead to the ability to compare results across raters and clients. Finally, the person's summary score or measure can be compared to an expected criterion or norm, thereby placing the client's performance in a more meaningful context for interpretation of the results.

A disadvantage of using standardized assessments is that formal training (and unpaid time away from work) is often required. While such practices are common in other fields, they are not always widely accepted in occupational therapy.

Standardized assessments can also be more time consuming and lacking in the flexibility needed to observe any daily life task performance. Finally, while not always viewed as a disadvantage, modern test theory[3,6] demands that each scale be designed to assess only one domain (e.g., work, play, ADLs).

To date, only three standardized performance assessments have been published. The most developed and widely researched is the *Assessment of Motor and Process Skills* (AMPS), an evaluation of personal and instrumental ADLs.[16,18] The AMPS international standardization sample now comprises over 103,000 persons from more than 30 countries ranging in age from 3 to 103 years. Closely related to the AMPS is the *School Version of the Assessment of Motor and Process Skills* (School AMPS).[25] The occupational therapist uses the School AMPS to evaluate the quality of a student's schoolwork task performance as observed in the natural classroom context. Finally, the *Assessment of Communication and Interaction Skill* (ACIS) can be used to evaluate communication/interaction skills in the context of social tasks.[27]

All three of these instruments have several features in common, including the basic principle that the occupational therapist should observe the client in the context of his or her performance of a daily life task. They also share the same rating scale format, and scoring is based on representative scoring examples that are listed in the test manuals. Finally, all three have been developed using preferred modern measurement theory, specifically Rasch measurement methods.[3,47,66] I will describe the AMPS in more detail in the following section to provide a more thorough description of a standardized performance analysis and its use in planning and evaluating the effectiveness of our interventions.

ASSESSMENT OF MOTOR AND PROCESS SKILLS

The *Assessment of Motor and Process Skills* (AMPS)[16,18] is a standardized performance analysis. The AMPS was developed in response to the need for a valid, reliable, sensitive, and clinically useful evaluation tool for evaluating the quality of a person's personal and instrumental activities of daily living (PADL and IADL) task performances. Hereafter, I will refer to

PADLs and IADLs collectively as ADLs. Unlike more global assessments of ADLs that are composed of a limited number of items, each of which represents a single ADL task (e.g., Functional Independence Measure[37]), the items that comprise the AMPS are the smallest observable units of the ADL performance. More specifically, the items on the AMPS are the performance skills that are the links, that when connected together, construct the chain of actions that becomes an ADL task performance. Thus, when the occupational therapist uses the AMPS to evaluate a person's quality of ADL task performance, he or she simultaneously evaluates the quality of the individual actions (performance skills) and the quality of the overall task performance. The AMPS, therefore, offers a standardized way of examining the naturalistic transaction between the person, the ADL task, and the environment, while evaluating the quality of a person's ADL task performance.

AMPS Tasks and Item Bank

A unique feature of the AMPS is that there are 85 standardized ADL tasks in the AMPS manual to meet the demand for task choices appropriate for persons from diverse cultural backgrounds and with diverse needs and interests. Each task has associated with it the 16 motor and 20 process skill items shown in Boxes 17-5 and 17-6. If we consider 85 tasks and 16 motor items that are scored for each task, it means that the AMPS is actually an item bank of 1360 motor items. Similarly, with 85 tasks and 20 process items that are scored for each task, the AMPS item bank contains a total of 1700 process items.

Of course, each person evaluated is not expected to perform all 85 tasks. The advantage of an item bank that ranges from very easy items to difficult items is that each person need only be scored on a selected set of items that are of some challenge, but not too hard. To accomplish this, when the occupational therapist administers the AMPS, each person only performs two tasks that offer a challenge (i.e., are occupational problems). The occupational therapist then scores only 32 of the 1360 motor items and 40 of the 1700 process items included in the total item bank.[16,18,20] Therefore, each of the skills listed in Boxes 17-5 and 17-6 is scored twice during each AMPS administration, once for each of the two tasks performed.

The 85 AMPS tasks range from simple to complex, and have been calibrated using the many-faceted Rasch analysis[46,47] to create a linearized hierarchy of task challenges and parallel item difficulties. The administration procedures of the AMPS are designed to allow the person evaluated to choose which two ADL tasks to perform for an AMPS evaluation. Because all of the AMPS tasks and items are calibrated on the same linear scales (motor and process), it does not matter which task performances are observed and which two sets of 16 motor and 20 process items are rated, provided the tasks offer the client a challenge. The client's final motor and process ability measures are adjusted statistically by the AMPS computer-scoring program so as to equalize the challenge of the tasks the client performs.[19,20,22]

Flexible and Client-Centered Assessment

When the occupational therapist administers the AMPS, it is important that he or she ensures that the tasks the client performs are familiar, have current or future relevance to the person's daily life routine, and are ones that the person has had at least some prior experience performing. As I noted earlier, it is also important that they are ones that present the person with an occupational challenge. Since the occupational therapist scores the quality of the person's motor and process skills in the context of performance of client-chosen tasks, the result is **client-centered assessment.**

Further allowing for flexible and client-centered assessment, the 85 standardized PADL and IADL tasks in the AMPS have been operationally defined and described only in terms of the essential goal and client-specified objects or materials that are to be used. Incorporating the concept of client-specified objects and materials has meant that the AMPS task descriptions are flexible enough to allow each person to perform the tasks in his or her usual manner using the tools and materials he or she typically would use. Such flexibility allows for the diversity of methods people use cross culturally to perform otherwise comparable tasks. For example, if a client chooses to perform the AMPS task of brewing a pot of coffee or tea, he or she is then free to specify whether to brew coffee or tea (i.e., client-specified task material). And, if the client chooses to brew coffee, he or she is free to specify whether to boil the coffee (typical in northern Sweden and Alaska), use a French press, or make the coffee in an electric percolator or coffee maker (i.e., client-specified task tool).

What is critical is that the client recognizes that he or she is to perform the tasks in the usual manner, using the tools and materials he or she usually uses. The flexibility of the AMPS, therefore, avoids the usual standardized test demands for meeting pre-established, externally imposed or contrived performance criteria. Instead, the effectiveness of the person's performance is judged based on what is logical or appropriate given the person's culture and the constraints of each task performed.

As the AMPS was developed, new tasks have continually been added based on the expressed needs of occupational therapists living in different world regions and working with persons with diverse cultural backgrounds. Whenever we add new tasks to the AMPS, we always attempt to design the tasks so that they can be used to evaluate persons from as many different cultures as possible. One feature of the AMPS that makes this possible is that everyone is encouraged to perform the task in his or her typical way and not according to strictly defined criteria. The coffee-making task discussed earlier provided one such example:

> I usually brew coffee in an electric coffee maker. When I first observed a man in northern Sweden making boiled coffee, I was quite surprised to see him put water into a metal coffee kettle (shaped like a copper tea kettle), and place the kettle on a hot wood-burning stove. When the water began to boil, he scooped several spoonsful of ground coffee into the kettle and waited until the water once again came to a boil. He then set the kettle aside, away from the hot stove. After awhile, he poured some coffee into a cup and then poured the coffee in the cup back into the kettle. He repeated this process two more times before he served the coffee in individual coffee cups.

> Had I been in the United States and evaluated an American who had said that he usually brewed coffee in an electric coffee maker, I would have been quite concerned. I likely would have given the man a number of lowered scores, for example Chooses and Uses (choosing and using an inappropriate tool to brew coffee), and Sequences (inappropriately and repeatedly pouring coffee into a cup and then back into the cup). But, because this is a typical way of making coffee in Sweden, his method would have been recognized by another Swede as a logical process for making coffee.

To ensure cross-cultural equivalency of the AMPS ability measures, we have implemented research studies to ensure that the difficulties of the performance skills (skill items) and challenges of the tasks do not vary from culture to culture, even though the specific tools and methods may vary.[2,9,29,30,48,62]

As another way of demonstrating the cross-cultural applicability of the AMPS tasks, all of the AMPS tasks that were developed for a particular world region (e.g., North America, Scandinavia, Asia) have also often been used to test persons in other world regions. Similarly, the AMPS skill items and tasks are designed to be free of gender bias.[12,51] While many people view several of the AMPS tasks as being "women's work," we have found that both men and women choose to perform most AMPS tasks equally often. Moreover, among the tasks we originally developed to target men,[4] at least 40% of the persons who have chosen to perform those tasks have been women.[51]

Administration Procedures

The administration of the AMPS begins with an occupational therapy interview with the client to identify what type of ADL tasks the client feels are problematic. This interview is part of a collaborative process between the occupational therapist and the client that provides the foundation for effective, client-centered occupational therapy assessment and intervention focused on the priorities of the client.[21]

Through this informal interview between the client and the occupational therapist, AMPS task choices that are matched to the abilities, needs, interests, and cultural background of the client are narrowed by the occupational therapist to a small subset of relevant tasks that provide the client a sufficient level of challenge. This subset of tasks is then offered to the client, and, from this subset, the client chooses which two tasks to perform.

Once the occupational therapist and the client agree on the tasks that will be performed, the next step is to establish a task contract. The task contract evolves as the occupational therapist and client discuss in more detail specific tasks the client will perform.

Once the client has chosen the tasks to be performed, and is fully familiarized (as well as the occupational therapist) with the test environment, the occupational therapist observes the client's AMPS task performances. After the client is observed, the occupational therapist rates the client's ADL task performance in terms of the quality (ease, efficiency, safety, and independence) of the universal, goal-directed motor and process skills that were observed as he or she performed each ADL task. That is, the AMPS-trained occupational therapist then scores each of the 16 motor and each of the 20 process skill items according to the quality of each action as observed during each of the client's ADL task performances.

More specifically, the client's performance on each of the motor and process skill items for each task is scored by the AMPS-trained occupational therapist using a 4-point scale as follows:

4 = *Competent* performance without evidence of increased effort, decreased efficiency, or lack of safety

3 = *Questionable* performance in which the examiner questions the effectiveness of the observed performance

2 = *Ineffective* performance that slows the task progression or otherwise interferes with effective task completion (e.g., increased effort, decreased efficiency, decreased safety)

1 = *Markedly deficient* performance as indicated by (a) the need for the examiner to intervene or provide assistance, or (b) performance that results in task breakdown, unacceptable delay, or imminent risk of damage to task objects or danger to the client.

The scoring criteria in the AMPS user's manual[18] are designed to allow the occupational therapist to consider the client's level of effort, degree of efficiency, degree of safety, and need for assistance.

Following scoring, the AMPS-trained occupational therapist enters the client's raw scores into his or her personal copy of the AMPS computer-scoring software[63] (a specialized application of the many-faceted Rasch analysis).[46,47] The AMPS computer-scoring software is used to convert a person's ordinal raw AMPS skill item scores into linear measures of ADL ability that can be placed on the linear AMPS motor and process scales.[20,22] The ADL ability measures are adjusted by the AMPS computer-scoring software to account for (1) skill item difficulty, (2) task challenge,

---

 **THREADED CASE STUDY: JOHN, PART 2**

When Kim first met John, she implemented an in-depth occupational therapy interview during which John clarified his interests, concerns, goals, and priorities.[1,21,23] One of his primary concerns was to be able to prepare meals with less assistance since he wanted to be able to live alone in his own apartment. After further discussion, it became clear that preparing a pot of coffee each day, making sandwiches, heating frozen meals in a microwave oven, and preparing his breakfast were very important to John.

Kim reasoned that these tasks were all appropriate challenges for John. She was also aware that if she was to work with him to design an effective intervention program, she would need to have a clearer sense of what actions within each task performance were most difficult for John, as well as what actions he could do well. Therefore, she explained to John that as part of her occupational therapy evaluation she would like to observe and evaluate him actually performing some of the tasks he had prioritized. Based on his preliminary priorities, Kim suggested to John that he choose to begin with those tasks he wanted to work on first. John chose to perform two tasks: prepare a pot of coffee and make a sandwich. Kim was aware that when she observed John, she would observe occupation: preparing a pot of coffee and making a sandwich.

As Kim continued to talk with John, she was aware that he had already indicated that he wanted to make a pot of coffee, not a pot of tea. Thus, the use of coffee was part of his self-determined contract for that task.

She also learned that he makes coffee using an electric coffee maker and that he adds sugar and milk to his coffee. Thus, John and Kim agreed that using an electric coffee maker and adding milk and sugar to his coffee would also be part of John's self-specified task contract.

When Kim talked with John about sandwiches, she learned that he preferred to make a ham sandwich with mustard on rye bread. Thus, ham, mustard, and rye bread became part of the task contract for John's second task. Kim was aware that she would observe him in a naturalistic kitchen that would, therefore, have in the refrigerator other spreads and butter. She also knew that there would be cheese in the refrigerator. Thus, if he chose any of those instead of or in addition to the ham and mustard, she would be aware that he did not perform according to the task contract they had established. Likewise, if he did not add sugar or milk to his coffee, she would be aware that he also did not perform the first task according to the task contract they had established.

Kim, based on her observations of John's performance, and after careful comparison of what she had observed with the scoring examples in the AMPS manual, was able to objectively score the quality of each motor and process skill using the 4-point rating scale in the AMPS manual. Kim scored Stabilizes, Positions, Reaches, Moves, and Transports = 1. She scored Paces, Continues, and Gathers = 2, and she scored Grips, Coordinates, Lifts, and Chooses = 4. She scored all of the other motor and process skills in a similar manner, once for each task performed (see Boxes 17-5 and 17-6 for the skill item definitions; the specific scoring criteria Kim used are in the AMPS scoring manual).

and (3) rater severity.[19,20,22] A higher ADL motor or ADL process ability measure indicates that the person is more able, or higher on the continuum of the AMPS motor and process ADL scales.

AMPS Computer-Generated Reports

The trained and calibrated AMPS rater can also use AMPS computer-scoring software to generate a number of reports that the occupational therapist can then use to interpret and document the results of the AMPS evaluation, and to plan appropriate occupational therapy interventions.

After Kim had entered John's raw scores into her copy of the AMPS computer-scoring software, she generated the following reports:

- *Raw Score Report*: Provides a table of John's raw scores that can be used to verify the accuracy of data entry and to compare his raw scores across tasks (Figure 17-1).
- *Performance Skill Summary*: Provides an overall summary of John's skill item strengths and problems (Figure 17-2).
- *Graphic Report*: Provides a visual representation of John's linearized motor and process ADL ability measures plotted in relation to the AMPS scale cutoffs. ADL ability measures below these cutoffs indicate that there was diminished quality or effectiveness of performance of instrumental and/or personal activities of daily living (Figure 17-3). John's ADL measures can be used to document his baseline performance, and later, to document the outcomes of Kim's occupational therapy interventions.
- *Occupational Therapy Evaluation of ADL Ability*: Provides a narrative report that, when used in combination with the graphic report, is suitable for documentation of the results and interpretation of John's AMPS evaluation. The report provides both a criterion-referenced and a norm-referenced interpretation of John's results (Figure 17-4).

Interpretation of the AMPS

The results of the AMPS can be used to answer four initial questions:

1. *With what performance skills (actions within an overall task performance) does the client experience difficulty?* The answer is based on the examination of the AMPS profile of that person's motor and process raw scores (see Figures 17-1 and 17-2).
2. *Can the client perform typical ADL tasks without increased effort, decreased efficiency, safety risk, or need for assistance?* The answer to this question is based on examination of where that person's ADL motor and ADL process ability measures are located in relation to the AMPS scale cutoff measures (see Figure 17-3).
3. *Is the client's level of ADL motor and ADL process ability within age expectations?* The answer to this question is based on comparison of that person's ADL motor and ADL process ability measures to the expected range for their healthy, well peers (see Figure 17-4).
4. *Is the client a candidate for restorative interventions based on the use of restorative occupation or compensatory*

interventions based on the use of adaptive occupation?[21,23] The answer to this question is determined based on where that person's motor and process ADL ability measures are located on the AMPS scales (see Figure 17-3). How to do this is discussed in more detail in the next section.

Planning Intervention Based on the Results of an AMPS Evaluation

An important feature of the AMPS is that the results of an AMPS evaluation facilitate the process of planning and implementing intervention.[16,21,24,45] There are two types of occupation-based interventions: adaptive occupation and restorative occupation.[21,23] **Adaptive occupation** involves the use of education and consultation in combination with (1) the provision of technical aids and assistive technology, (2) teaching the client alternative ways of doing (e.g., one-handed shoe tying), and (3) modification of the task or the physical or social environment. Adaptive occupations are most indicated when the evidence suggests that the most cost-effective intervention is to enable the client to compensate for ineffective performance skills.[21,23]

Restorative occupation involves the use of education and consultation in combination with the engagement of the client in occupations that can gradually be graded or modified so as to develop or restore performance skills.[21,23] The use of restorative occupation is indicated when the evidence suggests that the client has the potential to develop or restore needed performance skill in the time available for intervention. In many cases, adaptive occupation and restorative occupation can be provided simultaneously.

When the occupational therapist uses the results of an AMPS evaluation to facilitate the planning of cost-effective occupational therapy interventions, he or she must consider two aspects of the client's AMPS evaluation results: identifying core performance skill clusters and determining whether a specific occupational intervention is indicated.

In other words, first, the occupational therapist identifies clusters of performance skills that had the greatest impact on the client's occupational performance. After the occupational therapist identifies and prioritizes clusters of performance skills to consider addressing in intervention, he or she can use the graphic report (see Figure 17-3) to then determine if adaptive occupation and/or restorative occupation are indicated (recall that this was the fourth question related to the interpretation of the results of an AMPS evaluation). Very low ability measures on the ADL motor scale often indicate that restorative occupation to develop or restore motor skills is not cost effective.

Perhaps most importantly, the position of the client's ADL process ability on the graphic report (see Figure 17-3) can be used by the occupational therapist to facilitate a decision as to what type of adaptive occupation might be most appropriate. More specifically, if the client's ability measure is above zero logits on the ADL process scale, the client likely will do well learning to use new strategies or technical aids.

Text continued on p. 398

ASSESSMENT OF MOTOR AND PROCESS SKILLS (AMPS)
RAW SCORE REPORT BY ENTRY ORDER

Caution: Item and total raw scores are not valid representations of client performance, and they cannot be used for documentation or statistical analyses. Raw scores must be analyzed using the AMPS computer-scoring software to create ADL ability measures. Only ADL ability measures are valid for measuring change.

Client:	John S	Evaluation date:	01/10/2005
ID:	1111JS	Occupational therapist:	Kim A

Task 1:	A-3: Pot of boiled/brewed coffee or tea
Task 2:	F-2: Luncheon meat or cheese sandwich

Motor skills	Task A-3	Task F-2
Stabilizes:	1	1
Aligns:	4	4
Positions:	1	1
Reaches:	1	1
Bends:	2	2
Grips:	4	2
Manipulates:	2	2
Coordinates:	4	2
Moves:	1	1
Lifts:	4	4
Walks:	1	1
Transports:	1	1
Calibrates:	4	2
Flows:	4	4
Endures:	2	2
Paces:	2	2
Task challenge*	**Average**	**Average**

* Task challenges often vary between ADL motor skills and ADL process skills.

Figure 17-1 John's AMPS raw score report.

Continued

ASSESSMENT OF MOTOR AND PROCESS SKILLS (AMPS)
RAW SCORE REPORT BY ENTRY ORDER

Caution: Item and total raw scores are not valid representations of client performance, and they cannot be used for documentation or statistical analyses. Raw scores must be analyzed using the AMPS computer-scoring software to create ADL ability measures. Only ADL ability measures are valid for measuring change.

Client:	John S	**Evaluation date:**	01/10/2005
ID:	1111JS	**Occupational therapist:**	Kim A

Task 1: A-3: Pot of boiled/brewed coffee or tea

Task 2: F-2: Luncheon meat or cheese sandwich

Process skills	Task A-3	Task F-2
Paces:	2	2
Attends:	4	2
Heeds:	4	4
Chooses:	4	2
Uses:	4	4
Handles:	2	2
Inquires:	4	2
Initiates:	2	2
Continues:	2	1
Sequences:	4	4
Terminates:	4	2
Searches/locates:	4	2
Gathers:	2	2
Organizes:	2	2
Restores:	2	2
Navigates:	4	2
Notices/responds:	4	4
Adjusts:	4	2
Accommodates:	1	1
Benefits:	1	1
Task challenge*	**Average**	**Average**

* Task challenges often vary between ADL motor skills and ADL process skills.

Figure 17-1, Cont'd

ASSESSMENT OF MOTOR AND PROCESS SKILLS (AMPS) PERFORMANCE SKILL SUMMARY

Caution: Item and total raw scores are not valid representations of client performance, and they cannot be used for documentation or statistical analyses. Raw scores must be analyzed using the AMPS computer-scoring software to create ADL ability measures. Only ADL ability measures are valid for measuring change.

Client: John S
ID: 1111JS

Evaluation date: 01/10/2005
Occupational therapist: Kim A

Task 1: A-3: Pot of boiled/brewed coffee or tea (Average)

Task 2: F-2: Luncheon meat or cheese sandwich (Average)

Overall performance in each skill area is summarized below using the following scale:

A = Adequate skill, no apparent disruption was observed

I = Ineffective skill, moderate disruption was observed

MD = Markedly deficient skill, observed problems were severe enough to be unsafe or to require therapist intervention

MOTOR SKILLS: Skills observed when client moved self and objects during task performance	**A**	**I**	**MD**
Body Position			
STABILIZES: does not lose balance when interacting with task objects			X
ALIGNS: does not persistently support oneself during task performance	X		
POSITIONS the arm or body effectively in relation to task objects			X
Obtaining and Holding Objects			
REACHES effectively for task objects			X
BENDS or twists the body appropriate to the task		X	
GRIPS: securely grasps task objects		X	
MANIPULATES task objects as needed for task performance		X	
COORDINATES two body parts to securely stabilize task objects		X	
Moving Self and Objects			
MOVES: effectively pushes/pulls task objects and opens/closes doors or drawers			X
LIFTS task objects effectively	X		
WALKS effectively about the task environment			X
TRANSPORTS task objects effectively from one place to another			X
CALIBRATES the force and speed of task-related actions		X	
FLOWS: uses smooth arm and hand movements when interacting with task objects	X		
Sustaining Performance			
ENDURES for the duration of the task performance		X	
PACES: maintains an effective rate of task performance		X	

Figure 17-2 John's AMPS performance skill summary.

Continued

ASSESSMENT OF MOTOR AND PROCESS SKILLS (AMPS)
PERFORMANCE SKILL SUMMARY

Caution: Item and total raw scores are not valid representations of client performance, and they cannot be used for documentation or statistical analyses. Raw scores must be analyzed using the AMPS computer-scoring software to create ADL ability measures. Only ADL ability measures are valid for measuring change.

Client:	John S	Evaluation date:	01/10/2005
ID:	1111JS	Occupational therapist:	Kim A

Task 1:   A-3: Pot of boiled/brewed coffee or tea (Average)

Task 2:   F-2: Luncheon meat or cheese sandwich (Average)

Overall performance in each skill area is summarized below using the following scale:

A   = Adequate skill, no apparent disruption was observed

I   = Ineffective skill, moderate disruption was observed

MD   = Markedly deficient skill, observed problems were severe enough to be unsafe or to require therapist intervention

PROCESS SKILLS: Skills observed when client (a) selected, interacted with, and used task tools and materials; and (b) modified task actions, when needed, to complete the	A	I	MD
Sustaining Performance			
PACES: maintains an effective rate of task performance		X	
ATTENDS: does not look away from task performance		X	
HEEDS the goal of the specified task	X		
Applying Knowledge			
CHOOSES appropriate tools and materials needed for task performance		X	
USES task objects according to their intended purposes	X		
HANDLES task objects with care		X	
INQUIRES: asks for needed task-related information		X	
Temporal Organization			
INITIATES actions or steps of task without hesitation		X	
CONTINUES task actions through to completion			X
SEQUENCES the steps of the task in a logical manner	X		
TERMINATES task actions or steps appropriately		X	
Organizing Space and Objects			
SEARCHES and effectively LOCATES task tools and materials		X	
GATHERS tools and materials effectively into the task workspace		X	
ORGANIZES tools and materials in an orderly and spatially appropriate fashion		X	
RESTORES: puts away tools and materials and cleans the workspace		X	
NAVIGATES: maneuvers the hand and body around obstacles in the task environment		X	
Adapting Performance			
NOTICES and RESPONDS to task-relevant cues from the environment	X		
ADJUSTS: changes workplaces or adjusts switches and dials to overcome problems		X	
ACCOMMODATES: modifies one's actions to overcome problems			X
BENEFITS: prevents task-related problems from persisting			X

Figure 17-2, Cont'd

ASSESSMENT OF MOTOR AND PROCESS SKILLS (AMPS)
GRAPHIC REPORT

			Date	MOTOR	PROCESS
Client:	John S				
Occupational therapist:	Kim A				
		Evaluation 1	01/10/2005	−0.38	0.27

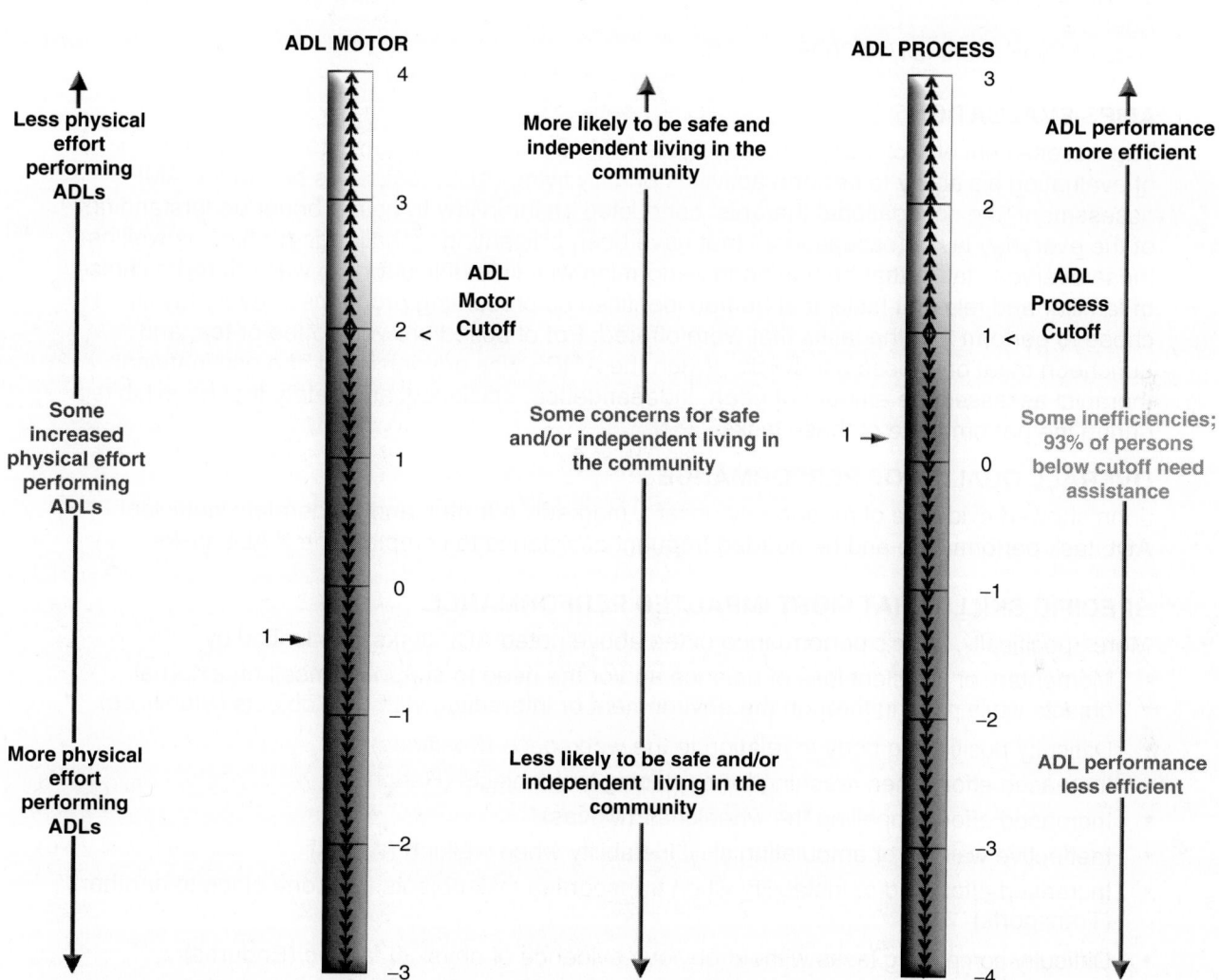

The numbers on the ADL motor and ADL process scales are units of ADL ability (logits). The results are reported as ADL motor and ADL process measures plotted in relation to the AMPS scale cutoffs. Measures below the cutoffs indicate that there was diminished quality or effectiveness of performance of instrumental and/or personal activities of daily living (ADLs). See the AMPS Narrative Report for further information regarding the interpretation of a single AMPS evaluation.

Figure 17-3 John's AMPS graphic report.

OCCUPATIONAL THERAPY EVALUATION OF ADL ABILITY

Results and Interpretation of an Assessment of Motor and Process Skills (AMPS) Evaluation

Therapist: Kim A, OTR
Client: John S
Age: 72
Date of Evaluation: 01/10/2005

AMPS EVALUATION

The Assessment of Motor and Process Skills (AMPS) was administered to John S as a means of evaluating his ability to perform activities of daily living (ADL) tasks. As part of the AMPS assessment, the occupational therapist conducted an interview to gain a better understanding of the everyday tasks (occupations) that have been presenting a challenge for him, as well as those everyday tasks that he has been performing with little difficulty. He was offered a choice of familiar and relevant tasks that he had identified as presenting problems in everyday life. He chose to perform 2 of the tasks that were offered: Pot of boiled/brewed coffee or tea, and Luncheon meat or cheese sandwich. When the AMPS was administered, the occupational therapist assessed the amount of effort, independence, efficiency, and safety that he exhibited during the performance of these tasks.

OVERALL QUALITY OF PERFORMANCE

John showed evidence of moderately unsafe, markedly effortful, and moderately inefficient ADL task performance and he needed frequent assistance to complete the 2 ADL tasks.

SPECIFIC SKILLS THAT MOST IMPACTED PERFORMANCE

More specifically, John's performance of the above noted ADL tasks was limited by:
- Momentary or transient loss of balance and/or the need to support himself on external objects while moving through the environment or interacting with task objects (Stabilizes)
- Difficulty positioning body in relation to the workspace (Positions)
- Increased effort when reaching for or placing task objects (Reaches)
- Increased effort propelling the wheelchair (Moves)
- Ineffective walking or ambulating skill; instability when walking (Walks)
- Increased effort and/or instability when transporting task objects from one place to another (Transports)
- Difficulty completing tasks without obvious evidence of physical fatigue (Endures)
- Failure to maintain a consistent and effective rate of performance (Paces)
- Pauses during actions or task steps, delaying task progression (Continues)
- Decreased skill accommodating for and preventing problems from occurring, and problems persisted or recurred during task performances (Accommodates and Benefits)

OVERALL ADL MOTOR ABILITY

ADL motor ability is an overall measure of a person's observed skill when moving oneself or task objects as needed for ADL task performance. John's ADL motor ability measure of -0.38 logits is plotted in relationship to the AMPS motor cutoff measure on the AMPS Graphic Report. His ADL motor ability is below the AMPS motor cutoff. This indicates that he has increased effort when he performs ADL tasks. To put this in perspective, approximately 95% of well, healthy persons of John's age have ADL motor ability measures between 1.07 and 3.27 logits. This indicates that his ADL motor performance is lower than age expectations.

Figure 17-4   John's occupational therapy evaluation of ADL ability report.

OVERALL ADL PROCESS ABILITY

ADL process ability is a global measure of a person's observed skill in efficiently (a) selecting, interacting with, and using tools and materials; (b) carrying out individual task actions and steps; (c) and modifying performance when problems are encountered. On the AMPS Graphic Report, John's ADL process ability measure of 0.27 logits is below AMPS process scale cutoff. This indicates that he is experiencing decreased safety, independence and/or efficiency when he performs familiar ADL tasks. As a basis for comparison, 95% of well, healthy persons of John's age have ADL process ability measures between 0.59 and 2.55 logits, thus his ADL process ability measure is lower than age expectations.

SUMMARY OF MAIN FINDINGS

- John's ADL motor and ADL process ability measures are both below the AMPS process cutoff and below age expectations, indicating that he is experiencing increased effort, decreased efficiency, decreased safety, and/or the need for assistance when performing chosen, familiar, and life relevant ADL tasks.
- Occupational therapy services may be indicated to enhance and/or prevent further decline of John's ADL task performance.

If there are any questions regarding this evaluation, please do not hesitate to contact me.

Kim A, OTR

Figure 17-4, Cont'd

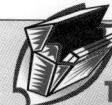

THREADED CASE STUDY: JOHN, PART 3

Performance Skill Clusters

When Kim examined John's raw score and performance skill summary reports (see Figures 17-1 and 17-2), she noted that stabilizes, positions, reaches, moves, walks, and transports were the motor skills that most affected John's performances. She reasoned that these six skills represented two clusters. First, John was unstable and at risk of a fall when he stood up and reached for task objects from overhead cupboards (stabilizes, reaches, walks). Second, he had marked increase in effort when he attempted to move his wheelchair. As a result, he had increased effort transporting task objects and positioning himself at the counter (moves, transports, positions). Kim felt that these two clusters would be critical to target in any intervention she and John planned.

Kim also noted a third cluster: paces, continues, and gathers. Here, she reasoned that John's increased effort when moving his wheelchair and transporting objects resulted in an overall slow pace and interruptions in his ongoing performance and gathering related task objects to the closest counter rather that into the same workspace. If, she reasoned, she could address the first two clusters, this third one would also likely be positively affected.

When Kim examined John's process skills, her greatest concern was accommodates and benefits. Again, she felt that they were related to the first two clusters; John demonstrated problems adapting his performances to overcome his motor skill deficits and prevent them from recurring. Kim was convinced that the key to success was to target the first two clusters.

Graphic Report

When Kim looked at John's graphic report, she saw that his ADL motor ability was below zero logits (log-odds probability units). Combined with the fact that he was 3 months post bilateral CVAs, she reasoned that restorative occupation-based interventions (e.g., neurodevelopmental, biomechanical) may not be indicated. Therefore, Kim tended to think that she would avoid using restorative occupation with John.

Kim noted that John's ADL process ability measure was 0.27 logit and above the critical value of zero. She reasoned that when she talked with John and reviewed the results of his AMPS evaluation and discussed options for intervention, she likely would want to recommend that John consider working with her to design adaptations and compensatory strategies that would enable him to return home. Perhaps, she reasoned, John might be open to placing needed task objects (e.g., his coffee mugs, plates) on lower shelves or the counter so that he did not have to stand up from his wheelchair and be at risk for a fall.

With regard to his moving the wheelchair, Kim felt that he needed another type of mobility device. While aware that this may be an issue of cost, she felt that an electric scooter might be a good option. If John agreed, she planned to contact the local distributor of electric scooters to find out more about what might be available, the cost, and what options might be available for reimbursement from John's medical insurance providers.

If, however, the client's ADL process ability is below zero logits, caregiver training and environmental modifications may be more appropriate and cost effective.[16]

Using the AMPS to Evaluate the Effectiveness of Intervention

The results of an AMPS evaluation can also be used to answer an important fifth question: *Has this person's ADL performance improved as a result of our interventions?* The answer to this question is based on the comparison of two sets of motor and process ADL ability measures (before and after intervention). The difference in the two sets of ADL ability measures provides an objective basis for measuring change. They are reported in the AMPS progress report (Figure 17-5). Changes in client ADL ability measures are used in research and quality assurance programs to provide us with an objective method to demonstrate to our clients, colleagues, healthcare administrators, and healthcare payers that occupational therapy services are cost effective and also improve the functional status of our clients.

THREADED CASE STUDY: JOHN, PART 4

When Kim talked with the local sales representative of electric scooters, he said that he had one in stock that he felt might be a good option for Kim's client. Kim and the sales representative arranged for him to bring the scooter to the clinic so that John would have an opportunity to try it.

The next week, after the scooter had been delivered, Kim and the sales representative oriented John to the controls and offered him the opportunity to practice managing the controls and driving around the clinic area, including the kitchen and bathroom. In fact, John was able to maneuver the scooter around a smaller, more crowded space than he would have when he returned home.

Kim reasoned that if she now used the AMPS to reevaluate John performing two familiar ADL tasks while seated in the electric scooter, she would be able to obtain objective evidence of how much its use changed John's ADL task performance. If the use of the scooter did result in an improvement in his ADL ability, Kim planned to present evidence to John's medical insurance providers.

When Kim re-administered the AMPS, John chose to make another sandwich and prepare a bowl of cereal (served with a glass of juice). Kim readily noted that while John still demonstrated a moderate increase in effort, he was able to perform both tasks independently. John, therefore, continued to receive several scores = 2, but he no longer received any scores = 1.

After entering John's scores into the AMPS computer-scoring software, Kim generated an AMPS Progress Report (see Figure 17-5). Clearly, the scooter had been an effective intervention. His ADL motor ability improved by 1.08 logit and his ADL process ability improved 0.68 logit despite no change in his underlying body functions.

Validity and Reliability

Over its 20-year history, the AMPS has been subjected to numerous evaluations of validity and reliability. Briefly, the AMPS has been shown to consist of two unidimensional scales of personal and domestic ADL ability.[19,20,22] The use of Rasch measurement methods has enabled the addition of new ADL tasks to the AMPS measurement system over time.[4,20] A number of studies have been published supporting the use of the AMPS ability measures cross-culturally,[2,9,29,30,48,62] across age groups,[8,36] and between genders.[12,51] AMPS motor and process ADL ability measures have been shown to remain stable when clients are tested using different pairs of AMPS tasks (alternate-forms reliability),[13,42] as well as between raters and over time.[16] Research has also demonstrated the usefulness of the AMPS with persons with a variety of diagnoses.[5,10,11,28,35,43,44,49,53,57,59-60] Finally, the AMPS is able to detect differences in ADL performance between clinic and home environments[7,52,58] and has been shown to be a sensitive outcome measure.[24,31,34,41,45,54,55,63]

PERFORMANCE ANALYSES VS. TASK ANALYSES

Performance analyses should not be confused with task analyses that are implemented for purposes of identifying the underlying impairments or contextual factors that limit occupational performance.[21]

Compare Kim's description of the quality of John's task performance presented at the beginning of this chapter with that of her supervisor, Maria, who had also observed John making a pot of coffee.

> John has limited active movement in his left arm; when he attempts to use it, his arm flexes slightly at the elbow and his shoulder abducts about 10°. He has full active range of motion of his right arm.
>
> As part of my occupational therapy evaluation, I observed John prepare himself a pot of coffee. He demonstrated decreased trunk rotation and very limited control of his left arm. He was unable to independently propel his wheelchair around the kitchen and had very poor standing balance. His judgment was poor, and he demonstrated limited insight into his disability. He needed standby assistance and verbal cues to prepare his coffee.

Maria used bottom-up reasoning and a bottom-up evaluation process, while Kim had started her occupational therapy evaluation of John by asking him about his concerns, priorities, interests, and goals. While Kim determined which areas of occupation were of greatest concern for John, her supervisor, Maria, still used bottom-up reasoning and evaluation. That is, knowing John's priorities, she observed him preparing a pot of coffee, but she immediately jumped to implementing a task analysis without first implementing a performance analysis. She observed exactly the same task performance that Kim had observed, but she reported her

ASSESSMENT OF MOTOR AND PROCESS SKILLS (AMPS)
PROGRESS REPORT

Client:	John S		Date	MOTOR	PROCESS
Occupational therapist:	Kim A	Evaluation 1	01/10/2005	−0.38	0.27
	Kim A	Evaluation 2	01/20/2005	0.70	0.95

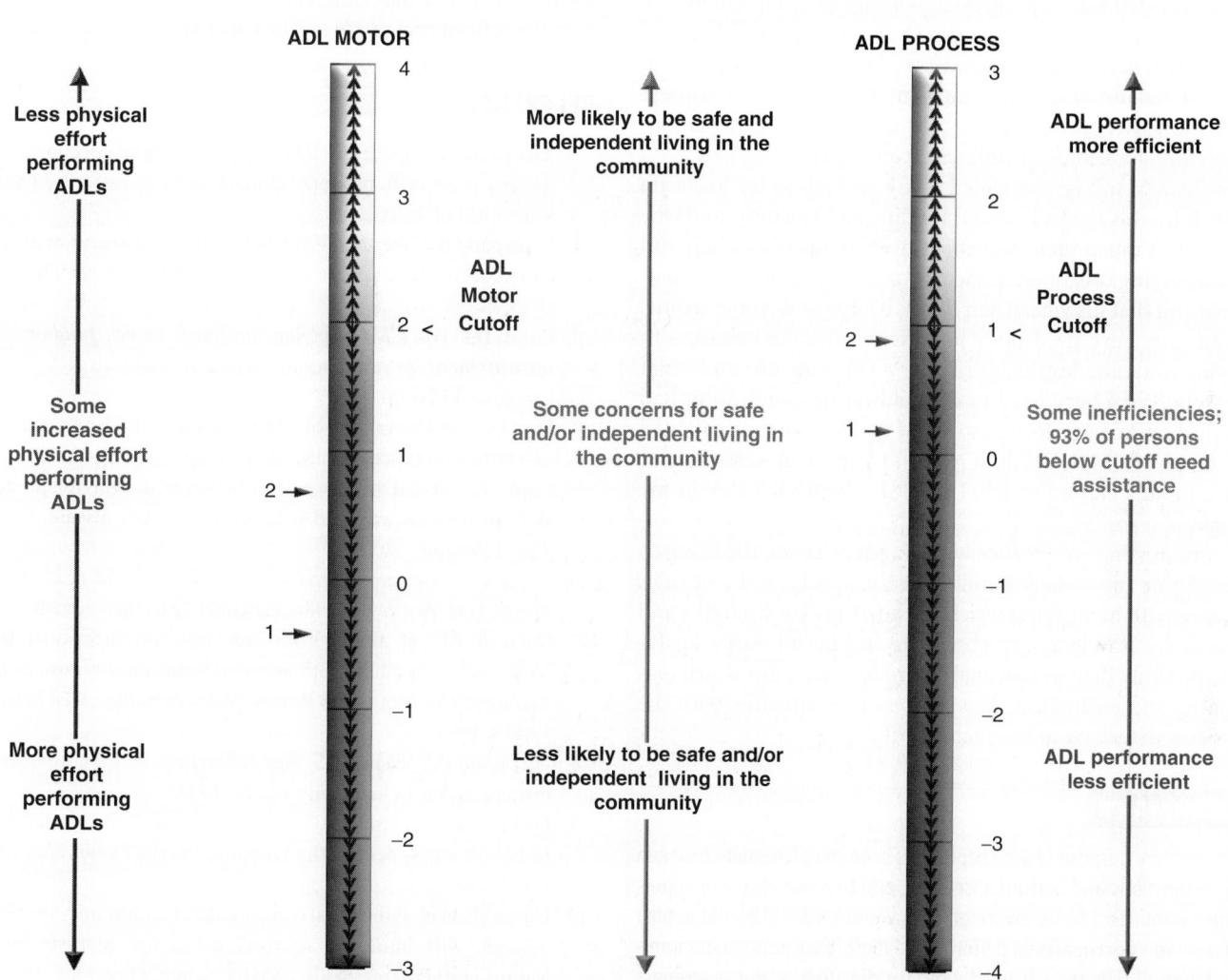

The numbers on the ADL motor and ADL process scales are units of ADL ability (logits). The results are reported as ADL motor and ADL process measures plotted in relation to the AMPS scale cutoffs. Measures below the cutoffs indicate that there was diminished quality or effectiveness of performance of instrumental and/or personal activities of daily living (ADLs).

John S was evaluated on two occasions, 01/10/2005 and 01/20/2005. The change in his ADL ability was 1.08 logits on the ADL motor scale, and 0.68 logit on the ADL process scale. His ADL motor and ADL process ability measures have improved since the initial evaluation. Two ADL measures must differ by at least 0.50 logits to indicate that a person's ADL ability has changed between two test sessions. If two ADL measures differ by at least 0.30 logit but less than 0.50 logit, there is still a possibility that the person's ADL ability has changed in a clinically meaningful way.

Figure 17-5   John's AMPS progress report.

interpretation of what she saw (task analysis), not her actual observations (performance analysis).

In contrast, Kim used a true top-down process.[21,23] Kim first interviewed John to determine his priorities. She too then observed his task performance. But she first implemented a performance analysis and documented what it was she actually had observed: first the quality of his overall task performance and then the quality of his performance skills. Her next step was to progress downward and implement her task analysis. This is what enabled her to interpret and understand why she observed what she did. In that process, she considered not only John's impairments, but also the context and the activity demands.[1,21,23] The results of her task analysis, therefore, looked quite different from Maria's.

When Maria implemented a task analysis to try to clarify why John was unstable when standing and reaching, and why he had so much increased effort moving his wheelchair and transporting task objects, she reasoned that he had poor balance and that his wheelchair was too large and cumbersome. John may have used poor judgment when he persisted in trying to stand, despite his risk for a fall. Kim also knew that he was trying very hard to do the best he could. John had said, "I know I was foolish to stand up like that, but I wanted to try to see if I could do it myself. I knew you were there to save me if I started to fall. I think it's better if I stay in my chair."

Progressing systematically from interviewing the client to determine his or her overall concerns, goals, and priorities (along with identifying which occupations are strengths and which are problems), to observing and performance analysis, and only then to task analysis, reflects true top-down reasoning and evaluation. This process is compatible with the process described in the Framework.

SUMMARY

The primary purpose of this chapter has been to differentiate between body functions and performance skills, and to make clear the importance of our first being aware of what we observed (i.e., the quality of a person's occupational performance) before we jump to our interpretation of why we observed what we did (that is, our awareness of the importance of implementing performance analyses before we implement task analyses). Our follow-up task analyses help us to understand the "whys" of what we observed. These whys can be related to body functions, contextual factors, activity demands, or some combination thereof.[1,65] In contrast, when we implement performance analyses and evaluate performance skills, we bring to consciousness the quality of what we observed.

In a true top-down reasoning and evaluation process, implementing a performance analysis must always follow our information gathering related to the person's unique occupational profile[1] or client-centered performance context.[21,23] When we progress from there to our performance analyses and then to our task analyses, we can begin to think about and interpret why we observed what we did. Perhaps we conclude that contextual factors (e.g., environmental,

societal) hindered task performance. Perhaps we conclude that personal factors (e.g., age, life experience) hindered task performance. And perhaps we conclude that impairments of body functions hindered task performance (see Table 17-2).

If we skip the important step of implementing a formal or informal performance analysis, we risk reverting to bottom-up reasoning and evaluation that is very much like the reasoning and evaluation process Maria used. She started with the occupational profile, but she lost the flow of true top-down reasoning and evaluation and jumped from the occupational profile to a task analysis.

REFERENCES

1. American Occupational Therapy Association: Occupational therapy practice framework: domain and process, *Am J Occup Ther* 56(6):609, 2002.
2. Bernspång B, Fisher AG: Validation of the Assessment of Motor and Process Skills for use in Sweden, *Scand J Occup Ther* 2:3, 1995.
3. Bond TG, Fox CM: *Applying the Rasch model: fundamental measurement in the human sciences*, Mahwah NJ, 2001, Lawrence Erlbaum.
4. Bray K, et al: The validity of adding new tasks to the Assessment of Motor and Process Skills, *Am J Occup Ther* 55:409, 2001.
5. Cooke KZ, et al: Differences in activities of daily living process skills of persons with and without Alzheimer's disease, *Occup Ther J Res* 20:87, 2000.
6. Crocker L, Algina J: *Introduction to classical and modern test theory*, Fort Worth TX, 1986, Harcourt Brace Jovanovich.
7. Darragh AR, et al: Environment effect on functional task performance in adults with acquired brain injuries: use of the Assessment of Motor and Process Skills, *Arch Phys Med Rehabil* 79:418, 1998.
8. Dickerson AE, Fisher AG: Age differences in functional performance, *Am J Occup Ther* 47:686, 1993.
9. Dickerson AE, Fisher AG: Culture-relevant functional performance assessment of the Hispanic elderly, *Occup Ther J Res* 15:50, 1995.
10. Doble SE, et al: Functional competence of community dwelling persons with multiple sclerosis using the Assessment of Motor and Process Skills (AMPS), *Arch Phys Med Rehabil* 75:843, 1994.
11. Doble SE, et al: Measuring functional competence in older persons with Alzheimer's disease, *Int Psychogeriatr* 9:25, 1997.
12. Duran L, Fisher AG: A comparison of male and female performance on the Assessment of Motor and Process Skills, *Arch Phys Med Rehabil* 77:1019, 1996.
13. Ellison S, Fisher AG, Duran L: The alternate forms reliability of the new tasks added to the Assessment of Motor and Process Skills, *J Applied Meas* 2:120, 2001.
14. Englund B: *BSI: Bedömning av social interaktion, Version 2 [ASI: Assessment of Social Interaction]*, unpublished test manual, 1997, Umeå University, Sweden.
15. Fisher AG: *Assessment of motor and process skills*, research ed., 1989, unpublished manuscript.

16. Fisher AG: *Assessment of motor and process skills,* vol 1, ed 6, Ft. Collins CO, 2005, Three Star Press.

17. Fisher AG: *Assessment of motor and process skills,* vol 2, ed 5, Ft. Collins, CO, 2003, Three Star Press.

18. Fisher AG: *Assessment of motor and process skills,* vol 2, ed 6, Ft. Collins, CO, 2005, Three Star Press.

19. Fisher AG: Development of a functional assessment that adjusts ability measures for task simplicity and rater leniency. In Wilson, M, editor: *Objective measurement: theory into practice,* vol 2, p. 145, Norwood NJ, 1994, Ablex.

20. Fisher AG: Multifaceted measurement of daily life task performance: conceptualizing a test of instrumental ADL and validating the addition of personal ADL tasks, *Phys Med Rehab: State Art Rev* 11:289, 1997.

21. Fisher AG: *Occupational Therapy Intervention Process Model: a model for planning and implementing top-down, client-centered, and occupation-based occupational therapy interventions,* manuscript in preparation, 2005.

22. Fisher AG: The assessment of IADL motor skills: an application of many-faceted Rasch analysis, *Am J Occup Ther* 47:319, 1993.

23. Fisher AG: Uniting practice and theory in an occupational framework, 1998 Eleanor Clarke Slagle Lecture, *Am J Occup Ther* 52:509, 1998.

24. Fisher AG, et al: *The effectiveness of occupational therapy with community living older adults,* manuscript in preparation, 2005.

25. Fisher AG, et al: *School AMPS: School version of the Assessment of Motor and Process Skills,* ed 2, Ft. Collins CO, 2005, Three Star Press.

26. Fisher AG, Kielhofner G: Skill in occupational performance. In Kielhofner G, editor: *A model of human occupation: theory and application,* ed 2, p. 113, Baltimore, MD, 1995, Williams & Wilkins.

27. Forsyth K, et al: *The Assessment of Communication and Interaction Skill (ACIS),* version 4.0, Chicago, 1998, University of Illinois at Chicago Model of Human Occupation Clearinghouse.

28. Girard C, et al: Occupational performance differences between psychiatric groups, *Scand J Occup Ther* 6:119, 1999.

29. Goldman SL, Fisher AG: Validation of the cross-cultural universality of the Assessment of Motor and Process Skills, *Br J Occup Ther* 60:77, 1997.

30. Goto S, et al: AMPS applied cross-culturally to the Japanese, *Am J Occup Ther* 50:798, 1996.

31. Graff MJL, et al: Occupational therapy at home for older individuals with mild to moderate cognitive impairments and their primary caregivers: a pilot study, *OTJR: Occup Participation Health* 23:155, 2003.

32. Hagedorn R: *Foundations for practice in occupational therapy,* ed 2, New York, 1997, Churchill Livingstone.

33. Hagedorn R: *Occupational therapy: perspectives and processes,* Edinburgh, Scotland, 1995, Churchill Livingstone.

34. Hariz GM, et al: Assessment of ability/disability in patients treated with chronic thalamic stimulation for tremor, *Movement Dis* 13:78, 1998.

35. Hartman ML, et al: Assessment of functional ability of people with Alzheimer's disease, *Scand J Occup Ther* 6:111, 1999.

36. Hayase D, et al: Age-related changes in activities of daily living (ADL) ability, *Austral Occup Ther J,* in press, 2005.

37. Keith RA, et al: The Functional Independence Measure: a new tool for rehabilitation. In Eisenberg MG, Grzesiak RC, editors: *Advances in clinical rehabilitation,* vol 1, p. 6, New York, 1987, Springer Publishers.

38. Kielhofner G: *A model of human occupation: theory and application,* ed 2, Baltimore, MD, 1995, Williams & Wilkins.

39. Kielhofner G: *A model of human occupation: theory and application,* ed 3, Philadelphia, 2002, Lippincott, Williams & Wilkins.

40. Kielhofner G: *Model of human occupation: theory and application,* Baltimore, MD, 1985, Williams & Wilkins.

41. Kinnman J, et al: Cooling suit for multiple sclerosis: functional improvement in daily living? *Scand J Rehabil Med* 32:20, 2000.

42. Kirkley KN, Fisher AG: Alternate forms reliability of the Assessment of Motor and Process Skills, *J Outcome Meas* 3:53, 1999.

43. Kottorp A, et al: Validity of a performance assessment of activities of daily living for persons with developmental disabilities, *J Intellectual Dis Res* 47:597, 2003.

44. Kottorp A, et al: IADL ability measured with the AMPS: relation to two classification systems of mental retardation, *Scand J Occup Ther* 2:121, 1995.

45. Kottorp A, et al: Client-centered occupational therapy for persons with mental retardation: implementation of an intervention programme in activities of daily living tasks, *Scand J Occup Ther* 10:51, 2003.

46. Linacre JM: *Facets: many-faceted Rasch measurement computer program,* Chicago, 1987-2004, MESA.

47. Linacre JM: *Many-faceted Rasch measurement,* ed 2, Chicago, 1993, MESA.

48. Magalhães LC, et al: Cross-cultural assessment of functional ability, *Occup Ther J Res* 16:45, 1996.

49. McNulty MC, Fisher AG: Validity of using the Assessment of Motor and Process Skills to estimate overall home safety in persons with psychiatric conditions, *Am J Occup Ther* 55:649, 2001.

50. *Merriam Webster's collegiate dictionary,* ed 10, Springfield, MA, 1993, Merriam Webster.

51. Merritt BK, Fisher AG: Gender differences in performance of activities of daily living, *Arch Phys Med Rehab* 84:1872, 2003.

52. Nygård L, et al: Comparing motor and process ability of persons with suspected dementia in home and clinic settings, *Am J Occup Ther* 48:689, 1994.

53. Oakley F, et al: Differences in activities of daily living motor skills of persons with and without Alzheimer's disease, *Austral Occup Ther J* 50:72, 2003.

54. Oakley F, et al: Improvement in activities of daily living in elderly following treatment for post-bereavement depression, *Acta Psychiatrica Scand* 105:231, 2002.

55. Oakley F, Sunderland T: The Assessment of Motor and Process Skills as a measure of IADL functioning in pharmacologic studies of people with Alzheimer's disease: a pilot study, *Int Psychogeriatr* 9:197, 1997.

56. *Oxford English dictionary*, ed 2, Oxford, 1989, Clarendon Press.

57. Pan AW, Fisher AG: The Assessment of Motor and Process Skills of persons with psychiatric disorders, *Am J Occup Ther* 48:775, 1994.

58. Park S, et al: Using the Assessment of Motor and Process Skills to compare occupational performance between clinic and home settings, *Am J Occup Ther* 48:697, 1994.

59. Robinson SE, Fisher AG: A study to examine the relationship of the Assessment of Motor and Process Skills (AMPS) to other tests of cognition and function, *Br J Occup Ther* 59:260, 1996.

60. Robinson SE, Fisher AG: Functional and cognitive differences between cognitively-well people and people with dementia, *Br J Occup Ther* 62:466, 1999.

61. Sellers SW, et al: Validity of the Assessment of Motor and Process Skills with students who are visually impaired, *J Vis Impair Blind* 95:164, 2001.

62. Stauffer LM, et al: ADL performance of black and white Americans on the Assessment of Motor and Process Skills, *Am J Occup Ther* 54:607, 2000.

63. Tham K, et al: Training to improve awareness of disabilities in clients with unilateral neglect, *Am J Occup Ther* 55:46, 2001.

64. Three Star Press: *AMPS 2005: Assessment of Motor and Process Skills computer-scoring program*, Ft. Collins CO, 2005, Three Star Press.

65. World Health Organization: *International classification of functioning, disability, and health: ICF*, Geneva, 2001, WHO.

66. Wright BD, Stone MH: *Best test design*, Chicago, 1979, MESA Press.

18 EVALUATION OF MOTOR CONTROL

LINDA ANDERSON PRESTON*

KEY TERMS

Motor control	Hypertonus	Decerebrate rigidity	Coordination
Plasticity	Spinal hypertonia	Decorticate rigidity	Serial casting
Paresis	Spasticity	Hypertonic stretch reflexes	Nerve blocks
Flaccidity	Clonus	Intrathecal baclofen pump	
Hypotonus	Rigidity	Postural mechanism	

LEARNING OBJECTIVES

After studying this chapter the student or practitioner will be able to do the following:

1. Differentiate between upper and lower motor neuron pathological conditions.
2. List the components of motor control.
3. Compare and contrast spasticity and hypertonia.
4. Recognize four types of rigidity.
5. Differentiate between spinal and cerebral hypertonus.
6. Identify all categories of the Ashworth Scale.
7. List standardized assessments designed for evaluating function after cerebrovascular accident.
8. Describe normal muscle tone.
9. List and describe at least four different states of abnormal tone.
10. Describe how to assess muscle tone.
11. List the components of the postural mechanism.
12. List and describe at least four types of cerebellar disorders.
13. List and describe at least four extra-pyramidal disorders.
14. Describe how to assess coordination.
15. Name several current medical and surgical treatment options for management of hypertonia.
16. List at least three conservative occupational therapy interventions for hypertonia.

CHAPTER OUTLINE

Performance assessments
Normal muscle tone
Abnormal muscle tone
  Flaccidity
  Hypotonus
  Hypertonus
  Spasticity
  Clonus
  Rigidity
Muscle tone assessment
  Guidelines for muscle tone assessment
  Manual rating scales for spasticity and hypertonicity
  Mechanical and computer rating systems for spasticity and hypertonicity
  Range of motion assessment in tone assessment
  Other considerations in tone assessment
  Assessing movement and control
  Sensation
  Medical assessment of muscle tone
Normal postural mechanism

Righting reactions
Equilibrium reactions
Protective reactions
  Assessment of righting, equilibrium, protective reactions, and balance
  Primitive reflexes
  Trunk control assessment
Coordination
Incoordination
  Cerebellar disorders
  Extra-pyramidal disorders
Assessment of coordination
  Medical assessment of coordination
  Occupational therapy assessment of coordination
Occupational therapy intervention
  Intervention for hypertonicity and spasticity
  Treatment of rigidity
  Treatment of flaccidity
  Treatment of incoordination
  Surgical intervention for movement disorders
Summary

*The author would like to thank Crystal Edwards, OTR/L and Jessica Dye, OTR/L.

THREADED CASE STUDY: JUAN

A 44-year-old man, Juan was referred to outpatient occupational therapy 2 weeks status, post right middle cerebral artery CVA with residual left upper extremity hemiparesis. He is right hand dominant with a history of hypertension. An occupational profile provided the following background information on Juan. He is married and has three adopted children, ages 17, 16, and 11. He is responsible for driving his children to school in the morning. His wife is a homemaker. He is the sole financial provider for his family. His job is very demanding, and commission-based. Premorbidly, he would work 12- to16-hour days and averaged 4 to 6 hours of sleep per night. His physician has not yet released him to return to work.

The Canadian Occupational Performance Measure (COPM) was administered to prioritize areas of occupation the client was no longer able to perform, and to ensure client-centered goal setting. With his left hand, he was unable to type on a keyboard, carry a plate or glass without spilling the contents, retrieve coins from a drive-through window cashier, or open his car door. He was most concerned about his ability to keyboard, as this was an essential job function. He would usually carry his drink in his right hand and his plate in his left hand to take to the table. He would open his car door with his left hand, as he often carried his laptop computer in his right hand. His morning routine on workdays included a stop at a fast-food drive-through window for a breakfast sandwich. It was frustrating for him to have to cross his body with his right hand to receive his food and change from the cashier, as it was more convenient for him to use his left hand as he had done premorbidly.

The occupational therapist assessed his proximal motor control first. The client's trunk, scapular, shoulder and elbow tone, ROM, motor control, and strength were considered within normal limits.

His active range of motion in supination was limited to 20° (normal is 80°-90°). The supination muscle group was rated 4-/5 on the strength grade scale. His pronation and finger flexor hypertonia was rated moderate on the Preston's Hypertonia Scale (Box 18-3). His extrinsic finger extension strength rated as 3-, and his lumbrical strength (proximal interphalangeal joint extensors) was 2-/5. His static two-point discrimination and kinesthesia tests were normal. His Modified Brunnstrom Stages of Motor Recovery Score was 4 (Table 18-1).

His Graded Wolf Motor Function Test total timed score was 470 seconds with his left upper extremity, and 40 seconds with his right upper extremity. The maximum total time on this test is 1560 seconds, which would mean the client could not complete any of the test items. The functional ability score mean was 5.5 (normal is 7) with his left upper extremity. His right upper extremity test score was 7 out of 7.

Critical Thinking Questions

As you read the following chapter, answer these questions about Juan.

1. Name the 3 main reasons why he cannot operate a keyboard with his left hand.
2. Describe 3 primary reasons why he cannot open his car door, receive change in his hand from the drive-though window cashier, or carry a glass without spilling the contents with his affected upper extremity.
3. Name 3 activities you would prescribe as a part of a home program to improve the motor control of his left finger extensors and forearm supinators. What lifestyle changes would you recommend for this client?

Motor control is the ability to make dynamic postural adjustments and direct body and limb movement in purposeful activity.[101] Components necessary for motor control include normal muscle tone, normal postural tone and postural mechanisms, selective movement, and coordination. Complex neurological systems (i.e., the cerebral cortex, basal ganglia, and cerebellum) collaborate to make motor control possible. A neurological insult such as *cerebrovascular accident* (stroke or brain attack), brain injury, or a disease such as multiple sclerosis or Parkinson's disease, affects motor control. Functional recovery depends on the initial amount of neurological damage, prompt access to medical treatment that limits the extent of neurological damage,[90] the nature of the neurological damage, whether it is static or progressive, and therapeutic intervention that can facilitate motor recovery.

Plasticity is an important concept in neurological rehabilitation because it helps explain why recovery is possible after brain injury or lesion. Plasticity is defined as "anatomical and electrophysiological changes in the central nervous system."[101] In some instances the *central nervous system* (CNS) is able to reorganize and adapt to functional demands after injury.[18] Motor relearning can occur through the use of existing neural pathways (*unmasking*) or through the development of new neural connections (*sprouting*).[79] In the case of unmasking, it is believed that seldom-used pathways become more active after the primary pathway has been injured. The adjacent nerves take over the function of the damaged nerves. In the case of sprouting, dendrites from one nerve form a new attachment or synapse with another (Figure 18-1).[24] It has also been demonstrated that new axonal processes develop in sprouting.[79]

Observing movements during occupational performance is a way to assess motor control. Following an evaluation of occupational performance, it may be necessary to evaluate the specific components that underlie motor control. These components are muscle tone, postural tone and the postural mechanism, reflexes, selective movement, and coordination.

OT PRACTICE NOTE

A comprehensive assessment can help the client and occupational therapist plan appropriate treatment intervention.

This chapter focuses on the functional effects of lesions in the *upper motor neuron system* (UMNS). The UMNS includes any nerve cell body or nerve fiber in the spinal cord (other than the anterior horn cells) and all superior structures. These structures include descending nerve tracts and brain cells of both gray and white matter that subserve motor function.

The lower motor neuron system includes the anterior horn cells of the spinal cord, the spinal nerves, the nuclei and axons of cranial nerves III through X, and the peripheral nerves. Lower motor neuron dysfunction results in diminished or absent deep tendon reflexes and muscle flaccidity. Figure 18-2 illustrates the influence of the upper motor neuron system over the lower motor neuron system.[70]

PERFORMANCE ASSESSMENTS

The occupational therapist has the challenge of maximizing the client's ability to return to purposeful and meaningful

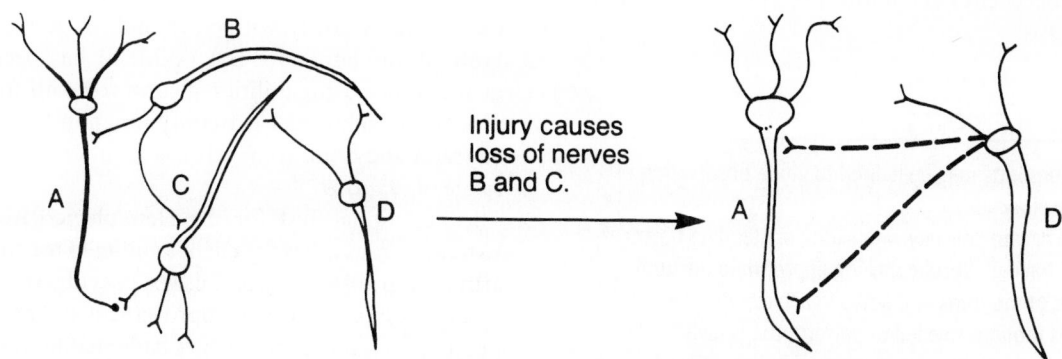

Injury causes loss of nerves B and C.

New dendrite connections "sprout" from nerve D to reestablish contact with nerve A.

Figure 18-1   Sprouting theory of nerve cell replacement. Injury causes loss of nerves B and C. New dendrite connections "sprout" from nerve D to re-establish contact with nerve A. (From DeBoskey DS, et al: *Educating families of the head injured,* Rockville, MD, 1991, Aspen Publishers.)

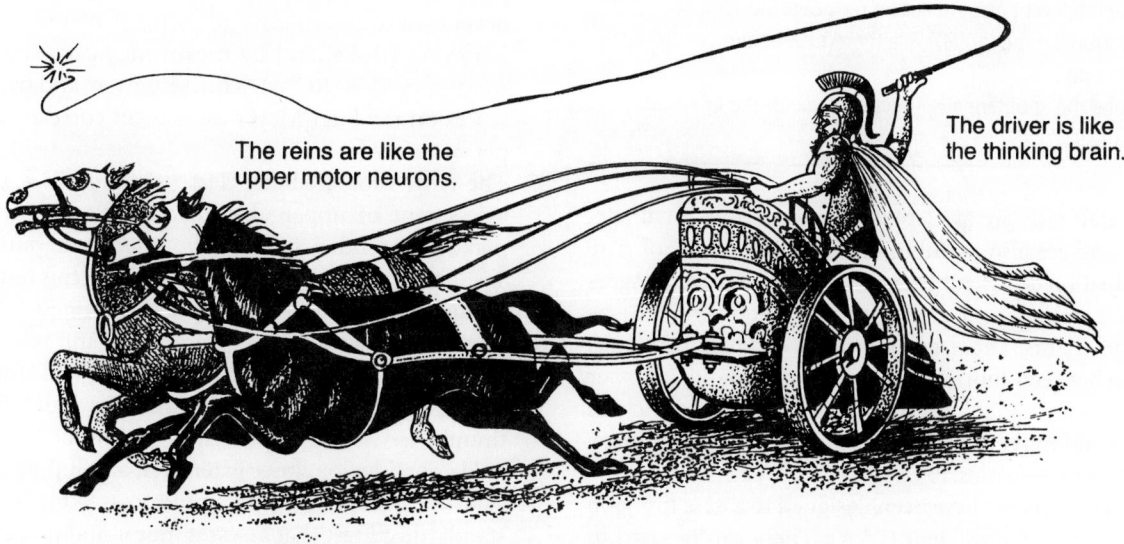

The reins are like the upper motor neurons.

The driver is like the thinking brain.

The horses are like lower motor neurons and muscles.

Figure 18-2   Control of movement is comparable with a chariot driver with a team of horses. The upper motor neuron system facilitates or inhibits the lower motor neuron system. The driver is like the brain, the reins are like the descending nerve tracts, the horses are like lower motor neurons and muscles. (From DeBoskey DS, et al: *Educating families of the head injured,* Rockville, MD, 1991, Aspen Publishers).

occupation within his or her physical, cultural, and social environment.[97] Therefore, evaluating functional performance is primary in helping clients to set realistic goals. The Canadian Occupational Performance Measure[62] is an assessment tool that ensures client-centered therapy. This tool helps prioritize the client's functional activity goals in the areas of self-care, leisure, and productivity.[62]

The *occupational therapist* (OT) can observe the client for motor control dysfunction during assessment of *basic activities of daily living* (BADLs) and *instrumental activities of daily living* (IADLs), along with productive and leisure activities. The therapist must observe how problems in motor control affect occupational performance. The therapist must also consider the client's sensation, perception, cognition, and medical status.

OT PRACTICE NOTES

The following questions may be helpful to guide observation of motor control dysfunction.
1. Is the client having difficulty with sitting or standing balance?
2. Is the client having difficulty making appropriate postural adjustments of the trunk and limbs to achieve the best position and motions needed to perform the activity?
3. Is there adequate trunk control to perform the activity?
4. Do changes in body and head position affect muscle tone?
5. Are primitive reflexes evoked during performance?
6. Is there hypertonicity limiting antagonist movement?
7. Are spatial or temporal sequencing problems interfering with coordinated movement?
8. Is there weakness that prohibits antigravity activity?
9. Are tremors, athetoid, or choreiform movements apparent?
10. Is there apparent incoordination (i.e., overshooting or undershooting the target)? Are there extraneous movements?
11. Describe the spontaneous, functional use of the involved extremities.

Many ADL tests are available to assess occupational performance and are also useful to observe motor control. The Test d'Evaluation des Membres Superieurs de Personnes Agees (TEMPA) is an upper extremity functional activity performance test for clients. The test was developed to help therapists distinguish between "normal and pathological aging in upper extremity performance."[26] Some of the test items include picking up and moving a jar, writing on an envelope, tying a scarf, and handling coins.[26]

Several assessments have been designed to assess function after cerebrovascular accident (CVA). These can be used to observe for motor control problems.
1. The Graded Wolf Motor Function Test (GWMFT) is a new assessment developed to measure functional gains after a hemiparetic event from cerebrovascular accident or traumatic brain injury.[76] This test was based on the Wolf Motor

Function Test.[9] It is called "Graded" because there are two levels of difficulty for each task; level A is more advanced, level B is easier (Figure 18-3). Gorman[40] investigated the inter-reliability and intra-reliability of the GWMFT with a sample of eight physical therapist investigators and three subjects. The intra-rater and inter-rater reliability was .935 on the timing scores. The intra-rater reliability was .897 and the inter-rater reliability was .879 on the functional ability scores. This is a very useful test that can be used on a wide variety of clients with hemiparesis with varying degrees of motor recovery. More research is needed to confirm the validity and reliability of this test.

In the aforementioned case study, Juan's mean functional ability score was 5.5 (Figure 18-3). He performed the test items slowly, with effort and a lack of precision.
2. Wolf Motor Function Test (WMFT) has been used to quantify the motor abilities of chronic clients from a population of high upper extremity function following CVA or traumatic brain injury. It has an inter-rater reliability range of .95 to .97.[9]
3. The Functional Test for the Hemiplegic/Paretic Upper Extremity[107] assesses the client's ability to use the involved arm for purposeful tasks. This test provides objective documentation of functional improvement and includes tasks ranging from those that involve basic stabilization, to more difficult tasks requiring fine manipulation and proximal stabilization. Examples include holding a pouch, stabilizing a jar, wringing a rag, hooking and zipping a zipper, folding a sheet, and putting in a light bulb overhead.[107]
4. The Fugl-Myer[57] assessment is based on the natural progression of neurological recovery after CVA. Low scores on the Fugl-Myer have been closely correlated with the presence of severe spasticity. Fugl-Meyer and associates developed a quantitative assessment of motor function following stroke, and by measuring such parameters as *range of motion* (ROM), pain, sensation, and balance. The scores on the Fugl-Meyer assessment correlate with ADL performance.[57]
5. The Arm Motor Ability Test (AMAT)[60] is a functional assessment of upper extremity function. Cutting meat, making a sandwich, opening a jar, and putting on a T-shirt are some of the tasks included in this test. This test has high inter-rater reliability and test-retest reliability.[60]
6. The Motricity Index (MI)[21] is a valid and reliable test of motor impairment that can be performed quickly. The test assesses pinching a cube with the index finger and thumb, as well as elbow flexion, shoulder abduction, ankle dorsiflexion, knee extension, and hip flexion.[21]
7. The Assessment of Motor and Process Skills (AMPS)[7] is a standardized test that assesses motor and process skills in IADLs. The test was created by occupational therapists. Although the test is not diagnosis specific, it has been widely used with clients who have had a CVA. Occupational therapy practitioners are eligible to become certified in the use of this test, through a five-day training course.[7]

GRADED WOLF MOTOR FUNCTION TEST
DATA COLLECTION FORM
Subject's Name: _____ Date: _____
Test (check one):   Pretreatment _____   Posttreatment _____   Follow-up ____
Arm tested (check one):   More affected _____   Less affected _____
Tasks (circle appropriate level)   Time (from level circled)   Functional Ability
Comments

---

1. Forearm to table (side)   0 1 2 3 4 5 6 7
    a. chair alone
    b. chair with platform and cushion

2. Forearm to box (side)   0 1 2 3 4 5 6 7
    a. box (full height)
    b. box (1/2 height)

3. Extend elbow (to the side)   0 1 2 3 4 5 6 7
    a. 40-cm line
    b. 28-cm line

4. Extend elbow (to the side) with weight   0 1 2 3 4 5 6 7
    a. 40-cm line
    b. 28-cm line

5. Hand to table (front)   0 1 2 3 4 5 6 7
    a. chair alone
    b. chair with platform and cushion

6. Hand to box (front)   0 1 2 3 4 5 6 7
    a. box (full height)
    b. box (1/2 height)

7. Reach and retrieve   0 1 2 3 4 5 6 7
    a. 40-cm line
    b. 28-cm line

8. Moving foam stick   0 1 2 3 4 5 6 7
    a. supination then pronation
    b. pronation only

9. Lift washcloth   0 1 2 3 4 5 6 7
    a. appropriate grasp
    b. inappropriate grasp

10. Flip light switch   0 1 2 3 4 5 6 7
    a. appropriate grasp
    b. inappropriate grasp

Figure 18-3 Graded Wolf Motor Function Test. (From Morris DM et al: *Graded Wolf Motor Function Test*. Dr. Edward Taub, Department of Psychology, University of Alabama at Birmingham, 415 CH, 1530 8th Avenue South, Birmingham, AL 35294-1770. Revision date 5/6/02.)

Continued

11. Lift pen   0 1 2 3 4 5 6 7
    a. appropriate grasp
    b. inappropriate grasp

12. Lift cotton balls   0 1 2 3 4 5 6 7
    a. appropriate grasp
    b. inappropriate grasp

13. Lift basket   0 1 2 3 4 5 6 7
    a. full height
    b. table-level height

Level B

0   Does not attempt with involved arm.
1   Involved arm does not participate functionally; however, attempt is made to use the
        arm. In unilateral tasks the uninvolved extremity may be used to move the involved
        extremity.
2   Does, but requires assistance of uninvolved extremity for minor readjustments or
        change of position, or requires more than two attempts to complete, or accomplishes
        very slowly.
3   Does, but movement is performed slowly, and/or with effort, and/or with excessive
        compensatory movements.
        Level A
4   Does, but requires assistance of uninvolved extremity for minor readjustments or
        change of position, or requires more than two attempts to complete, or accomplishes
        very slowly.
5   Does, but movement is performed slowly, and/or with effort, and/or with excessive
        compensatory movements.
6   Does; movement is close to normal, but slightly slower; may lack precision, fine
        coordination, or fluidity.
7   Does; movement appears to be normal.

Figure 18-3, cont'd

After observing functional performance, the occupational therapist usually will find it necessary to assess the performance components that underlie motor control: muscle tone, the postural mechanism, reflexes, sensation, and coordination.

NORMAL MUSCLE TONE

Normal muscle tone, a component of the normal postural mechanism, is a continuous state of mild contraction, or a state of preparedness in the muscle.[91] Tone is the resistance felt by the examiner as he or she passively moves a client's limb. It is dependent on the integrity of peripheral and CNS mechanisms and the properties of muscle. When normal muscle tone is present, a tension between the origin and insertion of a muscle is felt as resistance by the therapist when passively manipulating the limb. It is high enough to resist gravity, yet low enough to allow movement. The tension is determined partly by mechanical factors such as connective tissue and viscoelastic properties of muscle, and partly by the degree of motor unit activity. When passively stretched, the normal muscle offers a small amount of involuntary resistance.

Normal muscle tone relies on normal function of the cerebellum, motor cortex, basal ganglia, midbrain, vestibular system, spinal cord functions, and neuromuscular system (including the mechanical-elastic features of the muscle and connective tissues),[56] and on a normally functioning stretch reflex. The stretch reflex is mediated by the *muscle spindle*, a sophisticated sensory receptor continuously reporting sensory information from muscles to the CNS.

Normal muscle tone varies from one individual to another. Within the range that is considered normal, the degree of normal tone depends on such factors as age, sex, and occupation. Normal muscle tone is characterized by the following:

1. Effective co-activation (stabilization) at axial and proximal joints
2. Ability to move against gravity and resistance
3. Ability to maintain the position of the limb if it is placed passively by the examiner and then released
4. Balanced tone between agonist and antagonistic muscles
5. Ease of ability to shift from stability to mobility and reverse as needed

6. Ability to use muscles in groups or selectively with normal timing and coordination
7. Resilience or slight resistance in response to passive movement

Hypertonicity (increased tone) interferes with performance of normal selective movement because it affects the timing and smoothness of agonist and antagonist muscles groups. Normalization of muscle tone and amelioration of **paresis** (slight or incomplete paralysis/weakness) are desirable when striving for selective motor control. Some function can be achieved even though tone may not be normal.[87]

ABNORMAL MUSCLE TONE

Abnormal muscle tone is usually described with the following terms: *flaccidity, hypotonus, hypertonus, spasticity,* and *rigidity.* To plan appropriate treatment interventions, the therapist must recognize the differences among these tone states and identify them during the clinical assessment, to plan the appropriate intervention.

FLACCIDITY

Flaccidity refers to the absence of tone. The client will have absent deep tendon reflexes. Active movement is absent as well. Flaccidity can result from spinal or cerebral shock immediately after a spinal or cerebral insult. In traumatic upper motor neuron lesions of cerebral or spinal origin, flaccidity is usually present initially and then changes to hypertonicity within a few weeks.[66]

Flaccidity also can result from lower motor neuron dysfunction, such as a peripheral nerve injury or a disruption of the reflex arc at the alpha motor neuron level. The muscles feel soft and offer no resistance to passive movement. If the flaccid limb is moved passively, it will feel heavy. If moved to a given position and released, the limb will drop because the muscles are unable to resist gravity.[100]

HYPOTONUS

Hypotonus is considered by many to be a decrease of normal muscle tone (i.e., low tone). Deep tendon reflexes are diminished or absent. Van der Meche and Van der Gijn[104] suggested that hypotonus could be an erroneous clinical concept. They performed *electromyography* (EMG) analysis on the quadriceps muscles in "hypotonic" clients (e.g., peripheral neuropathy, cerebral infarction, and other diagnoses) and in relaxed normal subjects in a lower leg free-fall test. They concluded in their study that if a client's limb feels hypotonic or flaccid, it is the result of weakness, not long-latency stretch reflexes.[104]

HYPERTONUS

Hypertonus is increased muscle tone. Hypertonicity can occur when there is a lesion in the premotor cortex, the basal ganglia, or descending pathways. Damage to upper motor neuron systems increases stimulation of the lower motor neurons, with a resultant increased alpha motor activity. Any neurological condition changing the upper motor neuron pathways that directly or indirectly facilitate alpha motor neuron activity may result in hypertonicity. Other spinal or brainstem reflexes may become hyperactive, which leads to hypertonus patterns like the flexor withdrawal or the re-emergence of tonic neck reflexes.[66]

Hypertonicity often occurs in a synergistic neuromuscular pattern, particularly seen after CVA or traumatic brain injury. Synergies are defined as patterned movement characterized by co-contraction of flexors and extensors. A typical synergy seen in the upper extremity after CVA or traumatic brain injury is a flexion synergy.[65] In contrast, an extension synergy is seen in the lower extremity.

There is considerable energy cost in moving against hypertonicity. It takes a great deal of effort for clients with moderate to severe hypertonicity to move against this drawing force. There may not be enough antagonist power to overcome the spastic agonist muscle groups. Even clients with mild hypertonicity report frustration during functional activities. There is a loss of reciprocal inhibition between spastic agonists and antagonists. Clients are unable to rapidly turn off their muscles. The client with an upper motor neuron lesion will have dysfunction in spatial and temporal timing of movement. This makes his/her movements very uncoordinated.[108] This frustration, coupled with the fatigue, decreased dexterity, and paresis associated with UMNS, can influence therapy participation.[84] Furthermore, the architecture of hypertonic muscles changes over time. The muscles lose their ability to lengthen and shorten because of viscoelastic changes that result from the hypertonia.[18,56]

The abnormal timing of Juan's distal upper extremity muscles, particularly between the finger flexors and extensors, impaired his coordination so much that he could not keyboard with his left hand.

Hypertonicity can increase as a result of painful or noxious stimuli. These stimuli can often be reduced with good medical care. Stimuli that can increase tone are pressure sores, ingrown toenails, tight elastic straps on a urine collection leg bag, tight clothing, an obstructed catheter, urinary tract infections, constipation, and fecal impaction.[29,53] Other triggering factors include fear, anxiety, environmental temperature extremes, heterotopic ossification, and sensory overload. These factors are true for both cerebral and spinal hypertonicity; however, they are more pronounced in spinal hypertonia. Therapeutic intervention should be designed to reduce, eliminate, or cope with these extrinsic factors.

Clients with hypertonicity often have difficulty initiating movement, especially rapid movement.[56] Although hypertonic muscles appear to be able to take a lot of resistance, they do not function as normal, strong muscles do. Through the mechanism of reciprocal inhibition, hypertonic muscles inhibit activity of their antagonists and thus can mask potentially good or normal function of antagonists.[87,101] There are four types of hypertonia described below.

Cerebral Hypertonia

Cerebral hypertonia is caused by traumatic brain injury, stroke, anoxia, neoplasms (brain tumors), metabolic disorders, cerebral palsy, and diseases of the brain. In multiple sclerosis, hypertonia is produced from both spinal and cerebral lesions. Tone fluctuates continuously in response to extrinsic and intrinsic factors. Cerebral hypertonia usually occurs in definite patterns of flexion or extension, causing the limb to be pulled in one direction (Figure 18-4). Typically, the patterns occur in the antigravity muscles of the upper and lower extremities (e.g., flexors of the upper extremities, extensors of the lower extremities).

The re-emergence of primitive reflexes and associated reactions alters postural tone. When an individual is lying supine, muscle tone is less than when the individual is sitting or standing. The tone is at its highest during ambulation. Thus, attention to postural tone is important when positioning a client for splinting or casting. A cast or splint fabricated on a client in a supine position may not fit when the client is

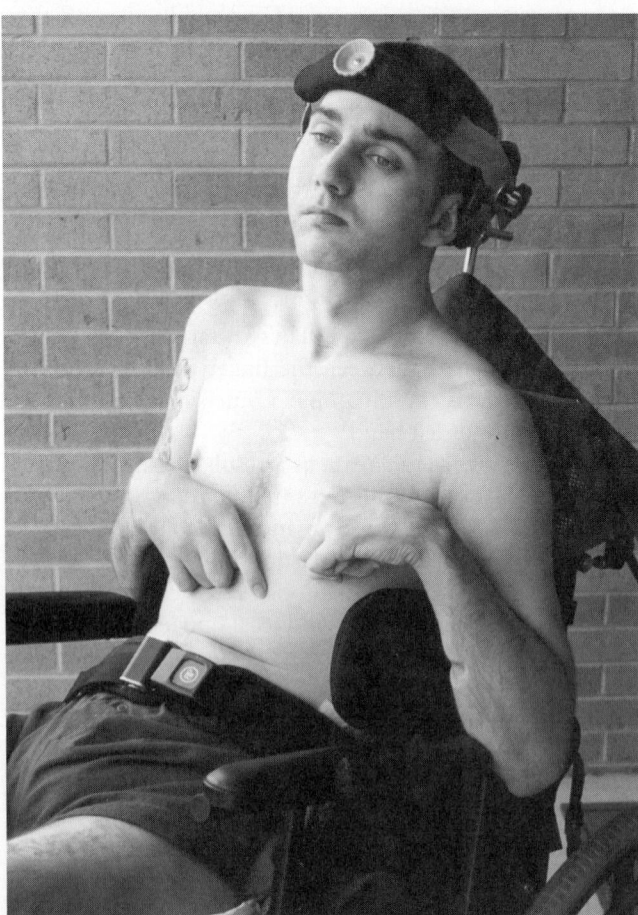

Figure 18-4   A client with right upper extremity dystonic posturing of the wrist and finger extensors. His left wrist shows severe hypertonicity. The tone abnormalities are a result of a traumatic brain injury.

sitting up, because of the influence of gravity and posture on increasing muscle tone.[87]

Spinal Hypertonia

Spinal hypertonia results from injuries and diseases of the spinal cord. In slow-onset spinal disease (e.g., spinal stenosis or tumor), there is no period of spinal shock. In traumatic spinal cord injury, spinal shock occurs and is characterized by flaccidity. With time (weeks or months) the flaccidity diminishes and hypertonus develops. The affected extremities first develop flexor and adductor tone.[110] Over time, extensor tone develops and becomes predominant in the lower extremities. Spinal hypertonia can lead to muscle spasms severe enough to cause an individual to fall out of a wheelchair, off a gurney, or out of bed. The degree of hypertonicity in incomplete spinal lesions varies, depending on the degree of damage to the spinal cord. The tone tends to be more severe in incomplete spinal cord lesions than in complete lesions.[87]

SPASTICITY

There has been much controversy in recent years about the difference between **spasticity** and hypertonia. Lance's[61] definition of spasticity is still accepted by many physicians and therapists. He defined spasticity as "a motor disorder characterized by a velocity-dependent increase in tonic stretch reflexes (muscle tone) with exaggerated tendon jerks resulting from hyperexcitability of the stretch reflex as one component of the upper motor neuron syndrome."[61]

Little and Massagli[65,66] believe that pure spasticity is a subset of hypertonia. It is possible that Lance's definition does not adequately distinguish between the presence of phasic and tonic stretch reflexes, which present different clinical scenarios. This chapter attempts to clarify the differences using current physiatry literature.

Spasticity has three characteristics:

1. Hyperactivity of the muscle spindle's phasic stretch reflex with hyperactive firing of the IA afferent nerve.
2. Velocity dependence, meaning the stretch reflex is only elicited by the examiner's rapid passive stretch.[65,66]
3. The "clasp-knife" phenomenon. This means that when the examiner takes the extremity through a quick passive stretch, a sudden catch or resistance is felt, followed by a release of the resistance. What actually happens is that the initial high resistance of spasticity is suddenly inhibited.[56]

One of the main systems that has been affected when spasticity is present is the *pyramidal system*, which consists of the corticospinal and corticobulbar tracts. The corticospinal tract controls goal-directed, voluntary movement by influencing LMN. The corticobulbar tract influences the voluntary action of the cranial nerves.[18]

Therapists often confuse *hypertonia* with spasticity. These two conditions are similar because they both pull the limb into a unilateral direction.

Hypertonia is different from spasticity in two ways:

1. Hypertonia is typically not velocity dependent; that is, rapid movement does not evoke it; rather, slow joint movement elicits them. The hypertonus persists as long as the muscle stretch is maintained because of the firing of group II muscle spindle afferents (tonic stretch reflex).[65,66]
2. During passive movement, there is no catch felt with hypertonia, as there is with the clasp-knife phenomenon of spasticity. It is objectively measurable with EMG.[57]

CLONUS

Clonus is a specific type of spasticity. This condition is often present in clients with moderate to severe spasticity. Clonus is characterized by repetitive contractions in the antagonistic muscles in response to rapid stretch. There are recurrent bursts of IA afferent activity, which result in a cyclical oscillation of phasic stretch reflexes.[56,66] Clonus is most commonly seen in the finger flexors and ankle plantar flexors.[66] The occurrence of clonus can interfere with participation in purposeful activity, transfers, and mobility. Therapists should educate clients and their families about how to bear weight actively, because this usually will stop the clonus. Therapists and physicians record clonus by counting the number of beats.[56] A three-beat clonus can be rated as mild and is less likely to interfere with ADLs than clonus that is 10-beat or more. Clonus may be elicited during quick stretch tone evaluation or may become apparent during assessment of occupation (e.g., grasping or ambulation). If clonus greatly interferes with ADLs, the client may be a candidate for a referral to a physiatrist or neurologist for oral medication, Botox[12] injection, Myobloc[77] injection, or alcohol or phenol motor point block.[84]

RIGIDITY

Rigidity is an increase in muscle tone of agonist and antagonist muscles simultaneously (i.e., muscles on both sides of the joint). Both groups of muscles contract steadily, leading to increased resistance to passive movement in any direction and throughout the ROM. Rigidity signals involvement of the extra-pyramidal pathways in the circuitry of the basal ganglia, diencephalon, and brainstem. It occurs in isolated forms in disorders such as Parkinson's disease, traumatic brain injury, some degenerative diseases, encephalitis, tumors,[25] and after poisoning from certain toxins and carbon monoxide. Rigidity is also seen in conjunction with spasticity in those with stroke and traumatic brain injury. Rigidity is not velocity dependent.[100]

Rigidity is evaluated during muscle tone evaluation (Figure 18-4). Four types of rigidity are commonly seen:

1. Lead pipe rigidity
2. Cogwheel rigidity
3. Decorticate rigidity
4. Decerebrate rigidity

Both lead pipe and cogwheel rigidity can occur in Parkinson's disease. In lead pipe rigidity, constant resistance is felt throughout the ROM when the part is moved slowly and passively in any direction. The rigidity feels similar to the feeling of bending solder or a lead pipe, thus, its name. In cogwheel rigidity, a rhythmic give occurs in the resistance throughout the ROM, much like the feeling of turning a cogwheel. It is thought that cogwheel rigidity is lead pipe rigidity with concomitant tremor, which results in the ratchety pattern.[74] Deep tendon reflexes are normal or only mildly increased in Parkinson's rigidity.

OT PRACTICE NOTE

It is crucial for the therapist to document the type of rigidity during initial assessment and how it affects the client's performance.

Decerebrate and decorticate rigidity can occur after severe traumatic brain injury with diffuse cerebral damage or anoxia. These abnormal postures occur immediately after injury and can last a few days or weeks if recovery occurs, or persist indefinitely if there is little or no recovery.

Decerebrate rigidity results from lesions in the bilateral hemispheres of the diencephalon and midbrain. It appears as rigid extension posturing of all limbs and the neck. Bilateral cortical lesions can result in decorticate rigidity, which appears as flexion hypertonus in the upper extremities and as extension tone in the lower extremities. Supine positioning increases the abnormal tone, and with either type of rigidity it may be extremely difficult to position clients in a sitting position.[66]

MUSCLE TONE ASSESSMENT

Objective assessment of muscle tone in the client with cerebral spasticity is difficult because the tone fluctuates continuously in response to extrinsic and intrinsic factors. The postural reflex mechanism, the position of the body and head in space, the position of the head in relation to the body, and stereotypical reflexes and associated reactions all influence the degree and distribution of abnormal muscle tone.[91]

GUIDELINES FOR MUSCLE TONE ASSESSMENT

The following steps describe correct procedures for assessing muscle tone.

It is helpful to rate the spasticity and hypertonia with the client in the same position, preferably at the same time of day, to enhance reliability, because body and head position influence cerebral hypertonus. The client's upper extremity muscle tone is usually evaluated with the client sitting on a mat table when possible. Remember that the client's trunk posture (e.g., the seated client bearing weight symmetrically versus slumped or leaning to one side) will affect the results of the tone evaluation. Tone fluctuates from hour to hour and day to day because of the intrinsic and extrinsic factors that influence it. This fluctuation makes accurate measurement difficult, particularly for cerebral hypertonia. Rating tone is still worthwhile, especially in the managed care environment, in which objective measures of progress are needed to justify the continuation of therapy.

Grasp the client's limb proximal and distal to the joint to be tested and move the joint slowly through its range to determine the free and easy ROM available. Note the presence and location of pain. If there is no active movement and if the limb feels heavy, record that the limb is flaccid or "0" in strength. If the limb has some active movement and no evidence of increased tone, the affected muscle or muscle group may be labeled "paretic" instead of "hypotonic." The paretic antagonist muscle can then be graded in strength (usually the strength grade will fall between 1 and 4-). Grading the paretic antagonist muscles provides more objective clinical information than merely labeling the muscles as hypotonic. Strength grading antagonists can help the occupational therapist triage phenol block and botulinum toxin type A or B injection candidates who have potential to improve function; for example, a client with elbow extension strength grade of 2- (in the presence of elbow flexor tone) would be a better block candidate than a client with a triceps strength grade of 0.

Juan did not have sufficient strength in his supinators [4-/5] or in his finger extensors (extrinsic 3-/5, intrinsic 2-/5) to counteract the pull of moderate finger flexor and pronator hypertonia.

Hold the limb on the lateral aspects to avoid giving tactile stimulation to the muscle belly of the muscle being tested.

Clinical assessment of spasticity involves holding the client's limb as just described and moving it rapidly through its full range while the client is relaxed. Label the tone "mild," "moderate," or "severe." (Refer to tone rating scales defined in the next section.)

Clinical assessment of rigidity and hypertonia involves moving the limb slowly during the range, noting the location of first tone or resistance to movement in degrees, and labeling it "mild," "moderate," or "severe." Some physicians find goniometric measuring of the location of the first tone helpful pre and post long-acting nerve block. Others find documentation of the limb's resting position helpful pre- and postinjection.[69]

Record findings for various muscle groups or movements.

MANUAL RATING SCALES FOR SPASTICITY AND HYPERTONICITY

Ashworth Scale

The Ashworth Scale[4] (Box 18-1) and the Modified Ashworth Scale[10] (MAS) are the two most widely used scales to manually rate spasticity.[79,93] These scales were not designed to differentiate between pure spasticity and **hypertonic**

OT PRACTICE NOTE

It is important to note the client's overall posture during the evaluation of muscle tone. Is the client's posture symmetrical, with equal weight bearing on both hips (if sitting) or on both feet (if standing)? Note how the client moves in general. Is the head aligned or tilted to one side? Is one shoulder elevated? Is the trunk rotated or elongated on one side and shortened on the other? Such abnormalities will affect the client's ability to move the limbs normally. Current intervention focuses heavily on quality of movement, achieving as normal motor control as possible during occupation.

Box **18-1** ASHWORTH SCALE

0 = Normal muscle tone
1 = Slight increase in muscle tone, "catch" when limb moved
2 = More marked increase in muscle tone, but limb easily flexed
3 = Considerable increase in muscle tone
4 = Limb rigid in flexion or extension[2]

Ashworth B: Preliminary trial of carisoprodol in multiple sclerosis, *Practitioner* 192:540, 1964.

---

stretch reflexes. These scales are used to quantify the degree of the hypertonus. There is controversy in the literature about the validity and reliability of these scales. Brashear et al. concluded that in upper limb spasticity the Ashworth Scale had good intra- and inter-rater reliability when used by trained medical professionals.[14] However, Seghal and McGuire[92] believe that the Ashworth scale lacks reliability. Pandyan et al.[80,82] noted that the Ashworth Scale and the Modified Ashworth scales should be used as an ordinal scale of resistance to passive movement, however they are not valid for assessing spasticity. Preston believes both scales should be considered nominal because the last stage of each scale is describing rigidity, not spasticity. Rigidity is an extrapyramidal phenomenon and spasticity is pyramidal; therefore both should not be measured on the same scale.[85]

Three studies have demonstrated that the MAS is a reliable scale for assessment of spasticity.[10,42,43] Four studies have demonstrated that it is not reliable.[3,8,32,65] Therapists familiar with the Ashworth Scale can help physicians evaluate candidates for neurosurgical procedures. For example, part of the selection criteria for the Synchromed Intrathecal Baclofen Pump (ITB)[73] implantation is based on the presence of a two-point reduction on the Ashworth Scale after the test dose of medication is given.[87] The resistance encountered during passive muscle stretching is described in Box 18-1.

Tardieu Scale

The Modified Tardieu Scale (MTS)[13] and the Tardieu Scale[45] both measure spasticity.[35] The Tardieu Scale is in French,

Mild: The stretch reflex (palpable catch) occurs at the muscle's end range (i.e., the muscle is in a lengthened position).
Moderate: The stretch reflex (palpable catch) occurs in midrange.
Severe: The stretch reflex (palpable catch) occurs when the muscle is in a shortened range.

Farber S: *Neurorehabilitation: a multisensory approach*, Philadelphia, 1982, Saunders.

Box **18-3**   PRESTON'S HYPERTONICITY SCALE

0: No abnormal tone detected during slow, passive movement.
1 or Mild: First tone or resistance is felt when the muscle is in a lengthened position during slow, passive movement.
2 or Moderate: First tone or resistance is felt in the midrange of the muscle during slow, passive movement.
3 or Severe: First tone or resistance occurs when the muscle is in a shortened range during slow, passive movement.

and was not reviewed. The MTS had an inter-rater reliability coefficient of .7 and was shown to be more reliable than the aforementioned MAS.[41]

Mild-Moderate-Severe Spasticity Scale

Some therapists and physicians find a mild-moderate-severe scale easier to use than the aforementioned scales. The scale in Box 18-2 is suggested as a guide for estimating the degree of spasticity.[31]

Preston's Hypertonicity Scale

Some therapists and physicians find a mild-moderate-severe hypertonia scale easier to use. The scales in Box 18-3 are suggested as a guide for estimating the degree of hypertonicity.

One of the reasons Juan could not keyboard with his left hand is the presence of moderate hypertonia in his finger flexors. He could not retrieve change in his left hand from the drive-through window cashier because moderate hypertonia in his forearm pronators limited full active supination. One needs to have close to normal supination and functional grasp/release to obtain change from a drive-through cashier.

MECHANICAL AND COMPUTER RATING SYSTEMS FOR SPASTICITY AND HYPERTONICITY

Mechanically determined parameters of assessing hypertonia may be more reliable than the aforementioned manual methods. McCrea et al. concluded that using a linear spring damper model to assess the hypertonic elbow was reliable and valid.[71] This model is not widely used in clinical practice,

or even research practice, because of time constraints and difficulty accessing certain muscle groups; e.g., it is easier to set up and measure elbow hypertonia than hip hypertonia in a mechanical tone rating device.

Leonard et al. investigated the construct validity of the Myotonometer™, a newly developed computerized, electronic device with a probe (that looks similar to an ultrasound transducer) that is placed on top of the skin over the muscle belly. Measurements were taken over the biceps brachii at rest and during maximum voluntary muscle contraction. It revealed a significant difference between affected and unaffected extremities in subjects with upper motor neuron spasticity. The authors concluded that the Myotonometer™ could provide objective data about the tone reduction efficacy of various tone-reducing procedures.[63]

Clearly, there needs to be more research in the areas of manual, mechanical, and computer rating systems for assessment of hypertonia. Sehgal and McGuire summed up the controversy over hypertonia/spasticity rating scales quite well, "A uniformly acceptable, reliable and practical measure of spasticity continues to elude the clinician."[92]

RANGE OF MOTION ASSESSMENT IN TONE ASSESSMENT

Passive ROM (PROM) assessment supplements and often correlates with tone assessment. For example, if a client with acute CVA (1 month after onset) has a wrist ROM measurement of 20° extension (normal is 70°) and if orthopedic etiology (e.g., arthritis or fixed contracture) has been ruled out, the therapist should assess the tone in the wrist flexors and extrinsic finger flexors. Hypertonicity of any of these muscles can prohibit full wrist extension. An assessment of PROM can reveal possible signs of joint changes (e.g., subluxation, dislocation, or contracture) that have occurred from chronic hypertonus, such as PIPs that measure −45° to 125° instead of 0° to 100°. Some physicians find PROM measurements useful in documenting the location of the first tone, or resting position, before and after Botox[12] or Myobloc[77] injections.

Juan only had 20° of active supination. His passive range of motion was not limited. He has a soft tissue limitation of active supination due to paresis of the supinator and hypertonicity of the pronators; 20° of supination is not enough to orient his hand palm up to hold coins.

OTHER CONSIDERATIONS IN TONE ASSESSMENT

Changes in bone or other peripheral structures can lead to ROM limitations. For example, the presence of heterotopic ossification can limit joint ROM. Heterotopic ossification is the formation of new bone in soft tissue or joints, which can lead to joint anklyosis. Heterotopic ossification can occur in individuals with traumatic brain injury and spinal cord injury, along with severe spasticity, or in other types of severe injuries.[11,55,106] Conversely, the presence of fixed contractures may be incorrectly labeled as hypertonus. Physiatrists or other physician specialists can aid in the diagnosis of contractures with the use of diagnostic short-term nerve blocks, EMG, and/or X-rays.[87]

Incidentally, Juan did not have any passive range of motion deficits so he did not have contractures.

ASSESSING MOVEMENT AND CONTROL

Along with the assessment of muscle tone previously described, the occupational therapist performs an assessment of upper extremity movement and control. The therapist identifies where and how much the client's motor control is dominated by synergies, and where selective, isolated movement is present. The degree to which abnormal tone interferes with selective control is identified. Also, determining in which direction of movement hypertonicity occurs and how it affects function helps determine the need for intervention.

Manual muscle testing usually is not appropriate for clients who exhibit moderate to severe hypertonicity or rigidity because the relative tone and strength of the muscles are not normal and movement is not voluntary or selective. Tone and strength are influenced by the position of the head and body in space, abnormal contraction, deficits in tactile and proprioceptive sensation, and impaired reciprocal inhibition.[108] However, if hypertonia is mild and selective movements are possible, it is helpful to grade the strength of the antagonists to measure progress objectively.[87]

Position change, spinal reflexes, the reticular formation, and supraspinal reflexes influence muscle tone and motor control. Because the level and distribution of muscle tone change as the position of the head in space and of the head in relation to the body change, tone cannot be assessed in isolation from postural mechanisms, motor function, synergies present, task specificity, and other factors related to motor control.[50]

SENSATION

The following sensibility tests are recommended for clients with damage to the central nervous system: static two-point discrimination, kinesthesia, proprioception, pain, and light touch using the Semmes-Weinstein Monofilaments test.[5] The therapist can assess light touch more accurately with the Semmes-Weinstein monofilaments because they have better pressure control than a cotton ball. (Chapter 22 provides procedures for administration of these sensory tests).

MEDICAL ASSESSMENT OF MUSCLE TONE

Physiatrists, orthopedic surgeons, and neurologists are some of the physicians who may specialize in assessment of muscle tone. They may use static or dynamic surface or *percutaneous* (needle) EMG. Multiple channels are used in dynamic

EMG to evaluate the hypertonicity of many contributing muscles.[65] EMG helps the physician determine abnormal, excessive electrical activity in muscles. EMG can help physiatrists and neurologists plan and implement short- and long-acting nerve blocks to treat hypertonia. Clients who have local muscle wasting, flaccidity, numbness, or unexplained paresis should receive EMG assessment to rule out peripheral neuropathy.[106]

NORMAL POSTURAL MECHANISM

The normal **postural mechanism** is composed of automatic movements that provide an appropriate level of stability and mobility. These automatic reactions develop in the early years of life and allow for trunk control and mobility, head control, midline orientation of self, weight bearing and weight shifting in all directions, dynamic balance, and controlled voluntary limb movement. The components of the normal postural mechanism include normal postural tone and control, integration of primitive reflexes and mass movement patterns, righting reactions, equilibrium and protective reactions, and selective movement.

In clients who have suffered UMNS damage, the normal postural mechanism is disrupted. Abnormal tone and mass patterns of movement dominate the client's movements, and these clients have impaired balance and stability. Movements are slow and uncoordinated. Therapists must assess the extent of damage to the postural mechanism in clients with CNS trauma or disease.

Normal postural tone allows automatic and continuous postural adjustment to movement. Postural control is the ability to control or regulate specific postural outputs. It is important to assess the following automatic reactions, which are part of the postural mechanism, in clients with CNS trauma or disease.

RIGHTING REACTIONS

Righting reactions direct the head to an upright position. Righting reactions help one assume a position. Automatic reactions maintain and restore the normal position of the head in space and the normal relationship of the head to the trunk, as well as the normal alignment of the trunk and limbs. Without effective righting reactions, the client will have difficulty getting up from the floor, getting out of bed, sitting up, and kneeling.[96]

EQUILIBRIUM REACTIONS

Equilibrium reactions help one sustain or keep a position. They are the "first line of defense against falling."[91] Equilibrium reactions are elicited by stimulation of the labyrinths within the inner ear, and are used to maintain and regain balance in all activities. These reactions ensure sufficient postural alignment when the body's center of gravity is altered by a change in the supporting surface.[54] Without equilibrium reactions, the client will have difficulty maintaining and recovering balance in all positions and activities.

PROTECTIVE REACTIONS

Protective reactions are the second line of defense against falling if the equilibrium reactions cannot correct a balance perturbation. They consist of protective extension of the arms and hands, which is used to protect the head and face when one is falling. Stepping and hopping are examples of lower extremity protective reactions. Without protective reactions, the client may fall or be reluctant to bear weight on the affected side during normal bilateral activities.[91]

Assessment of Righting, Equilibrium, Protective Reactions, and Balance

Formal testing of these reactions may be difficult because of the cognitive and physical limitations of the client or time constraints of the therapist. The therapist can evaluate righting reactions, however, during transfers and ADL. Equilibrium and protective reactions can be observed when the client shifts farther out of midline than necessary during functional activities, such as lower extremity dressing.

Balance depends on normal equilibrium and protective reactions. Balance is "the ability to maintain the center of gravity over the base of support, usually while in an upright position."[58] Balance involves a complex interaction between many systems, including the vestibular, proprioceptive, visual, and motor modulation from the cerebellum, basal ganglia, and cerebral cortex. Occupational and physical therapists must also observe the client's ankle, hip, and step strategies and note areas of breakdown in the kinetic chain.[28,100]

When assessing a client with CNS dysfunction, the therapist should assess the client's static and dynamic balance before leaving the client unattended on a mat table, in a wheelchair, or during ambulatory ADLs. Dynamic balance involves maintaining balance while moving, and static balance involves maintaining equilibrium while stationary.

The Physical Performance Test assesses physical function during activity. Seven of the nine tested items involve static and dynamic balance.[105] The test only takes 10 minutes to complete.[89] Figure 18-5 shows the test form and test protocol. Two other noteworthy balance assessments are the Tinetti Balance Test of the Performance-Oriented Assessment of Mobility Problems[98] and the Berg Balance Scale.[6]

PRIMITIVE REFLEXES

The dominance of primitive reflex movement patterns can interfere with the client's occupational performance. Difficulties that may be encountered are described below. Observation of these motor behaviors is a way of evaluating for the presence of primitive reflexes.

Brainstem Level Reflexes

Asymmetrical tonic neck reflex (ATNR)

The ATNR is tested with the client positioned in supine or sitting. Stimulus: actively or passively turn the client's head to 90° to one side. Response: increase of extensor tone of the limb on the face side and an increase of flexor tone on the skull side of the limb.[39] The client with an asymmetrical tonic neck reflex may have difficulty maintaining the head in midline while moving the eyes toward or past midline. The client may be unable to (1) extend an arm without turning the head or (2) flex the arm without turning the head the other way. The client may be unable to move either or both arms to midline, especially when in the supine position, because movement of the arms is dependent on head positioning. This positioning causes asymmetry in the arms. Thus, this reflex makes it difficult or impossible to bring an object to the mouth, hold an object in both hands, or grasp an object in front of the body while looking at it.

Symmetrical tonic neck reflex (STNR)

The STNR is tested with the client positioned in sitting or quadruped. Stimulus 1: flex the client's head and bring his/her chin toward the chest. Response: flexion of the upper extremities and extension of the lower extremities. Stimulus 2: extend the client's head. Response: extension of the upper extremities and flexion of the lower extremities.[59] The client with the STNR will be unable to support the body weight on hands and knees, maintain balance in a quadruped position, or crawl normally without fixating the head. The client will have difficulty moving from lying to sitting because when the head is lifted to initiate the task, increased hip extension resists the movement. As he or she struggles to sit up, increased leg extension can also interfere. The client will have difficulty with transfers from bed to wheelchair and wheelchair to bed because as the arms and neck are extended to initiate the transfer, one or both legs may show increased flexion, which may cause the client to slide under the bed or wheelchair. Additionally, the affected leg may actually lift off the floor, causing an inability to bear weight on that extremity.[23]

Tonic labrinthine reflex (TLR)

The TLR can be tested with the client supine with his or her head in mid-position. The stimulus is the test position. The response is an increase of extension tone or extension of the extremities. The TLR can also be tested with the client prone with the head in mid-position; again, the test position is the stimulus. The response is an increase in flexor tone or flexion of the extremities. The client exhibiting poorly integrated tonic labyrinthine reflex will be severely limited in the ability to move. A few examples of functional limitations are the inability to lift the head in the supine position, initiate flexion to sit up independently from the supine position, roll over, or sit in a wheelchair for long periods.

PHYSICAL PERFORMANCE TEST SCORING SHEET

		Time*	Physical Performance Test Scoring
	Score		

1. Write a sentence
(Whales live in the blue ocean.)

_____ sec

≤10 sec = 4
10.5-15 sec = 3
15.5-20 sec = 2
>20 sec = 1
unable = 0   _____

2. Simulated eating

_____ sec

≤10 sec = 4
10.5-15 sec = 3
15.5-20 sec = 2
>20 sec = 1
unable = 0   _____

3. Lift a book and put it
on a shelf

_____ sec

≤2 sec = 4
2.5-4 sec = 3
4.5-6 sec = 2
>6 sec = 1
unable = 0   _____

4. Put on and remove
a jacket

_____ sec

≤10 sec = 4
10.5-15 sec = 3
15.5-20 sec = 2
>20 sec = 1
unable = 0   _____

5. Pick up penny from floor

_____ sec

≤2 sec = 4
2.5-4 sec = 3
4.5-6 sec = 2
>6 sec = 1
unable = 0   _____

6. Turn 360°

discontinuous steps
continuous steps
unsteady
(grabs, staggers)
steady

0
2

0
2   _____

7. 50-foot walk test

_____ sec

≤15 sec = 4
15.5-20 sec = 3
20.5-25 sec = 2
>25 sec = 1
unable = 0   _____

8. Climb one flight of stairs

_____ sec

≤5 sec = 4
5.5-10 sec = 3
10.5-15 sec = 2
>15 sec = 1
unable = 0   _____

9. Climb stairs†

Number of flights of stairs   _____
up and down (maximum 4)

TOTAL SCORE (maximum 36 for nine-item, 28 for seven-item)

_____ nine-item
_____ seven-item

*For timed measurements, round to nearest 0.5 seconds.
†Omit for seven-item scoring.

Figure 18-5 Physical performance test: scoring sheet (From Reuben DB, Siu AL: An objective measure of physical function of elderly outpatients—the physical performance test, *J Am Geriatr Soc* 38(10):1111, 1990.)

In attempting to move from a supine to sitting position, extensor tone will dominate until the client is halfway up, when flexor tone begins to take over. Flexor tone continues until full sitting is reached, causing the head to fall forward, the spine to flex, and the client to fall forward. Sitting in a wheelchair for extended periods can lead to increased extensor tone as the client hyperextends the head to view the environment. The knee is extended, the foot is pushed forward off the wheelchair footrest, and eventually the client may slip or remain in a half-lying asymmetrical position.[59]

Positive supporting reaction

The positive supporting reaction is caused by pressure on the ball of the foot. This stimulus elicits the following response: rigid extension of the lower extremities due to co-contraction of the flexors and extensors of the knee and hip joints.[59] One may also see internal rotation of the hip, ankle plantar flexion, and foot inversion. The client with a positive supporting reaction will have difficulty placing the heel on the ground for standing, putting the heel down first in walking, and having normal body weight transference in walking. The client will have difficulty getting up from a chair, sitting in a chair, or walking down steps because the leg remains in rigid extension and it is not possible to move the joints while weight bearing. The rigid leg can carry the client's body weight but is unable to contribute to any balance reactions. All balance reactions therefore are compensated for with other parts of the body.[59]

Spinal Level Reflexes

Spinal reflexes can occur after an upper motor neuron lesion. They appear because of a lack of integration with higher centers. Some examples of exaggerated spinal reflexes are hyperactive deep tendon reflexes, the Babinski sign, flexor withdrawal reflex, crossed extension, and grasp reflex.[52] Three spinal reflexes are reviewed.[59]

Crossed extension reflex

The crossed extension reflex causes increased extensor tone in one leg when the other leg is flexed. Therefore, if the client with hemiplegia who is influenced by this reflex flexes the unaffected leg for walking, a strong extensor hypertonicity occurs in the affected leg and interferes with the normal pattern of ambulation. By the same token, the client can bridge (lift buttocks) in bed with the weight supported by both legs. If the unaffected leg is lifted (with hip flexed), however, a total extension pattern occurs in the affected leg and the bridge cannot be maintained.[59]

Flexor withdrawal

The client with flexor withdrawal will exhibit flexion of the ankle, knee, and hip when the sole of the foot is touched (swiped heel to ball of foot). This reflex clearly interferes with gait pattern and transfers.[59]

Grasp reflex

The client with a grasp reflex will not be able to release objects placed in the hand, even if active finger extension is present. The reflexes just discussed are rarely seen in isolation.[53]

TRUNK CONTROL ASSESSMENT

Collin and Wade[21] designed a quick and easily administered test of trunk control that is valid and reliable in clients with a diagnosis of CVA. It involves four timed tests: rolling to the weak side, rolling to the sound side, moving from supine to sitting, and sitting on the side of the bed with the feet off the floor for 30 seconds.[21]

To accurately assess trunk control, the therapist must evaluate strength and control in the following muscle groups: trunk flexors, extensors, lateral flexors, and rotators. The client should be sitting upright on a mat table, with the feet supported for all tests. Again, the client should not be left unattended on the mat table until the therapist determines that the client has adequate trunk control and sitting balance. The procedures described in the following sections are condensed from Gillen and Burkhardt's *Stroke Rehabilitation: A Function-Based Approach*.[37,38]

Trunk Flexors

The examiner asks the client to sit upright, slowly move his or her shoulders behind the hips (eccentric control), and hold the end-range posture (isometric control) (Figure 18-6, *A*). The client is then asked to move forward (concentric control) to resume the initial upright posture (Figure 18-6, *B*).

The examiner should observe for evidence of unilateral weakness, potential for falls, and symmetry of weight shift.

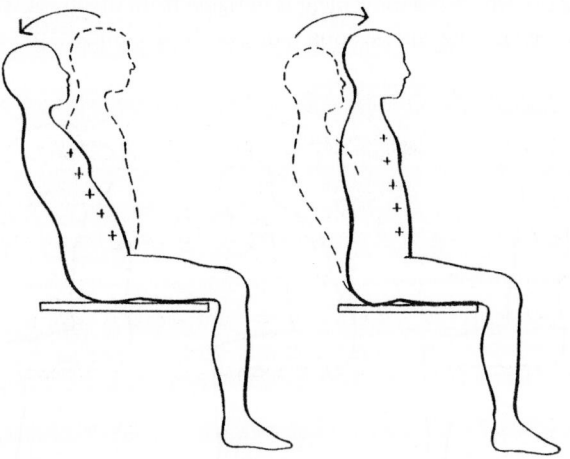

Figure 18-6 Trunk flexor control. Dotted lines indicate trunk starting position, solid lines indicate trunk final position, arrows indicate movement direction, and plus symbols indicate muscle groups primarily responsible for control of pattern. (Skeletal muscle activity occurs on both sides of the trunk [reciprocal innervation].) (From Gillen G, Burkhardt A: *Stroke rehabilitation: a function-based approach*, ed 2, St Louis, 2004, Elsevier Mosby.)

A functional test for trunk flexor control is to observe the client move from supine to sitting.

Trunk Extensors

Test 1

The client is sitting in a position of spinal flexion with a posterior pelvic tilt and moves into trunk extension while simultaneously moving the pelvis into neutral or into a slight anterior tilt. This test assesses concentric trunk extensor control, which is a prerequisite for lower extremity dressing and forward reach (Figure 18-7, *A*).

Test 2

The client is seated in an upright posture. The examiner asks the client to maintain an erect spine and lean forward. This test evaluates eccentric trunk extensor control (Figure 18-7, *B*). For both trunk extensor tests the examiner should observe signs of unilateral weakness and note end-range control.

Test 3

The client is asked to move his or her shoulders back to assume a seated, aligned, upright position. The trunk extensors are contracting concentrically (Figure 18-7, *C*).

Lateral Flexors

The client sits in an upright posture. The pelvis is stationary, and the upper trunk laterally flexes toward the mat table. Figure 18-8, *A* shows eccentric contraction of the left side and muscle shortening of the right side. The client is then asked to return to the original test position (concentric control of the left side) (Figure 18-8, *B*).

Figure 18-8, *C* shows assessment of trunk and pelvis lateral flexion, where the movement is initiated from the lower trunk and pelvis. The end position is one of trunk elongation on the

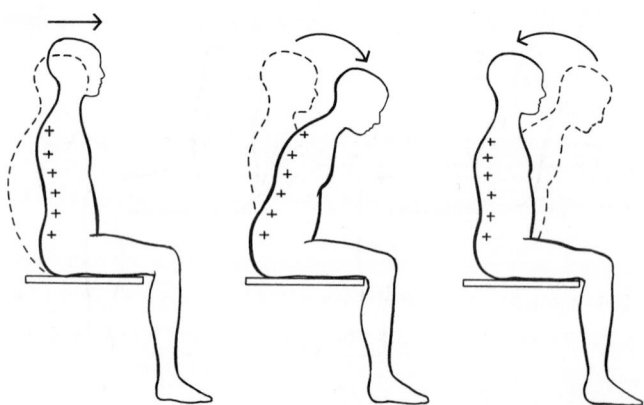

Figure 18-7   Trunk extensor control. Dotted lines indicate trunk starting position, solid lines indicate trunk final position, arrows indicate movement direction, and plus symbols indicate muscle groups primarily responsible for control of pattern. (Skeletal muscle activity occurs on both sides of the trunk [reciprocal innervation].) (From Gillen G, Burkhardt A: *Stroke rehabilitation: a function-based approach*, ed 2, St Louis, 2004, Elsevier Mosby.)

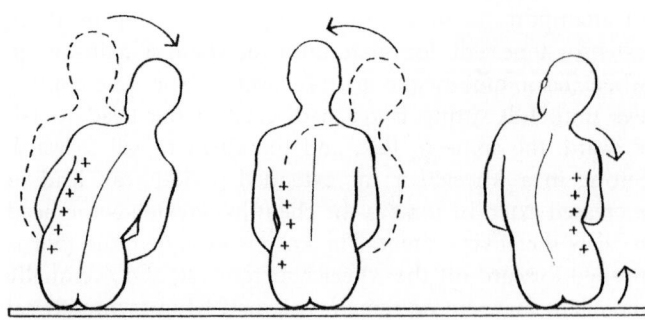

Figure 18-8   Lateral flexor control. Dotted lines indicate trunk starting position, solid lines indicate trunk final position, arrows indicate movement direction, and plus symbols indicate muscle groups primarily responsible for control of pattern. (Skeletal muscle activity occurs on both sides of the trunk [reciprocal innervation].) (From Gillen G, Burkhardt A: *Stroke rehabilitation: a function-based approach*, ed 2, St Louis, 2004, Elsevier Mosby.)

weight-bearing side and shortening on the non–weight-bearing side, which involves concentric contraction of the right side.

Lateral flexion is needed for fall prevention when a client is reaching to the side (e.g., shutting a car door).[38]

Trunk Rotation

The primary muscles responsible for rotation are the obliques. When a person rotates the trunk to the left, the right external and the left internal obliques are recruited. Rotational control is a prerequisite for upper extremity dressing and reaching across the midline. The following three movement patterns are evaluated:

1. The client sits upright and the pelvis is in a neutral, stable position. The client reaches with his or her right arm, across the body, in the direction of the floor. This motion helps assess concurrent flexion and rotation. The motion tests concentric control of the obliques and the back extensors (particularly the thoracic region). Both sides need to be tested.

2. The second movement pattern involves trunk extension with rotation. The upper trunk remains stable, and the lower trunk and pelvis move forward on one side (i.e., shifting forward). Again, both sides are tested.

3. The client is positioned supine for the third movement. The client initiates a "segmental roll by lifting the shoulders from the support surface and toward the opposite side of the body. This pattern is controlled by a concentric contraction of the abdominals (obliques)."[37]

COORDINATION

Coordination is the ability to produce accurate, controlled movement. Characteristics of coordinated movement are smoothness, rhythm, appropriate speed, refinement to the minimum number of muscle groups needed, and appropriate muscle tension, postural tone, and equilibrium. Coordination of muscle action is under the control of the cerebellum and influenced by the extra-pyramidal system.

For coordinated movement, all of the elements of the neuromuscular mechanism must be intact. Coordinated movement depends on the contraction of the correct agonist muscles with simultaneous relaxation of the correct antagonist muscles, together with the contraction of the joint fixator and synergist muscles. In addition, proprioception, body scheme, and the ability to judge space accurately and to direct body parts through space with correct timing to the desired target must be intact.

INCOORDINATION

Many types of lesions can produce disturbances in coordination. Disturbances of coordination often stem from cerebellar and extra-pyramidal disorders. Noncerebellar causes include diseases and injuries of muscles and peripheral nerves, lesions of the posterior columns of the spinal cord, and lesions of the frontal and post-central cerebral cortex. Paralysis of the limbs caused by a peripheral nervous system lesion prevents carrying out tests for coordination, even though CNS mechanisms are intact.

CEREBELLAR DISORDERS

Cerebellar dysfunction can cause incoordination that can affect any body region and cause a variety of clinical symptoms. For example, the client may have postural difficulties that include slouching or leaning positions (caused by bilateral lesions) or spinal curvature (caused by unilateral lesions) and wide-based standing. Eye movements, both voluntary and reflexive, may be affected, as well as the resting position of the eye. The following are common signs of cerebellar dysfunction that the therapist may encounter.[102]

Ataxia

Ataxia is manifested as delayed initiation of movement responses, errors in range and force of movement, and errors in the rate and regularity of movement. There is poor coordination between the agonist and antagonist muscle groups. This results in jerky, poorly controlled movements. When a client with ataxia reaches for an object, it is apparent that the shortest distance between the client and object is not a straight line. The client with gait ataxia has a staggering, wide-based gait with reduced or no arm swing. Step length may be uneven, and the client may have a tendency to fall. The client with cerebellar dysfunction isolated to only one cerebellar hemisphere will have a tendency to fall on the side of the lesion or dysfunction due to the ipsilateral influence of the cerebellum on the lower motor neurons. Ataxia will result in poor postural stability.[28,74]

Adiadochokinesis

Adiadochokinesis is an inability to perform rapid alternating movements such as pronation and supination or elbow flexion and extension. Preston tests this by counting how many cycles a client can perform in a 10-second time frame. A cycle

consists of one full repetition of supination and pronation. It is best to test the unaffected (or lesser affected side) first. The affected side is then compared with the unaffected side.[84]

Dysmetria

Dysmetria is an inability to estimate the ROM necessary to reach the target of the movement. There are two types of dysmetria. Hypermetria involves the limb overshooting the target. Conversely, hypometria involves the limb undershooting the target.[74]

Dyssynergia

Literally, *dyssynergia* is a "decomposition of movement" in which voluntary movements are broken up into their component parts and appear jerky. Dyssynergia can also cause problems in articulation and phonation.[25,74]

Rebound Phenomenon of Holmes

The *rebound phenomenon of Holmes* is the lack of a *check reflex*—that is, the inability to stop a motion quickly to avoid striking something. For example, if the client's arm is flexed against the resistance of the examiner and the resistance is released suddenly, the client's hand will hit the client's face or body.[25]

Nystagmus

Nystagmus is an involuntary movement of the eyeballs in an up-and-down, back-and-forth, or rotating direction. It interferes with the head control and fine adjustments required for balance. Nystagmus can occur as a result of vestibular system, brainstem, or cerebellar lesions.[25]

Dysarthria

Dysarthria is explosive or slurred speech caused by an incoordination of the speech mechanism. The client's speech may also vary in pitch, seem nasal and tremulous, or both.[25]

EXTRA-PYRAMIDAL DISORDERS

Extra-pyramidal disorders are characterized by hypokinesia or hyperkinesia. Parkinson's disease is characterized by hypokinesia (bradykinesia), cogwheel and lead pipe rigidity, a decrease or loss of postural mechanisms, and a resting, pill-rolling tremor.[27]

"Parkinson's Plus" is the name given to a group of movement disorders that have signs of Parkinson's disease with concomitant neurological deficits. *Progressive supranuclear palsy* (PSP) is one such disease.[52] Clients affected with PSP have "loss of vertical ocular gaze, rigidity of the neck and trunk muscles, dementia, and parkinsonian signs,"[51] usually in the absence of tremor. Life expectancy is shorter than in Parkinson's disease. Death often occurs within 6 to 10 years.[51]

Chorea

Chorea is irregular, purposeless, involuntary, coarse, quick, jerky, and dysrhythmic movements of variable distribution.

These movements may occur during sleep.[25] Two diagnoses often presenting with chorea are tardive dyskinesia and Huntington's disease. *Tardive dyskinesia* is a drug-induced disorder, often associated with neuroleptic drug use. Occupational therapists most often see clients who have tardive dyskinesia in psychiatric settings. *Huntington's disease* is an inherited, autosomal dominant disease. Clients with Huntington's disease have an ataxic gait with choreoathetoid movements. As the disease progresses, rigidity develops. Choreiform movements are faster than athetoid.[52]

Athetoid Movements

Athetoid movements are continuous, slow, wormlike, arrhythmic movements that primarily affect the distal portions of the extremities. These movements occur in the same patterns in the same subject and are not present during sleep.[25] Adult athetosis can occur after cerebral anoxia and Wilson's disease. Movement patterns include alternating "extension and flexion of the arm, supination and pronation of the forearm, and flexion and extension of the fingers."[51] Athetosis that occurs with chorea is termed "choreoathetosis."[52]

Dystonia

Dystonia results in persistent posturing of the extremities (e.g., in hyperextension or hyperflexion of the wrist and fingers) often with concurrent torsion of the spine and associated twisting of the trunk.[1] Dystonic movements are often continuous and are often seen in conjunction with spasticity. Figure 18-9 shows a client with a traumatic brain injury, with his right wrist and fingers exhibiting dystonia. Dystonia can be primary or secondary, the latter occurring with other CNS disorders (e.g., hypoxic brain injury or tumor). Segmental dystonia involves two or more adjacent body parts. Generalized and multifocal dystonia also exist. Focal dystonia involves only one limb, as seen in writer's cramp, musician's cramp, and spasmodic torticollis.[51]

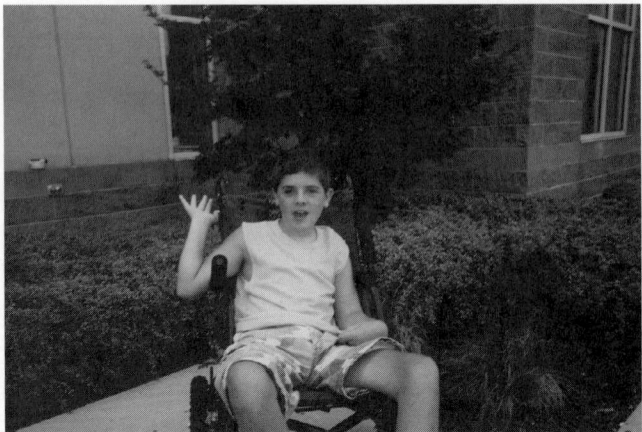

Figure 18-9 A client with right upper extremity dystonic posturing of the wrist and finger extensors. His left wrist shows severe hypotonicity. The tone abnormalities are a result of a traumatic brain injury.

Ballism

Ballism is a rare symptom that is produced by continuous, abrupt contractions of the axial and proximal musculature of the extremity. Ballism causes the limb to fly out suddenly. It occurs on one side of the body (hemiballism) and is caused by lesions of the opposite subthalamic nucleus.[25,74]

Tremor

The following are three common types of tremor:
1. *Intention tremor,* associated with cerebellar disease, occurs during voluntary movement. It is intensified at the termination of the movement and is often seen in multiple sclerosis. The client with intention tremor may have trouble performing tasks that require accuracy and precision of limb placement (e.g., drinking from a cup or inserting a key in a lock).
2. *Resting tremor* occurs at rest and subsides when voluntary movement is attempted. It occurs as a result of damage or disease of the basal ganglia and is seen in Parkinson's disease.
3. *Essential familial tremor* is inherited as an autosomal dominant trait. It is most visible when the client is carrying out a fine precision task.[51]

ASSESSMENT OF COORDINATION

MEDICAL ASSESSMENT OF COORDINATION

Incoordination consists of errors in rate, rhythm, range, direction, and force of movement.[36] Therefore, observation is an important element of the clinical examination. The neurological examination for incoordination may include the nose-finger-nose test, the finger-nose test, the heel-knee test, the knee pat (pronation-supination) test, hand pat and foot pat tests, finger wiggling, and drawing a spiral. Such tests can reveal dysmetria, dyssynergia, adiadochokinesis, tremors, and ataxia. Usually the neurologist or physiatrist performs these examinations. Magnetic resonance imaging and computerized tomography scans may also be ordered. Tremors are frequency rated with EMG, which helps the physician accurately diagnose tremor type.[51]

OCCUPATIONAL THERAPY ASSESSMENT OF COORDINATION

Selected activities and specific performance tests can reveal the effect of incoordination on function. The occupational therapist can observe for coordination difficulties during ADL assessment. The therapist can prepare simulated tasks that require coordinated muscle function, such as writing, opening containers, tossing and catching a bean-bag or ball, or playing a board game.[94] The therapist should observe for irregularity in the rate of movement and for sudden, corrective movements in an attempt to compensate for incoordination. Movement during the performance of various activities may appear irregular and jerky and overreach the mark. The following general guidelines and questions can be used when evaluating incoordination:

1. Assess the muscle tone and joint mobility first in a sitting position.
2. Observe for ataxia, proximal to distal, during functional upper extremity movement. Are movements away from or toward the body more difficult for the client? Where, within the ROM, is ataxia most prevalent?
3. Stabilize joints proximally to distally during the functional task and note differences in client performance, as compared with performance without stabilization. (Stabilization can be by splinting or stabilizing the affected body part against a wall.) Weighted cuffs may be applied to the extremity during task performance to determine if weighting or resistance decreases the tremor (use caution). Note the amount of resistance provided. Observe whether the weights make the coordination worse. Sometimes the use of weights increases tremor.
4. Observe for tremor. Are the eyes and speech affected?
5. Does the client's emotional status affect coordination?
6. How do the client's ataxia or coordination problems affect participation in occupation?
7. Perform an occupational profile as well as a performance patterns interview, asking about the client's roles, routines, goals, and environment to determine which functions are important for the client.

Numerous standardized tests of motor function and manual dexterity are available and can be used to evaluate coordination. Some of these tests are the Purdue Pegboard,[88] the Minnesota Rate of Manipulation Test,[75] the Lincoln-Oseretsky Motor Development Scale,[64] the Pennsylvania Bimanual Work Sample,[83] the Crawford Small Parts Dexterity Test,[22] the Jebsen-Taylor Hand Function Test,[53] and The 9-Hole Peg Test.[67] The standardized functional assessments for CVA, e.g., the GWMFT, mentioned earlier in this chapter, may also be useful for measuring the efficacy of occupational therapy intervention for impaired coordination.[76]

OCCUPATIONAL THERAPY INTERVENTION

INTERVENTION FOR HYPERTONICITY AND SPASTICITY

Hypertonicity is only one part of the UMNS. It is very important to treat other performance deficits of the UMNS such as paresis, fatigue, and decreased dexterity. These deficits can impede function more than hypertonia.[14]

Before treating hypertonus, the therapist and physician need to closely evaluate the function of the tone. Hypertonicity can have beneficial effects, such as aiding in standing and transfers, maintaining muscle bulk, and preventing deep vein thrombosis, osteoporosis, and edema. Intervention is necessary when spasticity interferes with ADLs, gait, sleep, or wheelchair positioning or when it causes severe pain and limits hygiene (e.g., the client is unable to wash hand or axilla)

or leads to contractures or decubitus ulcers. Hypertonicity or spasticity may be treated with conservative therapeutic interventions, pharmacological agents, or surgery.[87]

Conservative Treatment Approaches

Weight bearing

For hypertonicity reduction and paresis remediation in the upper extremity, therapists have been using weight-bearing skills/activities for many years when treating clients with upper motoneuron lesions. When researching the neuropsychological benefits of weight bearing, only three current (over the past 10 years) studies were found via an English language CINAHL and Medline Search.

Brouwer and Ambury concluded that corticospinal facilitation of motor units occurred during upper extremity weight bearing. They believed that afferent input from weight bearing increased motor cortical excitability.[15] Chakerain and Larson studied the effects of upper extremity weight bearing on hand opening and prehension in children with spastic cerebral palsy. Computer calculations of the clients' hand surface area were measured. There was an increase in surface area after weight bearing, and an increase in the maturity of movement components needed for prehension.[19] McIllroy and Maki demonstrated that if the affected arm is used when weight bearing, postural responses occur throughout the weight bearing extremity and occur during other perturbations of posture.[72]

Despite the fact that there are not very many well-controlled studies that document how and why weight bearing works physiologically, it certainly is a requirement for improving functional performance. Clients need upper extremity postural support when reaching to the floor to pick up an object while seated, to prevent falling. When standing, upper extremity weight bearing is needed to reach into a high cabinet to aid the clients' balance.[38]

Traditional Sensorimotor Approaches

Proprioceptive neuromuscular facilitation (PNF; see Chapter 30) has been shown to be effective in gaining motor control for a variety of diagnoses.[95] According to the Neuro-Developmental Treatment (NDT) Association,[78] therapists who follow an NDT approach:

- "Utilize an in-depth analysis of the intricacies of movement and how the details relate to the whole to allow for functional movement in a wide variety of environments.
- Believe that control of movement is based on a complex interaction of many body systems, which are plastic and adaptable, as well as on the tasks presented and the environments in which the tasks are performed. Therefore, function can be altered by changing one or more of these elements.
- Utilize an understanding of the development of atypical movement, as well as the compensations to help minimize the impact of CNS pathology and prevent the emergence of contractures and deformities which contribute to the functional problems."[78]

TABLE 18-1 Modified Brunnstrom Stages of Motor Recovery as a Guideline for Interdisciplinary Spasticity Management in Subjects with CVA or Hemiparesis from Traumatic Brain Injury

Brunnstrom Stage	Brunnstrom Motor Recovery of Arm and Hand	Interdisciplinary Spasticity Management Options
Stage 1	Flaccidity. No active movement.	Prevent contractures with PROM and splinting. Risk for metacarpophalangeal extension contractures.
Stage 2	Beginning development of spasticity, weak synergistic movement of scapular retractors, scapular elevators, elbow flexors, and forearm pronators.	Prevent contractures with PROM and splinting. Risk for shoulder, elbow, forearm, and finger flexion contractures. Promote active movement in gravity-reduced planes.* Blocks or surgery are generally not indicated at this stage.
Stage 3	Spasticity increasing. Synergy pattern can possibly be useful for carrying objects. Synergy patterns or some of their components can be performed voluntarily. Gross grasp is developing, however no finger release. Lateral pinch possible via thumb adduction tone and flexor pollicis longus tone.	Acute: Good candidate for nerve or motor point blocks to prevent contractures. There may be a possibility of facilitating recovery by unmasking movement in antagonists if the spastic agonists are weakened through blocks. See text for occupational therapy treatment suggestions. Chronic: After all conservative measures have failed, orthopedic surgery to release contractures to improve hygiene in the hand and ease UE dressing.
Stage 4	Spasticity declining, movement combinations from synergies are now possible. Elbow extension, wrist and finger extension are emerging; however are not to full range.	Acute: Good to excellent nerve block candidate. Better chance of gaining motor control of antagonists with blocks to the spastic agonists. See text for occupational therapy treatment suggestions. Chronic: Ongoing blocks three to four times per year if the risk/benefit ratio for orthopedic surgery is not acceptable to the client. Orthopedic surgery options include procedures to gain function as well as ameliorating contractures.
Stage 5	Synergies are no longer dominant. Finger extension is full range. Isolated finger extension is possible. Three-jaw chuck pinch is possible, but has poor motor control. Emergence of intrinsic function.	Excellent candidate for fine-tuning motor control via blocks, e.g., blocking the extrinsic flexor pollicis longus with the goal of facilitating intrinsic motor control of the thumb, opponens pollicis, abductor pollicis brevis, and flexor pollicis brevis.
Stage 6	Isolated joint movements are performed with ease. Intrinsic function is normal. All types of prehension.	The client is not a candidate for blocks or surgery. Discharge occupational therapy, as goals were met.

*Blocks refer to chemical denervation with botulinum toxin type A or B or neurolysis or motor point blocks with phenol or alcohol.
Note: Upper extremity recovery is variable owing to varying degrees of paralysis. Some clients may never progress through all the stages.
Adapted from Brunnstrom S: *Movement therapy in hemiplegia*, Philadelphia, 1970, Lippincott Williams & Wilkins.

Another occupational therapy objective is to have the client manage muscle tone to engage in and complete basic and instrumental activities of daily living. Positioning and movement in patterns opposite to hypertonic or synergistic patterns are important to expand the motor repertoire and develop movement that is as close to normal as possible. At times it is appropriate to facilitate synergistic movements in the client with chronic disease (or if the client does not recover beyond Modified Brunnstrom's Stage 3) (Table 18-1). The synergy patterns can be facilitated to improve lateral pinch or elbow flexion function. The client should be taught how to modulate the abnormal tone or how to instruct others to do so. The client should also be taught how to incorporate the affected upper extremity as much as possible into all ADLs. ADLs, crafts, games, and work activities can be used to teach incorporation of the extremities for a total approach to treatment.[99] Refer to Chapter 30 for a more detailed review of traditional sensorimotor treatment strategies.

Juan was recovering from an acute CVA. His Modified Brunnstrom Stages of Motor Recovery Score was 4 (see Table 18-1). He had good rehabilitation potential to restore the client factors needed for ADL tasks. The therapist will work with him on acquiring full finger extension and dexterity for keyboarding, and supination activities for opening doors and holding change.

Even when motor control is adequate for participation in occupation, the sensory, cognitive, and perceptual abilities of the client may affect the achievement of functional goals. Perceptual dysfunction may alter the client's abilities, requiring the therapist to focus on perceptual training as well.[7]

Casting

In some cases unilateral hypertonicity is severe enough to necessitate serial inhibitive casting or splinting (see Chapter 29). Casting in inhibitive postures has been shown to be effective in tone reduction.[46,110] The beneficial effect of casting on hypertonia and upper extremity contractures has also been well documented in the literature.[8,31,33]

Casting in inhibitive postures is effective because it provides neutral warmth, maintained pressure, and constant joint positioning with static lengthening of muscle.[49] **Serial casting** is most successful when a contracture has been present for less than 6 months. The cast may be bivalved (cut in half) and worn as a splint. This helps protect the skin and allows the therapist to work with the extremity out of the cast. However, many clinicians believe that a nonbivalved cast is more effective and actually causes less skin breakdown. A dropout cast, which can be used as part of the serial casting process, includes a cutout area, allowing movement of the joint in the desired direction. For example, for an elbow that has flexor hypertonicity, the dorsal upper arm portion of a long arm cast can be cut out to allow the triceps to be facilitated to extend the arm.

Serial casting should cease when desired position is achieved and tone is manageable with the last cast or splint. If there is no evidence of increased passive ROM after two to three casts are removed, serial casting must cease; however, the last cast should be kept, bivalved, and used as a "retainer" splint to prevent further contractures, similar to retainer use in orthodontics. Many innovations have occurred in commercially available spasticity reduction splints that are used to place the wrist and hand in inhibitive postures. The client and family need to be educated in continuing to incorporate the extremity in occupation, and to bear weight on the extremity as much as possible to retain the ROM gains achieved during casting.[87]

Physical Agent Modalities

Physical agent modalities such as cold, superficial heat, ultrasound, and neuromuscular electrical stimulation can be used as preparation for or in conjunction with purposeful activity and muscle re-education, provided the therapist has the appropriate training and can prove competency. Ultrasound can help inhibit or reduce hypertonicity temporarily and increase tendon and muscle extensibility. It is helpful to provide concurrent stretch during the ultrasound procedure.[87] Neuromuscular electrical stimulation has been shown to strengthen paretic muscles.[17,47]

Juan actually did gain strength and range of motion in his finger extensors with the help of neuromuscular electrical stimulation to the extensor digitorum communis muscle group, the extrinsic finger extensors. His extrinsic strength improved from 3-/5 to 4/5 within one month.

Distal to Proximal Approach

The *Functional Tone Management* (FTM) Arm Training Program was developed by Saebo Inc. to address the weaknesses of therapeutic interventions currently applied to the neurologically impaired upper extremity (UE) and hand. The occupational therapists that founded Saebo, theorized that because grasp and release capabilities are pivotal to re-integrating the UE into daily activities, a paradigm shift for UE neurological rehabilitation was needed. While traditional therapeutic interventions such as Bobath-based programs are based on a proximal to distal recovery pattern, Saebo developed their FTM Arm Training Program based on a distal activation model, focusing on the key point of early initiation of UE movements that incorporate grasp and release. In order to incorporate the hand into the FTM Arm Training, Saebo developed a dynamic orthosis for the hand, called the SaeboFlex (Figure 18-10).

The SaeboFlex orthosis assists an individual who exhibits hypertonia in the hand to place the hand in an open,

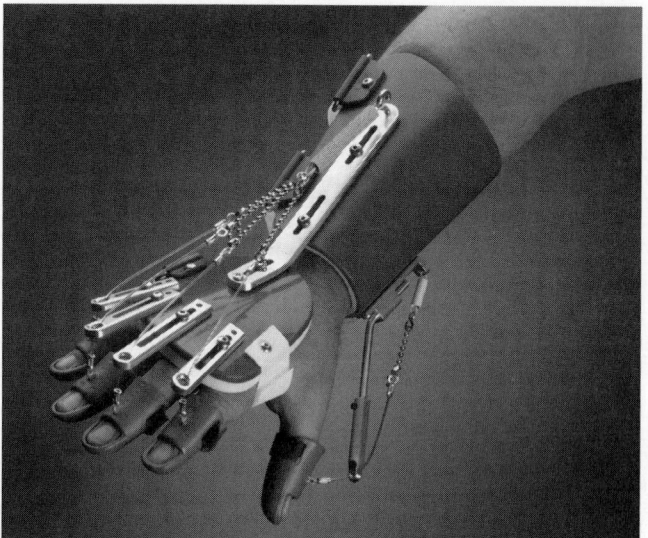

Figure 18-10   Saeboflex dynamic orthosis. (Courtesy Saebo, Inc., Charlotte, NC.)

functional position. This positioning is accomplished by means of a fixed wrist support and a variable strength finger and thumb spring system. Once the hand is open, the client can begin to retrain the finger flexors for improved motor control of the hand. While wearing the SaeboFlex, the client relearns to produce a graded muscle contraction of the finger flexors in order to grasp an object. The finger and thumb spring system, coupled with the client's own efforts to relax muscle activation, allows the hand to open enough for the object held in the hand to be released.

Once the client is comfortable using the SaeboFlex, the FTM Arm Training Program can begin. The FTM program combines high repetition grasp and release with task-specific arm training drills to progress the client toward a functional goal. A significant body of research supports the FTM Arm Training Program;[16,34,103] however, the program does not require the wrist or finger extension typically needed to participate in a constraint-induced program. Clinically observed improvements with the FTM Arm Training Program include increased AROM at the shoulder elbow and wrist, improved UE Fugl-Meyer scores, and decreased Modified Ashworth scores.[32] Clients as far as 20 years post-insult have shown improvements. Independent research studies using the SaeboFlex and FTM Arm Training Program are underway.

Pharmacological Agents

Pharmacological agents prescribed and administered by physicians include oral medication, short-term nerve blocks, and long-term blocks.

Clients with severe hypertonicity accompanied by severe pain may need evaluation of the cause of the pain. Drug therapy and other pain management techniques may be part of the treatment approach. The four commonly used oral medications for spasticity of UMN origin are diazepam, baclofen, dantrolene sodium, and tizanidine. Dantrolene sodium acts at the skeletal muscle. Dantrolene sodium is preferred in cerebral spasticity because it is less apt to cause sedation. However, it can cause weakness and liver damage. Diazepam's side effects include drowsiness, fatigue, and possible addiction. Baclofen is more effective with spinal cord injuries than with cerebral injuries. Its potential side effects are confusion, drowsiness, and hallucinations. Neither diazepam nor baclofen can be discontinued suddenly because to do so may cause seizures. Tizanidine HCl is labeled for spasticity reduction in multiple sclerosis and spinal cord injury. Its side effects may include hypotension, sedation, and visual hallucinations. No matter which drug is used, it is crucial for the occupational therapist to communicate to the medical staff any noted side effects that interfere with the client's overall function.[87]

Nerve blocks and motor point blocks are injections of a chemical agent to diminish or obliterate tone. There are short- and long-term blocks. Short-term blocks are injections of an anesthetic (e.g., bupivacaine) to temporarily reduce pain and muscle tone. These short-term blocks help the physician differentiate between hypertonus and contracture.[86] The short-term blocks last from 1 to 7 hours, depending on which anesthetic is used.

Long-term blocks, usually injections of phenol or botulinum toxin-type A (Botox) or botulinum toxin type B (Myobloc®), generally last several months. Botox® lasts for 2 to 5 months with spastic hypertonia. Botulinum toxin type B has been shown to quell cervical dystonia for 12-16 weeks.[2] Phenol blocks last from 2 to 8 months, depending on whether the motor points (2 to 3 months) or the motor branch (8 months) is injected. Phenol and the botulinum toxins type A and B have different mechanisms of action. Botulinum toxins type A and B exert their effect via chemical denervation, and phenol works via motor point or motor branch neurolysis. Both blocks can be used to diminish or obliterate hypertonicity in the agonist. The blocks help to prevent contractures and render the hypertonic muscle weak or flaccid.[20,44,81] The effect and time interval of the long-term block provide therapists the opportunity to increase antagonistic strength and function. A combination of long-acting blocks and casting or splinting is often used to treat hypertonicity. Long-term blocks in the upper extremities are commonly used in the subscapularis, brachioradialis, and flexor digitorum superficialis.[87]

Surgical Methods

Surgery to control hypertonicity is also an option. Dynamic EMG can help orthopedic surgeons plan surgery. Orthopedic surgical intervention can improve function or release contractures. Examples of upper extremity functional surgery include lengthening of the biceps tendon to reduce elbow flexion and gain elbow extension, thumb-in-palm release, and transfer of the flexor carpi ulnaris tendon to the extensor carpi radialis longus or brevis tendons to decrease the deforming force of wrist flexion while simultaneously augmenting wrist extension.[84] An example of a contracture release procedure is the flexor digitorum superficialis to profundus transfer to gain length in the extrinsic finger flexors.[48]

Therapists will encounter clients with severe spasticity who have had a neurosurgical procedure performed called *intrathecal baclofen pump* (ITB) implantation. This enables baclofen to enter the body at the spinal level and avoids the centrally mediated side effects of oral baclofen. The ITB provides baclofen, a spasticity-reducing medication, directly into the intrathecal (subarachnoid) space via a catheter attached to a subcutaneous implantable pump in the abdomen. A client must undergo a lumbar puncture test dose of intrathecal baclofen to determine candidacy before pump implantation.[73]

ITB has been shown to be very effective in the reduction of severe spinal spasticity and spasticity associated with multiple sclerosis and is also effective for cerebral spasticity. For further details of medical and surgical treatments and their relation to occupational therapy, the reader is referred to Preston and Hecht's *Spasticity Management: Rehabilitation Strategies.*[87]

TREATMENT OF RIGIDITY

Decerebrate and decorticate rigidity can wax and wane. When the rigidity is waning, it is recommended that the client be transferred to a wheelchair or reclining chair because the rigidity decreases in sitting. The rigidity is worse during episodes of agitation.[59] Parkinson's rigidity responds temporarily to heat, massage, stretching, and ROM exercises. Rocking back and forth before standing can aid in the transition.[65] See Chapter 35 discussing Parkinson's disease for additional treatment strategies for rigidity.

TREATMENT OF FLACCIDITY

Flaccidity stemming from upper motor neuron dysfunction (e.g., recovering from spinal or cerebral shock resulting from acute CNS insult) is treated with facilitation techniques such as weight bearing, high-frequency vibration, tapping, quick stretch, bed positioning with weight on the flaccid side the majority of the time, and functional neuromuscular electrical stimulation. Splinting the hand and wrist may be indicated for support. Therapists should closely supervise splinting, since contractures can result from excessive splint wear. Passive ROM exercises also are indicated. The arm can be passively positioned as normally as possible during ADL tasks to provide sensory and proprioceptive feedback. When the client is eating, have him or her place his or her arm on the dining room table, resting on top of a piece of Dycem.[29] Client and family education in proper positioning and joint protection is important to protect over-lengthening of soft tissues and prevent trauma, e.g., having his or her arm fall off of the lap and bump the wheel of their wheelchair.[87]

TREATMENT OF INCOORDINATION

Admittedly, treatment of incoordination is difficult. Activities graded on the basis of motor learning and control may be helpful for attaining proximal stability and then mobility.

Therapy directed toward the modulation of reflexes and abnormal synergy patterns and the enhancement of postural control mechanisms, such as the righting and equilibrium reactions, can help to improve coordination. Weight bearing, joint approximation, placing and holding techniques, and fixed points of stability (having the client stabilize his elbow or wrist on the tabletop) can be helpful.

It is critical that the therapist encourage the client to use his or her vision to help direct their upper extremity movements. The therapist should begin with small ranges of movement and gradually increase them as the client progresses. Initially, work is done in the plane and direction of movement that are easiest for the client, and the work progresses toward more difficult areas. Some of the involuntary movements of cerebellar or extra-pyramidal origin, particularly primary movement disorders, are difficult to manage or change. Therapists have more influence over the movement disorders that are associated with traumatic brain injury and stroke.

Methods and devices to compensate for incoordination may be necessary to make BADLs and IADLs safer, more possible, and more satisfying. Obtaining a thorough occupational profile is necessary to make appropriate activity and equipment choices and determine adaptive strategies that the client can carry over to the home environment. The physician may employ pharmacological agents or surgical intervention in an effort to dampen tremors or other involuntary movement patterns.[74]

SURGICAL INTERVENTION FOR MOVEMENT DISORDERS

Neurosurgical intervention for movement disorders may include stereotactic thalatomy for ballismus, chorea (Huntington's), Parkinson's disease, essential tremor, and athetosis. Surgical treatment for dystonia may include rhizotomy, neurectomy, cryothalotomy, or ITB implantation.[51] Deep brain stimulation has been effective in tremor reduction in essential tremor and Parkinson's disease.[74,97]

Because of the current managed care system, occupational therapists are receiving more referrals than ever before from primary care physicians. Occupational therapists who have a basic knowledge of the medical and surgical options in ameliorating motor control problems can play a triage role in suggesting referral to physician specialists.

THREADED CASE STUDY: JUAN, PART 2

Juan has experienced motor control dysfunction secondary to his CVA. The resultant effects have impaired his performances areas of occupation, performance patterns, and performance motor skills, and have affected many client factors. Fortunately, his proximal motor control was not affected by the CVA. His distal motor

control was affected enough to impair resuming the premorbid role of primary breadwinner for his family.

Juan cannot operate a keyboard with his left hand for three reasons: (1) the moderate finger flexion hypertonia pulled his fingers into flexion when he tried to keyboard, (2) the antagonist muscles (the finger extensors with the intrinsics being weaker than the extrinsics) are too weak to counteract the finger flexion hypertonia, and (3) he experienced abnormal timing of the agonist/antagonist muscles that impaired his coordination needed for keyboarding. His high timed score (left upper extremity) on the Graded Wolf Motor Function Test provided an objective measure of his coordination deficit.

Juan cannot open his car door, receive change in his hand from the drive-though window cashier, or carry a glass without spilling the contents due to moderate pronator hypertonia. The pronation hypertonia limited his available active range of motion for supination. Furthermore, his supination strength was weak, 4- out of 5, not quite enough to counteract the pronation hypertonicity. This, coupled with impaired dexterity from the stroke, interferes with the performance of these activities.

To improve the motor control of his finger extensors, a home program could include releasing a 5-inch foam ball while playing catch. Using his left hand to help wash his face with a washcloth would also help him obtain full finger extension. A good intrinsic motor control activity is flipping paper footballs with combined PIP and DIP finger extension. For his supinators, one could start having him control a lightweight hammer in his lap, turning it back and forth into supination and pronation. He could start opening lightweight interior doors with his left hand, then progress to heavier doors like his car door. He could start carrying an empty glass with his left hand and gradually progress to filling it 1/4 full, 1/2 full, then 3/4 full. Occupational therapists trained in neuromuscular electrical stimulation can expedite recovery of range of motion and strength by placing electrodes on his wrist extensors and extensor digitorum communis while the client actively performs composite wrist and finger extension. Another suggested electrode placement would be on the biceps and supinator muscle. For the latter placement, the negative electrode would be placed on the supinator and the positive on the biceps. (An asymmetrical waveform would be utilized.) Again, active recruitment of the supination motion would be encouraged.

Clearly, Juan was working too many hours premorbidly. He was not getting enough sleep and his hypertension was not controlled. Occupational therapy needs to include educating him in balancing work, rest, and leisure activities. While he is recovering, his wife can take over the duty of driving his children to school.

Incidentally, Juan is working full time now, 8- to 9-hour days, and keyboards at 75% of his premorbid speed. All of his goals listed during the COPM interview were met. He has full range of motion in all of his fingers and his strength grade is 4/5 in the extrinsic finger extensors. His two remaining motor deficits are decreased index finger (PIP) extension strength (3+ to 4−) and decreased speed of his PIP extension; it is much slower than his other three fingers. His blood pressure is now well controlled. He sleeps 8-10 hours per day.

SUMMARY

As one can determine from reading the aforementioned case study, the presence of abnormal elements of motor control affects the quality of movement and the ability to perform in areas of occupation. The occupational therapist assesses muscle tone, upper extremity recovery, and coordination, using standardized tests and observation of movement during occupational performance. The results of the motor control assessment can help the client and therapist collaborate on appropriate intervention. Ameliorating motor control can be a rewarding experience for the client and the therapist.

Review Questions

1. Define plasticity.
2. When would a physician recommend a long-term nerve block or motor point block?
3. Describe the characteristics of rigidity.
4. Compare and contrast spasticity and hypertonia.
5. Why should the assessment of muscle tone be performed in conjunction with the client's overall motor function?
6. Demonstrate how to perform an upper extremity muscle tone evaluation.
7. Describe equilibrium reactions and the functional implications of their presence in motor control.
8. Describe functional difficulties encountered when the asymmetrical tonic neck reflex is present.
9. Compare and contrast chorea and athetosis.
10. Describe ataxia.
11. Compare and contrast the following tremors: essential familial, resting, and intention.

REFERENCES

1. Adams RD, Victor M, editors: *Principles of neurology,* ed 5, New York, 1993, McGraw-Hill.
2. Albany K: Physical and occupational therapy considerations in adult patients receiving botulinum toxin injections for spasticity. In Mayer NH, Simpson DM, editors: *Spasticity: etiology, evaluation, management and the role of botulinum toxin,* New York, 2002, We Move™
3. Allison SC, et al: Reliability of the Modified Ashworth Scale in the assessment of plantar-flexor muscle spasticity in patients with traumatic brain injury, *Int J Rehabil Res* 19(1):67, 1996.
4. Ashworth B: Preliminary trial of carisoprodol in multiple sclerosis, *Practitioner* 192:540, 1964.
5. Bell-Krotoski JA, et al: Threshold detection and Semmes-Weinstein monofilaments, *J Hand Ther* 8(2):155, 1995.
6. Berg KO, et al: Measuring balance in the elderly: preliminary development of an instrument, *Physiother Can* 41:304, 1989.
7. Bernspang B, Fischer AG: Differences between persons with right or left CVA on the Assessment of Motor and Process Skills, *Arch Phys Med Rehabil* 76:1114, 1995.
8. Blackburn M, et al: Reliability of measurements obtained with the modified Ashworth scale in the lower extremity of people with stroke, *Phys Ther* 82(1):25, 2002.
9. Blanton S, Wolf S: An application of upper extremity constraint-induced movement therapy in a patient with sub-acute stroke, *Phys Ther* 79(9):847, 1999.
10. Bohannon RW, Smith MB: Interrater reliability of a modified Ashworth scale of muscle spasticity, *Phys Ther* 67(2):206, 1987.
11. Bontke CF, Boake C: Principles of brain injury rehabilitation. In Braddom R, editor: *Physical medicine and rehabilitation,* Philadelphia, 1996, WB Saunders.
12. Botox®, Allergan pharmaceuticals, Inc. 2525 Dupont Drive, P.O. Box 19534, Irvine, CA 92713-9534.
13. Boyd R, Graham H: Objective measurement of clinical findings in the use of botulinum toxin for the management of children with cerebral palsy, *Eur Journal of Neurol* 6:523, 1999.
14. Brashear A, et al: Inter- and intrarater reliability of the Ashworth Scale and the Disability Assessment Scale in patients with upper limb poststroke spasticity, *Arch Phys Med Rehabil* 83(10):1349, 2002.
15. Brouwer BJ, Ambury P: Upper extremity weight bearing effect on corticospinal excitability following stroke, *Arch Phys Med Rehabil* 75:861, 1994.
16. Butefisch C, et al: Repetitive training of isolated movements improves the outcome of motor rehabilitation of centrally paretic hand, *J Neur Sci* 130:59, 1995.
17. Carmick J: Clinical use of neuromuscular electrical stimulation for children with cerebral palsy *Phys Ther* 73(8):514, 1993.
18. Carr JH, Shepherd RB: *Neurological rehabilitation: optimizing motor performance,* Oxford, 1998, Butterworth-Heinemann.
19. Chakerian DL, Larson MA: Effects of upper-extremity weight bearing on hand-opening and prehension patterns in children with cerebral palsy, *Dev Med Child Neurol* 35:216, 1993.
20. Chironna RL, Hecht JS: Subscapularis motor point block for the painful hemiplegic shoulder, *Arch Phys Med Rehabil* 71(6):428, 1990.
21. Collin C, Wade D: Assessing motor impairment after a stroke: a pilot reliability study, *J Neurol Neurosurg Psychiatry* 53(7):576, 1990.
22. *Crawford Small Parts Dexterity Test,* New York, Psychological Corporation.
23. Cruickshank DA, O'Neill DL: Upper-extremity inhibitive casting in a boy with spastic quadriplegia, *Am J Occup Ther* 44(6):552, 1990.
24. DeBoskey DS, et al: *Educating families of the head injured,* Gaithersburg, MD, 1991, Aspen Publishers.
25. deGroot J: *Correlative neuroanatomy,* ed 21, Norwalk, CT, 1991, Appleton & Lange.
26. Desrosiers J, et al: Upper extremity performance test for the elderly (TEMPA): normative data and correlates with sensorimotor parameters, *Arch Phys Med Rehabil* 76(12):1125, 1995.
27. Dombovy ML: Rehabilitation concerns in degenerative movement disorders of the central nervous system. In Braddom RL, editor: *Physical medicine and rehabilitation,* Philadelphia, 1996, WB Saunders.
28. Donato S, Pulaski KH: Overview of balance impairments: functional implications. In Gillen G, Burkhardt A, editors: *Stroke rehabilitation: a function-based approach,* St. Louis, 1998, Mosby.

29. Dycem®, Sammons Preston Roylan. An Ability One Company. P.O. Box 5071, Bolingbrook, IL 60440-5071.

30. Eltorai I, Montroy R: Muscle release in the management of spasticity in spinal cord injury, *Paraplegia* 28(7):433, 1990.

31. Farber S: *Neurorehabilitation: a multisensory approach,* Philadelphia, 1982, WB Saunders.

32. Farrell J, et al: *Orthotic aided training of the paretic limb in chronic stroke: results of a phase 1 trial,* unpublished manuscript, 2003.

33. Feldman PA: Upper extremity casting and splinting. In Glenn MB, White J, editors: *The practical management of spasticity in children and adults,* Philadelphia, 1990, Lea & Febiger.

34. Feys H, et al: Early and repetitive stimulation of the arm can substantially improve the long-term outcome after stroke: a 5-year follow-up study of a randomized trial, *Stroke* 35:924, 2004.

35. Fosang AL, et al: Measures of muscle and joint performance in lower limbs of children with cerebral palsy, *Dev Med Child Neurol* 45(10): 664, 2003.

36. Ghez C: The cerebellum. In Kandel ER, Schwartz JH, Jessel TM, editors: *Principles of neural science,* ed 3, New York, 1991, Elsevier.

37. Gillen G: Trunk control: a prerequisite for functional independence. In Gillen G, Burkhardt A, editors: *Stroke rehabilitation: a function-based approach,* St Louis, 1998, Mosby.

38. Gillen G: Trunk control: a prerequisite for functional independence. In Gillen G, Burkhardt A, editors: *Stroke rehabilitation: a function-based approach,* ed 2, St Louis, 2004, Elsiever Mosby.

39. Goldberg C, VanSant A: Normal motor development. In Tecklin JS, ed: *Pediatric physical therapy,* ed 3, Philadelphia, 1999, Lippincott, Williams & Wilkins.

40. Gorman IG: personal communication, June 2004.

41. Gracies JM, Marosszeky JE, Renton R, et al: Short-term effects of dynamic lycra splints on upper limb in hemiplegic patients, *Arch Phys Med Rehabil* 81:1547, 2000.

42. Gregson JM, et al: Reliability of measurements of muscle tone and muscle powering in stroke patients, *Age Ageing* 29(3):223, 2000.

43. Gregson JM, et al: Reliability of the tone assessment scale and the Modified Ashworth Scale as clinical tools for assessing poststroke spasticity, *Arch Phys Med Rehabil* 80(9):1013, 1999.

44. Hecht JS: Subscapular nerve block in the painful hemiplegic shoulder, *Arch Phys Med Rehabil* 73(11):1036, 1992.

45. Held JP, Pierrot-Deseilligny E: *Reeducation motrice des affections neurologiques,* Paris, 1969, Bailliere.

46. Hill J: The effects of casting on upper extremity motor disorders after brain injury, *Am J Occup Ther* 48(3):219, 1994.

47. Hines AE, et al: Functional electrical stimulation for the reduction of spasticity in the hemiplegic hand, *Biomed Sci Instrum* 29:259, 1993.

48. Hisey MS, Keenan MAE: Orthopedic management of upper extremity dysfunction following stroke or brain injury. In Green DP, Hotchkiss RN, Pederson WC, editors, *Operative hand surgery,* ed 4, New York, 1999, Churchill Livingstone.

49. Hylton N: Dynamic casting and orthotics. In Glenn MB, Whyte J, editors: *The practical management of spasticity in children and adults,* Philadelphia, 1990, Lea & Febiger.

50. Iyer MB et al: Motor 1: lower centers. In Cohen H: *Neuroscience for rehabilitation,* ed 2, Philadelphia, 1999, Lippincott Williams & Wilkins.

51. Jain SS, Francisco GE: Parkinson's disease and other movement disorders. In DeLisa JA, Gans BM, editors: *Rehabilitation medicine: principles and practice,* ed 3, Philadelphia, 1998, Lippincott-Raven.

52. Jain SS, Kirshblum SC: Movement disorders, including tremors. In Delisa JA, editor: *Rehabilitation medicine: principles and practice,* ed 2, Philadelphia, 1993, JB Lippincott.

53. Jebsen RH, et al: An objective and standardized test of hand function, *Arch Phys Med Rehabil* 50(6):311, 1969.

54. Jewell MJ: Overview of the structure and function of the central nervous system. In Umphred DA, editor: *Neurological rehabilitation,* ed 2, St Louis, 1990, Mosby.

55. Jordan CL, Allely RR: Burns and burn rehabilitation. In Pedretti LW, editor: *Occupational therapy: practice skills for physical dysfunction,* ed 4, St Louis, 1996, Mosby.

56. Katz RT: Management of spasticity. In Braddom RL, editor: *Physical medicine and rehabilitation,* Philadelphia, 1996, WB Saunders.

57. Katz RT, et al: Objective quantification of spastic hypertonia: correlation with clinical findings, *Arch Phys Med Rehabil* 73(4):339, 1992.

58. Kisner C, Colby LA: *Therapeutic exercise foundations and techniques,* ed 3, Philadelphia, 1996, FA Davis.

59. Kohlmeyer K: Evaluation of performance skills and client factors. In Crepaeau EB, Cohn ES, Boyt-Shell BA, editors: *Willard and Spackman's occupational therapy,* ed 10, Philadelphia, 2003, Lippincott Williams & Wilkins.

60. Kopp B, et al: The Arm Motor Ability Test: validity, and sensitivity to change of an instrument for assessing disabilities in activities of daily living, *Arch Phys Med Rehabil* 78(6):615, 1997.

61. Lance JW: Symposium synopsis. In Feldman, Young, Koella, editors: *Spasticity: disordered motor control,* Chicago, 1980, Year Book.

62. Law M et al: *Canadian Occupational Performance Measure,* ed 3, Ottawa, 1998, Canadian Association of Occupational Therapists.

63. Leonard CT, et al: Assessing the spastic condition of individuals with the upper motoneuron involvement: validity of the myotonometer, *Arch Phys Med Rehabil* 82:1416, 2001.

64. *Lincoln-Oseretsky Motor Development Scale,* Chicago, CH Stoelting Company.

65. Little JW, Massagli TL: Spasticity and associated abnormalities of muscle tone. In Delisa JB, editor: *Rehabilitation medicine: principles and practice,* ed 2, Philadelphia, 1993, JB Lippincott.

66. Little JW, Massagli TL: Spasticity and associated abnormalities of muscle tone. In Delisa JA, Gans BM, editors: *Rehabilitation medicine: principles and practice,* ed 3, Philadelphia, 1998, Lippincott Raven.

67. Mathiowetz V et al: Adult norms for the nine hole peg test of finger dexterity, *Occup Ther J Res* 5(1):25, 1985.

68. Mayer NH: Clinicophysiologic concepts of spasticity and motor dysfunction in adults with an upper motoneuron lesion. In Mayer NH, Simpson DM, editors: *Spasticity: etiology,*

evaluation, management and the role of botulinum toxin, 2002, We Move™.

69. Mayer NH, Simpson DM, editors: *Spasticity: etiology, evaluation, management and the role of botulinum toxin*, New York, 2002, We Move™.

70. McCormack G, Pedretti LW: Motor unit dysfunction. In Pedretti LW, editor: *Occupational therapy practice skills for physical dysfunction*, ed 4, St Louis, 1996, Mosby.

71. McCrea PH, et al: Linear spring-damper model of the hypertonic elbow: reliability and validity, *J Neurosci Methods* 128 (1-2):121, 2003.

72. McIllroy WE, Maki BE: Early activation of arm muscles follows external perturbation of upright stance, *Neurosci Centers* 148:177, 1995.

73. Medtronic ITB™ Therapy, Medtronic Neurological, 710 Medtronic Parkway, Minneapolis, MN 55432.

74. Melnick ME, Oremland B: Movement dysfunction associated with cerebellar problems. In Umphred DA, editor: *Neurological rehabilitation*, ed 4, St Louis, 2001, Mosby.

75. *Minnesota Rate of Manipulation Test*, Circle Pines, Minn, American Guidance Service.

76. Morris DM et al: *Graded Wolf Motor Function Test.* Dr. Edward Taub, Department of Psychology, University of Alabama at Birmingham, 415 CH, 1530 8th Avenue South, Birmingham, AL 35294-1770. Revision date 5/6/02.

77. Myobloc®, Elan pharmaceuticals, 7475 Lusk Boulevard, San Diego, CA 92121.

78. Neurodeveopmental Treatment Association, Inc. (NDTA): Process in motion (Brochure).

79. Nudo RJ et al: Neural substrates for the effects of rehabilitative training on motor recovery after ischemic infarct, *Science* 272(5269):1791, 1996.

80. Pandyan AD, et al: A review of the properties and limitations of the Ashworth and Modified Ashworth scales as a measure of spasticity, *Clin Rehabil* 13(5):373, 1999.

81. Pandyan AD, et al: A biomechanical investigation into the validity of the modified Ashworth Scale as a measure of elbow spasticity, *Clin Rehabil* 17(3):290, 2003.

82. Pandyan AD, et al: Biomechanical examination of a commonly used measure of spasticity, *Clin Biomech* 16(10):859, 2001.

83. Pennsylvania Bi-Manual Work Sample: Educational Test Bureau, Circle Pines, MN, American Guidance Service.

84. Preston LA: *Effects of botulinum toxin type B on shoulder pain*, Master's thesis, Nashville TN, 2003, Belmont University.

85. Preston LA: Interdisciplinary upper-extremity spasticity management, *Physical Disabilities Special Interest Section Quarterly* 27(1):1, 2004.

86. Preston LA: OT's role in enhancing nerve blocks for spasticity, *OT Practice* 3(10):28, 1998.

87. Preston LA, Hecht JS: *Spasticity management: rehabilitation strategies*, Bethesda, MD, 1999, American Occupational Therapy Association.

88. Purdue Pegboard: Science Research Associates, Inc, 259 East Erie Street, Chicago, Ill, 60611.

89. Reuben DB, Siu AL: An objective measure of physical function of elderly outpatients, *J Am Geriatr Soc* 38:1105, 1990.

90. Roth EJ, Harvey RL: Rehabilitation of stroke syndromes. In Braddom RL, editor: *Physical medicine and rehabilitation*, Philadelphia, 1996, WB Saunders.

91. Ryerson SD: Hemiplegia. In Umphred DA, editor: *Neurological rehabilitation*, ed 4, St Louis, 2001, Mosby.

92. Sehgal N, McGuire JR: Beyond Ashworth electrophysiologic quantification of spasticity, *Phys Med Rehabil Clin N Am* 9(4):949, 1998.

93. Skold C, et al: Simultaneous Ashworth measurements and electromyographic recordings in tetraplegic patients, *Arch Phys Med Rehabil* 79(8):959, 1998.

94. Smith HD: Occupational therapy assessment and treatment. In Hopkins HL, Smith HD, editors: *Willard & Spackman's occupational therapy*, ed 8, Philadelphia, 1997, JB Lippincott.

95. St. John K, Stephenson J: *PNF I: the functional approach to proprioceptive neuromuscular facilitation*, Steamboat Springs, Colorado, 2002, The Institute of Physical Art, Inc.

96. Szklut SE, Breath DM: Learning disabilities. In Umphred DA, editors. *Neurological rehabilitation*, ed 4, St Louis, 2001, Mosby.

97. Tasker RR: Deep brain stimulation is preferable to thalamotomy for tremor suppression, *Surg Neurol* 49:145, 1998.

98. Tinetti ME: Performance oriented assessment of mobility problems in elderly patients, *J Am Geriatr Soc* 34:119, 1986.

99. Tomas ES, et al: Nonsurgical management of upper extremity deformities after traumatic brain injury, *Phys Med Rehabil* (state of the art reviews), 7(3), October 1993.

100. Umphred DA: Classification of treatment techniques based on primary input systems. In Umphred DA, editor: *Neurological rehabilitation*, ed 3, St Louis, 1995, Mosby.

101. Umphred DA, editor: *Neurological rehabilitation*, ed 3, St Louis, 1995, Mosby.

102. Urbscheit NL: Cerebellar dysfunction. In Umphred DA, editor: *Neurological rehabilitation*, St Louis, 1990, Mosby.

103. Van der Lee JH, et al: Exercise therapy for arm function in stroke patients: a systemic review of randomized controlled trials, *Clin Rehabil* 15:20, 2001.

104. Van der Meche F, Van der Gijn J: Hypotonia: an erroneous clinical concept? *Brain* 109(pt 6):1169, 1986.

105. Whitney SL, et al: A review of balance instruments for older adults, *Am J Occup Ther* 52(8):666, 1998.

106. Whyte J, Rosenthal M: Rehabilitation of the patient with traumatic brain injury. In DeLisa JA, editor: *Rehabilitation medicine: principles and practice*, ed 2, Philadelphia, 1993, JB Lippincott.

107. Wilson DJ, Baker LL, Craddock JA: *Functional test for the hemiplegic/paretic upper extremity*, Downey, CA, 1984, Los Amigos Research and Education Institute.

108. Winkler PA: Traumatic brain injury. In Umphred DA, editor: *Neurological rehabilitation*, ed 4, St Louis, 2001, Mosby.

109. Yasukawa A: Upper extremity casting: adjunct treatment for a child with cerebral palsy hemiplegia, *Am J Occup Ther* 44(9):840, 1990.

110. Young RR: Spasticity: a review, *Neurology* 44(suppl 9):S12, 1994.

19

OCCUPATION-BASED FUNCTIONAL MOTION ASSESSMENT

AMY PHILLIPS KILLINGSWORTH

KEY TERMS

Occupation-based functional
   motion assessment

Functional motion assessment
Individual activity analysis

Objective activity analysis
Clinical observation

LEARNING OBJECTIVES

After studying this chapter the student or practitioner will be able to do the following:

1. Define occupation-based functional motion assessment.
2. Describe why it is desirable to assess motor function through observation of engagement in occupation and activity performance.
3. State two circumstances under which assessment of performance skills is indicated.
4. Define individual activity analysis, or "dynamic performance analysis."
5. Describe why it is not possible to do an accurate objective activity analysis.
6. List at least three questions that can guide the clinical observation and clinical reasoning of the occupational therapy practitioner while conducting an occupation-based functional motion assessment.

7. List factors other than range of motion (ROM), strength, and motor control that can affect motor performance.
8. Discuss how information gained from the occupation-based functional motion assessment differs from that gained during assessment of specific client factors.
9. State the minimum level of strength required throughout the lower extremity for normal stance and positioning.
10. Compare levels of muscle strength and associated endurance in the upper extremities.
11. List areas of occupation that can be used to assess functional motion in the upper extremities and in the lower extremities.

CHAPTER OUTLINE

Clinical observation
Occupation-based functional motion assessment
   Lower extremity

Upper extremity
Summary

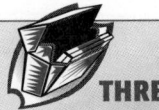

THREADED CASE STUDY: RAYMOND, PART I

Raymond is a 60-year-old foreman of several lineman crews of the telephone company. He has been with the company for more than 40 years; although he could have moved into a more administrative position over the years, he has always enjoyed working out in the field, being a mentor to the younger workers, and dealing with emergencies. He is known throughout his neighborhood as the person to call when help is needed with home repair tasks whether it is carpentry, plumbing, or electrical work. He is a member of a championship senior softball team and plays most weekends during the season, sometimes traveling out of town to participate in tournaments. He does quite a bit of volunteering through the outreach program at his church, participating in such activities as collecting, preparing, and delivering food to home-bound elderly and driving new immigrants to various appointments. He shares household duties with his wife and enjoys cooking for her.

Raymond was first diagnosed with rheumatoid arthritis 10 years ago when he began experiencing pain and stiffness in his shoulders, hips, and knees. His symptoms were managed with medication and except for occasional exacerbations he was able to fully engage in those occupations that were meaningful to him. In the last 6 months, he has experienced an exacerbation of his symptoms. The pain in his shoulders, hips, and knees has increased and he also began experiencing pain in his wrist and hands. His wife began to notice Raymond's change in mood as he became increasingly reluctant to engage in occupations in which he always took the lead, such as helping his neighbors with home projects, preparing food in his church outreach program, and participating in the softball games.

Since he could not do things the way he used to, he did not want to do them at all. He stated that he did not want people seeing him fumbling as he attempted to hold tools or cooking utensils because his grip was so weak, nor did he want to let his teammates down because of the decreased power in his batting swing and speed in running the bases. At work he found himself giving more verbal instructions to his crew rather than demonstrating techniques as he had always done before. His frustration with the increased amount of time it was taking him to complete ADLs such as shaving, buttoning his shirt, and putting on the boots he was required to wear at work was making him irritable. The fatigue he was experiencing at the end of the day "just from trying to move my body around" was also adding to the depression of this client.

The occupational therapy practitioner to whom he was referred, began anticipating the needs of this client based on the profile she developed. Evaluating this client as he engaged in occupations in specific contexts would provide the best information for determining intervention strategies that would be most helpful, such as adaptive equipment and joint protection techniques. Getting information underlying those client factors (muscle strength, ROM) contributing to his decrease in function was critical. Arrangements were made to assess the client in his home and to make a job site visit. By observing the client perform occupation-based tasks and motions at work and home, important information concerning his range of motion, strength and endurance, and motor control could be assessed.

Critical Thinking Questions

1. What is the advantage of administering an occupation-based functional motion assessment versus more specific assessments, such as joint measurement and manual muscle testing?
2. What information about the client's muscle strength and joint range of motion can be determined through the occupation-based functional motion assessment? What cannot be determined?
3. What is the value of administering the occupation-based functional motion assessment in different environmental contexts?

Many physical disabilities cause limitations in performance skills and client factors including joint range of motion (ROM), muscle strength, or motor control. These physical impairments in body functions and motor skills result in movement limitations that can cause slight to substantial deficits in performance of areas of occupation and prevent pursuit of self-care, work, leisure, and educational and social activities. The **occupation-based functional motion assessment** is a way of assessing ROM, strength, and motor control available for task performance by observing the client during performance of functional occupations (activities of daily living [ADLs], instrumental activities of daily living [IADLs], work, or leisure activities) in varied contexts.

Since the primary responsibility of the occupational therapist is to assess occupational performance, identify performance problems, and plan intervention strategies that will improve the client's ability to fully engage in occupations, sensorimotor limitations first should be assessed through observation of functional activities. When improvement of performance skills is a goal of the intervention program, assessment of performance skills, occupation demands, and client factors in a variety of environmental contexts such as home, work place, or school may be indicated to make an objective assessment of physical limitations and gains (see Chapters 18, 20, and 21 for additional information).

Mental functions including cognitive and perceptual abilities, such as motivation or the ability to sequence complex movement patterns or interpret incoming stimuli, can also affect motor function. These client factors must be considered in any performance evaluation (Chapters 24 and 25). However, this chapter is limited to consideration of motor function (i.e., ROM, strength, and motor control) during the occupation-based functional motion assessment.

OT PRACTICE NOTE

Except for a few diagnoses, specific assessments of ROM, muscle strength,[4] and motor control are seldom necessary. For example, performing a full ROM assessment or manual muscle test is time consuming, can be tiring to the client, and may duplicate other services, whereas assessing these factors while the client is engaging in occupation yields the most comprehensive picture of the client's actual abilities and limitations.

CLINICAL OBSERVATION

It is possible to administer a gross assessment of joint mobility and muscle strength by having the client perform those motions associated with functional tasks, i.e., a **functional motion assessment**. The occupational therapy (OT) practitioner could observe as the client reaches overhead as would happen when putting dishes away in an overhead cupboard, or taking a step to the side as when stepping into a bathtub.[7] This will give the practitioner some basic, although nonspecific, information about those factors that affect function.

In occupation-based practice, muscle strength, ROM, and motor control can be observed during the performance of ordinary ADLs,[2] IADLs, work, and leisure tasks. For example, while assessing ADLs, the therapist can observe for performance difficulties and movement patterns that may signal limited ROM, muscle weakness, muscle imbalance, poor endurance, limited motor control, and compensatory motions used for function. An occupation-based functional motion assessment has an advantage over the functional motion assessment because, while the client will perform motions as described above, there is the added resistance unto body structures that will occur as the result of using equipment such as a sliding door, manipulating objects such as cards, or resisting fatigue and having endurance during repetitive activities such as bouncing a ball. Also, because the client is performing these tasks in contexts that are meaningful, the client's full participation and engagement in the task may be heightened.

Essentially, when observing a client perform selected tasks, the occupational therapist is doing an **individual activity analysis** or "dynamic performance analysis"[7] to diagnose the occupational performance problems of that client. Because people perform the same task in a variety of ways and because there are so many variables in task performance, it is not possible to do an **objective activity analysis,** one that can be applied universally, and describe the sensorimotor requirements of the myriad of ADLs. The purpose of observation is to understand the client's occupational performance problems in the context of the interaction between the person, the task, and the environment.[2] This type of screening will serve the occupational therapy practitioner well in deciding a course of intervention for Raymond, who because of the current exacerbation status of his disease is not a candidate for more specific muscle strength assessment (see Chapter 21).

While observing Raymond in his home as he performs the functional tasks described later in this chapter, the therapist will not only be able to assess available ROM but also make some determination of the client's muscle strength.

The therapist's scientific knowledge of the particular dysfunction and an analysis of the ways in which activities are generally performed (activity demands) influence the assessment of performance problems and aid in the development of plans to remediate those problems.[2]

The following are questions to guide the **clinical observation** and clinical reasoning processes:

1. Does the client have adequate ROM to perform the task?
   a. Where are the joint limitations?
   b. What are some possible causes of the limitations?
   c. Are there true ROM limitations or are apparent limitations actually caused by decreased muscle strength?
2. Does the client have enough strength to perform the task?
   a. In which muscle groups is there apparent weakness?
   b. If strength appears inadequate to perform a task because the client cannot complete the ROM, is there truly muscle weakness or is there actually limited ROM?
3. Does the client have enough motor control to perform the task?
   a. Is the movement smooth and rhythmic?
   b. Is movement slow and difficult (e.g., as seen in spasticity and rigidity)?
   c. Are there extraneous movements when the client performs the task (e.g., tremors, athetoid, or choreiform movements)?

The observing occupational therapy practitioner must also consider the client's understanding of the instructions and perception of task importance, as well as the possibility of sensory, perceptual, and cognitive deficits. An analysis of the results of the occupation-based functional motion assessment may indicate that formal assessment of performance skills or body functions is needed. For example, such an assessment may be needed to differentiate muscle weakness from limited ROM or to quantify (with a muscle grade) muscle weakness in specific muscle groups.

Assessing ROM, strength, and motor control by observing the client perform functional activities can aid in selecting meaningful intervention goals relative to improving occupational performance. The therapist can ask the client about his or her ability to perform the tasks of daily living but should also observe the client performing such activities as dressing, walking, standing, and sitting to make an accurate assessment.[1] Having the client perform ADLs in addition to other tasks associated with his or her habits and routines while interacting in varied environmental contexts can also add to the depth of information concerning the client's ROM and muscle strength. The practitioner delivering occupational therapy services to Raymond has determined that doing both a home visit and job site visit will enhance her understanding of the demands on this client. Observation of Raymond interacting with materials, equipment, tools, and products in these environments will provide information about those critical motions and complex motor patterns required for him to fully engage in those occupations most meaningful to him. Completion of the tasks by Raymond in the timely manner required in these contexts will also give information about the client's endurance, thus giving more information about his muscle strength.

Joint ROM, manual muscle testing, and motor control assessments (Chapters 18, 20, and 21) will give the therapist specific information about the function of the musculoskeletal, neurophysiological, and sensorimotor systems. Although the tests require minimum to maximum active output by the client, the therapist will not be able to determine the client's ability to integrate these systems to perform specific goal-directed tasks based on the results of these assessments. Rather, the therapist will have information about movements of a specific limb or a combination of limbs. Under carefully controlled conditions, the therapist will know about the flexibility of the components of the joint and the strength of muscles to create movements such as flexion, abduction, and external rotation. However, the client's motor performance capabilities are not measured by these assessments. For example, the manual muscle test cannot measure muscle endurance (number of times the muscle can contract at its maximum level and resist fatigue), motor control (smooth rhythmic interaction of muscle function), or the client's ability to use the muscles for functional activities.[1]

OT PRACTICE NOTE

While observing a client performing functional activities, it would be most helpful if a therapist could also estimate the client's existing ROM, muscle strength, and motor control.

OCCUPATION-BASED FUNCTIONAL MOTION ASSESSMENT

The activities listed in the following sections for the occupation-based functional motion assessment are suggested as a general starting place for the student or beginning practitioner. Only upper and lower extremity activities are included. Movements of the face, mouth, neck, and spine are beyond the scope of this chapter. Many more motions and tasks could be suggested in each category. The reader is referred to *Musculoskeletal Assessment*, second edition, by Clarkson[1] for a comprehensive and detailed discussion of musculoskeletal assessment and its functional application.

LOWER EXTREMITY

Because of the somewhat stereotypical movements of the lower extremity, the arrangement of the large muscle groups, and the nature of the overall functions of weight bearing and ambulation, assumptions can be made about muscle strength during functional activities. For example, to assume a normal stance pattern, ambulate without any compensatory gait patterns, or position the lower extremities (without the assistance of the upper extremities) during dressing, a minimum of *fair plus* (F+) muscle strength is required in the musculature of the hips, knees, ankles, and feet. If muscle strength in the lower extremities is only F throughout the lower extremity, ambulation without aids will not be possible.[5] Good to normal muscle strength is required for the endurance to perform the small postural adjustments needed for maintained standing, repetitive movement patterns inherent in walking, and the lifting, maneuvering, and balancing on the lower limbs that usually occur during dressing.

Hip Complex

The hip joints support the body weight. Each joint acts as a fulcrum when a person is standing on one leg. Hip movement makes it possible to move the body closer to or farther from the ground, bring the foot closer to the trunk, and position the lower limb in space.[1]

During functional activities, lumbar-pelvic movements accompany hip movement, which extends the functional capabilities of the hip joint. The hip is capable of flexion, extension, adduction, abduction, and internal and external rotation.[1]

Flexion and extension

Full flexion and extension are required for many ADLs and IADLs. Standing requires full hip extension. Squatting, bending to tie a shoelace with the foot on the ground, and toenail care done with the foot on the edge of the chair all require full or near full hip flexion. Other activities that require moderate to full flexion and extension are donning panty hose or socks, bathing the feet in a bathtub, ascending and descending stairs or a step stool, sitting and rising in a standard chair, and riding a stationary bicycle.[1]

Abduction and adduction

Most ordinary ADLs and IADLs do not require full ranges of abduction and adduction. The main function of the hip abductors is to keep the pelvis level when one foot is off the ground. For ADLs, hip abduction may be used when stepping sideways into a shower or bathtub, donning trousers when sitting, squatting to pick up an object, sitting with the foot across the opposite thigh, getting on a bicycle, or, as in the case of Raymond, shifting weight from one foot to the other as he steps out when swinging the bat.[1,6]

Hip adduction brings the foot across the front of the body. An individual uses this motion when kicking a ball, moving an object on the floor with the foot, or crossing one thigh over the other for donning or removing shoes and socks.[1]

Internal and external rotation

Internal rotation occurs when a person is pivoting medially on one foot. When a person is sitting, there is internal rotation when the person reaches to the lateral side of the foot for washing or donning socks. Internal rotators are active in walking.[1]

External rotation with hip flexion and abduction brings the foot across the opposite thigh for donning shoes or socks, or examining the sole of the foot.[1,6]

Knee

The knee joint supports the body weight. With the foot fixed on the ground, knee flexion lowers the body toward the ground and knee extension raises the body. If the foot is off the ground, as in sitting, the knee and hip are used to orient the foot in space.[1]

Daily living activities that require moderate to full ranges of knee flexion and extension are standing and walking, squatting to lift an object from the floor, crossing the ankle of one foot over the thigh of the opposite leg, sitting down and rising from a chair, and dressing the feet.

Ankle and Foot

The foot is a flexible base of support when a person is on rough terrain. It functions as a rigid lever during terminal stance in the walking pattern. It absorbs shock when transmitting forces between the ground and the leg. The foot and ankle function to elevate the body from the ground when the foot is fixed. Dorsiflexion and plantar flexion occur at the ankle joint. Foot inversion and eversion occur at the subtalar joint.[1]

Plantar flexion

Full plantar flexion is used when a person is rising on the toes to reach upward to a high shelf. Some plantar flexion is used to depress the accelerator in an automobile or the control pedal on a sewing machine and when donning socks or shoes.

Dorsiflexion

Full range of dorsiflexion is needed to descend stairs. Dorsiflexion is used in such activities as positioning the foot to cut the toenails or tying shoe laces.[1]

Inversion and eversion

Inversion and eversion function to provide flexibility when an individual is walking on uneven ground. Inversion is used when the foot is crossed over the opposite thigh and the sole is inspected.[1]

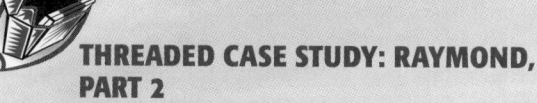

THREADED CASE STUDY: RAYMOND, PART 2

In administering an occupation-based functional motion assessment at Raymond's home, the occupational therapy practitioner was able to observe that in his attempt to don his shoes and socks, Raymond was unable to abduct and externally rotate his hip sufficiently enough

in combination with full flexion of the knee, in order to place the ankle of one foot over the opposite thigh.

At his job site Raymond had difficulty stepping up into his truck (the cab of which was somewhat elevated due to the oversize tires), not having enough hip and knee flexion range of motion. The OT also observed that if the truck was parked near a curb or he could step first on a box and then onto the step of the truck thus requiring less flexion range of motion, he had less difficulty. However, in both instances, he lacked sufficient strength in hip and knee extension to launch himself into the truck without compensating with his upper extremities.

UPPER EXTREMITY

By simply observing a client engaging in functional activities, the therapist cannot make general assumptions as easily about muscle strength in the upper extremities as in the lower extremities. There are three reasons why this is the case: (1) the variety of ways in which the upper extremity can be positioned to complete any given task (i.e., there is not one right way to do the task), (2) the complexity of motor patterns possible requiring gross motor and fine motor skill, and (3) the dependency of the distal joints and musculature on the more proximal joints for positioning.

If several people are observed donning shirts, it will be apparent that different techniques are used by each. One person may lift the arm out to the side, increasing shoulder abduction as the shirt is drawn onto the arm. Another person might prefer to dress with the arm more in front of the body, thus positioning the humerus in flexion. A third person might hyperextend the humerus as the shirt is pulled on. The difficulty, of course, is determining exactly how much ROM and muscle strength is minimally required at all of the joints involved when so many options are available to perform one task.

In the first two examples of donning a shirt, the musculature of the shoulder complex would certainly have to create more tension than if the humerus were in the adducted position. It would be inappropriate for the therapist to instruct the client on how to don the shirt if the therapist's goal was to attain some information regarding the client's level of independence in dressing and secondarily to make assumptions about ROM and muscle strength.

When observing a client perform occupation-based tasks and motions with the upper extremities, it is important to remember that even when it is not obvious or readily apparent, the muscles of the shoulder complex are contracting with varying degrees of tension. They may have to contract with enough force to position the hand in space and maintain it there, such as when a person is combing hair. At other times, the humerus must be held close to the body to provide a stable base from which the forearm, wrist, and hand can maneuver, such as when hitting the keys on a keyboard, cutting food with a knife, or writing. It would be an inaccurate assumption that the extremity is just hanging passively at the side when, in fact, the static contractions around the proximal joints make it possible for the musculature of the distal extremity to work effectively. Conversely, the shoulder complex may have to be a moving unit, as opposed to a positioning one, such as when moving groceries from a countertop to shelves in a kitchen cabinet.

General guidelines exist for assessing strength for function in the upper extremities. With good to normal endurance, the client with *good* (G) to *normal* (N) muscle strength throughout the upper extremity will be able to perform all ordinary ADLs and IADLs, work, play, and enjoy leisure and social participation occupations without undue fatigue.[5] The client with *fair plus* (F+) muscle strength usually will have low endurance and will fatigue more easily than a client with G to N strength. The client will be able to perform many basic ADLs and IADLs independently, but may need frequent rest periods. Work, play, and some social participation occupations may prove to be too strenuous, as in the case of Raymond attempting to hit a ball with force.

The client with muscle grades of *fair* (F) will be able to move parts against gravity and perform light tasks that require little or no resistance.[3,5] Low endurance is a significant problem and will limit the amount of activity that can be done. The client with low endurance probably will be able to eat finger foods and perform light hygiene if given the time and rest periods needed to reach the goals.[5] *Poor* (P) strength is considered below functional range, but the client with poor strength will be able to perform some ADLs with mechanical assistance and can maintain ROM independently.[5] (See Chapter 29, Section 2, Mobile Arm Supports.) Clients with muscle grades of *trace* (T) and *zero* (0) will be completely dependent, and unable to perform ADLs without externally powered devices. Some activities will be possible with special controls on equipment. Examples include power wheelchairs and electronic communication devices such as voice recognition computers or environmental control systems.[5]

Individuals use a variety of motor patterns when performing a functional task, and no one way is the right way to perform the task. These facts make it impossible for the therapist to predetermine the level of muscle strength, amount of ROM, and degree of motor control needed in the upper extremity to perform any given task. Individual styles of moving, numerous possibilities for compensatory movements when faced with loss of joint flexibility, poor endurance, lack of motor control, impaired sensation, and pain are all factors that may affect the client's ability to generate tension in a muscle or muscle group and sustain muscle activity. The pain Raymond experiences in his hands may be the primary cause of his inability to manipulate objects such as the buttons on his shirt.

Shoulder Complex

The shoulder complex is the most mobile joint complex in the body. Its function is to move the arm in space and position the hand for function. The shoulder complex is composed of the acromioclavicular, sternoclavicular, scapulothoracic, and glenohumeral joints and the muscles, ligaments, and other structures that move and support these joints. In the performance of functional activities, scapular, clavicular, and trunk motions normally accompany glenohumeral motion. These associated movements increase the range of glenohumeral motion for function. The shoulder complex functions in a coordinated manner that is accomplished through scapulothoracic and glenohumeral movement. This coordinated function is called *scapulohumeral* rhythm. Thus, movements at the shoulder are actually combinations of several joint motions and are dependent on scapulohumeral rhythm in the performance of any given activity.[1] Activities such as placing an object (e.g., book, box, or cup) on an overhead shelf or reaching overhead to pull on a light cord require these movements.[1]

Shoulder flexion and abduction with scapula upward rotation (overhead movements)

Activities such as placing an object (e.g., book, box, or cup) on an overhead shelf or reaching overhead to pull on a light cord require these movements.

Shoulder extension and adduction with scapula downward rotation

Activities such as reaching back for toilet hygiene, Raymond swinging his arm backward when preparing to pitch the softball, reaching backward to put an arm through the sleeve of a coat, and pulling open a refrigerator door require these movements.[1]

Horizontal adduction and abduction

These movements allow the arm to be moved around the body. Reaching the opposite axilla or opposite ear for hygiene activities, opening and closing a sliding door, combing the opposite side of the hair, and reaching the upper back while bathing are some activities that use horizontal adduction and abduction.[1]

Internal and external rotation

Some degree of either internal or external rotation accompanies every glenohumeral motion. The ROM varies in various positions of the arm. Full range of external rotation is required for reaching the back of the head for combing or washing hair. External rotation is often associated with supination when the elbow is extended, as when rotating a doorknob in a clockwise direction.[1]

Internal rotation is used when buttoning a shirt, eating, and drinking from a cup. Full range of internal rotation with scapulothoracic motion is used to reach into a back pocket, fasten a bra, put a belt through the belt keepers on trousers, or do toilet hygiene. Internal rotation is often associated with forearm pronation, as when putting a pillow behind the low back, turning a screwdriver to unfasten a screw, rotating a doorknob in a counterclockwise direction, and pouring water from a vessel.[1]

Extension and adduction

Extension and adduction are used to return the arm to the side of the body from shoulder flexion and abduction, as after reaching overhead. These motions are also used when quick movement or force is required, as when an individual is closing a vertically oriented window, crutch walking, or pushing off to rise from an armchair or when stabilizing the humerus to the lateral trunk as when carrying a basket of laundry.[1]

Flexion and adduction

Flexion and adduction are used in activities that require reaching the same side of the body, such as washing the cheek or ear and combing hair on the same side. Slight shoulder flexion with adduction is used for hand-to-mouth activities and putting on an earring back.

Elbow and Forearm

Elbow and forearm movements serve to place the hand for function. Elbow flexion moves the hand toward the body, and elbow extension moves the hand away from the body. Forearm pronation or supination usually accompanies elbow flexion and extension. Pronation and supination position the hand precisely for the requirements of the given activity. The elbow and forearm support skilled and forceful movements of the hand that are used during performance of ADLs and work activities.[1]

Full or nearly full range of elbow flexion, usually with some humeral flexion and forearm supination, is used to bring food to the mouth, shave the face or underarms, hold a telephone receiver, place an earring on the ear, and reach the neck level of a back zipper.

Full range of elbow extension, usually with pronation, is used when an individual is reaching to the feet to tie shoes, throwing a ball overhand, and using the arms to push off from a chair. Many other ADLs and IADLs require less than full range of these movements.[1]

Wrist and Hand

The wrist controls the length-tension relations of the extrinsic muscles of the hand. It positions the hand relative to the forearm for touch, grasp, or manipulation of objects. Wrist extension and ulnar deviation are most important in performance of ADLs.[1] It is possible to perform some ADLs when there is a loss of wrist ROM by using compensatory movements of the proximal joints.

The primary functions of the hand are to grasp and manipulate objects and to discriminate sensory information about objects in the environment. The arches of the hand make it possible to adapt the hand to the shape of the object being manipulated.

Power grip and precision grip are the bases of all hand activities. Power grip is used when force is required for grasping, such as holding a hammer handle, a full glass, or the handle of a purse or suitcase. Precision grip is used when an object is pinched and when it is being manipulated between the thumb and one or more fingers. Precision grip is used for holding a pencil, moving checkers or chess pieces, turning a key, threading a needle, and opening the cap of a medicine bottle.[1]

The occupational therapy practitioner observed Raymond in his home as he was preparing to make homemade soup. She noted that Raymond easily accessed ingredients that were on the first two shelves of above-counter cabinets, but displayed quite a bit of facial grimacing and two attempts reaching overhead to the top shelf. He was observed being able to fully open his fingers but not able to make a tight fist. When chopping vegetables, he was able to manage the less resistive ones like tomatoes and celery but could not exert enough force to cut through the carrots. While he could carry an empty pot to the sink without difficulty he was not able to stabilize his wrists to carry a full pot of water to the stove. At his job site, the occupational therapy practitioner again noted Raymond having difficulty holding some of the heavier tools in position and exerting appropriate force, such as with the large wire cutters.

SUMMARY

Many physical disabilities cause deficits in ROM, strength, and motor control that limit occupational performance. The occupational therapy practitioner is primarily responsible for assessing occupational performance, identifying performance problems, and planning intervention that will improve the client's occupational performance.

Because people perform the same activity in a variety of ways, the level of ROM, strength, or motor control needed to do a task is variable. Assessment of physical limitations can be made through observation of a client's performance while engaged in a variety of occupations. Therefore, as in the case of Raymond, the therapist must observe the client performing selected tasks in the person-task-environment interaction.[2]

While assessing the client's ability to perform ADLs, IADLs, work, or leisure occupations, the therapist should observe for sensorimotor problems. An analysis of the results of observation may indicate that an assessment of specific body factors or performance skills is needed.

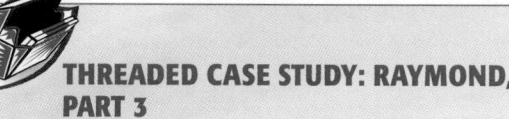

THREADED CASE STUDY: RAYMOND, PART 3

Due to the difficulty Raymond experienced when donning his socks and shoes, getting in and out of his truck, reaching overhead, and manipulating and applying needed force to kitchen and work tools, the occupational therapist has determined that range of

Continued

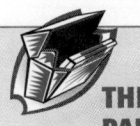

THREADED CASE STUDY: RAYMOND, PART 3—cont'd

motion and muscle testing assessments should be administered to some of this client's specific joints and muscles.

After the occupation-based functional motion assessment, the next step in the occupational therapy process would be for the OT to plan the intervention. The reader should refer to Chapter 38 on Arthritis for some ideas for interventions that could be implemented to return Raymond to participation in his customary rounds of occupation. The reader should also refer back to the beginning of this chapter and reflect upon the three probative questions posed at the end of Raymond's case study and be able to describe the advantages of using the occupation-based functional motion assessment, the amount and type of information that was gleaned regarding Raymond from this assessment, and the value to the OT of conducting this assessment in both the home and work contexts.

Questions to guide clinical observation and clinical reasoning and suggested activities to assess function of the upper and lower extremities are outlined in this chapter.

Review Questions

1. Compare and contrast functional motion assessment versus occupation-based task and motion assessment.
2. In occupation-based practice, how are sensorimotor functions first assessed?
3. What is meant by individual activity analysis?
4. Why is it not possible to do an objective activity analysis?
5. List three major questions that can guide the clinical observation and clinical reasoning of the occupational therapy practitioner when doing a occupation-based functional motion assessment.
6. Which factors, other than strength, ROM, and motor control, can affect the functional task-motion assessment?
7. How is the information gained from assessment of specific body factors different from that gained in an occupation-based functional motion assessment?
8. What is the minimum level of strength required throughout the lower extremity for normal stance and positioning?
9. List some activities or occupations that can be used to assess general function in the lower extremities: hip, knee, ankle, and foot.
10. Compare levels of muscle strength with endurance in the upper extremities.
11. List some activities that can be used to assess general function in the upper extremities: shoulder complex, elbow and forearm, and wrist and hand.

REFERENCES

1. Clarkson HM: *Musculoskeletal assessment*, ed 2, Philadelphia, 2000, Lippincott Williams & Wilkins.
2. Crepeau EB: Activity analysis: a way of thinking about occupational performance. In Crepeau EB, Cohn ES, Schell BA: *Willard and Spackman's occupational therapy*, ed 10, Philadelphia, 2003, Lippincott Williams & Wilkins.
3. Crepeau EB, et al: *Willard & Spackman's occupational therapy*, ed 10, Philadelphia, 2003, Lippincott Williams & Wilkins.
4. Hislop HJ, Montgomery J: *Daniels' and Worthingham's muscle testing*, ed 7, Philadelphia, 2002, WB Saunders.
5. Killingsworth A: *Basic physical disability procedures*, San Jose, CA, 1987, Maple Press.
6. Latella D, Meriano C: *Occupational therapy manual for evaluation of range of motion and muscle strength*, Clifton, New York, 2003, Delmar Thomson Learning.
7. Polatajko HJ, et al: Dynamic performance analysis: a framework for understanding occupational performance, *Am J Occup Ther* 54(2):65, 2000.

20 JOINT RANGE OF MOTION

AMY PHILLIPS KILLINGSWORTH
LORRAINE WILLIAMS PEDRETTI

KEY TERMS

Range of motion
Active range of motion
Passive range of motion

Joint measurement
Palpation
End-feel

Goniometer
Functional range of motion

LEARNING OBJECTIVES

After studying this chapter the student or practitioner will be able to do the following:

1. Define active, passive, and functional range of motion (ROM).
2. List the purposes of measuring ROM.
3. Name two methods used to screen for ROM limitations.
4. Name disabilities for which joint measurement is often an assessment tool.
5. Describe how ROM measurements are used to select intervention goals and methods.
6. Describe how to establish ROM norms for the client with unilateral involvement.
7. Describe what the therapist should do before actually measuring the joints with the goniometer.
8. Describe proper positioning of the therapist and methods to support limbs.
9. List precautions and contraindications for joint measurement.
10. List and describe the steps in the joint measurement procedure in correct order.
11. Describe how to record results of the joint measurement.
12. Measure all the joints of a typical practice subject, using the 180-degree method and correct procedure.
13. Describe at least three intervention strategies that can be used to increase ROM.

CHAPTER OUTLINE

Joint measurement
Principles and procedures in joint measurement
  Visual observation
  Palpation
  Positioning of therapist and support of limbs
  Precautions and contraindications
  End-feel
  Two-joint muscles
Methods of joint measurement
  The 180-degree system
  The 360-degree system

Goniometers
Recording measurements
Results of assessment as the basis for intervention planning
Procedure for measuring passive ROM
  General procedure—180-degree method of measurement
Directions for joint measurement—180-degree system
  Spine
  Upper extremity
  Lower extremity
Summary

THREADED CASE STUDY: EVELYN, PART 1

Evelyn is an 83-year-old woman who sustained a Colles' fracture when she fell on her outstretched, nondominant left hand in an attempt to break her fall after tripping on a doorstop as she exited a building. The fracture was reduced, and Evelyn was placed in a hand-to-below-elbow cast for 6 weeks. Upon removal of the cast, Evelyn's wrist and hand appeared swollen. She complained of pain and stiffness in the carpometacarpal and metacarpal joints of her thumb and the metacarpophalangeal and proximal interphalangeal joints of her fingers. She was unable to make a fist or oppose her thumb to her fingers.

Evelyn is a widow; her two grown children live nearby. Before her injury, she was independent in all activities of daily living (ADLs) and the majority of instrumental activities of daily living (IADLs). She used public transportation to move around her community, although her children and friends usually drove her to appointments. Evelyn volunteered at the local hospital weekly in its telecare program, calling elderly home-bound persons. She is an accomplished seamstress, makes all of her own clothing, and attends a weekly sewing class, primarily for the camaraderie of the other students, although she states, "There is always something new to learn." She also enjoys baking for her family, gardening, and generally engaging in tasks that contribute to the upkeep of her home. She attends church regularly and enjoys dining out with friends and family members.

Since her injury, her ability to participate in those occupations that are meaningful to her has been curtailed. She requires moderate to maximal assistance to hold a eating utensil in her left hand while cutting food with her right, wash and groom her hair, put on jewelry, bathe the right side of her body, transfer out of the bathtub, and engage in home maintenance tasks (e.g., changing bed linen). At her volunteer work site, she is unable to hold the telephone with her left hand while writing with her right hand. When cooking, she has difficulty stabilizing bowls, pots, and pans with her left hand while manipulating a cooking utensil with her right. Evelyn is experiencing a great deal of frustration with her loss of independence and inability to fully engage in those occupations that got her out in the community and facilitated interaction with others.

In reviewing Evelyn's occupational profile, the occupational therapist must focus on those client factors that are interfering with function. Loss of range of motion (ROM) in the left upper extremity, especially the inability to flex the fingers to make a fist and oppose the thumb to the fingers, which is required for fine motor activities, is prohibiting the client from fully engaging in the physical, social, personal, cultural, and spiritual contexts that bring meaning to her life. Before determining intervention goals and strategies, the therapist must assess ROM limitations to establish a baseline for treatment. While reading and studying this chapter, keep in mind Evelyn's ROM limitations and the restrictions they impose on her engagement in occupation.

Critical Thinking Questions

1. Why should the occupational therapist proceed with caution when assessing the ROM limitations of this client?
2. What is the appropriate sequencing of joint measurement assessment for this client? What methods should be applied first?
3. What is the advantage of joint measurement in evidence-based practice?

Joint **range of motion** (ROM) is the amount of movement that is possible at a joint.[3] It is the arc of motion through which a joint passes when moving within a specific plane. When the joint is moved by the muscles that act on the joint, it is called **active range of motion** (AROM). When the joint is moved by an outside force such as the therapist, it is called **passive range of motion** (PROM).[3] In normal individuals, PROM is slightly greater than AROM because of the slight elasticity of soft tissue.[3,10] The additional passive ROM that is available at the end of the normal active ROM helps to protect joint structures because it allows the joint to give and absorb extrinsic forces. If PROM is significantly more than AROM for the same joint motion, it is likely that there is muscle weakness.[13]

Decreased ROM can cause limited function and interfere with performance in areas of occupation. Limitations to ROM may occur as the result of injury or disease to the joint itself or to the surrounding joint tissue structures, joint trauma, or joint immobilization. These limitations may restrict the client's ability to perform successfully in chosen day-to-day occupations. Inflexibility at a joint may adversely affect both speed and strength of movement. A client who constantly has to work to overcome the resistance of an inflexible joint will probably demonstrate decreased endurance and fatigue during activity. The functional motion test (see Chapter 19), screening tests, and measurement of joint ROM with a goniometer can all be used to assess ROM.

OT PRACTICE NOTE

The primary concern of the occupational therapist is whether ROM is adequate for the client to engage in meaningful occupations.

Methods used to screen ROM limitations involve the observation of AROM and PROM. To screen for AROM, the therapist asks the client to perform all the active movements that occur at the joint.[3] To screen for PROM, the therapist moves the joint passively through all of its motions. The purpose of this is to estimate ROM, detect limitations, and observe quality of movement, end-feel, and the presence of pain.[3]

The therapist can then decide at which joints precise ROM measurement is indicated.

JOINT MEASUREMENT

Body function is a client factor that the occupational therapist must consider when classifying the client's underlying abilities. The therapist will be concerned with the client's ability to retrieve dishes in a cupboard, reach above shoulder level to shampoo hair, or depress gas and brake pedals in an automobile. **Joint measurement** is an assessment tool often used for physical disabilities that cause limited joint motion. These include skin contracture caused by adhesions or scar tissue; arthritis, fractures, burns, and hand trauma; the displacement of fibrocartilage or the presence of other foreign bodies in the joint; bony obstruction or destruction; and soft tissue contractures, such as tendon, muscle, or ligament shortening. Limited ROM can also be secondary to spasticity, muscle weakness, pain, and edema.[8,13]

ROM measurements help the therapist select intervention goals, appropriate intervention modalities, positioning techniques, and other strategies to reduce limitations. Specific purposes for measuring ROM are to determine limitations that interfere with function or may produce deformity, determine additional range needed to increase functional capacity or reduce deformity, determine the need for splints and assistive devices, measure progress objectively, and record progression or regression. The use of formal joint measurement will assist in determining the efficacy of intervention modalities and may also serve as evidence in assisting the client to see the outcome of the intervention through quantifiable data.

Normal ROM varies from one person to another. The occupational therapist can establish norms for each individual by measuring the analogous uninvolved part if possible.[3,4] Otherwise, the therapist uses average ranges listed in the literature as a guide.[3] The therapist should check records and interview the client to detect the presence of fused joints and other limitations caused by old injuries. Joints should not be forced when resistance is met on passive ROM. Pain may limit ROM, and crepitation may be heard on movement in some conditions. Therefore, before beginning joint measurement procedures, the therapist must explain what will be done and ask the client if he or she is experiencing any joint pain and, if so, where it is located and how severe it is. So as not to cause undue pain, the occupational therapist further explains to the client the importance of indicating any changes in pain throughout the procedure.

PRINCIPLES AND PROCEDURES IN JOINT MEASUREMENT

Before measuring ROM, the therapist should be familiar with average normal ROM ranges, joint structure and function, normal end-feels, recommended positioning for self and client, and bony landmarks related to each joint and joint axis.[3,4,10] The therapist should be skilled in correct positioning and stabilization for measurements, **palpation**, alignment and reading of the goniometer, and accurate recording of measurements.[10] For the most reliable measurements, the same therapist should assess and reassess the client at the same time of day, using the same instrument and the same measurement protocol.[3]

VISUAL OBSERVATION

The joint to be measured should be exposed, and the therapist should observe the joint and adjacent areas.[3] The therapist asks the client to move the part through the available ROM, if muscle strength is adequate, and observes the movement.[4] The therapist should look for compensatory motions, posture, muscle contours, skin color and condition, and skin creases and compare the joint with the noninjured part, if possible.[3] The therapist should then move the part through its range to see and feel how the joint moves and to estimate ROM.

PALPATION

Feeling the bony landmarks and soft tissue around the joint is an essential skill, gained with practice and experience. The pads of the index and middle fingers are used for palpation. The thumb is sometimes used. The therapist's fingernails should not make contact with the client's skin. Pressure is applied gently but firmly enough to detect underlying muscle, tendons, or bony structures. For joint measurement, the therapist must palpate to locate bony landmarks for placement of the goniometer.[3]

POSITIONING OF THERAPIST AND SUPPORT OF LIMBS

The therapist's position varies, depending on the joints being measured. When measuring fingers or wrist joints, the therapist may sit next to or opposite the client. If sitting next to the client, the therapist should measure the wrist and finger joints on that side and then move to the other side to measure the joints on the client's opposite side. This procedure makes the client more comfortable (eliminating the need to stretch across the midline) and ensures more accurate placement of the goniometer. When measuring the larger joints of the upper or lower extremity, the therapist may stand next to the client on the side being measured. The client may be seated or lying down. The therapist needs to employ good body mechanics in posture and in lifting and moving heavy limbs. The therapist should use a broad base of support and stand with the head upright, keeping the back straight. The feet should be shoulder width apart, with the knees slightly flexed. The therapist's stance should be in line with the direction of movement. The limb should be supported at the level of its center of gravity, approximately where the upper and middle third of the segment meet. The therapist's hands should be in a relaxed grasp that conforms to the contours of the part. The therapist can provide additional support by resting the part on his or her forearm.[3]

PRECAUTIONS AND CONTRAINDICATIONS

In some instances, measuring joint ROM is contraindicated or should be undertaken with extreme caution. It is contraindicated if there is a joint dislocation or unhealed fracture, immediately after surgery of any soft tissue structures surrounding joints, in the presence of myositis ossificans, or when ectopic ossification is a possibility.[3]

Joint measurement must always be done carefully. The following situations call for extreme caution:
1. The client has joint inflammation or an infection.
2. The client is taking either medication for pain or muscle relaxants.
3. The client has osteoporosis, hypermobility, or subluxation of a joint.
4. The client has hemophilia.
5. The client has a hematoma.
6. The client has just had an injury to soft tissue.
7. The client has a newly united fracture.
8. The client has undergone prolonged immobilization.
9. Bony ankylosis is suspected.
10. The client has carcinoma of the bone or any fragile bone condition.[3, 9]

END-FEEL

Passive ROM is normally limited by the structure of the joint and surrounding soft tissues. Thus, ligaments, the joint capsule, muscle and tendon tension, contact of joint surfaces, and soft tissue approximation may limit the end of a particular ROM. Each of these structures has a different end-feel as the therapist moves the joint passively through the ROM. **End-feel** is the normal resistance to further joint motion because of stretching of soft tissue, stretching of ligaments and joint capsule, approximation of soft tissue, and the contact of bone on bone. End-feel is normal when full ROM is achieved and the motion is limited by normal anatomical structures. Abnormal end-feel occurs when the ROM is increased or decreased or when ROM is normal but structures other than normal anatomy stop the ROM.[3] Practice and sensitivity are required for the therapist to detect different end-feels and to distinguish the normal from the abnormal.[3,10]

End-feel is normally hard, soft, or firm. An example of hard end-feel is bone contacting bone when the elbow is passively extended and the olecranon process comes into contact with the olecranon fossa. Soft end-feel can be detected on knee flexion when there is soft tissue apposition of the posterior aspects of the thigh and calf. A firm end-feel has a firm or springy sensation that has some give, as when the ankle is dorsiflexed with the knee in extension and the ROM is limited by tension in the gastrocnemius muscle.[3]

In pathological states, end-feel is abnormal when passive ROM is increased or decreased or when PROM is normal but movement is stopped by structures other than normal anatomy.[3] Practice and experience are required to detect end-feel accurately. Normal end-feel for each joint is noted with the directions for joint measurement that are listed in the following sections.

TWO-JOINT MUSCLES

When the ROM of a joint that is crossed by a two-joint muscle is measured, the ROM of the joint being measured may be affected by the position of the other joint because of passive insufficiency.[3] In other words, joint motion is limited by the length of the muscle. A two-joint muscle feels taut when it is at its full length over both joints it crosses and before it reaches the limits of the normal ROM of both joints.[7] For example, when the wrist is in full extension, passive finger extension is normally limited because of the passive insufficiency of the finger flexors that cross the wrist and finger joints. When the joints crossed by two-joint muscles are being measured, it is necessary to place the joint not being measured in a neutral or relaxed position to place the two-joint muscle on slack. For example, when finger extension is being measured, the wrist should be placed in the neutral position to avoid full stretch of the finger flexors over all of the joints they cross. Similarly, when hip flexion is being measured, the knee should also be flexed to place the hamstrings in the slackened position.[3]

METHODS OF JOINT MEASUREMENT

THE 180-DEGREE SYSTEM

In the 180-degree system of joint measurement, 0 degree is the starting position for all joint motions. For most motions, the anatomical position is the starting position. The body of the measuring instrument, the goniometer, is a half-circle protractor with an axis and two arms. It is superimposed on the body in the plane in which the motion is to occur. The axis of the instrument is aligned with the axis of the joint. All joint motions begin at 0 degree and increase toward 180 degrees.[3,5,10] The 180-degree system is used most often and is the one used later in this chapter to describe procedures for joint measurement.

THE 360-DEGREE SYSTEM

The 360-degree system of joint measurement is used less frequently than the 180-degree system. The goniometer is a full-circle, 360-degree protractor with two arms. Movements occurring in the coronal and sagittal planes are related to the full circle. When the body is in the anatomical position, the circle is superimposed on it in the same plane in which the motion is to occur, with the joint axis as the pivotal point. "The 0-degree (360-degree) position will be overhead and the 180-degree position will be toward the feet."[5] Thus, for example, shoulder flexion and abduction are movements that proceed toward 0 degree, and shoulder adduction and extension proceed toward 360 degrees. The average normal ROM for shoulder flexion is 170 degrees. Therefore, in the 360-degree system, the movement would start at 180 degrees and progress toward 0 to 10 degrees. The ROM recorded would be 10 degrees. On the other hand, shoulder extension that has a normal ROM of 60 degrees would begin at 180 degrees and progress toward 360 to 240 degrees, and 240 degrees would be the ROM recorded.[5] The total ROM of extension to flexion would be 240 to 10 degrees—that is, 230 degrees.[5,6]

Some motions cannot be related to the full circle. In these instances, a 0-degree starting position is designated, and the movements are measured as increases from 0 degree. These motions occur in a horizontal plane around a vertical axis. They are forearm pronation and supination, hip internal and external rotation, wrist radial and ulnar deviation, and thumb palmar and radial abduction (carpometacarpal flexion and extension).[5]

GONIOMETERS

Usually made of metal or plastic, goniometers come in several sizes and types and are available from medical and rehabilitation equipment companies.[5,10,12] The word **goniometer** is derived from the Greek *gonia*, which means angle, and

metron, which means measure.[9,14] Thus, *goniometer* literally means "to measure angles."

The universal goniometer (Figure 20-1) consists of a body, a stationary (proximal) bar, and a movable (distal) bar.[3,10] The stationary bar is attached to the body of the goniometer. The body is a half-circle or a full-circle protractor printed with a scale of degrees from 0 to 180 for the half-circle and 0 to 360 for the full-circle goniometer.[3,4] The movable bar is attached at the center, or axis, of the protractor and acts as a dial. As the movable bar rotates around the protractor, the dial points to the number of degrees on the scale.

Two scales of figures are printed on the half circle. Each starts at 0 degree and progresses toward 180 degrees, but in opposite directions. Because the starting position in the 180-degree system is always 0 degree and increases toward 180 degrees, the outer row of figures is read if the bony segments being measured are end to end, as in elbow flexion. The inner row of figures is read if the bony segments being measured are alongside one another, as in shoulder flexion.

Figure 20-1 shows five styles of goniometers. The first (Figure 20-1, *A*) is a full-circle goniometer that has calibrations for both the 360-degree and the 180-degree systems printed on its face. This goniometer has longer arms and is convenient for use on the large joints of the body. Figure 20-1, *B*, shows a half-circle instrument used for the 180-degree system. This goniometer is radiopaque and could be used during radiographic examinations if necessary. Its dial is notched at two places for accurate motion reading, regardless of whether the convexity of the half circle is directed toward or away from the direction of motion. Thus, the evaluator does not have to reverse the goniometer, obscuring the scale. A special

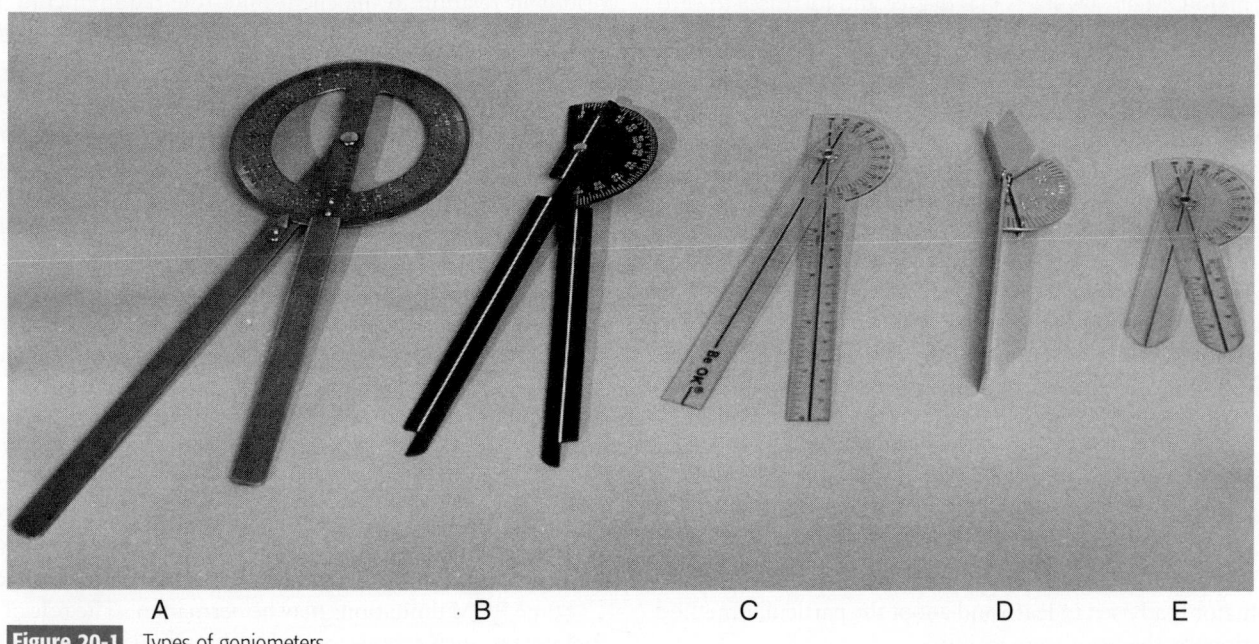

A   B   C   D   E

Figure 20-1   Types of goniometers.

finger goniometer is shown in Figure 20-1, *D*. Its arms are short and flattened. It is designed to be used over the finger joint surfaces rather than on their lateral aspects, as is done in most of the larger joint motions. Small plastic goniometers are shown in Figure 20-1, *C* and *E*. These are inexpensive and easy to carry. The longer one can be used with both large and small joints. The smaller is simply a larger one that has been cut for use as a finger goniometer. The dials of transparent goniometers are marked or notched in two places.

One important feature of the goniometer is the fulcrum. The nut or rivet that acts as the fulcrum must move freely yet be tight enough to remain where it was set when the goniometer is removed after joint measurement.[4] For easy, accurate readings, some goniometers have a locking nut that is tightened just before the goniometer is removed.[5]

Other types of goniometers are available. Some have a fluid indicator that provides the reading after the motion is completed.[5] Others can be attached to a body segment and have dials that register ROM. There are special goniometers for cervical and spine ROM measurements and for forearm rotation.[12] A tape measure or metric scale may also be used on some joints by measuring the distance between two segments—for example, the distance between the chin and chest when measuring cervical flexion and extension, the distance between the center of the tips of two fingers for finger abduction, and the distance between the thumb tip and little finger tip for opposition.[3]

RECORDING MEASUREMENTS

When using the 180-degree system, the evaluator should record the number of degrees at the starting position and the number of degrees at the final position after the joint has passed through the maximally possible arc of motion.[10] Normal ROM always starts at 0 degree and increases toward 180 degrees. When it is not possible to start the motion at 0 degree because of a limitation of motion, the ROM is recorded by writing the number of degrees at the starting position followed by the number of degrees at the final position.[3] For example, elbow ROM limitations can be noted as follows:

Normal: 0 to 140 degrees
Extension limitation: 15 to 140 degrees
Flexion limitation: 0 to 110 degrees
Flexion and extension limitation: 15 to 110 degrees

Abnormal hyperextension of the elbow may be recorded by indicating the number of degrees of hyperextension below the 0-degree starting position with a minus sign, followed by the 0-degree position and then the number of degrees at the final position.[10] This may be noted as follows:

Normal: 0 to 140 degrees
Abnormal hyperextension: −20 to 0 to 140 degrees

There are alternative methods of recording ROM. The evaluator is advised to learn and adopt the particular method required by the healthcare facility.

A sample form for recording ROM measurements is shown in Figure 20-2. Average normal ROM for each joint motion is listed on the form and in Table 20-1. When measurements are being recorded, every space on the form should be filled in. If the joint was not tested, "NT" should be entered in the space.[3]

It should be noted that scapula movement accompanies movements of the shoulder (glenohumeral) joint as outlined. Range of glenohumeral joint motion is highly dependent on scapula mobility, which gives the shoulder its flexibility and wide ranges of motion. Although it is not possible to measure scapula movement with the goniometer, the evaluator should assess scapula mobility by observation of active motion or passive movement before proceeding with shoulder joint measurements. Scapular ROM is noted as *full* or *restricted*.[3] If scapular motion is restricted, as when musculature is in a state of spasticity or contracture, and the shoulder joint is moved into extreme ranges of motion (for example, above 90 degrees of flexion or abduction), glenohumeral joint damage can result.

When joint measurements may be performed in more than one position (e.g., as in shoulder internal and external rotation), the evaluating occupational therapist should note on the record the position in which the measurement was taken. The therapist should also note any pain or discomfort experienced by the client, the appearance of protective muscle spasm, whether active or passive ROM was measured, and any deviations from recommended testing procedures or positions.[10]

RESULTS OF ASSESSMENT AS THE BASIS FOR INTERVENTION PLANNING

After joint measurement, the therapist should analyze the results in relation to the client's life-role requirements. The therapist's first concern should be to correct ROM that is below functional limits. Many ordinary activities of daily living (ADLs) do not require full ROM. **Functional range of motion** refers to the amount of joint range necessary to perform essential ADLs and instrumental activities of daily living (IADLs) without the use of special equipment. The first concern of intervention is to attempt to increase any ROM that is limiting performance of self-care and home-maintenance tasks to functional levels.[8] For example, a severe limitation of elbow flexion affects eating and oral hygiene. Therefore, it is important to increase elbow flexion to nearly full ROM for function. Likewise, a severe limitation of forearm pronation affects eating, washing the body, telephoning, caring for children, and dressing. Because sitting comfortably requires hip ROM of at least 0 to 100 degrees, a first goal might be to increase flexion to 100 degrees if it is limited. Of course, if additional ROM can be gained, the therapist should plan the progression of intervention to increase the ROM to the normal range.

Some ROM limitations may be permanent. The role of the therapist in such cases is to work out methods to compensate

JOINT RANGE MEASUREMENTS

Client's name _____ Chart no. _____

Date of birth _____ Age _____ Sex _____

Diagnosis _____ Date of onset _____

Disability _____

LEFT				RIGHT		
3	**2**	**1**	**SPINE**	**1**	**2**	**3**
			Cervical spine			
			Flexion 0-45			
			Extension 0-45			
			Lateral flexion 0-45			
			Rotation 0-60			
			Thoracic and lumbar spine			
			Flexion 0-80			
			Extension 0-30			
			Lateral flexion 0-40			
			Rotation 0-45			
			SHOULDER			
			Flexion 0 to 170			
			Extension 0 to 60			
			Abduction 0 to 170			
			Horizontal abduction 0-40			
			Horizontal adduction 0-130			
			Internal rotation 0 to 70			
			External rotation 0 to 90			
			ELBOW AND FOREARM			
			Flexion 0 to 135-150			
			Supination 0 to 80-90			
			Pronation 0 to 80-90			
			WRIST			
			Flexion 0 to 80			
			Extension 0 to 70			
			Ulnar deviation 0 to 30			
			Radial deviation 0 to 20			
			THUMB			
			MP flexion 0 to 50			
			IP flexion 0 to 80-90			
			Abduction 0 to 50			
			FINGERS			
			MP flexion 0 to 90			
			MP hyperextension 0 to 15-45			
			PIP flexion 0 to 110			
			DIP flexion 0 to 80			
			Abduction 0 to 25			
			HIP			
			Flexion 0 to 120			
			Extension 0 to 30			
			Abduction 0 to 40			
			Adduction 0 to 35			
			Internal rotation 0 to 45			
			External rotation 0 to 45			
			KNEE			
			Flexion 0 to 135			
			ANKLE AND FOOT			
			Plantar flexion 0 to 50			
			Dorsiflexion 0 to 15			
			Inversion 0 to 35			
			Eversion 0 to 20			

Figure 20-2   Form for recording joint ROM measurement.

TABLE **20-1**　**Average Normal Range of Motion (180-Degree Method)**

Joint	ROM	Associated Girdle Motion	Joint	ROM
CERVICAL SPINE			**WRIST**	
Flexion	0° to 45°		Flexion	0° to 80°
Extension	0° to 45°		Extension	0° to 70°
Lateral flexion	0° to 45°		Ulnar deviation (adduction)	0° to 30°
Rotation	0° to 60°		Radial deviation (abduction)	0° to 20°
THORACIC AND LUMBAR SPINE			**THUMB**	
Flexion	0° to 80°		DIP Flexion	0° to 80-90°
Extension	0° to 30°		MP flexion	0° to 50°
Lateral flexion	0° to 40°		Adduction, radial and palmar	0°
Rotation	0° to 45°		Palmar abduction	0° to 50°
			Radial abduction	0° to 50°
			Opposition	Thumb pad to touch pad of little finger
SHOULDER			**FINGERS**	
Flexion	0° to 170°	Abduction, lateral tilt, slight elevation, slight upward rotation	MP flexion	0° to 90°
Extension	0° to 60°	Depression, adduction, upward tilt	MP hyperextension	0° to 15°-45°
Abduction	0° to 170°	Upward rotation, elevation	PIP flexion	0° to 110°
Adduction	0°	Depression, adduction, downward rotation	DIP flexion	0° to 80°
Horizontal abduction	0° to 40°	Adduction, reduction of lateral tilt	Abduction	0° to 25°
Horizontal adduction	0° to 180°	Abduction, lateral tilt	**HIP**	
Internal rotation		Abduction, lateral tilt	Flexion	0° to 120° (bent knee)
Arm in abduction	0° to 70°		Extension	0° to 30°
Arm in adduction	0° to 40°		Abduction	0° to 40°
External rotation		Adduction, reduction of lateral tilt	Adduction	0° to 35°
Arm in abduction	0° to 90°		Internal rotation	0° to 45°
Arm in abduction	0° to 60°		External rotation	0° to 45°
ELBOW			**KNEE**	
Flexion	0° to 135-140°		Flexion	0° to 135°
Extension	0°			
FOREARM			**ANKLE AND FOOT**	
Pronation	0° to 80°-90°		Plantar flexion	0° to 50°
Supination	0° to 80°-90°		Dorsiflexion	0° to 15°
			Inversion	0° to 35°
			Eversion	0° to 20°

Data adapted from American Academy of Orthopaedic Surgeons: *Joint motion: method of measuring and recording*, Chicago, 1965, The Academy; Esch D, Lepley M: *Evaluation of joint motion: methods of measurement and recording*, Minneapolis, 1974, University of Minnesota Press.
DIP, Distal interphalangeal; *MP*, metacarpophalangeal; *PIP*, proximal interphalangeal.

for the loss of ROM. Possibilities include assistive devices, such as a long-handled comb, brush, shoehorn, and a device to apply stockings, or adapted methods of performing a particular skill. (See Chapter 10 for further suggestions of ADL techniques for those with limited ROM.)

In many diagnoses, such as burns and arthritis, the loss of ROM can be anticipated. The goal of intervention is to prevent joint limitation with splints, positioning, exercise, activity, and application of the principles of joint protection.

Limited ROM, its causes, and the prognosis for increasing ROM will suggest intervention approaches. Some of the specific methods used to increase ROM are discussed elsewhere in this text (see Chapters 28 and 39). These include stretching exercise, resistive activity and exercise, strengthening of antagonistic muscle groups, activities that require active motion of the affected joints through the full available ROM, splints, and positioning. To increase ROM, the physician may perform surgery or manipulate the part while the client is under anesthesia. The physical therapist or certified hand therapist may use joint mobilization techniques such as manual stretching with heat and massage.[8]

PROCEDURE FOR MEASURING PASSIVE ROM

Average normal ROM for each joint motion is listed in Table 20-1, in Figure 20-2, and before each of the following procedures for measurement. The reader should keep in mind that these are averages; ROM may vary considerably among individuals. Normal ROM is affected by age, gender, and other factors, such as lifestyle and occupation.[10] Therefore, the client (*C*) in the illustrations may not always demonstrate the average ROM listed for the particular motion.

In the illustrations, the goniometer is shown in such a way that the reader can most easily see its positioning. However, the occupational therapist may not always be in the best position for the particular measurement. For the purposes of clear illustration, the therapist is necessarily shown off to one side and may have one hand, rather than two, on the instrument. Many of the motions require that the therapist actually be in front of the client or that the therapist's hands obscure the goniometer. How the therapist holds the goniometer and supports the part being measured is determined by factors such as the position of the client, amount of muscle weakness, presence or absence of joint pain, and whether active or passive ROM is being measured. Both the therapist and the client should be positioned for the greatest comfort, correct placement of the instrument, and adequate stabilization of the part being tested to ensure the desired motion in the correct plane.

GENERAL PROCEDURE—180-DEGREE METHOD OF MEASUREMENT[3,10]

1. The client should be comfortable and relaxed in the appropriate position (described later) for the joint measurement.
2. Uncover the joint to be measured.
3. Explain and demonstrate to the client what you are going to do, why, and how you expect him or her to cooperate.
4. If there is unilateral involvement, assess the PROM on the analogous limb to establish normal ROM for the client.
5. Establish and palpate bony landmarks for the measurement.
6. Stabilize joints proximal to the joint being measured.

7. Move the part passively through ROM to assess joint mobility and end-feel.
8. Return the part to the starting position.
9. To measure the starting position, place the goniometer just over the surface of and lateral to the joint. Place the axis of the goniometer over the axis of the joint, using the designated bony prominence or anatomical landmark. Place the stationary bar on or parallel to the longitudinal axis of the proximal or stationary bone and the movable bar on or parallel to the longitudinal axis of the distal or moving bone. To prevent the indicator on the movable bar from going off the protractor dial, always face the curved side away from the direction of motion, unless the goniometer can be read after movement in either direction.
10. Record the number of degrees at the starting position and remove the goniometer. Do not attempt to hold the goniometer in place while moving the joint through ROM.
11. To measure PROM, hold the part securely above and below the joint being measured and gently move the joint through ROM. Do not force the joints. Watch for signs of pain and discomfort. (NOTE: PROM may also be measured by asking the client to move actively through ROM and hold the position. The therapist then moves the joint through the final few degrees of PROM.)
12. Reposition the goniometer and record the number of degrees at the final position.
13. Remove the goniometer and gently place the part in resting position.
14. Record the reading at final position and any notations on the evaluation form.

DIRECTIONS FOR JOINT MEASUREMENT— 180-DEGREE SYSTEM

SPINE
Cervical Spine

Measurements of neck movements are the least accurate because the neck has few bony landmarks and much soft tissue overlying bony segments.[4] A radiographic examination is the best means to make an accurate measurement of the specific joints.[11] Measurements may be taken with a tape measure to record the distance between the chin and chest for flexion and extension, chin and shoulder for neck rotation, and mastoid process and shoulder for lateral flexion.[3]

Approximate estimates of cervical flexion, extension, rotation, and lateral flexion may be made by using the goniometer or by estimating the number of degrees of motion, using a fixed axis and estimating the arc of motion from that point (see Figures 20-3 to 20-10).[1,4]

Cervical Flexion

0 to 45 degrees (Figure 20-3).

Position of the client

Sitting or standing erect.

Measurement

The client is asked to flex the neck so that the chin moves toward the chest. The number of degrees of motion may be estimated, or the therapist may measure the number of inches or centimeters from the chin to the sternal notch.[1,3,10] If a goniometer is used, the axis is placed over the angle of the jaw.

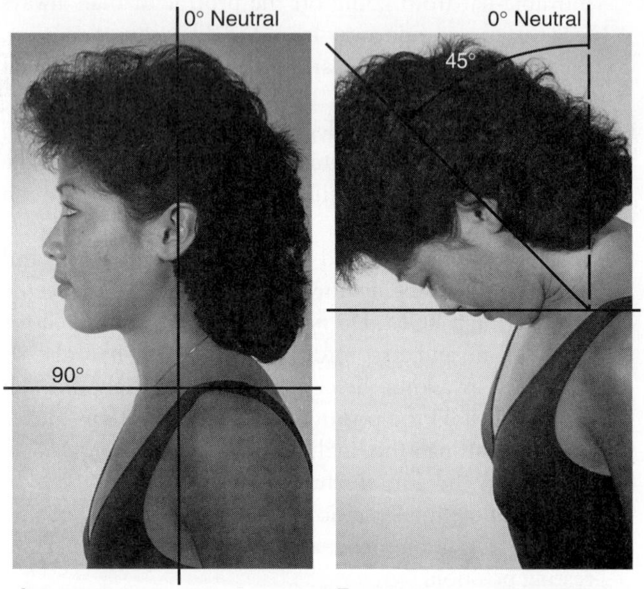

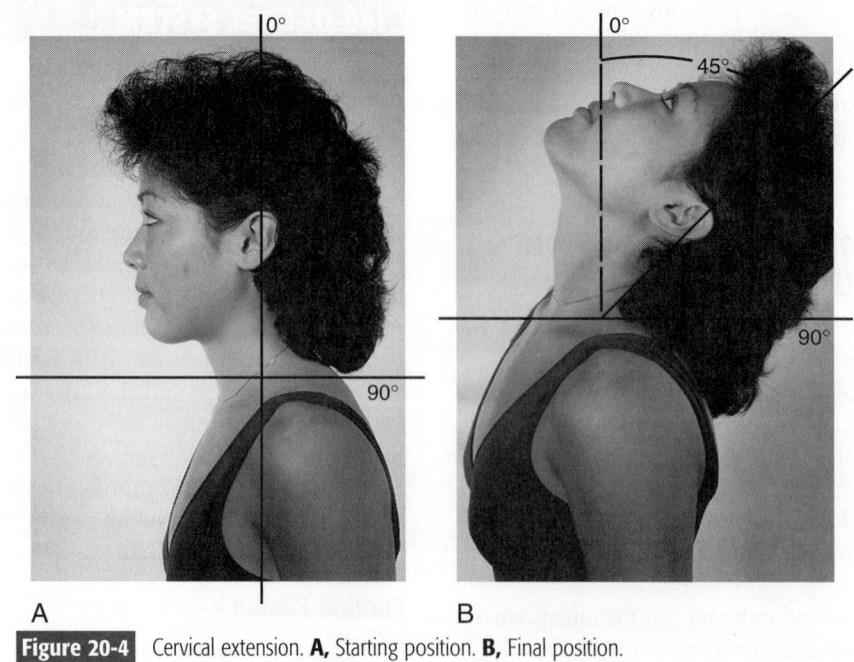

Figure 20-3   Cervical flexion. **A,** Starting position. **B,** Final position.

The therapist grasps the corner of the protractor, which is positioned with the arc upward, and steadies his or her arm by resting it against the client's shoulder. The arms of the goniometer are aligned with a tongue depressor, which the client is holding between the teeth. As the client performs neck flexion, the movable bar of the goniometer is adjusted downward to align with the new position of the tongue depressor.[4,10]

Cervical Extension

0 to 45 degrees (Figure 20-4).

Position of the client

Sitting or standing erect.

Measurement

The client is asked to extend the neck as if to look at the ceiling, so that the back of the head approaches the thoracic spine. The number of degrees of motion may be estimated, or the number of inches or centimeters from the chin to the sternal notch may be measured.[3] If a goniometer is used, the axis is placed over the angle of the jaw. The therapist grasps the corner of the protractor, which is now positioned with the arc downward, and steadies his or her arm against the client's shoulder. The movable bar of the goniometer is moved upward to align with the tongue depressor as the client extends the neck.[4,10]

Lateral Flexion

0 to 45 degrees (Figure 20-5).

Position of the client

Sitting or standing erect.

Figure 20-4   Cervical extension. **A,** Starting position. **B,** Final position.

Measurement

The client is asked to flex the neck laterally without rotation, moving the ear toward the shoulder. The number of degrees of motion may be estimated, or the therapist may measure the number of inches or centimeters between the mastoid process and the acromion process of the shoulder.[1,3] If a goniometer is used, the axis is placed over the spinous process of the seventh cervical vertebra. The stationary bar may be over the shoulder and parallel to the floor so that the motion begins at 90 degrees, or it may be aligned with the thoracic vertebra for a starting position of 0 degree. The movable bar is aligned with the external occipital protuberance.[1,10]

Cervical Rotation

0 to 60 degrees (Figure 20-6).

Position of the client

Lying supine or seated.

Measurement

The client is asked to rotate the head right or left without rotating the trunk. The amount of rotation may be estimated in degrees from the neutral position,[1] or a tape measure may be used to measure the distance from the tip of the chin to the acromion process of the shoulder. The measure is taken first in the anatomical position and then again after the neck has been rotated.[3] In the supine position, if a goniometer is used, it is set at 90 degrees and the axis is placed over the vertex of the head. The stationary bar is held steady, parallel to the floor or to the acromion process on the side being tested. The movable bar is aligned with the tip of the nose.[4,10]

Thoracic and Lumbar Spine

Flexion

0 to 80 degrees and 4 inches (Figure 20-7).

Position of the client

Standing erect.

Measurement

Four methods of estimating the range of spinal flexion are as follows: measuring trunk forward flexion in relation to the longitudinal axis of the body (therapist must hold the pelvis stable with the hands and observe any change in the client's normal lordosis); recording the level of the fingertips along the front of the client's leg; measuring the number of inches or centimeters between the client's fingertips and the floor; and measuring the length of the spine from the seventh cervical vertebra to the first sacral vertebra when the

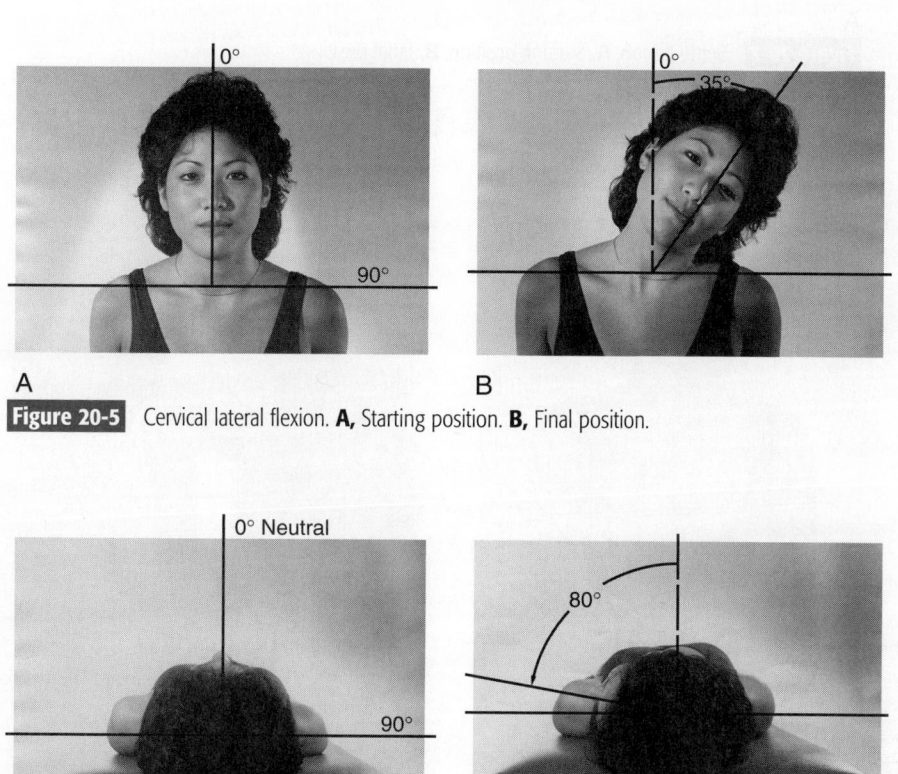

Figure 20-5   Cervical lateral flexion. **A,** Starting position. **B,** Final position.

Figure 20-6   Cervical rotation. **A,** Starting position. **B,** Final position.

client is erect and again after the client has flexed the spine (see Figure 20-7).[3,10] The fourth is probably the most accurate of these clinical methods.[1] In a normal adult, the average increase in length in forward flexion of the spine is 4 inches (10 cm).[3] If the client bends forward at the hips with a straight back, no difference in length will occur.

Lateral Flexion

0 to 40 degrees (Figure 20-8).

Position of the client

Standing erect.

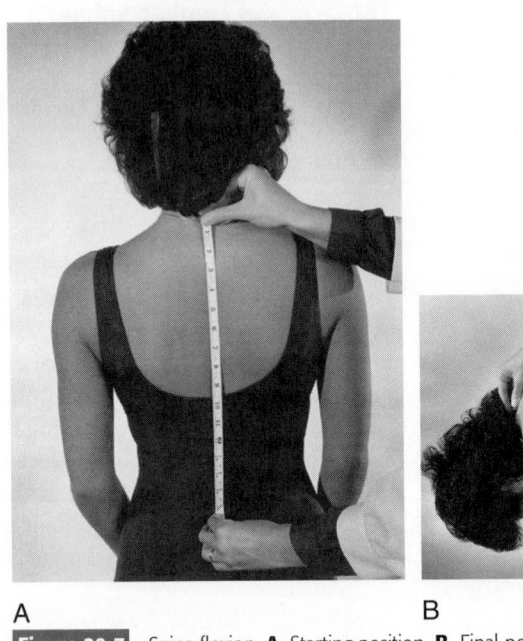
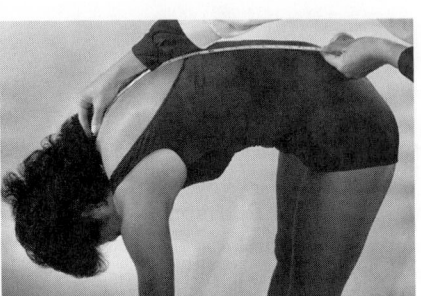

A   B

Figure 20-7   Spine flexion. **A,** Starting position. **B,** Final position.

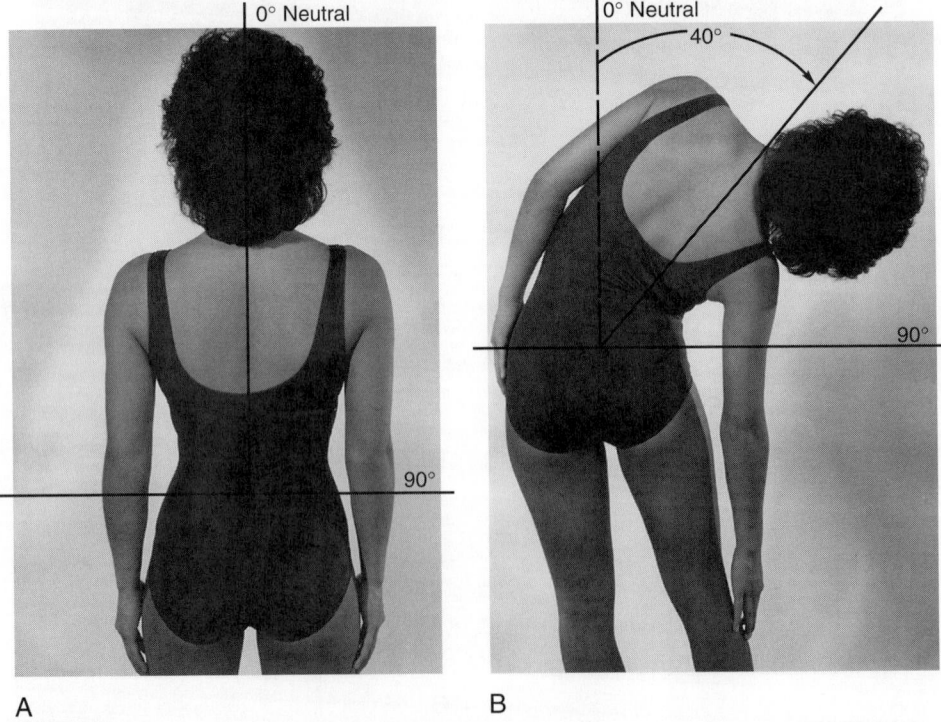

A   B

Figure 20-8   Spine lateral flexion. **A,** Starting position. **B,** Final position.

Measurement

Several methods may be used to estimate the range of lateral flexion of the trunk. The steel tape measure may be held in place during the motion and used to estimate the number of degrees of lateral inclination of the trunk compared with the vertical position. Other methods include estimating the position of the spinous process of C7 in relation to the pelvis (Figure 20-8); measuring the distance of the fingertips from the knee joint in lateral flexion; measuring the distance between the tip of the third finger and the floor[3]; and using a long-arm goniometer, placing the axis on S1, the stationary bar perpendicular to the floor, and the movable bar aligned with C7.[1,10]

Extension

0 to 30 degrees (Figure 20-9).

Position of the client

Standing erect or lying prone.

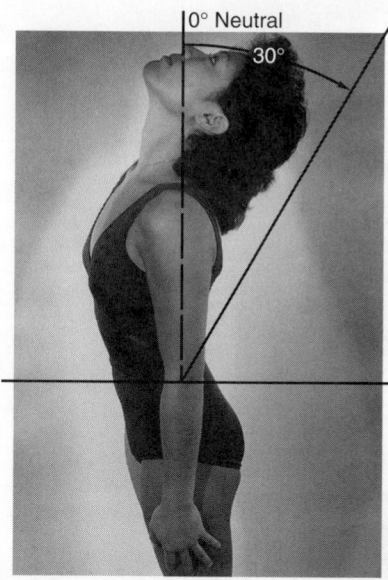

Figure 20-9   Spine extension.

Measurement

The client is asked to bend backward while maintaining stability of the pelvis. If necessary, the therapist stabilizes the pelvis from the anterior when the measurement is taken in the standing position. The range of extension is estimated in degrees from the vertical, using the superior iliac crest as the pivotal point in relation to the spinous process of C7. With the client in the supine position, a pillow is placed under the abdomen and the client's hands are placed at shoulder level on the treatment table. The pelvis is stabilized with a strap or by an assistant, and the client extends the elbows to raise the trunk from the table. A perpendicular measurement is taken of the distance between the suprasternal notch and the supporting surface at the end of the ROM.[3]

Rotation

0 to 45 degrees (Figure 20-10).

Position of the client

Supine or standing.

Measurement

The client is asked to rotate the upper trunk while maintaining a neutral position of the pelvis. The therapist may fix the pelvis firmly to maintain the neutral position. This step is especially important if the client is in the standing position. This motion is recorded in degrees, using the center of the crown of the head as a pivotal point and the arc of motion made by the shoulder as it moves upward or forward.

UPPER EXTREMITY[1-3,5,10,11]

Shoulder

Flexion

0 to 170 degrees (Figure 20-11).

Position of the client

Seated or supine with the humerus in neutral rotation.

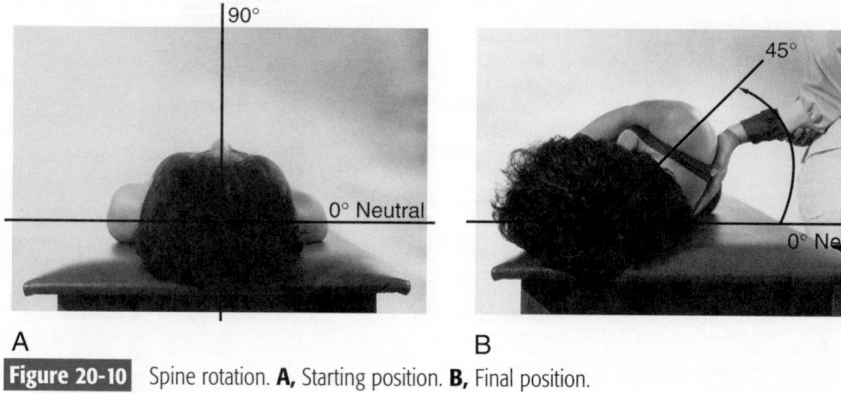

Figure 20-10   Spine rotation. **A,** Starting position. **B,** Final position.

Position of goniometer

The axis is in the center of the humeral head, just distal to the acromion process on the lateral aspect of the humerus. The stationary bar is parallel to the trunk, and the movable bar is parallel to the humerus. Note that when the shoulder is flexed, the axis point moves upward and backward to the posterior surface of the shoulder. Thus, to take the measurement of the final position, the therapist should place the goniometer on the lateral surface of the shoulder, aligned with the imaginary axis through the center of the humeral head, which is just slightly superior to the crease formed by the deltoid mass.

End-feel

Firm.[3]

Extension

0 to 60 degrees (Figure 20-12).

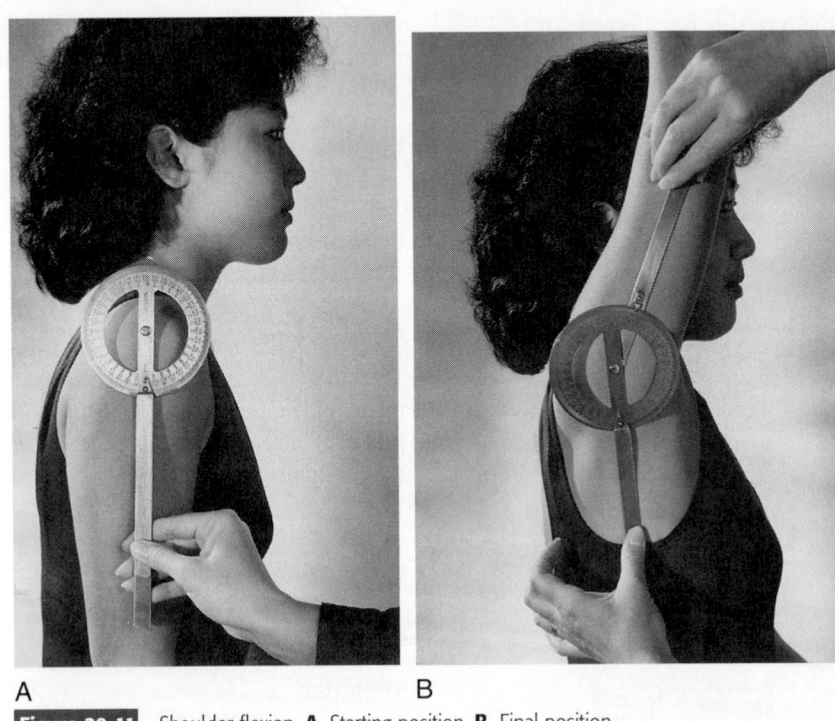

Figure 20-11   Shoulder flexion. **A,** Starting position. **B,** Final position.

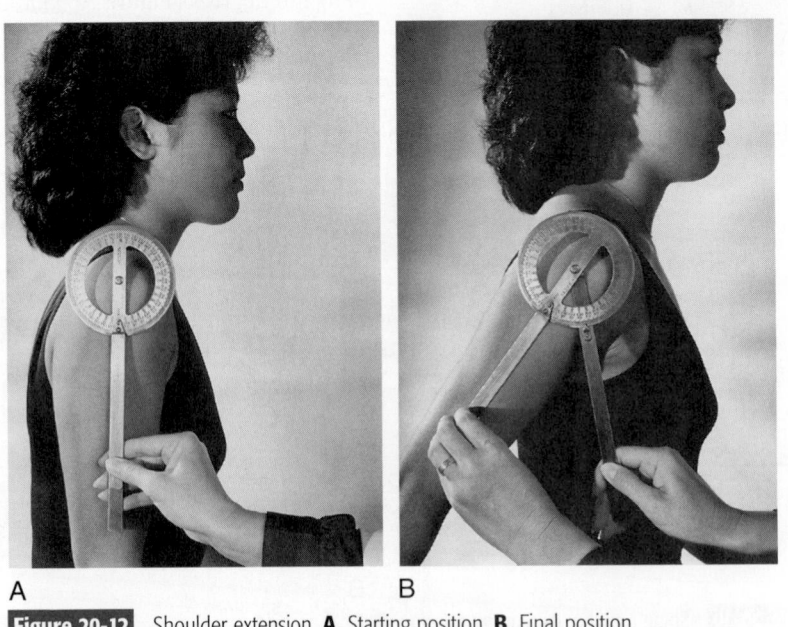

Figure 20-12   Shoulder extension. **A,** Starting position. **B,** Final position.

Position of the client

Seated or prone, with no obstruction behind the humerus and the humerus in neutral rotation.

Position of goniometer

Same as for flexion, but the axis point remains the same for starting and final positions. Movement should be accompanied by a slight upward tilt of the scapula. Excessive scapular motion should be avoided.

End-feel

Firm.[3]

Abduction

0 to 170 degrees (Figure 20-13).

Position of the client

Seated or lying prone, with the humerus in adduction and external rotation. Measure on the posterior surface.

Position of goniometer

The axis is on the acromion process on the posterior surface of the shoulder. The stationary bar is parallel to the trunk, and the movable bar is parallel to the humerus.

End-feel

Firm.[3]

Internal Rotation

0 to 60 degrees (Figure 20-14).

Position of the client

The following position is used if abduction cannot be achieved: seated with humerus adducted against trunk, elbow at 90 degrees, and forearm at midposition and perpendicular to body.[3]

Position of goniometer

The axis is on the olecranon process of the elbow, and the stationary bar and movable bar are parallel to the forearm.

Internal Rotation (Alternative Position)

0 to 70 degrees (Figure 20-15).

Position of the client

The following position is used if there is no danger of posterior dislocation and if abduction is possible: prone or supine with the humerus abducted to 90 degrees, the elbow flexed to 90 degrees, and the forearm in pronation, perpendicular to the floor.

Position of goniometer

The axis is on the olecranon process of the elbow, and the stationary bar and movable bar are parallel to the forearm.

End-feel

Firm.[3]

External Rotation

0 to 80 degrees (Figure 20-16).

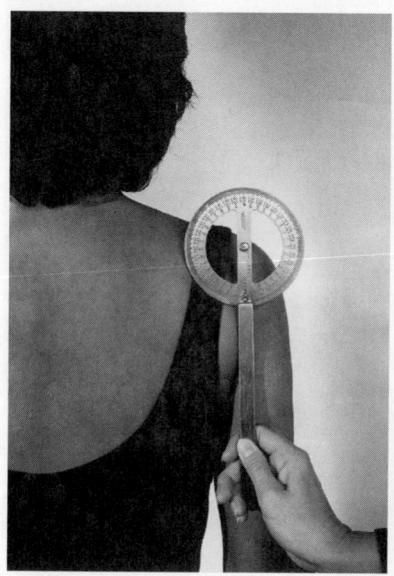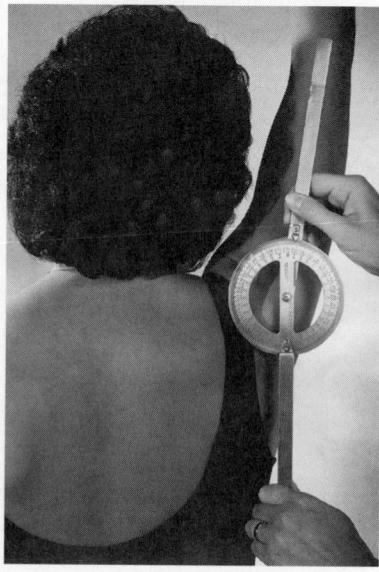

A   B

Figure 20-13 Shoulder abduction. **A,** Starting position. **B,** Final position.

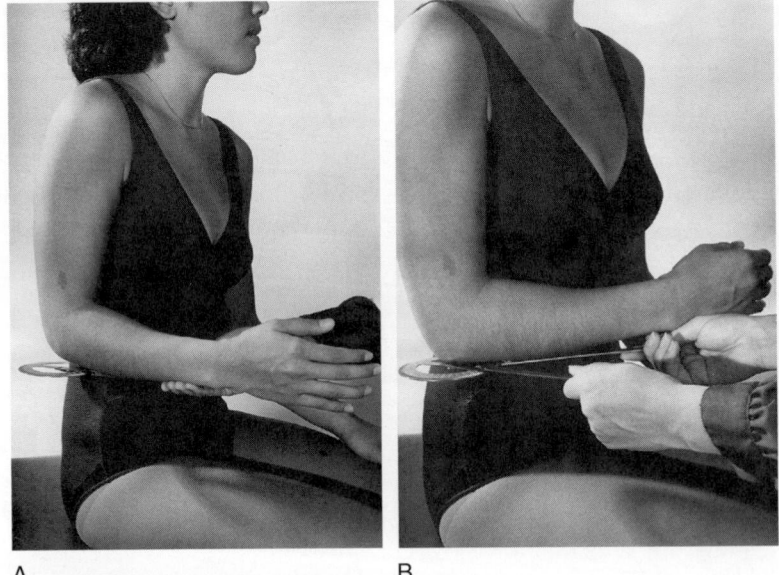

A   B

Figure 20-14   Shoulder internal rotation, shoulder adducted. **A,** Starting position. **B,** Final position.

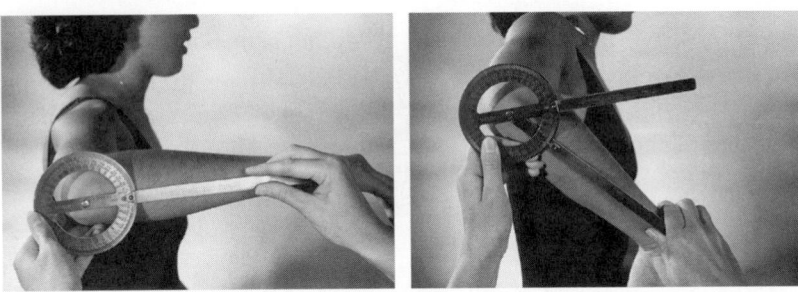

A   B

Figure 20-15   Shoulder internal rotation, shoulder abducted (alternative position). **A,** Starting position. **B,** Final position.

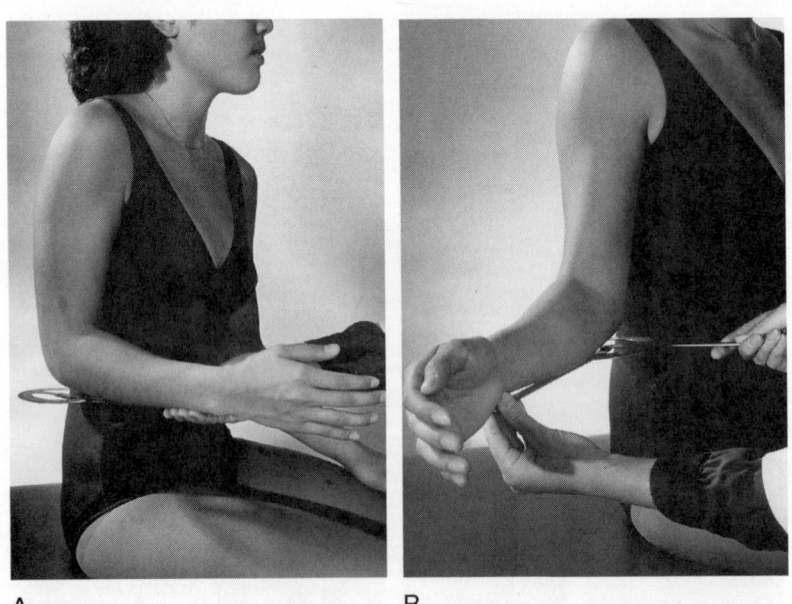

A   B

Figure 20-16   Shoulder external rotation, shoulder adducted. **A,** Starting position. **B,** Final position.

Position of the client

This position is used if abduction is not possible: seated, the humerus adducted, the elbow at 90 degrees, and the forearm in midposition, perpendicular to the body.

Position of goniometer

The axis is on the olecranon process of the elbow. The stationary bar and movable bar are parallel to the forearm.[3]

External Rotation (Alternative Position)

0 to 90 degrees (Figure 20-17).

Position of the client

The following position is used if there is no danger of anterior dislocation of the humerus[3]: seated or supine with the humerus abducted to 90 degrees, the elbow flexed to 90 degrees, and the forearm pronated.

Position of goniometer

The axis is on the olecranon process of the elbow, and the stationary bar and movable bar are parallel to the forearm.

End-feel

Firm.[3]

Horizontal Abduction

0 to 40 degrees (Figure 20-18).

Position of the client

Seated erect with the shoulder to be tested abducted to 90 degrees, the elbow extended, and the palm facing down. The therapist may support the arm in abduction.[3]

Position of goniometer

The axis is over the acromion process. The stationary bar is parallel over the shoulder toward the neck, and the movable bar is parallel to the humerus on the superior aspect.

End-feel

Firm.[3]

Horizontal Adduction

0 to 130 degrees (Figure 20-19).

Position of client and goniometer

Same as for horizontal abduction.

End-feel

Firm or soft.[3]

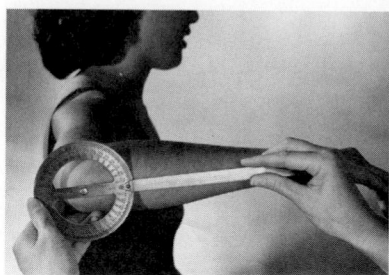
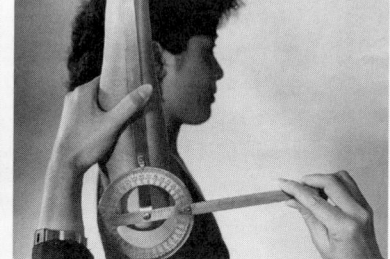

A   B

Figure 20-17 Shoulder external rotation, shoulder abducted (alternative position). **A,** Starting position. **B,** Final position.

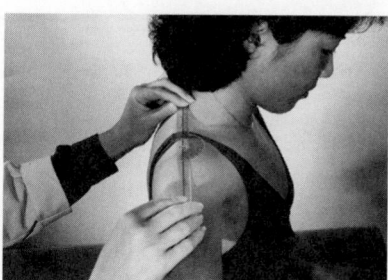
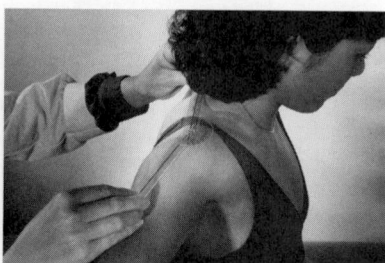

A   B

Figure 20-18 Shoulder horizontal abduction. **A,** Starting position. **B,** Final position.

Elbow

Extension to Flexion

0-135-150 degrees (Figure 20-20).

Position of the client

Standing, sitting, or supine with the humerus adducted and externally rotated and the forearm supinated.

Position of goniometer

The axis is placed over the lateral epicondyle of the humerus at the end of the elbow crease. The stationary bar is parallel to the midline of the humerus, and the movable bar is parallel to the radius. After the movement has been completed, the position of the elbow crease changes in relation to the lateral epicondyle because of the rise of the muscle bulk during the motion. The axis of the goniometer should be repositioned so that it is over, although it will not be directly on, the lateral epicondyle.

End-feel

Soft, hard, and firm: flexion. Hard or firm: extension and hyperextension.[3]

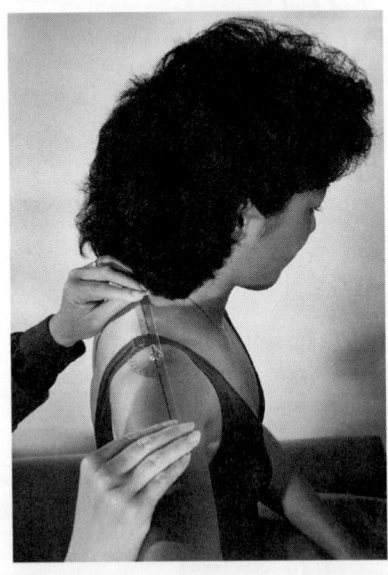
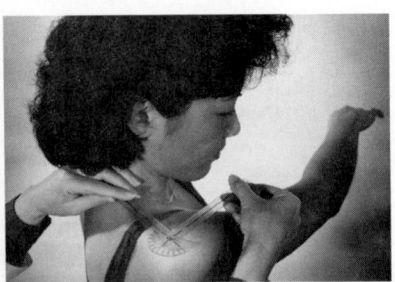

A   B

Figure 20-19   Shoulder horizontal adduction. **A,** Starting position. **B,** Final position.

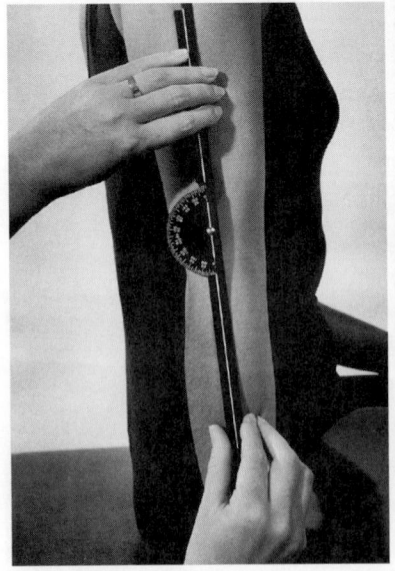
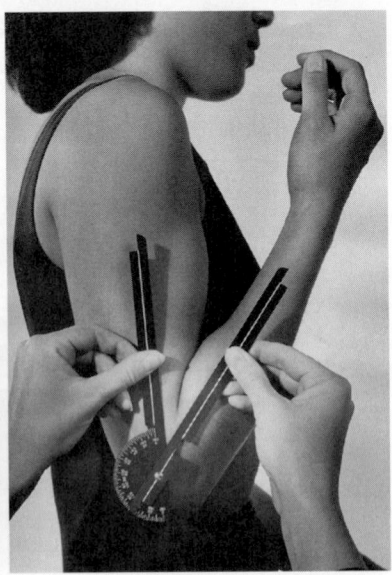

A   B

Figure 20-20   Elbow flexion. **A,** Starting position. **B,** Final position.

Forearm

Supination

0 to 80 degrees or 90 degrees (Figure 20-21).

Position of the client

Seated or standing with the humerus adducted, the elbow at 90 degrees, and the forearm in midposition.

Position of goniometer

The axis is at the ulnar border of the volar aspect of the wrist, just proximal to the ulna styloid. The movable bar is resting against the volar aspect of the wrist, and the stationary bar is perpendicular to the floor. After the forearm is supinated, the goniometer should be repositioned so that the movable bar rests squarely across the center of the distal forearm.

Supination (Alternative Method)

0 to 80 degrees or 90 degrees (Figure 20-22).

Position of the client

Seated or standing with the humerus adducted, the elbow at 90 degrees, and the forearm in midposition. Place a pencil in the client's hand so that it is held perpendicular to the floor.

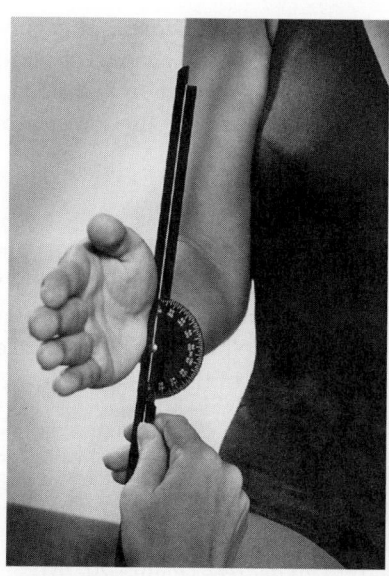
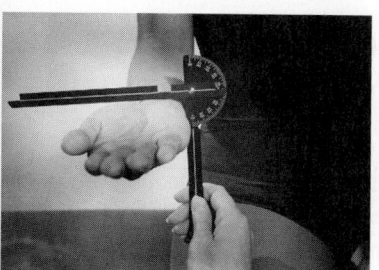

A   B

Figure 20-21   Forearm supination. **A,** Starting position. **B,** Final position.

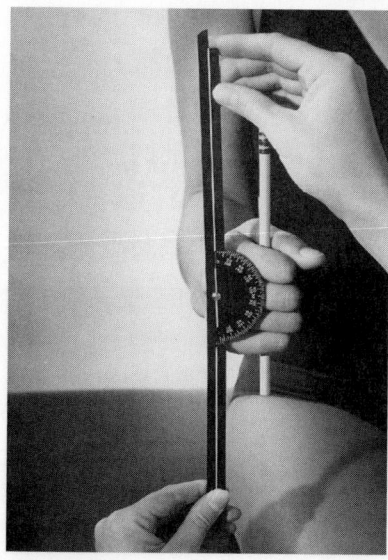
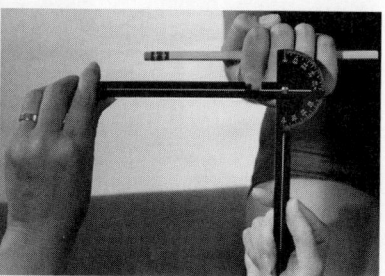

A   B

Figure 20-22   Forearm supination (alternate method). **A,** Starting position. **B,** Final position.

Position of goniometer

The axis is over the head of the third metacarpal, and the stationary bar is perpendicular to the floor. The movable bar is parallel to the pencil.

End-feel

Firm.[3]

Pronation

0 to 80 degrees or 90 degrees (Figure 20-23).

Position of the client

Seated or standing with the humerus adducted, the elbow at 90 degrees, and the forearm in midposition.

Position of goniometer

The axis is at the ulnar border of the dorsal aspect of the wrist, just proximal to the ulnar styloid. The movable bar is resting against the dorsal aspect of the wrist, and the stationary bar is perpendicular to the floor. After the forearm is pronated, reposition the goniometer so that the movable bar rests squarely across the center of the dorsum of the distal forearm.

Pronation (Alternative Method)

0 to 80 degrees or 90 degrees (Figure 20-24).

Position of the client

Seated or standing with the humerus adducted, the elbow at 90 degrees, and the forearm in midposition. A pencil is placed in the hand so that it is held perpendicular to the floor.

Position of goniometer

The axis is over the head of the third metacarpal, the stationary bar is perpendicular to the floor, and the movable bar is parallel to the pencil.

End-feel

Hard to firm.[3]

Wrist

Flexion

0 to 80 degrees (Figure 20-25).

Position of the client

Seated with the forearm in midposition and the hand and forearm resting on a table on the ulnar border. The fingers are relaxed or extended. This measurement may also be taken with the forearm pronated and resting on a table.[3]

Position of goniometer

The wrist is measured with the forearm in midposition, and the axis is on the lateral aspect of the wrist just distal to the radial styloid in the anatomical snuffbox. The stationary bar is parallel to the radius, and the movable bar is parallel to the metacarpal of the index finger.

End-feel

Firm.[3]

Extension

0 to 70 degrees (Figure 20-26).

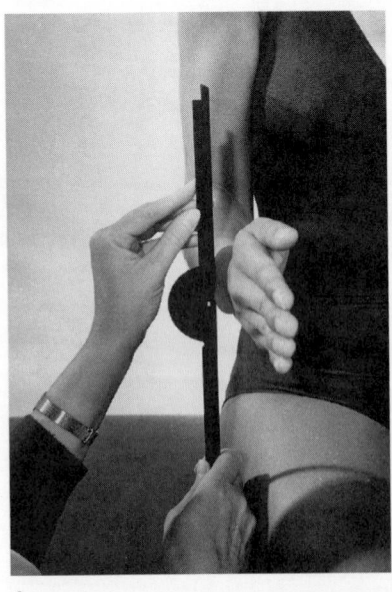
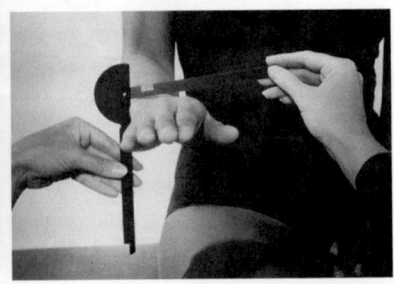

A   B
Figure 20-23   Forearm pronation. **A,** Starting position. **B,** Final position.

Position of the client and goniometer

The same as for wrist flexion, except that the fingers should be flexed.

End-feel

Firm or hard.[3]

Ulnar Deviation

0 to 30 degrees (Figure 20-27).

Position of the client

Seated with the forearm pronated, the wrist at neutral, the fingers relaxed in extension, and the palm of the hand resting flat on the table surface.

Position of goniometer

The axis is on the dorsum of the wrist at the base of the third metacarpal, over the capitate bone. The movable bar is

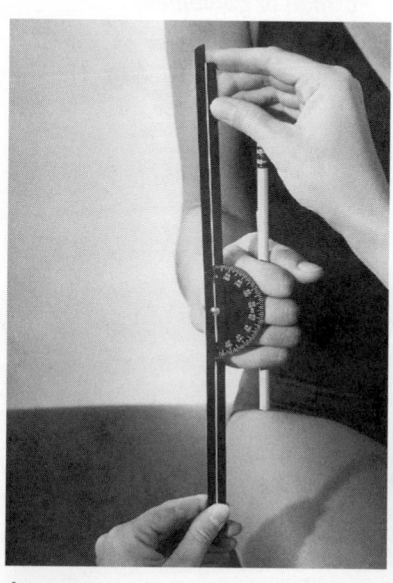
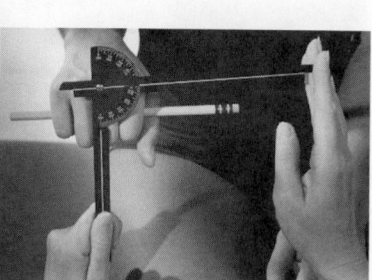

A   B

Figure 20-24 Forearm pronation (alternate method). **A,** Starting position. **B,** Final position.

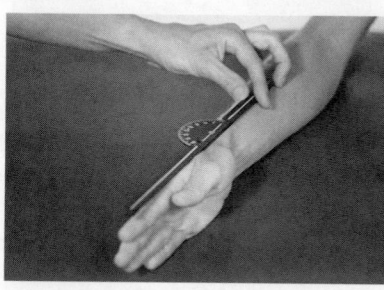
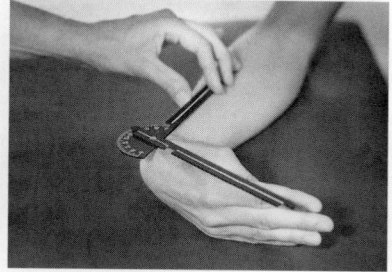

A   B

Figure 20-25 Wrist flexion. **A,** Starting position. **B,** Final position.

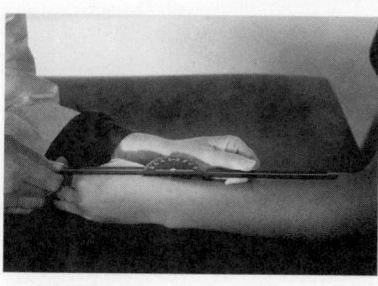
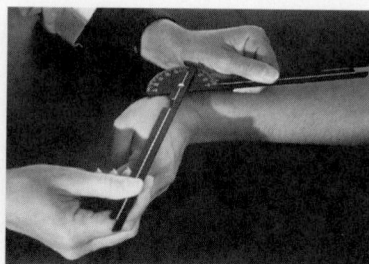

A   B

Figure 20-26 Wrist extension. **A,** Starting position. **B,** Final position.

parallel to the third metacarpal, and the stationary bar is over the midline of the dorsal forearm.

End-feel

Firm.[3]

Radial Deviation

0 to 20 degrees (Figure 20-28).

Position of the client and goniometer

Same as for ulnar deviation.

End-feel

Firm or hard.[3]

Fingers

Metacarpophalangeal Flexion

0 to 90 degrees (Figure 20-29).

Position of the client

Seated with the elbow flexed, the forearm in midposition, the wrist at 0-degree neutral, and the forearm and hand supported on a firm surface on the ulnar border.

Position of goniometer

The axis is centered on the dorsal aspect of the metacarpophalangeal (MP) joint. The stationary bar is on top of the metacarpal, and the movable bar is on top of the proximal phalanx.

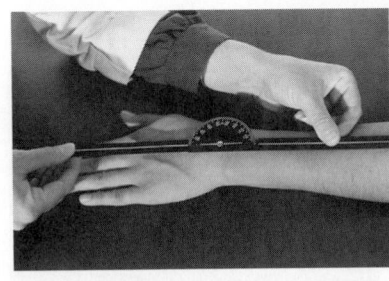
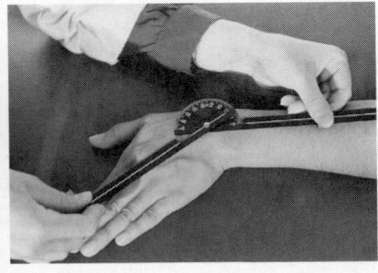

A   B

Figure 20-27 Wrist ulnar deviation. **A,** Starting position. **B,** Final position.

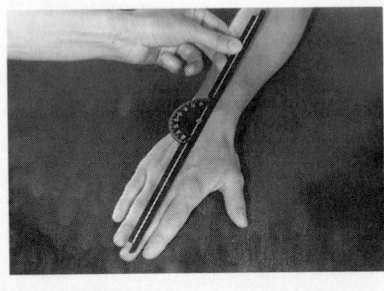
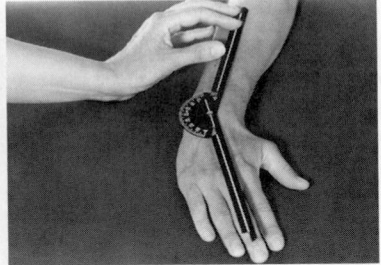

A   B

Figure 20-28 Wrist radial deviation. **A,** Starting position. **B,** Final position.

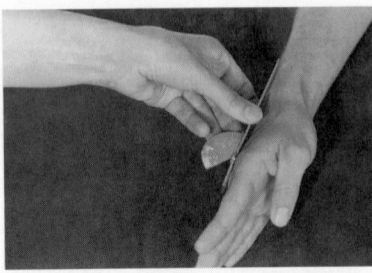
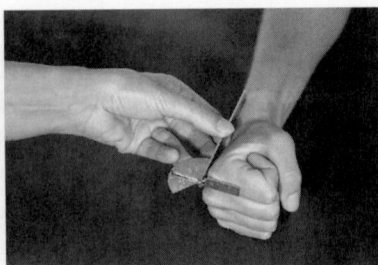

A   B

Figure 20-29 Metacarpophalangeal flexion. **A,** Starting position. **B,** Final position.

End-feel

Hard or firm.[3]

Metacarpophalangeal Joint Hyperextension

0 to 45 degrees (Figure 20-30).

Position of the client

Seated with the forearm in midposition, the wrist at 0-degree neutral, the interphalangeal joints relaxed or in flexion, and the forearm and hand supported on a firm surface on the ulnar border.

Position of goniometer

The axis is over the lateral aspect of the MP joint of the index finger. The stationary bar is parallel to the metacarpal, and the movable bar is parallel to the proximal phalanx. The little finger's MP joint may be measured similarly. ROM of the long and ring fingers can be estimated by comparison.

An alternative is to place the goniometer on the volar aspect of the hand. With use of the edge of the goniometer, the axis is aligned over the MP joint being measured, the stationary bar is parallel to the metacarpal, and the movable bar is parallel to the proximal phalanx.

End-feel

Firm.[3]

Metacarpophalangeal Abduction

0 to 25 degrees (Figure 20-31).

Position of the client

Seated with the forearm pronated, the wrist at 0-degree neutral deviation, the fingers straight, and the hand resting on a firm surface.

Position of goniometer

The axis is centered over the MP joint being measured. The stationary bar is over the corresponding metacarpal, and the movable bar is over the proximal phalanx.

End-feel

Firm.[3]

Proximal Interphalangeal Flexion

0 to 110 degrees (Figure 20-32).

Position of the client

Seated with the forearm in midposition, the wrist at 0-degree neutral, and the forearm and hand supported on a firm surface on the ulnar border.

Position of goniometer

The axis is centered on the dorsal surface of the proximal interphalangeal (PIP) joint being measured. The stationary bar is placed over the proximal phalanx, and the movable bar is over the middle phalanx.

Alternative Method

Measurement with a ruler can also be taken. The IP and MP joints of the fingers are flexed toward the palm. A ruler is

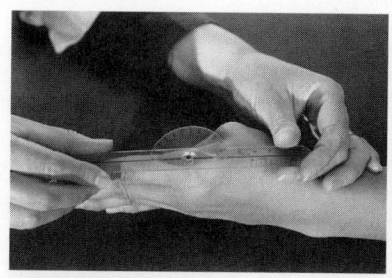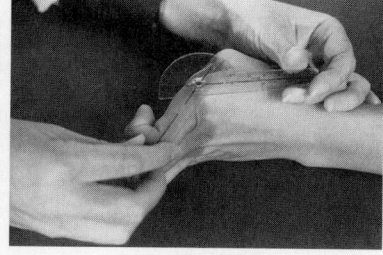

Figure 20-30 Metacarpophalangeal hyperextension. **A,** Starting position. **B,** Final position.

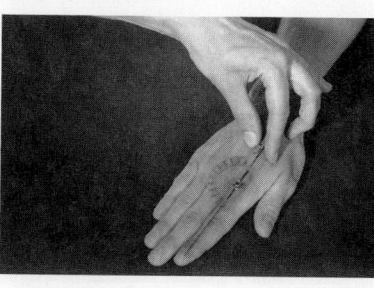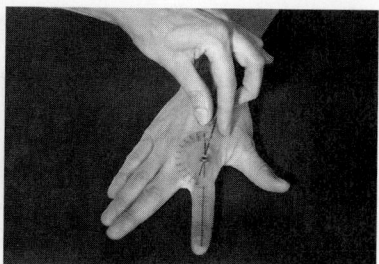

Figure 20-31 Metacarpophalangeal abduction. **A,** Starting position. **B,** Final position.

used to measure from the pulp of the middle finger to the proximal palmar crease.[3]

End-feel

Usually hard; may be soft or firm.[3]

Distal Interphalangeal Flexion

0 to 80 degrees (Figure 20-33).

Position of the client

Seated with the forearm in midposition, the wrist at 0-degree neutral, and the forearm and hand supported on the ulnar border on a firm surface.

Position of goniometer

The axis is on the dorsal surface of the distal interphalangeal (DIP) joint. The stationary bar is over the middle phalanx, and the movable bar is over the distal phalanx.

Alternative Method

With the MP joints in 0-degree extension, the client flexes the interphalangeal and PIP joints toward the palm. With a ruler, a measurement is taken from the pulp of the middle finger to the distal palmar crease.[3]

End-feel

Firm.[3]

Thumb

Metacarpophalangeal Flexion

0 to 50 degrees (Figure 20-34).

Position of the client

Seated with the elbow flexed, the forearm in 45 degrees of supination, the wrist at 0-degree neutral, the MP and interphalangeal joints in extension, and the hand and forearm supported on a firm surface.

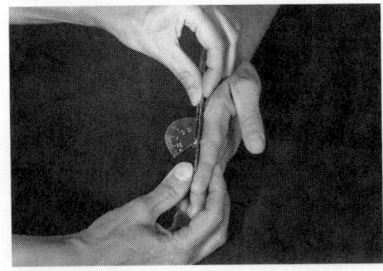
A

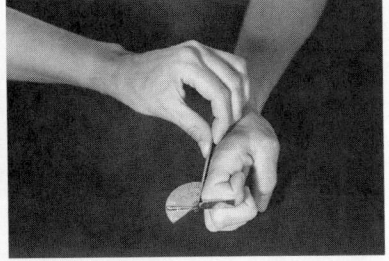
B

Figure 20-32   Proximal interphalangeal flexion. **A,** Starting position. **B,** Final position.

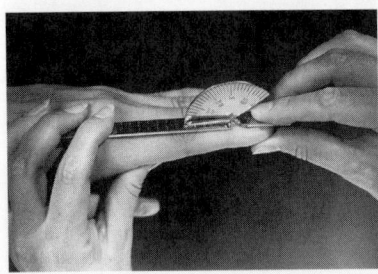
A

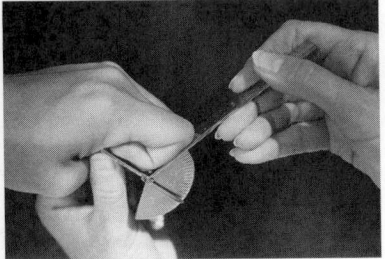
B

Figure 20-33   Distal interphalangeal flexion. **A,** Starting position. **B,** Final position.

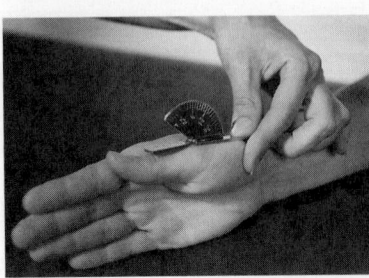
A

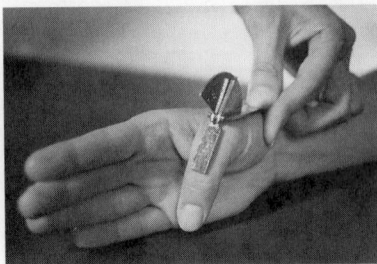
B

Figure 20-34   Thumb metacarpophalangeal flexion. **A,** Starting position. **B,** Final position.

Position of goniometer

The axis is on the dorsal surface of the MP joint. The stationary bar is over the thumb metacarpal, and the movable bar is over the proximal phalanx.

End-feel

Hard or firm.[3]

Interphalangeal Flexion

0 to 90 degrees (Figure 20-35).

Position of the client

Same as described for PIP and DIP finger flexion.

Position of goniometer

The axis is on the dorsal surface of the interphalangeal joint. The stationary bar is over the proximal phalanx, and the movable bar is over the distal phalanx.

Radial Abduction (Carpometacarpal Extension)

0 to 50 degrees (Figure 20-36).

Position of the client

Seated with the forearm pronated and the hand palm down, resting flat on a firm surface.

Position of goniometer

The axis is over the carpometacarpal (CMC) joint at the base of the thumb metacarpal. The stationary bar is parallel to the radius, and the movable bar is parallel to the thumb metacarpal.

Radial Abduction (Alternative Method)

0 to 50 degrees (Figure 20-37).

Position of the client and goniometer

The client is positioned the same as described in the first method. The axis is over the CMC joint at the base of the thumb metacarpal. The stationary and movable bars are together and parallel to the thumb and the first metacarpals. Neither will be directly over these bones.

End-feel

Firm.[3]

Palmar Abduction (Carpometacarpal Flexion)

0 to 50 degrees (Figure 20-38).

Position of the client

Seated with the forearm at 0-degree midposition, the wrist at 0 degree, and the forearm and hand resting on the ulnar border. The thumb is rotated so that it is at right angles to the palm of the hand.

Position of goniometer

The axis is at the junction of the thumb and index finger metacarpals. The stationary bar is over the radius, and the movable bar is parallel to the thumb and index finger metacarpals.

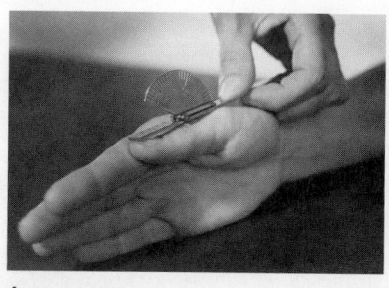 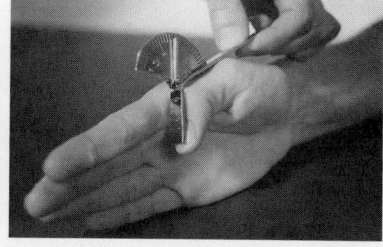

A   B

Figure 20-35 Thumb interphalangeal flexion. **A,** Starting position. **B,** Final position.

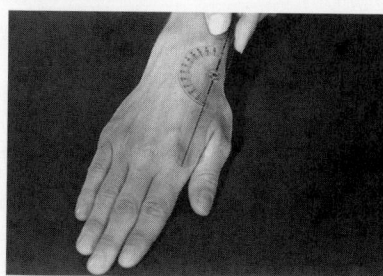 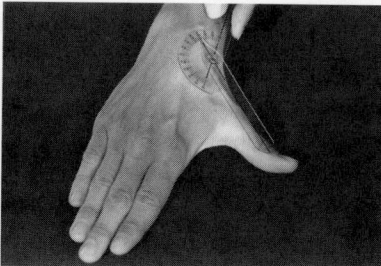

A   B

Figure 20-36 Thumb radial abduction. **A,** Starting position. **B,** Final position.

Palmar Abduction (Alternative Method)

0 to 50 degrees (Figure 20-39).

Position of the client and goniometer

The client is positioned in the same way described in the first method. The axis is at the junction of the thumb and index finger metacarpals. The stationary and movable bars are lined up together, parallel to the thumb and the index finger metacarpals.

End-feel

Firm.[3]

Opposition

Deficits in opposition may be recorded by measuring the distance between the centers of the pads of the thumb and the fifth finger with a centimeter ruler (Figure 20-40).

End-feel

Soft or firm.[3]

LOWER EXTREMITY[3,5,6,10]

Hip

Flexion

0 to 120 degrees (Figure 20-41).

Position of the client

Supine, lying with the hip and knee in 0-degree neutral extension and rotation.

Position of goniometer

The axis is on the lateral aspect of the hip, over the greater trochanter of the femur. The stationary bar is centered over the middle of the lateral aspect of the pelvis, and the

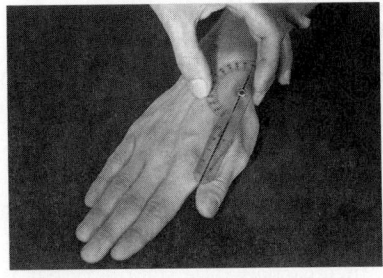
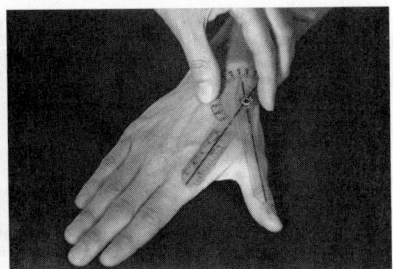

A   B

Figure 20-37   Thumb radial abduction (alternative method). **A,** Starting position. **B,** Final position.

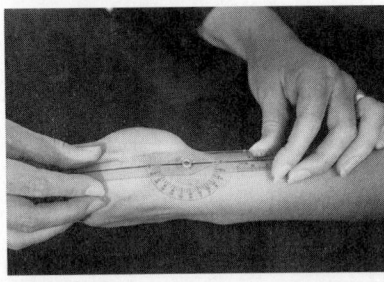
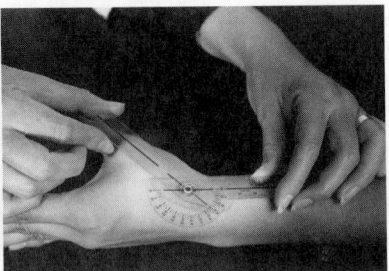

A   B

Figure 20-38   Palmar abduction. **A,** Starting position. **B,** Final position.

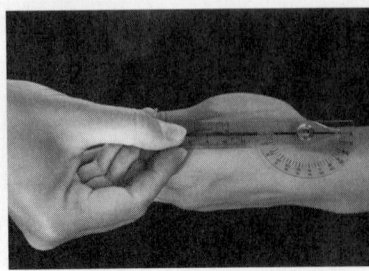
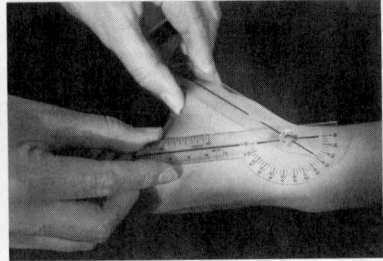

A   B

Figure 20-39   Palmar abduction (alternative method). **A,** Starting position. **B,** Final position.

movable bar is parallel to the long axis of the femur on the lateral aspect of the thigh. The knee is bent during the motion.

End-feel

Soft.[3]

Extension (Hyperextension)

0 to 30 degrees (Figure 20-42).

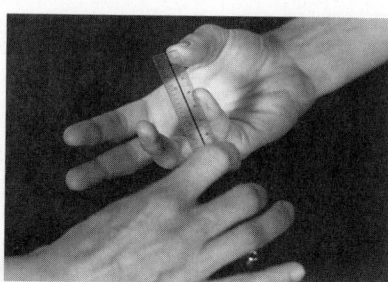

Figure 20-40   Thumb opposition to fifth finger.

Position of the client

The client is prone, lying with the hip and knee at 0-degree neutral extension and rotation and the feet over the end of the table.

Position of goniometer

Same as for hip flexion.

End-feel

Firm.[3]

Abduction

0 to 40 degrees (Figure 20-43).

Position of the client

The client is supine, lying with the legs extended and the hip in 0-degree neutral rotation. The pelvis is level.

Position of goniometer

The axis is placed on the anterior superior iliac spine. The stationary bar is placed on a line between two anterior

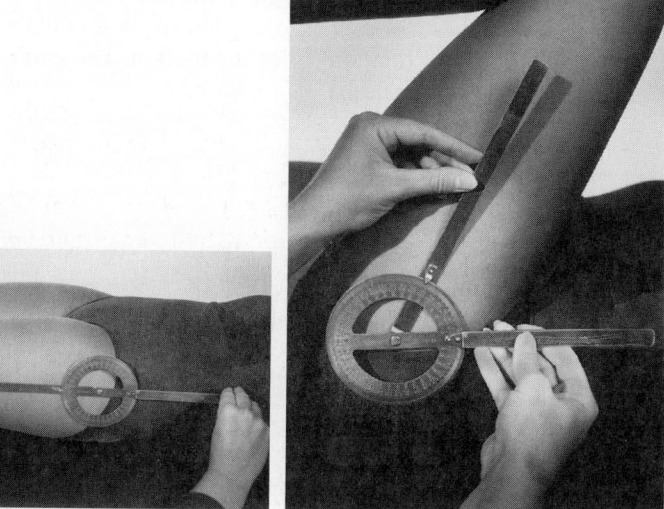

A   B

Figure 20-41   Hip flexion. **A,** Starting position. **B,** Final position.

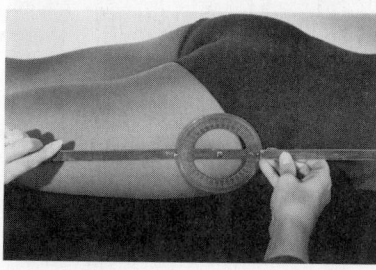
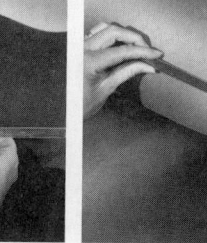

A   B

Figure 20-42   Hip extension. **A,** Starting position. **B,** Final position.

superior iliac spines, and the movable bar is parallel to the longitudinal axis of the femur over the anterior aspect of the thigh. Note that the starting position is at 90 degrees for this measurement and that the recording of the measurement should be adjusted by subtracting 90 degrees from the total number of degrees obtained in the arc of joint motion.

End-feel

Firm.[3]

Adduction

0 to 35 degrees (Figure 20-44).

Position of the client and goniometer

The client is supine, lying with the hip and knee of the leg to be tested in extension and neutral rotation. The leg not being tested should be abducted. The goniometer is positioned the same as for hip abduction.

End-feel

Firm or soft.[3]

Internal Rotation

0 degree to 45 degrees (Figure 20-45).

Position of the client

The client is seated with the hip in 0-degree neutral rotation and the hip and knee flexed to 90 degrees. The knee is flexed

over the end of the treatment table. A small roll or towel may be placed under the distal end of the femur to maintain it in a horizontal plane. The contralateral hip is abducted, and the foot may be supported on a stool.

Position of goniometer

The axis is on the center of the patella. The stationary and movable bars are parallel to the longitudinal axis of the tibia on the anterior aspect of the lower leg. The stationary bar remains in this position, perpendicular to the floor, while the movable bar follows the tibia as the hip is rotated.

End-feel

Firm.[3]

External Rotation

0 to 45 degrees (Figure 20-46).

Position of the client and goniometer

The client is seated with the hip in 0-degree neutral rotation and the hip and knee of the leg to be tested flexed to 90 degrees. The other leg should be (1) flexed at the knee so that the lower leg is back under the table or (2) flexed at the hip and knee so that the foot is resting on the table. These positions allow the motion to take place without obstruction. The trunk should remain erect during the performance of the motion. The goniometer is positioned as for internal rotation.

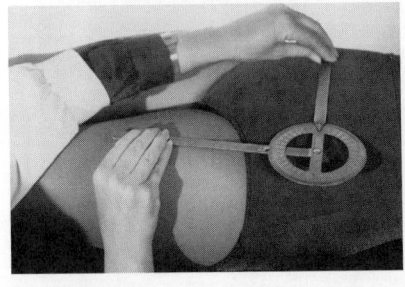
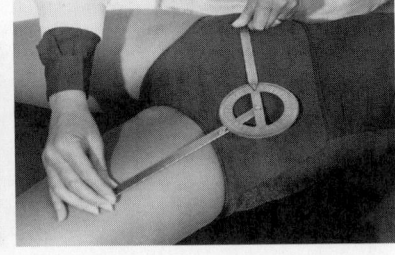

A   B

Figure 20-43 Hip abduction. **A,** Starting position. **B,** Final position.

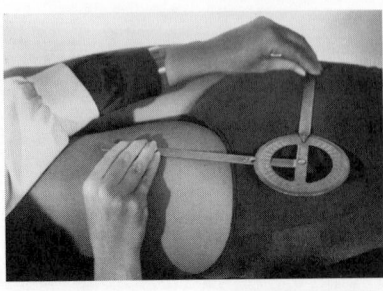
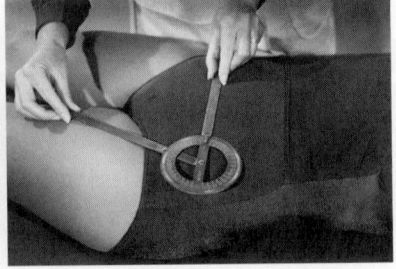

A   B

Figure 20-44 Hip adduction. **A,** Starting position. **B,** Final position.

End-feel

Firm.[3]

Knee

Extension-Flexion

0 to 135 degrees (Figure 20-47).

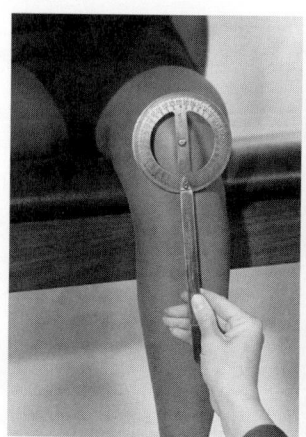 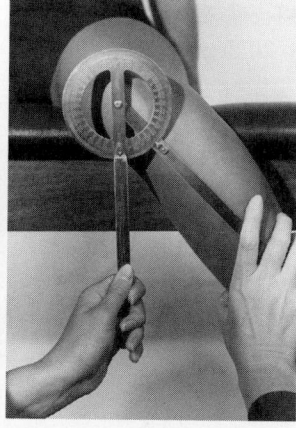

A   B

Figure 20-45 Hip internal rotation. **A,** Starting position. **B,** Final position.

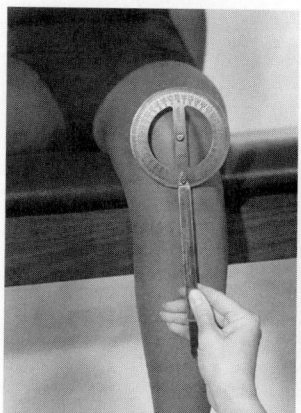 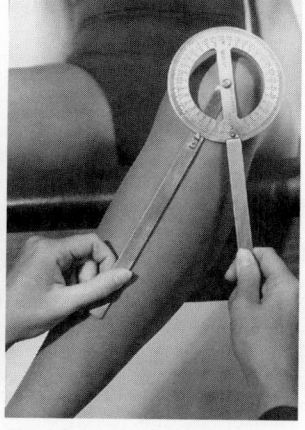

A   B

Figure 20-46 Hip external rotation. **A,** Starting position. **B,** Final position.

Position of the client

The client should be prone or supine, lying with the knees and hips extended and the hip in 0-degree neutral rotation.

Position of goniometer

With the client in the prone position, the axis is centered on the lateral aspect of the knee joint at the lateral epicondyle of the femur. The stationary bar is on the lateral aspect of the thigh, parallel to the longitudinal axis of the femur. The movable bar is parallel to the longitudinal axis of the fibula, aligned with the lateral malleolus, on the lateral aspect of the leg.

End-feel

Soft.[3]

Ankle

Dorsiflexion

0 to 15 degrees (Figure 20-48).

Position of the client

The client should be supine or seated with the knee flexed at least 30 degrees. The ankle is at 90-degree neutral position and the foot is in 0 degree of inversion and eversion.

Position of goniometer

The axis is placed below the medial malleolus.[3] The stationary bar is parallel to the longitudinal axis of the tibia, and the movable bar is parallel with the first metatarsal. (This measurement may also be taken on the lateral side of the foot.) Note that measurement begins at 90 degrees, so 90 degrees must be subtracted when recording the joint measurement.

End-feel

Firm or hard.[3]

Plantar Flexion

0 to 50 degrees (Figure 20-49).

Position of the client and goniometer

Same as for dorsiflexion.

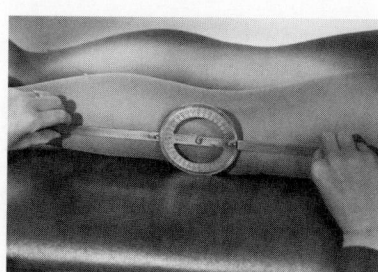 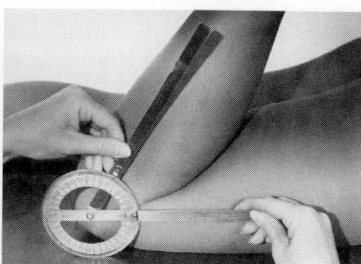

A   B

Figure 20-47 Knee flexion. **A,** Starting position. **B,** Final position.

End-feel

Firm or hard.[3]

Inversion

0 to 35 degrees (Figure 20-50).

Position of the client

The client is supine with the knee and hip extended and in 0-degree neutral rotation, the ankle in the 90-degree neutral position, and the foot extended over the edge of the table. A small roll is placed under the knee to maintain slight flexion. The alternative position is sitting with the knee flexed to 90 degrees, the leg over the edge of the supporting surface, and the ankle in 90-degree neutral position.

Position of goniometer

The axis is placed at the lateral border of the foot near the heel. The stationary bar is parallel to the longitudinal axis of the fibula on the lateral aspect of the leg. The movable bar is parallel to the plantar surface of the heel.

End-feel

Firm.[3]

Eversion

0 to 20 degrees (Figure 20-51).

Position of the client

Same as for inversion.

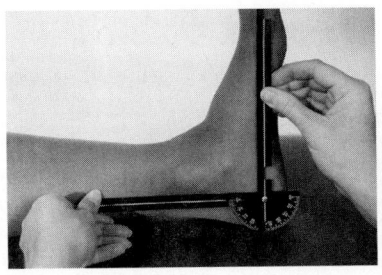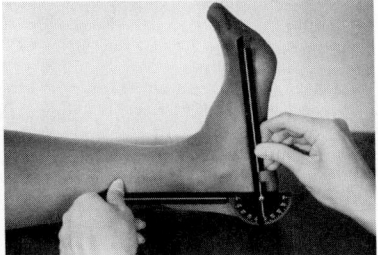

A B

Figure 20-48 Ankle dorsiflexion. **A,** Starting position. **B,** Final position.

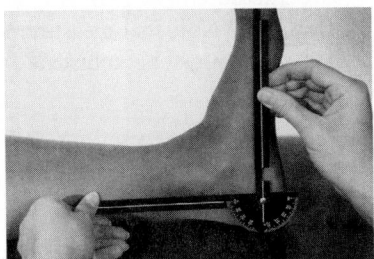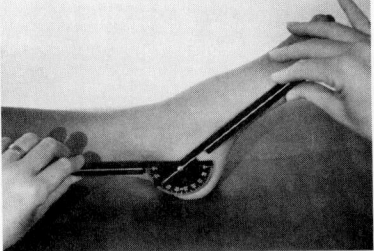

A B

Figure 20-49 Ankle plantar flexion. **A,** Starting position. **B,** Final position.

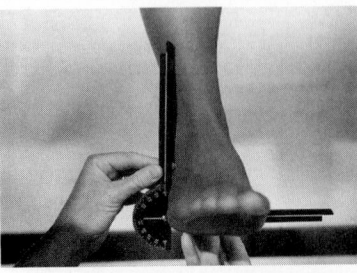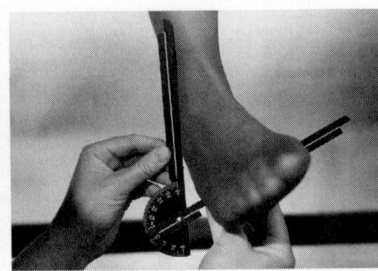

A B

Figure 20-50 Ankle inversion. **A,** Starting position. **B,** Final position.

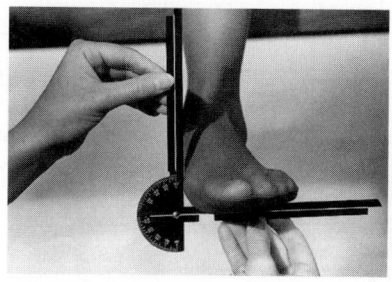 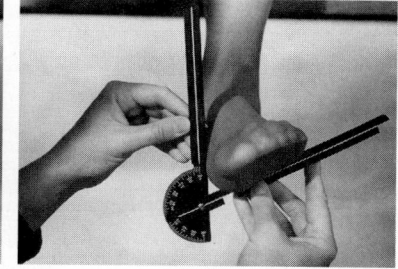

A B

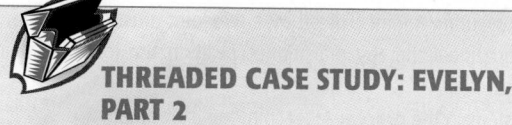

Figure 20-51 Ankle eversion. **A,** Starting position. **B,** Final position.

Position of goniometer

The axis is on the medial border of the foot, just proximal to the metatarsophalangeal joint. The stationary bar is parallel to the longitudinal aspect of the fibula on the medial aspect of the lower leg. The movable bar is parallel to the plantar surface of the sole. Note that measurements for inversion and eversion both begin at 90 degrees. Therefore, this amount must be subtracted from the total when measurements are recorded.

End-feel

Hard or firm.[3]

SUMMARY

Joint measurement is used to evaluate ROM in persons whose physical dysfunction affects joint mobility. Measurements of ROM are used in setting intervention goals, selecting intervention methods, and making objective assessments of progress that allow the therapist to select those intervention methods most likely to target the affected joints.

Before measuring ROM, the therapist should know any precautions or contraindications concerning the client's condition that may determine how extensive the joint measurement procedure can be. The therapist should also know the principles of joint measurement. The procedure for measuring joint ROM involves correct positioning for client and therapist, exposure of joints to be measured, palpation, appropriate stabilization and handling of parts, and correct placement of the goniometer at the beginning and end of the ROM. In order to support the efficacy of intervention strategies and modalities, the therapist must also consider which method of reporting will best serve as evidence of effective intervention.

Directions and illustrations for measuring all of the major joint motions in the neck, trunk, and upper and lower extremities are included in this chapter. The content is designed for the development of the fundamental techniques of joint measurement. The reader is referred to the references for more comprehensive treatment of the topic.[3,9,10]

THREADED CASE STUDY: EVELYN, PART 2

At the beginning of the chapter, Evelyn's case study was introduced. She is an active 83-year-old woman with a rich occupational life who sustained a Colles' fracture to her left nondominant upper extremity, had recently had her cast removed, and was experiencing residual problems (including joint ROM deficits). Readers were asked to consider three questions while studying the chapter:

Why should the therapist proceed with caution when assessing the range of motion limitations of this client?

The therapist should proceed with caution with all clients; in the case of Evelyn, heightened caution is necessary during joint measurement because of the edema, pain, and stiffness that she is experiencing in the thumb and fingers of her recently injured left wrist. Failure to proceed with caution during measurement of ROM could exacerbate each of these symptoms.

What is the appropriate sequencing of joint measurement assessment for this client? What methods should be applied first?

It is important for the therapist to first have Evelyn actively move her joints through all available pain-free (or within tolerable pain) ROM throughout both her left affected upper extremity as well as her unaffected right upper extremity (for comparison purposes). Next, the therapist should passively move Evelyn's affected joints through the available pain-free (tolerable) range of motion, noting the end-feel and estimating the ROM in those joints. Finally, the therapist measures the affected joints, using a goniometer and following the specific sequential directions for measuring each of the joints.

What is the advantage of joint measurement in evidence-based practice?

An advantage to joint measurement in evidence-based practice is that the client's ROM baselines are recorded and the effectiveness of interventions can be determined or substantiated on the basis of the results of follow-up joint measurements. Once these outcome data are collected by the therapist (along with similar data from other clients), a body of evidence regarding intervention effectiveness is compiled, which in turn can be used to select effective treatment for future clients with similar problems.

Review Questions

1. Describe general rules for positioning the goniometer when measuring joint ROM.
2. With which diagnoses is joint measurement likely to be used?
3. List and discuss four purposes of joint measurement.
4. Is formal joint measurement necessary for every client? If not, how may ROM be assessed?
5. What is the benefit of conducting precise joint measurement with a goniometer?
6. What is meant by *palpation*? How is palpation done?
7. What should the therapist look for when observing joints and joint motions?
8. List at least five precautions or contraindications to joint measurement.
9. What is meant by *end-feel*?
10. When measuring a joint crossed by a two-joint muscle, how should the occupational therapy practitioner position the joint not being measured?
11. List the steps in the procedure for joint measurement.
12. How is joint ROM measurement recorded on the evaluation form?
13. List the average normal ROM for elbow flexion, shoulder flexion, finger MP flexion, hip flexion, knee flexion, and ankle dorsiflexion.
14. Describe how to read the goniometer when using the 180-degree system of joint measurement.
15. What is meant by *functional range of motion*?
16. List three intervention methods that could be used to increase ROM.

Exercises

1. Measure all of the upper extremity joint motions of a normal client. Record the findings on the form in Figure 20-2.
2. Repeat the first exercise, but the client should play the role of someone with several joint limitations.
3. Observe joint motions used in ordinary ADL/IADL (e.g., self-care and home management). Estimate the functional ranges of motion for the following joint motions: shoulder flexion, external rotation, internal rotation, abduction, elbow flexion, wrist extension, hip flexion and extension, knee flexion, and ankle plantar flexion.

REFERENCES

1. American Academy of Orthopaedic Surgeons: *Joint motion: method of measuring and recording*, Chicago, 1965, The Academy.
2. Baruch Center of Physical Medicine: *The technique of goniometry* (unpublished manuscript), Richmond, VA, Medical College of Virginia.
3. Clarkson HM: *Musculoskeletal assessment, joint range of motion and manual muscle strength*, ed 2, Philadelphia, 2000, Lippincott, Williams & Wilkins.
4. Cole T: Measurement of musculoskeletal function: goniometry. In Kottke FJ, Stillwell GK, Lehmann JF, editors: *Krusen's handbook of physical medicine and rehabilitation*, ed 3, Philadelphia, 1982, WB Saunders.
5. Esch D, Lepley M: *Evaluation of joint motion: methods of measurement and recording*, Minneapolis, 1974, University of Minnesota Press.
6. Hurt SP: Considerations of muscle function and their application to disability evaluation and treatment: joint measurement, reprinted from *Am J Occup Ther* 1:69, 1947; 2:13, 1948.
7. Kendall FP, et al: *Muscles, testing and function*, ed 5, Baltimore, 2005, Williams & Wilkins.
8. Killingsworth A: *Basic physical disability procedures*, San Jose, Calif, 1987, Maple Press.
9. Latella D, Meriano C: Occupational therapy manual for evaluation of range of motion and muscle strength, Clifton, NY, 2003, Delmar Thomson Learning.
10. Norkin CC, White DJ: *Measurement of joint motion: a guide to goniometry*, ed 3, Philadelphia, 2003, FA Davis.
11. Rancho Los Amigos Hospital: *How to measure range of motion of the upper extremities* (unpublished manuscript), Rancho Los Amigos, CA, The Hospital.
12. Sammons Preston Ability One: Rehabilitation Catalog 2000, Bolingbrook, Ill.
13. Smith HD: Assessment and evaluation: an overview. In Hopkins HL, Smith HD, editors: *Willard and Spackman's occupational therapy*, ed 8, Philadelphia, 1993, JB Lippincott.
14. Venes D, Thomas CL, editors: *Taber's cyclopedic medical dictionary*, ed 19, Philadelphia, 2001, FA Davis.

21 EVALUATION OF MUSCLE STRENGTH

AMY PHILLIPS KILLINGSWORTH
LORRAINE WILLIAMS PEDRETTI

KEY TERMS

Screening tests
Against gravity
Resistance

Manual muscle test
Muscle grades
Muscle endurance

Muscle coordination
Gravity-minimized
Substitutions

LEARNING OBJECTIVES

After studying this chapter the student or practitioner will be able to do the following:

1. Describe screening tests for muscle strength assessment.
2. Identify what is measured by the manual muscle test (MMT).
3. List diagnoses for which the MMT is appropriate and those for which it is not appropriate, with the rationale for each.
4. List the steps of the MMT procedure in correct order.
5. Describe the limitations of the MMT.
6. Define muscle grades by name, letter, and number.
7. Administer an MMT, using the directions in this chapter, on a normal practice subject.
8. Describe how the results of the muscle strength assessment are used in intervention planning.

CHAPTER OUTLINE

Causes of muscle weakness
Screening tests
Manual muscle test
  Purposes of manual muscle testing
  Methods of assessment
  Results of assessment as a basis for intervention planning
  Relationship between joint range of motion and muscle weakness
  Limitations of the manual muscle test
  Contraindications and precautions
  Knowledge and skill of the occupational therapist
General principles of manual muscle testing
  Preparation for testing
  Gravity influencing muscle function
  Muscle grades
  Substitutions
  Procedure for testing
Manual muscle testing of the upper extremity
  Scapula elevation, neck rotation, and lateral flexion
  Scapula depression, adduction, and upward rotation
  Scapula abduction and upward rotation
  Scapula adduction
  Scapula adduction and downward rotation
  Shoulder flexion
  Shoulder extension

Shoulder abduction to 90 degrees
Shoulder external rotation
Shoulder internal rotation
Shoulder horizontal abduction
Shoulder horizontal adduction
Elbow flexion
Elbow extension
Forearm supination
Forearm pronation
Wrist extension with radial deviation
Wrist extension with ulnar deviation
Wrist flexion with radial deviation
Wrist flexion with ulnar deviation
Metacarpophalangeal flexion with interphalangeal extension
Metacarpophalangeal extension
Proximal interphalangeal flexion, second through fifth fingers
Distal interphalangeal flexion, second through fifth fingers
Finger abduction
Finger adduction
Thumb metacarpophalangeal extension
Thumb interphalangeal extension
Thumb metacarpophalangeal flexion
Thumb interphalangeal flexion
Thumb palmar abduction

Thumb radial abduction
Thumb adduction
Opposition of the thumb to the fifth finger
Manual muscle testing of the lower extremity
Hip flexion
Hip extension
Hip abduction
Hip adduction
Hip external rotation

Hip internal rotation
Knee flexion
Knee extension
Ankle plantar flexion
Ankle dorsiflexion with inversion
Foot inversion
Foot eversion
Summary

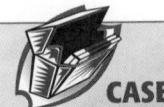

CASE STUDY: SHARON

After a week of experiencing increasing numbness and weakness in her extremities and shortness of breath, Sharon, a 32-year-old woman, was admitted to an intensive care unit at a local hospital with acute respiratory distress, generalized musculoskeletal weakness, decreased sensory processing, and difficulty swallowing. Sharon complained of pain and tenderness in her muscles and was very agitated and fearful. She was diagnosed as being in the acute phase of Guillain-Barré syndrome and was placed on a ventilator.[11] The OT practitioner fitted her with resting splints to support her weakened hands and minimize her muscle belly tenderness. When Sharon was moved from intensive care as the progression of the syndrome began to plateau, the therapist was able to greatly reduce her fear by adapting an environmental system that gave Sharon more control of her environmental context, allowing her to operate her call button, room lights, bed, and television.[19]

Sharon is a senior editor for a monthly food magazine. She has two children, ages 2 and 6. She has been married for eight years; her husband is a sales representative for a computer company. They live in a two-story town house in an urban community. Sharon primarily works at home, going into the magazine's office once or twice a week. However, once a month, during the week the magazine is being published, her life "becomes a bit crazy," and she may go into the office 5 days. She feels fortunate that she is able to employ a housekeeper/childcare person. In addition to caring for her home and family, Sharon is an avid photographer, exercises at a gym three times per week, and enjoys hiking and camping. She is a regular volunteer at her eldest child's school. She and her husband enjoy an active social life.

Six months after onset, Sharon is now being seen as an outpatient by an occupational therapist. Her disorder is in the recovery phase, with remyelination and axonal degeneration resulting in a generalized increase in muscle strength.[11] Sharon continues to be unable to fully engage in occupations that are meaningful to her, primarily because of residual weakness in her distal extremities and moderate limitation in endurance. She is usually in a wheelchair, but she uses a walker in her home. She has an aide that comes in the morning to assist her with bathing and personal grooming and to drive her to her outpatient appointments. She states that "although I can do things for myself, it takes so long that I end up being tired before my day even begins. I need help to safely shave my underarms and legs. Curling and blow-drying my hair can be exhausting." Sharon has also indicated that she cannot complete home maintenance tasks such as meal preparation (chopping foodstuff, managing pots and pans) and grocery shopping without assistance. She is also unable to fully provide for the care and supervision of her children, especially the 2-year-old, nor can she access the second story of her home on a regular basis. She is limited in her ability to participate in outdoor and community occupations, which formerly brought her a great deal of satisfaction. She has recently been able to resume some of her job responsibilities at home on a limited basis with a voice activated computer and is "grateful my employer still wants me and has been willing to make accommodations." She also indicated that with all of the progress she has made, she and her husband are trying to be realistic but are feeling more and more hopeful about her making a full recovery.

In reviewing the above occupational profile, the therapist must focus on those client factors that are interfering with body function—namely, decreased muscle strength and endurance.[9] Maintaining her arms at and above shoulder level without taking several rest breaks when vigorously brushing her back teeth, for example, remains a problem. Also a problem is applying enough force to open jars or perform fine motor activities, such as manipulating coins. These deficits are prohibiting the client from fully engaging in occupation for participation in the physical, social, personal, cultural, and spiritual contexts that bring meaning to her life.

Critical Thinking Questions

1. At what stage in this client's recovery should the occupational therapist first administer a muscle strength assessment?
2. There are several methods for assessing muscle strength; what are they? What information regarding the client's status could be gained from each of these methods?
3. What is the relationship between MMT and graded activity with this client?

Many physical disabilities cause muscle weakness. Slight to substantial limitations of performance in areas of occupation, such as bringing food to one's mouth, lifting a child, removing items from a grocery store shelf, and getting in and out of bed, can result from loss of strength, depending on the degree of weakness and whether the weakness is permanent or temporary. If improvement is expected, the occupational therapist must assess the muscle weakness and plan an intervention that will enable occupational performance and increase strength.

CAUSES OF MUSCLE WEAKNESS

A loss of muscle strength is a primary symptom or a direct result of the following diseases or injuries:

1. The lower motor neuron disorders, such as peripheral neuropathies and peripheral nerve injuries, spinal cord injury (because those muscles innervated at the level[s] of the lesion generally have a lower motor neuron paralysis), Guillain-Barré syndrome, and cranial nerve dysfunctions
2. Primary muscle diseases, such as muscular dystrophy and myasthenia gravis
3. Neurological diseases in which the lower motor neuron is affected, such as amyotrophic lateral sclerosis or multiple sclerosis

Disabilities in which a loss of muscle strength is caused by disuse or immobilization rather than being a direct effect of the disease process include burns, amputation, hand trauma (unless there is an accompanying nerve injury), arthritis, fractures, and a variety of other orthopedic conditions.

Muscle weakness can restrict or prevent performance in areas of occupation including activities of daily living (ADLs), instrumental activities of daily living (IADLs), education, work, play, leisure, and social participation. These limitations are assessed by observation of performance (see Chapter 19), screening tests, and manual muscle testing (MMT), when indicated.

SCREENING TESTS

Screening tests are useful for observing areas of strength and weakness and for determining which areas require specific MMT.[6,10,12,18] The screening tests can help the therapist avoid unnecessary testing or duplication of services.[12] The tests are used by occupational therapists in some healthcare facilities in which MMT is the responsibility of the physical therapy service. Like the occupation-based functional motion assessment described in Chapter 19, screening tests are also used to assess muscle strength. These tests are not as precise as MMT, and their purpose is to make a general evaluation of muscle strength and to determine areas of weakness, performance limitations, and the need for more precise testing. Screening may be accomplished by the following means:

1. Examination of the medical record for results of previous muscle test and range of motion (ROM) assessments
2. Observing the client entering the clinic and moving about
3. Observing the client perform functional activities, such as removing an article of clothing and shaking hands with the therapist[6,12,13]
4. Performing a gross check of bilateral muscle groups[13]

The last method can be performed while the client is comfortably seated in a sturdy chair or wheelchair. The client is asked to perform the motions **against gravity** (movements away from the floor) or in the gravity-minimized plane (parallel to the floor) if moving against gravity is not possible. Active range of motion (AROM) is observed, and **resistance** (application of force) can be given to the test motions to obtain a gross estimate of strength.

In the case of Sharon, who during the acute stage of her illness had very limited muscle strength, the occupational therapy (OT) practitioner would be able to observe changes by observing this client as she moved around her bed in an attempt to position herself. Initially she might require maximal assistance for any bed repositioning or for food intake. The therapist will notice a gradual increase in automatic movements of the limbs as Sharon raises her arms to her forehead to brush back her hair with her forearm, cups her hands around the water glass being held by her husband as she sips through a straw, bends and straightens her legs in an attempt to get comfortable, or momentarily lifts her trunk away from the surface of the bed. Observation of these spontaneous movements as Sharon begins to engage within the context of her environment can serve as preliminary and informal screening of this client's muscle strength.

MANUAL MUSCLE TEST

MMT is a means of evaluating muscle strength. MMT measures the maximal contraction of a muscle or muscle group.[6,7] The criteria used to measure strength are evidence of muscle contraction, amount of ROM through which the joint passes when the muscle contracts, and amount of resistance against which the muscle can contract. Gravity is considered a form of resistance.[6,7,13] MMT is used to determine the amount of muscle power and record gains and losses in strength.

PURPOSES OF MANUAL MUSCLE TESTING

The specific strength measurement of individual muscles through MMT can be essential for diagnosis of some neuromuscular conditions, such as peripheral nerve lesions and spinal cord injury. In peripheral nerve or nerve root lesions, the pattern of muscle weakness may help determine which nerve or nerve roots are involved and whether the involvement is partial or complete. Careful evaluation can help determine the level(s) of spinal cord involvement and provide an indication of whether the cord damage is complete or incomplete.[14] Along with sensory evaluation, MMT can therefore be an important diagnostic aid in neuromuscular conditions.

The purposes for assessing muscle strength are to determine the amount of muscle power available and thus establish a baseline for intervention, to discern how muscle weakness is limiting performance in meaningful occupations such as ADLs and IADLs, to prevent deformities that can result from imbalances of strength, to determine the need for assistive devices as compensatory measures, to aid in the selection of occupations within the client's capabilities, and to evaluate the effectiveness of intervention strategies and modalities.[15]

METHODS OF ASSESSMENT

Muscle strength can be assessed in several ways. The most precise method is a test of individual muscles. In this procedure the muscle is carefully isolated through proper positioning, stabilization, and control of the movement pattern, and its strength is graded. This type of muscle testing is described by Kendall and McCreary[14] and Cole, Furness, and Twomey.[8] Another, and perhaps more common, method of MMT is to assess the strength of groups of muscles that perform specific motions at each joint. This type of testing was described by Daniels and Worthingham,[10] Hislop and Montgomery,[12,13] the Rancho Muscle Testing Guide,[20] and, for the most part, is the form that is presented later in this chapter.

RESULTS OF ASSESSMENT AS A BASIS FOR INTERVENTION PLANNING

When planning intervention for the maintenance or improvement of strength, the OT practitioner considers several factors in the clinical reasoning process before determining intervention priorities, goals, and modalities. The results of the muscle strength assessment will suggest the progression of the intervention program. What is the degree of weakness? Is it generalized or specific to one or more muscle groups? Are the muscle grades generally the same throughout, or is there significant disparity in muscle grades? If there is disparity, is there an imbalance of strength between the agonist and antagonist muscles that necessitates protection of the weaker muscles during OT intervention or when performing ADLs and IADLs? When there is substantial imbalance between an agonist and antagonist muscle, intervention goals may be directed toward strengthening the weaker group while maintaining the strength of the stronger group. Muscle imbalance may also suggest the need for an orthosis to protect the weaker muscles from overstretching while recovery is in progress. Examples of such orthoses are devices such as the bed footboard to prevent overstretching of the weakened ankle dorsiflexors and the wrist cock-up splint to prevent overstretching of weakened wrist extensors.

Muscle grades will suggest the level of therapeutic activity or exercise that can help to maintain or improve strength. Is the weakness mild (G range), moderate (F to F+), or severe (P to 0)?[15] Muscles graded F−, for example, could be strengthened by active assisted exercise or light activity against gravity. Likewise, muscles graded *P* will require activity or exercise in the gravity-minimized plane, with little or no resistance, to increase strength. (See Chapter 28 for further discussion of appropriate exercise and activity for specific muscle grades.)

The endurance of the muscles (i.e., how many repetitions of the muscle contraction are possible before fatigue sets in) is an important consideration in intervention planning. A frequent goal of the therapeutic activity program is to increase endurance as well as strength. Because MMT does not measure endurance, the therapist should assess endurance by engaging the client in periods of exercise or activity graded in length to determine the amount of time that the muscle group can be used in sustained activity. There is usually a correlation between strength and endurance. Weaker muscles will tend to have less endurance than stronger ones. When selecting intervention modalities for increasing endurance, the therapist may elect not to tax the muscle to its maximal ability but rather to emphasize repetitive action at less than the maximal contraction to increase endurance and prevent fatigue.[15]

Sensory loss, which often accompanies muscle weakness, complicates the ability of the client to perform in an activity program. If there is little or no tactile or proprioceptive feedback from motion, the impulse to move is decreased or lost, depending on the severity of the sensory loss. Thus, the movement may appear weak and ineffective even when strength is adequate for performance of a specific activity. With some diagnoses, a sensory reeducation program (see Chapter 22) may be indicated to increase the client's sensory awareness and feedback from the part. In other instances, the therapist may elect to teach compensation techniques to address the sensory loss. These techniques include the use of mirrors, video playback, and biofeedback, which can be used as adjuncts to the strengthening program.

Other important considerations in the therapist's clinical reasoning are the diagnosis and expected course of the disease. Is strength expected to increase, decrease, or remain about the same? If strength is expected to increase, what is the expected recovery period? What is the effect of exercise or activity on muscle function? Will too much activity delay the progress of recovery? If muscle power is expected to decrease, how rapid will the progression be? Are there factors to be avoided, such as a vigorous activity or an exercise program that can accelerate the decrease in strength? If strength is declining, is special equipment practical and necessary? How much muscle power is needed to operate the equipment? How long will the client be able to operate a device before a decrease in muscle power makes it impracticable?[15] In the case of Sharon, the therapist must be aware of the change in muscle strength of this client. It is expected that muscle return will occur in a proximal to distal pathway and the need to protect the intrinsic muscles of the hand against overexertion is critical to ensure the possibility of full recovery.

Frequent muscle testing of select muscle groups will serve as a means to monitor the progression of the disease and to assist in the introduction of appropriate intervention strategies.[11,19]

The therapist should assess the effect of the muscle weakness on the ability to perform ADLs, which can be observed during the assessment. Which tasks are most difficult to perform because of the muscle weakness? How does the client compensate for the weakness? Which tasks are most important for the client to be able to perform? Is special equipment necessary or desirable for the performance of some ADLs, such as the mobile arm support for independence in eating (see Chapter 29)?

If the client is involved in a total rehabilitation program and receiving several other healthcare services, the activity and exercise programs must be synchronized and balanced to meet the client's needs rather than the needs of the professionals, their schedules, and possibly their competition. The occupational therapist must be aware of the nature and extent of the programs in which the client is engaged in physical therapy, recreation therapy, and any other services. Ideally, all members of the healthcare team should plan the exercise and activity programs together to ensure that they complement one another.

OT PRACTICE NOTE

The therapist must consider the following questions: What is the client doing in each of the therapies? How long is each treatment session? Are the goals of all of the therapies similar and complementary, or are they divergent and conflicting? Is the client being overfatigued in the total program? Are the various treatment sessions in rapid succession, or are they well spaced to meet the client's need for rest periods?

On the basis of these considerations and others pertinent to the specific client, the occupational therapist can select enabling and purposeful activities designed to maintain or increase strength, improve performance of ADLs, and enable the use of special equipment, while protecting weak muscles from overstretching and overfatigue.

RELATIONSHIP BETWEEN JOINT RANGE OF MOTION AND MUSCLE WEAKNESS

One of the criteria used to grade muscle strength is the joint ROM of the joint on which the muscle acts—that is, did the muscle move the joint through complete, partial, or no ROM? Another criterion is the amount of resistance that can be applied to the part once the muscle has moved the joint through the partial or complete AROM. In this context, ROM is not necessarily the full average normal ROM for the given joint; rather, it is the ROM available to the individual client. When the therapist measures joint motion (discussed in

Chapter 20), it is the passive ROM (PROM) that is the measure of the range available to the client. PROM, however, is not an indication of muscle strength.

When performing muscle testing, the occupational therapist must know the client's PROM to assign muscle grades correctly. It is possible that PROM would be limited or less than the average for a joint motion but that the muscle strength would be normal. Therefore, it is necessary for the therapist either to have measured joint ROM or to move joints passively to assess available ROM before administering the muscle test. For example, the client's PROM for elbow flexion may be limited to 0 to 120 degrees because of an old fracture. If the client can flex the elbow joint to 120 degrees and withstand moderate resistance during the muscle test, the muscle would be graded *G(4)*. In such cases the occupational therapist should record the limitation with the muscle grade—for example, 0 to 120 degrees/G.[10] Conversely, if the client's available ROM for elbow flexion is 0 to 160 degrees and he or she can flex the elbow against gravity through only 120 degrees, the muscle would be graded F– because the part moves through only partial ROM against gravity. When the therapist determines the client's available ROM before performing the muscle test, he or she can grade muscle strength on that basis rather than by using the average normal ROM as the standard. When assessing Sharon's muscle strength during the recovery phase of her illness, the OT practitioner most likely will find a disparity between the client's PROM and muscle strength, with limitation in strength preventing Sharon from moving her body parts through full available ROM, especially against gravity. The discrepancy will decrease as remyelination and axonal regeneration occur.

LIMITATIONS OF THE MANUAL MUSCLE TEST

The limitations of MMT are that it cannot measure **muscle endurance** (the number of times the muscle can contract at its maximal level and resist fatigue),[6] **muscle coordination** (the smooth, rhythmic interaction of muscle function), or motor performance capabilities of the client (the use of the muscles for functional activities).[8]

MMT is not appropriate for and cannot be used accurately with clients who have spasticity caused by upper motor neuron disorders such as cerebrovascular accident (stroke) or cerebral palsy. In these conditions, muscles are often hypertonic. Muscle tone and ability to perform movements are influenced by primitive reflexes and the position of the head and body in space. Also, movements tend to occur in gross synergistic patterns that make it impossible for the client to isolate joint motions, which is demanded in the MMT procedures.[2,3,6,7,16]

However, when administered during the final recovery stage, when spasticity and synergy patterns have disappeared and the client has achieved isolated control of voluntary muscle function, MMT may reveal some residual weakness. In these instances, some assessment of strength can be of value in designing a treatment program. (See Chapters 18, 31, and 32 for methods of evaluating motor function of clients with upper motor neuron disorders.)

CONTRAINDICATIONS AND PRECAUTIONS

Assessment of strength using MMT is contraindicated when the client has inflammation or pain in the region to be tested; a dislocation or unhealed fracture; recent surgery, particularly of musculoskeletal structures; myositis ossificans; or bone carcinoma or any fragile bone condition.[7,15]

Special precautions must be taken when resisted movement could aggravate the client's condition, as might occur with osteoporosis, subluxation or hypermobility of a joint, hemophilia or any type of cardiovascular risk or disease, abdominal surgery or an abdominal hernia, and fatigue that exacerbates the client's condition.[6,7]

Unlike the PROM assessment discussed in Chapter 20, MMT requires the client's complete involvement in the testing procedure. Therefore, the therapist must also be mindful of the client's willingness to expend true effort (especially when resistance is applied), to endure some discomfort, and to understand the requirements of the test. Results of MMT should not be compromised as a result of cognitive and language barriers or the client's ability to produce the motor skills required for the test.[13]

KNOWLEDGE AND SKILL OF THE OCCUPATIONAL THERAPIST

The validity of MMT depends on the OT practitioner's knowledge and skill in using the correct testing procedure. Careful observation of movement, careful and accurate palpation, correct positioning, consistency of procedure, and experience of the therapist are critical factors in accurate testing.[10,12-14]

To be proficient in manual muscle testing, the OT practitioner must have detailed knowledge about all aspects of muscle function. Joints and joint motions, muscle innervation, origin and insertion of muscles, action of muscles, direction of muscle fibers, angle of pull on the joints, and the role of muscles in fixation and substitution are important considerations. The therapist must be able to locate and feel contraction of the muscles; recognize whether the contour of the muscle is normal, atrophied, or hypertrophied; and detect abnormal movements and positions. The OT practitioner must use consistent methods in the application of test procedures. Knowledge and experience are necessary to detect substitutions and interpret strength grades with accuracy.[12-14]

It is necessary for the OT practitioner to acquire skill and experience in testing and grading muscles of normal persons of both genders and of all ages. Many factors affect muscle strength. The age, gender, and lifestyle of the client; the muscle size and type and speed of contraction; the effect of previous training for the testing situation; the joint position during the muscle contraction; previous training effect; and time of day, temperature, and fatigue all can affect muscle strength.[6,7] Experience can help the therapist differentiate among strength grades if these factors are taken into account.[18]

GENERAL PRINCIPLES OF MANUAL MUSCLE TESTING

PREPARATION FOR TESTING

If several tests are to be administered, they should be organized to avoid frequent repositioning of the client.[12,13] The OT practitioner should observe contour of the part, comparative symmetry of the muscle on both sides, and any apparent hypertrophy or atrophy. During PROM the therapist can estimate muscle tone. Is there less or greater than normal resistance to passive movement? During AROM the therapist can observe quality of movement, such as movement speed, smoothness, rhythm, and any abnormal movements such as tremors.[18]

Correct positioning of the client and the body part is essential to effective and correct evaluation. The client should be positioned comfortably on a firm surface. Clothing should be arranged or removed so that the therapist can see the muscle or muscles being tested. For maximal comfort to the client, administer the assessment to all the muscles possible in a given position (upright, prone, supine, sidelying) before changing the position of the client. If the client cannot be placed in the correct position for the test, the OT practitioner must adapt the test and use clinical judgment in approximating strength grades.[18] In addition to correct positioning, test validity depends on careful stabilization, palpation of the muscles, and observation of movement.[10]

GRAVITY INFLUENCING MUSCLE FUNCTION

Gravity is a form of resistance to muscle power. It is used as a grading criterion in tests of the neck, trunk, and extremities. In other words, the muscle grade is based on whether a muscle can move the part against gravity.[14] Movements against gravity are in a vertical plane (i.e., away from the floor or toward the ceiling) and are used with grades F (3), G (4), and N (5). Movements against gravity and resistance are performed in a vertical plane with added manual or mechanical resistance and are used with F+ (3+) to N (5) grades. Tests for the weaker muscles (O, T [1], P [2], and P+ [2+] grades) are often performed in a horizontal plane (i.e., parallel to the floor) to reduce the resistance of gravity on muscle power. This position has been referred to as the *gravity-eliminated, gravity-minimized,* or *gravity-lessened test position.*[10,14,18] *Gravity-eliminated* is the common term to designate this position.[16] Because the effect of gravity on muscle function cannot be eliminated completely, **gravity-minimized** or gravity-lessened may be more accurate terms. The term *gravity-minimized* is used in this chapter.[10,14]

In many muscle tests the effect of gravity on the ability to perform the movement must be considered in grading muscle power. It is of lesser importance, however, in tests of the forearm, fingers, and toes because the weight of the part lifted against gravity is insignificant compared with the muscle strength.[10,14] Therefore, the OT practitioner may choose to do the tests for F (3) to N (5) in the gravity-minimized plane. In other tests, positioning for movements in the gravity-decreased position or the against-gravity position may not be feasible. For example, in the test for scapula depression, positioning to perform the movement against gravity would require the client to assume an inverted position. In individual cases, positioning for movement in the correct plane may not be possible because of confinement to bed, generalized weakness, trunk instability, immobilization devices, and medical precautions. In these instances the OT practitioner must adapt the positioning to the client's needs and use clinical judgment in modifying the grading. If tests of the forearm, fingers, and toes are performed against gravity rather than in the gravity-minimized plane, the standard definitions of muscle grades can be modified when muscle grades are recorded. The partial ROM against gravity is graded *P (2)*, and the full ROM against gravity is graded *F (3)*.[10] Such modifications in positioning and grading should be noted by the therapist when results of the muscle test are recorded.

For consistency in procedure and grading, the gravity-minimized positions and against-gravity positions are used in the manual muscle tests described later, except in cases in which the positioning is not feasible or would be awkward or uncomfortable for the client. Modifications in positioning and grading have been cited with the individual tests.

MUSCLE GRADES

Although the definitions of the muscle grades are standard, the assignment of muscle grades during MMT depends on the clinical judgment, knowledge, and experience of the OT practitioner,[10] especially when determining slight, moderate, or maximal resistance. Age, gender, body type, occupation, and leisure activities all influence the amount of resistance

that a particular client can take.[9,10,12-14] Normal strength for an 8-year-old girl will be considerably less than that for a 25-year-old man, for example. Additionally, strength tends to decline with age, and full resistance to the same muscle group will vary considerably from an 80-year-old man to a 25-year-old man.[7,14] Therefore, the amount of resistance that can be applied to grade a particular muscle group as *N (5)* or *G (4)* varies among individual clients.[9,10,12-14]

The amount of resistance that can be given also varies among muscle groups. Muscle strength is relative to the cross-sectional size of the muscle. Larger muscles have greater strength.[7,10] For example, the flexors of the wrist are larger and therefore have more power and can take much more resistance than the abductors of the fingers. The OT practitioner must consider the size and relative power of the muscles and the leverage used when giving resistance.[15] The amount of resistance applied should be modified accordingly. When only one side of the body is involved in the dysfunction causing the muscle weakness, the OT practitioner can establish the standards for strength by testing the unaffected side first.

Because weak muscles fatigue easily, the results of MMT may not be accurate if the client is tired. There should be no more than three repetitions of the test movement because fatigue can result in grading errors if the muscle becomes tired as a result of low endurance.[7,8] Pain, swelling, or muscle spasm in the area being tested may also interfere with the testing procedure and accurate grading. Such problems should be recorded on the evaluation form.[18] Psychological factors must be considered in interpreting muscle strength grades. When interpreting strength, the therapist must assess the motivation, cooperation, and effort put forth by the client.[10]

In MMT, muscles are graded according to the criteria listed in Table 21-1.[6,10,12,13,20]

The purpose of using "plus" or "minus" designations with the muscle grades is to "fine grade" muscle strength. These designations are likely to be used by the experienced OT practitioner. Two OT practitioners testing the same individual

TABLE **21-1** **Muscle Grades and Their Definitions**

Number Grade	Word/Letter Grade	Definition
0	Zero (0)	No muscle contraction can be seen or felt.
1	Trace (T)	Contraction can be observed or felt, but there is no motion.
2−	Poor minus (P−)	Part moves through incomplete ROM with gravity minimized.
2	Poor (P)	Part moves through complete ROM with gravity minimized.
2+	Poor plus (P+)	Part moves through less than 50% of available ROM against gravity or through complete ROM with gravity minimized against slight resistance.[10]
3−	Fair minus (F−)	Part moves through more than 50% of available ROM against gravity.[10]
3	Fair (F)	Part moves through complete ROM against gravity.
3+	Fair plus (F+)	Part moves through complete ROM against gravity and slight resistance.
4	Good (G)	Part moves through complete ROM against gravity and moderate resistance.
5	Normal (N)	Part moves through complete ROM against gravity and maximal resistance.

ROM, Range of motion.

may vary up to a half grade in their results, but there should not be a whole grade difference.[18]

SUBSTITUTIONS

The brain thinks in terms of movement and not in terms of contraction of individual muscles.[10] Thus, a muscle or muscle group may attempt to compensate for the function of a weaker muscle to accomplish a movement. These movements are called *trick movements,* or **substitutions**.[6,7,14] Substitutions can occur during MMT. To test muscle strength accurately, the therapist must give careful instructions; eliminate substitutions in the testing procedure by correct positioning, stabilization, and palpation of the muscle being tested; and ensure careful performance of the test motion without extraneous movements. To prevent substitutions, the correct position of the body should be maintained and movement of the part performed without shifting the body or turning the part.[6,7,14] The therapist must palpate contractile tissue (muscle fibers or tendon) to detect tension in the muscle group under examination. It is only through correct palpation that the therapist can be certain that the motion observed is not being performed by substitution.[6,10] Undetected trick movements can mask the client's problems and result in inaccurate treatment planning.[6]

In the tests that follow, possible substitutions are described at the end of the directions. The OT practitioner should be familiar with these substitutions to detect them and correct the procedure. Detecting substitutions is a skill gained with time and experience.

PROCEDURE FOR MANUAL MUSCLE TESTING

Testing should be performed according to a standard procedure to ensure accuracy and consistency. The tests that follow are each divided into these steps: (1) position, (2) stabilize, (3) palpate, (4) observe, (5) resist, and (6) grade.

First, the client should be positioned for the specific muscle test. The occupational therapist should position himself or herself in relation to the client. Then, the therapist stabilizes the part proximal to the part being tested to eliminate extraneous movements, isolate the muscle group, ensure the correct test motion, and eliminate substitutions. The therapist should then demonstrate or describe the test motion to the client and ask him or her to perform the test motion and return to the starting position. The therapist makes a general observation of the form and quality of movement, looking for substitutions or difficulties that may require adjustments in positioning and stabilization. The therapist then places his or her fingers (typically the tips of the index and long fingers—avoid using the thumb because it has its own pulse) for palpation of one or more of the prime movers, or its tendinous insertion, on the muscle group being tested and asks the client to repeat the test motion. While simultaneously palpating the muscle group, the therapist again observes the

movement for possible substitution and the amount of range completed. When the client has moved the part through the available ROM, the therapist asks the client to hold the end position. The therapist removes the palpating fingers and uses the free hand to resist in the direction opposite that of the test movement. For example, when elbow flexion is tested, the therapist applies resistance in the direction of extension. The therapist usually must maintain stabilization when resistance is given. Manual muscle tests use the "break test"—that is, the resistance is applied after the client has reached the end of the available ROM.[12,13]

The client should be allowed to establish a maximal contraction (set the muscles) before the resistance is applied.[10,15] In most tests the OT practitioner applies the resistance near the distal segment to which the muscle is attached after preparing the client by giving the command to hold. Resistance should be applied gradually in a direction opposite to the line of pull of the muscle or muscle group being tested.[12] The break test should not evoke pain, and resistance should be released immediately if pain or discomfort occurs.[10] Finally, the therapist grades the muscle strength according to the preceding standard definitions of muscle grades. This procedure is used for the tests of strength of grades *F+ (3+)* and above. Resistance is not applied for tests of muscles from *F (3)* to *0*. Slight resistance is sometimes applied to a muscle that has completed the full ROM in the gravity-minimized plane to determine if the grade is *P+*. Figure 21-1 shows a sample form for recording muscle grades.

The following directions do not include tests for the face, neck, and trunk. Refer to the references for these tests, as well as a comprehensive treatment of the topic of manual muscle testing.[6, 8,10,12-14]

MANUAL MUSCLE TESTING OF THE UPPER EXTREMITY

SCAPULA ELEVATION, NECK ROTATION, AND LATERAL FLEXION

Muscles[10]	Innervation: nerve, nerve roots[10,14]
Upper trapezius	Accessory nerve (CN 12), C2-4
Levator scapula	Dorsal scapular nerve, C3-5

Procedure for Testing Grades Normal (N or 5) to Fair (F or 3)[10,12,13]

1. *Position:* The client is seated erect with arms resting at sides of body. The OT practitioner stands behind the client toward the side to be tested.
2. *Stabilize:* A chair back can offer stabilization to the trunk, if necessary.
3. *Palpate:* Palpate the upper trapezius parallel to the cervical vertebrae, near the shoulder-neck curve.[10]
4. *Observe:* Observe the elevation of the scapula as the client shrugs the shoulder toward the ear and rotates and laterally

MUSCLE EXAMINATION

Client's name _____ Chart no.

Date of birth_____ Name of institution_____

Date of onset_____ Attending physician_____ MD

Diagnosis:

LEFT									RIGHT			
				Examiner's initials								
				Date								
			NECK	Flexors			Sternocleidomastoid					
				Extensor group								
			TRUNK	Flexors			Rectus abdominis					
				Rt. ext. obl. / Lt. int. obl.	Rotators		Lt. ext. obl. / Rt. int. obl.					
				Extensors			Thoracic group / Lumbar group					
				Pelvic elev.			Quadratus lumb.					
			HIP	Flexors			Iliopsoas					
				Extensors			Gluteus maximus					
				Abductors			Gluteus medius					
				Adductor group								
				External rotator group								
				Internal rotator group								
				Sartorius								
				Tensor fasciae latae								
			KNEE	Flexors			Biceps femoris / Inner hamstrings					
				Extensors			Quadriceps					
			ANKLE	Plantar flexors			Gastrocnemius / Soleus					
			FOOT	Invertors			Tibialis anterior / Tibialis posterior					
				Evertors			Peroneus brevis / Peroneus longus					
			TOES	MP flexors			Lumbricales					
				IP flexors (first)			Flex. digit. br.					
				IP flexors (second)			Flex. digit. l.					
				MP extensors			Ext. digit. l. / Ext. digit. br.					
			HALLUX	MP flexor			Flex. hall. br.					
				IP flexor			Flex. hall. l.					
				MP extensor			Ext. hall. br.					
				IP extensor			Ext. hall. l.					

Measurements:

Cannot walk	Date	Speech	
Stands	Date	Swallowing	
Walks unaided	Date	Diaphragm	
Walks with apparatus	Date	Intercostals	

KEY

5	N	Normal	Complete range of motion against gravity with full resistance.
4	G	Good*	Complete range of motion against gravity with some resistance.
3	F	Fair*	Complete range of motion against gravity.
2	P	Poor*	Complete range of motion with gravity eliminated.
1	T	Trace	Evidence of slight contractility. No joint motion.
0	0	Zero	No evidence of contractility.
S or SS			Spasm or severe spasm.
C or CC			Contracture or severe contracture.

*Muscle spasm or contracture may limit range of motion. A question mark should be placed after the grading of a movement that is incomplete from this cause.

Figure 21-1 Muscle examination. (Adapted from March of Dimes Birth Defects Foundation.)

Continued

LEFT   RIGHT

				Examiner's initials							
				Date							
			SCAPULA	Abductor	Serratus anterior						
				Elevator / Depressor	Upper trapezius / Lower trapezius						
				Adductors	Middle trapezius / Rhomboids						
			SHOULDER	Flexor	Anterior deltoid						
				Extensors	Latissimus dorsi / Teres major						
				Abductor	Middle deltoid						
				Horiz. abd.	Posterior deltoid						
				Horiz. add.	Pectoralis major						
				External rotator group							
				Internal rotator group							
			ELBOW	Flexors	Biceps brachii / Brachioradialis						
				Extensor	Triceps						
			FOREARM	Supinator group							
				Pronator group							
			WRIST	Flexors	Flex. carpi rad. / Flex. carpi uln.						
				Extensors	Ext. carpi rad. l. & br. / Ext. carpi uln.						
			FINGERS	MP flexors	Lumbricales						
				IP flexors (first)	Flex. digit. sub.						
				IP flexors (second)	Flex. digit. prof.						
				MP extensor	Ext. digit. com.						
				Adductors	Palmar interossei						
				Abductors	Dorsal interossei						
				Abductor digiti quinti							
				Opponens digiti quinti							
			THUMB	MP flexor	Flex. poll. br.						
				IP flexor	Flex. poll. l.						
				MP extensor	Ext. poll. br.						
				IP extensor	Ext. poll. l.						
				Abductors	Abd. poll. br. / Abd. poll. l.						
				Adductor pollicis							
				Opponens pollicis							
			FACE								

Additional data:

Figure 21-1, cont'd

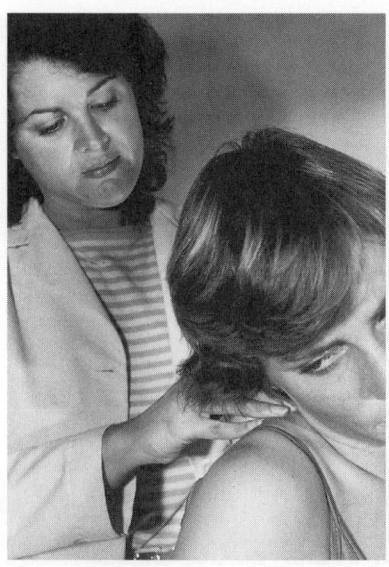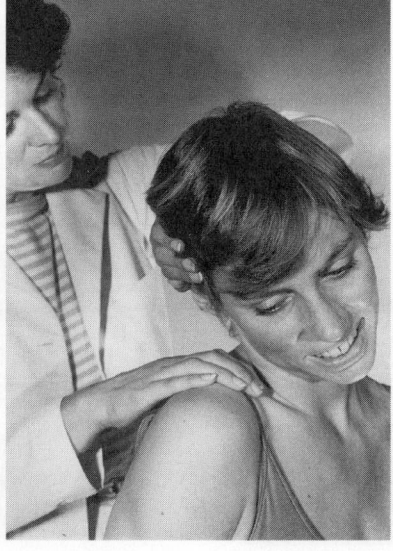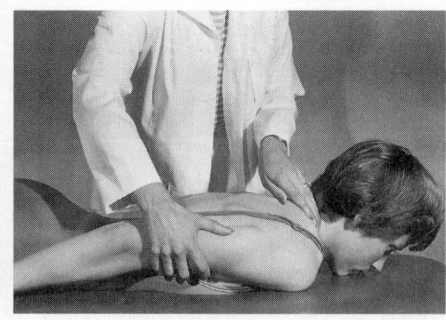

A   B   C

Figure 21-2   Scapula elevation. **A,** Palpate and observe. **B,** Resist. **C,** Gravity-minimized position.

flexes the neck toward the side being tested at the same time (Figure 21-2, *A*).[14]

5. *Resist:* Provide resistance by placing one hand on top of the shoulder toward scapula depression and the other hand on the side of the head toward derotation and lateral flexion to the opposite side (Figure 21-2, *B*).[14]

Procedure for Testing Grades Poor (P or 2), Trace (T or 1), and Zero (0)[10]

1. *Position:* The client should be prone with head in midposition. The OT practitioner stands opposite the side being tested.
2. *Stabilize:* The weight of the trunk on the supporting surface provides adequate stabilization.
3. *Palpate:* Palpate the upper trapezius, as described in the previous procedure, while observing the client elevating the shoulder being tested. Because of the positioning, the neck rotation and lateral flexion components are omitted for these grades (Figure 21-2, *C*).
4. *Grade:* The standard definitions of muscle grades should be used.

   Substitutions: Rhomboids and levator scapula can elevate the scapula if the upper trapezius is weak or absent. In the event of substitution, some downward rotation of the acromion will be observed during the movement.[4,15,20]

SCAPULA DEPRESSION, ADDUCTION, AND UPWARD ROTATION

Muscles[1,4]	Innervation[6,7]
Lower trapezius	Spinal accessory nerve, C3,4
Middle trapezius	
Serratus anterior	Long thoracic nerve, C5-7

Procedure for Testing Grades N (5) to F (3)

1. *Position:* The client is prone with arm positioned overhead in 130 to 165 degrees of abduction and resting on the supporting surface. The forearm is in midposition with the thumb toward the ceiling.[12] The therapist stands next to the client on the opposite side[7,10] or on the same side.[12,13]
2. *Stabilize:* The weight of the body provides adequate stabilization. This test is given in the gravity-minimized position, because it is not feasible to position the client for the against-gravity movement (head down). If the deltoid is weak, the arm may be supported and passively raised by the therapist while the client attempts the motion.[10]
3. *Palpate:* Palpate the lower trapezius distal to the medial end of the spine of the scapula and parallel to the thoracic vertebrae, approximately at the level of the inferior angle of the scapula.[10]
4. *Observe:* Observe the client while he or she lifts the arm off the supporting surface to ear level.[12] During this movement, there is strong downward fixation of the scapula by the lower trapezius (Figure 21-3, *A*).[10]
5. *Resist:* Provide resistance at the lateral angle of the scapula, toward elevation and abduction (Figure 21-3, *B*).[10] Resistance may be applied on the humerus just above the elbow in a downward direction if shoulder and elbow strength are adequate.[12-14]

Procedure for Testing Grades P (2), T (1), and 0

1. *Position and stabilize:* Position and stabilize the client as described in the previous test. No stabilization is required. The therapist may support the client's arm if the posterior deltoid muscles and triceps are weak.[12]

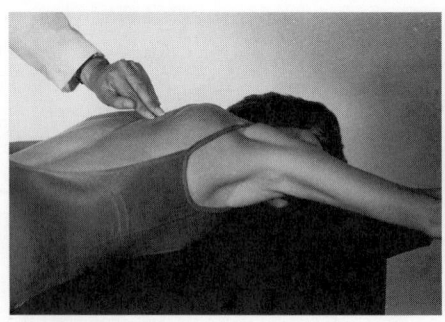 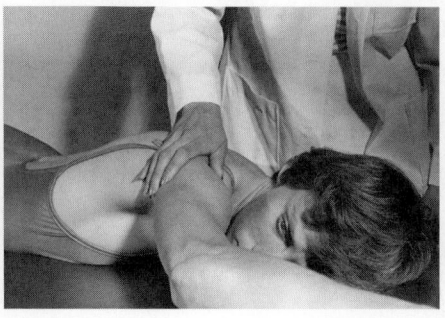 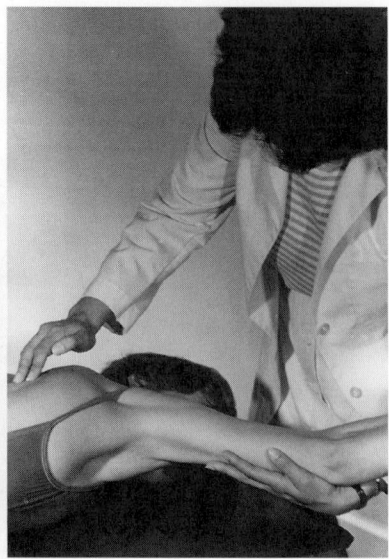

A   B   C

Figure 21-3   Scapula depression. **A,** Palpate and observe. **B,** Resist. **C,** Test for grades *P* to *O*.

2. *Palpate and observe:* Palpate and observe the client in the same manner as described for the previous test (Figure 21-3, *C*).
3. *Grade:* The client receives a grade of *P* if he or she can complete full scapular ROM without the weight of the arm.[12]

Substitutions: Middle trapezius or rhomboids may substitute.[6] Rotation of the inferior angle of the scapula toward the spine is evidence of substitution.[20]

SCAPULA ABDUCTION AND UPWARD ROTATION

Muscles[10,14]   **Innervation**[10,14]
Serratus anterior   Long thoracic nerve, C5-7

Procedure for Testing Grades N (5) to F (3)

1. *Position:* The client is supine with the shoulder flexed to 90 degrees and slightly abducted, elbow extended or fully flexed. The therapist stands next to the client on the side being tested.[6,7,10,13,14]
2. *Stabilize:* Provide stabilization over the weight of the trunk or over the shoulder.[6]
3. *Palpate:* Palpate the digitations of the origin of the serratus anterior on the ribs, along the midaxillary line and just distal and anterior to the axillary border of the scapula.[6,10] Note that muscle contraction may be difficult to detect in women and overweight clients.
4. *Observe:* Observe the client reaching upward as if pushing the arm toward the ceiling, abducting the scapula (Figure 21-4, *A*).[6,10]
5. *Resist:* Provide resistance at the distal end of the humerus, and push the client's arm directly downward toward

scapula adduction (Figure 21-4, *B*).[6,7,10,13] If there is shoulder instability, the therapist should support the arm and not apply resistance. In this instance, only a grade of *F (3)* can be tested.[7]

Procedure for Testing Grades P (2), T (1), and 0

1. *Position:* The client is seated with the arm supported by the therapist in 90 degrees of shoulder flexion and the elbow extended.[6,10,13]
2. *Stabilize:* Provide stabilization over the shoulder to be tested.
3. *Palpate:* The client is palpated in the same manner as described in the previous section.
4. *Observe:* The therapist should note any abduction of the scapula as the arm moves forward (Figure 21-4, *C*).[10] Weakness of this muscle produces "winging" of the scapula.[8]
5. *Grade:* The client is graded according to standard definitions of muscle grades.

Substitutions: The pectoralis major and minor may pull the scapula forward into abduction at its insertion on the humerus; the upper and lower trapezius and contralateral trunk rotation may also substitute.[6] The therapist observes for humeral horizontal adduction followed by scapula abduction.[7,14]

SCAPULA ADDUCTION

Muscles[10,14]   **Innervation**[6,10]
Middle trapezius   Spinal accessory nerve, C3,4
Rhomboids   Dorsal scapular nerve, C4,5

Procedure for Testing Grades N (5) to F (3)

1. *Position:* The client is prone with the shoulder abducted to 90 degrees and externally rotated and the elbow flexed

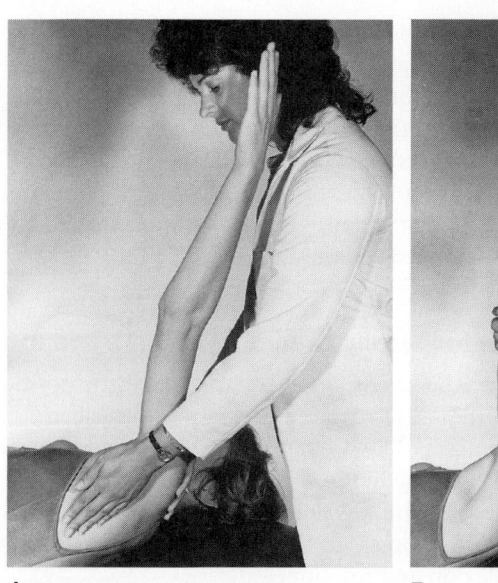
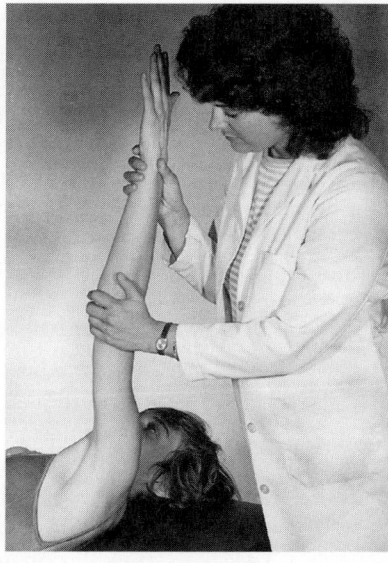
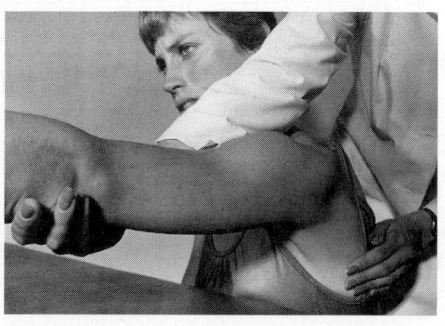

A   B   C

Figure 21-4 Scapula abduction. **A,** Palpate and observe. **B,** Resist. **C,** Gravity-minimized position.

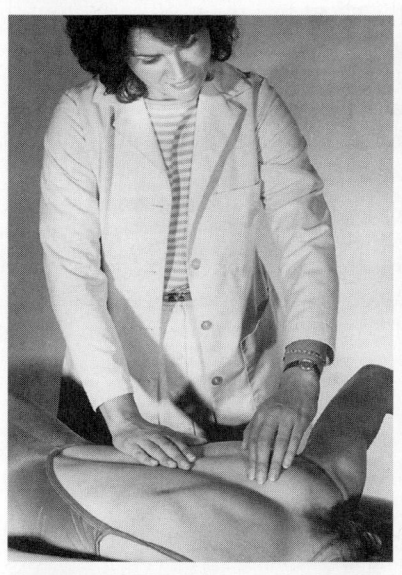
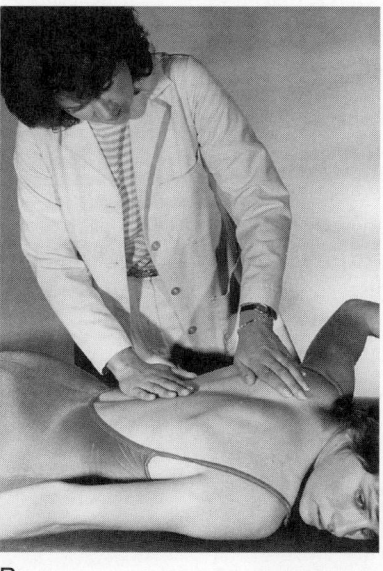
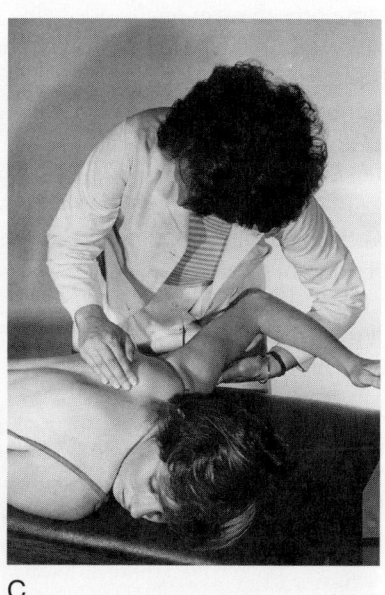

A   B   C

Figure 21-5 Scapula adduction. **A,** Palpate and observe. **B,** Resist. **C,** Test for grades *P* to *0*.

to 90 degrees, shoulder resting on the supporting surface. The therapist stands on the side being tested.[10,12-14]

2. *Stabilize:* The weight of the trunk on the supporting surface usually provides adequate stabilization, or stabilization can be provided over the midthorax to prevent trunk rotation if necessary.

3. *Palpate:* Palpate the middle trapezius between the spine of the scapula and the adjacent vertebrae in alignment with the abducted humerus.

4. *Observe:* Observe the client lifting the arm off the table, and note any movement of the vertebral border of the scapula toward the thoracic vertebrae (Fig. 21-5, *A*).

5. *Resist:* Provide resistance at the vertebral border of the scapula toward abduction (Figure 21-5, *B*).[6,7,10,13]

Procedure for Testing Grades P (2), T (1), and 0

1. *Position and stabilize:* The therapist positions and stabilizes the client in the same way as described in the previous test but now supports the weight of the arm by cradling it under the humerus and forearm.[14] The client may also be positioned sitting erect, with arm resting on a high table and the shoulder midway between 90-degree flexion and abduction.[10] The therapist stands behind the client in this instance.

2. *Palpate and observe:* Palpate and observe the middle trapezius. Ask the client to bring the shoulders together as if assuming an erect posture. Observe scapula adduction toward the vertebral column (Figure 21-5, *C*).
3. *Grade:* The client is graded according to standard definitions of muscle grades.

Substitutions: The posterior deltoid can act on the humerus and produce scapula adduction.[6] Observe for humeral extension being used to initiate scapula adduction. Rhomboids may substitute, but scapula will rotate downward.[7,15,20]

SCAPULA ADDUCTION AND DOWNWARD ROTATION

Muscles[7,8]	Innervation[6-8]
Rhomboids major and minor	Dorsal scapular nerve, C4,5
Levator scapula	
Middle trapezius	Spinal accessory nerve, C3,4

Procedure for Testing Grades N (5) to F (3)

1. *Position:* The client is prone with the head rotated to the opposite side; the arm on the side being tested is placed in shoulder adduction and internal rotation, with the elbow slightly flexed and the dorsum of the hand resting over the lumbosacral area of the back.[6,12] The therapist stands opposite the side being tested.[7,8,10]
2. *Stabilize:* The weight of the trunk on the supporting surface offers adequate stabilization.[7,14]
3. *Palpate:* Palpate the rhomboid muscles between the vertebral border of the scapula and the second to fifth thoracic vertebrae.[10,14] (They may be more easily discerned toward the lower half of the vertebral border of the scapula, because they lie under the trapezius muscle.)

4. *Observe:* Observe the client raising the hand up off the back while maintaining the position of the arm.[7,12] During this motion, the anterior aspect of the shoulder must lift from the table surface. Observe scapula adduction and downward rotation while the shoulder joint is in some extension (Figure 21-6, *A*).[10]
5. *Resist:* Provide resistance over the scapula toward abduction and upward rotation[6] (Figure 21-6, *B*).

Procedure for Testing Grades P (2), T (1), and 0

1. *Position:* The client sits erect with the arm positioned behind the back in the same manner described for the previous test. The therapist stands behind the client, slightly opposite to the side being tested.[10]
2. *Stabilize:* The trunk is stabilized by placing one hand over the shoulder, opposite the one being tested, to prevent trunk flexion and rotation.
3. *Palpate:* The rhomboids are palpated as described previously.
4. *Observe:* Scapula adduction and downward rotation are observed as the client lifts the hand away from the back (Figure 21-6, *C*).
5. *Grade:* The client is graded according to standard definitions of muscle grades.

Substitutions: The middle trapezius may substitute, but the movement will not be accompanied by downward rotation.[12] The posterior deltoid acting to perform horizontal abduction or glenohumeral extension can produce scapula adduction through momentum. Scapula adduction would be preceded by extension or abduction of the humerus.[15,20] The pectoralis minor could tip the scapula forward.[7]

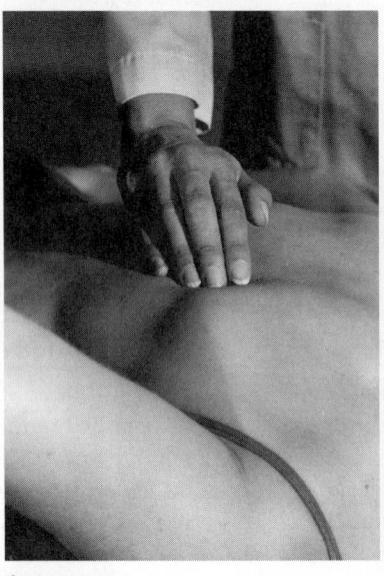 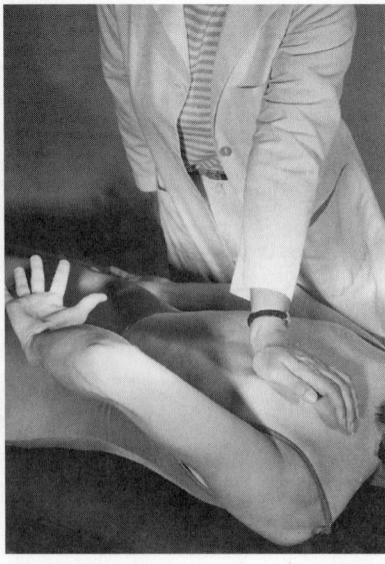 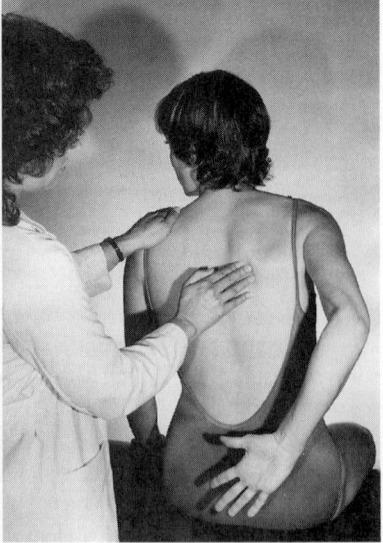

A   B   C

Figure 21-6   Scapula adduction and downward rotation. **A,** Palpate and observe. **B,** Resist. **C,** Gravity-minimized position.

SHOULDER FLEXION

Muscles[10]   Innervation[6,10]
Anterior deltoid   Axillary nerve, C5,6
Coracobrachialis   Musculocutaneous nerve, C5-7

Procedure for Testing Grades N (5) to F (3)

1. *Position:* The client is seated with the arm relaxed at the side of the body and the hand facing backward.[12] A straight-backed chair may be used to offer trunk support. The therapist stands on the side being tested and slightly behind the client.[7,10,20]

2. *Stabilize:* Provide stabilization over the shoulder being tested, but allow the normal abduction and upward rotation of the scapula that occurs with this movement.[10,13]

3. *Palpate:* Palpate the anterior deltoid just below the clavicle on the anterior aspect of the humeral head.[7]

4. *Observe:* Observe the client flexing the shoulder joint to 90-degree flexion (parallel to the floor; Figure 21-7, *A*).[6,10,12]

5. *Resist:* Provide resistance at the distal end of the humerus downward toward shoulder extension (Figure 21-7, *B*).[6,7,8,12]

Procedure for Testing Grades P (2), T (1), and 0

1. *Position:* The client is placed in a side-lying position. The side being tested is superior. If the client cannot maintain weight of the arm against gravity, the therapist can support it.[6,12] If the side-lying position is not feasible, the client may remain seated, and the test procedure described above can be performed with the grading modified.[10]

2. *Palpate and observe:* The therapist should palpate and observe the client in the same manner as described in the previous test. The arm is moved toward the face to 90-degree shoulder flexion (Figure 21-7, *C*).

3. *Grade:* The client is graded according to standard definitions of muscle grades. If the seated position was used for the tests of grades *poor* to *zero*, partial ROM against gravity should be graded *poor*.[10,13]

Substitutions: Clavicular fibers of the pectoralis major can perform flexion through partial ROM while performing horizontal adduction. The biceps brachii may flex the shoulder, but the humerus will first be rotated externally for the best mechanical advantage. The upper trapezius will assist flexion by elevating the scapula. Observe for flexion accompanied by horizontal adduction, external rotation, or scapula elevation.[10,15,20]

NOTE: Arm elevation in the plane of the scapula, about halfway between shoulder flexion and abduction, is called *scaption*. This movement is more commonly used for function than either shoulder flexion or abduction. Scaption is performed by the deltoid and supraspinatus muscles. It is tested in a way similar to that used for shoulder flexion, described previously, except that the arm is elevated in a position 30 to 45 degrees anterior to the frontal plane.[6,12]

SHOULDER EXTENSION

Muscles[4,10,14]   Innervation[6,10]
Latissimus dorsi   Thoracodorsal nerve, C6-8
Teres major   Lower subscapular nerve, C5-7
Posterior deltoid   Axillary nerve, C5,6

Procedure for Testing Grades N (5) to F (3)

1. *Position:* The client is prone, with the shoulder joint adducted and internally rotated so that the palm of the hand is facing up.[6,7,12] The therapist stands on the opposite side or on the test side.

2. *Stabilize:* Provide stabilization over the scapula on the side being tested.

3. *Palpate:* Palpate the teres major along the axillary border of the scapula. The latissimus dorsi may be palpated slightly below this point or closer to its origins parallel to the thoracic and lumbar vertebrae.[7,10] The posterior deltoid may be found over the posterior aspect of the humeral head (Figure 21-8, *A*).

4. *Observe:* Observe the client extending the shoulder joint.

5. *Resist:* Provide resistance at the distal end of the humerus in a downward and outward direction, toward flexion and slight abduction (Figure 21-8, *B*).[6,7,10,12-14]

Procedure for Testing Grades P (2), T (1), and 0

1. *Position:* The client is placed in the side-lying position; the therapist stands behind the client.[6]

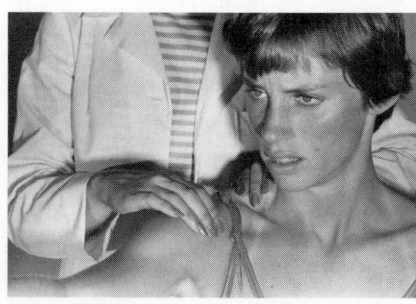
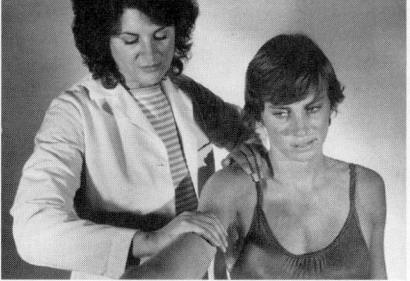
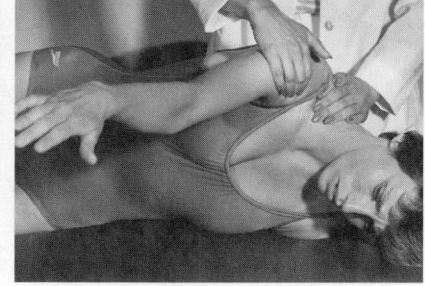

A   B   C

Figure 21-7 Shoulder flexion. **A,** Palpate and observe. **B,** Resist. **C,** Gravity-minimized position.

2. *Stabilize:* Provide stabilization over the scapula. If the client cannot maintain the weight of the part against gravity, the therapist should support the client's arm.[6] If the side-lying position is not feasible, the client may remain in the prone position and the test may be performed as described for the previous test with modified grading.[10]

3. *Palpate:* Palpate the teres major or latissimus dorsi as described for the previous test.

4. *Observe:* Observe the client extending the arm backward in a plane parallel to the floor (Figure 21-8, *C*).

5. *Grade:* Grade the client according to standard definitions of muscle grades. If the tests for grades *poor* to *zero* was done in the prone-lying position, completion of partial ROM should be graded *poor*.[10]

Substitutions: Scapula adduction can substitute. Observe for flexion of the shoulder or adduction of the scapula preceding extension of the humerus.[15]

SHOULDER ABDUCTION TO 90 DEGREES

Muscles[10,14]	Innervation[10]
Middle deltoid	Axillary nerve, C5,6
Supraspinatus	Suprascapular nerve, C5

Procedure for Testing Grades N (5) to F (3)

1. *Position:* The client is seated, with arms relaxed at the sides of the body. The elbow on the side to be tested should be slightly flexed and the palms facing toward the body. The therapist stands behind the client.[6,7,12]

2. *Stabilize:* Provide stabilization over the scapula on the side to be tested.[6,10,14]

3. *Palpate:* The middle deltoid over the middle of the shoulder joint from the acromion to the deltoid tuberosity.[6,10,14,15] The supraspinatus is too deep to palpate.[6]

4. *Observe:* Observe the client abducting the shoulder to 90 degrees. During the movement, client's palm should remain down and the therapist should observe that there is no external rotation of the shoulder or elevation of the scapula[6,10,12-15] (Figure 21-9, *A*).

5. *Resist:* Provide resistance at the distal end of the humerus toward adduction (Figure 21-9, *B*).[12]

Procedure for Testing Grades P (2), T (1), and 0

1. *Position:* The client is in the supine position, lying with the arm to be tested resting at the side of the body, palm facing in and the elbow slightly flexed. The therapist stands in front of the supporting surface toward the side to be tested.[10,12]

2. *Stabilize:* Provide stabilization over the shoulder to be tested.

3. *Palpate and observe:* Follow the technique described for the previous test. The therapist asks the client to bring the arm out and away from the body, abducting the shoulder to 90 degrees (Figure 21-9, *C*).

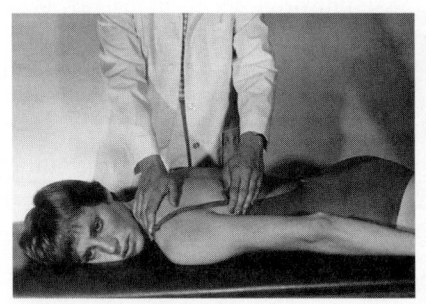
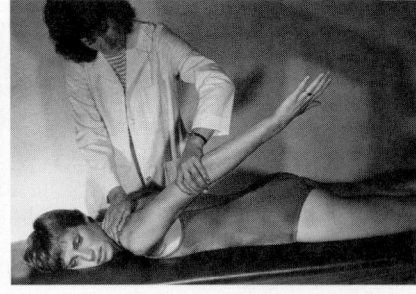
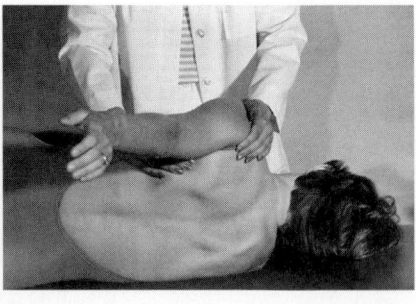

A   B   C

Figure 21-8   Shoulder extension. **A,** Palpate and observe. **B,** Resist. **C,** Gravity-minimized position.

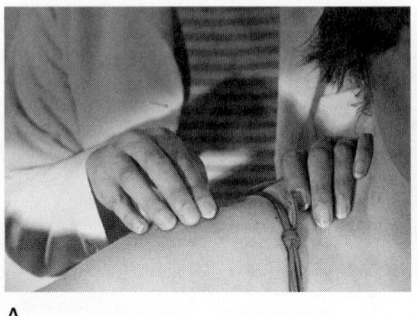
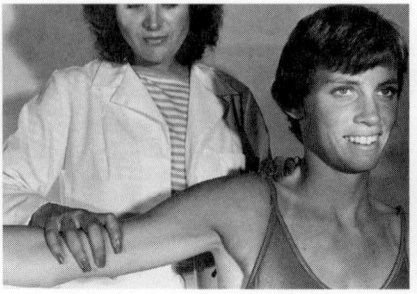
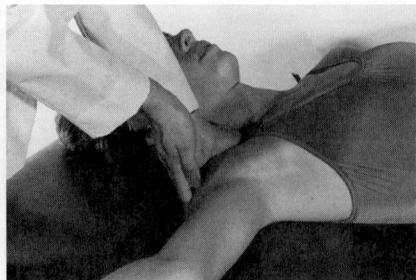

A   B   C

Figure 21-9   Shoulder abduction. **A,** Palpate and observe. **B,** Resist. **C,** Gravity-minimized position.

4. *Grade:* The client is graded according to standard definitions of muscle grades.

Substitutions: The long head of the biceps may attempt to substitute. Observe for elbow flexion and external rotation accompanying the movement.[12] The anterior and posterior deltoids can act together to effect abduction. The upper trapezius may attempt to assist. Observe for scapula elevation preceding the movement.[7,15,20]

SHOULDER EXTERNAL ROTATION

Muscles[4,10,14]	Innervation[4,10,14]
Infraspinatus	Suprascapular nerve, C5,6
Teres minor	Axillary nerve, C5,6

Procedure for Testing Grades N (5) to F (3)

1. *Position:* The client is prone, with the shoulder abducted to 90 degrees and the humerus in neutral (0-degree) rotation, elbow flexed to 90 degrees. Forearm is in neutral rotation, hanging over the edge of the table, perpendicular to the floor.[6-8,12] The therapist stands in front of the supporting surface, toward the side to be tested.[10,14]
2. *Stabilize:* Provide stabilization at the distal end of the humerus by placing a hand under the arm on the supporting surface to prevent shoulder abduction.[7,14]
3. *Palpate:* Palpate the infraspinatus muscle just below the spine of the scapula on the body of the scapula[6] or the teres minor along the axillary border of the scapula.[10]
4. *Observe:* Observe the client rotating the humerus so that the back of the hand is moving toward the ceiling (Figure 21-10, *A*).[6,7,10,12-14]
5. *Resist:* Provide resistance on the distal end of the forearm toward the floor in the direction of internal rotation (Figure 21-10, *B*).[6,10,12-14] Apply resistance gently and slowly to prevent injury to the glenohumeral joint, which is inherently unstable.[12]

Procedure for Testing Grades P (2), T (1), and 0

1. *Position:* The client is seated, with arm adducted and in neutral rotation at the shoulder. The elbow is flexed to 90 degrees, with the forearm in neutral rotation.

The therapist stands in front of the client toward the side to be tested.[6,7]

2. *Stabilize:* Provide stabilization on the arm against the trunk at the distal end of the humerus to prevent abduction and extension of the shoulder, and over the shoulder to be tested.[5,7,20] The hand stabilizing over the shoulder can be used to palpate the infraspinatus simultaneously.
3. *Palpate:* Palpate the infraspinatus and teres minor as described for the previous test.
4. *Observe:* Observe the client moving the forearm away from the body by rotating the humerus while maintaining neutral rotation of the forearm (Figure 21-10, *C*).[6,20]
5. *Grade:* The client is graded according to standard definitions of muscle grades.

Substitutions: If the elbow is extended and the client supinates the forearm, the momentum could aid external rotation of the humerus. Scapular adduction can pull the humerus backward and into some external rotation. The therapist should observe for scapula adduction and initiation of movement with forearm supination.[15,20]

SHOULDER INTERNAL ROTATION

Muscles[10,14,15]	Innervation[4,5,10]
Subscapularis	Subscapular nerve, C5,6
Pectoralis major	Medial and lateral pectoral nerves, C5-T1
Latissimus dorsi	Thoracodorsal nerve, C6-8
Teres major	Subscapular nerve, C5-7

Procedure for Testing Grades N (5) to F (3)

1. *Position:* The client is prone, with the shoulder abducted to 90 degrees, the humerus in neutral rotation, and the elbow flexed to 90 degrees. A rolled towel may be placed under the humerus. The forearm is perpendicular to the floor. The therapist stands on the side to be tested, just in front of the client's arm.[6-8,12]
2. *Stabilize:* Provide stabilization at the distal end of the humerus by placing a hand under the arm and on the supporting surface, as for external rotation.[6,7,10,14]
3. *Palpate:* Palpate the teres major and latissimus dorsi along the axillary border of the scapula toward the inferior angle.

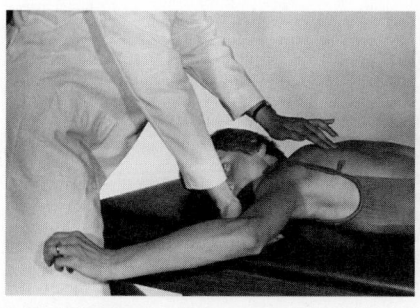
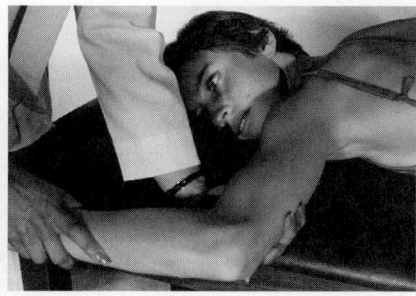
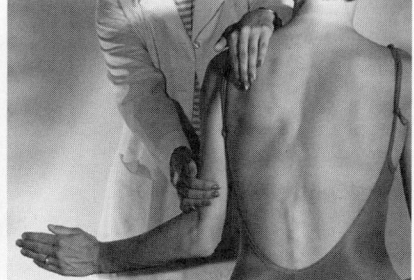

A   B   C

Figure 21-10 Shoulder external rotation. **A,** Palpate and observe. **B,** Resist. **C,** Gravity-minimized position.

4. *Observe:* Observe the client internally rotating the humerus, moving the palm of the hand upward toward the ceiling (Figure 21-11, *A*).[6,10]

5. *Resist:* Provide resistance at the distal end of the volar surface of the forearm anteriorly toward external rotation (Figure 21-11, *B*).[7,10,12-14]

Procedure for Testing Grades P (2), T (1), and 0

1. *Position:* The client is seated, with the shoulder adducted and in neutral rotation, elbow flexed to 90 degrees with the forearm in neutral rotation. The therapist stands on the side to be tested.[6,20]

2. *Stabilize:* Provide stabilization on the arm at the distal end of the humerus against the trunk to prevent abduction and extension of the shoulder.

3. *Palpate:* Palpate the teres major and latissimus dorsi, as described for the previous test.

4. *Observe:* Observe the client moving the palm of the hand toward the chest, internally rotating the humerus (Figure 21-11, *C*).

Substitutions: If the trunk is rotated, gravity will act on the humerus, rotating it internally.[6] The therapist should observe for trunk rotation. When the elbow is in extension, pronation of the forearm can substitute.[10,15,20]

SHOULDER HORIZONTAL ABDUCTION

Muscles[4,10,15]	Innervation[10,13]
Posterior deltoid	Axillary nerve, C5,6
Infraspinatus	Suprascapular nerve, C5,6

Procedure for Testing Grades N (5) to F (3)

1. *Position:* The client is prone, with the shoulder abducted to 90 degrees and in slight external rotation, elbow flexed to 90 degrees, and forearm perpendicular to the floor. The therapist stands on the side being tested.[14,15]

2. *Stabilize:* Provide stabilization over the scapula.[6,10]

3. *Palpate:* Palpate the posterior deltoid below the spine of the scapula and distally toward the deltoid tuberosity on the posterior aspect of the shoulder.[10]

4. *Observe:* Observe the client horizontally abducting the humerus, lifting the arm toward the ceiling (Figure 21-12, *A*).[12]

5. *Resist:* Provide resistance just proximal to the elbow obliquely downward toward horizontal adduction (Figure 21-12, *B*).[6,12-14]

Procedure for Testing Grades P (2), T (1), and 0

1. *Position:* The client is seated, with the arm in 90-degree abduction, the elbow flexed to 90 degrees, and the palm down, supported on a high table or by the therapist.[6,12] If a table is used, powder may be sprinkled on the surface to reduce friction.

2. *Stabilize:* Provide stabilization over the scapula.

3. *Palpate:* Palpate the posterior deltoid, as described for the previous test.

4. *Observe:* Observe client pulling arm backward into horizontal abduction (Figure 21-12, *C*).

5. *Grade:* Client is graded according to standard definitions of muscle grades.

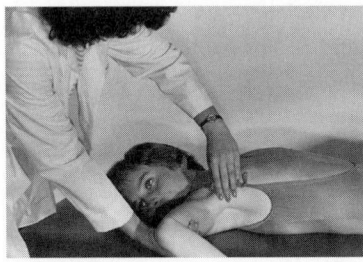 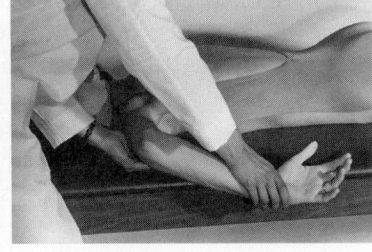 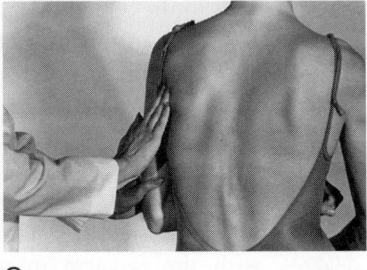

Figure 21-11 Shoulder internal rotation. **A,** Palpate and observe. **B,** Resist. **C,** Gravity-minimized position.

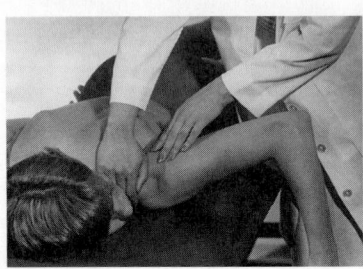 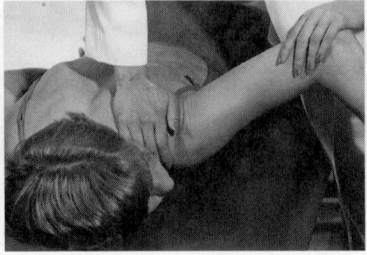 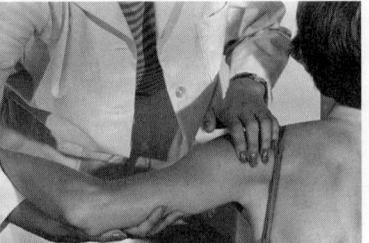

Figure 21-12 Shoulder horizontal abduction. **A,** Palpate and observe. **B,** Resist. **C,** Gravity-minimized position.

Substitutions: Latissimus dorsi and teres major may assist the movement if the posterior deltoid is very weak. Movement will occur with more shoulder extension rather than at the horizontal level. Scapula adduction may produce slight horizontal abduction of the humerus, but trunk rotation and shoulder retraction would occur.[6,15,20] The long head of the triceps may substitute. Maintain some flexion at the elbow to prevent this.[12]

SHOULDER HORIZONTAL ADDUCTION

Muscles[4,12-14]	Innervation[4,10,12,13]
Pectoralis major	Medial and lateral pectoral nerves, C5-T1
Anterior deltoid	Axillary nerve, C5,6
Coracobrachialis	Musculocutaneous nerve, C6,7

Procedure for Testing Grades N (5) to F (3)

1. *Position:* The client is supine, with the shoulder abducted to 90 degrees, elbow flexed or extended. The therapist stands next to the client on the side being tested or behind C's head.[4,6,7,9,10,12]
2. *Stabilize:* Stabilize the trunk by placing one hand over the shoulder on the side being tested to prevent trunk rotation and scapula elevation.
3. *Palpate:* Palpate over the insertion of the pectoralis major at the anterior aspect of the axilla.[6]
4. *Observe:* Observe the client horizontally adducting the humerus, moving the arm toward the opposite shoulder to a position of 90 degrees of shoulder flexion.[14] If the client cannot maintain elbow extension, the therapist may guide the forearm to prevent the hand from hitting the client's face (Figure 21-13, *A*).
5. *Resist:* Provide resistance at the distal end of the humerus, in an outward direction toward horizontal abduction (Figure 21-13, *B*).[6,7,10]

Procedure for Testing Grades P (2), T (1), and 0

1. *Position:* The client is seated next to a high table, with the arm supported in 90 degrees of shoulder abduction and slight flexion at the elbow.[4,12,20] Powder may be sprinkled

on the supporting surface to reduce the effect of resistance from friction during the movement, or the therapist may support the arm.[6]
2. *Stabilize:* Provide stabilization over the shoulder on the side being tested, simultaneously using the stabilizing hand to palpate the pectoralis major muscle.[6]
3. *Palpate:* Palpate the pectoralis major, as described for the previous test.
4. *Observe:* Observe the client horizontally adducting the arm toward the opposite shoulder, in a plane parallel to the floor (Figure 21-13, *C*).

Substitutions: Muscles may substitute for one another. If the pectoralis major is not functioning, the other muscles will perform the motion, which will be considerably weakened.[15] Contralateral trunk rotation, the coracobrachialis, or the short head of the biceps may substitute.[6]

ELBOW FLEXION

Muscles[10,12-14]	Innervation[12-14]
Biceps brachii	Musculocutaneous nerve C5,6
Brachialis	
Brachioradialis	Radial nerve C5,6

Procedure for Testing Grades N (5) to F (3)

1. *Position:* The client is seated, with the arm adducted at the shoulder and extended at the elbow and held against the side of the trunk. The forearm is supinated to test for the biceps, primarily (forearm should be positioned in pronation to test for the brachialis, primarily, and in midposition to test for brachioradialis).[10,12,13] The therapist stands next to the client on the side being tested or directly in front of the client.
2. *Stabilize:* Provide stabilization at the humerus (in adduction).
3. *Palpate:* Palpate the biceps brachii over the muscle belly, on the middle of the anterior aspect of the humerus. Its tendon may be palpated in the middle of the antecubital space.[6,7,10] (Brachioradialis is palpated over the upper third of the radius on the lateral aspect of the forearm, just below the elbow. The brachialis may be palpated lateral to

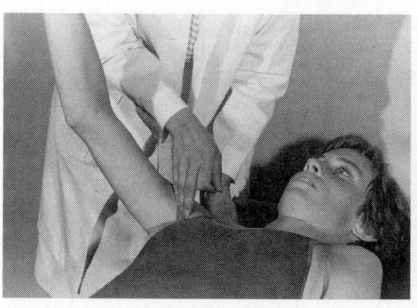 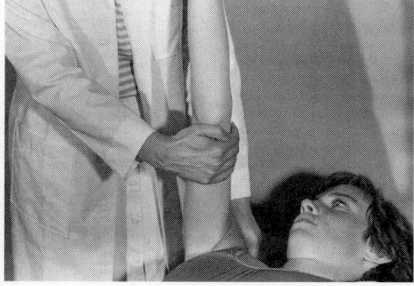 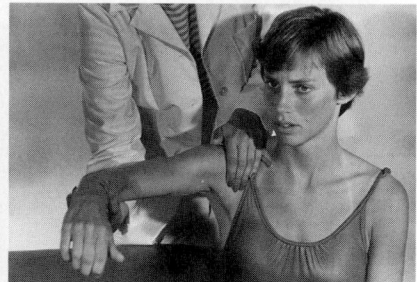

Figure 21-13 Shoulder horizontal adduction. **A,** Palpate and observe. **B,** Resist. **C,** Gravity-minimized position.

the lower portion of the biceps brachii if the elbow is flexed and in the pronated position.)[15]

4. *Observe:* Observe the client flexing the elbow, hand toward the face. The therapist should observe for maintenance of forearm in supination (when testing for biceps) and for relaxed or extended wrist and fingers (Figure 21-14, *A*).[6,15]

5. *Resist:* Provide resistance at the distal end of the volar aspect of the forearm, pulling downward toward elbow extension (Figure 21-14, *B*).[7,10,14]

Procedure for Testing Grades P (2), T (1), and 0

1. *Position:* The client is supine, with the shoulder abducted to 90 degrees and externally rotated, elbow extended, and forearm supinated. The therapist stands at the head of the table on the side being tested. (The client may also be seated, side being tested resting on the treatment table, which is at axillary height, humerus in 90-degree abduction, elbow extended, and forearm in neutral position.)[7]

2. *Stabilize:* Provide stabilization at the humerus. The stabilizing hand can be used simultaneously for palpation here.

3. *Palpate:* Palpate the biceps as described for the previous test.

4. *Observe:* Observe the client flexing the elbow, the hand toward the shoulder.[10] Watch for maintenance of forearm supination and relaxation of the fingers and wrist (Figure 21-14, *C*).[15]

5. *Grade:* The client is graded according to standard definitions of muscle grades.

Substitutions: The brachioradialis will substitute for the biceps, but the forearm will move to midposition during flexion of the elbow. Wrist and finger flexors may assist elbow flexion, which will be preceded by finger and wrist flexion.[10,12,13,15] The pronator teres may assist. Forearm pronation during the movement may be evidence of this substitution.[15]

ELBOW EXTENSION

Muscles[6,10,12]	Innervation[10,12-14]
Triceps	Radial nerve, C6-8
Aconeus	Radial nerve, C7,8

Procedure for Testing Grades N (5) to F (3)

1. *Position:* The client is prone, with the humerus abducted to 90 degrees, the elbow flexed to 90 degrees, and the forearm in neutral rotation and perpendicular to the floor. The therapist stands next to the client, just behind the arm to be tested.[7,14,20]

2. *Stabilize:* Provide stabilization at the humerus by placing one hand for support under it, between the client's arm and the table.[12,14]

3. *Palpate:* Palpate the triceps over the middle of the posterior aspect of the humerus or the triceps tendon just proximal to the olecranon process on the dorsal surface of the arm.[6,7,10,15]

4. *Observe:* Observe the client extending the elbow to just less than maximal range. The wrist and fingers remain relaxed (Figure 21-15, *A*).

5. *Resist:* Provide resistance at the distal end of the forearm into elbow flexion. Before resistance is given, be sure that the elbow is not locked. Resistance to a locked elbow can cause joint injury (Figure 21-15, *B*).[6,10]

Procedure for Testing Grades P (2), T (1), and 0

1. *Position:* The client is supine, with the humerus abducted to 90 degrees and in external rotation, the elbow fully flexed, and the forearm supinated. The therapist is standing next to the client, just behind the arm to be tested.[10] An alternate position is with the client seated, shoulder

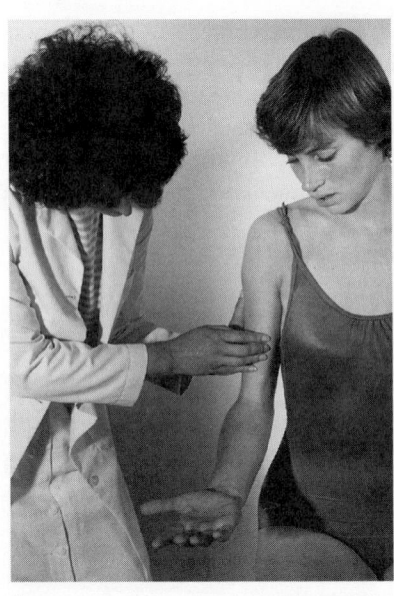
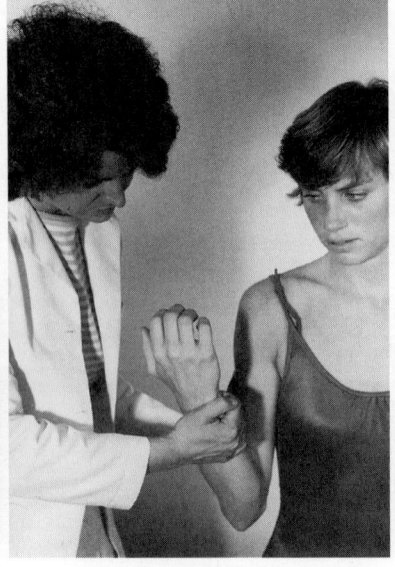
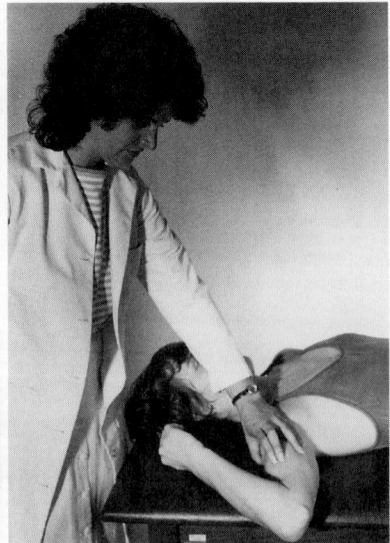

A   B   C

Figure 21-14 Elbow flexion. **A,** Palpate and observe. **B,** Resist. **C,** Gravity-minimized position.

abducted to 90 degrees in neutral rotation, elbow flexed, and forearm in neutral position, supported by the therapist.[7,10,12]

2. *Stabilize:* Provide stabilization at the humerus by holding one hand over the middle or distal end to prevent shoulder motion.

3. *Palpate:* Palpate the triceps as described for the previous test.

4. *Observe:* Observe the client extending the elbow, moving the hand away from the head (Figure 21-15, *C*).

5. *Grade:* The client is graded according to standard definitions of muscle grades.

Substitutions: Finger and wrist extensors may substitute for weak elbow extensors. Observe for the presence of finger and wrist extension preceding elbow extension. When the client is upright, gravity and eccentric contraction of the biceps will effect elbow extension from the flexed position.[15] Scapula depression, and shoulder external rotation, aided by gravity is another effective substitution pattern for elbow extension.[6]

FOREARM SUPINATION

Muscles[4,10,13]	Innervation[6,10,13]
Biceps brachii	Musculocutaneous nerve, C5,6
Supinator	Radial nerve, C5-7

Procedure for Testing Grades N (5) to F (3)

1. *Position:* The client is seated, with the humerus adducted, the elbow flexed to 90 degrees, and the forearm pronated. The therapist stands in front of the client or next to the client on the side to be tested.[6,7,10,12,13]

2. *Stabilize:* Provide stabilization at the humerus just proximal to the elbow.[6,10]

3. *Palpate:* Palpate the client over the supinator muscle on the dorsal-lateral aspect of the forearm, below the head of the radius. The muscle can be best felt when the radial muscle group (extensor carpi radialis and brachioradialis) is pushed up out of the way.[4] The therapist may also palpate the biceps on the middle of the anterior surface of the humerus.[6,7]

4. *Observe:* Observe the client supinating the forearm, turning the hand palm up. Because gravity assists the movement,

after the 0-degree neutral position is passed, the therapist may apply slight resistance equal to the weight of the forearm (Figure 21-16, *A*).[6,7]

5. *Resist:* Provide resistance by grasping around the dorsal aspect of the distal forearm with the fingers and heel of the hand, turning the arm toward pronation (Figure 21-16, *B*).[6]

Procedure for Testing Grades P (2), T (1), and 0

1. *Position:* The client is seated, shoulder flexed to 90 degrees and the upper arm resting on the supporting surface, elbow flexed to 90 degrees; the forearm is in full pronation in a position perpendicular to the floor.[6,7,20] The therapist stands next to the client on the side to be tested.

2. *Stabilize:* Provide stabilization at the humerus just proximal to the elbow.[6]

3. *Palpate:* Palpate the supinator or biceps as described for the previous test.

4. *Observe:* Observe the client supinating the forearm, turning the palm of the hand toward the face (Figure 21-16, *C*).

5. *Grade:* The client is graded according to standard definitions of muscle grades.

Substitutions: With the elbow flexed, external rotation and horizontal adduction of the humerus will effect forearm supination. With the elbow extended, shoulder external rotation will place the forearm in supination. The brachioradialis can bring the forearm from full pronation to midposition. Wrist and thumb extensors, assisted by gravity, can initiate supination. The therapist should note any external rotation of the humerus, supination to midline only, and initiation of motion by wrist and thumb extension.[10,13,15,20]

FOREARM PRONATION

Muscles[4,12,13,15]	Innervation[12,14]
Pronator teres	Median nerve, C6,7
Pronator quadratus	Median nerve, C6-8

Procedure for Testing Grades N (5) to F (3)

1. *Position:* The client is seated, with the humerus adducted, the elbow flexed to 90 degrees, and the forearm in full supination. The therapist stands beside the client on the side to be tested.[6,7,10,13]

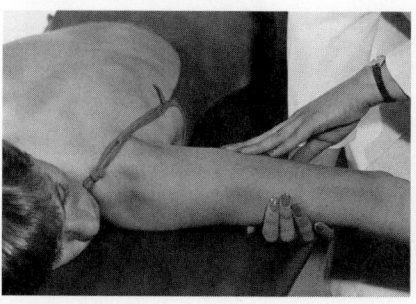
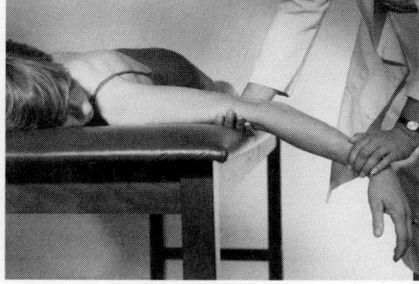
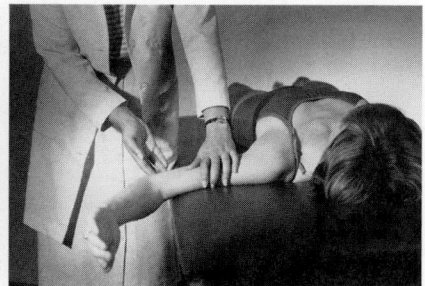

A   **B**   **C**

Figure 21-15 Elbow extension. **A,** Palpate and observe. **B,** Resist. **C,** Gravity-minimized position.

2. *Stabilize:* Provide stabilization at the humerus just proximal to the elbow to prevent shoulder abduction.[6,7,10,14]

3. *Palpate:* Palpate the pronator teres on the upper part of the volar surface of the forearm, medial to the biceps tendon and diagonally from the medial condyle of the humerus to the lateral border of the radius.[7,10,14,15]

4. *Observe:* Observe the client pronating the forearm, turning the hand palm down (Figure 21-17, *A*).[10] Slight resistance may be applied after the arm has passed midposition to compensate for the assistance of gravity after that point.[6]

5. *Resist:* Provide resistance by grasping over the dorsal aspect of the distal forearm, using the fingers and heel of the hand and turning toward supination (Figure 21-17, *B*).

Procedure for Testing Grades P (2), T (1), and 0

1. *Position:* The client is seated, shoulder flexed to 90 degrees, elbow flexed to 90 degrees, and the forearm in full supination. The upper arm is resting on the supporting surface, and the forearm is perpendicular to the floor.[20] The therapist stands next to the client on the side to be tested.

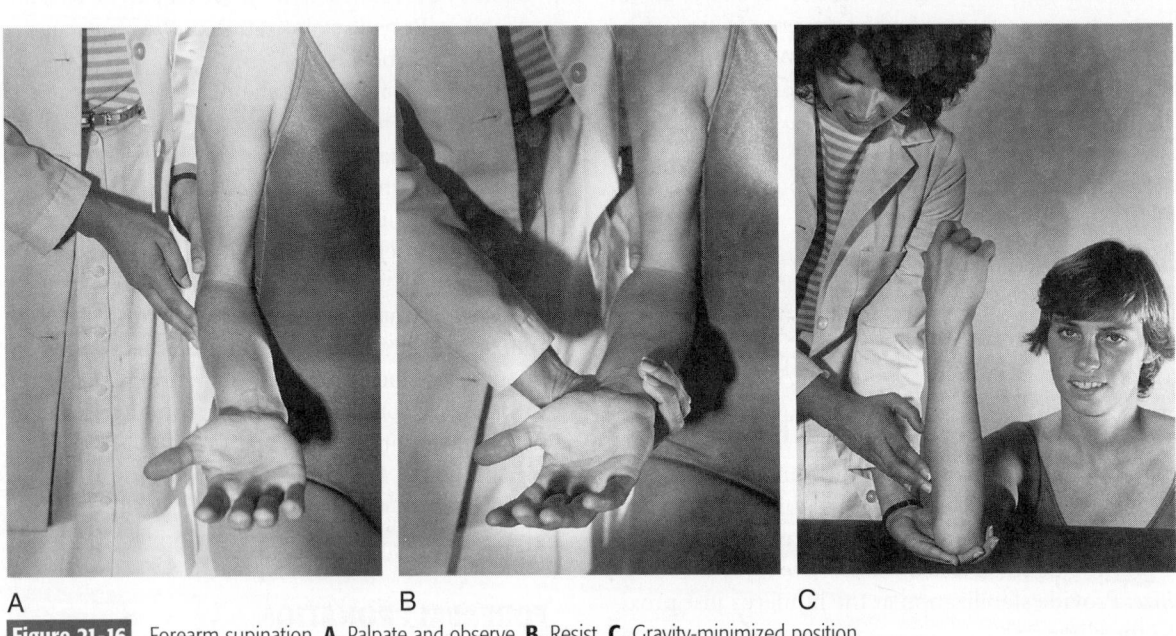

Figure 21-16   Forearm supination. **A,** Palpate and observe. **B,** Resist. **C,** Gravity-minimized position.

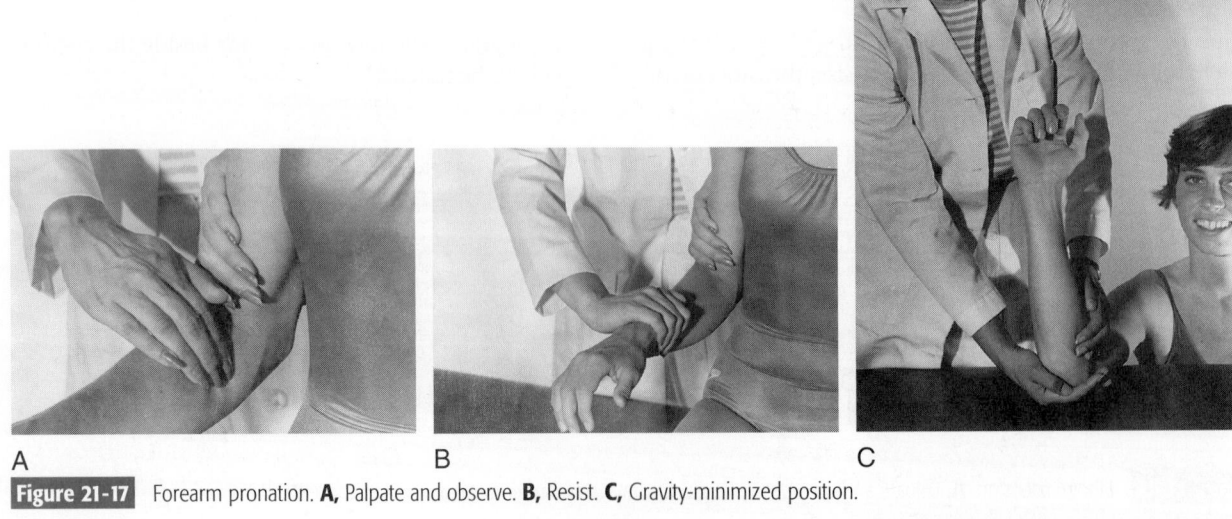

Figure 21-17   Forearm pronation. **A,** Palpate and observe. **B,** Resist. **C,** Gravity-minimized position.

2. *Palpate:* Palpate the pronator teres as described for the previous test.

3. *Observe:* Observe the client pronating the forearm, turning the palm of the hand away from the face (Figure 21-17, *C*).

4. *Grade:* The client is graded according to standard definitions of muscle grades.

Substitutions: With the elbow flexed, internal rotation and abduction of the humerus will produce apparent forearm pronation. With the elbow extended, internal rotation can place the forearm in a pronated position. Brachioradialis can bring the fully supinated forearm to midposition. Wrist flexion, aided by gravity, can effect pronation.[6,7,10,12,13,15,20]

WRIST EXTENSION WITH RADIAL DEVIATION

Muscles[10,12,14]	**Innervation**[6,12]
Extensor carpi radialis longus (ECRL)	Radial nerve, C5-7
Extensor carpi radialis brevis (ECRB)	Radial nerve, C6-8
Extensor carpi ulnaris (ECU)

Procedure for Testing Grades N (5) to F (3)

1. *Position:* The client is seated or supine, with the forearm resting on the supporting surface in pronation, the wrist at neutral, and the fingers and thumb relaxed. The therapist

sits opposite to or next to the client on the side to be tested.[10,14]

2. *Stabilize:* Provide stabilization over the volar or dorsal aspect of the distal forearm.[6,10,14]

3. *Palpate:* Palpate the ECRL and ECRB tendons on the dorsal aspect of the wrist at the bases of the second and third metacarpals, respectively.[6,7,10] The tendon of the ECU may be palpated at the base of the fifth metacarpal, just distal to the head of the ulna (Figure 21-18, *A*).[4,6,10,15]

4. *Observe:* Observe the client extending and radially deviating the wrist, lifting the hand from the supporting surface and simultaneously moving it medially (to the radial side). The movement should be performed without finger extension, which could substitute for the wrist motion (Figure 21-18, *B*).[6,10,15]

5. *Resist:* Provide resistance over the dorsum of the second and third metacarpals, toward flexion and ulnar deviation (Figure 21-18, *C*).[6,10,12-14]

Procedure for Testing Grades P (2), T (1), and 0

1. *Position:* The client is placed in the same manner as described for the previous test, except that the forearm is resting in midposition on its ulnar border.[10,20]

2. *Stabilize:* Provide stabilization at the ulnar border of the forearm, supported slightly above the table surface.[10]

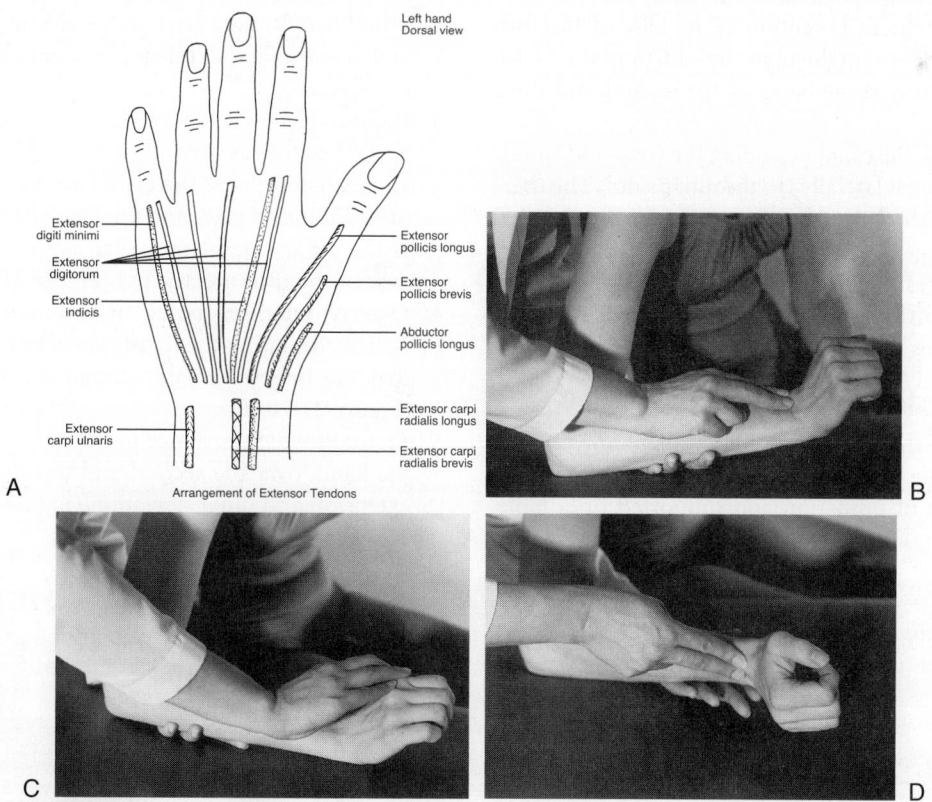

Figure 21-18   **A,** Arrangement of extensor tendons at wrist. **B,** Wrist extension with radial deviation. Palpate and observe. **C,** Resist. **D,** Gravity-minimized position.

3. *Palpate:* Palpate radial wrist extensors as described for the previous test.
4. *Observe:* Observe client extending the wrist, moving the hand away from the body (Figure 21-18, *D*).
5. *Grade:* The client is graded according to standard definitions of muscle grades.

Substitutions: Wrist extensors can substitute for one another. In the absence of the extensor carpi radialis muscles, the extensor carpi ulnaris will extend the wrist, but in an ulnar direction. The combined extension and radial deviation will not be possible. The extensor digitorum communis muscle and the extensor pollicis longus can initiate wrist extension, but finger or thumb extension will precede wrist extension.[6,7,12,13,15,20]

WRIST EXTENSION WITH ULNAR DEVIATION

Muscles[10,12-14]	Innervation[10,14]
Extensor carpi ulnaris (ECU)	Radial nerve, C6-8
Extensor carpi radialis brevis (ECRB)	
Extensor carpi radialis longus (ECRL)	Radial nerve, C5-7

Procedure for Testing Grades N (5) to F (3)

1. *Position:* The client is seated, forearm pronated, wrist neutral, fingers and thumb relaxed, supported on a table. The therapist sits opposite or next to the client on the side to be tested.
2. *Stabilize:* Provide stabilization under the distal forearm.[10,12-14]
3. *Palpate:* Palpate the ECU tendon at the base of the fifth metacarpal, just distal to the ulnar styloid,[6] and the ECRL and ECRB tendons at the bases of the second and third metacarpals.
4. *Observe:* Observe the client extending the wrist and simultaneously moving it laterally (to the ulnar side). The therapist should observe that the movement is not preceded by thumb or finger extension (Figure 21-19, *A*).[6,10,12,13,15]
5. *Resist:* Provide resistance over the dorsal-lateral aspect of the fourth and fifth metacarpals toward flexion and radial deviation (Figure 21-19, *B*).[6,10,14]

Procedure for Testing Grades P (2), T (1), and 0

1. *Position:* The client is placed in the same manner as that described for the previous test, except that the forearm is in 45 degrees of pronation and supported on a table.

The wrist is flexed and radially deviated, and the thumb and fingers are flexed.[6]

2. *Stabilize:* Provide stabilization under the distal forearm, supporting it slightly above the supporting surface.[10,14]
3. *Palpate:* Palpate the extensor tendons as described previously.
4. *Observe:* Observe client extending the wrist and moving it ulnarly at the same time (Figure 21-19, *C*).
5. *Grade:* The client is graded according to standard definitions of muscle grades.

Substitutions: In the absence of the ECU muscle, the ECRL and ECRB muscles can extend the wrist but will do so in a radial direction. The ulnar deviation component of the test motion will not be possible. Long finger and thumb extensors can initiate wrist extension, but the movement will be preceded by finger or thumb extension.[6,7,12,13,15,20]

WRIST FLEXION WITH RADIAL DEVIATION

Muscles[12,14]	Innervation[5,6,10]
Flexor carpi radialis (FCR)	Median nerve, C6-8
Flexor carpi ulnaris (FCU)	Ulnar nerve, C7-T1
Palmaris longus	Median nerve, C7-T1

Procedure for Testing Grades N (5) to F (3)

1. *Position:* The client is seated or supine, with the forearm resting in nearly full supination on the supporting surface, fingers and thumb relaxed.[7,12,15] The therapist is seated next to the client on the side to be tested.
2. *Stabilize:* Provide stabilization over the volar aspect of the midforearm.[6,10,14]
3. *Palpate:* The FCR tendon can be palpated over the wrist at the base of the second metacarpal bone. The palmaris longus tendon is at the center of the wrist at the base of the third metacarpal, and the FCU tendon can be palpated at the ulnar side of the volar aspect of the wrist, at the base of the fifth metacarpal (Figure 21-20, *A*).[4]
4. *Observe:* Observe the client simultaneously flexing and radially deviating the hand. The therapist should observe that the fingers remain relaxed during the movement[6] (Figure 21-20, *B*).
5. *Resist:* Provide resistance in the palm at the radial side of the hand, over the second and third metacarpals toward extension and ulnar deviation (Figure 21-20, *C*).[6]

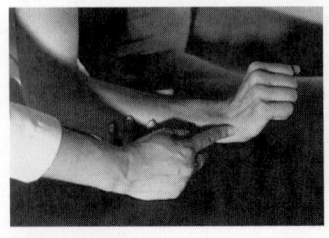 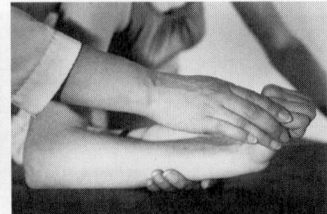 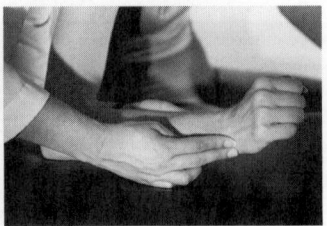

A   B   C

Figure 21-19   Wrist extension with ulnar deviation. **A,** Palpate and observe. **B,** Resist. **C,** Gravity-minimized position.

Procedure for Testing Grades P (2), T (1), and 0

1. *Position:* The client is seated with the forearm in midposition and the ulnar border of the hand resting on the supporting surface.[10,20] The therapist sits next to the client on the side to be tested.
2. *Stabilize:* Provide stabilization under the ulnar border of the forearm, supporting the wrist slightly above the supporting surface.
3. *Palpate:* Palpate the wrist flexor tendons as described for the previous test.
4. *Observe:* Observe the client flexing and radially deviating the wrist. Movement should not be initiated with finger flexion (Figure 21-20, *D*).
5. *Grade:* The client is graded according to standard definitions of muscle grades.

   Substitutions: Wrist flexors can substitute for one another. If flexor carpi radialis is weak or nonfunctioning in this test, flexor carpi ulnaris will produce wrist flexion, but in an ulnar direction, and the radial deviation will not be possible. The finger flexors can assist wrist flexion, but finger flexion will occur before the wrist is flexed. The abductor pollicis longus, with the assistance of gravity, can initiate wrist flexion.[6,7,15]

WRIST FLEXION WITH ULNAR DEVIATION

Muscles[10,13]	Innervation[5,10,13]
Flexor carpi ulnaris (FCU)	Ulnar nerve, C7-T1
Palmaris longus	Median nerve, C7-T1
Flexor carpi radialis (FCR)	Median nerve, C6-8

Procedure for Testing Grades N (5) to F (3)

1. *Position:* The client is seated or supine, with the forearm resting in nearly full supination on the supporting surface, fingers and thumb relaxed. The therapist is seated opposite or next to the client on the side to be tested.[10,14]
2. *Stabilize:* Provide stabilization over the volar aspect of the middle of the forearm.[10,14]
3. *Palpate:* Palpate the flexor tendons on the volar aspect of the wrist, the FCU at the base of the fifth metacarpal, the FCR at the base of the second metacarpal, and the palmaris longus at the base of the third metacarpal.[4]
4. *Observe:* Observe the client simultaneously flexing the wrist and deviating it ulnarly (Figure 21-21, *A*).
5. *Resist:* Provide resistance in the palm of the hand over the hypothenar eminence toward extension and radial deviation (Figure 21-21, *B*).[6,7,14]

Procedure for Testing Grades P (2), T (1), and 0

1. *Position:* The client is seated, with the forearm in neutral rotation and resting in 45 degrees of supination on the ulnar border of the arm and hand.[10] The therapist sits opposite or next to the client on the side being tested.
2. *Stabilize:* The client's arm can be supported slightly above the supporting surface and stabilized at the dorsal-medial aspect of the forearm to prevent elbow and forearm motion.
3. *Palpate:* Palpate the wrist flexor tendons as described for the previous test.

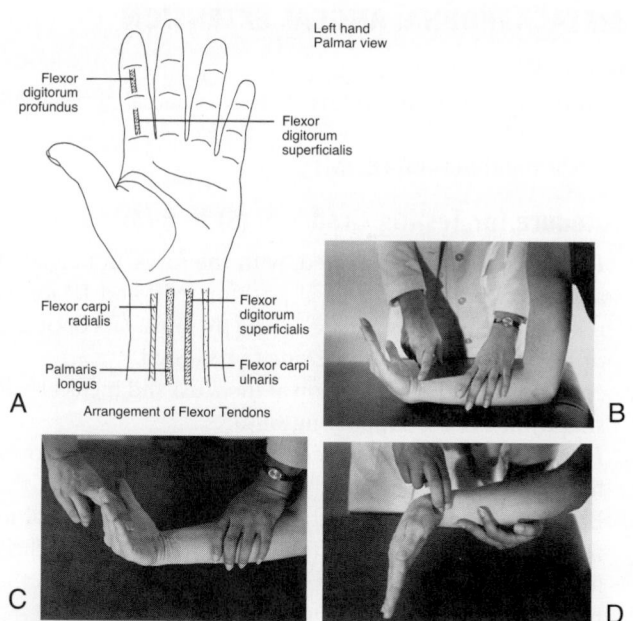

Figure 21-20 **A,** Arrangement of flexor tendons at wrist. **B,** Wrist flexion with radial deviation. Palpate and observe. **C,** Resist. **D,** Gravity-minimized position.

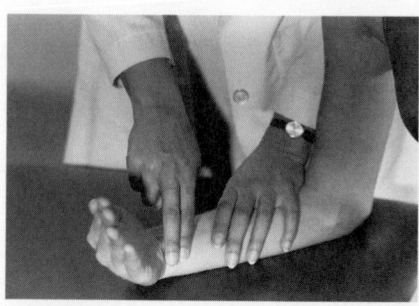
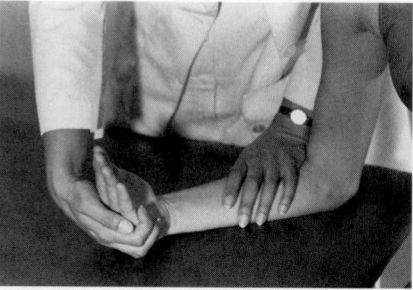
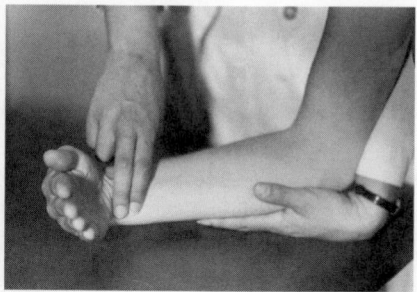

Figure 21-21 Wrist flexion with ulnar deviation. **A,** Palpate and observe. **B,** Resist. **C,** Gravity-minimized position.

4. *Observe:* Observe the client simultaneously flexing and deviating the wrist toward ulnar side (Figure 21-21, *C*).
5. *Grade:* The client is graded according to standard definitions of muscle grades.

Substitutions: Wrist flexors can substitute for one another. If the FCU is weak or absent, the FCR can produce wrist flexion in a radial direction and the ulnar deviation will not be possible. The finger flexors can also assist wrist flexion, but the motion will be preceded by flexion of the fingers.[6,15,20]

METACARPOPHALANGEAL FLEXION WITH INTERPHALANGEAL EXTENSION

Muscles[1,4]	Innervation[10,12]
Lumbricals 1 and 2	Median nerve, C8,T1
Lumbricals 3 and 4	Ulnar nerve, C8,T1
Dorsal interossei	
Palmar interossei	

Procedure for Testing Grades N (5) to F (3)

1. *Position:* The client is seated, with forearm in supination, wrist at neutral, resting on the supporting surface.[8] The metacarpophalangeal (MP) joints are extended, and the interphalangeal (IP) joints are flexed.[12,20] The therapist sits next to the client on the side being tested.
2. *Stabilize:* Provide stabilization over the metacarpals, proximal to the MP joints in the palm of the hand to prevent wrist motion.
3. *Palpate:* Palpate the first dorsal interosseous muscle just medial to the distal aspect of the second metacarpal on the dorsum of the hand. The remainder of these muscles are not easily palpable because of their size and deep location in the hand.[15,20]
4. *Observe:* Observe the client flexing the MP joints and extending the IP joints simultaneously (Figure 21-22, *A*).[12,14]
5. *Resist:* Provide resistance to each finger separately by grasping the distal phalanx and pushing downward on the finger into the supporting surface toward MP extension and IP flexion, or apply pressure first against the dorsal surface of the middle and distal phalanges toward flexion, followed by application of pressure to the volar surface of the proximal phalanges toward extension (Figure 21-22, *B*).[14]

Procedure for Testing Grades P (2), T (1), and 0

1. *Position:* The client is seated or supine, with the forearm and wrist in midposition and resting on the ulnar border on the supporting surface. MP joints are extended, and IP joints are flexed.[10,13] The therapist sits next to the client on the side being tested.
2. *Stabilize:* Provide stabilization at the wrist and palm of the hand.
3. *Palpate:* Palpate the client as described for the previous test.
4. *Observe:* Observe the client flexing the MP joints and extending the IP joints simultaneously (Figure 21-22, *C*).
5. *Grade:* The client is graded according to standard definitions of muscle grades.

Substitutions: Flexor digitorum profundus and superficialis may substitute for weak or absent lumbricals.[12] In this case, MP flexion will be preceded by flexion of the distal and proximal IP joints.[15,20]

METACARPOPHALANGEAL EXTENSION

Muscles[10,13]	Innervation[10,13]
Extensor digitorum communis (EDC)	Radial nerve, C7,8
Extensor indicis	
Extensor digiti minimi (EDM)	

Procedure for Testing Grades N (5) to F (3)

1. *Position:* The client is seated, with the forearm pronated and the wrist in the neutral position, MP and IP joints relaxed in partial flexion.[7,10,12] The therapist sits opposite or next to the client on the side to be tested.
2. *Stabilize:* Provide stabilization at the wrist and metacarpals slightly above the supporting surface.[10,12-14]
3. *Palpate:* Palpate the EDC tendons where they course over the dorsum of the hand.[6,7,10] In some individuals the EDM tendon can be palpated or visualized just lateral to the EDC tendon to the fifth finger. The extensor indicis tendon can be palpated or visualized just medial to the EDC tendon to the first finger.[6]
4. *Observe:* Observe the client extending the MP joints but maintaining the IP joints in some flexion (Figure 21-23, *A*).[6,12]

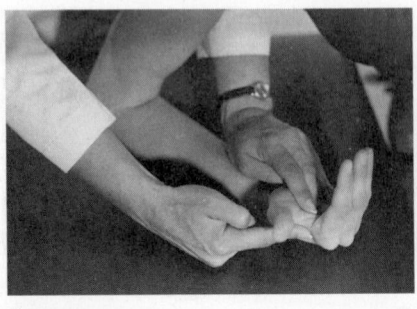 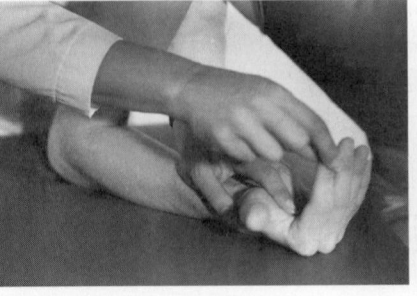 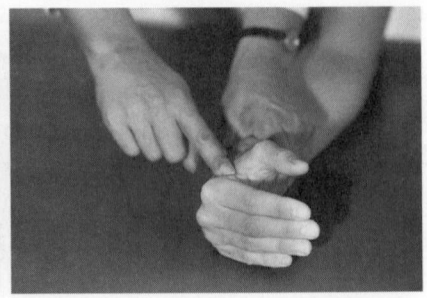

A   B   C

Figure 21-22   Metacarpophalangeal flexion with interphalangeal extension. **A,** Palpate and observe. **B,** Resist. **C,** Gravity-minimized position.

5. *Resist:* Provide resistance to each finger individually on the dorsum of the proximal phalanx toward MP flexion (Figure 21-23, *B*).[6,10,14]

Procedure for Testing Grades P (2), T (1), and 0

1. *Position:* The patient should be placed in a position similar to that described for the previous test, except that the client's forearm is in midposition and the hand and forearm are supported on the ulnar border.[10,12]
2. *Stabilize:* Provide stabilization in the same manner as described for the previous test.
3. *Palpate:* Palpate the patient in the same manner as described for the previous test.
4. *Observe:* Observe the client extending the MP joints while keeping the IP joints somewhat flexed (Figure 21-23, *C*).
5. *Grade:* The patient is graded according to standard definitions of muscle grades.

Substitutions: With the wrist stabilized, no substitutions are possible. When the wrist is not stabilized, wrist flexion with tendon action can produce MP extension.[6,7,10,13,15,20]

PROXIMAL INTERPHALANGEAL FLEXION, SECOND THROUGH FIFTH FINGERS

Muscles[10,14]
Flexor digitorum superficialis (FDS)

Innervation[6,10,12]
Median nerve, C7,8,T1

Procedure for Testing Grades N (5) to F (3)

1. *Position:* The client is seated, with the forearm supinated, wrist at neutral, fingers extended, and hand and forearm resting on the dorsal surface.[6,10,12] The therapist sits opposite or next to the client on the side being tested.
2. *Stabilize:* Provide stabilization at the MP joint and proximal phalanx of the finger being tested (Figure 21-24, *A*).[6,7,9,14]

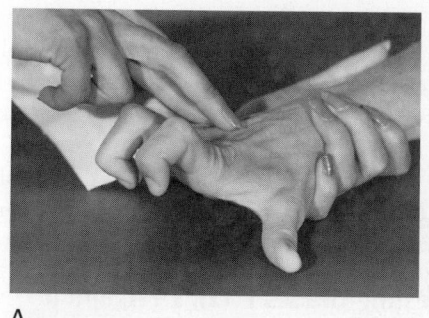
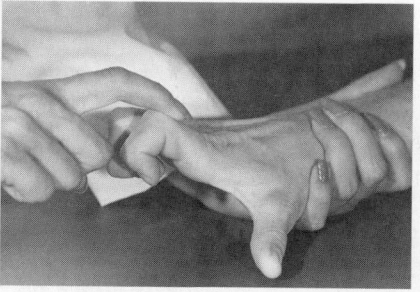
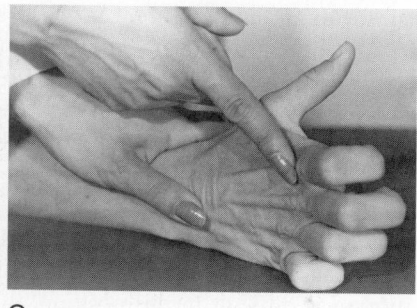

Figure 21-23 Metacarpophalangeal extension. **A,** Palpate and observe. **B,** Resist. **C,** Gravity-minimized position.

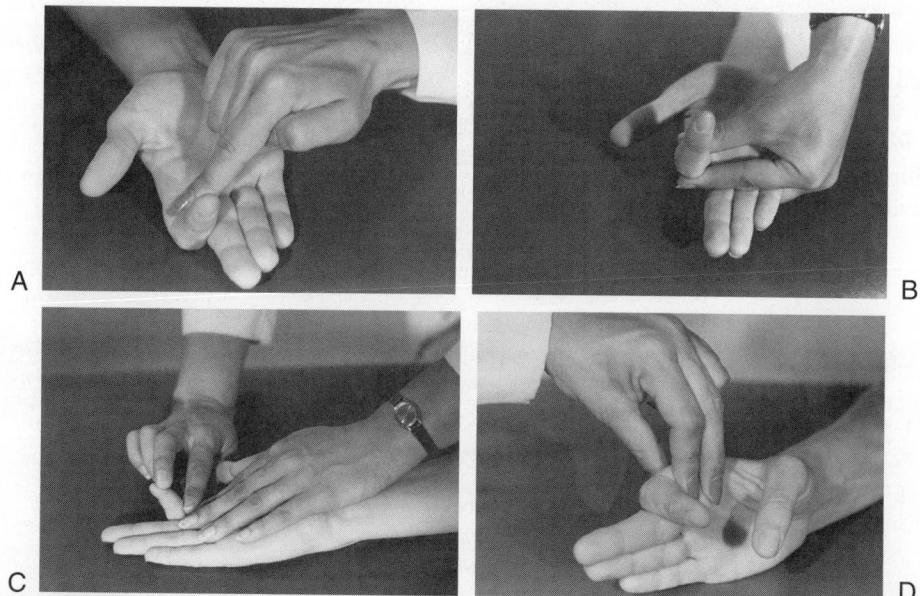

Figure 21-24 Proximal interphalangeal flexion. **A,** Palpate and observe. **B,** Position to assist with isolation of proximal interphalangeal joint flexion. **C,** Resist. Therapist checks for substitution by flexor digitorum profundus. **D,** Gravity-minimized position.

If it is difficult for the client to isolate PIP flexion, hold all of the fingers not being tested in MP hyperextension and PIP extension. This maneuver inactivates the flexor digitorum profundus so that the client cannot flex the distal joint (Figure 21-24, *B*).[4,6,12,20] Most individuals cannot perform isolated action of the PIP joint of the fifth finger, even with this assistance.[15]

3. *Palpate:* Palpate the FDS tendon on the volar surface of the proximal phalanx.[6] A stabilizing finger may be used to palpate in this instance.[15] The tendon supplying the fourth finger may be palpated over the volar aspect of the wrist between the flexor carpi ulnaris and the palmaris longus tendons, if desired.[4,6]
4. *Observe:* Observe the client flexing the PIP joint while maintaining DIP extension (Figure 21-24, *A*).
5. *Resist:* Provide resistance with one finger at the volar aspect of the middle phalanx toward extension.[6,10,14] If the therapist uses the index finger to apply resistance, the middle finger may be used to move the DIP joint to and fro to verify that the flexor digitorum profundus (FDP) is not substituting (Figure 21-24, *C*).

Procedure for Testing Grades P (2), T (1), and 0

1. *Position:* The client is seated, with the forearm in mid-position and the wrist at neutral, resting on the ulnar border.[12,20] The therapist sits opposite or next to the client on the side to be tested.
2. *Stabilize:* Provide stabilization at the MP joint and proximal phalanx of the finger.[10,14] If stabilization during the motion is difficult in this position, the forearm may be returned to full supination because the effect of gravity on the fingers is not significant.
3. *Palpate and observe:* The therapist palpates and observes the client in the same manner as described for the previous test, except that the movement is performed in the gravity-minimized position (Figure 21-24, *D*).
4. *Grade:* The client is graded according to standard definitions of muscle grades. If the test for grades *poor* and below is done with the forearm in full supination, partial ROM against gravity may be graded *poor*.[10]

Substitutions: The FDP may substitute for the FDS. DIP flexion will precede PIP flexion.[7,12,13,15,17,20] Tendon action of the long finger flexors accompanies wrist extension and can produce an apparent flexion of the fingers through partial ROM.[10,13,20]

DISTAL INTERPHALANGEAL FLEXION, SECOND THROUGH FIFTH FINGERS

Muscles[10,13]	Innervation[10,13]
Flexor digitorum profundus (FDP)	Median and ulnar nerves, C8, T1

Procedure for Testing Grades N (5) to F (3)

1. *Position:* The client is seated, with the forearm supinated, the wrist at neutral, and the fingers extended.[10] The therapist sits opposite or next to the client on the side being tested.[12]
2. *Stabilize:* Provide stabilization at the wrist at neutral and the PIP joint and middle phalanx of the finger being tested.[6,20]
3. *Palpate:* Use the finger stabilizing the middle phalanx to simultaneously palpate the FDP tendon over the volar surface of the middle phalanx.[6,10,15]
4. *Observe:* Observe the client flexing the DIP joint (Figure 21-25, *A*).
5. *Resist:* Provide resistance with one finger at the volar aspect of the distal phalanx toward extension (Figure 21-25, *B*).[6,7,10,14]

Procedure for Testing Grades P (2), T (1), and 0

1. *Position:* The client is seated, with the forearm in midposition and with the wrist at neutral, resting on the ulnar border.[12,20] The client may be positioned with the forearm supinated, if necessary.
2. *Stabilize:* The client is stabilized in the same manner as described for the previous test.
3. *Palpate:* The client is palpated in the same manner as described for the previous test.
4. *Observe:* Observe the client flexing the DIP joint (Figure 21-25, *C*).

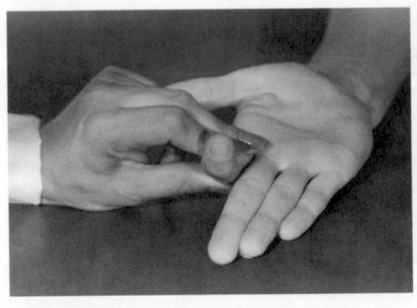 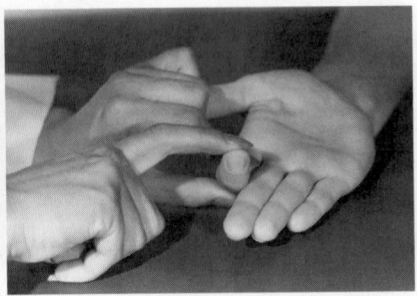 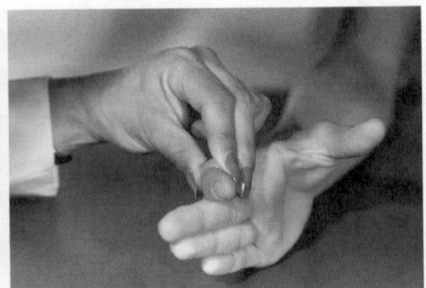

A   B   C

Figure 21-25 Distal interphalangeal flexion. **A,** Palpate and observe. **B,** Resist. **C,** Gravity-minimized position.

5. *Grade:* The client is graded according to standard definitions of muscle grades, except that if the test for grades *poor* and below was done with the forearm in full supination, movement through partial ROM may be graded *poor*.[10]

Substitutions: None possible during the testing procedure if the wrist is well stabilized because the FDP is the only muscle that can act to flex the DIP joint when it is isolated. During normal hand function, however, wrist extension with tendon action of the finger flexors can produce partial flexion of the DIP joints.[10,15,20]

FINGER ABDUCTION

Muscles[10,12]
Dorsal interossei
Abductor digiti minimi

Innervation[10,12]
Ulnar nerve, C8,T1

Procedure for Testing Grades N (5) to F (3)

1. *Position:* The client is seated or supine, with the forearm pronated, wrist at neutral, and fingers extended and adducted. The therapist is seated opposite or next to the client on the side to be tested.[10,13]
2. *Stabilize:* Provide stabilization at the wrist and metacarpals slightly above the supporting surface.
3. *Palpate:* Palpate the first dorsal interosseous muscle on the radial side of the second metacarpal or of the abductor digiti minimi on the ulnar border of the fifth metacarpal. The remaining interossei are not palpable.[6,7,10]
4. *Observe:* Observe the client spreading the fingers; abduction of the little finger, the ring finger toward the little finger, the middle finger toward the ring finger, and the index finger toward the thumb (Figure 21-26, *A*).[12]
5. *Resist:* Provide the first dorsal interosseous by applying pressure on the radial side of the proximal phalanx of the second finger in an ulnar direction (Figure 21-26, *B*); the second dorsal interosseous on the radial side of the proximal phalanx of the middle finger in an ulnar direction; the third dorsal interosseous on the ulnar side of the proximal phalanx of the middle finger in a radial direction; the fourth dorsal interosseous on the ulnar side of the

proximal phalanx of the ring finger in a radial direction; and the abductor digiti minimi on the ulnar side of the proximal phalanx of the little finger in a radial direction.[6,14] An alternative mode of resistance is to flick each finger toward adduction. If the finger rebounds, the grade is *N (5)*.[12]

Procedure for Testing Grades P (2), T (1), and 0

The tests for these muscle grades are the same as described for the previous test.

1. *Grade:* Because the test motions were not performed against gravity, the therapist must exercise professional judgment when grading. For example, partial ROM in the gravity-minimized position may be graded *poor* and full ROM graded *fair*.[10,13]

Substitutions: EDC can assist weak or absent dorsal interossei, but abduction will be accompanied by MP extension.[6,15,20]

FINGER ADDUCTION

Muscles[10-14]
Palmar interossei, 1, 2, 3

Innervation[10,13]
Ulnar nerve, C8,T1

Procedure for Testing Grades N (5) to F (3)

1. *Position:* The client is seated, with forearm pronated, wrist in neutral, and fingers extended and abducted.[10,13]
2. *Stabilize:* Provide stabilization at the wrist and metacarpals slightly above the supporting surface.[6]
3. *Palpate:* The condition is not palpable.[6] The muscle cannot be palpated.
4. *Observe:* Observe the client adducting the first, fourth, and fifth fingers toward the middle finger (Figure 21-27, *A*).
5. *Resist:* Provide resistance at the index finger at the proximal phalanx by pulling it in a radial direction, the ring finger at the proximal phalanx in an ulnar direction, and the little finger likewise (Figure 21-27, *B*).[6,14] These muscles are very small, and resistance must be modified to accommodate their comparatively limited power. Fingers can also be grasped at the distal phalanx and flicked in the direction of abduction. If the finger snaps back to the adducted position, the grade is *N (5)*.[12]

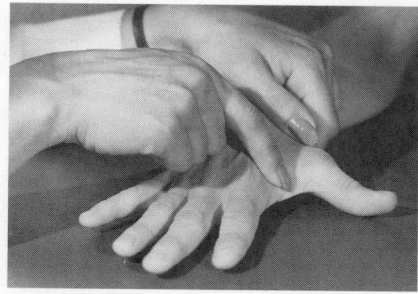
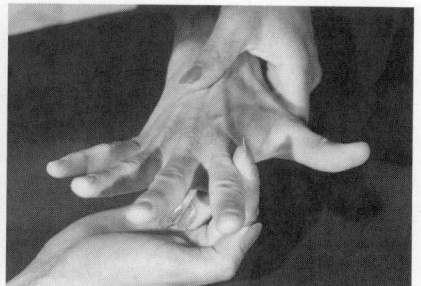

A   B

Figure 21-26   Finger abduction. **A,** Palpate and observe. **B,** Resist.

Procedure for Testing Grades P (2), T (1), and 0

The test for these muscle grades is the same as described for the previous test. The therapist's judgment must be used in determining the degree of weakness. Achievement of full ROM may be graded *fair* and partial ROM graded *poor*.[10,12]

Substitutions: FDP and FDS can substitute for weak palmar interossei, but IP flexion will occur with finger adduction.[13,15,20]

THUMB METACARPOPHALANGEAL EXTENSION

Muscles[10,12-14]	Innervation[10,12-14]
Extensor pollicis brevis (EPB)	Radial nerve, C6-8

Procedure for Testing Grades N (5) to F (3)

1. *Position:* The client is seated or supine, forearm in midposition, wrist at neutral, and hand and forearm resting on the ulnar border.[6,10,13] The thumb is flexed into the palm at the MP joint, and the IP joint is extended but relaxed. The therapist sits opposite or next to the client on the side to be tested.
2. *Stabilize:* Provide stabilization at the wrist and the thumb metacarpal.[6]
3. *Palpate:* Palpate the EPB tendon on the dorsoradial aspect of the base of the first metacarpal. It lies just medial to the abductor pollicis longus tendon on the radial side of the anatomical snuffbox, which is the hollow space created between the EPL and EPB tendons when the thumb is fully extended and radially abducted.[4,6,7]
4. *Observe:* Observe the client extending the MP joint. The IP joint remains relaxed (Figure 21-28, *A*). It is difficult for many individuals to isolate this motion.
5. *Resist:* Provide resistance on the dorsal surface of the proximal phalanx toward MP flexion (Figure 21-28, *B*).[6,10,12-14]

Procedure for Testing Grades (P), (T), and (0)

1. *Position and stabilize:* Positioning and stabilizing are the same as described for the previous test, except that the forearm is fully pronated and resting on the volar surface.[20] The therapist may stabilize the first metacarpal, holding the hand slightly above the supporting surface. The test may also be performed in the same manner as for grades *normal* to *fair*, with modified grading.[10]
2. *Palpate and observe:* The client is palpated and observed in the same way as described for the previous test. MP extension is performed in a plane parallel to the supporting surface (Figure 21-28, *C*).
3. *Grade:* The client is graded according to standard definitions of muscle grades. If midposition of the forearm was used, partial ROM is graded *poor* and full ROM is graded *fair*.[10,12]

Substitutions: Extensor pollicis longus may substitute for extensor pollicis brevis. IP extension will precede MP extension.[6,7,13,15,20]

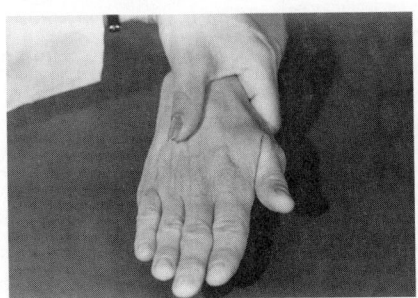 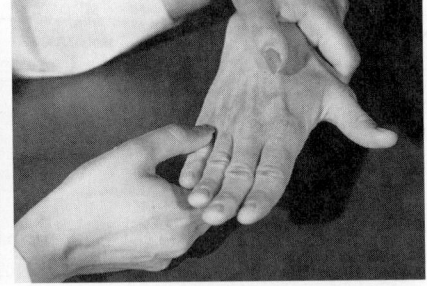

A   B

Figure 21-27   Finger adduction. **A,** Therapist observes movement of fingers into adduction. Palpation of these muscles is not possible. **B,** Resist.

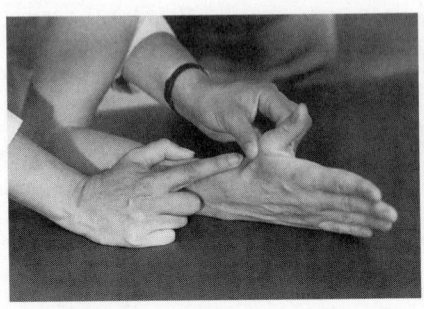 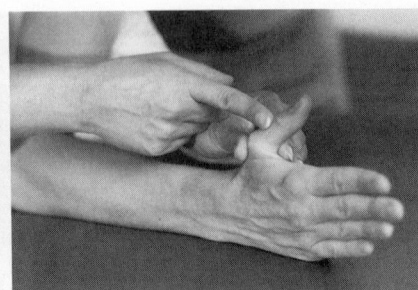 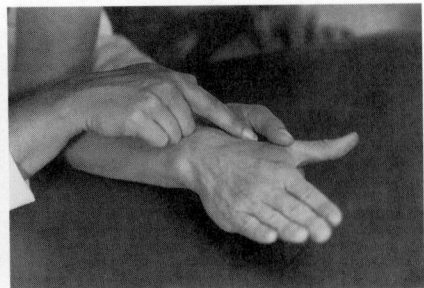

A   B   C

Figure 21-28   Thumb metacarpophalangeal extension. **A,** Palpate and observe. **B,** Resist. **C,** Gravity-minimized position.

THUMB IP EXTENSION

Muscles[10,12-14]
Extensor pollicis longus (EPL)

Innervation[10,12-14]
Radial nerve, C6-8

Procedure for Testing Grades N (5) to F (3)

1. *Position:* The client is seated or supine, forearm in midposition, wrist at neutral, and hand and forearm resting on the ulnar border.[6,10,13] The thumb is adducted, the MP joint is extended or slightly flexed, and the IP is flexed.[6] The therapist sits opposite or next to the client on the side being tested.

2. *Stabilize:* Provide stabilization at the wrist in neutral position, the first metacarpal, and the proximal phalanx of the thumb.[6]

3. *Palpate:* Palpate the EPL tendon on the dorsal surface of the hand medial to the EPB tendon, between the head of the first metacarpal and the base of the second on the ulnar side of the anatomical snuffbox.[4,6,10]

4. *Observe:* C extend the IP joint (Figure 21-29, *A*).

5. *Resist:* Provide resistance on the dorsal surface of the distal phalanx, down toward IP flexion (Figure 21-29, *B*).[6,10,14]

Procedure for Testing Grades P (2), T (1), and 0

1. *Position and stabilize:* Positioning and stabilizing are the same as described for the previous test, except that the forearm is fully pronated.[20] The therapist may stabilize so that the client's hand is held slightly above the supporting surface. The test may also be performed in the same position as for grades *normal* to *fair* with modification in grading.

2. *Palpate and observe:* The patient is palpated and observed in the same manner as described for the previous test. IP extension is performed in the plane of the palm, parallel to the supporting surface (Figure 21-29, *C*).

3. *Grade:* The client is graded according to standard definitions of muscle grades. If the test was performed with the forearm in midposition, partial ROM is graded P (2).[10]

Substitutions: A quick contraction of the flexor pollicis longus followed by rapid release will cause the IP joint to rebound into extension.[6] IP flexion will precede IP extension.[7,15] The abductor pollicis brevis, flexor pollicis brevis,

the oblique fibers of the adductor pollicis, and the first palmar interosseous can extend the IP joint because of their insertions into the extensor expansion of the thumb.[14,20]

THUMB METACARPOPHALANGEAL FLEXION

Muscles[10,12-14]
Flexor pollicis brevis (FPB)

Innervation[10,12-14]
Median and ulnar nerves, C8, T1

Procedure for Testing Grades N (5) to F (3)

1. *Position:* The client is seated or supine, the forearm supinated, the wrist in the neutral position, and the thumb in extension and adduction.[6,12] The therapist is seated next to or opposite the client.[7,10,14]

2. *Stabilize:* Provide stabilization at the first metacarpal and the wrist.[12]

3. *Palpate:* Palpate the client over the middle of the palmar surface of the thenar eminence just medial to the abductor pollicis brevis muscle.[6,10] The hand that is used to stabilize may also be used for palpation.

4. *Observe:* Observe the client flexing the MP joint while maintaining extension of the IP joint (Figure 21-30, *A*).[6] It may not be possible for some individuals to isolate flexion to the MP joint. In this instance, both MP and IP flexion may be tested together as a gross test for thumb flexion strength and graded according to the therapist's judgment.

5. *Resist:* Provide resistance on the palmar surface of the first phalanx toward MP extension (Figure 21-30, *B*).[6,7,10,14]

Procedure for Testing Grades P (2), T (1), and (0)

Positioning, stabilizing, and palpating are the same as described for the previous test.

1. *Observe:* Observe the client flexing the MP joint so that the thumb moves over the palm of the hand.

2. *Grade:* Full ROM is graded *fair*; partial ROM is graded *poor*.[10,13]

Substitutions: FPL can substitute for FPB. In this case, isolated MP flexion will not be possible and MP flexion will be preceded by IP flexion.[7,12,13,15,20]

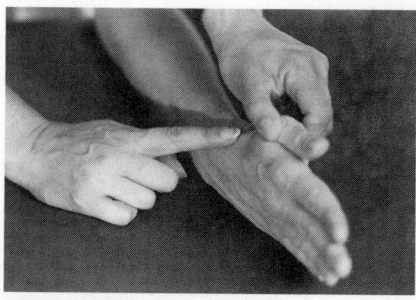
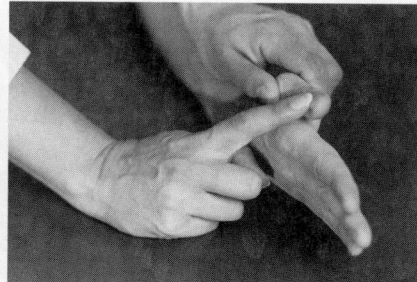
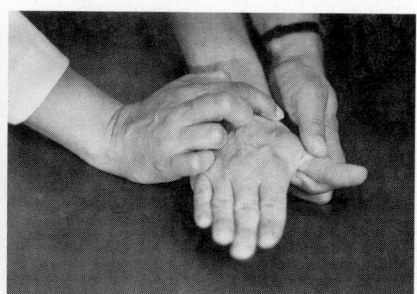

A   B   C

Figure 21-29 Thumb interphalangeal extension. **A,** Palpate and observe. **B,** Resist. **C,** Gravity-minimized position.

THUMB INTERPHALANGEAL FLEXION

Muscles[6,10,12]   **Innervation**[10,13]
Flexor pollicis longus (FPL)   Median nerve, C7-T1

Procedure for Testing Grades N (5) to F (3)

1. *Position:* The client is seated, with the forearm fully supinated, wrist in neutral position, and thumb extended and adducted.[10,13] The therapist is seated next to or opposite the client.
2. *Stabilize:* Provide stabilization at the wrist, thumb metacarpal, and proximal phalanx of the thumb in extension.[6,7,10,14]
3. *Palpate:* Palpate the FPL tendon on the palmar surface of the proximal phalanx.[6] In this instance, the palpating finger may be the same one used for stabilizing the proximal phalanx.
4. *Observe:* Observe the client flexing the IP joint in the plane of the palm (Figure 21-31, *A*).[10,12]
5. *Resist:* Provide resistance on the palmar surface of the distal phalanx, toward IP extension (Figure 21-31, *B*).[6,10,12-14]

Procedure for Testing Grades P (2), T (1), and 0

The test for these muscle grades is the same as that described for the previous test. The occupational therapist's judgment must be used in determining the degree of weakness. Achievement of full ROM may be graded *fair* and partial ROM graded *poor.*[10,13]

Substitutions: A quick contraction and release of the EPL may cause an apparent flexion of the IP joint. The therapist should observe for IP extension preceding IP flexion.[6,7,12,13,15,20]

THUMB PALMAR ABDUCTION

Muscles[13,14]   **Innervation**[13,14]
Abductor pollicis brevis (APB)   Median nerve, C8,T1

Procedure for Testing Grades Fair (F) to Normal (N)

1. *Position:* The client is seated or supine, forearm in supination, wrist at neutral, thumb relaxed in adduction against the volar aspect of the index finger. The OT sits opposite or next to the client on the side to be tested.[6,7,10,12-14]
2. *Stabilize:* Provide stabilization at the metacarpals and wrist.
3. *Palpate:* Palpate the APB muscle on the lateral aspect of the thenar eminence, lateral to the flexor pollicis brevis muscle.[10]
4. *Observe:* Observe the client raising the thumb away from the palm in a plane perpendicular to the palm (Figure 21-32, *A*).[6,14]
5. *Resist:* Provide resistance at the lateral aspect of the proximal phalanx, downward toward adduction (Figure 21-32, *B*).[6,14]

Procedure for Testing Grades P (2), T (1), and 0

1. *Position:* The client is positioned in the same manner as described for the previous test, except that the forearm and hand are supported on the ulnar border.[12,20]

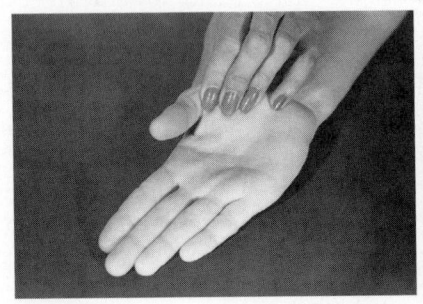
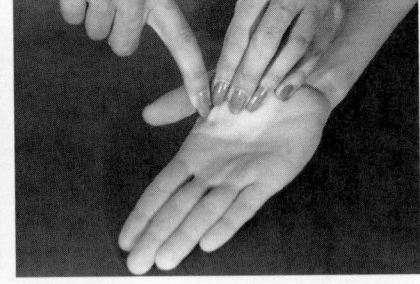

A   B

Figure 21-30 Thumb metacarpophalangeal flexion. **A,** Palpate and observe. **B,** Resist.

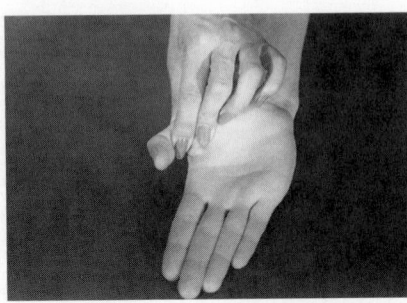
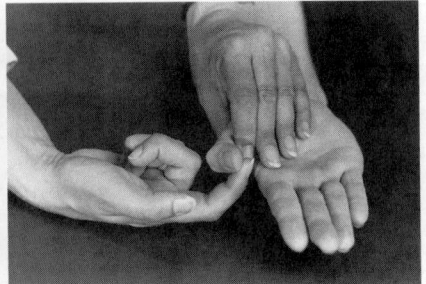

A   B

Figure 21-31 Thumb interphalangeal flexion. **A,** Palpate and observe. **B,** Resist.

2. *Stabilize:* Provide stabilization at the wrist and metacarpals.
3. *Palpate:* Palpate the APB muscle on the lateral aspect of the thenar eminence.
4. *Observe:* Observe the client moving the thumb away from the palm in a plane at right angles to the palm of the hand and parallel to the supporting surface (Figure 21-32, *C*).
5. *Grade:* The client is graded according to standard definitions of muscle grades.

Substitutions: APL can substitute for APB. Abduction will take place more in the plane of the palm, however, rather than perpendicular to it.[13,15,20]

THUMB RADIAL ABDUCTION

Muscles[12,14]   **Innervation**[12,14]
Abductor pollicis longus (APL)   Radial nerve, C6-8

Procedure for Testing Grades N (5) to F (3)

1. *Position:* The client is seated or supine, forearm in neutral rotation, wrist at neutral, thumb adducted and slightly flexed across the palm. Hand and forearm are resting on the ulnar border.[14] The therapist sits opposite or next to the client on the side being tested.
2. *Stabilize:* Provide stabilization at the wrist and metacarpals of the fingers.[10,14]

3. *Palpate:* Palpate the APL tendon on the lateral aspect of the base of the first metacarpal. It is the tendon immediately lateral (radial) to the EPB tendon.[4,6,10]
4. *Observe:* Observe the client moving the thumb out of the palm of the hand, abducting away from the index finger at an angle of about 45 degrees (Figure 21-33, *A*).[6]
5. *Resist:* Provide resistance at the lateral aspect of the thumb metacarpal toward adduction (Figure 21-33, *B*).[6,10,14]

Procedure for Testing Grades P (2), T (1), and 0

1. *Position:* The client is positioned in the same manner as described for the previous test, except that the forearm is in supination.[10]
2. *Stabilize:* Provide stabilization at the wrist and palm of the hand.
3. *Palpate:* The client is palpated in the same manner as described for the previous test.
4. *Observe:* Observe the client moving the thumb out away from the palm of the hand in the plane of the palm (Figure 21-33, *C*).
5. *Grade:* The client is graded according to standard definitions of muscle grades.

Substitutions: APB can substitute for APL. Abduction will not take place in the plane of the palm but rather in a more ulnar direction.[15,20] EPB can substitute for APL. The movement will be more toward the dorsal surface of the forearm.[12]

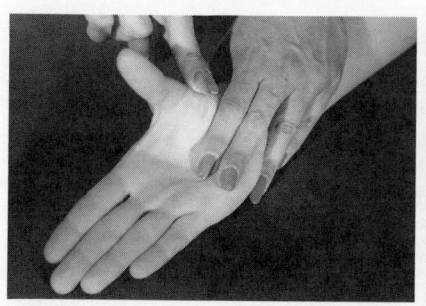 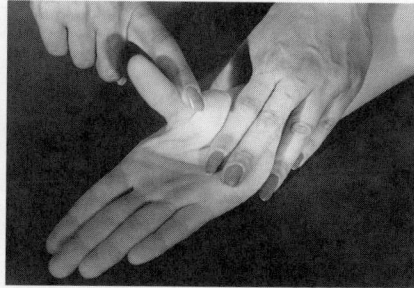 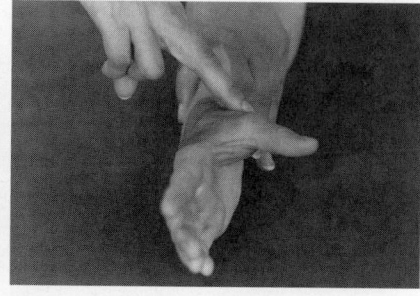

A   B   C

Figure 21-32   Thumb palmar abduction. **A,** Palpate and observe. **B,** Resist. **C,** Gravity-minimized position.

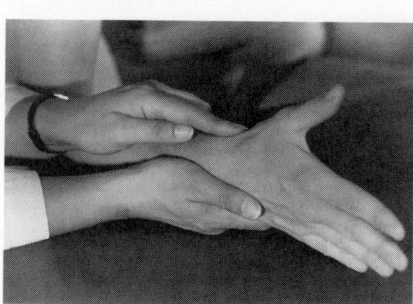 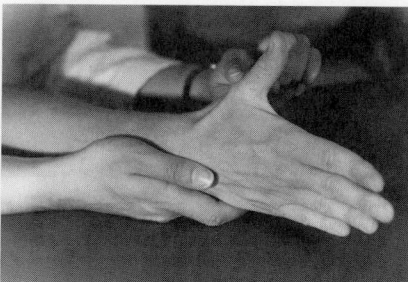 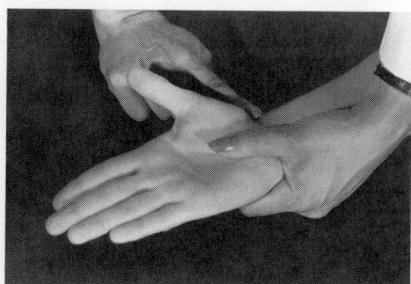

A   B   C

Figure 21-33   Radial abduction. **A,** Palpate and observe. **B,** Resist. **C,** Gravity-minimized position.

THUMB ADDUCTION

Muscles[10,12-14]   Innervation[10,12-14]
Adductor pollicis (AP)   Ulnar nerve, C8,T1

Procedure for Testing Grades N (5) to F (3)

1. *Position:* The client is seated or supine, forearm pronated, wrist at neutral, thumb relaxed and in palmar abduction.[10,13,20] The therapist is sitting opposite or next to the client on the side to be tested.
2. *Stabilize:* Provide stabilization at the wrist and metacarpals by grasping the hand around the ulnar side and supporting it slightly above the resting surface.[10,13]
3. *Palpate:* Palpate the AP on the palmar side of the thumb web space.[6,15]
4. *Observe:* Observe the client adducting the thumb to touch the palm (Figure 21-34, *A*).[10,12] (The palm is turned up in the illustration to show the palpation point.)
5. *Resist:* Provide resistance by grasping the proximal phalanx of the thumb near the metacarpal head and pulling downward, toward abduction (Figure 21-34, *B*).[10]

Procedure for Testing Grades P (2), T (1), and 0

1. *Position:* The client is positioned in the same manner as described for the previous test, except that the forearm is in midposition and the forearm and hand are resting on the ulnar border.[20]
2. *Stabilize:* Provide stabilization over the wrist and palm of the hand.
3. *Palpate:* Palpate the client in the same manner as described for the previous test.
4. *Observe:* Observe the client adducting the thumb to touch the radial side of the palm of the hand or the second metacarpal (Figure 21-34, *C*).

5. *Grade:* The client is graded according to standard definitions of muscle grades.
   Substitutions: FPL or EPL may assist weak or absent AP. If one substitutes, adduction will be accompanied by thumb flexion or extension preceding adduction.[13,15,20]

OPPOSITION OF THE THUMB TO THE FIFTH FINGER

Muscles[10,13]   Innervation[10,13]
Opponens pollicis   Median nerve, C8, T1
Opponens digiti minimi   Ulnar nerve, C8, T1

Procedure for Testing Grades N (5) to F (3)

1. *Position:* The client is seated or supine, with forearm supinated, wrist at neutral, thumb in palmar abduction, and fifth finger extended.[6,7,10,14] The therapist sits opposite or next to the client on the side to be tested.
2. *Stabilize:* Provide stabilization at the forearm and wrist.
3. *Palpate:* Palpate the opponens pollicis along the radial side of the shaft of the first metacarpal, lateral to the APB; the opponens digiti minimi on the shaft of the fifth metacarpal.[6,10,15]
4. *Observe:* Observe the client opposing the thumb to touch the thumb pad to the pad of the fifth finger, which flexes and rotates toward the thumb (Figure 21-35, *A*).[6,7]
5. *Resist:* Provide resistance at the distal ends of the first and fifth metacarpals toward derotation of these bones and flattening of the palm of the hand (Figure 21-35, *B*).[10,12]

Procedure for Testing Grades P (2), T (1), and 0

The procedure described for the previous test may be used for these grades, if grading is modified to compensate for the movement of the parts against gravity. For example,

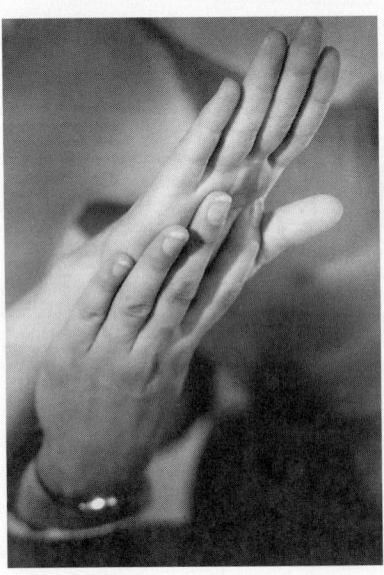

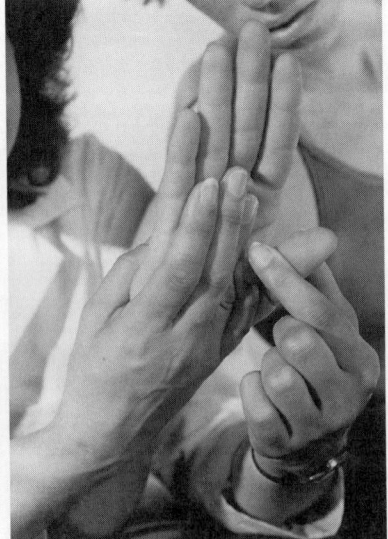

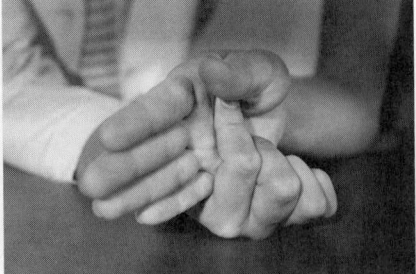

A   B   C

Figure 21-34   Thumb adduction. **A,** Palpate and observe. **B,** Resist. **C,** Gravity-minimized position.

movement through full ROM would be graded *fair* and through partial ROM would be graded *poor.*[10,12]

Substitutions: APB will assist with opposition by flexing and medially rotating the CMC joint, but the IP joint will extend. The FPB will flex and medially rotate the CMC joint, but the thumb will not move away from the palm of the hand. The FPL will flex and slightly rotate the CMC joint, but the thumb will not move away from the palm and the IP joint will flex strongly.[15,20] The DIP joints of the thumb and little finger may flex to meet, giving the appearance of full opposition.[7,12]

MANUAL MUSCLE TESTING OF THE LOWER EXTREMITY

HIP FLEXION

Muscles[4,7,10]	Innervation[4,6,10]
Psoas major	Lumbar plexus, L1-3
Iliacus	Femoral nerve, L2,3
Rectus femoris	Femoral nerve, L2-4
Tensor fasciae latae	Superior gluteal nerve, L4,5,S1
Sartorius	Femoral nerve, L2-S1
Pectineus	Femoral nerve, L2,3

Procedure for Testing Grades N (5) to F (3)

1. *Position:* The client is seated, with knees flexed over the edge of the table and feet above the floor.[12] The therapist stands next to the client on the side being tested.[7]

2. *Stabilize:* Provide stabilization at the pelvis at the iliac crest on the side being tested. The client may grasp the edge of the table or fold arms across chest.[6,7,10,12-14]

3. *Palpate:* The psoas and iliacus are difficult to palpate.[6] The rectus femoris may be palpated on the middle anterior aspect of the thigh, just lateral to the sartorius muscle.[4,15]

4. *Observe:* Observe the client flexing the hip so that the femur rises above the table surface (Figure 21-36, *A*).

5. *Resist:* Provide resistance just proximal to the knee on the anterior surface of the thigh, down toward the table into hip extension (Figure 21-36, *B*).[6,7,10,12-14]

Procedure for Testing Grades P (2), T (1), and 0

1. *Position:* The client assumes a side-lying position. The therapist stands behind the client, supporting the upper leg in neutral rotation and slight abduction, with the knee extended.[10,12,13] The lower leg (to be tested) is extended at the hip and knee.

2. *Stabilize:* The weight of the trunk may provide adequate stabilization, or the therapist may stabilize the pelvis.[10]

3. *Palpate:* The client is palpated in the same manner as described for the previous test.

4. *Observe:* Observe the client bringing the lower leg up toward the trunk, flexing the hip and knee (Figure 21-36, *C*).[10]

5. *Grade:* The client is graded according to standard definitions of muscle grades.

Substitutions: Observe for internal rotation, external rotation, and abduction accompanying the flexion as signs of

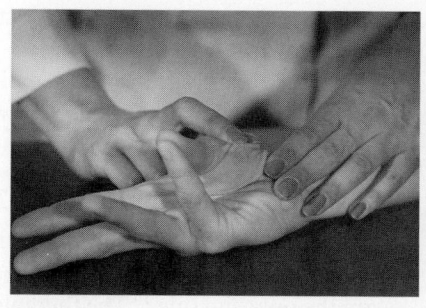
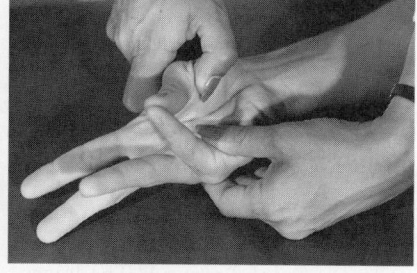

Figure 21-35 Thumb opposition. **A,** Palpate and observe. **B,** Resist.

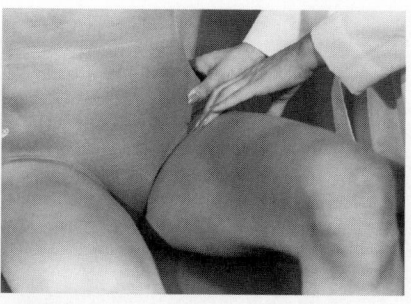
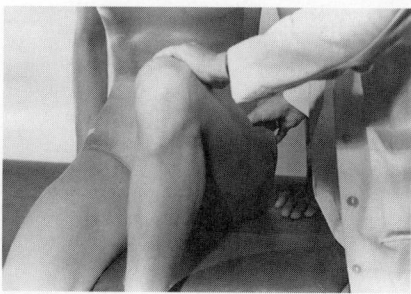
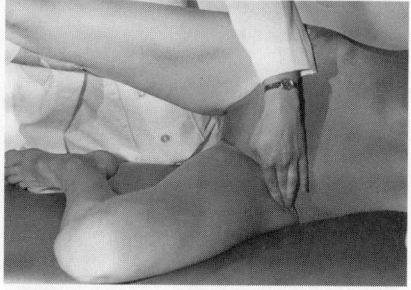

Figure 21-36 Hip flexion. **A,** Palpate and observe. **B,** Resist. **C,** Gravity-minimized position.

substitution or muscle imbalance in this muscle group.[6,7,13,14] The hip flexors can substitute for one another. If the iliacus and psoas major muscles are weak or absent, hip flexion will be accompanied by other movements: abduction and external rotation (sartorius), abduction and internal rotation (tensor fasciae latae), and adduction (pectineus).[10,12,13] If the anterior abdominal muscles do not stabilize the pelvis, it will flex on the thighs; the hip flexors may hold against resistance but not at maximal ROM.[14]

HIP EXTENSION

Muscles[6,12,14]	Innervation[10,13]
Gluteus maximus	Inferior gluteal nerve, L5-S2
Semitendinosus	Sciatic nerve, L5-S2
Semimembranosus	
Biceps femoris (long head)	Sciatic nerve, L5-S3

Procedure for Testing Grades N (5) to F (3)

1. *Position:* The client is prone, with the hip at neutral and the knee flexed to about 90 degrees. This position is used to isolate the gluteus maximus.[6,12] The client may also be prone with the knee extended.[12] The therapist stands next to the client on the opposite side.[14] Two pillows may be placed under the pelvis to flex the hips.[6,7]
2. *Stabilize:* Provide stabilization over the iliac crest on the side being tested.[10,12]
3. *Palpate:* Palpate the gluteus maximus on the middle posterior surface of the buttock.[15]
4. *Observe:* Observe the client extending the hip while keeping the knee flexed to minimize action of the hamstring muscles on the hip joint (Figure 21-37, *A*).
5. *Resist:* Provide resistance at the distal end of the posterior aspect of the thigh, downward, toward flexion (Figure 21-37, *B*).[10,12-14]

Procedure for Testing Grades P (2), T (1), and 0

1. *Position:* The client assumes a side-lying position. The therapist stands in front of the client, supporting the upper leg in extension and slight abduction.[10] The lower leg (to be tested) is flexed at the hip and knee.
2. *Stabilize:* Provide stabilization at the pelvis over the iliac crest.[10]

3. *Palpate:* The client is palpated in the same manner as described for the previous test.
4. *Observe:* Observe the client extending the hip, bringing the lower leg backward, while maintaining flexion of the knee (Figure 21-37, *C*).
5. *Grade:* The client is graded according to standard definitions of muscle grades.

Substitutions: Elevation of the pelvis and extension of the lumbar spine can produce some hip extension. In the supine position, gravity and eccentric contraction of the hip flexors can return the flexed hip to extension.[15] Hip external rotation, abduction, or adduction may be used to substitute.[7]

HIP ABDUCTION

Muscles[6,10,12]	Innervation[10,12-14]
Gluteus medius	Superior gluteal nerve, L4-S1
Gluteus minimus	

Procedure for Testing Grades N (5) to F (3)

1. *Position:* The client assumes a side-lying position, with the upper leg (to be tested) with the knee extended and hip extended slightly beyond the neutral position and slight forward rotation of the pelvis[12]; the lower leg is flexed at the hip and knee to provide a wide base of support.[7] The therapist stands behind or in front of the client.[6,7,10,12-14]
2. *Stabilize:* Provide stabilization at the pelvis over the iliac crest.[10,14]
3. *Palpate:* Palpate the gluteus medius on the lateral aspect of the ilium above the greater trochanter of the femur.[6,10]
4. *Observe:* Observe the client abducting the hip, lifting the leg upward (Figure 21-38, *A*).
5. *Resist:* Provide resistance at the point just proximal to the knee in a downward direction, toward adduction (Figure 21-38, *B*).[6,10,12]

Procedure for Testing Grades P (2), T (1), and 0

1. *Position:* The client is supine, with both legs extended and in neutral rotation. The therapist stands next to the client on the opposite side.[10] The therapist may use one hand to support at the ankle and slightly lift the test leg off the surface, being careful to offer no resistance or assistance to the movement.[12]

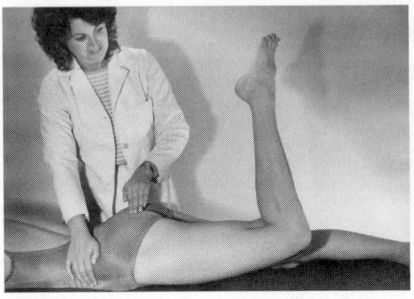
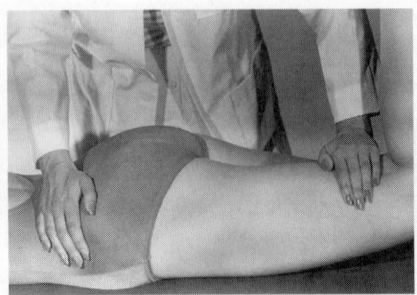
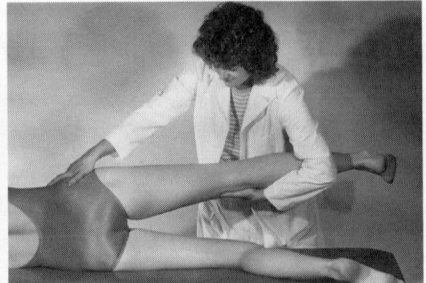

A   B   C

Figure 21-37   Hip extension. **A,** Palpate and observe. **B,** Resist. **C,** Gravity-minimized position.

2. *Stabilize:* Provide stabilization at the pelvis at the iliac crest on the side to be tested and at the opposite limb at the lateral aspect of the calf.[10]

3. *Palpate:* Use the hand stabilizing over the pelvis to palpate the gluteus medius muscle simultaneously by adjusting the position of the hand so that the fingers are touching the lateral aspect of the ilium, above the greater trochanter, as described for the previous test.

4. *Observe:* Observe the client abducting the hip, moving the free leg sideward, while maintaining neutral rotation during this movement (Figure 21-38, *C*).[10]

5. *Grade:* The client is graded according to standard definitions of muscle grades.

Substitutions: Lateral muscles of the trunk may contract to bring the pelvis toward the thorax, effecting partial abduction at the hip.[10] If the hip is externally rotated, the hip flexors may assist in abduction.[6,7,10,15]

HIP ADDUCTION

Muscles[4,10,12]	Innervation[4,10,12]
Adductor magnus	Obturator L2-4
Adductor brevis	
Adductor longus	
Gracilis	
Pectineus	Femoral L2-4

Procedure for Testing Grades N (5) to F (3)

1. *Position:* The client assumes a side-lying position, with the test limb lowermost; the therapist supports the uppermost limb in 25 degrees of abduction and stands behind the client.[12] This test may also be done with the client in the supine position.[6,8,10]

2. *Stabilize:* Support the client's upper leg in partial abduction while the client grasps the supporting surface for stability.[5,6,10,14]

3. *Palpate:* Palpate any of the adductor muscles as follows: adductor magnus at the middle of the medial surface of the thigh; adductor longus at the medial aspect of the groin; gracilis on the medial aspect of the posterior surface of the knee, just anterior to the semitendinosus tendon.[15]

4. *Observe:* Observe the client adducting the hip by raising the lower leg from the table until it meets the upper leg. Observe that there is no rotation, flexion, or extension of the hip or pelvic tilting (Figure 21-39, *A*).[12,14]

5. *Resist:* Provide resistance over the medial aspect of the leg, just proximal to the knee, downward toward abduction or outward if tested in supine position (Figure 21-39, *B*).[6,7,10,12-14]

Procedure for Testing Grades P (2), T (1), and 0

1. *Position:* The client is supine; the limb to be tested is abducted to 45 degrees. The therapist stands next to the client on the opposite side.

2. *Stabilize:* Provide stabilization over the iliac crest on the side to be tested.[10]

3. *Palpate:* The client is palpated in the same manner as described for the previous test.

4. *Observe:* Observe the client adducting the leg toward midline (Figure 21-39, *C*).

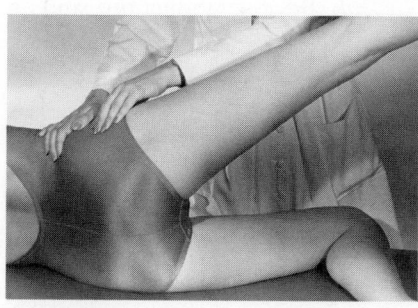 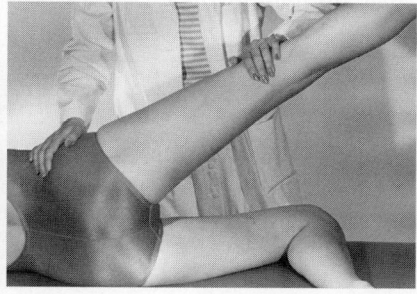 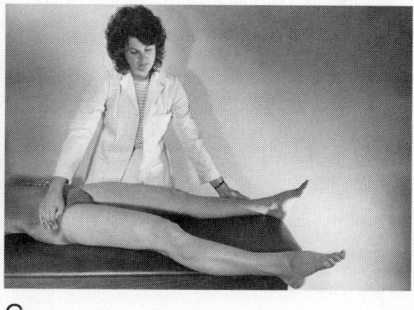

A   B   C

Figure 21-38   Hip abduction. **A,** Palpate and observe. **B,** Resist. **C,** Gravity-minimized position.

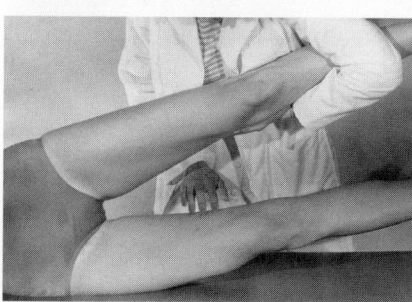 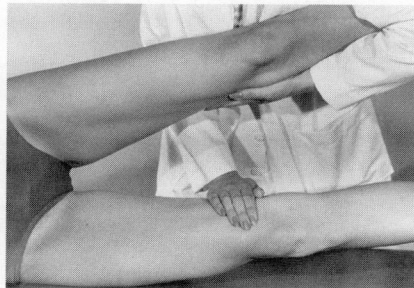 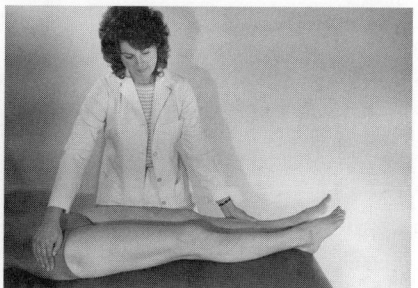

A   B   C

Figure 21-39   Hip adduction. **A,** Palpate and observe. **B,** Resist. **C,** Gravity-minimized position.

5. *Grade:* The client is graded according to standard definitions of muscle grades.

Substitutions: Hip flexors may substitute for adductors. The client will internally rotate the hip and tilt the pelvis backward. Hamstrings may be used to substitute for adduction. The client will externally rotate the hip and tip the pelvis forward.[12-15]

HIP EXTERNAL ROTATION

Muscles[10,12]	Innervation[10,12]
Quadratus femoris	Sacral plexus, L5, S1
Piriformis	Sacral plexus, S1,2
Obturator internus	Sacral plexus, L5-S2
Obturator externus	Obturator nerve, L3,4
Gemellus superior	Sacral plexus, L5-S2
Gemellus inferior	Sacral plexus, L4-S1

Procedure for Testing Grades N (5) to F (3)

1. *Position:* The client is seated, with knees flexed over the edge of the table. A small pad or folded towel is placed under the knee on the side to be tested. The therapist stands in front of the client toward the side to be tested.[6,10,12-14]
2. *Stabilize:* Provide stabilization at the lateral aspect of the knee on the side to be tested. The client may grasp the edge of the table to stabilize the trunk and pelvis.[6,10,14]
3. *Palpate:* These deep muscles are difficult or impossible to palpate.[6] Action of the external rotators may be detected by palpating deeply posterior to the greater trochanter of the femur.[10]
4. *Observe:* Observe the client rotating the thigh outwardly, moving the foot medially (Figure 21-40, *A*).
5. *Resist:* Provide resistance at the medial aspect of the lower leg, just proximal to the ankle in a lateral direction, toward internal rotation.[6,7,10,12-14] Resistance should be given carefully and gradually, because the use of the long lever arm can cause joint injury if sudden forceful resistance is given. Clients with knee instability should be tested in the supine position (Figure 21-40, *B*).[7,10]

Procedure for Testing Grades P (2), T (1), and 0

1. *Position:* The client is supine, with hips and knees extended; the hip to be tested is internally rotated. The therapist is standing next to the client on the opposite side.[10,12]
2. *Stabilize:* Provide stabilization at the pelvis on the side to be tested.
3. *Palpate:* Action of the external rotators may be detected by palpating deeply posterior to the greater trochanter of the femur.[10]
4. *Observe:* Observe the client externally rotating the thigh (roll laterally). Gravity may assist this motion once the client has passed the neutral position. The therapist may use one hand to palpate and the other to offer slight resistance during the second half of the movement to compensate for the assistance of gravity. If the range can be completed with slight resistance, a grade of *poor* can be given (Figure 21-40, *C*).[10]
5. *Grade:* The client is graded according to standard definitions of muscle grades for fair to normal muscles. Muscles are graded *poor* if ROM in the gravity-minimized position can be achieved against slight resistance during the second half of the ROM. A grade of *trace* can be assigned if contraction of external rotators can be detected by the deep palpation, described for the previous test, when the movement is attempted in the gravity-minimized position.[10]

Substitutions: The gluteus maximus may substitute for the deep external rotators when the hip is in extension. The sartorius may substitute, but external rotation will be accompanied by hip flexion, abduction, and knee flexion.[7,15]

HIP INTERNAL ROTATION

Muscles[4,10,14]	Innervation[10,14]
Gluteus minimus	Superior gluteal nerve, L4-S1
Gluteus medius	
Tensor fasciae latae	

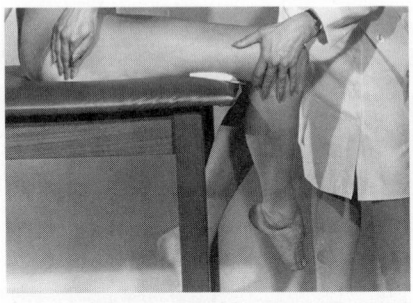 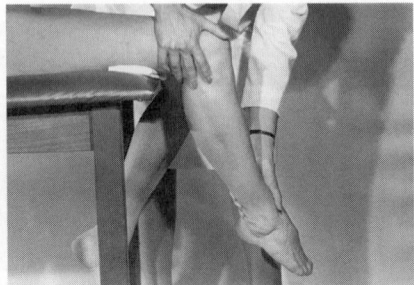 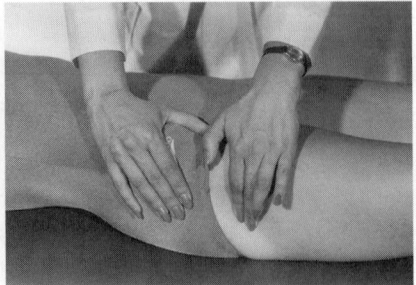

A   B   C

Figure 21-40 Hip external rotation. **A,** Palpate and observe. **B,** Resist. **C,** Gravity-minimized position.

Procedure for Testing Grades N (5) to F (3)

1. *Position:* The client is seated on a table, with the knees flexed over the edge and with a small pad placed under the knee. The therapist stands in front of or next to the client on the side to be tested.[6,10] (The therapist is shown on the opposite side in the illustration so that the palpation and stabilization will be apparent.)
2. *Stabilize:* Provide stabilization at the medial aspect of the knee. The client may grasp the edge of the table to stabilize the pelvis and trunk.[6,10,14]
3. *Palpate:* Palpate the gluteus medius between the iliac crest and the greater trochanter.[4]
4. *Observe:* Observe the client internally rotating the thigh, moving the foot laterally. The therapist should observe that the client does not lift the pelvis on the side being tested (Figure 21-41, *A*).[6,9,10]
5. *Resist:* Provide resistance at the lateral aspect of the lower leg, pushing the leg medially and, therefore, the thigh toward external rotation. The resistance is stressful to the knee joint. Clients with knee instability should be tested in the supine position described for the next test (Figure 21-41, *B*).[7,10,14]

Procedure for Testing Grades P (2), T (1), and 0

1. *Position:* The client is supine, with hips and knees extended; the hip to be tested is in external rotation. The therapist stands on the opposite side.[10,12]
2. *Stabilize:* Provide stabilization over the iliac crest on the side to be tested.[10]
3. *Palpate:* The client is palpated in the same manner as described for the previous test.
4. *Observe:* Observe the client rotating the thigh inwardly or medially. As in external rotation, gravity may assist the motion once the neutral position is passed but to a lesser degree than in the test for external rotation (Figure 21-41, *C*).
5. *Grade:* The client is graded according to standard definitions of muscle grades.
   Substitutions: Hip adduction and knee flexion may substitute; trunk medial rotation may also cause some internal rotation of the hip.[7,15]

KNEE FLEXION

Muscles[4,10,14]	Innervation[4,10,12,13]
Biceps femoris	Sciatic nerve, L5-S2
Semitendinosus	
Semimembranosus (hamstrings)	

Procedure for Testing Grades N (5) to F (3)

1. *Position:* The client is prone, with knees and hips in extension and neutral rotation with the foot in midline and toes hanging over the end of the table.[5,7,10,12-14] The therapist stands next to the client on the opposite side, or the same side, toward the lower end of the supporting surface.[10]
2. *Stabilize:* Provide stabilization firmly over the posterior aspect of the thigh, above the tendinous insertion of the knee flexors.[6,10]
3. *Palpate:* For the biceps femoris tendon proximal to the knee joint, palpate on the lateral aspect of the popliteal fossa; for the semitendinosus tendon proximal to the knee joint, palpate medial to the popliteal fossa.[4,6,15]
4. *Observe:* Observe the client flexing the knee to slightly less than 90 degrees (Figure 21-42, *A*).[13,15]
5. *Resist:* Provide resistance over the posterior aspect of the ankle downward toward knee extension.[6,10,13] Note that not as much resistance can be applied to knee flexion in this position as when tested in sitting position with the hip flexed (Figure 21-42, *B*).[14]

Procedure for Testing Grades P (2), T (1), and 0

1. *Position:* The client assumes a side-lying position, with knees and hips extended and in neutral rotation. The therapist stands next to the client and supports the upper leg in slight abduction to allow testing of the lower leg.[10]
2. *Stabilize:* Provide stabilization over the medial aspect of the thigh.
3. *Palpate:* Palpate the semitendinosus as described for the previous test.
4. *Observe:* Observe the client flexing the knee of the lower leg (Figure 21-42, *C*).
5. *Grade:* The client is graded according to standard definitions of muscle grades.

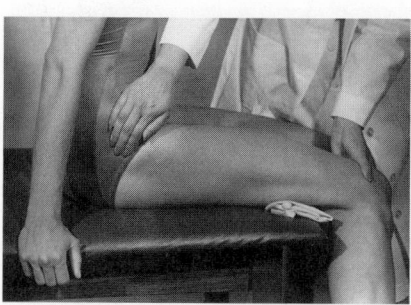 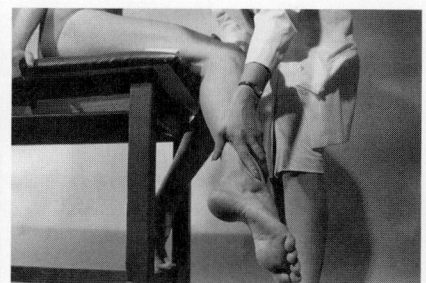 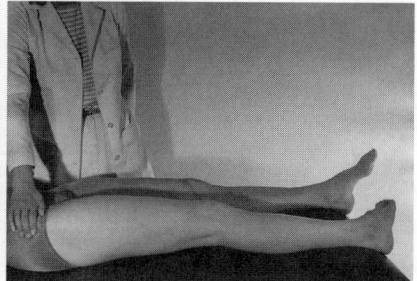

A   B   C

Figure 21-41 Hip internal rotation. **A,** Palpate and observe. **B,** Resist. **C,** Gravity-minimized position.

Substitutions: The sartorius may substitute or assist the hamstrings, but hip flexion and external rotation will occur simultaneously.[10,12,13,15] The gracilis may substitute, causing hip adduction with knee flexion.[12] The gastrocnemius may assist or substitute if strong plantar flexion of the ankle occurs during knee flexion.[10,12,13]

KNEE EXTENSION

Muscles[10]	Innervation[10]
The quadriceps group:	
Rectus femoris	Femoral nerve, L2-4
Vastus intermedius	
Vastus medialis	
Vastus lateralis	

Procedure for Testing Grades N (5) to F (3)

1. *Position:* The client is seated, with knees flexed over the edge of the table and feet suspended off the floor. The client may lean backward slightly to release tension on the hamstrings and grasp the edge of the table for stability.[6,10,12] The therapist stands next to the client on the side to be tested.[6,12]

2. *Stabilize:* Provide stabilization at the thigh by holding hand firmly over it, or place one hand under the client's knee to cushion it from the edge of the table. The client may grasp the edge of the table.[7,10, 12-14]

3. *Palpate:* Any of the muscles in the quadriceps femoris group can be palpated as follows: the rectus femoris on the anterior aspect of the midthigh; the vastus medialis on the medial aspect of the distal thigh; the vastus lateralis on the lateral aspect of the midthigh. The vastus intermedius cannot be palpated.[6,15]

4. *Observe:* Observe the client extending the knee to slightly less than full ROM. Observe for hip movements that may betray evidence of substitutions (Figure 21-43, *A*).

5. *Resist:* Provide resistance on the anterior surface of the leg, just above the ankle, with downward pressure toward knee flexion.[6,10,14] The client should not be allowed to lock the knee joint at the end of the ROM when full extension is achieved.[7,10] Maintenance of a slight amount of knee flexion will prevent this condition. Resistance to a locked knee can cause joint injury (Figure 21-43, *B*).[10]

Procedure for Testing Grades P (2), T (1), and 0

1. *Position:* The client assumes a side-lying position on the side to be tested. The lower leg is positioned with the hip extended and the knee flexed to 90 degrees. The therapist stands behind the client.

2. *Stabilize:* Provide stabilization at the upper leg in slight abduction with one hand, with the other hand over the anterior aspect of the thigh on the leg to be tested.[10]

3. *Palpate:* Any of the muscles can be palpated, as described for the previous test, with the same hand used to stabilize the

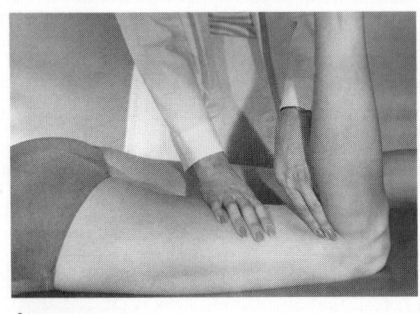 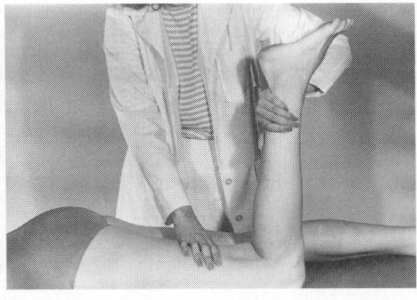 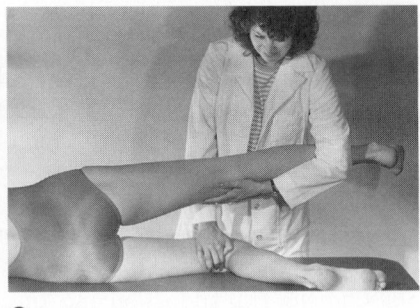

Figure 21-42 Knee flexion. **A,** Palpate and observe. **B,** Resist. **C,** Gravity-minimized position.

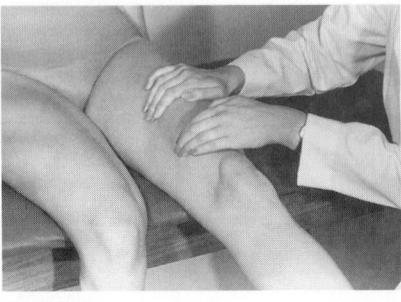 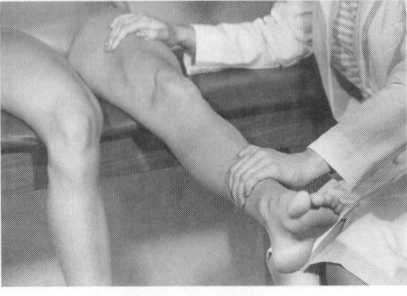 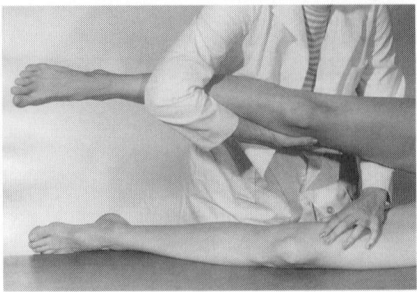

Figure 21-43 Knee extension. **A,** Palpate and observe. **B,** Resist. **C,** Gravity-minimized position.

client's thigh. Then ask the client to straighten the leg, extending the knee. Observe for hip movements that may betray signs of substitution (Figure 21-43, *C*).

4. *Grade:* The client is graded according to standard definitions of muscle grades.

Substitutions: Tensor fasciae latae may substitute for or assist weak quadriceps. In this case, hip internal rotation will accompany knee extension.[6,10,14]

ANKLE PLANTAR FLEXION

Muscles[4,10,14]
Gastrocnemius
Soleus

Innervation[14]
Tibial nerve, S1,2
Tibial nerve, L5-S2

Procedure for Testing Grades N (5) to F (3)

1. *Position:* The client is prone, with the hips and knees extended and the feet projecting beyond the edge of the table. The therapist stands at the lower end of the table, facing the client's feet.[6,7,13,14]
2. *Stabilize:* The weight of the leg is usually adequate stabilization. The client may stabilize the leg proximal to the ankle.[6]
3. *Palpate:* Palpate the gastrocnemius on the posterior aspect of the calf of the leg or the soleus, which is slightly lateral to and beneath the lateral head of the gastrocnemius.[15] The gastrocnemius tendon above the calcaneus may also be palpated.[10]
4. *Observe:* Observe the client flexing the plantar portion of the ankle. Observe for flexion of the toes and forefoot before movement of the heel, which may indicate substitutions (Figure 21-44, *A*).[6,14,15]
5. *Resist:* Provide resistance on the posterior aspect of the calcaneus as if pulling downward and on the forefoot as if pushing forward.[12] If there is considerable weakness, pressure to the calcaneus may be sufficient (Figure 21-44, *B*).[14]

Procedure for Testing Grades P (2), T (1), and 0

1. *Position:* The client assumes a side-lying position on the side to be tested; the hip and knee of the lower limb are extended, and the ankle is in midposition. The upper limb may be flexed at the knee to keep it out of the way. The therapist stands at the lower end of the table.[6,10]
2. *Stabilize:* Provide stabilization over the posterior aspect of the calf.[10]
3. *Palpate:* Palpate the client in the same manner as described for the previous test.
4. *Observe:* Observe the client pulling the heel upward, pointing the toes down. Observe for toe flexion, inversion, or eversion of the foot, which may indicate substitutions (Figure 21-44, *C*).
5. *Grade:* The client is graded according to standard definitions of muscle grades.

Substitutions: The flexor digitorum longus and flexor hallucis longus can substitute for plantar flexors, producing toe flexion and flexion of the forefoot, with incomplete movement of the calcaneus. Substitution by the peroneus longus and brevis will cause foot eversion, and substitution by the tibialis posterior will cause foot inversion. Substitution by all three will effect plantar flexion of the forefoot, with limited movement of the calcaneus.[10,12,13,15]

ANKLE DORSIFLEXION WITH INVERSION

Muscles[6,10,12]
Tibialis anterior

Innervation[6,10,14]
Peroneal nerve, L4-S1

Procedure for Testing Grades N (5) to F (3)

1. *Position:* The client is seated, with the legs flexed at the knees, over the edge of the table. The therapist sits in front of the client, slightly to the side to be tested.[6,10,12-14]
2. *Stabilize:* Provide stabilization at the leg, just above the ankle. The client's heel can rest in the therapist's lap.[6,12]
3. *Palpate:* Palpate the tibialis anterior tendon on the anterior medial aspect of the ankle joint.[6,7,10] Muscle fibers may be palpated on the anterior surface of the leg, just lateral to the tibia.[15]
4. *Observe:* Observe the client dorsiflexing and inverting the foot, keeping the toes relaxed.[12] Watch for extension of

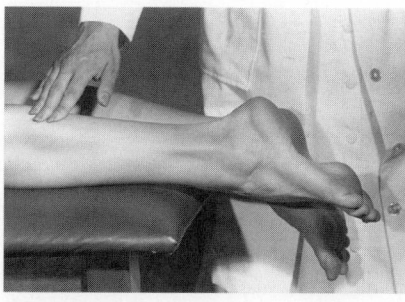
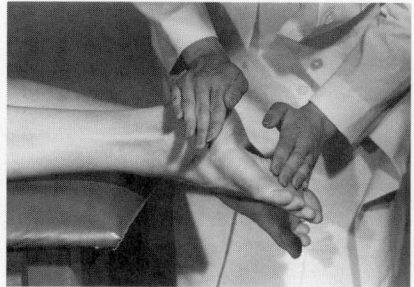
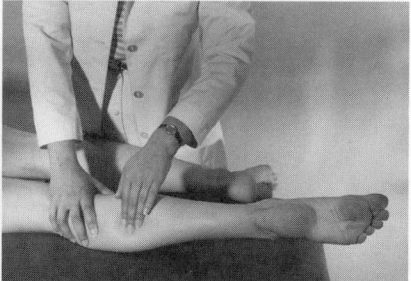

A   B   C

Figure 21-44 Ankle plantar flexion. **A,** Palpate and observe. **B,** Resist. **C,** Gravity-minimized position.

the great toe preceding the ankle motion, which may be a sign of muscle substitution (Figure 21-45, *A*).[9,12]

5. *Resist:* Provide resistance on the medial dorsal aspect of the foot, toward plantar flexion and eversion (Figure 21-45, *B*).[6,10,14]

Procedure for Testing Grades P (2), T (1), and 0

The same position and procedure described for the previous test may be used, with modified grading. The test may also be performed with the client in a side-lying or supine position.[7,10]

1. *Grade:* If the against-gravity position is used in the procedure for grades *P* to *0*, the therapist must exercise clinical judgment to determine muscle grades. Partial ROM against gravity can be graded *poor*.[12] If the test is performed in the supine position for these grades, standard definitions of muscle grades may be used.[10]

   Substitutions: The extensor hallucis longus and extensor digitorum longus may assist or substitute. Movement will be preceded by extension of the great toe or by all of the toes.[7,10,12-15]

FOOT INVERSION

Muscles[10,14]
Tibialis posterior

Innervation[7,8]
Tibial nerve, L5, S1

Procedure for Testing Grades N (5) to F (3)

1. *Position:* The client assumes a side-lying position on the side to be tested, with the hip in neutral rotation, the knee slightly flexed, and the foot and ankle in a neutral position.[6] The upper leg may be flexed at the knee to keep it out of the way. The therapist stands at the end of the table.

2. *Stabilize:* Provide stabilization at the leg to be tested above the ankle joint on the dorsal surface of the calf, being careful not to put pressure on the tibialis posterior muscle.[6,10]

3. *Palpate:* Palpate the tendon of the tibialis posterior muscle between the medial malleolus and navicular bone or above and just posterior to the medial malleolus.[6,7,10]

4. *Observe:* C invert the foot, keeping the toes relaxed. There normally will be some plantar flexion as well (Fig. 21-46, *A*).[10,14]

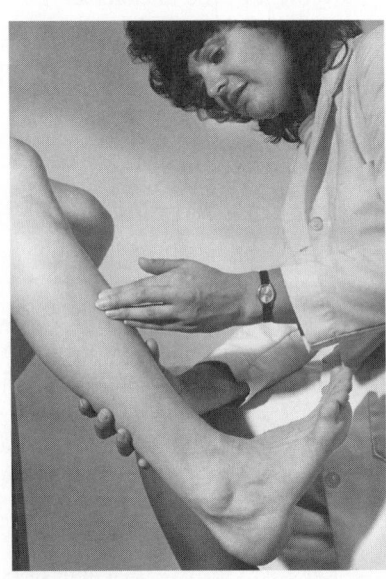
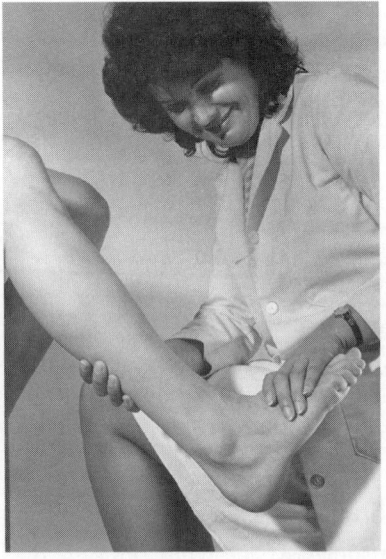

A   B

Figure 21-45 Ankle dorsiflexion with inversion. **A,** Palpate and observe. **B,** Resist.

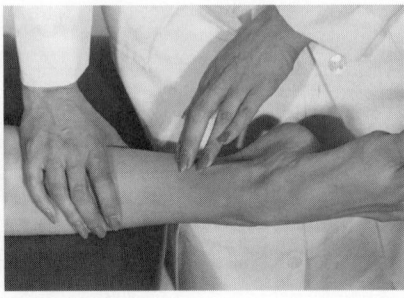
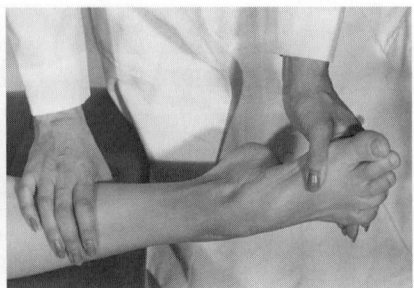

A   B

Figure 21-46 Foot inversion. **A,** Palpate and observe. **B,** Resist.

5. *Resist:* Provide resistance on the medial border of the forefoot toward eversion (Fig. 21-46, *B*).[6,7,10,14]

Procedure for Testing Grades P (2), T (1), and 0

1. *Position:* The client is supine, with the hip extended and in neutral rotation, the knee extended, and the ankle in midposition.
2. *Stabilize:* The client is stabilized in the same manner as described for the previous test.
3. *Palpate:* The client is palpated in the same manner as described for the previous test.
4. *Observe:* Observe the client moving the foot inward (medially), inverting it while keeping the toes relaxed.
5. *Grade:* The client is graded according to standard definitions of muscle grades.

   Substitutions: The flexor hallucis longus and flexor digitorum longus can substitute for the tibialis posterior. Movement will be accompanied by toe flexion, or toes will flex when resistance is applied.[10,12,13]

FOOT EVERSION

Muscles[10,14]	Innervation[10,14]
Peroneus longus	Peroneal nerve, L4-S1
Peroneus brevis	

Procedure for Testing Grades Normal (N) and Fair (F)

1. *Position:* The client assumes a side-lying position, with the lower leg flexed at the knee to keep it out of the way. The upper test leg is in hip extension with neutral rotation, knee extension, and ankle plantar flexion with foot inversion.[6]
2. *Stabilize:* Provide stabilization medially or laterally, above the ankle.[6]
3. *Palpate:* Palpate the peroneus longus over the upper half of the lateral aspect of the calf, just distal to the head of the fibula. Its tendon can be palpated on the lateral aspect of the ankle, above and behind the lateral malleolus. The peroneus brevis tendon may be palpated on the lateral border of the foot, proximal to the base of the

fifth metatarsal.[6,10,15] Its muscle fibers can be found on the lower half of the lateral surface of the leg, over the fibula.[10]
4. *Observe:* Observe the client everting the foot. (Note that this movement is normally accompanied by some degree of plantar flexion.[14,15]) Observe for dorsiflexion or toe extension, which may indicate substitutions (Figure 21-47, *A*).
5. *Resist:* Provide resistance against the lateral border and the plantar surface of the foot toward inversion and dorsiflexion (Figure 21-47, *B*).[6,14]

Procedure for Testing Grades P (2), T (1), and 0

1. *Position:* The client is supine, hip extended and in neutral rotation.[10] The knee is extended, and the ankle is in midposition.
2. *Stabilize:* Provide stabilization at the leg, under the calf.
3. *Palpate:* The client is palpated in the same manner as described for the previous test.
4. *Observe:* Observe the client everting the foot (Figure 21-47, *C*).
5. *Grade:* Grade according to standard definitions of muscle grades.

   Substitutions: The peroneus tertius, while everting the foot, also dorsiflexes it. If it is substituting for the peroneus longus and peroneus brevis, dorsiflexion will accompany eversion. The extensor digitorum longus can also substitute for the peroneals, and toe extension will precede or accompany eversion.[7,15]

SUMMARY

Many diseases and injuries result in muscle weakness. Screening tests can be used to assess the general level of strength available for the client to engage in ADLs; IADLs; and educational, work, and leisure occupations. These tests can also help determine which clients and muscle groups might require MMT.

MMT evaluates the level of strength in a muscle or muscle group. It is used with clients who have motor unit (lower motor neuron) disorders and orthopedic conditions. It does not measure muscle

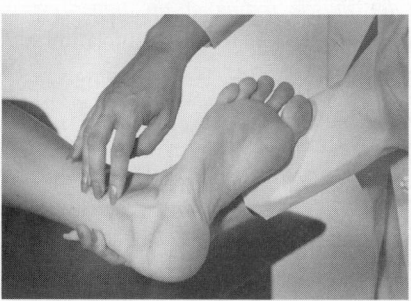
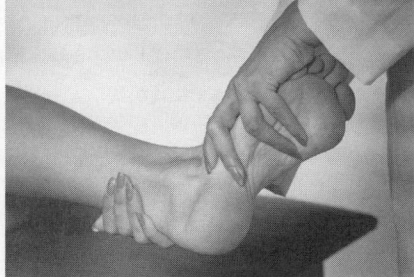
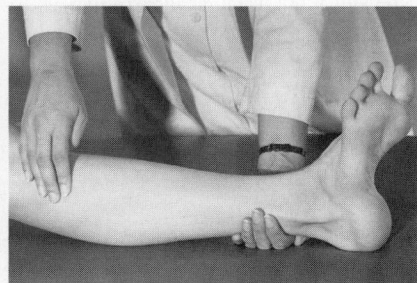

A   B   C

Figure 21-47 Foot eversion. **A,** Palpate and observe. **B,** Resist. **C,** Gravity-minimized position.

endurance or coordination, and it cannot be used accurately in upper motor neuron disorders when spasticity is present.

Accurate assessment of muscle strength depends on the knowledge, skill, and experience of the occupational therapist. Although there are standard definitions of muscle grades, clinical judgment is important in accurate evaluation.

Muscle test results are used to plan intervention strategies to improve occupational performance, compensate for muscle weakness, and increase strength. In some cases, the muscle test results can also be used to track the expected course and progression of the disease or disorder, which can assist the OT practitioner when choosing intervention modalities, strategies, and setting goals, as in the case of Sharon.

Review Questions

1. List three general classifications of physical dysfunction in which muscle weakness is a primary symptom.
2. List at least three purposes for assessing muscle strength.
3. Discuss five considerations and their implications in intervention planning that are based on the results of the muscle strength assessment.
4. Define *endurance*.
5. How can muscle weakness be differentiated from joint limitation?
6. If there is joint limitation, can muscle strength be measured accurately? How is strength recorded when available ROM is less than normal?
7. What does MMT measure?
8. What are the limitations of MMT?
9. When is MMT contraindicated?
10. What are the criteria for determining muscle grades?
11. In relation to the floor as a horizontal plane, describe or demonstrate what is meant by the terms "with gravity assisting," "with gravity minimized," "against gravity," and "against gravity and resistance."
12. List five factors that can influence the amount of resistance against which a muscle group can hold.
13. Define the muscle grades: N (5), F- (3-), F (3), P (2), P- (2-), T (1), and zero (0).
14. Explain what is meant by *substitution*.
15. How are substitutions most likely to be ruled out in the muscle testing procedure?
16. List the steps in the muscle testing procedure.
17. Is it always necessary to perform MMT to determine level of strength? If not, what alternatives may be used to make a general assessment of strength?
18. List the purposes of screening tests.

REFERENCES

1. Basmajian JF: *Muscles alive,* ed 4, Baltimore, 1978, Williams & Wilkins.
2. Bobath B: *Adult hemiplegia: evaluation and treatment,* ed 2, London, 1978, William Heinemann Medical Books.
3. Brunnstrom S: *Movement therapy in hemiplegia,* New York, 1970, Harper & Row.
4. Brunnstrom S: *Clinical kinesiology,* Philadelphia, 1972, FA Davis.
5. Chusid J: *Correlative neuroanatomy and functional neurology,* ed 19, Los Altos, CA, 1985, Lange Medical Publications.
6. Clarkson HM: *Musculoskeletal assessment,* ed 2, Philadelphia, 2000, Lippincott Williams & Wilkins.
7. Clarkson HM, Gilewich GB: *Musculoskeletal assessment,* Baltimore, 1989, Williams & Wilkins.
8. Cole JH, Furness AL, Twomey LT: *Muscles in action,* New York, 1988, Churchill Livingstone.
9. Crepeau EB, Cohn ES, Schell BA: *Willard and Spackman's occupational therapy,* ed 10, Philadelphia, 2003, Lippincott.
10. Daniels L, Worthingham C: *Muscle testing,* ed 5, Philadelphia, 1986, WB Saunders.
11. Hallum A: Neuromuscular diseases. In Umphred DA: *Neurological rehabilitation,* ed 4, St. Louis, 2001, Mosby.
12. Hislop HJ, Montgomery J: *Daniels and Worthingham's muscle testing,* ed 6, Philadelphia, 1995, WB Saunders.
13. Hislop HJ, Montgomery J: *Daniels and Worthingham's muscle testing,* ed 7, Philadelphia, 2002, WB Saunders.
14. Kendall FP, McCreary EK: *Muscles: testing and function,* ed 2, Baltimore, 1983, Williams & Wilkins.
15. Killingsworth A: *Basic physical disability procedures,* San Jose, CA, 1987, Maple Press.
16. Landen B, Amizich A: Functional muscle examination and gait analysis, *J Am Phys Ther Assoc* 43:39, 1963.
17. Latella D, Meriano C: *Occupational therapy manual for evaluation of range of motion and muscle strength,* Clifton, NY, 2003, Thomson Delmar Learning.
18. Pact V, Sirotkin-Roses M, Beatus J: *The muscle testing handbook,* Boston, 1984, Little, Brown.
19. Pulaski KH: Adult neurological dysfunction. In Creapeau EB, Cohen ES, Schell BA, editors: *Willard and Spackman's occupational therapy,* ed 10, Philadelphia, 2003, Lippincott Williams & Wilkins.
20. Rancho Los Amigos Hospital, Department of Occupational Therapy: *Guide for muscle testing of the upper extremity,* Downey, CA, 1978, Professional Staff Association of the Rancho Los Amigos Hospital.

22 | EVALUATION OF SENSATION AND INTERVENTION FOR SENSORY DYSFUNCTION

CYNTHIA COOPER
MICHELLE PRESSMAN ABRAMS

KEY TERMS

Mechanoreceptors	Nociceptors	Sensory threshold	Desensitization
Chemoreceptors	Neuropathy	Stereognosis	
Thermoreceptors	Proprioception	Habituation	

LEARNING OBJECTIVES

After studying this chapter the student or practitioner will be able to do the following:

1. Describe how sensation is positioned within the OTPF.
2. Describe and compare the difference in sensory loss due to a CVA versus a peripheral nerve repair.
3. Perform sensory mapping and sensory screening of the hand.
4. Interpret sensory findings in terms of client safety and identify compensatory strategies.
5. Instruct a client in an appropriate program for desensitization, describe ways to upgrade the program, and name the criteria that reflect client readiness to have the program upgraded.
6. Explain why people who lack protective sensation are at risk for serious injury and what types of injuries are possible.
7. Identify whether a client is a candidate for protective sensory reeducation or discriminative sensory reeducation based on sensory evaluation findings.

CHAPTER OUTLINE

Neuroplasticity
Somatosensory system
  Superficial sensation
  Proprioception
  Somatotopic arrangement
Sensory evaluation
Sensory assessment components
  History
  Sympathetic phenomena
  Sensory mapping of the hand
Sensory screening of the hand
Specific sensory tests

Proprioception
Stereognosis
Point localization
Semmes-Weinstein monofilaments
Threshold tests
Functional tests
Sensory reeducation
  Desensitization
  Protective sensory reeducation
  Discriminative sensory reeducation
Summary

THREADED CASE STUDY: MINSOO AND LAYLA, PART 1

Minsoo

Minsoo is a 70-year-old, right-hand-dominant male who survived a left *middle cerebral artery* (MCA) infarct on March 11, 2004. Minsoo was a very social man who liked to participate in community activities. As is typical with an MCA stroke, his early clinical symptoms included contralateral paralysis and sensory deficit, unilateral neglect, apraxia and impaired ability to judge distance, and limb-kinetic apraxia. These problems resulted in occupational limitations in self-feeding. The lack of sensation in his dominant hand caused Minsoo to either drop or "crush" the cup. Minsoo's occupational limitation in feeding had restricted his desire to participate in social gatherings where eating and drinking occurred. Being very sociable in nature, this marked decline in attending community functions was devastating to Minsoo's role as a social individual.

At the onset of the stroke, Minsoo demonstrated right hemiplegia. His tactile and proprioceptive sensations were absent, and he had loss of stereognosis in his right upper extremity. Functional recovery following a stroke can evolve over months or even years.[20] Throughout the first few months following the stroke, Minsoo began to recover some motor and sensory function in his right arm, but proprioception, stereognosis, and light touch discrimination remained grossly absent in his hand.

Critical Thinking Questions

1. Why does sensation affect Minsoo's occupational roles?
2. How can an occupational therapist incorporate purposeful activity that promotes sensory recovery into Minsoo's intervention?

Layla

Layla is a 12-year-old, right-hand-dominant female sixth-grader who fell against a glass tabletop and sustained a laceration of the ulnar nerve and ulnar artery at the right proximal forearm. Along with muscle imbalance associated with the motor loss of a high ulnar nerve injury, Layla also had sensory impairment of the right hand and forearm in the distribution of the ulnar nerve. In addition, she had dysesthesia and hypersensitivity so that she could not tolerate being touched along the ulnar forearm.

It was difficult for Layla to pull up a sleeve over this arm because of nerve pain. She could not perform the occupations of holding her school books on her forearm because of sensory pain. She said she felt self-conscious about not being able to simply use her arm normally in school, and she felt socially limited for this reason. She loved to play basketball and was not able to perform this occupation due to the sensory and motor impairment, so her role as an active and social preteen was disrupted. Her handwriting was impaired due to her injury, and she and her parents were concerned about keeping up with her role as a student.

Critical Thinking Questions

1. What sensory findings would substantiate Layla's need to accommodate her activities in order to protect her arm from further injury?
2. What sequence of sensory recovery is expected based on Layla's diagnosis?

People with normal sensation probably take for granted all that sensation contributes to their daily occupational performance. In contrast, people with sensory dysfunction may be acutely aware of the lost picture that normal sensation provides.[15] This chapter discusses the impact of somatosensory system dysfunction on occupational performance. It explores sensation in terms of touch, temperature, pain, and proprioception, and presents techniques for sensory testing, desensitization, and sensory reeducation. This chapter offers cases illustrating sensory loss secondary to both upper motor neuron (e.g., *cerebrovascular accident*, CVA) and lower motor neuron (e.g., peripheral nerve injury) deficits and stimulates clinical reasoning that guides evaluation, intervention, and outcomes appropriate to various diagnoses.

Sensation and sensory dysfunction affect clients' performance in areas of occupation such as *activities of daily living* (ADLs) or education. More specifically, *sensibility* is a body function, a component of the client factors that influences both motor and processing aspects of performance skills.

For example, Minsoo has deficits in body function (*proprioception*) resulting in diminished motor skills (inappropriate manipulation of grip force while holding a cup). These deficits in body function and motor skill lead to decreased performance in the occupation of drinking from a cup as part of his ADLs. All clients with sensory dysfunction, regardless of the etiology, should be evaluated to determine the occupational impact of the loss. The specific sensory tests and interventions may vary, according to the diagnosis and prognosis for recovery. The battery of tests selected may depend on whether the diagnosis is either *central nervous system* (CNS) or *peripheral nervous system* (PNS) in origin. For example, it is more likely for a person with CNS injury to have deficits in proprioception and stereognosis and for a person with PNS injury to have deficits in pressure threshold and two-point discrimination. A person with a history of CVA who then sustains a wrist fracture should be evaluated for proprioception and stereognosis, as well as pressure threshold, two-point discrimination, etc.

NEUROPLASTICITY

The brain has the plasticity to mechanically cause neuronal reorganization.[19] One aspect of this phenomenon, called neuroplasticity, includes the processes of habituation, learning and memory, and cellular recovery following an injury.[4] Along with changes in synaptic connections, there are also changes in non-neuronal cells such as astrocytes, associated with neuroplasticity.[4] Recent research is elucidating the role of glial cells in learning, memory, and repair of nerve damage.[11] Some concepts of neuroplasticity are as follows:[15]

- Sensory perception is a dynamic process that is experienced by the central nervous system.
- Receptor morphology is affected by hand use. Immobilization or disuse contributes to retrogressive modifications in receptors. Conversely, promoting normal use may stimulate new receptors.
- Because there is overlap of receptive fields of various nerve fibers, a single stimulus can excite different receptors.

Neurons may die following CNS injuries such as spinal cord injuries and strokes. The nervous system accommodates injuries by way of behavioral, physiological, and anatomical changes. Over time, the CNS can adapt by altering the strength of neural transmission through modifications in the structure and function of neurons and synapses. Occupational therapists can facilitate recovery through functional activities and involvement in occupation resulting in somatosensory reeducation.[21]

SOMATOSENSORY SYSTEM

The somatosensory system handles sensory input from superficial sources such as the skin, and from deep sources such as the musculoskeletal system. Sensation is stimulated by receptors in the periphery of the body. The sensory information then travels to the brain by way of the spinal cord.

Somatosensory receptors are specialized to respond to stimulation of a specific nature. These receptors are categorized as mechanoreceptors, chemoreceptors, and thermoreceptors. **Mechanoreceptors** respond to touch, pressure, stretch, and vibration and are stimulated by mechanical deformation. **Chemoreceptors** respond to cell injury or damage and are stimulated by substances that the injured cells release. **Thermoreceptors** respond to the stimulation of heating or cooling. Each of these three types of receptors has a subset called **nociceptors,** which sense pain when stimulated.[14]

A *dermatome* is the area of skin supplied by one spinal dorsal root and its spinal nerve. The affected dermatome correlates with the level of the spinal cord lesion. However, some peripheral nerves have innervation patterns that differ from dermatome patterns. This is due to regrouping of sensory axons in the brachial plexus and in the lumbosacral plexus[14] (Figure 22-1). Clinically, this is significant because sensory assessment along a dermatomal pattern is more appropriate in clients with central lesions, not peripheral lesions.

Afferents, which are peripheral axons, are categorized by the diameter of the axon. Axons with larger diameters transmit their information more quickly, in part because they are myelinated.[14]

Disturbances of somatosensation may present as paresthesia, hyperalgesia, dysesthesia, or allodynia. *Paresthesia* is described as a tingling, electrical, or prickling sensation. Tapping the volar aspect of the wrist may elicit paresthesias in the distribution of the median nerve in a person who has carpal tunnel syndrome. When this tapping elicits paresthesia, it is referred to as a *Tinel's sign. Hyperalgesia* is increased pain and may occur during nerve regeneration.[7] *Dysesthesia* is an unpleasant sensation that may be spontaneous or stimulated. *Allodynia* is pain in response to a stimulus that is not normally painful.[13] An example of allodynia is seen when a person with complex *regional pain syndrome* (also referred to as RSD) experiences pain with the mere movement of air wafting over the involved arm.

Neuropathy is dysfunction of the peripheral nervous system. The typical order of sensory impairment associated with peripheral neuropathy is loss in this sequence: discriminative touch and proprioception; cold; heat; and pain. This order is reversed for sensory recovery.[13]

SUPERFICIAL SENSATION

Superficial sensation is also referred to as cutaneous sensation. Compared to the proximal parts of our bodies, the distal parts have a higher density of receptors and smaller receptive fields. This arrangement contributes to enhanced fingertip sensation such as the ability to distinguish between one and two stimuli that are close together.[14] In terms of daily occupation, normal two-point discrimination enables a person to distinguish the edge of a dime from a penny with vision occluded. Figure 22-2 shows normal two-point discrimination values over different locations of the body.

Touch, pain, and temperature are aspects of superficial sensation. Touch encompasses both pressure and vibration. The sensation of touch is described as fine or coarse.[14]

Fine Touch

Superficial fine touch receptors include the following:[14]

- Meissner's corpuscles (light touch and vibration)
- Merkel's disks (pressure)

Subcutaneous fine touch receptors have larger receptor fields and therefore provide less discriminating information. Subcutaneous fine touch receptors include the following:[14]

- Pacinian corpuscles (touch and vibration)
- Ruffini's corpuscles (stretch of the skin)

Hairy skin transduces or converts the input of the same stimuli as glabrous (i.e., non-hairy) skin.[8] Hair follicle receptors sense hair displacement, which may explain the client

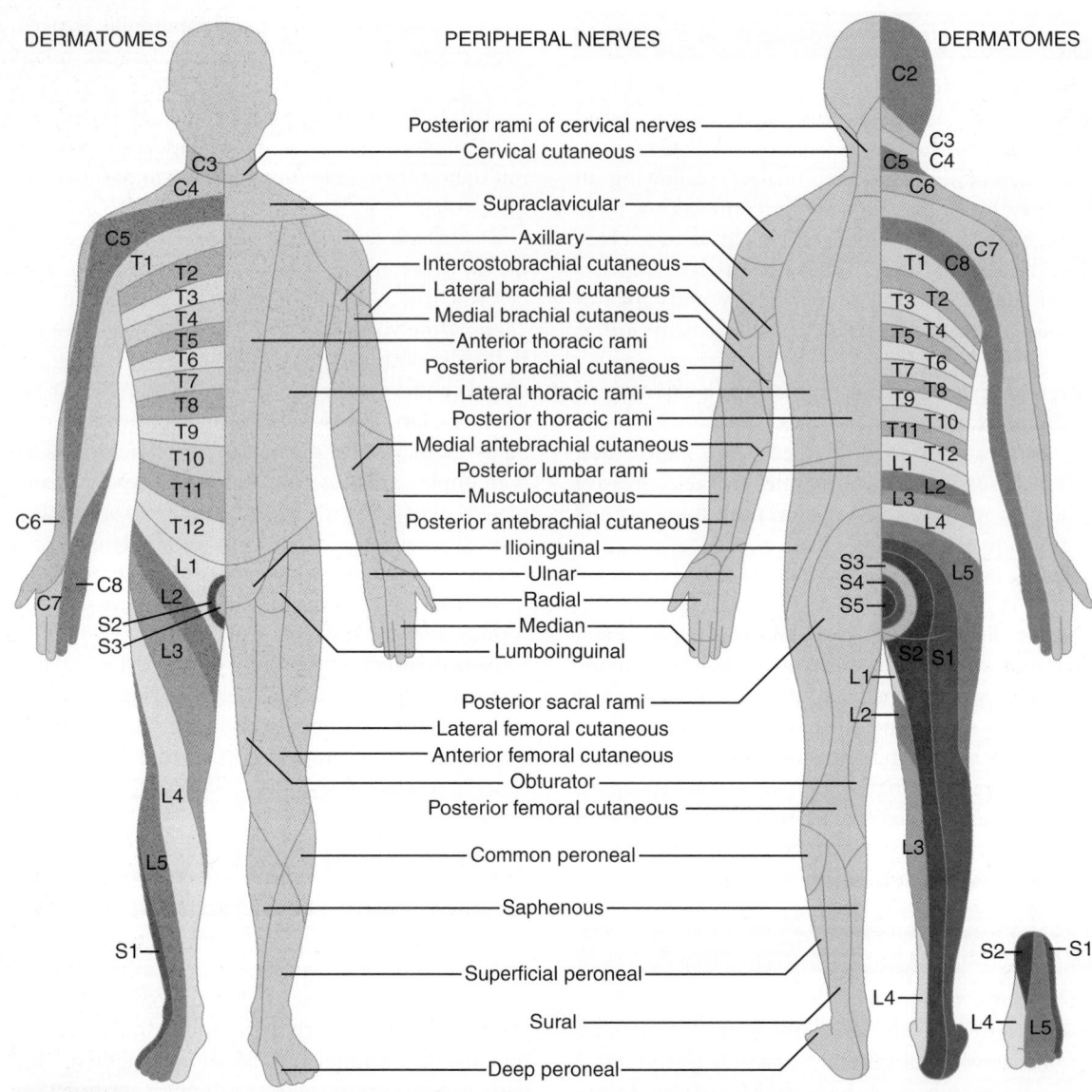

Figure 22-1 Cutaneous sensory distribution and dermatomes. (From Lundy-Ekman L: *Neuroscience: fundamentals for rehabilitation*, ed 2, Philadelphia, 2002, WB Saunders.)

with forearm hypersensitivity who said to her therapist, "My arm hair hurts." This is also why, for clients with hypersensitivity, application of splint straps and the intervention of desensitization should be implemented *in the direction of arm hair growth*, not against it.

Coarse Touch

Throughout the skin there are free nerve endings that provide sensations perceived as itch and tickle. Other free nerve endings include nociceptors that provide sensations perceived as pain, and thermal receptors that provide nonpainful sensations perceived as cold or warmth.[14]

Temperature

Thermal receptors detect warmth and cold. C fibers are associated with information about heat. A-delta fibers are associated with information about cold.[14] In the clinic, it is important to test temperature sensation prior to applying heat or cold modalities in order to avoid burn injuries. Thermal receptors are also critical for a person to be able to determine safe water temperature for bathing. The client with thermal sensory loss may need to learn compensatory strategies such as testing the water temperature with an unaffected body part.

Pain

Pain is an unpleasant sensory and perceptual experience that is associated with either actual or potential cellular damage. The experience of pain is subjective and multidimensional.[9]

Free nerve endings perceive pain, which is transmitted along small myelinated (covered with protective sheath) A-delta fibers. This fast pain is characterized as sharp in nature. When tissue has been damaged, there is onset of slow

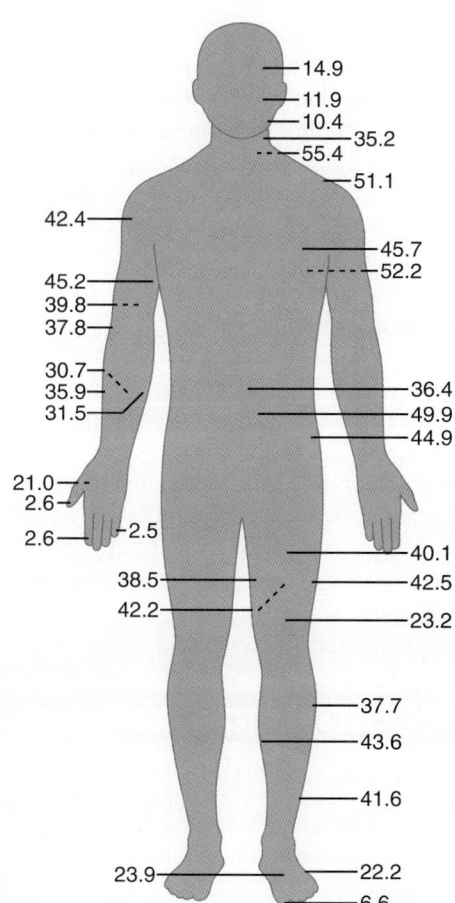

Figure 22-2 Normal two-point discrimination values over different locations of the body. (From Lundy-Ekman L: *Neuroscience: fundamentals for rehabilitation,* ed 2, Philadelphia, 2002, WB Saunders.)

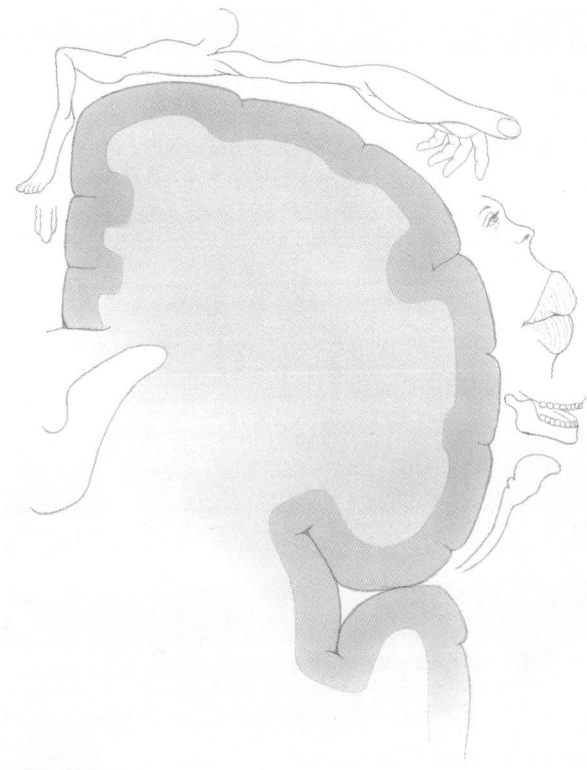

Figure 22-3 Homunculus. (From Lundy-Ekman L: *Neuroscience: fundamentals for rehabilitation,* ed 2, Philadelphia, 2002, WB Saunders.)

or aching quality of pain after the fast pain. Slow pain occurs by way of C fibers, which are smaller and unmyelinated, so the conduction velocities are slower. Slow pain is hard to localize because it uses various pathways. Fear and anxiety may contribute to worsening of pain. It is important to remember that edema also worsens pain, in part because edema increases pressure, aggravating free nerve endings.[13] Therefore, treating edema can help reduce pain.

PROPRIOCEPTION

Proprioception and pain are aspects of musculoskeletal sensation. **Proprioception** is the awareness of joint position.[8] Proprioception encompasses joint position, muscle stretch, and deep vibration. It has a direct effect at the spinal cord level through muscle spindles. Proprioception also has significant connections to the cortical and cerebellar pathways, with resulting impact on motor learning and motor adaptation.[24]

Following CVA and with other neurological disorders, proprioception is commonly affected.[12] Proprioceptive loss in the ankles can lead to diminished functional balance since the body relies on proprioception to sense if it is leaning

anteriorly or posteriorly. In Minsoo's case, he was unable to modulate the appropriate amount of grip force on the cup because of his deficits in proprioception in his right hand. When putting on a shirt, Minsoo would have to see the arm hole before inserting his right hand because he lacked awareness of where his arm was in space. Normal proprioception allows a person to locate a shirt armhole that is behind him and out of visual field.

SOMATOTOPIC ARRANGEMENT

The cerebral cortex receives information about the type and location of sensory stimulation (touch, proprioception, pain, and temperature) by way of conscious relay pathways. Discriminative touch, conscious proprioception, and stereognosis, on the other hand, travel a three-neuron pathway: (1) receptors to medulla; (2) medulla to thalamus; (3) thalamus to cerebral cortex.[14]

Information is received and organized somatotopically in the primary somatosensory cortex. The homunculus (Figure 22-3) is a diagram that shows the arrangement and proportions of cortical areas representing the surface of the body. Areas with large cortical representation indicate high density of receptors. As indicated in Figure 22-3, somatotopic arrangement is such that axons providing information from the index finger are situated closer to those from the thumb than those from the foot.[14]

SENSORY EVALUATION

The client's vision should be occluded for all sensory testing. This is accomplished by asking the client to keep the eyes closed, or by occluding the area with other means (Figure 22-4). A hand grid worksheet is used to record findings (Figure 22-5).

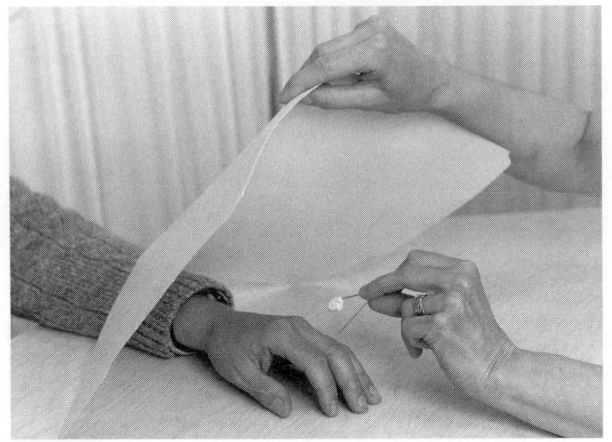

Figure 22-4   One method to occlude vision while performing sensory testing.

It is important to support the client's hand fully, using either the examiner's hand or resting the client's hand against putty to prevent it from moving, which could provide sensory information that interferes with the test being administered. Figure 22-6 demonstrates these options.

In order to create a conducive clinical setting and to promote accuracy in sensory evaluation, the following variables should be controlled:[7]

- Environment: background noise; try to have a quiet secluded room for sensory testing
- Client: ability to concentrate, anxiety, skin calluses, possible secondary agendas (e.g., incentives to have poorer status documented, such as litigation. Inconsistencies in response may occur).
- Instrument: calibration possibilities, manufacturer's quality
- Method: standard instructions, supporting and immobilizing the hand, consistency of stimulus application parameters, varying the timing and spacing of stimulus application, good documentation
- Examiner: skill, experience, concentration

SENSORY ASSESSMENT COMPONENTS

The components of a sensory assessment include a history, sympathetic phenomena, and sensory mapping of the hand.[7]

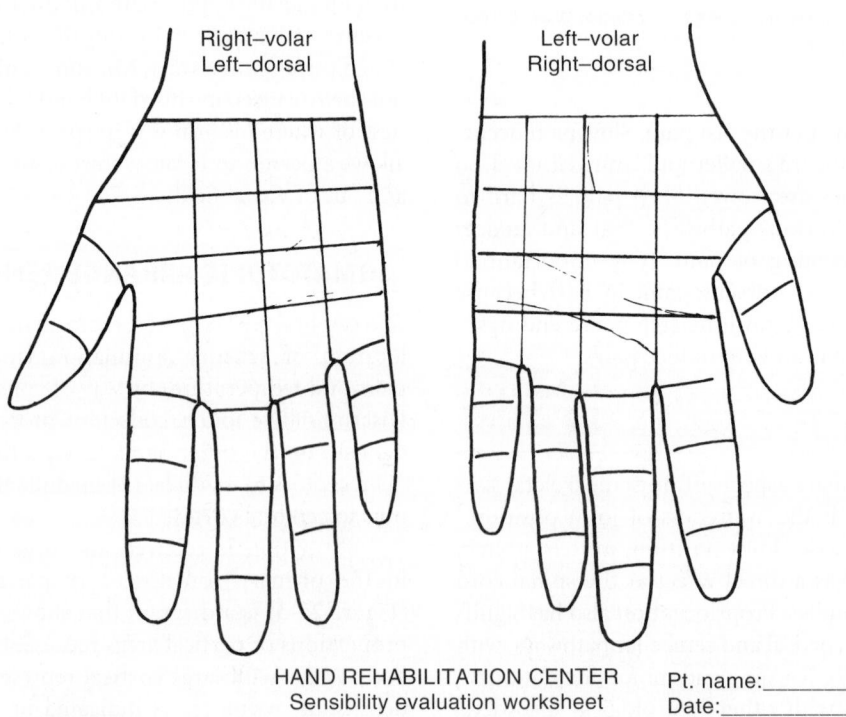

Right–volar
Left–dorsal

Left–volar
Right–dorsal

HAND REHABILITATION CENTER
Sensibility evaluation worksheet

Pt. name:_____
Date:_____

Figure 22-5   Hand grid worksheet. (From Callahan AD: Sensibility assessment for nerve lesions-in-continuity and nerve lacerations. In Mackin EJ, et al, editors: *Rehabilitation of the hand and upper extremity*, ed 5, St. Louis, 2002, Mosby.)

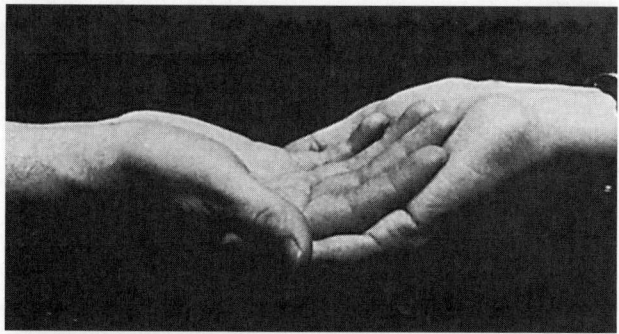

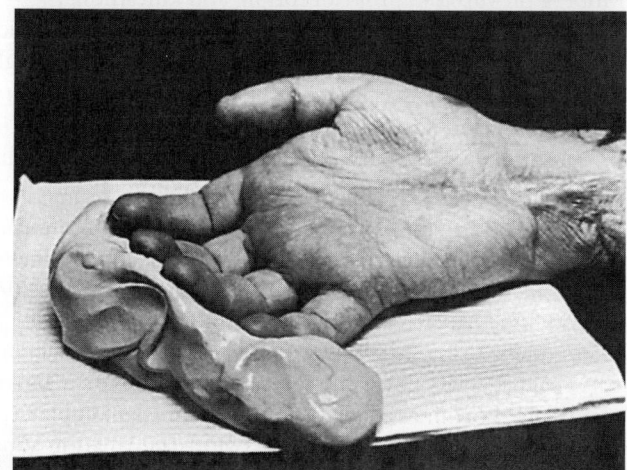

Figure 22-6 Ways to support the hand during sensory testing. **A,** In the examiner's hand, or **B,** in putty. (From Callahan AD: Sensibility assessment for nerve lesions-in-continuity and nerve lacerations. In Mackin EJ, editors: *Rehabilitation of the hand and upper extremity*, ed 5, St. Louis, 2002, Mosby.)

HISTORY

The history consists of the client interview and a review of medical reports. The following information should be included in the history:

- Name
- Age
- Hand dominance
- Sex
- Occupation
- Date of injury
- Nature of injury
- Client description of sensory problem
- Screening of motor function
- Grip and pinch if appropriate

SYMPATHETIC PHENOMENA

Sympathetic phenomena may correlate with sensory function because upper extremity cutaneous sensory fibers and sympathetic fibers follow the same pathways. In the upper extremity, the median nerve has more sympathetic fibers than the ulnar nerve, which may explain the increased risk

for developing complex RSD among clients with median nerve injury.

It is important to note the following:
- Vasomotor function: skin temperature, color, cold intolerance
- Sudomotor function: abnormal sweating: lack of sweating correlates with lack of discriminative sensation
- Pilomotor changes: no goose bumps
- Trophic changes: decrease in nutrition with atrophy of nails, finger pulps, slower healing, hair changes
- Increased risk for injury and slowness of healing

SENSORY MAPPING OF THE HAND

It may be helpful to begin with sensory mapping and sensory screening of the hand. Before testing, the client points out the area of sensory impairment using a finger of the unaffected hand. Some therapists draw this map right on the client's arm or hand (Figure 22-7). Show the client what a Semmes-Weinstein monofilament feels like when it is applied to a normal area, while the client's eyes remain open. Then with the client's eyes closed, repeat the application of the filament to the normal area (Figure 22-8).[2]

To first identify normal areas, test the volar surface and progress testing from distal to proximal and mark the normal areas (where filament number 2.83 is identified). Repeat this on the dorsum as appropriate. Then return to the volar surface and proceed with the filaments for the next levels.[2] If the examiner prefers, clients can map their area of involvement themselves. The probe should be moved over the hand slowly using a light pressure.[7] In the case of Layla, sensory

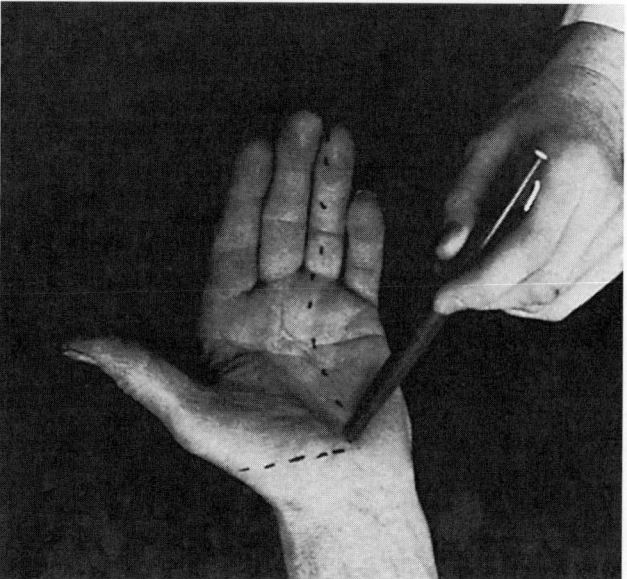

Figure 22-7 Sensory mapping on the patient's hand. (From Callahan AD: Sensibility assessment for nerve lesions-in-continuity and nerve lacerations. In Mackin EJ, et al, editors: *Rehabilitation of the hand and upper extremity*, ed 5, St. Louis, 2002, Mosby.)

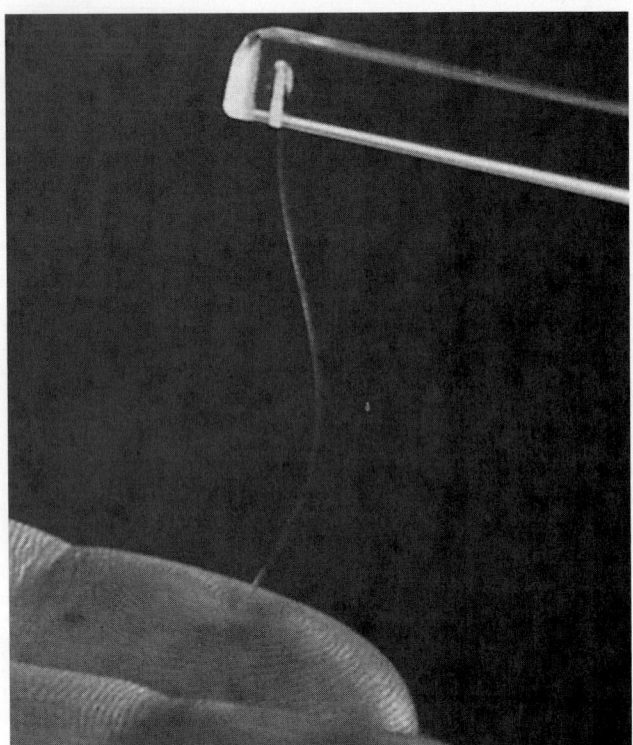

Figure 22-8 Application of Semmes-Weinstein monofilament to patient's finger tip. (From Fess EE: Documentation: essential elements of an upper extremity assessment battery. In Mackin EJ, et al, editors: *Rehabilitation of the hand and upper extremity*, ed 5, St. Louis, 2002, Mosby.)

mapping delineated the ulnar distribution of the hand to be impaired.

SENSORY SCREENING OF THE HAND

Sensory screening is a timesaving method to determine some parameters of sensory loss. When screening the hand, specific sites can be used to reflect larger portions of the hand. For screening median nerve function, test the thumb tip, index tip, and index proximal phalanx. For screening ulnar nerve function, test the distal and proximal small finger and the proximal ulnar palm. For screening the radial nerve, test the thumb web space.[2]

The existence of blisters, altered sweat patterns, calluses, shiny or dry skin, blanching of skin, scars, or wounds should be documented.[2] These features can affect the results of sensory testing and help identify factors to monitor during daily occupations. Healing is slowed due to decrease of vascularity and nutrition. Absence of "wear" marks, such as calluses and dirt or grease stains, suggests that the hand is not being used.[7] When there is nerve damage, the resulting atrophy of the soft tissue leads to increased susceptibility of the tissue. Therefore, pinprick testing might elicit a drop of blood unexpectedly. It is mandatory that the occupational therapist follows universal precautions.

SPECIFIC SENSORY TESTS

It is important to know what you are testing and what you are not testing, and to interpret findings correctly. Some techniques for sensory testing are standardized. These include touch-pressure, moving and static two-point discrimination, point localization, vibration threshold, and Dellon's modification of the Moberg pickup test. Nonstandardized techniques for sensory testing include awareness of touch, pain or pinprick, temperature, vibration, stereognosis, the Moberg pickup test, proprioception, and kinesthesia.[3]

Sensory threshold is the least stimulus needed to elicit responses. Examples of threshold tests are tests for light touch, vibration, and cutaneous pressure thresholds. *Tactile discrimination* refers to the amount or number of sensory receptors in an area. Both moving and static two-point discrimination tests evaluate tactile discrimination.

Vibration thresholds can be tested qualitatively using a tuning fork. A high-frequency tuning fork tests higher-frequency quickly adapting receptors, known as Pacinian corpuscles. A low-frequency tuning fork tests lower-frequency quickly adapting receptors, known as Meissner corpuscles.[18] Findings from use of these hand-held instruments lack worthiness due to problems of instrument control and other procedural discrepancies. More information about vibration testing can be found in the hand therapy literature.[7]

PROPRIOCEPTION

Conscious proprioception is defined as the awareness of joint position in space. It is through cerebral integration of information about touch and proprioception that objects can be identified by tactile cues and pressure.

To evaluate proprioception, the tester should minimize the amount of tactile input provided to the volar or dorsal surface. Hold the lateral aspects of the body part and move the joint in flexion or extension with vision occluded. The client indicates if the body part is moving "up" or "down" to correspond with flexion or extension (Figure 22-9). Minsoo's proprioception was intact at the level of the wrist but absent at the fingers, which is consistent with the proximal-to-distal pattern of recovery.

STEREOGNOSIS

The use of both proprioceptive information and touch to identify an item with vision occluded is called **stereognosis**. Without stereognosis, it is impossible to pick out a specific object, such as a coin or a key, from one's pocket, or use a zipper that fastens on your back, or pick up a plate from a sink of sudsy water.

To test stereognosis, the client's vision should be occluded. Typical familiar items such as a pen, a spoon, a key, a closed large safety pain, or sunglasses are placed in the palm of the affected hand. The client manipulates the item to identify it

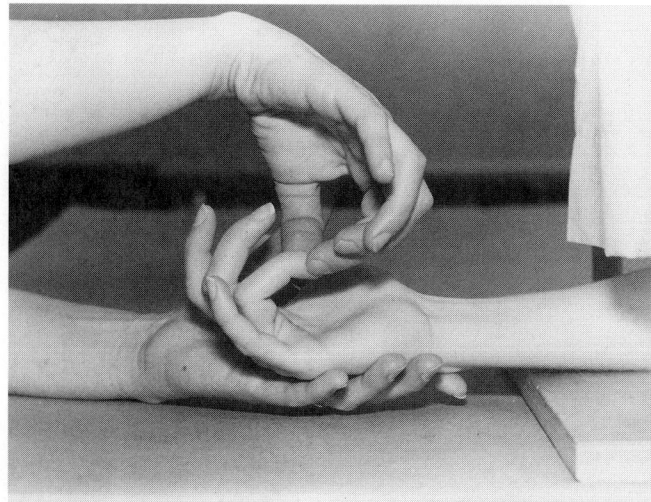

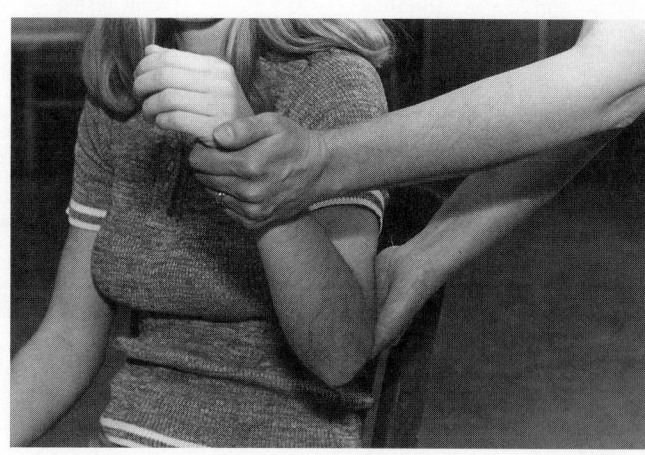

Figure 22-9 Testing proprioception of **A,** the fingers and **B,** of the elbow.

or its characteristics. If the motor function of the hand is impaired, the evaluator should assist by moving the item in the client's hand to provide adequate tactile input. (See Chapter 24 for more on stereognosis.)

POINT LOCALIZATION

Vibration and localization of touch are aspects of discriminative touch. The perception of point localization varies greatly. This test is thought by many to reflect a cognitive component of the client's abilities. For this reason, it is categorized as a tactile discrimination that requires cortical processing. To administer the point localization test, the client points with a small dowel to identify the area that was touched by a monofilament. The response is correct if the dowel is within one centimeter of accurate placement.[2]

SEMMES-WEINSTEIN MONOFILAMENTS

The Semmes-Weinstein monofilament test assesses pressure threshold.[2] It is a versatile and valid test that is easy to administer. The entire body can be assessed with this test, but it is more typical to use it on the hands. Testing technique must be consistent; otherwise there will be questions about intra-tester (from one test to the next with the same tester) and inter-tester (among various testers) reliability. Moderate correlation of the Semmes-Weinstein monofilaments with tests for object identification has been reported.[18] (See testing procedure under Threshold Tests.)

Pressure threshold categories for the monofilament test are as follows:
- Normal touch: light touch and deep pressure within normal limits.
- Diminished light touch: reduced recognition of light touch; however, the client probably has nearly normal

stereognosis and graphesthesia, good temperature awareness and protective sensation, and fair-to-good two-point discrimination.
- Diminished protective sensation: may tend to drop objects. Use of hands for object manipulation is diminished, but temperature and pain awareness are probably functional. May perceive two-point discrimination in the 7-10 mm range. This is a good level to begin sensory reeducation, which is addressed later in this chapter.
- Loss of protective sensation: difficulty using hands; temperature and pain awareness are likely to be absent; vision is required in order to handle objects. This client is at risk for injury despite the fact that deep pressure sensation and perception of pinprick may be intact. Instruct clients at this level in protective strategies to avoid injury.
- Untestable: No discrimination of levels of feeling except may possibly feel a pinprick. Instruct this client in protection and care of the hand. Layla initially fit this category but over many months, she regained diminished protective sensation of her ulnar digits.

THRESHOLD TESTS

Tests of sensory threshold[7] (Table 22-1) ask the question: What is the minimum stimulus that the client is able to perceive? Threshold tests evaluate pain, heat, cold, touch-pressure, and vibration.

Pinprick

Pinprick tests protective sensation. Client discerns between sharp or dull sides of the safety pin with random stimulation of sharp versus dull. Stimulate each area at least once with each stimulus.

TABLE 22-1 **Sensory Threshold and Functional Tests**

Test Category	Question	What Tested	Equipment	Results
Sensory Threshold	What is the minimum stimulus that the patient is able to perceive?	Pain	Sterilized safety pin	Intact protective sensation Absent protective sensation Hyperalgesic Pressure awareness only
		Heat/cold	Test tubes or cylinders	Intact protective sensation Absent protective sensation
		Touch-pressure	Semmes-Weinstein Pressure aesthesiometer (monofilaments)	Normal Diminished light touch Diminished protective sensation Loss of protective sensation Loss of all sensation except deep pressure Absence of all sensation
		Vibration	256-cps tuning fork	Abnormal or normal
Functional Tests	How functional is the patient's sensibility? Is there fine discriminative sensation or only gross sensation?	Static Two-Point Discrimination or Moving Two-point discrimination	Disk-Criminator or Boley Gauge	Normal Fair Poor Protective Anesthetic
		Localization of touch or localization of moving touch	Smallest diameter of the Semmes-Weinstein monofilament kit that patient can feel	No norms
		Moberg Pickup Test or Dellon modification of the Moberg Pickup Test	Everyday items such as coins, key, paper clip	No norms but allows observations about hand function
		Nine-Hole Peg Test	Nine-Hole Peg Test and stopwatch	Time in seconds

Equipment

A separate, sterilized safety pin is used for each individual client.

Results

- Intact protective sensation: correct response to both sharp and dull
- Impaired protective sensation: incorrect response to both sharp and dull
- Absent protective sensation: inability to perceive being touched
- Hyperalgesic: heightened pain reaction to the stimulus

Comments

Hyperalgesia may make this an unpleasant test for the client. Also, this test may cause discomfort to the client and there is concern for contamination/wounding related to the prospect of drawing blood. Some authorities do not advocate this test because it does not correlate with actual functional sensation. Yet, this test does help confirm that a nerve is not completely transected (i.e., cut).

Temperature Awareness

Temperature awareness is a test for protective sensation (Figure 22-10). If thermal sensation is impaired, heat modalities are likely to be contraindicated.

Equipment

Metal cylinders or test tubes with cold and warm water are needed.

Results

- Intact protective sensation: correct response to both hot and cold
- Absent protective sensation: inability to discern hot from cold

Comments

Test conditions are difficult to control. Some authorities are concerned about lack of research correlating temperature awareness with functional sensation. On a clinical level, the results of temperature awareness can be useful in determining the person's kitchen safety with use of the stove and bathroom safety with testing water temperature.

Touch-Pressure

Light touch is perceived by receptors in the superficial skin. Pressure (or deeper touch) is perceived by receptors in subcutaneous and deeper tissues. While light touch is important for fine discriminatory hand use, deep pressure is important as a form of protective sensation. Touch-pressure testing examines the spectrum from light touch to deep pressure.

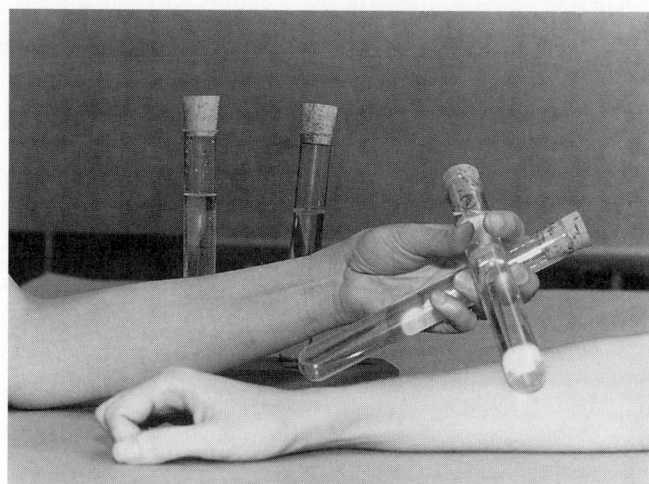

Figure 22-10 Test for temperature awareness.

Equipment

The Semmes-Weinstein pressure aesthesiometer consists of 20 probes (Figure 22-11). Each nylon filament has a number that "represents the logarithm of 10 times the force in tenths of milligrams (log 10 force 0.1 mg) required to bow the monofilament when it is applied perpendicular to the skin."[7]

Testing procedure

To administer the monofilament test, begin with the filaments for testing normal pressure threshold and then continue with filaments of increasing pressure until the client can identify being touched. The filaments are labeled from 1.65 to 6.65.

Because the finest filaments are difficult to feel, it is normal to need up to three stimulations at the same area before expecting the client to perceive being touched by these finer monofilaments, which are labeled 1.65 to 4.08. According to procedure, the tester applies those filaments three times at the same site. Filaments labeled higher than 4.08 are applied one time only. Always apply the filament in intervals of 1 to 1.5 seconds with the filament positioned perpendicularly; maintain the pressure for 1 to 1.5 seconds and lift the filament away in 1 to 1.5 seconds. The specific amount of pressure being exerted (tested) is reached once the filament bends. The client is instructed to respond by saying "touch." If the client gives one response, this is a positive response. After completing the volar surface of the hand, progress to the dorsal surface of the hand as appropriate.[2]

Results

See Table 22-2 for results.

Comments

Touch-pressure testing is the gold standard for clients with possible nerve entrapment such as carpal tunnel syndrome.

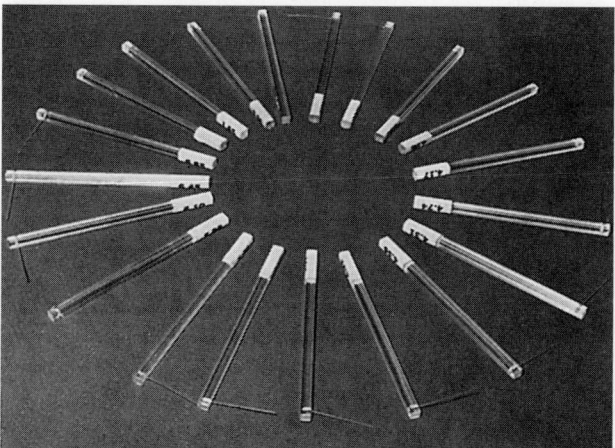

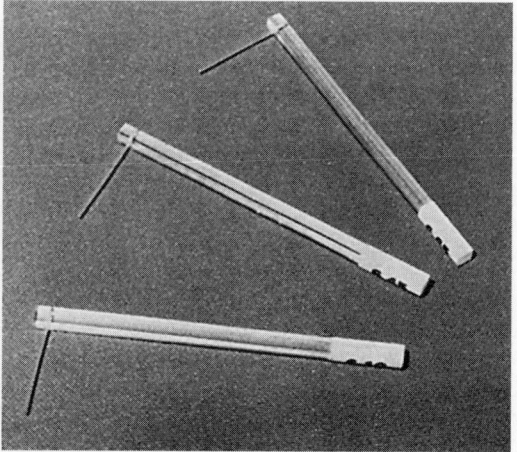

A   B

Figure 22-11 Semmes-Weinstein aesthesiometer monofilament set. **A,** A complete set and **B,** three monofilaments seen close up. (From Bell-Krotoski JA: Sensibility testing with the Semmes-Weinstein monofilaments. In Mackin EJ, et al, editors: *Rehabilitation of the hand and upper extremity*, ed 5, St. Louis, 2002, Mosby.)

Impaired pressure threshold compromises fine motor coordination in ADLs, such as donning earrings.

FUNCTIONAL TESTS

Functional sensory tests answer the question: How functional is the client's sensibility? Is there fine discriminative sensation or only gross sensation, a condition that would limit the client's ability to perform occupations?[2]

Static Two-Point Discrimination

While static two-point discrimination is considered to be the classic test of functional sensibility, there are differing opinions about the correlation of this test with fine hand-task use.

TABLE **22-2** **Semmes-Weinstein Monofilaments Interpretation Scale**

Color	Interpretation	Measurement
Green	Normal	1.65-2.83 marking
Blue	Diminished light touch	3.22-3.61 marking
Purple	Diminished protective sensation	3.84-4.31 marking
Red	Loss of protective sensation	4.56-6.65 marking
Red-lined	Untestable	>6.65 marking

One criticism has been about the potential variability in the force of application during testing. Despite this, good inter-tester reliability has been reported using the Disk-Criminator tool.[18]

Equipment

The Disk-Criminator or Boley Gauge (Figure 22-12) is needed. Instruments should be lightweight and the ends should not be sharp.

Testing procedure

Test only the pads of the fingers and thumb. Begin with 5 mm distance and test using a longitudinal orientation with light pressure only. This means to stop at the point of blanching the skin.

Results

Seven out of ten responses are required to be considered an accurate response. Increase the distance between the two points as needed until an accurate response is achieved. Stop testing after 15 mm distance between points and at less distance between points if the finger pulp length does not accommodate 15 mm. The norms are listed in Table 22-3.

Moving Two-Point Discrimination

Dellon reported that moving two-point discrimination returns before static two-point discrimination, so this test

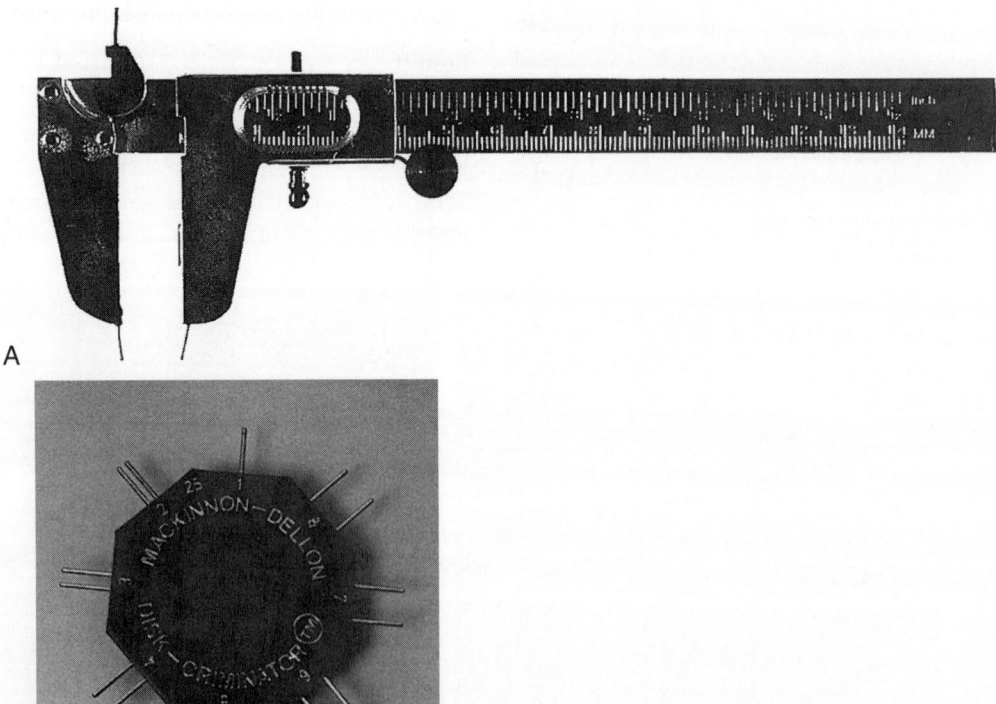

Figure 22-12   **A,** Boley Gauge and **B,** Disk-Criminator for testing static and moving two-point discrimination. (From Callahan AD: Sensibility assessment for nerve lesions-in-continuity and nerve lacerations. In Mackin EJ, et al, editors: *Rehabilitation of the hand and upper extremity*, ed 5, St. Louis, 2002, Mosby.)

TABLE 22-3 **Norms for the Static Two-Point Discrimination Test**

Classification	Distance
Normal	<6 mm
Fair	6-10 mm
Poor	11-15 mm
Protective	One point perceived
Anesthetic	No points perceived

provides an earlier assessment of return of discriminative sensation than does the static two-point discrimination test.

Testing procedure

Begin with the distance of the two points at 8 mm. Move the instrument proximally to distally on the fingertip using light pressure, keeping it in contact with the skin at all times. Maintain the two points parallel to the longitudinal axis so as not to stimulate the adjacent digital nerve. Normal moving two-point discrimination is 2 mm.

Localization of Touch

Localization of touch is considered to be a test of functional sensation because there is high correlation between this test and the test for two-point discrimination. This is an important test to perform following nerve repair as it helps to determine the client's baseline and projected functional prognosis.

Equipment

The smallest diameter of the Semmes-Weinstein monofilament kit that the client can feel is needed.

Testing procedure

Use the same filament over the entire area of involvement. Use the hand grid and test the center of the squares or zones on the hand grid documentation form. When the client feels the touch, they open their eyes and point to that exact area. Place a dot on the grid for correct responses. Stimulate each zone only one time.

Localization of Moving Touch

The localization of moving touch is the same as the localization of touch except the stimulus is moved for each zone along its midline, longitudinally.

Moberg Pickup Test

The Moberg Pickup Test is good for use with injuries involving the median and/or ulnar nerves. This test requires the ability to participate motorically.

Equipment

A sampling of everyday items such as coins, a key, or a paper clip is needed (Figure 22-13). The items are not standardized.

Testing procedure

Items are placed on the table in front of the client. Instruct the client to pick the items up as quickly as possible, one at a time, and place them in a box using the involved extremity. The time the task takes is recorded, and the examiner also observes which digits are used for the task. Then repeat the test with the uninvolved hand. Follow this with the involved hand, but with the eyes closed, noting the way in which the hand is used and the time the task takes.

Results

There are no norms for this test, but it allows for observations about hand function. This test is quick and easy to administer.

Dellon Modification of the Moberg Pickup Test

Dellon standardized the items used for the test and added the requirement that the client identify the items.

Testing procedure

If the ulnar nerve is not involved, try taping the ulnar digits to the client's palm if able. If the client is able to do the test with vision occluded, the examiner places items into the radial digits one at a time, and the client identifies the items. The examiner records the time it takes to identify each item, but 30 seconds is the maximum time allowed per item. Each item is placed in the client's hand two times.

Nine Hole Peg Test

The Nine Hole Peg Test assesses finger dexterity and can be especially helpful in looking at median nerve function and hand use.[16] It is commercially available.

Equipment

A Nine Hole Peg Test and stopwatch are needed.

Testing procedure

Follow test instructions.

Comments

There is high inter-rater reliability and normative data for this standardized evaluation tool.

The sensory tests above are used to identify impairments that warrant occupational therapy intervention. These interventions often include adaptation, compensation, and/or sensory reeducation.

SENSORY REEDUCATION

Within the somatosensory cortex, there is an inherent capacity for plasticity involving the circuitry.[5] Topographical reorganization of the cerebral cortex occurs following injury and can be influenced by sensory input and by learning and experience. This has been described eloquently by the neurologist and author, Frank R. Wilson, as a dynamic interplay of the

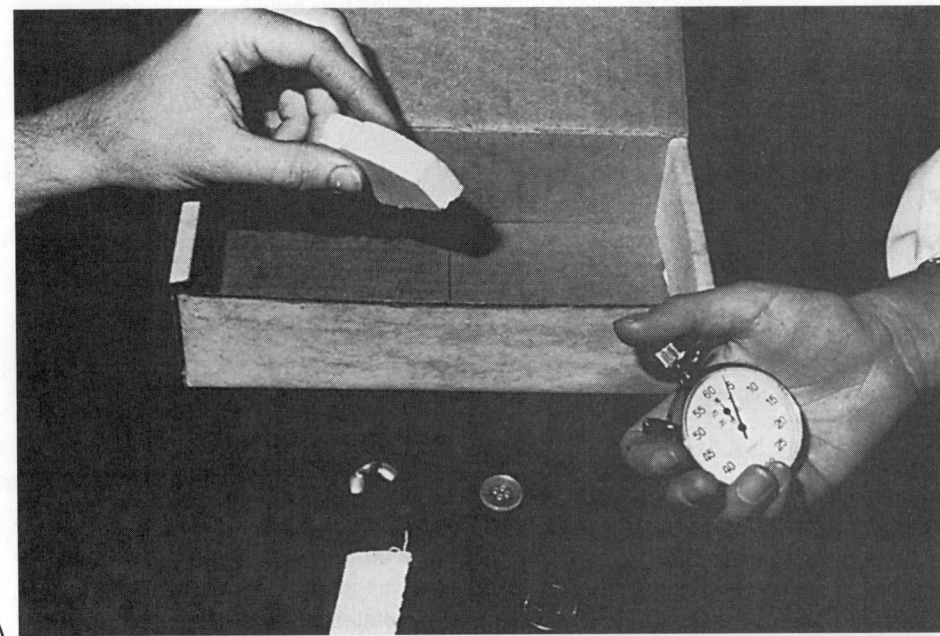

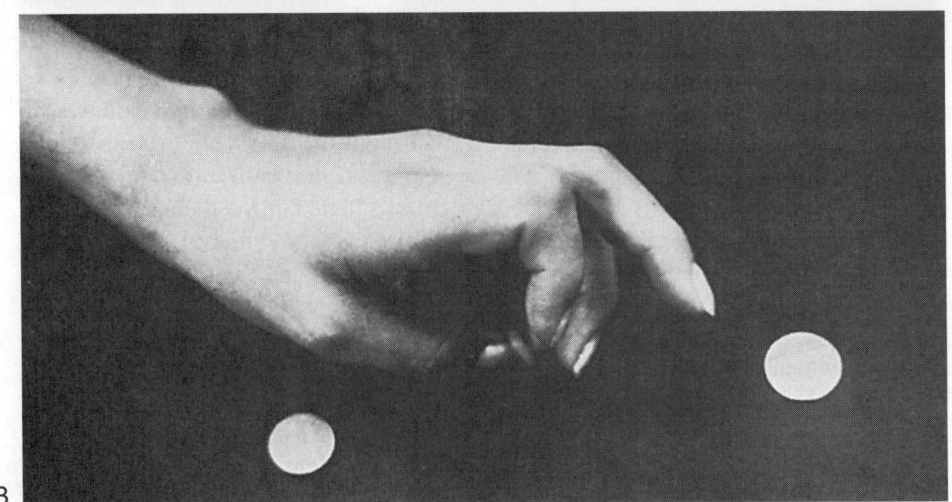

Figure 22-13 Everyday items used in Moberg Pickup Test. **A,** Performing the test and **B,** patient relying on portions of hand with better sensation to manipulate the objects. (From Callahan AD: Sensibility assessment for nerve lesions-in-continuity and nerve lacerations. In Mackin EJ, et al, editors: *Rehabilitation of the hand and upper extremity*, ed 5, St. Louis, 2002, Mosby.)

sensorimotor and cognitive worlds.[25] Referred sensations or phantom pain (pain felt in a part removed from its point of origin) among amputees are examples of cortical reorganization.

Stimulation and use of a body part affect the cortical map.[17] The passage of time, use of the involved hand, and training all help promote improved functional sensibility.[10] Children have greater capacity for neural regeneration and neuroplasticity than older people. Motivation and ability to concentrate enhance the results with sensory reeducation.

The concept of sensory reeducation has evolved over time, and there are multiple versions of intervention. All versions involve tasks stimulating localization, tasks of graded stimulus, and tasks of recognition.[10] Ordinary items found around the home can be used for sensory reeducation, making this training experience accessible and purposeful to clients. Training sessions work well if they are not too lengthy. Ten- or fifteen-minute intervals are recommended because of the high degree of concentration required of the client.[6] An example would be to instruct the client to reach into a bowl of uncooked beans and retrieve small items such as nuts, bolts, and pennies. In treating a client with a hypersensitive extremity, it is important to normalize that hypersensitivity through desensitization in order to maximize the tolerance to and benefits of sensory reeducation.

DESENSITIZATION

Habituation is a decrease in a response following repeated benign stimulus. There is a reduction in the excitatory neurotransmitters released, and if the stimulation continues over a prolonged period of time, a permanent change will occur with reduction in the number of synaptic connections.[4] **Desensitization** for hypersensitivity is a form of treatment that aims to elicit habituation, and therefore reduce the client's hypersensitivity and improve function.

Desensitization uses graded stimulation with procedures and modalities that are slightly aversive but tolerable. The stimuli are upgraded to be slightly more noxious as the client's tolerance increases.[23] Lois Barber, an occupational therapist and pioneer in hand splinting and hand therapy, developed a desensitization approach that exposes the hypersensitive area to textures such as sandpaper, contact particles such as rice, and vibration. Treatment is done for 10-minute intervals, 3 or 4 times a day (Figure 22-14).[1] Clients can be very creative at incorporating desensitization into their daily routine. For example, they may find that rubbing the hand on their textured shirt or corduroy pants is desensitizing and can be performed easily throughout the day.

In our second case study, Layla was so hypersensitive that she tolerated only silk-like materials against her skin to initiate desensitization. By comparison, Minsoo was instructed to incorporate weighted objects and more textured materials such as heavy ceramic mugs or silverware with a textured pattern into his ADL routine to promote sensory reeducation in conjunction with proprioceptive restoration.

The existence or persistence of hypersensitivity will often limit the use of the affected body part and may prevent

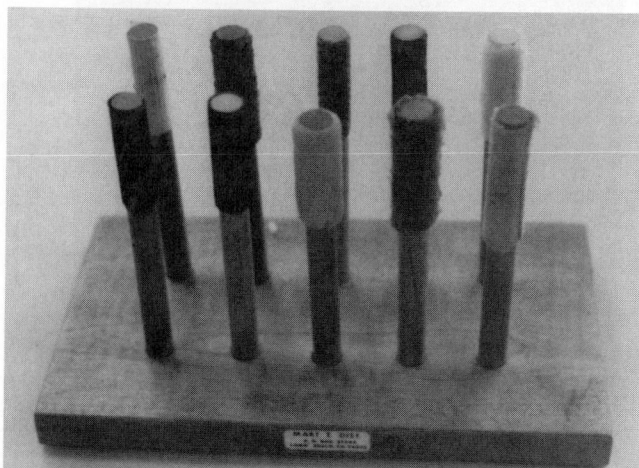

Figure 22-14 Dowels with graded textures used in desensitization. (From Stanley BG, Tribuzi SM, editors: *Concepts in hand rehabilitation*, Philadelphia, 1992, FA Davis.)

sensory reeducation from proceeding, so it is important to address this problem early if possible. Anne Callahan, an occupational therapist and prolific author in the field of hand therapy, identifies two groups of clients for sensory reeducation, with guidelines that differ according to the group.[6] The two groups are those who are candidates for protective sensory reeducation and those who are candidates for discriminative sensory reeducation.

PROTECTIVE SENSORY REEDUCATION

People who lack protective sensation are at risk for serious injury since they cannot feel pinprick or hot or cold exposures. They may develop blisters after holding objects and not realize this until they visually examine the hand. Following a CVA, a person with left hemiparesis and left neglect may inadvertently move their left hand on top of a stove burner during a cooking task. Given the lack of protective sensation, the client will be burned without sensing the painful stimulus of the hot stove. The same thing frequently happens to individuals with C6 tetraplegia. The protective sensation in their thumb, index, and long finger may be intact while the sensation in their ring and little finger is absent.

Callahan identifies the following protective instructions for sensory reeducation of these clients:[6]
- Protect from being exposed to sharp items or to cold or heat.
- Try to soften the amount of force used when gripping an object.
- Use built-up handles on objects whenever possible to distribute gripping pressure over a greater surface area.
- Do not persist in an activity for prolonged periods of time. Instead, change the tool used and the work task often.
- Visually examine the skin for edema, redness, warmth, blisters, cuts, or other wounds (tissue heals more slowly when there has been a nerve injury).
- If there is tissue injury or damage, be very careful in treating and try to avoid infection.
- Maintain skin suppleness as much as possible by soaking and applying moisturizing agents.

Layla's sensory status warranted learning and implementing these precautions into her daily round of occupations. However, given the severity of injury and recent onset, she was not yet a candidate for discriminative sensory reeducation.

DISCRIMINATIVE SENSORY REEDUCATION

Clients are candidates for discriminative sensory training if they have protective sensation intact, with recognition of at least 4.31 on the Semmes-Weinstein monofilaments test. The client who is not able to localize the stimulus is still a candidate for discriminative sensory reeducation. A client with a brain insult or nerve injury resulting in reduced discriminative sensation will be unable to fasten a bra in the back, braid her own hair, or locate a wallet in a bag or pocket with vision occluded. Discriminative sensory reeducation can be graded by initially using grossly dissimilar objects such as a spoon and a penny, progressing over time to more similar objects such as a dime and a penny.

When planning discriminative sensory reeducation intervention, it works best to identify short-term goals that are achievable and that will enhance function despite the sensory loss. If the client has motor involvement and cannot manually manipulate the stimulus, the stimulus can be moved over the hand instead. Discriminative sensory reeducation involves training in both localization and graded discrimination.[6]

Localization

Localization of moving touch tends to return before localization of constant touch. Retraining is done for both. With the client's eyes closed, the eraser end of a pencil or the therapist's hand is touched to the client's hand in the midline of one zone of the hand grid. This makes the documentation easier and the intervention more accurate and consistent, and minimizes afferent activity from adjacent areas of the skin. The stimulus is applied with either a moving or a constant touch. The client is told to open their eyes and point to the area that was touched. Interestingly, it has been shown that activity in the visual cortex is enhanced when touch of the hand is added to the visual stimulation, if the touch is provided on the same side as the visual stimulation.[22] The process is repeated while the client watches if the answer was incorrect. The steps are repeated again with eyes closed. The full process is then repeated in a new area. As the client improves, the stimulus is changed to a lighter and smaller touch.[6]

Graded Discrimination

Stimulation is graded from that requiring gross discrimination to that requiring fine discrimination. Levels of difficulty in discrimination are represented by the sequencing of these three categories: (1) same or different, (2) how they are the same or different, and (3) identification of the material or object.

The stimulus is applied to the skin in an area corresponding to the hand grid. Either the hand or the stimulus is moved to provide input. As above, the eyes are closed, then opened, and then closed for the retraining steps. Various textures can be used, such as different grades of sandpaper (Figure 22-15, *A*), fabrics, or objects such as nuts and bolts or coins (Figure 22-15, *B*).

Another version of discriminative training involves tracing a geometric shape or a letter or number on the fingertip or small area of the hand. This can be applied with a fingertip or the end of an instrument such as a small dowel or a pencil eraser. The client tries to identify the figure.

 OT PRACTICE NOTE

Games and puzzles make good discriminative activities and can be upgraded in the level of challenge provided. Block letters, three-dimensional shapes, and designs in Braille (not to be read, but rather to discriminate the pattern of dots) are often used.

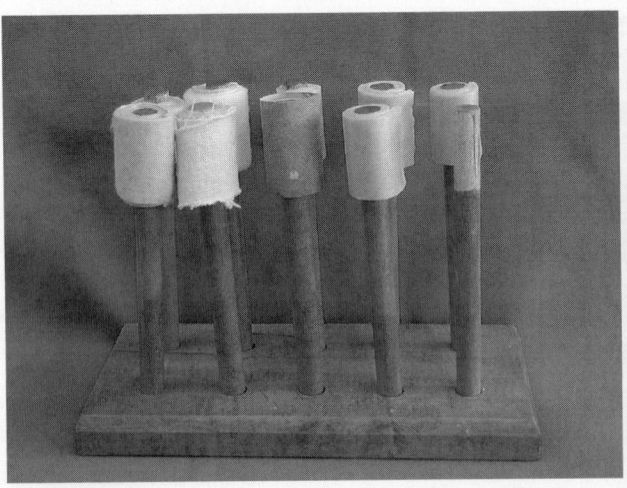
A

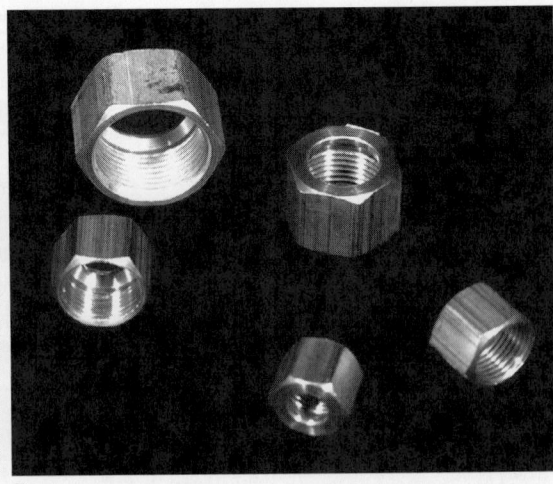
B

Figure 22-15   **A,** Different grades of sandpaper and **B,** nuts and bolts used in graded discrimination sensory reeducation. (**A** From Skirven TM, Callahan AD: Therapist's management of peripheral-nerve injuries. In Mackin EJ, et al, editors: *Rehabilitation of the hand and upper extremity*, ed 5, St. Louis, 2002, Mosby; **B** From Fess EE: Sensory reeducation. In Mackin EJ, et al, editors: *Rehabilitation of the hand and upper extremity*, ed 5, St. Louis, 2002, Mosby.)

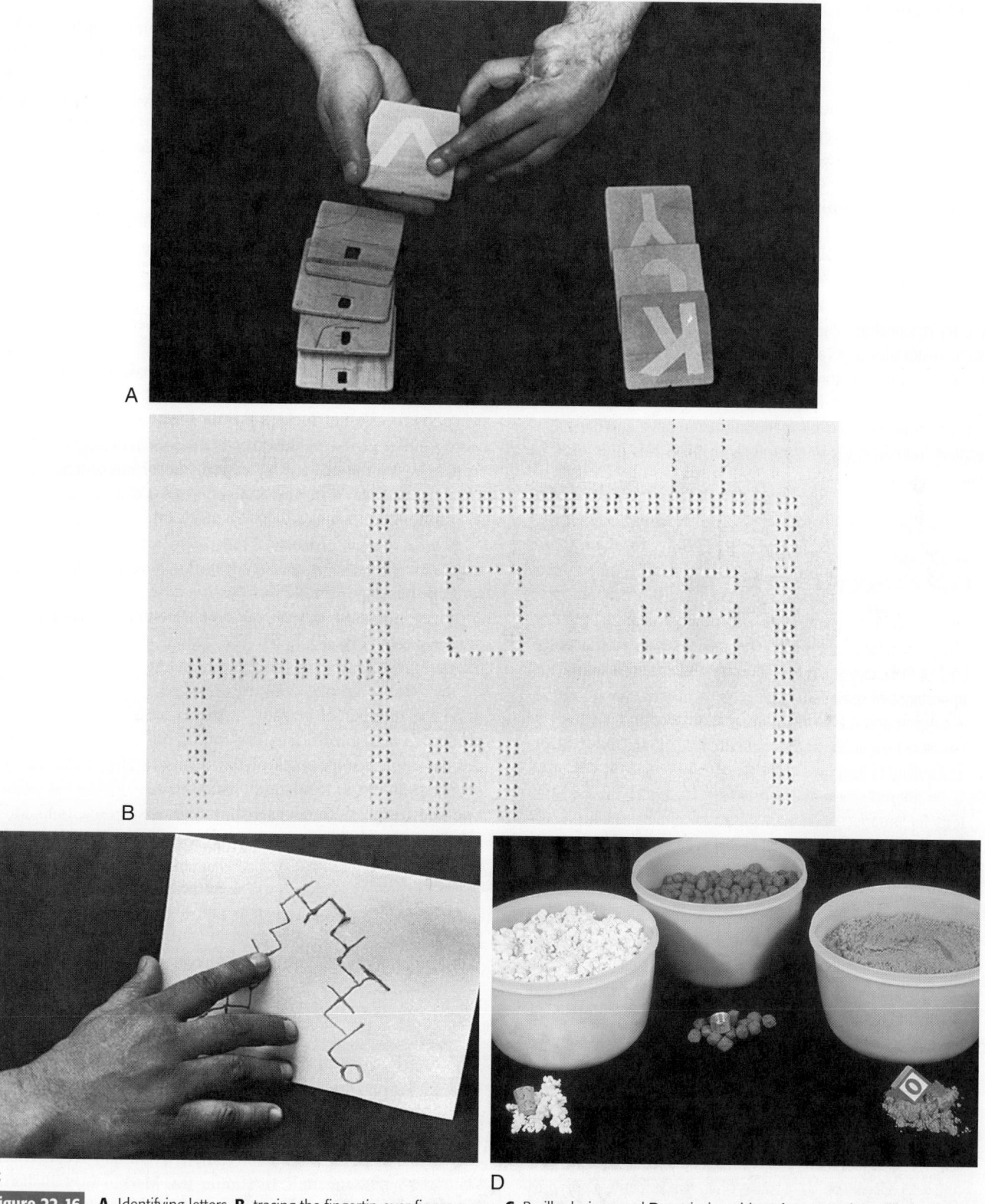

Figure 22-16 **A,** Identifying letters, **B,** tracing the fingertip over finger mazes, **C,** Braille designs, and **D,** retrieving objects from containers filled with contact particles such as rice or beans for graded sensory reeducation. (**A-C** From Skirven TM, Callahan AD: Therapist's management of peripheral-nerve injuries. In Mackin EJ, et al, editors: *Rehabilitation of the hand and upper extremity*, ed 5, St. Louis, 2002, Mosby; **D** From Fess EE: Sensory reeducation. In Mackin EJ, et al, editors: *Rehabilitation of the hand and upper extremity*, ed 5, St. Louis, 2002, Mosby.)

Difficulty is increased by adding the requirement of fingering for motor stimulation if appropriate, and by occluding vision. Discriminative training can include identifying objects out of a box, retrieving objects from rice or sand, or performing ADLs with the eyes closed (Figure 22-16). Progress can be determined by improvement in the number of accurate responses, better mapping of areas of localization, increased speed of completing motor tasks, better status of two-point discrimination, and improved level of function with ADLs overall.[6]

SUMMARY

Sensory dysfunction hinders occupational performance. Intervention can be restorative or it can be adaptive. Desensitization has a restorative effect because through repeated exposure, noxious stimuli become tolerable. This is also referred to as habituation. Protective and discriminative sensory reeducation can have an adaptive effect because training leads to cortical remapping. This is an example of neuroplasticity.

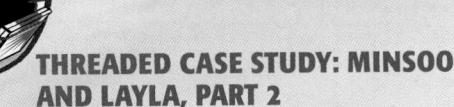

THREADED CASE STUDY: MINSOO AND LAYLA, PART 2

When considering the two case studies presented at the beginning of this chapter, it is interesting to think about the impact and importance of sensation on people's occupational lives. Accurate evaluation and the provision of appropriate intervention may be crucial to their ability to engage in occupations that give meaning and quality to their lives.

In Minsoo's case, the appropriate sensory tests initially are tests for proprioception and light touch discrimination because these are the deficits that limit his occupation of self-feeding. The performance skills to be addressed are coordination, and strength and effort (motor skills) and adaptation (process skills). Occupational therapy intervention approaches for Minsoo are to establish and restore sensation and to modify the methods he uses to complete a task by compensating with the use of intact systems as needed. For example, Minsoo could be taught to use visual cues to determine the amount of force applied while holding a paper cup. Minsoo could also be instructed to avoid using paper cups in public. These strategies would enable him to feel more successful in recovering his social role.

For 12-year-old Layla, the sensory tests initially should include mapping, testing for Tinel's sign, and assessing pain with pinch. The sequence of recovery following peripheral nerve repair is as follows: pain with pinch–positive Tinel sign, tenderness with pressure; and to pinprick–moving touch, light touch, and discriminative touch. The Semmes-Weinstein monofilament test result of "untestable" status indicates the need for training in protective sensory reeducation and use of visual cues to protect from further injury. Interventions based on the results of her sensory tests

emphasized desensitization so she could carry her school books on her arm. Sensory reeducation enhanced her ability to feel the ulnar aspect of her hand on the desk while writing homework assignments. These treatment interventions assisted her in returning to her student role.

Review Questions

1. Why do some peripheral nerves have innervation patterns that differ from dermatome patterns?
2. What is Tinel's sign?
3. What is the typical order of sensory recovery following peripheral nerve repair?
4. What are two reasons that our fingertips have enhanced sensation compared to most other areas of the body?
5. What compensatory strategies are advisable for testing water temperature in a person with impaired temperature awareness?
6. Name four functions of the sympathetic nervous system.
7. Describe how to perform sensory mapping of the hand.
8. What is sensory reeducation and how is it performed?
9. What is desensitization and when is it appropriate to use?
10. Give two examples of how impaired stereognosis would affect ADL functioning.
11. During bathing, what are the safety concerns for a client who lacks hot-cold awareness?

REFERENCES

1. Barber LM: Desensitization of the traumatized hand. In Hunter JM, Schneider LH, Mackin EJ, et al, editors: Rehabilitation of the hand, p. 721, ed 3, St. Louis, 1990, Mosby.
2. Bell-Krotoski JA: Sensibility testing with the Semmnes-Weinstein monofilaments. In Mackin EJ, Callahan AD, Skirven TM, et al, editors: Rehabilitation of the hand and upper extremity, ed 5 ed, p. 194, St. Louis, 2002, Mosby.
3. Bentzel K: Assessing abilities and capacities: sensation. In Trombly CA, Radomski MV, editors: Occupational therapy for physical dysfunction, ed 5, p. 159, Philadelphia, 2002, Lippincott Williams & WIlkins.
4. Burleigh-Jacobs A, Stehno-Bittel L: Neuroplasticity. Neuroscience: fundamentals for rehabilitation, ed 2, p. 67, Philadelphia, 2002, W.B. Saunders.
5. Calford MB: Mechanisms for acute changes in sensory maps, Adv Exp Med Biol 508:451, 2002.
6. Callahan AD: Methods of compensation and reeducation for sensory dysfunction. In Hunter JM, Mackin EJ, Callahan AD, editors: Rehabilitation of the hand: surgery and therapy, ed 4, p. 701, St. Louis, 1995, Mosby.
7. Callahan AD: Sensibility assessment for nerve lesions-in-continuity and nerve lacerations. In Mackin EJ, Callahan AD, Skirven TM, et al, editors: Rehabilitation of the hand and upper extremity, ed 5 ed, p. 214, St. Louis, 2002, Mosby.

8. Dellon AL: *Somatosensory testing and rehabilitation*, Bethesda, MD, 1997, American Occupational Therapy Association.

9. Engel JM: Pain management. In Pedretti LW, Early MB, editors: *Occupational therapy: practice skills for physical dysfunction*, ed 5, St. Louis, 2001, Mosby.

10. Fess EE: Sensory reeducation. In Mackin EJ, Callahan AD, Skirven TM, et al, editors: *Rehabilitation of the hand and upper extremity*, ed 5 ed, p. 635, St. Louis, 2002, Mosby.

11. Fields RD: The other half of the brain, *Scientific Am* April:54, 2004.

12. Kim JS, Choi-Kwon S: Discriminative sensory dysfunction after a unilateral stroke, *Stroke* 27:677, 1996.

13. Lundy-Ekman L: Somatosensation: clinical applications. In *Neuroscience: fundamentals for rehabilitation*, ed 2, p. 123, Philadelphia, 2002, WB Saunders.

14. Lundy-Ekman L: Somatosensory system. In *Neuroscience: fundamentals for rehabilitation*, ed 2, pp. 99-122, Philadelphia, 2002, WB Saunders.

15. Malaviya GN: Sensory perception in leprosy: neurophysiological correlates, *Internat J Leprosy* 71(2):119, 2003.

16. Mathiowetz V, et al: Adult norms for the Nine Hole Peg Test of finger dexterity, *Occup Ther J Res* 5(1):24, 1985.

17. Merzenich MM, Jenkins WM: Reorganization of cortical representations of the hand following alterations of skin inputs induced by nerve injury, skin island transfers, and experience, *J Hand Ther* 6(2):89, 1993.

18. Novak CB: Evaluation of hand sensibility: a review, *J Hand Ther* 14(4):266, 2001.

19. Rossini PM, et al: Post-stroke plastic reorganisation in the adult brain, *Lancet Neurology* 2(8):493, 2003.

20. Ryerson SD: Hemiplegia. In Umphred DA, editor: *Neurological rehabilitation*, ed 3, p. 681, ed 3, St. Louis, 1995, Mosby.

21. Selzer ME: Regeneration and plasticity in neurological dysfunction. In Lazar RB, editor: *Principles of neurologic rehabilitation*, p. 37, San Francisco, 1998, McGraw-Hill.

22. Shimojo S, Shams L: Sensory modalities are not separate modalities: plasticity and interactions, *Curr Opinion Neurobiology* 11:505, 2001.

23. Skirven TM, Callahan AD: Therapist's management of peripheral nerve injuries. In Mackin EJ, Callahan AD, Skirven TM, et al, editors: *Rehabilitation of the hand and upper extremity*, p. 599, ed 5, St. Louis, 2002, Mosby.

24. Umphred DA: Classification of treatment technique based on primary input systems. In Umphred DA, editor: *Neurological rehabilitation*, p. 118, ed 3 ed, St. Louis, 1995, Mosby.

25. Wilson FR: *The hand: how its use shapes the brain, language, and human culture*, New York, 1998, Pantheon Books.

23 EVALUATION AND TREATMENT OF VISUAL DEFICITS FOLLOWING BRAIN INJURY

MARY WARREN

KEY TERMS

Visual perception
Visual perceptual hierarchy
Visual cognition
Visual memory
Pattern recognition

Visual scanning
Search
Visual attention
Oculomotor control
Visual fields

Visual acuity
Visual field deficit
Hemi-inattention
Visual neglect
Binocular vision

Sensory fusion
Diplopia

LEARNING OBJECTIVES

After studying this chapter the student or practitioner will be able to do the following:

1. Describe the role vision plays in enabling the person to complete daily occupations.
2. Describe how visual input is processed within the CNS to turn raw visual data into cognitive concepts of space and form through the process of visual perception.
3. Describe the concept and features of the visual perceptual hierarchy as a framework for assessment and treatment of visual perceptual dysfunction.
4. Describe how assessment is used to link visual performance and process deficits to limitations in daily occupations.
5. Describe how the sensory functions of visual acuity, visual field, oculomotor control, visual attention, and visual scanning change following brain injury.
6. Describe how the sensory functions of visual acuity, visual field, oculomotor control, visual attention, and visual scanning contribute to engagement in daily occupations.
7. Describe how to assess and develop intervention plans for deficits in visual acuity, visual field, oculomotor control, visual attention, and visual scanning.
8. Describe how to modify the client's environment to increase visibility and facilitate engagement in daily occupations.

CHAPTER OUTLINE

THREADED CASE STUDY: PENNY, PART 1

Penny, age 70, sustained a right cerebrovascular accident (CVA). The stroke was caused by an occlusion in the right middle cerebral artery. The CVA resulted in left hemiparesis, left visual field deficit, and hemi-inattention. Penny was hospitalized for 1 week and then transferred to a rehabilitation hospital where she received 3 weeks of intensive inpatient rehabilitation including twice daily sessions of occupational and physical therapy.

Following inpatient discharge, she received an additional 6 weeks of therapy from both disciplines and then was discharged. It has now been 4 months since the onset of the stroke. Penny has been referred to University Low Vision Rehabilitation Clinic by her primary care physician after complaining that she is still having difficulty reading and expressing a desire to resume driving. She was evaluated by a low vision optometrist at the center and found to have normal visual acuity and contrast sensitivity function and a complete left homonymous hemianopsia. The optometrist also noted that Penny has a 5-year history of insulin-dependent diabetes. The optometrist referred Penny to the clinic's occupational therapy (OT) practitioner to address her reading limitations and other deficits in daily living activities and evaluate her potential to resume driving.

Prior to analyzing her occupational performance, the OT practitioner completed an occupational profile on Penny and gathered the following information. Penny has been married for 45 years. She has one grown, unmarried son who lives several states away and no other family in the area. Her husband, Pot, sustained a severe stroke 5 years ago. He has right hemiplegia and global aphasia. He is able to ambulate short distances using a 3-point cane and requires assistance for completion of all basic and instrumental ADLs. They live alone in a one-story home in a suburb. Penny is the primary caregiver for her husband. After her stroke, Penny hired a home care aide to assist in caring for Pot. The aide comes three days a week for 2 hours to help Pot complete bathing and other personal ADLs. Penny is unable to afford more service. Penny is a retired art teacher and well-known local artist, famous for her detailed ink drawings of local architecture. Penny describes herself as fiercely independent. Although her friends have been very kind, it has been extremely difficult to ask them for help and she would prefer to find ways to accomplish tasks by herself. She expresses pride that she has been able to care for Pot even though her physicians advised her to place him in a nursing home. Although he does not comprehend language and cannot speak, they have found a way to communicate through, gestures, music, and art that they both find spiritually satisfying. She states openly that his needs come first.

Penny states that she is having difficulty reading because of the visual field deficit and this is particularly problematic in completing financial management: paying bills and managing their retirement income. A friend now comes over once a month to proofread her checks and bank deposits and balance her checkbook. She also likes to read books to Pot because even though he doesn't understand the language he enjoys the cadence and she feels it is therapeutic. She also expresses a strong desire to resume driving so that she can run errands and take Pot to doctor appointments. There is no mass transit available in her suburb and she is reluctant to continuously ask friends. She states that she no longer sees well enough to complete her ink drawings, and has not attempted to complete any art since she returned home, although she misses it a great deal. She reports that she is independent in basic ADLs and completes meal preparation and home management activities independently but with difficulty. When shopping, Penny requires assistance from a friend for community mobility and locating items. She has difficulty locating objects and is fearful of collisions on the left side when moving about her environment.

Critical Thinking Questions

1. How does the presence of a left homonymous hemianopsia affect Penny's ability to complete reading and other daily living activities?
2. Does Penny actually have hemi-inattention or does she have an uncompensated left hemianopsia?
3. What intervention approach will be most beneficial in increasing Penny's independence in daily occupations?

An understanding of visual perceptual dysfunction after *cerebrovascular accident* (CVA) and traumatic brain injury must be preceded by the realization that visual perception is a process used by the *central nervous system* (CNS) to adapt to context and complete daily occupations. Visual perception is not a series of discrete perceptual skills or the function of a single sensory modality, but rather a process that integrates vision with other sensory input for adaptation and survival.[55,81,120] The activities a person completes in a day dictates the visual perceptual processing needed. Whether a client has a visual perceptual deficit after brain injury will depend on whether the ability to process visual information has been altered so that it prevents completion of a necessary daily activity or occupation.

ROLE OF VISION IN THE ADAPTATION PROCESS

According to Ayres,[6] the overall function of the brain is to filter, organize, and integrate sensory information to make an adaptive response to the context surrounding the person. The brain or CNS receives a variety of sensory information, including visual, proprioceptive, tactile, vestibular, and auditory. Vision is used with information from these other sensory systems to adapt to the situational context—to act on it and to manipulate, mold, and improve it. In adapting, the CNS combines the isolated bits of sensory information it receives, integrating them to form a picture. This picture, created by sensory input, becomes the context of a situation, and an individual uses this context to make decisions and formulate plans to respond to various situations.

Successful adaptation depends on the ability to anticipate situations and contexts. The key to survival is to stay one step ahead of circumstances, whether working with clients or navigating rush-hour traffic. Anticipation enables an individual to plan for situations and increases the chance of a successful outcome. Anticipation and planning are driven by the sensory context of a person's circumstances, for example, "It looks like rain, I'd better take an umbrella," or "It's dark in there, I'd better take a flashlight." When visual input is present, it dominates the sensory context for the simple reason that vision takes us farther into the environment than any of our other senses. We can see lightning before we hear thunder, see a car careening towards us before we hear the squeal of the tires or smell the exhaust. By warning us of changes in our environment, vision enables us to anticipate developing situations and formulate a plan to handle them. So when an object is unexpectedly flung in our direction, we duck, or when we see the banana peel on the floor we walk around it.

The decision-making process guided by vision is not limited to avoiding objects. We also rely on vision to "size up" situations. We say to ourselves, "He looks harmless," or "That looks delicious." Our language is peppered with phrases that reflect the importance of vision in decision making such as, "I'll believe it when I see it," "I'll keep an eye out for it," or "I can see what you mean." Vision plays an important role in social communication, enabling a person to "read" and respond to the subtle gestures and facial expressions used to communicate emotional content in conversations. Vision also plays an important role in motor and postural accommodation by warning of upcoming challenges to postural control, such as the presence of a curb or a curb cut and by alerting us to needed information such as the "exit" sign.

Vision has the power to convey large amounts of detailed information in milliseconds of time. Whereas we are able to instantly identify an object using vision, we would require many more milliseconds to identify the same object tactually or by hearing a verbal description of it. This explains the power of television as a medium for conveying information and why we rush to view the television when we hear about a significant event such as the fall of the World Trade Towers on September 11th.

The speed of information processing supplied by vision also enables us to successfully adapt to dynamic environments. In contrast to static environments in which we are the only moving object, dynamic community environments often contain several objects moving independent of ourselves and each other. In these environments, to successfully

adapt, we must not only monitor our own movement but adapt it to the movement of other objects to avoid collisions and potential harm.

Much of our success in adaptation depends on the rapid processing of information. It does no good to recognize the car after it has struck you; you must be ready for the event before it occurs. Only vision supplies us with sufficient information quickly enough to match our movement to the objects surrounding us. The daily occupations most affected by visual impairment take place in dynamic, unpredictable environments such as those found in the community and workplaces. Reintegrating a person with a visual impairment into the stable environment of the home is a relatively easy process, but reintegrating a person into community environments is much more difficult.

Visual impairment can occur secondary to disease, trauma, and aging.[8,36,71,106] Often a combination of at least two of these causes is observed, especially in older clients. Visual impairment can alter the quality and amount of visual input into the CNS or alter how the CNS is able to process and use incoming visual input. Either way, the result is a decrease in the ability to use vision to complete daily occupations. Changes are observed in those occupations dependent on vision. Clients with visual impairment may process visual information so slowly that they are unable to navigate a dynamic environment or play a card game with friends. Changes in decision making may be observed in which the client makes errors because insufficient visual information was received or because the received information was faulty. Because of the pervasive use of vision in adaptation, visual impairment has the potential to change the client's interaction with all aspects of the environment and the persons and objects in it.

Recall, for example, the many daily activities that Penny is having difficulty completing both in the home and community. Yet, despite its significance, the effect of visual impairment on occupational performance is often attributed to other causes because visual impairment is a hidden disability. Unlike a physical impairment, which can be easily observed, there are few outward signs of visual impairment. As a result, the limitations produced by visual impairment are often attributed to other causes such as motor or cognitive impairment especially when a brain injury has occurred.

AN OVERVIEW OF VISUAL PROCESSING WITHIN THE CENTRAL NERVOUS SYSTEM

For vision to be used for occupation, the raw material of vision (i.e., the pattern of light that falls on the retina) must be transformed into images of the surrounding environment that can be compared with stored memories, combined with other sensory input and knowledge, and used for decision making. The process is known as visual perception and the journey encompasses many of the major structures of the CNS. The processing route is a circular one, transporting visual information from the retina in the anterior of the brain to the occipital pole in the posterior brain and then back again to the prefrontal cortex in the anterior brain. Along the way visual input is sorted out, fine tuned, combined, and repackaged with other sensory input to provide a product which can be used for adaptation.[17,55,81]

The process begins as light enters the eye and passes through the cornea and lens to focus on the retina. The retina conveys this information over the optic nerve and tract to the *lateral geniculate nucleus* (LGN) of the thalamus.[54] Because of the crossing of the retinal nasal fibers (of the optic nerve) at the optic chiasm, the LGN receives information from the retinal hemifields of both eyes.[54,81] After synapsing in the LGN, visual information travels over the geniculocalcarine tracts to the V-1 area of the visual cortex (found within the occipital lobe).[54] Figure 23-1 shows these pathways. The visual cortex sorts through the incoming visual information, sharpening and fine tuning features such as orientation of line and color, then disperses this information for cortical processing.[54,55,128] From the visual cortex, visual information is processed by temporal and parietal circuitry and eventually sent to the prefrontal circuitry to be used in decision making.[55] Before it can be used by the prefrontal areas, visual information must be combined (integrated) with other incoming sensory information to establish images and relationships between the body and the environmental surround.[55,56,81]

To integrate vision with other sensory input, visual information is sent from the visual cortex to the prefrontal area over two routes: a "northern" or superior route, which takes it through the posterior parietal circuitry, and a "southern" or inferior route through the posterior temporal circuitry.[44,55,56,81] This process is known as *parallel-distributed sensory processing* (Figure 23-2). Visual information traveling the southern route through the posterior temporal circuitry is combined with language and auditory input and processed for visual object information and recognition.[55,81] The purpose of this processing is to identify objects and classify them. Neural processes in the posterior temporal lobe use precise visual input from the macular-foveal area of the retina to tune into the visual details of objects. Processing by posterior temporal circuitry is critical to the ability to distinguish discrete features of objects, such as the difference between the style of a can of diet Coke and regular Coke or particular facial features.[55]

Visual information traveling simultaneously through the northern route to the prefrontal circuitry is processed in the posterior parietal lobe. The parietal lobe is a synthesizer of sensory information, receiving input from all of the sensory systems and integrating the input to create internal sensory maps that are used to orient the body in space.[9,44,55,56,81,98,100] Visual information traveling through the parietal circuits is used to tune the CNS in to the presence of objects surrounding the body and to determine the spatial relationship of these objects to the body and to each other. Visual information

must be integrated with other sensory information to provide this orientation. Tactile, proprioceptive, kinesthetic, vestibular, and auditory information is necessary, along with visual input, to accurately assess the relationship between the self and surrounding objects. The map created by information synthesized in the parietal circuitry is body centered and dynamic, changing in shape and content as the body moves through space.[9,44,79,81,98,100]

The posterior parietal circuitry in each hemisphere contains a map of the space on the contralateral side of the body. Thus, the right hemisphere contains a map of the left side of the body and surrounding space, and the left hemisphere contains a map of the right side of the body and surroundings.[9,44,100] This map is not a detailed representation of space but provides a general impression of objects in space on that side of body. The CNS relies on visual information from the peripheral areas of the retinal fields to create and maintain these maps. This area of the brain participates in directing general attention to and awareness of space.[79]

The final destination for visual information traveling through the posterior temporal and parietal circuitry is the prefrontal area of the brain, where the information is used for cognitive processing to make decisions and formulate plans. This area, in conjunction with premotor circuitry and other areas, is responsible for planning skilled body movements, including eye movements.[43,44,55,81] Important visual structures located in the prefrontal lobes are the frontal eye fields, which are responsible for voluntary visual search of the space on the contralateral side of the body.[11,44,92,101,103] The frontal eye fields in the right hemisphere direct visual search towards the left visual space, and vice versa. The frontal eye fields conduct visual search based on an expectation of where visual information will be found in the environment.[42] For example, if you were looking for a light switch in a room, you would direct your visual search towards the walls, because that is where you expect to find a light switch. You would not waste time searching the floor or the ceiling. By directing visual search based on the expected location of crucial visual information, the CNS is able to process visual information quickly. This arrangement enables us to engage successfully in activities that require rapid visual processing, such as driving.

Not all visual information travels over the geniculocalcarine tracts for cortical processing. Many neural pathways leave the optic nerve and tract and travel to subcortical areas, including the hypothalamus and brainstem.[54,71,81] The brainstem contains important neural structures involved in visual processing. The superior colliculi, located in the midbrain of the brainstem, are primary brainstem processing centers for visual input. The superior colliculi are responsible for the detection of moving visual stimuli appearing in the peripheral visual fields.[44,54,71,77] When motion is detected, the colliculi automatically initiate eye movement towards the direction of the detected motion. In performing this function, the colliculi serve as an early warning system to prevent the CNS

PARALLEL-DISTRIBUTED PROCESSING OF THE VISUAL SYSTEM-I

Schematic inferior view of a horizontal slice of the brain

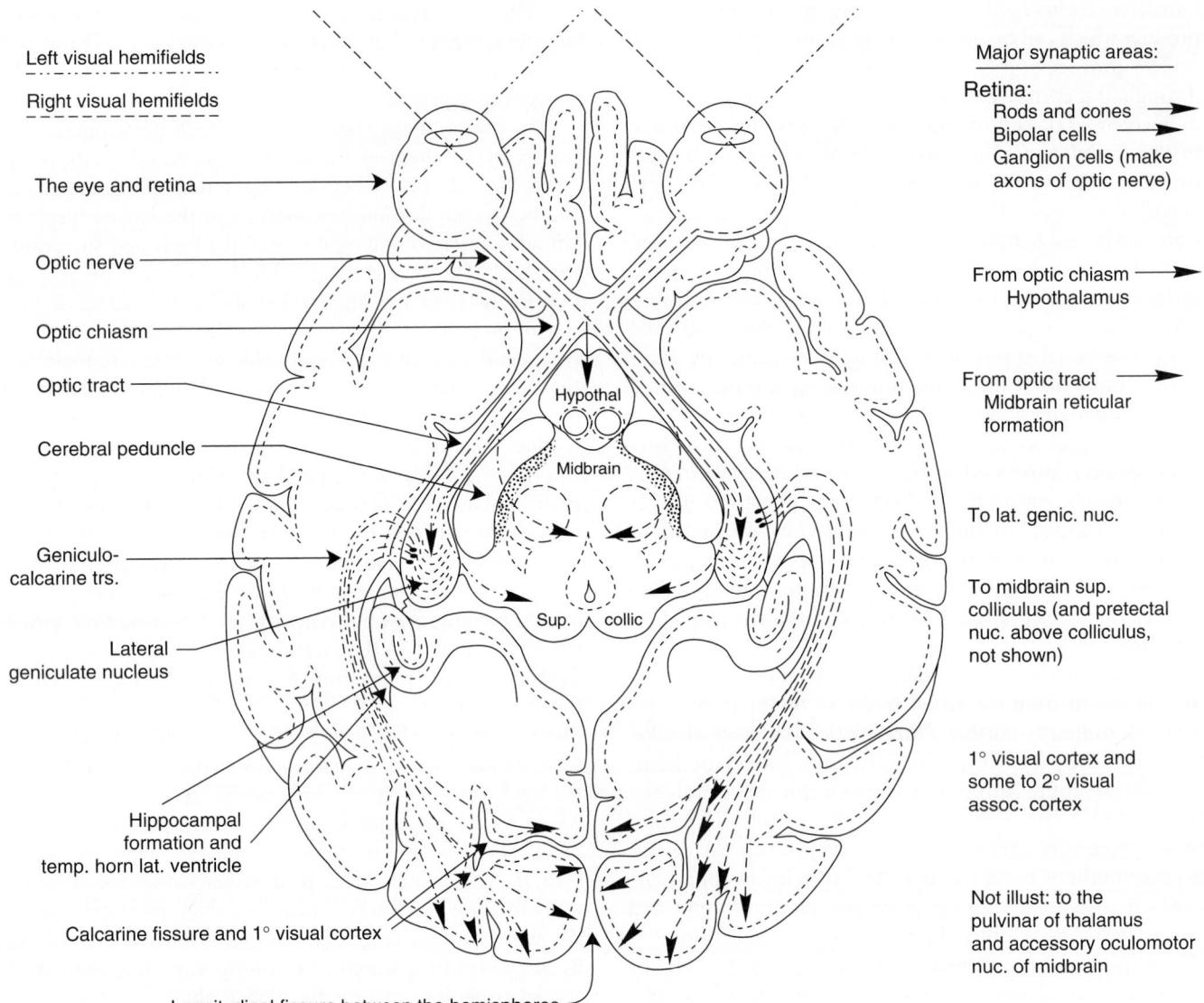

Left visual hemifields

Right visual hemifields

The eye and retina

Optic nerve

Optic chiasm

Optic tract

Cerebral peduncle

Geniculo-
calcarine trs.

Lateral
geniculate nucleus

Hippocampal
formation and
temp. horn lat. ventricle

Calcarine fissure and 1° visual cortex

Longitudinal fissure between the hemispheres

Hypothal

Midbrain

Sup.   collic

Major synaptic areas:

Retina:
    Rods and cones ⟶
    Bipolar cells ⟶
    Ganglion cells (make
    axons of optic nerve)

From optic chiasm ⟶
    Hypothalamus

From optic tract ⟶
    Midbrain reticular
    formation

To lat. genic. nuc.

To midbrain sup.
colliculus (and pretectal
nuc. above colliculus,
not shown)

1° visual cortex and
some to 2° visual
assoc. cortex

Not illust: to the
pulvinar of thalamus
and accessory oculomotor
nuc. of midbrain

The visual system is our most important sense in regard to:

A. Learning, memory, and recall including our ability to see color and fine
    details as well as the visual surround and global relationships.
B. Communication: use of symbolic language, speaking, and body language.
C. Spatiotemporal orientation in concert with vestibular-proprioceptive systems.
D. Early warning system to pleasure or danger, i.e., vision is our farthest
    reaching distance receptor and movement detector par excellence.
E. Visual-manual and visual-motor activities.

1°, Primary.
2°, Secondary.

Figure 23-1   Pathways from retina to LGN to visual cortex. (Courtesy of Josephine C. Moore, PhD, OTR.)

PARALLEL-DISTRIBUTED PROCESSING OF THE VISUAL SYSTEM

Two parallel routes carry visual information from the occipital lobe to the prefrontal lobe and frontal eye field (FEF). Fibers from these two routes distribute to many areas along each route (not illustrated) before terminating in the prefrontal cortex and FEF as illustrated.

(N) = "Northern" or superior route via parietal and frontal lobes.

(S) = "Southern" or inferior route via temporal and frontal lobes.

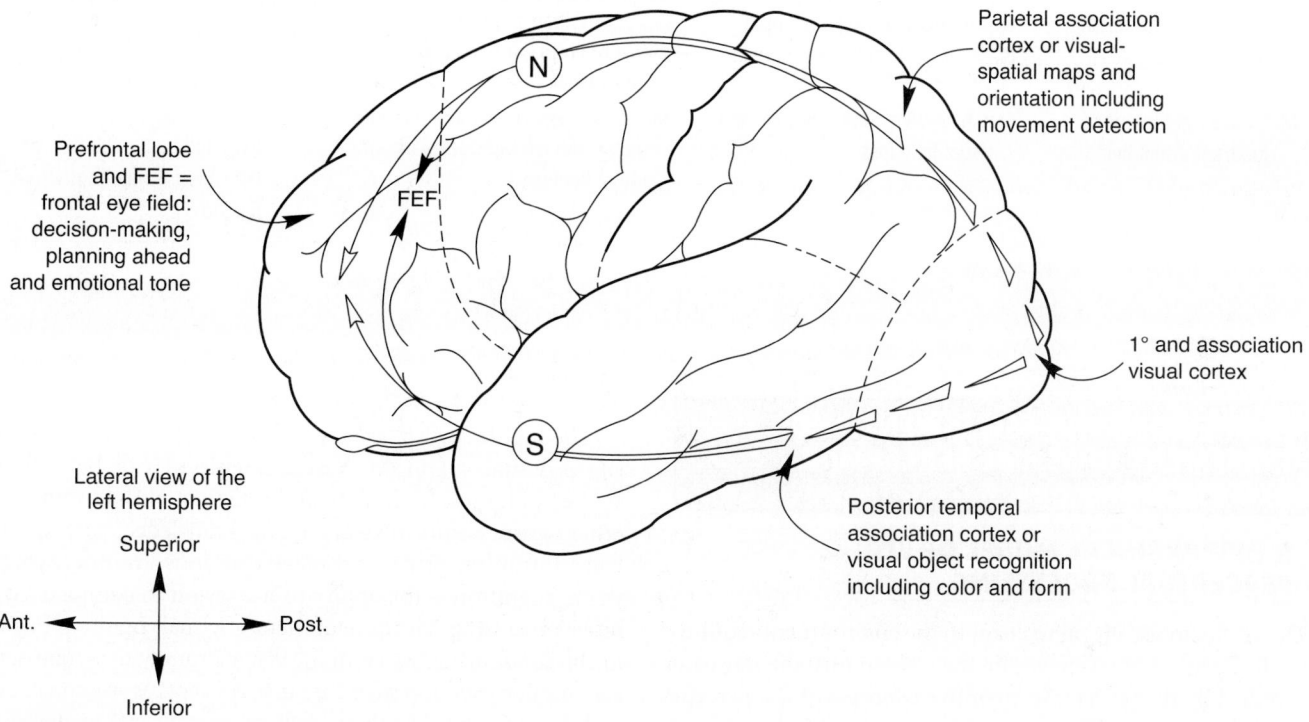

Parietal association cortex or visual-spatial maps and orientation including movement detection

Prefrontal lobe and FEF = frontal eye field: decision-making, planning ahead and emotional tone

1° and association visual cortex

Lateral view of the left hemisphere

Superior

Ant. ← → Post.

Inferior

Posterior temporal association cortex or visual object recognition including color and form

1°, Primary.

Figure 23-2   Visual input travels from the visual cortex through parietal and posterior temporal circuitry to the prefrontal lobe to complete cortical visual processing. (Courtesy of Josephine C. Moore, PhD, OTR.)

from being caught off guard by events occurring in the environment.[44,90] The nuclei of cranial nerves III, IV, and VI, which control the extraocular muscles of the eyes, are also located in the brainstem, along with basic visual functions such as the light (pupillary) reflex and the accommodation reflex.[54]

Many CNS areas are responsible for processing visual information, but all areas must work together for a person to make sense of what is seen, and thus use visual information to adapt.[44,55,79,81,99] Millions of long and short neural fibers tie the various cortical and subcortical structures to ensure effective and efficient visual processing. Like a car in which the fuel-injection system is as critical to performance as the spark plugs, the visual system will not run efficiently unless all of its components are working together. When brain injury or disease occurs, this communication system is

disrupted and the organization of visual processing breaks down. Table 23-1 lists effects of various CNS lesions on different aspects of the visual system. In reviewing the table, remember that a client will exhibit limitations only in those daily occupations that require the type of visual processing compromised by the lesion. For example, a deficit in the ability to process visual detail caused by a lesion in the left posterior temporal lobe would significantly affect the ability of a proofreader to return to work but might have little effect on a piano tuner's ability to return to work.

Penny's CVA occurred in the middle cerebral artery feeding the left hemisphere of the cortex and affected an area known as the internal capsule. As a result of the stroke, the temporal and parietal loops of the geniculocalcarine tracts were damaged along with areas in the posterior parietal lobe and the motor strip controlling the left upper and lower extremities.

TABLE 23-1   **Summary of Cortical Hemispheric Functions for Visual Processing and Deficits Secondary to Lesion Site**

Left Hemisphere Advantage		*Right Hemisphere Advantage*	
More detail-oriented in relation to persons, places, and things		More global or holistic	
Takes in minute details and compares and contrasts these details		Takes a general view of the environment	
Processes visual information sequentially in a systematic item-by-item, serial search strategy		Processes multiple visual inputs simultaneously, grouping them into meaningful categories	
Attends only to right visual fields		Attends globally to both left and right visual fields	
Parietal Lesion	*Post. Temp. Lesion*	*Parietal Lesion*	*Post. Temp. Lesion*
Biases attention to detail	Biases attention to global input	Biases attention to detail	Biases attention to global input
Biases brain to right hemisphere advantages	Biases brain to right hemisphere advantages	Biases brain to left hemisphere advantages	Biases brain to left hemisphere advantages
May have right inferior quadrant visual field loss	May have right superior quadrant visual field loss	May have neglect or hemi-inattention along with left inferior quadrant visual field loss	May have neglect or hemi-inattention along with left superior quadrant visual field loss

Modified with permission of Josephine C. Moore.

FRAMEWORK FOR ASSESSMENT AND TREATMENT OF VISUAL PERCEPTUAL DYSFUNCTION

A HIERARCHICAL MODEL OF VISUAL PERCEPTUAL PROCESSING

The ability to use vision to adapt to the environment requires the integration of vision within the CNS to turn the raw data supplied by the retina into cognitive concepts of the perception of space and objects that can be manipulated and used for decision making. The process by which this occurs is known as **visual perception.** Visual perceptual function can be conceptualized as an organized hierarchy of processes that interact with and subserve each other.[120] Figure 23-3 illustrates this hierarchy. Within the hierarchy, each process is supported by the one that precedes it and cannot properly function without the integration of the lower level process. As Figure 23-3 shows, the **visual perceptual hierarchy** consists of the processes of visual cognition (visuocognition), visual memory, pattern recognition, visual scanning, and visual attention. These perceptual processes are supported by three basic visual functions that form the foundation of the hierarchy: oculomotor control, visual fields, and visual acuity.

The ability to use visual perception to adapt to the environment is the result of the interaction of all of the processes in the hierarchy in a unified system. Although each perceptual process is discussed individually in this section, the reader should remember that the ability to adapt through vision is a result of the processes working in synergy. Although discrete perceptual processes can be identified, they do not operate independently of one another.

The highest order visual perceptual process in the hierarchy is visual cognition. **Visual cognition** can be defined as the ability to manipulate and integrate visual input with other sensory information to gain knowledge, solve problems, formulate plans, and make decisions. In other words, visual cognition is the ability to use vision to complete cognitive processing. The development of visual cognition begins in childhood when we combine visual input with somatosensory input to develop such cognitive concepts as size constancy and permanence. We then apply these concepts to decision making. For example, if we see a 12-inch-tall adult, we assume that the adult must be several yards away because by applying size constancy we know that adults are not 12 inches high. Because visual cognition enables complex visual analysis, it serves as a foundation for all academic endeavors, including reading, writing, and mathematics, and many vocations, such as artist, engineer, surgeon, architect, and scientist.

Visual cognition cannot occur without the presence of **visual memory,** the next process level in the hierarchy. Mental manipulation of visual stimuli requires the ability to create and retain a picture of the object in the mind's eye while the visual analysis is being completed. In addition to being able to store visual images temporarily in short-term memory, a person must also be able to store and retrieve images from long-term memory. For example, to interpret the illustration in Figure 23-4, one must be able to access visual memories of the shape of both a goose and a hawk. Adults and older children can easily resolve this illusion, but most toddlers cannot because they have not yet stored memories of the shapes of these birds.

Before a visual image can be stored in memory, an individual must recognize the pattern making up the image.

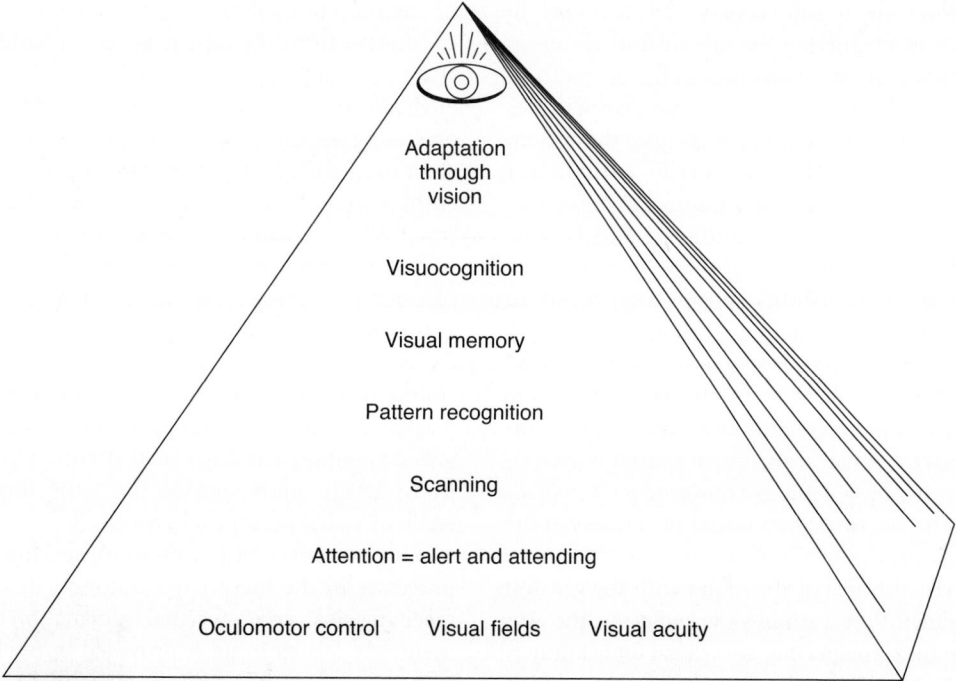

Figure 23-3   Hierarchy of visual perceptual development in central nervous system. (Courtesy of Josephine C. Moore, PhD, OTR. From Warren M: A hierarchical model for evaluation and treatment of visual perceptual dysfunction in adult acquired brain injury, part I, *Am J Occup Ther* 47[1]:55, 1993.)

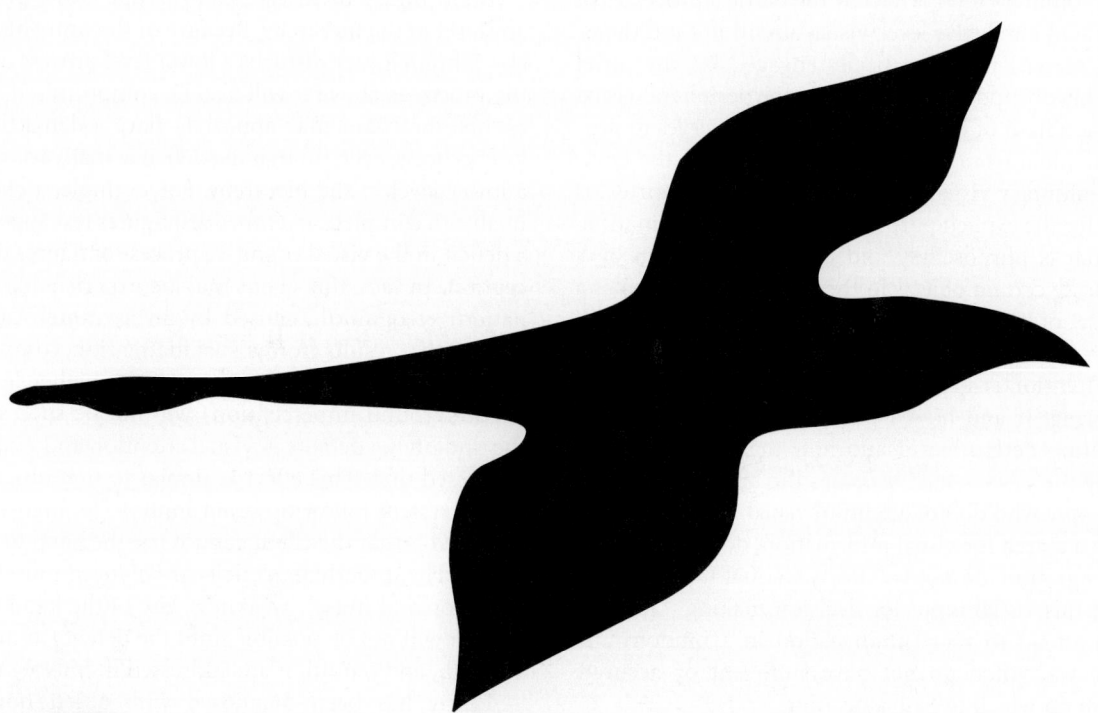

Figure 23-4   Is this a goose or a hawk? (From Warren M: A hierarchical model for evaluation and treatment of visual perceptual dysfunction in adult acquired brain injury, part I, *Am J Occup Ther* 47[1]:55, 1993.)

Pattern recognition, which subserves visual memory in the hierarchy, involves identifying the salient features of an object and using these features to distinguish the object from its surroundings.[37] A salient feature is one that distinguishes a particular object from another. For example, the salient feature that differentiates an "E" from an "F" is the lower horizontal line on the "E." Pattern recognition involves two abilities: the ability to identify the configural and holistic aspects of an object—to see its general shape, contour, and features—and the ability to identify specific features of an object, such as details of color, shading, and texture.[18] Both aspects of recognition must occur for accurate identification.[8]

Pattern recognition cannot be accomplished without the next process in the hierarchy: organized and thorough scanning of the visual array. **Visual scanning** or **search** is accomplished through the use of saccadic eye movements. A *saccade* is a movement of the eye toward an object of interest in the environment. The purpose of a saccade is to focus on the object with the *fovea*, the area of the retina with the greatest ability to process detail.[42] In scanning a visual array, the eyes selectively focus on the elements that are critical for accurately interpreting the array.[35,48,83,95] The most important details are reexamined several times through a series of cyclic saccades to ensure that correct identification is made. Unessential elements in the scene are ignored.[35,95,131]

Visual scanning is actually a product of **visual attention.**[35,48,45,90] The saccadic eye movements observed in scanning reflect the engagement of visual attention as it is shifted from object to object. Visual search occurs on two levels: an automatic or reflexive level largely controlled by the brainstem and a voluntary level driven by the cortical processes of cognition.[79] On a reflexive level, visual attention (and therefore visual search) is automatically engaged by any novel object moving or suddenly appearing in the peripheral visual field, such as a flash of light.[54,77] This response serves to protect an individual from unexpected intrusions in the environment. Voluntary visual search, directed by the cortex, is completed for the explicit purpose of gathering information. Visual search is purposefully and consciously driven by a desire to locate certain objects in the environment, such as a misplaced set of keys, or to obtain certain information, such as where an exit is located.[35,79]

Visual attention is a critical prerequisite for visual cognitive processing. If and how a person attends to an object or information determines if and how that visual input is analyzed by the CNS, which becomes the basis for decision making. People who do not attend to visual information do not initiate a search for visual information, do not complete pattern recognition, do not lay down a visual memory, and cannot use this visual input for decision making. Likewise, those who attend to visual information in a random and incomplete way often do not have sufficient or accurate information on which to base a decision.

The type of visual attention engaged by the CNS depends on the type of visual analysis needed. For example, the type of attention needed for awareness that a chair is in the room is different from the type needed to identify the style of the chair. The first instance requires a global awareness of the environment and the location of objects within it; the second requires selective visual attention to the details of the chair to identify its features. Also, it is necessary to be able to employ more than one type of visual attention at the same time. When crossing a crowded room to talk to a friend, a person must be aware of the movement of people and the placement of obstacles in the room to avoid collisions, while at the same time focusing on the friend (or target). The CNS employs several types of visual attention simultaneously and shifts constantly between types and levels of attention.[79] A large amount of neural processing is devoted to directing visual attention, causing visual attention to be disrupted easily by brain injury, but at the same time to be a highly resilient visual perceptual process.[79]

Engagement of visual attention and the other higher level processes in the hierarchy cannot occur unless the CNS is receiving clear, concise visual information from the environment.[21,120] Visual input is provided through the visual functions of oculomotor control, visual field, and visual acuity. **Oculomotor control** enables eye movements to be completed quickly and accurately and ensures perceptual stability. The **visual fields** register the visual scene and ensure that the CNS receives complete visual information. **Visual acuity** ensures that the visual information sent to the CNS is accurate. Without these prerequisite visual functions, an inadequate image is generated, preventing engagement of higher level visual perceptual processing.

Brain injury or disease can disrupt visual processing at any level in the hierarchy. Because of the unity of the hierarchy, if brain injury disturbs a lower level process or function, the processes above it will also be compromised. When this occurs, the client may appear to have a deficit in a higher level process, even though the deficit actually has occurred at a lower level in the hierarchy. For example, a client who is unable to complete an embedded figures test appears to have a deficit in the visual cognitive process of figure-ground perception. In fact, this client may be experiencing inaccurate pattern recognition, caused by an asymmetrical scanning pattern that results from visual inattention, compounded by a visual field deficit. Treatment of the higher level process (figure-ground imperception) will not be successful unless the underlying deficits in visual attention and visual field are addressed first. This effect is similar to that observed in the motor system following brain injury. The high-level deficit observed is that the client cannot use the hand to pick up an object. The underlying deficits are reduced muscle tone and sensation and muscle weakness. Use of the hand for manipulation will not be possible until the deficits in muscle tone, strength, and sensation are addressed in intervention.

Penny has been diagnosed with a left homonymous hemianopsia. Because of this deficit, she does not see objects in the left half of her visual field. This visual field defect

OT PRACTICE NOTE

Effective assessment and treatment of visual perceptual dysfunction require an understanding of how brain injury affects the integration of vision at each process level and how the levels interact to enable visual perceptual processing.

compromises her ability to attend to objects on her left side and she fails to search for objects on her left side. Failure to search for objects on her left side limits her ability to complete pattern recognition and form visual memory of objects on her left side. Because she has no visual memory of objects on the left side, she is more likely to experience disorientation and collide with objects on the left when navigating environments.

INTERVENTION

In working with the client with visual impairment following brain injury, the **occupational therapy** (OT) practitioner often encounters and works closely with two medical disciplines: ophthalmology and optometry. Both of these eye care specialists diagnose, manage, and treat visual impairment and both may serve as a referral source to OT practitioners. However, there are distinctions between the two professions of which OT practitioners must be aware in order to collaborate effectively and benefit from their input. Ophthalmologists are medical doctors (MDs) who complete a residency in ophthalmology. As physicians, ophthalmologists are primarily responsible for diagnosing and treating the medical conditions that cause the visual impairment. Neuro-ophthalmologists are board certified in this specialty and often treat the largest number of persons with visual impairment from brain injury. Consequently they often work with OT practitioners and serve as referral sources and consultants to OT practice.

Optometrists are independent healthcare providers who have a doctorate of optometry from a postgraduate university program. Like OT practitioners, optometrists specialize in a variety of areas following training including neurorehabilitative, developmental, and behavioral optometry. While they are not medical doctors, they also diagnose and treat medical conditions causing vision loss and provide nearly two thirds of primary eye care in the United States. Neither discipline, at this time, routinely serves as a member of the rehabilitation team and both provide mainly consultative services. Which specialty the team uses depends primarily on availability and reimbursement.

OCCUPATIONAL THERAPY EVALUATION

To develop an intervention plan, the OT practitioner must link limitations in activity and participation to the presence of a visual impairment. Establishing this relationship is the

purpose of the assessment of visual performance completed by an occupational practitioner. This process also is known as establishing "medical necessity," which is the prerequisite to receiving third party reimbursement for OT services. To achieve the link, the practitioner must be able to identify the limitation in occupation and then connect it to the presence of a visual impairment. This often requires that the OT practitioner also complete assessments to identify visual impairment. However, whereas an ophthalmologist or optometrist evaluates visual impairment for the purpose of diagnosing a visual disorder, occupational practitioners assess visual impairment to explain the presence of a limitation in occupation and participation.

OT PRACTICE NOTE

OT assessment has three purposes: (1) to identify the limitation in activity or occupation, (2) to link that limitation to the presence of a visual impairment, and (3) to develop an appropriate intervention plan based on the results of the assessment. In addressing evaluation and intervention, it is important to remember that a client's visual performance is significant not in terms of how it deviates from an established norm but in how it interferes with occupational performance. A client is considered to have a visual impairment that requires intervention if the impairment interferes with performance of a necessary daily occupation.

In an ideal treatment setting, the OT practitioner would work in partnership with an ophthalmologist or optometrist to identify the client's visual impairment. These eye care professionals would serve as members of the rehabilitation team and screen the client's vision at several intervals during the recovery period. They would provide the other rehab professionals on the team information regarding the health of the eyes and the status of visual acuity, visual field, and oculomotor control along with information on prognosis and medical and optical management. In reality, these two eye care specialists are rarely integrated into rehab teams and the process of obtaining a referral to either one is time consuming and difficult.

To succeed, the OT often must first convince the physician or case manager managing the client's recovery that a visual deficit exists and is limiting occupational performance. This requires the OT practitioner to be well versed in completing basic visual assessments such as acuity, contrast sensitivity function, and visual field to screen for visual impairment. Whereas the eye care specialist would use the information obtained from these evaluations to diagnose the client's visual impairment, the OT practitioner will use the information to justify referral to these specialists and to link the presence of an occupational limitation to visual impairment.

Several tests are available to occupational practitioners to assess visual performance. Subtests from the *Brain Injury Visual Assessment Battery for Adults* (biVABA) developed by the author are used in this chapter to describe assessment techniques.[121] The biVABA was designed specifically as a tool to assist OT practitioners to develop effective intervention plans for adults with visual impairment caused by brain injury. The biVABA consists of 17 subtests designed to measure visual processing ability. The assessments include evaluation tools used by ophthalmologists and optometrists to measure basic visual function, along with subtests designed specifically for occupational practitioners.

OCCUPATIONAL THERAPY INTERVENTION

The focus of OT intervention is to change the outcome in the categories of visual disability and visual handicap. Two primary approaches are used in providing intervention. A remediation approach may be used, in which intervention attempts to establish or restore the client's ability to complete visual processing by improving aspects of visual performance such as increasing the efficiency of visual search or improving visual attention. A compensatory approach is also used, in which the emphasis of intervention is on changing the context of the environment or task to enable the client to successfully use his or her current level of visual processing. These two approaches may be used alone or together depending on the needs of the client. Education of the client and family is always used in conjunction with the two approaches to increase their insight into how the client's visual processing has changed and how it has affected occupational performance. Education is a critical component of the intervention process because insight is crucial to the ability to learn compensatory strategies.[1,110]

OT ASSESSMENT AND INTERVENTION OF SPECIFIC VISUAL IMPAIRMENTS

The concept of a visual perceptual hierarchy provides the framework for the discussion of assessment and intervention. It is assumed that many changes in visual perceptual function after brain injury occur because of the alteration of the lower level processes within the perceptual hierarchy, including visual acuity, visual field, oculomotor control, and visual attention and scanning. Deficits in these functions prevent the CNS from accurately completing complex visual processing and using vision for adaptation. Identification of deficiencies in these processes, followed by treatment to remediate the deficits, enables the CNS to process visual input more efficiently and facilitates adaptation. This section focuses on assessment and intervention for these processes within the visual perceptual hierarchy and examines how brain injury disrupts the functioning of each process, how the process is assessed, and how the implementation of intervention is provided.

VISUAL ACUITY

Visual acuity is the ability to see small visual detail. Acuity contributes to the capability of the CNS to recognize objects. The dictionary defines acuity as "keenness or sharpness," and with regard to vision, acuity ensures that clear and precise visual information is provided to the CNS for processing.[2,109] The greater the quality of the visual input, the more precise the image created by CNS processing. The more precise the image, the faster and more accurate the ability of the CNS to recognize the object and discriminate it from other features in the environment. Good acuity therefore enables speed and accuracy of information processing and facilitates decision making.

Acuity occurs through a multi-step process that begins with the focusing of light onto the retina. Light rays enter the eye through the pupil and are focused on the retina by the anterior structures of the eye: the cornea, lens, and optic media (Figure 23-5).[109] The retina, acting like film in a camera, processes the light and records a "picture" that is relayed to the rest of the CNS via the optic nerve and pathway.[55] Although the concept is simple, the process is complex and involves many factors. These factors include the ability to focus light precisely onto the retina, the ability to maintain sharp focus over various focal distances, the ability to obtain sufficient illumination of the retina to capture a quality image, and the ability of the optic nerve to transmit the image through the CNS for perceptual processing.[54,55] Any compromise of the structures involved in this process will result in degradation of the image and reduced acuity.[106]

Visual acuity is most commonly measured by having the client read progressively smaller optotypes on a chart. The optotypes may be letters, numbers, or symbols. The most common acuity measurement unit used in the United States is the Snellen fraction (20/20, 20/50, etc.).[17] The fraction represents a ratio of distance to size of the optotype.[26] In layman's terms, a measurement of "20/20" means that standing at a distance of 20 feet, the viewer can see the letter that a person with normal vision can see at 20 feet, and 20/200 would indicate that a person standing at a distance of 20 feet can see a letter that a person with normal vision could identify at 200 feet. In reality, 20/20 means that the person can identify an optotype that subtends 1 minute of arc at a distance of 20 feet compared to a 20/200 optotype that subtends 10 minutes of arc at the same distance.

Visual acuity typically is associated with the ability to see high-contrast, black-on-white optotypes. However, visual acuity actually is a continuum of visual function ranging from the ability to detect high-contrast features on one end of the continuum to the ability to detect low-contrast features (such as beige on white) on the other end.[50] Low contrast acuity, known as *contrast sensitivity function* (CSF), is the ability to detect the borders of objects reliably as they decrease in contrast (rather than size) from their backgrounds.[50] CSF makes it possible to distinguish and identify

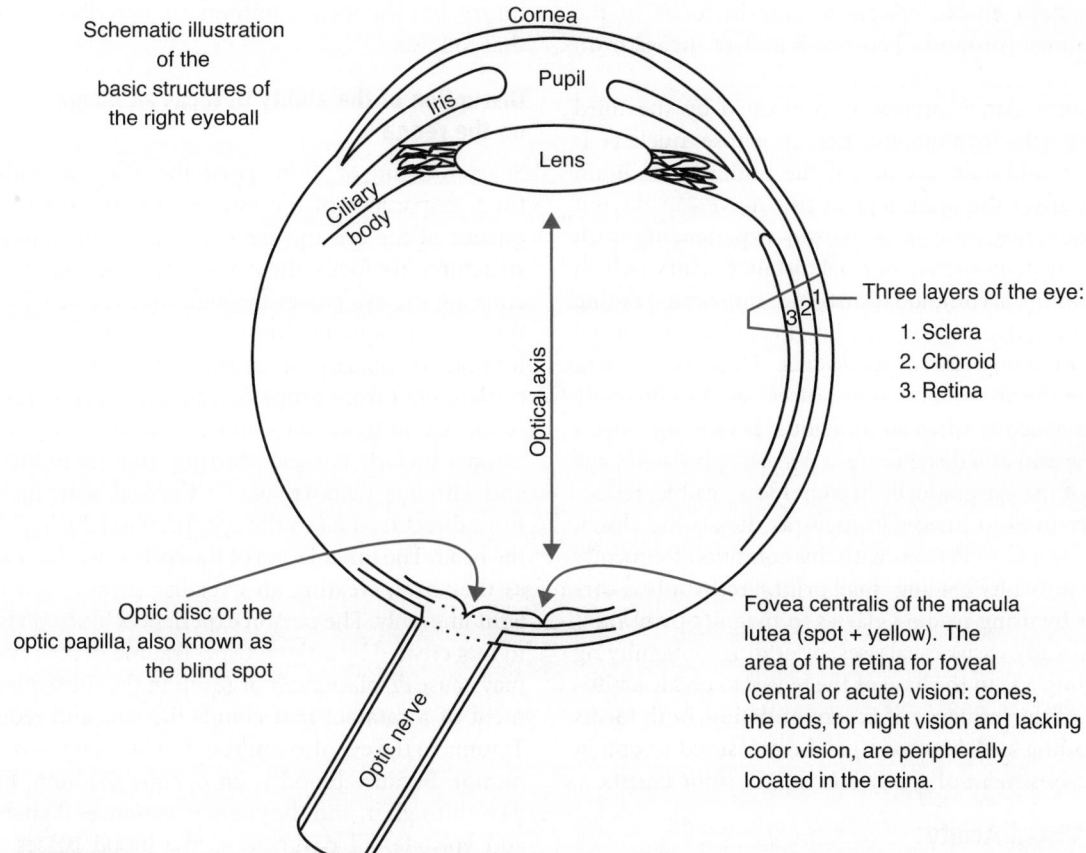

Schematic illustration of the basic structures of the right eyeball

Cornea

Pupil

Iris

Lens

Ciliary body

Optical axis

Three layers of the eye:
1. Sclera
2. Choroid
3. Retina

Optic disc or the optic papilla, also known as the blind spot

Optic nerve

Fovea centralis of the macula lutea (spot + yellow). The area of the retina for foveal (central or acute) vision: cones, the rods, for night vision and lacking color vision, are peripherally located in the retina.

Figure 23-5   Anterior structures of the eyeball. Light passes through these transparent structures to focus on the receptor cells of the retina. (Courtesy of Josephine C. Moore, PhD, OTR.)

faint features of objects, such as the curve of a concrete curb or the protrusion of the nose on the face.[50] Because much of the environment is made up of low-contrast features (gradations of colors between objects rather than stark contrasts), CSF is a critical visual function underlying the ability to negotiate an environment safely.[50]

For example, curbs and steps are routinely the same color throughout; without CSF, it would not be possible to see the depth in the curb or step. Carpets, walls, doors, door frames, and furniture also are often monochromatic in color; without the ability to distinguish low-contrast features, it would not be possible to locate the door or avoid the chair jutting out into the pathway in monochromatic environments. One of the most common low-contrast objects is the human face. Human faces contain very little differentiation in contrast between the facial features. That is, the nose is the same color as the forehead, cheeks, and chin, and eye and hair color are designed to blend with skin tones. To see the unique features of a human face requires very good contrast sensitivity function. Research has shown that CSF can be impaired in clients even when their high-contrast acuity is within normal limits.[16,19,48] Therefore both forms of acuity (high- and

low-contrast) must be measured to obtain an accurate assessment of acuity function.

Two forms of high-contrast visual acuity are measured: distance acuity and reading (near) acuity. Distance acuity is the ability to see objects at a distance. Near acuity is the ability to see objects clearly as they come close to the eye. Near acuity is most accurately called "reading acuity" because reading is the primary activity enabled by near acuity. Reading acuity is measured by having the client read sentences in progressively smaller sizes of print. Reading acuity is dependent on the brainstem neural process of accommodation. Accommodation enables the eye to maintain clear focus on objects as they come closer.[42] When an object approaches the eye, its point of focus on the retina is pushed farther back, eventually causing the image to go out of focus. The CNS adjusts for this situation through the three-step process of accommodation. As the object comes closer, (1) the eyes converge (turn inward) to ensure that the light rays entering the eye stay parallel and in focus, (2) the crystalline lens of the eye thickens to refract the light rays more strongly and shorten the focal distance, and (3) the pupil constricts to reduce scattering of the light rays.

These three steps enable objects to stay in focus in the near vision range (distances between 3 and 16 inches from the eyes).

The accommodative process is controlled by the third cranial nerve (the oculomotor nerve) whose nucleus is located in the midbrain portion of the brainstem.[42] Brain injuries that affect the brainstem or this nerve can disrupt the accommodative process. A person experiencing such disruption may demonstrate normal distance acuity (which does not require accommodation) and impaired reading acuity. Accommodation can also be affected by a normal by-product of aging called *presbyopia*. Until the fourth decade of life the accommodation process works efficiently to ensure equal acuity when an individual is viewing objects both up close and at a distance. As a person approaches age 50, the lens of the eye gradually becomes less flexible, reducing its ability to keep images in focus as they come closer, creating presbyopia.[102] Persons with this condition frequently complain of difficulty reading small print. Presbyopia is corrected either by using reading glasses to magnify print or, if the person already wears eyeglasses, by adding a magnifying lens or "reading ad" to the base of the lenses to create a bifocal. Because of the influence of accommodation, both forms of acuity, reading and distance, must be measured to obtain an accurate assessment of acuity function in some clients.

Deficits in Visual Acuity

In the normal eye, most deficiencies in visual acuity are caused by defects in the optical system (the cornea or lens or even the length of the eyeball), which cause images to be focused poorly on the retina.[102] The three most common optical defects reducing acuity are *myopia* (nearsightedness), *hyperopia* (farsightedness), and *astigmatism*. In myopia, the image of an object is focused at a point in front of the retina and is therefore blurred when it reaches the retina. Myopia is corrected by placing a concave lens in front of the eye. In hyperopia the image comes into focus behind the retina, causing the image to remain out of focus on the retina. Hyperopia is corrected by placing a convex lens in front of the eye. Figure 23-6 illustrates these defects. In astigmatism light is focused differently by two meridians 90° apart. A cornea that is not perfectly spherical and smooth but is more spoon-shaped or dimpled usually causes this defect. The defect results in a blurring of the image because both meridians cannot be focused on the retina. Astigmatism is corrected by placing a cylindrical lens in front of the eye.

Visual acuity deficits primarily occur as a result of impairment in three areas of visual processing: disruption of the ability to focus light onto the retina, inability of the retina to accurately process the image, and inability of the optic nerve to transmit the information to the rest of the CNS for processing.[106] These impairments may be the direct result of a brain injury, a disease process, or a change in the eye occurring incidental to the injury. It is not possible to describe all of the conditions that can result in reduced acuity after brain injury, but the most common are described in the sections that follow.

Disruption of the ability to focus an image on the retina

Sharp focusing of an image on the retina depends largely on the transparency of the intervening structures between the outside of the eye and the retina and on the ability of these structures to focus the light rays entering the eye. Light entering the eye passes through four transparent mediums: the cornea, aqueous humor, crystalline lens, and vitreous humor. An opacity or irregularity in these structures will prevent light from properly reaching the receptor cells in the retina. Conditions that can occur in conjunction with head trauma include corneal scarring, trauma-induced cataract, and vitreous hemorrhage.[106] Corneal scarring may occur from direct trauma to the eye sustained during an assault to the head. The inner layers of the cornea are damaged and scar as they heal, creating an irregular surface that refracts the light unevenly. The person experiences blurred vision similar to that created by astigmatism. Trauma to the crystalline lens may cause displacement or result in the subsequent development of a cataract that clouds the lens and reduces acuity. Trauma to the eye also can result in bleeding into the vitreous humor. Because blood is an opaque medium, light cannot pass through it, and the client experiences floaters, shadows, and episodes of darkness as the blood passes in front of the retina. Of these conditions, only vitreal hemorrhage is temporary and resolves without treatment.

Impairment of accommodation is another condition that affects the focusing ability of the eye. This condition is associated with brainstem injury, either from head trauma or from stroke.[53,71,72,102,106] As stated previously, brainstem injury can affect the functioning of one or all of the components of accommodation: convergence of the eyes, thickening of the lens, and pupillary constriction. When accommodation is impaired, the client has difficulty achieving and sustaining focus during near-vision tasks. The most frequent complaint voiced by the client is a difficulty maintaining focus during reading, which may cause the print to blur and swirl on the page.[25]

Disruption of the ability of the retina to process the image

The health and integrity of the retina also influence the quality of the image sent on to the CNS. The receptor cells of the retina can be damaged directly by injury or disease, preventing them from responding to light. Diseases that affect retinal function, such as macular degeneration and diabetic retinopathy, are associated with age and significantly increase in incidence in the seventh and eighth decades of life.[36] With damage to the retina (especially the macular area), both high- and low-contrast visual acuity are diminished, making accurate identification of features and objects difficult. It is estimated that approximately one in four persons over the age

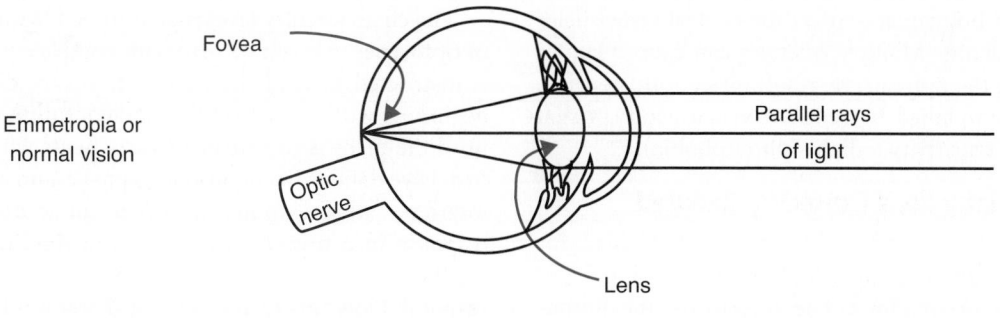

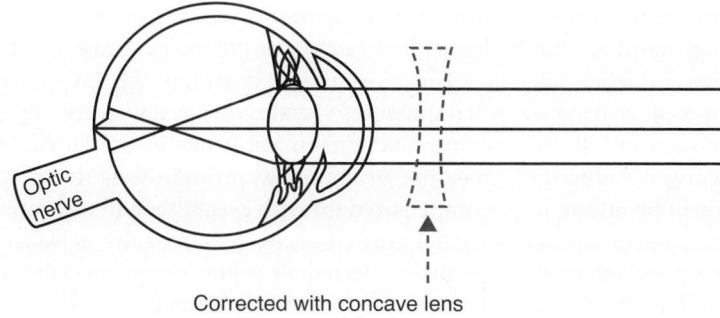

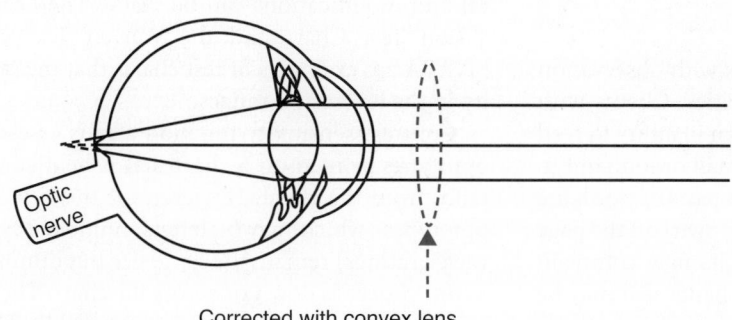

Figure 23-6   Normal, myopic, and hyperopic optical refraction of light coming into the eye and the type of lens used to correct myopic and hyperopic optical refractive errors. (Courtesy of Josephine C. Moore, PhD, OTR.)

of 80 years has a visual impairment that affects the retina significantly enough to prevent reading standard print. It is not uncommon for an older adult who has been referred for treatment of a *cerebrovascular accident* (CVA) (such as stroke) also to demonstrate reduced visual acuity secondary to eye disease. Too often the vision loss resulting from the disease is either overlooked or misdiagnosed as an impairment in attention or cognition associated with the CVA.

Disruption of the ability of the optic nerve to send the retinal image

The most common cause of optic nerve damage in brain injury is trauma.[53] Damage can occur from a direct penetrating injury to the nerve, such as a missile wound to the head from a gunshot.[53] Indirect trauma can also occur from an optic canal fracture associated with facial or blunt forehead fractures. These fractures are most common in children and young adults and usually result in unilateral injuries.[53] Severe closed head injuries can cause stretching or tearing of the optic nerve, resulting in significant and usually bilateral damage to the nerves. Bilateral optic nerve injury can also result from compression of the nerves secondary to intracranial swelling or hematoma.[53]

Other common conditions that can cause optic nerve damage are glaucoma and multiple sclerosis. Glaucoma typically damages the optic nerve fibers carrying peripheral visual field input but can also affect the central visual field, reducing visual acuity. Multiple sclerosis can cause plaques to develop along the optic nerve, resulting in optic neuritis, a condition accompanied by reduced visual acuity, visual field deficit, and sensitivity to light (photophobia).[106]

Occupational Limitations Caused by Reduced Visual Acuity

Reduced visual acuity can cause limitations in a significant number of daily occupations. The severity of the limitation depends on the extent of the acuity loss and whether there has been a loss of central acuity, peripheral acuity, or both. A loss of central acuity results in an inability to discriminate small visual details and to distinguish contrast and color. Activities dependent on reading, writing, and fine motor coordination (e.g., reading recipes and labels on foodstuffs, dialing a telephone, completing a check, paying a bill, applying makeup, shaving, identifying money, and shopping) will be affected. When peripheral acuity is reduced, as occurs with visual field deficit, mobility will be affected. The client may be unable to identify landmarks, see obstacles in the path of travel, or accurately detect motion, which may impair his or her ability to ambulate safely and maintain orientation in the environment. This may reduce independence in driving, shopping, and participation in community activities.

Assessment of Performance Skills

All assessment of performance skill begins with observation of the client's performance in daily activities. Clients with deficits in visual acuity often complain of an inability to read print and may state that the print is too small or too faint to read. Complaints that print is distorted, that parts of words are missing, or that the words run together and swirl on the page are also common. Clients with CSF deficits may complain of an inability to see faces clearly. These clients also may be unable to distinguish between colors of similar hue, such as navy blue and black, or to detect low-contrast substances such as water spilled on the floor.

If a decrease in visual acuity is suspected, a screening is completed to determine how acuity has changed. To obtain a complete picture of the client's visual acuity, both high- and low-contrast acuity are measured. High-contrast acuity is measured both for distance, using a test chart at a distance of 1 m or greater, and for reading, using a text card at 40 cm (16 inches). When measuring visual acuity, the practitioner must be sure that the chart is well illuminated and held at the specified distance from the client. Adequate illumination is important because as illumination decreases, so does acuity (no one can read a letter chart in the dark). Because acuity is depicted as a fraction of distance over letter size (e.g., 20/20 or 20/200), the measurement is not accurate unless the viewing distance is accurate. All test charts specify a distance at which they are to be used, and this should not be altered.

The client's acuity level is determined by the smallest line of optotypes that can be read with good accuracy. The client is instructed to read the optotypes on the chart out loud, beginning with the largest line and continuing to lower lines until the print is too small to see. Clients with brain injury may have deficits in cognition, language, and perception that interfere with the ability to provide an accurate and timely response in a testing situation. Extra time may be needed for the client to locate the optotype, process the image, and respond. Slowness in responding therefore does not necessarily indicate that the client lacks the acuity to identify the optotype. If the client struggles with the identification of optotypes on each line but is accurate, the test should proceed until a line is reached on which the client can no longer accurately identify the majority of the optotypes.

The most useful chart for the OT practitioner is one that measures visual acuity as low as 20/1000 so that significant reductions in acuity can be measured. Standard charts measure visual acuity primarily in the range that can be compensated for with eyeglasses and measure nothing below 20/200 Snellen acuity. When acuity is below that level, the client is referred to a low vision specialist for evaluation. Because some conditions such as optic nerve damage or macular diseases can result in profound vision loss (less than 20/400 acuity), it is important for a practitioner to be able to measure acuity in the lower ranges so that appropriate referral and modifications can be made. The LeaNumbers Low Vision Test Chart and the Warren Text card from the biVABA are examples of test charts that measure visual acuity in the low vision ranges.

Contrast sensitivity function also is assessed by viewing optotypes printed on a chart that is held at a specified distance from the client. However, for this type of testing, the optotypes (which may be letters, numbers, symbols, or sine wave gratings) remain the same size but diminish in contrast as one proceeds down or across the chart. The client is asked to identify as many optotypes as possible. There are many forms of CSF tests. The least expensive and most portable test charts are those designed by Dr. Lea Hyvarinen, and include the LeaNumbers Low Contrast Screener (part of the biVABA), the LeaSymbols Low Contrast Screener, and the LeaNumbers and LeaSymbols Low Contrast Tests. When contrast sensitivity function is measured, the client is asked to read down the chart as far as possible until the optotype is too faint to be identified. As with high-contrast acuity testing, the test chart must be held at a specific distance and must be well illuminated to obtain an accurate measurement.

In assessing visual acuity, the OT practitioner is not responsible for diagnosing the cause of the deficiency, but rather linking the presence of the deficiency to a limitation in occupational performance. This is a subtle but important distinction that affects the assessment procedure. When a client has reduced visual acuity, the ophthalmologist or optometrist uses the results of the assessment to determine the cause of the reduction (e.g., damage to the retina or cornea or the presence of a refractive error). With this information, the eye care specialist determines how to manage the condition to restore optimum sight using optical devices (glasses or contact lenses), a surgical procedure, or the prescribing of medications. In contrast, when a practitioner determines that a client has reduced visual acuity, the information is used to modify activities and the environment so that the client can compensate for the loss and successfully complete daily activities. For example, if a client cannot read the size of print on a medication label, the practitioner determines whether the print can be enlarged to a size that the client can read or determines another way for the client to identify the medication bottle.

Intervention

If a significant reduction in visual acuity is noted, the client should be referred to an ophthalmologist or optometrist to determine the nature and cause of the vision loss and whether vision can be restored. Referring clients to specialists can take days, weeks, and even months to complete. The client's intervention program cannot be placed on hold while the referral is being processed; therefore the practitioner uses the information obtained from the assessment to modify the environment and activities and enable the client to use his or her remaining visual acuity. This is achieved by increasing the visibility of the environment and tasks through manipulation of physical context.

Increase background contrast

Changing background color to contrast with an object can help the client see objects more clearly. The application of this technique can be as simple as using a black cup for milk and a white cup for coffee. In cases in which background color cannot be changed, such as on carpeted steps, color can be applied to provide a marker. For example, a line of bright fluorescent tape can be applied to the end of each step riser on the carpeted stairs to distinguish between them.[33]

Increase illumination

Increasing the intensity and amount of available light enables objects and environmental features to be seen more readily and reduces the need for high contrast between objects. For example, facial features can be identified more easily if a person's face is fully illuminated. The challenge in providing light is to increase illumination without increasing glare. Halogen, fluorescent, and full-spectrum lights provide the best sources of bright illumination with minimum glare and are generally recommended over standard incandescent lighting for both room and task illumination. Lighting should be strategically placed to provide full, even illumination without areas of surface shadow. For example, if a 50-W halogen lamp is used for reading, it should be positioned behind the client's shoulder so that the page of print is fully illuminated without the light shining directly in the client's eyes.

Reduce background pattern

Patterned backgrounds have the effect of camouflaging the objects lying on them. The detrimental effect of pattern on object identification can be minimized by using solid colors for background surfaces such as bedspreads, place mats, dishes, countertops, rugs, towels, and furniture coverings. Objects in the environment also create background pattern. Cluttered environments with haphazardly placed objects create challenges even for persons with good acuity. If possible, the number of objects in the environment should be reduced and those remaining arranged in an orderly fashion. Closets, drawers, shelves, and countertops should be reorganized and simplified, as should such areas as sewing baskets, desks, and refrigerators.

Enlarge objects or features that need to be seen

When possible, objects should be enlarged to make them more visible. Instructions can be reprinted in larger print, medications and other items relabeled, and calendars enlarged. The last line of print that is easily read on the reading acuity test card indicates the minimum size that print should be enlarged for the client. Contrast should also be increased because it does little good to enlarge print if the print is faint. Black on white or white on black print is usually more visible than any other color combination. Many items now are manufactured with larger print, including calculators, clocks, watches, telephones, check registers, glucose monitors, scales, playing cards, games, and puzzles. These items can be purchased through specialty catalogs.

Organize

Items used daily should be arranged on accessible shelves in single rows. Rarely used items should be stored on upper and lower shelves or removed. Commercially available organizing systems can be used to store similar items together to create workstations. Once closets and shelves are rearranged and simplified, every effort should be made to keep them organized. Putting items back where they belong and maintaining organization reduce frustration and facilitate independence. Establishing routines for tasks such as filing nails and paying bills prevents these tasks from becoming overwhelming. Task steps requiring vision to complete can be eliminated by using such items as pre-chopped and pre-measured food ingredients, wrinkle-free clothing, electronic funds transfer, and voice-activated telephone dialing.

Access community services

In addition to environmental modification, the client may benefit from the variety of services available to assist persons with vision loss. These services are generally free of charge and can be found in the resource section of the public library or by contacting an advocacy organization such as the American Foundation for the Blind (*www.afb.org*) or the

Lighthouse Information and Resource Center (www.lighthouse.org). The following are some examples of available services:

1. The National Library Service for the Blind and Physically Handicapped offers books, magazines, and music on cassette tape through its Talking Books program.
2. Most states offer radio reading services in conjunction with a university-sponsored public radio station.
3. Local telephone companies often offer free directory assistance to persons with disabilities; most pharmacies will provide large print medication labels, and many businesses will provide large print bills.

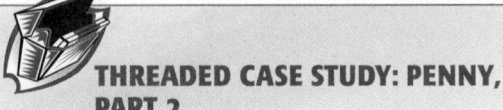

THREADED CASE STUDY: PENNY, PART 2

The location of Penny's stroke in the middle cerebral artery would not cause a change in visual acuity. However, Penny's medical condition of insulin-dependent diabetes may cause diabetic retinopathy and other eye conditions that can cause significant vision loss. After learning she was a diabetic, the optometrist carefully evaluated the health of Penny's eyes and checked her acuity. The optometrist saw changes on the retina that indicated Penny has early stage background diabetic retinopathy. The disease has not yet caused a reduction in visual acuity. The optometrist reinforced to Penny that she must maintain her blood glucose levels at the level prescribed by her physician, monitor her diet, and check her blood glucose levels several times a day. She conveyed this information to the occupational practitioner and instructed the OT to assess Penny's ability to compensate for her visual field deficit in completing diabetes self-management including drawing insulin and using a glucometer to monitor blood glucose levels and completing meal preparation according to her prescribed meal plan.

VISUAL FIELD

The visual field is the external world that can be seen when a person looks straight ahead. It is analogous to the dimensions of a picture imprinted on the film in a camera (with the retina representing the film). The normal visual field extends approximately 60° superiorly, 75° inferiorly, 60° to the nasal side, and 100° to the temporal side.[3,106] As Figure 23-7 shows, most of the visual field is binocular and is seen by both eyes. A small portion of the peripheral temporal field in each eye is monocular and can be seen only by one eye because the bridge of the nose occludes vision in the other eye. At the very center of the retinal visual field is the fovea, an area approximately 8° to 10° in diameter that records the visual details for object identification. The fovea is located in the macular area of the field, also referred to as the central visual field (Figure 23-7). This area, which is packed with cone receptor cells, is approximately 20° to 30° in diameter and is used for object identification.[81,109] The rest of the visual field is the peripheral field. The peripheral visual field is comprised of rod receptor cells that detect general shapes and movement in the environment. On the border between the central and peripheral visual fields on the temporal side is the blind spot, so called because the optic disc pierces the retina here and there are no sensory receptor cells.

Visual Field Deficits

Damage to the receptor cells in the retina or to the optic pathway that relays retinal information to the CNS for processing results in a **visual field deficit** (VFD).[3,54,80,106,129] Figure 23-1 illustrates this pathway as it changes from the optic nerve to the optic tract to the *geniculocalcarine tracts* (GCT). The location and extent of the visual field deficit depends on where damage occurs on the pathway. Although any type of visual field deficit is possible after brain injury, homonymous hemianopsia occurring from a lesion along the geniculocalcarine tracts, is the most commonly occurring deficit.[134] *Hemianopsia* (hemi = half, anopsia = blindness) means that there has been a loss of vision in one half of the visual field in the eye. *Homonymous* means that the deficit is the same in both eyes. A lesion along the GCT in the right hemisphere causes a left homonymous hemianopsia; a lesion along the GCT in the left hemisphere causes a right homonymous hemianopsia. In stroke, most hemianopsias are caused by occlusions of the posterior cerebral artery,[40,134] although a middle cerebral artery stroke such as that experienced by Penny in the case example can also cause this deficit.

Occupational Limitations Caused by Visual Field Deficits

Although a VFD is often considered a mild impairment in comparison with the dramatic loss of use of the limbs, it can create changes in visual processing that significantly limit daily performance.[40] The most important change occurs in the search pattern used by the person with VFD to compensate for the blind portion of the visual field. Instead of spontaneously adopting a wider search strategy (turning the head farther to see around the blind field) the person tends to narrow their scope of scanning.[89,132] The person typically turns the head very little and limits visual search to areas immediately adjacent to the seeing side of the body. The reason for this odd strategy is the influence of a visual process known as perceptual completion.[48,73,91,99,105] *Perceptual completion* is a process whereby the CNS samples a visual array and internally completes a visual scene based on an expectation of the visual information that would be found in the array as illustrated in Figure 23-8. The perceptual outcome of this process is that the viewer perceives that he or she is seeing a complete visual scene, even though part of the visual information in the scene was not recorded.[55,105]

Perceptual completion provides speed in information processing by enabling an individual to construct a complete visual scene based on partial visual input. As such, it plays an

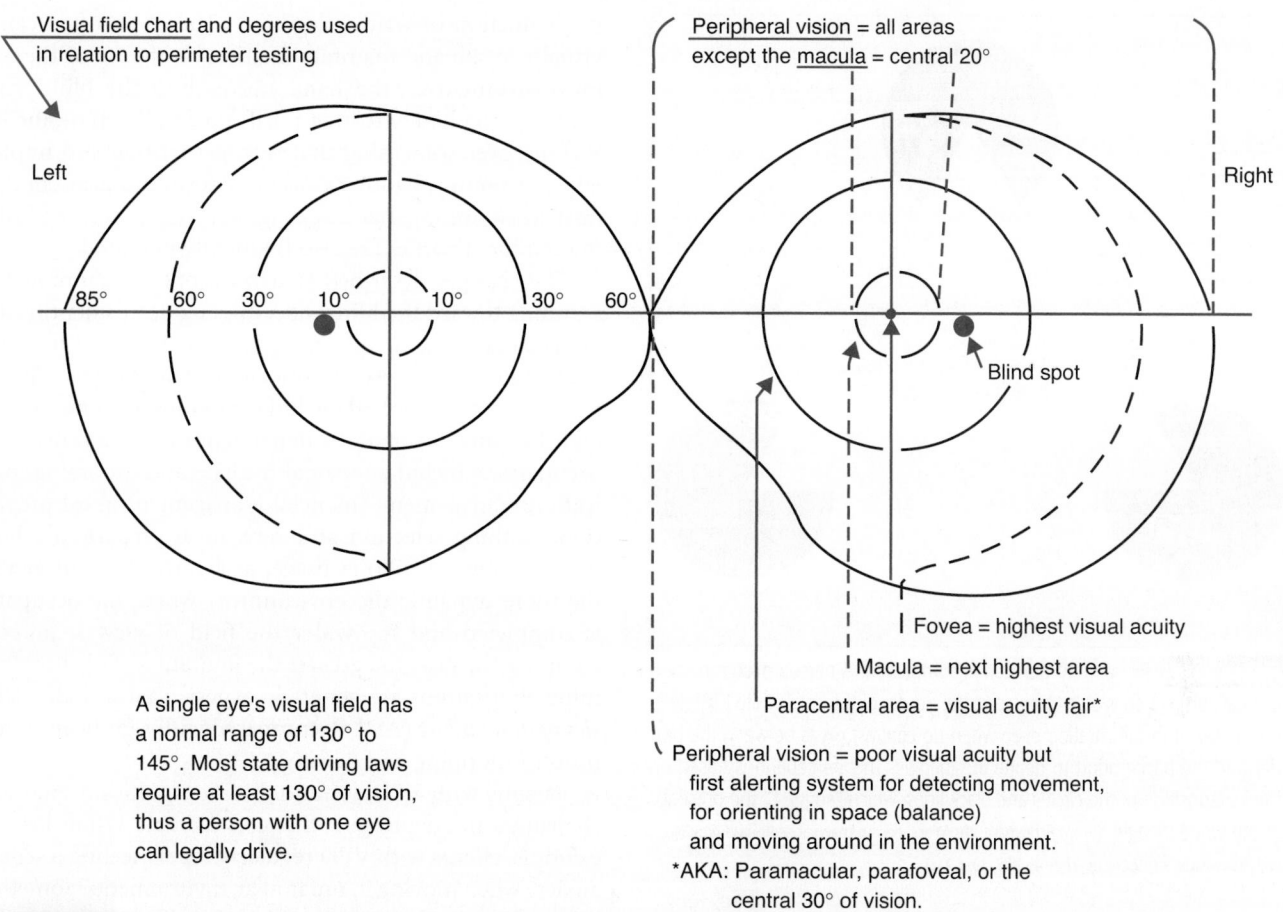

Visual field chart and degrees used in relation to perimeter testing

Left

Peripheral vision = all areas except the macula = central 20°

Right

85° 60° 30° 10° 10° 30° 60°

Blind spot

A single eye's visual field has a normal range of 130° to 145°. Most state driving laws require at least 130° of vision, thus a person with one eye can legally drive.

Fovea = highest visual acuity

Macula = next highest area

Paracentral area = visual acuity fair*

Peripheral vision = poor visual acuity but first alerting system for detecting movement, for orienting in space (balance) and moving around in the environment.
*AKA: Paramacular, parafoveal, or the central 30° of vision.

Figure 23-7   Visual field chart illustrating the divisions of the visual field related to visual acuity. (Courtesy of Josephine C. Moore, PhD, OTR.)

important role in the person's ability to adapt to fast-paced and dynamic environments. However, in the case of significant visual field loss, the presence of perceptual completion makes it difficult for the client to determine how his or her visual field has changed.[73,99] Because of perceptual completion, the client with a VFD is not immediately aware of the absence of vision after onset of the deficit.[71,73,105] He or she perceives the presence of a complete visual field without gaps or missing information. However, the CNS cannot place objects in a visual scene that it does not actually see. Therefore the client may not be aware of unanticipated objects on the blind side. As a result, the client may run into a recently placed chair or other obstacles on the blind side or may not be able to find items placed within the blind field. Until the client becomes aware of the VFD, he or she will have the odd perception of a complete visual scene in which objects always seem to be appearing, disappearing, and reappearing, without warning, on the affected side. Uncertainty regarding the accuracy of visual input on the affected side causes the client to adopt a protective strategy, in which he or she attends only to visual input from the intact visual field.[89,132] This creates narrowed scope of scanning restricted to the midline of the body and seeing side. The restriction creates significant

limitations in occupations that require monitoring of the entire visual field, such as driving a car or traversing a busy environment.

Even when the person becomes aware of the presence of a VFD, visual search into the blind field often is slow and delayed.[51,78,89,132] Again, the culprit is perceptual completion, which eliminates the presence of a marker to indicate the boundary between the seeing and non-seeing fields. Unable to determine the actual border of the seeing field or where a target might be within the non-seeing field, the client naturally slows down when scanning toward the blind field. The slow visual search towards the affected side increases the difficulties the client has navigating and finding objects within the environment and also reduces reading speed.

If the hemianopsia affects the macular portion of the visual field, especially the fovea, a client may miss or misidentify visual details when viewing objects because part of the object falls into the blind area of the field. This can create significant challenges in reading.[13,18,29,30,32,68,69,114,133-135] Normal readers view words through a "window" or perceptual span that allows them to see approximately 18 characters (letters) with each fixation of the eye.[133] The reader typically moves from word to word using a series of consecutive saccadic eye movements

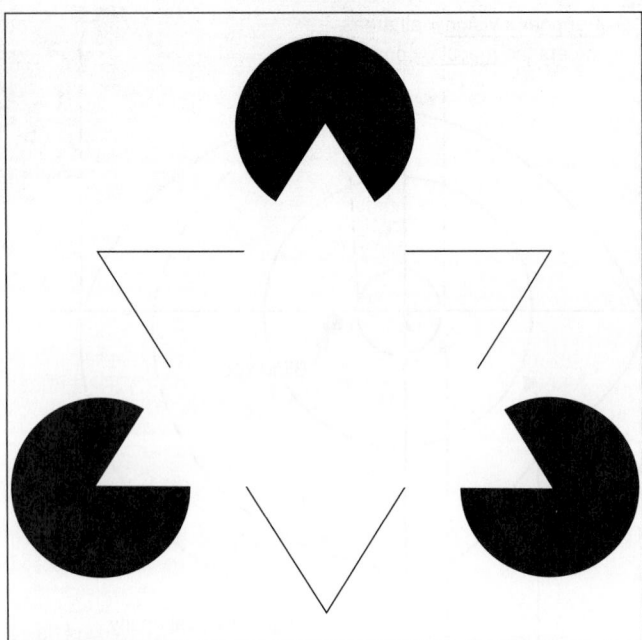

Figure 23-8 Example of perceptual completion. A person exercising perceptual completion is able to perceive the border of the solid white triangle in the center of this illustration even when no contrast exists between the border and the background to define the triangle. This perception is based on the juxtaposition of the circles and black lines, which "suggest" the presence of the white triangle. (From Schuchard RA: Adaptation to macular scotomas in persons with low vision, *Am J Occup Ther* 49:873, 1995.)

to cross the line of print. Presence of a hemianopsia can reduce the width of the perceptual span from 18 characters to as few as 3 to 4 characters. This may cause the client to view only part of a word during a fixation and even skip over small words, often resulting in the misidentification and omission of words.

For example, a client with a left hemianopsia may read the sentence, "She should not shake the juice" as "He should make juice," transforming "she" into "he" and "shake" into "make" and leaving out "not" and "the." Errors such as these cause the client to have to stop and reread sentences, reducing reading speed and comprehension. Accuracy in reading numbers generally creates more challenge for the client than reading words. Whereas context alerts the client to an error when reading sentences (the sentence does not make sense), numbers appear without precise context, causing mistakes to go unnoticed. For example, a bill for $28.00 may be misread as $23.00 and the error missed until a notice of insufficient payment is received. Clients making these kinds of errors quickly lose confidence in their ability to pay bills and manage their checkbook, and turn over these important daily occupations to someone else.

If the VFD has occurred on the same side as the dominant hand, the client may have difficulty visually guiding the hand in fine motor activities. The most common functional change

is a reduction of writing legibility. The client often cannot visually locate and maintain fixation on the tip of the writing instrument as the hand moves into the blind visual field, causing handwriting to drift up and down on the line. Writing over something that was just written and improperly positioning handwriting on a form are also common mistakes. Quilting, hand sewing, pouring liquids, and other fine motor activities are also frequently impaired.

The changes described (narrow scope of scanning, slow scanning toward the blind side, missing or misidentification of visual detail, and reduced visual monitoring of the hand) contribute to a variety of performance limitations. The primary activities affected include mobility, reading, writing, and the daily occupations dependent on these skills. These occupations include personal hygiene and grooming, medication management, financial management, meal preparation, clothing selection and care, meal preparation, home management, telephone usage, and yard work. In general, the more dynamic the environment where the occupation is completed and the wider the field of view required to complete the task, the greater the limitation. Therefore, only minor limitations are generally experienced in basic *activities of daily living* (ADLs), compared with significant limitations in shopping and driving.

Persons with VFD commonly face significant emotional challenges in adapting to this considerable vision loss. For example, clients with VFD regularly report feeling a sense of anxiety when moving in unfamiliar environments. Sometimes the anxiety can be so severe that the client experiences an autonomic nervous system reaction, becoming nauseated and short of breath and breaking out into a sweat in crowded environments. One individual with VFD described this sensation as "crowditis," reporting that he became physically ill if he had to go into a department store or other crowded environment. This anxiety can become debilitating, leading to a withdrawal from community activities and to social isolation. Other clients report a tremendous loss of self-confidence because of the numerous mistakes they make during the course of a day, and many express that they experience depression because of their limitations, especially in the ability to drive a car and read accurately.

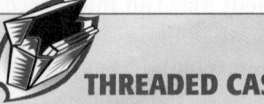

THREADED CASE STUDY: PENNY, PART 3

Penny reported to the occupational practitioner that she is able to successfully complete *basic activities of daily living* (BADLs) but has difficulty completing several *instrumental activities of daily living* (IADLs). She has difficulty reading and states that she reads very slowly and makes frequent mistakes especially when reading numbers. Because of these deficiencies in reading, she has difficulty reading bills and financial statements and disclosed that

THREADED CASE STUDY: PENNY, PART 3—CONT'D

she did not pay her Visa bill correctly one month and was charged a financing fee. She also has difficulty reconciling her checkbook as she may read entries incorrectly and then be unable to find her errors. She estimates that it takes her approximately three times as long to pay bills as it did before her vision loss and she always has a headache when she is finished. Her difficulty reading numbers also creates other challenges when renewing prescriptions for herself and for Pot. She frequently gives the wrong number to the pharmacist and because of this can no longer use the automated renewal line and must wait until she can get someone in person. This is very embarrassing. She also misread her blood glucometer incorrectly once and injected insulin when she did not need it, which caused her a reaction lasting several hours. She was an avid newspaper reader and read the metro and sports pages to Pot daily, an activity they both enjoyed, as he would recognize some of the names of local teams and players. She can no longer do this, nor can she read novels to him, which she felt was very therapeutic.

She reports that she is able to complete meal preparation although she spends a great deal of time scanning shelves trying to locate items. She also has difficulty seeing well enough to pour and measure items and will sometimes misread a recipe or set the microwave at the wrong time setting. She recalled a time when she was melting chocolate to put in a cake batter and set the microwave on 8 minutes rather than 3 and burned the chocolate.

She reports that her greatest limitations revolve around mobility. She is unable to drive, and must depend on others for transportation. When a friend takes her on a shopping outing, she has difficulty locating the items she needs and reading the labels. Because she does not want to inconvenience her friend and slow her down, she often comes home with the wrong item or without items because she could not find them. She also admits to feeling very uncomfortable in crowded environments, especially with people moving on her left side. She states that her heart pounds and she feels an overwhelming desire to leave. She is afraid that she will collide with someone she has experienced several instances of this and she also at times experiences disorientation. She and Pot attended church services regularly before her stroke and the deacons will provide transportation but she feels too uncomfortable to go.

She did not bring up her art but when asked about it, she became very quiet and finally stated that she felt that was behind her now. She stated that she had tried drawing again but could not see well enough and that she could not find the supplies she needed and was very frustrated. She does not want to resume drawing if she cannot do it well.

When asked to prioritize her goals for therapy, she stated driving as the number one goal and reading as the second goal. She also wanted to accurately complete financial management, meal preparation, and diabetes self-management.

Assessment

The process of measuring the visual field is known as *perimetry*.[3] Several types of perimeters are available. These range from simple bedside assessments (such as the confrontation test), which give a gross indication of field loss, to the very precise imaging of a *scanning laser ophthalmoscope* (SLO).[3,46,102,105,116] The perimetry test selected depends on the availability and cost of the test and the ability of the client to participate in testing. For example, confrontation testing does not incur any expense and can be performed nearly anywhere, whereas SLO imaging must be completed by a specially trained technician in a center that has purchased the $120,000 instrument. In between these two extremes are the tangent screen, Damato Campimeter, manual bowl perimeters (the Goldmann), and automated bowl perimeters (the Humphrey), ranging in cost from $100 to $20,000. In general, the more expensive the apparatus, the more precise the measurement provided.

All perimetry testing involves three parameters: fixation on a central target by the client while the testing is completed, presentation of a target of a specific size and luminosity in a designated area of the visual field, and acknowledgment of the second target without breaking fixation on the central target.[3] Testing is done with either static or kinetic presentation of the target. In static presentation, the target appears in a specified area of the visual field without being shown moving to that location. In kinetic testing the target moves in from the periphery until it is identified.[3,102]

The most accurate perimetry test available to clinicians is computerized, automated perimetry, which is completed by either an ophthalmologist or optometrist.[3] During automated perimetry, the client places his or her chin on a chin rest and fixates on a central target inside a bowl-shaped device. As the person fixates on the central target, lights are displayed inside the bowl in varying locations and intensities. The client responds to each seen light by pushing a small button. The test can be very thorough, presenting lights in over a hundred locations within the field and increasing the intensity of the light in a step threshold sequence if the target is not appreciated the first time. The result is an accurate measurement of the areas of absolute loss (no response) and relative loss (decreased retinal sensitivity) within the field. An ophthalmologist or optometrist may also use a simpler screening test, the tangent screen, to assess the integrity of the central visual field. The tangent screen consists of a black felt screen with a grid stitched into the felt in black thread so that the grid is visible only to the examiner.[3] The client sits directly in front of the screen at a distance of 1 m. The client is instructed to fixate on the center of the screen as the examiner moves or places a white target attached to a black wand in a certain area of the screen. Without breaking fixation on the center of the screen, the client indicates when the target is seen. If the client does not see the target when it is presented, that point in the visual field is recorded as a loss. The examiner uses the grid to determine the location of the field deficit.

OT practitioners can screen for VFD using simple perimetry testing in combination with careful observation of client performance in daily occupations. Confrontation testing is a bedside examination that provides a crude indication of visual field loss.[102,116] To complete a static confrontation test, the examiner sits in front of the client at a meter distance and has the client fixate on a centrally placed target (the examiner's eye). The examiner then holds up two targets in each of the four quadrants of the visual field (right upper, right lower, left upper, and left lower). The client indicates whether the targets are seen.[57,102,106] For a kinetic test the examiner stands behind the client and moves a target (generally a penlight) in from the periphery while the client fixates on a central target. The client indicates as soon as the target is noticed. Standardized versions of these tests are included in the biVABA. Because confrontation testing has been shown to be unreliable in detecting all but gross defects, OT practitioners using this form of testing must be careful to correlate their findings with observations of client performance.[116] If the confrontation test shows no deficit but the clinical observations suggest that a deficit is present, the clinical observations should carry the greater weight in deciding if a deficit exists.

Assessment using perimetry devices such as the Damato 30-Point Multifixation Campimeter (biVABA) enables OT practitioners to obtain a more accurate measurement of central visual field function. The Damato Campimeter, shown in Figure 23-9, is a portable test card that provides a precise measurement of the central 30° of the visual field. The test grid consists of 30 numbered targets that place the test stimulus at known points in the visual field by moving the eye rather than the target. The test stimulus is a 6-mm black circle that is shown in the center part of the card. The client is instructed to fixate on one of the numbered targets. The test stimulus is then shown in the central window, and the client indicates if the circle is seen. If the client does not see the black circle, that point in the visual field is recorded as a loss. The test proceeds with the client successively moving

the eye to view the numbered targets until the entire field is mapped out.

Clinical observation of the client's behavior is especially important to confirm the presence of VFD because of the limitations of perimetry testing.[102] Clients with fluctuating or limited attention, language, and cognition may give unreliable perimetry results. It also may be difficult to distinguish between VFD and a deficit in visual attention. However, the client's performance of daily activities will strongly indicate the presence of a VFD. For example, the presence of a visual field deficit may be indicated if any of the following are observed: the client changes head position when asked to view objects placed in a certain plane; the client consistently bumps into objects on one side; the client misplaces objects in one field; or the client makes consistent errors in reading.

Perimetry tests establish only whether a VFD is present and the size and location of the deficit. To determine whether intervention is needed, the practitioner must determine whether the client is able to compensate for the VFD in performing daily activities, as well as the quality and consistency of that compensation. The presence of a VFD can cause significant limitations in daily occupations. The level of impairment will depend on whether the VFD occurs alone or in conjunction with visual inattention. An analysis of occupational performance should be completed to identify limitations in basic and instrumental ADLs. If the client demonstrates difficulty completing an activity, the visual requirements of the activity should be analyzed to determine if the VFD is interfering with performance. For example, if the client is unable to locate a toothbrush during grooming, is it because the toothbrush is stored on the side of the client's field deficit?

Reading is another daily activity often affected by VFD. *The Visual Skills for Reading Test* (VSRT) provides an effective way to measure the interference of the VFD on reading performance. The VSRT is designed to assess the influence of a *scotoma* (or field loss) in the macula on the visual components of reading, including visual word recognition and eye movement control.[124] The client is asked to read single letters and words printed on a card. Three different versions of the test card in four font sizes are included in the test to accommodate clients with low vision and to permit retest. The words are not in context and are designed so that they can be misread and still make sense (e.g., "shot" can be mistakenly read as "hot"). The test measures reading accuracy and corrected reading rate and provides information on the prevalent types of reading errors made by the client. The client's performance on the letter and reading charts used to measure visual acuity also may indicate the influence of a VFD on reading performance. Because of the wider visual field, a client with a VFD may have more difficulty reading the larger symbols and words on the chart and may be able to read faster and more accurately as the optotypes (and field) decrease in size. Telephone Number Copy, part of the

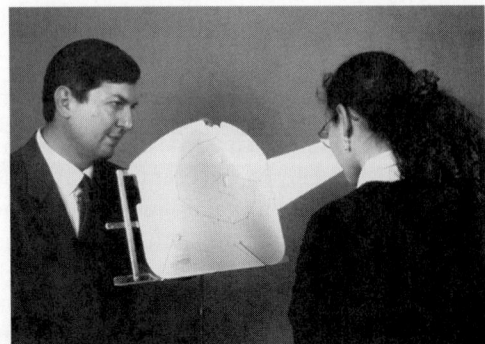

Figure 23-9 Position of examiner and client for completion of perimetry testing using the Damato 30-point Campimeter from the Brain Injury Visual Assessment Battery for Adults. (Courtesy of Precision Vision, LaSalle, IL.)

biVABA, provides information about the client's accuracy in reading numbers. In this test, the client is required to copy down telephone numbers that include numbers easily misread by persons with VFD, such as 6, 8, 9, and 3.

To effectively compensate for the VFD, the client must execute an organized and thorough search of the blind field, using the seeing portion of the visual field. This means that a client with a left visual field deficit must use the right visual field to search both the left and right fields. Clients with VFD demonstrate difficulty searching both *peripersonal space* (the space immediately around the body) and *extrapersonal space* (the space extending from the body into the environment). Deficiencies in searching peripersonal space affect performance of basic ADLs such as grooming, dressing, reading, and writing, as well as instrumental ADLs requiring monitoring of a wider visual field, such as meal preparation or leisure activities. Deficiencies in searching extrapersonal space

have a pronounced impact on mobility and affect activities in outside and community environments, such as driving, shopping, and mowing the yard.

To navigate dynamic community environments, the client must use a wide scanning strategy that is initiated on the side of the deficit and executed quickly and efficiently. The client also must be able to shift attention and search rapidly between the central visual field and the peripheral visual field. A variety of observational tests can be used to measure the ability to compensate for the VFD during mobility. An objective assessment of the client's ability to execute compensatory search strategies can be made using a Dynavision 2000, an apparatus increasingly used in rehabilitation to assess and train visual motor performance (Figure 23-10).[63-66] OT practitioners without access to a Dynavision can use a laser pointer to observe the client's search capability. The beam of light from the pointer is projected onto various

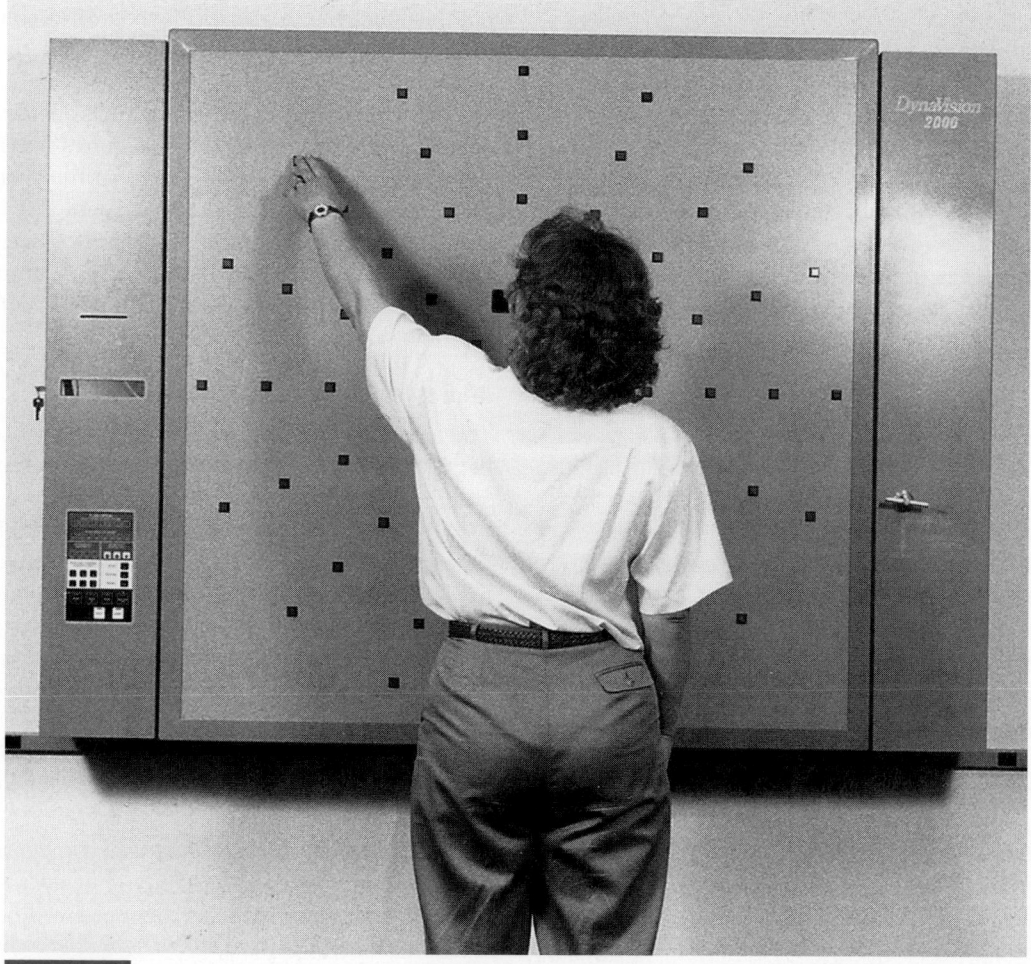

Figure 23-10 Example of a visual search task using the Dynavision 2000. The lights on the board are illuminated one at a time in random patterns. The client must locate the illuminated light and press it to turn it off. As a light is pressed, another light is illuminated. The client strikes as many lights as possible within a specified time. The activity can be used to teach and reinforce efficient search patterns to compensate for visual field deficits and visual inattention. (Courtesy Dynavision 2000, manufactured by Performance Enterprises, Ontario, Canada.)

areas of a blank white wall, and the client is instructed to locate and touch the projected red dot. The strategy used by the client to locate the dot and the efficiency of the strategy is noted. Integration of visual scanning with ambulation is the final component of the mobility assessment and must be completed to determine whether the client will be able to compensate for the deficit during body movement. This can be assessed by using such tests as the ScanCourse from the biVABA. To complete a ScanCourse, the client is instructed to walk through a course and identify targets placed in various locations on the left and right sides. The client's ability to locate the targets to each side during ambulation is noted.

THREADED CASE STUDY: PENNY, PART 4

Penny's left hemianopsia was identified by the optometrist using a Humphrey Visual Field Analyzer. This perimetry test showed that Penny has a complete left hemianopsia in both eyes affecting both the central and peripheral fields. Of particular importance is the finding that the border of the hemianopsia comes into the fovea and splits this area of the field. This observation indicates to the OT that Penny's perceptual span for reading has probably been significantly reduced on the left side, causing her to miss words and letters on the left. The practitioner confirms this using the VSRT, which shows that Penny does miss both letters and words on the left, reducing her reading accuracy to 83%. Her corrected reading rate is also significantly reduced, 32 words per minute, indicating that she reads text at a rate of approximately 51 words per minute (persons read approximately 1.6 times faster). Because of her stated difficulty accurately reading numbers, Penny was also given the Telephone Number Copy from the biVABA. She misread three numbers on this test, misidentifying a 3 as an 8, a 4 as a 1 and 9 and a 5 as an 8. She was able to find her errors on the test and correct her mistakes.

The Dynavision 2000 was used to observe Penny's ability to search for targets in her visual field. Analysis of the Dynavision performance showed that Penny demonstrated a reaction time of 2.35 seconds to locate targets in the left half of the board compared to 1.1 seconds in the right half of the board. In observing her locate targets on the board, the OT noted that Penny moved her head very slowly to the left side of the board to locate targets and did not turn her head far enough to see the lighted targets on the outer ring of lights. Penny also completed a ScanCourse. On the first pass through the course, she missed 4 of 10 targets located on the left side (60%) but easily identified 10/10 targets on the right side (100%). After receiving feedback on her performance, on the second pass through the course (going the reverse direction) she identified 9/10 targets (90%) on the left and 10/10 targets (100%) on the right.

Intervention

The performance limitations experienced by persons with VFD generally fall into two categories: difficulties with mobility and difficulties with reading. Because of the mobility limitation, clients will experience the limitations in daily occupations that must be completed in dynamic environments, such as shopping and participating in community events. Resumption of driving may or may not be a goal, depending on the driving statutes of the state in which the client resides. Some states do not specify a minimum degree of visual field for licensure. In these states a client may be able to safely resume driving if given the proper training. Challenges in completing reading will cause difficulty in completing such activities as financial management and meal preparation.

Although a limited body of research shows that some restitution of visual field may be possible with intensive rehabilitation[7,58,59,86] return of visual field function is unlikely.[106] Therefore, the major focus of intervention is to improve compensation for the visual field loss. Compensation for VFD requires adopting a conscious, cognitive strategy of using head movement to search and broaden the visual field. Because the CNS exercises perceptual completion, the client often lacks insight into the extent and boundaries of the field deficit. Successful compensation requires the client to believe firmly that the deficit exists and that the visual input from the blind side cannot be trusted. A client able to develop this level of insight will usually learn to effectively compensate for the deficit. Every effort must be made through activities and educational materials to make the client aware of the location and extent of the deficit.

Addressing limitations in mobility

The limitations experienced in mobility occur primarily because the client does not turn his or her head far enough, fast enough, or often enough towards the blind field to take in the information needed for safe mobility in the allotted time. If the inferior visual field has been affected, as occurs with a hemianopsia, the client may also experience difficulty monitoring the support surface on the deficit side. This can result in hesitancy in walking and a tendency to keep the head down and the eyes fixed on the floor directly in front of the client. Although this strategy may keep the client from colliding with objects, it also prevents the client from monitoring the surrounding environment and can cause disorientation during ambulation.

A combination of remediation and compensation strategies is used to address these mobility deficiencies. Remediation strategies focus on increasing the speed, width, and organization of the search pattern.[49,61,63,66,104,115] The client must learn to quickly turn the head and completely search the blind visual field. The desired outcome behaviors include the following:

1. Initiation of a wide head turn towards the blind field
2. An increase in the number of head and eye movements toward the blind field

3. Faster completion of head and eye movement toward the blind field
4. Execution of an organized and efficient search pattern that begins on the blind side
5. Attention to and detection of visual detail on the blind side
6. Ability to quickly shift attention and search between the central visual field and the peripheral visual field on the blind side

To achieve these outcomes, the client must complete activities where these performance skills are required within the performance of an occupation. This is difficult to achieve in the restricted environment of the clinic. The Dynavision 2000 apparatus has been shown to be effective in teaching these components of effective search patterns and is strongly recommended as an intervention tool.[43]

 OT PRACTICE NOTES

Other therapeutic activities that may facilitate development of these performance skills include the following:
1. Ball games in which balls are passed quickly from player to player
2. Balloon batting
3. Projection of light from a laser pointer onto various locations on a white wall for the client to search and find
4. Adhesive stick-on notes with numbers and letters printed on them, widely scattered over a wall for the client to search and find
5. Use of the strategy in completion of daily activities such as finding clothes in a closet or locating items needed for meal preparation

As the basic components of the search strategy are developed, they should be incorporated into activities that require combining search with ambulation. Indoor activities can include completing scan courses using cards with letters taped onto walls in various locations along hallways. Two examples are activities such as "find red" where the client points out every red item while walking towards a destination within the rehab center, and "narrated walks" where the client points out landmarks and changes in the environmental surroundings while ambulating towards a destination. These activities reinforce keeping the head up during ambulation, improving orientation. As skill is developed, practice in dynamic and in unfamiliar environments should be incorporated. The client completes activities in stores and malls where he or she identifies the number of persons standing in an aisle or inside a store on the blind side while ambulating by, and locates stores within a mall and specific items within stores using landmarks and organized search strategies.

Integrated into the intervention plan is instruction in compensatory strategies. The client is taught to identify features in the environment that could cause harm, such as steps, curb cuts, and other changes in the support surface. The client also is taught to be more observant of landmarks such as a picture on a wall or a change in wall color to assist in maintaining orientation.

Addressing limitations in reading

The client's primary challenges in reading occur because his or her present saccade strategy doesn't match the new restricted size of the perceptual span. That is, the client is trying to read using a saccade strategy designed for a wider unrestricted perceptual span. To improve reading speed and accuracy, the client must learn how to adapt a saccade strategy to the new perceptual span. This requires significant practice and can be extremely frustrating for the client. To address this, a remediation approach is used. Pre-reading exercises such as those designed by Warren[123] or Wright and Watson[130] and commercially available word and number searches are used to provide the practice the client needs to learn to make the precise eye movements required to see words completely again. These exercises are designed so that the client searches for specified letters, numbers, or words on worksheets (Figure 23-11). As the client's performance skill improves, large print books of familiar stories are used to provide the needed practice and transition the client into reading continuous text.

A compensatory intervention approach is also used to address reading and writing challenges. Clients with left hemianopsia often have difficulty accurately locating the next line of print on the left margin of the reading material and lose their place. Drawing a bold red line down the left margin provides the client with a visual cue to use as an "anchor" to find the left margin.[125] The same technique used on the right margin helps the client with right VFD who may be uncertain about the location of the end of the line of print. If the client has difficulty staying on line or moving from line to line, a ruler or card can be used to underline the line of print and keep the client's place.

Difficulty staying on line when writing is addressed by teaching the client to monitor the pen tip and maintain fixation as the hand moves across the page and into the side of field loss. Activities that require the client to trace lines towards the side of the VFD are effective in reestablishing eye-hand coordination. Practice in completing blank checks, envelopes, and check registers is also helpful.

Occupational performance can be enhanced by increasing the visibility of tasks and environments. Adding color and contrast to the key structures in the environment needed for orientation (e.g., door frames and furniture) will help the client locate these structures. Using black felt-tip pens can heighten the contrast in writing materials, and bold-lined paper can be used to help the client monitor handwriting. The simple addition of more light often increases reading speed and reduces errors. Reducing pattern in the environment by reducing clutter and using solid-colored objects enhances the client's ability to locate items.

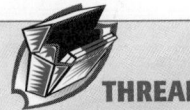

THREADED CASE STUDY: PENNY, PART 5

Penny received ten 1-hour sessions of outpatient occupational therapy intervention over a 10-week period. To address her limitations in reading, Penny was given pre-reading exercises involving letters, numbers, and words to help her modify her saccade strategy to match her reduced perceptual span. She completed the exercises at home for 45 minutes a day. During therapy sessions, she completed timed reading drills that showed the practitioner how she was progressing in speed and accuracy on the pre-reading exercises. The VSRT was repeated at 5 weeks and showed that her reading accuracy had increased to 92% and her reading rate increased to 72 words per minute. The Telephone Number Copy was also repeated with 100% accuracy. Penny was progressed to reading large print books with familiar content. Penny and Pot were fans of the Sue Grafton alphabet murder mysteries, so Penny's friend took her to the local library to check out a large print copy of one of the books she had read before. She read the book to Pot for an hour daily. At discharge, the VSRT was repeated and Penny demonstrated100% accuracy with a reading rate of 124 words per minute.

To address mobility and driving, the OT began by having Penny complete a succession of exercises on the Dynavision for the first 20 minutes of each treatment session. The exercises focused on increasing the speed and efficiency of the search pattern she executed to the left and on her ability to shift attention between the center and peripheral areas of the board and complete scanning with cognitive distractions. Scan courses using targets taped along the hallways of the center were used along with "find red" and narrated scanning. As Penny improved on indoor activities, the OT moved outdoors and had Penny navigate sidewalks and areas adjacent to the clinic. Prior to navigating an unfamiliar environment she was instructed to consciously turn her head widely and survey her surroundings, locating any potential obstacles and identifying landmarks. As her comfort in these environments increased, she was taken on a community outing to her local grocery store to practice the skills she had learned and receive instruction in how to quickly and efficiently scan shelves to locate needed items. Additional community outings were completed in her local mall and in her church.

Two weeks prior to discharge, Penny excitedly reported that she and Pot had attended church and lunch with friends afterward with no difficulty. Three weeks after therapy was initiated, the OT completed a home visit to assess Penny's environment and to meet Pot. Penny's friend and fellow artist who had been taking her to therapy also attended the session. The home assessment showed that Penny's home generally had sufficient lighting, contrast, and organization. However, the small kitchen had only a single small round ceiling light, leaving the countertops and work surfaces poorly lit. In addition she had deep cupboards packed with food and cookware and her countertops were also cluttered. Penny's studio, located in a bedroom, was cluttered and had only overhead lighting and a small table lamp.

Following the assessment, the OT suggested replacing the overhead lighting fixture in the kitchen with a large fluorescent fixture, adding fluorescent under-counter lighting, and reorganizing the shelves and countertops to remove rarely used items.

Although Penny was still resistant to resuming her art, suggestions were made to improve the lighting in her studio by adding a 50-W halogen task lamp on her work table along with increasing organization and decreasing clutter. A low-power magnifying lamp was also recommended to assist her to see details more clearly. Penny was initially resistant to these suggestions because she did not feel she could complete them but her friend stated that she would help her and within 2 weeks all recommendations were implemented.

The friend was also very interested in getting Penny to resume her art and asked for suggestions in how to accomplish this. The OT suggested that if the detailed drawings Penny had previously completed were still too difficult even with the studio modifications, maybe she could explore other forms of artistic expression that were not so visually demanding. The next week Penny reported in therapy that she and her friend had attended an art fair on the weekend and she thought she might experiment with watercolor landscapes, something she had done early in her career. Her friend was coming over to assist her that week.

Driving was addressed throughout this intervention period. The Dynavision exercises Penny completed were designed to improve the visual skills needed for driving, especially speed, flexibility, and width of the search strategy to the left. Limitations experienced by drivers with VFD were discussed in conjunction with strategies to compensate for these limitations and vehicle modifications. When Penny had shown sufficient improvement, the 4-minute test on the Dynavision was administered. This test has been shown to be predictive of behind the wheel performance.[65] A person scoring above 195 on the test is likely to successfully complete an on-road driving assessment. Penny scored 230 on the test and was referred to a driver's program for an assessment with an occupational practitioner credentialed as a *certified driver rehabilitation specialist* (CDRS). Penny passed the driving assessment and was released to resume driving during daylight hours over familiar routes.

Penny's ability to complete meal preparation, financial management, and diabetes self-management was addressed through improvement of reading and visual search skills, task and environmental modification, and adaptive equipment. A talking calculator to verify numbers assisted her to reconcile her checkbook. Because of the critical need for accuracy in drawing insulin and monitoring blood glucose levels, she was trained to use a nonvisual adaptive device to draw her insulin and a talking glucometer. The environmental modifications implemented following the home assessment greatly improved her ability to complete meal preparation along with instruction in how to increase contrast.

Cross out all of the double numbers 1.5M

```
8 1 2 6 7 2 3 1 2 2 4 5 6 8 8 7 5 6 8 8 4 5 3 2 6 7 8 5 6 7 7 4 5 6 6
5 8 8 3 4 5 2 8 8 3 4 5 8 8 2 1 9 9 4 5 2 3 8 8 5 6 7 6 5 9 9 7 6 5 4
8 9 8 6 3 4 5 8 8 2 3 4 5 2 7 7 9 9 8 7 8 9 5 6 8 8 3 4 5 7 6 8 5 5 4
8 8 6 5 3 4 2 3 7 8 8 6 9 0 3 4 8 8 4 5 2 3 4 5 6 7 8 8 4 6 6 5 4 6 9
3 2 8 8 9 3 4 2 8 8 4 5 7 2 3 5 5 7 8 9 0 0 3 8 3 9 2 3 3 4 3 2 2 1 5
4 8 5 7 3 6 6 7 4 3 2 5 5 3 4 7 8 9 9 2 3 4 2 2 4 5 6 4 3 6 7 8 8 5 4
1 1 2 3 4 5 6 6 5 4 4 4 5 6 7 7 8 8 9 0 0 6 5 6 7 7 4 5 3 4 5 3 3 2 5
4 5 6 6 5 4 4 4 3 3 2 2 5 6 4 7 2 3 4 5 5 9 8 7 6 7 8 8 8 4 5 6 2 2 1
3 4 5 6 5 5 4 6 6 5 4 6 5 6 7 8 4 2 4 5 2 2 4 4 9 9 8 8 7 7 8 6 6 6 4 3
6 6 4 6 3 7 8 8 5 3 3 3 6 7 7 5 5 4 4 1 1 6 6 9 5 5 3 3 7 1 4 2 3 4 4
5 5 3 3 2 5 7 3 1 1 1 4 4 6 6 8 4 3 5 5 6 6 7 7 3 6 8 5 7 6 5 4 3 2 2
2 3 4 4 5 6 6 7 5 8 7 7 9 8 9 0 0 1 1 1 2 3 4 4 4 3 3 5 6 3 5 4 3 2 2
3 3 4 4 5 4 6 3 7 5 5 7 8 9 0 1 1 8 7 6 5 4 4 1 1 4 5 3 9 6 8 5 4 7 3
4 4 5 3 7 5 5 7 9 9 7 0 9 6 4 5 6 6 8 0 8 0 1 2 2 3 4 4 5 7 8 9 0 1 1
5 5 6 4 5 5 5 4 3 2 2 1 2 4 9 8 9 9 0 0 7 6 5 5 6 7 5 8 4 8 4 4 3 8 3
2 3 4 2 2 1 3 2 5 7 6 8 5 4 4 5 7 3 4 3 2 1 3 5 6 7 7 8 0 0 6 3 2 3 2
3 3 4 4 2 2 5 7 7 8 9 9 0 7 6 5 5 4 4 3 7 7 5 4 3 3 2 2 1 2 3 3 4 5 6
3 3 4 4 4 5 5 6 6 7 4 2 2 5 8 0 7 6 8 6 5 3 3 3 3 7 8 0 6 4 2 4 5 6 6
6 6 4 6 3 7 8 8 5 3 3 3 6 7 7 5 5 4 4 1 1 6 6 9 5 5 3 3 7 1 4 2 3 4 4
5 5 3 3 2 5 7 3 1 1 1 4 4 6 6 8 4 3 5 5 6 6 7 7 3 6 8 5 7 6 5 4 3 2 2
2 3 4 4 5 6 6 7 5 8 7 7 9 8 9 0 0 1 1 1 2 3 4 4 4 3 3 5 6 3 5 4 3 2 2
8 8 6 5 3 4 2 3 7 8 8 6 9 0 3 4 8 8 4 5 2 3 4 5 6 7 8 8 4 6 6 5 4 6 9
3 2 8 8 9 3 4 2 8 8 4 5 7 2 3 5 5 7 8 9 0 0 3 8 3 9 2 3 3 4 3 2 2 8 5
```

© 1996 vis**ABILITIES** Rehab Services Inc.

Figure 23-11 Example of a pre-reading exercise. The client is instructed to cross out all of the double numbers on the page. (From Warren M: *Prereading and writing exercises for persons with macular scotomas*, Birmingham AL, 1996, visAbilities Rehab Services.)

VISUAL ATTENTION AND SCANNING

Visual attention is the ability to observe objects closely and carefully to discern information about their features and their relationship to oneself and other objects in the environment. It requires the ability to ignore irrelevant sensory input and random thought processes and to sustain focus for several seconds to several minutes. Visual attention also entails being able to shift visual focus from object to object in an organized and efficient manner. Engagement of visual attention is accomplished through visual scanning or search (these two terms are used interchangeably). Although these two processes are separated within the visual perceptual hierarchy to assist in understanding them, they cannot be separated in assessment and treatment of the client. Any change in visual attention will be observed in the client as a change in the scanning pattern used for visual search.

Visual attention can be divided into two categories: focal, or selective visual attention, and ambient, or peripheral,

visual attention.[37,55,85,94] *Focal attention* is used for object recognition and identification. Visual input from the macular area of the retina is used to complete this processing. Focal, or selective, attention enables an individual to accurately distinguish visual details such as differences between letters, numbers, and faces. *Ambient*, or *peripheral*, *attention* is concerned with the detection of events in the environment and their location in space and proximity to the person. It relies on input from the peripheral visual field. Peripheral attention ensures that a person is able to move safely through space and maintain orientation in space. Without peripheral attention, collisions with objects and disorientation when moving would be the norm. To have a fully operational and efficient visual system, these two modes of visual attention must work together. The contribution of each is equally important to perceptual processing.

In adults without brain injury, visual search is completed using an organized, systematic, and efficient pattern.[34,38,48,90,122,126] The type of search pattern used depends on the demands of the task. In reading English, for example, a left-to-right and top-to-bottom linear strategy is used. In scanning an open array (such as a room), a circular, left-to-right strategy generally is used, following either a clockwise or a counterclockwise pattern.

Deficits in Visual Attention and Scanning

Studies have shown that disruption in the normal visual search strategy can occur after brain injury. The characteristics of the disruption vary, depending on which hemisphere was damaged. Visual search deficits associated with right hemisphere injury are characterized by avoidance in searching the left half of the visual space.[10,22,24,37,38,45,47,90] This condition is known as **hemi-inattention.** Instead of initiating the normal left-to-right visual search pattern, clients with right hemisphere injuries often begin and confine search to the right side of a visual array. This creates an asymmetrical search pattern instead of the normal symmetrical pattern. The client misses visual information on the left side and, as a result, may be deprived of information needed to make accurate identification and decisions.

Hemi-inattention is associated with right hemisphere injuries and probably occurs because of a difference in the way the hemispheres are programmed to direct visual attention.[47,107] As illustrated in Figure 23-12, the left hemisphere directs attention toward the right half of the visual space surrounding the body. In contrast, the right hemisphere directs visual attention toward both the right and left halves of the space surrounding the body. If a lesion occurs in the left hemisphere, visual attention and search toward the right side are diminished, but some attentional capability is still provided by the right hemisphere. A similar lesion in the right hemisphere may completely eliminate attentional capability toward the left because there is no other area directing attention toward the left side.

Hemi-inattention often is confused with the presence of left VFD in the client. Although both conditions may cause the client to miss visual information on the left side, they are distinctly different conditions and do not have the same effect on performance. When left VFD occurs, the client

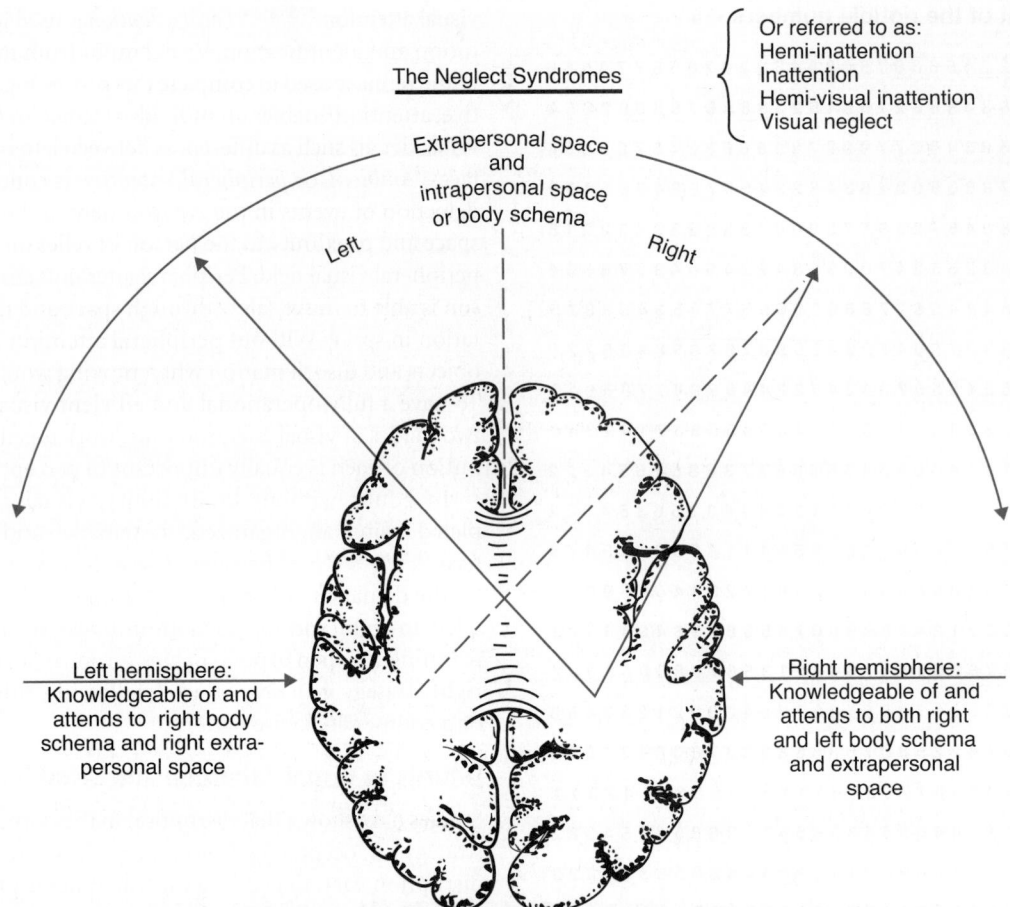

In relation to **movement** and **sensory perceptions** such as vision (visual-spatial and visual-object awareness and recognition), auditory and somesthetic (including body image or schema) cognition and awareness, it appears that the left hemisphere primarily attends to the right extrapersonal space and/or body image parameters while the right hemisphere attends to both right and left extrapersonal space and body image. Thus **left hemisphere lesions** of the 1°, 2° or 3° areas of the cerebral cortex or associated subcortical fiber tracts concerned with visual, auditory, somesthetic, or motor functions rarely result in a neglect syndrome because the right hemisphere can attend to and compensate for the left hemisphere deficit. However, **right hemisphere lesions** of one or more of these functional areas leave the brain unable to attend to or be aware of the left extrapersonal space and body schema. visual field deficits (especially left homonymous hemianopsia) always compound the neglect syndrome.

Figure 23-12   Difference between the right and left hemispheres in the direction of visual attention and the relationship of hemisphere lesions to hemi-inattention and neglect syndrome. (Courtesy of Josephine C. Moore, PhD, OTR.)

attempts to compensate for the loss of vision by engaging visual attention.[10,11,51,75] The client directs eye movements toward the blind left side in an attempt to gather visual information from that side. Because of the field deficit, however, the client may not move the eyes far enough to acquire the needed visual information from the left side and as a result may appear inattentive. In contrast, the client with hemi-inattention has lost the attentional mechanisms in the CNS that drive the search for visual information on the left.

No attempt will be made by the inattentive client to search for information on the left side of the visual space, and no eye movement or head turns will be observed toward the left side.[22,51] The most significant change in visual search happens when the two conditions occur together in the client.[10,20] In this case the client is not receiving visual input from the left side because of VFD and does not compensate for the loss of visual input by directing attention toward the left side. The combination of hemi-inattention and left VFD creates severe inattention, often called **visual neglect.** Clients with this condition show exaggerated inattention toward the left half of the visual space surrounding the body and often do not move the eyes past midline toward the left or turn the head toward the left side. Visual neglect may be compounded by neglect of the limbs on the left side of the body or neglect of auditory input from the left side.[45,61] The presence of neglect is associated consistently with poor rehabilitation outcomes.[51]

Another change in visual search associated with right hemisphere lesions is a tendency to fixate first on the most peripheral visual stimuli occurring in the right visual field.[45] If two visual stimuli simultaneously appear in the right visual field, the client will attend first to the most peripheral stimulus.[31] The client with this tendency makes frequent head turns to attend to events occurring in the right peripheral field, giving the impression of being distractible. Yet another change in visual search is a reluctance to rescan for additional information once an area has been viewed, especially if the area is on the left side.[90] This may cause the client to miss certain visual details when viewing complex visual arrays.

Although several distinct changes in visual search have been observed with right hemisphere lesions, only one has been observed following left hemisphere lesions. Clients with left hemisphere injury may show a symmetrical decrease in searching for detail when viewing a visual array.[15,45,117] These clients symmetrically scan the visual array for information but do not examine specific aspects of the visual scene to gather additional information. Because of this, they may miss visual details and often cannot accurately interpret or identify the objects around them. Left hemisphere injury does not result in hemi-inattention or neglect.

In general, clients with injuries to either hemisphere are slower in scanning and show more erratic fixation patterns, compared with persons without brain injury.[74,126] They also have greater difficulty engaging selective attention and executing an organized and efficient visual search strategy. Research has shown that when persons with brain injuries are asked to search complex visual arrays for specific targets, they have difficulty maintaining attention on the salient features of the target and mistakenly select targets with similar features.[93,126] They also demonstrate an inability to superimpose an organized, efficient structure for visual scanning when asked to search an array with randomly displayed objects. For example, if asked to locate a certain individual seated among others on rows of benches (a structured visual array), the injured person would be able to accomplish the task. However, if asked to find the same individual standing in a jumbled crowd of persons (a random visual array), the injured person would display a random approach to searching the array and would likely miss the target.

Occupational Limitations Caused by Visual Inattention

Disruption of visual attention creates asymmetry and gaps in the visual information gathered through visual search.

The quality of an individual's adaptation to the environment decreases because the CNS is not receiving complete visual information in an organized fashion and therefore is unable to effectively use this information to make appropriate decisions. Reduction in visual attention will affect all aspects of the performance of daily occupations. However, the most affected activities will be those that require inspection and integration of significant amounts of visual detail and those completed in dynamic environments. Driving and reading are two diverse examples of tasks often significantly affected by inattention.

Because visual attention is modulated through an extensive neural network involving the entire CNS, some capacity for visual attention generally is retained even in cases of severe brain trauma.[81] Conversely, because so many neural structures contribute to attention, changes in visual attention occur even with mild injuries.[99] Whether a change in visual attention affects occupational performance depends on the task to be completed. Tasks such as reading can require enormous amounts of selective visual attention if an individual is reading a highly technical textbook, and less selective attention if the individual is reading an advertisement. The task of driving requires continuous global attention to monitor the speed and position of other vehicles and objects, and sporadic selective attention to landmarks, street signs, and traffic lights. Whether a deficiency in visual attention manifests after brain injury depends on the circumstances and requirements of the tasks the client completes.

Assessment

As a process found at the intermediate level of the visual perceptual hierarchy, visual attention can be affected by deficits in lower level visual functions (visual acuity, oculomotor function, and visual field). Therefore, these functions should be assessed before visual attention is measured. The presence of aphasia and motor impairment can also affect performance on assessments for visual attention. How efficiently and completely a person attends to and takes in visual information determines the ability to use the information for adaptation. Therefore, the emphasis in assessment is on observing how a client initiates and carries out visual scanning to complete a task requiring visual search. During the assessment the practitioner should answer the following questions: Does the client initiate an organized search strategy? Can the client carry out the search strategy in an organized and efficient manner? Does the client obtain complete visual information from visual search? Is the client able to identify visual detail correctly? Does the client's ability to search for information decrease as the visual complexity of the task increases?

Research shows that persons with good visual attention demonstrate specific characteristics of search patterns that make them effective in obtaining visual information.[48,122,131] These characteristics include strategies that are organized, symmetrical, thorough, resilient, and consistent. The use of these strategies usually results in good accuracy and speed in completion of visual search tasks. In contrast, persons with significant VFD or inattention often demonstrate ineffective search strategies. These individuals demonstrate incomplete or abbreviated patterns in which only a portion of the visual array is searched, usually in a random, unpredictable fashion.[15,23,37,48,51,74,78,93,126] The organization and accuracy of the pattern often break down when the person is challenged to search more complex visual arrays. Figure 23-13 provides examples of some of the ineffective search strategies used on

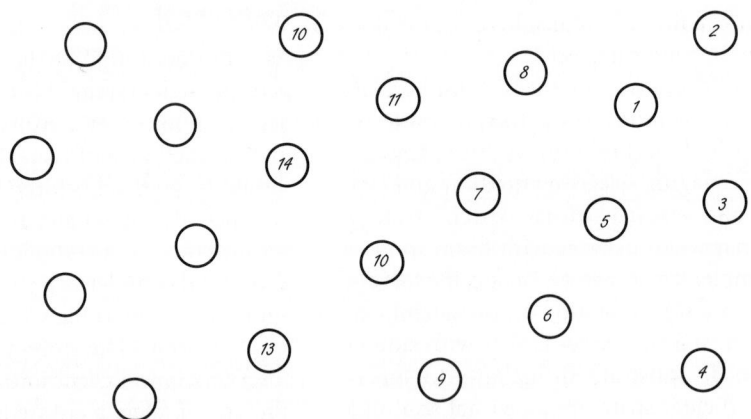

NAME: _____B.D._____ DATE:_____

P   F

GJHℙGOEITKGHⵝQOWⵝTUIEⵝRⵝITOOIⵝWQ

UIℙGℙNKJELSGHNⵝRⵝMVNGⵝWZXⵝRNOIM

TUEIOℙTHVNCJEⵝZMENⵝUIⵝVNOLⵝQTRNB

CVDℙMGJBⵝQWIDKRⵝGJⵝWKSⵝBNVRⵝLKI

QWIℙKBNGⵝCJⵝNVHⵝKWIEJDTIHⵝVNCNJⵝ

UTRHℙOBKVNPSLDKEIXKRⵝGHBNⵝLGJⵝN

OℙLNRIOWEⵝCNDⵝOMGNⵝRODⵝZXCⵝBMT

SINGLE LETTER SEARCH-CROWDED • 1997, visABILITIES Rehab Services Inc.

A

NAME: _____C.T._____ DATE:_____

RANDOM PLAIN CIRCLES-SAMPLE   ©1997, visABILITIES Rehab Services Inc.

B

Figure 23-13 Examples of ineffective search patterns used by clients to complete two visual search subtests of the Brain Injury Visual Assessment Battery for Adults. **A,** An abbreviated search pattern used by a client with left hemianopsia when crossing out the letters P and F on the subtest; the client executed an organized left-to-right linear search pattern but failed to locate the beginning of the line on the left side, and as a result failed to cross out targets on that side (the circled letters). **B,** An asymmetrical and abbreviated search pattern executed by a client with hemi-inattention and left hemi-anopsia. The client was asked to number the circles consecutively, choosing any pattern desired. The client began numbering the circles from the right rather than the left and failed to number circles on the left side of the array.

the visual search subtests of the biVABA by persons with brain injury. A client who employs ineffective search strategies may not acquire sufficient visual information to complete perceptual processing accurately. The client may acquire the information in such a way that it cannot be used to complete perceptual processing, or the person may not acquire the information rapidly enough to enable adaptation. The subsequent disruption of perceptual processing may cause errors in decision making and adversely affect performance of a variety of daily living activities.

When measuring visual attention, the practitioner must be aware that visual search can be significantly affected by both the presence of a VFD and hemi-inattention. Because VFD and hemi-inattention are not the same condition, it is necessary to distinguish between the two conditions to establish an effective intervention plan. This can be difficult, both because similar errors are observed with the two conditions on search tasks and because the two can also occur together in the same client. However, differentiation can be accomplished by observing the strategies used by the client to complete visual search tasks such as those on the biVABA (Figure 23-13). Although both VFD and hemi-inattention can result in decreased accuracy in identifying targets on a visual search task, the characteristics of the search deficiencies are different.[10,22,27,28,41,51]

For example, a client with a left hemianopsia may demonstrate a left-to-right linear search pattern that is abbreviated on the blind side. The search pattern is organized but results in a number of errors on the left because the client did not see that side of the array. In contrast, a client with hemi-inattention may demonstrate an asymmetrical pattern, initiating and confining visual search to the right side using a disorganized and random search pattern. The pattern also results in a large number of errors on the left. Although accuracy on the search task may be similar for these two clients, the cause of the errors is different. By observing the strategy used by the client to complete the search task, it is possible to distinguish between the two conditions. Table 23-2 compares the characteristics of search patterns used by persons with hemianopsia and persons with hemi-inattention. When the two conditions occur together, it is important to determine the severity of the inattention because this will determine whether the client is able to learn the strategies needed to compensate for the VFD.

The visual search tests that have been described are pencil-and-paper tasks presented in a restricted and well-defined personal space. Determining how the client applies a search strategy to broader extrapersonal space requires the use of a test such as the ScanBoard described by Warren.[122] The test, part of the biVABA, consists of a large (20 by 30 inch) board with a series of 10 numbers displayed in an unstructured pattern. The board is placed at eye level and centered at the client's midline. The client is asked to scan the board and point out all of the numbers that he or she sees. The examiner records the pattern the client follows in identifying the numbers. Research using this test has shown that adults with normal visual search employ an organized, sequential search pattern, beginning on the left side of the board and proceeding in either a clockwise or counterclockwise fashion until all of the numbers are identified. In contrast, adults with deficits in visual attention demonstrate disorganized, random, and often abbreviated search strategies, frequently missing numbers on one side of the board. Those with hemi-inattention often show an asymmetrical pattern, initiating and confining visual search to the right side of the board. Clients with VFD may miss numbers on the blind side but demonstrate an organized search strategy.

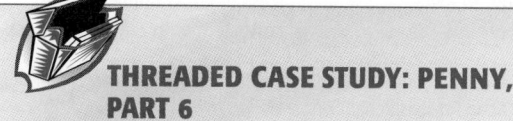

THREADED CASE STUDY: PENNY, PART 6

The physician referring Penny to the low-vision center noted that she had hemi-inattention in addition to the left hemianopsia. Because hemi-inattention can significantly interfere with completion of ADLs, especially driving, it was important to determine how much, if any, of Penny's difficulty scanning was due to inattention.

To assess this, Penny was given the visual search subtests from the biVABA. On three of the subtests involving searching for letter and words, she missed several of the targets located on the left side indicating an abbreviated search pattern towards the left. However, on each of the seven subtests, she consistently used an organized left to right and top to bottom search strategy. She also carefully looked at each target and rechecked her work for accuracy. These observations suggested normal attentional capability, which was verified by her performance on other assessments. For example, although she made mistakes in copying numbers on the Telephone Number Copy test, she was able to search and correct her mistakes without assistance. She also missed targets on the left side during her first pass through the ScanCourse, but after receiving feedback, made no errors on her second trial on the course. On the Dynavision assessment, she was also able to switch attention easily between the left and right sides of the board and her ability to search the left side of the board rapidly improved with practice.

After analyzing Penny's performance on these assessments, the OT concluded that because of the severity of her VFD, Penny may have appeared to be inattentive towards the left side during the first several weeks after her stroke when she was unaware of the VFD. But as she gained awareness of the deficit, she was able to use attention to help compensate for the loss of vision on the left. If Penny's performance had suggested the presence of the hemi-inattention, it would not have been appropriate to set a goal to resume driving and it would have been necessary to explore alternative forms of transportation.

TABLE 23-2 **Comparison of Search Patterns: Persons with Visual Field Deficit vs. Persons with Hemi-Inattention**

Visual Field Deficit	Hemi-Inattention
Search pattern is abbreviated toward blind field	Search pattern is asymmetrical; initiated/confined to the right side
Attempts to direct search toward blind side	No attempt to direct search toward left side
Search pattern is organized and generally efficient	Search pattern is random and generally inefficient
Client rescans to check accuracy of performance	Client does not rescan to check accuracy of performance
Time spent on task is appropriate to level of difficulty	Client completes task quickly; level of effort applied is not consistent with difficulty of task

From Warren M: *Brain Injury Visual Assessment Battery for Adults Test Manual,* Lenexa, KS, 1998, visAbilities Rehab Services.

Intervention

Information gathered from observing the client complete visual search tests should reveal specific deficiencies in the scanning pattern the client uses to acquire visual information during completion of daily tasks. For example, it may be observed that the client does not search toward the left side of visual arrays. If this deficiency is significant, a similar performance should be observed when the client completes a daily activity. This could be an inability to locate items placed to the left side of the sink in grooming or a tendency to begin reading a recipe in the middle of the line of print instead of at the left margin.

Depending on the severity of the deficit, some clients with inattention are able to complete basic and habitual daily activities and experience difficulty only on tasks that are unfamiliar or require search of a complex visual array.[76] Others, especially those with neglect, may have difficulty with such a simple task as finding all the food on their plate. By combining information from visual search tests with that gained from observation of ADL performance, it is possible to determine if and how the client's performance of daily activities has been affected by impairment of visual search. The goals on the intervention plan should be worded to reflect the specific daily activities compromised by the inattention. For example, the intervention plan could include such goals as, "The client will be able to complete grooming independently" or "The client will be able to prepare a simple meal independently."

The goals established for independent ADL performance are achieved by ensuring that the client learns to take in visual information in a consistent, systematic, and organized manner. Before a client can learn to reorganize a visual search,

he or she must understand how his or her visual search and attention have changed. To facilitate the development of this insight, the OT practitioner should carefully review the results of the client's performance on the visual search tests and show the client how his or her search pattern differed from the norm and caused errors. If, after receiving this feedback, the client wishes to retake one of the tests, he or she should be allowed to do so. If the client's performance improves on the retest, this is an indication of capability to benefit from therapy intervention and serves as a justification for intervention. Likewise, if the client's performance does not improve, this helps to verify the significance of the deficit and also may indicate reduced rehabilitation potential.

The intervention plan should incorporate compensatory strategies and environmental modification. The primary compensatory strategy taught to the client with hemi-inattention is to reorganize the scanning pattern to begin visual search on the left side of a visual array and progress left to right.[5,28,88,125,127] The use of this pattern will counteract the client's tendency to restrict all visual search to the right side and will increase the symmetry of the search pattern. Clients with left hemisphere injuries do not demonstrate asymmetry in visual search but often fail to notice details when searching visual arrays. These clients should be taught to initiate careful item-by-item search of visual arrays. Two scanning strategies are taught with all clients: a left-to-right linear pattern for reading and inspection of small visual detail, and a left-to-right clockwise or counterclockwise pattern for viewing unstructured and extra-personal visual arrays.[4] Activities should be selected that encourage and reinforce the use of these patterns.

Compensatory strategies can be taught more effectively if intervention activities are designed using the following guidelines:

1. Intervention activities should require the client to scan as broad a visual space as possible. Most daily activities require orientation to a broad visual space. To help the client complete a wide visual search, the working field of the activity should be large enough to require the client either to turn the head or to change body positions to accomplish the task.[127] Many activities and games can be enlarged to require head turning for scanning. For example, a deck of playing cards can be laid out, facing up, in rows 2 to 3 feet wide. The client is given another deck of playing cards and instructed to match the cards in hand to the cards on the table. The practitioner ensures that the client initiates a left-to-right, top-to-bottom, organized scanning pattern when searching for the matching cards to complete the task.

2. Intervention activities will be more effective if the client is required to interact physically with the target once it is located. Research has shown that a stronger mental representation of a visual image is formed if what is seen is verified by tactual exploration.[4,67] Whenever possible, the intervention activity should be designed to be interactive.

Games such as solitaire, dominoes, ball games, or activities such as putting together large puzzles are examples of activities with interactive qualities.

3. Intervention activities should emphasize conscious attention to visual detail and careful inspection and comparison of targets. Because complex visual processing is dependent on initiation of the item-by-item search strategy of selective visual attention, it is important to include scanning activities that require discrimination of subtle details and matching. Clients should be taught consciously to study objects for their relevant features, with emphasis placed on attending to detail in the impaired space. Many games such as solitaire, double solitaire, Concentration, Connect Four, checkers, Scrabble, and dominoes have these qualities. Large 300- to 500-piece puzzles, word or number searches, crossword puzzles, and needlecrafts such as latch hook also require these performance skills. Throughout performance of these tasks, clients should be encouraged to recheck their work to make sure that critical details are not missed.

4. Facilitate attention to the left half of visual space by occluding vision in the right half of the visual space. Occlusion of the right half of the visual field has been shown to be effective in increasing the client's attention toward the left.[14] The occluder, made by placing opaque tape over the right side of a pair of safety lenses, is worn while the client completes a therapeutic activity to facilitate attention. The lenses are removed once the activity is completed.

5. Practice the search strategy within context to ensure carryover of application to daily living activities. Clinic activities provide a starting place to begin teaching the strategies needed for successful visual perceptual processing. Research has shown, however, that clients with brain injury often do not spontaneously transfer skills from one learning situation to the next. Toglia[113] suggests that having the client apply the learned strategy in different contexts of daily living can facilitate transfer of learning. For example, the client can be required to use a left-to-right search strategy when selecting clothes from a closet, searching for items in a refrigerator, or shopping for groceries. The more often the strategy is repeated under varied circumstances, the more the skill is generalized and transferred to new situations. There is no substitute in therapy for the practice of real-life situations to help the client develop insight into abilities and compensation for limitations. Cafeterias, gift shops, and office areas within the hospital, and fast food restaurants and shops surrounding the hospital can be used to expose the client to more realistic and demanding visual environments.

Insight on the part of the client into the nature of the visual deficit and how it has affected functional performance is critical to learning compensation.[110-112] According to Toglia,[113] one of the reasons clients with brain injury do not spontaneously recognize their limitations and the need to compensate, is that their concept of their capabilities is based on pre-morbid experiences. This causes these clients to overestimate their abilities after injury. Without a realistic understanding of limitations, the client may be unwilling to use compensatory strategies. To increase insight, Abreu and Toglia[1] advocate teaching a client to monitor and control his or her performance by learning to recognize and correct for errors in performance. Giving the client immediate feedback about the performance and pointing out deficiencies facilitate this process of error detection. The process can also be facilitated by teaching the client to use self-monitoring techniques such as activity prediction, in which the client predicts how successfully an activity will be performed and identifies the aspects of the activity in which errors are likely to occur. The client then compares actual performance with predicted performance. This technique helps the client develop anticipatory skills and increase awareness of how the deficit affects functional capabilities. The use of video feedback has also been shown to be useful in enabling the client to understand how their neglect behavior affects occupational performance.[112]

Some clients, because of the severity of their deficits, lack the cognition to benefit from training in compensatory strategies. Although treatment intervention is limited, such clients may benefit from a modification of the environment to help the client use his or her limited attentional capabilities. The environment can be made more visible and "user friendly" by reducing factors that place stress on visual processing. Suggested environmental modifications include the following:

1. Reduce background pattern so that objects in the foreground can be seen more easily. The more densely packed the background pattern, the greater the amount of selective attention needed to locate the desired object. Clients with severe brain injuries may not be able to sustain the effort needed to complete this level of processing and may view their environments as filled with "visual noise" rather than meaningful objects. Backgrounds can be simplified by eliminating patterned designs and using solid colors on surfaces. Eliminating superfluous objects such as knickknacks and old magazines and organizing frequently used items on shelves and in containers also simplify the background. As a general rule, environments should be sparse and contain only the items needed by the client for completion of daily activities. Items that contain a lot of intrinsic pattern, such as reading materials, can be enlarged to decrease the density of the pattern.

2. Ensure that room and task illumination is adequate. Both too little and too much illumination can impair visual processing. However, environments usually contain too little rather than too much light. The type of lighting used should provide bright, even illumination without glare.

3. Increase contrast between background and foreground objects to enhance the visibility of items in the environment that need to be noticed. For example, the edge of a white plate placed on a black place mat is more visible

than it would be if placed on a white place mat, and milk in a black cup is more visible than in a white cup. The use of glass or clear plastic items should be avoided because these items reduce contrast by absorbing whatever pattern or color is around them.

OCULOMOTOR FUNCTION

The purpose of oculomotor function is to achieve and maintain *foveation* of an object.[42] That is, oculomotor function ensures that the object the person wishes to view is focused on the fovea of both retinas (to ensure a clear image) and that focus is maintained as long as needed to accomplish the desired goal. This is a daunting task because human beings interact within dynamic, moving environments. An image focused on the fovea is always in danger of slipping off as the head or object is moved. Foveation is achieved and maintained by eye movements that keep the target stabilized on the retina during fixation, gaze shift, and head movement.[42,70,77,97]

Another function of oculomotor control is to provide **binocular vision.** Binocular vision ensures perception of a single image even though the CNS is receiving two separate visual images (one from each eye). The process of combining two visual images into one is called **sensory fusion.** For sensory fusion to occur, corresponding points (or receptor cells) on the two retinas must be stimulated with the same image. If the retinas are thus stimulated, and if the images match in size and clarity, the CNS is able to fuse the two images perceptually into one. If the eyes do not align with each other or if there is a significant difference between the eyes in acuity, a double image (**diplopia**) may occur.[42,71,119]

Deficits in Oculomotor Function

Deficits in oculomotor control following brain injury generally result from either of two types of disruption: specific cranial nerve lesions causing paresis or paralysis of one or more of the extraocular muscles that control eye movements, or disruption of central neural control of the extraocular muscles affecting the coordination of eye movements.[5,60,72,74,96,97] In the first case, the message to the extraocular muscles through the cranial nerve is blocked; in the second case the message comes through but is scrambled. In both cases, the functional results are decreased speed, control, and coordination of eye movements. Three pairs of *cranial nerves* (CN) control the extraocular muscles: the oculomotor nerve (CN III), the trochlear nerve (CN IV), and the abducens nerve (CN VI). Among them, these nerves are responsible for controlling seven pairs of striated muscles that surround and attach to the two eyeballs.

When a cranial nerve lesion occurs, the muscles controlled by that cranial nerve are weakened or paralyzed, a condition known as paralytic strabismus.[82,119] As a result, the eye is unable to move in the direction of the paretic muscles and may even be unable to maintain a central position in the eye socket (i.e., it drifts in or out). Because the eyes must always move in synergy and line up evenly to maintain a single visual image, an individual sees a double image when the movement of one eye is impeded or when the eye's position changes and does not match that of the other. This condition, diplopia or double vision, is the primary functional disruption observed with cranial nerve lesions.[82,119]

Occupational Limitations Caused by Oculomotor Deficits

The presence of diplopia creates perceptual distortion, which may affect eye-hand coordination, postural control, and binocular use of the eyes. The performance limitations experienced by the client depend on where the diplopia occurs within the focal range (the range in which a person can keep objects in focus). Diplopia occurring within 20 inches of the face will disrupt reading and activities requiring eye-hand coordination, such as pouring liquids, writing, and grooming. Diplopia occurring at a distance (greater than 4 feet) will affect walking, driving, television viewing, and playing sports such as golf and tennis.

To eliminate the double image, the client will often assume a head position that avoids the field of action of the paretic muscle.[8,72,119] For example, a client with a left lateral rectus palsy (CN VI) will turn the head toward the left to avoid the need to abduct the eye. A client with paralysis of the right superior oblique muscle (CN IV) will tilt the head to the right and downward to avoid the action of that muscle.[8] Unless oculomotor function is carefully assessed, these alterations in head position may be interpreted as resulting from changes in muscle tone in the neck rather than as a functional adaptation purposely assumed to stabilize vision.

Often it is not the cranial nerves that are damaged during brain injury, but the neural centers that coordinate their actions. These structures are scattered throughout the brainstem and communicate extensively with cortical, cerebellar, and subcortical areas of the CNS and the spinal cord.[52,77] In cases of traumatic brain injury, diffuse damage may take place throughout the brainstem, affecting these control centers. If the centers are damaged, the person will have difficulty executing eye movements even though the cranial nerves are intact.[72,96,97,107] Disconjugate eye movements may occur, causing the client to have difficulty using the eyes together in a coordinated fashion. Dysmetric eye movement, in which the eye undershoots or overshoots a target, also may be observed.[106]

Damage to the pretectal nuclei in the brainstem can cause convergence insufficiency; a condition in which the client is unable to obtain or sustain convergence of the eyes.[25,72] Convergence is the muscle action of moving the eyes inward in adduction. It is one of the three components of accommodation, the process that keeps objects in focus as they come into close view. When convergence insufficiency occurs, clients have difficulty obtaining or sustaining adequate focus during near vision tasks (tasks within 20 inches of the face). Clients with this condition often complain of fatigue, eye pain, or headache after a period of sustained viewing in near tasks such as reading. As the eye muscles fatigue from the exertion of sustaining convergence during reading, clients may begin to complain that the print is swirling and moving on the page. The condition often is overlooked in evaluation because cranial nerve function usually is intact and clients' complaints instead are attributed to inattention, lack of effort, or dyslexia.[25,72]

These disturbances in ocular motility can create a variety of functional deficits for the client.[72,84] The speed and range of eye movement may be diminished. This will reduce the speed at which the client is able to scan the environment and take in visual information, causing delays in responding to the environment. The client may have difficulty maintaining a clear image and may experience doubling and blurring of visual images.[53,72] There may be difficulty focusing at different distances from the body. Depth perception may be diminished. These conditions will create significant visual stress for the client, reducing concentration and endurance for activities. The client may respond to this increased stress by becoming agitated and uncooperative in therapy sessions or by complaining of headaches, eyestrain, or neck strain.

Because a number of factors can disrupt the control of eye movements, much skill and expertise is needed to accurately diagnose the oculomotor deficit and design an appropriate treatment intervention. Practitioners who treat this type of dysfunction should do so with the guidance of an optometrist or ophthalmologist who specializes in visual impairment caused by neurological conditions.[39,84]

Assessment

The purpose of an assessment completed by the OT practitioner is to determine whether the client is experiencing limitations in daily occupations due to dysfunction within the oculomotor system. It is not to determine whether the oculomotor dysfunction is the result of cranial nerve lesion, brainstem injury, or other conditions. Determining the etiology of the dysfunction is the responsibility of the ophthalmologist or optometrist. However, the OT practitioner is often one of the first members of the rehabilitation team to observe that the client may have an oculomotor impairment affecting occupational performance. This frequently places the OT in the position of requesting further evaluation by an eye care specialist. To make an appropriate referral, it is necessary to complete a screening to identify patterns of oculomotor dysfunction that may account for the functional limitations observed in the client.

In assessing the client, a "listen and look" approach is used, wherein the practitioner listens to the complaints being voiced by the client or the rehabilitation staff working with the client and looks for deviations in oculomotor control that may contribute to these complaints. This approach is described in the biVABA, and the following steps in evaluation are from that assessment.

The first step in assessment is to obtain a visual history from the client. The history is necessary because adults with childhood histories of oculomotor dysfunction or reduced acuity often display oculomotor abnormalities that do not affect functional performance. These individuals frequently wear eyeglasses to correct for the deficiencies; in this case the eyeglasses must be worn during the assessment to obtain accurate results. Areas addressed in this part of the evaluation include whether the client had good vision before brain injury, whether the client wears eyeglasses, and whether the client has a history of conditions that may affect oculomotor control, such as congenital strabismus, lazy eye, or amblyopia.

Next, the client is asked whether he or she is experiencing diplopia. If the response is affirmative, the client should be questioned about the characteristics of the diplopia. Does the diplopia disappear when one eye is closed? This indicates impairment of the extraocular muscles. Do objects double side-to-side or on top of one another? Is the diplopia present at near distances or at far distances? Is there any area within the range of focus where the client is able to achieve single vision? The answers to these questions may suggest which cranial nerve has been injured (Table 23-3) and also supply important information about limitations the client may experience in daily activities. The practitioner concludes the interview by identifying activities the client has difficulty performing that could be caused by oculomotor dysfunction. The practitioner should look for a pattern in the client's response, such as difficulty with activities that require sustained focus in near space (reading, writing, and quilting). The practitioner should pay attention to whether the client's visual difficulty seems to change with the focal length of the task and whether the client's fatigue and reduced concentration appear to be related to activities requiring sustained focusing.

The next part of the assessment is observing the client's eyes and eye movements for deficiencies. First, the eyes are observed for asymmetries in pupil size, eyelid function, and eye position as the client focuses on a distant object.

TABLE **23-3** **Summary of Oculomotor Deficits Associated with Cranial Nerve Lesions**

Oculomotor Nerve III	Trochlear Nerve IV	Abducens Nerve VI
Impaired vertical eye movements	Impaired downward and lateral eye movements	Impaired lateral eye movements
Lateral diplopia for near vision tasks	Vertical diplopia for near vision tasks	Lateral diplopia for far vision tasks
Dilation of pupil and impaired accommodation	With bilateral lesion assumes downward head tilt	
Ptosis of eyelid		

Asymmetries such as a dilated pupil in one eye or a droopy eyelid (ptosis) may indicate cranial nerve involvement and suggest difficulty adjusting to light (light sensitivity) and reading. Next, movement of the eyes is observed by asking the client to track a moving object (such as a penlight) through the nine cardinal directions of gaze plus convergence.[87] This test can be thought of as an active *range of motion* (ROM) test of the eyes because the nine cardinal directions represent the directions through which the eyes move. The test is used to determine if there are deviations in strength and function of the extraocular muscles and is completed by observing the eyes move in a binocular test.

During the test, the practitioner observes the following: (1) the symmetry of the eye movement; (2) whether the eyes move the same distance in each direction; (3) whether the eyes are able to stay on target with a minimum of jerking movements; and (4) whether the client is able to hold the eyes in a deviated position at the end of the range for 2 to 3 seconds. Restriction of eye movement in a specific direction or difficulty moving the eyes in a specific direction may indicate impaired oculomotor function.[82] Observing the eyes as they track an object moving toward the bridge of the nose tests convergence. Most adults can maintain focus and track an object to a distance of approximately 3 inches from the bridge of the nose. At that point one eye usually breaks fixation and moves outward. The point at which convergence is broken is known as the *near point of convergence*.[82]

Although the near point of convergence is 2 to 3 inches from the bridge of the nose, few adults ever view objects that closely. Therefore, limitations in convergence are generally not functionally significant unless the client is unable to converge the eyes and easily maintain convergence to a distance of 12 to 16 inches from the bridge of the nose. An inability to converge the eyes to this distance and maintain convergence for several seconds while focusing on an object may cause the client to have difficulty performing tasks in near vision that require a sustained focus. Observation of convergence insufficiency may explain complaints made by the client regarding such tasks as reading, writing, quilting, or sewing.

The final component of the assessment is diplopia testing, which is completed only if the client is complaining of diplopia.[106] Diplopia testing is used to determine the severity of the diplopia and whether it is caused by a tropia or a phoria. *Tropia* is the suffix applied when there is a noticeable deviation of the position of one eye in relation to the other when the client is viewing an object.[106,119] *Phoria* is the suffix used when there is a deviation of the eye that is held in check by fusion and is therefore not noticeable when the client is focusing on an object. These terms are used in conjunction with a prefix describing the direction of the deviation. Four prefixes are used: eso-, meaning a turning in of the eye; exo-, a turning out of the eye; hypo-, a turning downward of the eye; and hyper-, a turning upward of the eye. Esotropia therefore describes an observable, inward deviation of the

eye commonly described as "crossed eyes," whereas esophoria indicates that the eye drifts inward when the client is not focusing on an object but is held in check when the client is focusing on an object.[72]

Diplopia testing is based on the principle that when an eye is required to fixate on an object, it will do so with the fovea. If an eye that is not fixating on a target is suddenly required to foveate, it will achieve foveation by making a saccade toward the target. By requiring the client to fixate with both eyes on a target and then covering one of the client's eyes during fixation, the examiner can determine whether both eyes are aligned in focusing on the target and, if not, which eye is the deviant (strabismic) eye.[87,118] Two tests are used: a cover/uncover test, which is completed when a tropia is suspected, and a cross or alternate-cover test, which is completed when a phoria is suspected.[87,118] If both eyes are aligned equally and fixating on the target, no movement of either eye will be observed when one is covered. If the eyes are not aligned, the deviating eye will move to take up fixation when the non-affected eye is covered. Clients with tropias generally complain of constant diplopia when viewing objects and must have one eye occluded to eliminate the diplopia. Clients with phorias often complain of diplopia only intermittently, usually when fatigued or stressed by sustained viewing of a target. Although the phoric client may complete most activities without diplopia, he or she may experience significant visual stress, which can manifest as headaches, eye strain, or decreased concentration.

The information gathered from the assessment should be compared with the client's visual complaints and observations of his or her occupational performance to determine if the oculomotor dysfunction is contributing to the client's functional limitations. For example, the presence of convergence insufficiency may help explain the difficulty the client is having in maintaining concentration when reading. As another example, the observation of downward movement of the left eye during the cover/uncover test may explain why the client complains of feeling off balance and unsure when descending stairs. If oculomotor deficiencies are observed that appear to limit occupational performance, referral should be made to an ophthalmologist or optometrist for further evaluation to determine the cause of the deficiency, the prognosis for improvement, and treatment options.

Intervention

The presence of oculomotor dysfunction usually does not prevent completion of daily occupations; however, it does make completion of daily activities both tedious and fatiguing. The client may express reluctance to perform some activities, or even stop performing them, because of the constant visual stress. Motor and postural control also may be compromised, reducing safety in navigation of the environment. For these reasons, oculomotor dysfunction must be addressed in intervention, although it is not specifically identified as a goal on the intervention plan. That is, the goal remains a functional goal such as safe and accurate completion of meal preparation, shopping, or bill paying, and management of the oculomotor dysfunction becomes one of the methods used to achieve the goal.

Intervention can be divided into four types: occlusion, application of prism, eye exercises, and surgery.[12,19,108,119] The last three interventions are used to reestablish fusion and binocularity and are completed only by ophthalmologists or optometrists. OT practitioners, under the direction of a physician, may apply occlusion. Most oculomotor dysfunction clears up without intervention within 6 to 12 months after the brain injury.[97,119] Because of this, ophthalmologists generally do not believe that it is necessary to provide any intervention other than to eliminate the diplopia for the client's comfort during the recuperation period. If the diplopia persists and becomes chronic, surgery can be used to reestablish fusion. Optometrists often choose a remediation approach and prescribe eye exercises to reestablish binocularity, in addition to using occlusion and prism.[12,102] Brief descriptions of these interventions follow. The treatment option selected for a client depends on the prognosis for recovery, the client's ability to participate in therapy, family and financial resources, and the eye specialist providing consultation.

Occlusion

The presence of diplopia causes perceptual distortion. This distortion creates confusion for the client and limits participation in daily activities. Therefore, diplopia must be eliminated if the client is to benefit fully from rehabilitation. Diplopia is eliminated by occluding the image presented to one eye. Occlusion can be achieved by assuming a head position or by covering one eye. Because assuming a deviant head position often affects motor and postural control, the preferred method is to cover one eye. Occlusion of the eye can be achieved through either full or partial occlusion.[12,19,102,108,119]

With full occlusion, vision is completely occluded in one eye by application of a "pirate patch," a clip-on occluder, or opaque tape. The challenge with complete occlusion is that it eliminates peripheral visual input, disrupting normal CNS mechanisms for control of balance and orientation to space.

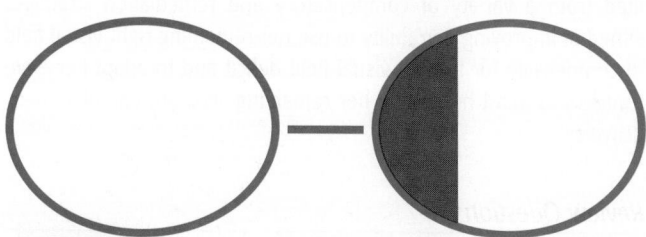

Figure 23-14 Example of partial occlusion to eliminate diplopia. Translucent tape is applied to the nasal portion of the eyeglass lens on the side of the non dominant eye. (From Warren M: *Brain Injury Visual Assessment Battery for Adults Test Manual*, Birmingham AL, 1998, visAbilities Rehab Services.)

This often causes the client to feel off balance and disoriented and reduces depth perception. Another challenge is that the client generally cannot tolerate long periods of occlusion of an eye, especially of the dominant eye. Therefore, for the comfort of the client, the period of occlusion is alternated between the eyes every hour. Alternating occlusion between the eyes also reduces the likelihood of the development of secondary contracture of the muscles antagonistic to the paretic muscle.

For partial occlusion, a strip of opaque material (such as 3M Transpore surgical tape) is applied to a portion of the eyeglass lens to block visual stimulation in the central visual field, while the peripheral visual field is left unoccluded (Figure 23-14). The client is instructed to view a target within the diplopic field. Tape is applied from the nasal rim toward the center of the lens until the client reports that the diplopia is gone when viewing the target. The tape is applied to the non-dominant eye for the greater comfort of the client. The width of the tape is gradually reduced as the muscle paresis resolves. An advantage of partial occlusion is that the client is more comfortable and therefore compliance is increased. Another advantage is that peripheral vision is left intact and available for use in orientation to space and balance. The main disadvantage of this type of occlusion is that the client must either wear prescription lenses or have tape applied to a pair of frames with plano (nonrefractive) lenses.

Prisms

Ophthalmologists and optometrists may use a prism to reestablish single vision in the primary directions of gaze: looking straight ahead and looking down. Application of a prism displaces the image, causing the disparate images created by the strabismus to fuse into a single image.[12,19,102] The prism can be ground into the eyeglass lenses worn by the client or temporarily applied to the lens of the glasses using a plastic Fresnel press-on prism. A prism is used only as long as it is needed to maintain fusion. If the paresis is resolving, the client is gradually weaned from the prism by reducing the dioptic strength of the prism over a period of time commensurate with the rate of recovery.

Eye exercises

There has yet to be objective research unequivocally demonstrating that the use of eye exercises will restore binocular function following paretic strabismus. Eye exercises do not appear to adversely affect muscle function, however, and the use of eye exercises can empower the client by increasing his or her participation in the recovery process. An optometrist directs the use of eye exercises in this aspect of the rehabilitation program.[102]

Surgery

Surgery is recommended when the degree of strabismus is too large to be overcome consistently and easily by fusional effort, or when there is a significant strabismic condition that does not resolve in 12 to 18 months.[119] The general approach in surgery is to make the action of one of the extraocular muscles either weaker or stronger by changing the position of its attachment on the eyeball. The position of the eye in the socket is changed by the procedure, and the image is realigned. Surgery is completed by an ophthalmologist specially trained in strabismus surgery.

Because Penny sustained a posterior cerebral artery occlusion, the lesion was confined to the right cerebral hemisphere. Subsequently she did not experience any oculomotor deficits.

COMPLEX VISUAL PROCESSING

The processes of pattern recognition, visual memory, and visual cognition involve complex processing and integration of vision with other sensory information, past experiences, and cognitive function. To complete this sophisticated level of processing requires not only organized, high-quality sensory input, but also good cognitive ability such as the ability to categorize information and complete abstract reasoning. Complex visual processing, like other cognitive functioning, is elicited by the demands of a particular event. It is a learned skill, established by one's experiences in mastering the environment. With few exceptions, complex visual processing always is applied within context—used to solve a problem, formulate a plan, or make a decision regarding a specific situation. Because of the contextual nature of complex visual processing, the best way to assess it is not to ask the client to complete some abstract, two-dimensional visual task, but rather to observe the client complete daily tasks requiring this level of processing. For example, if the client is an architect planning to return to work, his or her ability to design and execute building plans or other aspects of the job should be assessed, preferably at the client's place of employment. If the client wants to return to driving, his or her ability to handle complex traffic situations should be assessed with a behind-the-wheel assessment.

Visual input that is of poor quality or is incomplete or inaccurate will affect the ability to complete complex visual processing. Therefore visual acuity, visual field, oculomotor control, and visual attention and search should be assessed first to determine whether deficits exist that might contribute to deficiencies in complex processing. If deficits are identified, their effect on the client's performance of daily occupations requiring complex visual processing should be observed. For example, after having determined that a client has left VFD and an incomplete search pattern indicative of hemi-inattention, the OT practitioner should observe the client complete a daily occupation requiring attending, planning, and decision making. The activity may be preparing a meal, sorting and completing laundry, shopping for groceries, measuring the oil level in the car, or completing a job-related task. In observing the client, the practitioner should make special note of how the client's visual deficit affects his or her ability to process the more complex visual information needed to complete the task. If the client has difficulty successfully completing the task and if the visual deficit appears to be the cause, the practitioner should determine if it is possible to improve the client's performance with treatment of the visual deficit.

SUMMARY

The CNS relies on visual information to anticipate and plan adaptation to the environment and complete daily occupations. Brain injury or disease disrupts the processing of visual information, creating gaps in the visual input sent to the CNS. The quality of a person's occupational performance decreases, because the CNS does not have sufficient or accurate visual information to make decisions. Penny's left hemianopsia, for example, caused her to misread words and sentences because she did not always see letters and words on the left side; she also collided with persons and objects and experienced disorientation because of missing information on the left side. Whether a person's deficit in visual perceptual processing necessitates therapeutic intervention depends on the person's lifestyle and whether the visual deficit prevents successful completion of daily living activities. In Penny's case, as the primary caregiver for an ailing husband, she needed to be able to complete the family finances, drive, and shop; if her husband had been fit, she may not have needed to complete these activities.

The framework for assessment and intervention rests on the concept of a hierarchy of visual perceptual processing levels that interact with and subserve one another. Because of the unity of the hierarchy, a process cannot be disrupted at one level without an adverse effect on all perceptual processing. Assessment must be directed at measuring function at all process levels, with particular emphasis on the foundation of visual functions and visual attention and scanning. The absence of visual input on the left side caused Penny to appear to ignore visual stimuli on the left, giving the impression of hemi-inattention. Assessment demonstrated that she has normal attentional capability but had not yet learned to compensate for the hemianopsia.

Intervention focuses on increasing the accuracy and organization of visual input into the system through manipulation of the environment and by providing the client with strategies to compensate for or minimize the effect of the deficit in daily occupations. Penny benefited from a variety of compensatory and remediation strategies aimed at improving her ability to use her remaining right visual field to compensate for the left visual field deficit and to adapt her environment to assist her to use her remaining vision to complete daily activities.

Review Questions

1. What determines whether treatment intervention is needed for a client with a visual impairment?
2. What three aspects of environments/tasks can be modified to increase their visibility for the client with visual impairment?

3. What prevents a client from automatically compensating for VFD by turning the head farther to see around the blind field?

4. What kind of protective behaviors do persons adopt following onset of visual field deficit? Why do they adopt these strategies?

5. What is the normal search pattern executed by most adults when viewing an unstructured visual array? A structured array?

6. What is the primary compensatory strategy taught to the client with hemi-inattention?

7. What is the most crucial lower level visual process contributing to the ability to complete visual cognitive processing?

8. What changes occur in the visual search pattern of a client with hemi-inattention?

9. When would partial occlusion be used with the client? Describe the technique used to apply partial occlusion.

10. How does convergence insufficiency affect reading performance?

REFERENCES

1. Abreu BC, Toglia JP: Cognitive rehabilitation: a model for occupational therapy, *Am J Occup Ther* 41:439, 1987.

2. *American Heritage dictionary of the English language*, New York, 1969, Houghton Mifflin.

3. Anderson BR: *Perimetry with and without automation*, ed 2, St Louis, 1987, Mosby

4. Andrews TJ, Copolla, DM: Idiosyncratic characteristics of saccadic eye movements when viewing different visual environments, *Vision Research* 39:2947, 1999.

5. Antonucci G, et at: Effectiveness of neglect rehabilitation in a randomized group study, *J Clin Exp Neuropsychol* 17:383, 1995.

6. Ayres AJ: *Sensory integration and learning disorders*, Los Angeles, 1972, Western Psychological Services.

7. Azzopardi P, Cowey A: Is blindsight like normal, near-threshold vision? *Proc Natl Acad Sci* 94:14190, 1997.

8. Baker RS, Epstein AD: Ocular motor abnormalities from head trauma, *Surv Ophthalmol* 36:245, 1991.

9. Barinaga M: The mapmaking mind, *Science* 285:189, 1999.

10. Barton JJ, et al: Ocular search during line bisection. The effects of hemi-neglect and hemianopsia, *Brain* 121:1117, 1998.

11. Barton JJ, Black SE: Line bisection in hemianopsia, *J Neurol Neurosurg Psychiatry* 66:122, 1998.

12. Bedrossian EH: Non surgical management: acquired ocular muscle paralysis. In *The surgical and non surgical management of strabismus*, Springfield, IL, 1969, Charles C Thomas.

13. Behrmann M, et al: The eye movements of pure alexic patients during reading and nonreading tasks, *Neuropsychologia* 39: 983, 2001.

14. Beis JM, et al: Eye patching in unilateral spatial neglect: efficacy of two methods, *Arch Phys Med Rehabil* 80:71, 1999.

15. Belleza T, et al: Visual scanning and matching dysfunction in brain damaged patients with drawing impairment, *Cortex* 15:19, 1979.

16. Bodis-Wollner I, Diamond SP: The measurement of spatial contrast sensitivity in cases of blurred vision associated with cerebral lesions, *Brain* 99:695, 1976.

17. Bower B: Joined at the senses: perception may feast on a sensory stew, not a five-sense buffet, *Science News* 160:204, 2001.

18. Brendler K, Trauzettel-Klosinski S, Sadowski B: Reading disability in hemianopic field defects: the significance of clinical parameters, *Invest Ophthalmol Vis Sci* 37:S1079, 1996.

19. Bulens C et al: Spatial contrast sensitivity in unilateral cerebral ischaemic lesion involving the posterior visual pathway, *Brain* 112:507, 1989.

20. Cassidy TP, et al: The association of visual field deficits and visuo-spatial neglect in acute right hemisphere stroke patients, *Age Ageing* 28:257, 1999.

21. Cate Y, Richards L: Relationship between performance on tests of basic visual functions and visual perceptual processing in persons after brain injury, *Am J Occup Ther* 54:326, 2000.

22. Chedru F, et al: Visual searching in normal and brain damaged subjects, *Cortex* 9:94, 1973.

23. Chen Sea MJ, et al: Patterns of visual spatial inattention and their functional significance in stroke patients, *Arch Phys Med Rehabil* 74:355, 1993.

24. Chokron S, et al: The role of vision in spatial representation, *Cortex* 40:281, 2004.

25. Cohen M, et al: Convergence insufficiency in brain-injured patients, *Brain Injury* 2:187, 1989.

26. Colenbrander A: The functional vision score, a coordinated scoring system for visual impairments, disabilities and handicaps. In Kooijan AC, et al, editors: *Low vision: research and new development in rehabilitation*, Amsterdam, 1994, IOS Press.

27. Daini R, et al: Exploring the syndrome of spatial unilateral neglect through an illusion of length, *Exp Brain Res* 144: 224, 2002.

28. Delis DC, Robertson LC, Balliet R: The breakdown and rehabilitation of visuospatial dysfunction in brain injured patients, *Int Rehabil Med* 5:132, 1983.

29. DeLuca M, et al: Eye movement patterns in reading as function of visual field defects and contrast sensitivity loss, *Cortex* 32:491, 1996.

30. Demb JB, et al: Brain activity in visual cortex predicts individual differences in reading performance, *Proc Natl Acad Sci* 94:13363, 1997.

31. DeRenzi E, et al: Attentional shift towards the rightmost stimuli in patients with left visual neglect, *Cortex* 25:231, 1989.

32. Di Pace E, et al: Selective reading slowness in a traumatic patient with impairment in basic visual processes, *J Clin Exp Neuropsychol* 17:878, 1995.

33. Duffy M: *Making life more livable: simple adaptations for living at home after vision loss*, New York, 2002, American Foundation for the Blind Press.

34. Festinger L: Eye movements and perception. In Bach Y, Rita P, Collins CC, editors: *The control of eye movements*, New York, 1971, Academic Press.

35. Findlay JM, Kapoula Z: Scrutinization, spatial attention, and the spatial programming of saccadic eye movements, *Q J Experimental Psychol* 45:633, 1992.

36. Fletcher D, et al: Low vision rehabilitation: finding capable people behind damaged eyeballs, *West J Med* 154:554, 1991.

37. Gainotti G, et al: Contralateral and ipsilateral disorders of visual attention in patients with unilateral brain damage, *J Neurol Neurosurg Psychiatry* 53:422, 1990.

38. Gianutsos R, Matheson P: The rehabilitation of visual perceptual disorders attributable to brain injury. In Meier MJ, Benton AL, Diller L, editors: *Neuropsychological rehabilitation*, New York, 1987, Guilford Press.

39. Gianutsos R, et al: Rehabilitative optometric services for survivors of acquired brain injury, *Arch Phys Med Rehabil* 69:573, 1988.

40. Gilhotra JS, et al: Homonymous visual field defects and stroke in an older population, *Stroke* 33:2417, 2002.

41. Glass I, et al: Impersistent execution of saccadic eye movements after traumatic brain injury, *Brain Injury* 9:769, 1995.

42 Goldberg, ME: The control of gaze. In Kandel ER, Schwartz JH, Jessell TM, editors: *Principles of neural science*, ed 4, New York, 2000, McGraw-Hill.

43. Graziano MSA, et al: Coding of visual space by premotor neurons, *Science* 266:1054, 1994.

44. Gross CG, Graziano MSA: Multiple representations of space in the brain, *Neuroscientist* 1:40, 1995.

45. Halligan PW, et al: Visuo-spatial neglect: qualitative difference and laterality of cerebral lesion, *J Neurol Neurosurg Psychiatry* 55:1060, 1992.

46. Harrington DO: *The visual fields: a textbook and atlas of clinical perimetry*, ed 2, St Louis, 1964, Mosby.

47. Heilman K, Van Den Abel T: Right hemisphere dominance for attention: the mechanism underlying hemispheric asymmetries of inattention (neglect), *Neurology* 30:3, 1980.

48. Hess RF, Pointer JS: Spatial and temporal contrast sensitivity in hemianopsia: a comparative study of the sighted and blind hemifields, *Brain* 112:871, 1989.

49. Holt LJ, Anderson SF: Bilateral occipital lobe stroke with inferior altitudinal defects, *Optometry* 71:690, 2000.

50. Hyvarinen L: *Vision testing manual*, Villa Park, IL, 1996, Precision Vision.

51. Ishial S, et al: Eye fixation patterns in homonymous hemianopsia and unilateral spatial neglect, *Neuropsychologia* 25:675, 1987.

52. Jung DS, Park KP: Post traumatic bilateral internuclear ophthalmoplegia with exotropia, *Arch Neurol* 60:429, 2004.

53. Kahn J: Blunt trauma to orbital soft tissues. In Shingleton BJ, editor: *Eye trauma*, St Louis, 1991, Mosby.

54. Kandel E, Wurtz R: Central visual pathways, In Kandel ER, Schwartz JH, Jessell TM, editors: *Principles of neural science*, ed 4, New York, 2000, McGraw-Hill.

55. Kandel E, Wurtz R: Constructing the visual image. In Kandel ER, Schwartz JH, Jessell TM, editors: *Principles of neural science*, ed 4, New York, 2000, McGraw-Hill.

56. Kandel E, Wurtz R: Perception of motion, depth and form, In Kandel ER, Schwartz JH, Jessell TM, editors: *Principles of neural science*, ed 4, New York, 2000, McGraw-Hill.

57. Kanski JJ: *Clinical ophthalmology*, Toronto, 1984, Mosby.

58. Kasten E, et al: Computer-based training of stimulus detection improves color and simple pattern recognition in the defective field of hemianopic subjects, *J Cogn Neurosci* 12:1001, 2000.

59. Kasten E, et al: Computer-based training for the treatment of partial blindness, *Nature Med* 4:1083, 1998.

60. Keane JR: Fourth nerve palsy: historical review and study of 215 patients, *Neurology* 43:2439, 1993.

61. Kerkhoff G, et al: Contrasting spatial hearing deficits in hemianopsia and spatial neglect, *Neuroreport* 10:3555, 1999.

62. Kerkhoff G, et al: Neurovisual rehabilitation in cerebral blindness, *Arch Neurol* 51:474, 1994.

63. Klavora P, et al: Rehabilitation of visual skills using the Dynavision: a single case experimental design, *Can J Occup Ther* 62:37, 1995.

64. Klavora P, et al: The effects of Dynavision rehabilitation on behind-the-wheel driving ability and selected psychomotor abilities of persons post-stroke, *Am J Occup Ther* 49:534, 1995.

65. Klavora P, et al: Driving skills in elderly persons with stroke: comparison of two new assessment options, *Arch Phys Med Rehabil* 81:701, 2000.

66. Klavora P, Warren M: Rehabilitation of visuomotor skills in poststroke patients using the Dynavision apparatus, *Percept Motor Skills* 86:23, 1998.

67. Ladavas E, et al: Neglect as a deficit determined by an imbalance between multiple spatial representations, *Exp Brain Res* 116:493, 1997.

68. Leff AP, et al: The functional anatomy of single-word reading in patients with hemianopic and pure alexia, *Brain* 124:510, 2001.

69. Leff AP, et al: Impaired reading in patients with right hemianopia, *Ann Neurol* 47:171, 2000.

70. Leigh RJ, Brandt T: A reevaluation of the vestibulo-ocular reflex: new ideas of its purpose, properties, neural substrate and disorders, *Neurology* 43:1288, 1993.

71. Leigh RJ, Zee DS: *Neurology of eye movements*, ed 2, Philadelphia, 1991, FA Davis.

72. Lepore FE: Disorders of ocular motility following head trauma, *Arch Neurol* 52:924, 1995.

73. Levine DH: Unawareness of visual and sensorimotor deficits: a hypothesis, *Brain Cognition* 13:233, 1990.

74. Locher PJ, Bigelow DL: Visual exploratory activity of hemiplegic patients viewing the motor-free visual perception test, *Percept Mot Skills* 57:91, 1983.

75. Marshall JC, Halligan PW: Imagine only half of it, *Nature* 364:193, 1993.

76. Marshall SC, et al: Attentional deficits in stroke patients: a visual dual task experiment, *Arch Phys Med Rehabil* 78:7, 1997.

77. Marx P: Supratentorial structures controlling oculomotor functions and their involvement in cases of stroke, *Eur Arch Psychiatry Clin Neurosci* 239:3, 1989.

78. Meinenberg V, et al: Saccadic eye movement strategies in patients with homonymous hemianopia, *Ann Neurol* 9:537, 1981.

79. Mesulam MM: Spatial attention and neglect: parietal, frontal and cingulate contributions to the mental representation and attentional targeting of salient extrapersonal events, *Phil Trans Royal Soc London* 354:1325, 1998.

80. Miki A, et al: Functional magnetic resonance imaging in homonymous hemianopsia, A*m J Ophthalmol* 121:258, 1996.

81. Moore JC: *The visual system*, Course syllabus for OT Australia national CPE program, Melbourne, 1997, Australian Occupational Therapy Association.

82. Neger RE: The evaluation of diplopia in head trauma, *J Head Trauma Rehabil* 4:31, 1989.

83. Noton D, Stark L: Scanpaths in eye movements during pattern perception, *Science* 171:308, 1971.

84. Padula WV: *A behavioral vision approach for persons with physical disabilities*, Santa Anna, CA, 1988, Optometric Extension Program Foundation.

85. Palmer T, Tzeng OJL: Cerebral asymmetry in visual attention, *Brain Cogn* 13:46, 1990.

86. Pambakian ALM, Kennard C: Can visual function be restored in patients with homonymous hemianopia? *British J Ophthalmol* 81:324, 1997.

87. Park M: Eye movements and positions. In Duane TD, editor: *Clinical ophthalmology: strabismus, refraction, the lens*, Philadelphia, 1981, Harper & Row.

88. Paul S: Effects of computer assisted visual scanning training in the treatment of visual neglect: three case studies, *Phys Occup Ther Geriatrics* 14:33, 1996.

89. Pommerenke K, Markowitsch HJ: Rehabilitation training of homonymous visual field defects in patients with postgeniculate damage of the visual system, *Restorative Neurol Neurosci* 1:47, 1989.

90. Posner MI, Rafal RD: Cognitive theories of attention and the rehabilitation of attentional deficits. In Meier MJ, Benton AL, Diller L, editors: *Neuropsychological rehabilitation*, New York, 1987, Guilford Press.

91. Ramachandran VS, Blakeslee S: *Phantoms in the brain: probing the mysteries of the human mind*, New York, 1998, William Morrow.

92. Rao SC, et al: Integration of what and where in the primate prefrontal cortex, *Science* 6:821, 1997.

93. Rapesak SZ, et al: Selective attention in hemispatial neglect, *Arch Neurol* 46:178, 1989.

94. Reuter-Lorenz PA, Kinsbourne M: Hemispheric control of spatial attention, *Brain Cognition* 12:240, 1990.

95. Robinson DL, Petersen SE: The pulvinar and visual salience, *Trends Neurosci* 15:1, 1992.

96. Ron S, Gur S: Gaze and eye movement disorders, *Curr Opin Neurol Neurosurg* 5:711, 1992.

97. Ron S, et al: Eye movements in brain damaged patients, *Scand J Rehabil Med* 10:39, 1978.

98. Rubin N, et al: Enhanced perception of illusory contours in the lower versus upper visual hemifields, *Science* 1:651, 1996.

99. Safran AB, Landis T: Plasticity in the adult visual cortex: implications for the diagnosis of visual field defects and visual rehabilitation, *Curr Opin Ophthalmol* 7:53, 1996.

100. Sasaki Y, et al: Local and global attention are mapped retinoptically in human cortex, *PNAS* 98:2077, 2001.

101. Schall JD, Hanes DP: Neural basis of saccade target selection in frontal eye field during visual search, *Nature* 2:467, 1993.

102. Scheiman M: *Understanding and managing vision deficits: a guide for occupational practitioners*, Thorofare NJ, 1997, Slack Publishers.

103. Schiller PH, Chou IH: The effects of frontal eye field and dorsomedial frontal cortex lesions on visually guided eye movements, *Nat Neurosci* 1:248, 1998.

104. Schoepf D, Zangemeister WH: Target predictability influences the distribution of coordinated eye-head gaze saccades in patients with homonymous hemianopia, *Neurol Res* 18:425, 1996.

105. Schuchard RA: Adaptation to macular scotomas in persons with low vision, *Am J Occup Ther* 49:870, 1995.

106. Simon RP, et al: Disturbances of vision. In *Clinical neurology*, Norwalk, CT, 1989, Appleton & Lange.

107. Spier PA, et al: Visual neglect during intracarotid amobarbital testing, *Neurology* 40:1600, 1990.

108. Sterk CC: The conservative management of diplopia. In Sanders EACM, DeKeizer RJW, Zee DS, editors: *Eye movement disorders*, Boston, 1987, Martinus Nijhoff/Dr W Junk Publ.

109. Tessier-Lavigne M: Visual processing by the retina. In Kandel ER, Schwartz JH, Jessell TM, editors: *Principles of neural science*, ed 4, New York, 2000, McGraw-Hill.

110. Tham K, et al: The discovery of disability: a phenomenological study of unilateral neglect, *Am J Occup Ther* 54:398, 2000.

111. Tham K, et al: Training to improve awareness of disabilities in clients with unilateral neglect, *Am J Occup Ther* 55:46, 2001.

112. Tham K, Tegner R: Video feedback in the rehabilitation of patients with unilateral neglect, *Arch Phys Med Rehabil* 78:410, 1997.

113. Toglia J: Generalization of treatment: a multicontext approach to cognitive perceptual impairment in adults with brain injury, *Am J Occup Ther* 45:505, 1991.

114. Trauzettel-Klosinski S, Brendler K: Eye movements in reading with hemianopic field defects; the significance of clinical parameters, *Arch Clin Exp Ophthalmol* 236:91, 1998.

115. Trexler LE: Volitional control of homonymous hemianopsia, *Neuropsychologia* 36:573, 1998.

116. Trobe JD, et al: Confrontation visual field techniques in the detection of anterior visual pathway lesions, *Ann Neurol* 10:28, 1981.

117. Tyler HR: Defective stimulus exploration in aphasic patients, *Neurology* 19:105, 1969.

118. Van Vliet AGM: Beside examination. In Sanders EACM, De Keizer RJW, Zee DS, editors: *Eye movement disorders*, Boston, 1987, Martinus Nijhoff/Dr W Junk Publishers.

119. Von Noorden GK: Paralytic strabismus. In *Binocular vision and ocular motility: theory and management of strabismus*, ed 3, St Louis, 1985, Mosby.

120. Warren M: A hierarchical model for evaluation and treatment of visual perceptual dysfunction in adult acquired brain injury. I, II, *Am J Occup Ther* 47:42, 1993.

121. Warren M: *Brain injury visual assessment battery for adults test manual*, Birmingham, AL, 1998, visAbilities Rehab Services.

122. Warren M: Identification of visual scanning deficits in adults after cerebrovascular accident, *Am J Occup Ther* 44:391, 1990.

123. Warren M: *Prereading and writing exercises for persons with macular scotomas*, Birmingham AL, 1996, visAbilities Rehab Services.

124. Watson G, et al: The validity and clinical uses of the Pepper Visual Skills for Reading Test, *J Visual Impair Blind* 84:119, 1990.

125. Weinberg J, et al: Visual scanning training effect on reading—related tasks in acquired right brain damage, *Arch Phys Med Rehabil* 60(11):491, 1979.

126. Weintraub S, Mesulam MM: Visual hemispatial inattention: stimulus parameters and exploratory strategies, *J Neurol Neurosurg Psychiatry* 51:1481, 1988.

127. Wiart L, et al: Unilateral neglect syndrome rehabilitation by trunk rotation and scanning training, *Arch Phys Med Rehabil* 78:424, 1997

128. Winckelgren I: How the brain "sees" borders where there are none, *Science* 256:1520, 1992.

129. Wong AM, Sharpe JA: Representation of the visual field in the human occipital cortex: a magnetic resonance imaging and perimetric correlation, *Arch Ophthalmol* 117:208, 1999.

130. Wright V, Watson G: *Learn to use your vision for reading workbook.* LUV reading series, Trooper, PA, 1995, Homer Printing.

131. Yarbus AL: Eye movements during perception of complex objects. In Yarbus AL: *Eye movements and vision*, New York, 1967, Plenum Press.

132. Zangemeister WH, et al: Eye head coordination in homonymous hemianopsia, *J Neurol* 226:243, 1982.

133. Zihl J: Eye movement patterns in hemianopic dyslexia, *Brain* 118:891, 1987.

134. Zihl J: Rehabilitation of visual impairments in patients with brain damage. In Kooijan AC, et al, editors: *Low vision: research and new development in rehabilitation*, Amsterdam, 1994, IOS Press.

135. Zihl J: Visual scanning behavior in patients with homonymous hemianopia, *Neuropyschologia* 33:287, 1995.

RESOURCES

Brain Injury Visual Assessment Battery for Adults, visAbilities Rehab Services, Inc., 210 Lorna Square, #208, Birmingham, AL 35216; (888)752-4364; *www.visabilities.com.*

LeaNumbers and LeaSymbols Low Contrast Tests, Precision Vision, 944 First St., LaSalle, IL 60301; (815)223-2022.

Visual Skills for Reading Test, Lighthouse International, Professional Low Vision Products, 938-K Andreasen Drive, Escondido, CA 92029; (800)826-4200; *www.lowvision.com.*

Dynavision 2000, Performance Enterprises, 76 Major Buttons Drive, Markham, ONT L3P3G7, Canada; (905) 472-9074; *www.dynavision2000.com.*

Warren Pre-reading and Writing Exercises for Persons with Macular Scotomas, visAbilities Rehab Services, Inc., 210 Lorna Square, #208, Birmingham, AL, 35216; (888)752-4364; *www.visabilities.com.*

Learn to Use Your Vision for Reading Workbook, Lighthouse International Professional Low Vision Products, Escondido, CA 92029; *www.lowvision.com.*

24

ASSESSMENT AND INTERVENTION OF PERCEPTUAL DYSFUNCTION

SHAWN C. PHIPPS

KEY TERMS

Perception	Prosopagnosia	Stereopsis	Praxis
Adaptive approaches	Simultanognosia	Stereognosis	Apraxia
Remedial approaches	Visual-spatial perception	Astereognosis	Ideational apraxia
Agnosia	Figure-ground discrimination	Graphesthesia	Ideomotor apraxia
Color agnosia	Form constancy	Agraphesthesia	Dressing apraxia
Color anomia	Spatial relations	Body scheme	Constructional disorder
Metamorphopsia	Right-left discrimination	Finger agnosia	

LEARNING OBJECTIVES

After studying this chapter the student or practitioner will be able to do the following:

1. Describe how perceptual dysfunction affects participation in occupational performance.
2. Identify standardized and functional assessments for visual perception, visual-spatial perception, tactile perception, body schema perception, and perceptual motor skills.
3. Differentiate between remedial and adaptive approaches to treatment of perceptual dysfunction and how they facilitate engagement in occupation.

4. Describe specific occupational therapy interventions for targeted perceptual motor deficits that facilitate improved performance skills, client factors, and participation in areas of occupation.

CHAPTER OUTLINE

General principles of the OT assessment
General approaches to OT intervention
  Remedial approaches
  Adaptive approaches
Assessment and intervention of specific perceptual impairments

Visual perception disorders
Visual-spatial perception disorders
Tactile perception disorders
Motor perception disorders
Behavioral aspects of perceptual dysfunction

THREADED CASE STUDY: WALT, PART 1

Walt is a 38-year-old male who sustained a traumatic brain injury from a motor vehicle accident, resulting in right frontal, parietal, temporal, and occipital lobe damage. His occupational profile included a rich occupational history that consisted of full-time work as a graphic artist in a prestigious marketing firm. Walt is a husband and father of two young children, as well as an accomplished painter.

After the brain injury, Walt's roles as worker, husband, father, and artist were affected due to impairments with motor and process performance skills and client factors, such as perceptual and cognitive dysfunction. Walt was unable to participate in his most valued areas of occupation, including painting, using a computer, sketching, or playing catch with his children. His visual foundation skills, including visual acuity, oculomotor control, and visual field function, were found to be intact during the evaluation process. However, he demonstrated difficulty initiating motor actions when playing with his children and interpreting visual information for meaningful visual-spatial relationships when painting, sketching, or using the computer. In addition, he exhibited signs of unilateral neglect to the left half of his body and was unable to discriminate between different types of materials through touch alone.

During the initial assessment, the occupational therapist elected to use the Canadian Occupational Performance Measure[57] to obtain client-centered goals that would assist Walt in achieving his occupational performance goals. Walt identified as his main goals in occupational therapy to submit a painting to a local art gallery, play with his children, drive, and regain computer skills in preparation for resumption of part-time work as a graphic artist.

Critical Thinking Questions

1. How would you best assess Walt's occupational performance?
2. How would you best assess Walt's perceptual function?
3. How would you assist Walt in achieving his occupational performance goals using remedial and adaptive approaches for his perceptual dysfunction?

"Perception is the gateway to cognition"[14]

Perception is the mechanism by which the brain interprets sensory information received from the environment. The perceived information is then further processed by the various cognitive functions (described in Chapter 25), and the individual may choose either to respond with a verbal expression or motor act, or to simply perceive and think about the observed stimuli. For example, when waiting in a checkout line in a grocery store, a person may observe the array of brightly wrapped candy lining the aisle, may remember the sweet taste of the chocolate, may remember a recent resolution to lose weight, and may choose to resist adding any candy bars to the grocery cart. The person may look over to the next aisle, recognize a neighbor, and begin a conversation. In a few minutes, the person may notice that another register has a shorter line and may choose to move over to that line to be able to complete grocery shopping in a shorter amount of time. Perception of the environment provides the information to enable these response options.

In early development, tactile, proprioceptive, vestibular, and visual perception provide an internalized sense of the body scheme, which is basic to all motor function.[6,62,100] Highly developed spatial skills are critical to an architect, plumber, or designer, or an artist like Walt.[35] The process of interpreting visual input is a learned skill, as evidenced by blind individuals who, when sight is restored later in life, have difficulty making sense of what they see.[82]

Acquired perceptual deficits are noted in persons with *cerebrovascular accident* (CVA), *traumatic brain injury* (TBI), and later stages of degenerative disorders, such as multiple sclerosis and Parkinson's disease.[58,73] Spatial disorders and apraxia of a progressive nature are also seen in Alzheimer's disease.[5,13]

Severe perceptual deficits, frequently combined with cognitive impairments, can affect every area of occupation (e.g., ADLs, IADLs, education, work, play, leisure, and social participation) and can present serious safety concerns. For example, the individual who cannot judge distance and the spatial relationship of his foot to the top step of his stairwell may be in danger of a serious fall. Another person who cannot judge the position of the dial on the stove when preparing a meal may cause a fire. It is often the occupational therapist's role to evaluate safe and independent functioning in valued occupations and to assess visual, perceptual, and cognitive skills using both standardized instruments along with observations of occupational performance in context.

This chapter describes the client factors of visual perception, visual-spatial perception, tactile perception, body schema perception, motor perception, and the potential deficits in occupational performance that result from impairment to these client factors. Suggestions for standardized and functional testing are provided. General approaches to intervention are reviewed, and suggestions for treatment are presented.

GENERAL PRINCIPLES OF THE OT ASSESSMENT

When assessing perceptual abilities several assessment tools may be required. The optimal battery of standardized tests includes assessment tools that require a verbal response (e.g., naming a picture) or motor response (e.g., drawing or construction) or have flexible response requirements of either mode (multiple choice indicated by verbalizing the number or letter or by pointing to the chosen item). This enables the therapist to assess visual perceptual function in a client with severe physical impairments or with significant limitations in communication ability. With a variety of such tests, the therapist can gather information to discriminate between a deficit in the reception of information and a deficit in the verbal or motor output. This, in turn, influences the intervention approach. Observations of occupational performance and analysis of the perceptual-motor demands of functional activities further complement standardized assessment tools and enable the determination of underlying causes of deficits in occupational performance. Assessment methods should be conducted in the specific context of the occupation being performed.

Warren[90,91] emphasizes the importance of using a bottom-up approach to evaluate for impairments in visual foundation skills, such as visual acuity, oculomotor function, visual field function, visual attention, and visual scanning prior to evaluating the higher-level perceptual skills covered in this chapter. For example, a deficit in visual acuity could be the underlying cause of poor performance on a test of perceptual processing. The normal aging process also results in a decline in visual efficiency, and a variety of age-related eye diseases such as macular degeneration, glaucoma, diabetic retinopathy, and cataracts can affect visual acuity or visual field function.[55] It is also possible that performance on global perceptual tests may be affected by deficits in cognitive areas such as attention, memory, or executive function (see Chapter 25). For example, an individual with severely limited attention and concentration is unlikely to perform well on many standardized assessments, regardless of the modality or nature of the task. Tsurumi and Todd also analyzed the cognitive skills involved in the commonly used tests of visual perceptual functions and warn that an individual's performance using two-dimensional representations of visual stimuli may not be predictive of the person's performance in a three-dimensional world.[89]

Arnadottir[4] recommends the use of *activities of daily living* (ADLs) to assess neurobehavioral dysfunction, including perceptual dysfunction, and its effect on the performance of tasks essential to functional independence. She maintains that it is preferable for occupational therapists to assess neurobehavioral deficits directly from the ADL evaluation. She developed the Arnadottir OT-ADL Neurobehavioral Evaluation (A-ONE), which evaluates perceptual and perceptual-motor dysfunction in the context of ADL and functional mobility tasks, including ideational apraxia, ideomotor apraxia, unilateral neglect, body scheme disorders, organization/sequencing dysfunction, agnosias, and spatial dysfunction.[2,3,4]

Toglia's Multicontext Treatment Approach focuses on remediating and compensating for perceptual and cognitive impairments by promoting generalization of functional skills across multiple contexts.[88] Visual processing strategies, task analysis, incorporating the specific learning needs of the client, establishment of criteria for transfer of learning, metacognitive training, and practice in multiple environments are key components of Toglia's approach. This approach also assists the client with TBI to gain self-awareness of perceptual and cognitive strengths and weaknesses to promote the use of strategies for remediation or compensation of skills across multiple contexts.[89] Toglia's Dynamic Object Search Test is one assessment that can be utilized to assess visual processing, visual scanning, and visual attention.[88]

Another occupation-based assessment tool that can be used to assess the impact of deficient performance skills on functional tasks is the Assessment of Motor and Process Skills (AMPS).[33] This standardized assessment evaluates the performance skills necessary for engagement in areas of occupation by assessing 16 motor skills and 20 process skills (e.g., temporal organization, organizing space and objects). Each performance skill is evaluated in the context of client-identified and culturally relevant *instrumental activities of daily living* (IADL) occupations from a list of standardized activities at various levels of difficulty. The AMPS has a high rate of reliability and validity, and the evaluator must be an occupational therapist who has received advanced training and certification to administer this assessment.

The Loewenstein Occupational Therapy Cognitive Assessment (LOTCA)[50] and Rivermead Perceptual Assessment Battery[27,94] provide a comprehensive profile of visual perceptual and motor skills and involve both motor-free and constructional functions. A variety of other assessment tools require either a verbal or a simple pointing response. The Motor-Free Visual Perceptual Test-Revised (MVPT-R)[20] assesses basic visual perceptual abilities. An alternative version of the test presents the multiple choices in a vertical format (MVPT-V) to reduce the interference of hemianopsia or visual inattention.[64] The MVPT-V has been shown to be predictive of on-the-road driving performance and can be used as a screening tool to identify persons who would not be safe drivers.[63] The Test of Visual Perceptual Skills-Upper Level (TVPS-UL)[37] also provides a multiple-choice format and has been normed for adults. Test items require a higher level of visual analysis compared with the MVPT, and the test is untimed. The Hooper Visual Organization Test[47] requires that the individual mentally assemble fragmented drawings of common objects. The Minnesota Paper Form Board Test[59] is a high-level assessment of visual organization, requiring mental rotation of fragmented geometric shapes.

GENERAL APPROACHES TO OT INTERVENTION

An underlying assumption about perceptual-motor function is that perceptual deficits will adversely affect occupational performance. Further, it is assumed that remediation of or compensation for perceptual deficits will improve occupational performance.[65] In her critical analysis of approaches to treatment for perceptual deficits, Neistadt[65] described two general classifications of approaches: the adaptive and the remedial. **Adaptive approaches** provide training in daily living behaviors to facilitate adaptation to the client's unique contextual environment. In contrast, the **remedial approaches** seek to cause some change in *central nervous system* (CNS) functions.[65] The effectiveness of the various approaches to the remediation of perceptual deficits has not been well documented and requires further scientific investigation.[28,65,81]

A therapist may use one approach or a combination of approaches when designing an intervention plan to address the effects of perceptual dysfunction. The remedial and adaptive approaches can be used in a continuum, beginning with attempts to improve the basic skills and gradually incorporating compensatory techniques as the deficits persist.[51] The occupational therapy (OT) literature suggests specific activities for the intervention of perceptual deficits, but protocols for the use of such activities require further research.[100] For measuring effectiveness of treatment, criteria are needed for successful performance, task grading, objective methods of evaluating performance, and guidelines for task modification.[66] In the absence of such objective criteria, the occupational therapist relies on empirical methods to measure and document functional improvement. The relationship between perceptual deficits and functional performance has been demonstrated in several studies.[7,27,79,81]

REMEDIAL APPROACHES

Remedial, or transfer of training, approaches assume that practice in a particular perceptual task carries over to performance of similar activities or tasks requiring the same perceptual skills.[65] For example, practice in reproducing pegboard designs for spatial relations training could carry over to dressing skills that require spatial judgment (such as matching blouse to body and discriminating between right and left shoes). The capacity for persons to improve their performance on perceptual tests following perceptual training has been documented.[41] However, other studies have also shown that remediative strategies for optimizing perceptual skills may not be as effective as using engagement in occupation to promote changes in perceptual awareness and abilities.[28,61,67,68,100]

ADAPTIVE APPROACHES

Adaptive, or functional, approaches are characterized by the repetitive practice of particular tasks that help the person become more independent in areas of occupation.[65] These approaches are frequently used because current reimbursement for therapy services is based on functional outcome.[80] The therapist does not retrain specific perceptual skills. Rather, the person is made aware of the problem and taught methods of adapting to or compensating for the deficit during occupational performance. For example, if the individual has difficulty with dressing because of a body schema

perceptual impairment, the therapist may set up a regular dressing routine and provide cues with repetitive practice. With these adaptations, the person may learn to dress. Adaptation of the physical environment or the specific activity demands (e.g., objects used and their properties) is another way to compensate for a perceptual deficit. For example, if an individual has difficulty discriminating a white shirt against the white sheets of the bed, the therapist may encourage the person to select a patterned shirt or may lay the white shirt on a colored towel or bedspread to provide a contrasting background.

ASSESSMENT AND INTERVENTION OF SPECIFIC PERCEPTUAL IMPAIRMENTS

VISUAL PERCEPTION DISORDERS

Walt has difficulty recognizing the faces of his two children and identifying the difference between the brushes he uses for painting. He requires verbal cues to identify the unique features that distinguish the faces of his two children and to identify the appropriate painting utensil to use during an art project. He also has difficulty identifying and recognizing the significance of various traffic signs, which would prevent him from driving safely.

Walt presents with a visual perception disorder, which impairs the person's ability to recognize and identify familiar objects and people.[99] While these individuals have intact visual anatomical structures, objects and people may appear distorted, or larger or smaller than they actually are. They also have difficulty interpreting the meaning of objects in their environment, such as signs and maps. In addition, they can have difficulty recognizing, identifying, or remembering the names of colors in their environment. These visual perception disorders can lead to safety problems in dynamic environments and may affect social skills, as the person has difficulty recognizing family members, friends, and co-workers.

Agnosia

Visual object recognition refers to the ability to identify objects via visual input. An impairment in this area is called **agnosia,** and is caused by lesions in the right occipital lobe or posterior multimodal association area.[48,58] The individual with agnosia demonstrates normal visual foundation skills, as indicated by the person's ability to ambulate around furniture through a room; further, the inability to name objects is not caused by a language deficit in naming the object, as noted in aphasic disorders. Rather, the person is unable to recognize and identify an item using only visual means. If the person holds the object, he or she can identify it via tactile input, or by olfactory means if the object has a distinguishable odor, such as a flower.[83]

Assessment is performed by asking the individual to identify five common objects by sight, such as a pencil, comb, keys, a watch, and eyeglasses. If the client demonstrates word-finding difficulties, offer the client a choice of three answers. Ask the client to indicate the correct choice through a head nod ("yes" or "no"). If the client is unable to name four out of the five objects, visual agnosia may be indicated.

OT intervention for visual agnosia will focus on adaptive or compensatory methods of keeping frequently used objects, such as a hairbrush, in consistent locations, and teaching the client to rely more heavily on intact sensory modalities, such as stereognosis, to seek and find desired items.[48] Remediation approaches can include having the client practice identifying objects that are needed for occupational performance (e.g., paintbrush for Walt) or using nonverbal, tactile-kinesthetic guiding during occupations.[99] Following the activity, have the client practice naming the items that were used. Current research has found that efforts to remediate object recognition have met with limited success.[49]

Color Agnosia and Color Anomia

Color agnosia refers to the client's inability to remember and recognize the specific colors for common objects in the environment.[44] For example, Walt was unable to recognize the color of the paints he was using during his landscape painting. He confused the green paint he was using to paint the grass with the blue paint he intended to use for the sky. Alternatively, **color anomia** refers to the client's inability to name the color of the objects. While the client understands the differences between the different colors of objects, they are unable to name the object accurately. For example, Walt was able to recognize the color red, but was not able to name it as such.

To assess color agnosia, present the client with two common objects that are accurately colored and two objects that are not accurately colored. Ask the client to pick out those common objects that are not accurately colored. If the client is unable to choose the objects that are inaccurately colored, color agnosia may be indicated.

To assess color anomia, ask the client to name the color of various objects in their environment. If the patient has aphasia, ask them to nod their head "yes" or "no" after offering them choices of colors. If the client is unable to correctly name the colors of various objects, color anomia may be indicated.

OT intervention for color agnosia and color anomia will focus on providing the client with opportunities to recognize, identify, and name various colors of objects in their environment. Intervention is best provided in a familiar context and can be incorporated functionally during occupational performance. For example, while Walt is painting a landscape, the therapist would provide verbal cues that assist him in recognizing, identifying, and naming the various colors of paint he is using.

Metamorphopsia

Metamorphopsia refers to the visual distortion of objects, such as the physical properties of size and weight.[99]

For example, when Walt was playing sports with his two children, he could not distinguish between the basketball, the football, the baseball, or the volleyball. Each of the balls appeared heavier, lighter, larger, or smaller than they actually were, making it difficult to distinguish the differences between them through observation alone.

Assessment for metamorphopsia includes presenting the client with various objects of different weights and sizes (e.g. balls, drinking glasses filled with water, puzzle pieces). Ask the client to place each object in order according to size or weight through observation alone. Metamorphopsia may be indicated if the client is unable to determine the weight and size of the various objects.

OT intervention for metamorphopsia includes providing the client with opportunities to practice distinguishing objects in the natural environment through intact sensory modalities (e.g., tactile-kinesthetic). The functional use of objects during occupational performance will provide feedback to the client about the sizes and shapes of different objects. The therapist should also provide specific verbal descriptors of the object when using this approach. Other treatment modalities include puzzles, board games, and computer games that help the client to gain experience distinguishing the sizes and shapes of different objects.

Prosopagnosia

Prosopagnosia refers to an inability to recognize and identify familiar faces caused by lesions of the right posterior hemisphere.[15,48,83] The individual with prosopagnosia may have difficulty recognizing his or her own face, faces of family members and friends, and/or of famous individuals because they cannot recognize the unique facial expressions that make each face different. When attempting to identify family members and acquaintances, the person tends to compensate by relying on auditory cues such as the sound of the family member's voice or a distinctive feature such as long, blond hair.

Brain lesions can also impair the ability to interpret facial expressions, which can have significant social consequences.[17,97] For example, one individual tended to be very suspicious of others. He was observed to have difficulty describing the expressions of various persons depicted in photographs. Because he had emigrated to the United States from another country, it was considered that his difficulty could be a result of cultural differences. He was asked to bring in a newspaper that he regularly received from his native country. The captions of the photographs were occluded, and he was asked to describe the emotional expressions of the persons shown. He was then asked to translate the photo captions and became aware that he was unable to discriminate the emotions apparent on the faces.

A standardized Test of Facial Recognition[11] is available, which presents a multiple-choice matching of faces presented in front view and side view and under various lighting conditions. Informal functional assessments could include having the client identify the names of the people in photographs, with family members at a dinner table (e.g., Walt's two children side by side), or by having the client identify his or her own face in a mirror. Photographs of famous people could also be used. If aphasia is present, have the client communicate through gestures, such as head nodding (e.g., "yes" or "no") in response to different choices. If the client is unable to identify self or family members, prosopagnosia may be indicated. A formal test of facial expression discrimination is not available in the literature,[58] but an informal assessment is also possible using pictures and photographs of familiar people.

OT interventions for prosopagnosia include remedial approaches such as providing face matching exercises.[99] Adaptive approaches include providing pictures of family members and famous people with names and assisting the client to associate the family member's face with other unique characteristics and features, such as weight, height, mannerisms, accents, and hairstyle.

Simultanognosia

Simultanognosia refers to the inability to recognize and interpret a visual array as a whole, and is caused by lesions to the right hemisphere of the brain.[30] Clients with simultanognosia are able to identify the individual components of a visual scene, but are unable to recognize and interpret the gestalt of the scene. For example, Walt is able to identify the flowers and the trees in one of his paintings, but he is not able to recognize and interpret this painting as the landscape surrounding the family home where he grew up.

Assessment includes presenting the client a photograph of a detailed visual array (e.g., Walt's family photograph at the beach), asking the client to describe the scene in detail, and assessing whether or not the client can describe the scene as a whole. Many clients will be able to identify specific features of the visual array (e.g., the sand castle), but cannot describe the context or meaning of the whole scene (e.g., a family trip to the beach). Simultanognosia is indicated when the client cannot recognize and interpret a visual array as a whole.

OT intervention will focus on assisting the client to construct meaning of a visual array through verbal cues and therapeutic questions to facilitate abstract reasoning. Intervention is best provided in familiar contexts, such as a client's home, work setting, or during a community outing to the shopping mall.

VISUAL-SPATIAL PERCEPTION DISORDERS

Walt presents with difficulty distinguishing the right and left side of his body and often confuses right and left when given directions. He often gets lost and requires a family member to be with him at all times when he is in unfamiliar community environments. When painting, Walt has also been observed to have difficulty with distinguishing the foreground and

the background in his paintings and is unable to determine the differences between the amounts of paint in each of the cups next to him. In addition, he is often observed missing the canvas in front of him when attempting to apply the paint.

Walt presents with visual-spatial perception dysfunction. **Visual-spatial perception** refers to the capacity to appreciate the spatial arrangement of one's body, objects in relationship to oneself, and relationships between objects in space. Various efforts have been made to subdivide spatial skills into components, but recent writers acknowledge that spatial skills cannot be isolated easily from one another.[18] It is generally acknowledged that the right hemisphere, which controls spatial abilities, tends to function in the gestalt (whole), whereas the left hemisphere, which is responsible for linguistic operations, tends to focus on discrete details.[58]

Visual-spatial perception often occurs instantaneously, and it is because of this rapid processing of information that, when operating a motor vehicle, it is possible to react quickly to another driver's actions to avoid a collision. An individual with a mild visual-spatial perception impairment may need additional time to perform a task, but processes the information correctly, possibly by compensating with verbal analysis of the perceptual components. Severe impairment may result in the incorrect response despite additional time used in attempting to solve the problem.

Visual-spatial skills are not limited to the visual domain.[56] Sounds can be localized in space, and the mobility and daily occupations of blind individuals are heavily dependent on the tactile appreciation of the spatial arrangements of objects.[74] For example, a blind person's ability to navigate through a familiar room requires awareness of the layout of each piece of furniture in the physical environment, and continual shifting of the individual's "cognitive map" while changing position in the room.

As a pencil rolls across a desktop, it is the skill of visual-spatial perception that enables a person to appreciate the relative orientation of the pencil to the table surface as the pencil nears the edge and is about to fall to the floor. Figure 24-1 illustrates many of these visual-spatial functions.

Figure-Ground Discrimination Dysfunction

Figure-ground discrimination allows a person to perceive the foreground from the background in a visual array.[99] For example, Walt is unable to locate a particular painting utensil from the other writing utensils in the pencil holder, thereby distinguishing the targeted object from the background.

Figure-ground discrimination can be assessed functionally in a variety of contexts. During a dressing activity, you may ask the client to identify the white undershirt that is located on top of his or her white sheets. In the kitchen, you can ask the client to pick out all of the spoons from a disorganized utensil drawer. Figure-ground discrimination

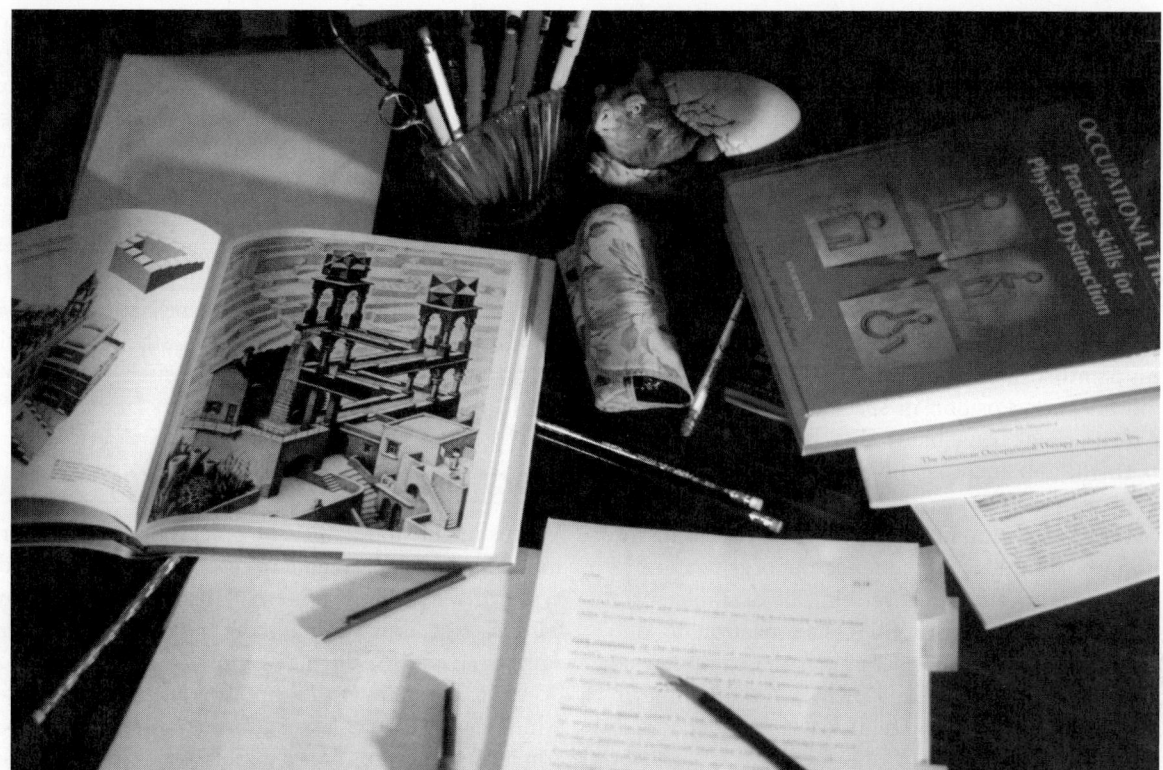

Figure 24-1   Visual-spatial functions in real life. Note that all components of spatial functions can be found in this scene.

dysfunction may be indicated if the client is unable to discriminate the foreground from the background in a complex visual array.

Using a remedial approach, intervention for figure-ground discrimination dysfunction should focus on challenging the client to localize objects of similar color in a disorganized visual array.[99] The task could be incorporated contextually into meaningful occupation. For example, the therapist working with Walt may have him localize the exact pencil he would like to use for his sketch drawings. The task can be downgraded by making the visual array less complex and upgraded by making the visual array more complex.

An adaptive approach to intervention would focus on modifying the environment to increase the organization of common functional objects (e.g., placing only the most necessary objects needed for self-care), decreasing the complexity of the visual array that the client has to discriminate (e.g., have only one paintbrush in front of Walt at a given time), or marking common objects with colored tape so that objects are easily distinguished from one another, particularly when the objects are of a similar color.[98]

Toglia's Multicontextual Approach may be used to help the client gain self-awareness of his or her figure-ground discrimination dysfunction and develop effective organizational and visual scanning strategies for discriminating the foreground and background in their environment.[88]

This intervention approach also focuses on the generalization of skill to multiple functional contexts by using strategies that the client has identified as effective in locating objects in their environment.

Form-Constancy Dysfunction

Form constancy is the recognition of various forms, shapes, and objects, regardless of their position, location, or size.[99] For example, a person can perceive all of the pencils on a desk, in various sizes or in various positions in the pencil holder.

To assess form constancy, ask the client to identify familiar objects in their environment through observation alone when those objects are placed upside down or on their side. For example, in the kitchen, you may ask Walt to identify a cup that is turned upside down or a toaster oven that is placed on its side. Form-constancy dysfunction may be indicated if the client is unable to identify objects in a position that varies from the norm.

Intervention for form-constancy dysfunction would include using tactile cues to feel objects in various positions so that the client learns the constancy of them despite their position, size, or location. Activities can be graded from positioning all objects in an upright position to placing objects in odd positions. Intervention is best provided with common objects that the client utilizes in everyday occupational performance.

Position in Space

Position in space, or **spatial relations,** refers to the relative orientation of a shape or object to the self. It is this component of perception that allows a person to recognize that the tip of the pencil is pointed away from him, and so directs the hand to effectively grasp the pencil.

To assess position in space, have the client place common objects in relation to the self or other objects using the following directional terms: top/bottom, up/down, in/out, behind/in front of, and before/after. For example, ask Walt to place his paintbrush on top of his computer or his basketball behind his back. Position in space dysfunction may be indicated if the client is unable to discern the relationships of objects to the self or other objects through directional terms.

Intervention for position in space includes providing the client with opportunities to experience the organization of objects in the environment to the self. For example, Walt could practice placing various objects in relation to one another in a graphic design program on the computer so that directional concepts of up/down, in/out, behind/in front of, and before/after can be reinforced.

Right-Left Discrimination Dysfunction

Right-left discrimination is the ability to accurately use the concepts of right and left.[99] An individual with right-left discrimination dysfunction may confuse the right and left side of his or her body or confuse right and left in directional terms when navigating through their environment.

To assess right-left discrimination, ask the client to point to various body parts (e.g., left ear) or assess the client's ability to accurately navigate their environment through verbal commands using right and left (e.g., turn right at the end of the hallway). Right-left discrimination dysfunction may be indicated if the client is unable to differentiate between right and left in relation to their body and their environment.

Intervention for right-left discrimination will focus on assisting the client to practice reciting right and left as they are interacting with their own body (e.g., "I am now placing my right arm into the shirt sleeve") or their environment (e.g., "I am now turning left at the stop sign"). Remediation of right-left discrimination can significantly improve topographical orientation as the client learns to navigate in a more dynamic home and community environment.

Stereopsis

Stereopsis is the inability to perceive depth in relation to the self or in relation to various objects in the environment.[99] Depth perception is critical to function in a three-dimensional world and to safety in driving and community mobility. Clients with visual dysfunction in one eye or who wear an eye patch to compensate for double vision may demonstrate stereopsis, because visual input from both eyes is required to perceive depth.

To assess depth perception, place a variety of common objects on a table surface and ask the client to identify which object is closer and farther away. In a community context, the client may also be assessed functionally by asking him or her to identify buildings or landmarks that are closer or farther away. Stereopsis may be indicated if the client is unable to judge the distance between objects in the environment.

Computer-assisted software has been developed that assists the client with developing depth perception by judging the relative distance of objects in relation to one another on a computer screen.[99] Tactile-kinesthetic approaches also help the client judge distances through the use of tactile input.[1]

TACTILE PERCEPTION DISORDERS

Walt is unable to identify the objects he uses for painting by touch alone. He is unable to discriminate between different types of materials or different forms and shapes by tactile means, and must compensate visually to determine the objects he is using during occupational performance.

Walt presents with an impairment in tactile perception, which involves tactile discriminative skills of the second somatosensory area of the parietal lobes. These skills require a higher level of synthesis than the basic tactile sensory functions of light touch and pressure described in Chapter 22.

Astereognosis

Stereognosis, also known as tactile gnosis,[22] is the perceptual skill that enables an individual to identify common objects and geometric shapes through tactile perception without the aid of vision. It results from the integration of the senses of touch, pressure, position, motion, texture, weight, and temperature and is dependent on intact parietal cortical function.[39] Stereognosis is essential to occupational performance because the ability to "see with the hands" is critical to many daily activities. It is the skill that makes it possible to reach into a handbag and find a pen and to find the light switch in a dark room. Along with proprioception, stereognosis enables the use of all hand tools and performance of hand activities without the need to concentrate visually on the implements being used. Examples are knitting while watching television, reaching into a pocket for house keys, and using a fork to eat while engaged in conversation. A deficit in stereognosis is called **astereognosis.** Persons who have astereognosis but retain much of their motor function must visually monitor their hands' activities. Thus, they must be very slow and purposeful in their movements and tend to be generally less active.

The purpose of a stereognosis test is to assess a client's ability to identify common objects and perceive their tactile properties.[9,21,43,53] A means to occlude the person's vision is needed, such as a curtain or folder as described in Chapter 22. Typical objects that could be used for identification include a pencil, fountain pen, pair of sunglasses, key, nail, safety pin, paper clip, metal teaspoon, quarter, nickel, button, and small leather coin purse. Any common objects may be used, but it is important to consider the client's social and ethnic background to ensure that he or she has had previous experience with the objects. Three-dimensional geometric shapes (e.g., square, sphere, and pyramid) can also be used to test shape and form perception.

The test should be conducted in privacy in an environment with minimal distractions. The client should be seated at a table in a position that accommodates the affected hand and forearm comfortably. The therapist should sit opposite the person being tested. If the client is unable to manipulate test objects because of motor weakness, the therapist should assist him or her to manipulate them in as near normal a manner as possible. The client's vision is occluded, with the dorsal surface of the hand resting on the table. Objects are presented in random order. Manipulation of objects is allowed and encouraged. The therapist assists with the manipulation of items if the person's hand function is impaired. The client should be asked to name the object, or, if he or she is unable to name the object, to describe its properties. Clients with aphasia may view a duplicate set of test objects after each trial and point to a choice. The person's response to each of the items presented is scored. The therapist notes if the object is identified quickly and correctly, if there is a long delay before the identification of the object, or if the individual can describe only properties (e.g., size, texture, material, and shape) of the object. The therapist also notes if the person cannot identify the object or describe its properties.

A graded intervention program for astereognosis has been described by Eggers.[29] Initially, the client manipulates the object while looking at it and making noise with the object such as tapping it on the tabletop. This approach allows the client to see and hear an object while feeling it for the benefit of intersensory facilitation; then vision is occluded during the tactile exploration. Finally, a pad is placed on the tabletop so that both auditory and visual clues are eliminated and the person relies on tactile-kinesthetic input alone. The program for tactile-kinesthetic reeducation begins with gross discrimination of objects that are very dissimilar—for example, smooth and rough textures or round and square shapes. Next, the client is asked to estimate quantities (such as the number of marbles in a box) through touch. Then the client must discriminate between large and small objects hidden in sand and progress to discriminating between two- and three-dimensional objects. Finally, the client is required to pick a specific small object from among several objects.

Farber also described a treatment approach to retrain stereognosis for adults and children with CNS dysfunction.[32] First, the client is allowed to examine the training object visually as it is rotated by the therapist. The client is then allowed to handle the object in the less affected hand while observing the hand. In the next step, the client is allowed to manipulate the object with both hands while looking. Then the object is placed in the affected hand and the client manipulates the object while looking at it. The individual may place the hand in a mirror-lined, three-sided box to increase visual input during these manipulations. This sequence is then repeated with the vision occluded. Once several objects can be identified consistently, two of the objects may be hidden in a tub of sand or rice. The client is then asked to reach into the tub and retrieve a specific object. If the sensation of the sand or rice is over-stimulating or disturbing, the objects can be placed in a bag.[32]

Agraphesthesia

An additional test of tactile perception that measures parietal lobe function is the test for **graphesthesia,** the ability to recognize numbers, letters, or forms written on the skin.[19,39,71] The loss of this ability is called **agraphesthesia.** To test graphesthesia, the examiner occludes the client's vision and traces letters, numbers, or geometric forms on the fingertips or palm with a dull-pointed pencil or similar instrument. The client tells the therapist which symbol was written.[71] If the client has aphasia, pictures of the symbols may be provided for the individual to indicate a response after each test stimulus. Agraphesthesia is indicated if the client is unable to state or identify the symbol written on the palm of the hand.

OT intervention for agraphesthesia will focus on providing the client with opportunities for tactile discrimination through the use of the hands. The therapist can grade the intervention from tracing letters and numbers to words and geometric forms on the palm of the hand. With their vision occluded, the client can also practice writing their name in their opposite palm.

Body Schema Perception Disorders

Walt demonstrates unilateral inattention to the left side of his body and his environment. He demonstrates asymmetrical visual scanning to the left side of his environment, misses details in his drawings on the left, and routinely neglects the functional use of his left upper extremity during functional tasks. He often states that his left arm is owned by someone else, and has difficulty with holding a painting utensil due to impairments with spatial relationships between his fingers.

Following a CVA or TBI, a person's sense of his or her body's shape, position, and capacity frequently is distorted. This is known as a disorder of **body schema,** or autotopagnosia.[10] This can be noted in attempts to draw a human figure (Figure 24-2) or in a person's unrealistic expectations of performance abilities.[58] For example, an individual with left hemiplegia after a TBI expressed his intention to return to his previous manual labor job of installing garage doors. The disorder can affect egocentric perception of one's own body or allocentric orientation of another person's body.[70,73] A person may neglect one side of the body or demonstrate generally distorted impressions of the body's configuration.

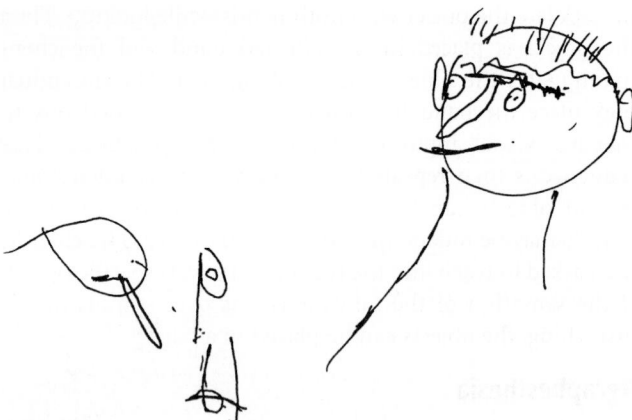

Figure 24-2 Example of a body schema perception disorder. Drawing on left is the person's first attempt to draw a face. Therapist asked the person to try again. Second effort is drawing on right.

The person may confuse his or her body with that of another, such as the person who thought that her wedding ring had been stolen by the therapist, not realizing that the hand she was viewing was her own. **Finger agnosia,** or the inability to discriminate the fingers of the hand, can also be part of the disorder.[10] An impaired body scheme will also affect participation in occupation and performance skills.[81]

Body schema perception disorders can be assessed by asking the individual to draw a human figure (Figure 24-2) or point to body parts on command (e.g., "Touch your left hand" and "Touch your right knee"). Finger agnosia is evaluated by occluding the person's vision and asking him or her to name each finger as it is touched by the therapist. Unilateral body neglect can be observed functionally during occupational performance as the client ignores the affected limb and/or states that a body part is not his or her own. A body schema perception disorder may be indicated if the client is unable to correctly identify parts of his or her body.

A remedial approach to intervention for body schema perception disorders should focus on providing the client with opportunities to reinforce body knowledge through tactile and proprioceptive stimulation.[99] For example, while Walt is dressing or painting, have him incorporate his left upper extremity into the activity and verbally acknowledge that this is in fact *his* left arm and hand being used. Tactile-kinesthetic guiding or constraint-induced movement therapy techniques can also be used if the client has difficulty initiating the use of their affected limb. As the client incorporates the use of their affected limb into occupational performance, the client will begin to gain perceptual awareness of their body and the relationship of various body parts.

MOTOR PERCEPTION DISORDERS

When given a shirt to don, Walt attempts to put his legs through the sleeves of the shirt. During drawing and painting activities, he seems to hesitate and is unable to initiate a motor plan without physical cues. He knows that he is painting and knows what he would like to paint, but is unable to translate this idea into a motor action. Walt is also unable to operate the mouse on the computer for a graphic design activity due to difficulty with motor planning. In addition, when given a three-dimensional craft project, he is unable to use effective problem solving strategies during the construction of the design.

Praxis is the ability to plan and perform purposeful movement. Walt presents with a motor perception disorder that affects his motor planning. **Apraxia** has been classically defined as a deficit in "the execution of learned movement which cannot be accounted for by either weakness, incoordination, or sensory loss, or by incomprehension of or inattention to commands."[38] The disorder can result from damage to either side of the brain or to the corpus callosum[45,96] but is more frequently noted with left hemisphere damage.[46] Apraxia is often seen in persons with aphasia; however, not all aphasic persons are apraxic, nor are all apraxic persons aphasic.[42,45] This type of dysfunction may occur after CVA or TBI. Progressive apraxia is often noted with degenerative disorders such as Alzheimer's disease.[45,72] See also Chapters 33 to 35 in this text.

Apraxia has been strongly correlated with dependence in areas of occupation.[85,92] For example, in a severe case of apraxia, an individual, Ms. S, initially required full assistance with *basic activities of daily living* (BADLs). Ms. S was fully cognizant of ongoing events but could not even direct her arm and leg movements in a way that would assist the nursing staff during dressing. When asked to pick up a pencil, Ms. S walked around all four sides of the table in an attempt to position her hand correctly to grasp the object. She could describe the desired action in words ("I want to pick up the pencil between my thumb and index finger, with the lead point of the pencil close to the tips of my fingers") but reported after returning to her seat that her hand never "looked like it was in the right position" to take hold of the pencil.

The categories of apraxia are difficult to differentiate, and authors differ in their use of terms.[86] The principal types are ideational apraxia, ideomotor apraxia, dressing apraxia, and constructional disorder. Because the distinction between ideational and ideomotor apraxia is often perplexing, some authors recommend simply using the term *apraxia*.[54,58]

Ideational Apraxia

Ideational apraxia is a conceptual deficit, seen as an inability to use real objects appropriately.[23,26,42] More recent authors suggest the use of the term *conceptual apraxia*.[46,72] The individual also may have difficulty sequencing acts in the proper order,[45] such as with folding a sheet of paper and inserting it into an envelope. The individual may use the wrong tool for the task or may associate the wrong tool with the object to be acted on, such as by attempting to write with a spoon.[45] This deficit has significant functional implications in a variety of areas of occupation.

Ideomotor Apraxia

Ideomotor apraxia is an inability to carry out a motor act on verbal command or imitation. However, the person with ideomotor apraxia is able to perform the act correctly when asked to use the actual object.[25,45] For example, a person is unable to mime the action of brushing his teeth on request but is observed using a toothbrush correctly when he is performing grooming activities in context. Observation of the person in areas of occupation is critical to the identification of ideomotor apraxia. Impairments are demonstrated only in the testing environment and appear to have little functional impact, as compared with ideational apraxia.[86]

Dressing Apraxia

Another category of motor perception disorders seen in the literature is **dressing apraxia.** The classification of dressing impairment as a form of apraxia has been questioned in recent years because the difficulties in ADLs are considered to be caused by perceptual or cognitive dysfunction[16,92,100] (if apraxia is not noted in other activities), or are seen as an extension of an ideational or ideomotor apraxic disorder.

General Principles in the Assessment and Treatment of Apraxia

It is important that assessments of sensory function, muscle strength, and dexterity are completed before the test of praxis because deficits in these areas would complicate any assessment of apraxia. If a person has a hemiplegia, the unaffected hand is used for testing. Input from the speech-language pathologist is important for establishing an individual's capacity for basic comprehension via words or gestures. Because of the frequent association of apraxia with aphasia and left hemisphere brain damage, an apraxia screening is included as a part of many aphasia batteries[86] used by speech-language pathologists.

The literature[16] offers several apraxia assessments used in research, such as the Florida Apraxia Screening Test (FAST),[78,79] the Movement Imitation Test,[24,25] and the Use of Objects Test.[24] The Loewenstein Occupational Therapy Cognitive Assessment (LOTCA)[50] includes a praxis subsection, as does the Rivermead Perceptual Assessment Battery,[94] both of which serve as screening tools for the disorder. The Santa Clara Valley Medical Center Praxis Test and the Solet Test for Apraxia are two additional evaluation tools developed by occupational therapists.[99]

A thorough assessment includes items presented, such as those shown in Table 24-1,[45] and involves both transitive movements (action involving both tool and use, such as writing with an imaginary pen) and intransitive movements (movements for communication, such as waving farewell). Lists of gestures used in assessment are noted in several studies.[16,45,76,78,95]

Returning to the case of Ms. S, who has severe apraxia, she was first treated by practicing basic motor movements,

TABLE **24-1** **Elements of a Comprehensive Apraxia Assessment**

Test Condition	Example
Gesture to command	"Show me how you would take off your hat." (transitive)
	"Show me how you would throw a kiss." (intransitive)
Gesture to imitation	"Copy what I do."
	Therapist shrugs shoulders. (intransitive)
	Therapist flips an imaginary coin. (transitive)
Gesture in response to seeing the tool	"Show me how you would use this object."
	Therapist provides screwdriver for display.
Gesture in response to seeing the object upon which the tool works	"Show me how you would use this object."
	Therapist provides screwdriver and block of wood with screw partially inserted.
Actual tool use	"Show me how you would use this object."
	Therapist provides screwdriver for use.
Imitation of the examiner using the tool	"Copy what I do."
	Therapist makes stirring motion, using a spoon.
Discrimination between correct and incorrect pantomimed movements	"Is this the correct way to blow out a match?"
	Therapist pantomimes holding match in unsafe manner (e.g., match held upside down, with head of match near palm of hand).
Gesture comprehension	"What object am I using?"
	Therapist pantomimes shaving face with a razor.
Serial acts	"Show me how you would open an imaginary can of soda, pour it into a glass, and take a drink."

From Heilman KM, Rothi LJG: Apraxia. In Heilman KM, Valenstein E, editors: *Clinical neuropsychology*, New York, 1993, Oxford University Press.

then following a developmental sequence, to more advanced functional motor activities. For example, following repetition of basic movement patterns, the client with apraxia progressed to coloring geometric shapes on note cards (felt-tip markers were initially placed in a vertical stand for easy grasp) and gradually to writing exercises. Independent telephone use was important to Ms. S, so a large calculator was used for keystroke practice. She gradually progressed to a disconnected telephone and then to a functional telephone. By the termination of the intervention program, Ms. S was independent in most areas of occupation, although additional time was needed for each activity.

For another client with apraxia, the clinical reasoning process was used in planning the treatment, beginning with spoken instruction for each sequence in the task, written or pictorial instructions, and visual monitoring of her limbs throughout each aspect of the task.[16] Another case study of apraxia treatment involved conductive education—that is, breaking the task into smaller units and verbally guiding (conducting) the sequence.[67] The individual improved on targeted tasks, but minimal generalization was noted in everyday occupations.

The intervention for dressing impairment involves teaching a set pattern for dressing and giving cues that help the person distinguish right from left or front from back. A helpful method is to have the individual position the garment the same way each time (e.g., positioning a shirt with the buttons face-up and pants with the zipper face-up). Labels, small buttons, or ribbons can be used as cues to differentiate the front from the back of the garment.[99,100]

Constructional Disorder

The term **constructional disorder** is now favored over the previously used term of two- and three-dimensional constructional apraxia since the deficit does not clearly fall within the definition of apraxia.[12,16,58] Many occupations depend on visuoconstructional skills, or the ability to organize visual information into meaningful spatial representations. Constructional deficits refer to the inability to organize or assemble parts into a whole, as in putting together block designs (three-dimensional) or drawings (two-dimensional). Constructional deficits can result in significant dysfunction in occupations that require constructional ability, such as dressing, following instructions for assembling a toy, and stacking a dishwasher.[69,87] Figure 24-3, which shows evidence of left inattention, also demonstrates constructional deficits. An individual acts on his or her contextual environment based on the information he or she perceives. Therefore, deficits in perception become more apparent when a person interacts with the environment in maladaptive ways.

Traditional tests of constructional abilities in a two-dimensional mode are the Test of Visual-Motor Skills for adults,[36] the copy administration of the Benton Visual Retention Test,[84] and the Rey Complex Figure.[58] The latter two tests also are used to evaluate visual memory skills. Use of the Rey Complex Figure has been suggested for a quick screening of visual perceptual functions.[60] The Three-Dimensional Block Construction[8] involves the use of various blocks to copy a design from a three-dimensional model. Nonstandardized tests that may be used are drawing, constructing matchstick designs, assembling block designs, or building a structure to match a model.[99] In daily living, occupations such as dressing or setting the table require constructional skills. To perform such tasks successfully, an

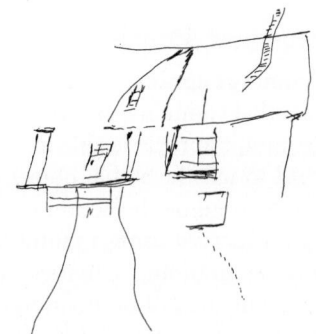

Figure 24-3 Example of two-dimensional constructional disorder and left-sided inattention in a drawing of a house by a retired architect who had had a right CVA.

individual must have integrated visual perception, motor planning, and motor execution.[8,40,66,93,100]

Several studies have gathered data on the constructional skills of unimpaired subjects for use as a normative reference for persons with CVA and TBI.[31,66] In a study of constructional abilities in the well elderly, Fall[31] demonstrated that results are influenced by the type of test administration. Subjects tended to score higher on tests that used three-dimensional models as guides for construction than on those that used photographs or drawings. The implications of this finding for occupational therapists are that (1) the type of test administration affects scores, and (2) in teaching persons with constructional disorders, models or demonstrations of desired performance are likely to produce better results than would photographs or drawings.[31]

The remedial approach to intervention involves the use of perceptual tasks such as paper and pencil activities, puzzles, and three-dimensional craft projects to improve constructional skills. The adaptive approach would include participation in occupational performance and developing compensatory approaches to the functional performance skill deficits. Many areas of occupation are suitable for treatment of constructional deficits, such as folding towels, setting the dinner table, and weeding the garden.

BEHAVIORAL ASPECTS OF PERCEPTUAL DYSFUNCTION

Some degree of accurate self-awareness and recognition of the effect of the disability on one's functioning is needed if the person is to invest energy in the therapy process.[34] An individual who is unaware of perceptual deficits may be a serious safety risk and may attempt occupations that are well beyond present physical abilities. Denial is often noted in early stages of recovery from CVA or TBI and may serve as a protective coping mechanism that allows the individual to gradually absorb the effect of the injury on his or her functioning. A person's innate trust of the accuracy of perceptions often is a basis for unrealistic self-confidence;

demonstrating to the individual that his or her perceptions are now distorted and no longer trustworthy can profoundly affect the person's sense of self. A therapist needs to respect and be sensitive to the individual's sense of self and be prepared to aid the client in understanding the changes in perceptual capacity and in re-establishing an accurate sense of self-awareness. Several questionnaires are available to assess an individual's self-awareness.[52] The questionnaires typically are issued to the person with deficits as well as to a family member or close acquaintance. The discrepancies in the two questionnaires are used as a measure of the accuracy of the individual's insight and serve as the basis for intervention. The individual's behavior may also be the result of a disorder in executive function.[52] See Chapter 25 for additional discussion of this possibility.

An individual who has some degree of awareness of the disability often is depressed, which seems an appropriate response to the gravity of the situation. The therapist needs to recognize and appreciate this emotional response and help the person achieve an emotional balance to re-establish quality of life through celebrating progress in therapy while acknowledging the impact of the disability.[34,77] (See also Chapter 6 on social and psychological aspects.)

THREADED CASE STUDY: WALT, PART 2

1. How would you best assess Walt's occupational performance?

Walt's performance in his most valued occupations has been affected due to perceptual impairment. A combination of skilled observation and formal assessments, such as the A-ONE[2,3,4] and the AMPS,[33] could be used to assess Walt's occupational performance in a variety of functional contexts. In addition to assessing occupational performance, these assessments can also assess Walt's perceptual functioning. The COPM[57] can also be used to evaluate the client's primary goals in occupational therapy and set the stage for an occupation-based approach to intervention.

2. How would you best assess Walt's perceptual function?

Throughout the chapter, a variety of assessment tools have been presented to evaluate visual perception, visual-spatial perception, tactile perception, body schema perception, and motor perception. In addition, other comprehensive perceptual tests, such as the MVPT-R,[20] the Dynamic Object Search Test,[88] the TVPS-UL,[37] the Lowenstein Occupational Therapy Cognitive Assessment,[50] the Rivermead Perceptual Assessment Battery,[27,94] the Minnesota Paper Form Board Test,[59] and the Hooper Visual Organization Test[47] could be used to assess global areas of visual processing and perceptual functioning.

3. How would you assist Walt in achieving his occupational performance goals using remedial and adaptive approaches for his perceptual dysfunction?

In order to assist Walt in achieving his occupational performance goals of submitting a painting to a local art gallery, playing with his children, driving, and regaining computer skills in preparation for resumption of part-time work as a graphic artist, the therapist would need to use a combination of remedial and adaptive approaches to treat his perceptual impairments. This chapter outlines a variety of intervention possibilities for Walt. The evidence shows that the most successful outcomes for treating perceptual impairments are through occupation-based activities that have meaning and offer the client the opportunity to generalize skills to multiple contexts.[28,61,67,68,100]

Review Questions

1. Describe the effects of visual perception, visual-spatial perception, tactile perception, body schema perception, and motor perception on occupational performance.
2. Compare the advantages and disadvantages of formal perceptual testing and functional assessment in the context of occupational performance.
3. Describe one assessment used to test perceptual impairments in the following areas: visual perception, visual-spatial perception, tactile perception, body schema perception, and motor perception.
4. Describe the two approaches to treatment of perceptual deficits and give one example of an occupational therapy intervention for each.
5. Describe an intervention for each of the following types of perceptual dysfunction: visual perception, visual-spatial perception, tactile perception, body schema perception, and motor perception.

REFERENCES

1. Affolter FD: *Perception, interaction, and language: interaction of daily living: the root of development*, Berlin, 1987, Springer-Verlag.
2. Arnadottir G: Evaluation and intervention with complex perceptual impairment. In Unsworth C: *Cognitive and perceptual dysfunction: a clinical reasoning approach to evaluation and intervention*, Philadelphia, 1999, FA Davis.
3. Arnadottir G: Impact of neurobehavioral deficits on activities of daily living. In Gillen G, Burkhardt A, editors: *Stroke rehabilitation: a function-based approach*, ed 2, St Louis, 2004, Mosby.
4. Arnadottir G: *The brain and behavior: assessing cortical dysfunction through activities of daily living*, St Louis, 1990, Mosby.
5. Ashford JW, et al: Diagnosis of Alzheimer's disease. In Kumar V, Eisdorfer C, editors: *Advances in the diagnosis and treatment of Alzheimer's disease*, New York, 1998, Springer-Verlag.
6. Ayres AJ: *Sensory integration and learning disorders*, Los Angeles, 1972, Western Psychological Services.

7. Baum B, Hall K: Relationship between constructional praxis and dressing in the head injured adult, *Am J Occup Ther* 35:438, 1981.

8. Benton AL, Fogel ML: Three-dimensional constructional praxis: a clinical test, *Arch Neurol* 7:347, 1962.

9. Benton AL, Schultz LM: Observations of tactile form perception (stereognosis) in pre-school children, *J Clin Psychol* 5:359, 1949.

10. Benton AL, Sivan AB: Disturbances of the body schema. In Heilman KM, Valenstein E: *Clinical neuropsychology*, New York, 1993, Oxford University Press.

11. Benton AL, et al: *Contributions to neuropsychological assessment: a clinical manual*, Oxford, 1983, Oxford University Press.

12. Benton AL, Tranel D: Visuoperceptual, visuospatial, and visuoconstructive disorders. In Heilman KM, Valenstein E, editors: *Clinical neuropsychology*, New York, 1993, Oxford University Press.

13. Binetti G, et al: Visual and spatial perceptions in the early phase of Alzheimer's disease, *Neuropsychology* 12(1):29-33, 1998.

14. Blakemore C, Movshon JA: Sensory system: introduction. In Gazzaniga MS, editor: *The cognitive neurosciences*, London, 1996, MIT Press.

15. Bruce V, Young A: *In the eye of the beholder: the science of face perception*, Oxford, 1998, Oxford University Press.

16. Butler JA: Evaluation and intervention with apraxia. In Unsworth C: *Cognitive and perceptual dysfunction: a clinical reasoning approach to evaluation and intervention*, Philadelphia, 1999, FA Davis.

17. Calder AJ, et al: Facial emotion recognition after bilateral amygdala damage: differentially severe impairment of fear, *Cogn Neuropsychol* 13:699, 1996.

18. Caplan BM, Romans S: Assessment of spatial abilities. In Goldstein G, Nussbaum PD, Beers SR, editors: *Neuropsychology*, New York, 1998, Plenum Press.

19. Chusid JG: Correlative neuroanatomy and functional neurology, ed 19, Los Altos, CA, 1985, Lange Medical Publications.

20. Colarusso RP, Hammill DD: *Motor-Free Visual Perception Test—Revised (MVPT-R)*, Novato, CA, 1996, Academic Therapy Publications.

21. DeJong R: *The neurologic examination*, New York, 1958, Paul B. Hoeber.

22. Dellon AL: Evaluation of sensibility and re-education of sensation in the hand, Baltimore, MD, 1981, Williams & Wilkins.

23. De Renzi E: Methods of limb apraxia examination and their bearing on the interpretation of the disorder. In Roy EA, editor: *Neuropsychological studies of apraxia and related disorders*, Amsterdam, 1985, North-Holland.

24. De Renzi E, et al: Modality-specific and supramodal mechanisms of apraxia, *Brain* 105:301, 1982.

25. De Renzi E, et al: Imitating gestures: a quantitative approach to ideomotor apraxia, *Arch Neurol* 37:6, 1980.

26. De Renzi E, et al: Ideational apraxia: a quantitative study, *Neuropsychologia* 6:41, 1968.

27. Donnelly SM, et al: The Rivermead Perceptual Assessment Battery: its relationship to selected functional activities, *Br J Occup Ther* 61:27, 1998.

28. Edmans JA, Lincoln NB: Treatment of visual perceptual deficits after stroke: single case studies on four patients with right hemiplegia, *Br J Occup Ther* 54:139, 1991.

29. Eggers O: *Occupational therapy in the treatment of adult hemiplegia*, Rockville, MD, 1984, Aspen Systems.

30. Ellis AW, Young AW: *Human cognitive neuropsychology*, Hillsdale, NJ, 1988, Lawrence Erlbaum Assoc.

31. Fall CC: Comparing ways of measuring constructional praxis in the well elderly, *Am J Occup Ther* 41:500, 1987.

32. Farber SD: *Neurorehabiliation, a multisensory approach*, Philadelphia, 1982, WB Saunders.

33. Fisher AG: *Assessment of motor and process skills*, Fort Collins, CO, 1995, Three Star Press.

34. Fleming J, Strong J: Self-awareness of deficits following acquired brain injury: considerations for rehabilitation, *Br J Occup Ther* 58:55, 1995.

35. Gardner H: *Frames of mind: the theory of multiple intelligences*, New York, 1983, Basic Books.

36. Gardner MF: *The Test of Visual-Motor Skills (TVMS)*, Burlingame, CA, 1992, Psychological and Educational Publications.

37. Gardner MF: *The Test of Visual Perceptual Skills—Revised (TVPS-R)*, Hydesville, CA, 1997, Psychological and Educational Publications.

38. Geschwind N: *The apraxias: neural mechanisms of disorders of learned movement*, *Am Sci* 63:188, 1975.

39. Gilroy J, Meyer JS: Medical neurology, London, 1969, Macmillan.

40. Goodglass H, Kaplan E: *Assessment of aphasia and related disorders*, ed 2, Philadelphia, 1972, Thomas Publishers.

41. Gordon WA, et al: Perceptual remediation in patients with right brain damage: a comprehensive program, *Arch Phys Med Rehabil* 66:353, 1985.

42. Haaland KY, Harrington DL: Neuropsychological assessment of motor skills. In Goldstein G, Nussbaum PD, Beers SR, editors: *Neuropsychology*, New York, 1998, Plenum Press.

43. Head H, et al: *Studies in neurology*, London, 1920, Oxford University Press.

44. Hecaen H, et al: The syndrome of apractognosis due to lesions of the minor cerebral hemisphere, *Arch Neurol Psychiat* 75:400, 1956.

45. Heilman KM, Rothi LJG: Apraxia. In Heilman KM, Valenstein E, editors: *Clinical neuropsychology*, New York, 1993, Oxford University Press.

46. Heilman KM, et al: Conceptual apraxia from lateralized lesions, *Neurology* 49:457, 1997.

47. Hooper HE: *Hooper Visual Organization Test*, Los Angeles, 1983, Western Psychological Assoc.

48. Humphreys GW, Riddoch MJ: *To see but not to see: a case study of visual agnosia*, Hove, UK, 1987, Lawrence Erlbaum Assoc.

49. Humphreys GW, Riddoch MJ: Visual object processing in normality and pathology: implications for rehabilitation. In Riddoch MJ, Humphreys GW, editors: *Cognitive neuropsychology and cognitive rehabilitation*, Hove, UK, 1994, Lawrence Erlbaum Assoc.

50. Itzkovich M, et al: *The Loewenstein Occupational Therapy Cognitive Assessment (LOTCA) manual*, Pequannock, NJ, 1990, Maddock.

51. Katz N, editor: *Cognition and occupation in rehabilitation*, ed 2, Bethesda, MD, 2005, AOTA Press.

52. Katz N, Hartman-Maeir A: Metacognition: the relationships of awareness and executive functions to occupational performance. In Katz N, editor: *Cognition and occupation in rehabilitation: cognitive models for intervention in occupational therapy*, Bethesda, MD, 1998, American Occupational Therapy Association.

53. Kent BE: Sensory-motor testing: the upper limb of adult patients with hemiplegia, *Phys Ther* 45:550, 1965.

54. Kimura D, Archibald Y: Motor functions of the left hemisphere, *Brain* 97:337, 1974.

55. Kline DW, Scialfa CT: Visual and auditory aging. In Birren JE, Schaie KW, editors: *Handbook of the psychology of aging*, ed 4, San Diego, CA, 1996, Academic Press.

56. Kritchevsky M: The elementary spatial functions of the brain. In Stiles-Davis J, Kritchevsky M, Bellugi U, editors: *Spatial cognition: brain bases and development*, Hillsdale, NJ, 1988, Lawrence Erlbaum Assoc.

57. Law M, et al: *The Canadian Occupational Performance Measure*, ed 3, Ottawa, ONT, 1998, CAOT Publications.

58. Lezak MD: *Neuropsychological assessment*, New York, 1995, Oxford University Press.

59. Likert R, Quasha WH: *The revised Minnesota Paper Form Board Test*, New York, 1970, Psychological Corporation.

60. Lincoln NB, et al: The Rey figure copy as a screening instrument for perceptual deficits after stroke, *Br J Occup Ther* 61:33, 1998.

61. Lincoln NB, et al: An evaluation of perceptual retraining, *Internat Rehabil Med* 7:99, 1985.

62. MacDonald J: An investigation of body scheme in adults with cerebral vascular accident, *Am J Occup Ther* 14:72, 1960.

63. Mazer BL, et al: Predicting ability to drive after stroke, *Arch Phys Med Rehabil* 79:743, 1998.

64. Mercier L, et al: *Motor-free visual perception test—vertical (MVPT-V)*, Novato, CA, 1997, Academic Therapy Publications.

65. Neistadt ME: A critical analysis of occupational therapy approaches for perceptual deficits in adults with brain injury, *Am J Occup Ther* 44:299, 1990.

66. Neistadt ME: Normal adult performance on constructional praxis training tasks, *Am J Occup Ther* 43:448, 1989.

67. Neistadt ME: Occupational therapy treatments for constructional deficits, *Am J Occup Ther* 46:141, 1992.

68. Neistadt ME: Perceptual retraining for adults with diffuse brain injury, *Am J Occup Ther* 48:225, 1994.

69. Neistadt ME: The relationship between constructional and meal preparation skills, *Arch Phys Med Rehabil* 74:144, 1993.

70. Newcombe F, Ratcliff G: Disorders of visuospatial analysis. In Boller F, Grafman J, editors: *Handbook of neuropsychology*, vol 2, Amsterdam, 1989, Elsevier Science Publishers.

71. Occupational Therapy Department, Rancho Los Amigos Hospital: *Upper extremity sensory evaluation: a manual for occupational therapists*, Downey, CA, 1985.

72. Ochipa C, et al: Conceptual apraxia in Alzheimer's disease, *Brain* 115:1061, 1992.

73. Ogden JA: Spatial abilities and deficits in aging and age-related disorders. In Boller F, Grafman J, editors: *Handbook of neuropsychology*, vol 4, Amsterdam, 1990, Elsevier Science Publishers.

74. Pick HL: Perception, locomotion, and orientation. In Welsh RL, Blasch BB, editors: *Foundations of orientation and mobility*, New York, 1980, American Foundation for the Blind.

75. Pilgrim E, Humphreys GW: Rehabilitation of a case of ideomotor apraxia. In Riddoch MJ, Humphreys GW: *Cognitive neuropsychology and cognitive rehabilitation*, Hove, UK, 1994, Lawrence Erlbaum Assoc.

76. Poole JL, et al: The mechanisms for adult-onset apraxia and developmental dyspraxia: an examination and comparison of error patterns, *Am J Occup Ther* 51:339, 1997.

77. Radomski MV: There is more to life than putting on your pants, *Am J Occup Ther* 49:487, 1995.

78. Rothi LJG, Heilman KM: Acquisition and retention of gestures by apraxic patients, *Brain Cogn* 3:426, 1984.

79. Rothi LJG, Heilman KM: Ideomotor apraxia: gestural discrimination, comprehension, and memory. In Roy EA, editor: *Neuropsychological studies of apraxia and related disorders*, Amsterdam, 1985, North-Holland.

80. Rubio KB, Gillen G: Treatment of neurobehavioral deficits: a function-based approach. In Gillen G, Burkhardt A, editors: *Stroke rehabilitation: a function-based approach*, ed 2, St Louis, 2004, Mosby.

81. Rubio KB, Van Deusen J: Relation of perceptual and body image dysfunction to activities of daily living after stroke, *Am J Occup Ther* 49:551, 1995.

82. Sacks O: *An anthropologist on Mars*, New York, 1995, Knopf.

83. Sacks O: *The man who mistook his wife for a hat and other clinical tales*, New York, 1985, Summit Books.

84. Sivan AB: *The Benton Visual Retention Test*, San Antonio, TX, 1992, Psychological Corporation.

85. Sundet K, et al: Neuropsychological predictors in stroke rehabilitation, *J Clin Exp Neuropsychol* 10:363, 1988.

86. Tate RL, McDonald S: What is apraxia? The clinician's dilemma, *Neuropsychol Rehabil* 5:273, 1995.

87. Titus MN, et al: Correlation of perceptual performance and activities of daily living in stroke patients, *Am J Occup Ther* 45:410, 1991.

88. Toglia J: A dynamic interactional approach to cognitive rehabilitation. In Katz N, editor: *Cognition and occupation across the lifespan: models for intervention in occupational therapy*, ed 2, Bethesda, MD, 2005, AOTA Press.

89. Toglia J: Generalization of treatment: a multi-contextual approach to cognitive-perceptual impairment in the brain-injured adult, *Am J Occup Ther* 45:505, 1991.

89a. Tsurumi K, Todd V: Theory and guidelines for visual task analysis and synthesis. In Scheiman M, editor: *Understanding and managing vision deficits: a guide for occupational therapists*, Thorofare, NJ, 1997, Slack Publ.

90. Warren M: A hierarchical model for evaluation and treatment of visual perceptual dysfunction in adult acquired brain injury: Part I, *Am J Occup Ther* 47:42, 1993.

91. Warren M: A hierarchical model for evaluation and treatment of visual perceptual dysfunction in adult acquired brain injury: Part II, *Am J Occup Ther* 47:55, 1993.

92. Warren M: Relationship of constructional apraxia and body scheme disorders to dressing performance in adult CVA, *Am J Occup Ther* 35:431, 1981.

93. Warrington E, et al: Drawing ability in relation to laterality of lesion, *Brain* 89:53, 1966.

94. Whiting S, et al: *RPAB—Rivermead Perceptual Assessment Battery*, Windsor, UK, 1985, NFER-Nelson Publishers.

95. Willis L, et al: Ideomotor apraxia in early Alzheimer's disease: time and accuracy measures, *Brain Cogn* 38:220, 1998.

96. York CD, Cermack SA: Visual perception and praxis in adults after stroke, *Am J Occup Ther* 49:543, 1995.

97. Young AW, et al: Face perception after brain injury: selective impairments affecting identity and expression, *Brain* 116(Pt 4):941, 1993.

98. Zoltan B: Remediation of visual-perceptual and perceptual-motor deficits. In Rosenthal M, Griffith ER, Bond MR, et al, editors: *Rehabilitation of the adult and child with traumatic brain injury*, Philadelphia, 1990, FA Davis.

99. Zoltan B: *Vision, perception, and cognition*, ed 3 (rev), Thorofare, NJ, 1996, Slack Publishers.

100. Zoltan B, et al: *Perceptual and cognitive dysfunction in the adult stroke patient*, ed 2, Thorofare, NJ, 1986, Slack Publishers.

SUGGESTED READING

Gentile M: *Functional visual behavior in adults: an occupational therapy guide to evaluation and treatment options*, ed 2, Bethesda, MD, 2005, AOTA Press.

Scheiman M: *Understanding and managing vision deficits: a guide for occupational therapists*, Thorofare, NJ, 1977, Slack Publishers.

Zoltan B: Vision, perception, and cognition: a manual for the evaluation and treatment of the neurologically impaired adult, Thorofare, NJ, 1996, Slack Publishers.

25 EVALUATION AND TREATMENT OF COGNITIVE DYSFUNCTION

CAROLYN GLOGOSKI
NANCY V. MILLIGAN
CAROL J. WHEATLEY

KEY TERMS

Metacognition
Cognition
Self-awareness
Executive functions
Sensory-perceptual component
Higher-level cognition
Anosognosia

Central executive
Short-term memory
Primary memory
Working memory
Long-term memory
Explicit memory
Episodic memory

Semantic memory
Implicit memory
Procedural memory
Orientation
Abstract thinking
Concrete thinking
Convergent thinking

Divergent thinking
Deductive reasoning
Inductive reasoning
Dyscalculia

LEARNING OBJECTIVES

After studying this chapter the student or practitioner will be able to do the following:

1. Define *cognition.*
2. Explain the way that information is processed during cognition.
3. Explain the effect of higher-level cognition on occupation and functional performance.
4. Describe the process by which an individual might forget information.

5. Identify and briefly discuss the major cognitive treatment approaches in the field of occupational therapy.
6. Cite standardized assessment tools for each of the higher-level areas of cognition.
7. Describe specific treatment efforts for targeted cognitive deficits.
8. Describe the effects of the aging process on cognitive skills.

CHAPTER OUTLINE

THREADED CASE STUDY: SABRINA, PART 1

Sabrina is a 17-year old African-American woman who suffered a bilateral frontal lobe traumatic brain injury (TBI) as a result of a high-speed motor vehicle crash 8 weeks ago. She was unconscious at the accident scene. She was intubated and quickly transported to a trauma center hospital 40 miles away, where a bilateral frontal craniotomy was performed to relieve intracranial pressure. She was then hospitalized in the intensive care unit (ICU). During an interview with Sabrina's mother, the occupational therapist documented the following information while completing the occupational profile. Sabrina is an eleventh grader at a suburban Catholic high school, where her mother teaches English. Sabrina was described as an above-average student who swam competitively on the swim team and played on the women's soccer team. Sabrina's mother stated that Sabrina was very outgoing and participated in many school activities. She is the youngest of four children and is the only child currently living at home with her parents.

During the first 3 weeks of Sabrina's hospitalization, her mother, who had taken a leave of absence from her job, slept at the hospital every night to be close to her daughter. Sabrina's parents frequently expressed their desire to be actively involved in all aspects of their daughter's rehabilitation, with the desired goal to have Sabrina return home and go back to her high school as soon as possible but no later than next fall for senior year.

The preceding description is the introductory portion of a case study describing a client with a traumatic brain injury (TBI). This case will be mentioned throughout the chapter to help the reader understand cognition and cognitive rehabilitation as it is embedded in the Occupational Therapy Practice Framework. Clients with injuries such as Sabrina's that compromise cognitive function allow us to better understand the role of cognition in supporting occupational performance and the role of occupational therapists in cognitive rehabilitation.

Critical Thinking Questions

1. In continuing to compile information for the occupational therapy evaluation's analysis of occupational performance, the therapist should consider what client factors, contextual features, and activity demands that will support or inhibit Sabrina's desired occupational performance outcomes?
2. Which assessments will help us to further define Sabrina's occupational performance strengths and weaknesses as we analyze her occupational performance?
3. How does the cognitive information-processing model help us understand what areas are priorities for us to target for evaluation and intervention, and what three types of occupational therapy interventions will help us address these targeted areas?

The ability to satisfactorily and competently engage in our usual daily tasks; go to work or school; experience leisure, interpersonal, and social relationships; and participate in our treasured occupations is highly dependent on cognition. In the case study, Sabrina's impaired cognitive functioning will significantly interfere with her desired occupation of returning to school and socializing with her friends.

In many instances, cognitive impairment can be quite subtle and not easily recognized until the person has difficulty performing occupational tasks. Even then, persons who have cognitive impairment may not be aware of the extent of the functional consequences of their injury. We often take cognition for granted because it is so efficient. Cognitive dysfunction is identified in persons with traumatic brain injury, stroke, dementia and other neurological conditions, schizophrenia, developmental disabilities, learning disabilities, and many other conditions. In some clients, we might call it a hidden disability. Family members and significant others often focus on the physical appearance of their loved ones after a traumatic event and may not that realize that clients who have cognitive deficits are unable to perform various tasks that they say they can do.

A traditional, bottom-up approach to rehabilitation is often focused on basic cognitive abilities (orientation, attention, memory, concentration, visual perception, visuospatial processing, language, and simple problem solving) that

are impaired. Actual occupational performance is a much more complex phenomenon that requires integration and synthesis of several skills and other levels of processing that are not captured when a cognitive skill is assessed in isolation. Therefore, although these basic abilities serve as the foundation of higher-level cognitive function, intervention should address higher-level cognitive skills instead of focusing just on the basic skills for restoration or compensation.

More complex higher-level cognitive skills, including self-awareness and executive functions, have recently been identified as the essential components for purposeful, proactive interactions and complex decision making.[44,54,85] Deficits in these higher-level skills are not consistently identified using standard cognitive assessments[91] but are essential for promoting occupational performance.

Knowledge in the area of cognition has expanded significantly in recent years. Increasingly, cognition is seen as a multilevel, multifaceted, integrative process. This is especially true of higher-level cognitive functions.[44] Other terms sometimes used to describe aspects of higher-level cognition include *metacognitive knowledge* and *metacognitive process*,[18] *metacognitive monitoring*, and *metacognitive control*,[41] all phrases that pertain to knowing about knowing and knowing how to know.[15,29] The term **metacognition** has also been used to refer to the ability to know and monitor a variety of basic cognitive skills. Metacognition allows an individual the flexibility to select and employ various memory strategies, problem-solving approaches, and reasoning skills to complete a cognitive task.[65]

The focus of this chapter is the concept of **cognition**. *Cognition* refers to the acquisition and use of knowledge involving a number of mental components. When these components are taken together, they form a complex system of interdependent mental processes.[50] Under the broad category of cognition are basic cognitive skills (attention, memory, and perception) and higher-level cognitive skills (awareness and executive functions).[44] Basic cognitive skills and higher-level cognitive skills are classified in the Occupational Therapy Practice Framework under the heading "client factors" as body function categories of global and specific mental function.[2] This chapter will also describe the actual workings of cognition by describing a model of information processing.[50] This model will help us understand how input from the environment is effectively or ineffectively taken in, processed, stored, and later retrieved to produce satisfactory or unsatisfactory behavioral outputs.

COGNITIVE FUNCTION OVERVIEW

DEFINING AND CONCEPTUALIZING COGNITION

Cognition, as viewed by Toglia,[91] is the outcome of an ongoing dynamic interaction between the person, an activity, and the environment. It is suggested that occupational therapists are uniquely qualified, by nature of their training, to focus on occupational performance and performance skills using activity analysis in offering unique rehabilitative services.[44] Cognition is the process by which the individual acquires and uses information. This occurs through complex, interdependent mental processes that help the person adapt to environmental demands and expectations.[50,56,91]

What follows is a brief overview of two widely used models of cognition in occupational therapy (OT) and in cognitive rehabilitation. These models have at their core the concept of cognitive information processing. Each of these models highlights the importance of receptiveness to sensory-perceptual input, the basic mental abilities that underlie aspects of actual performance, and the higher-level cognitive functions that consciously direct behavior toward selected goals crucial for occupational performance.

The dynamic interactional approach[89-91] suggests that higher-level cognitive processes are not hierarchical, fixed, or stable but are instead dynamic, changing with our interactions in the environment and in response to contextual factors. Cognition involves information-processing skills, learning, and the ability to generalize. The underlying processes and strategies and the potential of the individual to learn are analyzed when assessing and treating cognitive deficits. Knowledge acquired before the task and feedback used during and after completion of occupational performance are

integrated with many factors, including other people and the environment. These influence the individual's self-perceptions, beliefs, use of processing strategies, activity demands, and selected performance environment when engaging in occupations. Toglia's model draws from cognitive and educational psychology and has been used with all populations in the treatment of developmental, psychological, and neurological deficits.

A hierarchical feedback–feedforward model, describing higher-level cognitive processes, comes from the perspective of neurorehabilitation[85] and is explained in Katz and Hartman-Maeir.[44] This model has three parts, with self-awareness at the top of the hierarchy, executive functions in the middle of the hierarchy, and sensory-perceptual components at the base of the hierarchy:

- **Self-awareness** is the ability to perceive the self in relative objectivity while still maintaining a subjective sense of self through one's thoughts and feelings.[71]
- **Executive functions** are directed, effective activity involving volition to take action; planning to reach a goal by identifying and organizing steps; taking purposive action and actually implementing a plan; and finally ensuring effective performance by monitoring, self-correcting, and regulating aspects of the performance to achieve success.[54]
- **Sensory-perceptual component** involves the registration of sensory information from the environment (through taste, smell, touch, sound, sight) and internal stimuli that affect the sensory receptors. This function will be discussed at greater length later in this chapter, in relation to the information-processing model.

Katz and Hartman-Maeir state that, although there is a strong relationship among the three processes of the hierarchical feedback–feedforward model, they may not operate together at all times.[44] Executive functions most likely depend on and control multiple cognitive processes from many different regions of the brain. This helps to explain why executive dysfunction is not localized to frontal lobe damage alone but also involves disturbances in diffuse neural networks, such as the disturbance of corticostriatal circuits (the connections between the cortex and corpus striatum) seen in persons with Alzheimer's disease, Parkinson's disease, or schizophrenia.[27,44,86] Aspects of the hierarchical feedback–feedforward model serve as the main basis for the discussion of higher-level cognition that immediately follows and the information-processing model discussed later in the chapter.

HIGHER-LEVEL COGNITION

Katz and Hartman-Maeir use the terms *awareness* and *executive functions* to describe the main mechanisms of **higher-level cognition**.[44] In most cases, awareness and executive function are interrelated and interdependent. Lack of awareness, whether it is neurogenic (a breakdown in the neurological monitoring system as a result of brain damage or disease mechanisms) or psychogenic (related to psychological coping mechanisms to protect the individual from painful reality), operates at multiple levels. Different approaches to assessment and intervention are suggested for each, although it is likely that both origins of unawareness operate at the same time or at different stages in recovery.[43,44,47] Two major approaches are used in the cognitive rehabilitation of dysfunction in awareness and executive function. One involves a remediation or process-oriented approach (restoring impaired areas of cognitive function). The second approach uses compensatory substitution or environmental modification to achieve successful performance and maximize participation despite the cognitive deficits present.[59,83]

Awareness, sometimes termed *self-awareness,* involves the ability to see oneself objectively while still retaining a subjective sense of self that is attuned to one's thoughts and feelings. This requires knowledge of when and how much one's abilities and behaviors deviate from what is typical. Awareness calls for an ongoing capacity to monitor the self. Individuals whose awareness capacities are unimpaired can realistically understand their cognitive strengths and weaknesses regardless of the particular task or context in which they are performing. For example, a student knows that her capacity for speed-reading for comprehension is a strength on which she can rely whether she is reading a novel for pleasure, using a cookbook, or studying for school.

Lack of awareness, or **anosognosia** (lack of knowledge or denial of deficits or disease process and the implications of the deficit), is another descriptor often used in reference to aphasia; cognition; visual disturbances; and other sensory, motor, or perceptual deficits found in persons with neurological disorders.[44] In psychiatry the terms *poor insight* and *impaired insight* refer to the person's lack of awareness about the presence of the psychiatric disorder, symptoms, consequences, or need for intervention. The severity of anosognosia for persons with traumatic brain injury (TBI) or dementia is frequently related to the severity and progression of the disease and the location of brain lesions.[25,63] Manifestation of a severe deficit in awareness can create serious obstacles for the rehabilitation process. A client may persistently deny the problem exists and refuse intervention designed to address the deficit.

After a cerebrovascular accident (CVA), a person may have ansognosia and lack awareness of visual field deficits, weakness in the extremities, or language disturbances. The individual may deny memory deficits, perceptual difficulties, and even functional deficits. Impaired mobility and other safety issues, such as the person's insistence that driving abilities are intact, are frequently a concern to family and others. This type of dysfunction may also be seen in persons with dementia.

Impaired awareness after a TBI can result in the lack of recognition or denial of deficits or the implications of the deficits on occupational performance. This impairment can be seen in the client who has deficits related to memory and orientation to time. The client may not be aware of the memory impairment or its affect on the ability to manage time (e.g., to come to dinner on time), relate socially (e.g., to meet and talk with friends), and engage in many occupational performance areas of activities of daily living (ADLs) and instrumental activities of daily living (IADLs).

The particular location of lesions in the brain is thought to explain the specific ways in which unawareness is manifested and the severity of the deficit.[44,71] Bilateral damage to both brain hemispheres is associated with complete lack of awareness, occipital lobe damage with blindness, temporal damage with impairments related to auditory perception and memory, frontal lobe damage with planning and interpersonal deficits, and parietal lobe damage with unawareness of hemiplegia or unilateral neglect. Partial unawareness is thought to be related to psychological factors involving coping mechanisms.

Evaluation of Awareness

Awareness can be assessed in several ways, which often presents challenges for direct, objective measurement.[44] One method asks clients a series of questions about their perception of their condition, deficits, and performance when completing ADLs (e.g., Prigatano Competency Rating Scale).[72,73] This self-rating is then compared with the therapist's rating of the client using a functional measure. Another method asks clients to predict ability before performance and to estimate their actual performance after completing the activity (e.g., Assessment of Awareness of Disability).[88] A number of other assessments of awareness with targeted populations have been identified.[44]

Intervention for Awareness

A compensatory approach is used for persons with severe unawareness deficits, the rationale being that the neurogenic mechanisms of unawareness are not open to change. Modification of the physical and human environment, through use of a nonconfrontational approach, is employed to improve performance in natural settings.[28] In persons with mild to moderate unawareness who are able to integrate information and experience, a remedial approach is suggested.[82] Interventions are targeted at facilitating feedback on task performance and allowing integration of the information so that the client can discover deficits and disabilities. An educational and experiential approach has been found to be effective.

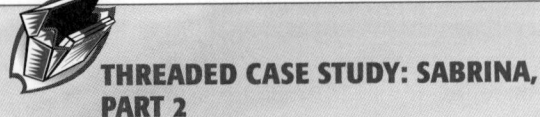

THREADED CASE STUDY: SABRINA, PART 2

At several points during her recovery, Sabrina had unrealistic expectations regarding her abilities in activities of daily living (ADLs) and instrumental activities of daily living (IADLs). Approximately 6 weeks after her injury, Sabrina continued to lack awareness of

THREADED CASE STUDY: SABRINA, PART 2—cont'd

potential problems. She perceived that she was independent in completing her showering and personal care routines. When her awareness was assessed, it became apparent that she was not able to view her performance objectively and required cognitive retraining.

Sabrina was educated on the consequences of her injury and then given opportunities to share personal experiences. She was asked to analyze the required skills of the target task of washing her hair and to predict her performance. When beginning a new ADL, Sabrina first had to ask, "What do I need to do to achieve this goal?" Then she had to break down the goal into specified tasks or subgoals and identify the steps in each. For example, when given the task of taking a shower, Sabrina identified the tasks of washing hair, rinsing shampoo out of her hair, applying conditioner, rinsing her hair, washing all body parts with soap, and rinsing. Sabrina then had to identify the necessary items she required to complete the task and obtain them before starting to shower. She learned to ask herself questions about her performance before (predicting), during, and after ADLs to improve her awareness.

Executive function makes a central contribution to the performance of novel and complex tasks. *Executive function* has been used to refer to those functions that consciously control and direct behavior toward selected goals. It has been further defined as "... complex cognitions such as solving novel problems, modifying behavior in light of new information, generating strategies, or sequencing complex actions".[27] Another definition has been offered by Ylvisaker, Szerkeres, and Feeney and includes self-awareness, goal selection, planning steps to achieve goal, initiating implementation behavior, inhibiting interfering behavior, monitoring and evaluating performance, and using strategic problem solving when faced with challenges.[104] Broader, more comprehensive definitions of executive function (such as the one just described and the one used by Lezak[54]) emphasize the way that self-awareness is interconnected with executive function.

The mechanism of executive function is explained in many ways, but the working memory model[9] has promise as a practical method to understand the way in which executive function can be applied to intervention. This model proposes that the mechanism of working memory allows access to previously stored memory for comparison with current information. Working memory is able to further process the new information using selected and divided attention mechanisms. This mechanism is referred to as a **central executive** (CE) or an attentional control system. The CE is an oversight system that "orchestrates the selection, initiation, planning, monitoring, and termination of all processing routines ... and overrides (i.e., inhibits) automatic patterns of thought ... when

these processes seem unwarranted".[50] The CE coordinates two subordinate systems in working memory (phonological loop—storage of language-based information and visuospatial template—nonverbal and position-in-space information) and allows coordination between simultaneous tasks of the two subordinate systems. The CE is involved in the ability to reason, make decisions, and comprehend and for long- and short-term memory.[11] However, Baddeley et al.[11] and others[3,16,27,85,87] argue that the CE is not the only system underlying executive functions and that there are multiple executive functions. These executive functions comprise a multicomponent system of diffuse cortical neural networks (in prefrontal cortex and frontal-striatal structures and cortical circuitry) mediated by neurotransmitters such as dopamine. These diffuse cortical networks help us to understand the ways in which executive functions can control separate cognitive processes in different brain regions. It also explains why executive dysfunctions are not only identified with frontal lobe damage to the brain but also evident in clients with Alzheimer's disease and schizophrenia in whom frontal lobe damage has not been identified.

Executive disorders are frequently demonstrated in clients who have sustained TBIs and strokes. In a large study of clients who had strokes,[94] 40% of stroke survivors experienced executive dysfunction. Deficits in executive function have been consistently identified in persons with dementias and schizophrenia.[44] In both of these populations, executive dysfunction has shown a significant relationship to poorer functional outcomes with ADLs and IADLs and can have a negative outcome on rehabilitation outcomes.

With a brain injury (e.g., TBI), the delicate balance between brain structures is not related merely to a localized lesion in the brain.[44] The functional system as a whole (in the brain) can be disturbed by one lesion that affects several areas in the brain through extensive connections, or specific function can be disturbed by localized lesions in the brain.[58] Symptoms may also appear because of disinhibition (lack of an inhibiting effect) of an undamaged or intact area of the brain caused by damage elsewhere in the brain. This interconnectedness explains why cognitive interventions aim to regain a balance between brain structures and create compensatory strategies in the hope that remaining circuits in the brain can reorganize in areas directly and indirectly affected by the brain injury.[46]

Executive Function Evaluation

Executive functions can be assessed[44] using screening instruments (e.g., Executive Clock Drawing Test[77]), tabletop tests (e.g., Behavioral Assessment of Dysexecutive Syndrome [BADS][66,98]), functional tasks (e.g., Kitchen Task Assessment[12]; Executive Function Performance test [EFPT][43]), and questionnaires and rating scales (e.g., Profile of Executive Control System [PRO-EX][14]). Assessments often consist of structured tasks. Such tasks offer limited opportunity to evaluate executive function. Some newly developed tests assess all components of executive function, whereas others are targeted to more specific functions. Executive functions consist of so many unique properties that a combination of assessment tools is recommended. It may even be necessary to develop a frontal-executive battery to address the level of complexity encountered with executive function.

Executive Function Interventions

In remediating executive function, occupational therapists provide clients with experiences allowing them to choose, select, plan, and self-correct so that they can become as independent as possible in problem solving. An intervention method used in self-instructional training coaches the client to use strategies of inner speech, beginning with self-talk or verbalization of the plan, and then the plan is whispered and finally internally verbalized by the client as the behavior becomes self-regulated.[22] Other remedial strategies target specific executive function components. For example, time management could be addressed by using an exercise that asks clients to estimate time for completion of various daily tasks. Remedial techniques also include asking clients to formulate predictive questions about their performance, to write lists of steps, to ask themselves questions about the nature of the tasks to be performed, to give themselves verbal instructions by speaking aloud, and to check to see whether they have done what was planned.

Compensation intervention[44] for executive dysfunction could involve the training of certain behaviors that are adaptive for a specific setting so that they become automatic and do not require self-regulation and planning.[35] This behavioral method focuses on the acquisition of specific skills needed in a specific setting, and the client would be encouraged to rehearse those skills until they became habitual. A therapist could use environmental management by organizing the physical space with schedules, reminders, and pagers for task initiation. Another strategy would be to manipulate physiological factors to assist in regulating arousal and alertness through nutrition, stimulation, and medications.

In Sabrina's case, the therapist initially provided both verbal cueing and hand-over-hand guidance for Sabrina to attend to a particular task. The number and frequency of both types of cueing were decreased at regular intervals as Sabrina became more familiar with the task and routine. Eventually, Sabrina used enlarged laminated instructions, which she read aloud to promote safe effective performance.

Executive dysfunction and lack of awareness provide significant challenges to persons seeking full participation in ADLs and IADLs as well as other occupational performance areas. The body of current research supports the idea that higher-level cognitive deficits have a significant effect on function, and research in this area has experienced tremendous growth in recent years.[44] No rehabilitation program for cognition is complete without assessing and intervening with these higher-level cognitive components.

COGNITIVE INFORMATION-PROCESSING MODEL

Information is transformed, reduced, elaborated on, stored in memory, recovered from memory, and used in some way during cognition.[50,64,75] Cognition is a process by which sensations from the environment are transformed by the subject through the construction of personal representations of the experience. Some of this information is forgotten (reduced), and other information is elaborated on by integrating it with previous experiences using established neuronal pathways, forming the subject's perception. This information is stored in memory and can be retrieved later if needed. Information is used during decision making, problem solving, reasoning, goal setting, and meeting psychological needs to support occupational performance. According to Levy,[50] the information-processing model, based on concepts from the neurosciences, has its roots in an earlier model of memory[5] and was then further refined.[34,61,70]

HOW IT WORKS

Information is taken in from the environment and is preserved, transformed, and transferred. This processing of information uses three clearly defined stages of memory. First, information from the environment is taken into sensory-perceptual memory, transformed as it moves to short-term working memory, and then further encoded and stored in long-term memory, where it can be retrieved later. The following outline summarizes the memory systems in this model:

Stages of Memory: Encoding, Storage, and Retrieval
- Sensory-Perceptual Memory Stage
- Short-Term/Working Memory Stage
  - Primary Memory
  - Working Memory
    - Phonological Loop
    - Visuospatial Template
- Long-Term Memory Stage

Levy states that "like a computer, the mind takes in information, performs operations on it to change the form and content, stores the information, retrieves it when needed, and generates responses to it. Similarly, each of the three stages involves transforming information into a memory trace that can be stored (encoding), holding or maintaining the to-be-remembered information for immediate or later use (storage), and accessing the information when needed (retrieval)."[50]

The meaning that we construct as a result of the constant input of information from the environment is a dynamic process that makes use of the two-way flow of information. Levy has constructed a diagram of this model based on the work of several cognitive theorists (Figure 25-1). As demonstrated by the model, this flow goes from sensory-perceptual memory to short-term working memory to long-term memory. It may also flow from long-term memory to short-term

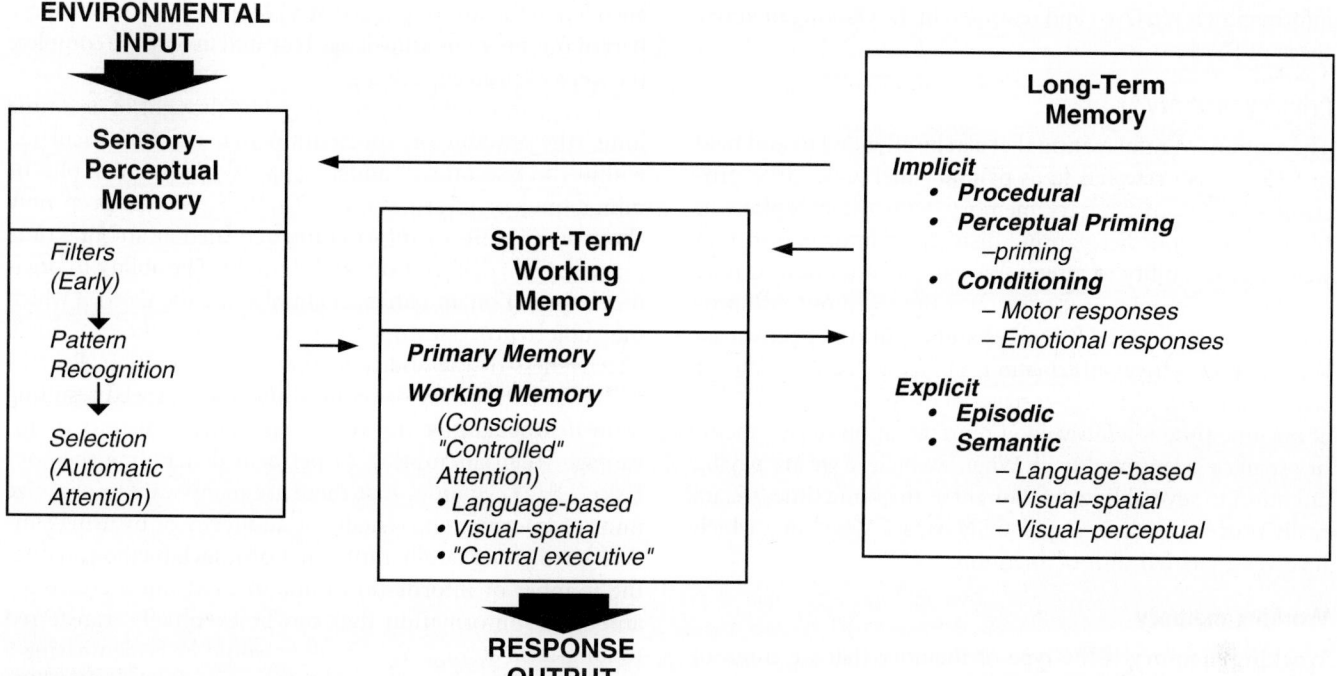

Figure 25-1   Cognitive information-processing model. (From Levy LL: Cognitive aging in perspective: information processing, cognition and memory. In Katz N: *Cognition and occupation across the life span: Models for intervention in occupational therapy*, ed 2, p. 307, Bethesda, MD, 2005, American Occupational Therapy Association.)

memory or from long-term memory to sensory-perceptual memory. Information could be forgotten, or memory impaired, if the sensory-input was never transformed into a memory trace (encoded) and not stored because of a lack of attention in the initial stage. Memory deficits can also occur during the transformation process as some information is lost. Finally, memory deficits may become apparent because the information cannot be retrieved (from long-term memory) when needed.

STAGES

Initial Phase: Sensory-Perceptual Memory

A physical stimulus (touch, taste, sound, smell, sight) from the environment is detected by specific sensory receptors. The massive amounts of primitive and short-lived sensations are encoded and filtered to form sensory-specific memory traces (visual-iconic memory, auditory-echoic memory). These memory traces exist long enough (i.e., 100 milliseconds to 5 seconds) to be stored. Stimuli are determined to be relevant or irrelevant through attentional processes that monitor and filter and through perceptual processes that organize the information into meaningful patterns. The information that was determined to be irrelevant decays over time and is not stored for long-term use. Perceiving and attending are automatically directed processes. These processes involve retrieval from stored memory to assist with further filtering and transformation of these trace memories. The process of

transformation is based on complex personal factors (e.g., knowledge, motivation, prior experience) that make use of associative neural networks from previously stored information. The transitory patterns or sensory codes constructed in sensory-perceptual memory are transferred to short-term working memory, which will be discussed in the next section.

Second Phase: Short-Term Working Memory

Activated information is a key term used when referring to the content of **short-term memory** (STM).[50] The information in STM is held in simple storage (the primary memory) and then processed by reflecting and thinking about the information in a working space (working memory).[10] The activation of information occurs as we reflect on information in the working memory area of STM. Activation is critical for retention of this information. If this information in STM is not activated (i.e., thought about and processed), it will disappear as a result of decay. The information in STM is transferred from sensory-perceptual memory and then transformed. This information consists of basic impressions that have been attended to and are held in mind (working memory).

The second source of information transferred into the working memory space in STM comes from long-term memory (LTM) stores and is a more complex process. This process involves retrieval of previous information to aid in comprehension and integration of the information just received. New ideas can also be formed when LTM information is retrieved and reworked in the working memory space of STM.

Primary memory

The amount of information that can be attended to and held in STM is also referred to as **primary memory.** Little processing occurs in primary memory, with the exception of filtering out and disregarding distracting information that weakens our ability to attend. We can pay attention to only one line of thought processing at a time without compromising our attentional resources and cognitive effectiveness (quantity of active information, ability to concentrate or reliably attend). The longest string of digits that we can recall at any one time is a fairly good representation of our memory span or attentional span. When we believe we are paying attention to several lines of thought at the same time, we are really processing them sequentially or task switching, which involves an actual shift of attention.

Working memory

Working memory is the type of memory that we think of most often when discussing STM. Information in working memory has been described as undergoing a process of activation.[50] This phase of memory involves the ability to keep information in a holding area of the mind, providing an opportunity for the information to be further processed. The amount of information that can be held at a given time is crucial in determining the quality and quantity of higher-order executive functions. Working memory has the important function of coordinating higher-level cognitive performance. These include being able to consciously attend and concentrate; to think abstractly, as opposed to concretely; to understand language; to identify goals and make plans; to respond flexibly to new circumstances; to reason, engage in problem solving, and make decisions; and to use judgment and think creatively.

Information undergoes further processing as the working memory space of STM overrides automatic reactions to problems and engages in the process of search and retrieval of needed information from the huge store of information available through the use of vast, rich, complex neural networks.[50] This process is guided or overseen by the CE system. The CE system provides oversight by selecting and regulating the flow of information in the working memory space. This system serves to override and coordinate the selection, initiation, planning, monitoring, and termination of all the encoding, storing, and retrieval processes.

Impairment in working memory is evident in individuals who have difficulty making decisions in ambiguous situations, solving complex problems, and performing IADLs.[50] The nature of this difficulty involves an inability to focus and track relevant information that must be coordinated while simultaneously inhibiting distracting information and automatic responses.

Encoding in working memory consists of semantic codes (chunked and elaborated material from LTM), sounds of words, and visuospatial images. Most of the information encoded in the working space of STM involves words that are part of our previous knowledge base and used as we complete the steps of problem solving.

Storage in working memory can be thought of as a time limit (the amount of information that can be articulated within 1 to 2 seconds)[10] and as capacity (seven units [plus or minus one] of information). Therefore, we can keep only about seven units of information activated at any one time for reflection, deliberation, and thought. The ability to organize information into units, or chunks, and the speed at which the subject processes information influence the functional effectiveness of the ability to process information. Persons with limited capacity or reduced processing speed resulting from neurocognitive disorders experience a distinct disadvantage when attempting to perform demanding memory tasks.[31,50,79] Levy notes that there are many ways to organize units of information (visually or auditorily or by using similarities to group familiar information); such methods reduce the number of information units in STM but increase the amount of information that can be eventually transferred to long-term storage. An example would be remembering a 10- or 11-digit personal number, such as a bank code. These numbers can be remembered in chunked units to reduce the number of information units but increase the amount of information stored.

Retrieval in working memory uses our conscious attention. Our STM contains only information that we have selected. Because we can hold only about seven units of information in STM, information is lost or damaged if our focus or attention shifts before this information has been processed for later retrieval. Sometimes, information enters STM so briefly that it is never processed. Eventual retrieval of information occurs only if we pay sufficient or conscious attention. Maintaining activation or paying sufficient attention for longer than 1 to 30 seconds requires rehearsing[23] or repeating information to self or others; this is sometimes called *rote memory*. Rote memory allows the individual to hold information for a period that is sufficient for further processing. Elaborative rehearsal is one such form of processing that focuses on the meaning of information and its relationship to information already in storage.

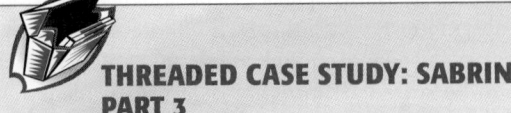

THREADED CASE STUDY: SABRINA, PART 3

To ensure that Sabrina could achieve safe and consistent performance of ADLs, the occupational therapist made use of a laminated plastic instruction poster as an external aid (cue) for the repetition of instructions as the therapist's assistance and direction were gradually withdrawn. Sabrina was trained to evaluate her performance before engaging in the performance by asking herself, "How well do I think I will do with this task?" before

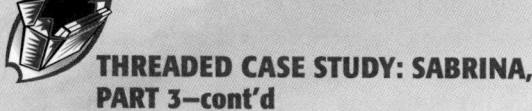

THREADED CASE STUDY: SABRINA, PART 3–cont'd

performance, "How well am I doing on this task?" during performance, and "How many errors did I make?" or "How well did I do?" after performance. This routine was part of an effort to keep activating this sequence of questions in short-term working memory and thereby facilitate some executive cognitive functions.

Third Phase: Long-Term Memory

Long-term memory is an unlimited permanent storage component of information processing. Information that is no longer in STM working memory or in conscious awareness can be stored in LTM for retrieval at a later time. LTM information includes information transferred minutes ago, hours ago, or years ago. Newly transferred information is fragile and can be more easily disrupted when it is in the hippocampal area of the brain.[50] This information becomes stable once it leaves this area because it has undergone a number of biochemical processes and further development in the hippocampus. Information readily moves between LTM and STM and back again so that we can easily shift prior information to working memory for elaboration, further understanding, or problem solving with new information.

Encoding in LTM occurs acoustically (i.e., through sound), visually (i.e., by way of images), and through spatial configuration and sequences of words. This information is organized as episodic memory, or according to its relationship to emotional states, time, or place; alternatively, it may be organized semantically in terms of important relationships. A visual image is more readily stored and retrieved because it is stored as both a word and an image. Semantic encoding is the predominant means of encoding in LTM. The storage system in LTM is organized as follows[50,81,84,93]:

- Explicit
  - Episodic: recent events, remote events, prospective events
  - Semantic: language-based, visuospatial, visual-perceptual
- Implicit
  - Procedural
  - Perceptual priming
  - Conditioning

Explicit memory is a conscious process whereby information is recalled. Explicit memory is involved with "factual knowledge of people, places, and things, and what these facts mean."[42] This form of memory, also referred to as *declarative memory,* is flexible and "involves the association of multiple bits and pieces of information"; it is called on through deliberate, conscious effort. Both episodic and semantic memory functions are considered types of explicit memory. Included in **episodic memory** are events that have been personally experienced and are connected to a particular place

and time (e.g., holiday events, celebrations, a luncheon date, where the scissors are stored) and relevant factual information (e.g., the names of nieces and nephews, the name of your state senator, a recent conversation).[50,81,84,93] Recent episodic memory covers facts and events that are learned on a daily basis or involve orientation to time and place. This information is reflected in the ability to remember something for 5 to 10 minutes and can be readily lost or forgotten if it is not emotionally significant or not related to previously acquired knowledge. Word lists are frequently used to assess this type of memory, and the quality of recent episodic memory is important in trying to determine a person's ability to learn. Remote episodic memory is information that is remembered concerning events that have happened in the past. Prospective memory is for events that will take place in the future (e.g., remembering to turn off the oven, remembering a doctor's appointment that is scheduled for a future date). The encoding of information for episodic memory is highly related to emotional states; by using the same emotional states or contextual cues, retrieval of information is enhanced.

Semantic memory, memory for words and factual information, builds on new information using prior knowledge.[42] Associated memory networks are created on the basis of the synthesis of new facts and concepts with preexisting knowledge. This integrated associated memory network is organized conceptually and provides the basis for knowledge, insight, and judgment. Semantic memory is constructed through use of visual-perceptual information, visuospatial perceptions, and language-based knowledge. This kind of memory has more permanence than episodic memories. The ways in which this kind of memory is assessed include vocabulary tests, the general information subtests of intelligence tests, and verbal fluency tests that require free recall of words in a particular category.

Implicit memory involves the automatic recall of information according to Levy.[50] Implicit memory is used during performance of many rote motor and overlearned perceptual tasks, such as starting a familiar car or riding a bicycle.[42] This form of memory is also referred to as *nondeclarative memory* and is often used without conscious effort. **Procedural memory** is the most extensive type of memory that we acquire and has the most permanence, remaining accessible even to persons with substantial cognitive deficits. This is memory for skill performance. Although they are based on semantic and episodic memory, these memories become automatic over time and with practice, no longer requiring conscious effort. Procedural memory is a blend of cognitive, motor, and perceptual skills involved in acquiring "how" or performance-based information. Procedural memories, by becoming automatic, make few demands on short-term memory because these memories become effortless and do not require conscious direction.[81,84,93] Perceptual priming is another process involved with implicit memory. Association networks are activated by a prior stimulus that in effect primes, or makes a memory more readily available for later processing of that perceptual stimulus without the awareness of the previous exposure; the mental process that occurs during subliminal learning would be a good example of this phenomenon. The process of acquiring implicit memory involves the use of conditioning. Motor and emotionally toned memories are formed automatically through operant and classical conditioning.

The occupational therapist used conditioning and perceptual priming with Sabrina as she was emerging from the coma. These methods were used to stimulate arousal in the areas of eye opening; auditory, visual, and motor responses; and verbal communication when Sabrina was in a minimally conscious state. Sabrina's parents and siblings provided stimulation using items that were familiar to Sabrina. Later, during Sabrina's cognitive retraining, the occupational therapist facilitated Sabrina's repetition of self-awareness techniques and safe performance of ADLs to eventually build procedural memories.

Storage of LTM occurs in a systematic way on account of the massive amounts of information that must be stored. The retrieval of information in LTM is highly dependent on the way that information was processed in the working memory space of STM. The construction of our own meaning of the new information in STM must occur by associating the new information with memories already stored in LTM. The processes of constructing meaning and associating it with information in LTM are greatly influenced through the use of four strategies: elaboration, organization, use of context, and repetition.[50] With elaboration we build a new understanding of recent information by enhancing or changing it as we associate it with previously stored information. Extra associations are built with the knowledge that we already have. Elaboration is a process that greatly facilitates later retrieval and the strength of our memory. Efficiently and meaningfully grouping, diagramming, or clustering information elaborated on in STM, using an organizational strategy, significantly enhances the amount of complex material that can be stored and later retrieved. Conceptual material that was embedded in an organized framework by an individual improves the retrieval process for that person. A third strategy is the association of episodic memories with contextual cues. Using the same subjective (emotional state) and objective (setting, time of day, odors) contextual cues experienced during initial encoding (learning) provides powerful cues for retrieval. Repetition is another storage strategy. The more frequently information is activated or used, the stronger the pattern of neuronal connection.[38,50,57] Repetition speeds retrieval time, and by practicing what we wish to remember, we often engage in elaboration, forming new associations.[50]

The occupational therapist repeatedly used all four of these strategies in treating Sabrina to enhance the transfer of the semantic and episodic memory material acquired in therapy sessions, allowing it to become permanently embedded in LTM for retrieval. This approach enhanced Sabrina's functional performance of many ADLs and IADLs.

Retrieval with LTM means having information in LTM accessible when it is needed or wanted. Activation of the association network of stored information in LTM relies on the retrieval cues that are used. These associations are the cues and links that activate the network for retrieval.[50] The generation of a thought in working memory produces activity in neuronal connections with the potential to spread to association networks. The association networks located in LTM can then transfer related information temporarily to working memory for further elaboration and enhancement. Retrieval of specific information can occur through free recall. A piece of information is transferred from LTM to working memory depending on the working memory's ability to use an effective search and retrieval for cues in LTM. For free recall to occur, no external associational cues are provided. A second retrieval process occurs through recognition recall. Externally provided associational cues activate relevant memories in LTM directly so that working memory is not required to engage in the search-and-retrieval process, which is much easier. The use of recognition memory is a very effective strategy to assist in the retrieval of information for persons with cognitive disability.[21-53] The OT sessions with Sabrina made extensive use of recognition memory through the use of external cues (e.g., therapist guidance, laminated posters, chart of behaviors).

SUMMARY

The information-processing model has been presented in an overview format in this chapter.[50] Levy's work is a definitive source for occupational therapists interested in additional information about this model. The information-processing model is an invaluable means of conceptualizing the complex component systems of cognition. The ability of persons to acquire or learn information and an understanding of why and how our clients seem to forget or experience marked difficulties learning new information are best explained by the information-processing model and an understanding of higher-level cognition. Cognition is central to occupational performance in its truest and most meaningful sense. What follows is an overview of the basic cognitive skills. These skills are frequently addressed in cognitive rehabilitation. The reader is encouraged, however, to bear in mind that evaluating and intervening with basic cognitive skills are not sufficient and represent an overly simplistic approach to understanding and addressing occupational performance.

COGNITIVE SKILLS

The basic cognitive abilities are orientation, attention, memory, concentration, visual perception, visuospatial[79] processing, language, and simple problem solving. Higher-level cognitive skills consist of awareness and executive functions. Executive functions include the concepts of volition, planning, purposive action, effective performance, and the ability to monitor and make effective changes.[54] These higher-level cognitive skills are part of the Occupational Therapy Practice Framework in the categories of body functions and client factors[2] and are categorized in the terminology of the International Classification of Functioning, Disability and Health (ICF).[102]

BASIC COGNITIVE ABILITIES

Orientation refers to an individual's ongoing attentiveness to situations, the environment, and the passage of time. An unimpaired person is oriented to person (i.e., able to name self and others), place (i.e., present location, in terms of city, state, county, address), and time (i.e., year, month, day, time of day, length of time in an event or sequence of events in time, the passage of time). Orientation involves an individual's explicit episodic memory capacity because a person must be able to remember past occurrences to place current events in their proper perspective.

After a severe TBI resulting in a period of coma, clients initially may be confused regarding their identity or confuse the identities of other individuals upon regaining consciousness. They may think that the therapist or nurse is a family member. They may not know the day, date, length of time that they have been hospitalized, or even where they are. A particular kind of orientation, topographical orientation, describes an individual's awareness of his or her position in relation to the environment (e.g., the room, building, or town). Examples of this type of disorientation may be seen when an individual becomes confused while attempting to leave a room. Familiar environments can help compensate for this deficit.

Attention requires a fluid, ever-changing focus on what is important internally and in the external environment. Attention involves the simultaneous engagement of alertness, selectivity, sustained effort, flexibility, and mental tracking.[92] An individual first must be alert and awake and then able to select a relevant focus of interest. The individual must be able to maintain focus for as long as needed, yet be able to shift focus if another event of interest or importance occurs. In addition, the individual must ignore information if it is not relevant and must be able to track multiple sequences of information simultaneously. Because these skills underlie all aspects of cognitive functioning, they are frequently affected by TBI or CVA. These deficits may hinder all higher skill levels. For example, a person who is unable to attend to a task for more than a few seconds cannot take in all the necessary information to incorporate information into working memory and use it to perform a higher-level reasoning task.

Information processing can occur through habits, using well established neuronal pathways; this is referred to as *automatic processing* or, when it is on a more conscious level, *controlled processing*.[101] A client undergoing rehabilitation often must use controlled processing to perform basic tasks

that were handled automatically before the injury. A client who has difficulty with divided attention, or simultaneous multiple attention, has impairment in short-term working memory with capacity or activation and may not be able to focus on and perform more than one task at a time. The client typically responds by reverting to focused attention. For example, during OT, the client with dementia who is asked a question while working on a table-top activity often stops working on the activity to engage in conversation and has difficulty initiating action again.

Concentration requires sustained attention, also referred to as *vigilance.* Clients may be highly distractible or very sensitive to events in the immediate environment, which pulls their focus away from the task at hand. It is important to note which types of stimuli (e.g., visual, auditory, tactile, or gustatory) distract the person easily and replace important information affecting working memory capacity. A low-stimulus environment, or "quiet room," may be beneficial. Such a room is designed for minimal visual stimuli and for insulation from nearby noise and activity.

Some clients have the opposite problem—that is, they can become very deeply focused on a given stimulus or activity and have difficulty maintaining a general awareness of events occurring around them. A client's brother once described him as tending to "get sucked into the computer," and a closer examination of his activity revealed that he was not performing any useful work, only rearranging his computer files day after day. Either extreme is undesirable. Normal functioning requires that a person be able to focus, sustain a low level of awareness of peripheral events, disengage, and then reengage concentration as needed.

MEMORY

Many of the processes of memory (Figure 25-2) were described earlier in this chapter. Other elements of memory not covered in the previous section are described in this section. The memory process can break down at any level. If a person is unable to maintain attention, the information may never enter the system. Some persons are able to process information in STM or working memory but never encode

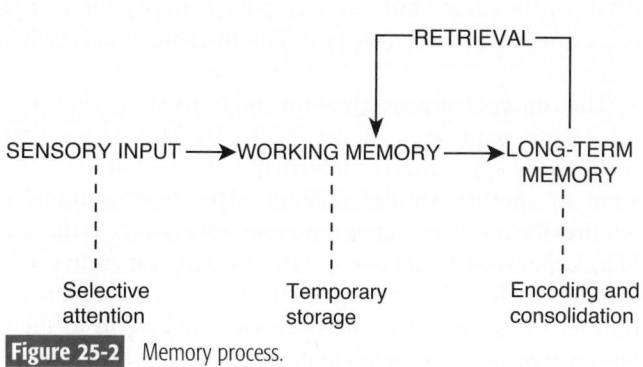

Figure 25-2   Memory process.

the material into long-term storage. Others can store the information but have a deficit in the retrieval process. Strategic testing, comparing tests requiring free recall (open-ended questions) with recognition (multiple-choice responses), may help the therapist determine the breakdown in the memory process, which can then guide the treatment approach.

The ability to recite information is generally taken as an indication of recall and is referred to as *explicit memory*. Tests often require a person to repeat a list of words or draw a set of geometrical designs, or a therapist may quiz a client about events occurring earlier in the day. Explicit memory is divided into two categories. *Episodic memory* refers to an individual's ability to recall personal history and life experiences. The general fund of knowledge shared by groups of people is called *semantic memory* and includes such information as language and rules of social behavior. Semantic memory is generally less affected than episodic recall after an injury.[39]

Some individuals have a considerable deficit in explicit memory but less impaired procedural memory, or memory for a skill or series of actions.[39] For example, a client may be unable to tell a therapist the steps in making a sandwich and a cup of coffee but may be able to perform the task correctly. The process of obtaining a driver's license requires both a written test (semantic memory) and a behind-the-wheel test (procedural recall). It is procedural learning that enables a person to consolidate the acquisition of new self-care techniques despite severe memory deficits on standardized memory tests. This phenomenon underscores the need for integration of test performance and observations made during functional activities.

Persons with memory deficits may confabulate information, filling in the gaps in memory with imaginary material.[17] They are not aware of adding erroneous information to the factual data and can therefore become confused about past events or may insist on the accuracy of their memory, to the confusion of others around them. Some persons with memory deficits pretend that they remember in an attempt to cover their embarrassment at the extent of their memory loss, but this practice is not considered confabulation.

Family members frequently report that the client recalls events from his or her life before the accident with great detail and accuracy but has very poor memory for events occurring in the immediate past. This phenomenon is called *Ribot's law.*[76]

The concepts of generalization and transfer are also critical to the acquisition of new skills. Transfer of learning refers to the application of information learned in one situation to another, similar situation. This type of transfer requires the use of executive functions. An example is the use of a clothes washer and dryer in the OT department to teach laundry skills; this training method requires that clients transfer skills learned in the clinic's laundry room to their homes. *Generalization* refers to the ability to apply knowledge and skills to a variety of similar but novel situations and requires use of executive skills.[68] A person who can generalize would be able to launder clothes even in a novel laundry setting. Individuals with cognitive deficits frequently have difficulty with transfer of learning and may be unable to generalize skills to novel situations. Transfer of new skills must be built into intervention planning because the client may not be able to transfer skills independently.

The principle of domain-specific learning is based on the assumption that generalization is not likely to be achieved by individuals who have severe memory impairments. However, a person may be able to learn specific skills relative to a particular situation and to continue to apply these skills in that specific environment.[80] Teaching one-handed cooking skills in the OT department kitchen may be ineffective if the client is unable to generalize those skills to the kitchen at home. This client may be better served if the instruction is provided in the home environment by an occupational therapist who can then make use of contextual cues to assist with retrieval. Job coaching, a type of supported employment, is based on this premise. The skills needed for the job are taught on the job site rather than being taught in advance in a setting other than the job site.[96]

REASONING AND PROBLEM SOLVING

Reasoning and problem-solving skills, briefly described in the basic cognitive skills section of this chapter, are executive functions and are not easily assessed by instruments that address basic mental status. **Abstract thinking** enables a person to see relationships between objects, events, or ideas; to discriminate relevant from irrelevant detail; and to recognize absurdities.[54] Cognitive deficits in this area and resultant behaviors create difficulty in the transfer of knowledge to new situations and in problem solving.[105] Persons with frontal and prefrontal lobe damage commonly lose abstract thinking ability and think only in the most concrete, literal manner. This literal thinking is often paired with mental inflexibility.

The following is an example of **concrete thinking.** A client is asked the interview question "What brought you to this hospital?" The client responds, "My parents' car." The person is interpreting the question literally, rather than understanding it as a reference to the accident that resulted in brain injury.

Problem solving is a complex process involving many cognitive skills. Problem solving can take the form of **convergent thinking,** which enables a person to arrive at a central idea, and **divergent thinking,** which is aimed at generating alternatives.[103] The process of grocery shopping provides an example of both types of thinking. An individual knows that milk, eggs, and butter are needed and, by convergent thinking, identifies them as dairy products. Divergent thinking is used to arrive at a list of stores that carry these items.

OT PRACTICE NOTES

The steps that compose the problem-solving process have been organized into the acronym SOLVE[69] for easy recall:

Specify the problem: Clients frequently have difficulty defining the problem and therefore tend to generate misdirected solutions.

Options: For those who focus narrowly on one solution, developing several possible solutions increases the likelihood of success.

Listen to advice: Obtaining another viewpoint encourages further exploration of the problem and reduces the risk that the critical element will be missed.

Vary the solution: Variety encourages expanded mental flexibility.

Evaluate: Clients are encouraged to assess what worked and what did not and use the new information for future situations

This sequence can be taught to the client, with instructions to use the steps when a problem is encountered in therapy or in functional tasks.[13,103] The therapist assists the client in transferring this technique to a variety of functional situations.

Various types of reasoning can be used in the problem-solving process. **Deductive reasoning** refers to the ability to arrive at conclusions. For example, a person notices that items grasped in the affected right hand tend to drop to the floor and concludes that the hand is not reliable for grasping and holding. **Inductive reasoning** enables a person to draw generalizations on the basis of specific experiences. For example, after a period of persistent right-hand incoordination, the person realizes that the ability to return to a previous occupation involving bilateral manual skills (e.g., assembly-line work) is now questionable.[13,103]

Reasoning deficits can be noted in a person's inability to recognize the long-term consequences of an action and a tendency to focus instead on the immediate effect. Persons with deficits in reasoning may have difficulty establishing priorities when faced with a number of tasks to be accomplished.

Dyscalculia is a deficit in the reasoning ability used to perform simple calculations (Figure 25-3). This deficit can have important implications for an individual's ability to function independently in the community. Various types of calculation disorders have been identified.[60] A person may also have difficulty reading (alexia) or writing (agraphia) numbers, and consultation should be sought with the speech-language pathologist or psychologist on the team.

RELATIONSHIP OF COGNITIVE DEFICITS TO PERFORMANCE

Because cognitive processes are interrelated, the therapist must assess a broad spectrum of skill areas, from basic sensory functions to complex processing, and compare findings

Figure 25-3 Examples of spatial dyscalculia.

with those of other members of the team. A poor score on a test of complex cognitive function may be caused or complicated by a deficiency in a more basic skill. For example, a person with a left-sided visual field loss may select a lightweight garment on a cold day simply because he or she failed to scan the full contents of the closet to see the sweater hanging to the left. In addition, the individual who does not remember the selection of clothing brought to the rehabilitation facility will not search for the sweater among his or her belongings.

INTELLECTUAL CAPACITY BEFORE INJURY

The client's family should be interviewed and existing records reviewed to determine the client's level of functioning before the injury or CVA. For example, clients who were below average in intellectual level before injury cannot be expected to perform at a higher level on tests administered after the injury. Similarly, if a client's previous learning disability affects the ability to read and write, the therapist should recognize that the quality of the client's written responses on a given test may be the result of factors other than the CVA. Another example is the client who functioned at a very high level before brain injury and who now scores in the average range. Although the person's functioning may be sufficient for daily activities, this is still a significant drop from previous capacity. The client may need to learn new ways to cope with this change in functional level.

IMPACT OF SUBSTANCE ABUSE

Individuals with cognitive impairments caused by head trauma, CVA, or other causes may also have a history of substance abuse.[8] The long-term effects of use and abuse of illegal substances are widely recognized, but studies have been hindered by related factors of ongoing abuse, medical complications, and poor education.[62] It is important to know if a client has a history of alcoholism because prolonged use can lead to Korsakoff's syndrome, with significant loss of new learning capacity.[21]

COGNITION AND AGING

In the normal aging process, many older adults experience sensory and perceptual impairments. These impairments can influence cognitive processing if they prevent sensory information from registering correctly in the sensory cortex[50] and influencing the person's ability to fully attend to information. Medication side effects, sleep disorders, stress, depression, and the proper management of medical conditions such as hypertension, diabetes, and high cholesterol can be associated with cognitive deficits.[6,37,95] The decline noted in working memory is related to difficulty with inhibitory mechanisms of attending, reduced rate of information-processing speed, and slower learning. These factors may have implications for everyday functioning, such as the ability to remember a route, adhere to medication schedules, and recall the faces of new acquaintances. An older adult's performance is relatively higher for familiar tasks in familiar settings than for unfamiliar tasks in unfamiliar settings.[40] Because the speed of information processing is slower for older clients, the therapist must tailor the pacing of the activity to the client and allow for multiple repetitions and a longer response time.[51,97]

Some assessment tools, such as the Benton Visual Retention Test, adjust the interpretation of scores based on age. The Mini-Mental State Examination frequently is used as a screening tool to assess the cognitive skills of the older population but should be used with scoring adjusted for age and educational level.[30,49,51]

An area of growing concern to occupational therapists working in geriatric settings is providing appropriate services to clients with Alzheimer's dementia.[52] This disorder leads to progressive decline in behavior, attention, memory, visual perception, praxis, language, and executive functioning.[54,62] The goal of therapeutic intervention is to maximize the client's functional level, increase safety, minimize confusion, develop behavioral management strategies, and serve as a resource to families.[4,24,36] Rather than attempting to improve the client's recall with drills or internal mnemonic strategies, the therapist makes changes to the environment to stimulate memory and orientation. Alzheimer's units in skilled nursing facilities may be designed to minimize residents' confusion. An example is the placement of a small display case next to a client's doorway in which to store articles that have a strong personal meaning and thereby aid the client in recognizing which room is his or her own.[19,20]

COGNITIVE FUNCTION AND PERFORMANCE

Normal cognitive function results from a dynamic balance among all brain structures. Functional activity is not localized to a restricted section of the brain but depends on the reciprocal interconnections of organized neural networks or systems of working zones in the brain.[7,58] The ways in which specific tasks are accomplished are influenced by the circumstances around the performance. The networks of fibers in the brain that produce higher mental processes are open to change depending on environmental and developmental factors. When brain damage occurs, the rather fragile balance between the structures of the brain is disturbed.

Cognitive rehabilitation is directed at restoring the balance among brain structures and devising compensatory strategies to promote function. Because there are numerous ways to perform cognitive functions, there can be several strategies to help reorganize cognitive abilities, especially higher-level abilities that are impaired and central to fulfilling occupations that are desired by the client. It is believed that recovery of some functions may be possible as a result of plasticity, or the ability of neurons in cortical circuits to be modified. The remaining circuits that were directly or indirectly affected by injury can reorganize to support functional change.[7,46]

OCCUPATIONAL PERFORMANCE AND COGNITIVE REHABILITATION

EVALUATION

The initial step of the evaluation process begins with an understanding of the client's occupational history and experiences, patterns of daily living, interests, values, and needs. In this data-collection stage, one that involves the occupational profile, it is important to obtain information about the client's plans for the future using a collaborative approach that often involves family participation. This process is repeated at intervals as the client progresses.

Clients who have cognitive deficits may be unable to accurately identify problems and concerns regarding their performance of occupations and daily life activities. In these circumstances, spouses, parents, family members, and significant others can provide the necessary information for the occupational profile and the desired client/family outcome goals.

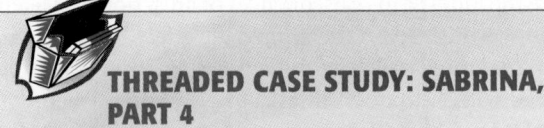

THREADED CASE STUDY: SABRINA, PART 4

Sabrina's family provided the initial information for her occupational profile. The analysis of Sabrina's occupational performance was an ongoing process that began with the JFK Coma Recovery Scale-Revised (CRS-R).[32] The CRS-R is a specialized assessment instrument designed for use with clients who have disorders in consciousness, including those who are in a coma, vegetative state, or minimally conscious state. Findings have shown this assessment tool to be an appropriate measure for characterizing the client's level of consciousness and monitoring recovery of neurobehavioral function.[33]

During the first 4 weeks of Sabrina's recovery, occupational therapy intervention focused on facilitation techniques from the standardized treatment procedures of the CRS-R Administration and Scoring Guidelines to stimulate arousal in the areas of eye

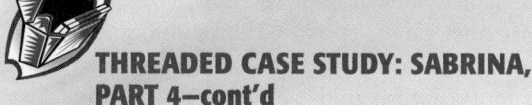

THREADED CASE STUDY: SABRINA, PART 4—cont'd

opening, and auditory, visual, motor, and oral motor/verbal communication because Sabrina was in a minimally conscious state. To ensure family involvement in the rehabilitation process, the therapist instructed Sabrina's parents and siblings in methods to provide stimulation using proper techniques in conjunction with items that were identified as being familiar to Sabrina. Sabrina's family felt included as members of the intervention team.

As a client emerges from the coma state, evaluation of the client's cognitive abilities is initially conducted to provide a baseline of the current cognitive skills. This evaluation allows the occupational therapist to determine the occupational performance level, identify preferred learning patterns, and assist with determining treatment goals and intervention strategies. Assessment results are also used to measure progress and plan further intervention.[7] Initial evaluation may begin with assessing the client's orientation.

The Test of Orientation for Rehabilitation Patients (TORP), an assessment tool designed to measure cognitive orientation, was administered to Sabrina 4 weeks after her injury, as she appeared to be in the emergent stage of awareness. The TORP contains 46 items and measures orientation to person and personal situation, place, time, schedule, and temporal continuity.

Test item responses are verbal, but they can be modified for nonverbal or aphasic clients. Each test item is written both as an open-ended question and as an auditory recognition task. The recognition task is used only if the client is unable to respond verbally or if the client responds incorrectly to open-ended questions.

In addition to orientation skills, other cognitive functions should also be evaluated. Additional cognitive assessment instruments can be used to assess the client's initial cognitive performance and provide a more in-depth assessment of specific cognitive skills. The following list describes several cognitive batteries and the cognitive functions that they assess:

- The Cognitive Assessment of Minnesota (CAM)[78] consists of 17 subset tests, including attention span, memory, orientation, mathematics, visual neglect, ability to follow directions, object identification, judgment, reasoning and safety. The CAM is designed and has norms for adults from ages 17 to 70.
- The Lowenstein Occupational Therapy Cognitive Assessment (LOTCA)[45] consists of 25 subtests and 6 areas of division: orientation, visual perception, spatial perception, praxis organization, visuomotor organization, and thinking operations. The LOTCA-Geriatric (LOTCA-G)[26] is recommended for use with the geriatric population with dementia.[7]

- The Neurobehavioral Cognitive Status Examination (Cognistat)[67] first assesses the client's level of consciousness, orientation, and attention, then five cognitive areas: language, constructions, memory, calculations, and reasoning.[7]
- The Rivermead Behavioral Memory Test, second edition (RBMT-II)[99] evaluates memory abilities in everyday tasks and assesses the client's capacity to perform normal life functions. Results from this assessment can help therapists identify areas of activities of daily living for treatment.[7]
- The Behavioral Inattention Test (BIT)[100] is designed to identify a wide variety of visual neglect behaviors. It consists of six conventional subtests, including line crossing, letter cancellation, star cancellation, figure and shape copying, line bisection, and representational drawing. The nine behavior subtests evaluate aspects of daily life, including telephone dialing, menu reading, article reading, telling time, coin sorting, address and sentence copying, map navigation, and card sorting. Scores on this assessment can provide a functional profile of neglect and a meaningful guide for treatment.[7]

Determination of the most appropriate assessment is guided by the normative data available for target populations, the treatment philosophy of the treatment team, the training of the occupational therapist, and, often, the limitations imposed by third-party payment systems and the institutional setting.

Occupational performance areas are best evaluated using observation of both ADLs and IADLs, with attention paid to specific behaviors. Structured observations can target the occurrence and frequency of behaviors without cueing and then with cueing and specific functions such as dressing, washing, transferring by observing, and noting the cues and compensations needed. More standardized assessments of performance skills may be necessary when deficits in functional skills are unclear. (See Chapter 17 for a discussion of the assessment of motor and process skills.)

ASSESSMENT OF MOTOR AND PROCESS SKILLS

INTERVENTION GOALS AND METHODS

The results from cognitive assessment instruments can provide crucial information about the client's cognitive abilities, functional skills, and deficits—information that is necessary when designing an individual's intervention plan. For example, Sabrina's performance on the CAM 6 weeks after her injury displayed the following cognitive deficits: limited attention span (3-4 minutes), moderate memory loss, lack of insight into and awareness of potential problems, and limited problem-solving capability. One of Sabrina's OT goals stated that she would be able to follow a personal care schedule and perform all personal care independently with 100% compliance and accuracy by her discharge date. This was one step in helping Sabrina and her family to meet their occupational performance goal for her to return home as quickly as possible and the longer-term goal of attending high school when it was feasible. The information from the CAM was used to help design and incorporate strategies that would allow Sabrina to stay focused on task.

Intervention approaches at this stage focus on restoring and maintaining performance skills, patterns, and body functions and making compensations in context, performance patterns, or activity demands. Various methods are incorporated depending on the client's status. Methods include the following:

- *Enhancing remaining abilities that focus on allowing the client to perform activities he or she is still able to perform through habit and procedural memory.* These tasks usually are basic activities of daily living (BADLs). The client's performance can be enhanced through human supports and compensation of the context through environmental supports until cognitive functioning improves.
- *Remedial cognitive training strategies that are specifically designed for the client's training level and performance needs.* Strategies can be used for impaired attention span, simplifying complexities of tasks by reducing the activity demands, and improving thinking operation strategies.
- *Learning strategies for self-mediated learning.* This helps the client to understand and perceive important information and be able to analyze, classify, and problem solve.

THREADED CASE STUDY: SABRINA, PART 5

The intervention methods used in Sabrina's occupational therapy cognitive rehabilitation combined all four strategies. The methods used focused on enhancing her remaining abilities by combining remedial cognitive training strategies, instructions, and applications of learning strategies with procedural strategies and compensatory aids. For example, Sabrina and her therapist developed a daily personal care schedule and routine that Sabrina followed every day. The therapist initially provided both verbal cueing and hand-over-hand guidance for Sabrina to attend to the task. The number and frequency of both types of cueing were decreased at regular intervals as Sabrina became more familiar with the task and routine. Eventually, Sabrina used enlarged laminated instructions, which she read aloud and later repeated silently to promote safe effective performance.

Retraining Sabrina to use learning strategies was incorporated into the ADL training sessions. The technique used was the action-goal strategy.[69] This metacognitive strategy used to develop increased awareness is a two-step approach that requires breaking complex problems into various parts or subgoals. An action-goal strategy was also used to help Sabrina solve common everyday problems that she encountered when performing her other ADLs. The laminated instruction poster was a useful aid until safe and consistent performance was achieved. A third strategy, used to enhance awareness,[1] prompted Sabrina to evaluate her performance by asking herself, "How well do I think I will do with this task?" before performance, "How well am I doing on this task?" during performance, and "How many errors did I make?" or "How well did I do?" after performance.

Sabrina was discharged from the hospital to her home 8 weeks after her injury. When Sabrina was initially evaluated at the hospital's outpatient day treatment program for clients with traumatic brain injuries, the occupational therapist used the *Canadian Occupational Performance Measure* (COPM).[48] The COPM is a semi-structured interview designed to measure the client's perceived occupational performance and level of satisfaction with performance. Sabrina identified and prioritized four problems on the COPM, which became the goals and focus of her occupational therapy day treatment intervention program. Cognitive retraining strategies were identified to assist Sabrina in achieving her goals. For example, Sabrina's first goal was to be independent in IADLs in the areas of community mobility, safety procedures, shopping, and simple meal preparation. To achieve Sabrina's desired goals, the following remedial cognitive methods and learning strategies were implemented over the course of Sabrina's outpatient rehabilitation.

Sabrina and the occupational therapist developed a list of four aspects of her life that she wanted to change. Sabrina identified attention, memory, thinking, and energy as the skills/behaviors that she wanted to improve. A 10-point rating scale was designed for each behavior so that Sabrina could rate her performance in each area every day. A chart was made with the four behaviors so that Sabrina could keep track of her progress and also see and compare how these different behaviors interacted with one another. The chart of behaviors showed Sabrina that everything she did potentially affected everything else. For example, she was able to recognize how her inattentiveness to listening to directions of a task also affected her performance in memory and problem solving when actually carrying out the task. Videotapes of initial therapy sessions were used so that Sabrina could watch and evaluate her performance.[69] Sabrina shared her list with her family so that they could also provide her with feedback on her performance and give her appropriate cues when indicated.

The kitchen at home was reorganized with signs, labels, pictures, and clear containers to assist Sabrina with meal preparation and safety procedures; this approach allowed Sabrina to more easily identify needed materials and transfer safe performance to the home setting. Sabrina was encouraged to continue use of self-talk during performance to maintain attention. She began using a memory book that also served as her diary to record positive and negative feelings encountered during the day and the levels of fatigue and energy that she experienced throughout the day. Sabrina reviewed her diary entries at the end of day and again, with her occupational therapist, at the end of the week to identify themes and analyze behaviors.

• *Procedural strategies.* The therapist trains the client to perform all the component parts of specific tasks, one step at a time, until all steps are performed independently in the correct sequence.[7]

As the client progresses, ongoing evaluation and revisions to the intervention plan are essential to the cognitive retraining process. Moreover, incorporating client-centered assessment measures allows clients to prioritize their goals and provide feedback regarding the intervention plan. Interventions should be modified and should include methods and strategies that will support and promote the client's progress.

SUMMARY

As a reader, you have been using your higher-level cognitive skills and the information-processing model in reading and understanding the preceding material. This chapter has described the information-processing model, higher-level cognitive skills, basic cognitive processing, aspects of cognitive evaluation, and suggested methods for remediation and compensation interventions using the case of Sabrina. The field of cognitive neuroscience is always changing as new mechanisms are developed to elucidate the complexity of the brain. To provide the optimal benefit to patients and clients, students and therapists are encouraged to continue to stay abreast of new developments.

Review Questions

1. Define *cognition,* and describe its relationship to occupational performance skills.
2. Describe higher–level cognitive functions and the methods by which these client factors are assessed.
3. What factors are influential in determining which assessment tool (or tools) are used in the evaluation of a client's performance skills?
4. Name and describe the four intervention approaches that can be used to restore and maintain performance skills, patterns, and body functions and make compensations in context, performance patterns, or activity demands.
5. Why is ongoing evaluation and intervention planning necessary to the cognitive retraining process?
6. List other areas of cognition that the occupational therapist should assess. What are the related factors of performance that the therapist should consider when evaluating cognitive function?
7. What are the implications of a deficit in attention and concentration for an individual's ability to function during everyday activities?
8. Describe the various types of memory functioning.

REFERENCES

1. Abreu BC: *The quadrophonic approach: evaluation and treatment of the brain injured patient,* New York, 1990, Therapeutic Services System.
2. American Occupational Therapy Association: Occupational therapy practice framework: domain and process, *Am J Occup Ther* 56(6):609, 2002.
3. Andres P: Frontal cortex as the central executive of working memory: time to revise our view, *Cortex* 39(4-5):871, 2003.
4. Aronson MK: Caring for the dementia patient. In Aronson MK, editor: *Understanding Alzheimer's disease,* New York, 1988, Charles Scribner's Sons.
5. Atkinson R, Schiffrin R: Human memory: a proposed system and its control processes. In Spence K, Spence J: *The psychology of learning and motivation,* vol. 2, pp. 89-195, New York, 1968, Academic Press.
6. Auperin A, et al: Ultrasonic assessment of carotid wall characteristics and cognitive functions in a community sample of 59- to 71-year-olds, *Stroke* 27(8):1290, 1996.
7. Averbuch S, Katz N: A cognitive retraining model for clients with neurological disabilities. In Katz N: *Cognition and occupation across the life span: models for intervention in occupational therapy,* pp. 113-138, Bethesda, MD, 2005, AOTA Press.
8. Babor TF: Substance use disorders and persons with physical disabilities: nature, diagnosis and clinical subtypes. In Heinemann AW, editor: *Substance abuse and physical disability,* New York, 1993, Hayworth Press.
9. Baddeley A: The concept of working memory. In Gathercole S: *Models of short-term memory,* pp. 1-28, Hove, UK, 1996, Psychology Press.
10. Baddeley A: Working memory: the interface between memory and cognition, *J Cognitive Neurosci* 4(3):281, 1992.
11. Baddeley A et al: Dual-task performance in dysexecutive and nondysexecutive patients with a frontal lesion, *Neuropsychology* 11(2):187, 1997.
12. Baum C, Edwards DF: Cognitive performance in senile dementia of the Alzheimer's type: the Kitchen Task Assessment, *Am J Occup Ther* 47(5):431, 1993.
13. Beyer BK: *Practical strategies for the teaching of thinking,* Boston, 1987, Allyn & Bacon.
14. Braswell, M et al: *Profile of executive control system: instructional manual and assessment,* Wake Forest, NC, 1993, Lash and Associates Publishing/Training.
15. Brown A: Metacognition, executive control, self-regulation and other more mysterious mechanisms. In Weinert F, Kluwe R: *Metacognition, motivation, and understanding,* Hillsdale, NJ, 1987, Erlbaum.
16. Burgess P: Strategy application disorder: the role of frontal lobe in human multi-tasking, *Psychological Res* 63:279, 2000.
17. Burgess PW, Shallice T: Confabulation and the control of recollection, *Memory* 4:359, 1996.
18. Butler D: Metacognition and learning disabilities. In Wong BYL: *Learning about learning disabilities,* ed 2, pp. 277-310, New York, 1998, Academic Press.
19. Calkins MP: Designing special care units: a systematic approach, *Am J Alzheimer's Care Res* March/April:16, 1987.
20. Calkins MP: Designing special care units: a systematic approach. Part II, *Am J Alzheimer's Care Res* May/June:16, 1987.
21. Cermack LS: Models of memory loss in Korsakoff and alcoholic patients. In Parsons OA, Butters N, Nathan PE, editors: *Neuropsychology of alcoholism,* London, 1987, Guilford Press.

22. Cicerone KD, Giacino JT: Remediation of executive function deficits after traumatic brain injury, *NeuroRehabil* 2:12, 1992.

23. Craik F, Lockhart R: Levels of processing: a framework for memory research, *J Verbal Learning Behavioral Brain Sciences* 11:671, 1972.

24. Davis CM: The role of the physical and occupational therapist in caring for the victim of Alzheimer's disease. In Taira ED: *Therapeutic interventions for the person with dementia,* New York, 1986, Hayworth Press.

25. Derouesne C, et al: Decreased awareness of cognitive deficits in patients with mild dementia of the Alzheimer type, *Int J Geriatr Psychiatry* 14(12):1019, 1999.

26. Elazar B, Itzkovich M, Katz N: Lowenstein occupational therapy cognitive assessment—geriatric (LOTCA-G), Pequannock, NJ, 1996, Maddak, Inc.

27. Elliott R: Executive functions and their disorders, *Br Med Bull* 65:49, 2003.

28. Flaherty, Wallat 1997

29. Flavell JH: *Cognitive development,* Englewood Cliffs, NJ, 1985, Prentice-Hall.

30. Folstein MF, Folstein SE, McHugh PR: Mini-mental state: a practical method for grading the cognitive state of patients for the clinician, *J Psychiatr Res* 12:189, 1975.

31. Fry AF, Hale S: Processing speed, working memory, and fluid intelligence: evidence for a developmental cascade, *Psychological Science* 7:237, 1996.

32. Giacino JT, Kalmar K: *Coma recovery scale-revised (CRS-R),* Edison NJ, 2004, Johnson Rehabilitation Institute.

33. Giacino JT, Kalmar K, Whyte J: The JFK coma recovery scale—revised, measurement characteristics and diagnostic utility, *Arch Phys Med Rehabil* 85(12):2020, 2004.

34. Giles CL, Horne BG, Lin T: Learning a class of large finite state machines with a recurrent neural network, *Neural Networks* 8(9):1359, 1995.

35. Giles GM: A neurofunctional approach to rehabilitation following severe brain injury. In Katz N, editor: *Cognition and occupation in rehabilitation: cognitive models for intervention in occupational therapy,* ed 2, Bethesda, MD, 2005, American Occupational Therapy Association.

36. Glickstein JK: *Therapeutic interventions in Alzheimer's disease,* Rockville, MD, 1988, Aspen.

37. Gregg EW, et al: Is diabetes associated with cognitive impairment and cognitive decline among older women? *Arch Internal Med* 160(2):174, 2000.

38. Haist F, Bowden Gore J, Mao H: Consolidation of memory over decades revealed by functional magnetic resonance imaging, *Nat Neurosci* 4(11):1139, 2001.

39. Harrell M, et al: *Cognitive rehabilitation of memory: a practical guide,* Gaithersburg, MD, 1992, Aspen.

40. Hess TM, Pullen SM: Memory in context. In Blanchard-Fields F, Hess TM: *Perspectives on cognitive change in adulthood and aging,* New York, 1996, McGraw-Hill.

41. Jarman RF, Vavrik J, Walton PD: Metacognitive and frontal lobe processes: at the interface of cognitive psychology and neuropsychology, *Genet Soc Gen Psychol Monogr* 121(2):153, 1995.

42. Kandel ER, Kupfermann I, Iversen S: Learning and memory. In Kandel ER, Schwartz JH, Jessell TM, editors: *Principles of neural science,* ed 4, p.1227, New York, 2000, McGraw-Hill.

43. Katz N, et al: Unawareness and/or denial of disability: implications for occupational therapy intervention, *Can J Occup Ther* 69(5):281, 2002.

44. Katz N, Hartman-Maeir A: Higher-level cognitive functions: awareness and executive functions enabling engagement in occupation. In Katz N, editor: *Cognition and occupation across the life span: models for intervention in occupational therapy,* ed 2, pp. 3-25, Bethesda, MD, 2005, American Occupational Therapy Association.

45. Katz N, et al: Loewenstein "occupational cognitive assessment (LOTCA) battery for brain injured patients: reliability and validity," *Am J Occup Ther* 43:184, 1989.

46. Kolb B, Gibb R: Neuroplasticity and recovery of function after brain injury. In Stuss D, Winocur G, Robertson I, editors: *Cognitive rehabilitation,* Cambridge, 1999, Cambridge University Press.

47. Kortte MT, Wegener ST, Chwalisz K. Anosognosia and denial: their relationship to coping and depression in traumatic brain injury, *Rehabil Psychol* 48(3):131, 2003.

48. Law M, et al: *Canadian occupational performance measure,* ed 4, Ottawa, 2005, Canadian Association of Occupational Therapists.

49. Levy LL: Cognitive aging in perspective: implications for occupational therapy practitioners. In Katz N: *Cognition and occupation across the life span: models for intervention in occupational therapy,* ed 2, pp. 327-344, Bethesda, MD, 2005, American Occupational Therapy Association.

50. Levy LL: Cognitive aging in perspective: information processing, cognition and memory. In Katz N: *Cognition and occupation across the life span: models for intervention in occupational therapy,* ed 2, pp. 305-325, Bethesda, MD, 2005, American Occupational Therapy Association.

51. Levy LL: Cognitive changes in later life: rehabilitation implications. In Katz N, editor: *Cognition and occupation in rehabilitation: cognitive models for intervention in occupational therapy,* Bethesda, MD, 1998, American Occupational Therapy Association.

52. Levy LL: The cognitive disabilities model in rehabilitation of older adults with dementia. In Katz N, editor: *Cognition and occupation in rehabilitation: cognitive models for intervention in occupational therapy,* Bethesda, MD, 1998, American Occupational Therapy Association.

53. Levy LL: Cognitive integration and cognitive components. In Larson K, et al: *The role of occupational therapy with the elderly,* Rockville, MD, 1996, American Occupational Therapy Association.

54. Lezak MD: *Neuropsychological assessment,* New York, 1995, Oxford University Press.

55. Lezak MD: Newer contributions to the neuropsychological assessment of executive functions, *J Head Trauma* 8:24, 1993.

56. Lidz C: Cognitive deficiencies revisited. In Lidz C, editor: *Dynamic assessment: evaluating learning potential,* New York, 1987, Guilford.

57. Lopez J: Shaky memories in indelible ink, *Nat Reviews Neurosci* 1:6, 2000.

58. Luria A: *The working brain*, London, 1973, Penguin Books.

59. Mateer C: The rehabilitation of executive disorders. In Stuss D, Winocur G, Robertson J, editors: *Cognitive neurorehabilitation*, Cambridge, 1999, Cambridge University Press.

60. McCarthy RA, Warrington EK: *Cognitive neuropsychology: a clinical introduction*, San Diego, 1990, Academic Press.

61. McClelland JL, McNaughton BL, O'Reilly RC: Why there are complementary learning systems in the hippocampus and neocortex: insights from the successes and failures of connectionist models of learning and memory, *Psychological Review* 102:419, 1995.

62. McGowin DF: *Living in the labyrinth: a personal journey through the maze of Alzheimer's*, New York, 1993, Delacorte Press.

63. Migliorelli R, et al: Anosognosia in Alzheimer's disease: a study of associated factors, *J Neuropsychiatry Clin Neurosci* 7(3):338, 1995.

64. Neisser U: *Cognitive psychology*, New York, 1967, Appleton-Century-Crofts.

65. Nelson TO, Narens LN: Why investigate metacognition? In Metcalfe J, Shimamura P, editors: *Metacognition: knowing about knowing*, pp. 1-26, Cambridge, 1994, MIT Press.

66. Norris G, Tate RL: Behavioural assessment of the dysexecutive syndrome (BADS): ecological, concurrent and construct validity, *Neuropsychol Rehabil* 10(1):33, 2000.

67. Northern California Neurobehavioral Group, Inc: *Manual for the neurobehavioral cognitive satus examination*, Fairfax, CA, 1995, Northern California Neurobehavioral Group, Inc.

68. Parente R, Anderson-Parente J: *Retraining memory: techniques and applications*, Houston, 1991, CSY Publishing.

69. Parente R, Herrmann DJ: *Retraining cognition: techniques and applications*, ed 2, Austin, 1996, Pro-Ed.

70. Parks RW, Levine DS, Long DL: *Fundamentals of neural network modeling: neuropsychology and cognitive neuroscience*, Cambridge, MA, 1998, MIT Press.

71. Prigatano G: Disturbance in self-awareness of deficit after traumatic brain injury. In Prigatano G, Schacter D, editors: *Awareness of deficit after brain injury*, pp. 111-126, New York, 1991, Oxford Press University.

72. Prigatano GP: *Neuropsychological rehabilitation after brain injury*, Baltimore, 1986, Johns Hopkins University Press.

73. Prigatano G, Ogano M, Amakusa B: A cross-cultural study on impaired self-awareness in Japanese patients with brain dysfunction, *Neuropsychiatry Neuropsychol Behav Neurol* 10(2):135, 1997.

74. Prigatano G, Wong JL: Cognitive and affective improvement in brain dysfunctional patients who achieve inpatient rehabilitation goals, *Arch Phys Med Rehabil* 80(1):77, 1999.

75. Reed S: *Cognition*, Belmont, CA, 2000, Wadsworth.

76. Ribot T: *Diseases of memory*, New York, 1882, Appleton-Century-Crofts. Cited in Schacter DL: *Searching for memory: the brain, the mind, and the past*, New York, 1996, Basic Books.

77. Royall DR, Mahurin RK, Gray KF: Bedside assessment of executive cognitive impairment: the executive interview, *J Am Geriatr Soc* 40(12):1221, 1992.

78. Rustad RA, et al: *The cognitive assessment of Minnesota*, Tucson, AZ, 1993, Therapy Skill Builders.

79. Salthouse T: The processing speed theory of adult age differences in cognition, *Psychol Rev* 103:403, 1996.

80. Schacter DL, Glisky EL: Memory remediation: restoration, alleviation, and the acquisition of domain-specific knowledge. In Uzzell BP, Gross Y, editors: *Clinical neuropsychology of intervention*, Boston, 1986, Martinus Nijihoff.

81. Schacter DL, Tulving E: What are the memory systems of 1994? In Schacter DL, Tulving E, editors: *Memory systems 1994*, Cambridge, 1999, MIT Press.

82. Sohlberg M: Assessing and managing unawareness of self, *Semin Speech Lang* 21(2):135, 2000.

83. Sohlberg M, Mateer C: Introduction to cognitive rehabilitation. In Sohlberg M, Mateer C, editors: *Cognitive rehabilitation: an integrative neuropsychological approach*, New York, 2001, Guilford Press.

84. Squire L: Declarative and nondeclarative memory: multiple brain systems supporting learning and memory. In Schacter DL, Tulving E, editors: *Memory systems 1994*, Cambridge, 1999, MIT Press.

85. Stuss D: Biological and psychological development of executive functions, *Brain Cognition* 20:8, 1992.

86. Stuss D, Alexander M: Executive functions and the frontal lobes: a conceptual view, *Psychol Res* 63:289, 2000.

87. Stuss D, Levine B: Adult clinical neuropsychology: lessons from studies in frontal lobes, *Ann Rev Psychol* 53:401, 2002.

88. Tham K, Bernspång B, Fisher AG: Development of the assessment of awareness of disabilities, *Scand J Occup Ther* 6:184, 1999.

89. Toglia J: *A dynamic interactional approach to cognitive rehabilitation*, Boston, 1992, Andover Medical.

90. Toglia JP: A dynamic interactional model to cognitive rehabilitation. In Katz N: *Cognition and occupation in rehabilitation*, pp. 5-50, Rockville, MD, 1998, American Occupational Therapy Association.

91. Toglia JP: A dynamic interactional model to cognitive rehabilitation. In Katz N: *Cognition and occupation across the life span models for intervention in occupational therapy*, p. 29, Bethesda, MD, 2005, American Occupational Therapy Association.

92. Toglia J: Attention and memory. In Royeen CB, editor: *AOTA self study series: cognitive rehabilitation*, Rockville, MD, 1993, American Occupational Therapy Association.

93. Tulving E: Introduction to memory. In Gazzaniga M, editor: *The new cognitive neurosciences*, p. 727, Cambridge, MA, 2000, MIT Press.

94. Vataja R, et al: MRI correlates of executive dysfunction in patients with ischaemic stroke, *Eur J Neurol* 10(6):625, 2003.

95. Waldstein SR: Health effects on cognitive aging. In National Research Council: *The aging mind: opportunities for cognitive research*, pp. 189-217, Washington DC, 2000, National Academy Press.

96. Wehman PH: Cognitive rehabilitation in the workplace. In Kreutzer JS, Wehman PH, editors: *Cognitive rehabilitation for*

persons with traumatic brain injury: a functional approach, Baltimore, 1991, Paul H Brookes Publishing.

97. West RL: Compensatory strategies for age-associated memory impairment. In Baddeley AD, Wilson BA, Watts FN, editors: *Handbook of memory disorders,* Chichester, UK, 1995, John Wiley & Sons.

98. Wilson BA, et al: *Behavioral assessment of dysexecutive syndrome,* Bury St Edmonds, England, 1996, Thames Valley Test Company.

99. Wilson BA, Cockburn J, Baddeley A: *Rivermead behavioral memory test,* ed 2, Bury St Edmonds, England, 2003, Thames Valley Test Company.

100. Wilson BA, Cockburn J, Halligan PW: *Behavioural inattention test,* Titchfield, Hants, England, 1987, Thames Valley Test Company.

101. Wood RL: Management of attention disorders following brain injury. In Wilson BA, Moffat N, editors: *Clinical management of memory problems,* Rockville, MD, 1984, Aspen Publishers.

102. World Health Organization: *International classification of functioning, disability and health,* Geneva, 2001, The Organization.

103. Ylvisaker M: Topics in cognitive rehabilitation therapy. In Ylvisaker M, Gobble EM: *Community re-entry for head injured adults,* Boston, 1987, Little, Brown.

104. Ylvisaker M, Szekeres SF, Feeney TJ: Cognitive rehabilitation: executive functions. In Ylvisaker M, editor: *Towards brain injury rehabilitation: children and adolescents,* pp. 221-269, Boston, 1998, Butterworth-Heinemann.

105. Zoltan B: *Vision, perception and cognition,* ed 3, Thorofare, NJ, 1996, Charles B Slack.

26

EATING AND SWALLOWING

KAREN NELSON JENKS

GIGI SMITH

KEY TERMS

Feeding	Sulcus	Pyriform sinuses	Tracheostomy
Eating	Bolus	Aspiration	Instrumental assessments
Dysphagia	Velum	Nasogastric tube	Videofluoroscopy
Deglutition	Velopharyngeal port	Gastrostomy tube	Fiberoptic endoscopy

LEARNING OBJECTIVES

After studying this chapter the student or practitioner will be able to do the following:

1. Name and locate oral structures concerned with eating and swallowing.
2. Name and describe the stages of normal eating and swallowing.
3. List the components of the swallowing assessment.
4. Name and describe normal and abnormal oral reflexes.
5. Describe the role of the occupational therapist in the clinical assessment of eating and swallowing.
6. Describe four steps in the swallowing assessment.
7. Describe the appropriate progression of foods and liquids in the assessment and intervention of deglutition and dysphagia.
8. Name two types of tracheostomy tubes, and list the advantages and disadvantages of each.
9. List symptoms of swallowing dysfunction.
10. Identify basic intervention goals for clients with eating and swallowing dysfunction.
11. Describe the roles of the dysphagia team members.
12. Describe proper positioning for safe feeding and swallowing.
13. Describe two methods of non-oral feeding.
14. List principles of oral feeding.
15. List and describe intervention techniques for management of eating and swallowing dysfunction.

CHAPTER OUTLINE

Anatomy and physiology of normal eating swallow
  Pre-oral phase
  Oral phase
  Pharyngeal phase
  Esophageal phase
Eating and swallowing assessment
  Medical chart review
  Occupational profile
  Cognitive-perceptual status
  Physical status
  Oral assessment
  Clinical assessment of swallowing
Instrumental assessment
  Assessment with videofluoroscopy
  Assessment with fiberoptic endoscopy

Intervention
  Goals
  Team management
  Positioning
  Oral hygiene
  Non-oral feedings
  Oral feedings
  Diet selection
  Diet progression
  Principles of oral feeding
  Techniques for the management of dysphagia
Summary

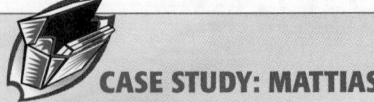

CASE STUDY: MATTIAS

Mattias, a 65-year-old man experienced a right cerebrovascular accident (RCVA) 3 days ago, which resulted in left hemiplegia. During his occupational therapy (OT) evaluation of activities of daily living (ADLs) it was determined that Mattias had difficulties with self-feeding, chewing, and swallowing at meals. He had frequent episodes of coughing, pocketing food in the left cheek, and frequently had food on his left side of his face. His oral intake is below the normal calorie range at this time. He complains that he chokes on many foods, including water.

An occupational profile provided the following background information on Mattias. He is married and has two daughters. Until onset, he was working full time as a vice president for marketing in the computer industry. He and his wife are active socially in their golf and tennis club. They also entertain with frequent dinner parties and both are exceptional cooks. Their oldest daughter is engaged and planning to be married in 4 months.

During the OT assessment, Mattias was asked to prioritize his concerns regarding his occupational performance. Mattias wants to be able to attend and participate in his daughter's wedding in 4 months. His goal is to be able to escort her down the aisle. He wants to be able to eat and drink without concerns about choking or coughing particularly because he and his wife were going to prepare the dinner for the wedding rehearsal party. He also wants to be able to make and drink a toast to his daughter and her new husband without risk of choking. He had planned to work to the end of the year and then retire. Upon retirement he and his wife planned to travel to Italy to attend a 1-week cooking class.

Critical Thinking Questions

1. What evaluations would you perform to develop an intervention plan for his eating and swallowing needs based on the information described above?
2. What interventions would you consider to address his goals of participating in his daughter's wedding?
3. How does context influence Mattias' need to eat safely and eat a variety of foods? How would you incorporate this knowledge into your intervention plan?
4. How would you systematically grade the challenges in the intervention program for Mattias?

Eating is the most basic activity of daily living, necessary for survival from birth until death. Eating occurs throughout life development in a variety of contexts and in every culture. Although eating and feeding are closely related, these terms are not synonymous. **Feeding** refers to the ability of the client to bring food or fluids to the mouth.[42] **Eating** or deglutition refers to the ability to manipulate and swallow food and liquids. Both feeding and eating are influenced by contextual issues.[6] **Dysphagia** is difficulty with swallowing or the inability to swallow.

Occupational therapists (OTs) are trained to assess and provide intervention for the performance issues involved in the task of eating. Performance skills include motor skills such as postural control of the trunk, head, and extremities, and endurance while the client is eating; client factors such as muscle strength and motor control, muscle tone, normal and abnormal reflexes, sensory, perceptual, and cognitive abilities; and performance patterns including the habits and routines that may interfere with the eating process. The contexts that may influence the client's successful engagement in eating are also assessed.[6]

ETHICAL CONSIDERATIONS

Continuing education and special training are required for competence in assessment of and intervention with dysphagia.

This chapter provides the OT with a foundation for the assessment and intervention process of the adult client with eating and swallowing dysfunction. Conditions that can result in eating and swallowing issues are cerebral vascular accident (CVA), head injury, brain tumor, anoxia, Guillain-Barré syndrome, multiple sclerosis, amyotrophic lateral sclerosis, Parkinson's disease, myasthenia gravis, poliomyelitis, and quadriplegia. Anatomical or developmental dysphagia is not included in this chapter.

ANATOMY AND PHYSIOLOGY OF NORMAL EATING SWALLOW

Deglutition, the normal consumption of solids or liquids, is a complex sensorimotor process involving the brainstem, the cerebral cortex, six cranial nerves, the first three cervical nerve segments, and 48 pairs of muscles.[10,30,40] A normal swallow requires all these structures to be intact (Figure 26-1). Therefore, the OT working with the client with eating and swallowing problems must have a thorough understanding of the anatomy, including the muscle origin and insertion and the physiology of all phases of the swallow (Table 26-1). The eating and swallowing process can be divided into four stages: pre-oral phase, oral phase, pharyngeal phase, and esophageal phase (Figure 26-2).[6,37]

PRE-ORAL PHASE

The pre-oral phase of eating and swallowing begins with the voluntary act of looking at and reaching for food.[6,37] This ability to search for, reach, and bring food to the mouth is considered feeding and serves as a key component for

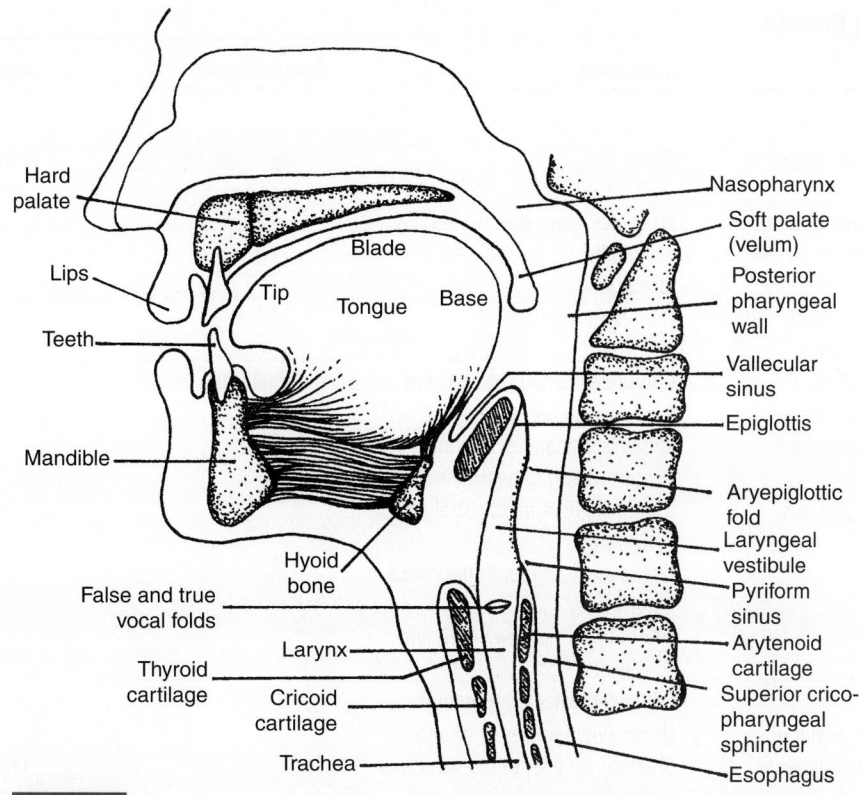

Figure 26-1   Oral structures, swallowing mechanism at rest. (Courtesy Rene Padilla, Occupational Therapy Department, Creighton University, 1994.)

successful initiation of this stage. Cognition and perception play important roles during this phase. Visual and olfactory information stimulates salivary secretions. Salivation plays an important role as a triggering mechanism for the entire swallowing process.[10,47] As tactile contact is made with the food, the jaw comes forward to open. The lips close around a glass or utensil to remove the food or liquid. The labial musculature forms a seal to prevent any material from leaking out of the oral cavity. This phase reflects the close relationship between feeding and eating. As Mattias brought food to his mouth, he did not have symmetrical lip closure on utensils or a glass and often food or fluid would dribble from the left side of his mouth.

As chewing begins, the mandible and tongue move in a strong, combined rotary and lateral direction. The upper and lower teeth shear and crush the food. The tongue moves laterally to push the food between the teeth. The buccinator muscles of the cheeks contract to act as lateral retainers, to prevent food particles from falling into the sulcus between the jaw and cheek.[37] The tongue sweeps through the mouth, gathering food particles and mixing them with saliva.[10] Recall that Mattias frequently had food remaining in his cheek after swallowing. This pocketing of food in the cheek may occur from diminished motor control of the tongue to manipulate the bolus or may indicate diminished sensory appreciation for food remaining in the **sulcus.** Sensory receptors

throughout the oral cavity carry information of taste, texture, and temperature of the food or liquid through the seventh and ninth cranial nerves to the brainstem. The chewing action of the mandible and tongue is repeated rhythmically, repositioning the food until a cohesive **bolus** is formed. The length of time needed to form a bolus one can safely swallow varies with the viscosity of the food. A short time is needed for soft foods, and a longer time is needed for more textured or dense foods.[29] Large amounts of thick liquids or thick and dense foods require the tongue to divide the food into smaller parts to be swallowed one at a time.[37] The posterior portion of the tongue forms a tight seal with the velum, preventing slippage of the bolus or liquid into the pharynx.[13,18,37] Respiration is inhibited during bolus formation to prevent food from falling into the open airway.[43]

In preparation for the next stage, the solid or liquid bolus, having been formed into a cohesive and swallowable mass, may be held between the anterior tongue and palate, with the tongue tip elevated or with the tongue tip dipped toward the floor of the mouth.[37] The tongue cups around the bolus to seal it against the hard palate. The larynx and the pharynx are at rest during this phase of the swallowing process. The airway is open.

Impairment of the pre-oral phase can lead to a disruption in the normal swallow sequence. Mattias has problems with this phase of the eating process. Of additional concern to

TABLE **26-1** **Swallowing Process**

Structure	Muscle	Movement	Cranial Nerve	Sensation
ORAL PREPARATORY STAGE				
Jaw	Pterygoideus medialis	Opens jaw	←Trigeminal (V)→	Face, temple, mouth, teeth, mucus
	Pterygoideus medialis and lateralis	Protrudes lower jaw; moves jaw laterally		
	Masseter	Closes jaw		
	Digastricus; mylohyoideus; geniohyoideus	Depresses lower jaw		
Mouth	Orbicularis oris	Compresses and protrudes lips	←Facial (VII)	
	Zygomaticus minor	Protrudes upper lip		
	Zygomaticus major	Raises lateral angle of mouth upward and outward (smile)		
	Levator anguli oris	Moves angle of mouth straight upward		
	Risorius	Draws angle of mouth backward (grimace)		
	Depressor labii inferioris	Draws lower lip downward and outward		
	Mentalis	Protrudes lower lip (pouting)		
	Depressor anguli oris	Draws down angles of mouth		
Tongue	Superior longitudinal	Shortens tongue; raises sides and tip of tongue	Facial (VII)→	Taste, anterior two thirds of tongue
	Transverse	Lengthens and narrows tongue	←Glossopharyngeal (IX)→	Taste, posterior third of tongue
	Vertical	Flattens and broadens tongue	←Hypoglossal (XII)	
	Inferior longitudinal	Shortens tongue; turns tip of tongue downward		
ORAL STAGE				
Tongue	Styloglossus	Elevates and pulls tongue posteriorly	←Accessory (XI)	
	Palatoglossus	Elevates and pulls tongue posteriorly; narrows fauces		
	Genioglossus	Depresses, protrudes, and retracts tongue; elevates hyoid	←Hypoglossal (XII)	
	Hyoglossus	Depresses and pulls tongue posteriorly		
Soft palate	Tensor veli palatini	Tenses soft palate	←Trigeminal (V)→	Mouth
	Levator veli palatini	Elevates soft palate	←Accessory (XI)	
	Uvulae	Shortens soft palate		
PHARYNGEAL STAGE				
Fauces	Palatoglossus	Narrows fauces	←Vagus (X)→	Membranes of pharynx
	Palatopharyngeus	Elevates larynx and pharynx		

From Bass N: The neurology of swallowing. In Groher M, editor: *Dysphagia: diagnosis and management,* ed 3, Newton, Mass, 1997, Butterworth-Heinemann Publishers; Davies P: *Steps to follow,* New York, 1985, Springer-Verlag; Hislop H, Montgomery J, Connelly B: *Daniels & Worthington's muscle testing: techniques of manual examination,* ed 6, Philadelphia, 1995. WB Saunders; Liebman M: *Neuroanotomy made easy and understandable,* Rockville, Md, 1986, Aspen Publishers; Netter F, Dalley A: *Atlas of human anatomy,* ed 2, 1998, Ciba-Geigy: ←, Movement function; →, sensory function.

TABLE **26-1**   **Swallowing Process—cont'd**

Structure	Muscle	Movement	Cranial Nerve	Sensation
Hyoid	Suprahyoideus	Elevates hyoid anteriorly, posteriorly	←Trigeminal (V)	
	Stylohyoideus			
	Sternothyroideus	Depresses thyroid cartilage	←Cervical segments 1,2,3	
	Omohyoideus	Depresses hyoid		
Pharynx	Salpingopharyngeus	Pharynx elevation	←Glossopharyngeal (IX)	
	Palatopharyngeus	Pharynx elevation		
	Stylopharyngeus	Pharynx and larynx elevation		
	Constrictor pharyngeus superior	Sequentially constricts the nasopharynx, oropharynx, laryngopharynx	←Vagus (X)→	Membranes of pharynx
	Constrictor pharyngeus medius			
	Constrictor pharyngeus inferior			
	Cricopharyngeus	Relaxes during swallow; prevents air from entering esophagus		
Larynx	Aryepiglotticus	Closes inlet of larynx	←Vagus (X)→	Membranes of larynx
	Thyroepiglotticus			
	Thyroarytenoideus	Closes glottis; shortens vocal cords		
	Arytenoid-oblique, transverse	Adducts arytenoid cartilages		
	Lateral cricoarytenoid	Adducts and rotates arytenoid cartilage		
	Vocalis	Controls tension of vocal cords		
	Postcricoary-tenoideus	Widens glottis		
	Cricothyroideus-straight, oblique	Elevates cricoid arch		
ESOPHAGEAL STAGE				
Esophagus	Smooth	Peristaltic wave	←Vagus (X)	

Mattias is the embarrassment of having food or fluid dribble from the left side of his mouth. His decreased sensory awareness compromises his ability to notice foods/fluids and use a napkin to wipe the remaining food from his face.

ORAL PHASE

The oral phase of swallowing begins when the tongue moves the bolus toward the back of the mouth.[4] The tongue elevates to squeeze the bolus up against the hard palate. The tongue forms a central groove to funnel the food posteriorly. The amount of food swallowed is inversely related to the viscosity of the food. For less viscous foods, such as thin liquids, larger amounts may be swallowed. In contrast, more viscous foods or thick liquids require that a smaller amount be swallowed. This is necessary to make it easier for the bolus to pass through the pharynx.[37]

The oral phase of the swallow is voluntary, requiring the person to be alert.[13,37,40] A normal voluntary swallow is necessary to elicit a strong swallow response during the pharyngeal stage that follows. Overall, the oral phase takes approximately 1 second to complete with thin liquids and slightly longer with thick liquids.

Mattias is alert but has difficulties maneuvering food within his mouth during the oral phase. His ability to chew textured foods is compromised, and he requires additional time to chew foods. This contributes to the decreased oral intake.

PHARYNGEAL PHASE

Voluntary and involuntary components are necessary for a normal swallow. Neither mechanism alone is sufficient to produce the immediate, consistent swallow necessary for

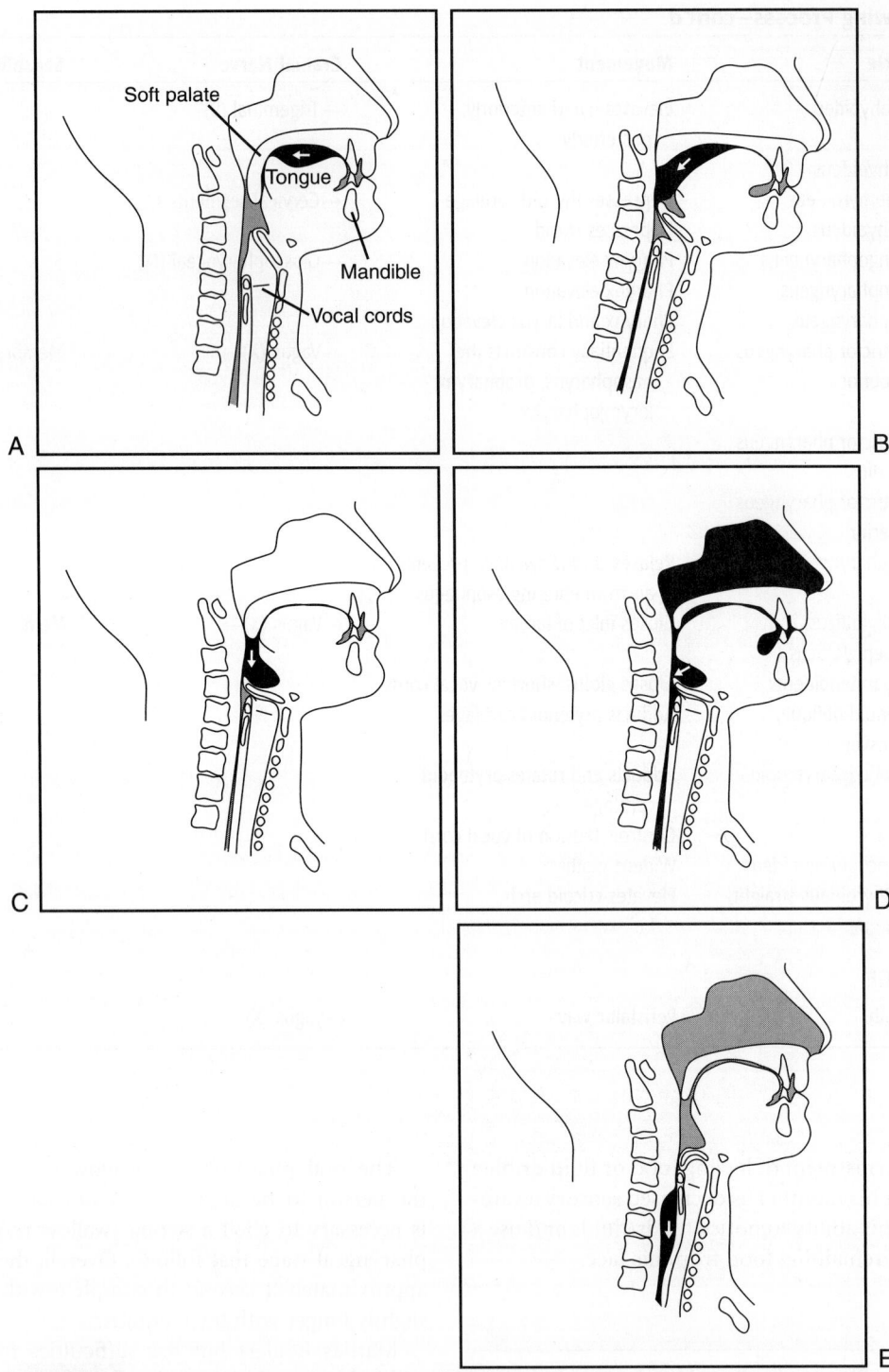

Figure 26-2   The normal swallow. **A,** Lateral view of bolus propulsion during the swallow, beginning with the voluntary initiation of the swallow by the oral tongue. **B,** Triggering of the pharyngeal swallow. **C,** Arrival of the bolus in the vallecula. **D,** Tongue base retraction to the anteriorly moving pharyngeal wall. **E,** Bolus in the cervical esophagus and the cricopharyngeal region. (From Logemann J: *Evaluation and treatment of swallowing disorders,* Austin, Texas, 1998, ProEd Publishers.)

normal eating.[37] The pharyngeal phase marks the beginning of the involuntary portion of the swallowing process.

This phase of swallowing begins when the bolus passes through the anterior faucial arches and the middle of the tongue base into the pharynx, marking the start of the involuntary component of the swallow. After the swallow response has been triggered, it continues with no pause in bolus movement until the total act is completed. The swallow response is controlled by the medulla oblongata of the brainstem.[40] Within the medulla oblongata the medullary reticular formation is responsible for screening out all extraneous sensory patterns and for responding only to those patterns that indicate the need to swallow. The reticular formation also assumes control of all motor neurons and related muscles needed to complete the swallow. Higher brain functions such as speech and respiration are preempted.[40,43]

When the swallow response is triggered, several physiological functions occur simultaneously. The **velum** elevates and retracts, closing the **velopharyngeal port** to prevent regurgitation of material into the nasal cavity. The tongue base elevates to direct the bolus into the pharynx. The entire pharyngeal tube elevates and contracts from the top to the bottom in the pharyngeal constrictors, carrying the bolus into and through both sides of the pharynx to the upper esophageal sphincter.[13] This movement must be rapid and efficient so that respiration is interrupted only briefly. The pharyngeal phase of the swallow takes approximately 1 second to complete for thin liquids. Mattias frequently coughs, indicating difficulties with the timing and coordination of the pharyngeal phase. His problems swallowing water may indicate diminished laryngeal elevation and decreased airway protection during the swallow.

Concurrently, the larynx elevates beneath the back of the tongue base, protecting the airway. Three actions facilitate closure of the larynx. These are soft palate elevation and retraction and closure of the nasopharynx; laryngeal displacement anteriorly and superiorly with obliteration of the laryngeal vestibule; closure of glottic and supraglottic structures (at the epiglottis and true vocal cords), before the arrival of the bolus at the upper esophageal sphincter, preventing food from entering the airway; and relaxation and opening of the upper esophageal sphincter (UES).[13,28,32,37] As the UES (sphincter) relaxes and opens, food passes through the pharynx, dividing in half at the valleculae and moving down each side through the **pyriform sinuses.** The bolus reforms into a whole at the top of the esophagus and then passes through the esophagus. If the involuntary swallow response does not occur, neither do these physiological functions, thus preventing a safe, normal swallow.[31,37]

ESOPHAGEAL PHASE

The esophageal phase of the swallow starts when the bolus enters the esophagus through the cricopharyngeal juncture or UES. The esophagus is a straight tube, about 10 inches long, that runs from the pharynx to the stomach. The pharynx is separated from the esophagus by the UES. The lower esophageal sphincter (LES) separates the esophagus from the stomach.[15,37] The upper third of the esophagus is composed of striated muscle and is innervated by the central nervous system. The middle section is made up of striated and smooth muscle and is innervated by the enteric nervous system that is visceral. The lower third of the tube is composed of smooth muscle.[15,28,40] The bolus is transported through the esophagus by peristaltic wave contractions. The overall transit time needed for the bolus to reach the stomach varies from 8 to 20 seconds. As the food enters the esophagus, the epiglottis returns to the relaxed position, in which the airway is open.

Mattias complains of frequently coughing and choking on food and fluid. This may be due to problems with the pre-oral, oral, pharyngeal, or esophageal phase of eating. As you read the following section, use the case presentation of Mattias and consider what assessment results you would look for to identify which phase is producing the episodes of coughing and choking.

EATING AND SWALLOWING ASSESSMENT

When a referral is received from a physician, a thorough eating and swallowing assessment for possible dysfunction must be completed. The OT reviews the client's medical history and assesses the client's visual, perceptual, and cognitive skills; physical control of head, trunk, and extremities; oral structures; and swallowing ability.

MEDICAL CHART REVIEW

A review of the client's medical chart before initiating the bedside assessment often reveals important information. The therapist should take note of the client's diagnosis, pertinent medical history (including prior incidents of aspiration), prescribed medications, and current hydration and nutritional status.

The medical diagnosis may help indicate the etiology or cause of eating and/or swallowing problems the client may be experiencing. For example, a diagnosis of a neurological disorder such as a CVA should alert the therapist that eating or swallowing problems may exist. It is important to know whether problems were sudden or gradual in onset. The therapist should seek information regarding duration of the client's eating swallowing difficulties and note any secondary diagnoses that could contribute to dysphagia such as gastrointestinal or respiratory problems, or head and neck surgeries. A diagnosis of dehydration or malnutrition may indicate a chronic problem with deglutition.

Particular attention should be paid to reported episodes of pneumonia or **aspiration** (entry of food or material into the airway below the level of the true vocal folds).[35,37,41] Aspiration pneumonia occurs when food or material enters into the lung and can be a serious complication, which is identified by X-ray and treated with antibiotics. Possible predictors of pneumonia include the need for frequent suctioning, COPD, CHF, use of a feeding tube, weight loss, swallowing problems, multiple medications, and eating dependence.[34] An elevated temperature may also indicate that a client is aspirating.

An examination of the client's current hydration and nutritional status provides valuable information about the client's ability to manage oral intake. This information can be found in the dietary section of the chart or in the nursing progress notes in the intake and output (I & O) record. An altered diet texture (pureed food or thickened liquids) alerts the therapist to a problem with the client's ability to safely eat a regular diet. The presence of an IV (intravenous fluid) may be indicative of dehydration. Weight loss is frequently a result of a swallowing problem. Consideration should be given to prescribed medications that may alter the client's alertness, orientation, and muscle control.[46] The nursing notes may also indicate whether the client coughs or chokes when taking medications. How the client is receiving nutrition is also important—for example, the presence of a non-oral feeding device such as a **nasogastric tube** (NG tube) or **gastrostomy tube** (G tube) is often an indication of a serious dysphagia problem.

OCCUPATIONAL PROFILE

In the beginning of the evaluation process, the therapist must obtain information from the client to develop the occupational profile. Information gathered for the profile is designed to help the therapist understand what is meaningful and important to the client.[5] Prior eating habits and routines and the importance of eating to the client (and his family and/or significant other) are essential to know so that interventions can be established to meet the client's needs. The client may have strong feelings about particular foods or food textures. The presentation of food may have a significant influence on the individual's desire to participate in eating. Most adults have firmly rooted routines surrounding the activity of eating. For example, an elderly person may eat a late breakfast, a larger meal at midday, and only a light meal in the evening. He or she may watch TV while eating. This routine can be severely interrupted in an institutionalized setting.

 OT PRACTICE NOTE

It is important to know the previous habits and routines of the individual and incorporate them into the intervention program. The therapist must also be sensitive to cultural issues revolving around eating and foods.

The intervention program is developed based on information provided to the therapist in the occupational profile. Mattias clearly identified his intervention priorities and discussed his concerns about participating in his daughter's wedding. The issues related to eating and drinking are closely tied to the cultural and social expectations for the father of the bride.

COGNITIVE-PERCEPTUAL STATUS

The client's cognitive and perceptual abilities are assessed to determine if the client can actively participate in an eating and swallowing assessment and intervention program. The therapist should establish whether the client is alert; oriented to name, day, and date; and able to follow simple directions, either verbal, with demonstration, or with manual guidance. The therapist should also assess the client's visual function, visual-perceptual skills, and motor planning skills. An individual who exhibits confusion, dementia, poor awareness of the eating task, poor attention span, or impaired perception will require close supervision during eating for safe consumption.[8,9,13,41]

PHYSICAL STATUS

Control of head and trunk is an important component of a safe swallow. To assess head control, the therapist asks the client to turn the head from side to side and up and down, while the therapist observes the range of motion and control available in addition to the smoothness of the movement. Assessment should include the quality of head movement without physical assistance or support initially and with assistance, if needed. The therapist should also gently move the client's head passively from side to side and up and down to look for stiffness or abnormal muscle tone. Poor head control may indicate decreased strength, decreased or increased muscle tone, or decreased awareness of posture. Appropriate head control is necessary to provide a stable base for adequate jaw and tongue movement, allowing an optimal swallow response. Head control is also necessary to anatomically position the client in the safest posture to reduce the risk of aspiration.

In assessing the client's trunk control, the therapist observes whether the client is sitting in midline with equal weight bearing on both hips. The therapist assesses whether the client can maintain the midline position independently when involved in eating or whether he or she requires the use of postural supports (such as wheelchair trunk supports or a lap board) and whether a return to midline is possible if loss of balance occurs. To participate in an eating and swallowing intervention program, the client must maintain an upright position with head and trunk in midline to provide correct alignment of the swallowing structures.[8,12] If the client has poor head or trunk control, the therapist may need to assist the client during assessment and intervention.

Mattias is able to independently sit in a chair and at the side of the bed. His head control appears adequate, but he tends to sit shifted to his right side, and his head is most often facing to the right side instead of positioned in midline. This indicates poor trunk and head alignment and can impact eating.

ORAL ASSESSMENT

Outer Oral Status

The face and mouth are sensitive areas to assess. Most adults are cautious about or even threatened by having another person touch their faces. Therefore, each step of the assessment process should be carefully explained, using terms that the individual understands. The therapist also should tell the client how long he or she will be touching the face; for example, "For a count of three." The therapist assesses the outer oral structures, including the facial musculature and mobility of the cheeks, jaw, and lips. Working within the client's visual field, the therapist moves his or her hand(s) slowly toward the client's face. This allows the individual time to process and acknowledge the approach. If the client is hypersensitive or resistant to the therapist's touch, the therapist can first guide the client's own hand to the face as needed to evaluate that area.

It is important for the client to feel comfortable with the therapist's touch during the assessment. If a client is not comfortable with the face or lips being touched, he or she will certainly be less inclined to allow the therapist's hand inside his or her mouth.

Sensation

Indications of poor oral sensation are drooling, food on the mouth, and food falling out of the mouth, of which the client is unaware. To assess the client's awareness of touch, the therapist occludes the client's vision and uses a cotton-tipped swab to touch the client gently with a quick stroke to different areas of the face. The person is asked to point to where he or she was touched. If pointing is difficult for the client, the client is asked to nod or say "Yes" or "No" when touched. The client with intact sensation responds accurately and quickly.

The client's ability to sense hot and cold should be assessed. The therapist may use two test tubes, one filled with hot water and one with cold water. A laryngeal mirror that is first heated and then cooled using hot and cold water may also be used. The client's face or lips are touched in several places, and the client is asked to indicate whether the touch was hot or cold. An aphasic client may have difficulty answering correctly. In this instance the therapist must make an assessment from clinical observations.

Poor sensory awareness affects the client's ability to move facial musculature appropriately. The client's self-esteem may be affected, especially in social situations, if decreased awareness causes the client to ignore saliva, food, or liquids remaining on the face or lips. Consider Mattias and his personal goal of eating at his daughter's wedding rehearsal dinner. The diminished sensation around Mattias' face will need to be addressed to avoid embarrassment during this important event. Strategies that promote compensatory habit formation should be used, such as having Mattias wipe his face after every second or third bite of food to remove any food on his face. This strategy provides additional sensory input to the face in addition to decreasing the potential embarrassment of having food remain on his face.

Musculature

An assessment of the facial muscles provides the therapist with information about the movement, strength, and tone available to the client for chewing and swallowing. The therapist first observes the client's face at rest and notes any visible asymmetry. If a facial droop is obvious, the therapist should observe whether the muscles feel slack or taut. A masked appearance, with little change in facial expression, may also be observed. The therapist should observe whether the client appears to be frowning or grimacing with the jaw clenched and the mouth pulled back. This facial posture may indicate increased or decreased muscle tone.

The therapist tests the facial musculature by asking the client to perform the movements listed in Table 26-2. The therapist should note how much assistance the client needs to perform these movements. As the client moves through each task, symmetry of movement is assessed. Asymmetry could indicate weakness or increased tone. Musculature is palpated for abnormal resistance to the movement. Resistance, which feels as if the client is fighting the movement, is caused by hypertonicity.

If the client is able to hold the position at the end of the movement, the therapist applies gentle pressure against the muscle to determine the muscle's strength. An individual with normal strength is able to hold the position throughout the applied resistance. The person who is able to hold the position briefly against pressure may have adequate strength for chewing and swallowing with assistance. The client who is unable to move into the testing position independently or requires assistance will have difficulty with eating and with facial expression.

Oral reflexes

A client with clearly documented neurological involvement may demonstrate primitive oral reflexes that interfere with a dysphagia retraining program. The rooting, bite, and suck-swallow reflexes, normal from 0 to 5 months of age, may interfere with the mature oral motor control in adults who have sustained damage to brainstem or cortical structures. The gag, palatal, and cough reflexes, which should be present in adults and act to protect the airway, may be impaired. Specific assessment techniques can be found in Table 26-3.

TABLE 26-2 **Outer Oral Motor Assessment**

Function	Instruction to Client	Testing Procedure*
Facial expression	"Lift your eyebrows as high as you can."	Place one finger above each eyebrow. Apply downward pressure.
	"Bring your eyebrows toward your nose in a frown."	Place one finger above each eyebrow. Apply pressure outward.
	"Wrinkle your nose upwards."	Place one finger on tip of nose and apply downward pressure.
	"Suck in your cheeks."	Apply pressure outward against each inside cheek.
Lip control	"Smile."	Observe for symmetrical movement. Palpate over each cheek.
	"Press your lips together tightly and puff out your cheeks."	Place one finger above and one finger below lips. Apply pressure, moving fingers away from each other; check for ability to hold air.
	"Pucker your lips as in a kiss."	Apply pressure inwardly against lips (toward teeth).
Jaw control	"Open your mouth as far as you can."	Help patient maintain head control. Apply pressure from under chin upward and forward.
	"Close your mouth tightly. Don't let me open it."	Help client maintain head control. Apply pressure on chin downward.
	"Push your bottom teeth forward."	Place two fingers against chin and apply pressure backward.
	"Move your jaw from side to side."	Place one finger on left cheek and apply pressure to right.

Data from Alta Bates Hospital Rehabilitation Services: *Bedside dysphagia evaluation protocol*, Berkeley, Calif, 1999; Community Hospital of Los Gatos, Rehabilitation Services: *Dysphagia protocol*, Los Gatos, Calif, 1999; Logemann J: *Evaluation and treatment of swallowing disorders*, Austin, Tex, 1998, Pro-Ed Publishers; Miller R: Clinical examination for dysphagia. In Groher M: *Dysphagia diagnosis and management*, ed 3, Newton, Mass, 1997, Butterworth-Heinemann Publishers.
*Apply resistance only in the absence of abnormal muscle tone.

TABLE 26-3 **Oral Reflexes**

Reflex	Assessment	Functional Implications
Rooting (0-4 months)	*Stimulus:* touch client on right or left corner of mouth	Limits isolated motor control of lip muscles
	Response: client moves lips and head in direction of stimulus	Moves head out of midline, which alters alignment of swallowing mechanism
Bite (4-7 months)	*Stimulus:* touch crowns of teeth with unbreakable object	Prevents normal forward, lateral, and rotary movements of jaw necessary for chewing
	Response: client involuntarily clamps teeth shut	
Suck-swallow (0-4 months)	*Stimulus:* introduction of food and liquid	Prevents development of normal voluntary swallow
	Response: sucking	
Tongue thrust (abnormal)	*Stimulus:* introduction of food and liquid	Interferes with ability to keep lips and mouth closed
	Response: tongue comes forward to front of teeth	Prevents tongue from propelling food to back of mouth in preparation for swallow; prevents formation of bolus, loss of tongue lateralization
Gag (0-adult)	*Stimulus:* pressure on back of tongue	Protects airway (not always present in normal adult); hypersensitive gag reflex can interfere with chewing, swallowing
	Response: tongue humping, pharyngeal constriction	
Palatal (0-adult)	*Stimulus:* stroke along faucial arches	Protects airway, closes off nasal passages, triggers swallow response
	Response: constriction of faucial arches; elevation of uvula	

Data from Avery-Smith W: Management of neurologic disorders: the first feeding session. In Groher M, editor: *Dysphagia: diagnosis and management*, ed 3, Newton, Mass, 1997, Butterworth-Heinemann; Farber S: *Neurorehabilitation, a multisensory approach*, Philadelphia, 1982, WB Saunders; Logemann J: *Evaluation and treatment of swallowing disorders*, Austin, Tex, 1998, Pro-Ed Publishers; Schulze-Delrieu K, Miller R: Clinical assessment of dysphagia. In Perlman A, Schulze-Delrieu K, editors: *Deglutition and its disorders: anatomy, physiology, clinical diagnosis and management*, San Diego, Calif, 1997, Singular Publishing; Silverman EH, Elfant IL: *Am J Occup Ther*, 1979.

Persistence of these primitive oral reflexes interferes with the client's isolated oral motor control, which is needed for chewing and swallowing.

Inner Oral Status

An assessment of the client's inner oral status includes an examination of oral structures, tongue musculature, palatal function, and swallowing. By performing the outer oral status assessment first, the therapist has established rapport and trust with the client. Each procedure is first explained to the client. The therapist works within the client's visual field and gives the person time to process the instructions found in Table 26-4.

Before beginning the assessment, use universal precaution techniques, such as appropriate hand washing and use of examination gloves. The therapist should check for allergies to latex before examining the person's mouth and use an examination glove of appropriate material for an inner oral examination. The therapist must place only a wet, gloved finger or dampened tongue blade into the client's mouth, because the mouth is normally a wet environment. A dry finger or tongue blade can be uncomfortable.[16] After a count of three, the therapist removes the finger and allows the client to swallow.

Dentition

Because the adult uses teeth to shear and grind food during bolus formation, the therapist needs to assess the condition and quality of the client's teeth and gums.[46] Poor dental status can contribute to dysphagia and may lead to pneumonia.[34]

For assessment purposes, the mouth is divided into four quadrants: right upper, right lower, left upper, and left lower. Each quadrant is assessed separately, as is each side (e.g., assess right upper side, then right lower side). First the therapist slides a wet fifth finger under the client's upper lip and moves it back toward the cheek, rubbing the gums three times.[16] The therapist notes whether the client's gums are bleeding, tender, or inflamed and whether the gums feel spongy or firm. Loose teeth and sensitive or missing teeth are also noted.

OT PRACTICE NOTE

The therapist should take caution to avoid placing his or her finger between the client's teeth until it has been determined that the client does not have a bite reflex.

After assessing the gums, the therapist turns over his or her finger and slides the pad of the finger against the inside of the client's cheek and gently pushes the cheek outward to feel the tone of the buccal musculature. The therapist notes whether the cheek is firm with an elastic quality, too easy to stretch, or tight without any stretch. The therapist observes the condition of the inside of the client's mouth, checking for bite marks on the tongue, cheeks, and lips. Next, the therapist should remove the finger from the client's mouth, allow or assist the client to swallow saliva, and assist the client to move the lip and cheek musculature into the normal resting position. This procedure is repeated for each quadrant. The therapist should avoid moving the finger across midline from the right to the left side of the client's gums because this practice can be annoying.

If the client has dentures, the therapist must discern whether the fit is adequate for chewing. Because dentures are held in place and controlled by normal musculature and sensation, changes in these areas, or marked weight loss, affect the client's ability to use dentures effectively.[19] Dentures should fit over the gums without slipping or sliding during eating or talking. Because the client needs to wear dentures throughout the dysphagia training period, necessary corrections or repairs should be completed quickly.[41,47] A dental consultation may be needed to ensure appropriate fit if dentures cannot be held firmly with commercial adhesive creams or powders. Clients who have gum or dental problems require appropriate follow-up and good oral hygiene to participate in a feeding and eating program. Poor oral hygiene may lead to the development of bacteria and build up of plaque, and if aspirated, contributes to the increased risk of pneumonia.[34] Loose dentures or teeth may necessitate changes in food consistencies that the client may have otherwise managed.

Tongue movement

The tongue has a critical role in the normal chewing and swallowing process. Controlled tongue movement is necessary for moving and shaping food in the mouth. The tongue propels the food back in preparation for swallowing; therefore, a thorough assessment of the tongue's strength, range of motion, control, and tone is needed.[13,46,51]

The client is asked to open the mouth, and the therapist can assess the appearance of the tongue with a flashlight and note whether the tongue is pink and moist, very red, or heavily coated and white in appearance. A heavily coated tongue may decrease the client's sensations of taste, temperature, and texture and may indicate poor tongue movement or may be a sign of infection.

When examining the shape of the tongue, the therapist notes whether it is flattened, bunched, or rounded. Normally, the tongue is slightly concave with a groove running down the middle. The therapist observes the tongue at rest in the mouth and determines whether it is in the normal position of midline, resting just behind the front teeth, retracted or pulled back away from the front teeth, or deviated to the right or left side. A retracted tongue may indicate an increase of abnormal muscle tone or a loss of range of motion as a result of soft-tissue shortening. The client exhibiting tongue

TABLE 26-4 **Inner Oral Motor Assessment**

Function	Instruction to Client	Testing Procedure*
TONGUE		
Protrusion	"Stick out your tongue."	Apply slight resistance toward the back of the throat with tongue blade after client exhibits full range of motion.
Lateralization	"Move your tongue from side to side."	Apply slight resistance in opposite direction of motion with tongue blade.
	"Touch your tongue to your inside cheek—right, then left; move your tongue up and down."	Using finger on outside of cheek, push against tongue inwardly.
Tipping	"Touch your tongue to your upper lip."	With tongue blade between tongue tip and lip, apply downward pressure.
	"Open your mouth. Touch your tongue behind your front teeth."	With tongue blade between tongue and teeth, apply downward pressure on tongue.
Dipping	"Touch your tongue behind your bottom teeth."	With tongue blade between tongue and bottom teeth, apply upward pressure.
Humping	"Say, 'ng'; say, 'ga.'"	Observe for humping of tongue against hard palate. Tongue should flow from front to back.
	"Run your tongue along the roof of your mouth, front or back."	Observe for symmetry and ease of movement.
SWALLOW		
Hard palate	"Open your mouth and hold it open."	Using flashlight, gently examine for sensitivity by walking finger from front to back.
Soft palate	"Say, 'ah' for as long as you can (5 seconds). Change pitch up an octave."	Observe for tightening of faucial arches, elevation of uvula. Using laryngeal mirror, stroke juncture of hard and soft palate to elicit palatal reflex. Observe for upward and backward movement of soft palate.
Hyoid elevation (base of tongue)	"Can you swallow for me?"	Place finger at base of client's tongue underneath the chin, and feel for elevation just before movement of the larynx.
LARYNGEAL		
Range of motion	"I am going to move your Adam's apple side to side."	Grasp larynx by placing fingers and thumb along sides. Move larynx gently side to side; evaluate for ease and symmetry of movement.
Elevation	"Can you swallow for me?"	Place fingers along the larynx: first finger at hyoid, second finger at top of larynx, and so on. Feel for quick and smooth elevation of larynx as the client swallows.
COUGH		
Voluntary	"Can you cough?"	Observe for ease and strength of movement, loudness of cough, swallow after cough.
Reflexive	"Take a deep breath."	As client holds breath, using palm of hand, push downward (toward stomach) on the sternum. Evaluate strength of reaction.

Data from Community Hospital of Los Gatos, Rehabilitation Services: *Dysphagia protocol*, Los Gatos, Calif, 1999; Coombes K: *Swallowing dysfunction in hemiplegia and head injury*, course presented by International Clinical Educators, Aug 24-27, 1986, and Aug 24-28, 1987, Los Gatos, Calif; Hislop H, Montgomery J, Connelly B: *Daniels & Worthington's muscle testing: techniques of manual examination*, ed 6, Philadelphia, 1995, WB Saunders; Miller R: Clinical examination for dysphagia. In Groher M: *Dysphagia diagnosis and management*, ed 3, Newton, Mass, 1997, Butterworth-Heinemann Publishers; Schulze-Delrieu K, Miller R: Clinical assessment of dysphagia. In Perlman A, Schulze-Delrieu K, editors: *Deglutition and its disorders: anatomy, physiology, clinical diagnosis and management*, San Diego, Calif, 1997, Singular Publishing.
*Apply resistance in absence of abnormal muscle tone.

deviation with protrusion may have muscle weakness on the affected side, causing the tongue to deviate toward the unaffected side because the stronger muscles dominate. The client also may have abnormal tone, which results in the tongue deviating toward the affected side.

Grasping the tongue gently between the forefinger and thumb, the therapist can pull the tongue slowly forward. A wet gauze square wrapped around the tip of the tongue may help the therapist to grip it.[16] Next, the therapist walks a wet finger along the tongue from front to back, to determine whether the tongue feels hard, firm, or mushy. The tongue should feel firm. An abnormally hard tongue may be the result of increased muscle tone, and a "mushy" tongue is associated with low muscle tone. The right side of the tongue is compared with the left side for symmetry.

While continuing to grip the tongue between forefinger and thumb, the therapist can assess the client's range of motion by moving the tongue forward, side to side, and up and down. The tongue with normal range will move freely in all directions without resistance.[46] Moving the tongue through its range, the therapist can simultaneously evaluate tone. As the therapist gently pulls the tongue forward, he or she determines whether it is easily moved or whether resistance is noted. A tongue pulling back against the movement indicates increased tone. A tongue that seems to stretch too far beyond the front teeth is indicative of decreased tone. When moving the tongue side to side, the therapist notes whether it is easier to move in one direction or the other direction. Increased tone makes it difficult for the therapist to move the tongue in any direction without feeling resistance against the movement. Clients who are confused or apraxic may resist this passive motion but not have an actual increase in tone.

To assess the tongue's motor control (strength and coordination), the therapist asks the client to elevate, stick out, and move the tongue laterally (see Table 26-4). If the client has difficulty following verbal directions, the therapist can use a wet tongue blade to guide the client through the desired movements. The client is asked to place the tongue against the tongue blade and to keep it there. The therapist then moves the tongue blade slowly, guiding the client's tongue in the testing direction.[16] Ease of movement, strength of movement, and coordination of movement are assessed for each direction.

Poor muscle strength or abnormal tone decreases the ability of the tongue to sweep the mouth and gather particles to form a cohesive bolus. If the tongue loses even partial control of the bolus, food may fall into the valleculae, the pyriform sinuses, or the airway, possibly leading to aspiration before the actual swallow.[37] The back of the tongue must also elevate quickly and strongly to propel the bolus past the faucial arch into the pharynx to trigger the swallow response.[16,46] The therapist must carefully assess the tongue's function. The client with poor tongue control may not be a candidate for eating. The therapist must first normalize tone

and improve tongue movement before attempting to feed the client. The correct selection of appropriate foods also facilitates motor control when the client is ready for eating. Close supervision by an experienced therapist is required for this type of client to participate in eating.

Mattias had decreased tongue mobility and control. When he protruded his tongue it was deviated towards the left, which indicates diminished motor control on the left side of his tongue. An additional indication of diminished tongue control is the pocketing of food in his mouth following a swallow.

CLINICAL ASSESSMENT OF SWALLOWING

Because aspiration is a primary concern in swallowing, the OT must carefully assess the client's ability to swallow safely. Before the therapist presents the client with material to swallow, he or she should assess the ability of the client to protect the airway. The client must have an intact palatal reflex, elevation of the larynx, and a productive cough. The purpose of a productive cough is to remove any food or liquid from the airway.[48] Directions for assessing all the components of the swallow are described in Table 26-4. The therapist should note the speed and strength of each component. The client with intact cognitive skills may accurately report to the therapist where and when difficulty occurs with the swallow.[37]

The OT assimilates all the information from the assessment process. Clinical judgment plays an important role in the accurate assessment of dysphagia.[4,8,16] The following are questions that should be asked:

1. Is the client alert and able to transition from forming the bolus to an immediate swallow when presented with food?
2. With assistance, does the client maintain adequate trunk and head control?
3. Does the client display adequate tongue control to form a partially cohesive bolus and to regulate the speed with which the bolus enters the pharynx?
4. Is the larynx mobile enough to elevate quickly and with sufficient force?
5. Can the client handle the saliva with minimal drooling?
6. Does the client have a productive cough, strong enough to expel any material that may enter the airway?

If the answer is yes to all of the above questions, the therapist may assess the client's oral and swallow control with a variety of food consistencies.

The therapist should request an assessment tray from dietary services. The following foods are merely suggestions and the therapist must consider cultural factors and medical conditions that influence the selection of foods. For example, an individual who is a vegetarian or a person who is lactose intolerant will require an appropriate selection of foods. The tray should contain a sample of foods of various textures including pureed food such as pudding or applesauce, soft foods such as a banana or macaroni and cheese, and ground tuna with mayonnaise or chopped meat with gravy. The tray should also include a thick drink such as nectar blended with one half banana for a 7-ounce drink, a semi-thick drink such as fruit nectar or a yogurt drink, and a thin liquid such as water.[1,11]

To minimize the risk of aspiration, pureed foods are chosen for clients with decreased oral motor control and chewing difficulties or apraxia. Clients who have poor endurance or have difficulty with attending to the task of eating may also require pureed foods. Soft foods are more easily formed into a bolus and require less chewing than regular or ground textures for clients who have impaired oral motor control. Soft foods are also easier for the client to keep in a cohesive bolus as they are moved through the oral cavity. Ground foods allow the therapist to assess a client's ability to chew, form a cohesive bolus, and move it in the mouth. Thick liquids move more slowly from the front of the mouth to back, giving the client with a delayed swallow more time to control the liquid until the swallow response is triggered. Thin liquids are the most difficult to control because they require intact oral motor strength, good coordination, and an intact swallow to prevent aspiration.

For the client who appears to have some ability to chew, the therapist should start with pureed and soft textures. Solid textures may be introduced next if the client is able to safely and efficiently swallow the pureed and soft food textures.[14,15,45,47] The following procedures should be completed after each swallow of food or liquid:

1. Using a fork, the therapist places a small amount (1/3 teaspoon) on the middle of the client's tongue. A fork allows the therapist greater control of food placement in the mouth.[14,16,37] Two to three bites are presented with each texture to check for fatigue in controlling that texture.

2. The therapist palpates for the swallow by placing the index finger at the hyoid notch, the second finger at the top of the larynx, and the third finger along the mid larynx. The therapist can feel the strength and smoothness of the swallow and can note whether the client requires subsequent or additional swallows to clear the bolus.[16,37] The therapist evaluates oral transit time by noting when food entered the mouth, when tongue movement was initiated, and when the elevation of the hyoid notch was felt, which indicates the beginning of the swallow process. The therapist can time the swallow from the time that hyoid movement begins to when laryngeal elevation occurs, indicating triggering of the swallow response.[37] A normal swallow takes only 1 second to complete for thin liquids.

3. The therapist asks the client to open the mouth to check for remaining food. Food is commonly seen in the lateral sulci, under the tongue, on the base of the tongue, and against the hard palate.[13,37] Food remaining in the mouth indicates decreased or impaired oral transit skills. The client who exhibits oral motor deficits has increasing difficulty with chewing, shaping a bolus, and channeling food backward as harder consistencies of food are introduced.[16]

4. The therapist asks the client to say, "ah." By listening carefully, the therapist can assess the client's voice quality and classify the sound production as strong, clear, gurgly, or gargling.[16,37]

A gurgly voice may result from a delayed swallow response, which allows material to collect in the larynx. The therapist asks the client to take a second "dry" swallow to clear any pooling of material. Asking the client to say, "ah" again enables the therapist to assess whether the voice quality remains gurgly or gargling for any length of time after the dry swallow. In addition, the therapist asks the client to pant for a few seconds. This will shake loose any material that may remain in the pyriform sinuses or valleculae.[14] If the voice is still gurgly, the therapist should be concerned with the possibility that material has come into contact with or is sitting on the vocal cords.[37]

If the client has significant coughing episodes, particularly before the therapist feels the initiation of the swallow (elevation of hyoid notch) with any consistency, the procedure should not be continued. When coughing is noted from food with a pureed consistency, the therapist may try a soft food such as a banana, if the client has good anterior to posterior tongue movement.[16] If problems persist, a videofluoroscopy may be indicated.

Although Mattias had frequent episodes of coughing during the bedside evaluation, no gurgly or raspy vocal quality was noted during speech. He is able to clear material from his vocal folds with a strong protective cough. He is able to swallow his secretions, but drooling was noted from the left corner of his mouth, which indicates diminished sensation.

A client with CNS damage and impaired sensation may have difficulty with a pureed food because it does not stay together as a bolus. The weight of soft foods, denser than a pureed food, may facilitate the triggering of the swallow response. If the client continues to cough even with soft foods, the swallow assessment should be discontinued. In this instance a videofluoroscopy swallow study is indicated. If a client is having difficulty at this level, only a pre-feeding intervention program should be considered. Because Mattias is able to safely manage a modified diet texture using positioning strategies and does not have signs and symptoms of aspiration, a videofluoroscopy was not deemed necessary.

A client who has difficulty managing solid consistencies may or may not have difficulty with liquids. To assess the client's swallow with liquids, the therapist starts with a thickened (thick) nectar, then a pure nectar (semithick), and finally a thin liquid such as water or juice (see Table 26-8). Small amounts of the liquid are placed on the middle of the client's tongue with a spoon. The therapist proceeds by following the four-step sequence described earlier for solid foods. The therapist assesses the client's skill at moving material from front to back, the time of oral transit and swallow, and the voice quality after each swallow. Each liquid consistency is assessed for two or three swallows to check for fatigability. If the client tolerates and swallows liquids by spoon without difficulty, the therapist assesses the ability to tolerate liquids from a cup or with a straw.[14] Again, the client's voice quality is checked following the swallow.

A client with a poor swallow may aspirate directly or pool liquids in the pyriform sinuses and valleculae, which, when full, overflow into the laryngeal vestibule and down into the trachea. If a client continues to have a gurgling or gargling voice after a second dry swallow or substantial coughing with any of the liquid consistencies, the assessment should be discontinued (Figure 26-3).

The therapist must also assess the client's ability to alternate between liquids and solids, which occurs naturally during meals. The therapist presents the client with an easily managed food bolus, followed by the safest type of liquid

tolerated, and then assesses the client for coughing when the consistency of the food is changed.

A client with a **tracheostomy** tube in place can be assessed as previously described. The same criteria must be met before the therapist assesses the client's eating and swallowing of food or liquids. The therapist must have a thorough understanding of the types of tracheostomy tubes and varied functions. The therapist must also be aware that clients who have had a tracheostomy tube, especially those on ventilation, for any length of time may experience changes in the swallowing mechanism such as muscle atrophy, decreased sensation, and laryngeal damage.[20]

Two main types of tracheostomy tubes exist: fenestrated and nonfenestrated (Figures 26-4 and 26-5).[23,37,52] A fenestrated tube is designed with an opening in the middle to allow increased air flow. This type of tube is frequently used

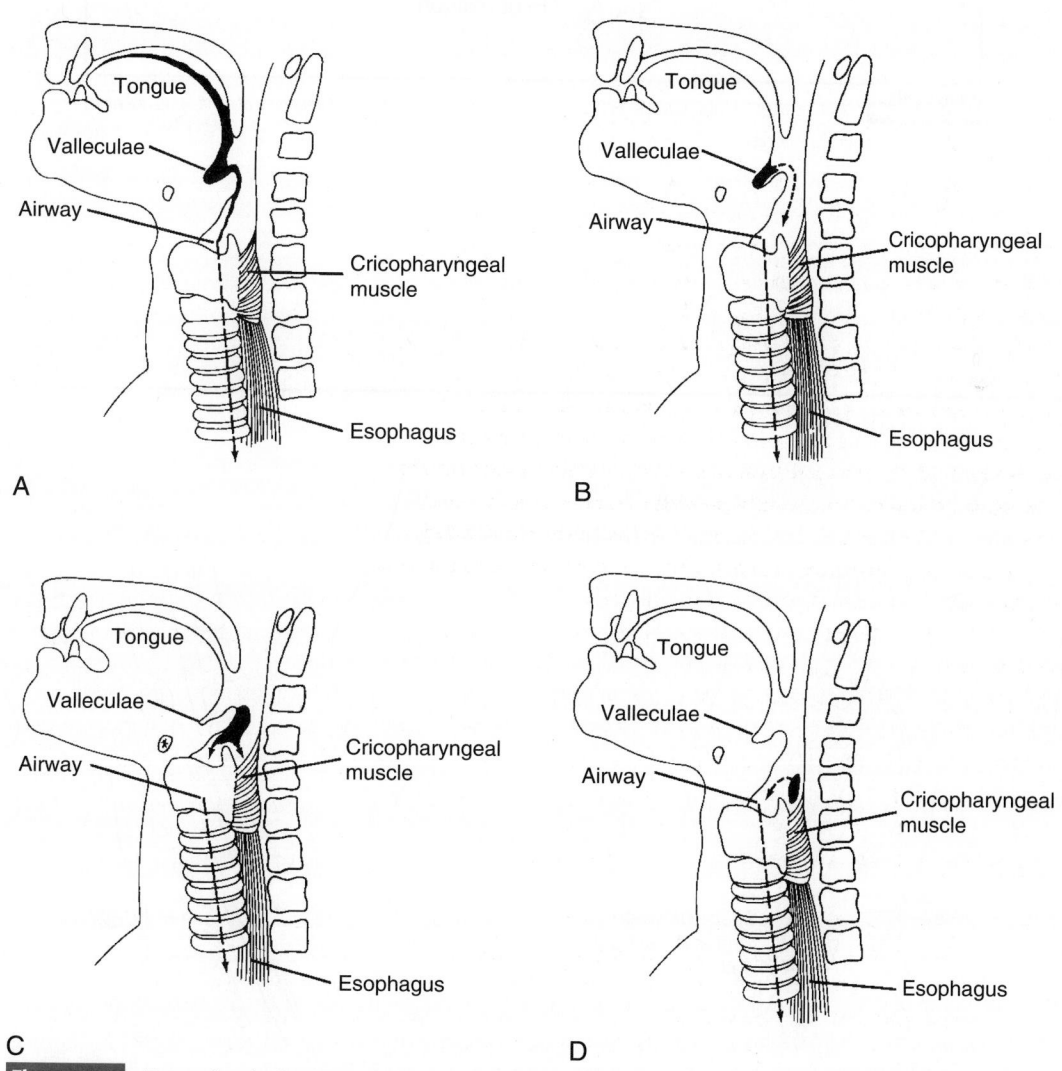

Figure 26-3 Types of aspiration. **A,** Aspiration before swallow caused by reduced tongue control. **B,** Aspiration before swallow caused by absent swallow response. **C,** Aspiration during swallow caused by reduced laryngeal closure. **D,** Aspiration after swallow caused by pooled material in pyriform sinuses overflowing into airway. (From Logemann J: *Evaluation and treatment of swallowing disorders,* San Diego, 1983, College-Hill Press.)

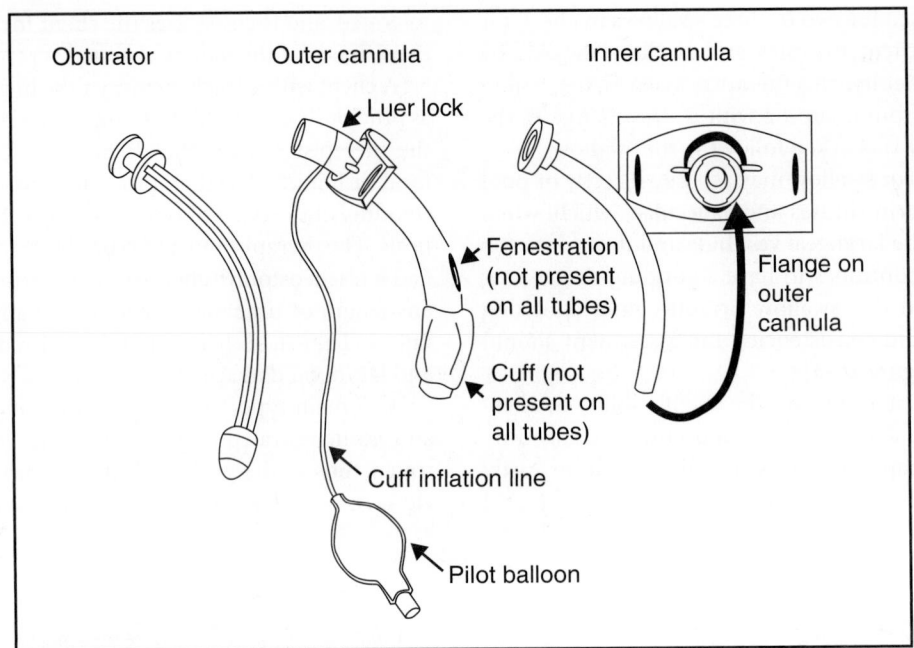

Figure 26-4 Tracheostomy tube components. (From Logemann J: *Evaluation and treatment of swallowing disorders,* Austin, Tex, 1998, ProEd Publications.)

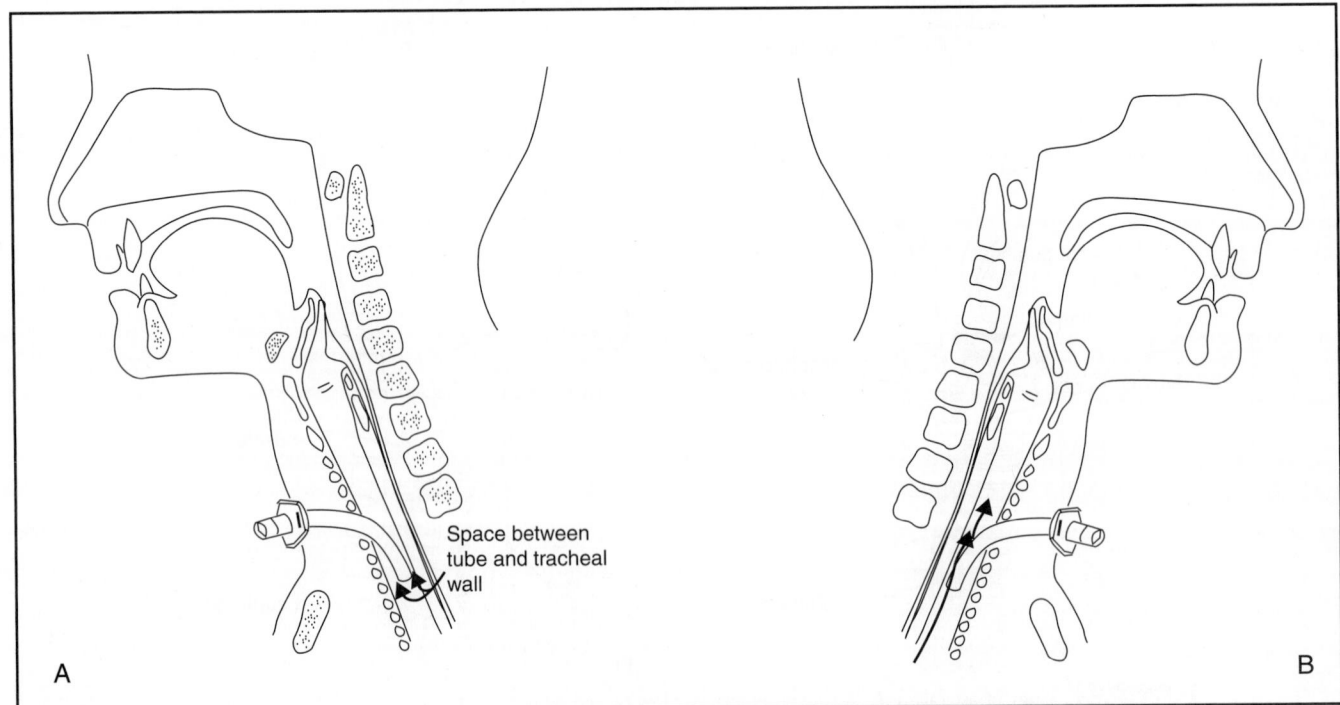

Figure 26-5 **A,** Midsagittal section of the head and neck showing the position of an uncuffed tracheostomy tube. **B,** Midsagittal section of the head and neck showing the passage of air between the tracheostomy tube and the tracheal wall. (From Logemann J: *Evaluation and treatment of swallowing disorders,* Austin, Tex, 1998, ProEd Publications.)

for clients being weaned from a tube because it allows a client to breathe nasally as he or she relearns a normal breathing pattern. Placement of an inner cannula piece into the tracheostomy tube allows the fenestrated opening to be closed off. With the inner cannula removed, a trachea button may be used to allow the client to talk. A nonfenestrated tube has no opening. A fenestrated tube is preferred for treating a client with dysphagia.

A tracheostomy tube may be cuffed or uncuffed. A cuffed tube has a balloon-like cuff surrounding the bottom of the tube.[23,37] When inflated, the cuff comes into contact with the trachea wall, preventing the aspiration of secretions into the airway. A cuffed tube is used in cases in which aspiration has occurred. The therapist should consult with the client's attending physician to see whether the client is still at risk of aspiration, or if it is safe to deflate the cuff for an eating and swallowing assessment.

Before the therapist presents any food to the client with a tracheostomy who has a fenestrated tube, the inner cannula should be in place. If the client has a cuffed tube, the therapist should thoroughly suction orally and around the cuff, present food, and slowly deflate the cuff while suctioning to prevent substances from penetrating the airway. The airway again needs to be suctioned orally and through the tracheostomy to ensure that all secretions have been cleared.[13,24,37] The nursing staff or a therapist who has been trained and is considered competent can perform the suctioning procedure.

After presenting food or liquids, the therapist should check for oral transit skills and swallow as previously described. Blue food coloring may be added to food or liquids presented orally if the client is not allergic to dyes and can help the therapist identify material in the trachea. Use of blue food coloring is contraindicated for critically ill clients.[22] The client can use a gloved finger to cover the trachea opening, to achieve a more normal tracheal pressure during the swallow.[37]

If the tracheostomy tube is cuffed, the cuff is slowly deflated. The airway is suctioned through the tracheostomy tube to determine whether any material entered the airway. The swallow assessment should not be continued if material is found in the trachea.[13,24,37] The presence of a tracheostomy tube may affect a client's swallow because secretions are increased and laryngeal mobility is decreased. When assessment is complete, the airway is thoroughly suctioned. The inner cannula is removed from the fenestrated tube, or the cuff inflated to the level prescribed by the physician.[23,24]

The client's performance on the swallowing assessment determines whether the client is able to participate in a feeding program and at which food and liquid consistencies he or she is able to function efficiently. The therapist must decide which consistency is the safest for the client. The safest consistency is that which the client is able to chew, move through the oral cavity, and swallow with the least risk of aspiration.

Indicators of Eating and Swallowing Dysfunction

The indicators of swallowing dysfunction include the following[13,16,37,46,48]:

1. Difficulty with bringing food to the mouth
2. The inability to shape food into a bolus
3. Coughing or throat clearing before, during, or after the swallow
4. Gurgling voice quality
5. Changes in breathing pattern
6. Delayed or absent swallow response
7. Poor cough
8. Reflux of food after meals

The presence of any swallowing dysfunction can lead to aspiration pneumonia. The following are acute symptoms of aspiration occurring immediately after the swallow[16,23,24,48]:

1. Any change in the client's color, particularly if the airway is obstructed
2. Prolonged coughing
3. Gurgling voice and extreme breathiness or loss of voice

During the 24 hours immediately after the swallow, the therapist and medical staff must observe the client for additional signs of aspiration. These may be a nasal drip, an increase in profuse drooling of a clear liquid, and temperatures of 100° F or greater, which may not have been evident during the clinical examination.[16,26,37] If aspiration pneumonia develops, the client must be reevaluated for a change in diet levels or taken off the feeding program, if necessary. An alternative feeding method may be necessary to ensure adequate hydration and nutrition.

INSTRUMENTAL ASSESSMENT

Instrumental assessments are important techniques for assessing a client's swallow. They are performed in conjunction with the clinical bedside assessment to rule out or identify silent aspiration. Silent aspiration may not always be accurately identified solely through a clinical bedside assessment. Between 40% and 60% of clients with neurological impairment who have dysphagia are found to be silent aspirators during instrumental assessment.[37,44,48] Aspiration can occur before the swallow because of poor tongue control, pooled material in the valleculae, or a delayed or absent swallow response. Poor laryngeal closure can result in aspiration during the swallow. Aspiration after the swallow is the result of pooled material in the pyriform sinuses or in the valleculae overflowing into the trachea. Knowing the reason why a client is aspirating can help the OT plan appropriate intervention.[37,38] Instrumental evaluations provide valuable information in a window of time. This information must be considered as part of the complete evaluation process, including the bedside assessment and client performance during intervention sessions and meal activities.[49,50]

The two most common instrumental evaluations used, videofluoroscopy (VSS) and fiberoptic endoscopy (FEES), are described below.

ETHICAL CONSIDERATIONS

Instrumental assessment procedures require advanced knowledge and training in techniques, purpose, and indications for use. Only OTs who have these advanced skills may use instrumental evaluation procedures.[6]

ASSESSMENT WITH VIDEOFLUOROSCOPY

Videofluoroscopy study (VSS) is a radiographic procedure using a modified barium swallow recorded on videotape.[37] This instrument allows the therapist to assess the stages of the swallow and the ability of the client to swallow various consistencies of food textures. The VSS allows the therapist to see the client's jaw and tongue movement, measure the transit times of the oral and pharyngeal stages, observe the swallow, note any residue in the valleculae and the pyriform sinuses, and check for any aspiration. With videofluoroscopy, the therapist can determine the anatomic or physiological cause of aspiration. Various compensatory techniques may also be assessed to determine if the airway can be protected, which may allow the therapist to initiate a feeding program.[37,38] Videofluoroscopy, used in conjunction with the clinical assessment, may be used to select appropriate intervention techniques and the safest diet level to help the client achieve a safe swallow.

A fluoroscopy machine has three components: a fluoroscopy tube, a monitor for viewing the picture, and an elevation table or platform. A television videocassette records the image. Other necessary pieces of equipment normally available in a radiology department are lead-lined aprons, lead-lined gloves, and foam positioning wedges.[37,38] Because it may not be possible to lower the fluoroscopy machine enough to view a client seated in a wheelchair, a special plywood seat system or wheelchair platform with a ramp may be needed. Commercially made seating systems are also available.

Three people are involved in performing videofluoroscopy: the radiologist, the OT, and the video technician. The client should be positioned to allow a lateral view, with the fluoroscopy tube focused on the lips, hard palate, and posterior pharyngeal wall. The lateral view is most frequently used because it allows the therapist to evaluate all four stages of the swallow. This view clearly shows the presence of aspiration. A posterior-anterior view also may be needed to evaluate asymmetry in the vocal cords and pooling of the valleculae or pyriform sinuses.

During a videofluoroscopy assessment, the therapist presents the client with food or liquid to which barium paste or powder has been added.[14,37,38] The therapist mixes or spreads small amounts of paste or powder onto or into each food or liquid consistency. Premixing the consistencies with the barium paste or powder prevents time-consuming interruptions during the actual assessment procedure.

Food and liquids are presented in the same sequence used for the clinical assessment. Starting with pureed foods, the client is given $1/2$ teaspoon at a time of each consistency and asked to swallow when instructed.[14] Liquids are tested separately, beginning with the thickened substance. Material is given in small amounts to reduce the risks of aspiration, if it occurs. An experienced dysphagia therapist may choose to use only foods or liquids that the client had difficulty with during the clinical examination, rather than to proceed through the entire sequence. The therapist continues to present each consistency to determine if the client can swallow safely and efficiently without aspirating. If aspiration occurs, the therapist should try a compensatory strategy and re-assess with the same texture. If aspiration occurs while using the strategy, then discontinue the assessment with that texture.

The videofluoroscopy procedure can also be used to observe for fatigue of the oral or pharyngeal musculature or the swallow reflex. The client is asked to take repeated, or *serial*, swallows of solids and liquids. The therapist should also assess the client's ability to control mixed consistencies of solids and liquids such as soups with broth and bits of vegetables, as well as the clients and to alternate between solids and liquids. The solid and liquid consistency that the client manages without aspiration is selected as the starting point for eating and swallowing intervention. A client aspirating on pureed or soft foods is not suited for an oral program. The client who is aspirating thick liquids is not a candidate for liquid intake.

VSS is a valuable tool to be used in conjunction with the clinical examination. It can provide the therapist with additional information regarding the client's difficulties. By identifying silent aspirators, the therapist can feel comfortable with the decisions made in determining a course of treatment. Because VSS exposes the client to radiation, the therapist should exercise good clinical judgment when deciding whether VSS is needed. The therapist must keep in mind that VSS records the client's performance in an isolated instance and is not a conclusive indicator of the client's potential ability in a feeding program. If a client continues to progress without difficulty, a second VSS is not necessary. A second VSS may be needed, however, to reevaluate a client who shows signs of readiness to participate in a feeding program or to determine whether a client can progress to thin liquids.[16,37] Contraindications to performing VSS include rapid progress of the client, a poor level of awareness or poor cognitive status, oral stage problems only, and the physical inability of the client to undergo the test.

When the results of a VSS test are documented, foods that were presented, problems that occurred at each stage, and the number of swallows taken to clear the food or liquid are recorded. The therapist also should document any facilitation techniques that worked effectively.[14,37,38]

ASSESSMENT WITH FIBEROPTIC ENDOSCOPY

Fiberoptic endoscopy (FEES) is an alternative technique used to assess swallowing. This technique is valuable when it is not possible for the client to participate in VSS or is used as a follow-up assessment for the client making rapid progress. It can be repeated as often as necessary without exposure to radiation.[33,36,45]

The equipment needed for a FEES includes a flexible fiberoptic nasopharyngolaryngoscope, a portable light source, a video camera, a video recorder, and a television monitor. Placed on a rolling cart, this system can be brought directly to the client. The therapist first topically anesthetizes one nasal fossa. After anesthetized, the therapist passes a flexible fiberoptic tube through the nasal fossa, positioning the tip just above the palate.[33] The therapist initially examines the oral cavity and swallowing structures. Food and liquids are then introduced as described previously. The therapist notes bolus formation, tongue movement, swallow, and aspiration, if it occurs. The FEES allows the therapist to see the pharynx and the larynx before and after the swallow, assessing for the possibility of aspiration.[36]

The results of a thorough assessment determine the course of intervention to increase a client's ability to eat. Upon completion of the entire dysphagia assessment, the therapist should clearly document the client's major problems, goals and objectives, and intervention plan. The objectives should be concise and measurable. The intervention plan should include the type of diet needed, the training and facilitation that the client requires, positioning techniques to be used during feeding, and the type of supervision that must be provided. Recommendations should be communicated to the appropriate nursing and medical staff.

INTERVENTION

Because a client may display more than one problem at each stage of deglutition, the intervention program for eating and swallowing problems is multifaceted. Intervention for the client with dysphagia involves trunk and head positioning and control, feeding skills, oral motor skills, and swallowing retraining. Perceptual and cognitive deficits that interfere with eating are also addressed. Effective intervention may require the OT to devote 35% to 45% of the client's total daily intervention time to oral motor and swallowing retraining.[26] Clients with severe problems can require up to 6 months of intense intervention before they reach optimal recovery. In preparing an intervention program for a person with acquired dysphagia, the therapist must first identify the symptoms and causes of the deficits.[7,9,16,19,37,39]

GOALS

The overall goals of OT in the remediation of eating and swallowing dysfunction are as follows*:

1. Facilitation of appropriate positioning during eating
2. Improvement of motor control at each stage of swallow, through normalization of tone and the facilitation of quality movement
3. Maintenance of an adequate nutritional intake
4. Prevention of aspiration
5. Reestablishment of oral eating to the safest, optimum level

TEAM MANAGEMENT

Because of the complex nature of dysphagia treatment, the client's optimal progress is facilitated by development of a team approach. The dysphagia team should consist of the client's attending physician, the OT, the dietitian, the nurse, the physical therapist, the speech-language pathologist, the radiologist, and the client's family. Each professional contributes expertise toward client improvement. All members of the dysphagia team should have a thorough working knowledge of treating clients with dysphagia. Interdepartmental inservice education is frequently required so that team members have a similar frame of reference.

The OT's role is to assess the client and implement the appropriate course of intervention. The OT is also responsible for coordinating the team effort, which includes obtaining physician's orders as needed, communicating with all other team members and staff, providing family education to ensure proper follow-through, and selecting the appropriate diet. The OT initiates changes in the client's program whenever necessary.[7,9,16,47]

The attending physician's role involves the medical management of the client's health and safety. The physician oversees all decisions regarding treatment for diet level selection, oral and non-oral feeding procedures, and the progression of treatment as recommended by the team. The physician should reinforce the course of treatment with the client and the family.[24,26,37,47]

The dietitian is responsible for monitoring the client's caloric intake. He or she makes recommendations to ensure that the client receives a balanced, nutritional diet in accordance with the medical condition. The dietitian is involved in suggesting types of feeding formulas for the non-oral client. Diet supplements to augment oral intake may be recommended. In conjunction with the OT, the dietitian ensures that the proper food and liquid consistencies are served to the client. Additional training may be necessary for the dietary staff because dysphagia diets vary from traditional medical diets.

---

*References 3,4,7,8,16,21,37.

The client's physical therapist is involved in muscle reeducation and tone normalization techniques of the trunk, neck, and face. The client receives treatment in balance, strength, and control. The physical therapist is involved in increasing the client's pulmonary status for breath support, chest expansion, and cough.[1]

The role of the speech-language pathologist involves the reeducation of the oral and laryngeal musculature used in speaking and voice production. Because these muscles are also used in swallowing, a therapist with dysphagia experience may participate in oral motor and swallowing training during pre-feeding and feeding sessions.[26]

The nurse is another key member of the dysphagia team. The nursing staff is responsible for monitoring the client's medical and nutritional status. The nurse usually is the first to notice changes in the client's condition, such as an elevated temperature; an increase in pulmonary congestion; and an increase in secretions, which indicates swallowing dysfunction.[24] The nurse informs the physician and OT of these changes. The client's oral and fluid intake is recorded in the nursing notes, and the nurse notifies the dysphagia team when the client's nutritional status is adequate or inadequate. Supplemental tube feedings that have been ordered by the physician are administered by the nursing staff, which also provides oral hygiene, tracheostomy care, and supervision for appropriate clients during meals.[1,14,24,37]

The client's family is included on the team to act as program supporters. The family frequently underestimates the danger of aspiration. Therefore, education of the family and the client must occur, beginning with the first day of assessment. The family and client should understand which food consistencies are safe to eat and which foods must be avoided.[3,45]

The roles of the team members may vary from one treatment facility to another. Designated roles must be clearly defined to ensure a coordinated team approach. Therapists who are responsible for direct treatment should have advanced knowledge and training in the treatment procedures.

POSITIONING

Proper positioning is essential when working with the client who has dysphagia. The client should be positioned symmetrically with normal alignment between the head, neck, trunk, and pelvis. The ideal position is as follows[4,8,9,11,19]:

1. The client is seated on a firm surface, such as a chair.
2. The client's feet are flat on the floor.
3. The client's knees are at 90-degree flexion.
4. There is equal weight bearing on both ischial tuberosities of the hips.
5. The client's trunk is flexed slightly forward (100-degree hip flexion) with the back straight.
6. Both of the client's arms are placed forward on the table.
7. The head is erect, in midline, and the chin is slightly tucked.

For the client who may be restricted to bed but is able to sit in a semi-reclined position, the same positioning principles apply: equal weight bearing on both ischial tuberosities for the hips, the trunk flexed slightly forward (100-degree hip flexion) with the back straight, knees slightly flexed, and both arms placed forward on a bedside table. The head and neck should be aligned appropriately to reduce the risk of aspiration.

For the client who must remain supine in bed, oral feeding is generally contraindicated. If the client can be positioned sidelying in bed, appropriate head and neck alignment must be achieved before assessment of feeding skills. The client's knees and hips should be slightly flexed and trunk aligned while supported in the sidelying position. The use of additional pillows, rolls, and supports may be required to maintain the appropriate alignment.

Mattias was able to sit in a chair and responded well to physical prompts to sit aligned with both arms supported on the tabletop. Although he was concerned that resting his arms on the table was impolite, his therapist suggested using a chair with armrests. He typically would slightly extend his neck when attempting to swallow foods, and using the technique of a slight chin tuck diminished the coughing and choking episodes when he ate textured foods.

Figure 26-6 shows two different supportive positions that allow the therapist to help the client maintain head control. Correct positioning allows more appropriate muscular action, which thereby facilitates quality motor control and function of the facial musculature, jaw and tongue movement, and the swallowing process, all of which minimize the potential for aspiration.

A client who has difficulty moving into the correct position or maintaining the position presents a challenge to the OT. A more careful analysis of the client is needed to determine the major problem preventing good positioning. Poor positioning may be a result of decreased control or balance secondary to hypertonicity or hypotonicity or poor body awareness in space secondary to perceptual dysfunction (Figure 26-7).[4,11,16,19] After the cause is identified, the therapist can treat it accordingly. Specific treatment suggestions are described later in this chapter. To assist in maintaining trunk position, the therapist may consider the use of an adaptive lateral trunk support. Seating the client at a table provides forward trunk support.

ORAL HYGIENE

Oral care by nursing and therapy team members prevents gum disease, the accumulation of secretions, the development of plaque, and the aspiration of food particles that remain after eating. The appropriate therapy team member begins the oral hygiene process by positioning the client upright and symmetrically. The client who is apprehensive or who displays a hypersensitive oral cavity may first require preparation by the therapist. Preparation steps may include

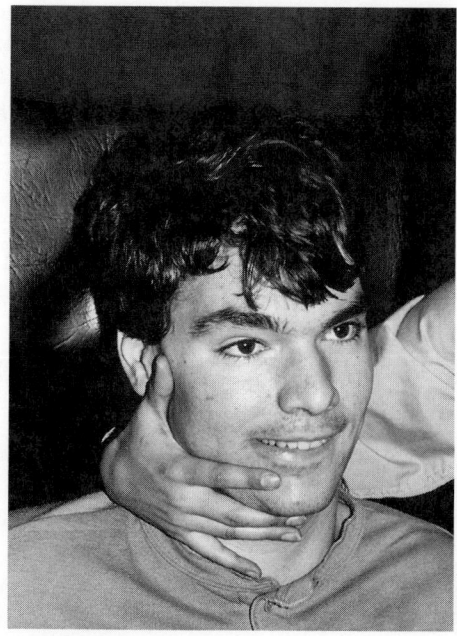
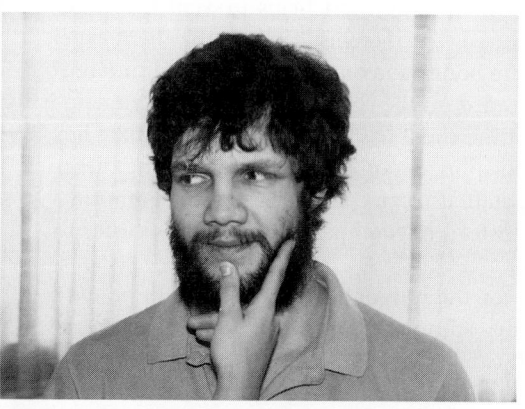

A   B

Figure 26-6   Head control. **A,** Side hold position for clients requiring maximum to moderate assistance. **B,** Front hold position for clients requiring minimal assistance. (Courtesy Meadowbrook Neurological Care Center, San Jose, Calif, 1988.)

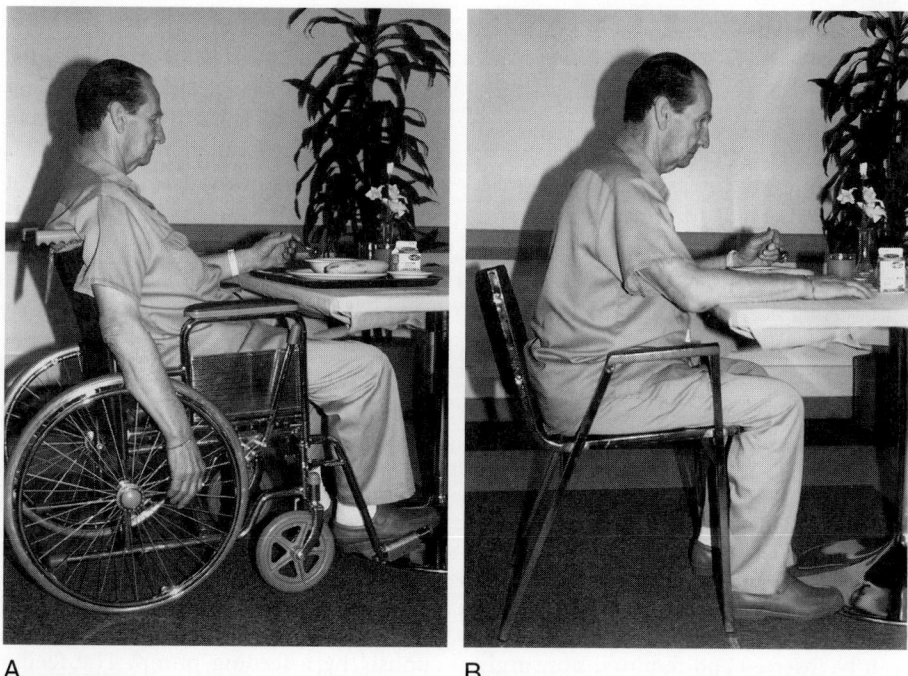

A   B

Figure 26-7   Positioning of the client with dysphagia. **A,** Incorrect positioning. **B,** Correct positioning. (Courtesy Meadowbrook Neurological Care Center, San Jose, Calif, 1988.)

firmly stroking outside the client's mouth or lips with the client's or therapist's finger. Sensitive gums can also be firmly rubbed, preparing the client for the toothbrush.

For cleaning purposes, the mouth can be divided into four quadrants. A toothbrush with a small head and soft bristles is used to clean each quadrant, starting with the top teeth and moving from front to back. When brushing the bottom teeth, the therapist brushes from back to front. Next, holding the toothbrush at a vertical angle, the therapist brushes the inside teeth downward from gums to teeth.

Finally, the cutting surfaces of the teeth are brushed. An electric toothbrush can be more effective, if the client can tolerate it.

After each procedure the client is allowed to dispose of secretions. After brushing, the client is carefully assisted in rinsing the mouth. If the client can tolerate thin liquids, small amounts of water can be given. Having the client flex the chin slightly toward the chest helps prevent the water from being swallowed. The therapist can help the client expel the water, by placing one hand on each cheek and simultaneously pushing inward on the cheeks while the chin remains slightly tucked. If the client has no ability to manipulate liquids, a dampened sponge toothette can be used. The therapist and nursing staff also can consider using small amounts of baking soda instead of toothpaste because it is easier to rinse out.[16,19]

Oral hygiene for the non-oral or oral client can be used as effective sensory stimulation of touch, texture, temperature, and taste. It can be used to facilitate beginning jaw and tongue movements and to encourage an automatic swallow.[17] Lack of oral stimulation over a prolonged time leads to hypersensitivity within the oral cavity. Clients who display poor tongue movement and who are eating frequently have food remaining on their teeth or dentures or between the cheek and gum. A client with decreased sensation is not aware of the remaining food. A thorough cleaning should follow each time the client eats.

NON-ORAL FEEDINGS

A client who is aspirating more than 10% of food or liquid consistencies or whose combined oral and pharyngeal transit time is more than 10 seconds, regardless of positioning or facilitation techniques, is an inappropriate candidate for oral eating.[17,37] Such a client needs a non-oral nutritional method until eating and drinking capability is regained. Clients who lack the endurance to take in sufficient calories also may require non-oral feedings or supplements.

The two most common procedures for non-oral feedings involve the NG tube and the G tube.[23,24] The NG tube is passed through the nostril, through the nasopharynx, and down through the pharynx and esophagus to rest in the stomach.[24] The NG tube is a temporary measure that should not be used for longer than 1 month.[37] Several advantages exist to using the NG tube:

1. The NG tube can be inserted and removed nonsurgically, if necessary.
2. The NG tube allows the physician to choose between continuous or bolus feedings (a feeding that runs no more than 40 minutes).
3. The NG tube allows the therapist to begin pre-feeding and feeding training while the tube is in place.
4. The NG tube provides full nutrition and hydration if necessary and keeps the digestive system active, which is important for moving to oral feedings.

Some disadvantages of the NG tube also exist[24,27,37,50]:

1. It can desensitize the cough reflex and the swallow response.
2. It can interfere with a positioning program (the client needs to be elevated to 30 degrees during feeding).
3. It can increase aspiration risk, pharyngeal secretions, and nasal reflux.
4. It can decrease the client's self-esteem.

Placement of a G tube is a minor surgical procedure. The client receives a local anesthetic, and a small skin incision is made to create an external opening in the abdominal wall for a percutaneous endoscopic gastrostomy (PEG) procedure. A tube is passed through the opening into the stomach. Several advantages exist to using a G tube:

1. Using a G tube allows the physician to choose between continuous or bolus feedings.
2. The G tube provides full nutrition and hydration if necessary and keeps the digestive system active, which is important for moving to oral feedings.
3. It allows the therapist to begin a pre-feeding or feeding program while the tube is in place.
4. It carries less risk of reflux and aspiration.
5. It does not irritate or desensitize the swallowing mechanisms.
6. It does not interfere with a positioning program.
7. It can be removed when the client no longer requires supplemental feedings or liquids.

Some disadvantages exist to using a G tube[24,27,52]:

1. The stoma site can become irritated or inflamed.
2. The family can perceive the tube as being permanent.

A G tube is the ideal choice for the client who may require tube feeding or supplemental feedings for longer than 1 month.[17,37]

A commercially prepared liquid formula that provides complete nutrition usually is used for tube feedings. Many types and brands are available. The physician and dietitian determine which formula is best suited to the client. The feedings are administered by either a bolus or a continuous method. A bolus feeding takes 20 to 40 minutes to run through either the NG tube or the G tube. It can be gravity assisted or run through a feeding pump. Bolus feedings can be scheduled at numerous times throughout a 24-hour period.

Continuous feedings, which may be better tolerated by the client, are smaller amounts that are administered continuously by a feeding pump. The feeding pump can be set to regulate the rate at which the formula is dripped into the tube. A disadvantage of continuous feedings is that the client is less mobile because the pump always accompanies the client.

While the client is on a non-oral program, the OT concentrates efforts on retraining the client in oral motor control and swallowing. The pre-feeding retraining can occur whether the client is on bolus or on continuous feedings. As a client begins to eat enough to require an adjustment in the intake amount of formula, however, bolus feedings become the preferred method. A bolus feeding allows the therapist to work with the physician to wean the client from formula feeding. A bolus feeding can be held back before a feeding session, and the number of bolus feedings per day can be decreased as the client improves. If satisfied by the tube feedings, the client will not have an appetite and will have decreased motivation to eat.

As the client improves, oral intake can be increased, and the formula feeding can be used to supplement the client's caloric intake. An accurate calorie count, determined by recording the percentage of oral intake, assists the physician in decreasing the calories received through the tube feedings as the client begins to meet nutritional needs orally. If the client has progressed only enough to handle solids, the NG or G tube can be used to meet the client's total or partial fluid requirements. Either tube can be removed when the client is safely able to eat and drink enough to meet caloric and fluid needs.[1,14,37]

ORAL FEEDINGS

For a client to be an appropriate candidate for oral feeding, several criteria must be met. The therapist can use the criteria for evaluating a client's swallow with foods or liquids. To participate in an oral feeding program, a client must (1) be alert, (2) be able to maintain adequate trunk and head positioning with assistance, (3) have beginning tongue control, (4) manage secretions with minimal drooling, and (5) have a reflexive cough. The therapist needs to identify the food or liquid consistency that is most appropriate for the client. The safest consistency with which to initiate the oral program is one that enables the client to complete the oral and pharyngeal stages combined in less than 10 seconds and to swallow with minimal aspiration (10% or less).[37] The ultimate goal of an oral feeding program is for the client to achieve swallowing without any aspiration.

DIET SELECTION

A dysphagia diet must be carefully selected to reflect the needs of the client. In general, foods chosen for dysphagia diets should (1) be uniform in consistency and texture, (2) provide sufficient density and volume, (3) remain cohesive, (4) provide pleasant taste and temperature, and (5) be easily removed or suctioned when necessary.[16,17,24] The following foods are contraindicated for dysphagia diets: foods with multiple textures, such as vegetable soup and salads; fibrous and stringy vegetables, meats, and fruits; crumbly and flaky foods; foods that liquefy, such as gelatin and ice cream; and foods with skins and seeds.[14]

The OT should work closely with the dietitian to identify the appropriate dysphagia diet for the client. Using established dysphagia diets develops a standard for consistently describing which food textures and what foods are allowed

at each level. This consistency is critical for client safety. Because many different disciplines are involved in the care of an individual with dysphagia, standardized language is needed when describing food and liquid textures to facilitate the diagnostic and nutritional management of the client.[2] The National Dysphagia Diet Task Force (NDDTF) has developed a science-based, multi-level, standardized diet for clients with dysphagia. Once the appropriate diet level has been determined by the therapist, all members of the team, including the family and the client, should be educated about which foods are acceptable in each level, and which foods should be avoided to ensure the client's safety. Liquid diet levels should also be established. When requesting a dysphagia diet, the therapist should specify both levels desired, liquid and solid, because a client may handle each differently.

DIET PROGRESSION

Tables 26-5 through 26-7 list foods in three progressive dysphagia levels. These levels reflect the food texture levels recommended by the National Dysphagia Diet Task Force.[1,2,14,17,45] After mastering Level 3 the client may progress to a regular diet. Level 1 foods are pureed. This food group is best for persons with little or no jaw or tongue control, a moderately delayed swallow, and a decreased pharyngeal transit, resulting in pooling in the valleculae and pyriform sinuses. This diet is designed for clients who have moderate to severe dysphagia and who have a reduced ability to protect their airway.[2,16,37] Pureed foods move more slowly past the faucial arches and into the pharynx, which allows time for the swallow response to trigger. Pureed foods should be homogenous, pudding-like in consistency. No coarse textures, raw fruits or vegetables, or nuts are allowed. Any foods that require mastication are not allowed.[2] Because pureed foods cannot be formed into an adequate bolus, they offer little opportunity for increasing oral motor control.[16] Level 1 foods are best used only to increase the client's oral intake. The client should be advanced to the next level as soon as possible. Mattias agreed to eat pureed foods to increase his caloric intake and joked with his wife that his OT gave him permission to eat ice cream. He was progressed to textured foods (Level 2) but continued to use the pureed foods as a supplement because of the effort required to eat a sufficient quantity of textured foods.

Level 2 items are soft foods that stay together as a cohesive bolus; thus, the possibility of particles spilling into the airway is decreased. Level 2 foods are best for clients with a beginning rotary chew, enough tongue control with assistance to propel food back toward the pharynx, and a minimally delayed swallow.[16,17] Mechanical soft foods reduce the risk of aspiration in individuals who have both a motor and a sensory loss, which affects the start of the swallow response.[8,25,48] Mechanical soft foods with a density provide increased proprioceptive input throughout the mouth. These foods also stay together as a cohesive bolus rather than crumbling and falling uncontrolled into the airway. Because clients who are

TABLE 26-5   **Dysphagia, Level 1: Dysphagia Pureed**

Food Groups	Recommended	Avoid
Cereals and breads	Pureed bread mixes, pregelled slurried breads, pancakes, or French toast Smooth, homogenous cooked cereals, creamed wheat or rice, Malto Meal. Cereals should have a pudding-like consistency	All other breads, rolls, crackers, muffins, etc. All dry cereals and any cereals with lumps Oatmeal
Eggs	Custard, pureed eggs	All others
Fruits	Pureed fruits or well-mashed bananas Applesauce	All others – Any whole fruits (fresh, frozen, canned)
Potatoes and starches	Mashed potatoes with gravy, pureed potatoes with gravy, butter, margarine, or sour cream Pureed well-cooked noodles, pasta or rice. Must be pureed to a smooth, homogenous consistency	All others
Soups	Soups that have been pureed in a blender or strained. May need to be thickened. Thickened, strained cream soups (to a consistency of pureed vegetables)	Soups that have chunks or lumps
Vegetables	Pureed vegetables without lumps, chunks, pulp, or seeds	All vegetables that have not been pureed
Meat and meat substitutes	Pureed meat Pureed poultry with gravy Softened tofu mixed with moisture Hummus or other pureed legume spread	Whole or ground meats, fish, or poultry Cottage cheese, cheese Peanut butter, unless pureed into foods
Desserts	Smooth puddings, custards, yogurt, pureed desserts and soufflés	Ices, gelatins, frozen juice bars, bread and rice pudding, yogurt with fruit All other desserts **These foods are considered thin liquids and should be avoided if thin liquids are restricted.** Frozen malts, milk shakes, frozen yogurt, ice cream, sherbet, gelatin
Fats	Butter, margarine, strained gravy, sour cream, mayonnaise, cream cheese, whipped topping	All fats with chunky additives

Data from American Dietetic Association: *National dysphagia diet: standardization for optimal care*, Chicago, 2002, American Dietetic Association; American Occupational Therapy Association: *AOTA resource guide: feeding and dysphagia*, Rockville, Md, 1997; Avery-Smith W: An occupational therapist coordinated dysphagia program, *Occup Ther Pract* 3:10, 1998; Community Hospital of Los Gatos, Rehabilitation Services: *Dysphagia protocol*, Los Gatos, Calif, 2003; Curran J: Nutritional considerations. In Groher M, editor: *Dysphagia: diagnosis and management*, ed 3, Newton, Mass, 1997, Butterworth-Heinemann Publishers; Rader T, Rende B: *Swallowing disorders: what families should know*, Tucson, Ariz, 1993, Communication Skill Builders Publishers.

at this diet level display improved tongue control, the swallow response may be triggered faster as the back of the tongue elevates toward the hard palate. For the client who is just beginning to chew, mashing the food with a fork enhances the ability to keep the food together as a bolus.[16]

Level 3, dysphagia advanced or chopped ground food items, requires chewing, controlled bolus formation, and a fair or delayed swallow. This food group offers a wider variety of consistencies. Meats should be finely cut to facilitate a controlled swallow. Smaller particles are less likely to obstruct the airway and are less of a health risk than large pieces, if minimal aspiration occurs. These foods are safer than items found on a regular diet yet require work on the part of the client. Level 3 foods work well for the client who has minimal problems with jaw or tongue control and a mildly delayed but intact swallow response. The client who has reached a

Level 3 diet needs to be concerned with a delayed swallow only when fatigued. After 3 weeks of intervention, Mattias progressed to a Level 3 diet, which greatly increased the variety of foods he could eat and increased his overall satisfaction with meal selections. He continued to support caloric intake using foods from both Level 1 and 2 because of motor coordination and fatigue issues. His daughter selected foods for the wedding meal that required minimal chewing including baked sole and crème brulee in addition to the wedding cake.

When a client is ready to progress to the next diet level, the therapist can adjust the meals by requesting one or two items from the higher group, which enables assessment at the new level. This technique is also appropriate for clients who become fatigued. The client is thus able to work with the therapist on the harder food item first and continue the meal with foods that are easier. The therapist also may consider

TABLE 26-6 Dysphagia, Level 2: Dysphagia Mechanically Altered Characteristics (Mechanical Soft)

Food Groups	Recommended	Avoid
Cereals and breads	Cooked refined cereals with little texture (e.g., oatmeal) Slightly moistened dry cereals with little texture (e.g., Corn Flakes, Rice Krispies) Soft pancakes with syrup French toast without crust Graham crackers	Very coarse cooked cereals that may contain seeds or nuts Whole-grain dry or coarse cereals All others
Eggs	Poached, scrambled or soft eggs (egg yolks should be moist and mashable with butter, not runny) Souffles–may have small chunks	Hard cooked or fried eggs
Fruits	Soft canned or cooked fruits without seeds or skill Soft, ripe bananas Baked apple (no skin)	Fruits with seeds, coarse skins, fibers; fruits with pits, raisins, grapes, all raw fruits except those listed
Potatoes and starches	Well-cooked, moistened, boiled, baked, or mashed potatoes Well-cooked noodles in sauce	Potato skins and chips, fried potatoes, rice
Soups	Soups with easy to chew or easy to swallow soft meats or vegetables (particle sizes $<\frac{1}{2}$ inch) Cream soups	Soups that have large chunks of meat or vegetables Soups with rice, corn, peas
Vegetables	Soft, well-cooked vegetables; should be easily mashed with a fork	All raw vegetables Cooked corn and peas Broccoli, cabbage, brussels sprouts, asparagus, or other fibrous, non-tender cooked vegetables
Meat and meat substitutes	Moistened ground or cooked meat, poultry, or fish. May be served with gravy Casseroles without rice Soft-moist lasagna, moist macaroni and cheese Moist meatballs, meat loaf, or fish loaf Tuna or egg salad without large chunks, celery, or onion Cottage cheese, smooth quiche Tofu All meats or protein substitutes should be served with sauces or moistened to help maintain cohesiveness in the oral cavity	Dry, tough meats (such as bacon, sausage, hot dogs) Peanut butter Dry casseroles Pizza Sandwiches All other cheeses
Desserts	Pudding and custard Soft fruit pies with bottom crust only Crisps and cobblers without seeds or nuts Canned fruit (excluding pineapple) Soft, moist cakes with icing Pregelled cookies or soft moist cookies "dunked" in milk, coffee, or other liquid	Dry, coarse cakes or cookies Anything with nuts, seeds, coconut, pineapple, or dried fruit Rice or bread pudding
Fats	Butter, margarine, strained gravy, sour cream, mayonnaise, cream cheese, whipped topping	All fats with chunky additives

Data from American Dietetic Association: *National dysphagia diet: standardization for optimal care*, Chicago, 2002, American Dietetic Association; American Occupational Therapy Association: *AOTA resource guide: feeding and dysphagia*, Rockville, Md, 1997; Avery-Smith W: An occupational therapist coordinated dysphagia program, *Occup Ther Pract* 3:10, 1998; Community Hospital of Los Gatos, Rehabilitation Services: *Dysphagia protocol*, Los Gatos, Calif, 2003; Curran J: Nutritional considerations. In Groher M, editor: *Dysphagia: diagnosis and management*, ed 3, Newton, Mass, 1997, Butterworth-Heinemann Publishers; Rader T, Rende B: *Swallowing disorders: what families should know*, Tucson, Ariz, 1993, Communication Skill Builders Publishers.

TABLE 26-7 **Dysphagia, Level 3: Dysphagia Advanced**

Food Groups	Recommended	Avoid
Cereals and breads	All well-moistened cereals Any well-moistened breads, muffins, pancakes, waffles, etc. Add butter, margarine, syrup, etc., to moisten	Coarse or dry cereals such as shredded wheat Dry toast, crackers Crusty bread such as French bread, hard rolls Popcorn
Eggs	Eggs, prepared any way	
Fruits	All canned and cooked fruit Soft, peeled fresh fruit, without seeds Soft berries	Difficult to chew fresh fruits such as apples or pears Stringy, high-pulp fruits such as papaya or pineapple Uncooked dried fruit Fruit with seeds or coarse skins
Potatoes and starches	All, including rice and fried potatoes	Potato skins Tough, crisp-fried potatoes
Soups	All soups except those on the Avoid list	Soups with tough meats Corn or clam chowders Soups with large chunks (>1 inch)
Vegetables	All cooked, tender vegetables Shredded lettuce	All raw vegetables, except shredded lettuce Cooked corn Non-tender, stringy, cooked vegetables
Meat and meat substitutes	Thin-sliced tender or ground meats and poultry Well-moistened fish Casseroles with small chunks of meat, ground meats, or tender meats	Tough, dry meats and poultry
Desserts	All except those on the Avoid list	Dry, coarse cakes or cookies Anything with nuts, seeds, coconut, pineapple, or dried fruit
Fats	All except those on the Avoid list	All fats with chunky additives

Data from American Dietetic Association: *National dysphagia diet: standardization for optimal care*, Chicago, 2002, American Dietetic Association; American Occupational Therapy Association: *AOTA resource guide: feeding and dysphagia*, Rockville, Md, 1997; Avery-Smith W: An occupational therapist coordinated dysphagia program, *Occup Ther Pract* 3:10, 1998; Community Hospital of Los Gatos, Rehabilitation Services: *Dysphagia protocol*, Los Gatos, Calif, 2003; Curran J: Nutritional considerations. In Groher M, editor: *Dysphagia: diagnosis and management*, ed 3, Newton, Mass, 1997, Butterworth-Heinemann Publishers; Rader T, Rende B: *Swallowing disorders: what families should know*, Tucson, Ariz, 1993, Communication Skill Builders Publishers.

arranging several small meals throughout the day for the client who fatigues, rather than three traditional meals.

A client should progress to a regular diet when oral motor control is within functional limits, allowing the client to chew and form any consistency into a bolus and propel it back toward the faucial arches. The client at this level should be able to swallow any food or liquid consistency with only occasional coughing. Continuing dietary precautions for a client with a history of dysphagia include avoiding raw vegetables, stringy foods, and foods containing nuts or seeds.[1,14,17]

Because a client may exhibit a difference in ability to manage different liquids, a progression of liquid levels, separate from the solid levels, should be developed. The liquid progression is divided into four groups: "thin," "nectar-like," "honey-like," and "spoon-thick."[2]

Examples of liquids in these levels are given in Table 26-8.

Thickened liquids are made by adding such thickening agents as banana, pureed fruit, yogurt, dissolved gelatin, baby cereal, cornstarch, or a commercial thickener to achieve the appropriate viscosity. A dietitian can provide the OT with specific recipes. These substances are usually added to the liquids and power-blended for smoothness. The thick drink or soup should stay blended and not be allowed to separate or liquefy. Thick liquids are the appropriate choice for clients with markedly delayed swallow. A thick liquid moves more slowly through the faucial arches, which gives some time for the swallow response to be triggered. Nectar-like liquids such as fruit nectars, buttermilk, tomato juice, and yogurt drinks, which have a natural medium viscosity, are used with those who have a moderate swallow delay of 3 to 5 seconds.[16,29,37] Thin or low-viscosity liquids, the highest liquid level, require intact swallowing ability.

PRINCIPLES OF ORAL FEEDING

The therapist should incorporate certain principles into the oral feeding program. First, an important aspect of the oral preparation stage is looking at, recognizing, and reaching

TABLE **26-8**   **Liquids**

Liquid Level	Examples
Thin liquids	Water, ice chips
	Coffee, tea
	Milk
	Hot chocolate
	Fruit juices
	Broth or consommé
	Gelatin dessert
	Ice cream
	Sherbet
Nectar-like	Nectars
	Extra thick milkshake
	Extra thick eggnog
	Strained creamed soups
	Yogurt and milk blended
	V-8 juice
Honey-like	Nectar thickened with banana
	Nectar thickened with pureed fruit
	Regular applesauce with juice
	Eggnog with baby cereal
	Creamed soup with mashed potatoes
	Commercial thickener
Spoon-thick	Commercial thickener

Data from American Dietetic Association: *National dysphagia diet: standardization for optimal care*, Chicago, 2002, American Dietetic Association; American Occupational Therapy Association: *AOTA resource guide: feeding and dysphagia*, Rockville, Md, 1997; Avery-Smith W: An occupational therapist coordinated dysphagia program, *Occup Ther Pract* 3:10, 1998; Community Hospital of Los Gatos, Rehabilitation Services: *Dysphagia protocol*, Los Gatos, Calif, 2003; Curran J: Nutritional considerations. In Groher M, editor: *Dysphagia: diagnosis and management*, ed 3, Newton, Mass, 1997, Butterworth-Heinemann Publishers; Rader T, Rende B: *Swallowing disorders: what families should know*, Tucson, Ariz, 1993, Communication Skill Builders Publishers.

for food. The client must actively participate in the eating process. Food should be presented within the client's visual field. If the client has a severe visual field deficit or unilateral neglect, the therapist must assist the client to scan the plate or tray visually.

When physically possible the client should feed himself or herself, even if assistance is necessary. If the client does not have a normal hand-to-mouth movement pattern, the therapist must help the client achieve one by guiding the extremity in the correct pattern. Abnormal movement of the upper extremity influences abnormal movement in the trunk, head, face, tongue, and pharynx and decreases the client's ability to safely swallow.

If the client is not capable of self-feeding, the therapist can keep the client actively involved by allowing the client to choose which food or liquid is preferred for each bite. Food is presented by moving the utensil slowly from the front, toward the mouth, so that the client can see the food

the entire time. The utensil should not be brought in from the side because the client will have less preparation time. The client should be allowed as much control of the eating situation as possible.

For adults, eating is a social activity shared with friends and family. A normal dining environment facilitates normal eating. The client can be redirected if distracted and can use environmental cueing when eating in a dining room with others. Adjustments, such as eating in the dining room but at a separate table, can be made to facilitate client concentration. The therapist must be conscious of how the client appears to others and help the client to eat in a normal manner. Cultural preferences must be taken into account when selecting foods and dining settings. The client's normal eating habits and routines should be considered in the development of the eating program. Special care must be taken to obtain this information during the initial assessment.

The OT must continually assess the client's positioning, upper extremity movement, muscle tone, oral control, and swallow. The therapist helps the client perform the task correctly and does not allow eating while the client exhibits an abnormal pattern. If the client displays poor oral motor skills, the therapist looks for food pocketing after every few bites. The rate of the client's intake is monitored. The therapist should determine when too much food is in the mouth and when the client puts food into the mouth before the previous bite has been cleared. The therapist feels for the swallow with a finger at the hyoid notch if the client displays abnormal laryngeal tone or a delayed swallow.[16,37] The therapist also assesses the client's voice quality upon completion of the swallow.

The frequency with which the therapist must check each component depends on the skill level and performance of the client. The more difficulty the client exhibits, the more frequent the assessment. The therapist may find it necessary to assess after each bite or sip, after a few bites or sips, or after each food item. Use of good observational skills allows the therapist to make the appropriate clinical decision. Specific techniques for assessment during feeding trials can be found in the swallowing assessment section of this chapter. After completing the feeding process, the client should remain in an upright position for 15 to 30 minutes to reduce the risk of refluxing food and of aspirating small food particles that may remain in the throat.[1,8,14]

The therapist also must continue to observe the client for signs of aspiration while eating and monitor for the development of aspiration pneumonia over time. Although a conservative estimate of aspiration is 10% of material swallowed, measurement is difficult while a client eats. Clients vary in the amount of aspiration they can tolerate before developing aspiration pneumonia, according to age, health, and pulmonary status. The signs of acute and chronic aspiration were outlined previously.

When a client is participating in oral feedings, careful monitoring of the nutritional status is necessary. The client's

TABLE **26-9** **Dysphagic Treatment: Oral Preparatory Stage**

Structure	Symptoms	Problem	Pre-feeding Technique	Feeding Technique
Trunk	Leaning to one side	Decreased trunk tone Ataxia Increased trunk tone Poor body awareness in space	Facilitate trunk strength Exercises at midline Have client clasp hands, lean down, and touch foot, middle, other foot; rotate trunk with hands clasped and shoulders flexed to decrease or normalize tone	Assist client to hold correct position; assist with head control Assist client to hold correct feeding position; provide with perceptual boundary; consider lateral trunk support
	Hips sliding forward out of chair	Increased tone in hip extensors Poor body awareness in space	See previous entry above Provide firm seating service	Adjust positioning so that client leans slightly forward at hips, arms forward on table
Head	Inability to hold head in midline	Decreased tone Weakness	Facilitate strength through neck and head exercises in flexion, extension, and lateral flexion	Assist with head control
	Inability to move head	Increased tone Poor range of motion	Tone reduction of head, shoulders, and trunk Facilitate normal movement Myofascial release techniques Soft tissue mobilization	Assist with head control
Upper extremity	Spillage of food from utensils	Decreased tone Apraxia Decreased coordination	Facilitate increased tone through weight bearing, sweeping, or tapping muscle belly of desired muscle	Guide client through correct movement pattern Provide adaptive equipment or utensils as needed
	Inability to self-feed	Increased tone Abnormal movement patterns Weakness or decreased motor control	Reduce proximal tone with scapula mobilization, weight bearing through arm Strengthening exercises Facilitation of normal movement	Guide client through correct movement pattern Provide adaptive equipment or utensils as needed
Face	Drooling, food spillage from mouth	Decreased lip control Poor lip closure secondary to decreased tone, poor sensation Apraxia	Place a wet tongue blade between client's lips; ask client to hold tongue blade while therapist tries to pull it out Vibrate lips with back of electric toothbrush down cheek and across lips Lip exercises: movements described in outer oral motor evaluation; client performs repetitions 2-3 times daily Blow bubbles into glass of liquid with straw	Using side handgrip for head control, the therapist approximates lip closure by guiding and assisting with jaw closure Have client use a straw when drinking liquids until control improves Place food to unimpaired side Use cold food or liquids
		Decreased sensation	Fan lips so that client feels drool or wetness on lips or chin to increase awareness	Teach client to pat mouth (versus wiping mouth) and chin every few bites or sips

Data from American Occupational Therapy Association: *Am J Occup Ther*, 1996; Avery-Smith W: Management of neurologic disorders: the first feeding session. In Groher M, editor: *Dysphagia: diagnosis and management*, ed 3, Newton, Mass, 1997, Butterworth-Heinemann Publishers; Bobath B: *Adult hemiplegia: evaluation and treatment*, ed 2, London, 1978, William Heinemann Medical Books; Community Hospital of Los Gatos, Rehabilitation Services: *Dysphagia protocol*, Los Gatos, Calif, 2003; Coombes K: *Swallowing dysfunction in hemiplegia and head injury.* Course presented by International Clinical Educators, Aug 24-27, 1986, and Aug 24-28, 1987, Los Gatos, Calif; Davies P: *Steps to follow*, New York, 1985, Springer-Verlag; Farber S: *Neurorehabilitation: a multisensory approach*, Philadelphia, 1982, WB Saunders; Logemann J: *Manual for the videofluorographic study of swallowing*, ed 2, Austin, Tex, 1993, Pro-Ed Publishers.

TABLE **26-9** **Dysphagic Treatment: Oral Preparatory Stage—cont'd**

Structure	Symptoms	Problem	Pre-feeding Technique	Feeding Technique
Tongue	Pocketing of food in cheeks or sulci Poor bolus formation	Poor tongue control for lateralization or tipping Decreased tone Poor sensation	Tongue exercises: use movements described in inner oral motor evaluation	Avoid crumbly foods Stroke client's outside cheek where pocketing occurs with index finger back and up toward client's ear; instruct client to check cheek for pocketing
	Retracted tongue	Increased tone Retracted jaw	Tongue range of motion: wrap tip of tongue in wet gauze; gently pull tongue forward, side to side and up and down; move slowly Pull tongue wrapped in wet gauze forward past front teeth, using index and middle fingers to vibrate tongue back and forth sideways to decrease tone and facilitate protrusion	Avoid crumbly foods Reduce tone as needed during meal Double swallow Resist head flexion to facilitate jaw closure Resist head extension to facilitate jaw opening

caloric needs are determined by the dietitian and the physician and depend on the client's height, weight, activity level, and medical condition.[17,37] Fluid intake is monitored by having the physician order a calorie count and a liquid intake and output hydration count (I and O).[14] Each person who supervises or works with the client should record, in percentages, the caloric amount of each item the client eats or drinks. The dietitian converts the percentages into a daily calorie total. The client also should be monitored for physical signs of nutritional deficiency and dehydration. These symptoms are weakness, irritability, decreased alertness, changes in eating habits, hunger, thirst, decreased turgor, and changes in amounts or color of urine.[17,27,47] If a client is not able to take in the necessary calories (50% of the determined total), supplemental feedings are necessary to make up the difference.[14] The physician and dietitian decide on the number of supplemental feedings.

TECHNIQUES FOR THE MANAGEMENT OF DYSPHAGIA

Tables 26-9 through 26-12 provide intervention techniques for the management of dysphagia. These techniques are not intended to be used in all situations. Each client presents a different clinical picture and may display one deficit or a combination of deficits. After careful assessment the therapist must determine the primary cause of the client's deficits and intervene accordingly. The occupational profile

determines the focus of OT services and identifies the importance of dysphagia intervention within the client's priorities.

Intervention with a client with dysphagia requires a logical and consistent approach.[4,16] Abnormal tone, for example, should be normalized before the therapist can expect good motor control. Motor control must be improved before a client can shape food into a cohesive bolus and achieve an effective swallow. Individualized pre-feeding techniques can prepare the client for eating. The therapist should strive toward facilitating the return of normal eating habits and routines for each client.

The therapist must continually assess the client's response to intervention and make necessary modifications to the eating and swallowing program. Therefore, the therapist must develop excellent clinical observation skills.[7,16,37] For difficult clients the clinician should seek a consultation with an experienced dysphagia therapist. To develop expertise in dysphagia management, it is recommended that the therapist seek continued education in this area.

SUMMARY

Eating is the most basic activity of daily living. Several performance components are required for the client to eat and swallow effectively. Dysphagia refers to difficulty with swallowing or an inability to swallow. The OT is trained to provide intervention for many of the problems that interfere with normal eating. An understanding of the normal anatomy and physiology of swallowing and advanced training in

TABLE 26-10 **Dysphagic Treatment: Oral Stage**

Structure	Symptoms	Problem	Pre-feeding Technique	Feeding Technique
Tongue	Slow oral transit Tongue retraction	Poor anterior to posterior movement; decreased tone, poor sensation Increased tone	Practice "ng-ga" sounds Grasping tongue wrapped in gauze, pull it forward past front teeth; use finger or tongue blade to vibrate base of tongue back and forth sideways Improve tongue range of motion	Tuck chin toward chest Position food in center, midtongue Avoid crumbly foods Use cold or hot foods instead of warm Correct positioning Place index finger at base of tongue under chin; stroke up and forward
	Slow oral transit time Inability to channel food back toward pharynx	Inability to form central groove in tongue Apraxia	Grasping tongue wrapped in gauze, pull forward to front teeth; stroke firmly down middle of tongue with edge of tongue blade	Tuck chin toward chest Position food in center, midtongue Avoid crumbly foods Use cold or hot foods instead of warm Correct positioning Place index finger at base of tongue under chin; stroke up and forward
	Repetitive movement of tongue; food is pushed out front of mouth	Tongue thrust	Facilitate tongue retraction to bring tongue back into normal resting position; vibrate on either side of the frenulum found inside the mouth, under the tongue with finger Increase jaw control; teach isolated tongue movements	Correct positioning Place food away from midline of tongue toward back of mouth Provide downward and forward pressure to back of tongue with spoon after food placement
	Food falls off tongue into sulci or food remains on tongue without client awareness	Poor sensation	Ice tongue with ice chips placed in gauze to prevent ice chips from slipping into pharynx Brush tongue with toothbrush to stimulate receptors	Use foods with high viscosity or density Alternate presentation of cold and hot foods during meal
	Slow oral transit time; food remains on hard palate; coughing before swallow	Poor tongue elevation; decreased tone	Ask client to practice "k," "g," "n," "d," and "t" sounds Lightly touch tongue blade or soft toothbrush to roof of mouth at back of tongue; instruct client to press spot with tongue; resist movement with blade or brush to increase strength Vibrate tongue at base below chin; provide quick stretch by pushing down on base of tongue	Correct positioning With finger under chin at base of tongue, move finger upward and forward to facilitate elevation Avoid crumbly foods Double swallow

Data from Community Hospital of Los Gatos, Rehabilitation Services: *Dysphagia protocol*, Los Gatos, Calif, 2003; Coombes K: *Swallowing dysfunction in hemiplegia and head injury*. Course presented by International Clinical Educators, Aug 24-27, 1986, and Aug 24-28, 1987, Los Gatos, Calif; Davies P: *Steps to follow*, New York, 1985, Springer-Verlag; Farber S: *Neurorehabilitation: a multisensory approach*, Philadelphia, 1982, WB Saunders; Logemann J: *Evaluation and treatment of swallowing disorders*, ed 2, Austin, Tex, 1998, Pro-Ed Publishers; Martin BJW: Treatment of dysphagia in adults. In Cherney L, editor: *Clinical management of dysphagia in adults and children,* Gaithersburg, Md, 1994, Aspen Publishers; Silverman EH, Elfant IL: *Am J Occup Ther*, 1979.

TABLE **26-10** **Dysphagic Treatment: Oral Stage—cont'd**

Structure	Symptoms	Problem	Pre-feeding Technique	Feeding Technique
	Slow oral transit time Food remains on back of tongue because client is unable to elevate tongue to push food to hard palate Coughing before the swallow Retracted tongue	Decreased sensation Increased tone Decreased range of motion Soft tissue shortening	Tone tongue with gauze reduction; grasping wrapped tongue forward with around tip, pull finger or tongue blade Apply pressure to base of tongue right to left Grasping base of tongue under chin between two fingers, move it back and forth to decrease tone Tone reduction Range of motion exercises Place a variety of tastes on lips to facilitate tongue-licking lips	Adjust correct positioning by increasing forward flexion at hips, arms forward to decrease tone Reduce tone as needed; give client breaks because tone increases with effort With finger under chin at base of tongue, move finger upward and forward to facilitate tongue elevation

TABLE **26-11** **Dysphagia Treatment: Pharyngeal Stage**

Structure	Symptoms	Problem	Pre-feeding Technique	Feeding Technique
Soft palate	Tight voice; nasal regurgitation Air felt through nose or mist seen on mirror when client says "ah" Decreased tone Nasal speech	Increased tone Decreased tone Rigidity	Facilitate normal head/neck positioning Have client tuck chin into therapist's cupped hand, then push into hand as therapist applies resistance; client says, "ah" afterward; speed and height of uvula elevation should increase; follow by thermal application	Facilitate normal head and neck positioning With head and neck in midline, have client tuck chin slightly to decrease rate of food entering into pharynx
	Delayed swallow	Decreased triggering of swallow response	Thermal application: using a laryngeal mirror #00 after being placed in ice water or chips for 10 seconds, touch base of faucial arch; repeat up to 10 times; process can be repeated several times a day	Alternate presentation of food; start very cold substance, then warm; cold substance can increase sensitivity of faucial arches; tuck chin slightly forward to prevent bolus entering airway
Hyoid	Delayed elevation of hyoid bone Poor tongue elevation Tongue retraction	Delayed swallow Incomplete swallow Abnormal tongue tone; poor range of motion	Increase tongue humping because elevation of tongue and hyoid stimulates triggering of response Tone reduction	Place index finger under chin at base of tongue and push up forward to facilitate tongue elevation
Pharynx	Coughing after swallow	Decreased pharyngeal movement Penetration into laryngeal vestibule	None	If appropriate, alternate presentation of liquid with stage II or stage III solids; liquid material moves solids through pharynx

Data from Community Hospital of Los Gatos, Rehabilitation Services, *Dysphagia protocol*, Los Gatos, Calif, 1999; Coombes K: *Swallowing dysfunction in hemiplegia and head injury*. Course presented by International Clinical Educators, Aug 24-27, 1986, and Aug 24-28, 1987, Los Gatos, Calif; Davies P: *Steps to follow*, New York, 1985, Springer-Verlag; Kaatzke-McDonald M, Post E, Davis P: *Dysphagia*, 1996; Logemann J: *Evaluation and treatment of swallowing disorders*, Austin, Tex, 1998, Pro-Ed Publishers; Martin BJW: Treatment of dysphagia in adults. In Cherney L, editor: *Clinical management of dysphagia in adults and children*, Gaithersburg, Md, 1994, Aspen Publishers; Schulze-Delrieu K, Miller R: Clinical assessment of dysphagia. In Perlman A, Schulze-Delrieu, editors: *Deglutition and its disorders: anatomy, physiology, clinical diagnosis and management*, San Diego, Calif, 1997, Singular Publishing; Smith C, Logemann J, Colangelo L, et al: *Dysphagia* 14(1):1, 1999.

Continued

TABLE 26-11   **Dysphagia Treatment: Pharyngeal Stage—cont'd**

Structure	Symptoms	Problem	Pre-feeding Technique	Feeding Technique
	Coating of pharynx seen on videofluoroscopy Gurgling voice	Pharyngeal weakness	Isometric or resistive head and neck exercises	Have client take second dry swallow to clear valleculae and pyriform sinuses Tilt head to stronger side Supraglottic swallow
	Seen on videofluoroscopy, anteroposterior view; material residue seen on one side; weak or hoarse voice	Unilateral pharyngeal movement	None	Compensatory technique for clients with low tone: have client turn head toward affected side during swallow to prevent pooling in affected pyriform sinuses; evaluate technique against its effect on client positioning and tone in trunk, upper extremities
Larynx	Coughing, choking after swallow	Decreased laryngeal elevation Decreased tone Weakness	Quickly ice up sides of larynx; ask client to swallow; assist movement by guiding larynx upward Vibrate laryngeal musculature from under chin, downward on each side to sternal notch	Teach client to clear throat immediately after swallow to move residual Use supraglottic swallow, Mendelsohn maneuver, effortful swallow
	Noisy or audible swallow	Increased tone Rigidity Uncoordinated swallow	Range of motion—place fingers and thumb along both sides of larynx and gently move it back and forth until movement is smooth and easy, tone decreased Using chipped ice, form pack in washcloth and place around larynx for 5 min	Placing fingers and thumb along both sides of larynx, assist client with upward elevation before swallow Double swallow
Trachea	Continuous coughing before, during, after swallow	Aspiration—before: poor tongue control; during: delayed swallow response; after: decreased pharyngeal movement	Teach client how to produce a voluntary cough; ask client to take a deep breath and cough while breathing out; therapist uses palm of hand to push downward (toward stomach) on the sternum	Encourage client to keep coughing; facilitate reflexive cough; push downward on sternum as client breathes out; suction client if problem increases Push into client's sternal notch to assist with cough
	Client grabs or reaches for throat Reddening in the face No voice or cough	Blocked airway	None	Perform Heimlich maneuver Seek medical assistance

eating and swallowing disorders are required to effectively treat dysphagia.

Assessment of the client with dysphagia includes testing of head and trunk control, sensation, perception, cognition, inner and outer oral structures, oral reflexes, and swallowing. Assessment may also include videofluoroscopy or fiberoptic endoscopy.

Several members of the rehabilitation team are involved in the treatment of the client with dysphagia. Positioning, selection of appropriate feeding procedures, diet texture selection, diet progression, and special techniques to facilitate normal patterns of swallowing are part of the intervention plan. The social, cultural, and psychological aspects of eating are also important considerations in the intervention program.

TABLE **26-12 Dysphagia Treatment: Esophageal Stage**

Structure	Symptoms	Problem	Pre-feeding Technique	Feeding Technique
Esophagus	Frequent regurgitation of food or liquid and coughing or choking after the swallow: material collecting in a side pocket in esophagus	Esophageal diverticulum	Requires a medical diagnosis; problem can be seen through traditional barium x-ray examination Surgical correction is needed	Report symptoms to medical staff (therapist cannot treat)
	Regurgitation of food, coughing, or choking on food after the swallow: inability of food to pass through the pharynx, esophagus, or stomach	Partial or total obstruction of the pharynx or esophagus Impaired esophageal peristalsis	Requires a medical diagnosis; problem can be seen through traditional barium X-ray examination Surgical correction is needed	Report symptoms to medical staff (therapist cannot treat)

Data from Coombes K: *Swallowing dysfunction in hemiplegia and head injury*. Course presented by International Clinical Educators, Aug 24-27, 1986, and Aug 24-28, 1987, Los Gatos, Calif; Davies P: *Steps to follow*, New York, 1985, Springer-Verlag; Logemann J: *Evaluation and treatment of swallowing disorders*, Austin, Tex, 1998, Pro-Ed Publishers; Smith C, Logemann J, Colangelo L, et al: *Dysphagia*, 1999; Martin B: Treatment of dysphagia in adults. In Cherney L, editor: *Clinical management of dysphagia in adults and children*, Gaithersburg, Md, 1994, Aspen. Workman J, Pillsbury H, Hulka G: Surgical interventions in dysphagia. In Groher M: *Dysphagia: diagnosis and management*, ed 3, Newton, Mass, 1977, Butterworth-Heinemann.

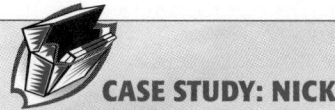

CASE STUDY: NICK

Nick is a 65-year-old man who suffered a right cerebrovascular accident (CVA) with left hemiplegia 2 weeks ago. He has a G tube in place for nutrition. He recently retired from his position as vice president of a local marketing company. Nick lives with his wife. He and his wife have two grown children living in the area. Before the onset of the CVA, Nick was independent in all ADLs and instrumental activities of daily living (IADLs). He was an active member of the community.

Results of the OT evaluation indicate that Nick needs moderate to maximum assistance in dressing, toileting, bathing, eating and swallowing, and transfers. The clinical assessment of eating indicates that the client has a mild to moderate increase in jaw and facial tone with poor rotary chew, poor isolated tongue control, and mild increase in laryngeal tone with delayed swallow.

The videofluoroscopy confirmed that the client had a mildly delayed swallow with minimal pooling in the valleculae and pyriform sinuses. Aspiration was less than 10% on pureed foods. The client was seen three times a day for 6 weeks by OT. A summary of evaluation results and a treatment plan are shown in Figure 26-8.

The client responded well to treatment. The G tube was removed after 5 weeks. The client achieved all treatment goals by the time of discharge. He went home with family supervision for correct diet, positioning, and swallowing techniques during meals. The client was referred to home health OT for 2 to 3 weeks for ADLs and home modification so that independence at home could be achieved. The client returned for follow-up outpatient visits.

Review Questions

1. List the components of dysphagia.
2. List the four stages of swallowing and the characteristics of each.
3. List the physiological functions that occur when the swallow response triggers, and explain why these functions are necessary.
4. Why is it necessary to assess a client's mental status during a dysphagia evaluation?
5. Describe what the therapist should look for when evaluating the trunk and head during the dysphagia evaluation.
6. What information can the therapist gain when assessing the client's facial motor control?
7. How does poor tongue control contribute to aspiration?
8. Name the components required to protect the airway.
9. What is the safest food sequence to follow for a swallowing evaluation?
10. Describe the finger placement that a therapist can use to feel the strength and smoothness of the swallow.
11. Why should the therapist assess voice quality after a swallow?
12. Will a client who has difficulty handling solids also have difficulty with liquids?
13. What options does the OT have when a client coughs?
14. List the indicators of swallowing dysfunction.
15. List the acute symptoms of aspiration.
16. When is videofluoroscopy necessary?
17. List the elements in treatment of the client with dysphagia.
18. Describe the position in which a client should be treated and give the rationale for this position.
19. What are the indications for placing a client on a non-oral treatment program?
20. Name five important criteria a client must meet to participate in an oral feeding program.

Dysphagia Evaluation and Treatment Plan

Pt: _65 y. male_

Dx: _Ⓡ CVA_

Onset: _2 weeks ago_

Medical hx: _Elevated BP — 5 years. Elevated blood lipids. Otherwise unremarkable. Independent in ADL & IADL prior to onset._

Current nutritional status: _gastrostomy tube, NPO_

	WNL	Adequate— without assistance	Unable	Comments
Mental status:				
Alert/oriented		c̄ assist		oriented to name, max assist for date
Direction following		c̄ assist		appropriate c̄ guiding
Physical status (symmetry, control, tone):				
Head control		c̄ assist		slight ↑'d tone c̄ head turning
Trunk control		c̄ assist		ataxic, TLR present
Endurance		c̄ assist		fatigues after 30 min.
Respiratory				
Suctioning required	N/A			
Tracheostomy	N/A			
Outer oral status:				
Facial expressions		c̄ assist		flat affect 2° ↑'d tone to moderate degree
Jaw movement			✓	poor rotary chew, poor jaw glide, pt. uses up & down movt.
Lip movement		c̄ assist		unable to purse & retract, poor lip compression
Sensation		c̄ assist		delayed 2° ↓'d attention
Abnormal reflexes		c̄ assist		suck-swallow present, others absent
Inner oral status (symmetry, control, tone):				
Dentition	✓			good, slightly inflammed gums
Tongue				slight white coating & mid Ⓡ tongue laceration
Appearance		c̄ assist		
Tone		c̄ assist		↑'d c̄ retraction
Movement: Protrusion		c̄ assist		deviated to Ⓡ
Lateralization		c̄ assist		mild weakness
"ng" → "ga"			✓	poor anterior to posterior
Soft palate/gag reflex:	✓			uvula rises symmetrically
Cough (reflexive/voluntary):	✓			
Swallow:				
Spontaneous	✓			intact
Voluntary		c̄ assist		delayed 2° to tone
Laryngeal movement				
Tongue		c̄ assist		requires tone reduction
Elevation		c̄ assist		delayed fatigue factor after serial swallows
Food management:				Overall pt. shows ↓'d cognitive awareness of food in mouth & requires cueing
Puree		c̄ assist		pt. uses suck-swallow
Mechanical soft		c̄ assist	}	pocketing assist
Chopped/ground		c̄ assist	}	needed c̄ rotary chew
Regular diet			N/A	
Liquids: Thick		c̄ assist		c̄ straw, 5 sec. delay, Ø cough
Semithick		c̄ assist		c̄ straw, 5 sec. delay, coughing
Thin			N/A	

Figure 26-8 Case study: dysphagia evaluation and treatment plan.

Dysphagia Evaluation and Treatment Plan

Major problems:

① ↓'d cognition for attention and awareness of food in mouth s̄ cueing.

② ↑'d jaw & facial tone resulting in poor rotary chew.

③ Poor isolated tongue movements for lateralization, humping.

④ ↑'d laryngeal tone resulting in delayed swallow.

⑤ Poor sitting balance.

Recommendations/treatment plan:
(positioning, diet level, environment, techniques)

① Positioning - upright on solid seating surface, slight forward lean.

② Tone reduction techniques for jaw, tongue, & larynx before & during meal.

③ Diet level - pureed & mechanical soft foods, thickened liquids 2x daily c̄ therapist only.

④ Therapeutic feeding in quiet setting.

⑤ No food or liquid in pts. room.

⑥ Monitor patient for signs of aspiration.

⑦ Videofluoroscopy for confirmation.

Long-term goals:

① Independent trunk and head control for self feeding.

② ↑ attention and awareness of food in mouth to WFL.

③ ↑ isolated motor control of facial expression to WNL.

④ ↑ isolated motor control of jaw, tongue, & larynx to WFL.

⑤ ↑ oral intake for solids from pureed to regular diet for all meals with family supervision.

⑥ ↑ oral intake for liquids from thick to thin.

⑦ Calorie and hydration count, wean from gastrostomy.

⑧ Family ① in swallowing & diet follow through.

Figure 26-8, cont'd

---

21. List the properties of food preferred for diets for clients with dysphagia.
22. Describe the effect that poor hand-to-mouth movements have on the client's swallow.
23. Why is it important to involve the client in the eating process?
24. What are the symptoms of nutritional deficiency?
25. Describe two possible treatment techniques used for a client who displays a masked appearance.
26. Name three treatment techniques the OT can use for poor rotary jaw movement and increased tone.
27. Describe two ways a therapist can decrease abnormally high tone in the tongue.
28. Describe thermal application as a treatment technique. For which problem is it used?
29. When is use of the dry swallow technique appropriate?
30. How can the therapist facilitate a cough?

REFERENCES

1. Alta Bates Hospital Rehabilitation Services: *Bedside dysphagia evaluation protocol*, Berkeley, Calif, 1999, the Hospital.
2. American Dietetic Association: *National dysphagia diet: standardization for optimal care*, Chicago, IL, 2002, American Dietetic Association.

3. American Occupational Therapy Association: *AOTA resource guide: feeding and dysphagia*, Rockville, Md, 1997, The Association.

4. American Occupational Therapy Association: Eating dysfunction: position paper, *Am J Occup Ther* 50(10):846, 1996.

5. American Occupational Therapy Association: Occupational therapy practice framework: domain and process, *Am J Occup Ther* 56(6):609, 2002

6. American Occupational Therapy Association: Specialized knowledge and skills in eating and feeding for occupational therapy practice, *Am J Occup Ther* 57:660, 2003.

7. Avery-Smith W: An occupational therapist coordinated dysphagia program, *Occup Ther Pract* 3(10):20, 1998.

8. Avery-Smith W: Management of neurologic disorders: the first feeding session. In Groher M, editor: *Dysphagia: diagnosis and management*, ed 3, Newton, Mass, 1997, Butterworth-Heinemann.

9. Avery-Smith W, Dellarosa D: Approaches to treating dysphagia in patients with brain injury, *Am J Occup Ther* 48(3):235, 1994.

10. Bass N: The neurology of swallowing. In Groher M, editor: *Dysphagia: diagnosis and management*, ed 3, Newton, Mass, 1997, Butterworth-Heinemann.

11. Bobath B: *Adult hemiplegia: evaluation and treatment*, ed 2, London, 1978, William Heinemann Medical Books.

12. Buchholz D, Bosma J, Donner M: Adaption, compensation, and decompensation of the pharyngeal swallow, *Gastrointest Radiol* 10(3):235, 1985.

13. Cherney L, Pannell J, Cantieri C: Clinical evaluation of dysphagia. In Cherney L, editor: *Clinical management of dysphagia in adults and children*, Gaithersburg, Md, 1994, Aspen Publishers.

14. Community Hospital of Los Gatos, Rehabilitation Services: *Dysphagia protocol*, Los Gatos, Calif, 2003.

15. Conklin JL: Control of esophageal motor function, *Dysphagia* 8(4):311, 1993.

16. Coombes K: *Swallowing dysfunction in hemiplegia and head injury*. Course presented by International Clinical Educators, Aug 24-27, 1986, and Aug 24-28, 1987, Los Gatos, Calif.

17. Curran J: Nutritional considerations. In Groher M, editor: *Dysphagia: diagnosis and management*, ed 3, Newton, Mass, 1997, Butterworth-Heinemann.

18. Curtis D, Cruess D, Wilgress E: Normal solid bolus swallowing: erect position, *Dysphagia* 1:63, 1986.

19. Davies P: *Steps to follow*, New York, 1985, Springer-Verlag.

20. Davis L, Stanton ST: Characteristics of dysphagia in elderly patients requiring mechanical ventilation, *Dysphagia* 19:7, 2004.

21. Farber S: *Neurorehabilitation: a multisensory approach*, Philadelphia, 1982, WB Saunders.

22. FDA Public Health Advisory: Reports of blue discoloration and death in patients receiving enteral feedings tinted with the dye, FD&C Blue No. 1, September 29, 2003.

23. Fleming S: Treatment of mechanical swallowing disorders. In Groher M, editor: *Dysphagia: diagnosis and management*, ed 3, Newton, Mass, 1997, Butterworth-Heinemann Publishers.

24. Griggs B: Nursing management of swallowing disorders. In Groher M, editor: *Dysphagia: diagnosis and management*, ed 3, Newton, Mass, 1997, Butterworth-Heinemann Publishers.

25. Groher M: Bolus management and aspiration pneumonia with pseudobulbar dysphagia, *Dysphagia* 1:215, 1987.

26. Groher M: Establishing a swallowing program. In Groher M, editor: *Dysphagia: diagnosis and management*, ed 3, Newton, Mass, 1997, Butterworth-Heinemann Publishers.

27. Groher M: Ethical dilemmas in providing nutrition, *Dysphagia* 5(2):102, 1990.

28. Hendrix TR: Coordination of peristalsis in pharynx and esophagus, *Dysphagia* 8(2):74, 1993.

29. Hiiemae K, Palmer JB: Food transport and bolus formation during complete feeding sequences on foods of different initial consistency, *Dysphagia* 14(1):31, 1999.

30. Hislop H, Montgomery J, Connelly B: *Daniels & Worthington's muscle testing: techniques of manual examination*, ed 6, Philadelphia, 1995, WB Saunders.

31. Kahrilas PJ: Pharyngeal structure and function, *Dysphagia* 8(4): 303, 1993.

32. Kendall K, Leonard R, McKenzie S: Airway protection: evaluation with videofluoroscopy, *Dysphagia* 19:65, 2004.

33. Langmore S, McCulloch T: Examination of the pharynx and larynx and endoscopic examination of pharyngeal swallowing. In Perlman A, Schulze-Delrieu K, editors: *Deglutition and its disorders: anatomy, physiology, clinical diagnosis, and management*, San Diego, Calif, 1997, Singular Publishing.

34. Langmore S, Skarupski K, Park P, et al: Predictors of aspiration pneumonia in nursing home residents, *Dysphagia* 17:298, 2002.

35. Leder S, Epinosa J: Aspiration risk after acute stroke: comparison of clinical examination and fiberoptic endoscopic evaluation of swallowing, *Dysphagia* 17:214, 2002.

36. Leder S, Sasaki C, Burrell M: Fiberoptic endoscopic evaluation of dysphagia to identify silent aspiration, *Dysphagia* 13(1):19, 1998.

37. Logemann J: *Evaluation and treatment of swallowing disorders*, Austin, Tex, 1998, Pro-Ed Publishers.

38. Logemann J: *Manual for the videofluorographic study of swallowing*, ed 2, Austin, Tex, 1993, Pro-Ed Publishers.

39. Martin BJW: Treatment of dysphagia in adults. In Cherney L, editor: *Clinical management of dysphagia in adults and children*, Gaithersburg, Md, 1994, Aspen Publishers.

40. Miller A, Bieger D, Conklin JL: Functional controls of deglutition. In Perlman A, Schulze-Delrieu K, editors: *Deglutition and its disorders: anatomy, physiology, clinical diagnosis, and management*, San Diego, Calif, 1997, Singular Publishing.

41. Miller R: Clinical examination for dysphagia. In Groher M: *Dysphagia diagnosis and management*, ed 3, Newton, Mass, 1997, Butterworth-Heinemann Publishers.

42. O'Sullivan N: *Dysphagia care: team approach with acute and long-term patients*, ed 2, Bolingbrook, IL, 1995, Sammons Preston.

43. Palmer J, Hiiemae K: Eating and breathing: interactions between respiration and feeding on solid food, *Dysphagia* 18:169, 2003.

44. Perry L, Love C: Screening for dysphagia and aspiration in acute stroke: a systematic review, *Dysphagia* 16:7, 2001.

45. Rader T, Rende B: *Swallowing disorders: what families should know*, Tucson, Ariz, 1993, Communication Skill Builders Publishers.

46. Schulze-Delrieu K, Miller R: Clinical assessment of dysphagia. In Perlman A, Schulze-Delrieu K, editors: *Deglutition and its disorders: anatomy, physiology, clinical diagnosis and management*, San Diego, Calif, 1997, Singular Publishing.

47. Silverman EH, Elfant IL: Dysphagia: an evaluation and treatment program for the adult, *Am J Occup Ther* 33(6):382, 1979.

48. Smith C, Logemann J, Colangelo L, et al: Incidence and patient characteristics associated with silent aspiration in the acute care setting, *Dysphagia* 14(1):1, 1999.

49. Stanford Hospital and Clinics Department of Rehabilitation Services: *Dysphagia/swallowing evaluation procedure*, Stanford, Calif, 2003.

50. Stanford Hospital and Clinics Department of Rehabilitation Services: *Swallowing disorders in adults: assessment and management*, Course presented by Stanford Hospital and Clinics, February 7-8, 2004, Stanford, Calif.

51. Stone M, Shawker T: An ultrasound examination of tongue movement during swallowing, *Dysphagia* 1(2):78, 1986.

52. Workman J, Pillsbury H, Hulka G: Surgical interventions in dysphagia. In Groher M: *Dysphagia: diagnosis and management*, ed 3, Newton, Mass, 1977, Butterworth-Heinemann Publishers.

27 EVALUATION AND PAIN MANAGEMENT

JOYCE M. ENGEL

KEY TERMS

Pain
Acute pain

Chronic pain
Biopsychosocial model

Pain evaluation
Pain interventions

LEARNING OBJECTIVES

After studying this chapter the student or practitioner will be able to do the following:

1. Discuss the differences between acute and chronic pain.
2. Explain the biopsychosocial model of pain.
3. Describe two common pain syndromes.
4. Summarize two approaches to pain assessment.
5. Describe three approaches to pain intervention.

CHAPTER OUTLINE

Definitions of pain
Biopsychosocial model of pain
Pain syndromes
  Headache pain
  Low back pain
  Arthritis
  Complex regional pain syndrome
  Myofascial pain syndrome
  Fibromyalgia
  Cancer pain
  Central pain syndrome
Evaluation
Intervention

Medication
Activity tolerance
Body mechanics and posture training
Energy conservation, pacing, and joint protection
Splinting
Relaxation
Adaptive equipment
Biofeedback
Distraction
Therapeutic modalities
Transcutaneous electrical nerve stimulation
Summary

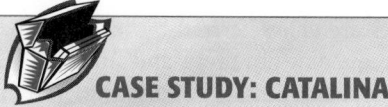

CASE STUDY: CATALINA

Catalina, a 34-year-old single woman, was injured 5 months ago when catching a heavy weight while employed as an electrician. She sustained a lumbar strain. Catalina was initially treated at an emergency room, where narcotics, muscle relaxants, heat application, and bed rest were prescribed. After persistent pain complaints, she was given pelvic traction and TENS. Catalina has not returned to work since her injury and described her current lifestyle as sedentary. She described her pain as severe (a "9" or "10" on a 10-point numerical scale, with "0" representing "no pain" and "10" indicating "pain as bad as could be") and almost constant. She identified prolonged sitting, standing, and ambulation as exacerbating pain factors. Catalina described occasional mild pain relief with ibuprofen use and bed rest. Her self-report on the Brief Pain Inventory revealed moderate to high pain interference with IADL and recreational, social, and work activities. Catalina described using pain-contingent rest and asking for assistance as the means of coping with her pain.

During evaluation, Catalina was found to have decreased active right shoulder range of motion and strength, decreased left lower extremity strength, and muscle spasms throughout the left lumbar paraspinal muscles and into the left buttocks. She demonstrated poor body mechanics, poor posture, and mild shortness of breath. Catalina offered numerous verbal complaints of pain and expressed fear that the pain would never go away.

Physical retraining and cognitive behavioral techniques were emphasized in intervention. Catalina participated in generalized mobility, strengthening, and cardiovascular endurance exercises as a means of increasing her occupational performance, minimizing fatigue, and increasing feelings of well-being. Functional tasks were incorporated into treatment. Catalina was instructed in how to monitor her daily routine (e.g., balance of rest, relaxation, and activity) and modify faulty thinking (e.g., catastrophizing, such as thinking nothing can stop the pain). Her daily routine included progressive relaxation rehearsal.

Catalina made good progress in her 4-week treatment program. She demonstrated normal mobility, strength, and endurance. Bed rest during the day was eliminated. Catalina was taught proper posture and body mechanics and was observed to use them in her routine activities. Her verbal complaints of pain remained unchanged, but she stated that she no longer felt the pain was controlling her. Catalina was now ready to progress to a work-hardening program.

Critical Thinking Questions

1. What occupational limitations would you expect as a result of Catalina's injury and pain?
2. How would you provide an occupation-based intervention program to meet Catalina's occupational performance needs?
3. What problems in social participation do you anticipate as a result of the level of pain Catalina experiences on a daily basis?

Dr. Albert Schweitzer[41] wrote, "Pain is a more terrible lord of mankind than even death itself." At least 75 million Americans live with chronic pain, and most are significantly disabled by it. More than 55% of the elderly report experiencing pain on a daily basis. Chronic pain accounts for at least 80% of all physician visits. Pain also causes more than 50 million lost workdays at a cost of more than $3 billion in lost wages and more than $100 billion in lost productivity.[36] No doubt Schweitzer would agree that the costs of human suffering cannot be estimated. The obligation to manage pain and relieve a consumer's suffering is now recognized by governing bodies as fundamental to healthcare.[18] Pain may coexist with a medical condition (e.g., arthritis) or rehabilitative procedure (e.g., stretching) or may be the primary complaint (e.g., low back pain). Occupational therapy (OT) practitioners may suspect that pain is impeding the patient's progress but feel unsure about how to approach evaluation and intervention. This chapter defines pain, discusses the biopsychosocial model of pain, describes common pain syndromes, outlines assessment procedures, and proposes interventions.

DEFINITIONS OF PAIN

Pain is defined as an unpleasant sensory and emotional experience associated with actual or potential tissue damage or described in terms of such damage.[33] This definition conveys that pain is a subjective experience and multidimensional. Individual variables such as mood, attention, prior pain experiences, and culture are known to affect one's experience of pain (See Box 27-1, p. 653).[1,30]

Most investigators agree in differentiation of acute from chronic pain, which is critical for selecting appropriate assessment and intervention strategies. Acute pain has a well-defined pain onset. It is associated with sympathetic nervous system arousal (e.g., increases in muscle tone). **Acute pain** serves a biological purpose, directing attention to injury, irritation, or disease and signaling the need for immobilization and protection of a body part.[31] Fortunately, acute pain usually responds to medication and treatment of the underlying cause of pain.[19]

In contrast, **chronic pain** may begin as acute pain or may be more insidious and endure beyond the point at which an underlying pathological condition can be identified. Increased sympathetic nervous system activity does not continue. Chronic pain does not appear to serve a biological purpose. It is not amenable to routine methods of pain control. Our client, Catalina, is now experiencing chronic pain, which negatively affects her occupational performance. Chronic pain often produces significant changes in personality, lifestyle, and functional ability.[19]

BIOPSYCHOSOCIAL MODEL OF PAIN

Occupational therapy (OT) has long embraced the biopsychosocial model for its emphasis on the interaction of the individual's body, mind, and environment.[34] A **biopsychosocial model** that conceptualizes the multilayered nature of pain can be critical to accurate evaluation and effective intervention. Loeser and Fordyce[27] suggested the phenomenon of pain could essentially be divided into four distinct domains: nociception, pain, suffering, and pain behavior. *Nociception* is the detection of tissue damage by transducers in the skin and deeper structures, and the central transmission of this information by A-delta and C fibers in the peripheral nerves. *Pain* is the perceived noxious input to the nervous system. *Suffering* is the negative affective response to pain. It may be difficult to differentiate suffering from fear, anxiety, isolation, or depression. Finally, *pain behavior* is what an individual says or does (e.g., taking pain medications) or does not say or do (e.g., job absenteeism), which leads others to believe that individual is experiencing noxious stimuli. Pain behaviors are observable and are influenced by cultural and environmental consequences. This model purports that one can experience or demonstrate some domains of the model in the absence of others. Return to our client, Catalina. She continues to experience pain but also expressed fear that the pain would never go away. In that sense she is captive to her pain experience. In chronic nonmalignant pain, pain behaviors and suffering often exist in the absence of nociception.[13,27,52]

PAIN SYNDROMES

Pain is a primary reason for seeking healthcare. The evaluation and treatment of pain resulting from trauma, disease, or unknown etiology are significant healthcare concerns. The following sections provide descriptions of common pain syndromes.

HEADACHE PAIN

Recurrent headaches are one of the most common pain problems. Approximately 28 million Americans experience recurrent migraine headaches.[15] More than half of the population of persons with headaches does not seek treatment because they perceive the problem as too trivial, have concerns about medication side effects, and believe no adequate treatment is available.[28]

Migraine headaches are characterized by recurrent pain episodes varying in frequency, duration, and intensity. The pain is typically unilateral and pulsatile (pulsating) and may be accompanied by anorexia, nausea, vomiting, neurological symptoms (e.g., photosensitivity and photophobia), and mood changes (e.g., irritability).[28] A strong genetic predisposition exists for migraines. Experimental evidence supports the role of serotonin in migraine. Stress, attention, and mood (e.g., anxiety) affect these headaches.

Tension-type headaches are the most common headache disorder. Approximately 73% of adult Americans experience one or more tension headaches in a year.[7] Tension headaches are generally considered to be muscular in origin. No sufficient evidence exists, however, for a specific pathophysiology.[3] These headaches are typically of mild to moderate intensity. The pain is bilateral and of a pressing character and does not have associated symptoms. Precipitating headache factors include situational stress, missed meals, sleep deprivation, and noxious stimuli (e.g., heat exposure).[28]

LOW BACK PAIN

Low back pain (LBP) is the second most common pain complaint among the adult population. Approximately 3% to 7% of the population in western industrialized countries experience chronic LBP. Job absenteeism, loss of productive activity, and decreased participation are common consequences of LBP.[50] The most common causes of LBP are injury (e.g., lifting) and stress, resulting in musculoskeletal and neurological disorders (e.g., muscle spasm and sciatica). Back pain also may result from infections, degenerative diseases (e.g., osteoarthritis), rheumatoid arthritis, spinal stenosis, tumors, and congenital disorders.[40] LBP tends to improve spontaneously over time.[51] Once significant back pain has lasted for 6 months, however, the chance of return to work is only 50%.[9]

Catalina's LBP has significantly compromised her ability to engage in occupations. She has not returned to work and is no longer able to engage in a preferred recreational activity of dancing and bowling. Her ability to care for her personal ADL is compromised, and she had difficulties stepping in and out of the tub and even bending over to turn the water faucet handles to regulate the water temperature. She must request assistance when grocery shopping because bending and reaching produce increased pain. Catalina even reports that getting in and out of her car is difficult and requires planning and care because of her fear of increasing the pain in her back.

ARTHRITIS

Approximately one third of all American adults experience joint pain, swelling, or limitation of motion because of arthritis.[25] Osteoarthritis (OA), the most common form of arthritis, is a degenerative joint disease characterized by a progressive, dull ache and swelling, typically affecting the fingers, elbows, hips, knees, and ankles. OA may be exacerbated by movement. Degeneration of the articular cartilage and swelling occur, typically affecting weight-bearing joints in persons after age 45.[45]

Rheumatoid arthritis (RA) usually has a slow, insidious onset, characterized by aches, pains, swelling, and stiffness. Any joint may be involved, but usually a symmetrical pattern affects the fingers, wrists, knees, ankles, and cervical spine. This systemic disease involves remissions and exacerbations of destructive inflammation of connective tissue, especially in the synovial joints.[45] See Chapter 38 for more information on arthritis.

COMPLEX REGIONAL PAIN SYNDROME

Complex regional pain syndrome (CRPS) pain is continuous, severe burning pain that results from trauma, postsurgical inflammation, infection, or laceration to an extremity and causes a cycle of vasospasm and vasodilatation. Pain, edema, shiny skin, coolness of the hand, and extreme sensitivity to touch occur. An individual experiencing CRPS may also have excessive sweating or dryness. The key feature of CRPS is continuous, intense pain out of proportion to the severity of the injury (if an injury has occurred), which gets worse over time. Exacerbating pain factors include movement, cutaneous stimulation, and stress.[23,54]

MYOFASCIAL PAIN SYNDROME

Myofascial pain refers to a large group of muscle disorders defined by the presence of "trigger points" (i.e., localized areas of deep muscle tenderness). Pressure on the trigger point elicits pain to a well-defined distal area. Myofascial pain is perceived as a continual dull ache often located in the head, neck, shoulder, and low back areas. The trapezius muscle is one of the most commonly affected muscles. The pain may result from sustained muscle contraction or from an acute strain caused by a sudden overload or overstretching of the muscles in the head, neck, shoulder, or lower back regions.[17,44]

FIBROMYALGIA

The prevalence of fibromyalgia ranges from 0.7% to 3.2% in the adult population. Fibromyalgia is widespread musculoskeletal pain in the muscles, ligaments, and tendons. Skeletal muscles have been implicated as the cause of fibromyalgia, but no specific abnormalities have been identified. Abnormalities of the neuroendocrine system, autoimmune dysfunction, immune regulation, cerebral blood flow difficulties, and sleep disturbances have been suggested.[20]

CANCER PAIN

Patients with cancer often have multiple pain problems that are frequently undertreated. Cancer pain varies greatly in its frequency, duration, and intensity. In the initial and intermediate stages 40% to 50% of patients experience moderate to severe pain. About 60% to 90% of patients with advanced cancer have pain. Cancer pain may result from tumor progression, interventions (e.g., surgery, chemotherapy, and radiation), infection, or muscle aches when patients decrease their activity.[47]

CENTRAL PAIN SYNDROME

Central pain syndrome is a neurological disorder caused by damage to or dysfunction of the central nervous system (e.g., stroke, Parkinson's disease, multiple sclerosis). The presentation of central pain syndrome varies widely as a result of the many potential causes. The pain is typically constant, moderate-to-severe in intensity, and perceived as a burning or "pins and needles" sensation. Exacerbating pain factors include touch, movement, temperature changes, and emotional distress. Numbness may accompany the areas of pain.[35]

EVALUATION

A referral for OT evaluation is made when pain interferes with the patient's occupational performance. As an interdisciplinary team member, the OT focuses the evaluation on the factors that contribute to the patient's pain perception and pain interference. Before the OT program is implemented and throughout the interventions,[18] objective measures of occupational performance should be obtained to assess the occupational profile of the patient and the value of those occupations. Factors that may contribute to pain perception, occupational role disruption, decreased occupational performance, and diminished quality of life should be identified.

The OT performs a **pain evaluation**, viewing pain as a complex phenomenon involving psychological arousal, sensations of noxious stimulation, tissue damage or irritation, behavioral avoidance, complaints of subjective distress, and the social environment. Self-report measures are the most common type of pain assessment because pain is considered to be primarily a subjective phenomenon. The clinical interview focuses on the patient's identification of pain location, frequency, duration, intensity, onset, exacerbating and relieving pain factors, past and present pain treatments, affect, and occupational performance. The single most reliable indicator of the existence and intensity of pain, and any resultant affective discomfort, is the patient's self-report.[49] A Verbal Rating Scale (VRS), 0-10 Numeric Pain Intensity Scale, or Visual Analog Scale (VAS) (Figure 27-1) may be used in assessing self-reports of pain intensity.[37,49] These instruments have strong psychometric properties and high utility. When OT services were initiated for Catalina, the therapist used a self-report scale to determine the existence and intensity of the pain she experienced on a daily basis.

Pain behaviors are commonly targeted in evaluation and intervention.[12] Pain behaviors include guarded movement,

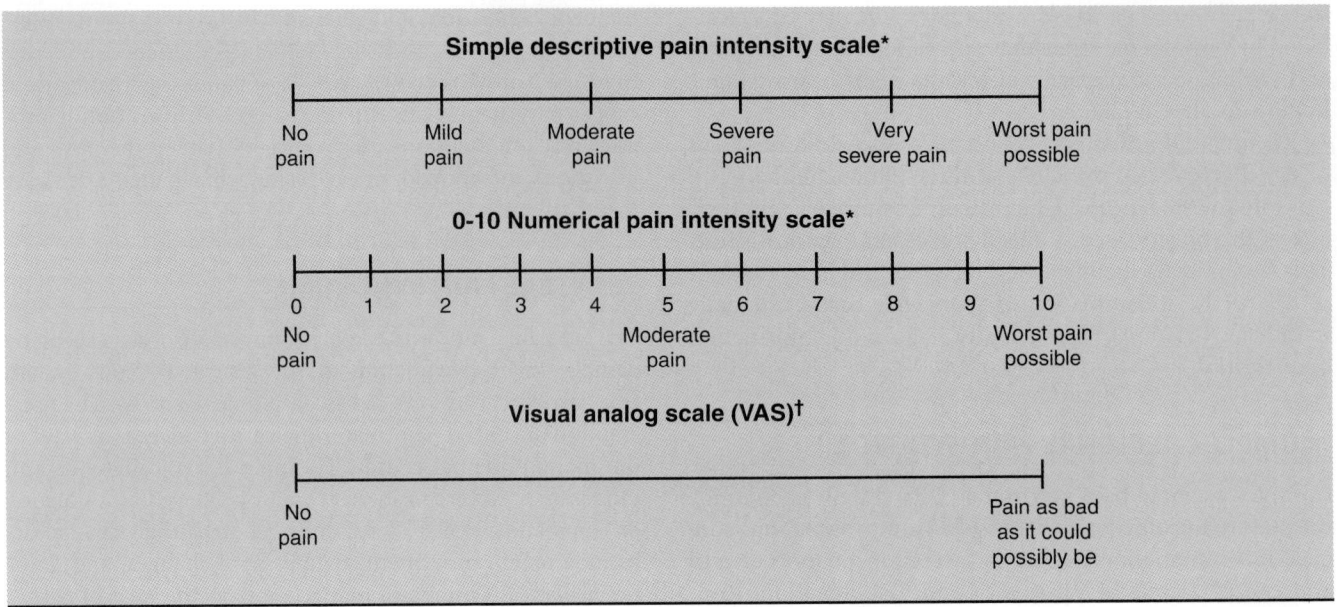

Figure 27-1   Examples of pain intensity scales. *If used as a graphic rating scale, a 10-cm baseline is recommended. †A 10-cm baseline is recommended for VAS scales. (From US Department of Health and Human Services, Acute Pain Management Guideline Panel: *Acute pain management in adults: operative procedures. Quick reference guide for clinicians*, AHCPR Pub No. 92-0019, Rockville, Md, 1995, US Government Printing Office.)

bracing, posturing, limping, rubbing, and facial grimacing.[24] The University of Alabama Pain Behavior Scale[39] is an example of a standardized rating scale that is reliable, valid, and an easy method for documenting overt behaviors. Analysis of the patient's pain behaviors before, during, and after intervention can provide valuable information about the role of situational and learned factors in the individual's pain perception, in addition to responses to intervention. Merskey[32] cautioned practitioners not to provide treatment for reduction of pain behaviors in lieu of attempts at pain alleviation. Evaluation that focuses solely on pain behavior may lead to the inaccurate conclusion that pain behavior suggests malingering, lack of motivation, or hypochondriasis.

Occupational performance is the primary focus of the OT. The patient may complete daily activity diaries as an assessment technique and outcome measure. With this technique, hourly entries of time spent in sitting, standing, reclining, and productive activities are recorded by the patient and may be corroborated by trained staff during treatment.[11] Activity diaries are highly reliable and valid.[11] The Brief Pain Inventory (BPI)[8] is a reliable and valid instrument that may also be used to measure pain interference. Patients rate on an ordinal scale how much their pain has interfered with general activity, mood, mobility, work, interpersonal relationships, sleep, enjoyment of life, self-care, and recreation (Figure 27-2). This information may be helpful in determining baseline tolerance levels for specific occupations that may be addressed in treatment. Catalina had indicated that her pain and the fear associated with the pain severely limited her ability to engage in several occupations. She had not returned to work and had severely limited social activities. Her contact with friends was limited to infrequent telephone conversations and occasionally a friend would stop by to visit. Before her injury she regularly went out with friends to movies, dancing, and bowling, but all those activities had been eliminated because of the pain.

INTERVENTION

The obligation to manage pain and relieve a patient's suffering is fundamental. An interdisciplinary team approach to chronic pain is common and includes the patient as an active and educated participant. The Joint Commission on Accreditation of Rehabilitation Centers[22] has identified pain management standards. The OT works in collaboration with the person served, a physician, and a psychologist. A physical therapist, nurse, vocational specialist, or dietitian may also provide evaluation and intervention. OT interventions focus on increasing physical capacities, productive and satisfying performance of life tasks and roles, mastery of self and environment through activities, and education.[21] Because the causes of pain are multifactorial, so are the approaches to treatment. Typical **pain interventions** are described below.

The effectiveness of pain interventions can be measured and documented in a variety of ways. Clinical improvement can be measured in occupational performance (e.g., BPI), increased participation (e.g., diary), lower pain intensity (e.g., VRS), reduction in pain behaviors (e.g., University of Alabama Pain Behavior Scale), improved mood (e.g., Sickness Impact Profile[2]), and decreased drug and healthcare utilization.

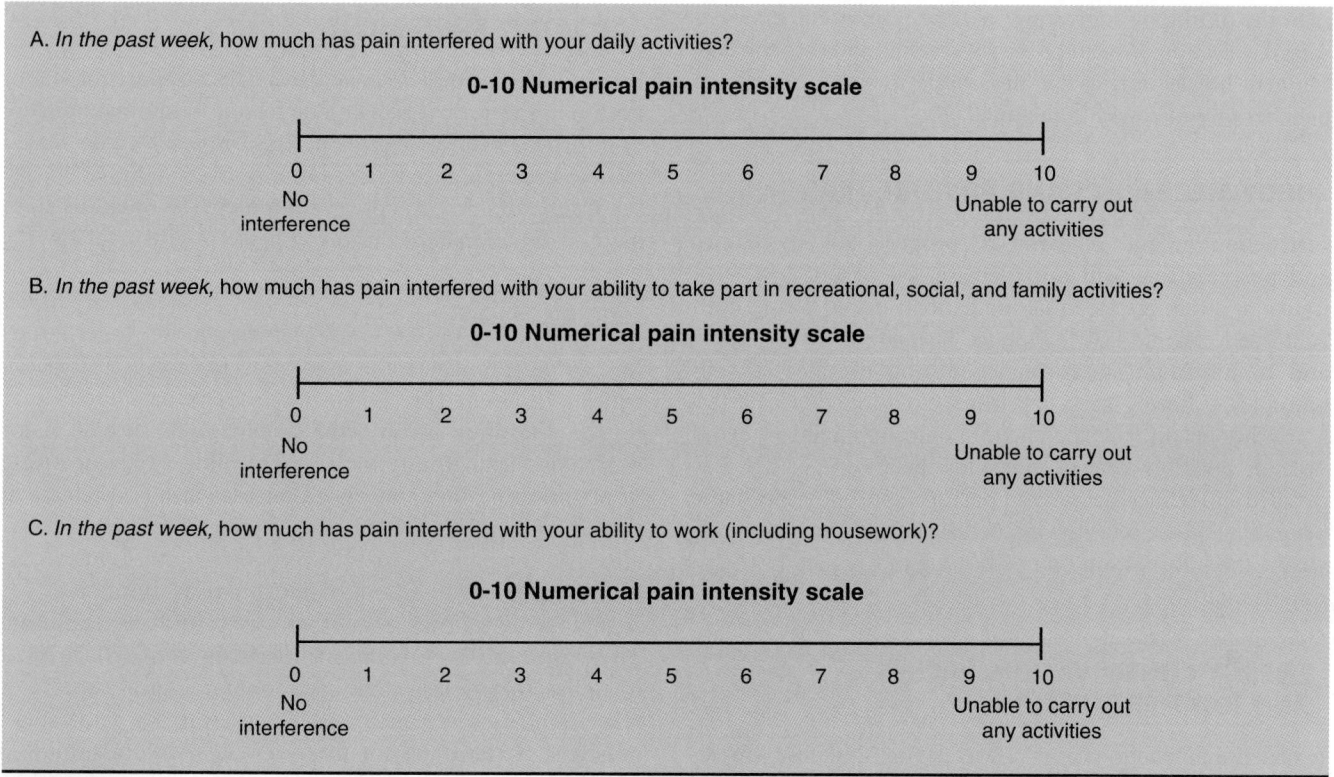

A. *In the past week,* how much has pain interfered with your daily activities?

0-10 Numerical pain intensity scale

0 1 2 3 4 5 6 7 8 9 10
No interference — Unable to carry out any activities

B. *In the past week,* how much has pain interfered with your ability to take part in recreational, social, and family activities?

0-10 Numerical pain intensity scale

0 1 2 3 4 5 6 7 8 9 10
No interference — Unable to carry out any activities

C. *In the past week,* how much has pain interfered with your ability to work (including housework)?

0-10 Numerical pain intensity scale

0 1 2 3 4 5 6 7 8 9 10
No interference — Unable to carry out any activities

Figure 27-2   Pain interference scales. (From National Institutes of Health, National Institute of Child Health and Human Development, National Institute of Neurological Disorders and Stroke: Ongoing research [Grant No. 1 PO1 HD/NS33988]).

MEDICATION

Medications are generally the treatment of choice for individuals experiencing acute pain. OTs need to observe patients for possible drug reactions. To reduce possible discomfort from rehabilitative procedures, practitioners should check that patients are adequately medicated in advance. The World Health Organization[53] analgesic ladder is well established in adult pain management as a stepwise approach for choosing an analgesic. Aspirin and acetaminophen are frequently used in the treatment of mild pain (e.g., backache) because of their high level of effectiveness, low level of toxicity, and limited abuse potential. Nonsteroidal anti-inflammatory agents have been used in the treatment of arthritis and inflammation of musculoskeletal origin. Codeine is often used for moderate-intensity pain that has not responded adequately to aspirin or acetaminophen. Morphine is the standard medication used in the relief of severe pain. The use of opioid analgesics (a newer term for narcotics) in chronic nonmalignant pain has been controversial because of concerns about addiction.[19]

ACTIVITY TOLERANCE

Although a few days of rest may be indicated for acute pain, therapeutic activity is important for the treatment of any underlying impairment. Activity levels are increased on a gradual basis, with the patient working to "tolerance" (i.e., gradual increase in task demands such as duration, mobility, strength, and endurance), as opposed to "pain," before a scheduled rest period. The patient should not initiate rest at the time of the pain onset or exacerbation because this may reinforce pain behaviors.[13] A gradual increase in activity also lessens the likelihood of an exacerbation of pain. Fordyce[13] provided guidelines for the use of quota programs for patients with chronic pain. Regular gentle exercise (e.g., walking, swimming, water aerobics) is recommended. Modalities (e.g., heat or cold) may be applied before activity as a means of enhancing functional performance. When an individual is engaged in interesting and purposeful activity, he or she may be more relaxed, less preoccupied with pain, and more fluid in movement.

 OT PRACTICE NOTE

Task selection based on occupational roles, interests, and abilities is a unique contribution of OT in pain management.[46]

The OT intervention program for Catalina considered her active lifestyle before the injury and began with simple activities such as accompanying a friend to a local shopping mall and walking in the complex. The OT helped Catalina plan the outing by suggesting that the walk occur during a weekday evening instead of busy weekends and that she take frequent breaks during the initial walk to sit on one of the benches provided within the mall.

BODY MECHANICS AND POSTURE TRAINING

Instruction in and rehearsal of proper body mechanics and postures that will not increase the risk of low back injury or strain are essential for patients experiencing both acute and chronic LBP.[29] Practice in using the body safely and to maximum performance during routine tasks in natural (i.e., home, work, or leisure) environments is particularly important.[43,46] The client should be taught to avoid tasks or positions that do not allow balanced posture. For detailed guidelines on proper posture and body mechanic principles, please refer to Chapter 41. For patients in wheelchairs, the information on positioning in Chapter 11 is also important.

ENERGY CONSERVATION, PACING, AND JOINT PROTECTION

Instruction in energy conservation, pacing, and joint protection may be beneficial for achieving recommended amounts of rest during task completion, recommended time spent physically active, and balance between rest and physical activity. Clients, especially those with rheumatoid arthritis, are taught to use these strategies before they experience pain and fatigue so that occupational performance can continue as long as possible without pain and fatigue.[14]

Catalina was able to employ strategies of energy conservation and pacing to return to many previous occupations such as doing her laundry using a portable table to place the laundry basket on the table when putting the clothes in her top-loading washer. The table was also used when she removed the clothes from the washer before she moved them to the side-opening dryer. This example illustrates the use of energy conservation and pacing that was employed throughout Catalina's daily life.

SPLINTING

Splinting of the upper extremity may be necessary if contractures or muscle imbalances occur. In complex regional pain syndrome static resting splints may provide pain relief. Splint use is alternated with tasks that require joints to be taken through range of motion, because total immobilization could lead to increased pain and dysfunction. Static resting splints maintain joint alignment and reduce inflammation and pain during flare-ups of rheumatoid arthritis. Splints that support the wrist in a functional position throughout the day and night may be necessary for 4 to 6 weeks.[4] People should use caution because orthoses may add to the stress on proximal joints when the wrist is confined.[6]

ADAPTIVE EQUIPMENT

Patients with acute LBP may use a back support for stabilization of the lumbar area and increased abdominal pressure to improve postural alignment. This can result in decreased muscle spasm, reduced pain, and improved ability to engage in occupations.[4,48] Adaptive equipment is often used to increase function and comfort in persons with arthritis.[45]

RELAXATION

Relaxation training can be used to decrease muscle tension, which is believed to precipitate or exacerbate pain. Progressive muscle relaxation involves the systematic tensing of major musculoskeletal groups for several seconds, passive focusing of attention on how the tensed muscles feel, and release of the muscles and passive focusing on the sensations of relaxation. As the patient learns to recognize muscle tension, he or she can direct attention to inducing relaxation.[38]

Autogenic training is another way to induce relaxation. This approach involves the silent repetition of self-directed formulas that describe the psychophysiological aspects of relaxation (e.g., "My arms and legs are warm"). The patient passively concentrates on these phrases while assuming a relaxed body posture, with eyes closed, in a quiet setting. Relaxation training has been used successfully to modify a variety of chronic pain complaints, including headache, LBP, myofascial pain, arthritis, and cancer pain.[16,38]

Relaxation strategies were very helpful to Catalina and allowed her to regain a "bit of her old self." When out shopping with friends, she would often pause briefly and appear to be studying the clothing item while employing the relaxation strategies rehearsed during her OT sessions. This allowed her to continue with the outing.

BIOFEEDBACK

Biofeedback is the use of instrumentation to provide visual or auditory signals that indicate some change in a biological process, such as skin temperature, as it occurs. The signals are used to increase the patient's awareness of these changes so that the changes may come under voluntary control. Biofeedback is based on the assumption that a maladaptive psychophysiological response results in chronic pain. Despite the questionable validity of this assumption, data do exist to support the use of biofeedback for the treatment of headache disorders, LBP, arthritis, myofascial pain, and CRPS.[16] Biofeedback for pain control is typically done in conjunction with relaxation training.

DISTRACTION

Distraction is often used to divert an individual's attention and concentration away from acute mild-to-moderate intensity pain and reduce distress, especially during medical and rehabilitative procedures. Distraction may have an internal focus (e.g., daydreaming, guided imagery) or external focus (e.g., listening to music, watching television).

THERAPEUTIC MODALITIES

Physical agent modalities (PAM) may be used by OTs as adjuncts to or preparation for purposeful activities. Appropriate postprofessional education is needed to ensure that the practitioner is competent in the use of these modalities.[5] Both heat and ice are useful in reduction of pain and muscle spasm of musculoskeletal and neurological pathologies. Superficial heat includes hot packs, heating pads, paraffin wax, fluidotherapy, hydrotherapy, whirlpool, and heat lamps. The application of heat results in an increase in local metabolism and circulation. Vasoconstriction occurs initially, followed by vasodilatation, resulting in muscle relaxation. The use of heat is indicated in the treatment of subacute and chronic traumatic and inflammatory conditions such as muscle spasms, arthritis of the small joints of the hands and feet, tendonitis, and bursitis.[5,11,26]

The use of heat is contraindicated in several instances. Heat is not to be used for patients who have acute inflammatory conditions, cardiac insufficiency, malignancies, or peripheral vascular disease. Preexisting edema may be aggravated. Heat may cause malignancies to spread.

Cold can improve pain control by elevating the pain threshold (i.e., the minimal level of noxious stimulation at which the patient first reports pain). Local vasoconstriction occurs in direct response to cold therapy (cryotherapy). When the area is subsequently exposed to air, vasodilatation occurs. Cold applications also result in decreased local metabolism, slowing of nerve conduction velocity, diminished muscle spasm secondary to joint or skeletal pathological conditions and spasticity, decreased edema, and lessened tissue damage. Cold can be applied via commercial packs, sprays, ice cups, or a massage stick.[5,26]

Several contraindications exist to the use of cryotherapy. Patients who are extremely sensitive may not be able to tolerate cold. If a patient has a history of frostbite in the area to be treated, another modality must be used. If a patient has Raynaud's disease, severe pain may occur in the treated area. Cryotherapy is contraindicated in the very young and elderly, because their thermoregulatory responses may not function sufficiently.[11]

TRANSCUTANEOUS ELECTRICAL NERVE STIMULATION

Transcutaneous electrical nerve stimulation (TENS) is a noninvasive pain relief measure that uses cutaneous stimulation. A TENS unit consists of a battery-powered generator that sends a mild electrical current through electrodes placed on the skin at or near the pain site, which stimulates A fibers. Some success has been demonstrated with using

TENS to relieve acute and chronic painful conditions caused by disease or injury of nervous system structures or the skeleton, muscle pain of ischemic origin in the extremities, and angina pectoris.[42]

SUMMARY

Pain is a complex phenomenon. OTs bring their understanding of anatomy, physiology, kinesiology, psychology, and function to the comprehensive evaluation and treatment of the patient with pain. Interventions focus on relieving pain, improving occupational performance, and developing coping strategies. Data are needed to support the use of the OT interventions described in this chapter.

Box **27-1** GLOSSARY

Nociception: The detection of potentially tissue-damaging thermal or mechanical energy by specialized nerve endings.
Pain: An unpleasant sensory *and* emotional experience associated with actual or *potential* tissue damage.
Pain behavior: Observable and measurable behaviors used by the patient to communicate the experience of pain to others.
Suffering: An unwanted condition and the corresponding negative emotion.

Review Questions

1. Contrast acute pain and chronic pain.
2. List and describe two different pain syndromes that may be present in persons referred for OT.
3. Identify the essential elements of a pain assessment.
4. Explain at least six interventions used in the treatment of pain.
5. Describe the role and define the scope of OT in the evaluation and treatment of pain.

REFERENCES

1. Baptiste S: Chronic pain, activity and culture, *Can J Occup Ther* 55:179, 1988.
2. Bergner M, Bobbitt RA, Carter WE, et al: The Sickness Impact Profile: development and final version of a health status measure, *Med Care* 19:787, 1981.
3. Biber MP: Headache. In Warfield CA, Fausett HJ, editors: *Manual of pain management*, ed 2, Philadelphia, 2002, Lippincott Williams & Wilkins.
4. Borrelli EF, Warfield CA: Occupational therapy for pain, *Hosp Pract*, August 15, 1986.
5. Breines EB: Therapeutic occupations and modalities. In Pedretti LW, Early MB, editors: *Occupational therapy: practice skills for physical dysfunction*, ed 5, St. Louis, 2001, Mosby.
6. Bulthaup S, Cipriani D, Thomas JJ: An electromyography study of wrist extension orthoses and upper-extremity function, *Am J Occup Ther* 53(5):434, 1999.

7. Cailliet R: *Headache and face pain syndromes*, Philadelphia, 1992, FA Davis.

8. Cleeland CS: Research in cancer pain: what we know and what we need to know, *Cancer* 67:823, 1991.

9. Ellis RM: Back pain, *BMJ* 310(6989):1220, 1995.

10. Follick MJ, Ahern DK, Laser-Wolston N: Evaluation of a daily activity diary for chronic pain patients, *Pain* 19(4):373, 1984.

11. Fond D, Hecox B: Superficial heat modalities. In Hecox B, Mehreteab TA, Weisberg J, editors: *Physical agents: a comprehensive text for physical therapists*, Norwalk, Conn, 1994, Appleton & Lange.

12. Fordyce WE: *Behavioral methods for chronic pain and illness*, St Louis, 1976, Mosby.

13. Fordyce WE: Contingency management. In Bonica JJ, editor: *The management of pain*, ed 2, Philadelphia, 1990, Lea & Febiger.

14. Furst GP, Gerber LH, Smith CC, et al: A program for improving energy conservation behaviors in adults with rheumatoid arthritis, *Am J Occup Ther* 41(2):102, 1987.

15. Gallagher RM: Primary headache disorders. In Weiner RS, editor: *Pain management: a practical guide for clinicians*, ed 6, Boca Raton, Fl, 2001, CRC Press.

16. Gaupp LA, Flinn DE, Weddige RL: Adjunctive treatment techniques. In Tollison CD, Satterthwaite JR, Tollison JW, editors: *Handbook of pain management*, ed 2, Baltimore, 1994, Williams & Wilkins.

17. Goldberg DL: Controversies in fibromyalgia and myofascial pain syndromes. In Arnoff GM, editor: *Evaluation and management of chronic pain*, ed 3, Baltimore, 1998, Williams & Wilkins.

18. Hamdy RC: The decade of pain control and research (Editorial), *Southern Med J* 94(8):753, 2001.

19. Hawthorn J, Redmond K: *Pain: causes and management*, Malden, Mass, 1998, Blackwell Science.

20. Hernandez-Garcia JM: Fibromyalgia. In Warfield CA, Fausett HJ, editors: *Manual of pain management*, ed 2, Philadelphia, 2002, Lippincott Williams & Wilkins.

21. International Association for the Study of Pain, ad hoc Subcommittee for Occupational Therapy/Physical Therapy Curriculum: Pain curriculum for students in occupational therapy or physical therapy, *IASP Newsletter* November/December, 1994, The Association.

22. Joint Commission on Accreditation of Healthcare Organization: *Comprehensive accreditation manual for hospitals: the official handbook*, Oak Brook Ill, 2003, Commission.

23. Kasch MC: Hand injuries. In Pedretti LW, editor: *Occupational therapy: practice skills for physical dysfunction*, ed 4, St Louis, 1996, Mosby.

24. Keefe FJ, Block AR: Development of an observation method for assessing pain behavior in chronic low back pain patients, *Behav Ther* 13:363, 1982.

25. Lawrence RC, et al: Estimates of the prevalence of arthritis and selected musculoskeletal disorders in the United States, *Arthritis Rheumatism* 41(5):778, 1998.

26. Lee MHM, et al: Physical therapy and rehabilitation medicine, In Bonica JJ, editor: *The management of pain*, ed 2, Philadelphia, 1990, Lea & Febiger.

27. Loeser JD, Fordyce WE: Chronic pain. In Carr JE, Dengerink HA, editors: *Behavioral science in the practice of medicine*, New York, 1983, Elsevier.

28. Mauskop A: Head pain. In Ashburn MA, Rice LJ, editors: *The management of pain*, New York, 1998, Churchill Livingstone.

29. McCauley M: The effects of body mechanics instruction on work performance among young workers, *Am J Occup Ther* 44(5):402, 1990.

30. Melzack R: *The puzzle of pain*, New York, 1973, BasicBooks.

31. Melzack R, Wall PD: *The challenge of pain*, London, 1988, Penguin Books.

32. Merskey H: Limitations of pain behavior, *APS* 1:101, 1992.

33. Merskey H, Bogduk N, editors: *Classification of chronic pain. Definitions of chronic pain syndromes and definition of pain terms*, ed 2, Seattle, 1994, International Association for the Study of Pain.

34. Mosey AC: An alternative: the biopsychosocial model, *Am J Occup Ther* 28:137, 1974.

35. National Institute of Neurological Disorders and Stroke, 2004.

36. National Pain Awareness: *Key messages about chronic pain* [on-line]. Available: http://www.painconnection.org/NationalPainAwareness/KeyMessagesAboutChronicPain.DOC, 2004.

37. Patterson DR, Jensen M, Engel-Knowles J: Pain and its influence on assistive technology use. In Scherer MJ, editor: *Assistive technology: matching device and consumer for successful rehabilitation*, Washington, DC, 2002, American Psychological Association.

38. Payne RA: *Relaxation techniques: a practical handbook for the health care professional*, New York, 2000, Churchill Livingstone.

39. Richards JS, et al: Assessing pain behavior: the UAB Pain Behavior Scale, *Pain* 14:393, 1982.

40. Rowlingson JC, Keifer RB: Low back pain. In Ashburn MA, Rice LJ, editors: *The management of pain*, New York, 1998, Churchill Livingstone.

41. Schweitzer A: *On the edge of the primeval forest*, p 62, New York, 1931, Macmillan.

42. Sjolund BH, Eriksson M, Loeser JD: Transcutaneous and implanted electrical stimulation of peripheral nerves. In Bonica JJ, editor: *The management of pain*, ed 2, Philadelphia, 1990, Lea & Febiger.

43. Smithline J, Dunlop LE: Low back pain. In Pedretti LW, Early MB, editors: *Occupational therapy: practice skills for physical dysfunction*, ed 5, St Louis, 2001, Mosby.

44. Sola AE, Bonica JJ: Myofascial pain syndromes. In Bonica JJ, editor: *The management of pain*, ed 2, Philadelphia, 1990, Lea & Febiger.

45. Spencer EA: Upper extremity musculoskeletal impairments. In Crepeau EB, Cohn ES, Schell BAB, editors: *Willard & Spackman's occupational therapy*, ed 10, Philadelphia, 2003, Lippincott.

46. Strong J: *Chronic pain: the occupational therapist's perspective*, New York, 1996, Churchill Livingstone.

47. Strong J, Bennett S: Cancer pain. In Strong J, Unruh AM, Wright A, et al, editors: *Pain: a textbook for therapists*, New York, 2002, Churchill Livingstone.

48. Tyson R, Strong J: Adaptive equipment: its effectiveness for people with chronic lower back pain, *Occup Ther J Res* 10:111, 1990.

49. U.S. Department of Health and Human Services: *Management of cancer pain*, Rockville, Md, 1994, AHCPR.

50. Van Tulder MW, Jellema P, van Poppel MNM, et al: Lumbar supports for prevention and treatment of low back pain (Cochrane Review). In *The Cochrane Library*, Issue 4. Oxford, 2000. Update Software.

51. Waddell G: A new clinical model for the treatment of low back pain, *Spine* 12:632, 1987.

52. Wolff M, Wittink H, Michel TH: Chronic pain concepts and definitions. In Wittink H, Michel TH, editors: *Chronic pain management for physical therapists*, Boston, 1997, Butterworth-Heinemann.

53. World Health Organization: *Cancer pain relief and palliative care.* Report of a WHO expert committee. World Health Organization Technical Report Series, 804, p 1, Geneva, Switzerland, 1990, World Health Organization.

54. Wright A: Neuropathic pain. In Strong J, Unruh AM, Wright A, et al, editors: *Pain: a textbook for therapists*, New York, 2002, Churchill Livingstone.

The Occupational Therapy Process: Implementation of Intervention

28 THERAPEUTIC OCCUPATIONS AND MODALITIES

ESTELLE B. BREINES

KEY TERMS

Active occupations
Egocentric realm
Exocentric realm
Consensual realm

Occupational genesis
Physical agent modalities
Grading
Simulated or enabling activity

Adjunctive modalities
Isotonic exercises
Isometric exercises
Active exercise

Resistive activity
Passive exercise

LEARNING OBJECTIVES

After studying this chapter the student or practitioner will be able to do the following:

1. Recognize the organizing concepts of occupational genesis as they relate to active occupation.
2. Discuss the role of activity analysis in the selection of therapeutic activity.
3. Understand the similarities and distinctions between the therapeutic activity and therapeutic exercise.
4. Identify the role of physical agent modalities in occupational therapy practice.
5. Describe how grading activity heightens functional performance.
6. Differentiate between the various types of therapeutic exercise.
7. Describe how and why simulated and enabling activities are used in practice.
8. Describe how and why adjunctive modalities are used in occupational therapy practice.
9. Identify the requirements established by the American Occupational Therapy Association for the use of adjunctive modalities in occupational therapy practice.
10. Perform an activity analysis appropriate for physical dysfunction.

CHAPTER OUTLINE

Active occupation
Philosophical foundations
  Egocentric realm
  Exocentric realm
  Consensual realm
  Relationships among realms
Evolving practice
Purposeful occupation and activity
Occupation and health
  Assessment of occupational role performance
Activity analysis
  Principles of activity analysis
Therapeutic approaches

  Biomechanical approach
  Sensorimotor approach
Adapting and grading activity
  Adaptation of activity
  Grading of activity
Selection of activity
Simulated or enabling activity
Adjunctive modalities
  Therapeutic exercise and activity
  Physical agent modalities
Selection of appropriate modalities in the continuum of care
Summary

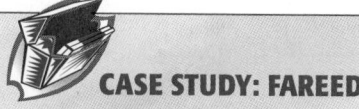

CASE STUDY: FAREED

Fareed is an 82-year-old retired bookkeeper whose primary diagnosis is s/p right CVA with residual shoulder/hand pain of his left upper extremity (LUE). The stroke resulted in his hospitalization and subsequent admission to a subacute facility. He has a past medical history of hypertension and prostate cancer, and he has exhibited reactive depression since his recent hospitalization.

Before the recent hospitalization, Fareed lived with his wife in a private home in a suburban neighborhood. One of his children lives in a nearby town and visits weekly. His other two children and their families live in cities within a day's drive and visit several times a year.

Since his retirement, which he had looked forward to, Fareed developed or expanded several interests, including woodworking, gardening, cooking, and traveling. He and his wife have taken a yearly vacation, traveling to various locations in the United States for periods of 3 weeks since his retirement. Fareed had also been responsible for managing the family finances. In all, Fareed had an active schedule before his recent hospitalization.

Initial evaluation revealed that Fareed is dependent in dressing, independent in feeding, and exhibits a mild left visual field cut.

He has limited active and passive ROM of the left shoulder, with pain on passive flexion of the left shoulder at the end of the range. Active ROM is limited in the LUE, but Fareed is able to grasp, pronate his forearm, flex the elbow, and internally rotate the shoulder. His balance and mobility are impaired. Although his prospects for recovery are positive, Fareed expresses feelings of dejection about regaining his ability to resume his independence, roles, and activities.

Focus of OT intervention included the following:

- Engage in meaningful occupations to reduce depression
- Adapt and grade activities (ADL; assistive, active, and resistive restorative activities) using unilateral, bilateral, and balance activities, to enable participation in life roles
- Reduce pain associated with movement to enable use of LUE in occupations; apply heat to left shoulder and provide analgesic 20 minutes before active occupation treatment.
- Increase ROM and strength of LUE
- Improve balance and mobility through participation in activity
- Prepare Fareed and family with skills needed for him to return home

Intervention was initiated at bedside with sitting balance activities as a preface for dressing training. The client was instructed in scanning techniques to reduce the effects of his visual field cut. Fareed learned one-handed techniques for upper extremity dressing, gradually shifting to bilateral dressing as his strength and ROM improved.

The client was further evaluated to identify an intervention activity that he would find meaningful. He decided to pursue a woodworking task, making a small bench for his youngest grandchild. Because he was not able to use his left arm actively at the initiation of OT services, the therapist set his project up by using an inclined sanding board. This permitted him first passive, then active-assistive, and then active motion to heighten performance. Before beginning the activity, to reduce pain in his LUE and heighten his tolerance for movement, heat was applied to his shoulder using hot packs. To improve his balance and standing tolerance, the sanding board was placed on a standing table. As his performance improved, Fareed was discharged to home and returned to the clinic as an outpatient three times per week. With encouragement from his family and his therapist, Fareed completed the bench, which resulted in feelings of self-satisfaction.

Acting on suggestions from the therapist, the family installed raised garden beds at home, enabling him to participate in an occupation at home, an activity he particularly loved. These efforts resulted in his gradual recognition that he was able to engage in some of his favorite activities, albeit in adapted form. As he recovered motor performance in his arm and his balance became safer, his depression lifted, aided by some medication. He and his wife began to use the Internet to find new recipes that they could cook together and Fareed began to write the checks again and explore potential travel opportunities.

Critical Thinking Questions

1. Identify occupations Fareed engaged in before his stroke, those in which he engaged during intervention, and those he assumed or resumed. Describe how his progress relied upon evaluation of his occupational performance.
2. Explore the contextual factors that influenced Fareed in resuming preferred activities. Describe roles he resumed as a consequence of these influences.
3. Describe how the activities in which Fareed engaged were adapted to provide an interface between activity demands and client factors.

ACTIVE OCCUPATION

Active occupations are the foundation of occupational therapy (OT) practice. Active occupations are those activities in which people engage as part of their life's roles. These include personal care; the constructional tasks that involve the use of hand and mechanical tools; technological activities that involve such tools as calculators, computers, and electronics; games of various sorts; and vocational skills. They function together in a complex process, stimulating growth and health throughout the life span.

When physical disability strikes and the ability to perform occupational roles and activities becomes impaired, the occupational therapist (OT) helps clients to regain their skills using active occupations as therapeutic tools to stimulate performance and gears intervention to enable clients to assume or resume their ability to engage in life's occupations.

Active occupation is the primary therapeutic modality of OT, designed to stimulate function and to lead to improved function, and is relevant throughout the life span.

Engagement in activity enhances performance beyond the given task. Learning to perform one activity skillfully leads to skillful performance in other activities. Therefore, active occupations are the objectives and the tools of practice. Activities are the means and the end to heightened performance. Whether related to personal care, work, or leisure, active occupations constitute an effective and substantial portion of any OT program and distinguish OT as a profession.

The needs and interests of clients guide the selection of occupations used for therapy. These needs are governed by the roles clients play in their worlds. As members of society, clients represent the societies in which they perform activities, and the activities in which they engage reflect their worlds. The clients' needs and interests are tied to the societies in which they live. Therefore, active occupations reflect society's values. In a society in which independence, leisure, and work all are valued, the interests of clients are variable and include self-care, hobbies, and work-related tasks.

Clients must assume their personal and social obligations to become effective members of society. To assume these responsibilities, clients must acquire the skills needed to perform their occupational roles. The roles people assume reflect their participation in occupations. For persons with disabilities, participation may require relearning skills, learning new skills, or learning to perform activities in new ways. Therefore, the OT must be prepared with a broad knowledge of activities and techniques that may then be used as tools of therapy in a client-centered approach. OTs must understand the roles and activities in which people engage in performing their life's tasks. As a consequence, OTs must be prepared to meet the challenges that ordinarily occur as people and societies evolve and change.

Just as society changes and adapts with the invention of new objects and methods, so do the activities clients use in their lives. Nowhere is this more readily observed than in an examination of the OT treatment environment. Just as the nature of activity has changed over time as societies have evolved and adapted, the scope of OT's intervention methods and modalities has changed and broadened considerably over the years.

When the field of OT became formalized in the early 1900s, the nature of human occupation was limited to the scope of activities that had been developed up to that time. Consequently, the use of handicrafts and early industrial tasks guided activity at the outset of the profession. Although commonly described as crafts, these activities can be viewed from an anthropological perspective, representing the times in which they were developed and in which they met people's personal and social needs. For example, making baskets and clay pots was not a frivolous activity when they were first designed. Rather, they were vital containers used to gather foods and other items, and the knowledge of how to make them was an important skill. However, times changed, and

along with these changes society developed new and different occupations, which require OTs to expand their skills to incorporate activities and techniques of the modern era.

OTs currently are qualified and competent in the use of a variety of therapeutic occupations and modalities, traditional and modern.[1] Their competence is derived from entry-level to advanced graduate education, specialty certification, continuing education, and work experience. The scope of practice is broad and addresses the continuum of intervention from wellness to acute care through advanced rehabilitation. Therefore, OT offers comprehensive services, and challenges the OT practitioner to keep pace with new developments in society and in practice.

PHILOSOPHICAL FOUNDATIONS

OTs organize intervention by integration of a comprehensive knowledge of the client's mind and body (the **egocentric realm**) with knowledge of the tangible world (the **exocentric realm**) and the social influences (the **consensual realm**) that contribute to function. The relationships among these three interactive forces are in constant flux in a lifelong developmental process that is stimulated by active occupation. These forces are evident in the various theories and models of practice OTs draw upon for practice. They can be noted within the various concepts of the Occupational Therapy Practice Framework.[2]

These foundational ideas stem from the work of John Dewey[19] and the other American philosophers of pragmatism whose work influenced the mental hygiene movement, which in turn influenced the founders of the profession.[13] Dewey's use of the terms *purposive activity* and *active occupation*, along with his renowned concept of learning through doing, are found in his text *Democracy and Education*,[19] published in 1916 in Chicago, a year before the establishment of the National Society for the Promotion of Occupational Therapy.

EGOCENTRIC REALM

Intensive training in the various client factors of motor, neurological, perceptual-cognitive, and emotional skills prepares the OT with a refined knowledge of what contributes to a client's performance in all aspects of the mind and body. Mind and body are seen as interactive and together govern performance. Our client, Fareed, has experienced a loss in motor function, due to a neurological insult, which contributes to a loss in occupational performance. This change in abilities has resulted in a reactive depression, which illustrates the interaction between the various egocentric factors.

EXOCENTRIC REALM

OTs have an equally refined understanding of the material world, the context in which people live, act, and react. Textures, weights, direction, location, time, and other tangible, contextual, and objective means regulate performance in the world. A person functions within a real world filled with objects and environments that must be manipulated in one manner or another. OTs are expert in adapting the tangible and durable elements of the world to enhance function. Returning to our client Fareed, we need to examine the exocentric realm of the world. The task demands of cooking, gardening, woodworking, and traveling require the client to control and manipulate the material world. The neurological insult Fareed experienced compromised his ability to control and manipulate the environmental features and objects necessary to engage in preferred activities.

CONSENSUAL REALM

OTs also bring their knowledge of the effects of society and social interactions on individual and group performance. This knowledge is used to enhance clients' function by effectuation of the roles they play in their social worlds. Recognizing and valuing the sociocultural contexts of occupation and their implications for client performance contribute to the OT's knowledge base and form a fundamental basis for formulation of the practice environment.

RELATIONSHIPS AMONG REALMS

The three major aspects of OT's knowledge base, the egocentric (mind and body), exocentric (time and space), and consensual (society) realms, are thoroughly integrated in active performance, regardless of interest, purpose, environment, or era.[12,13] OTs consider the interactions among these realms to influence or heighten the possibility of the client to engage in occupations (Figure 28-1). For example, a splint (exocentric) can be used to stabilize a wrist to reduce pain (egocentric), enabling the client to prepare a meal for the family (consensual). A walker can be adapted so that a client can carry her knitting (exocentric), allowing her to prepare gifts for her grandchild (consensual), and heighten her feelings of efficacy (egocentric).

Development and Evolution

The interaction among these three realms represents a developmental continuum. They influence one another

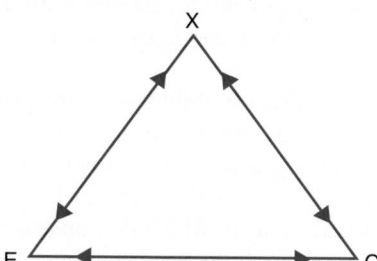

Figure 28-1 The egocentric *(E)*, exocentric *(X)*, and consensual *(C)* realms of the OT's knowledge base are related. (From Breines EB: *Occupational therapy from clay to computers: theory & practice*, Philadelphia, 1995, FA Davis.)

throughout the life span in a process defined as **occupational genesis**.[11] Interactions among physical and mental capacities, the tangible world, and the roles people play in their worlds are reflected and governed by the activities in which people engage throughout their lives.

Intensive preparation in these three realms and their interactions constitute the education and preparation of the OT practitioner and guide the therapist in developing an intervention plan. With this comprehensive foundation, OTs use various modalities to integrate these three realms, which enhances client performance and enables clients to meet life needs.

EVOLVING PRACTICE

Just as society and its occupations have evolved and continue to evolve, OT practice has evolved. New media and modalities (Box 28-1) have emerged to enable clients to become skilled in functional performance. In addition to therapeutic exercise and activity and the facilitation and inhibition techniques associated with various sensorimotor approaches to treatment, therapists have added adjunctive therapies to their repertoires, all designed to enhance clients' performance in purposeful occupation.

Although use of adjunctive therapies such as **physical agent modalities** is not considered to be an entry-level skill,[3,5] some therapists have become increasingly skilled in the application of these therapies. These modalities traditionally belonged to the field of physical therapy but have long since entered the realm of OT practice. They are used by trained OTs to enhance the development of the individual's ability to perform purposeful occupation, the primary objective of OT. Their use by OTs should be limited to the

---

Box **28-1** OCCUPATIONAL THERAPY MODALITIES

Modality: The employment of, or method of employment of, a therapeutic agent (Webster's New World College Dictionary, edition 2).[1] Traditionally, the modalities of OT were its crafts. The term has grown to be understood more broadly and defines active occupation as the primary therapeutic modality of OT. The term *modality* also includes media and methods.[43] Media are the means by which therapeutic effects are transmitted. For example, media can include a variety of objects, such as an article of clothing, a vestibular ball, or an adapted tool. Methods are the steps, sequence, or approaches used to activate the therapeutic effect of a medium, such as the movements required in the creation of a macramé plant hanger to heighten shoulder flexion or reduce edema, or the movements used with the vestibular ball to effect the desired motor responses. The modalities, media, and methods of OT are variable in their application and require considerable expertise to select, modify, adapt, and apply to elicit therapeutic effects.

role of an adjunct to or preparation for purposeful active occupation.

PURPOSEFUL OCCUPATION AND ACTIVITY

One of the first principles of OT, stated by Dunton in 1918, is that some useful end to occupation must exist for it to be effective in the treatment of mental and physical disability.[49] This principle implies that occupation has a purpose, and that purposeful activity has an autonomous or inherent goal beyond the motor function required to perform the task.[9] An individual engaged in purposeful activity focuses attention on the goal rather than on the processes required to reach the goal.[4,6]

Conversely, non-purposeful activity has been defined as activity that has no inherent goal other than the motor function used to perform the activity.[49] The person performing a non-purposeful activity is likely to be focused on the activity process or movements rather than a functional or meaningful goal. Therapeutic exercise and enabling activities such as moving cones and stacking blocks cannot be considered purposeful activity when they have no purpose for the client. This statement does not imply that such media have no place in the continuum of intervention. However, intervention must consider the inherent occupational objectives of the client so both tools of treatment and skills to be acquired are more readily tied to purpose, meaning, and therapeutic value and constitute the occupational nature of therapy.

Purposeful activity is the cornerstone of OT and is its primary intervention modality.[49,51] In a position paper on purposeful activity, the American Occupational Therapy Association (AOTA) defined purposeful activity as "goal-directed behaviors or tasks that comprise occupations. An activity is purposeful if the individual is an active, voluntary participant and if the activity is directed toward a goal that the individual considers meaningful."[6] Although some theorists have attempted to distinguish between purposefulness and meaningfulness, others use these terms interchangeably to indicate that the investment of the performer in either purpose or meaning determines its usefulness in therapy. The uniqueness of OT lies in its emphasis on the extensive use of purposeful or meaningful activity. This emphasis gives OT the theoretical foundation for its broad application to psychosocial, physical, and developmental dysfunction, in addition to health maintenance.[4]

Purposeful activity has inherent and therapeutic goals. For example, sawing wood (Figure 28-2) may have the inherent goal of securing parts for construction of a bookshelf, whereby the therapeutic objectives may be to strengthen shoulder and elbow musculature. The conscious effort of the client is focused on the ultimate outcome of the project and not on the movement itself.[9] The client directs and is in control of the movement; however, that control is ordinarily outside of conscious awareness as the client focuses on the goal aspects of performance. In fact, performance outside of conscious

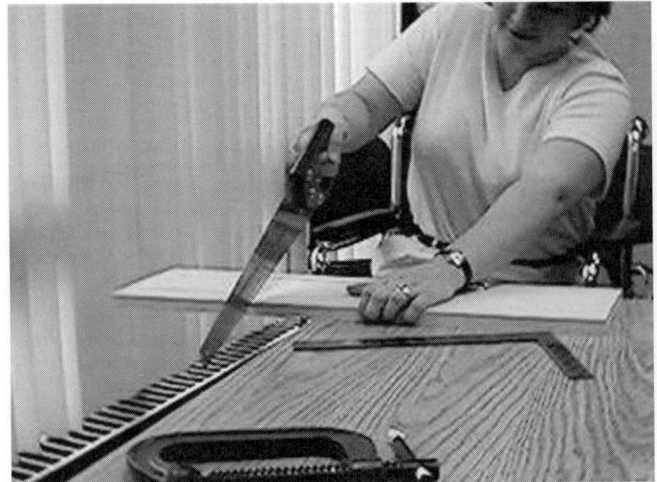

Figure 28-2   Sawing wood to strengthen shoulder and elbow musculature.

awareness distinguishes OT's therapeutic effectiveness. To enhance skill building, performance must become automatic and decrease reliance on cognitive monitoring.[13] Automatic performance serves as a subskill for more advanced performance. For example, Huss[24] suggested that the child who must attend to sitting is unable to focus on the task performance that automatic sitting would ordinarily enable. Consequently, the child cannot engage in active occupations essential to growth and the development of social roles. Ayres' emphasis on the interaction of subcortical regions of the brain as requisite to skilled performance affirms this same principle.[8,9]

The importance of purposeful activity is readily observed in goal-directed performance. As the client becomes absorbed in the performance of any given activity, affected parts are used more naturally and with less fatigue.[48] Concentration on motion has a detrimental effect on that motion, and muscles controlled by conscious attention and focused effort fatigue rapidly. The value of goal-oriented effort in purposeful tasks is clear. It is of greater therapeutic value to focus attention on an activity of interest to the client and its inherent goal than on the muscles or motions being used to accomplish the activity,[9] and that is what goal-directed OT effects.

A number of studies have shown the efficacy of purposeful activity.[39] Steinbeck[49] demonstrated that clients who do purposeful activity perform for a longer period than when they are engaging in non-purposeful activity. A study of motivation for product-oriented versus non–product-oriented activity by Thibodeaux and Ludwig[51] indicated the need to determine the client's level of interest in the process and the product and to incorporate his or her image of the activity in treatment planning. Rocker and Nelson[45] found that not being allowed to keep an activity product can elicit hostile feelings in normal subjects, which demonstrates the importance of tangible productivity for sustaining people's interest. Yoder, Nelson, and Smith[55] studied the effects of added-purpose versus rote exercise in female nursing home residents.

The added-purpose exercise resulted in significantly more movement repetitions than did rote exercise.[55] These studies suggest that goal-directed, purposeful activity increases motivation for participation in sustained activity and can therefore be assumed to heighten the willingness of clients to engage in therapeutic activity.

When an intervention plan is being developed, the inherent goals of the activity, the client's level of interest in the activity, and the meaning of the activity and its product are important considerations in the ultimate effectiveness of the media and methods selected for intervention. Purposeful activities are used, or adapted for use, to meet one or more of the following therapeutic objectives: (1) to develop or maintain strength, endurance, work tolerance, range of motion (ROM), and coordination; (2) to practice and use voluntary, automatic movement in goal-directed tasks; (3) to provide for purposeful use of and general exercise to affected parts; (4) to explore vocational potential or train in work skills; (5) to improve sensation, perception, and cognition; (6) to improve socialization skills and enhance emotional growth and development; and (7) to increase independence in occupational role performance. Some of these objectives alone may not be considered purposeful unless they relate to function. Arts, crafts, games, sports, leisure, self-care, home management, purposive mobility, and work-related activities are considered purposeful activities, and may hold occupational significance for the client.

OCCUPATION AND HEALTH

OT was founded on the concept that human beings have an occupational nature. That is, it is natural for humans to be engaged in activity, and the process of being occupied contributes to the health and well-being of the organism.[9,12,17,25] Activity is valuable for the maintenance of health in the healthy person and for the restoration of health after illness and disability. When the client engages in relevant, meaningful, and purposeful activity, change is possible and dysfunction is reversible.[17] The OT acts as facilitator of the change process.[16] Therefore, physical dysfunction can be ameliorated when the client participates in goal-directed (purposeful) and thus therapeutic activity.[9]

The value of purposeful activity lies in the client's simultaneous mental and physical involvement. Activity provides the exercise needed to help develop the use of affected parts and also provides an opportunity to meet emotional, social, and personal gratification needs.[9,48] Cynkin and Robinson[17] pointed out that, for the attainment of optimal function and health, the human being must be consciously involved in problem-solving and creative activity, processes that are linked with the use of the hands.[17]

The majority of occupational performance involves the hands or requires the substitution of methods that simulate the use of hands. The use of a computer-driven environmental control unit operated by a sip-and-puff mechanism is an example of an activity ordinarily performed by the hands but, in this case, a substitution for hand control is made using the sip-and-puff mechanism.

The activities that form the pattern of a person's life, which are performed routinely and automatically, are taken for granted until some dysfunction disrupts their performance. The OT's role is to adapt activity so that clients can resume their ability to perform life's tasks. OT is founded on the notion that dysfunction can be modified, altered, or reversed toward function through engagement in the activities of real life. Cynkin and Robinson[17] make several assumptions about activities that are summarized as follows:

- A wide variety of activities are important to the individual. Activities fulfill many of a person's needs and wants, and they are essential to physical and psychosocial growth and development and the attainment of mastery and competence.
- Activities are socioculturally regulated by the values and beliefs of the culture that defines acceptable behavior for groups of people in the culture. Whether a society is rigid or flexible in its interpretation of acceptable behaviors for various groups, at some point deviations in behavior or activity patterns are deemed unacceptable.
- Activity-related behavior can change from dysfunctional toward more functional. Persons can change and desire change.
- Changes in activity-related behavior take place through motor, cognitive, and social learning.[17]

ASSESSMENT OF OCCUPATIONAL ROLE PERFORMANCE

The therapist should establish the client's occupational goals and needs. A top-down, client-centered approach is recommended. Identifying appropriate and meaningful therapeutic activities should begin with obtaining and analyzing the client's occupational history and interests.[51]

The Canadian Occupational Performance Measure[30] and the Activity Configuration[16] are two examples of occupational performance assessments. See Chapter 3 for more information about assessment of occupational performance.

ACTIVITY ANALYSIS

Careful activity analysis is essential to the selection of appropriate treatment activities. It should yield information about various activities as intervention strategies for physical dysfunction and health maintenance. Activities should be analyzed from three perspectives: the contributions of the person or actor, the effects of the physical environment on performance, and the implications of the social environment. The therapist should recognize that these three elements are inextricable and form the context for intervention. The importance of context in intervention is widely recognized throughout the profession.[2,7]

Comprehensive guides to activity analysis have been developed by a number of theorists[12,30,52] and can serve as useful resources. A guide to activity analysis specifically relevant to practice in physical dysfunction can be found at the end of this chapter.

PRINCIPLES OF ACTIVITY ANALYSIS

Activities selected for therapeutic purposes should be goal directed; have some meaning to the client to meet individual needs in relation to social roles; require the mental or physical participation of the client at the "just right" level of challenge; be designed to prevent or reverse dysfunction; develop skills to enhance performance in life roles; relate to the client's interests; be adaptable, gradable, and age appropriate; and be selected through knowledge and professional judgment of the OT in concert with the interests and investment of the client.[22] A comprehensive activity analysis includes all aspects of performance that are potentially elicited by specific activities and reveals their potential for therapeutic application. Fareed had expressed an interest in returning to woodworking and selected a project that he could make for his youngest grandchild. This reflects client-centered activity selection. It is not merely activity for no or limited purpose, but the activity is selected by the client because it has meaning for the client.

THERAPEUTIC APPROACHES

A variety of therapeutic approaches are available to OTs. Although these approaches differ in their emphasis, all are consistent with an occupational approach to intervention. Aspects of activity analysis relevant to various therapeutic approaches are listed below.

BIOMECHANICAL APPROACH

The biomechanical approach to intervention is likely to be used in the treatment of lower motor neuron and orthopedic dysfunctions. Improvements in strength, ROM, and muscle endurance are the goals of OT for such dysfunctions. Thus, the emphasis of activity analysis is on muscles, joints, and motor patterns required to perform the activity. The outcome of OT service is focused on the engagement in the specified activity, but the approach is focused on the biomechanical client factors required to complete the task. Steps of the activity must be identified and broken down into the motions required to perform each step. ROM, degree of muscle strength, and type of muscle contraction to perform each step should be identified. The activity analysis format at the end of this chapter is based on the biomechanical approach.

SENSORIMOTOR APPROACH

Sensorimotor approaches to intervention are likely to be used for upper motor neuron disorders such as cerebral palsy,

stroke, and head injury. Activity analysis for these dysfunctions should focus on the sensory perception of the client and the movement patterns required in the particular treatment approach. The therapist must also consider the effect of the activity on balance, posture, muscle tone, and the facilitation or inhibition of abnormal reflexes and movements. For example, if the therapist is using the proprioceptive neuromuscular facilitation (PNF) approach, it is important to incorporate PNF patterns in the activity or to select activities that use these patterns naturally. For the neurodevelopmental (Bobath) approach, postures and movements that inhibit abnormal reflexes, reactions, and tone are important. These and other sensorimotor approaches and their applications to activity are discussed in Chapters 30 and 31.

Analysis of the perceptual and cognitive requirements of the activity is particularly important for clients with upper motor neuron disorders because these functions are often disturbed. The therapist must select activities that meet the requirements for motor performance and can be performed with some success.

Regardless of diagnosis or therapeutic approach, activity analysis should include the contextual aspects of performance. The tangible environment and the social environment dictate occupational performance to the same extent that physical and mental capacities do, and they must be considered in developing an intervention plan.

ADAPTING AND GRADING ACTIVITY

ADAPTATION OF ACTIVITY

It may be necessary to adapt activities to suit the special needs of the client or the environment. An activity may have to be performed in a special way to accommodate the client's residual abilities—for example, eating using a special splint with a utensil holder fitted to the hand (Figure 28-3).

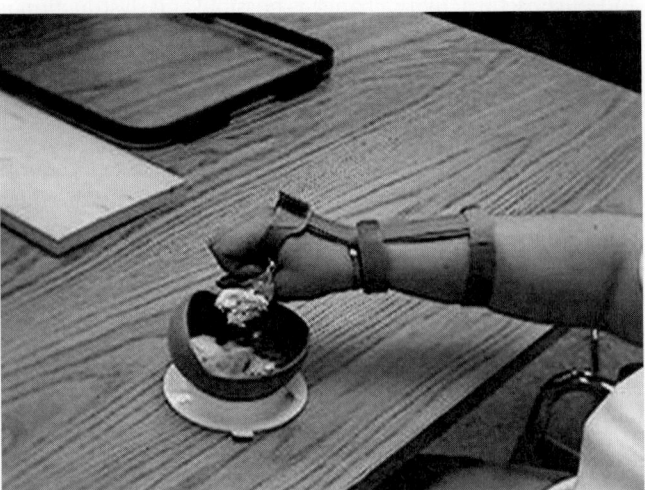

Figure 28-3 Eating using a special splint with a utensil holder fitted to the hand.

An activity may have to be adapted to the positioning of the client or to the environment—for instance, by setting up a special reading stand and providing prism glasses to enable a client to read while supine in bed. The problem-solving ability, creativity, and ingenuity of OTs in making adaptations are some of their unique skills.

The therapist should remember that for adaptations to be effective, the client must be able to use them in a comfortable position. The client must understand the need and purpose of the activity and the adaptations and be willing to perform the activity with the simple modifications. Peculiar and complicated adaptations that require frequent adjustment and modification should be avoided.[42,48]

GRADING OF ACTIVITY

Grading an activity means to pace it appropriately and modify it for the client's maximal performance. If movement patterns or degree of resistance cannot be attained when the activity is performed in the usual manner, simple modifications may be made. The client usually accepts changes if they are not complex and do not require strained and unnatural motions. The novice is cautioned that the value of the activity may be diminished if it is designed to be performed with artificial movements or excessive resistance. Such methods discourage participation and interfere with the development of coordination.[27,48] They also require that the client focus on movements rather than on the goal of the activity, which reduces satisfaction and defeats the primary purpose of purposeful activity as described earlier. The skilled OT adapts and grades activities so that they are easily accepted by the client and provide the "just right" demand upon performance.

Activities may be graded in many ways to suit the client's needs and meet the intervention objectives. Activities can be graded for increasing strength, ROM, endurance and tolerance, coordination, and perceptual, cognitive, and social skills. Activities may also be graded according to diminishing capacities of clients, as are expected to occur with such progressive diseases such as Parkinson's disease, multiple sclerosis, and amyotrophic lateral sclerosis.

Strength

Strength may be graded by an increase or decrease in resistance. Methods include changing the plane of movement from gravity-eliminated to against-gravity, by adding weights to the equipment or to the client, using tools of increasing weights, grading the texture of the materials from soft to hard or fine to rough, or changing to another more or less **resistive activity**.

For example, a weight attached to the wrist by a strap increases resistance to arm movements during needle or leatherwork (Figure 28-4). A pulley-and-weight system can be attached to an inclined plane sanding board to increase resistance to the biceps when the sanding block is pulled

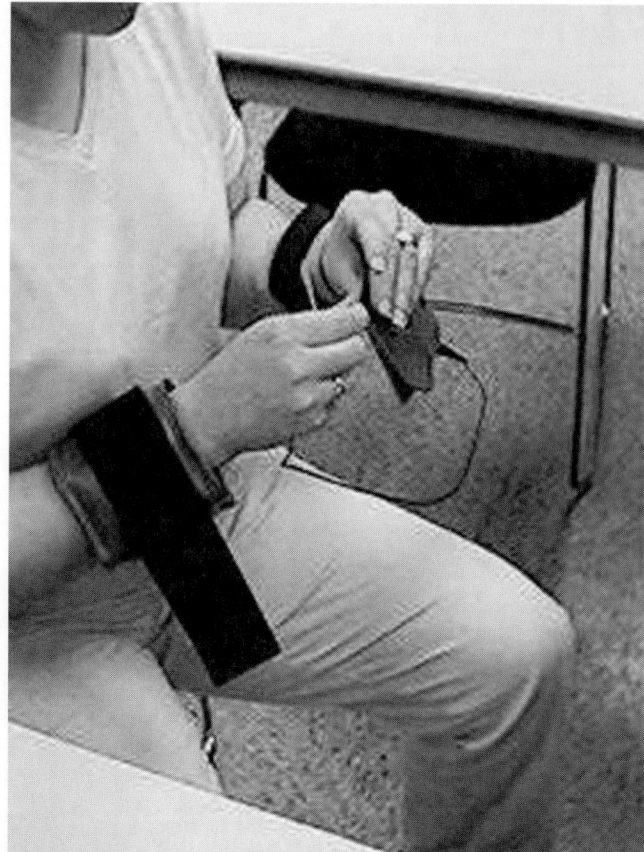

Figure 28-4 Weight attached to the wrist increases resistance during needlework or leatherwork.

downward, as the client sands a cutting board for use in one-handed cutting. Springs may be used to increase resistance on a block printing press. When grasp strength is inadequate, grasp mitts may be used to fasten the hand to a tool or equipment handle to assist grip strength and allow arm motion.

Range of Motion

Activities for increasing or maintaining joint ROM may be graded by positioning materials and equipment to demand greater reach or excursion of joints or by adapting equipment with lengthened handles to facilitate active stretching.

An example of a simple adaptation is positioning a weaving project in a vertical position to achieve the desired range of shoulder flexion while working. As the work progresses, the activity itself establishes increased demands on active range. Positioning objects, such as tiles used in a mosaic tile project, at increasing or decreasing distances from the client changes the range needed to reach the materials (Figure 28-5). Tool handles such as those used in woodworking may be increased in size by using a larger dowel or by padding the handle with foam rubber to accommodate limited ROM or to facilitate grasp (Figure 28-6). Reducing the amount of padding as range or grasp improves can facilitate grading.

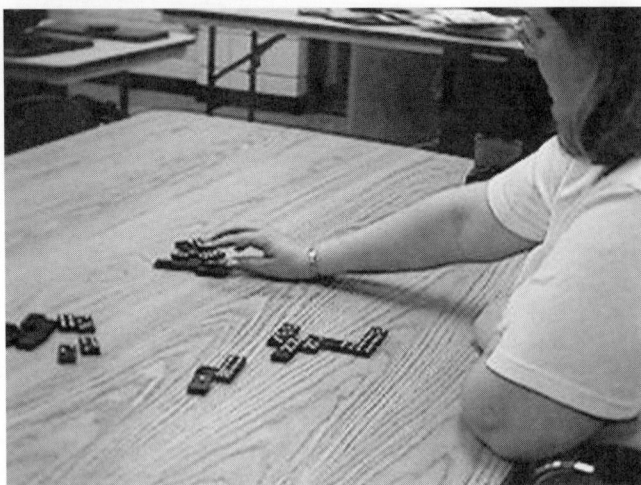

Figure 28-5 Placing objects at alternate distances changes the range needed to reach materials.

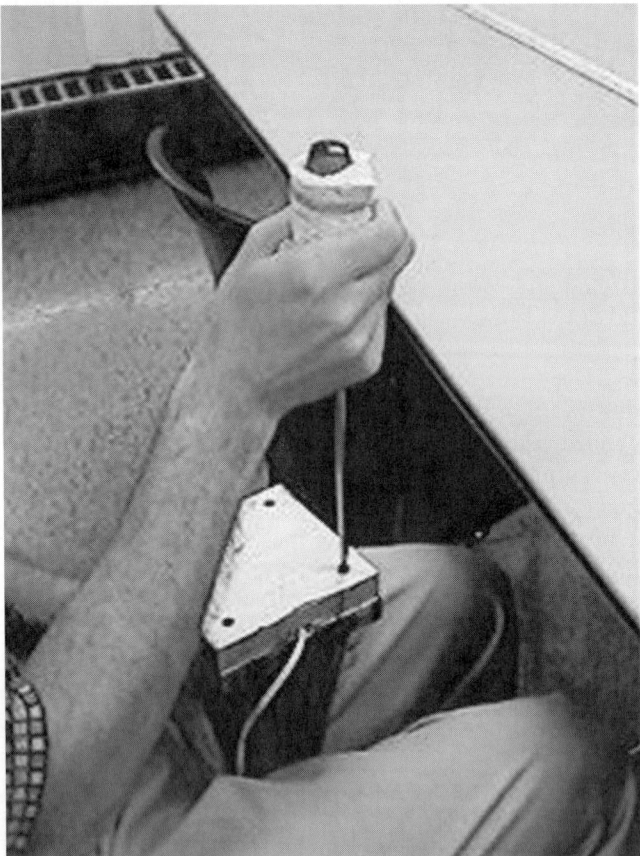

Figure 28-6 The size of tool handles may be increased by padding the handle with foam rubber.

Endurance and Tolerance

Endurance may be graded by moving from light to heavy work and increasing the duration of the work period. For example, an initial household task of folding paper napkins can be graded to sorting heavier and heavier objects, such as

the task of sitting to sort kitchen utensils, and then graded to a standing position to organize tools on a pegboard or to place household items onto shelves. Standing and walking tolerance may be graded by an increase in the time spent standing to work, perhaps at first at a stand-up table (Figure 28-7), and an increase in the time and distance spent in activities requiring walking, perhaps including home management and workshop activities.

When conditions that are progressively degenerative, such as muscular dystrophy, multiple sclerosis, or Parkinson's disease, require grading endurance in a negative direction to accommodate a diminishing physical condition, it is advisable to change the activity to one that requires less effort rather than reducing the demands of an existing project. The latter can have a negative psychological effect if the client readily recognizes the reduction in performance capacity.

Coordination

Coordination and muscle control may be graded by decreasing the gross resistive movements and increasing the fine controlled movements required. An example is progressing from sawing wood with a crosscut saw to using a coping saw to using a jeweler's saw. Dexterity and speed of movement

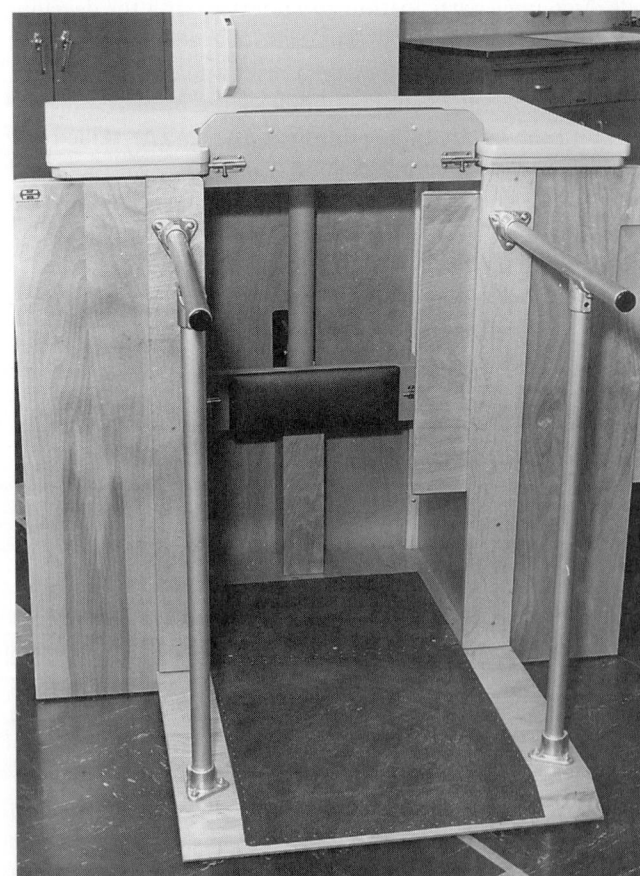

Figure 28-7 Stand-up table with sliding door, padded knee supports, and backrest.

may be graded by practicing at increasing speeds once movement patterns have been mastered through coordination training and neuromuscular education.

Perceptual, Cognitive, and Social Skills

In grading cognitive skills, the therapist can begin the treatment program with simple one- or two-step activities that require little judgment, decision making, or problem solving, and progress to activities with several steps that require some judgment or problem-solving processes. A client in a lunch preparation group may butter bread that has already been lined up on the work surface. This task could be graded to lining up the bread, then buttering it and placing a slice of lunch meat on it, and, ultimately, to making sandwiches.

For grading social interaction, the intervention plan may begin with an activity that demands interaction only with the therapist. The client can progress to activities that require dyadic interaction with another client and, ultimately, to small group activities. The therapist can facilitate the client's progression from the role of observer to that of participant and then to leader. Concomitantly, the therapist decreases his or her supervision, guidance, and assistance to facilitate more independent functioning in the client.

SELECTION OF ACTIVITY

In the treatment of physical dysfunction, activities are usually selected for their potential to improve sensorimotor and psychosocial components to ensure that clients' motivation to engage in activity is sustained. Activities selected for the improvement of physical performance should provide desired exercise or purposeful use of affected parts. They should enable the client to transfer the motion, strength, and coordination gained in adjunctive and enabling modalities to useful, normal daily activities. If activities are to be used for physical restoration, they should have certain characteristics, as follows:

- Activities should provide action rather than merely the position of involved joints and muscles; that is, they should allow alternate contraction and relaxation of the muscles being exercised and allow clients to course through their available ROM.
- Activities should provide repetition of motion. That is, activities should allow for a considerable number of repetitions of movement patterns sufficient to be beneficial to the client.
- Activities should allow for one or more kind of grading, such as for resistance, range, coordination, endurance, or complexity.[22,48]

The type of exercise needed must be considered when choosing an activity. Active and resistive exercises are most often used in the performance of purposeful activity.[48] Requirements for passive and active-assisted exercise are harder (although not impossible) to apply to purposeful activities, for example, bilateral sanding or using a sponge with both hands to wipe a surface. Other important considerations in the selection of activity are the objects and environment required to perform the activity; safety factors; preparation and completion time; complexity, type of instruction, and supervision required; structure and controls in the activity; learning requirements; independence, decision making, and problem solving required; social interaction potential and communication skills required; and potential gratification to the person.

If an activity is selected in which the client has an interest, the client is more likely to experience sufficient satisfaction to sustain performance. The therapist's job is to guide the client to suitable therapeutic activities at just the right level of challenge so that the client will achieve satisfaction by engaging in the activity. This satisfaction is an important characteristic of intrinsic motivation. Thus, purposeful activities meet the requirements for motor performance and can be performed with success, which provides positive personal and social feedback. When the OT evaluated Fareed, preferred activities and hobbies were explored. This allowed the OT to select from an array of activities that had been identified by Fareed and could be incorporated into the intervention plan.

SIMULATED OR ENABLING ACTIVITY

The clinical environment may not be fully equipped to meet the exact occupational needs of all clients. When this is the case, it may be necessary to simulate appropriate active occupation by adaptation of the environment or activity to meet the client's needs and retain his or her interest, called **simulated or enabling activity**.

OTs have developed a variety of methods to simulate active occupation. A number of these activities were devised initially from equipment and found materials used in other activities. A devised activity is the simulated inclined sanding board (Figure 28-8). The sanding board was designed to

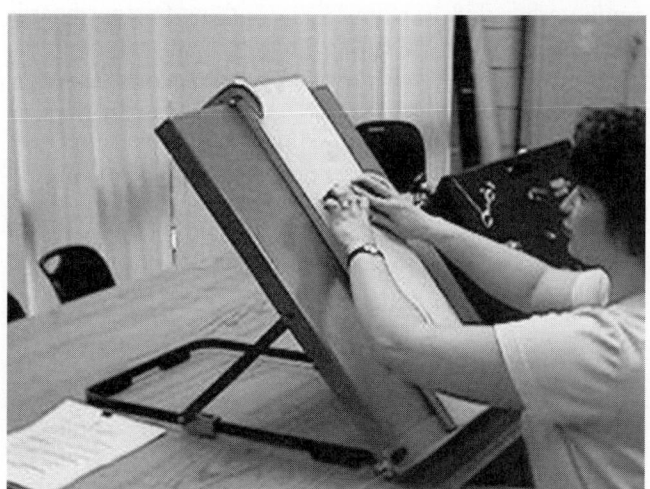

Figure 28-8 Inclined sanding board used to sand wood.

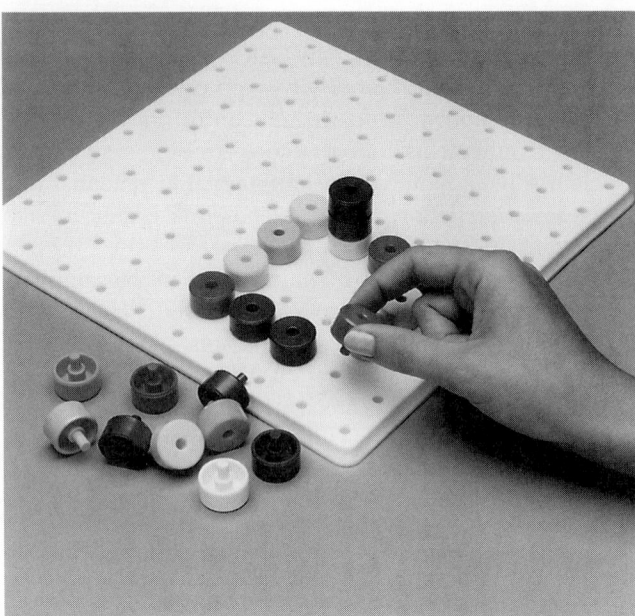

Figure 28-9 Puzzles and other perceptual and cognitive training media are used on the tabletop. (Courtesy North Coast Medical, Morgan Hill, Calif.)

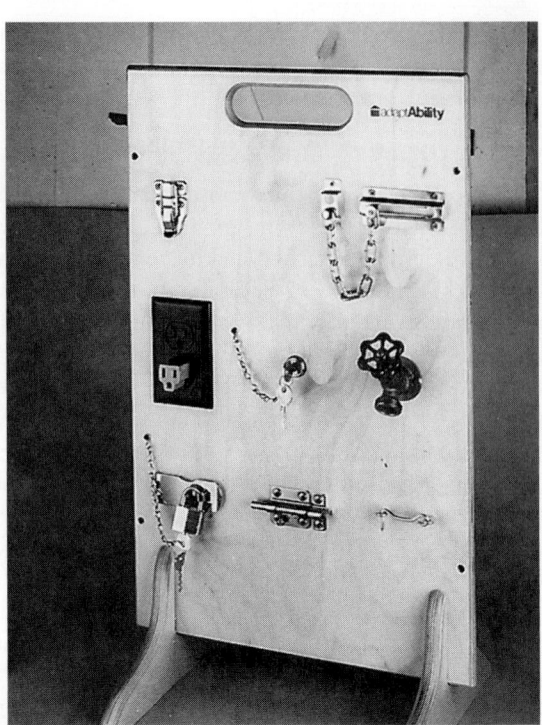

Figure 28-10 Boards built with household fasteners are simulations used for practicing manipulation and management of common household hardware. (Reprinted with permission, S & S Worldwide, adaptAbility, 1995.)

incline wood while the wood was being sanded. Therapists began using the board, without the wood, to exercise muscles of the elbow and shoulder. Without the wood, no end product results and thus no inherent purposefulness. However, incorporating wood for a project can turn this from a simulated to a meaningful activity. Our client, Fareed, had indicated that he wanted to pursue a woodworking task. Instead of having Fareed engage in rote exercise using an empty sanding board, his OT placed wood on the sanding board, which would later be used by Fareed to construct a bench for his grandchild.

Puzzles and other perceptual and cognitive training media are used to train clients in visual perceptual functions, motor planning skills, memory, sequencing, and problem solving, among other skills (Figure 28-9). Clothing fastener boards and household hardware boards may provide practice in the manipulation of everyday objects before the client is confronted with the real task (Figure 28-10). At a higher level of technological sophistication, commercial work simulators (see Chapter 13) and computer programs are used to improve physical and cognitive client factors.

Although many of these items are readily available in clinics, the nature and purpose of OT are best encompassed in an activity in which the client finds purpose and meaning. The therapist should take into consideration the needs and interests of the client in selecting activities, rather than relying on available objects that meet only physical needs.

Enabling activities are considered non-purposeful and generally do not have an inherent goal, but they may engage the mental and physical participation of the client. The purposes of engaging in enabling activities are to practice

specific motor patterns, to train in perceptual and cognitive skills, and to practice sensorimotor skills necessary for function in the home and community. Indeed, many enabling modalities used in OT practice facilitate perceptual, cognitive, and motor learning. Such activities may be appropriate for the skill acquisition stage of learning, when the client is getting the idea of the movement and practicing problem solving. Practice should be daily or frequent and feedback given often so that errors are decreased and skills refined to prepare for performance of real-life purposeful activity. These activities should be used judiciously, and their place in the sequence of the intervention program should be well planned. They may be used along with adjunctive modalities and purposeful activities as part of a comprehensive intervention program.

ADJUNCTIVE MODALITIES

Adjunctive modalities may be used as a preliminary to purposeful activity. When used by the OT, they are meant to prepare the client for occupational performance. Examples of adjunctive modalities are exercise, orthotics, sensory stimulation, and physical agent modalities.[40] Therapeutic exercise and physical agent modalities are described below. Many of the principles of therapeutic exercise are readily and customarily incorporated into therapeutic activity and consequently are inherent aspects of OT practice.

THERAPEUTIC EXERCISE AND ACTIVITY

The field of OT always has recognized that the mind and body are inextricably united in performance. The psychological and physical effects of purposeful activity were recognized in the treatment of individuals with mental conditions, in addition to in the treatment of persons with physical dysfunction.[10,13,20,25] Because it was recognized that physical benefits accrued from the performance of activity, kinesiological considerations were applied in the selection of appropriate therapeutic activities. To apply kinesiological considerations to purposeful activity, it was necessary to understand the principles of therapeutic exercise.

As intervention methods evolved, OTs began to use therapeutic exercise alone to prepare clients for purposeful activity and to expedite treatment in a healthcare system constrained by budget and time. The treatment of clients in acute stages of illness and disability imposed new demands and role responsibilities on OTs. Short therapy sessions in acute care settings, the extent of the client's physical incapacities, and shortened lengths of stay in hospital and rehabilitation facilities caused OTs to expand the range of modalities used in intervention.

The use of therapeutic exercise as an isolated modality raised considerable controversy.[21] It was feared that if OTs used exercise or other preparatory modalities, purpose would be forgotten. Exercise and activity tended to be seen by some as mutually exclusive; however, the principles of exercise had been applied to purposeful activity from early in the history of OT. Exercise and activity are complementary in the intervention continuum, and both may be used in a single intervention plan. However, if only pure exercise is used, the client has not received OT.[21]

When used by OTs, therapeutic exercise should be used to remediate sensory and motor dysfunction, augment purposeful activity, and prepare the client for performing a desired occupation.

A comprehensive understanding of the principles of exercise is basic to the application of therapeutic activity. Therapeutic exercise is defined as any body movement or muscle contraction to prevent or correct a physical impairment, improve musculoskeletal function, and maintain a state of well-being.[15,28] A wide variety of exercise options are available; each should be tailored to meet the goals of the intervention plan and the specific capacities and precautions relative to the client's physical condition.

Exercise can be used to increase ROM and flexibility, strength, coordination, endurance, and cardiovascular fitness.[28] Specific exercise protocols may be used to achieve specific goals. However, exercise without activity is apt to place the exercise in the realm of deliberate rather than automatic performance, which therefore violates essential principles of OT discussed earlier. Although judicious application of therapeutic exercise may have a limited place in the therapeutic program, the OT should structure treatment so that the client is engaged in activity primarily to take advantage of the automaticity generated by purposeful goal-directed therapeutic activity.

Purposes

The general purposes of therapeutic exercise, as with therapeutic activity, are as follows:

- To develop awareness of normal movement patterns and improve voluntary, automatic movement responses
- To develop strength and endurance in patterns of movement that are acceptable and necessary and do not produce deformity
- To improve coordination, regardless of strength
- To increase the power of specific isolated muscles or muscle groups
- To aid in overcoming ROM deficits
- To increase the strength of muscles that will power hand splints, mobile arm supports, and other devices
- To increase work tolerance and physical endurance through increased strength
- To prevent or eliminate contractures developing as a result of imbalanced muscle power by strengthening the antagonistic muscles[42]

Indications for Use

Therapeutic exercise is most effective when providing intervention for orthopedic disorders (such as contractures and arthritis) and lower motor neuron disorders that produce weakness and flaccidity. Examples of the latter are peripheral nerve injuries and diseases, poliomyelitis, Guillain-Barré syndrome, infectious neuritis, and spinal cord injuries and diseases.

The candidate for therapeutic exercise must be medically able to participate in the exercise regimen, able to understand the directions and purposes, and interested and motivated to perform. The client must have available motor pathways and the potential for recovery or improvement of strength, ROM, coordination, or movement patterns, as applicable. Some sensory feedback must be available to the client; that is, sensation must be at least partially intact so that the client can perceive motion and the position of the exercised part and sense superficial and deep pain. Muscles and tendons must be intact, stable, and free to move. Joints must be able to move through an effective ROM for those types of exercise that use joint motion. The client should be relatively free of pain during motion and should be able to perform isolated, coordinated movement. If the client has any dyskinetic movement, he or she should be able to control it so that the procedure can be performed as prescribed.[41] The type of exercise selected depends on muscle grade, muscle endurance, joint mobility, diagnosis and physical condition, treatment goals, position of the client, and desirable plane of movement. Each of these requirements is also applicable to the use of exercise-focused therapeutic activity and should underlie its selection as a therapeutic tool.

Contraindications

Therapeutic exercise and exercise-focused therapeutic activity are contraindicated for clients who have poor general health or inflamed joints or who have had recent surgery.[41] They may not be useful where joint ROM is severely limited as the result of well-established, permanent contractures. As defined and described here, they cannot be used effectively for those who have spasticity and lack voluntary control of isolated motion or those who cannot control dyskinetic movement. The latter conditions are likely to occur in upper motor neuron disorders.

Exercise Programs

Muscle strengthening

Active-assisted, active, and resistive **isotonic exercises** and **isometric exercises** are used to increase strength. After partial or complete denervation of muscle tissue and during inactivity or disuse, muscle strength decreases. When strength is inadequate, substitution patterns or "trick" movements are likely to develop.[54] A substitution is the attempt to achieve a functional goal by using muscle groups and patterns of motion not ordinarily used. Substitution is used when muscles normally used to perform the movements or restrictions in ROM are lost or weakened because of structural dysfunction. An example is using shoulder abduction to achieve a hand-to-mouth movement if elbow flexors cannot perform against gravity (Figure 28-11). When muscle loss is permanent, some substitution patterns may be desirable as a compensatory measure to improve performance of functional activities, such as the use of tenodesis to permit grasp that will enable self-feeding. Many substitute movements are not desirable, however, and it is often the aim of therapeutic exercise to prevent or correct substitution patterns.[54]

A muscle must contract at or near its maximal capacity and for enough repetitions and time to increase strength.

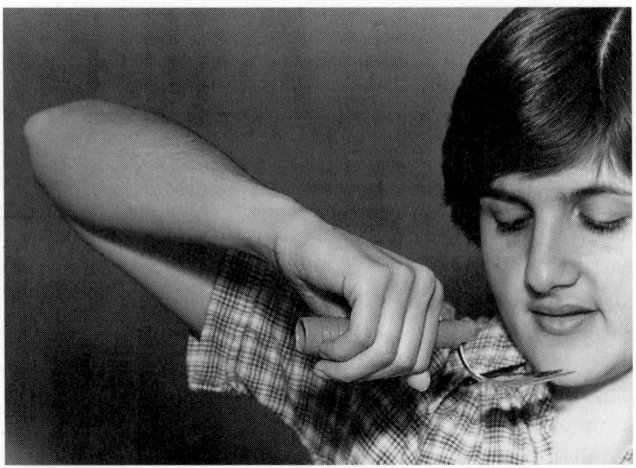

Figure 28-11 Using shoulder abduction as compensation to achieve hand-to-mouth movement.

Strengthening programs generally are based on having the muscle contract against a large resistance for a few repetitions. Strengthening exercises are not effective if the contraction is insufficient.[15,29] Excessive repetitions of strengthening exercises, however, may result in muscle fatigue, pain, and temporary reduction of strength. If a muscle is overworked, it becomes fatigued and is unable to contract. The type of exercise must suit the muscle grade and the client's fatigue tolerance level. Fatigue level varies from individual to individual, and the threshold for muscle fatigue decreases in pathological states.[29] Many clients may not be sensitive to fatigue or may push themselves beyond tolerance in the belief that this approach hastens recovery. Therefore, the therapist must carefully assess the client's muscle power and capacity for performance. The therapist must also supervise the client closely and observe for signs of fatigue. These signs may be slowed performance, distraction, perspiration, increase in rate of respiration, performance of exercise pattern through a decreased ROM, and inability to complete the prescribed number of repetitions.

Increasing muscle endurance

Endurance is the ability of the muscle to work for prolonged periods and resist fatigue. Although a high-load, low-repetition regimen is effective for muscle strengthening, a low-load and high-repetition exercise program is more effective for building endurance.[15,18] Having determined the client's maximum capacity for a strengthening program, the therapist can reduce the maximum resistance load and increase the number of repetitions to build endurance in specific muscles or muscle groups. The strength versus endurance training may be seen as a continuum. Resistance and the number of repetitions can be modulated so that gains in strength and endurance accrue.[15]

Physical conditioning and cardiovascular fitness

Improving general physical endurance and cardiovascular fitness requires the use of large muscle groups in sustained, rhythmic aerobic exercise or activity. Examples are swimming, walking, bicycling, jogging, and some games and sports. This type of activity is often used in cardiac rehabilitation programs in which the parameters of the client's physical capacities and tolerance for exercise should be well defined and medically supervised. To improve cardiovascular fitness, exercise should be done 3 to 5 days per week at 60% to 90% of maximum heart rate or 50% to 85% of maximum oxygen uptake. Between 15 and 60 minutes of exercise or rhythmic activities using large muscle groups is desirable.[15]

Range of motion and joint flexibility

Active and passive ROM are used to maintain joint motion and flexibility. **Active exercise** is performed solely by the individual. An outside force such as the therapist or a device can be used for performing passive ROM exercise. The continuous passive motion machine, a device that can be preset to provide continuous passive motion throughout the joint range, is an example. Application of any mechanical device requires caution and careful monitoring to prevent mishaps and possible deleterious effects.[15]

Stretching or forced exercise may be necessary to increase ROM. Some type of force is applied to the body part when soft tissue (muscles, tendons, and ligaments) is at or near its available length. The use of a low-resistance stretch of sustained duration is preferred to high resistance and repetitive, quick, bouncing movements. The former method is less likely to produce tissue tearing, trauma, and activation of stretch reflexes in hypertonic muscles. The use of thermal agents or neuromuscular facilitation techniques may enhance static stretching.[15]

Coordination and neuromuscular control

Coordination is the combined activity of many muscles into smooth patterns and sequences of motion. Coordination is an automatic response monitored primarily through proprioceptive sensory feedback. Kottke[27] defined control as "the conscious activation of an individual muscle or the conscious initiation of a pre-programmed engram." Control involves conscious attention to and guidance of an activity.

A preprogrammed pattern of muscular activity represented in the central nervous system (CNS) has been described as an *engram*. An engram is formed only if many repetitions of a specific motion or activity occur. With repetition, conscious effort of the client is decreased and the motion becomes more and more automatic. Ultimately the motion can be carried out with little conscious attention. It has been hypothesized that when an engram is excited, the same pattern of movement is produced automatically. Neuromuscular education or control training involves teaching the client to control individual muscles or motions through conscious attention. Coordination training is used to develop preprogrammed multimuscular patterns or engrams.[27]

Types of Muscle Contraction

Isometric or static contraction

During an isometric contraction no joint motion occurs, and the muscle length remains the same. The limb is set or held taut as agonist and antagonist muscles are contracted at a point in the ROM to stabilize a joint. This action may be without resistance or against some outside resistance, such as the therapist's hand or a fixed object. An example of isometric exercise of the triceps against resistance is pressing down against a tabletop with the ulnar border of the forearm while the elbow remains at 90-degree flexion. An example of an activity that requires isometric contraction is stabilizing the arm in a locked position when carrying a shopping bag slung over the forearm.[23,29]

Isotonic or concentric contraction

During an isotonic contraction the joint moves and the muscle shortens. This contraction may be done with or

without resistance. Isotonic contractions may be performed in positions with gravity decreased or against gravity, according to the client's muscle grade and the goal of the exercise or activity. An isotonic contraction of the biceps is used to lift a fork to the mouth for eating.[23,29]

Eccentric contraction

When muscles contract eccentrically, the tension in the muscle increases or remains constant, while the muscle lengthens. This contraction may be performed with or without resistance. An example of an eccentric contraction performed without resistance is the lowering of the arm to the table when placing a napkin next to a plate. The biceps contracts eccentrically in this instance. An example of eccentric contraction against resistance is the controlled return of a pail of sand lifted from the ground. In this example the biceps is contracting eccentrically to control the rate and coordination of the elbow extension in setting the pail on the ground.[23,29]

Exercise and Activity Classifications

Isotonic resistive exercise

Resistive exercise uses isotonic muscle contraction against a specific amount of weight to move the load through a certain ROM.[15,23,29] It is also possible to use eccentric contraction against resistance. Resistive exercise is used primarily for an increase in the strength of fair plus to normal muscles but may also be helpful for producing relaxation of the antagonists to the contracting muscles. This latter purpose can be useful if increased range is desired for stretching or relaxing hypertonic antagonists.

The client performs muscle contraction against resistance and moves the part through the available ROM. The resistance applied should be the maximum against which the muscle is capable of contracting. Resistance may be applied manually or by weights, springs, elastic bands, sandbags, or special devices. The source of resistance depends on the activity, and resistance is graded progressively with an increasing amount of resistance.[15,23,29] The number of possible repetitions depends on the client's general physical endurance and the endurance of the specific muscle.

Many types of strength training programs exist; most are based on the principle that to increase strength, the muscle must contract against its maximal resistance. The number of repetitions, rest intervals, frequency of training, and speed of movement vary with the particular approach and with the client's ability to accommodate to the exercise or activity regimen.[10] One specialized type of resistive exercise is the DeLorme method of progressive resistive exercise (PRE).[18,47] PRE is based on the overload principle: muscles perform more efficiently if given a warm-up period and must be taxed beyond usual daily activity to improve in performance and strength.[18] During the exercise procedure small loads are used initially and increased gradually after each set of 10 repetitions. The muscle is thus warmed up to prepare to exert its maximal power for the final 10 repetitions. The exercise procedure consists of three sets of 10 repetitions each, with resistance applied as follows: first set, 10 repetitions at 50% of maximal resistance; second set, 10 repetitions at 75% of maximal resistance; third set, 10 repetitions at maximal resistance.[15,18,47] The load must be sufficient so that the client can perform 10 repetitions. As strength improves, resistance is increased so that 10 repetitions can always be performed.[10] The client is instructed to inhale during the shortening contraction and exhale during the relaxation or eccentric contraction.[18,47]

An example of a PRE is a triceps, capable of 12 pounds maximal resistance, extending the elbow, first against 6 pounds for 10 repetitions, then against 9 pounds for 10 repetitions, and the final 10 repetitions against 12 pounds. Maximal resistance, the amount of resistance the muscle can lift through the ROM 10 times, is determined by contracting the muscle and moving the part through the full ROM against progressively increasing loads for sets of 10 repetitions, until the maximal load that can be lifted 10 times is reached.

At the beginning of the treatment program it is often difficult for the therapist to determine the client's maximal resistance. Reasons may be that the client may not know how to exert maximal effort, may be reluctant to exercise strenuously for fear of pain or reinjury, may be unwilling or unable to endure discomfort, and may have difficulty with the timing of exercises.

The experience of the therapist and trial and error aid in determination of maximal resistance. The therapist should estimate the amount of resistance the client can take based on the muscle test results and add or subtract resistance (weight or tension) until the client can perform the sets of repetitions adequately.

The exercises should be performed once daily, four or five times a week, and rest periods of 2 to 4 minutes should be allowed between each set of 10 repetitions. The exercise procedure may be modified to suit individual needs. Some possibilities are 10 repetitions at 25% of maximal resistance, 10 repetitions at 50%, 10 repetitions at 75%, and 10 repetitions at maximal resistance. Another possibility is five repetitions at 50% and 10 repetitions at maximal resistance. Still another possibility is to omit the second set of exercises. Adjustments in the first two sets of exercises may be made to suit the capacity of the individual.[18]

Another approach is the Oxford technique, essentially a reverse of the DeLorme method. The exercise sequence begins with 100% resistance and decreases to 75%, and then to 50% on subsequent sets of 10 repetitions each.[18,47] The greatest gains may be made in the early weeks of the intervention program, with smaller increases occurring at a slower pace in the subsequent weeks or months. During performance of the exercise, the therapist should be aware of joint alignment of the exercise device; proper fit and adjustment of the device;

ruling out of substitute movements; and clear instruction on speed, ROM, and proper breathing.[18,42]

OT PRACTICE NOTE

APPLICATION TO ACTIVITY

Many purposeful activities lend themselves well to resistive exercise. For instance, leather lacing can offer slight resistance to the anterior deltoid if the lace is pushed in an upward direction. Sanding wood with a weighted sand block can offer substantial resistance to the anterior deltoid and triceps if done on an inclined plane. Activities such as sawing and hammering offer resistance to upper extremity musculature. Kneading dough and forming clay objects offer resistance to muscles of the hands and arms.

Isotonic active exercise

Isotonic muscle contraction is used in active exercise. Eccentric contraction may also be used. Active exercise is performed when the client moves the joint through its available ROM against no outside resistance. Active motion through the complete ROM with gravity decreased or against gravity may be used for poor to fair muscles to improve strength, with the added benefit of maintaining ROM. It may be used with higher muscle grades for the maintenance of strength and ROM when resistance is contraindicated. Active exercise is not used to increase ROM because this purpose requires added force not present in active exercise.

In active exercise the client moves the part through the complete ROM independently. If the exercise is performed in a gravity-decreased plane, a powdered surface, skateboard may be used to reduce the resistance produced by friction on a supporting surface. A deltoid aid, or free-moving supension sling may be used to support the extremity when moving in a gravity-decreased plane of motion. The exercise is graded by a change to resistive exercise as strength improves.[23,29]

OT PRACTICE NOTE

APPLICATION TO ACTIVITY

Activities that offer little or no resistance can be used as active exercise. A needlework activity performed in the gravity-decreased plane provides active exercise to the wrist extensors. When a grade of fair, or 3, is reached, the activity can be repositioned to move against gravity, or an alternate activity may be selected such as latch hooking (Figure 28-12).

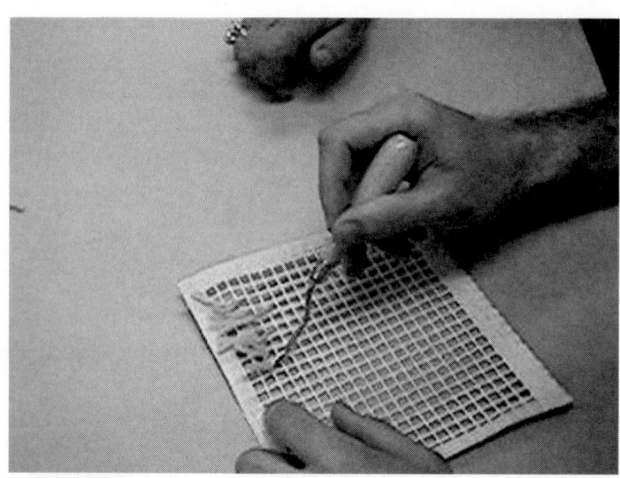

Figure 28-12 Latch hooking to provide active resistive exercise to the wrist extensors.

Active-assisted exercise

Isotonic muscle contraction is used in active-assisted exercise. The client moves the joint through partial ROM, and the therapist or a mechanical device completes the range. Slings, pulleys, weights, springs, or elastic bands may be used to provide mechanical assistance.[47] The goal of active-assisted exercise is to increase strength of trace, poor minus, and fair minus muscles while maintaining ROM. In the case of trace muscles the client may contract the muscle, and the therapist completes the entire ROM. This exercise is graded by decreasing the amount of assistance until the client can perform active exercises.[23,29]

OT PRACTICE NOTE

APPLICATION TO ACTIVITY

If assistance is required to complete the movement, an activity must be structured so that assistance can be offered by the therapist, the client's other arm or leg, or a mechanical device. Various bilateral activities lend themselves well to active-assisted exercise. Bilateral sanding, bilateral sponge wiping, using a sweeper, and sawing are some examples. In bilateral activities the unaffected arm or leg can perform a major share of the work, and the affected arm or leg can assist to the extent possible.

Passive exercise

In **passive exercise** *no* muscle contraction occurs. Therefore, passive exercise is not used to increase strength because no force is applied. The purpose of passive exercise is to maintain ROM, thereby preventing contractures, adhesions, and deformity. To achieve this goal, the person should perform exercise for at least three repetitions, twice daily.[28] It is used when absent or minimal muscle strength (grades 0 to 1) precludes the active motion or when active exercise is contraindicated because of the client's physical condition. During the exercise procedure the joint or joints to be exercised are moved through their normal ranges manually by the therapist or client, or mechanically by an external device such as a pulley or counterbalance sling. The joint proximal to the joint being exercised should be stabilized during the exercise procedure (Figure 28-13).[23]

OT PRACTICE NOTE

APPLICATION TO ACTIVITY

It is often possible to include a passive limb in a bilateral activity if the contralateral limb is unaffected. Several of the activities described previously for active-assisted exercise can also be used for passive exercise.

Passive stretch

For passive stretching, the therapist moves the joint through the available ROM and holds momentarily, applying a gentle but firm force or stretch at the end of the ROM. No residual pain should occur when the stretching is discontinued. Passive stretch or forced exercise is meant to increase ROM. It is used when a loss of joint ROM occurs and stretching is not contraindicated. If muscle grades are adequate, the client can move the part actively through the available ROM and the therapist can take it a little farther, thus forcing or stretching the soft-tissue structures around the joint.

Passive stretching requires a good understanding of joint anatomy and muscle function. It should be carried out cautiously under good medical supervision and with medical approval. Muscles to be stretched should be in a relaxed state.[29]

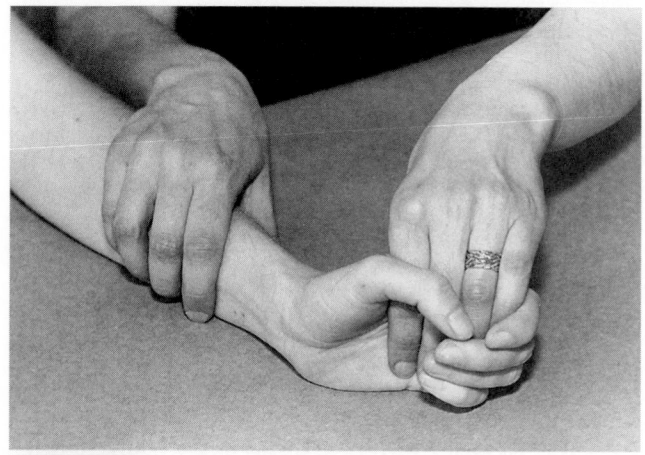

Figure 28-13 Passive exercise of the wrist with stabilization of the joint proximal to the one being exercised.

The therapist should never force muscles when pain is present, unless ordered by the physician to work through pain. Gentle, firm stretching held for a few seconds is more effective and less hazardous than quick, short stretching. The body parts around the area being stretched should be stabilized, and compensatory movements should be prevented. Incorrect stretching procedures can produce muscle tearing, joint fracture, and inflammatory edema.[28]

 OT PRACTICE NOTE

APPLICATION TO ACTIVITY

Passive stretching may be incorporated into an activity if an unaffected part guides the movement of the affected part and forces it slightly beyond the available ROM. One example is the passive stretch of wrist flexors during a block printing activity if the block is pressed down to stabilize the block with an open hand while the client is standing.

Active stretch

The purpose of active stretch is the same as for passive stretch: to increase joint ROM. In active stretching, the client uses the force of the agonist muscle to increase the length of the antagonist. This requires good to normal strength of the antagonist, good coordination, and motivation of the client. For example, forceful contraction of the triceps to stretch the biceps muscle can be performed. Because the exercise may produce discomfort, a natural tendency exists for the client to avoid the stretching component of the movement. Therefore, supervision and frequent evaluation of its effectiveness are necessary.

 OT PRACTICE NOTE

APPLICATION TO ACTIVITY

Many activities can be used to incorporate active stretching. For example, slowly sawing wood requires a forceful contraction of the triceps with a concomitant stretch of the biceps.

Isometric exercise without resistance

Isometric exercise uses isometric contractions of a specific muscle or muscle group. In isometric exercises a muscle or group of muscles is actively contracted and relaxed without producing motion of the joint that it ordinarily moves. The purpose of isometric exercise without resistance is to maintain muscle strength when active motion is not possible or is contraindicated. It may be used with any muscle grade above trace. It is especially useful for clients in casts, after surgery, and with arthritis or burns.[15]

The client is taught to set or contract the muscles voluntarily and to hold the contraction for 5 or 6 seconds.

Without offering resistance, the therapist's fingers provide a kinesthetic image of resistance and help the client learn to set the muscle. If needed, the therapist's fingers may be placed distal to the joint on which the muscles act. If passive motion is allowed, the therapist may move the joint to the desired point in the ROM and ask the client to hold the position.

Isometric exercise affects the cardiovascular system, which may be a contraindication for some clients. It may cause a rapid and sudden increase in blood pressure, depending on the age of the client, the intensity of contraction, and muscle mass being contracted. Therefore, it should be used with caution.[15]

Isometric exercise with resistance

Isometric exercise with applied resistance uses isometric muscle contraction performed against some outside resistance. Its purpose is to increase muscle strength in muscles graded fair, or 3, to normal, or 5. The client sets the muscle or muscle group while resistance is applied and holds the contraction for 5 or 6 seconds. Isometric exercises should be performed for one exercise session per day, 5 days a week. In addition to manual resistance, the client may hold a weight or resist against a solid surface, depending on the muscle group being exercised. A small weight held in the hand while the wrist is stabilized at neutral requires isometric contractions of the wrist flexors and extensors.

Exercise is graded by increasing the amount of resistance or the degree of force the client holds against. A tension gauge should be used to accurately monitor the amount of resistance applied. Isometric exercises are effective for increasing strength, but isotonic exercise is the method of choice. Isometric exercise has several specific applications, as in arthritis, when joint motion may be contraindicated but muscle strength must be increased or maintained.[23,42] The cardiovascular precautions stated previously are particularly important with isometric resistive exercise.

 OT PRACTICE NOTE

APPLICATION TO ACTIVITY

Any activity that requires holding or static posture incorporates isometric exercise. Holding tool handles and holding the arm in elevation while painting are examples. This type of exercise, if contraction is sustained, can be very fatiguing.

Neuromuscular control and coordination

Procedures for the development of neuromuscular control and neuromuscular coordination are briefly outlined in the following paragraphs. The reader is referred to original sources for a full discussion of the neurophysiological mechanisms underlying these exercises. Neuromuscular education or control training involves teaching the client to control individual muscles or motions through conscious attention. Coordination training is used to develop preprogrammed multimuscular patterns or engrams.[27]

Neuromuscular control

It may be desirable to teach control of individual muscles when they are so weak that they cannot be used normally. The purpose is to improve muscle strength and muscle coordination to new patterns. To achieve these ends, the person must learn precise control of the muscle, an essential step in the development of optimal coordination for persons with neuromuscular disease.

To participate successfully the client must be able to learn and follow instructions, cooperate, and concentrate on the muscular retraining. Before beginning, the client should be comfortable and securely supported. The exercises should be carried out in a nondistracting environment. The client must be alert, calm, and rested. He or she should have an adequate pain-free arc of motion of the joint on which the muscle acts, in addition to good proprioception. Visual and tactile sensory feedback may be used to compensate or substitute for limited proprioception, but the coordination achieved will never be as great as when proprioception is intact.[27]

The client's awareness of the desired motion and the muscles that produce it is first taught to the client using passive motion to stimulate the proprioceptive stretch reflex. This passive movement may be repeated several times. The client's awareness may be enhanced if the therapist also demonstrates the desired movement and if the movement is performed by the analogous unaffected part. The skin over the muscle belly and tendon insertion may be stimulated to enhance the effect of the stretch reflex. Stroking and tapping over the muscle belly may be used to facilitate muscle action.[27]

The therapist should explain the location and function of the muscle, its origin and insertion, line of pull, and action on the joint. The therapist should then demonstrate the motion and instruct the client to think of the pull of the muscle from insertion to origin. The skin over muscle insertion can be stroked in the direction of pull while the client concentrates on the sensation of the motion during the passive movement performed by the therapist.

The exercise sequence begins with instructions to the client to think about the motion, while the therapist carries it out passively and strokes the skin over the insertion in the direction of the motion. The client is then instructed to assist by contracting the muscle while the therapist performs passive motion and stimulates the skin as before. Next the client moves the part through ROM with assistance and cutaneous stimulation, while the therapist emphasizes contraction of the prime mover only. Finally the client carries out the movement independently, using the prime mover.

The exercises must be initiated against minimal resistance if activity is to be isolated to prime movers. If the muscle is very weak (trace to poor), the procedure may be carried out entirely in an active-assisted manner so that the muscle contracts against no resistance and can function without activating synergists. Progression from one step to the next depends on successful performance of the steps without substitutions. Each step is carried out three to five times per session for each muscle, depending on the client's tolerance.

Coordination training

The goal of coordination training is to develop the ability to perform multimuscular motor patterns that are faster, more precise, and stronger than those performed when control of individual muscles is used. The development of coordination depends on repetition. Initially in training, the movement must be simple and slow so that the client can be consciously aware of the activity and its components. Good coordination does not develop until repeated practice results in a well-developed activity pattern that no longer requires conscious effort and attention.

Training should take place in an environment in which the client can concentrate. The exercise is divided into components that the client can perform correctly. Kottke calls this approach *desynthesis*.[27] The level of effort required should be kept low, by reducing speed and resistance, to prevent the spread of excitation to muscles that are not part of the desired movement pattern. Other theorists offer contrary advice, which emphasizes the integration of movements that customarily occurs during activity. The therapist's experience and judgment are important in determining which method to use.

When the motor pattern is divided into units that the client can perform successfully, each unit is trained by practice under voluntary control, as described previously for training of control. The therapist instructs the client in the desired movement and uses sensory stimulation and passive movement. The client must observe and voluntarily modify the motion. Slow practice is imperative to make this monitoring possible. The therapist offers enough assistance to ensure precise movement while allowing the client to concentrate on the sensations produced by the movements. When the client concentrates on movement, fatigue occurs rapidly and the client should be given frequent, short rests. As the client masters the components of the pattern and performs them precisely and independently, the sequence is graded to subtasks or several components that are practiced repetitively. As the subtasks are perfected, they are linked progressively until the movement pattern can be performed.

The protocol can be graded for speed, force, or complexity, but the therapist must be aware that the increased effort put forth by the client may result in incoordinated movement. Therefore, the grading must remain within the client's capacity to perform the precise movement pattern. The motor pattern must be performed correctly to prevent the development of faulty patterns.

If CNS impulses are generated to muscles that should not be involved in the movement pattern, incoordinated motion results. Constant repetition of an incoordinated pattern reinforces the pattern, resulting in a persistent incoordination. Factors that increase incoordination are fear, poor balance, too much resistance, pain, fatigue, strong emotions, prolonged inactivity,[27] and excessively prolonged activity.

 OT PRACTICE NOTES

APPLICATION TO ACTIVITY

OT can be used to develop coordination, strength, and endurance. Active occupations have the advantage of engaging the client's attention and interest. Activities should be structured to enable the client to use the precise movement pattern and to work at speeds consistent with the maintenance of precision.

Therapists may initiate coordination training with neuromuscular education and progress to repetitious activities requiring desired coordinated movement patterns. Placing small blocks, marbles, cones, paper cups, or pegs is an enabling activity that demands repetitious patterns of nonresistive movement. Purposeful activities such as leather lacing, mosaic tile work, and needlecrafts, and household tasks such as wiping, sweeping, and dusting also provide such repetitious movements.

PHYSICAL AGENT MODALITIES

The introduction of physical agent modalities (PAMs) into OT practice generated considerable controversy.[50,53] The use of such modalities was initiated by OTs who specialize in hand rehabilitation, in which inclusion of physical agents in a comprehensive treatment program became expedient.[44,46] After much study and discussion, the AOTA published a position paper on physical agent modalities.[3,5] In this official document, physical agents were defined and their use as adjuncts to or preparation for purposeful activity was specified. "The exclusive use of physical agent modalities as a treatment method during a treatment session without application to a functional outcome is not considered occupational therapy."[5] Further, the use of PAMs is not considered entry-level practice: rather, appropriate postprofessional education is required to ensure competence of the OT practitioners using these modalities.[5] The AOTA stipulated that the practitioner must have documented evidence of the theoretical background and technical skills to apply the modality and integrate it into an OT intervention plan.[3,5] Generated from these notions, several states have required in their licensure laws that OTs have advanced training to use PAMs in treatment.

PAMs are used before or during functional activities to enhance the effects of the OT intervention program. This section introduces the reader to basic techniques and when and why they may be applied. Because modalities are most commonly used by OTs for treatment of hand injuries and diseases, the examples provided are focused on intervention to improve upper extremity function. The use of the techniques described is not limited to the treatment of hands, however.

Thermal Modalities

In a clinical setting heat is used to increase motion, decrease joint stiffness, relieve muscle spasms, increase blood flow, decrease pain, and aid in the reabsorption of exudates and edema in a chronic condition.[32] Collagen fibers have an elastic component and when stretched will return to their original length. Applying heat before a prolonged stretch, as in dynamic splinting, allows the permanent elongation of these fibers. The blood flow maintains a person's core temperature at 98.6° F. To obtain maximum benefits from heat, tissue temperature must be raised to 105° to 113° F. Precautions must be taken with temperatures above this range to prevent tissue destruction.

Contraindications to the use of heat include acute inflammatory conditions of the joints or skin, sensory losses, impaired vascular structures, malignancies, and application to the very young or very old. The use of heat may substantially enhance the effects of splinting and therapeutic activities that attempt to increase range of motion and functional abilities.

Conduction

Conduction is the transfer of heat from one object to another through direct contact. Paraffin and hot packs provide heat by conduction. Paraffin is stored in a tub that maintains a temperature between 125° and 130° F. The client repeatedly dips his or her hand into the tub until a thick, insulating layer of paraffin is applied to the extremity. The hand is then wrapped in a plastic bag and towel for 10 to 20 minutes.[32] This technique provides an excellent conforming characteristic, so it is ideal for use in hands and digits. Partial hand coverage is possible. The paraffin transfers its heat to the hand, and the bag and towel act as an insulator against dissipation of heat to the air.

Care must be taken to protect insensate parts from burns. To prevent excessive vasodilation, paraffin should not be applied when moderate to severe edema is present. It cannot be used if open wounds are present. Paraffin can be used in the clinic or incorporated into a home program. The tubs are small, and the technique is safe and easy to use in the home. It is an excellent adjunct to home programs that include dynamic splinting, exercises, or general ADLs. It may be used in the clinic before therapeutic exercises and functional activities.

Hot packs contain either a silicate gel or a bentonite clay wrapped in a cotton bag and submerged in a hydrocollator, a water tank that maintains the temperature of the packs at

160° to 175° F.[32] Because tissue damage may occur at these temperatures, the packs are separated from the skin by layers of towels. As with paraffin, precautions should be taken in application of hot packs to insensate tissue that has sustained vascular damage. Hot packs are commonly used for myofascial pain, before soft-tissue mobilization, and before any activities aimed at elongating contracted tissue.[14] For a client with a hand injury the packs may be applied to the extrinsic musculature to decrease muscle tone caused by guarding, without also heating the hand. Unless contraindicated, hot packs can be used (with precautions) when open wounds are present.

Convection

Convection supplies heat to the tissues by fluid motion around the tissues. Examples of convection are whirlpool and fluidotherapy. Whirlpool is used more commonly for wound management than for heat application. Fluidotherapy involves a machine that agitates finely ground cornhusk particles by blowing warm air through them. This device is similar to the whirlpool, but corn particles are used instead of water. The temperature is thermostatically maintained, with the therapeutic range extending to 125° F. Studies have shown this technique to be excellent for raising tissue temperature in the hands and feet.[14] An additional benefit is its effect on desensitization. The agitator can be adjusted to decrease or increase the flow of the corn particles, thus controlling the amount of stimulation to the skin. Because an extremity can be heated gradually, this technique is effective as a warm-up before exercises, dexterity tasks, functional activities, and work simulation tasks.

Conversion

Conversion occurs when heat is generated internally by friction, for example, by means of ultrasound. The sound waves penetrate the tissues, causing vibration of the molecules, and the resulting friction generates heat. The energy of sound waves is thus converted to heat energy. The sound waves are applied with a transducer, which glides across the skin in slow, continuous motions. Gel is used to improve the transmission of the sound to the tissues. Ultrasound is considered a deep heating agent. At 1 MHz (1 million cycles per second), it can heat tissues to a depth of 5 cm. The previous methods produce heating to 1 cm.[36] Many therapeutic ultrasound machines provide a 3-MHz option for treatment of more superficial structures, with the corresponding heating depth reduced to 3 cm. Ultrasound at frequencies higher than recommended standards can destroy tissue. In addition, precautions must be taken to avoid growth plates in the bones of children, an unprotected spinal cord, and freshly repaired structures such as tendons and nerves. Because of its ability to heat deeper tissues, ultrasound is excellent for treating problems associated with joint contractures, scarring with its associated adhesions, and muscle spasms.

When applying the ultrasound, the therapist should apply a stretch to the tissues while they are being heated, followed by activities, exercises, and splints to maintain the stretch.

Ultrasound may also be used in a nonthermal application, in which the ultrasound waves are used to drive antiinflammatory medications into tissues. This process is called *phonophoresis*. Ultrasound is thought to increase membrane permeability for greater symptom relief and may also be used after corticosteroid injections.

Cryotherapy, the use of cold in therapy, is often used in the treatment of edema, pain, and inflammation. The cold produces a vasoconstriction, which decreases the amount of blood flow into the injured tissue. Cold decreases muscle spasms by decreasing the amount of firing from the afferent muscle spindles. Cryotherapy is contraindicated for clients with cold intolerance or vascular repairs. The use of cryotherapy may be incorporated into intervention programs provided in the clinical setting; however, it is particularly useful in a home program.

Cold packs can be applied in a number of ways. Many commercial packs exist, which range in size and cost. An alternative to purchasing a cold pack is to use a bag of frozen vegetables or to combine crushed ice and alcohol in a plastic bag to make a reusable slush bag. Ice packs should be covered with a moist towel to prevent tissue injury. The benefit of commercial packs is that they are easy to use, especially if the client must use them frequently during the day. When clients are working, it is recommended that they keep cold packs at home and at work to increase the ease of use. The optimum temperature for storing a cold pack is 45° F.

Other forms of cryotherapy include ice massage and cooling machines. Ice massage is used when the area to be cooled is small and very specific—for example, inflammation of a tendon specifically at its insertion or origin. The procedure entails using a large piece of ice (water frozen in a paper cup) and massaging the area with circular motions until the skin is numb, usually for 4 to 5 minutes. Cooling devices, which circulate cold water through tubes in a pack, are available through vendors. These devices maintain their cold temperatures for a long time, but they are expensive to rent or purchase. They are effective in reducing edema immediately after surgery or injury, during the inflammatory phase of wound healing.

Contrast baths combine the use of heat and cold. The physical response is alternating vasoconstriction and vasodilation of the blood vessels. The client is asked to submerge the arm, for example, alternating between two tubs of water. One contains cold water (59° to 68° F), and the other contains warm water (96° to 105° F). The purpose is to increase collateral circulation, which effectively reduces pain and edema. As with the use of cold packs, contrast baths are a beneficial addition to a home therapy program. This technique is contraindicated for clients with vascular disorders or injuries.

Electrical Modalities

Electrical modalities are used to decrease pain, decrease edema, increase motion, and reeducate muscles. As with all PAMs, OTs use these modalities to increase a client's functional abilities. Many techniques are available; those most commonly used are presented here. Electrical modalities should not be used with clients with pacemakers or cardiac conditions.

Transcutaneous electrical nerve stimulation

Transcutaneous electrical nerve stimulation (TENS) employs electrical current to decrease pain. Pain is classified in three categories: physical, physiological, and psychological. When trauma occurs, an individual responds to the initial pain by guarding the painful body part, often by restricting motion of the body part or assuming a posture that limits use of the painful body part. This guarding may result in muscle spasms and fatigue of the muscle fibers, especially after prolonged guarding. The supply of blood and oxygen to the affected area decreases, and resultant soft-tissue and joint dysfunction occurs.[35] These reactions magnify and compound the problems associated with the initial pain response. The therapist's goal after an acute injury is to prevent this cycle. In the case of chronic pain, the goal is to stop the cycle that has been established. TENS is an effective technique for control of pain without the side effects of medications. Pain medications are frequently used in conjunction with TENS, which often reduces the duration of their use. TENS is safe to use, and clients can be educated in independent home use.

TENS provides constant electrical stimulation with a modulated current and is directed to the peripheral nerves through electrode placement. The therapist can control several attributes of the modulation waveform such as the frequency, amplitude, and pulse width. When TENS is applied at a low-fire setting, endogenous opiates are released. Endorphins, naturally occurring substances, reduce the sensation of pain. The effects of high-frequency TENS are based on the gate control theory originally proposed by Melzack and Wall in 1965. This theory describes how the electrical current from TENS, applied to the peripheral nerves, blocks the perception of pain in the brain. Nociceptors (pain receptors) transmit information to the CNS through the A-delta, and C fibers. A-delta fibers transmit information about pressure and touch. It is thought that TENS stimulates the A fibers, effectively saturating the gate to pain perception, and the transmission of pain signals via the A-delta, and C fibers is blocked at the level of the spinal cord.[34] TENS can be applied for acute or chronic pain. TENS is frequently used postsurgically, when it is mandatory that motion be initiated within 72 hours such as in tenolysis and capsulotomy surgeries or when it is important to maintain tendon gliding through the injured area after fractures. TENS can be especially helpful with clients who have a low threshold to pain, which makes exercising easier. TENS is also useful when working with clients with reflex sympathetic dystrophy because continued active motion is crucial.

TENS can be used to decrease pain from an inflammatory condition such as tendonitis or a nerve impingement; however, the client must be educated in tendon and nerve protection and rest, with a proper home program of symptom management, positioning, and ADL and work modification. Without the sensation of pain, the client may overdo and stress the tissues. Other techniques should be tried first to decrease pain for these clients. TENS is also used for treatment of trigger points, with direct electrode application to the trigger point to decrease its irritability.[37]

Neuromuscular electrical stimulation

Neuromuscular electrical stimulation (NMES) provides a continuous interrupted current. It is applied through an electrode to the motor point of innervated muscles to provide a muscle contraction. The current is interrupted to enable the muscle to relax between contractions, and the durations of the on and off times can be adjusted by the therapist. Adjustments can also be made to control the rate of the increase in current (ramp) and intensity of the contraction.

NMES is used to increase ROM, facilitate muscle contractions, and strengthen muscles.[38] It may be used postsurgically to provide a stronger contraction for released tendon gliding—for example, after a tenolysis. It also may be used later in the tendon repair protocol, once the tendon has healed sufficiently to tolerate stress, usually at a minimum of 6 weeks. NMES may be used to lengthen a muscle that has become weakened because of disuse. During the reinnervation phase after a nerve injury, this technique may be used to help stimulate and strengthen a newly innervated muscle. Care must be taken not to overfatigue the muscle. NMES can be applied during a dexterity or functional activity, which allows the muscle to be retrained in the purpose of its contraction. As with TENS, NMES may be incorporated into a home program with proper client education and follow-through.

Other techniques that use an electrical current include high-voltage galvanic stimulation (HVGS) and inferential electrical stimulation. These techniques are applied to treat pain and edema.[38] Electrical stimulation may be applied in conjunction with ultrasound through a single transducer to provide heat simultaneously with current. This approach is beneficial in treatment of trigger points and myofascial pain. Iontophoresis uses a current to drive ionized medication into inflamed tissue and scar tissue. The technique uses an electrode filled with the medication of choice. The medicine is transferred by applying an electric field that repels the ions into the tissues.

SELECTION OF APPROPRIATE MODALITIES IN THE CONTINUUM OF CARE

Many years ago professional roles and responsibilities were more specifically delineated. OTs initiated therapy with clients only after the clients were capable, at least to some degree, of performing purposeful activity.[19] Evolution of intervention methods, trends in healthcare, and medical technology have significantly altered the role of the respective therapists and expanded the repertoire of treatment modalities that therapists are competent to practice.

Clients are now referred to OT long before they are capable of performing purposeful activity. Therapists are treating clients in the very acute stages of illness and disability. Intervention is directed toward preparing the client for the time when purposeful activity is possible. This approach may mean that the OT applies a positioning splint to a client immediately after hand surgery, considering how the hand will be used in a later phase of the intervention program and in real life. It means the therapist may use sensory stimulation for the client who is comatose because arousal and interacting with persons and objects in the environment will make performance of purposeful activity possible in the future. It means the therapist may apply paraffin to decrease joint stiffness and increase mobility of finger joints before engaging in a macrame project. It also may mean preparing the client and family to plan for the future, when life skills may need to be performed in new ways, such as modified sexual positioning for clients with arthritis. The unique perspective of the OT is seeing the potential for performance and using modalities that lead incrementally to performance relevant to the lives clients wish to lead.

SUMMARY

Engagement in occupation is the primary tool and objective of OT practice. OTs use purposeful activity, activity analysis, adaptation, grading of activities, therapeutic exercise, simulated or enabling activities, and adjunctive modalities in the continuum of intervention, and they may use these methods simultaneously toward these ends. Through this breadth of practice skills, based on the client's personal and social needs, the OT helps the client apply newly gained strength, ROM, and coordination during the performance of purposeful activity, which prepares the client to assume or reassume life roles. Appropriate therapeutic activity is individualized and designed to be meaningful and interesting to the client while meeting therapeutic objectives.

Therapeutic activity may be adapted to meet special needs of the client or the environment. It may be graded for physical, perceptual, cognitive, and social purposes to keep the client functioning at maximal potential at any point in the treatment program. The uniqueness of OT lies in its extensive use of goal-directed purposeful activities as treatment modalities, making use of the mind-body continuum within the tangible and social context. Purposeful activity is the core of OT practice.

In practice, therapists' roles may not be sharply defined because they are subject to variations in expectations that stem from regional differences, health care developments, legislation, institutional philosophy, and the roles and responsibilities assigned by the treatment facility. In all instances, OTs must be well trained and well qualified to deliver all aspects of practice. They should not hesitate to refer clients to experts for treatment whenever appropriate.

ACTIVITY ANALYSIS

The activity analysis offers the reader one systematic approach for looking at the therapeutic potential of activities. This model includes some factors that must be considered about the performer, the environmental context, and the activity in the selection of purposeful, therapeutic activity. In the model, just two steps of a multi-step activity are analyzed for the sake of space and simplicity. The reader is encouraged to complete the motor analysis by considering movements of the shoulder, forearm, and wrist that accompany the pinch and release pattern analyzed.

I. **Preliminary Information**

   A. Name of activity: Pinch pottery

   B. Components of the task

     1. Roll some clay into a ball, 3 to 4 inches in diameter.

     2. Place the ball centered on the work table in front of the performer.

     3. Make a hole in the center of the ball with the right or left thumb (Figure 28-14).

     4. With the thumb and first two fingers of both hands, pinch around and around the hole from base to top of the ball.

       a. Pinch by pressing thumb against index and middle fingers.

       b. Release pinch by extending thumb and index and middle fingers slightly.

     5. Continue pinching in this way, gradually spreading the walls of the clay until a small bowl of the desired size is formed.

   C. Steps of activity being analyzed

     1. Pinch

     2. Release

   D. Equipment and supplies necessary

     1. Ball of soft ceramic clay

     2. Wooden table 30 to 32 inches high or a wooden work surface fastened to a table with C clamps

     3. Chair at the work table

     4. Sponge and bowl of water

     5. Ceramic smoothing tool

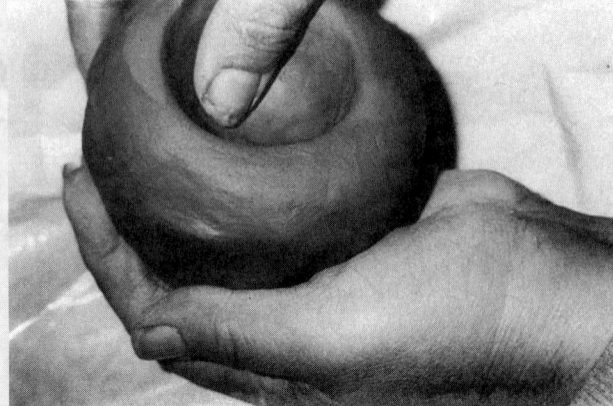

Figure 28-14 Opening pinch pot with thumb. (From Breines EB: *Occupational therapy from clay to computers: theory & practice*, Philadelphia, 1995, FA Davis.)

E. Environmental context[16,17]: OT workshop or craft activity room. A sink and damp storage area should be available in the work area. There should be ample room around the work table so that the performer is not crowded and can move freely between the table and the sink and damp storage closet. Lighting should be adequate for clear visualization of clay object and work area.

F. Position of the performer in relation to the work surface and equipment: The performer is seated in the chair at the table, at a comfortable distance for reaching and manipulating the clay and tools. The clay is centered in front of the performer, and the tool, sponge, and water bowl are to the right and near the top of the work area.

G. Starting position of the performer: Sitting erect with feet flat on the floor; shoulders are slightly abducted and in slight internal rotation, bringing both hands to the center work surface; elbows are flexed to about 90 degrees; forearms are pronated about 45 degrees; wrists are slightly extended and in ulnar deviation, thumbs are opposed to index and middle fingers, ready to pinch the posterior surface of the opened clay ball.

H. Movement pattern used to perform the steps under analysis: Flexion of the MP and IP joints of index and middle fingers; opposition and flexion of the thumb (pinch) followed by extension of the MP and IP joints index and middle fingers and extension and palmar abduction of the thumb (release). Repeat the pattern around ball of clay until a small bowl of desired size and thickness is formed.

II. **Motor Analysis[26]**

   A. Joint and muscle activity: List the joint motions for all movements used during performance of the activity. For each, indicate amount of ROM used (minimal, moderate, or full), muscle group used to perform the motion, strength required (minimal [P to F], moderate [F to G], and full [G to N]), and type of muscle contraction (isotonic, isometric, eccentric) (Table 28-1).

   B. Grading: Grade this activity for one or more of the following factors:

     1. ROM: Cannot be graded for ROM

     2. Strength: Grade for strength by increasing the consistency of the clay

     3. Endurance: Grade for sitting tolerance by increasing the length of activity sessions.

     4. Grade for sitting balance by decreasing sitting support

     5. Coordination: Requires fine coordination as performed; grade coordination by adding scored or painted designs to surface; grade to sculpture of small clay figures

   C. Criteria for activity as exercise

     1. Action of joints: Movement localized to flexion and extension of MP and IP joints of index and middle fingers; CMC, MP, and IP joint of thumb

     2. Repetition of motion: The pinch and release sequence is repeated until the bowl has reached the desired height and thickness

TABLE 28-1 **Motions for Pinch**

Joint Motion	Range of Motion	Muscle Group	Strength	Type of Muscle Contraction
INDEX AND MIDDLE FINGERS				
MP flexion	Minimal	FDP, FDS lumbricales	Moderate	Isotonic
PIP flexion	Minimal	FDP, FDS	Moderate	Isotonic
DIP flexion	Minimal	FDP	Moderate	Isotonic
Finger adduction	Maximal	Palmar interossei	Moderate	Isometric
THUMB				
Opposition	Full	Opponens pollicis, FPI, FPB	Moderate	Isotonic
MOTIONS FOR RELEASE INDEX AND MIDDLE FINGERS				
MP extension	Minimal	EDC, EIP	Minimal	Isotonic
PIP and DIP extension	Minimal	EDC, EIP	Minimal	Isotonic
Finger adduction	Maximal	Palmar interossei	Moderate	Isometric
THUMB				
Radial abduction	Moderate	APL, APB	Minimal	Isotonic
MP, IP extension	Full	EPL, EPB	Minimal	Isotonic

Adapted from Killingsworth A: *OT120 activity module*, San Jose, Calif, 1989, San Jose State University.

APB, Abductor pollicis brevis; *APL*, abductor pollicis longus; *DIP*, distal interphalangeal; *EDC*, extensor digitorum communis; *EIP*, extensor indicis proprius; *EPB*, extensor pollicis brevis; *EPL*, extensor pollicis longus; *FDP*, flexor digitorum profundus; *FDS*, flexor digitorum superficialis; *FPB*, flexor pollicis brevis; *FPL*, flexor pollicis longus; *IP*, interphalangeal; *MP*, metacarpophalangeal; *PIP*, proximal interphalangeal.

3. Gradable: The activity is gradable for strength and endurance

III. Sensory Analysis[33,34]

Check the sensory stimuli received by the person performing the activity. Include any sensory experience obtained from position, motion, materials, or equipment. Describe how sensation is received (Table 28-2).

IV. Cognitive Analysis[33]: Check All that Apply and Justify Your Answer (Table 28-3).

V. Safety Factors: What Are the Potential Hazards of this Activity? Describe Safety Precautions Necessary for this Activity. There Are Few Hazards in this Activity. Ingesting Clay or Using the Smoothing Tool Inappropriately Is Possible. Also, Sitting Balance Must be Adequate to Maintain Upright Posture to Perform the Activity. Precautions Must be Taken: Adequate Supervision Should be Provided to Ensure Appropriate Use of Clay and Tool, and the Task Should be Performed from a Wheelchair with Supports if Sitting Balance Is Impaired.

VI. Interpersonal Aspects of Activity

A. Solitary activity: May be done alone
B. Potential for dyadic interaction: May be done in parallel with one other person but does not require interaction

TABLE 28-2 **Sensory Analysis**

Sensory Modality		How Received
Tactile	X	Touching clay and tools
Proprioceptive (joint motion and position sense)	X	Being aware of joint position and motion during pinch/release
Vestibular (balance, sense of body, head motion)	X	Maintaining posture in chair while performing activity
Visual	X	Seeing clay object, environment
Olfactory (smell)	X	Smelling a slight odor of damp clay
Pain	O	
Thermal (temperature)	X	Hands sensing coldness of clay
Pressure	X	Fingertips and thumb tips pressing against walls of clay bowl
Auditory (hearing)	O	
Other		

O, Sensory stimuli not received; *X*, sensory stimuli received.

TABLE 28-3 **Cognitive Analysis**

Cognitive Skill		Justification
Memory	X	Remembers instruction
Sequencing (steps in order)	X	Performs steps in order
Problem-solving skills	X	Knows what to do if clay is too wet or too dry, if walls of bowl are too thin or too thick
FOLLOWING INSTRUCTIONS		
Spoken	X	Is able to comprehend and follow spoken instructions
Demonstrated	X	Is able to comprehend and follow demonstrated instructions
Written	O	
Concentration and attention required	X	Moderate: focuses on bowl and knows when its walls are thin enough and high enough

O, Cognitive skill not used; *X*, cognitive skill required in activity.

C. Potential for group interaction: May be done in a group but does not require interaction

VII. Psychological and Psychosocial Factors

A. Symbolism in performer's culture[16]: May be seen as more feminine than masculine in mainstream American culture; may be associated with the artistic, liberal, naturalist groups of people in American society

B. Symbolic meaning of activity to performer: May be seen as leisure skill rather than work: may be regarded as child's play by some persons

C. Feelings or reactions evoked in performer during performance of activity[33]: The soft, moist, pliable, and plastic properties of the clay may evoke soothing feelings in many persons. Others may regard it as messy or dirty. Potential for personal gratification is good because attractive end product is easy to achieve; activity is creative, individualistic, and useful.

VIII. Therapeutic Use of Activity

A. List the autonomous goal of the activity: To make a small clay bowl

B. List possible therapeutic objective(s) for the activity
   1. To increase pinch strength
   2. To improve coordination of opposition
   3. To increase sitting tolerance

Review Questions

1. Identify the three realms of occupational genesis and their relation to the concept of development.
2. Define modality.
3. What is required for an activity to be considered purposeful?
4. Name two reasons why activity is valuable.
5. Name a client-centered tool used to identify clients' goals, objectives, and lifestyles.
6. Name three perspectives of activity analysis.
7. What term best describes how activities and environments are modified to meet the individualized needs of clients?
8. What is used to create the "just right" challenge in performance?
9. What is the term that refers to activities that are contrived to elicit movements but are considered non-purposeful?
10. When are adjunctive modalities appropriately used by OTs?
11. For which types of disabilities would therapeutic exercise (as defined in this chapter) be inappropriate?
12. List and define three types of muscle contraction.
13. Identify an activity that can be used to provide resistive exercise, and describe how it could be done.
14. List four general categories of physical agent modalities.
15. What kinds of symptoms are treated with cryotherapy?

REFERENCES

1. American Occupational Therapy Association: Association policy: occupational therapists and modalities (Representative Assembly, April, 1983), *Am J Occup Ther* 37(12):816, 1983.
2. American Occupational Therapy Association: Occupational therapy practice framework: domain and process, *Am J Occup Ther* 56(6):609, 2002.
3. American Occupational Therapy Association: Official AOTA statement on physical agent modalites, *Am J Occup Ther* 45(12):1075, 1991.
4. American Occupational Therapy Association: Position paper on purposeful activities, *Am J Occup Ther* 37(12):805, 1983.
5. American Occupational Therapy Association: Position paper: physical agent modalities, *Am J Occup Ther* 46(12):1090, 1992.
6. American Occupational Therapy Association: Position paper: physical agent modalities, *Am J Occup Ther* 47(12):1081, 1993.

7. American Occupational Therapy Association: Uniform terminology for occupational therapy, ed 3, *Am J Occup Ther* 48(12):499, 1994.

8. Ayres AJ: Basic concepts of clinical practice in physical disabilities, *Am J Occup Ther* 12(8):300, 1958.

9. Ayres AJ: Occupational therapy for motor disorders resulting from impairment of the central nervous system, *Rehabil Lit* 21:302, 1960.

10. Barton G: *Teaching the sick: a manual of occupational therapy and reeducation*, Philadelphia, 1919, WB Saunders.

11. Breines EB: Genesis of occupation: a philosophical model for therapy and theory, *Aust Occup Ther J* 37:45, 1990.

12. Breines EB: *Occupational therapy from clay to computers: theory & practice*, Philadelphia, 1995, FA Davis.

13. Breines EB: *Origins and adaptations: a philosophy of practice*, Lebanon, NJ, 1986, Geri-Rehab.

14. Cannon NM, Mullins PT: *Manual on management of specific hand problems*, Pittsburgh, 1984, American Rehabilitation Educational Network.

15. Ciccone CD, Alexander J: Physiology and therapeutics of exercise. In Goodgold J, editor: *Rehabilitation medicine*, St Louis, 1988, Mosby.

16. Cynkin S: *Occupational therapy: toward health through activities*, Boston, 1979, Little, Brown.

17. Cynkin C, Robinson AM: *Occupational therapy: toward health through activities*, Boston, 1990, Little, Brown.

18. DeLateur BJ, Lehmann J: Therapeutic exercise to develop strength and endurance. In Kottke FJ, Stillwell GK, Lehmann JF, editors: *Krusen's handbook of physical medicine and rehabilitation*, ed 4, Philadelphia, 1990, WB Saunders.

19. Dewey J: *Democracy and education: an introduction to the philosophy of education*, Toronto, 1916, Collier-Macmillan.

20. Dunton WR: *Prescribing occupational therapy*, Springfield, Ill, 1928, Charles C Thomas.

21. Dutton R: Guidelines for using both activity and exercise, *Am J Occup Ther* 43(9):573, 1989.

22. Hopkins HL, Smith HD, Tiffany EG: The activity process. In Hopkins HL, Smith HD, editors: *Willard & Spackman's occupational therapy*, ed 7, Philadelphia, 1988, JB Lippincott.

23. Huddleston OL: *Therapeutic exercises*, Philadelphia, 1961, FA Davis.

24. Huss AJ: From kinesiology to adaptation, *Am J Occup Ther* 35(9):574, 1981.

25. Kielhofner G: A heritage of activity: development of theory, *Am J Occup Ther* 36(11):723, 1982.

26. Killingsworth A: *Activity module for OCTH 120, functional kinesiology*, 1989, San Jose State University, San Jose, California (unpublished).

27. Kottke FJ: Therapeutic exercises to develop neuromuscular coordination. In Kottke FJ, Stillwell GK, Lehmann JF, editors: *Krusen's handbook of physical medicine and rehabilitation*, ed 4, Philadelphia, 1990, WB Saunders.

28. Kottke FJ: Therapeutic exercise to maintain mobility. In Kottke FJ, Stillwell GK, Lehmann JF, editors: *Krusen's handbook of physical medicine and rehabilitation*, ed 4, Philadelphia, 1990, WB Saunders.

29. Kraus H: *Therapeutic exercise*, Springfield, Ill, 1963, Charles C Thomas.

30. Law M, Baptiste S, Carswell A, et al: *Canadian occupational performance measure*, ed 3, Ottowa, Canada, 1998, Canadian Association of Occupational Therapists.

31. Lamport NK, Coffey MS, Hersch GI: *Activity analysis & application: building blocks of treatment*, Thorofare, NJ, 1996, Slack.

32. Lehmann JF: *Therapeutic heat and cold*, ed 3, Baltimore, 1982, Williams & Wilkins.

33. Llorens LA: Activity analysis: agreement among factors in a sensory processing model, *Am J Occup Ther* 40(2):103, 1986.

34. Llorens L: *Activity analysis for sensory integration (CPM) dysfunction*, 1978 (unpublished).

35. Mannheimer JS, Lampe GN: *Clinical transcutaneous electrical nerve stimulation*, Philadelphia, 1990, FA Davis.

36. Michlovitz SL: *Thermal agents in rehabilitation*, ed 2, Philadelphia, 1990, FA Davis.

37. Moran CA, Saunders SR, Tribuzi SM: Myofascial pain in the upper extremity. In Hunter JM, et al, editors: *Rehabilitation of the hand*, ed 3, St Louis, 1990, Mosby.

38. Mullins PT: Use of therapeutic modalities in upper extremity rehabilitation. In Hunter JM, et al, editors: *Rehabilitation of the hand*, ed 3, St Louis, 1990, Mosby.

39. Nelson D, et al: The effects of occupationally embedded exercise on bilaterally assisted supination in persons with hemiplegia, *Am J Occup Ther* 50(8):639, 1996.

40. Pedretti LW, Smith RO, Hammel J, et al: Use of adjunctive modalities in occupational therapy, *Am J Occup Ther* 46(12):1075, 1992.

41. Rancho Los Amigos Hospital: *Muscle reeducation* (unpublished), Downey, Calif, 1963, the Hospital.

42. Rancho Los Amigos Hospital: *Progressive resistive and static exercise: principles and techniques* (unpublished), Downey, Calif, the Hospital.

43. Reed KL: Tools of practice: heritage or baggage? *Am J Occup Ther* 40(9):597, 1986.

44. Reynolds C: OTs and PAMs: a physical therapist's perspective, *OT Week* 8(37):17, Bethesda, Md, 1994, American Occupational Therapy Association.

45. Rocker JD, Nelson DL: Affective responses to keeping and not keeping an activity product, *Am J Occup Ther* 41(3):152, 1987.

46. Rose H: Physical agent modalities: OT's contribution, *OT Week* 8(37):16, Bethesda, Md, 1994, American Occupational Therapy Association.

47. Schram DA: Resistance exercise. In Basmajian JV, editor: *Therapeutic exercise*, ed 4, Baltimore, 1984, Williams & Wilkins.

48. Spackman CS: Occupational therapy for the restoration of physical function. In Willard HS, Spackman CS, editors: *Occupational therapy*, ed 4, Philadelphia, 1974, JB Lippincott.

49. Steinbeck TM: Purposeful activity and performance, *Am J Occup Ther* 40(8):529, 1986.

50. Taylor E, Humphrey R: Survey of physical agent modality use, *Am J Occup Ther* 45(10):924, 1991.

51. Thibodeaux CS, Ludwig FM: Intrinsic motivation in product-oriented and non-product-oriented activities, *Am J Occup Ther* 42(3):169, 1988.

52. Watson DE, Llorens LA: *Task analysis: an occupational performance approach*, Bethesda, Md, 1997, American Occupational Therapy Association.

53. West WL, Weimer RB: This issue is: should the representative assembly have voted as it did, on occupational therapist's use of physical agent modalities? *Am J Occup Ther* 45(12):1143, 1991.

54. Wynn-Parry CB: Vicarious motions. In Basmajian JV, editor: *Therapeutic exercise*, ed 3, Baltimore, 1982, Williams & Wilkins.

55. Yoder RM, Nelson DL, Smith DA: Added-purpose versus rote exercise in female nursing home residents, *Am J Occup Ther* 43(9):581, 1989.

29 ORTHOTICS

DONNA LASHGARI
LYNN YASUDA

KEY TERMS

Orthosis	Friction	Static splint	Immobilization splints
Tenodesis	Torque	Serial static splint	Mobilization splints
Axis of motion	Translational forces	Static progressive splints	Suspension arm devices
Force	Dynamic splints	Restriction splints	Mobile arm supports

LEARNING OBJECTIVES

After studying this chapter the student or practitioner will be able to do the following:

1. Identify basic hand anatomy.
2. Describe the difference between single-axis and multiaxis joints and explain how they relate to splinting.
3. Define torque and describe how a splint produces torque.
4. Discuss the relationship of angle of approach to dynamic splinting.
5. Describe the three major purposes and goals of splints and when they should be employed.
6. Demonstrate an understanding of the principles of making a splint pattern.
7. Identify three characteristics of low-temperature thermoplastic material.
8. Discuss two ways in which splints may apply force.
9. Demonstrate how to determine the proper length of a forearm-based splint.
10. List the purposes of suspension arm devices.
11. Describe the limitations of the suspension arm support.
12. List the elements of adjustment for suspension arm devices.
13. Briefly describe the evolution of the traditional mobile arm support (MAS) and name its parts.
14. List the benefits of the MAS to persons with severe upper extremity weakness.
15. List the criteria for use of the MAS and describe how it works.
16. List two special parts of the MAS.
17. Describe the advantages of the JAECO-Rancho Multilink Mobile Arm Support.

CHAPTER OUTLINE

Section 1: Hand Splinting: Principles, Practice, and Decision Making
  Role of the occupational therapist
  Anatomical structures of the hand
    Wrist
    Metacarpal joints
    Metacarpophalangeal joints
    Thumb
    Interphalangeal joints
    Forearm rotation
    Ligaments of wrist and hand
    Muscles and tendons of forearm, wrist, and hand
    Nerve supply
    Blood supply
    Skin
  Superficial anatomy and landmarks
  Prehension and grasp patterns
    Lateral prehension
    Palmar prehension
    Tip prehension
    Cylindrical grasp
    Spherical grasp
    Hook grasp
    Intrinsic plus grasp
  Mechanics of the hand and principles of splinting
    Axis of motion
    Force
  Splint classifications
    Splints classified by type

According to *Mosby's Medical, Nursing, & Allied Health Dictionary*, orthotics is "the design and use of external appliances to support a paralyzed muscle, promote a specific motion, or correct musculoskeletal deformities"; an orthosis is "a force system designed to control, correct, or compensate for a bone deformity, deforming forces, or forces absent from the body...[and] often involves the use of special braces"; and a splint is "an orthopedic device for immobilization, restraint, or support of any part of the body."[2] Splints and suspension arm devices can be considered orthoses. Occupational therapists (OTs) often design and construct splints. An orthotist usually designs and constructs suspension arm devices and OTs adjust them and train clients to use them. In practice, the term **orthosis** is more frequently used to refer to suspension arm devices than splints. Hand splinting is the topic of Section 1 of this chapter and suspension arm devices are described in Section 2.

SECTION 1: HAND SPLINTING: PRINCIPLES, PRACTICE, AND DECISION MAKING

Donna Lashgari

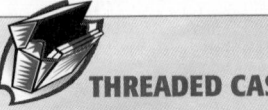

THREADED CASE STUDY: ALEXEI, PART 1

Alexei is a delightful, witty gentleman of 78 who resides in a nice retirement complex in the area since the passing of his wife 5 years ago. The complex offers three levels of care: independent apartment living, assisted living, and nursing care. At the time of his injury, Alexei was living in the independent area, had his own self-furnished apartment, took the van transportation provided

by the complex once a week for grocery shopping, and took public transportation to his weekly computer class at a nearby senior center. The complex offers some extra services for a fee, and Alexei paid for monthly housekeeping. He does his own laundry, cooking, and light cleaning. He has diabetes and takes care of his own testing and insulin injections. His beloved parakeet had recently died and he was shopping for another. He had trained the parakeet to do several tricks, and it was his pride and joy.

It was outside a pet store that he fell and suffered a comminuted distal radius and ulna fracture of his right dominant wrist. After open reduction and internal fixation (ORIF), he was discharged to the nursing care level of his complex for 2 days, then to the assisted living level. Unless he could quickly become independent with managing his activities of daily living (ADLs) and medical needs, in his case diabetic testing and injections, he would lose his apartment and be transferred to the assisted living level permanently. This level would not allow him a pet.

Alexei was 5 weeks post ORIF when he was referred to hand therapy for beginning active range of motion (ROM) and edema reduction. He was wearing a protective removable splint. Because of maximal edema in his hand, he had only 20% total active motion of his fingers and thumb and was assisted with most self-care and ADLs, was eating with his left, nondominant hand, and was dependent on nursing for his diabetic needs. Alexei's goal was to regain enough range of motion and dexterity in his right dominant hand to be independent with all ADLs and medical needs to return to his apartment, which would allow him to keep his own furniture, get another bird, and set his own schedule.

Although Alexei's insurance would cover any needed therapy, he was able to attend only once a week because of transportation issues. Because his therapy time would be limited, our focus in OT was to work toward his goals using dynamic splinting to regain ROM for functional grip and pinch and to collaborate with the nursing staff at his assisted living residence to help him meet his goal of managing his medical needs. Alexei attended therapy six times over the following 5 weeks. We worked closely by telephone with the nurse in assisted living who carried out our recommended contrast baths and nightly isotoner glove application to reduce edema. We fabricated a volar-based dynamic flexion splint for MP and PIP flexion and a dorsal-based finger extension splint, which he alternated during the day for approximately 2 to 3 hours each. We adjusted his splints each visit for greater ROM and proper 90-degree angle of pull on each finger, and he was quick to learn his exercise regimen and followed it religiously. By his third visit he was independent in all self-care and hygiene tasks using built-up utensil handles and a zipper pull. At this time, we were able to discontinue his extension splint and focus on flexion and dexterity.

At this point, Alexei became assertive with his wish to return to his own apartment and was allowed to move back with his assurance that soon he would once again be independent in all areas. He partnered with the nurse to work toward independence with medical needs, a difficult task because insulin needles are small and smooth. As his ROM and dexterity improved through dynamic splinting, he was able to test his sugar levels and walk to assisted living to receive insulin as needed. At 14 weeks post op, he was once again independent with his own injections using coban or rubber finger cots for traction on the needle and was once again shopping for a parakeet.

Critical Thinking Questions

1. What would have happened to Alexei if therapy had consisted of just the 45-minute ROM and edema reduction sessions once a week, without the addition of the dynamic splint for home use?
2. How critical was the team approach of the client, the therapist, and the nurse in achieving this client's ultimate goals?
3. What part did ascertaining the client's main goal during the initial interview play in using limited time and resources to achieve that goal?
4. What would have happened if weekly therapy were conducted without that goal as the primary focus?

A client-centered focus to any type of therapy is vital. The case of Alexei illustrates how splinting was used to achieve a good outcome in a difficult case.

The human hand is the brain's most important instrument with which to explore and master the world. It is the only body part that can substitute for other senses. We read with our hands if we suffer a loss of vision; we communicate with our hands in the absence of speech or hearing. Our hands give us expression and console us. We first explore our hands and explore with our hands as infants. The wonder of the human hand is the precision with which it functions and the extremes of abuse it tolerates. We can and do take our hands for granted as they complete a multitude of functional tasks such as dressing, cooking, or typing because they seem to function effortlessly—that is, until we experience some level of impairment or dysfunction.

The hand does not function independently of the whole human organism. It is connected to the brain via a complex tangle of nerves and is dependent on precise synaptic connections. The hand does not function independently of the upper extremity (UE); stability and control of the shoulder, elbow, and wrist are needed to position the hand in space. Dysfunction anywhere from the brain to the fingertips may cause impaired function of the hand.

Humans achieve mastery and independence over their environment because of the superiority of the human brain and the dexterity of the hand. Tying a knot, opening a necklace clasp, wielding a hammer, and throwing a ball are abilities unique to the human hand. That we can close a necklace with our vision occluded is testament to the sensibility of the hand. That we can wield a hammer to drive a nail is testament to the integrity of the skin and the strength of the muscles that power the hand. That we can speak volumes with a sweep of our hands or a caressing touch is testament to the aesthetics of the hand. It is a remarkable instrument indeed. As Mary Reilly, one of the profession's most recognized leaders, stated in her 1961 Slagle lecture, "Man through the use of his hand can creatively deploy his thinking, feeling, and purposes to make himself at home in the world and to make the world his home."

OTs deal with the human being as a whole, not as just a hand, a toe, or a shoulder. With the human hand, even the smallest impairment may affect function. Loss of placement of the hand may mean an inability to achieve a hand-to-mouth pattern, which makes independent feeding impossible. Pain and fear can and do accompany injury, and when independence or livelihood is threatened by hand dysfunction, the outcomes are often dramatic, affecting that person and the family members who rely on him or her. The hand is perhaps most valued only when it ceases to function and we must give it attention.

A splint is one of the most important tools therapists use to minimize or correct impairment and to restore or augment function. Little else so readily calls attention to the hand as a splint. An individual may not receive comments on a new ring or a recent manicure, but put a splint on the hand and all will take notice. The decision to provide or fabricate a splint requires an in-depth understanding of the pathological condition to be affected and of the many splinting choices available.

Section 1 of this chapter serves as an introduction to the anatomical and biomechanical principles necessary to the understanding of the basic concepts and models of splinting. This section briefly reviews the anatomy of the hand and its relationship to principles of splinting, introduces the biomechanical principles involved in splint design and fabrication, and introduces a splint fabrication process involving instruction in pattern making, material choices, types of traction, and techniques of fabrication.

ROLE OF THE OCCUPATIONAL THERAPIST

The education an OT receives in the analysis of activity and the assessment of human occupation and function leads naturally to the use of splinting as one therapeutic tool in the intervention regimen. OTs most commonly fabricate splints for the hand and upper extremity (UE), but they also may be called upon to design and fabricate splints for the lower extremity (LE) and even for the back or spine. The basic principles of splinting apply regardless of which body part is being splinted.

Involvement of the OT in all phases of splint fabrication is recommended from the initial assessment of need, through the design phase, the fabrication, and the training and follow-up necessary to ensure proper use and fit of the splint. This involvement requires an understanding of the anatomy and biomechanics of the normal, unimpaired hand and of the pathology of the impaired hand. Many excellent texts describe both hand anatomy and biomechanics in extensive detail and should be included in the library of any OT treating the hand. This chapter briefly reviews the anatomy and biomechanics of the hand most pertinent to splinting. The lists of references and suggested readings at the end of this chapter provide several excellent selections for further study.

One reference of note that should be included in every therapist's library is *Clinical Mechanics of the Hand*,[7] third edition, by Paul W. Brand and Anne Hollister. This text is an excellent source for a straightforward explanation of the mechanics of muscles, joints, and skeletal structures and how they contribute to the remarkable dexterity and strength of the hand. Brand and Hollister also discuss clinical approaches and how they affect the natural biomechanics of the hand.

ANATOMICAL STRUCTURES OF THE HAND

WRIST

The hand and wrist are a complex of 27 bones that contribute to the mobility and adaptability of the upper extremity; the 54 bones that make up both hands and wrists are approximately one fourth the total bones of the entire body. The wrist is a complex consisting of the distal ulna and radius and the eight carpal bones arranged in two rows. The carpal bones form the concave transverse arch and, with the configuration of the distal radius, contribute substantially to the

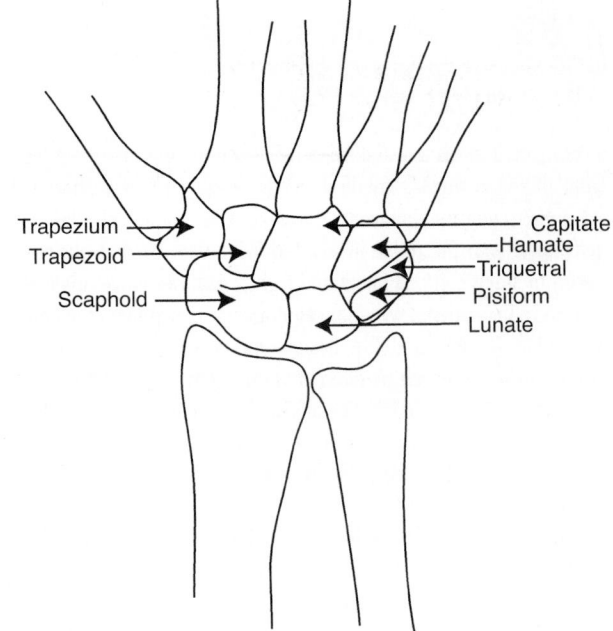

Trapezium
Trapezoid
Scaphold

Capitate
Hamate
Triquetral
Pisiform
Lunate

Figure 29-1 Skeletal structures of the wrist, dorsal view.

conformability of the hand.[22] The distal ulna does not articulate with any carpal bone and its contribution to wrist stability is through the attachments of the ulnar collateral ligament, which places a check on radial deviation (Figure 29-1).

The wrist complex allows a greater arc of motion than any other joint complex except the ankle. This mobility is a result of a unique skeletal configuration and an involved ligamentous system. All motion at the wrist is component motion that occurs in more than one anatomical plane; no pure or isolated motions occur. This concept is key in any treatment directed at the wrist. Extension occurs with a degree of radial deviation and supination. Wrist flexion includes ulnar deviation and pronation. The wrist is contiguous and continuous with the hand. The distal carpal row (the trapezium, trapezoid, capitate, and hamate) articulates firmly with the metacarpals. Motion is produced across these articulations by muscles that cross the carpals and attach to the metacarpals. The proximal carpal row (the scaphoid, lunate, and triquetrum) articulates distally with the distal carpal row and proximally with the radius and the triangular cartilage. Gliding motions occur between the carpal rows during flexion, extension, and deviation, with excessive motion checked by the carpal ligaments.

Placement of the hand for functional tasks is reliant on the stability, mobility, and precision of placement permitted by the wrist complex. Any mechanism of injury or disease that alters this complex system, such as rheumatoid arthritis, translates into some level of dysfunction. Even the simplest splint that crosses the wrist will in some way alter the functional abilities of the hand.

OT PRACTICE NOTE

Splint designs that attempt to augment or substitute for wrist motion are likely to limit component motions or be too complex to fabricate or wear.

Wrist Tenodesis

Tenodesis is the reciprocal motion of the wrist and fingers that occurs during active or passive wrist flexion and extension. Tenodesis is the action of wrist extension producing finger flexion and wrist flexion producing finger extension. It is caused by the lack of change in length of the long finger muscles during wrist flexion or extension (Figure 29-2). The extrinsic finger muscle tendon units have a fixed resting length and, because they cross multiple joints before inserting onto the phalanges, they can affect the position of several joints without any contraction or length change required of the muscles. This concept is crucial to understanding how passive positioning of the wrist affects the resting position of the digits. In the nerve-injured hand, tenodesis is often harnessed by splints to provide function. The client with spinal cord injury with sparing of a wrist extensor (C6 or C7 functional level) gains considerable function from a tenodesis, or wrist-driven flexor hinge hand splint. In a dynamic splint, such as a tenodesis splint, the effect that tenodesis has on tendon length will dictate in part the wrist position that will optimize forces directed at the digits.

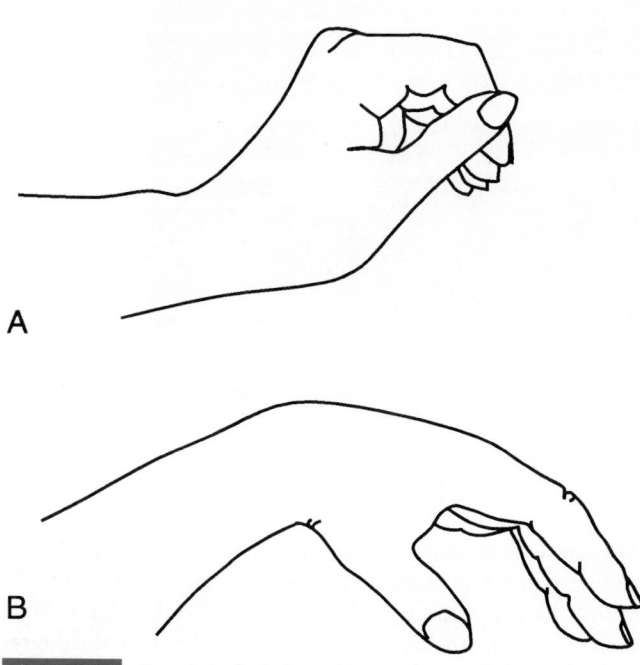

Figure 29-2 Tenodesis. **A,** Active wrist extension results in passive finger flexion. **B,** Active wrist flexion results in passive finger extension.

METACARPAL JOINTS

The metacarpals articulate with the carpal bones proximally and with the phalanges distally. The first metacarpal, the thumb, articulates with the saddle-shaped trapezium and is considered separately. The second metacarpal fits into the central ridge of the trapezoid and the third articulates firmly with the facets of the capitate. These articulations form the immobile central segment of the hand around which the other metacarpals rotate. The fourth and fifth metacarpals articulate with the concave distal surface of the hamate. The shorter length of the ulnar two metacarpals and their greater mobility form the flexible arches of the hand, which allows it to conform and fold around objects of various shapes.

The distal transverse arch of the hand lies obliquely across the metacarpal heads. This obliquity is critical to the hand's ability to adapt its shape to objects. The hand does not form a cylinder as it closes but instead assumes the position of a cone. In making a fist, the ulnar two digits of the hand contact the palm first and the radial two digits follow. This cascade of the fingers is a direct result of the oblique angle formed at the metacarpal heads (sloping angle, not parallel, to the wrist). This concept is most important in splinting in determining the distal trim lines for a wrist support when full metacarpophalangeal (MP) flexion is desired. The splint in Figure 29-3, *A* is improperly trimmed distal to the MP creases. Distal trim lines should be established proximal to the MP creases, as in Figure 29-3, *B*.

METACARPOPHALANGEAL JOINTS

The distal heads of the metacarpals articulate with the proximal phalanges to form the MP joints. Active motion is possible along an axis of flexion and extension and along an axis of abduction and adduction. In addition, a small degree of rotation is present at the MP joints. These axes of motion allow for expansion or spreading of the hand and contribute to the ability of the hand to conform to different shapes and sizes of objects. An attempt to hold a softball without abduction of the fingers shows the importance of this motion. A splint with trim lines along the ulnar border of the hand that extend too far distally limits flexion and abduction of the fourth and fifth digits. As a result, the hand will have a limited ability to grasp large objects and function will be restricted (Figure 29-4, *A*). Distal trim lines that fall proximal to the MP creases will allow for full MP flexion (Figure 29-4, *B*).

THUMB

The base of the first metacarpal articulates with the trapezium to form a highly mobile joint that is often compared with the shape of a saddle. The base of the first metacarpal is concave in the anteroposterior plane and convex in the lateral plane. This surface is met by reciprocal surfaces on

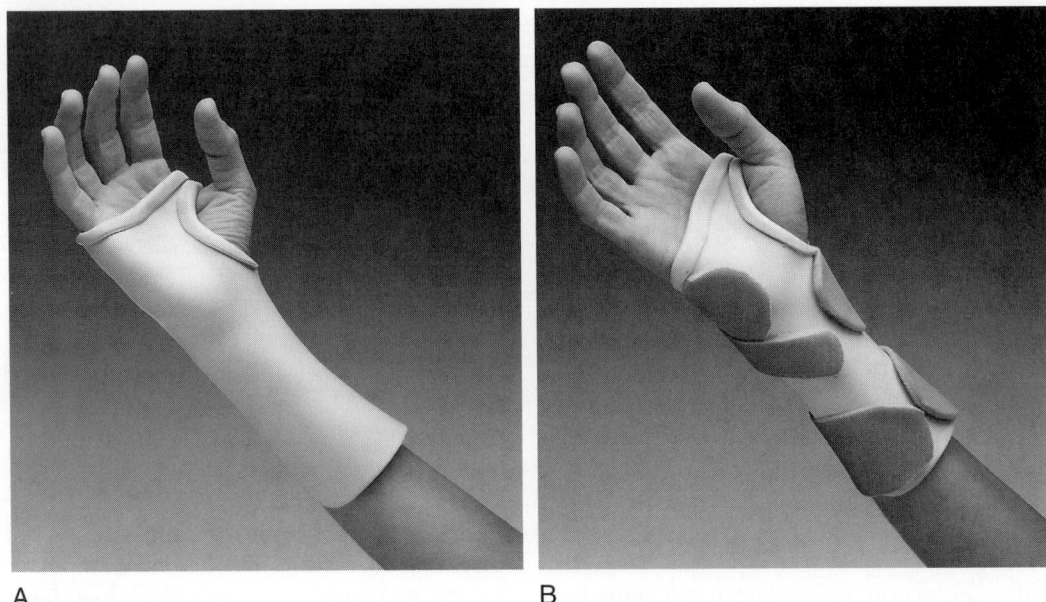

A   B

Figure 29-3   **A,** Trim lines of splint extend distal to metacarpophalangeal creases and limit finger flexion. **B,** Splint's distal trim lines fall proximal to metacarpophalangeal creases (following the oblique angle of the metacarpal heads) and permit full finger flexion.

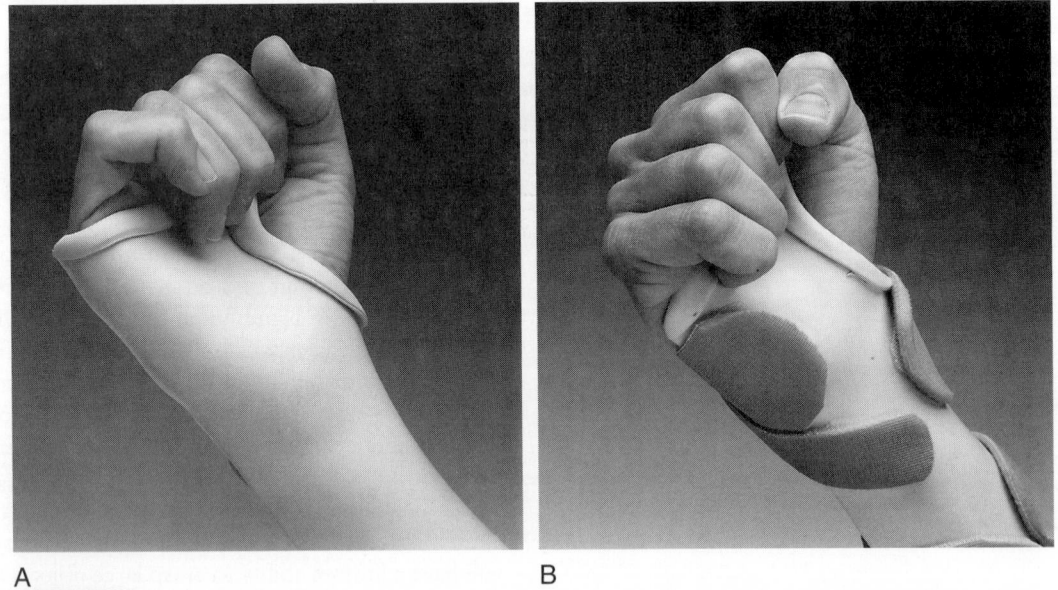

A   B

Figure 29-4   **A,** Fourth and fifth digits are prevented from full flexion. **B,** Full finger flexion is possible with proper trim lines.

the trapezium. This configuration allows for a wide arc of motion, with the thumb able to rotate not only for pad-to-pad opposition but also for full extension and abduction to move away from the palm.[22] Both motions are important to function. That is, a thumb posted in permanent opposition may make grasp possible but release of objects impossible.

This concept is crucial to the understanding of splints that augment the tenodesis action of the hand by posting the thumb in opposition to the index and long fingers. With such splints the therapist must carefully consider the degree of abduction and opposition in which the thumb is posted, to maximize both grasp and release.

INTERPHALANGEAL JOINTS

The proximal interphalangeal (PIP) and distal interphalangeal (DIP) joints are true hinge joints, with motion in only one plane. This limitation of motion ensures greater stability in these joints, which contributes to their ability to resist palmar and lateral stresses and so impart strength and precision to functional tasks.

FOREARM ROTATION

Close consideration of forearm rotation (i.e., supination and pronation) is necessary because of the importance of these motions to function and to the fitting of splints. Forearm rotation occurs at the elbow and at the distal forearm, with axes of rotation through the center of the radial head and capitulum and along a line extending through the base of the ulnar styloid (Figure 29-5). During pronation the ulnar styloid moves laterally as the radial styloid travels medially. During supination the opposite occurs, with the ulnar styloid

moving medially. This movement results in a displacement of the styloids, which in turn alters the architecture of the forearm in supination as compared with pronation.

The way in which this change in dimensions affects splint trim lines is shown in Figure 29-6. Lines drawn at midline along the supinated forearm shift dramatically upon pronation. Splints are generally used for function with the forearm in pronation, but they are easier to fabricate with the forearm in supination. Important to note is that if the forearm is not pronated before the splint material is set, the trim lines will be high on the radial border and low on the ulnar border.

One final active demonstration highlights the importance of forearm position on hand function. Place a coin of any size on a tabletop and, holding the forearm in neutral (thumb straight up), attempt to pick up the coin. It becomes rapidly apparent that the ability to position the hand for function relies in great part on the more proximal joints of the forearm.

LIGAMENTS OF WRIST AND HAND

The ligamentous structures of the hand act as checkreins for the hand and wrist, which limit extremes of motion and provide stability. The complex motions of the wrist depend in large part on the ligaments that restrain them, rather than on

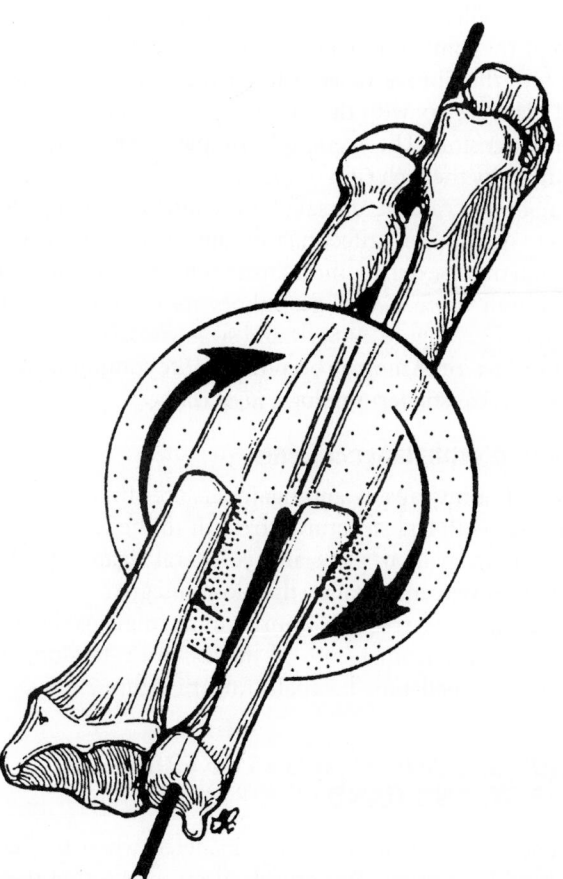

Figure 29-5   The axis of motion for supination and pronation extends the length of the forearm and is centered through the radial head and capitulum and the distal ulnar styloid. (From Colello-Abraham K: *Rehabilitation of the hand,* ed 3, St Louis, 1990, Mosby.)

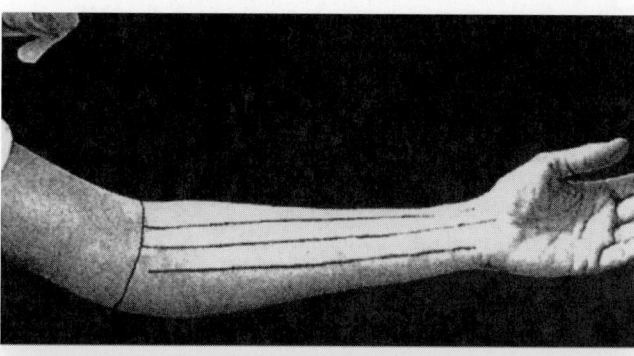
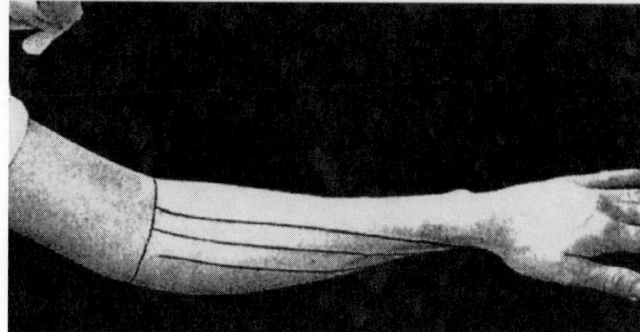

Figure 29-6   The shape of the forearm is altered as it moves from supination to pronation. Forearm-based splints must be repositioned to accommodate this if the forearm is rotated during the fabrication process. (From Wilton JC: *Hand splinting, principles of design and fabrication,* Philadelphia, 1997, WB Saunders.)

the contact surfaces between the carpals and metacarpals. Three groups of ligaments are discussed briefly to highlight their contribution to wrist stability and mobility.

The palmar ligaments include the radioscaphocapitate ligament, which contributes support to the scaphoid; the radiolunate ligament, which supports the lunate; and the radioscapholunate ligament, which connects the scapholunate articulation with the palmar surface of the distal radius. The stability and mobility of the thumb and radial carpus depend on the integrity of these ligaments. Disruption of the ligaments results in instability and pain at the wrist and in significant dysfunction of the thumb. Splinting is frequently the treatment of choice to supply stability for pain reduction.

The radial and ulnar collateral ligaments provide dorsal stability. These capsular ligaments, along with the radiocarpal and dorsal carpal ligaments, provide carpal stability and permit ROM. Disruption of any of these ligaments may result in pain, loss of strength, and functional impairment.

The triangular fibrocartilage complex (TFCC) includes the ligaments and the cartilaginous structures that suspend the distal radius from the distal ulna and the proximal carpus. Tears or strains in this complex are evidenced by pain and weakness with resultant loss of function in resistive tasks. The advent of new imaging techniques has made the diagnosis of TFCC tears more common, and splinting is often ordered for support and pain relief.

Metacarpophalangeal Joints

The soft tissue structures that surround the MP joints include the joint capsule, collateral ligaments, and an anterior fibrocartilage or volar plate. The capsule covers the head of the metacarpal and is reinforced by the collateral ligaments. The collateral ligaments are configured to allow side-to-side motion when the MP is in extension and to tighten as the MP is flexed. The volar plate is attached to the base of the proximal phalanx and loosely attached to the base of the neck of the metacarpal through the joint capsule. This configuration allows for sliding of the plate proximally during MP flexion. The plate returns to its lengthened state with the MP in extension and acts as a checkrein to volar displacement of the MP joint when it is extended.

When the MPs are immobilized in extension, a strong tendency exists for secondary shortening of the lax collateral ligaments, in addition to contraction and adherence of the volar plate, which results in limited MP flexion and loss of functional grasp patterns. The commonly accepted resting position splint, which places the wrist in 25 degrees to 35 degrees of extension, the MP joints at 60 degrees to 70 degrees of flexion, and the PIP and DIP at 10 degrees to 35 degrees of flexion, is designed to prevent shortening and maintain the joints in midrange for optimal function. An important consideration is to ensure that the mobile fourth and fifth digits are positioned in the splint to accommodate their additional degree of mobility by allowing somewhat greater flexion at their MP joints (Figure 29-7).

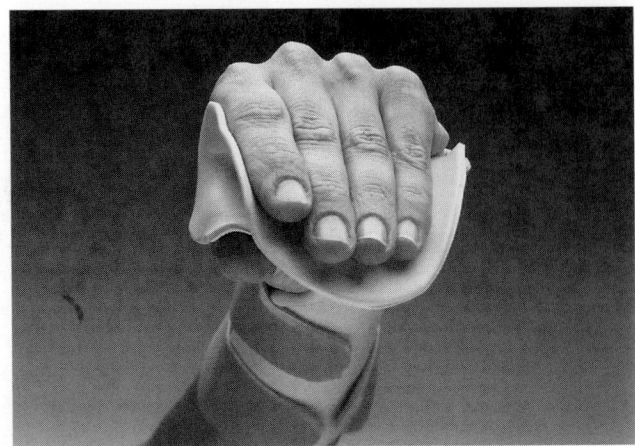

Figure 29-7 Oblique angle of transverse arch at metacarpophalangeal joints must be accommodated to ensure maintenance of more mobile fourth and fifth digits.

Proximal Interphalangeal Joints

The PIP joint capsule and ligaments provide stability and allow mobility in one plane only. Collateral ligaments on each side of the joint run in a dorsal-to-palmar direction, inserting into the fibrocartilage plate of the PIP. These ligaments and plate are lax with the PIP joint in flexion and taut with it in extension. The seemingly simple joint is made more complex by the inclusion of the extensor mechanism passing through the capsule dorsally and contributing slips to the system of ligaments affecting this joint. The potential for disruption of the extensor mechanism is high. Many of the most commonly fabricated finger splints are used to correct PIP boutonniere (Figure 29-8, *A*) and swan-neck (Figure 29-8, *B*) deformities, or as they are becoming more commonly referred to, in less caustic terminology, *joint changes.*

Distal interphalangeal joints

The DIP joint capsule and ligaments are similar to the PIP joint but with less structural strength to the terminal insertions of its palmar plate and collateral ligaments. As the structures become smaller, they lose integrity and strength. One of the most frequent injuries to the digits is the disruption of the terminal end of the extensor tendon, which results in a mallet or "baseball" finger (Figure 29-8, *C*).

MUSCLES AND TENDONS OF FOREARM, WRIST, AND HAND

Balance in the hand must be considered when the hand is assessed for a splint. Two groups of muscles act on the wrist and hand: (1) the extrinsic muscles that arise from the elbow and the proximal half of the midforearm and (2) the intrinsic muscles with origins and insertions entirely in the hand. The extrinsic muscles include both a flexor and extensor

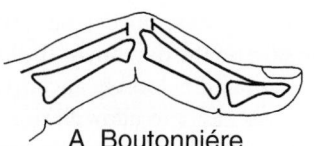

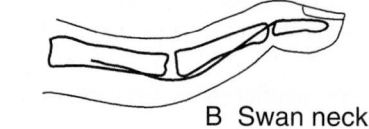

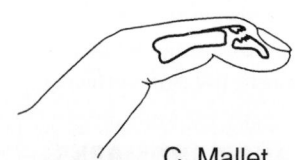

Figure 29-8   **A,** Boutonniere deformity, or joint change characterized by proximal interphalangeal joint flexion and distal interphalangeal joint hyperextension. **B,** Swan-neck deformity, or joint change, with proximal interphalangeal joint hyperextension and distal interphalangeal joint flexion. **C,** Mallet finger with distal interphalangeal joint flexion and loss of active extension.

group acting on the wrist and on the digits. The intrinsics include the lumbricals, the dorsal and palmar interossei, and the thenar and hypothenar groups. Smooth, coordinated motions of the hand in functional activities depend on a well-integrated balance between and within these two muscle groups. Many of the contractures OTs attempt to correct with splinting are caused by neurological dysfunction (central or peripheral), which results in imbalance of muscle tone or innervation.

NERVE SUPPLY

A discussion of the nerve supply to the hand should include mention of the continuity of the brachial plexus from its origins in the spinal cord to its terminal innervations in the hand. Injuries or compressions that occur anywhere along this continuum may result in motor or sensory dysfunction. When splinting the UE, the therapist must give attention to the pathways of the nerves that supply the UE and to the potential sites for nerve entrapment. In the fabrication of splints, care must be taken to avoid applying pressure over sites where the nerves are superficial and prone to compression. These sites include the ulnar nerve at the elbow and in Guyon's canal at the ulnar border of the wrist, the radial nerve at the elbow and in the thenar snuffbox, and the digital nerves along the medial and lateral borders of the digits (Figure 29-9).

Three peripheral nerves supply the motor and sensory function to the hand (Figure 29-10). The radial nerve is the

primary motor supplier to the extensor and supinator muscles. The sensory fibers of the radial nerve supply the dorsum and radial border of the hand. The median nerve provides motor supply to the flexor-pronator group, which includes most of the long flexors and the muscles of the thenar eminence. The sensory distribution of the median

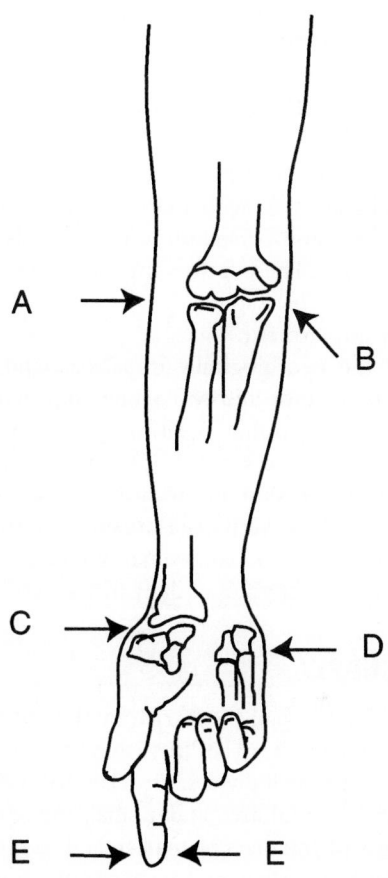

Figure 29-9   Potential sites for nerve compression from improperly fitted splints. **A,** Radial nerve. **B,** Ulnar nerve. **C,** Radial digital nerve in anatomical snuffbox. **D,** Ulnar nerve in Guyon's canal. **E,** Digital nerves.

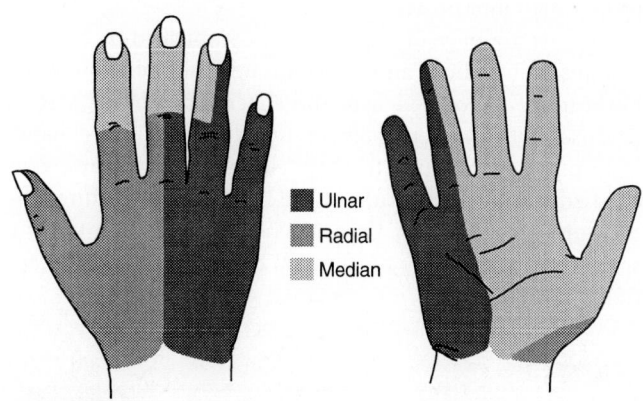

Ulnar
Radial
Median

Figure 29-10   Sensory distribution in hand. Median nerve distribution includes most of the prehensile surface of the palm.

nerve is functionally the most important because it includes the palmar surface of the thumb, index, and long fingers and the radial half of the ring finger. The ulnar nerve supplies most of the intrinsic muscles, the hypothenar muscles, the ulnarmost profundi, and the adductor pollicis brevis. The sensory supply of the ulnar nerve includes the palmar surface of the ulnar half of the ring finger, the little finger, and the ulnar half of the palm.

Nerve dysfunction presents a challenge to the splint maker. Muscle imbalance leads to dysfunctional posturing of the hand and muscle atrophy that reduces the natural padding of the hand. Abrasions or ulcerations may occur in persons who do not remove their splints because they do not feel pain caused by shearing forces or pressure areas inside the splint. Finally, skin with marked sensory impairment lacks natural oils and perspiration, which leads to dry skin that abrades easily. These factors must be assessed and considered carefully when splints are being fitted on persons with sensory impairment.

Splinting the neurologically impaired hand is directed at prevention of joint and soft-tissue contractures and at restoration of functional positioning. Splinting cannot restore sensibility and care must be taken to prevent damage to sensory-impaired skin and to limit further reduction of sensory feedback by covering sensate surfaces (those surfaces that have sensation) and consequently reducing functional use of the hand in activities of daily living (ADLs).

BLOOD SUPPLY

Blood supply to the hand is carried by the radial and ulnar arteries. The ulnar artery lies just lateral to the flexor carpi ulnaris tendon, where it divides into a large branch that forms the superficial arterial arch and a small branch that forms the lesser part of the deep palmar arch. The ulnar artery is vulnerable to trauma where it passes between the pisiform and the hamate (Guyon's canal). The radial artery divides at the proximal wrist crease into a small, superficial branch and a larger, deep radial branch. The superficial arterial arch further divides into common digital branches and then into proper digital branches.

Venous drainage of the hand is accomplished by two sets of veins: a superficial and a deep group. Therapists are more likely to be concerned with the superficial venous system because it lies superficially in the dorsum of the hand. Disruption of this superficial system may result in extensive fluid edema in the dorsum of the hand, which requires the therapist's intervention. Care must also be taken not to strap splints too tightly over the dorsum of the hand, which traps fluids from draining.

SKIN

The mobility of the hand is directly related to the type and condition of the skin. Anyone who has put on a ring that is slightly too small, only to be unable to remove it, has experienced the redundancy of the skin on the dorsum of the hand. The skin on the dorsum of the hand is loosely anchored to underlying structures and moves easily to allow flexion and extension of the digits. The ring "problem" occurs because of a greater degree of elasticity in the dorsal skin when it is pulled distally, as opposed to when it is pulled proximally. This fact should be considered when the use of finger splints is contemplated.

The palmar skin, by contrast, is thicker and relatively inelastic. It is firmly connected to the underlying palmar aponeurosis for stability and protection during prehension activities. Furthermore, the underlying fascia of the palmar skin is thicker and protects the nerve endings, while it acts to supply adequate moisture and oils to the skin surface.

SUPERFICIAL ANATOMY AND LANDMARKS

When fabricating a splint, therapists must consider where to apply force without causing further trauma. Despite its deftness and power, the hand's lack of protective fascia means that it tolerates external pressures poorly and shearing stresses not at all. The prominent ulnar styloid, the distal radial styloid, and the thumb carpometacarpal joint are common sites for pressure. A truism that will always hold in splinting is that padding adds pressure. The softest padding added to a too-tight splint will only add more pressure. Pressure is relieved by the creation of a relief in the splint or by application of padding and material molded over the pad to make it an integral part of the splint (Figure 29-11). Added padding to relieve pressure after the splint is formed should be avoided.

PREHENSION AND GRASP PATTERNS

The ability of the human hand to assume myriad functional positions and to apply only the precise amount of pressure necessary to hold an object is a result of the mobility and stability supplied by the skeleton, the power of the muscles,

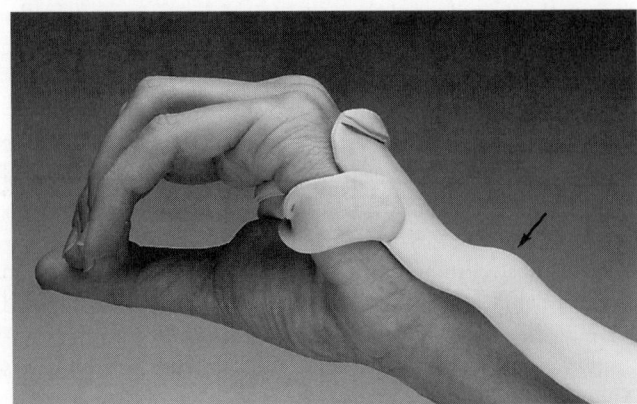

Figure 29-11   Relief "bubbled" over the ulnar styloid accomplished by molding plastic over a pad placed on the styloid.

and the remarkable degree of sensory feedback from the nerves. This sensory feedback is used to assess the size, shape, texture, and weight of an object. The brain then determines which type of prehension to use to complete a functional task using this object. The feedback used in the grasping and lifting of an object is dependent both on the brain's interpreting correctly what is seen and on the hand's responding appropriately. Once an object is in the hand, further adaptation in prehension will occur if the initial visual assessment was faulty.

Splints can maximize functional prehension. In achieving this goal the therapist must be aware of what a splint can and cannot do; a splint can stabilize an unstable part, position a thumb in opposition, and even assist or substitute for lost motion. A splint with added dynamic components can even gradually revise tissue along its lines of pull by applying slow gentle stretch to gain increased functional range of motion. The splint maker must be aware that a splint may also negatively limit mobility at uninvolved joints, reduce sensory feedback, add bulk to the hand, and transfer stresses to unsplinted joints proximal or distal to the part being splinted.

The prehension patterns the hand is able to achieve are as exhaustive as the objects that are available to grasp or pinch. Several authors have contributed to classifications of normal prehension, and the presentation by Flatt[10] is recommended for further study of the subject. It is possible to reduce the many patterns to two basic classifications, prehension and grasp, from which other patterns may be derived. Prehension is defined as a position of the hand that allows finger and thumb contact and facilitates manipulation of objects. Grasp is defined as a position of the hand that facilitates contact of an object against the palm and the palmar surface of the partially flexed digits.

The thumb is involved in all but one type of grip, that of hook grasp. Carpometacarpal and MP rotation is crucial to prehension and cannot be overstressed in its importance in splinting to achieve function. This rotation allows for full contact of the thumb in pad-to-pad prehension, and this motion is used in a normally active person hundreds of times daily in performance of all areas of occupation, including ADLs, instrumental activities of daily living (IADLs), work, leisure, and social participation.

LATERAL PREHENSION

In lateral prehension the pad of the thumb is positioned to contact the radial side of either the middle or distal phalanx of the index finger (Figure 29-12, *A*). Most commonly this

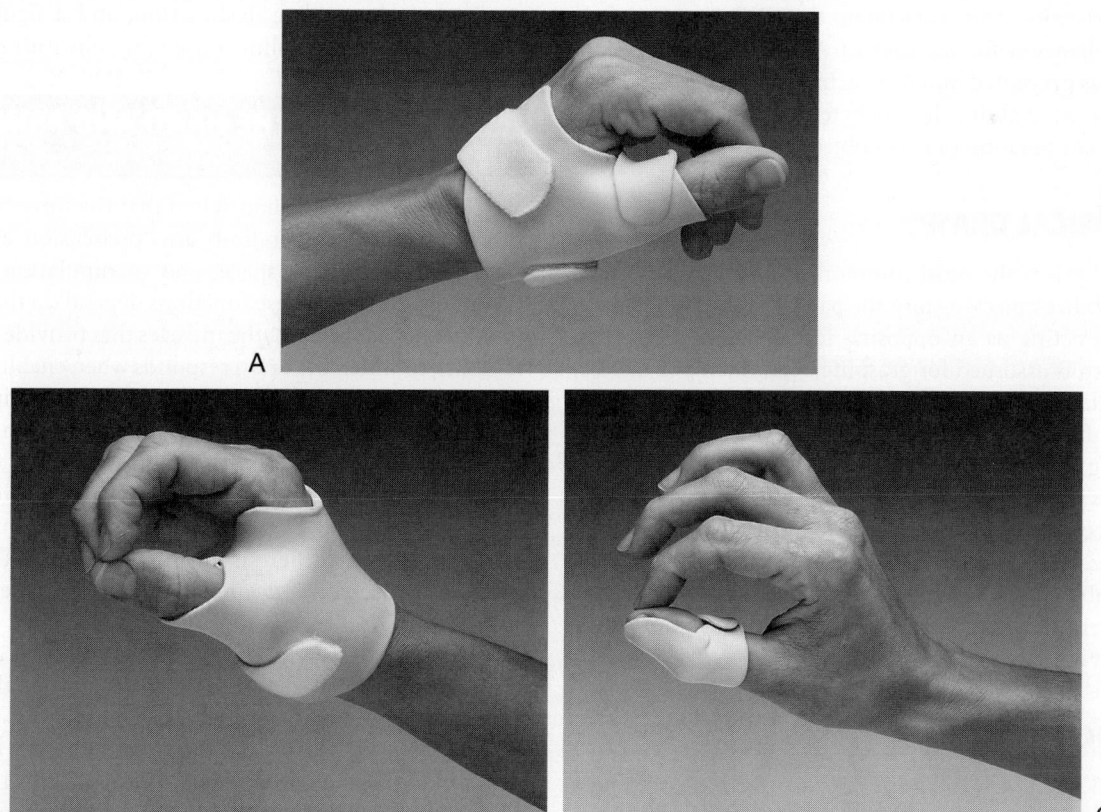

Figure 29-12   **A,** Lateral prehension or key pinch in short opponens splint that positions thumb in lateral opposition to index finger. **B,** Palmar prehension or three-jaw chuck pinch in short opponens that positions thumb in opposition to index and long fingers. **C,** Tip prehension with thumb and index finger in interphalangeal blocker that secures interphalangeal joint in slight flexion to assist tip prehension.

pattern of prehension is used in holding a pen or eating utensil and in holding and turning a key. The short or long opponens splint is used to stabilize the thumb to achieve this prehension pattern.

PALMAR PREHENSION

Palmar prehension is also called *three-jaw chuck pinch*. The thumb is positioned in opposition to the index and long fingers (Figure 29-12, *B*). The important component of motion in this pattern is thumb rotation, which allows for pad-to-pad opposition. This prehension pattern is used in lifting objects from a flat surface, in holding small objects, and in tying a shoe or bow. The short and long opponens splints may also be fabricated to position the thumb in palmar prehension.

TIP PREHENSION

In tip prehension the IP joint of the thumb and the DIP and PIP joints of the finger are flexed to facilitate tip-to-tip prehension (Figure 29-12, *C*). These motions are necessary to pick up a pin or a coin. It is difficult to substitute for tip prehension because it is rarely a static holding posture. Once a pin is in the hand, tip prehension will convert to palmar prehension to provide more skin surface area to retain a small object. A thumb IP hyperextension block is useful to limit IP hyperextension and to facilitate the IP flexion required for tip prehension. In the case of Alexei, maximal edema and stiffness prevented him from achieving the tip or palmar prehension needed for his diabetes management, which included manipulation of small objects.

CYLINDRICAL GRASP

Cylindrical grasp, the most common static grasp pattern, is used to stabilize objects against the palm and the fingers, with the thumb acting as an opposing force (Figure 29-13, *A*). This pattern is assumed for grasping a hammer, pot handle, drinking glass, or the handhold on a walker or crutch. Static splinting offers little to restore this grasp directly, although positioning the wrist in extension offers greater stability to the hand as it assumes this grasp pattern. However, a dynamic outrigger component can be added to a volar splint to gently gain increased MP and PIP flexion to increase cylindrical grasping ability, as was found to be successful for Alexei. A dorsal wrist stabilizer alone offers stability while minimizing palm coverage.

SPHERICAL GRASP

Also called *ball grasp*, this pattern is assumed for holding a round object, such as a ball or apple. It differs from cylindrical grasp primarily in the positioning of the fourth and fifth digits. In cylindrical grasp the two ulnar metacarpals are held in greater flexion. In spherical grasp the two ulnar digits are supported in greater extension to allow a more open hand posture (Figure 29-13, *B*). In splinting, to facilitate or support this pattern of grasp, the wrist-stabilizing splint must be trimmed proximal to the distal palmar crease and contoured to allow for the obliquity at the fourth and fifth metacarpal heads.

HOOK GRASP

Hook grasp is the only prehension pattern that does not include the thumb to supply opposition. The MPs are held in extension, and the DIP and PIP joints are held in flexion (Figure 29-13, *C*). This is the attitude the hand assumes when holding the handle of a shopping bag, a pail, or a briefcase. In the nerve-injured hand, splinting is more commonly directed at correcting this posture by flexing the MPs than at facilitating it.

INTRINSIC PLUS GRASP

Intrinsic plus grasp is characterized by the positioning of all the MPs of the fingers in flexion, the DIP and PIP joints in full extension, and the thumb in opposition to the third and fourth fingers (Figure 29-13, *D*). This pattern is used in grasping and holding large, flat objects such as books or plates. Intrinsic plus grasp is often lost in the presence of median or ulnar nerve dysfunction, and a figure-eight or dynamic MP flexion splint is used for substitution.

MECHANICS OF THE HAND AND PRINCIPLES OF SPLINTING

McCollough and Sarrafian stated that the three basic motor functions of the upper limb are "prehension and release, transfer of objects in space, and manipulation of objects within the grasp."[16] These functions depend on the structural integrity of the skeleton, the muscles that provide power, and feedback to which the brain responds when enabling the limb to meet functional demands. The task of restoring any one of these basic functions through the application of a splint is complex and relies on an understanding of the biomechanics of the hand and the mechanics involved in splinting. It is beyond the scope of this chapter to present this topic in depth. Presented here is an introduction to those tenets of clinical mechanics deemed necessary for the beginning splint maker.

Mechanics deals with the application of force, and biomechanics may be viewed as the body's response to those forces. In the hand the force required for producing motion is supplied by muscles. The force is then transmitted by the tendons to the bones and joints, with control supplied by the skin and pulp of the fingers and palm.[9] How the application of a splint affects the transmission of force to produce motion depends on the relationship between the axis of rotation of joints and anatomical planes and the forces imposed on the hand.

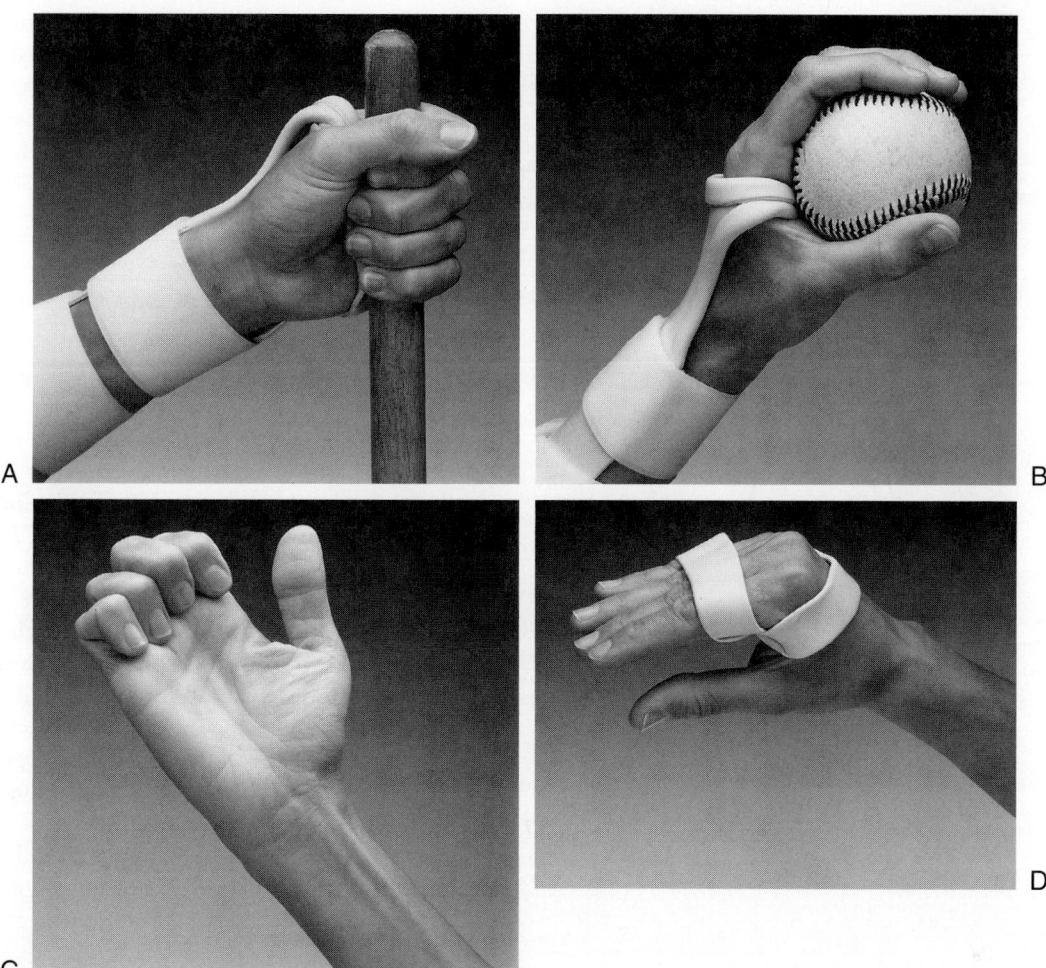

Figure 29-13 **A,** Cylindrical grasp in dorsal splint that stabilizes wrist to increase grip force and minimizes palm covering. **B,** Spherical grasp in dorsal splint. Splint stabilizes wrist to increase grip force and permits metacarpal mobility required for spherical grasp. **C,** Hook grasp does not involve thumb. Grasp pattern is seen in median and ulnar neuropathy; splinting is aimed at correcting rather than augmenting grasp. **D,** Figure-eight splint substitutes for loss of intrinsic function with median and ulnar neuropathy.

AXIS OF MOTION

Hollister and Giurintano[12] define **axis of motion** as a stable line that does not move when the bones of a joint move in relation to each other (Figure 29-14). This stable line is illustrated by Figure 29-14, *B,* which shows a tire perfectly balanced around its axis of motion. When a tire is perfectly balanced, it does not wobble; it has pure motion around a single point.

In a single-axis joint, motion occurs in only one plane. The PIP joint is an example of a single-axis joint in alignment with an anatomical plane. It moves only in the plane of flexion and extension.

Joints that have more than one axis of motion may move in more than one plane at a time. For example, the wrist complex has two axes of motion: flexion-extension and radial-ulnar deviation. A joint with multiple axes has conjoint motions that occur in addition to the primary motions described by the joint. Wrist flexion occurs with a moment of ulnar deviation and with a small degree of pronation. Wrist extension occurs with radial deviation and slight supination. These conjunct motions are what make circumduction of the wrist possible. They are also what make splinting the wrist with hinged joints a challenge.

A splint with a movable hinge or coil has a single axis. When used to splint a single-axis joint such as a PIP joint, a hinge can and should be properly aligned to avoid binding that will limit motion. If a single-axis hinge or coil is used to reproduce motion in a multiaxis joint, some binding or friction will always occur, no matter how well aligned, because the hinge or coil does not allow for, or reproduce, the conjunct motions available in the unsplinted joint.

A

B

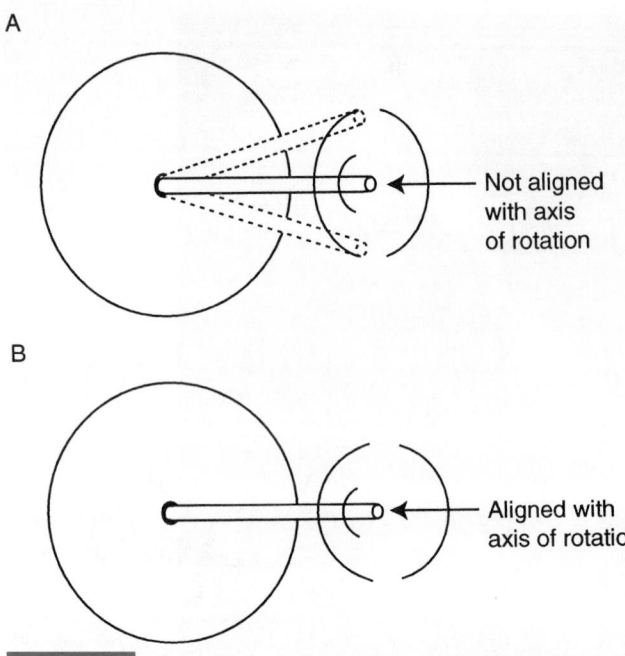

Figure 29-14 **A,** If a tire is not balanced around its axis, it wobbles. If a splint hinge is not aligned with joint axis, wobble is seen as binding of joint. **B,** Proper alignment of a tire or of a hinge with anatomical joint results in smooth, unimpeded motion.

FORCE

It is crucial to understand basic principles of force and apply them correctly in splinting. An understanding of the forces applied by levers and the stresses that occur between opposing surfaces can help explain what happens as forces are applied within the body by muscles and externally by splints.

Definitions

The use of the term **force,** as it relates to splinting, describes the effect materials and dynamic components have on bone and tissue. Force is a measure of stress, friction, or torque. Stress is resistance to any force that strains or deforms tissue. Shear stress occurs when force is applied to tissues at an angle or in opposing directions. Pinching skin between the surface of a splint and the underlying bony structures causes shear stress.

Friction occurs when one surface impedes or prevents gliding of a surface on another. Friction is produced in the stiff or contracted joint when soft-tissue restriction prevents gliding of the bones. Splints may contribute to friction if they are misaligned in relation to a joint axis. For example, a hinged splint that is not properly aligned with the axis of rotation will limit motion by producing friction as the joint attempts to move.

Torque is a measure of the force that results in rotation of a lever around an axis. The torque created when a lever rotates depends on the force used and the length of the lever employed. In the body, muscles are the levers that create torque when they act to move a joint. Externally, splints may act as levers to apply the force necessary to move a bone around its axis. The measure of torque is given by the following formula:

Torque = (amount of) Force × (length of) Lever arm

Internally, the length of the lever arm is measured as the perpendicular distance from the axis of the joint to the tendon. Externally, the length of the lever arm is measured as the estimated distance from the joint axis to the attachment of force. In splinting, the attachment point of the force is usually a soft or molded cuff. If the splint includes an outrigger with a finger cuff, as shown in Figure 29-15, the lever arm is the distance from the axis of the joint to the finger cuff, as indicated in line *M.*

Figure 29-15 demonstrates that the angle of approach of the force to the finger also affects the length of the lever arm and ultimately the torque applied. The angle of approach is the angle that the line of traction makes as it meets the part being splinted. When the angle of approach is at a right angle (90 degrees) to the long axis of the phalanx, the lever arm is *M.* When the cuff is at less than 90 degrees to the long axis of the phalanx, the lever arm is shortened to *M1.* This shorter lever arm will produce less torque and therefore less rotation unless greater force is applied.

Given an equal amount of resistance or load, a 2-foot lever will require half as much force to create motion around an axis as will a 1-foot lever. The important principle for splint makers is that the greater the distance between the

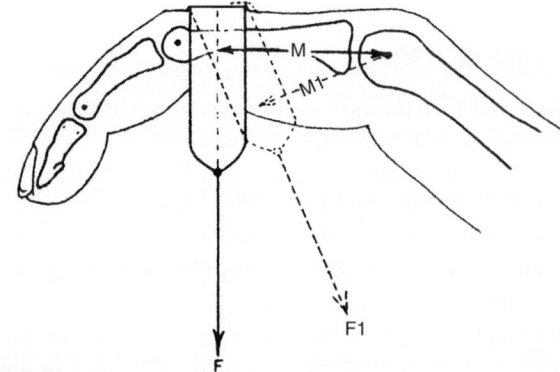

Figure 29-15 Tension *F* on the phalanx has a moment arm of *M* acting on the joint. Tension *F1* has a smaller moment arm, *M1,* (with less resulting torque) when the angle of approach is not 90 degrees. (From Brand PW, Hollister A: *Clinical mechanics of the hand,* ed 2, St Louis, 1993, Mosby.)

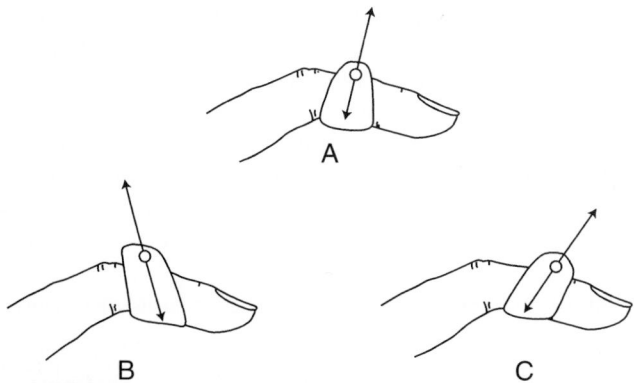

Figure 29-16   **A,** Angle of approach is 90 degrees to middle phalanx, ensuring force pulling proximal interphalangeal joint into extension is not causing distraction or compression. **B,** Angle of approach less than 90 degrees to middle phalanx causes joint compression. **C,** Angle of approach greater than 90 degrees distracts joint.

attachment of the cuff or strap to the joint axis, the less the force required to achieve motion.

Translational Forces

In addition to the angle of approach affecting the length of the lever arm, an approach of less than or greater than 90 degrees results in **translational forces.** The outrigger splint in Figure 29-16, *A*, shows a 90-degrees angle of approach between the nylon line and the phalanx demonstrating the correct angle of pull.

When force is applied at any angle other than 90 degrees, translational forces are created. This alteration of the angle of approach translates some of the rotational force away from producing joint extension and directs the force into joint compression or joint distraction (Figure 29-16, *B* and *C*). The greater the deviation from 90 degrees, the greater the translational force. Depending on the type of splint and the condition of the joint, the joint compression or distraction may lead to mere discomfort or to actual joint damage. Translational force also is undesirable because it undermines the effectiveness of the splint by shortening the lever arm.[7]

The challenge in splinting with an outrigger is to position the splint so that a 90-degree angle of approach exists. In the outrigger in Figure 29-17, as long as the finger does not move, the 90-degree angle will remain. As soon as the finger moves, however, the 90-degree angle changes. Because few outriggers allow for this automatic readjustment in position, the outrigger must be adjusted as the contracture lessens to maintain the 90-degree angle of approach.

Alexei required weekly adjustments of his flexion outrigger to maintain the 90-degree angle of approach as his MP and PIP flexion increased. As his finger flexibility and functional hand motion improved, he was able to lessen the time spent in the splint.

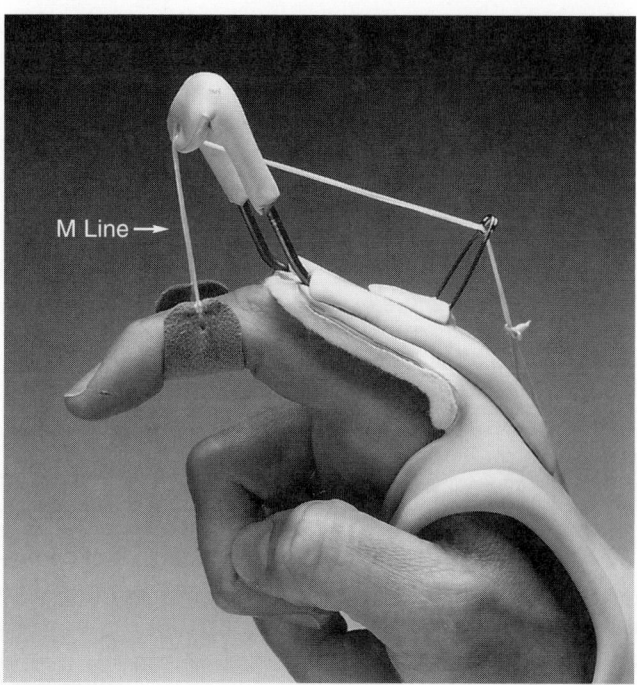

Figure 29-17   As dynamic traction acts on range of motion at the proximal interphalangeal joint, splint must be adjusted to maintain 90-degree angle of approach.

SPLINT CLASSIFICATIONS

Splints may be described in a number of ways. Terminology varies, and it is useful to understand some of the ways splints may be described. For purposes of clarity, splint classifications are described here according to type, purpose, and design.

One reference to be considered when discussing classification is the *Splint Classification System* (SCS)[1] published by The American Society of Hand Therapists (ASHT). The SCS describes splint nomenclature based on the functional requirement of a splint, as well as on the anatomy affected. This nomenclature is quite inclusive of the broad variety of UE splints fabricated by occupational therapists and is suggested for study.

SPLINTS CLASSIFIED BY TYPE

Dynamic splints include one or more resilient components (elastics, rubber bands, or springs) that produce motion. The force applied from the resilient component is constant even when tissues have reached end range. Dynamic splints are designed to increase passive motion, to augment active motion by assisting a joint through its range, or to substitute for lost motion. Dynamic splints generally include a static base on which to attach the movable, resilient components (Figure 29-18). A common use of dynamic splinting is to gain greater finger range of motion by adding dynamic MP extension and/or MP flexion components to a splint.

Figure 29-18 is the type of dynamic splint fabricated for Alexei to gain finger extension. Figure 29-19 shows the type of dynamic splint fabricated for Alexei to gain finger flexion.

A **static splint** has no movable components and immobilizes a joint or part. Static splints are fabricated to rest or protect, to reduce pain, or to prevent muscle shortening or contracture. An example of a static splint is a resting pan splint that maintains the hand in a functional or resting position (Figure 29-20).

A **serial static splint** achieves a slow, progressive increase in ROM by repeated remolding of the splint or cast. The serial static splint has no movable or resilient components, but rather is a static splint whose design and material allow repeated remoldings. Each adjustment repositions the part at the end of the available range to progressively gain passive motion. A cylindrical cast designed to reduce a PIP joint flexion contracture through frequent removal and recasting is a classic example of a serial static splint (Figure 29-21).

Static progressive splints include a static mechanism that adjusts the amount or angle of traction acting on a part. This mechanism may be a turnbuckle, cloth strap, nylon line, or buckle. The static progressive splint is distinguished from the dynamic splint by its lack of a resilient force. It is distinguished from a serial static splint in having a built-in adjustment mechanism so that the part can be repositioned at end range without the need to remold the splint. Generally the static progressive mechanism can be adjusted by the client as prescribed or as tolerated (Figure 29-22).

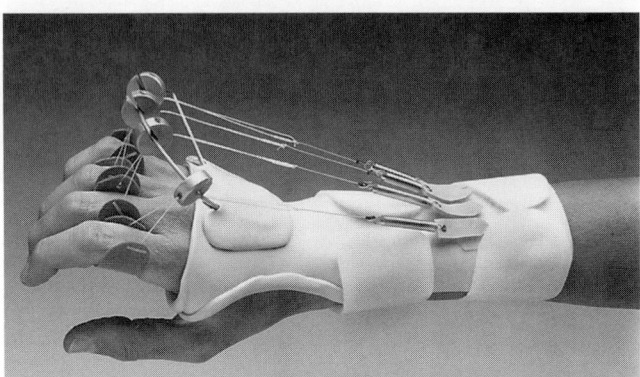

Figure 29-18 Forearm-based four-digit outrigger with dynamic extension assist supplied by springs.

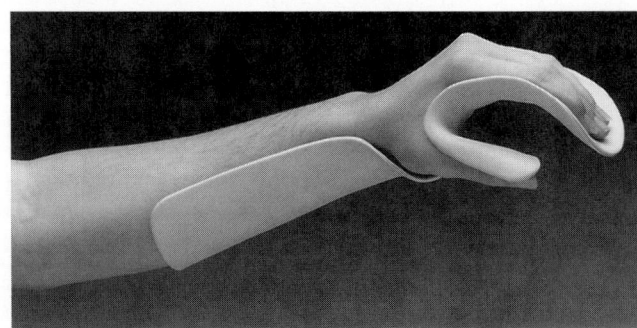

Figure 29-20 Single-surface static resting splint positions hand in 20-degree to 30-degree wrist extension, 45-degree to 60-degree metacarpophalangeal flexion, and 15-degree to 30-degree proximal interphalangeal and distal interphalangeal flexion.

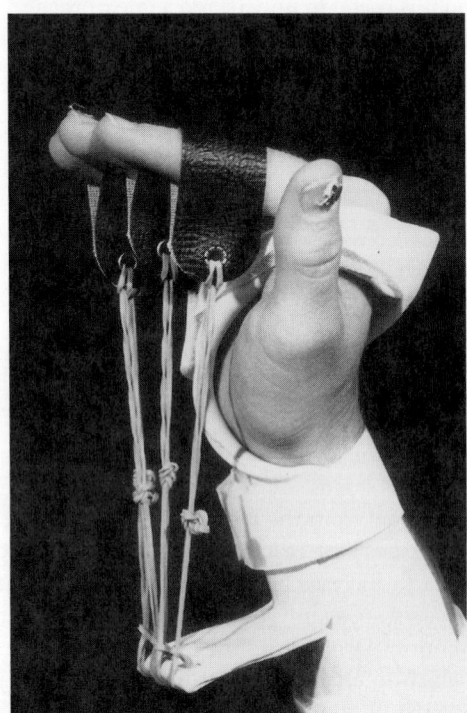

Figure 29-19 Dyamic splint for finger flexion. (From Fess EE, Gettle KS, Philips CA, et al: *Hand and upper extremity splinting: principles and methods*, ed 3, St Louis, 2005, Mosby.)

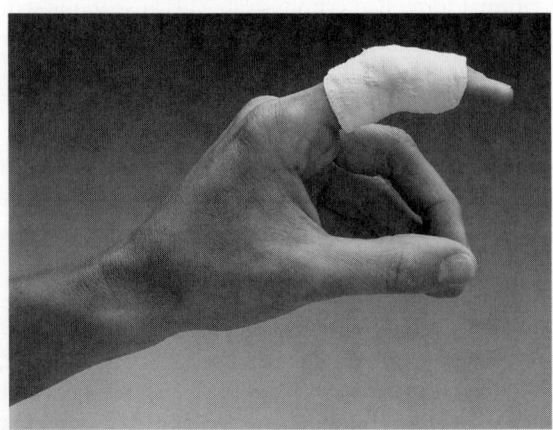

Figure 29-21 A series of cylindrical plaster casts is made to reduce flexion contracture at proximal interphalangeal joint.

SPLINTS CLASSIFIED BY PURPOSE

Although nomenclatures may vary, the categories presented in the splint classification system (SCS) describe splints in functional rather than in design terms.[1] The SCS describes three overriding purposes of splints: restriction, immobilization, and mobilization. The publication also lists many functions of splints, each of which is placed in one of three categories. Splints may fulfill more than one function or purpose, depending upon the method of fabrication and the problems they address.

Restriction Splints

Restriction splints limit joint ROM but do not completely stop joint motion. One example is the splint in Figure 29-23 that blocks PIP joint hyperextension while allowing unlimited PIP joint flexion. Semiflexible splints are available that limit motion at the extremes of range but allow motion in

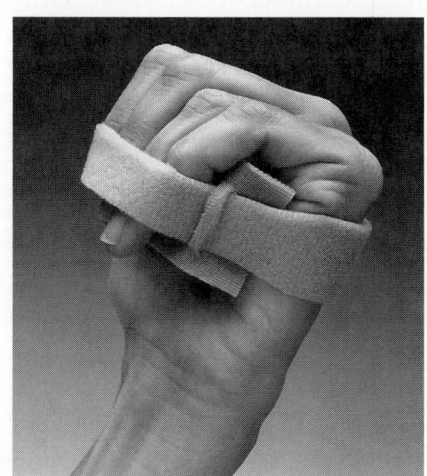

Figure 29-22   Static progressive web strap adjusts with hook closure. Client is taught to adjust strap as tolerance permits.

the middle of range. Although the splint may be restrictive, the goal or function of the splint may vary.

Immobilization Splints

Immobilization splints may be fit for protection to prevent injury, for rest to reduce inflammation or pain, or for positioning to facilitate proper healing after surgery. The classic example is the resting pan splint (see Figure 29-20), which serves two of the three functions. A resting splint fit for a client after a cerebrovascular accident (CVA) positions the wrist and digits to prevent contractures and can protect the desensate hand against damage.

Mobilization Splints

Mobilization splints are designed to increase limited ROM or to restore or augment function. A mobilizing splint may assist a weak muscle or substitute for motion lost because of nerve injury or muscle dysfunction (Figure 29-24). The splint may attempt to balance the pull of unopposed spastic muscles to prevent deformity or joint changes and to assist function. A splint may give resistance for a weak muscle to exercise against to improve its strength or to facilitate tendon gliding after tendon surgery. Frequently, mobilizing splints are used to increase the ROM of contracted joints, such as in the case of Alexei, who experienced severe finger stiffness as a result of the edema, which pooled in his hand after his forearm fracture.

SPLINTS CLASSIFIED BY DESIGN

After the purpose of the splint has been determined, the next decision relates to its design. Each of the types of splints described earlier (static, dynamic, serial static, and static progressive) may be fabricated as a single surface design, a circumferential design, or a three-point design. A final category, the loop design, is generally limited to acting on finger IP joints by providing a loop of material that wraps around the joints to restore the final degrees of joint flexion.

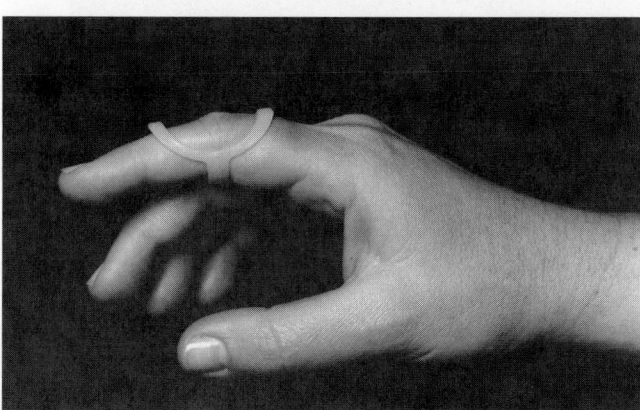

A

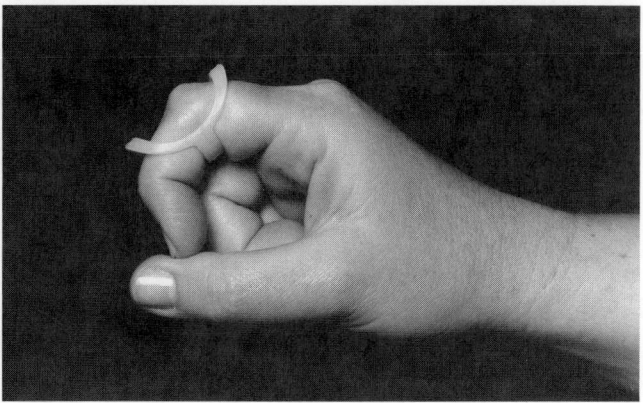

B

Figure 29-23   Oval-8 ring splints. **A,** Ring splint restricts proximal interphalangeal joint hyperextension. **B,** Ring splint allows full flexion.

All splints are designed to provide some degree of force. That force may be distributed as a continuous loop, with equal and opposing forces wrapping around two or more joints (Figure 29-25, *A*). More commonly the force is applied through three points of pressure (Figure 29-25, *B*). Although the loop design is generally used only on finger IP joints, some variation of the three-point pressure design is used in all other splints.

Three-point finger splints that incorporate springs, spring wire, or elastics are often used to correct DIP and PIP joint flexion contractures. A flexion contracture exists when a joint will not move passively out of a closed position into extension. These designs include two points of pressure, one proximal to the joint and one distal, and the third or central opposing force acting directly over or close to the joint, as in Figure 29-25, *B*. In a three-point finger splint the force of the central point is equal to the sum of the two forces of the correcting points. This fact is clinically important because tissue tolerance under this central point may be insufficient and may react with pain and inflammation. This problem is seen frequently at the PIP joint, where limited surface area exists over which to distribute pressure. Pressure must be distributed with contoured surfaces that are as broad as possible, and the spring or elastic force and the wearing time must be adjusted to the client's tolerance. Proper padding incorporated into the splint can also aid in distributing pressure.

The dynamic finger-based three-point splint just described is a unique design that does not adhere to the 90-degree rule. That is, when the splint is applied to a joint with a flexion contracture, the angle of approach of the line of traction is never 90 degrees. The more severe the contracture, the more translational force is present; therefore, it is less effective than a properly contoured outrigger splint that adheres to the 90-degree rule. This design should be fitted only in the presence of IP joint flexion contractures of 35 degrees or less. For finger contractures in excess of 35 degrees a hand- or forearm-based outrigger splint is recommended because it can be positioned to apply force at a 90-degree angle of attack. Alternatively, a conforming, serial static splint can be used, as described in the section on traction.

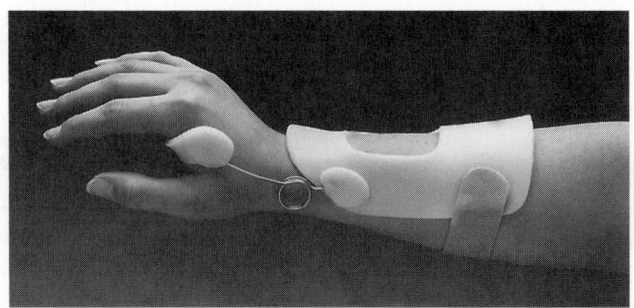

Figure 29-24   Spring coil splint substitutes for absent wrist extension in radial nerve injury.

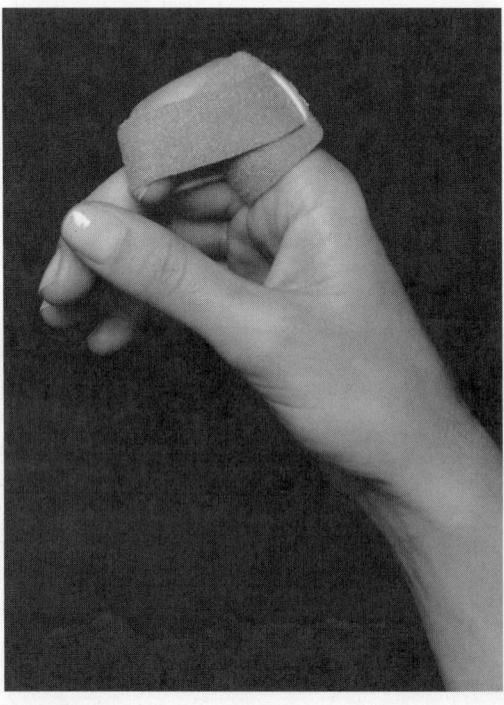

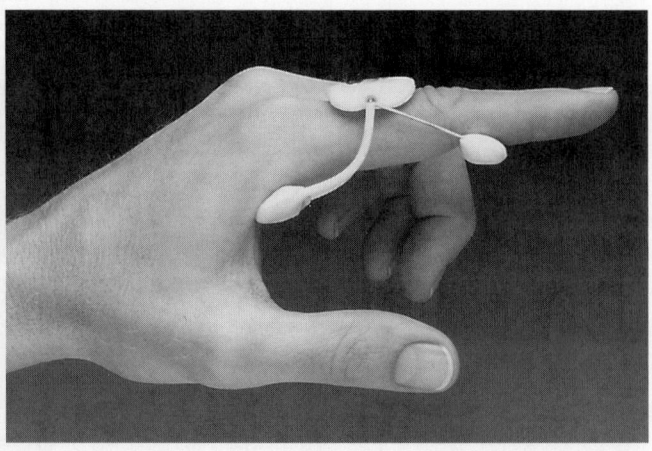

A   B

Figure 29-25   **A,** Final flexion strap designed to restore full interphalangeal joint flexion provides equal force on all surfaces of the digit.
B, Three-point pressure splint with spring wire reduces proximal interphalangeal joint flexion contractures of 35 degrees or less.

Single-Surface or Circumferential Design

If a molded splint is to be fabricated, the next decision is whether to use a circumferential or single-surface design. Single-surface splints are fabricated to cover only one surface, either the volar or dorsal surface of a limb or the ulnar or radial half of the hand or forearm. Straps are added to create the three points of pressure necessary to secure the splint (Figure 29-26, *A*).

Circumferential splints wrap around a part, covering all surfaces with equal amounts of pressure (Figure 29-26, *B*). Straps are used solely to close the splint or to create an overlap. Thinner materials can be employed in molding a circumferential splint, because the increased contours in the material add to the splint's rigidity. An example of added strength from contours is corrugated paper. Circumferential splints then can be made lighter and out of highly perforated materials for air circulation without a sacrifice of control.

Indications for single-surface splinting

Single-surface splinting is effective for supporting joints surrounded by weak or flaccid muscles, such as after a CVA or peripheral nerve injury. Because little or no active motion is available, the extra control given by circumferential splinting is not needed, and donning and doffing the splint will be easier. A single-surface splint is also effective as the base for attaching outriggers in dynamic splinting and for postoperative splints in which the fabrication of a circumferential splint may damage repaired structures.

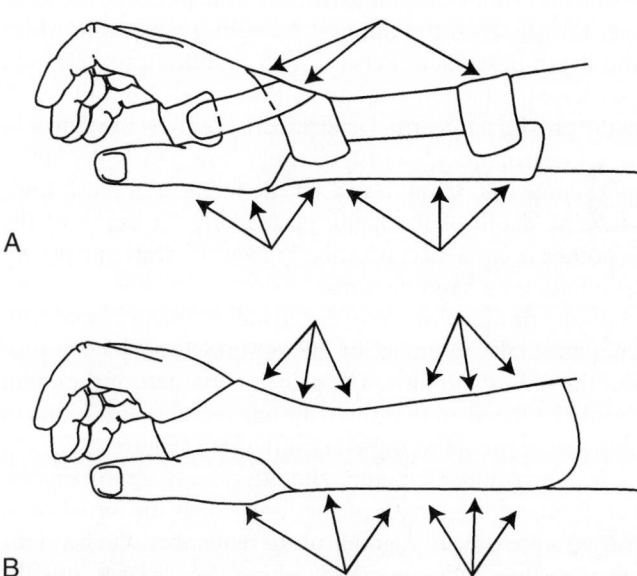

A

B

Figure 29-26 **A,** Single-surface splint requires properly placed straps to create three-point pressure systems to secure splint and ensure distribution of pressure. **B,** Circumferential splints create multiple three-point pressure systems to secure splint for immobilization.

Indications for circumferential splinting

Circumferential splinting is effective for immobilizing painful joints or for protecting soft tissue (Figure 29-25, *B*). Because the circumferential design gives comfortable, complete control, it is particularly helpful when the client will be wearing the splint during activity, when shear forces can be a problem. This comfortable, complete control also makes a circumferential design useful for serial static splints used to reduce contractures. The control a circumferential design supplies also makes it a good design for stabilizing proximal joints when outriggers are applied to act on more distal joints.

WHEN TO SPLINT AND WHEN NOT TO SPLINT

A first step in deciding which splint style and design to choose is to determine if the client is a good candidate for wearing a splint. Several issues should be examined in this regard.

COMPLIANCE ISSUES

First, the therapist must consider whether the client is likely to comply with the splinting program. The splint may have a negative effect on the client's ability to be independent in self-care or to function at work. Some clients are sensitive about their appearance and refuse to wear a splint if it offends their aesthetic sense or negatively affects their body image. Compliance with a splinting program may be poor if the client's general level of motivation to get better is low. On the other hand, some clients are so highly motivated that they will overdo the splinting program and cause themselves damage. Finally, the client's cognitive and perceptual ability to follow a splinting program should be considered, especially if no responsible care provider is available to supervise the splint-wearing precautions.

ABILITY TO DON AND DOFF A SPLINT

Even if compliance is not an issue, the client may have problems donning and doffing (putting on and removing) the splint. For example, the client may have no one at home to assist in donning and doffing a difficult splint. The hospitalized client may not have adequate staff help to follow the wearing schedule or apply the splint correctly.

SKIN TOLERANCE AND HYPERSENSITIVITY

The therapist must assess the skin condition of the client before deciding to fit a splint. Clients who experience diaphoresis and produce excessive perspiration that may lead to skin maceration need to be evaluated more carefully for splint consideration and type, such as ventilated plastics and absorbent padding. Some clients are intolerant of any pressure because of extremely fragile skin or sensory dysfunction. If these issues exist and cannot be ameliorated, safe alternative therapeutic interventions must be substituted for the splint.

WEARING SCHEDULE

If none of the preceding issues prevents the client from being a candidate for splinting, the therapist must decide on the best wearing schedule for the splint. Nighttime may be the optimal time for the client to wear a static splint designed to change ROM. It is also the time when clients need resting splints to prevent them from sleeping in positions that damage the hand. During the daytime the client may wear a dynamic splint or a splint designed to assist function. It is often best to minimize splinting during the day if possible so that the client can use his or her hand as normally as possible. For some who must wear positioning hand splints at night, it may be advisable to alternate wearing splints on one hand at a time so that the individual is not left without the sensory input and function of a splint-free hand. Such a splint-wearing schedule, although not ideal for meeting therapeutic goals, may at least offer a compromise for better compliance.

SPLINT FABRICATION PROCESS

STEP ONE: CREATING A PATTERN

Once the decision has been reached to fabricate a splint, arguably the most important step in the fabrication process is deciding on and creating a pattern. Although it may seem elementary even to the novice splint maker, this step can determine the success of the splint in terms of fit and function. Allowing the time to make a well thought-out and properly fitted pattern gives the splint maker the chance to deal with such issues as what he or she is trying to accomplish with the splint, why the splint is being made, and how and where that splint is going to fit. Ultimately a properly fitted pattern will make the entire fabrication process easier and faster and will increase the chance of success.

 OT PRACTICE NOTE

The process of making a pattern involves an understanding of the anatomy and biomechanics of the hand and the materials to be used, in addition to a bit of old-fashioned dressmaking. Understanding how positional changes alter length and how depth and width relate to the pattern is paramount to success.

The common technique of making a pattern starts with a tracing or outline of the hand. This is generally taken with the hand lying flat when possible, or by tracing the uninvolved hand if necessary. An amount is added to this outline to approximate the width and length needed for the splint. A common error in this technique is not taking into account the position in which the hand (or other body part) will ultimately be held in the splint.

Figure 29-27, *A* and *B*, shows a pattern taken with the hand lying flat, without adding any length to the pattern. In Figure 29-27, *C*, when the pattern is fit on the volar surface of the hand with the hand in functional position (the wrist in 35 degrees of extension, the MP joints at 70 degrees of flexion, and the IP joints in 10 to 20 degrees of flexion), the pattern extends beyond the fingertips and is in fact too long. The same pattern on the dorsum of the hand (Figure 29-27, *D*) with the wrist now in flexion illustrates that the pattern is now too short. Going from the volar surface of the hand to the dorsal surface is akin to driving around the inside of a curve as opposed to the outside of a curve. As any race car driver knows, the inside of a curve is the shorter distance. Altering the position of the hand and altering the surface to which the splint will be fit alters the length of the pattern. The splint maker must accommodate for this by checking the splint pattern on the hand in the position in which the hand will be splinted.

Depth is the second dimension that must be considered when a pattern is made. The ideal trim lines of a single-surface splint fall at midline along the arm, hand, leg, or foot. A splint trimmed at midline provides optimal support and allows for proper strapping to help secure the splint in place (Figure 29-28).

To determine how much to add to the outline to achieve midline trim lines, the maker must observe the width and depth of the arm or hand. The forearm is a cone shape, not a straight cylinder, and it graduates in depth over the forearm muscle. Even the thinnest forearm graduates in width and depth proximally. Persons with significant muscle bulk may have graduation at quite an acute angle from the wrist to the proximal forearm. Determination of how much to add to a forearm trough must consider how much the splint must come out, around, and up the forearm to reach midline. The depth of the hand, particularly the depth of the hypothenar eminence, must be known to create the proper trim lines for a hand platform.

In the fit of any forearm-based splint, the proximal trim lines must take advantage of the soft muscle bellies that protect the radius and ulna. The proximal borders of the splint should be flared so that the trim line remains at midline to help secure the splint in place on the arm (Figure 29-29).

A forearm-based splint should extend approximately two thirds of the length of the forearm, as measured from the wrist proximally. A good rule to remember is to bend the client's elbow fully and mark where the forearm and the biceps muscle meet. The splint should be trimmed ¼ inch below this point to avoid limiting elbow flexion and to prevent the splint from being pushed distally when the elbow is flexed (Figure 29-30).

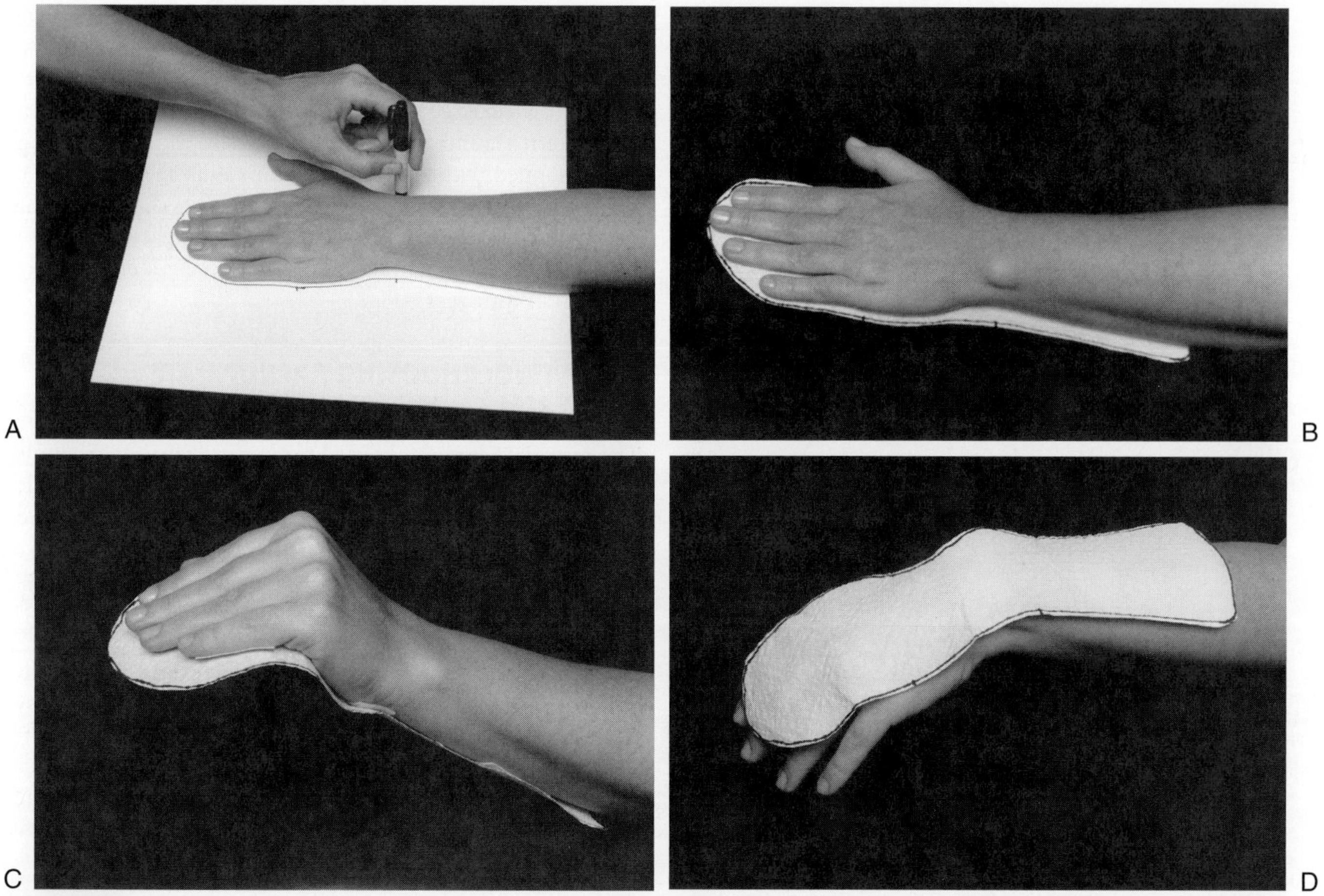

Figure 29-27   **A,** Tracing with pencil perpendicular to arm creates a true size pattern. **B,** Pattern is full length with hand flat. **C,** Pattern is too long when fit on the volar surface with hand in resting position. **D,** Pattern is too short when fit on dorsum of hand with wrist and fingers in flexion.

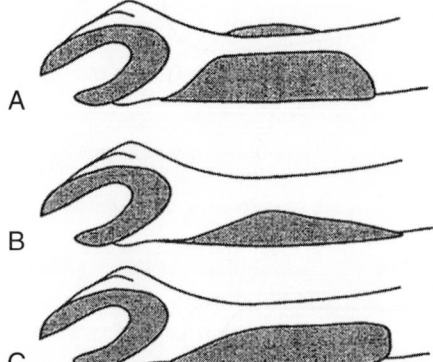

Figure 29-28   Forearm trim lines. **A,** Trim lines are too high, extending above forearm. Straps will bridge arm and be ineffective. **B,** Trim lines too low. Straps cannot substitute for too-low trim lines without applying excessive pressure. **C,** Midline trim lines ensure that straps properly secure splint on arm and hand.

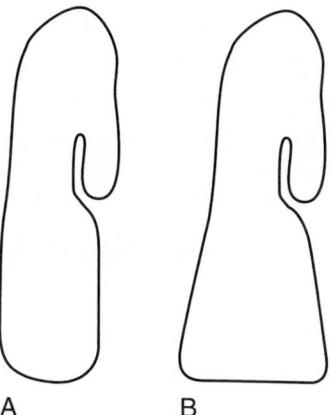

A   B

Figure 29-29   **A,** Narrowing the proximal pattern will cause trim lines to drop below midline. **B,** Flaring the proximal border of the splint maintains trim lines at midline.

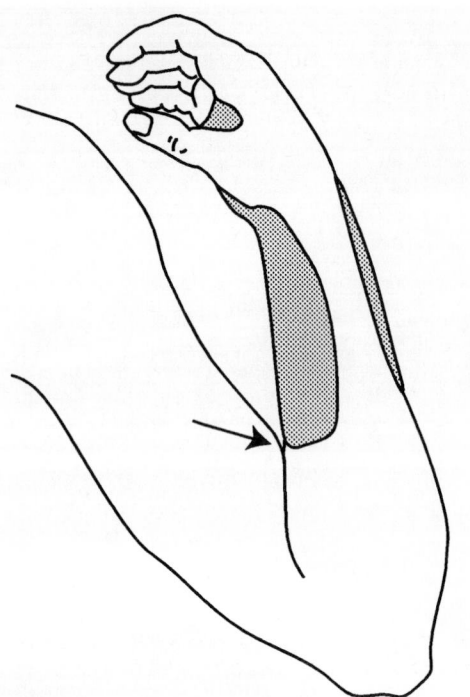

Figure 29-30 Length of forearm-based splint is checked by flexing elbow and noting where biceps meets forearm. Splint is trimmed $1/4$ to $1/2$ inch distal to point of contact.

Most low-temperature thermoplastics used to make splints will stretch to conform around angles and contours. When a pattern is created that will go around an acute angle, such as a 90-degree angle around a flexed elbow or wrist, the pattern should include a dart, where the material can be overlapped without causing undue bulk (Figure 29-31). The pattern may also be angled where necessary to accommodate acute angles. A well-fit and well-thought-out pattern translates to less material wasted, less expense, and shorter fabrication time.

STEP TWO: CHOOSING APPROPRIATE MATERIAL

The materials commonly used for custom fabricated splints are those in a family of plastic polymers that become pliable at a temperature low enough for the material to be molded directly on the skin. The low-temperature thermoplastics (LTTs) currently available have certain characteristics that can be defined according to how a material reacts or handles when warm and how it reacts once molded.

Choosing the optimal material for a given splint application can make the difference between a quick and easy splint-making process or one that requires extensive adjustments and reheating. It behooves every splint maker, novice to advanced, to sample a variety of materials and test for the

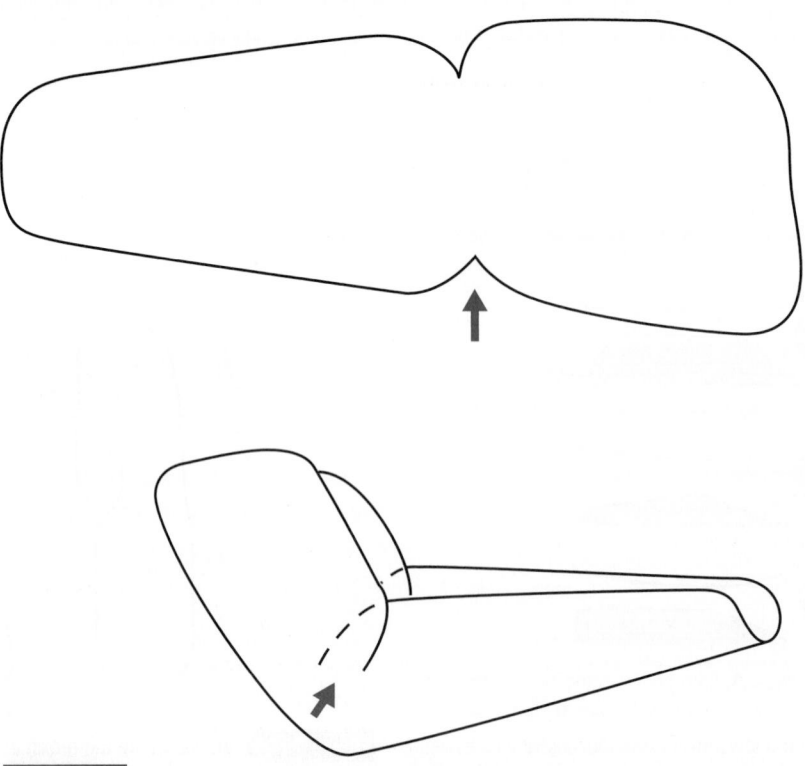

Figure 29-31 Drawing darts in elbow pattern allows material to be overlapped and contoured without excess material.

handling characteristics so that no surprises occur when a material is heated and ready to be cut and fitted to a client.

Characteristics of Splint Materials

Each LTT has some handling characteristics that apply when the materials are warm and pliable and some that apply when they are cold or molded. The following is a list of the most common characteristics and how they contribute to the choice of a material for a specific application.

Resistance to stretch

Resistance to stretch describes the extent to which a material resists pulling or stretching. The greater the resistance, the greater the degree of control the splint maker will have over the material. Materials that resist stretch tend to hold their shape and thickness while warm and can be handled more aggressively without thinning. The more resistive materials are recommended for large splints and for splints made for persons who are unable to cooperate in the fabrication process. In contrast, the less resistance to stretch a material has, the more the material is likely to thin during the fabrication process and the more delicately it must be handled. The advantage of stretch is seen in the greater degree of conformability obtained with less effort on the splint maker's part.

Conformability or drape

Resistance to stretch and conformability or drape describe nearly the same characteristic; that is, if a material stretches easily, it will have better drape and conformability. The great advantage of materials with a high degree of drape or conformability is that with a light, controlled touch or simply the pull of gravity, they readily conform around a part for a precise fit, with minimal effort on the splint maker's part. The disadvantage of materials with a high degree of drape (and generally also low resistance to stretch) is that they tolerate only minimal handling, and care must be taken to prevent overstretching and fingerprints in the material. Materials with a high degree of drape are not recommended for large splints or for uncooperative clients. They are ideal, however, for splinting postoperative clients when minimal pressure is desired and for dynamic splint bases, in which conformability secures the splint against migration (movement distally) when components are attached. Materials with a low degree of drape must be handled continuously until the materials are fully cooled to achieve a contoured fit and often will not conform intimately around small parts such as the fingers.

Memory

Memory is the ability of a material, when reheated, to return to its original, flat shape after it has been stretched and molded. The advantage of high memory in a material is that the splint can be remolded repeatedly without the material thinning and losing strength. Materials with memory require

handling throughout the splint-making process because until they are fully cooled and molded, they tend to return to a flat shape. This and the slightly longer cooling time of materials with high memory can be used to advantage with clients who require more aggressive handling to achieve the desired position. Disadvantages of materials with excellent memory are their tendency to return to a flat sheet state when an area is spot heated for adjustment and their need for longer handling to ensure that they maintain their molded shape until fully cooled.

Rigidity versus flexibility

Rigidity and flexibility in cold splint material are terms describing the amount of resistance a material gives when force is applied to it. A highly rigid material is very resistive to applied force and may, with enough force, break. A highly flexible material bends easily when even small force is applied to it, and it is not apt to break under high stress. Materials are available that fall all along this continuum. More rigid materials may be selected for clients with strong spasticity.

Generally, the thicker a thermoplastic and the more plastic its formula contains, the more rigid the material will be. Thermoplastics come in thicknesses from $1/8$ inch (3.2 mm) to as thin as $1/16$ inch (1.6 mm). The thinner materials and the thermoplastics that contain rubber-like polymers in their formula tend to have greater flexibility in their molded state. Flexibility in a material allows for easier donning and doffing of circumferential splints and may be desirable for clients unable to tolerate the more unforgiving rigid materials. Rigidity is also a factor of the number and depth of the contours included in the design. The same material may yield a semiflexible splint when used to make a single-surface splint with shallow contours and a rigid splint, when used to make a tightly filled circumferential splint.

Bonding

Bonding is the ability of a material to adhere to itself when warmed and pressed together. Many materials are coated to resist accidental bonding and require solvents or surface scraping to remove the coating to bond. Uncoated materials, which require no solvents or scraping, have very strong bonding properties when two warm pieces are pressed together. Self-bonding is helpful when outriggers or overlapping corners are applied to form acute angles but can be a problem if two pieces adhere accidentally.

Self-sealing edges

Self-sealing edges are edges that round and seal themselves when heated material is cut. This characteristic produces smooth edges that require no additional finishing, which adds time to the fabrication process. Materials with little or no memory and high conformability generally produce smooth, sealed edges when cut while warm. Materials with memory, or those that have a high resistance to stretch, resist sealing and require additional finishing.

Soft splint materials

Soft, flexible materials such as cotton duck, neoprene, knit elastics, and plastic-impregnated materials may be used alone or in combination with metal or plastic stays to fabricate semiflexible splints. These materials allow fabrication of splints that permit partial motion around a joint, yet still limit or protect the part. Semiflexible splints are sometimes used during sporting activities and to assist clients with chronic pain in returning to functional activity. Semiflexible splints are also used for geriatric clients and for clients with arthritis who often cannot tolerate rigid splints.

Neoprene splints can be fabricated with use of sealing glue or iron-on tapes. Careful attention must be given to the patterns for soft splints because the support they offer relies primarily on achieving a secure fit without gapping or excess material. Most other soft materials require sewing, and the fully equipped OT department should include a sewing machine. A sewing machine is useful for adapting and adjusting prefabricated soft splints to ensure that each splint that leaves the clinic is indeed custom fit, if not custom fabricated.

Choosing the Best Category of Material for the Splint

Although an experienced splint maker can make many types of splints from the same material, it is better to choose a material with the appropriate handling characteristics for the type of splint being made. The following list can be used as a guideline from which to start choosing materials for different applications. The availability of materials and the experience level of the therapist further determine the most appropriate material.

Forearm-based and hand-based splints

Splints need close conformability around a part when they serve as a base for a dynamic splint, stabilize a part of the body, reduce contractures, remodel scar tissue, or immobilize to facilitate healing of an acute condition. Such splints should be made from a material with a high degree of conformability to achieve a conforming fit. When conformability is not crucial, the splint can be made from a material with high resistance to stretch and low to moderate drape. Splints fabricated for burns and other acute trauma do not require as conforming a fit and can be made from low-drape materials. Materials that resist stretch and tolerate aggressive handling are also recommended for positioning of a spastic body part, because such a material will not stretch and thin during the splint-making process. Experienced OTs who work without a formal pattern choose a material with a higher degree of drape and conformability and allow gravity to assist in the splinting process.

Large upper and lower extremity splints

Long splints fabricated for the elbow, shoulder, knee, or ankle should generally be made of materials that have high resistance to stretch to provide the control necessary for dealing with large pieces of material. Such splints generally do not need to be highly conforming because they are molded over broad expanses of soft tissue. Care must be taken to provide relief for bony prominences or to provide padding to distribute pressure.

Circumferential splints

A splint designed to wrap all the way around the part should be fabricated from materials that have a high degree of memory and that tolerate stretching without forming thin spots. The materials should be highly perforated, thin, or able to be stretched evenly. After being stretched, these materials will cinch in around the body part but still allow sufficient flexibility for easy donning and doffing. These materials work very well for fracture bracing and for circumferential splints that are used for contracture reduction and for stabilizing or immobilizing joints. Another choice for making less restrictive circumferential splints is the use of semiflexible materials, which facilitate easy donning and doffing and allow limited motion within the available arc of motion.

Serial splints

Serial splints that require frequent remolding to accommodate increases in joint range of motion should be made from a material that has considerable memory or is highly resistant to stretch to avoid thinning with repeated remolding. The chosen material should have moderate to high rigidity when molded to resist forces from contracted joints or from spastic muscle tone.

STEP THREE: CHOOSING THE TYPE OF TRACTION

All splints provide some form of traction to move or stabilize a joint or joints. The traction mechanism may be dynamic, using a spring, hinge, or elastic. Traction may also be static, employing straps or turnbuckles or involving remolding of the splint base itself. If the mechanism moves or is resilient, the splint is called a *dynamic splint*, and if it does not move, the splint is called a *static splint*. The following section describes the various options for applying traction and discusses the appropriate uses of each option.

Dynamic Traction

The purpose of dynamic splints is the mobilization of a joint through the use of a resilient force attached to an outrigger or through the use of a spring coil. Each mechanism of force has advantages and disadvantages that make it suited for some uses and ill suited to others. The construction techniques differ substantially when spring coils are used, versus outriggers with elastic components. Thus, the indications for each style of splint vary.

Spring coils are best suited to assist weak muscles or substitute for paralyzed muscles (see Figure 29-24). Clients with weak or paralyzed muscles will likely require the splint for a long time and will wear it while working or performing their ADLs. The low-profile, lightweight construction of a coil splint is recommended because it is less likely to interfere with hand function. Spring coils retain their force and alignment over time, rarely require adjustment, and are ideal for long-term conditions.

Splints with outriggers are the optimal choice for splinting postoperative clients (Figure 29-32). These splints allow frequent adjustments to maintain correct positioning and to accommodate changes in bandage thickness and edema as the healing and rehabilitation progresses. The postoperative client will likely use the splint for only a short time, generally 4 to 6 weeks. Such a client will not be returning to normal functional activities with the affected hand during that time. Thus, the bulkiness and limitation of function with an outrigger splint are relatively unimportant, but it is vital that the splint be able to be self-donned, because it is usual for the client to remove it for periods of time or alternate it with other splints. Alexei's dynamic extension outrigger (see Figure 29-18) is an example of this. He alternated it with his dynamic flexion outrigger and discontinued it after 3 weeks as his extension goal was met.

Splints with outriggers are also used for contracture reduction. For this purpose they are generally most effective when used during the early stages of healing when the contracture feels soft and is easy to reduce.[8] Frequently clients at this stage still have pain and inflammation. They cannot tolerate a rigid, static splint, but they will tolerate a light force provided by an outrigger.

Static Traction

The overall purpose of static traction splints is to apply traction to immobilize or restrict motion. When static splints immobilize, they are protecting, resting, or positioning. When they restrict, they are blocking motion, aligning

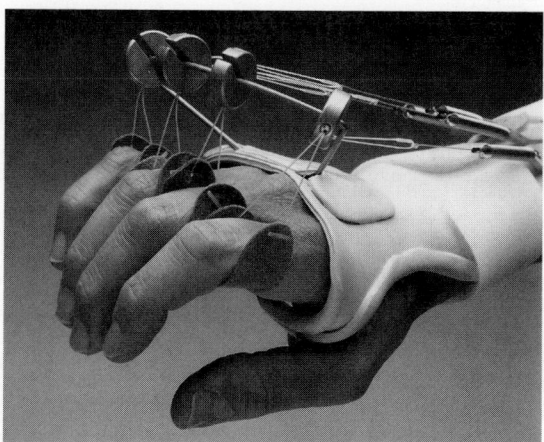

Figure 29-32 Easily adjustable Phoenix outrigger with slotted pulleys allows frequent changes in angle of approach.

joints, or limiting motion. When static splints are used to mobilize, they are used in either a serial static or static progressive fashion to reduce contractures and remodel scars.

Serial Static Traction

A serial static splint is fabricated by repeated adjustments that position a joint at its end range of motion each time to achieve slow, progressive increases in ROM. For example, a cylindrical cast made for gaining PIP extension must be remade after a time (usually 1 to 3 days) to reposition the joint at the end of its range of motion (see Figure 29-21).

Static Progressive Traction

A static progressive splint requires a built-in mechanism for adjusting the traction. Choosing which mechanism to use, be it a turnbuckle, Velcro strap, or buckle (see Figures 29-22 and 29-25, *A*), depends on availability, the therapist's experience, and the client's ability to manage the mechanism. A good rule to follow is to choose the simplest component that will achieve the desired goal.

Serial static splints and static progressive splints each have certain advantages and disadvantages. Serial static splints are useful for difficult clients who have high muscle tone or who are cognitively impaired and would have problems with the adjustment mechanisms. This splint choice also gives the therapist the control necessary for clients who are noncompliant or who would be overly zealous and apply too much force. The disadvantages are that the splint requires more therapist time because it must be remolded many times and that if the client does not remove it for several days, some ROM may be lost in the direction opposite to that in which the splint is applying force.

The advantages of a static progressive splint are that the therapist has to make only one splint and that reliable clients with normal muscle tone may make more rapid progress because they can tailor the adjustment to their own pace and tolerance. The disadvantage of a static progressive splint is that it cannot be used on the client who has abnormal tone or who is unreliable.

Implications of application of force

All splints, whether static or dynamic, apply force and to some degree stress on the structures they contact. The unimpaired hand tolerates a wide range of stresses by adaptation when possible and by avoidance when not. The client with sensory or cognitive impairment may lack the protective responses necessary to reposition the hand away from the stresses applied by splints.

Pressure causes ischemia (localized anemia caused by obstruction of blood supply to tissues), and pressure increases when splints are contoured too sharply, when they do not conform uniformly, or when they do not cover a broad enough area of soft tissue. Splints that migrate or move on the hand because of insufficient strapping or contouring may actually apply pressure in areas that the splint was designed to relieve.

Amount of force to apply

How much force can be applied safely? No absolute rules exist regarding the amount of force that can be applied for immobilization or to a restricted joint to produce motion. The splint maker must apply sufficient force to create motion, but not so much as to cause ischemia. Much depends on the degree of the contracture, how long the restriction has existed, the age of the client, and the location of the restriction. This leaves the therapist with several options when choosing which force and how much force to apply.

For example, external force in dynamic splints is generally applied through the addition of rubber bands, elastic, or springs. No option is ideal, and all require careful selection and frequent adjustment. The amount of force supplied by rubber bands and springs depends on their thickness and their length. The thickness of the band or spring determines its potential force, whereas the length of the band or spring (or the number of coils in the spring) determines the ROM through which the force can be applied. When either bands or springs are used, it is desirable to use the optimal force (i.e., the greatest tolerable force over the longest wearing time) that does not produce ischemia. To accomplish this, the midrange of the bands or springs should be used, rather than their end ranges, which are either too slack or too strong. A gauge is available for measuring the applied force of elastic, which should generally be between 100 and 300 grams.

Techniques are available for avoiding pressure areas and shear forces in a dynamic splint, particularly where traction is applied to mobilize a finger joint. First, the joint(s) proximal to the finger joint being splinted must be stabilized. For instance, to mobilize a PIP joint with an outrigger and cuff, the MP joint must be held securely so that no movement occurs to cause the splint to produce pressure points elsewhere on the hand or digits. Care must be taken in the contouring of the splint around the proximal phalanx to distribute pressure and prevent motion that could cause shearing over the dorsum of the finger. In this case, padding may be necessary to help distribute pressure over the small and thinly padded phalanx (Figure 29-33).

Duration of traction

Basic to answering the question, "How long should traction be applied?" is an understanding of theories of tissue stretching versus tissue growth. Three key concepts aid in the understanding of these two different tissue responses. First, all materials, including human tissue, respond to applied stress. If stress is applied over time and then relaxed, the tissue will no longer return to its original shape but will adapt to the new shape. This stretching phenomenon in skin is a result of its plastic behavior and is known as *creep*. The lengthening that occurs with creep is found to be the result of "a slippage of short collagen fibers on one another within

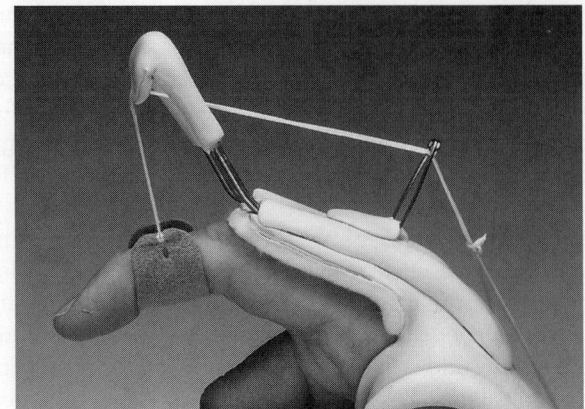

Figure 29-33 Felt padding distributes pressure over bony proximal phalanx.

the tissue. Some fibers may rupture while others just slide on each other."[7]

The second concept is that of the elastic limit of tissue. Think of pulling on a rubber band. As the band is pulled, tension increases until the elastic limit is reached. If pulled beyond its elastic limit, the rubber band will break. In clinical terms the end of the elastic limit is the point of tissue elongation at which pain will be felt and tissue damage may occur. Stretching tissue beyond its elastic limit does not lead to permanent lengthening, but instead to unwanted tearing and probable further tissue contracture.[7] For creep to occur in living tissue, traction must hold the skin with sufficient force to exceed the skin's elastic limit. This may cause tearing of small fibers, which leads to inflammation and additional scarring caused by fibrogen deposits.

The third concept is tissue growth. True growth occurs when "living cells will sense strain and collagen fibers will be actively and progressively absorbed and laid down again with modified bonding patterns with no creep and no inflammation."[7] This is the aim of splinting when the goal is contracture reduction or lengthening of restricted soft tissue.

Two approaches exist to the application of traction to lengthen soft tissue and reduce contractures. One approach is to position the tissue at the end range of its elastic limits and hold it statically for short periods, and then to relax and reposition it frequently. This approach is termed *stress relaxation*.[6] The second approach is to apply force within the elastic limits of the tissue, hold it for a long period, and then reposition it. The difference in these two approaches is one of time and of being able to judge the elastic limits of tissue. The first approach relies on principles of stress relaxation, which theorizes that tissues reach their elastic limit over a shorter period with frequent repositioning and will retain this newly set limit over time.[6] The second and more commonly used approach relies on the application of a low load over a long time to allow tissue growth to occur.

Both approaches have merit, and it is up to the therapist, who develops this skill with experience over time, and the prescribing physician to determine the appropriate approach in each instance.

STEP FOUR: CHOOSING A SPLINT DESIGN FOR A GIVEN PURPOSE

Mobilizing Splints to Remodel Scar Tissue and Reduce Contractures

Scar tissue is one of the major contributors to deformity or joint changes. Any time an insult to tissue occurs, as in after an open injury or after surgery, scar tissue is produced by the body to heal the wound. The scar may be subcutaneous, superficial, or both. When it is subcutaneous, it often results in loss of motion because scar tissue acts like glue, keeping tissue planes from gliding. Scar also contracts; when that contracture occurs over a joint, loss of joint motion results. To restore motion, scar tissue must be remodeled; that is, it must be softened and lengthened. If the contracture is caused by shortened soft tissue that is not scar, that soft tissue must also be lengthened. The process is the same for scar or soft tissue.

The effectiveness of splinting for remodeling scar and reducing contractures can be increased greatly by application of a deep heat modality, such as paraffin or moist heat, before application of the splint. When tissue is unheated it is less elastic, meaning it has a great deal of tension and is difficult to elongate. With the application of heat, tissue becomes temporarily more elastic, meaning that the tension in the tissue is reduced and the tissue is much easier to elongate.

Many approaches exist for splinting for remodeling scar and reducing contractures. Three-point splints can be used for flexion contractures (extension ROM is decreased), loop splints for IP joint extension contractures (flexion ROM is decreased), and outriggers for MCP extension contractures (lacks full flexion ROM at the MCPs). Dynamic outriggers can be used for reducing early, soft tissue contractures, particularly when the client cannot tolerate a static splint. Static progressive splints or static splints can be used in a serial fashion.

Immobilizing and Restrictive Splints for Pain Reduction

Of the many uses of splints, perhaps the most common is to limit or reduce pain by providing rest and support. The most common splint prescriptions are written for splints to reduce the pain caused by the inflammatory processes of tendinitis or after sprain or strain injuries.

Several questions help determine which splint will best serve the client's need. First, if the injury is caused by an acute sprain, the choice may be for an immobilizing splint until pain and edema have subsided. If the pain is chronic in nature and caused by the performance of a particular activity, a semiflexible splint may serve best. A semiflexible

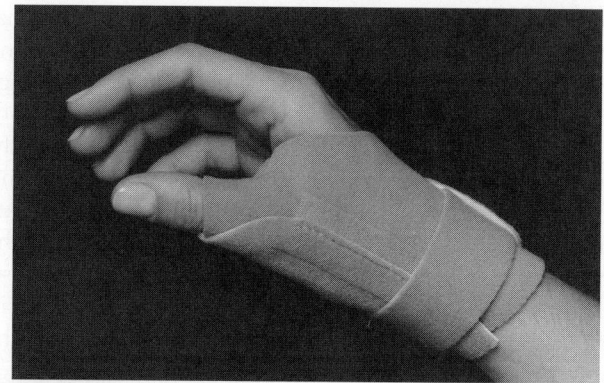

Figure 29-34 Flexible thumb splint provides support yet allows midrange movement.

restrictive splint may sufficiently reduce pain by limiting ROM yet still allow function without increasing stress on unaffected joints or tissue (Figure 29-34).

A second question concerns the need for full-time splinting versus intermittent wear. In the presence of an acute injury with orthopedic involvement or tissue damage, the splint may need to immobilize and to protect the part from further damage. Here, client tolerance and compliance will in part determine material and design choice. The therapist may also need to consider the integrity of tissue and the need to accommodate bandages and bandage changes. If the splint is indicated only for intermittent wear, the design choice may depend more on the client's ability to readily don and doff the splint. The choice of materials may be dictated by the functional needs of the client. For intermittent splints used for vocational activities, lightweight, well-aerated materials may be indicated. For intermittent splints used for positioning, such as a resting splint designed to maintain functional position between exercise sessions, stronger materials may be indicated and perforations may not be necessary.

A third important question in deciding on a splint design is, "What structures need to be immobilized or supported, and which should be left free?" When protective or pain-reducing splints are provided, care must be taken to splint only the involved structures and not impede motion elsewhere. If the purpose of the splint is to rest the tendons at the wrist to reduce inflammation, the splint must not limit CMC or MP joint motion if these structures are not symptomatic. If used during the performance of ADLs, splints that fully immobilize a joint may transfer stress to joints proximal or distal to the immobilized joint. For this reason semiflexible splints that restrict only end ranges of motion may be indicated during activity, whereas an immobilizing splint may be indicated for total rest at night.

Immobilizing Splints for Positioning

One of the splints most frequently fabricated by OTs is the resting pan (also known as the *resting hand* or *functional position splint*), used to maintain the hand in a functional position (see Figure 29-20). The purpose of this positioning splint is to keep the soft tissues of the hand in midrange to maintain optimal mobility and prevent shortening of the soft tissue structures around the joints. Occasionally, positioning splints are prescribed to position joints at end range to prevent contractures in the presence of severe tissue damage. Resting splints fitted on persons with burns are the prime example of this splint because the MP joints are positioned in full available flexion. The important decision in this case is determination of the optimal position for the most functional outcome.

Positioning splints may be fabricated for temporary use after surgery and may require frequent adjustment to accommodate changes in edema and bandages. The materials chosen for these splints should have memory to allow for remolding while keeping their thickness and strength. The choices of a dorsal versus a volar-based splint and a single-surface versus a circumferential splint depend on surgical and wound sites, need for ease of donning and doffing, client's available sensation, and therapist and physician preference and experience.

STEP FIVE: FABRICATION

The fabrication processes for single-surface and circumferential splints differ significantly. They do have a starting point in common: the pattern from which the splint will be made. Starting with a paper pattern is recommended, particularly for the novice splint maker. One very basic rule of splinting is to get the pattern right before beginning to work with plastic. It is far less expensive to discard a few pieces of paper than even a small piece of LTT. Also, if one saves the paper splint pattern in the client's chart, it is easy to use to fabricate another if the splint is lost, or enlarged if a pediatric client grows. Pattern making, design principles, and principles of fit are important knowledge for splint fabrication and can be learned by the novice splint maker by going online to the website associated with this publication or by referring to a book such as *Hand and Upper Extremity Splinting: Principles and Methods.*[9]

Fabrication Techniques for Single-Surface Splinting

Single-surface splints cover the volar surface, the dorsal surface, the ulnar half, or the radial half of the arm and hand. Generally, single-surface splints have gentle contours and cover as broad an area of tissue as is feasible to distribute pressure. The following steps should be used as a guideline in the process of creating a single-surface splint. For the sake of demonstration, the single-surface and the circumferential splints described and pictured are wrist extension (cock-up) splints (Figure 29-35, *A*).

1. Except for the fingers, 1/8-inch–thick material is recommended to obtain sufficient rigidity to hold the joint firmly in position. The broad contours of single-surface

splints require thicker materials to provide sufficient support.

2. Etch the pattern onto the cold thermoplastic material with a scratch awl or wax pencil before placing the material in a hot water bath. The water temperature for most materials to soften properly is approximately 160° F. Temperature and time will vary, depending on the material and its thickness, and this information is typically provided by the material's manufacturer in the accompanying literature. Most materials heat to the pliable stage in 2 to 3 minutes.

3. Carefully remove the material from the hot water bath and lay it flat on the table to cut. To prevent stretching, avoid holding material unsupported while cutting (Figure 29-35, *B*).

4. Starting in the neck of the scissors, cut with long, even strokes to prevent jagged edges.

5. Reheat the material if it has cooled too much to be formed. Place the material on the forearm and hand with the forearm in supination so that gravity can assist the initial molding. Some therapists prefer the elbow propped on a table with the hand in the air if the client is compliant. Check that the trim lines fall at midline. If they do not, mark where excess material needs to be removed. Trim the material before it cools. Note areas that will need to be folded for clearance and to create smooth edges. Fold and secure the edges firmly in place (Figure 29-35, *C*).

6. Reposition the splint on the forearm. Maintaining control on the wrist and forearm sections, carefully pronate the forearm. Maintain the wrist in extension at all times. The tendency for the wrist to drop into flexion when the forearm is pronated is universal. Controlling the wrist will ensure that the desired wrist position is maintained at all times (Figure 29-35, *D*). If necessary, rotate the forearm section to ensure that the trim lines are at midline. Refer to Figure 29-6 to review the importance of the changing shape of the forearm from a supinated to a pronated position.

7. Allow the splint to cool until it holds its shape. It does not have to be held in place until completely cold. Remove the splint. Heat and smooth any rough edges as needed and apply the straps.

8. Strapping is critical to secure the splinted part in the splint and to diminish shear forces and the possibility of pressure areas developing. The splint may require several straps, and wide or crossed straps are suggested to obtain the necessary control. Because the forearm may cone shaped, straps placed straight across the forearm will contact the skin effectively only on their proximal surface (Figure 29-36). To have the forearm straps apply effective and well-distributed pressure, you may consider placing them at an angle.

9. Single-surface splints rely on strapping to hold them in place and to create one or more three-point pressure systems to securely hold the joint or joints being splinted (see Figure 29-25, *B*). To ensure that straps function

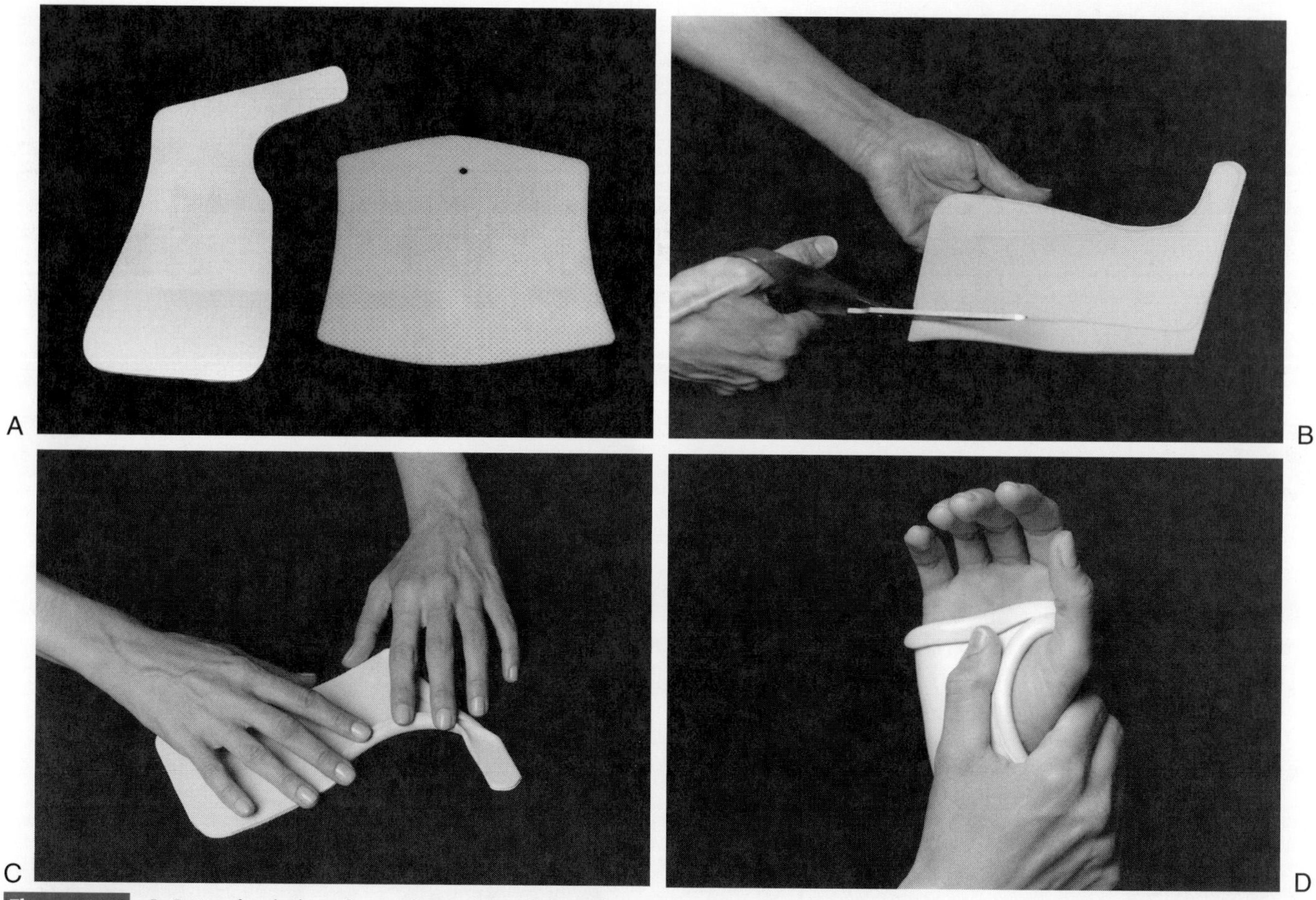

Figure 29-35   **A,** Pattern for single-surface cock-up splint on left requires precision for a proper fit. Pattern on right for circumferential splint does not need precise fit because material stretches and overlaps to achieve proper size. **B,** Support material on table to prevent stretching and cut with long strokes of scissors. **C,** Fold edges of material and gently press flat to create thin, smooth edges that distribute pressure better. **D,** Gently support the wrist at all times to achieve proper fit.

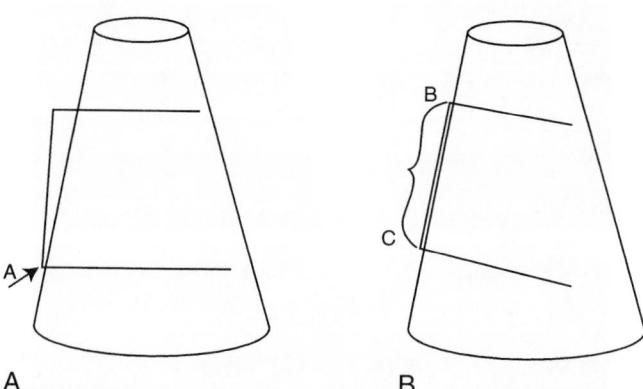

Figure 29-36   Forearm is cone shaped, gradually widening from wrist to elbow. **A,** Strap laced straight across broader proximal forearm contacts skin only at point *A* and does not secure splint. **B,** Strap placed at angle applies even pressure along line *BC* to secure splint.

properly, trim lines must fall midline along the arm and hand. If the trim lines are left too high, making the trough too deep for the part, the straps will bridge the part and sit up on the edge of the splint, where they are ineffective. The most effective way to secure a splint in place on the forearm is to apply pressure through the splint onto the soft tissue of the forearm muscle bellies. If the forearm trim lines angle below the muscle bellies, the splint will no longer be secured on the muscle bellies.

10. Instruct the wearer in the wearing schedule and in the proper care of the splint. To prevent ischemia and shear forces, check the fit of the splint regularly.

Fabrication Techniques for Circumferential Splints

1. Use a thin or highly perforated elastic material or flexible rubber material that has some memory. For hand and forearm-based splints, thin elastic materials ($\frac{1}{16}$-, $\frac{1}{12}$-, or

³/₃₂-inch) provide sufficient strength because of the rigidity provided by the curves of the splint. For splints covering larger areas, a highly perforated ⅛-inch material is recommended. Materials for circumferential splints should be coated to prevent permanent adherence when warm or should be able to be pulled apart once cooled.

2. Etch the pattern onto the material. Because the materials for circumferential splints are generally stretched to contour around the arm, the pattern does not need to be as precise as for a single-surface splint. It is important to know how much the material will be pulled and if it will be overlapped or finished edge to edge so that a piece of sufficient size is cut (Figure 29-37).

3. Wrap the material all the way around the part being splinted. Two techniques can be used to create a closure for a circumferential splint. The first is to pull the material around the part and pinch the remaining material together to create a seam. Gently tug on the seam to conform the material. When the material is cool, open the seam and trim the splint. The second technique is to overlap the two ends to form a flap (Figure 29-38). To prevent the flap from adhering (this may happen when the coating is thinned as the material is stretched), wait until it has cooled slightly before overlapping.

4. Smooth edges as necessary. The circumferential splint creates multiple three-point pressure systems by virtue of its design, and strapping is used only to hold the splint firmly closed.

Fabrication and Fitting of Semiflexible Splints and Prefabricated Splints

Materials used in the fabrication of semiflexible splints include neoprene, cotton duck, woven elastics, and thermoplastic-impregnated materials. Neoprene splints are generally fabricated with use of a special glue that adheres pieces together at the edges. The patterns for neoprene splints must be precise to achieve a conforming fit. Cotton duck and other woven materials require sewing and considerable skill in pattern creation and the addition of darts to ensure a good fit. Very thin thermoplastic materials can be used to create semiflexible splints, and certain patterns can be adapted to allow for partial range of motion within a splint.

Many of the commercially prefabricated splints are made from woven materials, because they present the broadest range of size adjustability and are less likely to require custom fabrication. It is highly recommended that even a prefabricated splint be custom fit by a therapist to ensure proper fit and adherence to an appropriate wearing schedule. A well-supplied splint department should include a sewing machine to custom fit all splints. Remember when fitting prefabricated supports that if a client comes to see a therapist with a prescription for a splint, it is the therapist's responsibility to take the time and develop the skills to be certain that even prefabricated splints fit as if they were custom made.

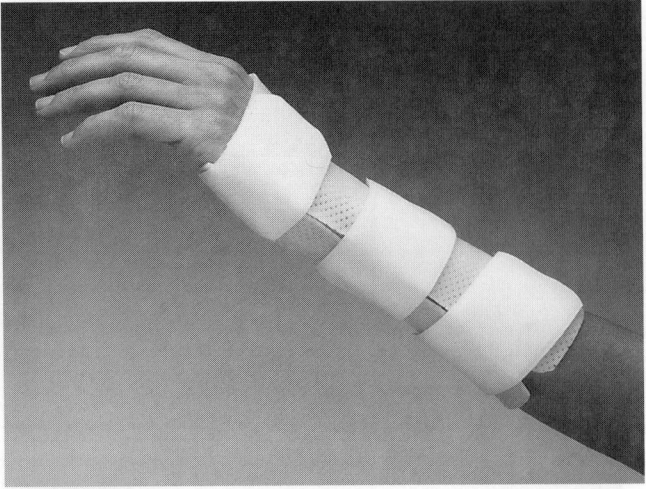

Figure 29-37 Circumferential splint trimmed to close edge to edge.

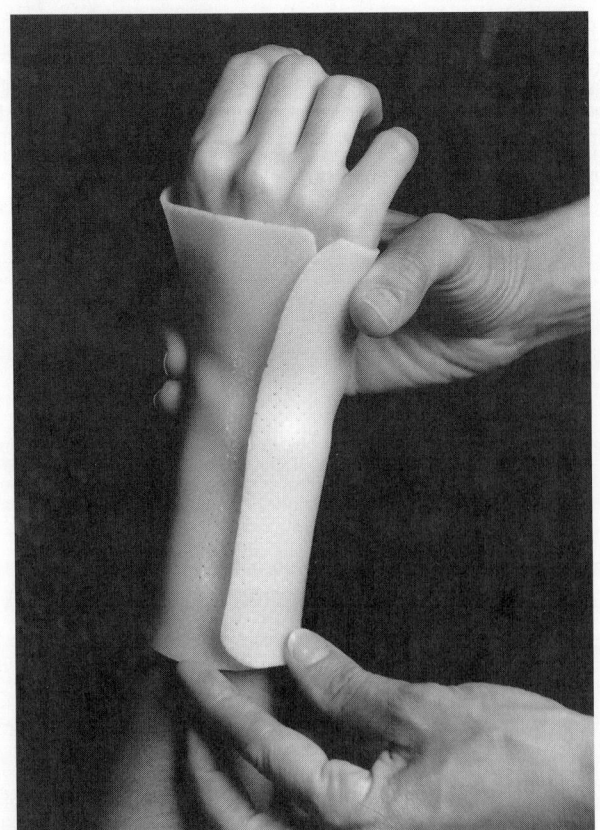

Figure 29-38 Circumferential splint made from flexible material with overlap for easy donning and doffing.

SUMMARY

Section 1 of this chapter introduces the basic concepts of splint design and problem solving that must precede the fabrication of a splint. The anatomy and biomechanics of the hand and types of grasp and prehension are reviewed. Splint classification and the purposes of splinting are described. The section presents a variety of splinting materials and their appropriate uses for different types of splints. Principles of safe and effective splinting and basic fabrication techniques are also described. The OT must bring to the splinting process a knowledge of anatomy and biomechanics, skills in assessing function, and the ability to determine the optimal intervention for each client.

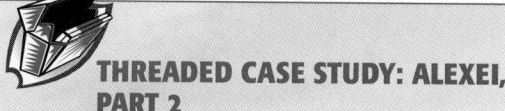

THREADED CASE STUDY: ALEXEI, PART 2

Using the Occupational Therapy Practice Framework, the evaluation of Alexei began with an occupational profile to establish his needs, priorities, and goals, which included the ability to administer his own medications and be independent in his ADLs to return to his independent living apartment. An analysis of his occupational performance identified his inability to grasp small objects such as his insulin syringes and glucose level tester and to perform ADLs such as grasping a normal eating utensil or toothbrush, zipping his pants, or taking money from his wallet. Alexei demonstrated problems within the performance skills category, including poor coordination of motion and difficulty manipulating objects. Under the category client factors, problems with his right dominant hand included lack of ROM and mobility required for successful task performance. The personal (or internal) contexts supporting Alexei identified during the evaluation revealed his flexibility and intelligence, his engaging and assertive communication style, his ability to learn an exercise regimen and use of complex splints, his history of successfully managing health-related problems such as his diabetes, his strong motivation to remain independent in his own apartment, and his psychological need to live in a place that would allow him to have a companion pet. His external contexts, including physical and social contexts, both supported and interfered with Alexei achieving his goals. The positive aspects included his living in a full-service senior housing complex, a supportive nursing staff at his complex willing to help him regain independence, and an administrator at the complex willing to modify the rules slightly to support Alexei's goal of returning to his apartment in the independent living section of the complex. The negative aspects of these contexts included lack of adequate transportation to therapy and the living site's strict procedural rules for residents staying in the least restrictive setting.

What would have happened to Alexei if OT intervention had consisted of just the therapy sessions but no dynamic splinting? ROM gains during therapy would probably not have been maintained.

The intervention plan of dynamic splinting was established based on Alexei's limited ability to get to therapy appointments, coupled with his ability to carry out much of his rehabilitation on his own or with the assistance of the nursing staff at the assisted living complex.

How critical was the team approach, and how important was ascertaining the client's main goal during the initial evaluation? The outcome was ultimately successful because of the collaborative relationship between the very motivated client, the OT, and the nursing staff all focusing on and working toward the goal of retraining Alexei in independent medical management, and the complex administrator agreeing to bend the rules for a month until his goal of complete independence could be achieved. Without a focused goal, much therapy time could have been lost working towards gains less important to the client and may have ultimately robbed him of his independence.

SECTION 2: SUSPENSION ARM DEVICES AND MOBILE ARM SUPPORTS

Lynn Yasuda

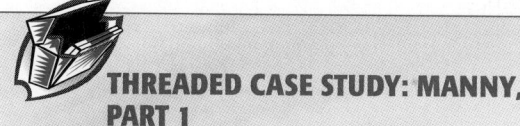

THREADED CASE STUDY: MANNY, PART 1

Manny is 31 years old. He has been married for 5 years and has a 3-year-old daughter. He had been working for 5 years in a law firm with 20 attorneys. He incurred a complete C5 level spinal injury in an auto accident 1 month ago. He is currently in a rehabilitation center in the city where he lives and worked. Upon arrival at the rehabilitation center, his early expectation was that he would recover from his spinal cord injury. However, as the medical staff described to him the evidence of a complete fracture dislocation in the cervical spine, he began to think that he would need the ability to perform selective occupations in an adaptive manner to resume life in the community where he resided before his injury.

In an OT assessment, using the Canadian Occupational Performance Measure, the client was asked what were his most important occupations in which he would like to participate upon his return home. The occupation of most importance was to resume his law practice. This occupation was of primary importance so that he could financially support his family and regain his sense of integration back in the community. This meant he must be able to manage the occupations of written communication, phone use, computer use, and essential activities and basic ADLs (i.e., self-feeding, provide pressure relief, and have mobility) in

Continued

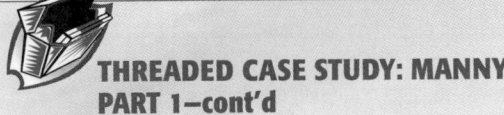

THREADED CASE STUDY: MANNY, PART 1—cont'd

the office. He also felt that he needed to resume the role of father by being able to play with his child, and he wanted to be able to participate in social activities with his wife, such as attending dinners in restaurants. Upon admission he was unable to participate in any of the occupations listed above. In his performance skills, his upper extremity strength was 2 in the proximal muscles, 2 in elbow flexion, 0 elbow extension, and 0 skeletal muscles distal to the forearm. Manny's sensation was also absent partially in the upper arm and completely from the elbow distally. Because of appropriate intervention during his admission to an acute facility, his passive range of motion throughout was within functional ranges.

Critical Thinking Questions

1. With Manny's performance skills, would any equipment enable him to resume his most important occupation of practicing law? What is this equipment?
2. How would you approach the discussion of equipment needs for return to work with this client?
3. What series of interventions will you provide to enable Manny to return to his law firm, where the partners were concerned about his ability to manage the many aspects of the job of an attorney?

Suspension arm devices and mobile arm supports are commonly used and can fulfill several treatment objectives for the person with severe physical disability. These devices can support the shoulder and forearm, encourage motion of weakened proximal musculature, prevent disuse atrophy, prevent loss of ROM, provide pain relief, provide proximal support for distal function, and enable occupational performance.

SUSPENSION ARM DEVICES

Suspension arm devices are suspended from above the head, generally on an overhead suspension rod that is most often attached to a wheelchair. They can also be attached to regular chairs, a child's highchair, a body jacket, and even an overhead track used for walking clients.[5] Without the suspension rod, they are also attached to over-bed frames to allow the client to use the device while in bed. These suspension arm devices were found in OT clinics as early as the 1940s. The ease of management, low cost, and ability to support proximal weakness of the upper limb contributed to their early popularity,[15] and they continue to be used for selected purposes.

PURPOSES

Suspension arm devices may be used to meet some of the following objectives:

- To position the shoulder girdle musculature to allow distal muscles to engage in occupational performance
- To assist and support below fair-grade (F or 3) shoulder girdle musculature
- To allow gravity-eliminated exercise for weak shoulder girdle musculature
- To encourage use of increased ROM through repetitive activities[15]
- To prepare clients to use MAS by encouraging weak proximal musculature to move
- To support a painful shoulder
- To position an edematous hand away from a dependent position
- To prevent loss of shoulder ROM

Suspension arm devices are generally more effective for positioning and exercise than for occupational performance because of the mechanical principles on which they operate. The upper limb swings as a pendulum from straps or springs attached to the suspension rod, which makes it difficult for fine adjustments in movement.[15]

VARIATIONS IN SUSPENSION ARM DEVICES

Several variations of suspension arm devices exist. The overhead rod may be the same, but the attachments to the rod identify the variation. The variations listed here are commercially available and are in current use.

Suspension Sling

The suspension sling (Figure 29-39) has a single strap (A) suspended from the suspension rod (B). A horizontal bar (adjustable balance bar, JAECO[13]) with holes for adjustment of the fulcrum (C) supports the two leather suspension slings (D). These slings provide support for the wrist and elbow separately. The adjustable suspension mount (E) is attached to the wheelchair and holds the suspension rod.

Suspension Arm Support

The suspension arm support (JAECO Orthopedic Inc.[13]) (Figure 29-40) has a forearm support that is the same as that used in the mobile arm support. It is suspended from a single point on the suspension rod. This device can be used as an initial step for the client who can benefit from an MAS and is easily applied to the wheelchair. It can be easily attached and adjusted to over-bed frames to allow clients who are confined to bed to perform tabletop activities in addition to hand-to-face occupations with this device (Figure 29-41). However, it does not have the fine adjustment capabilities of the MAS, which extremely weak clients need. With a special mount (Figure 29-42), the suspension arm support is easily adaptable to the reclining wheelchair.

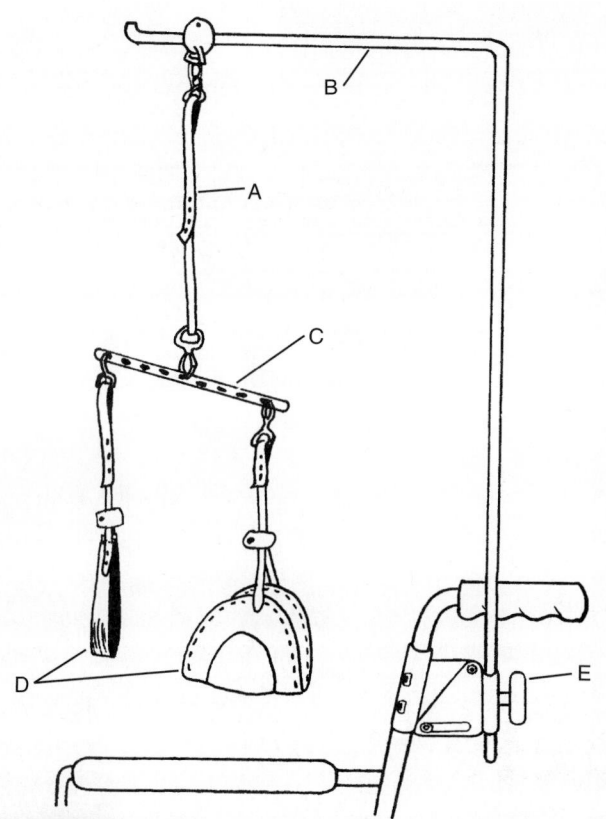

Figure 29-39 Suspension sling. **A,** Strap. **B,** Suspension rod. **C,** Horizontal bar (adjustable balance bar). **D,** Wrist and elbow suspension slings. **E,** Adjustable suspension mount. (Adapted with permission from Occupational Therapy Department, Rancho Los Amigos Hospital, Downey, Calif.)

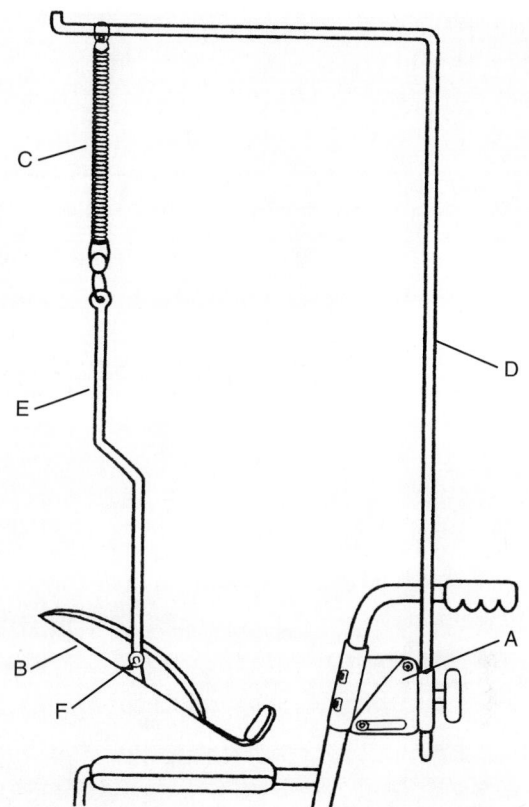

Figure 29-40 Suspension arm support. **A,** Adjustable suspension mount. **B,** Forearm support. **C,** Springs. **D,** Suspension rod. **E,** Suspension bar. **F,** Rocker arm (offset swivel).

This feature makes it useful during the rehabilitation of clients who cannot yet sit fully upright.

ADJUSTMENT OF SUSPENSION ARM DEVICES

Straps

The strap that connects the suspension rod to the limb directly or by the horizontal bar (adjustable balance bar) or forearm support attachment may be adjusted for length. This provides elevation control for the entire limb or for the wrist and elbow separately when separate supports are provided. Adjustments for height relative to the work surface or to the face are similar to those discussed in the later section on MAS.

Height

The suspension rod can be adjusted on the wheelchair suspension mount. The higher the suspension rod, the flatter the arc of pendulum swing when the arm is in motion. Usually the rod is kept as high as is possible while still allowing

the wheelchair to pass through doorways. Lowering the rod shortens the pendulum arc and causes the upper limb to move uphill at each extreme of the arc. Lowering the suspension rod can thus add undesirable resistance to a group of muscles during occupational performance.

Rotation

The shoulder can be placed in horizontal abduction and external rotation as the suspension rod is rotated outward or in horizontal adduction and internal rotation if the suspension rod is rotated inward. This gives mechanical advantage to those muscles held in shortened range and offers resistance to the opposing muscles.[3,15]

Springs

Springs of various tensions may be inserted in the straps supporting the upper limb. In early muscle reeducation, these springs allow the very weak client to produce and visualize some slight bouncing movement while upright by contracting available muscles, a motion not as easily possible with straps alone.

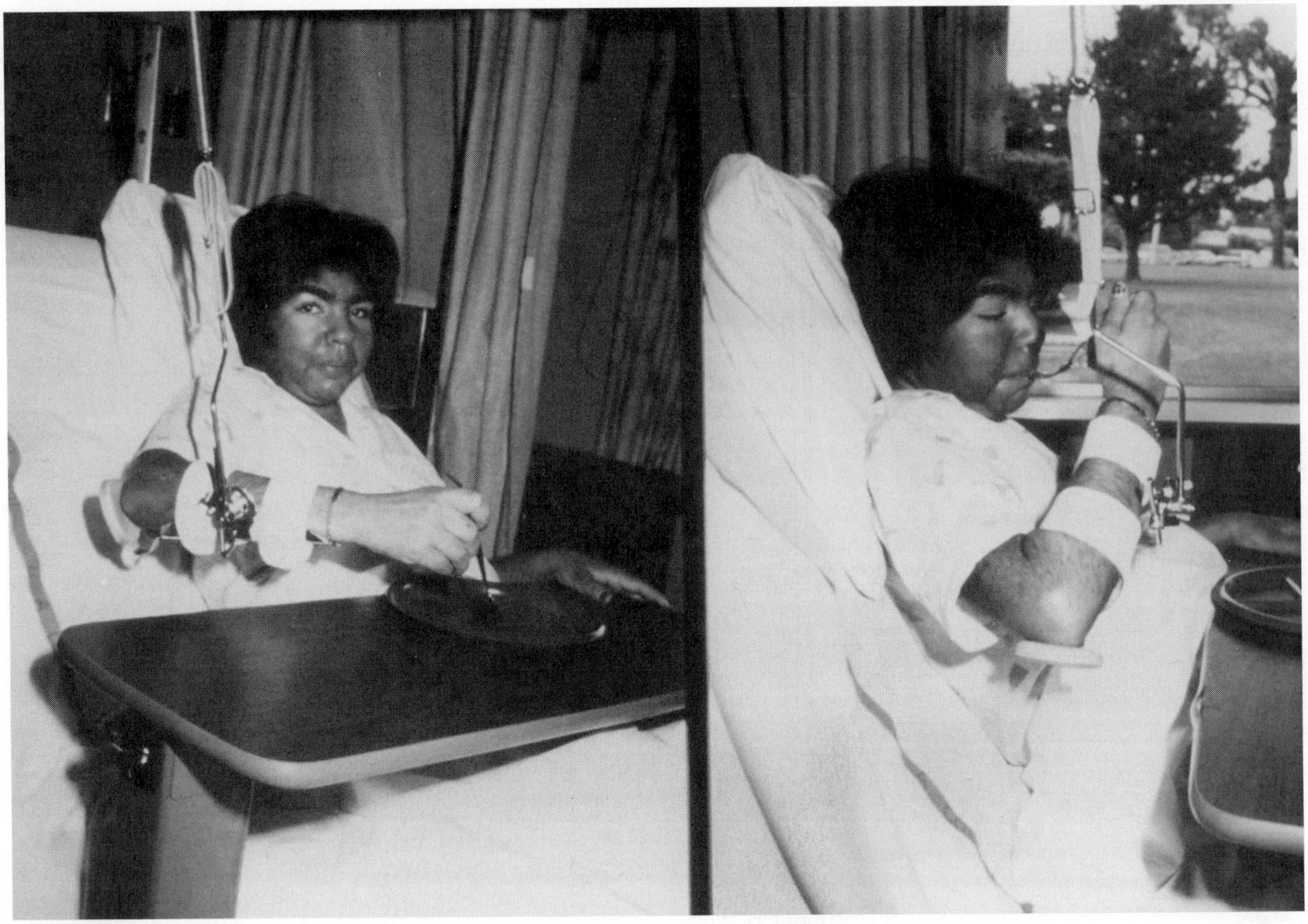

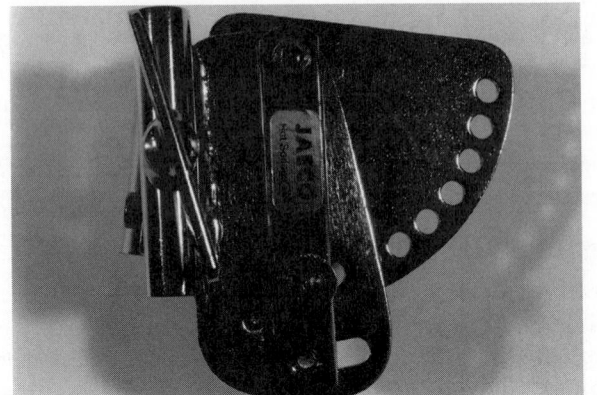

Figure 29-41   Suspension arm support attached to bed. (From ARHP Arthritis Teaching Slide Collection, American College of Rheumatology.)

Horizontal Bar

Moving the strap on the holes on the horizontal bar (also called *adjustable balance bar*, made by JAECO[13]) will position the elbow in greater or lesser degrees of flexion. The bar is often positioned for the comfort of the client, or, if edema is present, the hand is held higher than the elbow.

Forearm Support

The forearm support (manufactured by JAECO[13]) is the same one used in the MAS. However, this forearm support has a vertical metal suspension rod attached to the rocker arm (also called *offset swivel*). The rocker arm can be moved on the forearm support, which permits greater directional assistance for vertical motion, up or down, depending on the client's specific weakness in shoulder rotator or elbow musculature.

Reclining Suspension Mount

For all suspension devices, the suspension rod may be supported by a reclining suspension mount that permits the suspension to be perpendicular to the floor when the client is reclined in the wheelchair (see Figure 29-42).

Figure 29-42   Reclining suspension arm support mount– JAECO. (Courtesy Paul Weinreich, Rancho Los Amigos National Rehabilitation Center.)

TRAINING IN THE USE OF SUSPENSION ARM DEVICES

Suspension arm supports can be used as training for or as an interim device before using the MAS. Training can include exercises for the shoulder and elbow, including scapular protraction and adduction, shoulder flexion and extension, elbow flexion and extension, and shoulder internal and external rotation (especially with the use of the forearm support and rocker arm). Because the forearm support is easily attached to over-bed frames, occupational performance can be practiced using a table surface and any distal orthoses and adapted equipment that are needed[7] before the client is able to be upright in a wheelchair.

OT PRACTICE NOTE

Clients should recognize early in rehabilitation that they can manage an occupation of choice so that feelings of helplessness and hopelessness are not overwhelming.

THREADED CASE STUDY: MANNY, PART 2

When Manny first was admitted to rehabilitation, he was still hopeful that he would recover from his spinal cord injury without any physical loss. It could be difficult, at this time, to introduce the idea of arm supports, which may appear to him as taking away his hope for recovery. Manny was educated by the OT to understand that use of this equipment would facilitate any recovery that may be possible. He was confined to bed for the first few days in rehabilitation, but he was medically cleared to use his upper extremities and to partially sit in bed. The use of the suspension arm support in bed would allow him to participate in some occupation that he wishes to do and is not overly challenging. Manny decided that turning pages would be a good initial occupation because he liked to read and because it was a first step toward what he would need to do in his law practice. A suspension arm support was attached to overhead bars attached to his bed. An over-bed tray with a book rack held his book. A universal cuff with the eraser end of a pencil attached and a wrist support enabled Manny to turn pages with his suspension arm support and with his bed raised for partial sitting. This allowed Manny to start thinking early in his rehabilitation about occupations he could manage with arm supports in addition to working on the performance skill of strengthening upper extremity musculature, which otherwise would be underused while Manny was lying in bed.

MOBILE ARM SUPPORTS

Mobile arm supports are mechanical devices that support the weight of the arm and provide assistance to shoulder and elbow motions through a linkage of ball-bearing joints. They are used for persons with weakness of the shoulder and elbow that affects their ability to position the hand. Mobile arm supports are or have been known by other names. Among these are MASs, ball-bearing feeder, ball-bearing arm support, balanced forearm orthosis (BFO), and arm positioner.

The MAS in current use (Figure 29-43) has not changed significantly in design since 1952.[4] Earlier prototypes were reported as long ago as 1936, when a client at the Georgia Warm Springs Foundation was given a Barker feeder, a device that was bolted to the lap board of a wheelchair and that required shoulder depression to bring the hands toward the head. Several other models were subsequently reported in the literature, until the design of the 1952 segmented arm feeder, which has close similarities to that seen today.[4,21]

MASs have increased upper extremity function for persons with severe arm paralysis caused by conditions such as cervical spinal cord injury, muscular dystrophy, Guillain-Barré syndrome, amyotrophic lateral sclerosis, poliomyelitis, and polymyositis.[11,24] The MAS has also been used for pain relief in the upper arm during occupational performance for clients with arthritis and other painful conditions.

HOW MOBILE ARM SUPPORTS WORK

MASs compensate for proximal weakness in the upper extremities in three ways. They provide arm motion, which allows for active ROM in the shoulder and elbow; they allow weak muscles that cannot perform movement to allow for occupational performance; and they enable hand placement for occupational performance in a variety of positions.

The purposes of mobile arm supports can be for occupational performance (i.e., allowing the weak arm to perform tabletop and hand-to-face occupations, which otherwise are impossible or difficult) and therapeutic exercises (i.e., improving ROM, strength, and endurance). The devices can be temporary or permanent.[19]

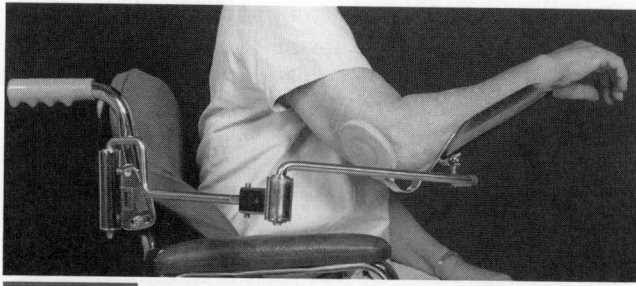

Figure 29-43   Traditional mobile arm support set up on a wheelchair. (Courtesy Paul Weinreich, Rancho Los Amigos National Rehabilitation Center.)

The mechanical principles of mobile arm supports are threefold. The MAS uses gravity to assist weak muscles, supports a weak arm to reduce the load on weak muscles, and reduces friction by using ball-bearing joints.[19]

CRITERIA FOR USE[19]

Occupational Performance Need

The person must have a need to perform specific occupations that cannot otherwise be accomplished because of weak shoulder and elbow musculature.

Adequate Source of Power

The source of power can be the muscles of the neck, trunk, shoulder, shoulder girdle, and elbow.

Adequate Motor Control

The person must be able to contract and relax functioning muscles. People with such conditions as cerebral palsy or significant elbow flexor tone are not usually good candidates for the mobile arm supports.

Sufficient Range of Motion

The preferred ROM for joints to use the MAS well is shoulder flexion and abduction (90 degrees), shoulder external rotation (30 degrees), shoulder internal rotation (normal), elbow flexion (normal), forearm pronation (80 degrees), and hip flexion (100 degrees).

Stable Trunk Positioning

An upright sitting posture is ideal. Good head and neck positioning is important.

Client Motivation

The client must want to use the device and have sufficient motivation for training to use it proficiently.

Supportive Environment

Generally, people who use this device cannot put it on themselves and will need support to help with the use of the device.

Manny meets all of the criteria listed above. He has occupations of interest that can be accomplished through the use of a mobile arm support. He has adequate performance skills (strength, ROM, stable sitting posture, and motor control) that will allow him to use the MAS. He is highly motivated to return to his law practice and has a very supportive wife. The support of the law firm is somewhat questionable as they wonder how he will be able to manage all aspects of the work of an attorney in their offices.

ADJUSTMENT OF MOBILE ARM SUPPORTS

The adjustment of MASs generally requires postgraduate hands-on training. However, having some knowledge of adjustment will give the reader a greater appreciation for the need to have additional training to learn how to make fine adjustments. One study has shown that even when the MAS is not adjusted correctly, a person with sufficient muscle power can overcome the lack of fine adjustment.[25] This does not negate the need for therapists to be trained to ensure the best possible adjustment and mechanical advantage possible for the client using the MAS.

Even with hands-on training, additional parts exist beyond the basic pieces that enhance the effectiveness of the device. The training needed to use these additional parts comes with practice, experience, and consultation with therapists familiar with the use of special parts.

Adjustment of Basic Parts

See Figure 29-44.

Forearm support

The forearm support is initially fitted by bending the dial to accommodate the left or right elbow (Figure 29-44, *D*).

Rocker arm

The rocker arm is attached to the support. The standard rocker arm is attached to the first and third holes closest to the elbow.

Semireclining mount, proximal arm, distal arm, and forearm support

The mount (Figure 29-44, *C*) is attached to the left or right wheelchair upright, the proximal arm (Figure 29-44, *B*) is placed in the mount, the distal arm (Figure 29-44, *A*) is placed in the proximal arm, and the forearm support is placed in the distal arm.

Balancing the mobile arm support at neutral

The mount is adjusted so that the ball bearings are parallel to the floor.

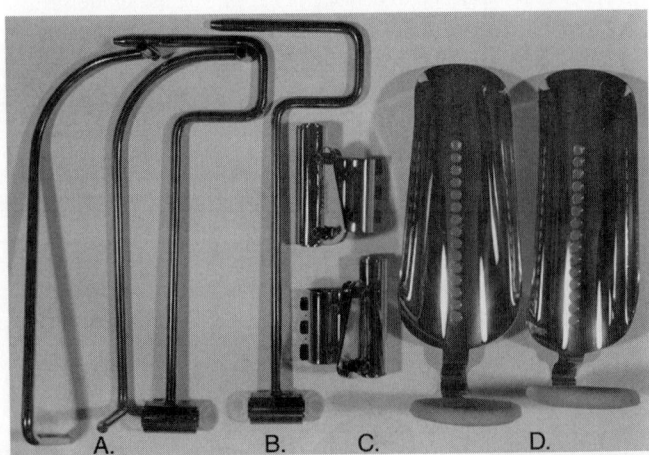

Figure 29-44   Parts of traditional mobile arm support. **A,** Distal arms, right and left; **B,** proximal arms; **C,** semireclining mounts, right and left; **D,** forearm supports

Checking the mount height

The client is placed in the MAS, and the therapist passively moves the hand to the mouth. If the shoulder is elevated or depressed, the height of the mount should be adjusted.

Assessing forearm support for fit and adaptations

The support is observed for forearm comfort and allowance of wrist flexion (if client has active motion). Measurements are taken to have the support cut if necessary to prevent discomfort and nonconformity to the size and shape of the forearm.

Adjusting for horizontal motion

The mount is rolled to assist horizontal abduction or adduction. The pitch of the mount or the distal bearing is adjusted to achieve maximum horizontal motion in front of the client.

Adjusting for vertical motion

The rocker arm is moved on the mount if up or down motion is difficult.

Readjusting for fine balance

The therapist reviews all the adjustments to ensure maximum motion.

Checking fit during occupational performance

Further adjustments may be needed with the weight of objects in the hand.[19]

TRAINING

Training includes practice in all occupations that interest the client and that need to be performed. Any of these occupations may require various adjustments until the final settings are achieved. If strength or ROM increases during the training period, further adjustments may be needed. Adapted equipment can be used in conjunction with the MAS. A wrist-hand orthosis may be required or adjusted for use with the MAS.[19]

Follow-up with clients is indicated, especially for a growing child. MASs can come out of adjustment over time. The questions in Box 29-1 are modified from an MAS appraisal form that was developed at Rancho Los Amigos National Rehabilitation Center in the polio era.[18] It can be a useful tool to check the adequacy of the fit of the MAS when the client returns to the clinic for follow-up visits.

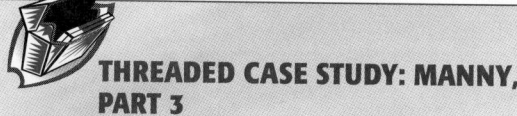

THREADED CASE STUDY: MANNY, PART 3

After 2 weeks in rehabilitation, Manny was able to sit in a wheelchair 2 to 3 hours daily. He was given a motorized wheelchair, which he operated with a chin switch for mobility and for reclining the wheelchair to obtain pressure relief every hour while he was awake. He was still unable to participate in any of his most important occupations necessary to return to his law practice.

He was given a traditional MAS and a lapboard on his wheelchair. He continued to turn pages, now with an MAS and his wrist-hand orthosis. Also, with the MAS, his wrist-hand orthosis, and a computer he began written communications, sending e-mails to his wife, his child, co-workers, and friends. Occupational performance activities that require hand-to-mouth are more complex than tabletop activities, so these occupations were introduced more slowly, by working on reaching higher and higher in vertical motions. Games, such as building pyramids with blocks, were used until he could reach his mouth with his hand and then eating activities were introduced, using a wrist-hand orthosis that could hold an adapted spoon and fork.

Although with Manny's available upper extremity strength, it was questionable whether he could use his MAS for driving his motorized wheelchair, Manny wanted to do so. He did not like the image of a chin switch to drive his wheelchair. He practiced using the MAS for driving his wheelchair until this task was accomplished. With practice, he could also efficiently operate his computer, turn pages, manage a speakerphone, and feed himself simple meals. He needed assistance in removing his MAS, when he reclined to have pressure on his ischium relieved.

When he was discharged, he returned to the outpatient OT clinic, where a plan was made to have the OT and Manny visit the law office to demonstrate how he could perform the occupations needed in the law office. In addition to the equipment obtained as an inpatient, it was recommended that Manny could benefit from a large round desk that acted as a turntable operated electrically. On this turntable he could access his special phone, computer, and reading matter. Manny would also show that through his oratory skills a positive image would be perceived by the public arriving to his office. This visit and the implementation of the resulting equipment recommendations resulted in Manny's return to his law practice 2 months after discharge.

SPECIAL PARTS OF THE MOBILE ARM SUPPORT

Some commonly used special parts include the outside rocker arm assembly (also known as an *offset swivel*) (Figure 29-45, *A*) and the elevating proximal arm (Figure 29-45, *B*).[13] The outside rocker assembly has a ball-bearing joint that allows greater freedom in vertical motion. The elevating proximal arm is useful for the person who has deltoid muscles that are between fair (F or 3) and poor (P or 2). The client initiates the elevating motion, and rubber band assists allow the client to flex and abduct the humerus to a higher level.

Many other useful, but not commonly used, special parts are commercially available for clients with special problems. Understanding the use and adjustment of these special parts generally requires training.[19] With the advent of new

1. Are the client's hips set back in the chair?
2. Is the spine in good vertical alignment?
3. Is there good lateral trunk stability?
4. Is the chair seat and back adequate for comfort and stability?
5. Is the client able to sit upright?
6. If the client wears wrist-hand orthoses, are they on?
7. Does the client have adequate passive ROM?
8. Is the mount tight on the wheelchair and positioned perpendicular to the floor?
9. Is the mount at the proper height so that the shoulders are not forced into elevation?
10. Is the proximal arm all the way down in the mount?
11. Does the elbow dial clear the lap surface when the trough is in the "up" position?
12. When the forearm support is in the "up" position, is the client's hand as close to the mouth as possible?
13. Can the client obtain maximal active reach?
14. Is the forearm support the correct length? Does the distal end of the forearm support stop at the wrist joint?
15. Are the forearm support edges rolled so that they do not contact the forearm?
16. Is the elbow secure and comfortable in the elbow support?
17. Is the forearm support balanced correctly?
18. In vertical motion, is the dial free of the distal arm?
19. Can the client control motion of the proximal arm from either extreme?
20. Can the client control motion of the distal arm from either extreme?
21. Can the client control vertical motion of the trough from either extreme?
22. Have stops been applied to limit range, if necessary?
23. Can the client lift a sufficient amount of weight to perform desired occupational performance?

designs for wheelchairs, it is sometimes necessary to adapt the MAS bracket to attach to the newer wheelchairs. Some wheelchair manufacturers can assist with providing solutions to these problems, and some centers have developed common solutions.[19]

CURRENT DEVELOPMENT AND FUTURE RESEARCH

Although the traditional MAS has been used effectively by some for more than 50 years, little evidence can be found in the literature during this period to show the development of the MAS to expand its use with those who have upper extremity weakness.

An example of development during this period was an attempt by engineers approximately 40 years ago to provide a powered arm for persons who had minimal strength in the upper extremities. The Rancho Electric Arm was developed to meet the needs of those who were too weak to use a conventional MAS.[23] It required the clients to use their tongues to operate seven tiny toggle switches in complex patterns to achieve motions at the joints of the arm and hand.[14]

In 1995 the Rehabilitation Engineering Program at Rancho Los Amigos National Medical Center received a National Institute on Disability and Rehabilitation Research (NIDRR) grant to design, develop, and test a new MAS.[17] During the 5 years of the grant, the project developed an entirely new MAS system. It incorporated a multi-link arm that has a low profile and a high-tech appearance (Figures 29-46 and 29-47, *A*). The new mount fits many current wheelchairs, has simple, intuitive adjustability without tools, and locks in position to retain adjustments (Figure 29-47, *B*). The forearm support includes a slide-lock to adjust its pivot point (Figure 29-47, *C*).[17] The new JAECO/Rancho Multilink Arm (MAS) was transferred to a manufacturer, JAECO

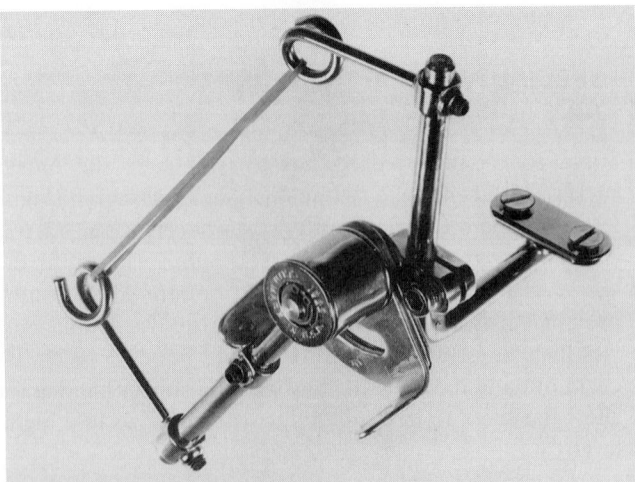

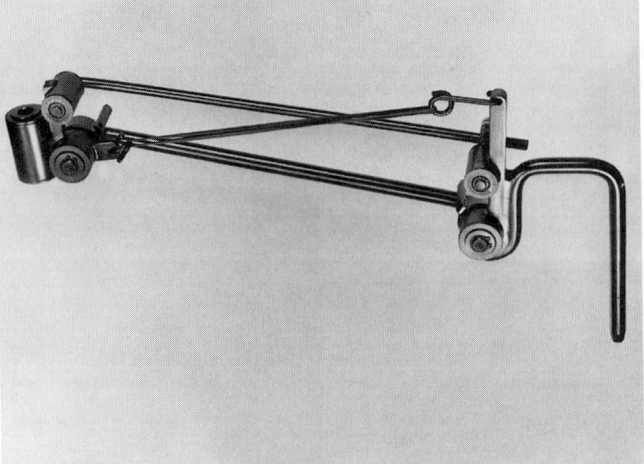

A   B

Figure 29-45   **A,** Offset swivel with up and down stops and humeral rotation assist (outside rocker arm with rubber band assist). **B,** Elevating proximal arm. (Courtesy JAECO Orthopedic Inc., Hot Springs, Ark.)

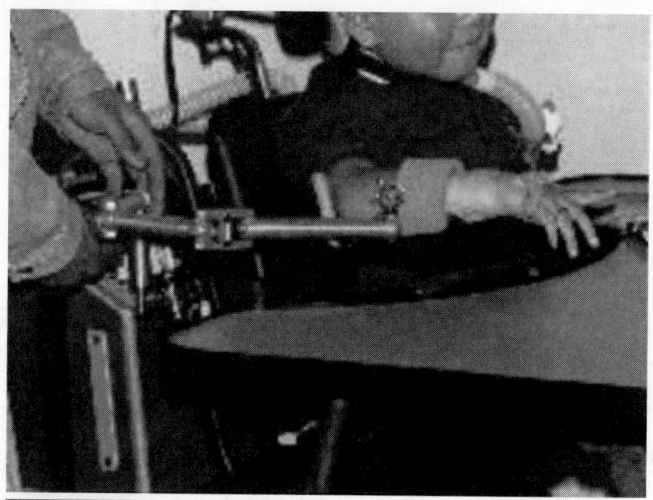

Figure 29-46 New multilink mobile arm support. (From Rancho Los Amigos National Rehabilitation Center, Rehabilitation Engineering Center, Downey, Calif.)

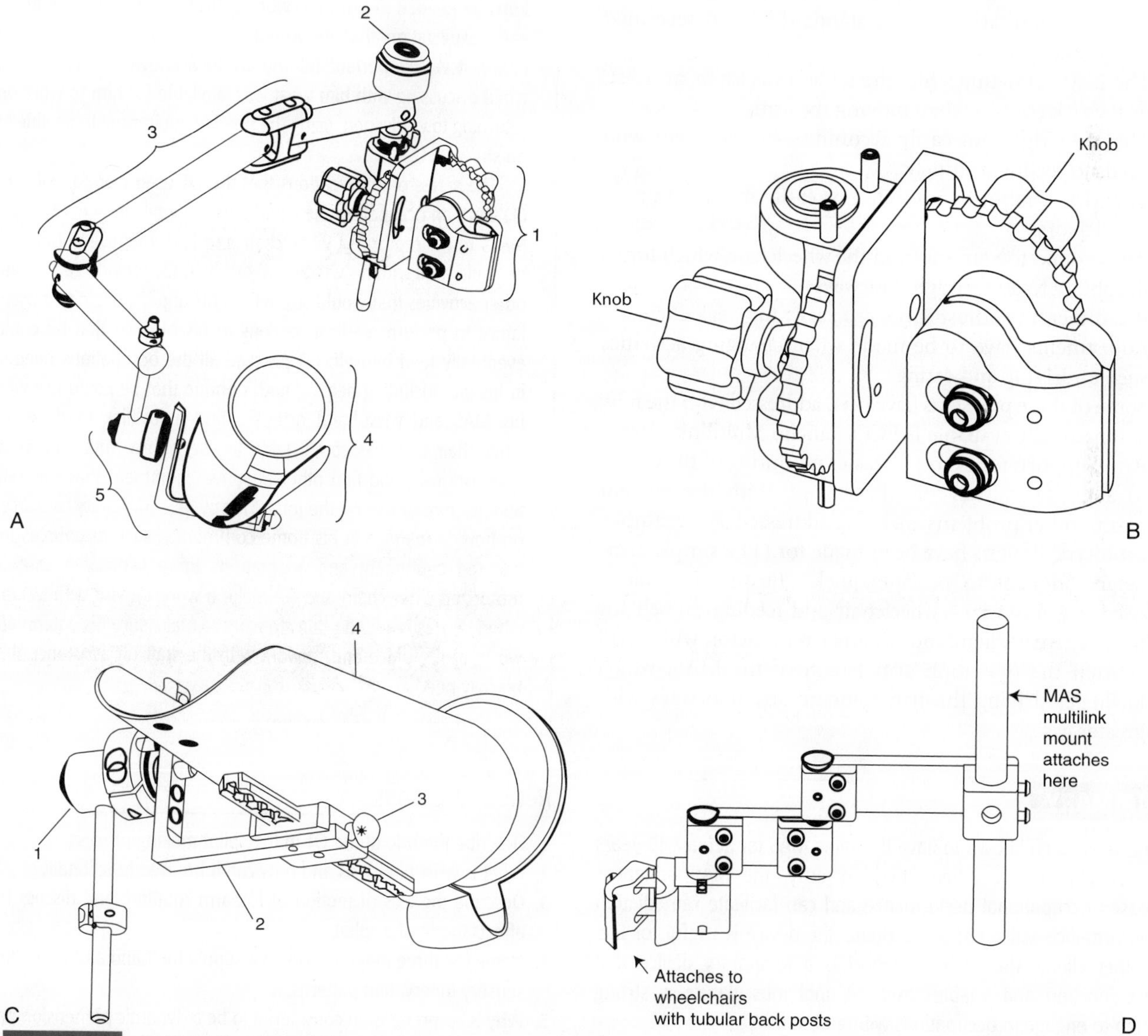

A

B

Knob

Knob

C

1

2

3

4

D

MAS multilink mount attaches here

Attaches to wheelchairs with tubular back posts

Figure 29-47 **A,** JAECO/Rancho Multilink Mobile Arm Support. (1) MAS mount. (2) Proximal shaft with bubble level. (3) Multilink. (4) Forearm support with elbow dial. (5) Offset swivel with adjustable slide. **B,** JAECO/Rancho Multilink Mobile Arm Support mount. Two knobs control adjustment without use of tools. **C,** JAECO/Rancho Multilink Mobile Arm Support offset swivel with adjustable slide. (1) Offset swivel with (2) adjustable slide. (3) Spring-loaded pull-out knob to adjust position on the forearm support (4). **D,** JAECO Mount Adaptor MR-10. Enables the JAECO/Rancho mount to attach to wheelchairs with tubular back posts. (Courtesy JAECO Orthopedic Inc., Hot Springs, Arkansas.)

Orthopedic, Inc., who opened it to mass marketing in 2003.[17] In addition, mount adaptors (Figure 29-47, *D*) are new devices provided by this manufacturer to enable either the new JAECO/Rancho MAS mount or the traditional MAS bracket to attach to an even greater variety of wheelchairs, which have exploded onto the market.

Within two current NIDRR research grants (NIDRR #2022-02 and NIDRR #1835-03), work on the MAS continues. Further solutions are being sought to the problems identified with the traditional MAS and the new Multilink MAS.

In one of these two grants, a survey was conducted with 17 OTs with an average of 15 years of experience working with clients with spinal cord injury in various parts of the United States and Canada.[25] One of the questions asked of the respondents was to identify problems with the traditional MAS. The following is a partial list of some of the more highly ranked limitations of the standard MAS determined by these therapists:

- The MAS sometimes hits the table, wheelchair armrest, or joystick control when moving the arm.
- The MAS does not easily accommodate the client who needs to recline routinely.
- The MAS cannot be mounted or easily mounted on all wheelchairs.
- Parts extend too far out from the wheelchair, which limits the ability to go through doorways.
- It is difficult to adjust MAS, especially for weak clients.
- Adjustments have to be made when changing activities such as driving and eating.
- Some of these problems have been addressed with the now commercially available JAECO/Rancho Multilink Mobile Arm Support; for example, easier mounting of the device to a greater variety of wheelchairs. With the current grants, other problems are being addressed. For example, prototype designs have been made for (1) a simple arm-height adjustor to provide quick adjustment to allow driving a motorized wheelchair and feeding oneself for the very weak client and (2) an arm retractor, which will shorten the operation arm length of the MAS, which facilitates driving through standard size doorways with greater ease.[20]

SUMMARY

Clients have been known to have the same MAS for at least 10 years and probably more. When fitted correctly, the MAS enhances increased occupational performance and can facilitate remediation of performance skills. For some clients the device is useful for life. For other clients the mobile support is a temporary device that allows function and enables exercise until musculature is strong enough to engage in occupations without them.

As the MAS continues to be developed, fitting and adjustment will become streamlined, the cosmetic appearance will be less conspicuous and more appealing to clients, and adjustments will be simplified for therapists. Thus, it is hoped that all clients who can

benefit will be fitted with an MAS to engage in occupations to support their participation in the home and communities to which they belong.

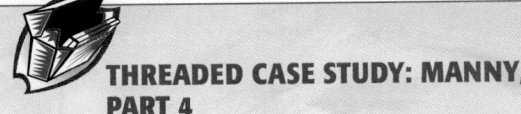

THREADED CASE STUDY: MANNY, PART 4

With Manny's performance skills, initially he was able to benefit from the use of suspension arm supports in bed, wearing a wrist-hand orthosis, and using adapted equipment to be able to read and turn pages. When he was up in a motorized wheelchair, he was given an MAS with which he continued to use his wrist-hand orthosis with other adapted equipment, to perform the occupations he needed to return to work in his law firm. Because of his early expectation that he would recover from his spinal cord injury, it was important for the OT to acknowledge his hopes, while discussing with him what was available for him to work on returning to work soon, using the needed equipment to be able to do so.

The series of interventions that the OT used were as follows: (1) work on occupations he could perform while in bed, (2) apply MASs to his motorized wheelchair and find adaptive equipment he could hold with his wrist-hand orthosis, (3) provide games and other activities that would strengthen his upper extremity musculature to perform vertical motions in his MAS so that he could eventually feed himself, (4) practice all the occupations needed in his job, including helping find a phone that he could use with his MAS and wrist-hand orthosis, find a joystick to drive his wheelchair that was comfortable to use with a MAS and wrist-hand orthosis, and find other adaptive equipment that was reliable for him to use on the job, (5) provide community resources on how to manage in his home community, such as sources for adapted equipment and adaptations for a vehicle to carry a motorized wheelchair, and (6) make a worksite visit with Manny when he was ready to return to work to make sure his equipment works in the office and to work with the staff on assistance that he may need.

Review Questions

1. Describe the role of the OT in the splint-making process.
2. What is wrist tenodesis and how can it be used functionally?
3. Describe the axis of motion of forearm rotation, and discuss how it affects the fit of a splint.
4. Name the three major nerves that supply the hand and describe their sensory innervation patterns.
5. Why is tip prehension considered to be a dynamic prehension pattern rather than static?
6. What is the one grasp pattern that does not include the thumb?
7. Define the terms *friction*, *torque*, and *stress*.
8. How is shear stress created and how can it best be avoided?

9. Why do translational forces minimize the effectiveness of a splint?
10. Describe the difference between a dynamic and a static splint.
11. How may a splint pattern vary if it is to be fitted on the dorsum of the hand, as compared with the volar surface?
12. How does the amount of drape in a low-temperature thermoplastic material affect the making of a splint?
13. What is the recommended type of material for small finger splints? Why?
14. What is the recommended type of material for large elbow and lower extremity splints? Why?
15. What is the importance of straps on a single-surface splint?
16. What are the purposes of suspension arm devices and MASs?
17. Where are suspension arm devices attached?
18. What are the limitations of suspension arm devices?
19. What is the difference between a suspension arm sling and a suspension arm support?
20. Who are good candidates for suspension arm devices?
21. How are suspension arm devices adjusted?
22. Approximately how long have traditional mobile arm supports been used?
23. Name the parts of the MAS.
24. What are the benefits of the MAS?
25. How does the MAS work?
26. What are the criteria necessary to use the MAS?
27. How is the MAS adjusted for each client?
28. What is the advantage of the JAECO/Rancho Multilink Mobile Arm Support?

REFERENCES

1. American Society of Hand Therapists: *Splint classification system*, Chicago, 1992, The Society.
2. Anderson KN, Anderson LE, Glanze WD, editors: *Mosby's medical, nursing, and allied health dictionary*, ed 4, St Louis, 1994, Mosby.
3. Bennett RL: Orthotics for function. I. Prescription, *Phys Ther Rev* 36(11):1, 1956.
4. Bennett RL: The evolution of the Georgia Warm Springs Foundation Feeder, *Artif Limb* 10(1):5, 1966.
5. Bennett RL, Stephens HR: Care of severely paralyzed upper extremities, *JAMA* 149(2):105, 1952.
6. Bonutti PM, Windau JE, Ables BA, et al: Static progressive stretch to reestablish elbow range of motion, *Clin Orthop* June(303):128, 1994.
7. Brand PW, Hollister A: *Clinical mechanics of the hand*, ed 3, St Louis, 1999, Mosby.
8. Colditz J: Dynamic splinting of the stiff hand. In Hunter J, Schneider L, Mackin E, et al: *Rehabilitation of the hand: surgery and therapy*, ed 3, St Louis, 1990, Mosby.
9. Fess EE, Gettle KS, Philips CA, et al: *Hand and upper extremity splinting: principles and methods*, ed 3, St Louis, 2005, Mosby.
10. Flatt AE: *Care of the arthritic hand*, St Louis, 1983, Mosby.
11. Haworth R, Dunscombe S, Nichols PJR: Mobile arm supports: an evaluation, *Rheumatol Rehabil* 17(4):240, 1978.
12. Hollister A, Giurintano D: How joints move. In Brand PW, Hollister A: *Clinical mechanics of the hand*, ed 3, St Louis, 1999, Mosby.
13. *JAECO Orthopedic Inc. Catalog*, Hot Springs, Ark (undated).
14. Landsberger SE: *Keep moving: RERC on technologies to enhance mobility and function for individuals with spinal cord injury NIDRR application*, Los Amigos Research and Education Institute, Rancho Los Amigos National Rehabilitation Center, Downey, Calif, 2002.
15. Long C: Upper limb bracing. In Licht S, editor: *Orthotics etcetera*, Baltimore, 1966, Waverly Press.
16. McCollough N, Sarrafian S: Biomechanical analysis system. In *Atlas of orthotics, biomechanical principles and application*, St Louis, 1975, Mosby.
17. McNeal D, et al: *Rehabilitation engineering program: annual report, RERC on technology for children*, Los Amigos Research and Education Institute, Rancho Los Amigos National Rehabilitation Center, Downey, Calif, 2000.
18. Rancho Los Amigos Medical Center, Occupational Therapy Department: *Mobile arm support appraisal*, Downey, Calif, 1969, the Center (unpublished).
19. Rancho Los Amigos National Rehabilitation Center, Occupational Therapy Department: *Mobile arm support workshop manual*, Downey, Calif, 1998.
20. Rehabilitation Engineering Program: *Quarterly report. Keep moving: RERC on technologies to enhance mobility and function for individuals with spinal cord injury*, Los Amigos Research and Education Institute, Rancho Los Amigos National Rehabilitation Center, Downey, Calif, 2004.
21. Snelson R, Conry J: Recent advancements in functional arm bracing correlated with orthopedic surgery for the severely paralyzed upper extremity, *Orthop Prosthet Appliance J*, 41, 1958.
22. Strickland JW: Anatomy and kinesiology of the hand. In Fess EE, Gettle KS, Philips CA, et al: *Hand and upper extremity splinting: principles and methods*, ed 3, St Louis, 2005, Mosby.
23. Trombly CA, Radomski MV: *Occupational therapy for physical dysfunction*, ed 5, Baltimore, 2002, Lippincott Williams & Wilkins.
24. Wilson DJ, McKenzie MW, Barber LM: *Spinal cord injury: a treatment guide for occupational therapists*, rev ed, Thorofare, NJ, 1984, Slack.
25. Yasuda YL: Unpublished document for NIDRR Grant: *Keep moving: RERC on technologies to enhance mobility and function for individuals with spinal cord injury*, Downey, Calif, 2004, Los Amigos Research and Education Institute, Rancho Los Amigos National Rehabilitation Center.
26. Yasuda YL, Bowman K, Hsu JD: Mobile arm supports: criteria for successful use in muscle disease clients, *Arch Phys Med Rehabil* 67(4):253, 1986.

30

Traditional Sensorimotor Approaches to Intervention

WINIFRED SCHULTZ-KROHN
CHARLOTTE BRASIC ROYEEN
GUY MCCORMACK
SARA A. POPE-DAVIS
JUDY M. JOURDAN

KEY TERMS

Lower motor neurons
Upper motor neurons
Information flow
Motivational urge
Conation
Ideation
Movement strategy
Motor program
Sensorimotor system
Reflex and hierarchical models
Sensory stimulation
Evolution in reverse
Mass movement patterns
Coeffect
Generalizability

Somatic marker
Meta-emotion
Reciprocal inhibition
Cocontraction
Heavy work
Skill
Supine withdrawal
Rollover
Pivot prone
Neck cocontraction
Ontogenetic development
  patterns
Proprioceptive stimulation
Vestibular stimulation
Inversion

Inhibitory techniques
Proprioceptive neuromuscular
  facilitation
Diagonal patterns
Stretch
Verbal commands
Verbal mediation
Manual contacts
Part-task practice
Whole-task practice
Stepwise procedures
Unilateral patterns
Bilateral patterns
Symmetrical patterns
Asymmetrical patterns

Reciprocal patterns
Combined movements
Traction
Approximation
Maximal resistance
Repeated contractions
Rhythmic initiation
Slow reversal
Stabilizing reversals
Rhythmic stabilization
Contract-relax
Hold-relax
Slow reversal-hold-relax
Rhythmic rotation

LEARNING OBJECTIVES

After studying this chapter the student or practitioner will be able to do the following:

1. Describe the four general processes of information flow related to control of movement.
2. Define *motivational urge,* and name the locus of this function in the brain.
3. Trace the flow of information in the central and peripheral nervous systems that leads to purposeful movement.
4. Define the *sensorimotor system*, its locus in the brain, and its function during motor performance.
5. List the structures that constitute the higher, middle, and lower levels of the central nervous system components for movement.
6. Name the four traditional sensorimotor approaches to intervention and the theorist responsible for each.
7. Name the two models of motor control that form the basis for the sensorimotor approaches to treatment.
8. Briefly describe each of the four traditional sensorimotor approaches to intervention; compare and contrast their similarities and their differences.

9. Identify the importance of Margaret Rood's work in respect to performance skills.
10. Define key concepts first proposed by Margaret Rood in respect to posture, mobility, and coordination within the domain of functional purposes.
11. Delineate how Rood's concepts have been redefined in light of current understanding of neuroscience.
12. Recognize the four components of motor control emphasized by Rood.
13. Describe the major motor patterns of development identified by Rood.
14. Delineate examples of how Rood's major motor patterns are used during occupation.
15. State reasons for caution when employing Rood's treatment techniques.
16. Give two examples of Rood techniques still used today.

17. Contrast the traditional Rood approach and the Rood approach reconstructed for the Occupational Therapy Practice Framework: Domain and Process.[3]
18. Understand and apply PNF as preparatory methods to facilitate client participation in desired occupations.
19. Define PNF and how this approach facilitates adaptive responses that are performed in daily occupations.
20. Understand the principles of PNF and how to apply them to enhance client performance.
21. Describe the influence of sensory input on motor learning.
22. Use the PNF evaluation to determine factors limiting clients' participation in their occupation.
23. Recognize upper and lower extremity (LE) diagonal patterns in daily performance skills.
24. Name the theorists who developed the proprioceptive neuromuscular facilitation (PNF) approach.

CHAPTER OUTLINE

OVERVIEW

Winifred Schultz-Krohn

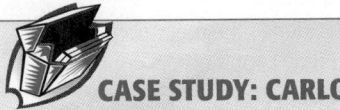

CASE STUDY: CARLOS

Carlos, a 59-year-old construction foreman, is 3 days after a right cerebrovascular accident (CVA) and currently requires maximum assistance for most self-care tasks. He is able to speak, recognizes his wife and two adult children, but appears easily confused when he is expected to participate in self-care activities. He has no functional motor control of his left arm or hand, and sensation is markedly impaired on his left extremities. He presents with decorticate posture in both left extremities with flexion tone dominating his arm and extensor tone dominating his leg. He is able to partially roll to the right side of the hospital bed and push up on his right arm to a sitting position, but at home he sleeps on the opposite side of the bed. He is able to stand using a quad cane in his right hand but is unable to safely walk from the bed to the bathroom in his hospital room.

As Carlos's occupational therapist (OT), you are expected to design and implement an intervention plan based on the best evidence available. OTs, who are working with clients who have sustained damage to the central nervous system (CNS) are often concerned with enhancing functional movement as a means to promote independence in occupational performance.[32] To achieve this objective, a variety of intervention approaches are available from which the therapist may choose. This chapter reviews the traditional sensorimotor approaches and presents a brief description of each.

Critical Thinking Questions

The following questions should be considered as you read this overview of the traditional sensorimotor approaches to intervention.

1. How can a traditional intervention approach improve Carlos's occupational performance?
2. What potential difficulties should be anticipated using a traditional intervention approach?
3. What current knowledge of CNS function could be used to support the selection and implementation of traditional sensorimotor intervention methods?

NEUROLOGICAL CONSIDERATIONS FOR TRADITIONAL SENSORIMOTOR APPROACHES TO INTERVENTION

Occupation performance frequently requires precise voluntary movement that is controlled and monitored by the nervous system. Various structures within the nervous system are coordinated to selectively activate specific muscles to initiate, perform, and complete a desired task or activity. If a movement is poorly performed and thereby compromises task performance, feedback occurs through knowledge of the results of the action, and the neurological commands to the muscles are modified so that accuracy of movement is achieved. Knowledge of the intricate working of the nervous system is of special importance to the OT concerned with refinement and improvement of the motor performance of clients with neurological conditions. A brief overview of the flow of information associated with the control of movement is described in the following sections.

CNS CONTROL OF MOVEMENT

The firing of motor neurons located in the anterior horn of the spinal cord produces all movements.[84] These neurons directly innervate the skeletal muscles. The activity of the spinal or **lower motor neurons** can be modulated by segmental spinal circuitry and by the descending influence of the motor neurons located in the motor cortex and brainstem. These neurons are referred to as **upper motor neurons.** Two other structures, the basal ganglia and the cerebellum, and their associated pathways, are also intimately involved with motor control. Lesions in these structures are associated with characteristic movement disorders.

Movement production does not begin and end with the upper or lower motor neurons. Many CNS structures contribute to the development of the signals that activate muscles. Although much about the control of movement is still unknown, animal and human research suggests that four general processes are related to the flow of information needed to control movement. The four general processes of **information flow** are motivation, ideation, programming, and execution.[12,21] A schematic diagram that indicates the main direction of information flow and connecting the various motor centers appears in Figure 30-1.

The motivation or emotive component of the movement is a function of the limbic system.[12,81] The **motivational urge** or *impulse* to act associated with the limbic system is transformed to ideas by the cortical association areas. This connection of knowledge and affective behavior is also referred to as **conation.**[47] Conation represents the intentional, deliberate, and goal-directed aspect of behavior and is related to the individual's reason for the motor performance. The association areas of the frontal, parietal, temporal, and occipital lobes are concerned with **ideation,** or the goal of the movement, and the programming or **movement strategy** (plan) that best achieves the goal. Programming of a movement strategy also involves the premotor areas, the basal ganglia, and the cerebellum. The **motor program** is the procedure or the spatiotemporal order of muscle activation that is needed for smooth and accurate motor performance. The execution level, represented by the motor cortex, the cerebellum, and the spinal cord, is concerned with the activation of the spinal motor neurons and interneurons

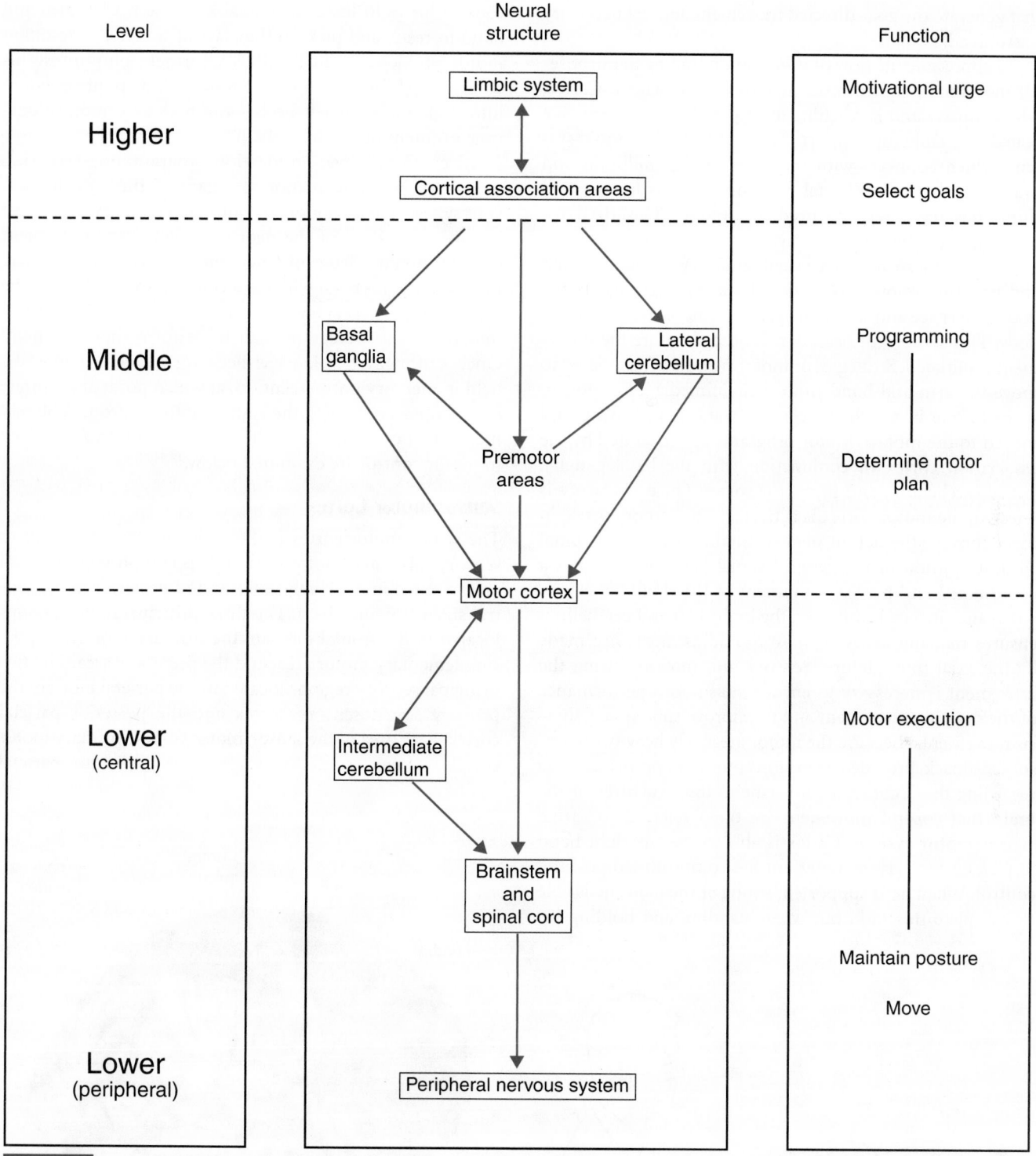

Figure 30-1   Schematic representation of the hierarchy of the neural structures involved in motor control. The left column indicates the hierarchical level and the right column the major function of the neural structures shown in the center column during motor performance. (Adapted from Cheney PD: Role of cerebral cortex in voluntary movements: a review, *Phys Ther* 65[5]:624, 1985.)

that generate the goal-directed movement and the necessary postural adjustments.

To appreciate the flow of information leading to purposeful movement, consider the actions of your client, Carlos, who is thirsty and is reaching out for a glass of water while seated at a table for support (Figure 30-2). The limbic system, which connects with the areas of the midbrain and brainstem that control vital functions such as hunger and thirst, has registered the need for water.[45] This need for drinking water has been conveyed to the cortical association areas, which also received visual, auditory, somatosensory, and proprioception information about precisely where the body is in space and where the glass of water is relative to the body. This sensory information is needed before the movement is initiated. Strategies or motor plans are formulated to move the arm and hand from their immediate location in space to one in which the glass of water is picked up and moved to the mouth. Motor programs are generated by the association cortex in conjunction with the basal ganglia, lateral cerebellum, and premotor cortex. Once a strategy is selected, the motor cortex is activated. The motor cortex, in turn, conveys the action plan to the brainstem and spinal cord. Activation of the cervical spinal neurons generates a coordinated and precise movement of the shoulder, elbow, wrist, and fingers. Input from the brainstem and cerebellum ensures that the necessary postural adjustments are made by the axial musculature. Sensory information during the movement is necessary to ensure the smooth performance of the ongoing movement and to improve subsequent similar movements. Because the motor areas rely heavily on sensory feedback, provided by exteroceptors and proprioceptors regarding the accuracy of movement, the structures of the brain that control movement are often referred to as the **sensorimotor system.** Carlos is able to use his right hand to pick up the glass of water but has compromised postural control. When he is supported, sitting at the table, he is able to complete this task, but when standing and holding his

cane in his right hand he is unable to use his left arm and hand to reach and pick up the glass of water. The resultant motor problems from the RCVA further compromise his ability to perform a bimanual task such as pouring liquid into a glass even when he has the necessary motivational urge or intention for movement.

Given the motivation-ideation-programming-execution scheme of how information is organized through the nervous system, it is obvious that control of voluntary movement involves almost all of the neocortex. Voluntary movement depends on knowledge of where the body is in space, where the body intends to go with respect to this external space, the internal and external loads that must be overcome, and formulation of a strategy or plan to perform the movement. Once a strategy or plan has been formulated, it must be held in memory until execution, at which point appropriate instructions are sent to the spinal motor neurons. The primary functional aspects of the sensorimotor areas involved in motor control are examined below.[12,54,81]

Sensorimotor Cortex

The sensorimotor cortex is the major integrating center of sensory input and motor output. It is composed of cortical areas located immediately anterior and posterior to the central sulcus (Figure 30-3). The three principal motor regions located in the frontal lobe are the primary motor area, the supplementary motor area, and the premotor area. The two principal sensory regions located in the parietal lobe are the primary somatosensory cortex and the posterior parietal cortex. Each area of the sensorimotor cortex (primary motor cortex, primary somatosensory cortex, posterior parietal

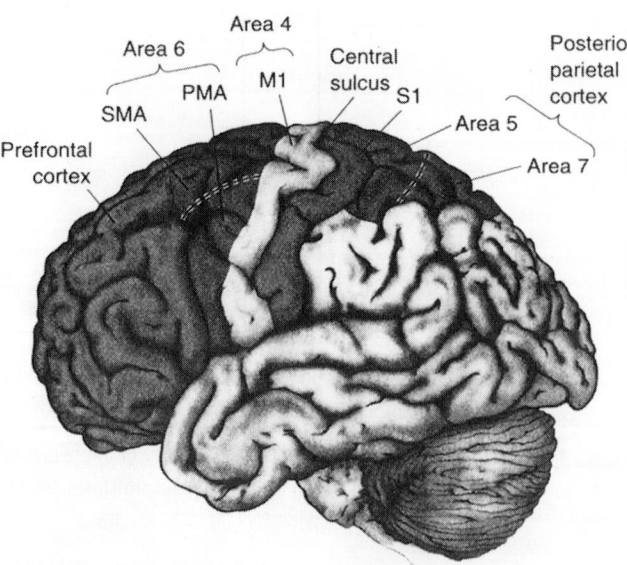

Figure 30-3   Areas of the neocortex intimately involved in planning and instruction of voluntary movement. Areas 4 and 6 constitute motor cortex. (From Bear MF, Connors BW, Paradiso MA: *Neuroscience: exploring the brain*, Baltimore, 1996, Williams & Wilkins.)

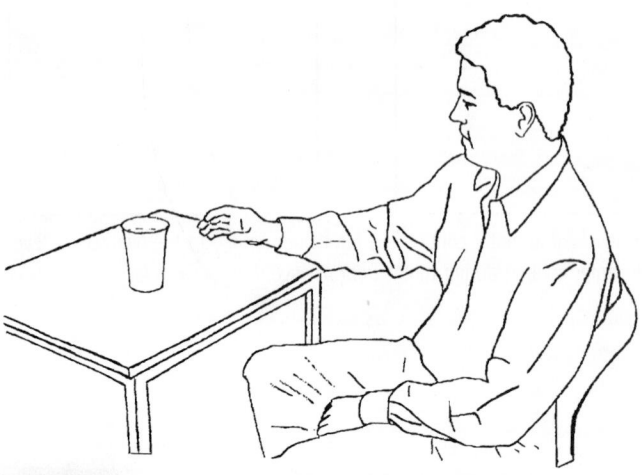

Figure 30-2   A person reaching out for a glass of water.

cortex, supplementary motor area, and premotor cortex) is arranged in a manner that provides a topographical representation of the contralateral body segments.[54,74] Each of these areas is responsible for certain aspects of movement generation. In the previous example of reaching out for the glass of water, Carlos had a mental image of his body and its relation to the surrounding space by integrating the information supplied through somatosensory, proprioceptive, and visual inputs to the posterior parietal cortex. Clients with a lesion in this area demonstrate impairment of body image and its relation to extrapersonal space, and, in the extreme situation, neglect of the contralateral body segments.

The posterior parietal cortex integrates and translates sensory information so that the ensuing movements are directed appropriately in extrapersonal space. It is extensively interconnected with the association areas of the frontal lobe that are considered involved in determination of the consequences of movement strategies such as moving the arm forward, curling the fingers around the glass, and lifting the glass to the mouth. The fingers begin to curl appropriately before any contact occurs with the glass; therefore, the size and shape of the glass must be recognized before grasping. The prefrontal association areas and the posterior parietal cortex project to the premotor area, which is thought to be concerned with orientation of body segments before initiation of movement. The input of the posterior parietal cortex to the premotor area may be important in the somatosensory guidance of movement.[21] Lesions of the premotor area or posterior parietal cortex have been demonstrated to result in the generation of inappropriate movement strategy.[51]

Planning of movement is considered to be the function of the supplementary motor area. In animal studies, the electrophysiological recordings of cells in this area indicate that the cells typically increase discharge rates about a second before the observable execution of movement of either hand.[87] The same findings have been corroborated in humans with use of imaging techniques to study patterns of cortical activation. Imaging studies using positron emission tomography (PET) monitor changes in local blood flow, because an increase in the local cerebral blood flow is associated with increased neuronal activity. Under these conditions, when subjects were asked to imagine a movement without actually moving the finger, the blood flow to the supplementary motor cortex increased and no comparable increase in blood flow was seen in the primary motor area.[77] When subjects were asked to perform a series of finger movements from memory, blood flow to the supplementary motor cortex increased in advance of the movement but not during the performance of the movement. Unilateral lesions of the supplementary motor area result in apraxia (the loss of the ability to perform movement in the absence of motor or sensory impairments). Another effect of such lesions is the inability to produce the correct sequence of muscle activation for complex motor activities such as speaking, writing, buttoning, typing, sewing, and playing the piano.

The primary somatosensory cortex projection to the primary motor cortex and association areas provides the sensory input needed for motor planning, movement initiation, and regulation of ongoing movement.[37] The primary motor cortex integrates the information it receives from other areas of the brain and generates the descending command for the execution of movement. Not only is this descending command sent to the brainstem and spinal cord, but a copy of it is also sent to the basal ganglia and cerebellum. The descending command specifies the muscles to be activated and the direction, speed, and required force.[21] Lesions of the primary somatosensory cortex typically result in contralateral sensory loss. Movements are uncoordinated because the ability to register sensory feedback during and after the movement is compromised. Damage to the primary motor area results in motor execution deficits. The client presents the classic picture of contralateral muscle weakness, spasticity, and poor isolation of movement with corresponding loss of function.

RELATION TO SENSORIMOTOR INTERVENTION APPROACHES

The CNS structures involved with movement can be grouped functionally into higher, middle, and lower levels. The higher level consists of the limbic system and association areas, where the motivation for action is generated. The sensorimotor areas, along with the basal ganglia and cerebellum, form the middle level, and the lower level consists of the nuclei in the brainstem and spinal cord. Under normal circumstances, an individual's repertoire of motor activity is large. After damage to the CNS regions involved with movement, the coordinated efforts between the various levels of motor control are disrupted, and the motor response may be limited or stereotyped. Traditional sensorimotor approaches to intervention can be viewed as targeting the middle sensorimotor level, the motor planning–strategy formulation process, and the lower-level execution process, with the aim of reintegrating, as far as possible, a complete motor control hierarchy. It easily can be seen that the motor relearning program should also be cognitively oriented and targeted toward achieving a goal or "occupational" task. This represents the inherent limitation of the traditional sensorimotor approaches. These approaches do not actively engage the client's volitional intent or motivation to perform a motor act.

Clients need to be taught motor strategies or compensatory mechanisms to adapt to the deficits produced by a lesion. Compensatory mechanisms and the shaping of motor programs are brought about by the use of sensory inputs. The sensorimotor approaches use sensory stimulation to elicit specific movement patterns. Early in the intervention phase, the emphasis is on the use of external sensory stimuli. Once a movement response is obtained, to reinforce and strengthen the response, the focus shifts to the use of intrinsic sensory information, which thereby encourages voluntary motor control.

The four traditional sensorimotor intervention approaches historically used by occupational therapy (OT) practitioners are the Rood approach, the Brunnstrom (movement therapy) approach, the proprioceptive neuromuscular facilitation approach (PNF), and the neurodevelopmental (Bobath or NDT) approach. These approaches, developed in the 1950s and 1960s, all have their theoretical basis in the **reflex and hierarchical models** of motor control. Although more contemporary models are currently being used to guide intervention with clients who demonstrate CNS dysfunction, an understanding of these traditional approaches is warranted to appreciate their contributions to clinical practice and to recognize the appropriate application of these approaches in selected populations.

REFLEX AND HIERARCHICAL MODELS OF MOTOR CONTROL

Reflex and hierarchical models of motor control view movement strategies along a developmental continuum. Two major fundamental assumptions underlie the reflex and hierarchical models:

The basic units of motor control are reflexes. Reflexes are motor responses that occur in response to specific sensory stimuli. Reflexes are automatic, predictable, and stereotypical; they are normal responses seen from early infancy. As the CNS matures, reflexes become integrated and are believed to form the foundation for volitional motor control. Volitional (purposeful) movement is the summation and integration of reflexive movement. When damage to the CNS occurs, a resurgence of reflexive motor activity occurs in addition to an inability to modulate these reflexive movements.

Motor control is hierarchically arranged. In a hierarchical model of motor control, the CNS is believed to have a specific organizational structure, and motor development and function depend on that structure. This hierarchical organization refers to a system in which the higher centers of the brain regulate and exert control over lower centers of the CNS. The higher centers, specifically the cortical and subcortical areas, are responsible for regulation and control of volitional, conscious movement. The lower levels regulate and control reflexive, automatic, and responsive movement. Based on this conceptualization, when damage occurs to the CNS, it is believed that the damaged area can no longer regulate and exert control over the underlying areas. Motor control, according to this belief, becomes a function of the next lower functioning level of the CNS. Typically this means a return to more reflexive and primitive movement patterns.

The four traditional sensorimotor intervention strategies rely heavily on these basic assumptions about motor development and motor control. Consequently, intervention strategies used in these approaches frequently involve the application of sensory stimulation to muscles and joints to evoke specific motor responses, handling and positioning techniques to effect changes in muscle tone, and the use of developmental postures to enhance the ability to initiate and carry out movements. Table 30-1 presents a comparison and summary of key treatment strategies used in each of the four traditional sensorimotor approaches.

OVERVIEW: THE TRADITIONAL SENSORIMOTOR INTERVENTION APPROACHES

ROOD APPROACH

Margaret Rood drew heavily from both the reflex and the hierarchical models in designing her intervention approach. Key components of the Rood approach are the use of **sensory stimulation** to evoke a motor response and the use of developmental postures to promote changes in muscle tone.[66] Sensory stimulation is applied to muscles and joints to elicit a specific motor response. Stimulation has the potential to have either an inhibitory or a facilitatory effect on muscle tone. Types of sensory stimulation described by Rood include the use of slow rolling, neutral warmth, deep pressure, tapping, and prolonged stretch. Examples of how this stimulation may be applied include tapping over a muscle belly to facilitate (increase) muscle tone and applying deep pressure to a muscle's tendinous insertion to elicit an inhibitory (decreased) effect. Rood also described the use of specific developmental sequences believed to promote motor responses. These sequences were proximal to distal and cephalocaudal. Treatment strategies move clients through these developmental sequences.

In current clinical practice, practitioners may use selected principles from Rood's work as adjunctive or preliminary interventions to prepare an individual to engage in a purposeful activity—for example, the application of quick stretch over the triceps before instructing a client to reach for a cup or glass to improve elbow extension. A client may be instructed in ways to apply his or her own sensory stimulation to enhance activities of daily living (ADL) performance. For example, during upper extremity dressing, the OT may ask Carlos to perform a prolonged stretch to the left biceps, which results in a reduction of muscle tone, which may, in turn, increase the ease with which the arm is moved through the sleeve of his shirt.

Limitations in the use of Rood's approach are numerous and include the passive nature of the sensory stimulation (it is applied "to" an individual) and the short-lasting and unpredictable effect of some of the sensory stimulation. Please refer to the discussion later in this chapter for additional details regarding the Rood approach to intervention.

THE BRUNNSTROM (MOVEMENT THERAPY) APPROACH

Signe Brunnstrom, a physical therapist (PT), developed an intervention approach specifically for individuals who had sustained a cerebrovascular accident (CVA).[14,15] The approach

TABLE 30-1 **Comparison of Key Treatment Strategies Used in the Traditional Sensorimotor Approaches**

Key Treatment Strategies	Rood Approach	Brunnstrom Approach (Movement Therapy)	Proprioceptive Neuromuscular Approach	Neurodevelopmental Treatment
Sensory stimulation used to evoke a motor response	YES (Uses direct application of sensory stimuli to muscles and joints)	YES (Movement occurs in response to sensory stimuli)	YES (Tactile, auditory, visual sensory stimuli promote motor responses)	YES (Abnormal muscle tone occurs, in part, because of abnormal sensory experiences)
Reflexive movement used as a precursor for volitional movement	YES (Reflexive movement achieved initially through the application of sensory stimuli)	YES (Move patient along a continuum of reflexive to volitional movement patterns)	YES (Volitional movements can be assisted by reflexive supported postures)	NO
Treatment directed toward influencing muscle tone	YES (Sensory stimuli used to inhibit or facilitate tone)	YES (Postures, sensory stimuli used to inhibit or facilitate tone)	YES (Movement patterns used to normalize tone)	YES (Handling techniques and postures can inhibit or facilitate muscle tone)
Developmental patterns/sequences used for the development of motor skills	YES (Ontogenic motor patterns used to develop motor skills)	YES (Flexion and extension synergies; proximal to distal return)	YES (Patterns used to facilitate proximal to distal motor control)	YES
Conscious attention is directed toward movement	NO	YES	YES	YES
Treatment directly emphasizes development of skilled movements for task performance	NO	NO	NO	YES

she designed draws strongly from both the reflex and hierarchical models of motor control. Brunnstrom conceptualized clients who had sustained a CVA as going through an **"evolution in reverse."** Spastic or flaccid muscle tone and the presence of reflexive movements that may be evident after a client sustains a CVA are considered part of the normal process of recovery and are viewed as necessary intermediate steps in regaining volitional movement.[83] Brunnstrom clearly detailed stages of motor recovery after a CVA (Table 30-2). These stages include the description of flexor synergy patterns and extensor synergy patterns for the upper and lower limbs. Carlos currently displays flexor tone dominating his left arm and extensor tone dominating his left leg. This dominating tone interferes with isolated control of his left extremities.

In the Brunnstrom approach emphasis is placed on facilitating the progress of the individual by promotion of movement, from reflexive to volitional. In the early stages of recovery this may include the incorporation of reflexes and associated reactions to change tone and achieve movement. For example, to generate reflexive movement in the arm,

resistance may be applied to one side of the body to increase muscle tone on the opposite side. This technique is applied until the client demonstrates volitional control over the movement pattern.

In current clinical practice most OT practitioners do not use Brunnstrom's treatment strategies for fear of increasing and encouraging the development of abnormal movement patterns, which may become habitual. However, the stages of recovery are used in some rehabilitation settings to describe motor recovery. Brunnstrom's contribution to neurorehabilitation is most often identified as the clear descriptions she provided for the stages of recovery from a CVA.

PROPRIOCEPTIVE NEUROMUSCULAR FACILITATION APPROACH

The PNF approach is grounded in the reflex and hierarchical models of motor control. Developed through the collaborative efforts of a physician, Dr. Herman Kabat, and two PTs, Margaret Knott and Dorothy Voss, in the 1950s, this intervention approach continues to be used but has not been

TABLE **30-2** **Motor Recovery After Cerebrovascular Accident***

		Characteristics	
Stage	Leg	Arm	Hand
1	Flaccidity	Flaccidity; inability to perform any movements	No hand function
2	Spasticity develops; minimal voluntary movements	Beginning development of spasticity; limb synergies or some of their components begin to appear as associated reactions	Gross grasp beginning; minimal finger flexion possible
3	Spasticity peaks; flexion and extension synergy present; hip-knee-ankle flexion in sitting and standing	Spasticity increasing; synergy patterns or some of their components can be performed voluntarily	Gross grasp, hook grasp possible; no release
4	Knee flexion past 90 degrees in sitting, with foot sliding backward on floor; dorsiflexion with heel on floor and knee flexed to 90 degrees	Spasticity declining; movement combinations deviating from synergies are now possible	Gross grasp present; lateral prehension developing; small amount of finger extension and some thumb movement possible
5	Knee flexion with hip extended in standing; ankle dorsiflexion with hip and knee extended	Synergies no longer dominant; more movement combinations deviating from synergies performed with greater ease	Palmar prehension, spherical and cylindrical grasp and release possible
6	Hip abduction in sitting or standing; reciprocal internal and external rotation of hip combined with inversion and eversion of ankle in sitting	Spasticity absent except when performing rapid movements; isolated joint movements performed with ease	All types of prehension, individual finger motion, and full range of voluntary extension possible

*Recovery of hand function is variable and may not parallel the six recovery stages of the arm.
From Brunnstrom S: *Movement therapy in hemiplegia,* New York, 1970, Harper & Row.

revised since its origins. Major emphasis in this approach is on the developmental sequencing of movement and the balanced interplay between agonist and antagonist in producing volitional movement.[94] PNF describes **mass movement patterns,** which are diagonal in nature, for the limbs and trunk. Intervention strategies use these patterns to promote movement. The use of sensory stimulation, including tactile, auditory, and visual inputs, is also actively incorporated into treatment to promote a motor response.

In OT clinical practice the inclusion of PNF patterns often can be seen in the way functional activities are designed, especially in the placement of objects during purposeful activities. For example, a client is asked to reach into a shopping bag placed on his left side to retrieve objects that will then be placed into a cabinet on the right side. Specific information regarding the application of PNF is discussed later in this chapter.

NEURODEVELOPMENTAL TREATMENT APPROACH

Neurodevelopmental treatment (NDT), also known as the Bobath treatment approach, is based on normal development and movement. Berta Bobath, a PT, and her husband, Karel Bobath, a physician, provided the initial theoretical

foundations of NDT in the 1950s.[46] At that time they drew from the hierarchical model of motor control. The primary objectives of neurodevelopmental treatment are to normalize muscle tone, inhibit primitive reflexes, and facilitate normal postural reactions.[9] Improving the quality of movement and helping clients relearn normal movement patterns are key objectives of this approach. To achieve these objectives, therapists employ numerous techniques, including handling techniques, weight bearing over the affected limb, the use of positions that encourage the use of both sides of the body, and the avoidance of any sensory input that may adversely affect muscle tone. In clinical practice today, many of these techniques and strategies are used within the context of purposeful activities.

NDT has continued to revise its theoretical framework in response to new evidence on the function of the CNS.[46] Discussions on the rationale for NDT include the current understanding of motor systems and motor learning. See Chapter 31 for further descriptions.

SUMMARY

Movement takes place within an occupational context. Emotional needs influence motor strategies. The spinal cord or brainstem can mediate reflexive responses, but interpretation and transformation of sensory signals by all areas of the sensorimotor system are essential for voluntary movement to occur with precision. The primary somatosensory cortex and posterior parietal cortex are primarily responsible for processing sensory information. The premotor area uses sensory information for the planning of movements, the supplementary motor area is important for bimanual coordination, and the motor cortex is important for execution.

The traditional sensorimotor intervention approaches have their theoretical basis in reflex and hierarchical models of motor control. These approaches offer a valuable link between neurophysiological principles and the rehabilitation treatment of clients with CNS dysfunction. In contemporary practice many of the techniques described in these approaches are used as adjunctive or preliminary techniques or are incorporated into more task-directed treatment activities.

SECTION 1: THE ROOD APPROACH: A RECONSTRUCTION

Charlotte Brasic Royeen*, Guy McCormack

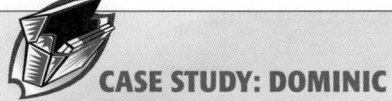

CASE STUDY: DOMINIC

The client, Dominic, was a divorced 57-year-old attorney who lived by himself in a hill community in a suburban neighborhood. His house was located on a steep lot with several steps to climb when going from the driveway to the front door of the house. One day while trimming bushes in the front yard, he lost his balance, fell, and hit his head and right shoulder on the pavement of the driveway. He did not lose consciousness but dislocated the acromioclavicular joint, which resulted in severe soft tissue contusion. He received a laceration to the forehead and encountered severe pain in the shoulder region of his dominant right arm. Dominic was referred to a clinic, where he was first seen by a PT for pain management, to regain range of motion, and to strengthen his shoulder muscles. He was referred by his physician to receive OT services to assist him with performance in areas of occupation such as ADLs, instrumental activities of daily living (IADLs), work, and leisure. OT services were also provided to address his performance patterns with an emphasis on habits and routines.

As consistent with the Occupational Therapy Practice Framework,[3] an evaluation was conducted to develop an occupational profile. The occupational profile revealed that Dominic liked to read, prepare gourmet dinners for friends, and watch college basketball on television. His ability to engage in these occupations was hampered by the pain in his right shoulder and concerns

were identified regarding client safety in the home during dressing, meal preparation, and getting in and out of the shower. During activity demands in the physical context, the client presented with what appeared to be a balance disturbance especially when trying to walk down stairs to go to his car.

As a result of this balance disturbance, he was seen by a neurologist for further examination. The neurologist surmised that when the client injured his head it caused compression to the trochlear nerve (CN IV). The trochlear nerve is the only cranial nerve that exits the dorsal aspect of the brainstem and runs a long course to the cavernous sinus into the orbit, where it supplies the superior oblique muscle. Because of its long intracranial course, the nerve root is often at risk during head trauma. The trauma to the root of the trochlear nerve resulted in weakness of the superior oblique muscle, which caused outward rotation of the affected eye, which caused double vision (diplopia) and weakness in downward gaze.[30,97] Most commonly, clients with trochlear nerve involvement experience deviation of the eye when looking downward and inward, which causes difficulty descending stairs.

The intervention plan was designed with Dominic to establish and restore the function of his shoulder so that he could dress, restore his capacity to prepare gourmet meals, and return to his role as an attorney with a reduced workload. Although the PT used some topical analgesic and manual techniques on his shoulder, the severe pain did not subside and prevented him from performing areas of occupation. Dominic was taught how to apply a 10-minute ice massage to his painful shoulder. Current knowledge of pain management suggests that the combination of cold and massage motion over painful soft tissue reduces the temperature in tissues, slows down metabolic rate, reduces inflammation, reduces the formation of edema, alters nerve conduction velocity, reduces sensitivity of pain receptors thereby altering the perception of pain and can reduce muscle spasms.[67] Studies have shown that ice massage not only reduces pain, but its analgesic effect lasts longer than the use of heat or ice alone.[4] The client was instructed in how to perform the ice massage, 10 minutes before receiving occupational therapy intervention. The reduced pain enabled the client to put on his shirt and reach downward to pull up his pants and socks with a "reacher." The client was also taught how to use a massage vibrator over bruised parts of the shoulder region to increase proprioceptive stimulation and to increase circulation in the soft tissues. The combination of ice massage and vibration as restoration of body functions enabled the client to participate in areas of occupation.

Because the compression of the trochlear nerve root has recovery potential as a peripheral nerve, the prognosis for recovery and eye function was rather good. Initially, Dominic was taught to compensate for the double vision and weakness in downward gaze by performing motions in developmental patterns. For example, the client was able to participate in weight bearing on elbows by first sitting at a table with his elbows and forearms supported on the tabletop and then progress to the

*The first author wishes to acknowledge the inspirational leadership of Virginia Scardina in promoting the work of Margaret Rood.

Continued

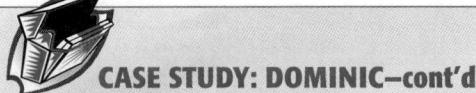

CASE STUDY: DOMINIC–cont'd

quadrupedal position. In this position, he was able to perform rocking and weight shift patterns, which helped to mobilize his shoulder, as he was looking at large printed reading material. The client learned to tilt his head toward the unaffected side, which thereby caused the uninvolved eye to turn and line up with the extorted or affected eye, which enabled him to regain biocular vision. By changing his head position to compensate for double vision, he was also able to actively shift his body weight in a safe position and receive vestibular stimulation through the movement of the hair cells in the vestibule and semicircular canals. Eventually, he was able to stand at the counter and sink and cut vegetables and meats in preparation for gourmet dinners. By using knowledge of sensory stimulation, neurophysiology, and basic pain management techniques, the client was able to regain the performance skills and patterns in the context of his home. As his vision improved and the pain subsided he was able to perform ADLs and IADLs independently. He was able resume many of his work responsibilities with a greater appreciation for maintaining a balance with work, play, and leisure.

Critical Thinking Questions

1. What justification would you offer for using the intervention methods described in this case study?
2. What would be your anticipated outcomes after using these methods?
3. What additional Rood techniques could be used to foster improved function?

Dominic's case was complicated, but it illustrates how Rood's techniques can be helpful for multiple problems of neurological or orthopedic origin. Much has changed in neuroscience and neurorehabilitation since Margaret Rood developed her original concepts. However, her contribution to the fields of OT and physical therapy (PT) has been substantial. This section has been revised with great care and respect for Rood's contributions. At the same time great care has been devoted to reviewing the current scientific evidence and research that both supports and refutes Rood's work. This section will review Rood's work from a new perspective.

Margaret S. Rood was formally educated in OT and PT. She originated her theory in the 1940s and revised it many times. Rood did not write extensively; she seemed to prefer clinical teaching for the dissemination of her ideas. Most of the literature that describes the Rood approach is based on interpretations by accomplished occupational and PTs such as Ayres,[6,7] Farber,[35] Heininger,[42] Randolph,[76] Huss,[49] and Stockmeyer.[85]

In the late 1960s, 1970s, and 1980s much interest was invested in the application of interventions from studies derived from animal models in neurophysiology.[16,33,65] Sensory physiology investigations were showing that sensory receptors had different thresholds for stimuli in laboratory models. Evidence showed that nerve impulses traveled along specific nerve fibers to specific laminae in the spinal cord, where the impulses would synapse and ascend in different pathways within the spinal cord.[39] For example, Rood believed that when the hair follicles on the skin were deflected or stimulated with a camel-hair brush over certain dermatomes, specific muscle groups (myotomes) could be facilitated through the gamma loop of the muscle spindle.[80] Rood believed that brushing hair follicles produced a lasting effect on muscle tone. This effect seemed to work on some muscle groups more than others. However, more recent evidence has shown that hair follicles adapt rapidly; therefore, their effect is short in duration. In contrast, pressure applied to the same area of skin activates the Ruffni endings, which are indeed slowly adapting.[39] Once again, one should not assume that a direct cause and effect relationship exists between stimuli and the response of cutaneous receptors.

The understanding of the nervous system during the time Rood developed her theory was based on a hierarchical model that was generated by systematic research on animals. In 1893 Sherrington performed segmental spinal and CNS lesions in frogs, cats, and monkeys and observed the motor deficits that ensued.[11,39] Head discovered that sensory distribution is segmentally oriented to spinal segments called *dermatomes*.[11,39,57] According to Rood's theory, sensory input can produce three different responses or reactions: (1) local reactions in the soft tissue matrix, (2) a regional reaction across two to three dermatomes through reflex arcs, and (3) a general reaction.[78-80] In summary, these early investigations developed a perception of the nervous system as being "hard wired" and its function was conceived to be hierarchical in nature.[30,42]

Current research continues to support Rood's premise that certain receptors in the skin carry impulses along unmyelinated C fibers and terminate in the substantia gelatinosa (lamina II), but we now know that fibers also terminate in other regions of the spinal cord. In addition, visceral C-afferents have disparate clusters of terminals in lamina II and their physiological significance is still unknown. Although a specific laminar distribution of terminal endings exists in the spinal cord, contrary to Rood's original thought, it does not mean that each lamina is dedicated to a single function. The majority of afferent fibers that synapse with dorsal horn cells are polysynaptic, which means they connect with divergent pathways. The primary afferents carrying impulses from the skin, muscles, tendons, and viscera influence cells in the CNS through both monosynaptic and polysynaptic connections.[13,16,30,39,40] At the same time, the impulses conveyed by afferent inputs may undergo greater or a lesser degree of modification and integration by synaptic connections within the spinal cord and from descending inhibitory neurons.[39,64] Furthermore, nerve fibers originating in muscles are not purely motor but are in part sensory (Ia afferent), and cutaneous nerve fibers are not purely sensory because they contain sympathetic efferents (unmyelinated pesudomotor) fibers.[64] In her clinical observations, Rood began to discover that cutaneous stimuli were less reliable, and brushing and icing was used with more caution on persons with neurological impairment.

On a systematic review of the literature, current thought in neurological rehabilitation suggests that long-term outcomes of neurophysiological techniques for children with cerebral palsy are best achieved when the intervention is applied at the appropriate developmental age and when the skills are associated with daily functional activities.[11,17,20,26,40] Current sensory physiology continues to support the proposition that each type of sensory receptor is sensitive to a particular modality (i.e. cold, heat, light pressure), yet many of these studies have been done on mechanoreceptors and proprioceptors in isolation. A general conclusion is that sensory receptors work in ensembles.[13,17,57,64,69] Therefore, it is unlikely that a single group of receptors can be exclusively activated by a stimulus. The stimulus response is multimodal and pervasive. A single stimulus can set off a cascade of impulses that affect the autonomic, endocrine, immune, and nervous systems.

Since the late 1980s, a large number of neuropeptides have been identified in primary sensory neurons and their central terminals.[39,64] We now know that these neuropeptides are capable of profoundly modifying the processing of somatosensory information in the dorsal horn of the spinal cord. These substances have a long-term modification or regulatory effect rather than the singular effect on an action potential that is produced by neurotransmitters. The neuropeptides are found in cells with unmyelinated axons in pelvic viscera. Neuropeptides are differentially distributed in the spinal cord and those fibers combined with autonomic nerve fibers. Neuropeptides have also been associated with emotions.[65,73]

As a result of these newly discovered substances, theories have given rise to the "wet brain theory," which suggests that neurotransmitters and neuropeptides play significant roles in transmission and modulation of neuronal activity. Researchers are also investigating the role of astrocytes, a type of glial cell, in the brain. Astrocytes are thought to play a greater role in affecting the action of neurons. Studies on levels of calcium and the amino acid glutamate suggest that astrocytes and neurons have a cell-to-cell communication. Astrocytes may produce trophic factors, specific molecules that nourish neurons and process information for memory.[8,95] Since the 1980s researchers have also found strong connections between the nervous, immune, and endocrine systems. Certain immune molecules known as cytokines may activate certain neurons by passing through leaky junctions in blood vessels or by triggering second messengers nitric acid and prostaglandins.[68] These active molecules suggests an evolving body-mind relationship that was unknown in Rood's time.

Rood used vibration as a proprioceptive stimulation to facilitate muscles. She found that when the tendon or muscle belly in a limb received vibratory stimuli, the underlying muscle was facilitated while the antagonist was inhibited (reciprocal innervation). However, current evidence suggests that the application of vibration to the skin has many other physiological effects. Vibration has been found to increase blood supply in soft tissues, and it has been shown to dissipate pain-mediating substances in tissues.[35,49,56] In a study on the effects of vibration on torticollis, vibration was found to cause lengthening of dystrophic neck muscles and was more effective than transcutaneous electrical nerve stimulation.[55] Another study showed that vibration releases substance P, causing inhibition of nociceptive neurons in the dorsal horn of the spinal cord.[27] Another study found that vibration stimulates large myelinated fibers in the skin, subcutaneous tissues, and muscles, but it can cause elevation of polypeptide hormones such as gastrin and cholecystokinin in the blood stream.[90] Gastrin is implicated in gastric acid secretion and cholecystokinin plays a role in facilitating digestion in the small intestine. However, the use of vibration as a therapeutic modality seems to have fallen out of favor in recent years. Electrical stimulation seems to be one of the most common modalities used in neurological rehabilitation today.* The use of modalities has also changed considerably in recent years. Practitioners are concerned with functional outcomes and use modalities mainly as adjunctive measures rather than the thrust of their intervention.[97]

As previously mentioned, theories and related frames of reference exist within the context of the time and level of knowledge from which they originate. Many would say that the work of Margaret Rood is out of date and thus not worthy of study. Some of the techniques and the hypotheses posed by Rood have never been adequately tested or researched. Nonetheless, to discount Rood's work as out of date is to discount an important historical perspective of OT and to dismiss the possibility of incorporating elements of her work into more recent understanding of CNS processing linked to therapeutic intervention. Thus, the purpose of this chapter is to offer a reconstruction of Rood's work based on current understanding of nervous system processing and occupation-based intervention.

A measure of the contribution of a scholar to a field is not whether he or she is ultimately determined to be right or wrong, but how much research and deliberation the person's work engendered. Rood's work continues to be valuable to OT in terms of orientation to the interaction of the nervous system with behavior, function, and, most significantly, occupation. For all of these reasons, the work of Margaret Rood is important for therapists to study.

The work of Margaret Rood was set in the context of the developmental and neurophysiological literature of the

---

*References 16,17,20,28,31,40,67,75.

1930s through the 1970s. In that context, the neuroscience literature was based on assumptions of the hierarchical nature of the nervous system that have subsequently been revised. In light of current understanding a reconstruction of Rood's work is executed based in part on current understanding of chaos theory and dynamic systems. Rood's main contribution has been to highlight the importance of interactions that occur between the nervous system and occupation (i.e., that the nervous system and occupation coeffect one another in a dynamic, nonlinear manner). **Coeffect** refers to the interaction of one or more forces upon the other force(s), which suggests a state or condition of active interdependence.

Specifically, Rood identified (1) that the feedback loops of motor and sensory signals coeffect each other, (2) that patterns of sensory-motor behaviors emerge over time, and (3) that the psychic, somatic, and autonomic functions operate within a system of coeffects or interrelationships.

RECONSTRUCTION OF ROOD'S THEORY FOR OCCUPATION-BASED PRACTICE

Rood's work has been synthesized into the essential concepts presented in Table 30-3, which provides a historical view with a reinterpretation of concepts that still apply.

As delineated in Table 30-3, six key concepts of Rood have been reconstructed (right column) from the traditional view (left column) in light of current knowledge and understanding

TABLE **30-3** **Summary of Main Concepts of Rood's Work**

Traditional Rood	Reconstruction of Rood
Normalization of muscle tone is a prerequisite for movement.	Muscle tone and motor control coeffect each other.
Treatment begins at the developmental level of functioning.	Flexion and extension patterns coeffect each other.
Reeducation of muscular responses occurs through repetition.	Repetition of muscular responses creates movement patterns.
Movement is directed toward functional goals.	Intention or goal direction coeffects movement.
Approximation of real life context increases treatment effectiveness and generalizability.*	Approximation of real life context increases treatment effectiveness and generalizability.
Therapeutic use of self should match client needs.*	Therapists use somatic markers to select interaction methods with clients.†

*This was a basic Rood premise taught to the first author by Margaret Rood during a 2-week training course in Cincinnati in the 1970s.
†See Chapter 8, "The Somatic Marker Hypothesis," in Damasio AR: *Descartes' error: emotion, reason and the human brain*, New York, 1994, Avon Books.

pertaining to the areas. Each of these reconstructed concepts is briefly discussed in the following paragraphs.

Muscle tone and motor control coeffect each other refers to the relationship that exists between the tone of the muscles and the execution of the motor act. These are but two parameters among a myriad of variables that influence movement. However, they are singled out for this special emphasis because Rood called for therapists to look at muscle tone as a contributor to movement. It is now known that muscle tone is not the only prerequisite for motor control and that those relative degrees of motor control can, in fact, exist in spite of poor or inadequate muscle tone. In electrical stimulation studies with clients who had sustained a stroke, it was found that the reduction of muscle tone is less important than muscle strength for functional motor control. However, grip strength was found to be a good marker for restoration of hand function.[10,20,22] In addition, current evidence suggests that neuroplasticity continues years after stroke and improvement in motor control is not a prerequisite for functional gain. Improvement in movement strategies and enhanced movement efficiency seem to be the keys for improved voluntary movement.*

Flexion and extension patterns coeffect each other refers to the dynamic relationship between flexion patterns experienced through everyday occupations and extension patterns also experienced through everyday occupations (e.g., sitting in a flexion pattern while reading this text). It is hypothesized that the balance or imbalance between flexion and extension patterns influence each other in a dynamic system of postural patterns. In all likelihood, humankind spends much more time in flexion patterns (sitting at work, sitting in front of the television, sitting while eating) than we were originally designed to do. Investigations using electrical stimulation to the extensors of the hand as compared with alternative stimulation of flexors and extensors did not show statistically significant differences on psychometric measures. However, participants reported that they gained functional improvements in the ability to grasp and release small objects and could use their affected arm in ADLs.[28,35]

Repetition of muscular response creates movement patterns refers to the learning that occurs through repeated neuromuscular actions that lay down the engrams for the repertoire of motor behavior available to a given individual. Functional neuroimaging studies of motor recovery after stroke show that cortical reorganization takes place in both hemispheres of the brain during recovery after stroke.[17,22,24] Recent studies support the assumption that repetition of muscular responses is efficacious. Rhythmic training has been shown to improve spatiotemporal arm control when compared with no rhythmic training.[89] In another randomized controlled trial, in clients with chronic motor impairment after stroke, specific repetitive bilateral arm training of

*References 17,22,28,61,63,86,88,89.

the upper extremities appeared to induce cortical reorganization in bilateral and contralesional hemisphere circuitry and in neurons in the cerebellum as shown through functional magnetic resonance imaging (MRI).[61] Preliminary findings in constraint induced movement techniques have shown positive findings in functional recovery and changes in functional MRI studies.[58,61,63,88] Furthermore, promising research evidence demonstrates that after a spinal cord injury, control of movement can be improved through repetition of body weight support and functional electrical stimulation techniques.[36]

Intention or goal direction coeffects movement refers to the developing research base that shows that intent of a motor action influences the nature and quality of motor action. Current studies on animal models (rhesus monkeys) show that tiny probes implanted into several regions of the brain can detect neural signals translated to a joystick and a cursor projected on a computer monitor. Through systematic operant conditioning the monkeys learned to guide the cursors and guide the movement of objects on the screen by thought process alone. The monkey was able to move a robotic arm with thoughts alone. This study has moved one step closer to a merger on mind and machine, which would be a major breakthrough for those who have severe motor deficits.[18,62]

Activities that provide approximation of real life context increase treatment effectiveness and **generalizability** refers to the supposition that performance in real life or simulated contexts increases the effectiveness of "practice" and, indeed, of therapy itself. Virtual reality systems are beginning to simulate occupations such as driving, sports, and negotiating environments such as crossing a busy street to promote neuronal activity in the motor cortex.[62]

In a more interpersonal manner, *therapists use somatic markers to select interaction methods with clients* refers to a working hypothesis that master clinicians intuitively and automatically "fit" their demeanor and emotional state to those of the client being served. **Somatic marker,** a term coined by Damasio,[25] is used here to refer to the collection of feelings or emotional tone of a person at any given time, in a learned response to a given situation. Somatic marker is a concept related to the larger conceptualization of meta-emotion. The term **meta-emotion** is used here to refer to the conceptualization and study of the interactions or coeffects between emotions, the body, and occupation (i.e., "feeling while doing"). Most precisely, meta-emotion of occupation refers to feeling/thinking about feeling/thinking while doing with meaning. Meta-emotion of occupation assumes the integration and shared variance between cognition and emotion.

ROOD'S FOUR COMPONENTS OF MOTOR CONTROL

Table 30-3 reveals that Margaret Rood's concepts pertaining to motor function were far ranging. An important contribution of her work is the emphasis she placed on components of motor control. She was a forerunner of current motor control theories in that she was among the first to identify and articulate the importance of components of motor control in the therapeutic context. Therapists can apply these same concepts today in occupation-based practice. Accordingly, the four components of motor control Rood emphasized are summarized below.

RECIPROCAL INHIBITION (INNERVATION)

Reciprocal inhibition is an early mobility pattern that serves a protective function. It is a phasic (quick) type of movement that requires contraction of the agonist muscle as the antagonist muscle relaxes. This basic movement pattern is primarily a reflex governed by spinal and supraspinal centers. It is, in fact, the underpinning for movement needed to engage in occupation. For example, the practitioner may apply a stimulus such as vibration on the agonist muscle as a client moves his or her arm toward an object for grasping or releasing. Recent evidence suggests that if the sensory stimulus is applied during the course of an ongoing movement, the quality of the action can be modulated and improved.[26,28]

COCONTRACTION (COINNERVATION)

Cocontraction, or coinnervation, provides stability and is considered a tonic (static) muscle pattern. This muscle pattern provides the ability to hold a position or an object for a longer duration. Cocontraction is the simultaneous contraction of the agonist muscle and antagonist muscle. It is the foundation of postural control, which provides the stability needed for engaging in occupation. For example, head control and postural control of the trunk are some of first areas where cocontraction is needed to perform valued occupations. Early activities using standing tables allowed for safe, upright positioning, which required cocontraction of muscles while the person performed simple tasks such as puzzle assembly to engage in occupation.

HEAVY WORK

Heavy work is described by Stockmeyer as "mobility superimposed on stability."[85] In this postural pattern the proximal muscles contract and move, whereas the distal segment is fixed. A good example of heavy work is creeping. In the quadruped position, the distal segments, wrists, and ankles are in a fixed position. The proximal joints, such as the neck and thorax, are stable, whereas the shoulder and hip girdles are free to move. Heavy work patterns may be associated with many of the occupations typically involved with agriculture and industry, such as lifting, moving, or pulling. It is hypothesized that modern society (Western civilization) lacks heavy work patterns, resulting in a functionally deficient neurophysiological state for members of this society.

SKILL

Skill is the highest level of motor control and combines the effort of mobility and stability.[78] In the execution of a skilled pattern the proximal segment is stabilized while the distal segment moves freely. The art of oil painting demonstrates this pattern. The artist stands back from the canvas, holds his or her arm at full length, and manipulates the brush freely in the hand. Skill is associated with many of the functions needed in the information age, such as typing and fine eye-hand coordination for computer work. It is further hypothesized that modern society has an excessive preponderance of skill demands, to the exclusion of heavy work patterns, with a resultant imbalance.

MOTOR PATTERNS

In this section the major motor patterns of development that Rood emphasized are reviewed. For each motor pattern photographs of humans engaged in the postural pattern as an activity or an occupation are shown.

SUPINE WITHDRAWAL (SUPINE FLEXION)

Supine withdrawal is a total flexion response toward the vertebral level of T10. This position is protective because the flexion of the neck and the crossing of the arms and legs protect the anterior surface of the body. This position is a mobility posture that requires reciprocal innervation, yet it also requires heavy work of the proximal muscles and the muscles of the trunk.[78] Therapeutically, supine withdrawal aids in the integration of the tonic labyrinthine reflex. Rood recommended this pattern for clients who lacked reciprocal flexion pattern and for individuals dominated by extensor tone (Figure 30-4).

ROLLOVER (TOWARD SIDE LYING)

When an individual is rolling over, the arm and leg flex on the same side of the body. This movement, **rollover,** is a mobility pattern for the extremities and activates the lateral trunk musculature.[88] Rollover is encouraged for individuals who are dominated by tonic reflex patterns in the supine position. The rolling action also stimulates the semicircular canals of the vestibular system, which in turn activate the neck and extraocular muscles (Figure 30-5).

PIVOT PRONE (PRONE EXTENSION)

The **pivot prone** position demands a full range of extension of the neck, shoulders, trunk, and lower extremities. This pattern has been called a mobility pattern and a stability pattern. The position is difficult to assume and hold against gravity. Therefore, the pivot prone position plays an important role

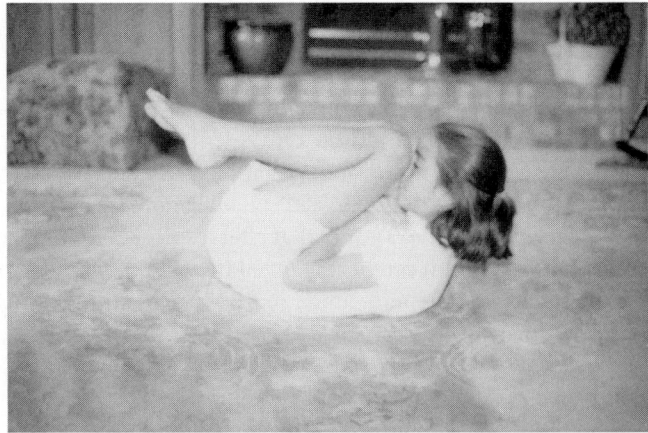

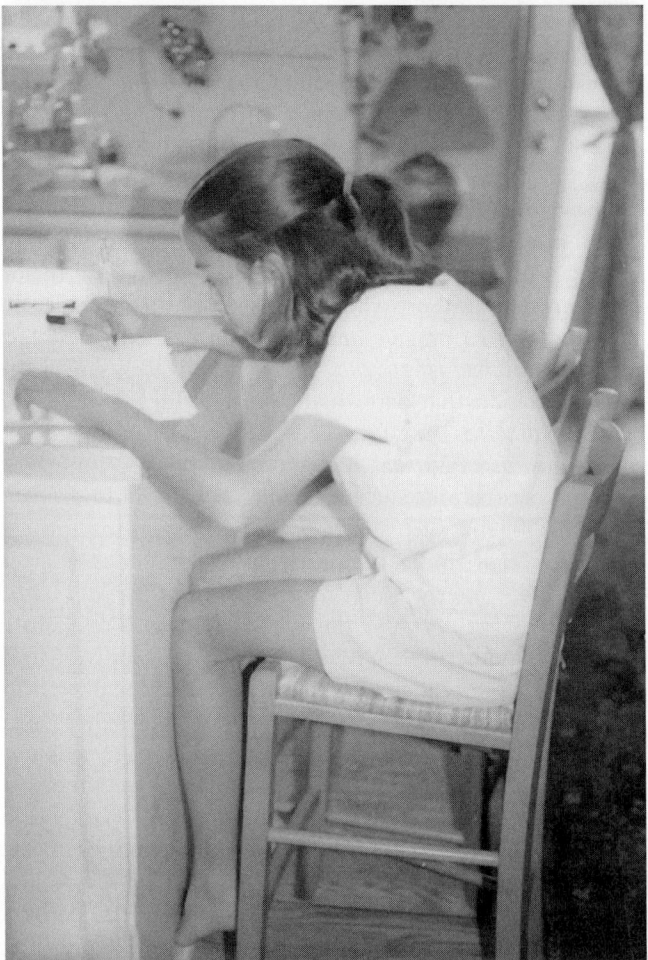

Figure 30-4 Supine withdrawal or supine flexion.

in preparation for stability of the extensor muscles in the upright position. The pivot prone position has been associated with the labyrinthine righting reaction of the head. The ability to maintain the position indicates integration of the symmetrical tonic neck reflexes and the tonic labyrinthine reflexes (Figure 30-6).

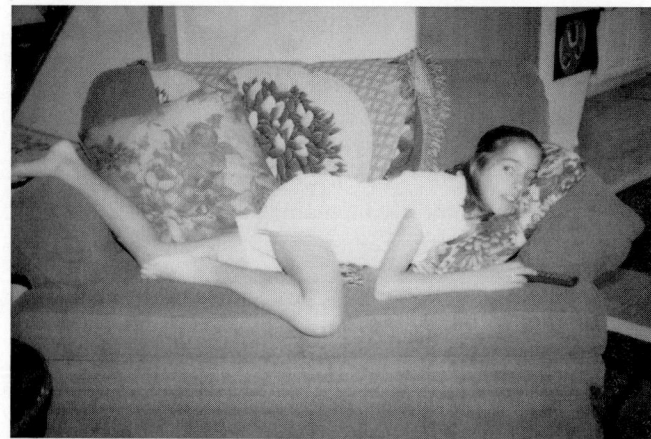

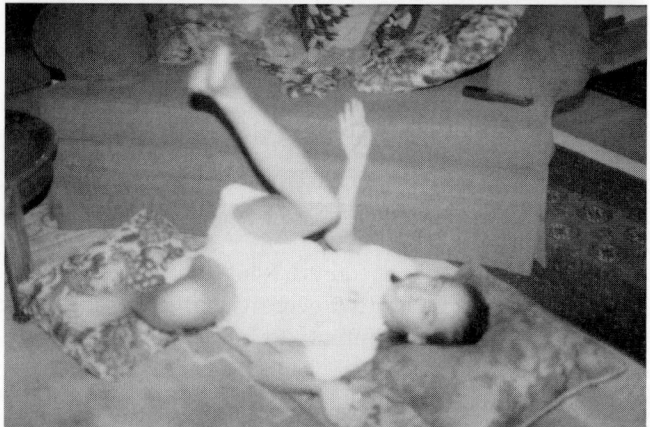

Figure 30-5 Rollover toward side lying.

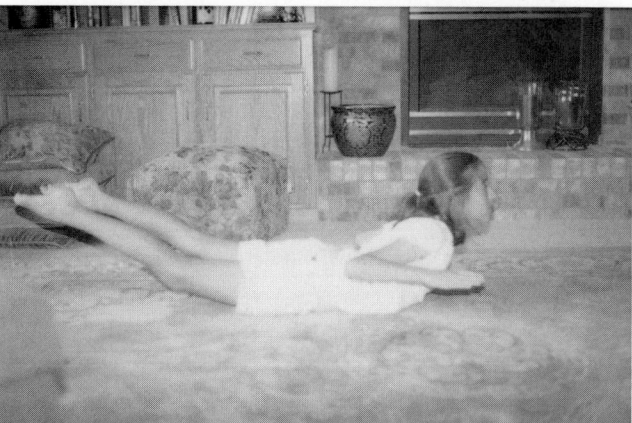

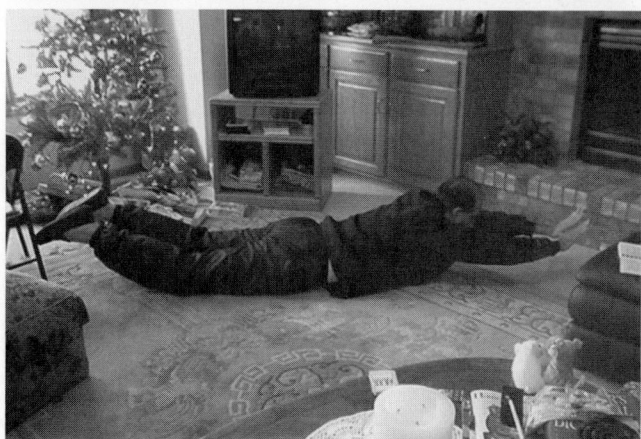

Figure 30-6 Pivot prone or prone extension.

NECK COCONTRACTION (COINNERVATION)

Neck cocontraction is the first genuine stability pattern. In keeping with the cephalocaudal and cephalorostral rules, cocontraction of the neck precedes cocontraction of the trunk and extremities. As the head bobs up and down, the extensors and rotators are stretched. This action is thought to activate flexors and deep tonic extensors of the neck.[78-80,85] It is important to make sure the neck flexors are well established, however, before the prone position is assumed. To raise the head against gravity, the client needs to have good cocontraction of the flexors and extensors of the neck.[35] Neurologically this pattern elicits the tonic labyrinthine righting reaction when the face is perpendicular to the floor. As the head flexes, it stretches the proprioceptors in the neck and upper trapezius, which causes them to contract against the forces of gravity.[42,49,80] This functional position also promotes neck stability and extraocular control (Figure 30-7).

ONTOGENETIC DEVELOPMENT PATTERNS

Ontogenetic development patterns observed in normal development are outlined in the following sections. In the past these patterns were used as a basis for therapy. It was assumed that motor control could be inhibited or facilitated by positioning in the patterns. It may be the case that these patterns have beneficial effects when combined with occupational engagement, but that these effects are not necessarily or exclusively on motor control. Future research will shed more light on these assumptions.[69]

ON ELBOWS (PRONE ON ELBOWS)

After cocontraction of the neck and prone extension, weight bearing on the elbows is the next pattern to be achieved. Bearing weight on the elbows stretches the upper trunk musculature to influence stability of the scapular and glenohumeral regions. This position gives the client better visibility of the environment and an opportunity to shift weight from side to side. It is also inhibitory to the symmetrical tonic neck reflex (Figure 30-8).

This method was used with Dominic to foster glenohumeral stability and mobilize his shoulder in a controlled situation. He was asked to sit at the kitchen table with his forearms and elbows resting on the table and then shift his body from side to side.

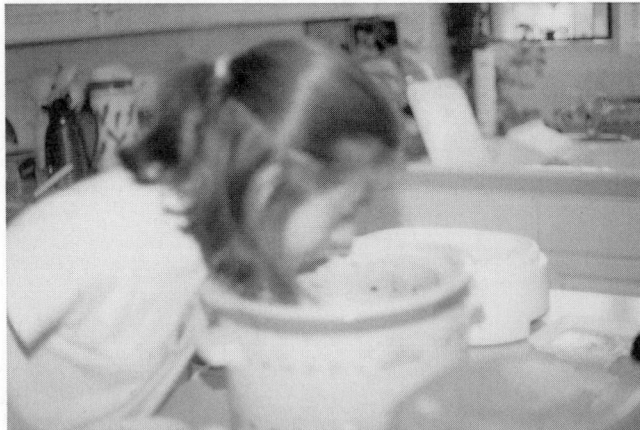

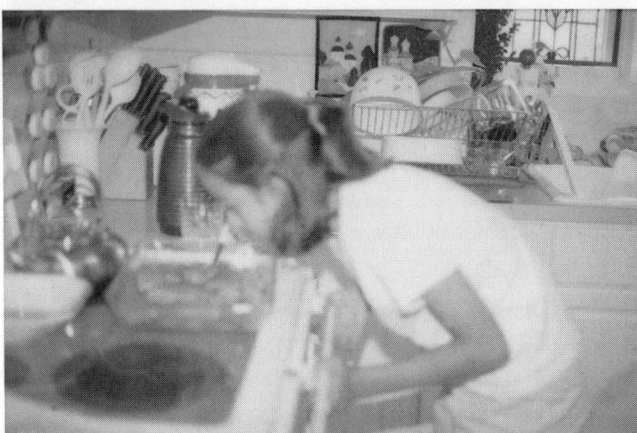

Figure 30-7 Neck cocontraction or coinnervation.

ALL FOURS (QUADRUPED POSITION)

The quadruped position follows stability of the neck and shoulders. The lower trunk and lower extremities are brought into a cocontraction pattern. Initially the position is static and the abdomen may sag at the T10 level, which causes stretching of the trunk and limb girdles. This stretching develops cocontraction of the trunk flexors and extensors. Eventually shifting weight forward, backward, side to side, and diagonally provides mobility superimposed on the stability phase. The weight shifting may be preparatory to equilibrium responses (Figure 30-9).

This was also used with Dominic as he gained control of his shoulder girdle and pain diminished. The movement was helpful in providing vestibular input while he worked on improving visual motor control.

STATIC STANDING

Assuming the upright bipedal position, static standing is thought to be a skill of the upper trunk because it frees the upper extremities for prehension and manipulation.[78,85] Weight is first equally distributed on both legs, and then

weight shifting begins. This position brings into play higher level neurological integration, such as righting reactions and equilibrium reactions (Figure 30-10).

WALKING

The gait pattern unites skill, mobility, and stability. Normal locomotion entails the ability to support the body weight, maintain balance, and execute the stepping motion.[4,31,61] Walking includes a stance phase, push off, swing, heel strike, and stride length.[31] Walking is a sophisticated process requiring coordinated movement patterns of various parts of the body, including weight shifting (Figure 30-11).

In addition to the theoretical emphasis Rood placed upon the previously discussed motor patterns, she developed many innovative treatment strategies and techniques, as described in the following section.

TRADITIONAL ROOD TREATMENT TECHNIQUES FOR OCCUPATION-BASED PRACTICE

The reader is likely to encounter Rood techniques in practice. Knowledge of advanced neuroscience is revealing that these techniques may continue to have value in practice. Table 30-4 presents a summary of traditional treatment techniques employed by Rood.

OT PRACTICE NOTE

Caution is urged in adopting any or all of these techniques in current occupation-based practice because these interventions are designed to specifically influence client factors such as muscle tone and not occupation per se. Thus, occupation-based practice would never include the provision of any of these treatment techniques isolated from an occupation. Also, these interventions unduly address motor function as isolated from the dynamic system of engagement in occupation.

Of the previously identified Rood intervention techniques, those most relevant to today's practice and those consistent with the current understanding of neuroscience were selected for summary presentation in this section. Further, only interventions appropriate for entry-level practice are discussed.

PROPRIOCEPTIVE FACILITATORY TECHNIQUES

Proprioceptive stimulation refers to the use of sensory input to improve movement of body parts by the facilitation of muscle spindles, Golgi tendon organs, joint receptors, and the vestibular apparatus.[59,65] In general, the goal of proprioceptive

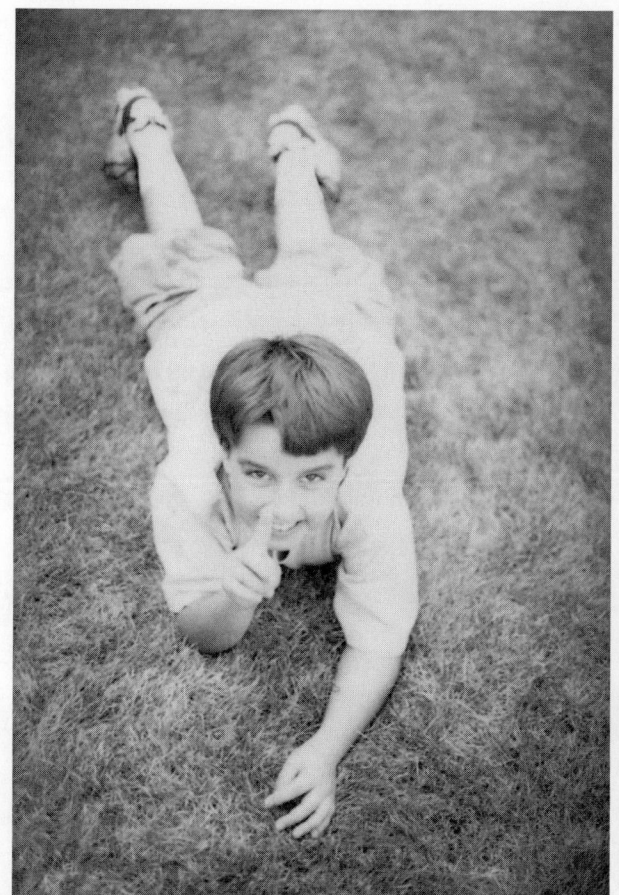
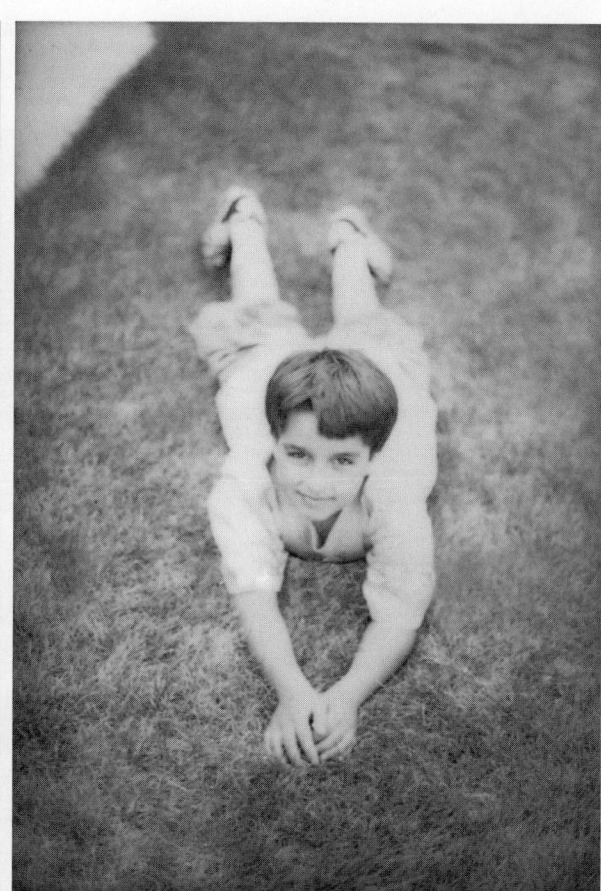

Figure 30-8 Prone on elbows.

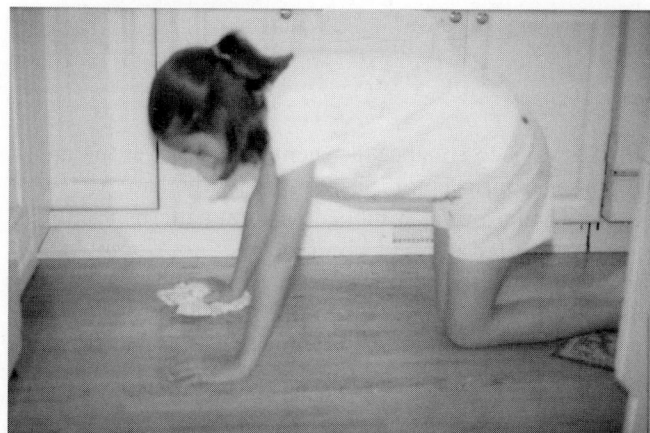
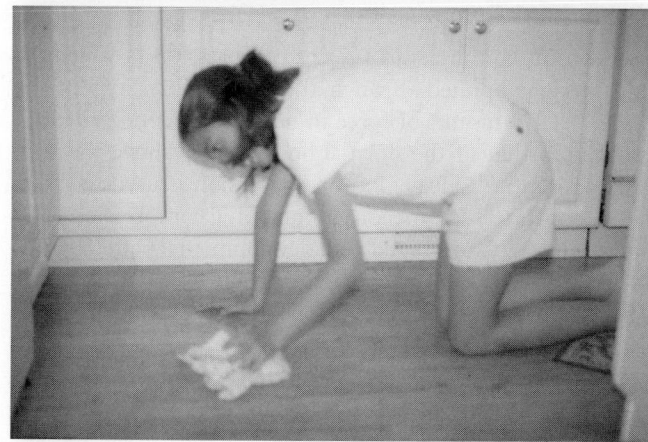

Figure 30-9 Quadruped (all fours).

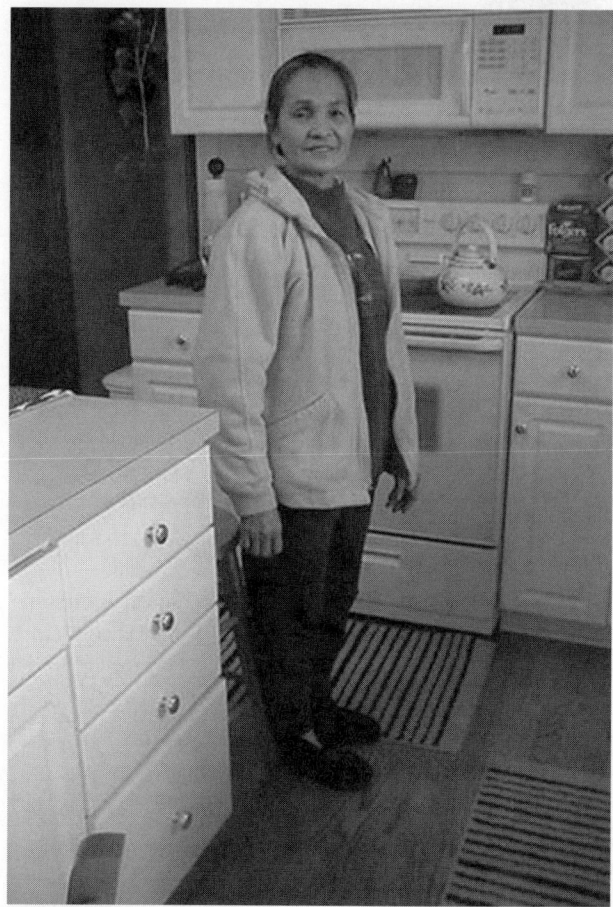

Figure 30-10 Static standing.

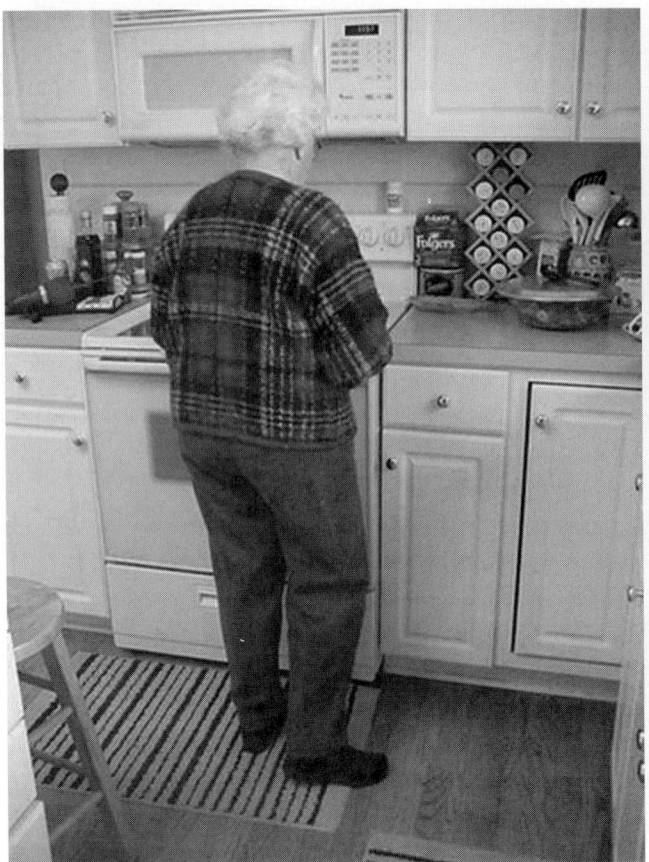
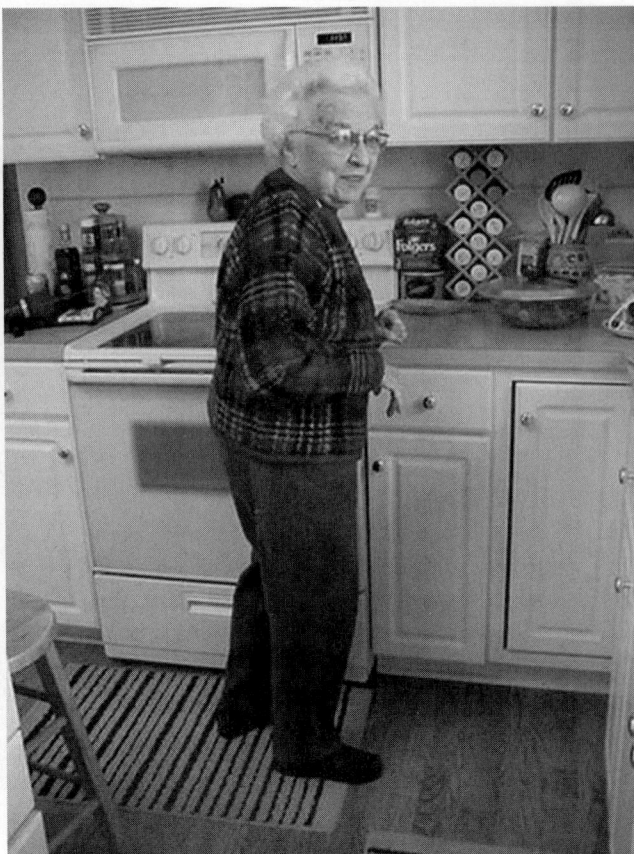

Figure 30-11 Weight shifting.

TABLE **30-4** **Summary of Rood Facilitatory and Inhibitory Techniques**

Cutaneous Facilitation Techniques	Proprioceptive Facilitation Techniques	Inhibitory Techniques
Light moving touch*	Heavy joint compression	Neutral warmth
Fast brushing*	Resistance	Joint approximation
Icing*	Vestibular stimulation	Slow stroking
	Inversion	Rocking
	Stretch pressure*	Gentle shaking or rocking*
	Stretch*	Tendinous pressure*
	Intrinsic stretch*	Maintained stretch*
	Secondary ending stretch*	Slow rolling*
	Tapping*	
	Therapeutic vibration*	
	Osteopressure*	

*These techniques are well beyond the scope of entry-level practice and are therefore not dealt with in this chapter.

stimulation is to enhance the client's control over the motor response. Proprioceptors adapt more slowly than exteroceptors and can produce sustained postural patterns.[64] Little or no neuronal recruitment occurs in the proprioceptive system. Therefore, the motor response is thought to last as long as the stimulus is applied.[64,98] Four types of proprioceptive facilitatory techniques are described in the following paragraphs: heavy joint compression, resistance, vestibular stimulation, and inversion.*

Heavy Joint Compression

Heavy joint compression is joint compression greater than body weight applied through the longitudinal axis of the bone.[6,7] The amount of force in heavy joint compression is more than that of the normal body weight above the supporting joint.[42,49] Heavy joint compression is used to facilitate cocontraction at the joint undergoing compression. This approach can be combined with developmental patterns, such as prone on elbows, quadruped, sitting, and standing positions. The joint compression may be done manually by the therapist

---

*References 33,35,40,75,76,78,79.

or with weighted wrist cuffs or sandbags. Clinically, joint compression is most effective when applied through the longitudinal axis of long bones such as the humerus (glenohumeral joint) and the femur (acetabulum).

Resistance

Rood used heavy resistance to stimulate primary and secondary nerve endings of the muscle spindle. Resistance is used in an isotonic fashion in developmental patterns to influence the stabilizer muscles. According to Stockmeyer,[85] resistance to contraction of muscles in the shortened range facilitates muscle spindle afferents in the deeper, tonic postural muscles. Farber[35] used quick stretch before resistance to increase the responsiveness of the muscle spindle. In addition, when a muscle contracts against resistance, it assumes a shortened length that causes the muscle spindles to contract to readjust to the shorter length. This is the process of biasing the muscle spindle so that it is more sensitive to stretch. Intermittent resistance graded to the desired motion is better than manual stretching for alleviating tight muscles.[35,42,80]

Vestibular Stimulation

Vestibular stimulation is a powerful sensory input.[7,29] The static labyrinthine system can be used to promote extensor patterns of the neck, trunk, and extremities.[38] The kinetic labyrinth can be used to elicit phasic subcortical responses such as protective extension.[38] Jones and Watt[52] studied muscular responses to unexpected falls in human subjects. Their findings demonstrate that the vestibular system activates the antigravity muscles and their antagonists before the stretch reflex of the muscle spindles. The vestibular system is a divergent system that affects tone, balance, directionality, protective responses, cranial nerve function, bilateral integration, auditory language development, and eye pursuits.[29,97,98] The vestibular system is stimulated during linear acceleration and deceleration in horizontal and vertical planes and during angular acceleration and deceleration, such as spinning, rolling, and swinging. Vestibular stimulation can be either facilitatory or inhibitory, depending on the rate of stimulation. Fast rocking tends to stimulate, whereas slow, rhythmic rocking tends to cause a generalized relaxation response.[6,7,35]

Inversion

Rood encouraged the use of the inverted position (**inversion**) to alter muscle tone in selected muscles. In the inverted position the static vestibular system produces increased tonicity of the muscles of the neck, midline trunk extensors, and selected extensors in the limbs.[42,79] In studies on human subjects the effects of head position on selected skeletal muscles have been measured. The findings indicate that extensor tone is maximized in certain muscles in the head-down position, whereas extensor tone is minimized in those muscles in the upright position. For best results, the head must be in normal alignment with the neck. If the neck is flexed or extended, the tonic neck reflex interferes with the response.[29,38,65] Inversion should be used with extreme care for individuals with cardiovascular disease. As the head approaches a point below the level of the shoulders, baroreceptors in the carotid sinus are stimulated by blood pressure changes. This positioning produces a physiological response through the parasympathetic nervous system, reducing blood pressure, decreasing muscle tone, and promoting generalized relaxation. Inversion techniques can be combined with vibration or neck compression to change tone in selected muscles.[6,7,35,42,85]

INHIBITORY TECHNIQUES

Four **inhibitory techniques** are neutral warmth, slow stroking, light joint compression, and rocking in developmental patterns.

Neutral Warmth

The neutral warmth technique most likely affects the temperature receptors of the hypothalamus and stimulates the parasympathetic nervous system.[30,40,42] Neutral warmth can be used for individuals with hypertonia, particularly those with spasticity and rigidity. It may also be helpful for children with attention deficit disorders.[7,35] The provision of neutral warmth can be accomplished by having the individual assume a recumbent position while the entire body is wrapped in a cotton blanket or comforter for approximately 5 to 10 minutes. Neutral warmth provides a moderate amount of heat that is homeostatically compatible with the receptors of the hypothalamus. The individual usually feels relaxed, and muscle tone is decreased.[49,73]

Slow Stroking

Slow stroking has been described as an inhibitory technique. The individual lies in the prone position while the therapist provides rhythmic, moving, deep pressure over the dorsal distribution of the primary posterior rami of the spine. The therapist applies fingertip pressure on both sides of the spinous process to affect the nerve endings and the sympathetic outflow of the autonomic nervous system. The stroking action is done slowly and continuously from the occiput to the coccyx. The hands are alternated so that as one hand reaches the bottom of the spine, the other is starting downward from the top.[35,42,49,73,76] Inhibition techniques have been found to be clinically beneficial when accompanied by soft music. Music also has been used as a closure technique following sensory integrative therapy to calm children after vestibular and proprioceptive facilitation. Slow stroking should not exceed 3 minutes because it may cause a rebound phenomenon, resulting in excitation of the sympathetic branch of the autonomic nervous system.[35,85]

Light Joint Compression (Approximation)

Joint compression of body weight or less than body weight can be used to inhibit spastic muscles around a joint.[78,80] This technique may be used with individuals who have hemiplegia to alleviate pain and temporarily offset the muscle imbalance around the shoulder joint.[35] The individual can be sitting or lying in the supine position. The therapist places one hand over the individual's shoulder and the other hand under the flexed elbow joint. The arm is abducted 35 degrees to 45 degrees, and a compression force of body weight or less is applied through the longitudinal axis of the humerus.[7] This procedure compresses the glenohumeral joint and the articulation between the humerus and ulna. Moreover, if applied properly, this technique compresses two joints but has the most dramatic effect on the shoulder. Once the muscles begin to relax, the therapist can slowly and gently circumduct the humerus in small circles to reduce pain and stiffness in the shoulder joint.[35] Joint compression of the shoulder and elbow joints can also be achieved when the client is in the on-elbows position. Light joint compression is also beneficial when applied through the longitudinal axis of the wrist and elbow joints.[35,73] The therapist places one hand behind the elbow and places the individual's forearm in midposition; the wrist joint is extended, and compression is applied through the heel of the client's hand. Joint compression has its greatest effect during the time that the stimulus is applied.[11,20,35,42,49]

Rocking in Developmental Patterns

In keeping with the developmental sequence and Rood's concept of mobility superimposed on stability, Rood encouraged movement as the individual gained mastery of the static position.[80,85] Developmentally, the individual first must assume and be able to achieve a static position and then integrate coordinated movements while maintaining the posture. Rood referred to this process as the development of "skill." For example, in the quadruped position, the client shifts weight to a three-point stance so that one hand is free to reach forward to grasp and explore the immediate environment. Movement may begin by shifting the weight forward and backward. The shifting may progress to side-to-side and diagonal patterns as the client becomes comfortable with the rhythmic movements.[35] In the quadruped position, individuals with hemiplegia are assisted by achieving stability of the involved elbow when the therapist applies pressure and stretch to the triceps brachii and anconeus. As the therapist applies compression that is greater than body weight to facilitate cocontraction, the pressure exerted on the extended wrist and heel of the hand inhibits the wrist flexors. Light, moving touch over the dorsum of the hand is performed to promote finger extension.[35,42,78] Rocking in the quadruped position should first be performed with the neck in a straight, normal relationship to the body so that the proprioceptors of the neck do not influence the tonicity of the limbs.[78-80] As the individual moves in an anteroposterior plane, the shoulder and pelvic girdles are mobilized. Later in treatment, the therapist may want to incorporate flexion, extension, and rotation of the neck as a reflex inhibition measure.[79]

RECONSTRUCTION OF THE ROOD APPROACH FOR OCCUPATION-BASED PRACTICE

Traditionally, OTs used the previously described techniques primarily to prepare an individual for purposeful activities. Hence, a basic tenet of the Rood approach is that activity should be purposeful—that is, occupation-based. The introduction of purposeful activities leading to occupation adds meaning and relevance to the endeavor. Rood's methods are most useful in preparation for engagement in occupation. Reconceptualization of her work in light of current research and knowledge is most useful in understanding and thinking about occupational performance in context. Specifically, Rood's conceptual framework is reconstructed in the next section.

ROOD'S CONCEPTUAL FRAMEWORK: A RECONSTRUCTION

Five key assumptions underlie thinking about occupation-based practice in context (Figure 30-12). These functions are adapted from Stockmeyer,[85] who presented Rood's initial work.

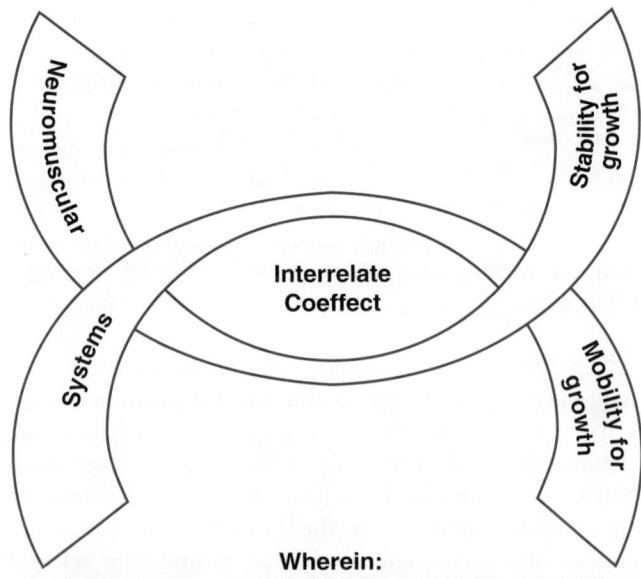

Wherein:
Stability based upon structural and functional design
Mobility for survival through protection and movement

Figure 30-12 A reconstruction of Rood's conceptual framework. (Figure designed by Rene Padilla, OTR-L.)

TABLE **30-5** **Heuristic of Rood Reconstructed**

Neuromuscular Network	Function	Key Control Parameter	Associated Outcome
Network I	Inspiration	Cranial nerve V	Supine flexion: body functions
	Suck	Medial longitudinal fasciculus (MLF)	
	Swallow		
	Flexion		
Network II	Extension	Vestibulospinal tract (VST)	Pivot prone: antigravity
Network III	Cocontraction	Muscle spindle	Joint stability: posture
Network IV	Mobility	Corticospinal tract (CST)	Movement through space: skill
Network V	Motivation	Limbic system	Engagement in occupation
		Frontal lobe	
		Cognition	
		Emotions	

Assumption 1: Neuromuscular function related to occupation is a chaotic system of multiple networks interacting and changing, based upon coeffects and sensitivity to initial conditions.

Assumption 2: As a chaotic system, neuromuscular function unfolds in a dynamic process.

Assumption 3: Key control parameters influencing the neuromuscular system are the somatic, autonomic, emotional, and cognitive or motivational variables.

Assumption 4: Motor and sensory systems coeffect each other.

Assumption 5: Occupation shapes function.

In the future, it is likely that others will elaborate on these key assumptions based on the work of Rood.

Finally, as a way to think about the networks that subserve motor function as a foundation for occupation, Table 30-5 is provided as a heuristic. Note that this heuristic links networks to function, control parameters, and associated outcomes and reflects the essence of Rood's thinking as updated with current neuroscientific knowledge and understanding. The reader is referred to Royeen[82] for more about integrating complexity and chaos theory with occupation.

SUMMARY

This chapter offers a reconstruction of Margaret Rood's work based on current understanding of CNS processing and therapeutic intervention. Chaos theory and dynamic systems theory are used to help reconstruct her theory for occupation-based practice. Rood's original components of motor control in therapeutic intervention provide the basis for engagement in occupation. Major motor patterns of development originally developed by Rood and their purpose in occupations are delineated. Traditional Rood treatment techniques for entry-level practice and the application of these techniques to occupation-based practice are summarized, based on current findings in neuroscience. In conjunction with Rood's tenet that activity should be purposeful; the context of occupational performance is emphasized. A conceptual framework is proposed based on Rood's important

concepts, which provided five key assumptions in occupation-based practice in context. Finally, a heuristic is provided to identify the networks that subserve motor function as a foundation for occupation.

SECTION 2: PROPRIOCEPTIVE NEUROMUSCULAR FACILITATION APPROACH

Sara A. Pope-Davis, Judy M. Jourdan

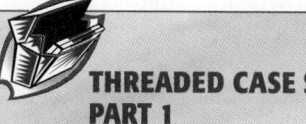

THREADED CASE STUDY: LETICIA, PART 1

Leticia, a 34-year-old married mother of two, was involved in an automobile accident in which she sustained a brain injury and fractures of her left wrist and several ribs. Leticia's injuries left her with diplopia, a rigid posture, and a lack of motor control resulting from ataxia. As a mother, Leticia had always been involved with her children and was a teacher's aide at their grade school. It is important to Leticia that she resume her parenting role, including caring for their home, driving a car, and resuming her work in the classroom. Unfortunately, she fatigues quickly and struggles to engage in the routine daily activities she used to enjoy with her family. She specifically references her desire to be able to play games with her children, prepare family meals, and tutor children in the third grade class in which she assisted before her accident.

Critical Thinking Questions

1. How do you know which movement patterns to select to help Leticia regain the ability to perform these family- and work-related occupations or tasks?

Continued

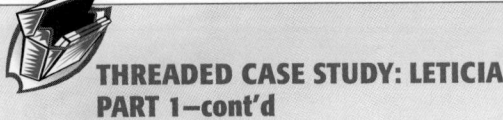

THREADED CASE STUDY: LETICIA, PART 1—cont'd

2. Which PNF techniques will most effectively address Leticia's impairments and how do you select a PNF technique to facilitate the desired performance of a task?

3. How do you determine the progression of intervention from a PNF perspective?

Based upon normal movement and motor development, **proprioceptive neuromuscular facilitation** (PNF) is more than a technique, it is a philosophy of intervention. Through the case study of Leticia we will discuss the application of PNF to the evaluation and intervention of occupational therapy. Basic principles, diagonal patterns, and more commonly used techniques will be introduced, and their application and presence in routine daily life skills will be demonstrated. PNF addresses the client factors of posture, mobility, strength, effort, and coordination. To use PNF effectively, it is necessary to understand normal development, learn the motor skills to use the techniques, and apply the concepts and techniques to OT activities. This section should form the basis for further reading and training under the supervision of a therapist experienced in PNF.

PNF is based on normal movement and motor development. In normal motor activity the brain registers total movement and not individual muscle action.[50] Encompassed in the PNF approach are mass movement patterns that are spiral and diagonal in nature and that resemble movement seen in functional activities. In this multisensory approach, facilitation techniques are superimposed on movement patterns and postures through the therapist's manual contacts, verbal commands, and visual cues. These facilitation techniques and movement patterns can be preparatory methods that prepare the client to participate more effectively in their daily occupations or applied within the performance of a task.

PNF is used as an intervention technique for numerous conditions, including Parkinson's disease, spinal cord injuries, arthritis, stroke, head injuries, and hand injuries.

HISTORY

PNF originated with Dr. Herman Kabat, physician and neurophysiologist, in the 1940s. He applied neurophysiological principles, based on the work of Sherrington, to the intervention of paralysis secondary to poliomyelitis and multiple sclerosis. In 1948 Kabat and Henry Kaiser founded the Kabat-Keiser Institute in Vallejo, California. Here Kabat worked with PT Margaret Knott to develop the PNF method of intervention. By 1951 the **diagonal patterns** and core techniques were established. PNF is now used to treat numerous neurological, musculoskeletal, and general medical conditions.

In 1952 Dorothy Voss, a PT, joined the staff at the Kaiser-Kabat Institute. She and Knott undertook the teaching and supervision of staff therapists. In 1954 Knott and Voss presented the first 2-week course in Vallejo. Two years later, the first edition of *Proprioceptive Neuromuscular Facilitation* by Margaret Knott and Dorothy Voss was published by Harper & Row.

During this same period several reports in the *American Journal of Occupational Therapy* described PNF and its application to OT intervention.[5,19,23,53,91,96] It was not until 1974 that the first PNF course for OTs, taught by Dorothy Voss, was offered. Since then, Beverly Myers, an OT, and others have offered courses for OTs throughout the United States. In 1984 PNF was first taught concurrently to both PTs and OTs at the Rehabilitation Institute in Chicago.[72,94] Today courses are offered throughout the United States as well as Europe, Asia, and South America.

PRINCIPLES OF INTERVENTION

Voss presented 11 principles of intervention at the Northwestern University Special Therapeutic Exercise Project in 1966. These principles were developed from concepts in the fields of neurophysiology, motor learning, and motor behavior and are still essential to the practice of PNF today.[92]

All human beings have potentials that have not been fully developed. This philosophy is the underlying basis of PNF. Therefore, in evaluation and intervention planning, the client's abilities and potentials are emphasized. For example, the client who has weakness on one side of the body can use the intact side to assist the weaker part. Likewise, the client who has hemiplegia with a flaccid arm can use the intact head, neck, and trunk musculature to begin reinforcement of the weak arm in weight-bearing activities.

Normal motor development proceeds in a cervicocaudal and proximodistal direction. The cervicocaudal and proximodistal direction is followed in evaluation and intervention. When severe disability is present, attention is first given to the head and neck region, with its visual, auditory, and vestibular receptors, and then to the upper trunk and extremities. If the superior region is intact, an effective source of reinforcement for the inferior region is available.[94] The proximodistal direction is followed by developing adequate function in the head, neck, and trunk before developing function in the extremities. This approach is of particular importance in intervention that facilitates fine motor coordination in the upper extremities. Unless adequate control exists in the head, neck, and trunk region, fine motor skills cannot be developed effectively. For example, Leticia needs to strengthen her head, neck, and trunk muscles to regain adequate postural control before she can adequately perform fine motor tasks required in her job such as cutting with scissors. This illustrates how addressing a specific client factor of postural control can influence occupational performance.

Early motor behavior is dominated by reflex activity. Mature motor behavior is supported or reinforced by postural reflexes. As the human being matures, primitive reflexes are integrated and available for reinforcement to allow for progressive development such as that of rolling, crawling, and sitting. Reflexes also have been noted to have an effect on tone changes in the extremities. Hellebrandt, Schade, and Carns[44] studied the effect of the tonic neck reflex (TNR) and the asymmetrical tonic neck reflex (ATNR) on changes in tone and movement in the extremities of normal adults. They found that head and neck movement significantly affected arm and leg movement. In applying this finding to intervention, for example, weak elbow extensors can be reinforced with the ATNR by having the client look toward the side of weakness. Likewise, the client can be assisted in assuming postures with the influence of reflex support. For example, Leticia can use the body-on-body righting reflex to support her ability to assume sitting upright on the edge of the bed from a side-lying position when she gets up in the morning.

Early motor behavior is characterized by spontaneous movement, which oscillates between extremes of flexion and extension. These movements are rhythmic and reversing in character. In intervention it is important to attend to both directions of movement. When the OT practitioner is working with the client on getting up from a chair, attention also must be given to sitting back down. Often with an injury, the eccentric contraction (e.g., sitting down) is lost and becomes very difficult for the client to regain. If not properly treated, the client may be left with inadequate motor control to sit down smoothly and thus may "drop" into a chair. This eccentric control would be particularly important for Leticia because she is required to sit in low chairs at her children's school. Similarly, in training for ADLs the client must learn how to get undressed and dressed.

Developing motor behavior is expressed in an orderly sequence of total patterns of movement and posture. In the normal infant the sequence of total patterns is demonstrated through the progression of locomotion. The infant learns to roll, to crawl, to creep, and finally to stand and walk. Throughout these stages of locomotion the infant also learns to use the extremities in different patterns and within different postures. Initially the hands are used for reaching and grasping within the most supported postures, such as supine and prone. As postural control develops, the infant begins to use the hands in side-lying, sitting, and standing positions. In intervention, to maximize motor performance, clients should be given opportunities to work in a variety of developmental postures. The use of extremities in total patterns requires interaction with component patterns of the head, neck, and trunk. For example, in swinging a tennis racquet in a forehand stroke, the arm and the head, neck, and trunk move in the direction of the swing. Without the interaction

of the distal and proximal components, movement becomes less powerful and less coordinated.

The growth of motor behavior has cyclic trends, as evidenced by shifts between flexor and extensor dominance. The shifts between antagonists help to develop muscle balance and control. One of the main goals of the PNF intervention approach is to establish a balance between antagonists. Developmentally the infant establishes this balance before creeping (i.e., when rocking forward [extensor dominant] and backward [flexor dominant] on hands and knees). Postural control and balance must be achieved before movement can begin in this position. In intervention it is important to establish a balance between antagonistic muscles by first observing where imbalance exists and then facilitating the weaker component. For example, if the client who has a stroke demonstrates a flexor synergy (flexor dominant), extension should be facilitated.

Normal motor development has an orderly sequence but lacks a step-by-step quality. Overlapping occurs. The child does not perfect performance of one activity before beginning another, more advanced activity. In trying to ascertain in which total pattern to position the client, normal motor development should be heeded. If one technique or developmental posture is not effective in obtaining the desired result, it may be necessary to try the activity in another developmental posture. For example, if a client who has ataxia, such as Leticia, is unable to perform a fine motor task while sitting, it may be necessary to practice skills in a more supported posture, such as prone on the elbows or with her elbows supported on a surface such as a table. Just as the infant reverts to a more secure posture when attempting a complex fine motor task, so must the client. On the other hand, if the client has not perfected a motor activity such as walking on level surfaces, he or she may benefit from attempting a higher-level activity such as walking up or down stairs, which in turn can improve ambulation on level surfaces. It is natural for the client to move up and down the developmental sequence, and this allows multiple and varied opportunities for practicing motor activities. The cognitive demands of the task in relation to the developmental posture also must be considered. When the client's position is varied, either by changing the base of support or by shifting weight on different extremities, the quality of visual and cognitive processing is influenced.[1]

Locomotion depends on reciprocal contraction of flexors and extensors, and the maintenance of posture requires continual adjustment for nuances of imbalance. Antagonistic pairs of movements, reflexes, and muscles and joint motion interact as necessary with the movement or posture. This principle restates one of the main objectives of PNF—to achieve a balance between antagonists. An example of imbalance is the client with a head injury who is unable to maintain adequate sitting balance for a tabletop cognitive activity because of a dominance of trunk extensor tone. Another example is the client who has hemiplegia with tight finger flexors secondary to flexor-dominant tone in the hand.

In intervention, emphasis is placed on correcting the imbalances. In the presence of spasticity, first the spasticity is inhibited and then the antagonistic muscles, reflexes, and postures are facilitated.

Improvement in motor ability is dependent upon motor learning. Multisensory input from the therapist facilitates the client's motor learning and is an integral part of the PNF approach. For example, the therapist may work with a client on a shoulder flexion activity such as reaching into the cabinet for a cup. The therapist may say, "Reach for the cup," to add verbal input. This approach also encourages the client to look in the direction of the movement to allow vision to enhance the motor response. Thus, tactile, auditory, and visual input are used. Motor learning has occurred when these external cues are no longer needed for adequate performance.

Frequency of stimulation and repetitive activity are used to promote and retain motor learning and to develop strength and endurance. Just as the therapist who is learning PNF needs the opportunity to practice the techniques, the client needs the opportunity to practice new motor skills. With practice, habits will be formed that support motor performance in occupation. In the process of development the infant constantly repeats a motor skill in many settings and developmental postures until it is mastered, as becomes apparent to anyone who watches a child learning to walk. Numerous attempts fail, but efforts are repeated until the skill is mastered. After the activity is learned, it becomes part of the child. He or she is able to use the activity automatically and deliberately as the occasion demands.[94] The same is true for the person learning to play the piano or to play tennis. Without the opportunity to practice, motor learning cannot successfully occur. Just as Leticia's students may be given homework to help them practice the material they learn in school, Leticia will also need to be given a home program that encourages her to practice the postures and movements facilitated in therapy.

Goal-directed activities coupled with techniques of facilitation are used to hasten learning of total patterns of walking and self-care activities. When facilitation techniques are applied to self-care, the objective is improved functional ability, but improvement is obtained by more than instruction and practice. The correction of deficiencies is accomplished by direct application of manual contacts and techniques to facilitate a desired response.[48] During an intervention session, this approach may mean applying **stretch** to finger extensors to facilitate release of an object or providing joint approximation through the shoulders and pelvis of a client who has ataxia to provide stability while the client is standing to wash dishes. With repetition of appropriate facilitation techniques, Leticia will have the opportunity to feel more normal movement and need to rely less on the therapist's external input.

MOTOR LEARNING

Motor learning requires a multisensory approach. Auditory, visual, and tactile systems are all used to achieve the desired response. The correct combination of sensory input with each client should be ascertained, implemented, and altered as the client progresses. The developmental level of the client and the ability to cooperate also should be taken into consideration.[94] The approach used with a client who has aphasia differs from the approach used with a client who has a hand injury. For example, verbal instructions would be better understood by the client with a hand injury than the client with aphasia. Less verbal and more tactile and gestural cues would be appropriate with the client who has aphasia. Similarly, the approach used with a child varies greatly from that used with an adult. Interventions with Leticia must take into consideration her visual deficits in addition to any cognitive impairment that remains as a result of her head injury.

AUDITORY SYSTEM

Verbal commands should be brief and clear. It is important to time the command so that it does not come too early or too late in relation to the motor act. Tone of voice may influence the quality of the client's response. Buchwald[16] states that tones of moderate intensity evoke gamma motor neuron activity and that louder tones can alter alpha motor neuron activity. Strong, sharp commands simulate a stress situation and are used when maximal stimulation of motor response is desired. A soft tone of voice is used to offer reassurance and to encourage a smooth movement, as in the presence of pain (e.g., when techniques are used to increase the mobility in Leticia's left wrist). When a client is giving the best effort, a moderate tone can be used.[94]

Another effect of auditory feedback on motor performance was studied by Loomis and Boersma.[60] They used a "**verbal mediation** strategy" to teach wheelchair safety before transferring out of the chair to clients with right CVA. Loomis and Boersma taught clients to say aloud the steps required to leave the wheelchair safely and independently. They found that only clients who used verbal mediation learned the wheelchair drill sufficiently to perform safe and independent transfers. These clients also had better retention of the sequence of steps, which suggests that verbal mediation is beneficial in reaching independence with better sequencing and fewer errors.

When Leticia first arrived in therapy, she suffered considerable pain at the site of her wrist fracture. Early PNF intervention should use soft verbal commands when activities that involve wrist mobility are performed. In contrast, when facilitating Leticia's ability to perform assumption of postures (i.e., moving from side-lying to tall kneeling), more forceful, sharp commands may be needed.

VISUAL SYSTEM

Visual stimuli assist in initiation and coordination of movement. Visual input should be monitored to ensure that the client is tracking in the direction of movement. For example, the therapist's position is important because the client often uses the therapist's movement or position as a visual cue. If the therapist desires Leticia to move in a forward direction, he or she should be positioned diagonally in front of the client. In addition to the therapist's position, placement of the OT activity also should be considered. Using one of her children's favorite board games, the therapist could place it in front and to the left of Leticia to achieve the goal of increased head, neck, and trunk rotation. Because OT is activity oriented, an abundance of visual stimuli is offered to the client.

Special consideration will need to be given to the use of vision when working with Leticia. Her stronger head and neck musculature can be used to reinforce oculomotor control. Total body and extremity diagonal patterns can be used to reinforce eye teaming.

TACTILE SYSTEM

Developmentally the tactile system matures before the auditory and visual systems.[34] Furthermore, the tactile system is more efficient. This is because it has temporal and spatial discrimination abilities, as opposed to the visual system, which can make only spatial discriminations, and the auditory system, which can make only temporal discriminations.[41] Affolter[2] states that during development, processing of tactile-kinesthetic information can be considered fundamental for building cognitive and emotional experience. Looking at and listening to the world do not result in change; however, the world cannot be touched without some change taking place. A Chinese proverb often cited at PNF courses reinforces this viewpoint: "I listen and I forget, I see and I remember, I do and I understand."

It is important for the client to feel movement patterns that are coordinated and balanced. This is particularly important for clients with ataxia, such as Leticia. With the PNF approach, tactile input is supplied through the therapist's **manual contacts** to guide and reinforce the desired response. This approach may involve gently touching the client to guide movement, using stretch to initiate movement, and providing resistance to strengthen movement. The type and extent of manual contacts depend on the client's clinical status, which is determined through evaluation and reevaluation. For example, the use of stretch or resistance in the presence of musculoskeletal instability may be contraindicated, as in the early healing phases of Leticia's fractures. Likewise, stretch or resistance should not be used if they cause increased pain or tone imbalance.

To increase speed and accuracy in motor performance, the client needs the opportunity to practice. Through repetition, habit patterns that occur automatically without voluntary effort are established. The PNF approach uses the concepts of **part-task practice** and **whole-task practice.** In other words, to learn the whole task, emphasis is placed on the parts of the task that the client is unable to perform independently. The term **stepwise procedures** is descriptive

of the emphasis on a part of the task during performance of the whole.[94] Performance of each part of the task is improved by combining practice with appropriate sensory cues and techniques of facilitation. For example, the client learning to transfer from a wheelchair to a tub bench may have difficulty lifting the leg over the tub rim. This part of the task should be practiced, with repetition and facilitation techniques to the hip flexors, during performance of the transfer. When the transfer becomes smooth and coordinated, it is no longer necessary to practice each part individually. It is also unnecessary for the therapist to provide continued facilitation.

Leticia has difficulty getting down on the floor to play games with her children. In intervention, she should be provided with facilitation and practice of moving from sitting on a chair to tall kneeling to side-sitting on the floor. She will initially require considerable manual facilitation by the therapist to move through and achieve these various movement patterns. As she develops more skill, the therapist will reduce and adjust the intensity of the tactile input.

In summation, several components are necessary for motor learning to occur. In the PNF intervention approach, these components include multisensory input from the therapist's verbal commands, visual cues, and manual contacts. Touch is the most efficient form of stimulation and provides the opportunity for the client to feel normal movement. Current motor-learning theory argues that for motor learning to occur, the client cannot be a passive recipient of intervention. Therefore, the client needs opportunities to practice motor skills in the context of functional life situations. Initially the therapist's manual contacts and sensory input are needed. These should be decreased, however, as the client demonstrates and learns skilled movement. The amount of feedback from the therapist should also be decreased as the client learns to rely on his or her own internal feedback system for error detection and correction.

ASSESSMENT

Assessment of the client requires astute observational skills and knowledge of normal movement. An initial assessment is completed to determine the client's abilities, deficiencies, and potential. After the intervention plan is established, ongoing assessment of the client is necessary to ascertain the effectiveness of intervention and to make modifications as the client changes.

The PNF assessment follows a sequence from proximal to distal. First, vital and related functions are considered, such as breathing, swallowing, voice production, facial and oral musculature, and visual-ocular control. Any impairment or weakness in these functions is noted. Because Leticia fatigues quickly, breathing patterns and efficiency need to be closely evaluated as she engages in her daily activities.

The head and neck region is observed after vital functions. Deficiencies in this area directly affect the upper trunk and extremities. Head and neck positions are observed in varying postures and total patterns during functional activities. It is important to note (1) dominance of tone (flexor or extensor), (2) alignment (midline or shift to one side), and (3) stability and mobility (more or less needed).[72]

After observation of the head and neck region, the assessment proceeds to the following parts of the body: upper trunk, upper extremities, lower trunk, and lower extremities. Each segment is assessed individually in specific movement patterns, in addition to in developmental activities in which the body segments interact. For example, shoulder flexion can be observed in an individual upper-extremity movement pattern, in addition to during a total developmental pattern such as rolling.

During assessment of developmental activities and postures, the following issues should be addressed:

- Is there a need for more stability or mobility?
- Is there a balance between flexors and extensors, or is one more dominant?
- Is the client able to move in all directions?
- What are the major limitations (e.g., weakness, incoordination, spasticity, and contractures)?
- Is the client able to assume a posture and to maintain it? If not, which total pattern or postures are inadequate?
- Are the inadequacies more proximal or distal?
- Which sensory input does the client respond to most effectively—auditory, visual, or tactile?
- Which techniques of facilitation does the client respond to best?

When applying these questions to Leticia's evaluation the following observations can be made. First, Leticia will need to work on developing stability to diminish the effects of her ataxia. She is not dominated by either flexor or extensor tone, but when fatigued has more difficulty maintaining upright posture. She will therefore need to have facilitation of head, neck, and trunk extensors when fatigued. She can move in all directions but has less stability when walking backwards. Her major limitations are poor motor control and rigidity, but prevention of a wrist contracture is also a concern. Leticia is having difficulty assuming kneeling, sitting, and standing postures because of her instability. Once in an upright posture, she can maintain it for a few minutes, but then fatigue sets in. She will therefore need to build endurance in more supported lower developmental postures. When moving into more upright postures, she will need PNF techniques to build strength and endurance. Her inadequate proximal control and trunk rigidity impact her ability to effectively use her extremities, especially in higher developmental positions. Visual sensory input may not be the best to start with because of her diplopia; however, facilitation of oculomotor control using PNF techniques will be of benefit as she progresses. Facilitation techniques that Leticia responds to best are rhythmic stabilization, stabilizing reversals, and approximation.

Finally the client is observed during self-care and other ADLs to determine whether performance of individual and total patterns is adequate within the context of a functional activity. The client's performance may vary from one setting to another. After the client leaves the structured setting of the OT or PT clinic for the less structured home or community environment, deterioration of motor performance is not unusual. Thus, the intervention plan must accommodate the practice of motor performance in a variety of settings in locations appropriate to the specific activity.

INTERVENTION IMPLEMENTATION

After assessment an intervention plan is developed that includes goals the client hopes to accomplish. The techniques and procedures that have the most favorable influence on movement and posture are used. Similarly, appropriate total patterns (developmental postures) and patterns of facilitation are selected to enhance performance.

DIAGONAL PATTERNS

The diagonal patterns used in the PNF approach are mass movement patterns observed in most functional activities. Part of the challenge in OT assessment and intervention is recognition of the diagonal patterns in ADLs. Knowledge of the diagonals is necessary for identifying areas of deficiency. Two diagonal motions are present for each major part of the body: head and neck, upper and lower trunk, and extremities. Each diagonal pattern has a flexion and extension component, together with rotation and movement away from or toward the midline.

The head, neck, and trunk patterns are referred to as (1) flexion with rotation to the right or left and (2) extension with rotation to the right or left. These proximal patterns combine with the extremity diagonals. The upper and lower extremity diagonals are described according to the three movement components at the shoulder and hip: (1) flexion and extension, (2) abduction and adduction, and (3) external and internal rotation. Voss[92] introduced shorter descriptions for the extremity patterns in 1967 and referred to them as diagonal 1 (D_1) flexion/extension and diagonal 2 (D_2) flexion/extension. The reference points for flexion and extension are the shoulder and hip joints of the upper and lower extremities, respectively.

The movements associated with each diagonal and examples of these patterns seen in self-care and other ADLs are presented in the following sections. Note that in functional activities, not all components of the pattern or full range of motion (ROM) are necessarily seen. Furthermore, the diagonals interact during functional movement, changing from one pattern or combination to another, when they cross the transverse and sagittal planes of the body.[71]

Unilateral Patterns

1. *Upper extremity (UE) D_1 flexion (shoulder flexion-adduction-external rotation):* Scapula elevation, abduction, and rotation;

shoulder flexion, adduction, and external rotation; elbow in flexion or extension; forearm supination; wrist flexion to the radial side; finger flexion and adduction; thumb adduction (Figure 30-13, *A*). Examples in functional activity: hand-to-mouth motion in feeding, tennis forehand, combing hair on the left side of the head with right hand (Figure 30-14, *A*), rolling from supine to prone.

2. *UE D₁ extension (shoulder extension-abduction-internal rotation):* Scapula depression, adduction, and rotation; shoulder extension, abduction, and internal rotation; elbow

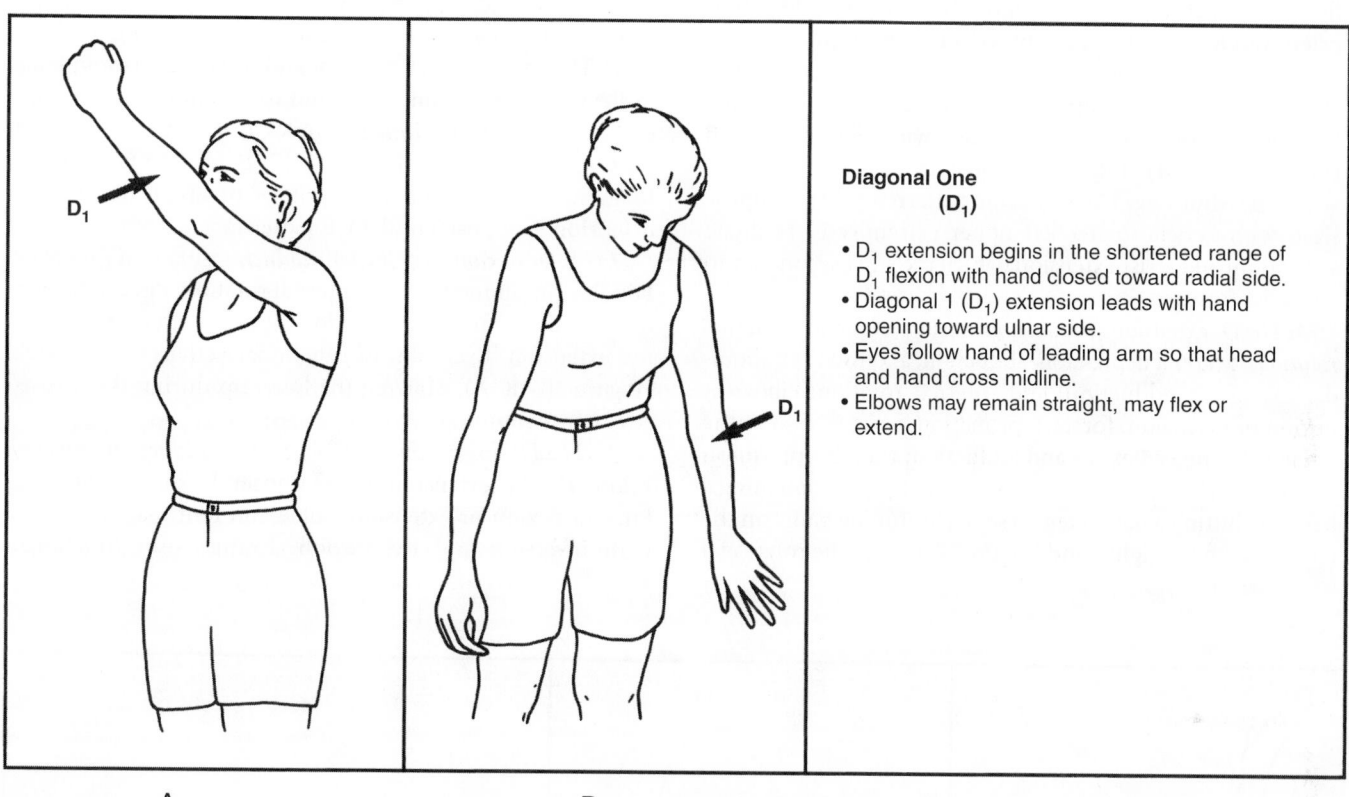

Diagonal One (D₁)

• D₁ extension begins in the shortened range of D₁ flexion with hand closed toward radial side.
• Diagonal 1 (D₁) extension leads with hand opening toward ulnar side.
• Eyes follow hand of leading arm so that head and hand cross midline.
• Elbows may remain straight, may flex or extend.

A   B

Figure 30-13   **A,** Upper extremity D₁ flexion pattern. **B,** Upper extremity D₁ extension pattern. (From Myers BJ: *Unit I: PNF diagonal patterns and their application to functional activities,* videotape study guide, Rehabilitation Institute of Chicago, 1982.)

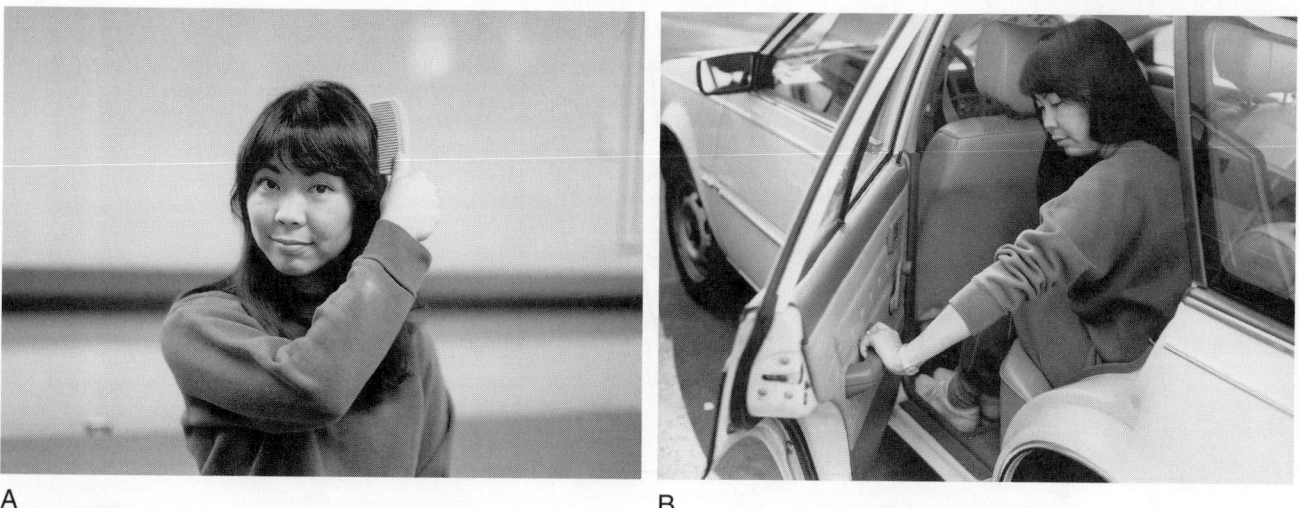

A   B

Figure 30-14   **A,** Upper extremity D₁ flexion pattern is used in combing hair, opposite side. **B,** Upper extremity D₁ extension pattern is used in pushing a car door open.

in flexion or extension; forearm pronation; wrist extension to the ulnar side; finger extension and abduction; thumb in palmar abduction (Figure 30-13, *B*). Examples in functional activity: pushing a car door open from the inside (Figure 30-14, *B*), tennis backhand stroke, rolling from prone to supine.

3. *UE D₂ flexion (shoulder flexion-abduction-external rotation):* Scapula elevation, adduction, and rotation; shoulder flexion, abduction, and external rotation; elbow in flexion or extension; forearm supination; wrist extension to the radial side; finger extension and abduction; thumb extension (Figure 30-15, *A*). Examples in functional activity: combing hair on the right side of the head with the right hand (Figure 30-16, *A*), lifting a racquet in tennis serve, back stroke in swimming. The D₂ flexion pattern would be emphasized with Leticia in her left upper extremity to facilitate supination and wrist extension, which are weak secondary to her wrist fracture.

4. *UE D₂ extension (shoulder extension-adduction-internal rotation):* Scapula depression, abduction, and rotation; shoulder extension, adduction, and internal rotation; elbow in flexion or extension; forearm pronation; wrist flexion to the ulnar side; finger flexion and adduction; thumb opposition (Figure 30-15, *B*). Examples in functional activity: pitching a baseball, hitting a ball in tennis serve, buttoning pants on the left side with the right hand (Figure 30-16, *B*). The rotational

component in LE D₁ flexion and extension parallels the UE patterns.

5. *LE D₁ flexion (hip flexion-adduction-external rotation):* Hip flexion, adduction, and external rotation; knee in flexion or extension; ankle and foot dorsiflexion with inversion and toe extension. Examples in functional activity: kicking a soccer ball, rolling from supine to prone, putting on a shoe with legs crossed (Figure 30-17, *A*).

6. *LE D₁ extension (hip extension-abduction-internal rotation):* Hip extension, abduction, and internal rotation; knee in flexion or extension; ankle and foot plantar flexion with eversion and toe flexion. Examples in functional activity: putting leg into pants (Figure 30-17, *B*), rolling from prone to supine. The rotational component of LE D₂ flexion and extension is opposite to the UE patterns.

7. *LE D₂ flexion (hip flexion-abduction-internal rotation):* Hip flexion, abduction, and internal rotation; knee in flexion or extension; ankle and foot dorsiflexion with eversion and toe extension. Examples in functional activity: karate kick (Figure 30-18, *A*), drawing the heels up during the breaststroke in swimming.

8. *LE D₂ extension (hip extension-adduction-external rotation):* Hip extension, adduction and external rotation: knee in flexion or extension; ankle and foot plantar flexion with inversion and toe flexion. Examples of functional

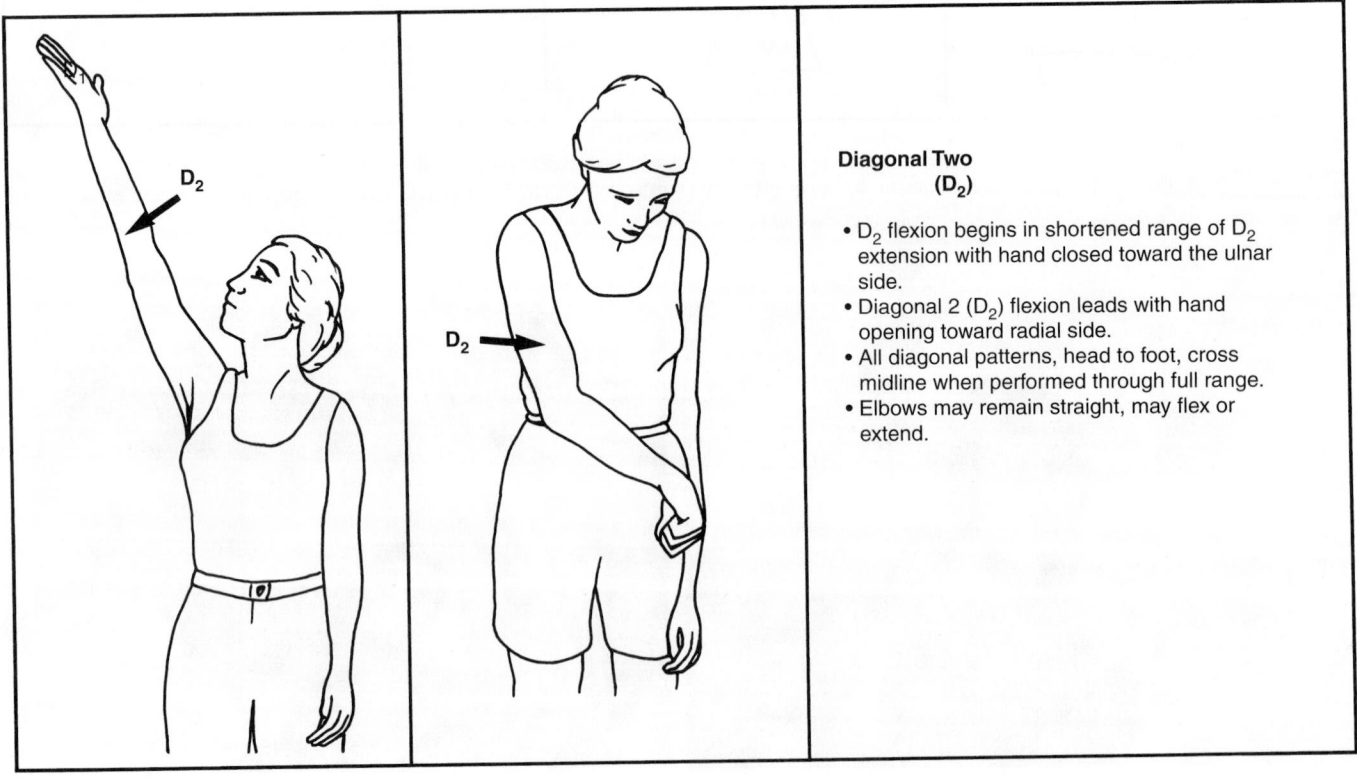

Diagonal Two (D₂)

- D₂ flexion begins in shortened range of D₂ extension with hand closed toward the ulnar side.
- Diagonal 2 (D₂) flexion leads with hand opening toward radial side.
- All diagonal patterns, head to foot, cross midline when performed through full range.
- Elbows may remain straight, may flex or extend.

A   B

Figure 30-15   **A,** Upper extremity D₂ flexion pattern. **B,** Upper extremity D₂ extension pattern. (From Myers BJ: *Unit I: PNF diagonal patterns and their application to functional activities,* videotape study guide, Rehabilitation Institute of Chicago, 1982.)

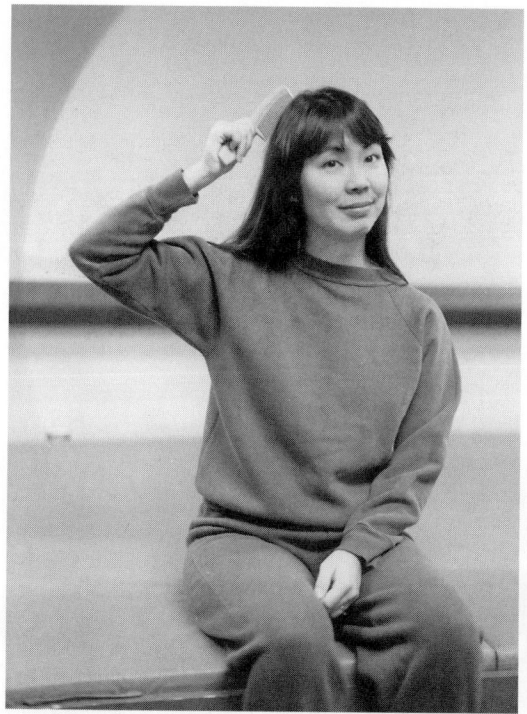
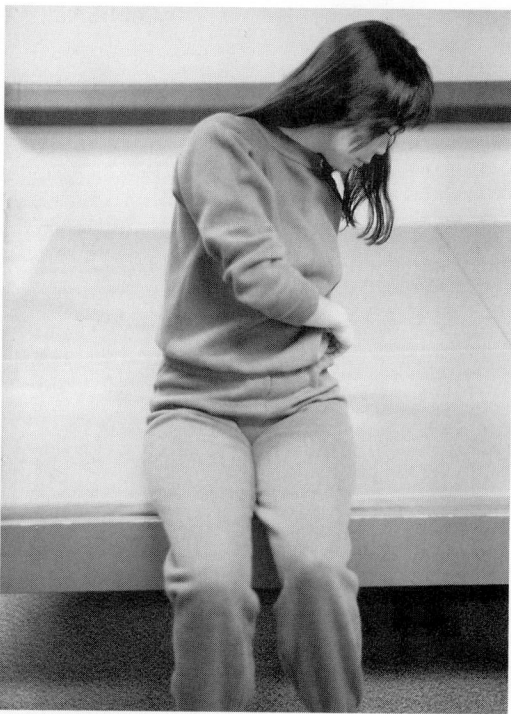

A   B

Figure 30-16 **A,** Upper extremity D₂ flexion pattern is used in combing hair, same side. **B,** Upper extremity D₂ extension pattern is used in buttoning trousers, opposite side.

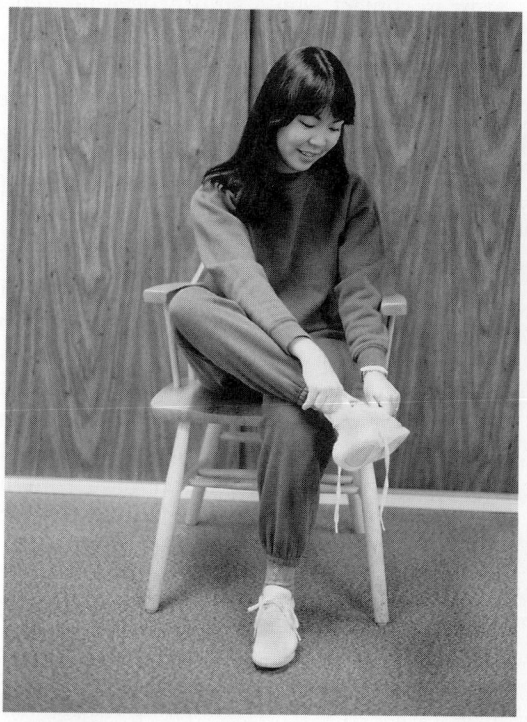
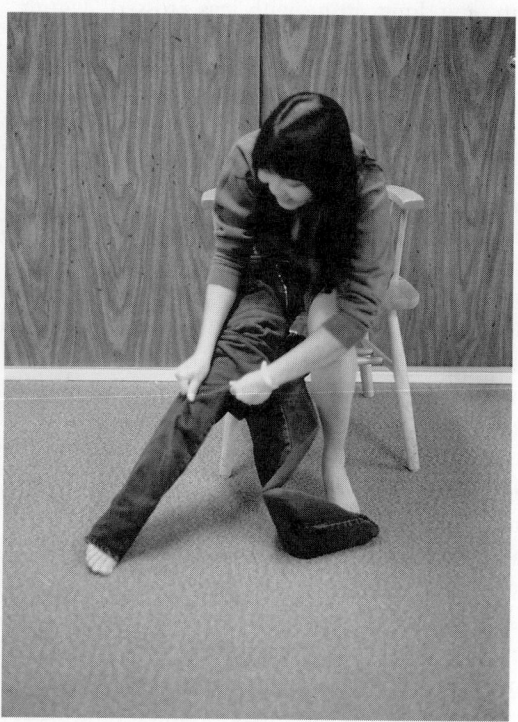

A   B

Figure 30-17 **A,** Lower extremity D₁ flexion pattern is demonstrated in crossed leg when putting on shoe. **B,** Lower extremity D₁ extension pattern is used when pulling on trousers.

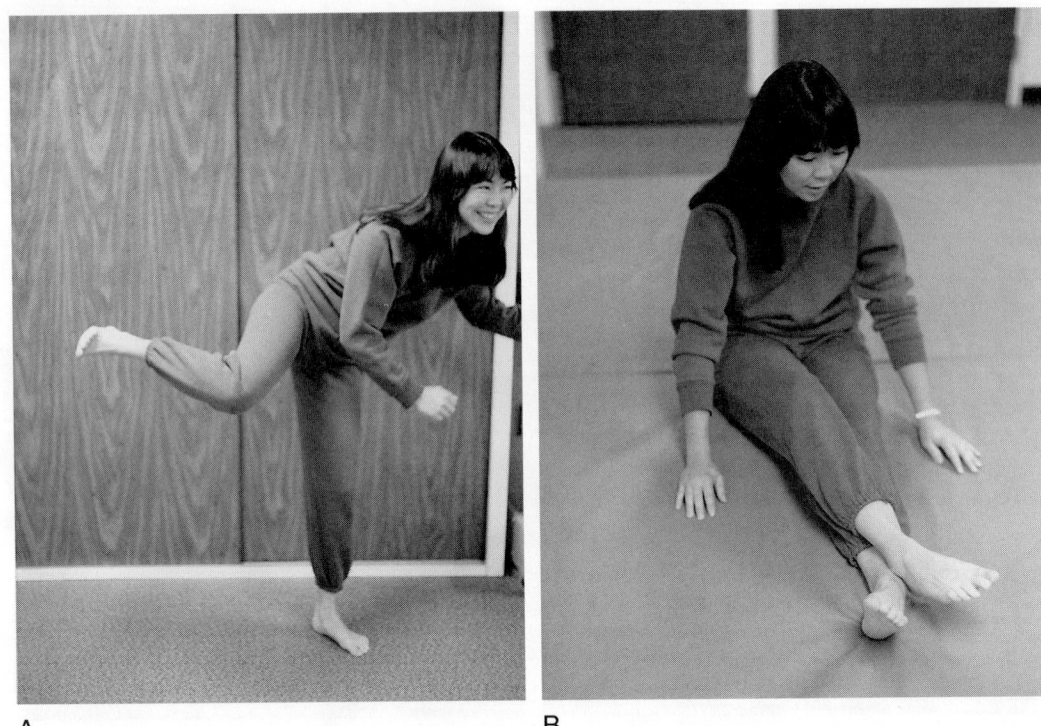

A   B

Figure 30-18 **A,** Lower extremity D_2 flexion pattern is shown in karate kick. **B,** Lower extremity D_2 extension pattern is used in long sitting with legs crossed.

activity: push-off in gait, the kick during the breast-stroke in swimming, long sitting with legs crossed (Figure 30-18, *B*).

Bilateral Patterns

Movements in the extremities may be reinforced by combining diagonals in **bilateral patterns** as follows:

1. *Symmetrical patterns:* Paired extremities perform similar movements at the same time (Figure 30-19, *A*). Examples: bilateral symmetrical D_1 extension, such as pushing off a chair to stand (Figure 30-20, *A*); bilateral symmetrical D_2 extension, such as starting to take off a pullover sweater (Figure 30-20, *B*); bilateral symmetrical D_2 flexion, such as reaching to lift a large item off a high shelf (Figure 30-20, *C*). Bilateral symmetrical UE patterns facilitate trunk flexion and extension.

2. *Asymmetrical patterns:* Paired extremities perform movements toward one side of the body at the same time, which facilitates trunk rotation (Figure 30-19, *B*). The asymmetrical patterns can be performed with the arms in contact, such as in the chopping and lifting patterns in which greater trunk rotation is seen (Figures 30-21 and 30-22). Furthermore, with the arms in contact, self-touching occurs. This is frequently observed in the presence of pain or in reinforcement of a motion when greater control or power is needed.[94] This phenomenon is observed in the baseball player at bat and in the tennis player who uses a two-handed backhand to increase control and power. Asymmetrical patterns with arms in contact would be beneficial for Leticia to control ataxia. Examples of asymmetrical patterns are bilateral asymmetrical flexion to the left, with the left arm in D_2 flexion and the right arm in D_1 flexion, such as when putting on a left earring (Figure 30-23), and bilateral asymmetrical extension to the left, with the right arm in D_2 extension and the left arm in D_1 extension, such as when zipping a left-side zipper.

3. *Reciprocal patterns:* Paired extremities move in opposite directions simultaneously, either in the same diagonal or in combined diagonals. If paired extremities perform movements in combined diagonals (Figure 30-19, *C*), a stabilizing effect occurs on the head, neck, and trunk because movement of the extremities is in the opposite direction while head and neck remain in midline. During activities requiring high-level balance, the reciprocal patterns with combined diagonals come into play with one extremity in D_1 extension and the other extremity in D_2 flexion. Examples of this are pitching in baseball, sidestroke in swimming, and walking a balance beam with one extremity in a diagonal flexion pattern and the other in a diagonal extension pattern (Figure 30-24). In contrast, reciprocal patterns in the same diagonal, such as D_1 in arm swing during walking, facilitate trunk rotation. Leticia needs to work with reciprocals of D_1 to improve rhythm of arm swing and trunk rotation during walking.

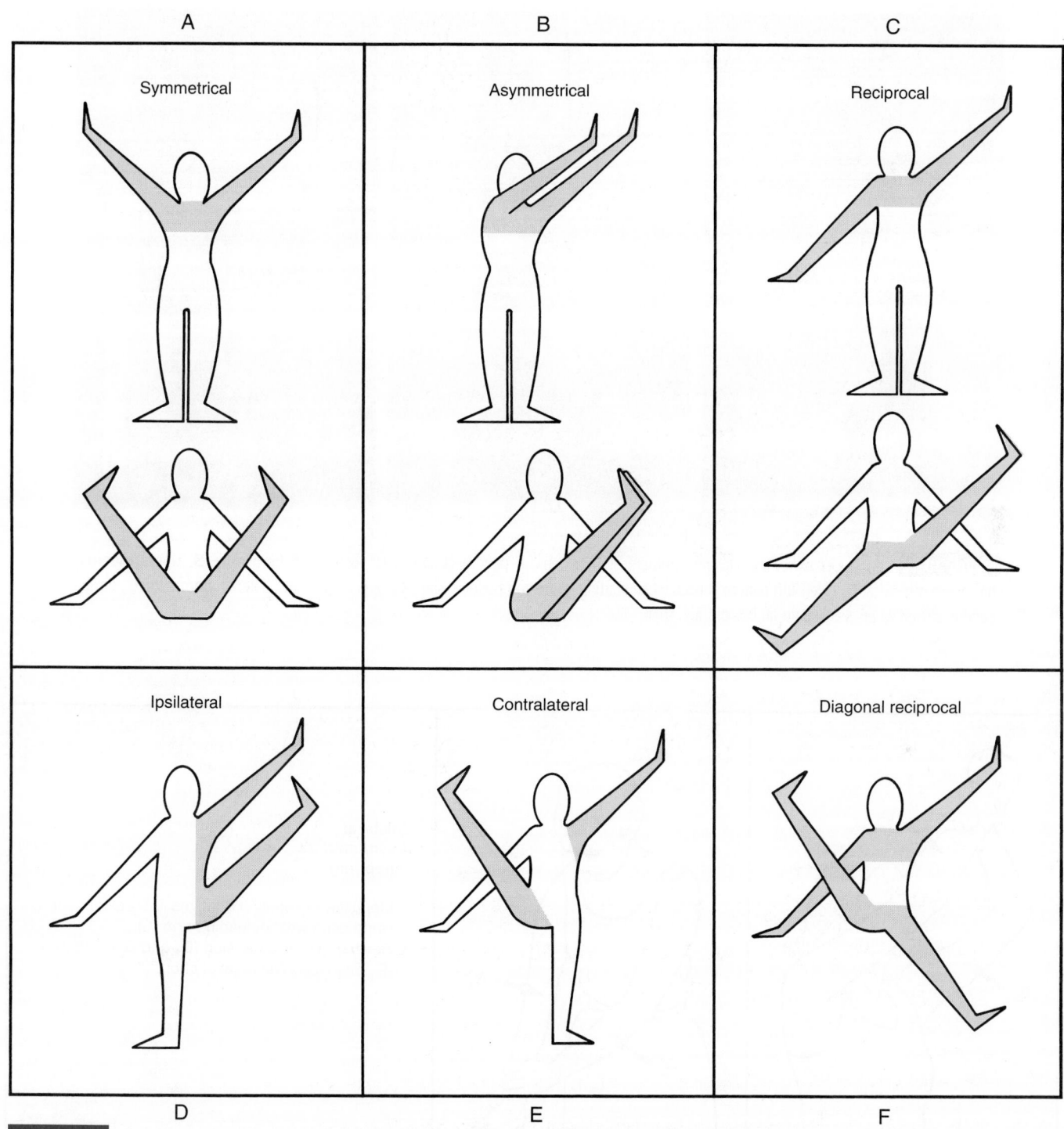

Figure 30-19 **A,** Symmetrical patterns. **B,** Asymmetrical patterns. **C,** Reciprocal patterns. **D,** Ipsilateral pattern. **E,** Contralateral pattern. **F,** Diagonal reciprocal pattern. (From Myers BJ: *Unit I: PNF diagonal patterns and their application to functional activities,* videotape study guide, Rehabilitation Institute of Chicago, 1982.)

Combined Movements of Upper and Lower Extremities

Interaction of the upper and lower extremities results in (1) ipsilateral patterns, with extremities of the same side moving in the same direction at the same time, (2) contralateral patterns, with extremities of opposite sides moving in the same direction at the same time, and (3) diagonal reciprocal patterns, with contralateral extremities moving in the same direction at the same time while opposite contralateral extremities move in the opposite direction (Figure 30-19, *D, E,* and *F*).

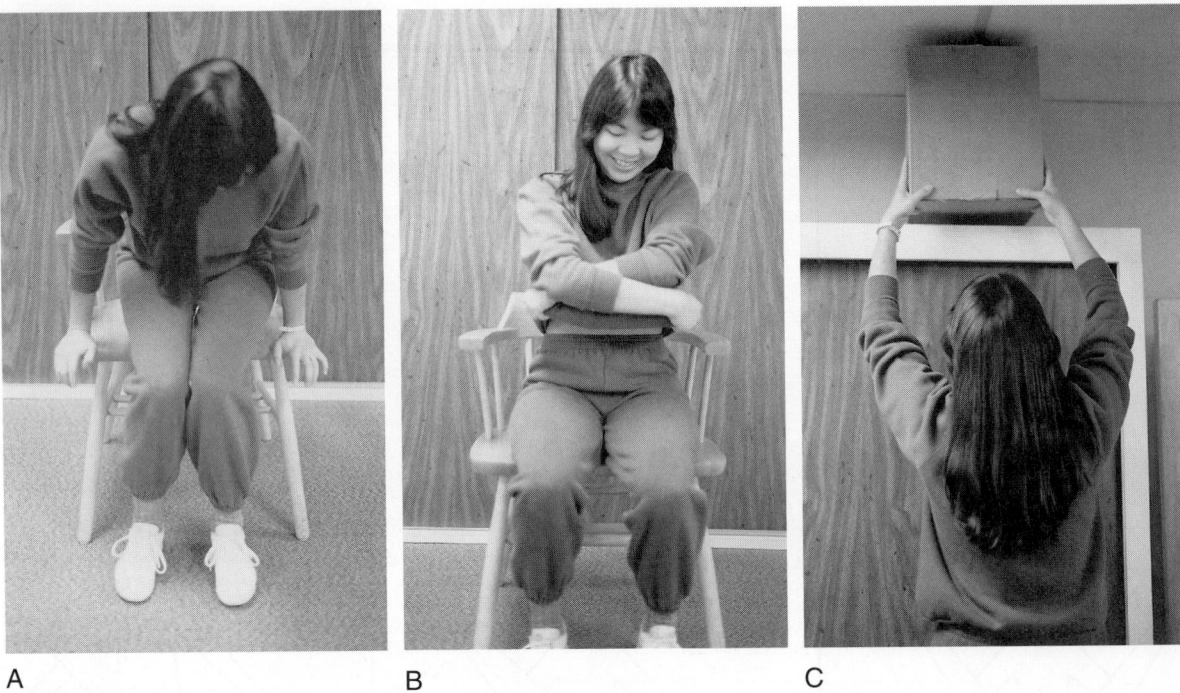

A   B   C

Figure 30-20 **A,** Upper extremity bilateral symmetrical D$_1$ extension pattern is shown in pushing off from chair. **B,** Upper extremity bilateral symmetrical D$_2$ extension pattern is used when starting to take off pullover shirt. **C,** Upper extremity bilateral symmetrical D$_2$ flexion pattern is used when reaching to lift box off high shelf.

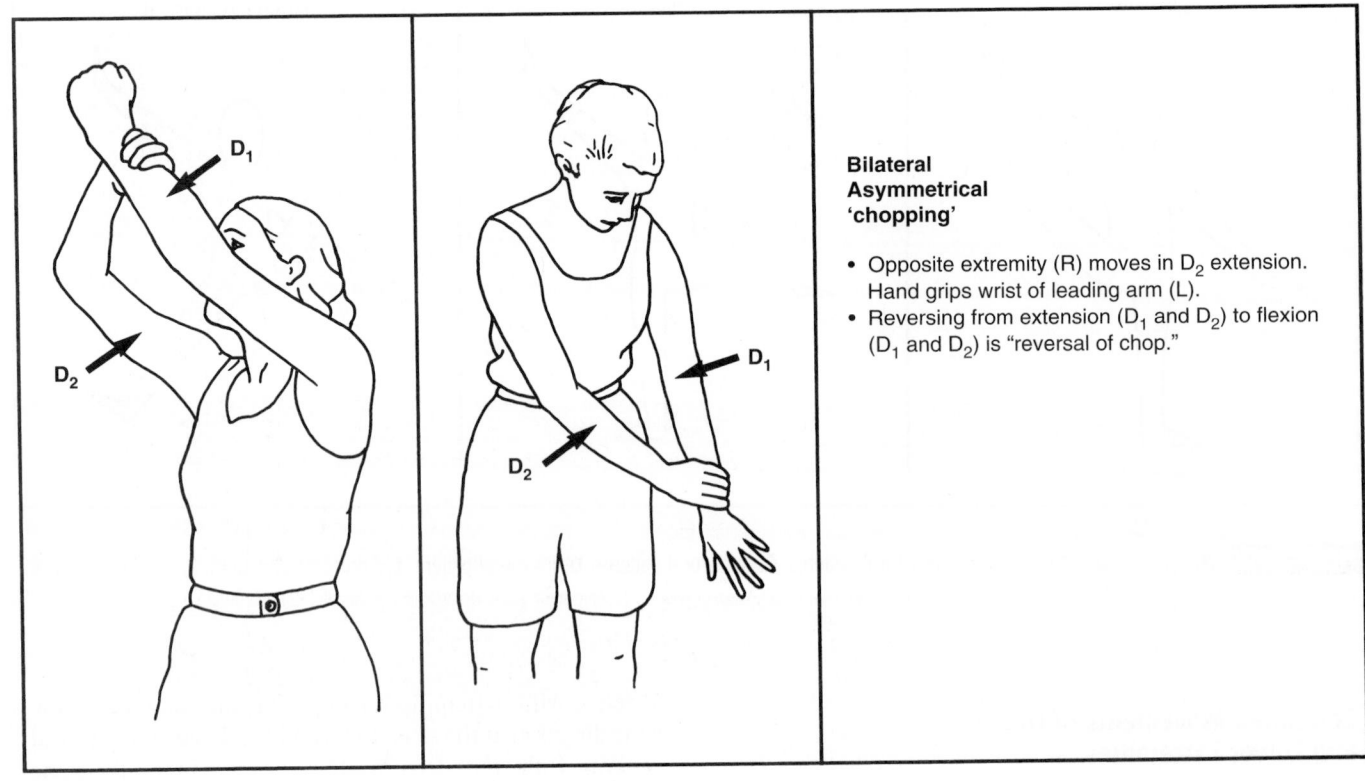

Bilateral Asymmetrical 'chopping'

- Opposite extremity (R) moves in D$_2$ extension. Hand grips wrist of leading arm (L).
- Reversing from extension (D$_1$ and D$_2$) to flexion (D$_1$ and D$_2$) is "reversal of chop."

A   B

Figure 30-21 Bilateral asymmetrical chopping. (From Myers BJ: *Unit I: PNF diagonal patterns and their application to functional activities,* videotape study guide, Rehabilitation Institute of Chicago, 1982.)

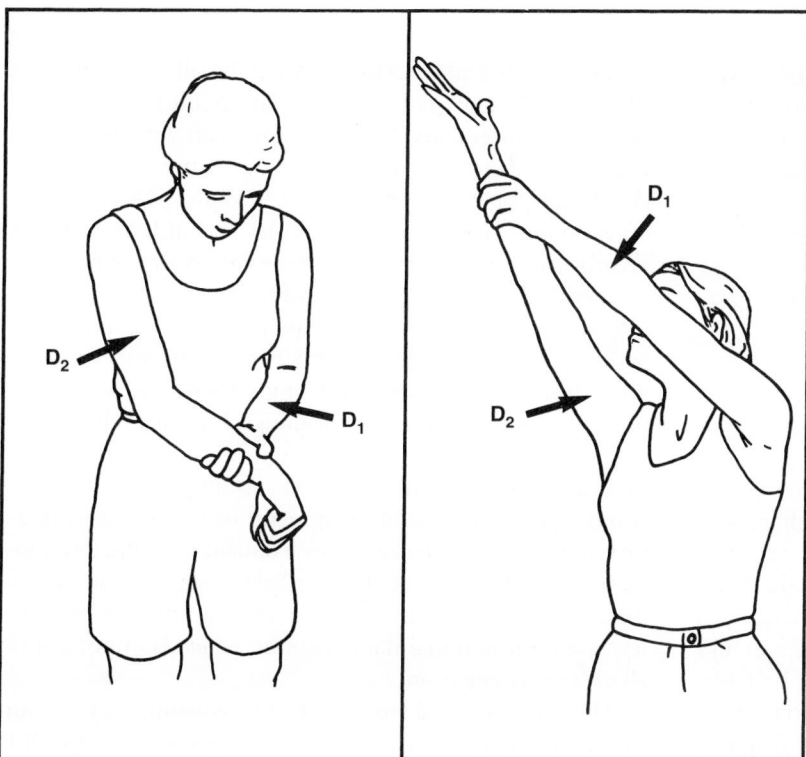

**Bilateral
Asymmetrical
'Lifting'**

- in lifting the hand opens with abduction, D_1 flexion, and D_2 flexion, and closes with adduction, D_1 extension and D_2 extension. Reversing from flexion (D_1 and D_2) to extension (D_1 and D_2) is "reversal of the lift."
- Contact with opposite extremity, self-touching, promotes stability and perception.

A   B

Figure 30-22 Bilateral asymmetrical lifting. (From Myers BJ: *Unit I: PNF diagonal patterns and their application to functional activities,* videotape study guide, Rehabilitation Institute of Chicago, 1982.)

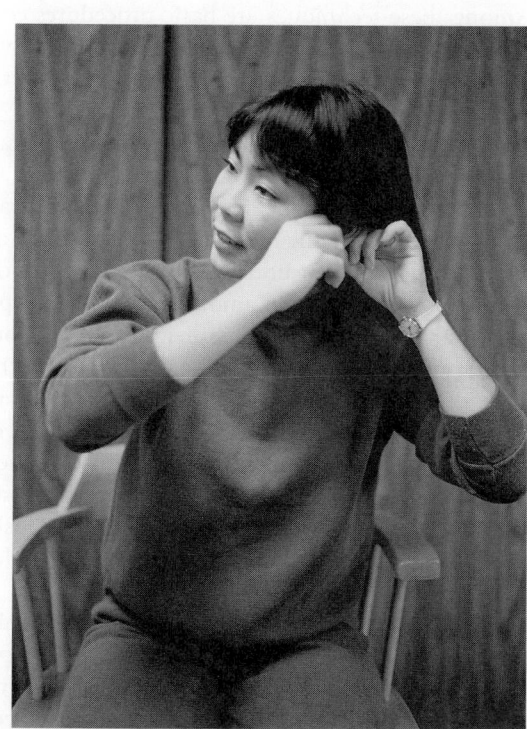

Figure 30-23 Putting on earring requires use of upper extremity bilateral asymmetrical flexion pattern.

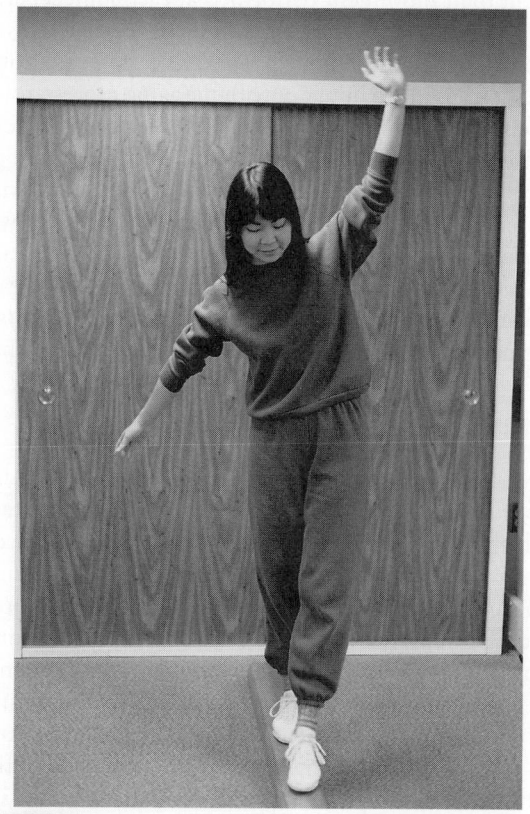

Figure 30-24 Bilateral reciprocal pattern of upper extremities is used to walk balance beam.

The **combined movements** of the upper and lower extremities are observed in such activities as crawling and walking. Awareness of these patterns is important in the assessment of the client's motor skills. The ipsilateral patterns are more primitive developmentally and indicate a lack of bilateral integration. Less rotation also is observed in ipsilateral patterns. Therefore, the goal in intervention is to progress from ipsilateral to contralateral to diagonal reciprocal patterns.

Several advantages exist to the use of the diagonal patterns in intervention. First, crossing of midline occurs. This movement is of particular importance in the remediation of perceptual motor deficits such as unilateral neglect, in which integration of both sides of the body and awareness of the neglected side are intervention goals. Second, each muscle has an optimal pattern in which it functions. For example, the client who has weak thumb opposition benefits from active movement in D_2 extension. Similarly, D_1 extension is the optimal pattern for ulnar wrist extension. Leticia should work in D_2 flexion after her Colles wrist fracture is stable. This pattern will increase range of motion and strengthen supination and radial wrist extension. Third, the diagonal patterns use groups of muscles, which is typical of movement seen in functional activities. For example, in eating, the hand-to-mouth action is accomplished in one mass movement pattern (D_1 flexion) that uses several muscles simultaneously. Therefore, movement in the diagonals is more efficient than movement performed at each joint separately. Finally, rotation is always a component in the diagonals (e.g., trunk rotation to the left or right and forearm pronation and supination). With an injury or with the aging process, rotation frequently is impaired and can be facilitated with movement in the diagonals. In intervention, attention should be given to the placement of activities so that movement occurs in the diagonal. For example, if the client is working on a wood-sanding project, trunk rotation with extension can be facilitated by placing the project on an inclined plane in a diagonal. Leticia can incorporate rotational movements into homemaking activities such as unloading the dishwasher.

TOTAL PATTERNS

In PNF, developmental postures also are called *total patterns of movement and posture*.[70] Total patterns require interaction between proximal (head, neck, and trunk) and distal (extremity) components. The assumption of postures is important, as is the maintenance of postures. When posture cannot be sustained, emphasis should be placed on the assumption of posture.[93] For example, before the client can be expected to sustain a sitting posture, he or she must have ability in lower developmental total patterns of movement, such as rolling and moving from side-lying to side-sitting.

The active assumption of postures can be included in OT activities. For example, a reaching and placing activity could be set up so that the client must reach for the object in the supine posture and place the object in the side-lying posture. The use of total patterns also can reinforce individual extremity movements. For example, in an activity such as wiping a tabletop, wrist extension is reinforced when the client leans forward over the supporting arm. This would be a way to make homemaking activities part of Leticia's home exercise program for her wrist in the later stages of recovery.

Several facts support the use of total patterns in the PNF intervention approach.[70] First, total patterns of movement and posture are experienced as part of the normal developmental process in all human beings. Therefore, recapitulation of these postures is meaningful to the client and acquired with less difficulty. Second, movement in and out of total patterns and the ability to sustain postures enhance components of normal development, such as reflex integration and support, balance between antagonists, and development of motor control in a cephalocaudal, proximodistal direction. Third, the use of total patterns improves the ability to assume and maintain postures, which is important in all areas of occupation.

The sequence and procedures for assisting clients with the developmental postures were developed by Voss. In 1981 Myers developed a videotape that shows the use of the sequence and procedures in OT.[70] This video demonstrates more information on the application of the total patterns and postures to OT.

PROCEDURES

PNF techniques are superimposed on movement and posture. Among these techniques are basic procedures considered essential to the PNF approach. Two procedures, verbal commands and visual cues, were discussed previously. Other procedures are described in the following sections.

Manual contacts refers to the placement of the therapist's hands on the client. These contacts are most effective when applied directly to the skin. Pressure from the therapist's touch is used as a facilitating mechanism and serves as a sensory cue to help the client understand the direction of the anticipated movement.[94] The amount of pressure applied depends on the specific technique being used and on the desired response. The location of manual contacts is chosen according to the groups of muscles, tendons, and joints responsible for the desired movement patterns. If the client is having difficulty reaching to comb the back of the hair because of scapular weakness, the desired movement pattern is D_2 flexion. Manual contacts should be on the posterior surface of the scapula to reinforce the muscles that elevate, adduct, and rotate the scapula.

Stretch is used to initiate voluntary movement and enhance speed of response and strength in weak muscles. This procedure is based on Sherrington's neurophysiological principle of reciprocal innervation.[84] When a muscle is stretched, the Ia and II fibers in the muscle spindle send excitatory messages to the alpha motor neurons, which innervate the stretched muscle. Inhibitory messages are sent to the antagonistic muscle simultaneously.[34]

When stretch is used in the PNF approach, the part to be facilitated is placed in the extreme lengthened range of the desired pattern (or where tension is felt on all muscle components of a given pattern). This range is the completely shortened range of the antagonistic pattern. Special attention is given to the rotatory component of the pattern because it is responsible for elongation of the fibers of the muscles in a given pattern. After the correct position for the stretch stimulus has been achieved, stretch is superimposed on the pattern. The client should attempt the movement at the exact time that the stretch reflex is elicited. The use of verbal commands also should coincide with the application of stretch, to reinforce the movement. Discrimination should be exercised with use of stretch to prevent an increase in pain or muscle imbalances.

Traction facilitates the joint receptors by creating a separation of the joint surfaces. It is thought that traction promotes movement and is used for pulling motion.[94] In activities such as carrying a heavy suitcase or pulling open a jammed door, traction can be felt on joint surfaces. Although traction may be contraindicated for clients with acute symptoms, such as after surgery or a fracture, it can sometimes provide relief of pain and promote greater ROM in painful joints.

Approximation facilitates joint receptors by creating a compression of joint surfaces. It promotes stability and postural control and is used for pushing motion.[94] Approximation is usually superimposed on a weight-bearing posture. For example, to enhance postural control in the prone on elbows posture, approximation may be given through the shoulders in a downward direction. As part of a home program to enhance proximal stability, Leticia could play board games on the floor with her children in weight-bearing positions such as prone on elbows or side-sitting. A weighted vest could be used in place of the therapist's manual contacts to provide approximation.

Maximal resistance is a procedure that involves Sherrington's principle of irradiation—namely, that stronger muscles and patterns reinforce weaker components.[84] This procedure is frequently misunderstood and applied incorrectly. The procedure is defined as the greatest amount of resistance that can be applied to an active contraction while allowing full ROM to occur, or to an isometric contraction without defeating or breaking the client's hold.[94] Maximal resistance is *not* the greatest amount of resistance that the therapist can apply. The objective is to obtain maximal effort on the part of the client because strength is increased by movement against resistance that requires maximal effort.[43]

If the resistance applied by the therapist results in uncoordinated or jerky movement or if it breaks the client's hold, too much resistance has been given. Movement against maximal resistance should be slow and smooth. To use this technique effectively, the therapist must sense the appropriate amount of resistance. For clients with neurological impairment or pain, the resistance may be very light, and light resistance is probably maximal for the client's needs. The therapist's manual contacts may offer light resistance that actually assists by providing the client with a way to track the desired movement. In the presence of spasticity, resistance may increase existing muscle imbalance and thus needs to be monitored. For example, if an increase in finger flexor spasticity is noted with resisted rocking in the hands-knees position, resistance should be decreased or eliminated or an alternate position should be used.

TECHNIQUES

Specific techniques are used in conjunction with these basic procedures. A few have been selected for discussion. These techniques are divided into three categories: those directed to the agonists, those that are a reversal of the antagonists, and those that promote relaxation.[94]

Techniques Directed to the Agonist

Repeated contractions is a technique based on the assumption that repetition of an activity is necessary for motor learning and helps develop strength, ROM, and endurance. The client's voluntary movement is facilitated with stretch and resistance, using isometric and isotonic contractions. Repeated contractions could be used to increase trunk flexion with rotation in the client who has difficulty reaching to put on a pair of shoes from the sitting position. The client bends forward as far as possible. At the point where active motion weakens, the client is asked to "hold" with an isometric contraction. This action is followed by isotonic contractions, facilitated by stretch, as the client is asked to "reach toward your feet." This sequence is repeated either until fatigue is evident or until the client is able to reach the feet. The pattern can be reinforced further by asking the client to hold with another isometric contraction at the end of the sequence.

Rhythmic initiation is used to improve the ability to initiate movement, which may be a problem with Parkinson's disease or apraxia. This technique involves voluntary relaxation, passive movement, and repeated isotonic contractions of the agonistic pattern. The verbal command is, "Relax and let me move you." As relaxation is felt, the command is, "Now you do it with me." After several repetitions of active movement, resistance may be given to reinforce the movement. Rhythmic initiation allows the client to feel the pattern before beginning active movement. Thus, the proprioceptive and kinesthetic senses are enhanced.

Reversal of Antagonists Techniques

Reversal of antagonists techniques employ a characteristic of normal development—namely, that movement is reversing and changes direction. These techniques are based on

Sherrington's principle of successive induction, according to which the stronger antagonist facilitates the weaker agonist.[84] The agonist is facilitated through resistance to the antagonist. The contraction of the antagonist can be isotonic, isometric, or a combination of the two. These techniques may be contraindicated for clients in whom resistance of antagonists increases symptoms such as pain and spasticity. For example, the facilitation of finger extension (agonist) would not be achieved effectively through resistance applied to spastic finger flexors (antagonist). In this situation, finger extension may be better facilitated through the use of repeated contractions, in which the emphasis is only on the extensor surface.

Slow reversal is an isotonic contraction (against resistance) of the antagonist followed by an isotonic contraction (against resistance) of the agonist. Slow reversal-hold is the same sequence, with an isometric contraction at the end of the range. For the client who has difficulty reaching his mouth for oral hygiene because of weakness in the D_1 flexion pattern, the slow reversal procedure is as follows: an isotonic contraction against resistance in D_1 extension with the verbal command, "Push down and out," followed by an isotonic contraction of D_1 flexion against resistance with the verbal command, "Pull up and across." An increase or buildup of power in the agonist should be felt with each successive isotonic contraction. Slow reversal used in conjunction with repeated contractions could be applied to trunk movement patterns to help Leticia overcome her rigidity and improve the balance of antagonists. This sequence of techniques could also be used to increase Leticia's wrist range of motion and strength once her fracture is stable.

Stabilizing reversals are characterized by alternating isotonic contractions opposed by enough resistance to prevent motion. In practice, the therapist gives resistance to the client in one direction while asking the client to oppose the force, allowing no motion. Once the client is fully resisting the force, the therapist gradually moves the resistance in another direction. Each time the client is able to respond to the new resistance, the therapist moves the hand to resist a new direction, reversing directions as often as needed to achieve the client's stability. This technique is used to increase stability, balance, and muscle strength.

Rhythmic stabilization is used to increase stability by eliciting simultaneous isometric contractions of antagonistic muscle groups. Cocontraction results if the client is not allowed to relax. This technique requires repeated isometric contractions, leading to increased circulation or the tendency for the client to hold his or her breath, or both. Therefore, rhythmic stabilization may be contraindicated for clients with cardiac involvement, and no more than three or four repetitions should be done at a time on any clients.

In rhythmic stabilization manual contacts are applied on both agonist and antagonist muscles, with resistance given simultaneously. The client is asked to hold the contraction against graded resistance. Without allowing the client to relax, manual contacts are switched to opposite surfaces. Rhythmic stabilization is useful with clients lacking postural control because of ataxia or proximal weakness. Used intermittently during an activity requiring postural stability, such as meal preparation in standing posture, this technique enhances muscle balance, endurance, and control of movement.

Because these two stabilizing techniques can be superimposed upon activity-based movements, they could be used to facilitate Leticia's ability to perform numerous daily activities. For example, rhythmic stabilization could be used to improve trunk endurance and stability when Leticia experiences fatigue while standing at the sink to do the dishes.

Relaxation Techniques

Relaxation techniques are an effective means of increasing ROM, particularly in the presence of pain or spasticity, which may be increased by passive stretch.

Contract-relax involves passive motion to the point of limitation in movement patterns. This is followed by an isotonic contraction of the antagonist pattern against maximal resistance, with only the rotational component of the diagonal movement allowed. This action is followed by relaxation, then by further passive movement into the agonistic pattern (e.g., contract-relax could involve passive motion to the point of limitation in D_2 flexion, which would be followed by an isotonic contraction of D_2 extension, then by further passive movement into D_2 flexion). This procedure is repeated at each point in the ROM in which limitation is felt to occur.[94] Contract-relax is used when no active range in the agonistic pattern is present. However, the ultimate goal is active movement through the full range. Therefore, once relaxation and increased ROM occur, active movement should be facilitated.

Hold-relax is performed in the same sequence as contract-relax but involves an isometric contraction (no movement allowed) of the antagonist, followed by relaxation and then active movement into the agonistic pattern. Because this technique involves an isometric contraction against resistance, it is particularly beneficial in the presence of pain or acute orthopedic conditions. For the client with reflex sympathetic dystrophy (RSD) who has pain with shoulder flexion, abduction, and external rotation, the therapist asks the client to hold against resistance in the D_2 extension pattern, then to initiate active movement into the D_2 flexion pattern. This technique is beneficial for the client with RSD during self-care activities such as shampooing hair and zipping a shirt in back.

Slow reversal-hold-relax begins with an isotonic contraction, followed by an isometric contraction, relaxation of the antagonistic pattern, and then by active movement of the agonistic pattern. When the client has the ability to move the agonist actively, the technique is preferred. For example, to increase active elbow extension in the presence of tight elbow flexors, the therapist asks the client to perform D_1 flexion with elbow flexion as resistance is applied. When the ROM is complete, the client is asked to hold with an isometric contraction, followed immediately by relaxation. When relaxation is felt, the client moves actively into D_1 extension with elbow extension. This technique helps increase elbow extension for such activities as reaching to lock the wheelchair brakes or picking up an object off the floor.

Rhythmic rotation is effective in decreasing spasticity and increasing ROM. The therapist passively moves the body part in the desired pattern. When tightness or restriction of movement is felt, the therapist rotates the body part slowly and rhythmically in both directions. After relaxation is felt, the therapist continues to move the body part into the newly available range. This technique is effective in preparing the paraplegic client with LE spasticity or clonus to put on a pair of pants. The technique is also effective in preparing for splint fabrication on a spastic extremity.

are assessed and addressed in intervention within total patterns of movement and posture. Carefully selected techniques are superimposed on these total patterns to enhance motor response and facilitate motor learning.

PNF uses multisensory input. The coordination and timing of sensory input are important in eliciting the desired response from the client. The client's performance should be monitored, and sensory input should be adjusted accordingly.

To use PNF effectively, the therapist must understand the developmental sequence and the components of normal movement. The therapist must learn the diagonal patterns and how they are used in ADL, must know when and how to use the techniques of facilitation and relaxation, and must be able to apply patterns and techniques of facilitation to OT evaluation and intervention. Attaining these skills requires observation and practice under the supervision of a therapist experienced in the PNF approach.

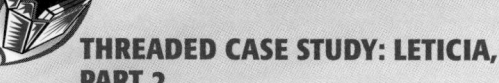

THREADED CASE STUDY: LETICIA, PART 2

To respond to the initial three questions at the beginning of this chapter, we need to review our assessment of Leticia. To determine the most effective movement patterns, we need to observe Leticia in her daily tasks in addition to her performance of specific diagonal patterns and total patterns of movement. Techniques and procedures that best address Leticia's key deficits of motor control and rigidity should be selected. In addition to a focus on these key areas, special attention should be given to whether more mobility or stability is needed. Trunk ataxia would respond best to stabilizing techniques such as rhythmic stabilization, stabilizing reversals, and approximation. Rigidity would need mobilizing techniques such as slow reversal, slow reversal hold, and repeated contractions. These techniques can be applied to clients during occupation-based activity.

The progression of intervention begins at the time of evaluation and considers the client's abilities as well as deficiencies. In Leticia's case, intervention will need to follow the PNF principles. Intervention should initially address proximal control and start in lower developmental positions where she has ability to perform coordinated movement. Once more proximal stability is achieved intervention can progress to work in higher developmental postures such as standing. Integrated into this progression of movement patterns and techniques are select procedures that facilitate desired motor response or activity performance.

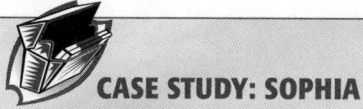

CASE STUDY: SOPHIA

Sophia, a 50-year-old woman, was referred for OT services with an RCVA resulting in left hemiplegia. Before the CVA she had a history of hypertension but otherwise good health. Referral to OT was made 10 days after onset of CVA for evaluation and intervention in ADL, visual perceptual skills, and left UE function.

Assessment

An initial assessment revealed intact vital and related functions, such as oral and facial musculature and swallowing. Voice production was good. Sophia had a tendency to hold her breath during activities and subsequent decreased endurance was noted. Visual tracking was impaired, with an inability to scan past midline and apparent left-side neglect.

The head and neck were observed to be frequently rotated to the right and slightly flexed because of weak extensors. The trunk was noted to be asymmetrical in sitting posture, with most of the weight supported on the right side. Sophia's posture was flexed because of weak extensors. Static sitting balance was fair and dynamic sitting balance was poor, with Sophia listing forward and left.

Sophia's right arm was normal in sensation and strength, although motor planning was impaired. The left arm was essentially flaccid, with impaired sensation of light touch, pain, and proprioception. Sophia complained of mild glenohumeral pain during passive movement at the end ranges of shoulder abduction and flexion. Scapular instability was noted. No active movement could be elicited in the left arm.

Perceptual testing showed apraxia (especially during activities requiring crossing of midline) and left-side neglect. Sophia was alert and oriented, with good attention span and memory. Carryover in tasks was adequate.

Continued

SUMMARY

The PNF approach emphasizes the client's abilities and potential so that strengths assist weaker components. Strengths and deficiencies

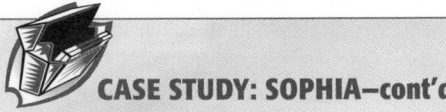

CASE STUDY: SOPHIA—cont'd

Sophia needed moderate assistance in ADLs and moderate to maximum assistance with transfers. Impaired balance and apraxia were the most limiting factors in performance of ADLs. She stated her immediate goal as being able to get herself ready in the morning with less time and effort.

Intervention Implementation

Following the cervicocaudal direction of development, alignment of the head and neck was the appropriate starting point for intervention. Left-side awareness, sitting posture, and trunk balance were directly influenced by the position of the head and neck. Before the start of self-care activities, Sophia performed head and neck patterns of flexion and extension with rotation. To reinforce rotation to left, the therapist was positioned to the left of Sophia. Clothing and hygiene articles also were placed to her the left.

A lack of trunk control was another problem. During bending activities while seated, Sophia reported a fear of falling and was unsure of her ability to return to the upright position. Consequently, she had difficulty leaning forward to transfer from wheelchair. Slow reversal-hold technique was used to reinforce trunk patterns during ADLs. For example, as a preparatory method to facilitate trunk control needed for donning pants over legs, the therapist was positioned in front and to the left of Sophia. Manual contacts were on the anterior aspect of either scapula. The therapist moved with Sophia and applied resistance as she leaned forward. At the end of the range, Sophia was instructed to hold with isometric contraction. Manual contacts were then switched to the posterior surface of either scapula. Resistance was applied as Sophia returned to the upright position. The verbal command was, "Look up and over your right shoulder." When she was upright, she was again instructed to hold with isometric contraction. In addition to reinforcing trunk control, this technique alleviated Sophia's fear of leaning forward, because the therapist was in continual contact with her.

An indirect benefit of the flexion and extension patterns of the head, neck, and trunk was the reinforcement of respiration. Sophia was encouraged to inhale during extension and exhale during flexion. This approach eliminated Sophia's tendency to hold her breath.

Intervention consisted of total patterns and techniques to facilitate proximal stability in the left UE and to provide proprioceptive input. Weight-bearing activities were selected because no active movement was available in the left arm. Sophia used the right UE in diagonal patterns to perform repetitive perceptual tasks such as a mosaic tile design, paper and pencil activities, and board games. These activities were performed to include the side-lying posture on the left elbow, the prone posture on elbows, the side-sitting posture with weight on the left arm, and on all fours. To reinforce stability at the shoulder girdle, approximation and rhythmic stabilization were used with manual contacts at both shoulders and then at the shoulder and pelvis. The performance of perceptual tasks in diagonals improved Sophia's motor planning, left-side awareness, and trunk rotation.

Sophia was instructed in bilateral asymmetrical chopping and lifting patterns to support the scapula and left UE in rolling and other activities. These patterns also enhanced left-side awareness and trunk rotation. To facilitate scapular movement during chop and lift patterns, the therapist applied stretch to initiate movement, followed by slow reversal technique. In preparation for the lift pattern, manual contacts were placed on the posterior surface of the scapula. Stretch was applied in lengthened range. As Sophia initiated the lifting pattern, resistance was given and maintained throughout the ROM. This procedure was repeated for antagonistic or reverse of lift pattern, with manual contacts switching to the anterior surface of the scapula.

About 3 to 4 weeks after the injury Sophia was able to initiate left UE movement in synergy with predominance of flexor tone. Weight-bearing activities and rhythmic rotation were helpful in normalizing tone, and both techniques were used with ADLs such as dressing and bathing. Wrist and finger extensions were facilitated in the D_1 extension and D_2 flexion patterns using repeated contractions.

Outcomes

Reevaluation after 5 weeks of OT revealed increased endurance and ability to coordinate breathing with activity, and consistency in crossing midline during visual scanning activities. Sophia was able to turn her head and neck to the left without cues from the therapist. The fear of falling forward with bending had diminished, and she automatically turned her head to look up and over her shoulder to reinforce assumption of the upright position. As trunk strength continued to improve, reinforcement with head and neck rotation was no longer necessary. Visual tracking alone, in the direction of movement, was sufficient to reinforce assumption of the upright position. Eventually Sophia was able to obtain an upright position without apparent visual or head and neck reinforcement. Sitting balance improved with bilateral weight bearing through both hips. Shoulder pain decreased and scapular stability improved during weight-bearing activities. Sophia initiated left UE movement out of flexor synergy pattern. Right UE motor planning was within functional limits for ADL. Transfers and self-care required only minimal assistance, and cues were no longer needed for left UE awareness.

Review Questions

1. What are the four general processes of information flow related to control of movement?
2. Define *motivational urge* and name the locus of this function in the brain.
3. Trace the flow of information in the central and peripheral nervous systems that leads to purposeful movement.
4. What is the sensorimotor system?
5. List the areas of the sensorimotor cortex.
6. List the structures that constitute the higher, middle, and lower levels of the central nervous system components for movement.
7. Name the four traditional sensorimotor approaches to treatment and the theorist responsible for each.
8. Which two models of motor control form the basis for the sensorimotor approaches to treatment?
9. Briefly describe each of the four traditional sensorimotor approaches to treatment. Compare and contrast their similarities and their differences.
10. List some techniques used by therapists to influence or modify motor responses in each of the traditional sensorimotor approaches.
11. How are the sensorimotor approaches used in current clinical practice?
12. Why is it important to study Margaret Rood's work?
13. How have key concepts identified by Rood been redefined today?
14. What were the four components of motor control emphasized by Rood?
15. What were the major motor patterns of development described by Rood?
16. Give examples of how Rood's major motor patterns are used during occupation.
17. It was stated that caution is needed when using traditional Rood treatment techniques in current occupation-based practice. What reasons are given for this caution?
18. List which Rood techniques are used today and why. Give examples of two techniques.
19. What are the similarities and differences of the traditional Rood approach and the Rood approach in occupation-based practice?
20. Name the five key assumptions underpinning the reconstruction of Rood.
21. Give examples of how the TNR and the ATNR reinforce motor performance.
22. Is rolling from prone to supine a flexor- or extensor-dominant activity?
23. In the presence of pain, what tone of voice should be used when giving verbal commands?
24. Discuss the significance of auditory, visual, and tactile input in motor learning.
25. Which UE diagonal pattern is used for the hand-to-mouth phase of eating? For zipping front-opening pants?
26. Discuss the advantages of using the chop and lift patterns.
27. Which trunk pattern is used when donning a left sock?
28. List three advantages of using the diagonal patterns.
29. What is the developmental sequence of total patterns?
30. If a client needs more stability, which of the following total patterns should be chosen: side-lying or prone posture on elbows?
31. Which PNF technique facilitates postural control and cocontraction?
32. Discuss the neurophysiological principles of Sherrington upon which the PNF techniques of facilitation are based.
33. What is an effective technique to prepare the client with UE flexor spasticity to don a shirt?
34. Define *maximal resistance*.
35. Name two PNF techniques that facilitate initiation of movement.

REFERENCES

1. Abreu BF, Toglia JP: Cognitive rehabilitation: a model for occupational therapy, *Am J Occup Ther* 41(7):439, 1987.
2. Affolter F: Perceptual processes as prerequisites for complex human behavior, *Int Rehabil Med* 3(1):3, 1981.
3. American Occupational Therapy Association: Occupational therapy practice framework: domain and process, *Am J Occup Ther* 56(6):609, 2002.
4. Andrews JR, Harrelson GL, Wilk K: *Physical rehabilitation of the injured athlete*, ed 3, p 51, 451, Philadelphia, 2004, Saunders.
5. Ayres JA: Proprioceptive neuromuscular facilitation elicited through the upper extremities. I. Background, II. Application, III. Specific application to occupational therapy, *Am J Occup Ther* 9(1):1, 1955.
6. Ayres JA: *Sensory integration and learning disorders*, Los Angeles, 1972, Western Psychological Services.
7. Ayres JA: *The development of sensory integrative theory and practice*, Dubuque, Iowa, 1974, Kendall/Hunt.
8. Blondel O, Collin C, McCarran WJ, et al: A glia-derived signal regulating neuronal differentiation, *J Neurosci* 20(21):8012, 2000.
9. Bobath B: *Adult hemiplegia: evaluation and treatment*, ed 3, London, 1991, Heinemann Medical Books.
10. Boissy P, Bourbonnais D, Carlotti MM, et al: Maximal grip force in chronic stroke subjects and its relationship to global upper extremity function, *Clin Rehabil* 13:334, 1999.
11. Bower E: Physiotherapy for cerebral palsy: a historical review. In Ward, CD editor: *Rehabilitation of motor disorders, Ballieris Clinical Neurology* vol 3, p 29, 1993.
12. Brooks VB: *The neural basis of motor control*, New York, 1986, Oxford University Press.
13. Brown PB, Koerber HR, Ritz LA: Somatotopic organization of primary afferent projections to the spinal cord. In Scott SD, editor: *Sensory neurons*, p 116, New York, 1992, Oxford Press.
14. Brunnstrom S: Motor behavior in adult hemiplegic patients, *Am J Occup Ther* 15(1):6, 1961.
15. Brunnstrom S: *Movement therapy in hemiplegia*, New York, 1970, Harper & Row.
16. Buchwald J: Exteroceptive reflexes and movement, *Am J Phys Med* 46(1):141, 1967.
17. Byl N, Roderick J, Mohamed O, et al: Effectiveness of sensory and motor rehabilitation of the upper limb following the principles of neuroplasticity: patients stable post stroke, *Neurorehabil Neural Repair* 17(3):196, 2003.
18. Carmena JM, Lebedev MA, Crist RE, et al: Learning to control a brain-machine interface for reaching and grasping in primates, *Public Library Sci Bio* 1(2):193, 2003.

19. Carroll J: The utilization of reinforcement techniques in the program for the hemiplegic, *Am J Occup Ther* 4(5):211, 1950.

20. Chae J, Bethoux F, Bohine T, et al: Neuromuscular stimulation for functional recovery in acute hemiplegia, *Stroke* 29:975, 1998.

21. Cheney PD: Role of cerebral cortex in voluntary movements: a review, *Phys Ther* 65(5):624, 1985.

22. Clautti C, Baron JC: Functional neuroimaging studies of motor recovery after stroke in adults: a review, *Stroke* 34:1553, 2003.

23. Cooke DM: The effects of resistance on multiple sclerosis patients with intention tremor, *Am J Occup Ther* 12(2):89, 1958.

24. Cramer SC, Bastings EP: Mapping clinically relevant plasticity after stroke, *Neuropharmacology* 39:842, 2000.

25. Damasio AR: *Descartes' error: emotion, reason and the human brain*, New York, 1994, Avon Books.

26. Dean CM, Shepherd RB: Task-related training improves performance of seated reaching tasks after stroke: a randomized controlled trail, *Stroke* 28:722, 1997.

27. DeKoninck Y, Salter MW, Henry JL: Substance P released endogenously by high intensity sensory stimulation, *Neuroscience Ltr* 176:128, 1994.

28. De Kroon JR, Iyzerman MJ, Lankhorst GJ: Electrical stimulation of the upper limb in stroke: stimulation of the extensors of the hand vs. alternate stimulation of flexors and extensors, *Am J Phys Med Rehabil* 83:592, 2004.

29. DeQuiros JB: Diagnosis of vestibular disorders in the learning disabled, *Learning Disabilities* 9:50, 1974.

30. Duus P: *Topical diagnosis in neurology*, ed 2, p 89, New York, 1989, Thieme Med Publishers.

31. Duysens J, Tax A, Narvijn S, et al: Gating of sensation and evoked potentials following foot stimulation during human gait, *Exp Brain Res* 105:423, 1995.

32. Eggers O: *Occupational therapy in the treatment of adult hemiplegia*, Rockville, MD, 1987, Aspen Publications.

33. Eldred E: Peripheral receptors: their excitation and relation to reflex patterns, *Am J Phys Med* 46(1):69, 1967.

34. Farber SD: *Neurorehabilitation: a multisensory approach*, Philadelphia, 1982, WB Saunders.

35. Farber S: *Sensorimotor evaluation and treatment procedures for allied health personnel*, Indianapolis, 1974, Indiana University and Purdue University Medical Center.

36. Field-Fote EC: Spinal cord control of movement: implications for locomotor rehabilitation following spinal cord injury, *Phys Ther* 80:477, 2000.

37. Fromm C, Wise SP, Evarts EV: Sensory response properties of pyramidal tract neurons in the precentral motor cortex and postcentral gyrus of the rhesus monkey, *Exp Brain Res* 54(1):177, 1984.

38. Fukuda T: Studies on human dynamic postures from the viewpoint of postural reflexes, *Acta Otolaryngol* 161(suppl):8, 1961.

39. Fyffe RE: Laminar organization of primary afferent terminals in the mammalian spinal cord. In Scott S: *Sensory neurons diversity, development and plasticity*, p 131, New York, 1992, Oxford University Press.

40. Greenwood RJ, Barnes MP, McMillan TM, et al: *Handbook of neurological rehabilitation*, ed 2, p 577, New York, 2003, Psychology Press.

41. Hagbarth KE: Excitatory and inhibitory skin areas for flexor and extensor mononeurons, *Acta Physiol Scand* 26(suppl 94):1, 1952.

42. Heininger M, Randolph S: *Neurophysiological concepts in human behavior*, St Louis, 1981, Mosby.

43. Hellebrandt FA: Physiology. In Delorme TL, Watkins AL: *Progressive resistance exercise*, New York, 1951, Appleton, Century, & Crofts.

44. Hellebrandt FA, Schade M, Carns ML: Methods of evoking the tonic neck reflexes in normal human subjects, *Am J Phys Med* 4(90):139, 1962.

45. Holstege G: The emotional motor system, *Eur J Morphol* 30(1):67, 1992.

46. Howle JM: *Neuro-developmental treatment approach: theoretical foundations and principles of clinical practice*, Laguna Beach, Calif, 2002, NDTA Association.

47. Huitt W: *Conation as an important factor of mind*. Educational Psychology Interactive, Valdosta, GA, 1999, Valdosta State University. Retrieved July 2005, from http://chiron.valdosta.edu/whuitt/col/regsys/conation.html.

48. Humphrey TL, Huddleston OL: Applying facilitation techniques to self care training, *Phys Ther Rev* 38(9):605, 1958.

49. Huss AJ: Sensorimotor approaches. In Hopkins H, Smith H, editors: *Willard and Spackman's occupational therapy*, Philadelphia, 1978, JB Lippincott.

50. Jackson JH: *Selected writings*, vol 1, London, 1931, Hodder & Staughton (edited by J Taylor).

51. Jeannerod M: *The neural and behavioral organization of goal-directed movements*, Oxford, 1988, Clarendon Press.

52. Jones GM, Watt D: Muscular control of landing from unexpected falls in man, *J Physiol* 219(3):729, 1971.

53. Kabat H, Rosenberg D: Concepts and techniques of occupational therapy for neuromuscular disorders, *Am J Occup Ther* 4(1):6, 1950.

54. Kandel ER, Schwartz JH, Jesell TM, editors: *Principles of neural science*, ed 3, New York, 1991, Elsevier.

55. Karnath H, Konczak J, Dichgans J: Effect of prolonged neck muscle vibration on lateral heald tilt in severe spasmodic torticollis, *J Neurological Neurosurgery Psychiatry* 69:658, 2000.

56. Kostopaulos D, Rizopoulos K: *The manual of triggerpoint and myofascial therapy*, p 51, Thorofare, 2001, Slack.

57. Lederman E: *Fundamentals of manual therapy*, p 69, New York, 1997, Churchill Livingstone.

58. Levy CE, Nichols DS, Schmalbrock PM: Functional MRI evidence of cortical reorganization in upper-limb stroke hemiplegia treated with constraint-induced movement therapy, *Am J Phys Med Rehabil* 80:4, 2000.

59. Loeb GE, Brown IE, Lan N, et al: The importance of biomechanics, *Adv Exp Med Biol* 508:481, 2002.

60. Loomis JE, Boersma FJ: Training right brain damaged patients in a wheelchair task: case studies using verbal mediation, *Physiother Can* 34(4):204, 1982.

61. Luft AR, McCombe-Waller S, Whitall J, et al: Repetitive bilateral arm training and motor cortex activation in chronic stroke: a randomized controlled trial, *J Am Med Assoc* 292(15):1853, 2004.

62. Maffat M: Braving new worlds: to conquer, to endure, *Phys Ther* 84:1056, 2004.

63. Majsak MJ: Application of motor learning principles to the stroke population, *Topics Stroke Rehabil* 3(2):27, 1996.

64. Mathews PB: Proprioceptors and their contribution to somatosensory mapping: complex messages require complex processing, *Canadian J Physiol Pharm* 66:430, 1988.

65. McCloskey DI: Kinesthetic sensibility, *Physiol Rev* 58:763, 1978.

66. McCormack G: The Rood approach to treatment of neuromuscular dysfunction. In Pedretti LW, editor: *Occupational therapy: practice skills for physical dysfunction,* ed 4, St Louis, 1996, Mosby.

67. Merrick M: Therapeutic modalities as an adjunct to rehabilitation. In Andrews J, Harrelson GL, Wilk KE: *Physical rehabilitation of the injured athlete,* ed 3, p 51, Philadelphia, 2003, Saunders.

68. Middekauff HR, Chin J: Cycloxygenases produces products that sensitize muscle mechano-receptors in health humans, *Am J Physiol Heart Circ Physiol* 287:1944, 2004.

69. Muir GD, Steeves JD: Sensory motor stimulation to improve locomotor recovery after spinal cord injury, *Trends Neurosci* 20:72, 1997.

70. Myers BJ: *Assisting to postures and application in occupational therapy activities,* Chicago, Rehabilitation Institute of Chicago, 1981 (videotape).

71. Myers BJ: *PNF: patterns and application in occupational therapy,* Chicago, Rehabilitation Institute of Chicago, 1981 (videotape).

72. Myers BJ: *Proprioceptive neuromuscular facilitation: concepts and application in occupational therapy as taught by Voss.* Notes from course at Rehabilitation Institute of Chicago, September 8-12, 1980.

73. Oken B: *Complementary therapies in neurology: an evidence based approach,* p 95, Boca Raton, 2004, The Parthenon Pub Co.

74. Penfield W: *The excitable cortex in conscious man,* Liverpool, 1958, Liverpool University Press.

75. Powell J, Pandyan AD, Granat M, et al: Electrical stimulation of wrist extensors in poststroke hemiplegia, *Stroke* 30:1384, 1999.

76. Randolph G: Therapeutic and physical touch: physiological response to stressful stimuli, *Nurs Res* 33(1):33, 1984.

77. Roland P, Larsen B, Lassen NA, et al: Supplementary motor area and other cortical areas in organization of voluntary movements in man, *J Neurophysiol* 43(1):118, 1980.

78. Rood M: Neurophysiological mechanisms utilized in the treatment of neuromuscular dysfunction, *Am J Occup Ther* 10:4, 1956.

79. Rood M: Occupational therapy in the treatment of the cerebral palsied, *Phys Ther Rev* 32:220, 1952.

80. Rood M: The use of sensory receptors to activate, facilitate and inhibit motor responses, automatic and somatic, in developmental sequence. In Sattely C, editor: *Approaches to the treatment of patients with neuromuscular dysfunction,* Dubuque, Iowa, 1962, William C Brown.

81. Rothwell JC: *Control of human voluntary movement,* ed 2, London, 1994, Chapman & Hall.

82. Royeen CB: The 2003 Eleanor Clark Slagle lecture—Chaotic occupational therapy: collective wisdom for a complex profession, *Am J Occup Ther* 57:609, 2003.

83. Sawner K, LaVigne J: *Brunnstrom's movement therapy in hemiplegia: a neurophysiological approach,* ed 2, Philadelphia, 1992, JB Lippincott.

84. Sherrington C: *The integrative action of the nervous system,* ed 2, New Haven, Conn, 1961, Yale University Press.

85. Stockmeyer S: An interpretation of the approach of Rood to the treatment of neuromuscular dysfunction, NUSTEP proceedings, *Am J Phys Med* 46(1):900, 1967.

86. Sullivan JE, Hedman LD: A home program of sensory and neuromuscular electrical stimulation with upper-limb task practice in a patient five years after a stroke, *Phys Ther* 84:1045, 2004.

87. Tanji J, Taniguchi K, Saga T: Supplementary motor area: neuronal response to motor instructions, *J Neurophysiol* 43(1):60, 1980.

88. Taub E, Wolf S: Constraint induced movement techniques to facilitate upper extremity use in stroke patients, *Topics Stroke Rehabil* 3(4):38, 1997.

89. Thaut MH, Kenyon GP, Hurt CP, et al: Kinematic optimization of spatiotemporal patterns in paretic arm training with stroke patients, *Neuropsychologia* 40:1073, 2002.

90. Uunas-Maberg K, Lundeberg T, Bruzelius P: Vagusly mediated release of gastrin and cholecystokinin following sensory stimulation, *Acta Physiol Scand* 146:349, 1992.

91. Voss DE: Application of patterns and techniques in occupational therapy, *Am J Occup Ther* 8(4):191, 1959.

92. Voss DE: Proprioceptive neuromuscular facilitation, *Am J Phys Med* 46(1):838, 1967.

93. Voss DE: Proprioceptive neuromuscular facilitation: the PNF method. In Pearson PH, Williams CE, editors: *Physical therapy services in the developmental disabilities,* Springfield, Ill, 1972, Charles C Thomas.

94. Voss DE, Ionta MK, Myers BJ: *Proprioceptive neuromuscular facilitation,* ed 3, Philadelphia, 1985, Harper & Row.

95. Watts RJ, Schuldiner O, Perrino J, et al: Glia engulf degenerating axons during developmental axon pruning, *Current Biol* 14:675, 2004.

96. Whitaker EW: A suggested treatment in occupational therapy for patients with multiple sclerosis, *Am J Occup Ther* 4(6):247, 1950.

97. Wilson-Panwells A, Akesson EJ, Stewart PA: *Cranial nerves: anatomy and clinical comments,* p 42, Toronto, 1988, BC Decker Inc.

98. Winward CE, Halligan PW, Wade DT: Current practice and clinical relevance of somatosensory assessment after stroke, *Clin Rehabil* 13:48, 1999.

SUGGESTED READINGS

Adler SS, Beckers D, Buck M: *PNF in practice: an illustrated guide,* Berlin, 1993, Springer-Verlag.

Goloszewski S, Kremser C, Wagner M, et al: Functional magnetic resonance imaging of the human motor cortex before and after whole-hand electrical stimulation, *Scand J Rehabil Med* 31:165, 1999.

Kunkel A, Kopp B, Muller G, et al: Constraint-induced movement therapy for motor recovery in chronic stroke patients, *Arch Phys Med Rehabil* 80:624, 1999.

Kwalkel GW, Wagenaar RC, Twisk JW, et al: Intensity of leg and arm training after primary middle-cerebral artery stroke: a randomized trial, *Lancet* 354:191, 1999.

Thornborough JR: *Pretest key concepts neuron function*, p 103, New York, 1994, McGraw-Hill Inc.

Weiss, PL, Naveh Y, Katz N: Design and testing of a virtual environment for patients with unilateral spatial neglect to cross a street safely, *Occup Ther Intl* 10:39, 2003.

31

Neuro-Developmental Treatment of Adult Hemiplegia

CATHY RUNYAN*

KEY TERMS

Principles of management
Neuro-Developmental
    Treatment (NDT)
Manual cues
Neuroplasticity

Functional activity
Functional activity limitation
Ineffective movement strategies
Missing components of
    movement

Impairments
Individualized functional
    outcomes
Problem solving

LEARNING OBJECTIVES

After reading this chapter the student or practitioner will be able to do the following:

1. Discuss the purpose and the evolution of the Neuro-Developmental Treatment (NDT) approach.
2. Describe how alignment of the trunk and limbs influences muscle activity.
3. Describe the importance of 24-hour management for adult clients with hemiplegia.
4. Discuss the need for appropriate use of manual cues for adult clients with hemiplegia.
5. Discuss current assumptions about acquisition of movement.
6. Discuss modeling of the central nervous system.
7. Describe the significance of neuroplasticity and the importance of increasing active use of the involved side for adult clients with hemiplegia.

8. Describe the core principles of management of the NDT approach.
9. Discuss individualized functional outcomes for adult clients with hemiplegia and factors that influence selection of those outcomes.
10. Describe the progressive identification of functional activity limitations, ineffective movement strategies, missing components of movement, and underlying impairments when individualizing functional outcomes for adult clients with hemiplegia.
11. Understand the importance of problem solving and manual cues and their relationship to the core principles of management of the NDT approach.

CHAPTER OUTLINE

* Copyright © 2005 by Cathy Runyan OTR/L (www.RecoveringFunction.com)

THREADED CASE STUDY: JOE, PART 1

This chapter describes use of the Neuro-Developmental Treatment (NDT) approach to promote occupational performance and collaboratively select outcomes for Joe, a 46-year-old male who experienced a right cerebral vascular accident (CVA) 5 months ago (Figure 31-1). Joe is a husband and a father of twin teenage boys. Joe is concerned that he may not be able to continue in his occupation as a real estate agent, which provides most of his family's financial support. Joe is now living at home and receiving interventions in a home care setting.

Critical Thinking Questions

Joe's occupational therapist, Cathy, posed the following questions to develop and implement an intervention plan:

1. What factors influence the selection of outcomes for Joe?
2. What physical limitations resulting from the CVA are preventing Joe from participating in his occupation as a real estate agent?
3. What are examples of appropriate outcomes for Joe?

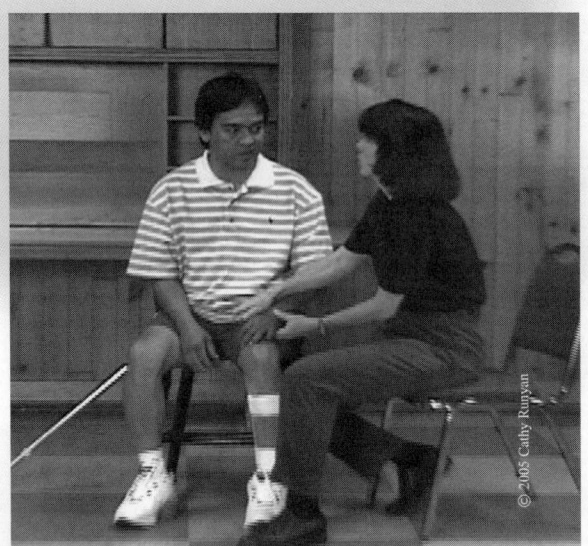

Figure 31-1 Joe is a 46-year-old husband, the father of twin, teenage boys, and a real estate agent. (Copyright © 2005 by Cathy Runyan OTR/L [www.RecoveringFunction.com].)

On average, someone in the United States has a stroke every 45 seconds. The number of stroke survivors in the United States is growing each year, making it one of the leading causes of disability in this country. This is due in part to advances in the acute management of stroke victims and in part to the increased incidence of stroke in younger individuals. As a consequence, the need for effective stroke rehabilitation has never been more critical.[2]

This chapter begins with a brief discussion of the evolution of the Neuro-Developmental Treatment (NDT) approach. A background in the origins of this approach allows therapists to better understand current applications of the approach. In the remainder of the chapter, the core principles of the approach are highlighted, and one of these principles, "Individualize Functional Outcomes," is presented in detail and is related to the case presentation of Joe.

This chapter provides the foundation necessary for continuing the development of your NDT expertise. You should view the information in this chapter as only the beginning of your evolution. There is much more to learn about providing interventions for adult clients with hemiplegia using the NDT approach. To competently apply this approach, occupational therapists are encouraged to participate in hands-on NDT coursework, since a unique aspect of the NDT approach is the appropriate use of manual cues.

EVOLUTION OF THE NEURO-DEVELOPMENTAL TREATMENT APPROACH

The sections below discuss the origins of the NDT approach as well as factors that have directly influenced its evolution. In addition, insight is given into thinking in the neurotherapies and the neurosciences at large during this evolution.

THE BOBATHS

The NDT approach was originated by Berta and Karel Bobath in England, beginning in the early 1940s. The **principles of management** they established for providing interventions for adult clients with hemiplegia and children with cerebral palsy have allowed therapists to improve the occupational performance of many clients. The Bobaths insisted that therapists using the NDT approach participate in the evolution of these principles as more is learned about the potential for recovery of function for these individuals. They believed that their approach would continue to be used only if it continued to evolve.

Teamwork

Berta was a physiotherapist, and Karel was a physician. Their respective backgrounds made them a very effective team for improving the functional abilities of adults with hemiplegia and children with cerebral palsy. Berta's role on the team was to provide the most effective therapeutic interventions for these clients, whereas Dr. Bobath's role was to investigate the neurosciences to better understand why Berta was able to achieve such remarkable results. The Bobaths dedicated their lives to helping these clients realize their full potential for recovery of function.[19]

Revolutionary Ideas

During early development of the NDT approach, prevailing attitudes were that paralysis resulting from a cerebrovascular accident (CVA) was a permanent condition. In contrast, the Bobaths argued that individuals with hemiplegia have the potential to recover function. Whereas the health professions at large were teaching these individuals to compensate for their loss of function by using residual movement strategies (i.e., by using the less involved side), the Bobaths argued that instead these individuals should *increase* active use of their involved side.[4]

Much more is known about brain function today than was known when the Bobaths were first developing their approach. Today we have the benefit of technologies that allow us to better understand brain function. For example, brain mapping continues to evolve as an increasingly accurate method for understanding brain function. Other technologies, such as functional magnetic resonance imaging, transcranial magnetic stimulation, positron emission tomography, and evoked potential, provide additional methods for better understanding brain function. But even without the technologies we have today, the Bobaths knew that individuals with a lesion of the central nervous system (CNS) have potential for recovery. They knew this because they were witnessing firsthand the functional outcomes resulting from their application of the NDT approach. Dr. Bobath wrote, "The outstanding quality of the higher CNS activity is its plasticity, its ability to learn, and perhaps one should also add the 'gift of forgetting,' the ability of forming temporary and constantly changing chains of synaptic connections in response to the many and various demands of the environment."[4]

Naming the Approach

Therapists outside the United States who study this approach refer to it as the *Bobath approach*. In the United States, the Bobaths decided to call this approach **Neuro-Developmental Treatment** because they were encouraged not to use their own name to identify the approach: *neuro* to mean brain function, *developmental* to mean components of movement required to develop, and *treatment* to mean management.

Their choice of the term *neuro* relates directly to the etiologies of hemiplegia and cerebral palsy. Their choice of the term *developmental* refers to the development of components of movement required for motor control. This term had historically been associated with the treatment of children; however, the Bobaths insisted that therapists provide all individuals, regardless of age, the opportunity to use the components of movement required for effective movement strategies. Therapists skilled in NDT refer to their use of manual cues for recovering functional use of components of movement as *accessing missing components of movement*. The Bobaths believed that skilled interventions that access missing components of movement give clients the opportunity to learn new movement strategies. Moreover, the Bobaths believed that when emphasis is placed on the quality of that movement, clients have the opportunity to achieve additional functional outcomes. The Bobaths intended that the term *treatment* connote ongoing management.

Only ongoing management can provide opportunities for the continued practice that results in increased retention, carryover, and improved function for the balance of the individual's life.

Early Influences on Berta Bobath

Berta was an instructor of gymnastics before she became a physiotherapist, which likely influenced her thinking during early development of the approach. The following sections discuss three areas important to the training of gymnasts that Berta also found to be important when treating clients with hemiplegia.

Alignment of body segments

Berta knew that proper alignment of body segments is important for postural control and active use of the involved side for clients with hemiplegia.[3] Alignment is a core element of movement that requires a base of support (BOS), a healthy soft tissue system, structural integrity of the joints, and adequate range of motion (ROM). Ideal alignment results in optimal length-tension relationships for muscle fibers, increasing the potential for muscle activation.[12] When musculoskeletal structures are ideally aligned, potential for muscle activation is increased. When the trunk and limb muscles on the involved side activate more immediately, then the client with hemiplegia will realize greater gains when practicing.

Twenty-four-hour management

Berta knew that clients with hemiplegia need to practice between intervention sessions to increase retention and carryover. She also knew that clients with hemiplegia need to manage their involved extremities, either through self-care or the assistance of others. To this end she pioneered the use of 24-hour management for the client with hemiplegia.[3] Therapists using the NDT approach today continue to emphasize the importance of practice between intervention sessions. In addition, these therapists teach 24-hour management for the client, the caregiver, and the professional team. When prescribing 24-hour management programs, it is important that therapists match expectations for retention and carryover to a client's cognitive, physical, and emotional capacities. It is also important that therapists teach the client's caregivers and professional team the specific management strategies to be used so they can assist with the management program.

The use of physical handling

During intervention sessions, Berta was accustomed to using just the right amount of physical handling to promote active use of the involved side for clients with hemiplegia. She found it necessary to use physical handling for clients with hemiplegia who could not perform movements when she used visual or verbal cues alone.[3] If the client with hemiplegia demonstrates the inability to move because of impairments resulting from CVA, the therapist should use specific physical handling to access missing components of movement. The therapist should continue to use verbal instructions and features of the environment to encourage movement as well, but physical handling should be used when necessary.

When Berta used physical handling to facilitate active use of missing components of movement, she knew there are certain key points of control (i.e., specific places on the trunk and limbs for manual input applied in specific directions), which promote motoric responses that lead to effective movement. Therapists today often refer to the use of physical handling of key points of control as the use of **manual cues** to access missing components of movement. It is important that the manual cues used to access missing components of movement activate the muscles responsible for those missing components. Manual cues must increase active use of these muscles in ways that are consistent with the synergies evident in effective movement strategies. This requires that the therapist use manual cues to simultaneously facilitate effective movements and inhibit ineffective ones.

Berta recognized that clients with hemiplegia achieve more functional outcomes if they actively use their involved side. For this reason, it is not sufficient to say that therapists skilled in NDT use manual cues to access missing components of movement. They also grade their use of manual cues to provide clients with hemiplegia just the right level of challenge in order to promote active use of the involved side. By grading their use of manual cues, they do not *guide* the client with hemiplegia through new movements; they facilitate the *learning* of new movements. In other words, overuse of manual cues can reduce challenge and actually impede progress because the client with hemiplegia must actively participate with the therapist in order to learn new options in movement.[3]

HISTORICAL ASSUMPTIONS IN THE NEUROTHERAPIES

The following sections review certain assumptions about acquisition of movement and functions of the CNS that were prevalent in the neurotherapies during the time the Bobaths were developing their approach as well as how those assumptions differ from present day thinking.

Acquisition of Movement

Assumptions were made that movements practiced by clients in one position would automatically become available to them in other positions. For example, it was assumed that movements practiced as a result of bridging in a supine position would automatically be used during the mid-stance phase of gait.[25]

Today we know that acquisition of skilled movement for a given activity requires practice of the movement strategies specific to that activity.[18] For example, to learn any sport you would need to practice the movement strategies required for that particular sport. If you wanted to become an Olympic diver, simply standing on the diving board and jumping up and down would not provide sufficient training. Instead, you would need to apply that component skill to the entire task of diving to improve your ability to dive. Similarly, if a client is made to practice flexion of the involved shoulder but that skill is not applied to reaching forward for a cup, or to pushing the upper extremity into the sleeve of a coat, the practice lacks functional application.[7] It is possible to strengthen the muscles required to flex the shoulder, and we know there could be some cross training (i.e., practiced movements for a given activity that might also contribute to other activities).[6] However, until a client is given practice for shoulder flexion while reaching, we cannot expect the client to generalize the movement strategy to the functional activity of reaching for a cup or pushing the involved upper extremity into the sleeve of a coat. Therapists using the NDT approach provide practice for specific components of movement in the context of a functional activity requiring those components of movement.

There was also an emphasis on applying developmental sequences to the treatment of adult clients with hemiplegia. These developmental sequences were derived from the movement typically observed during the stages of development of a normal child. This practice is no longer recommended in contemporary NDT courses that focus on adults with hemiplegia. Adult clients are not expected to roll in bed before they sit, half-kneel before they stand, sit before they walk, and so forth. Adult clients are not expected to assume certain positions, such as quadruped, simply for the sake of achieving a developmental milestone. However, if it is more functional for an adult client to practice quadruped because that client was a carpet installer before the onset of hemiplegia and now has the potential to return to work and reassume a life role, then practicing quadruped to develop the movement components required for installing carpet should be included in the intervention plan.

Modeling the Central Nervous System

Assumptions were also made that CNS behavior is hierarchical. This view was largely a result of the work of Sir Charles Sherrington, who was awarded a Nobel Prize for his work on the functioning of neurons. Sherrington was a principal proponent of the hierarchical model as a vehicle for explaining functions of the CNS.[21]

Today therapists who use the NDT approach recognize that the hierarchical model is inadequate for explaining the complexities of the CNS. Although there are hierarchical aspects of the CNS, a systems model gives us a more manageable view of CNS functions.[9] By using a systems model to describe functions of the CNS, we acknowledge that different parts of the CNS influence one another. An example of this can be seen by examining the relationship between the perceptual and neuromuscular systems. In healthy individuals, the neuromuscular system relies on the perceptual system to produce effective movement strategies. Conversely, the perceptual system relies on the neuromuscular system to provide information about movement experiences.[1] This information may be used immediately or integrated for future motoric responses (e.g., responses to changes in the environment or to changes in intent). A healthy neuromuscular system provides the ability to explore, which shapes the perceptual system, whereas a healthy perceptual system provides the neuromuscular system with information for adjusting to what it encounters. Each system influences the other.

As we learn more about the functions of the CNS, models will undoubtedly be revised; however, at present, the systems model provides us with the best working model for explaining CNS functions and investigating impairments in systems that influence an individual's movement strategies.

NEUROPLASTICITY

The U.S. government declared the 1990s to be "the decade of the brain," which spurred a significant increase in funding for brain research.[11] This increase in funding resulted in numerous discoveries that have influenced poststroke interventions. Among the most important research is that which is related to **neuroplasticity**, the ability of the CNS to shape and/or renew itself in response to practiced activities.

Research is providing substantial evidence that neuromechanical changes do occur based on what is practiced. In studies with healthy animals, scientists have demonstrated that neuroplasticity occurs in the sensory and motor cortices. Evidence of neuroplasticity following a lesion in the sensory cortex has been demonstrated by Michael Merzenick, PhD.[10] Evidence of neuroplasticity following a lesion of the motor cortex has been demonstrated by Randolph Nudo, PhD.[14,15] There is also clinical evidence of neuroplasticity in human subjects who have cortical lesions. Beth Fisher, PhD, PT, and Katherine Sullivan, PhD, PT, have demonstrated that neuroplasticity can occur on the lesioned side of the cerebral cortex in an adult client following a CVA 1 year after onset when provided appropriate practice for use of the involved side. They wrote, "Rehabilitation strategies that promote recovery rather than compensation are those that provide a structured behavioral experience that incorporates (a) active participation in motor skill learning, (b) specific skills training and strengthening that is directed to the hemiparetic limbs, and (c) intense, task-specific practice that optimizes the sensorimotor experience of the task training. The review of current intervention strategies…provides evidence that, in fact, manipulation of the same practice variables that have consistently promoted behavioral recovery and neuroplasticity in animals and in the growing body of literature on brain mapping and imaging in humans is the necessary ingredient for maximizing the tremendous potential for recovery in our patients with stroke."[8]

As a result of these and other, similar findings, attitudes in the medical community are changing. Physicians realize that more can and should be done to influence recovery for individuals who have experienced a CVA. Specifically, they are embracing the emphasis that the NDT approach places on active use of the involved side to promote neuroplasticity on the lesioned side of the cerebral cortex.

PRINCIPLES OF MANAGEMENT

The core principles of the NDT approach are outlined in Table 31-1. These core principles provide a foundation for developing problem-solving strategies and intervention methods. Because NDT is a problem-solving approach, understanding these core principles is a first and necessary step for occupational therapists interested in becoming skilled in NDT. In the next section, the principle "Individualize Functional Outcomes" is described in detail because therapists should have a thorough understanding of this principle before considering the others.

INDIVIDUALIZE FUNCTIONAL OUTCOMES

Adult clients with hemiplegia benefit from interventions that are specific to their life roles, support systems, medical condition, life environments, and physical limitations resulting from CVA. This requires the therapist to provide interventions specific to a client's functional activity limitations, ineffective movement strategies, missing components of movement, and underlying impairments while working toward individualized functional outcomes. These considerations are discussed in greater detail in the following sections.

LIFE ROLES AND SUPPORT SYSTEMS

A CVA is an event for which no one has the opportunity to plan. When an individual experiences sudden onset of hemiplegia, there can be significant and immediate loss of function. Not only does this individual experience functional loss, but those who rely on this individual also experience losses. In other words, there is a ripple effect throughout the social context when this individual can no longer participate in life roles such as parenting, helping older family members, coaching, working as a committee member, or providing financial support. In addition, this individual may need to rely on others to assist in activities of daily living (ADL) and home management.

Occupational therapists must consider the effects of the CVA on the client and society when developing functional outcomes in order to individualize them appropriately. Individualizing functional outcomes increases active participation by the client during interventions, and allows the client to return to important life roles following interventions.

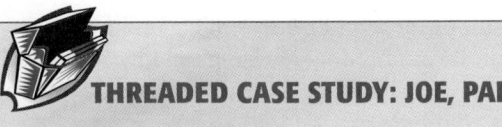

THREADED CASE STUDY: JOE, PART 2

Consider Joe, an adult client with hemiplegia. The occupational profile developed by Cathy revealed Joe's life roles to be those of a 46-year-old husband, the father of twin, 14-year-old boys, and a real estate agent. Since his stroke, Joe's life roles have changed. He is no longer able to provide financial support for his family by working as a real estate agent, and he is not able to help his sons. As a result, his wife's life roles have also changed. She now performs almost all household management activities, including many activities that Joe once managed, such as taking the boys to after-school activities. She is very concerned about her responsibilities at work because she must often leave work early to attend to Joe's needs. Joe now requires his wife's assistance for certain activities of daily living (ADL), including getting up from the dinner table, holding his hymnal at church, and pulling up his pants when dressing and after toileting. Joe revealed that he had recently fallen in the restroom, sliding down between the stall and the toilet, and had required assistance from his wife to get up.

MEDICAL CONDITION

It is essential to investigate the medical condition of adult clients with hemiplegia before developing interventions so that functional outcomes may be individualized appropriately. The following paragraphs discuss specific areas that should be investigated.

Therapists must be certain to adhere to medical precautions. For example, if a client has just returned from hip surgery for the involved lower extremity with the precaution of *non–weight-bearing with decreased hip flexion*, the therapist should avoid any weight bearing on the involved lower extremity.

OT PRACTICE NOTE

Medical precautions are *always* a primary concern when individualizing functional outcomes for adult clients with hemiplegia.

TABLE 31-1 **Core Principles of Management of the Neuro-Developmental Treatment Approach**

Principle	Synopsis	Action
Individualize Functional Outcomes	The adult client with hemiplegia will benefit from interventions that are specific to life roles, support systems, and underlying impairments.	Provide interventions specific to the client's functional activity limitations, ineffective movement strategies, and missing components of movement, while working toward individualized functional outcomes.
Emphasize Motor Control	Loss of motor control is the initial reason for use of ineffective movement strategies in adult clients with hemiplegia.	Focus on activities that require active participation by the client for problem solving and restore a balance of muscle activity, both of which are necessary for use of effective movement strategies. This will also contribute to increased muscle strength and ROM and to improved proprioception, balance, coordination, and perception.
Increase Active Use of the Involved Side	The adult client with hemiplegia must be encouraged to use the involved side. This allows the opportunity for neuroplasticity on the side of the cerebral cortex in which the lesion is located and reduces incidence of the behavior *learned non-use*.	Use manual cues and progressive challenge when accessing missing components of movement to provide opportunities for increased active use of the involved side.
Provide Practice to Improve Motor Performance Leading to Motor Learning	Motor learning for adult clients with hemiplegia requires use of appropriate schedules of practice, appropriate amounts of practice, and a logical progression of challenge.	Provide practice, which improves motor performance during client sessions and leads to motor learning across sessions.
Teach 24-Hour Management to Increase Retention and Carryover	Increasing retention and carryover for adult clients with hemiplegia encourages them to incorporate the involved side during functional activities between therapy sessions.	Provide specific instruction for component practice as well as management of the client on a 24-hour basis.
Use an Interdisciplinary Approach to Interventions	Each member of the therapy team should provide continued practice for all missing components of movement when providing interventions for adult clients with hemiplegia.	Access all missing components of movement while providing a discipline specific emphasis.

Therapists must ascertain the onset date of hemiplegia because this information will play an important role in determining potential for recovery. Although potential for recovery diminishes with time, effective interventions can be provided for individuals in a chronic condition if the therapist individualizes intervention activities and functional outcomes appropriately.[23]

THREADED CASE STUDY: JOE, PART 3

Joe's medical history and medical condition revealed that he had a heart attack 5 years before his stroke; however, he had no cardiovascular precautions at the time of intervention. His stroke occurred 5 months prior to the first intervention session with his home-based occupational therapist, Cathy (Figure 31-2). After his stroke, he was in a coma for 10 days. At that time, physicians told Joe's wife that he had a 5% chance for survival. He was admitted for approximately 4 weeks to a nursing home, where a gastrostomy tube was inserted to address significant swallowing problems. The tube was removed approximately 1 month later. Joe was transferred to a rehabilitation center for an additional 2 weeks of therapy, after which he was discharged to his home. Joe had no additional therapy in the 3 months preceding the home-based intervention. At the time of this first visit, Joe still has some difficulty swallowing certain liquid consistencies.

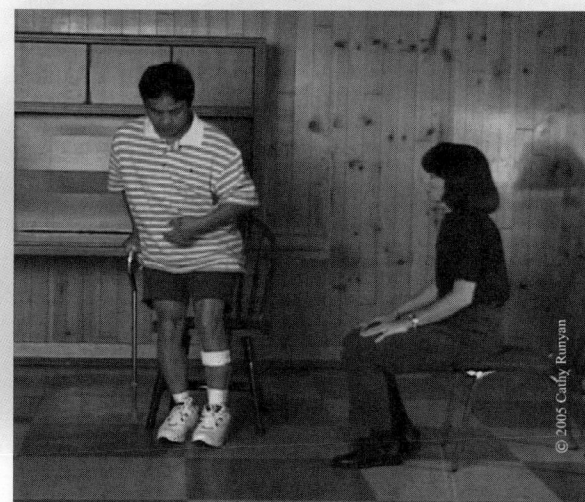

Figure 31-2 Joe experienced sudden onset of hemiplegia 5 months before his intervention session with Cathy. (Copyright © 2005 by Cathy Runyan OTR/L [www.RecoveringFunction.com].)

FUNCTIONAL ACTIVITIES

A **functional activity** is one that is consistent with an individual's life roles and life environments. Therapists can increase a client's interest and active participation during

interventions by employing features of the environment that relate to that client's life roles and life environments. Use of such features encourages the achievement of additional functional outcomes and promotes retention and carryover for those outcomes.[22] The occupational therapist must carefully consider features of the environment, whether NDT interventions are provided in the hospital, clinic, work, or home setting. Often, features of the clinical environment do not relate to the client's life roles and life environments. It is not difficult to understand why most clients are not inspired by activities such as stacking cones, threading beads on wire, or placing pegs in holes. These activities lack any relationship to the client's typical activities before the onset of the CVA. Similarly, a low mat surrounded by open floor space is not typical of the environments with which most clients interact. Effective use of NDT requires that movements are practiced in the context of functional activities.

Asking the client about life roles and life environments can help the therapist create a functional, individualized environment for interventions. For example, if the client worked as a librarian before onset of hemiplegia and desires to return to that job, the therapist could provide the activity of shelving books within a clinical setting. If the placement of furniture in the client's home environment requires specific movements, the therapist should attempt to replicate that environment in the clinic to encourage practice of those movements. In fact, in cases where it is possible, the therapist should consider using items during interventions that are owned by the client. To the extent that items used during interventions are similar to items typically encountered by the client, the interest and active participation of the client will be increased. This will also engage the client for longer periods of time, providing opportunities for repetition and therefore for increased retention of functional gains and carryover to a variety of situations.[20]

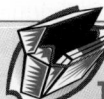

THREADED CASE STUDY: JOE, PART 4

Below are examples of items used to provide opportunities for Joe's participation in functional activities:

- *A heavy book.* This item was used to achieve functional outcomes that addressed Joe's concern about holding a hymnal at church (Figure 31-3, *A*).
- *An office chair with armrests on wheels.* This item was used to achieve functional outcomes that addressed Joe's concern about using the office chairs at his real estate office.

Continued

THREADED CASE STUDY: JOE, PART 4—cont'd

- *A standard height, 18-inch dinette chair without armrests.* This item was used to achieve functional outcomes that addressed Joe's concern about standing from the dinner table (Figure 31-3, *B*).

- *A high bookshelf with three shelves.* This item was used to achieve functional outcomes that addressed Joe's concern about reaching manuals on high shelves at his real estate office.

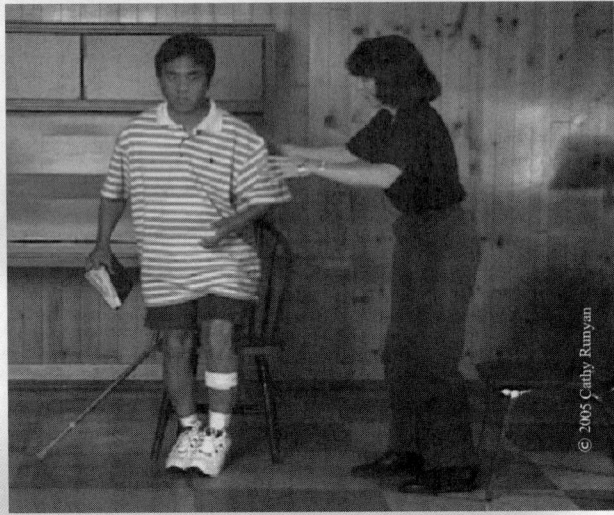

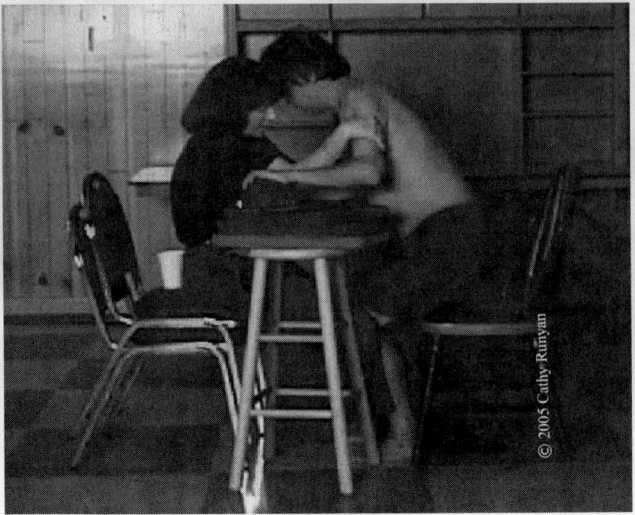

A   B

Figure 31-3   **A,** Joe's intervention session with Cathy included objects that were functional for Joe, for example, a book similar in size and weight to the hymnals he holds when standing to sing at church. **B,** Joe wants to be able to pull his chair toward the table when sitting and push it back when standing. He does not want to require his wife's help when having dinner with his family. (Copyright © 2005 by Cathy Runyan OTR/L [www.RecoveringFunction.com].)

FUNCTIONAL ACTIVITY LIMITATIONS

A **functional activity limitation** is one that prevents an individual from fully participating in activities consistent with the individual's life roles and life environments. For example, the inability to carry a child while walking is a functional activity limitation for an individual with hemiplegia who is the parent of an infant child, whereas that individual's inability to ice skate would not be a functional activity limitation if the individual has no interest in or need to ice skate. Examples of functional activity limitations related to basic ADL that are important to virtually all clients include the inability to dress, independently transfer to a bed, or stand at a sink to groom.

A functional activity limitation is relatively simple to identify, and its impact is easy to understand. However, identifying and understanding the factors that contribute to a functional activity limitation is a complex problem. Identification of functional activity limitations is the first step taken by skilled NDT therapists when progressively breaking down a client's large problems into smaller ones that are more easily understood and more efficiently addressed.

Specifically, observed functional activity limitations are broken into their ineffective movement strategies, which in turn are broken into their missing components of movement, which are then broken into their underlying impairments. By creating intervention activities for a client that access these missing components of movement, NDT-skilled therapists promote the use of effective movement strategies. Through an understanding of underlying impairments, these therapists are able to assess a client's potential for achieving certain functional outcomes. Subsequent sections of the chapter illustrate this process in detail, using the case presentation of Joe.

Identification of functional activity limitations also allows the occupational therapist to individualize functional outcomes that are reimbursable. Reimbursement criteria require the therapist to demonstrate that skilled intervention produced functional outcomes.[5] By documenting the client's functional activity limitations before intervention and comparing them to the client's functional abilities after intervention, the therapist can document improvements in the client's functional performance that are reimbursable.

THREADED CASE STUDY: JOE, PART 5

Below are examples of functional activity limitations for Joe:

- *Inability to sit down on and stand up from a variety of surfaces without use of his right, less involved upper extremity for support and balance during the ascent and descent.* Individuals with functional ability are able to sit down on and stand up from a variety of surfaces without use of their upper extremities for support and balance during the ascent and descent.
- *Inability to use his left, involved upper extremity for active support when sitting down on or standing up from an office chair.* Individuals with functional ability are able to use either upper extremity for active support when standing up from or sitting down on a variety of surfaces.
- *During stand to sit, inability to sustain symmetrical, active use of his lower extremities during the descent to an unstable surface (an office chair on wheels), which increased his risk

of falling (Figure 31-4, A).* Individuals with functional ability are able to use their lower extremities to sit down on a variety of unstable surfaces, including an office chair on wheels (Figure 31-4, B).
- *Inability to stand up from or sit down on a standard-height chair in a timely manner without using his right, less involved upper extremity in the lift off.* Individuals with functional ability are able to stand up from or sit down on a standard-height chair in approximately 2 seconds, as well as change their speed of movement according to the demand of the activity.
- *During sit to stand, or stand to sit, from a dinette chair, inability to maintain balance while carrying an object (Figure 31-5, A).* Individuals with functional ability are able to stand and sit and maintain balance while carrying various objects (Figure 31-5, B).

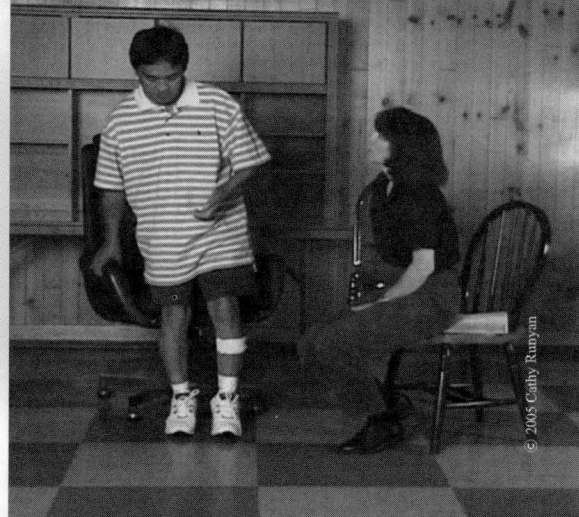

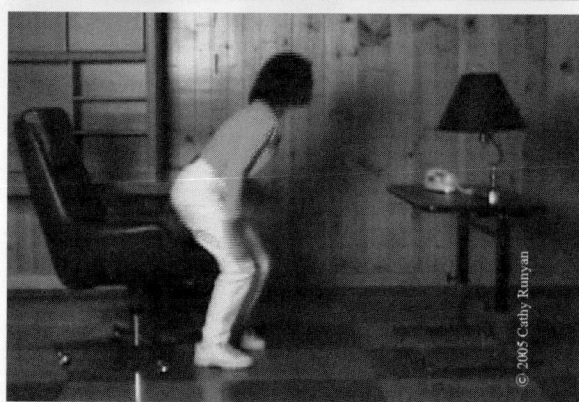

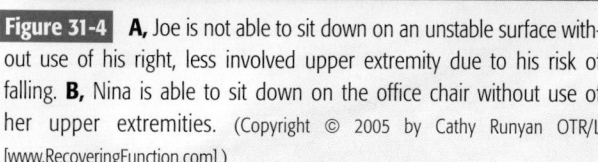

Figure 31-4 **A,** Joe is not able to sit down on an unstable surface without use of his right, less involved upper extremity due to his risk of falling. **B,** Nina is able to sit down on the office chair without use of her upper extremities. (Copyright © 2005 by Cathy Runyan OTR/L [www.RecoveringFunction.com].)

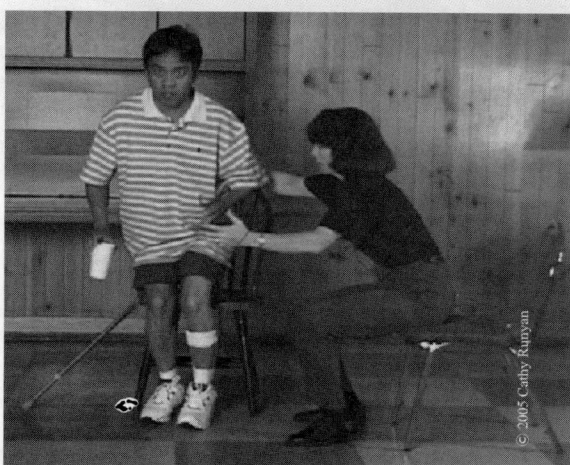

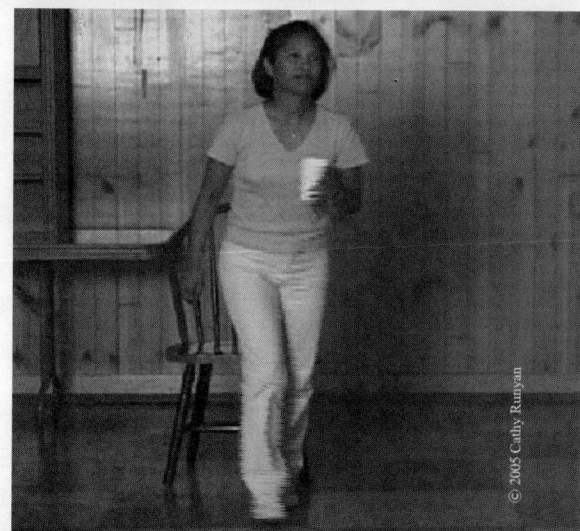

Figure 31-5 **A,** Joe is not able to maintain his balance when standing from a dinette chair while carrying an object. **B,** Elisa is able to stand up from a dinette chair while carrying an object in either hand. (Copyright © 2005 by Cathy Runyan OTR/L [www.RecoveringFunction.com].)

Continued

THREADED CASE STUDY: JOE, PART 5—cont'd

- *In standing, inability to bear weight equally on his lower extremities when reaching with his right, less involved upper extremity for an object on a high shelf (placed slightly to the left) while using his left, involved upper extremity to bear weight through his extended wrist and hand on a counter.* Individuals with functional ability are able to stand at a kitchen counter and bear weight through an extended hand and wrist on a counter while the other hand reaches to retrieve an object from a high shelf.
- *In standing, inability to bear weight equally on his lower extremities when reaching with his right, less involved upper extremity for an object on a high shelf placed slightly to the left.* Individuals with functional ability are able to stand at a kitchen counter and reach to retrieve an object from a high shelf placed slightly to the left.

- *In standing, inability to safely pull up his pants for lower body dressing using his right, less involved upper extremity.* Individuals with functional ability are able to safely pull up their pants while standing.
- *In standing, inability to actively bear weight through his left, involved lower and upper extremities while using his right, less involved upper extremity to move a chair toward or away from him (Figure 31-6, A).* Individuals with functional ability are able to stand on their left lower extremity and bear weight through the left upper extremity while using their right hand to move a chair toward themselves or away from themselves (Figure 31-6, *B* and *C*).

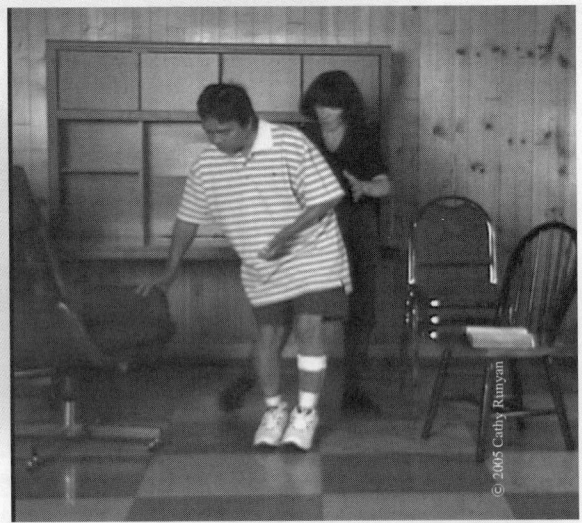

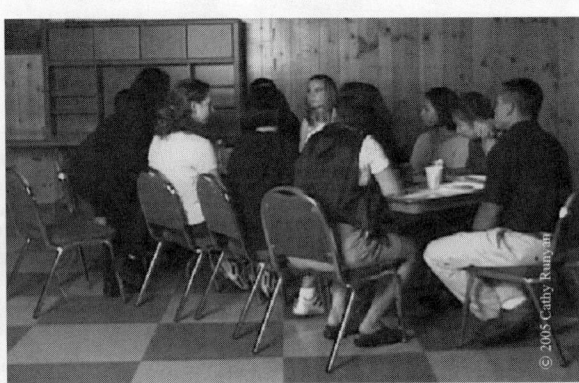

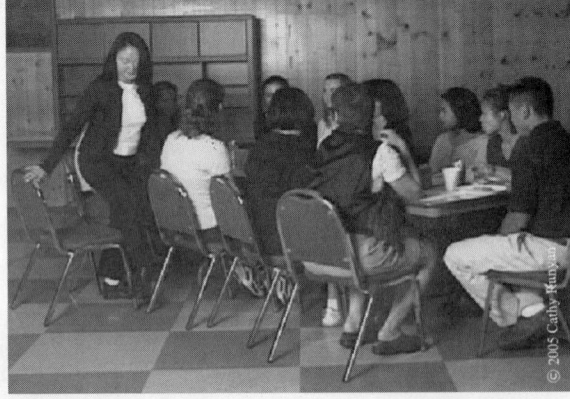

Figure 31-6 **A,** Joe is not able to easily pull the chair toward him. **B,** Ileana is able to pull her chair toward her when sitting from standing. **C,** Ileana is able to stand and push her chair away. (Copyright © 2005 by Cathy Runyan OTR/L [www.RecoveringFunction.com].)

INEFFECTIVE MOVEMENT STRATEGIES

Functional activity limitations result from the use of **ineffective movement strategies.** Understanding a client's ineffective movement strategies for a functional activity requires the therapist to first have a thorough understanding of the effective movement strategies required for that activity. Effective movement strategies are those used by an individual when all components of movement required for a specific activity are available. These are the strategies that healthy individuals use routinely. These strategies and the movements they produce are automatic, ingrained in the CNS as the result of years of repetition, but can also be evoked consciously.[13] The movements produced by effective movement strategies are efficient, allowing for increased endurance, and result in increased balance and safety. For example, a healthy individual is able to walk down a hallway while carrying a cup of coffee and talking to a colleague without thinking about each step taken.[17] In fact, this individual is able to easily maintain balance when moving aside to let someone pass by, or when bending over to retrieve a dropped coin from the floor. Furthermore, the availability of all components of movement allows this individual to change use of effective movement strategies dynamically—for example,

moving the coin to the left with one foot during the retrieval due to someone unexpectedly walking by. This ability to dynamically change movement strategies also allows for increased safety for the individual.[24]

To the contrary, ineffective movement strategies are those used by an individual when all components of movement required for a planned activity are not available. Ineffective movement strategies are not automatic but instead require the individual to concentrate on movement. The movements produced by ineffective movement strategies are not efficient, requiring excessive time and exertion, resulting in fatigue. For example, when walking down a hallway, the individual with hemiplegia often must concentrate intently on each step taken and stop walking in order to engage in conversation. This individual is not able to easily move aside to let someone pass by and in fact might experience a loss of balance if someone passes by too closely. Furthermore, the lack of availability of all components of movement does not allow this individual to change movement strategies dynamically in response to unpredicted changes in the environment, resulting in decreased safety for the individual. Without intervention by the skilled therapist, ineffective movement strategies can lead to falls. In addition, ineffective movement strategies can cause pain due to repetitive strain, nerve entrapment, or malaligned joints.

THREADED CASE STUDY: JOE, PART 6

Below are examples of ineffective movement strategies related to Joe's functional activity limitation "in standing, inability to bear weight equally on his lower extremities when reaching with his right, less involved upper extremity for an object on a high shelf (placed slightly to the left) while using his left, involved upper extremity to bear weight through his extended wrist and hand on a counter":

- *His left, involved foot was not part of his BOS. His midfoot excessively supinated, and his ankle plantarflexed (Figure 31-7, A).* Individuals using effective movement strategies are able to use their feet as part of their BOS. Their feet are mobile, not stiff, and adapt to the surface on which they are standing. A stable BOS provided by the foot influences the kinetic chain above the foot, including alignment and mobility of the knee, hip, pelvis, shoulders, head, and upper extremities. Individuals using effective movement strategies are able to use their feet as a BOS for lower extremity weight bearing during a variety of activities. As a result of using their feet to increase the BOS for active support in weight bearing, these individuals are safer and more functional when using their other extremities (Figure 31-7, B).
- *He did not actively use his left, involved lower extremity for weight bearing.* Individuals using effective movement strategies are able to align their limbs over their BOS and automatically adjust the use of muscle activity in weight bearing when standing.

They are able to use concentric, eccentric, and isometric muscle contractions of their lower extremities according to the demand of the activity. Individuals using effective movement strategies are able to use the following: (1) eccentric muscle activity of their extensors to descend into gravity, (2) concentric muscle activity of their extensors to ascend from gravity, (3) isometric muscle activity (appropriate co-contraction of muscle activity) to control a posture for the time it would take to complete an intended activity (Figure 31-8).

- *His hips remained flexed bilaterally.* Individuals using effective movement strategies are able to use a stable BOS with an appropriate alignment of their lower extremities in weight bearing and extend their hips appropriately for the activity.
- *His pelvis rotated posteriorly and tilted slightly upward on his left, involved side (Figure 31-9, A).* Individuals using effective movement strategies are able to use a stable BOS with the appropriate alignment of their lower extremities in weight bearing. They are able to rotate and tilt the pelvis in a variety of directions in all planes during sit to stand, stand to sit, and when standing. The alignment of the pelvis influences alignment of the lower extremities, including the foot that provides the BOS. The alignment of the lower trunk, including the pelvis, also influences the alignment of the upper trunk including the shoulders (Figure 31-9, B).

Continued

THREADED CASE STUDY: JOE, PART 6—cont'd

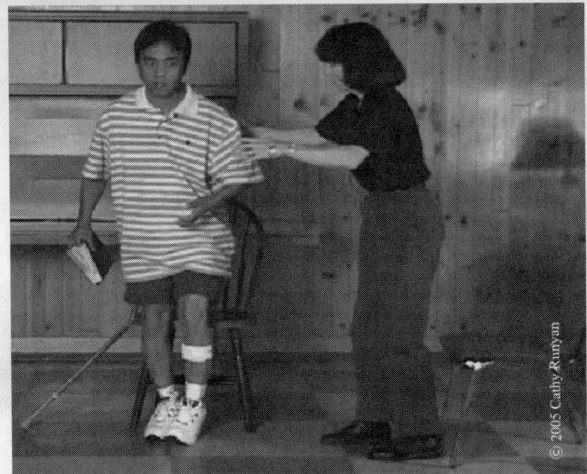

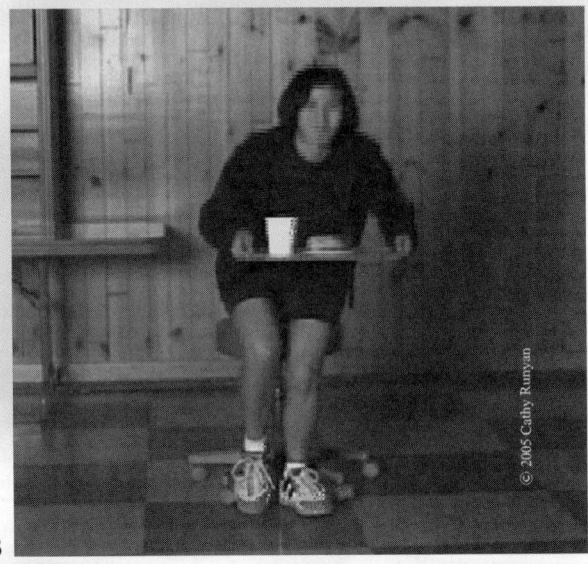

Figure 31-7   **A,** Joe's left, involved foot was not part of his BOS when standing. **B,** Melissa is able to use either foot as part of her BOS when standing. (Copyright © 2005 by Cathy Runyan OTR/L [www.RecoveringFunction.com].)

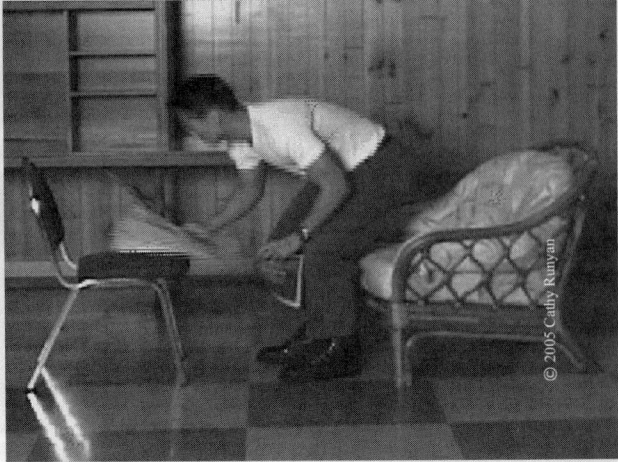

Figure 31-8   Vin is able to control his lower extremity extensors and control a posture for the time it takes to complete an intended activity. (Copyright © 2005 by Cathy Runyan OTR/L [www.RecoveringFunction.com].)

- *His trunk remained in a position of lumbar and thoracic flexion.* Individuals using effective movement strategies are able to move their trunk in a variety of positions in all planes. They are able to use concentric, eccentric, and isometric muscle contractions of their trunk extensors in response to gravity and according to the demand of the activity. Alignment of the trunk influences the alignment of the limbs, including the head.
- *His ribs were open in the posterior aspect and closed in the lateral aspect on his left, involved side.* Individuals using effective movement strategies are able to move their ribs so as to assume a variety of postures in all planes. Alignment of the ribs influences alignment of the thoracic spine, the pelvis, the scapula, and therefore the humerus.

- *His left, involved scapula was downwardly rotated.* Individuals using effective movement strategies are able to move their scapula through all planes. They also are able to stabilize their scapula against the ribcage to provide greater stability for the upper extremities when required. Alignment of the scapula influences alignment of the ribs and humerus. Alignment of the scapula also influences alignment of the ribs and pelvis.
- *His left, involved humerus remained in internal rotation.* Individuals using effective movement strategies are able to move their humerus in a variety of directions, in all planes, in and out of weight bearing (including external rotation).
- *His left elbow remained flexed.* Individuals using effective movement strategies are able to use their upper extremities for active support to bear weight through their hand. These individuals are able to use concentric, eccentric, and isometric muscle contractions to extend and flex their elbow when pushing weight away from their hand, to accept weight onto their hand, and to control their posture for the time it takes to complete the intended activity.
- *His left forearm remained supinated.* Individuals using effective movement strategies are able to actively pronate their forearm in and out of weight bearing. Pronation with approximation through the wrist is essential for the upper extremity to accept full weight bearing.
- *He did not initiate use of his left, involved hand as part of his BOS. His wrist and fingers remained flexed.* Individuals using effective movement strategies are able to use either hand as part of their BOS. They are able to bear weight through their extended hand and wrist. Their hand and wrist are mobile, not stiff or painful. A stable base provided by the hand influences the alignment and mobility of the forearm, elbow, humerus,

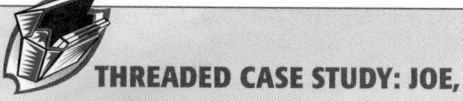

THREADED CASE STUDY: JOE, PART 6—cont'd

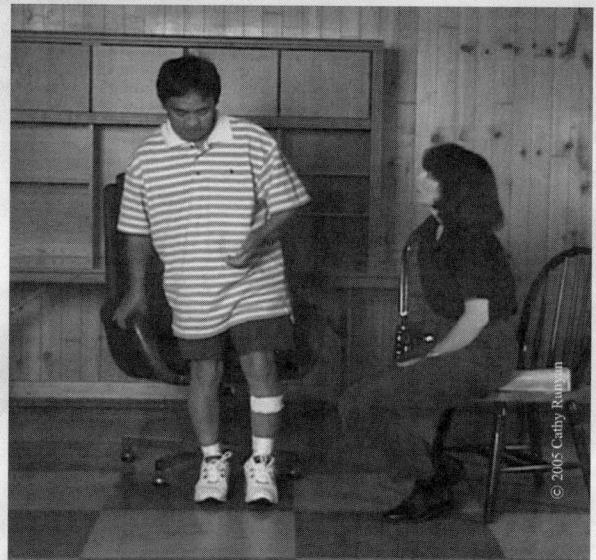

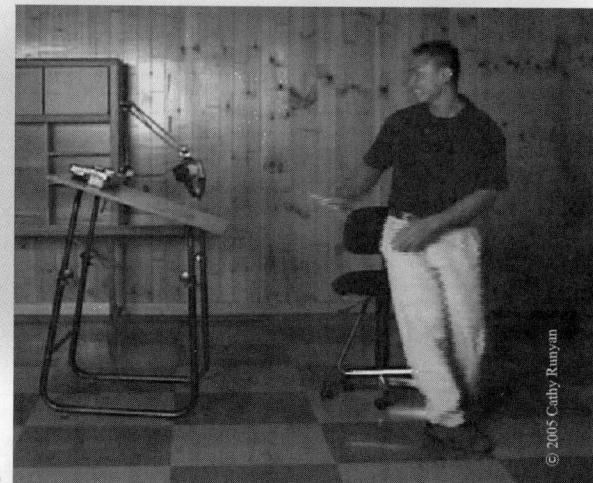

Figure 31-9 **A,** Joe's pelvis rotated posteriorly and tilted slightly upward on his left, involved side. **B,** Victor is able to move his pelvis in a variety of directions in all planes during the transition of sit to stand, or stand to sit, and when standing. (Copyright © 2005 by Cathy Runyan OTR/L [www.RecoveringFunction.com].)

scapula, clavicle and ribcage. Individuals using effective movement strategies are able to use either hand as a BOS for upper extremity weight bearing during a variety of activities. As a result of using their hand to increase their BOS for active support in weight bearing, these individuals are safer and more functional when reaching with their other extremities.

- *He experienced a loss of balance, using only his right, less involved foot as his BOS, when his right, less involved upper extremity was not included as part of his BOS.* Individuals using effective movement strategies are able to balance. They are able to organize their trunk and limbs around their center of mass related to the influences of gravity. They are able to use their trunk and limbs (including their head) as part of the BOS. They are also able to use their limbs to support, to reach, to pull, and to manipulate objects.

- *His weight was excessively shifted to the right in a lateral direction, and his left, involved shoulder was excessively rotated forward.* Individuals using effective movement strategies are able to shift their weight in a variety of directions, including the anterior/posterior direction (sagittal plane), the lateral direction, (frontal plane), and they are able to rotate body segments on either side in a posterior or anterior direction (transverse plane). Individuals using effective movement strategies are also able to weight shift in combinations of all of these directions over a stable BOS as well as a moving BOS.

- *Inadequate use of left lateral weight shift from full weight bearing on the right, less involved lower extremity to weight bearing on his lower extremities bilaterally to assume a symmetrical posture.* Individuals using effective movement strategies are able to weight shift laterally to the left when standing, moving from full weight bearing on their right lower extremity to weight bearing bilaterally on their lower extremities to assume a symmetrical posture.

- *Inadequate use of lateral weight shift to the left from a symmetrical posture to full weight bearing on the left, involved extremities.* Individuals using effective movement strategies are able to weight shift laterally to the left when standing, moving from a symmetrical posture to full weight bearing on their left extremities.

MISSING COMPONENTS OF MOVEMENT

Ineffective movement strategies result from **missing components of movement**. Understanding a client's missing components of movement requires the therapist to first have a thorough understanding of components of movement. Components of movement are the building blocks of movement from which effective movement strategies are built. A simple, effective movement strategy may require only one component of movement, whereas a complex effective movement strategy may require many components of movement.

Each component of movement required by an effective movement strategy contributes to its overall effectiveness. Specifically, a component of movement is a range of movement for a given body segment required for a particular effective movement strategy. Examples of the components of movement required by the effective movement strategy "active use of the left upper extremity in full weight bearing" are *extension of the left wrist, extension of the left elbow, and depression of the left scapula.*

A missing component of movement is one that is required by an effective movement strategy but is either absent or is available in a diminished capacity. A movement strategy becomes increasingly ineffective as its number of missing components of movement increases. For example, for the effective movement strategy "active use of the left upper extremity in weight bearing" mentioned in the preceding paragraph, absence of wrist extension would result in the inability to bear weight onto the involved hand. Similarly, limited range of wrist extension, rather than the full range required by this effective movement strategy, would result in limited ability to bear weight on the involved hand.

As described in the next section, assessment of missing components of movement allows assessment of the underlying impairments that are causing the loss of those components of movement. In addition, because many ineffective movement strategies may be due to the same missing components of movement, therapists can create an efficient set of intervention activities by aligning those activities with a client's missing components of movement, rather than aligning them with the client's ineffective movement strategies directly. By simultaneously assessing and accessing these missing components through the use of manual cues during intervention sessions, the therapist transforms ineffective movement strategies into more effective ones.

THREADED CASE STUDY: JOE, PART 7

Below are examples of missing components of movement related to Joe's ineffective movement strategy "in standing, decreased use of lateral weight shift to the left from a symmetrical posture, to full weight bearing on the left, involved extremities":

- *Dorsiflexion of his left, involved ankle and pronation of his left, involved midfoot.* Joe is not able to terminate muscle activity of his ankle plantar flexors and supinators of his midfoot. Once aligned in weight bearing, his left, involved foot stays in neutral on the floor.
- *Extension of his left, involved hip (Figure 31-10).* Joe is able to initiate but not sustain active use of his hip extensors.

- *Forward rotation of the left side of his pelvis (Figure 31-11).* Joe is able to initiate but not sustain active use of his abdominals to maintain a neutral position of the left side of his pelvis in synergy with the musculature controlling his left hip extensors.
- *Extension of his lumbar spine.* Joe is able to initiate but not sustain active use of his lumbar extensors.
- *Extension of his thoracic spine.* Joe is able to initiate but not sustain active use of his thoracic extensors.
- *Posterior rotation on the left side of his thorax.* Joe is able to initiate but not sustain active use of his thoracic extensors to maintain a neutral position of the left side of his thorax.

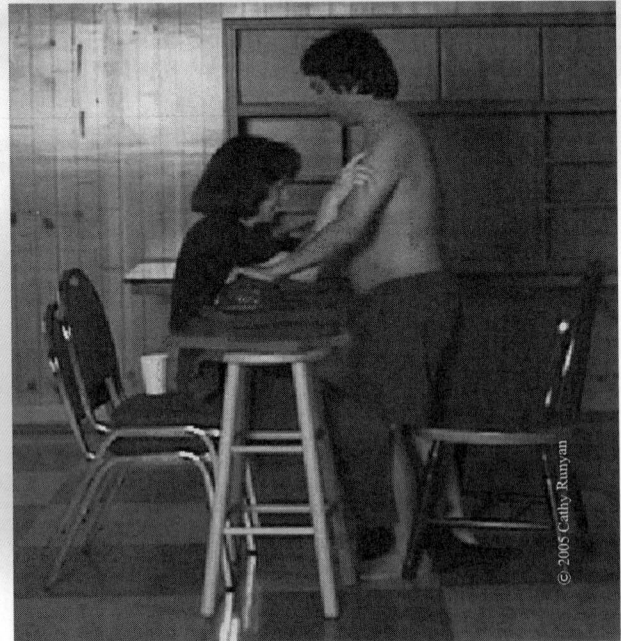

Figure 31-10 Joe is not able to initiate or sustain active use of his left, involved hip extensors when aligned in weight bearing while standing. (Copyright © 2005 by Cathy Runyan OTR/L [www.RecoveringFunction. com].)

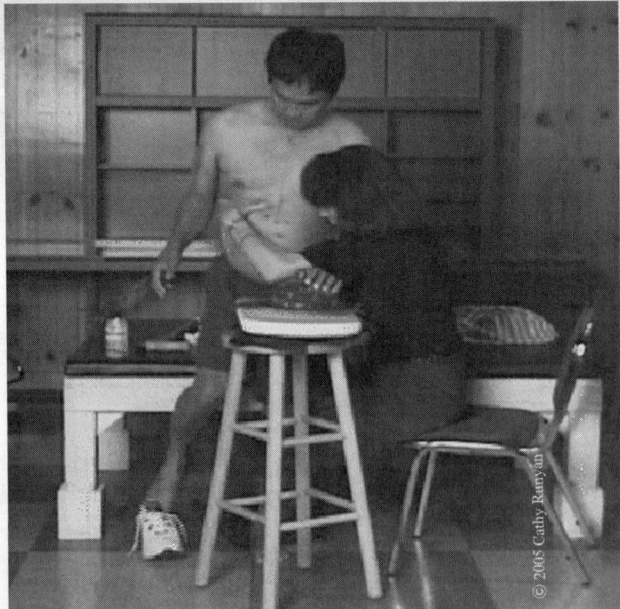

Figure 31-11 Joe is not able to initiate or sustain active use of his abdominals to bring the left, involved side of his pelvis forward to neutral while controlling his left, involved hip extensors. (Copyright © 2005 by Cathy Runyan OTR/L [www.RecoveringFunction.com].)

THREADED CASE STUDY: JOE, PART 7—cont'd

- *Expansion in the lateral aspect of the left side of his ribs.* Joe is not able to expand his ribs in the lateral aspect.
- *Adduction of his left, involved scapula.* With his scapula aligned in neutral, Joe is able to initiate adduction but he is not able to sustain it.
- *Depression of his left, involved scapula.* With his scapula aligned in neutral, Joe is not able to initiate or sustain active use of his scapular depressors.
- *External rotation of the left, involved humerus.* Joe is not able to terminate muscle activity of his internal rotators. Once his scapula is aligned in neutral and his left, involved upper extremity is in weight bearing, Joe is able to initiate active use of his humeral external rotators but cannot sustain it.
- *Extension of his left, involved elbow.* Joe is not able to terminate muscle activity of his elbow flexors. Once his elbow flexors are fully lengthened and his left, involved upper extremity is in weight bearing, Joe can initiate active use of his elbow extensors.
- *Pronation of his left, involved forearm.* Joe is not able to initiate or sustain active use of the forearm pronators. Once his upper extremity is aligned in weight bearing, his forearm remains pronated.
- *Extension of his left, involved wrist.* Joe is not able to initiate or sustain active use of wrist extensors. Once his upper extremity is aligned in weight bearing on an adapted surface, his wrist remains extended (Figure 31-12).
- *Extension of his left, involved fingers.* Joe is not able to initiate or sustain active use of finger extensors. He is not able to terminate muscle activity of his finger flexors. Once his upper extremity is aligned in weight bearing on an adapted surface allowing some flexion, his fingers remain extended.

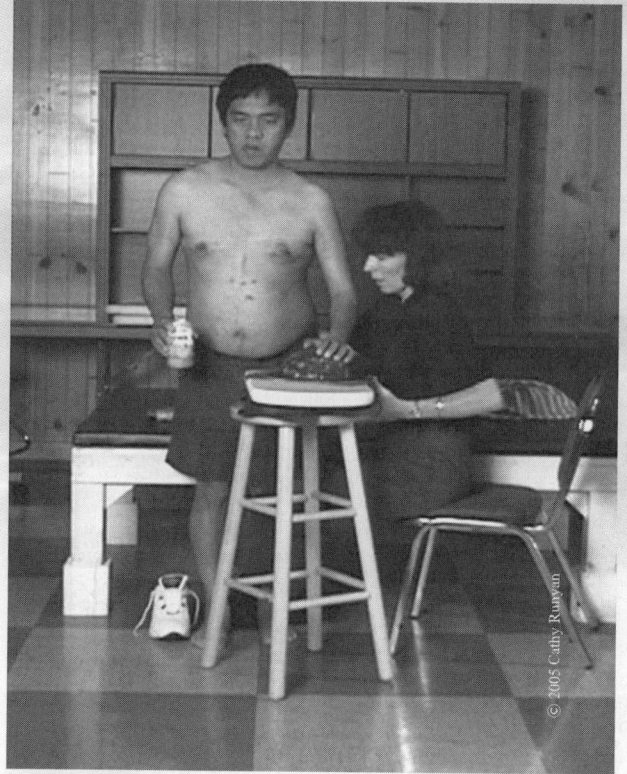

Figure 31-12   Once Joe's left, involved upper extremity is aligned in weight bearing, his left wrist stays in an extended position on the surface. (Copyright © 2005 by Cathy Runyan OTR/L [www.RecoveringFunction.com].)

Therapists skilled in NDT not only observe movement when assessing missing components of movement they also measure that movement in the context of a specific movement strategy. In particular, they measure both the required range of movement and the client's actual range of movement. This allows the client's progress during interventions to be documented for other members of the therapy team, as well as for reimbursement. For example, the required range for the missing component of movement *extension of his left involved wrist* for a specific movement strategy might be documented as *from neutral to full extension of his left, involved wrist.* Likewise, the client's actual range might be documented as *from neutral to ³/4 extension of his left, involved wrist.* The proper assessment of these ranges requires the skilled use of manual cues that is learned through hands-on NDT coursework.

IMPAIRMENTS

Missing components of movement are the result of underlying **impairments** in specific systems. Understanding underlying impairments requires the therapist to have a thorough understanding of the behavior of systems in healthy individuals. The proper functioning of these systems allows for the availability of the components of movement required by the use of effective movement strategies. A single impairment may affect many components of movement; conversely, a single component of movement may be affected by multiple impairments. By progressively breaking down a functional activity limitation into its ineffective movement strategies, then into its missing components of movement, and finally into its underlying impairments, the therapist ultimately arrives at the root causes of the functional activity limitation (i.e., the impairments in specific systems). An example of an impairment is *hypotonicity of the elbow extensors*. An example of impairments that could cause loss of the component of movement "extension of the left elbow" are *hypotonicity of the left elbow extensors, hypertonicity of the left elbow flexors, weakness of the left elbow extensors, loss of ROM for left elbow extension, sensory loss of the left upper extremity,* and *proprioceptive loss of the left upper extremity.* Assessing underlying impairments is critical to individualizing functional outcomes because this allows the therapist to determine the potential for achieving a given functional outcome.

THREADED CASE STUDY: JOE, PART 8

Below are examples of underlying impairments related to Joe's missing component of movement "adduction of the left, involved scapula" (Figure 31-13):

- *Neuromuscular system: Hypotonicity of left scapular adductors.* With his scapula aligned in neutral Joe is able to initiate adduction but not able to sustain it.
- *Neuromuscular system: Hypertonicity of left scapular abductors.* Joe is not able to terminate muscle activity of his scapular abductors.
- *Neuromuscular system: Weakness of the left scapular adductors.* With his left scapula aligned in neutral Joe is able to initiate adduction but not able to sustain it.
- *Musculoskeletal system: Decreased ROM for left scapular adduction.* Joe required soft-tissue stretch of his scapular abductors.
- *Sensory system: Diminished sensation of the left, involved upper extremity.* Joe's diminished sensation was evident when tested cortically and subcortically.
- *Proprioceptive system: Diminished position and kinesthetic sense of his left, involved upper extremity.* Joe's diminished position and kinesthetic sense were evident when tested cortically and subcortically.

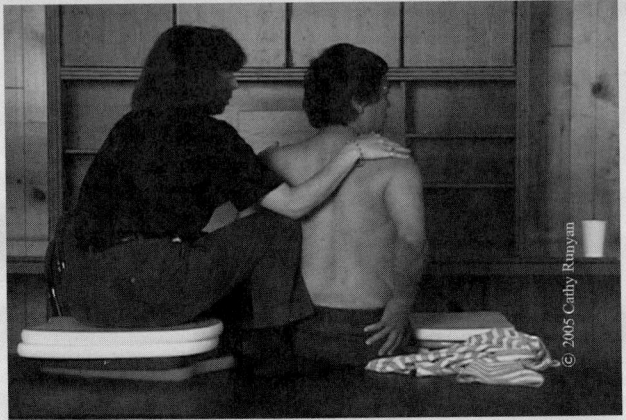

Figure 31-13   Cathy assessed Joe's underlying impairments associated with the missing component of movement "adduction of the left, involved scapula." (Copyright © 2005 by Cathy Runyan OTR/L [www.RecoveringFunction.com].)

INDIVIDUALIZED FUNCTIONAL OUTCOMES

Individualized functional outcomes are achievable, reimbursable, functional activities consistent with a client's life roles, support systems, medical condition, life environments, and physical limitations resulting from CVA. Therapists skilled in the NDT approach ascertain a client's potential for achieving functional outcomes by assessing the client's underlying impairments. They provide clients the opportunity to achieve functional outcomes by accessing missing components of movement, thereby promoting use of the effective movement strategies required by those outcomes. When using the NDT approach, therapists should always be working toward individualized functional outcomes.

As mentioned previously, it is important for the therapist to assess the client's potential for achieving a given functional outcome. For example, the functional outcome "while standing at the sink for grooming with symmetrical weight bearing of the lower extremities, the client is able to weight bear through the left, involved upper extremity onto the hand to increase the BOS for increased safety" requires the component of movement *extension of the left, involved elbow.* If a client is missing this component of movement because of a true contracture of the elbow flexors and that client has no potential for neutral extension of the elbow, then this functional outcome is not achievable by that client. If, however, the client is missing this component of movement because of a decreased ability to initiate and sustain active use of the elbow extensors but has potential for elbow extension, the therapist is responsible for helping the client achieve this outcome by accessing this missing component of movement.

THREADED CASE STUDY: JOE, PART 9

Below are examples of individualized functional outcomes achieved by Joe:

- Sit to stand, or stand to sit, with symmetrical use of his lower extremities from a variety of surfaces without use of his right, less involved upper extremity in the lift off or the descent (Figure 31-14).

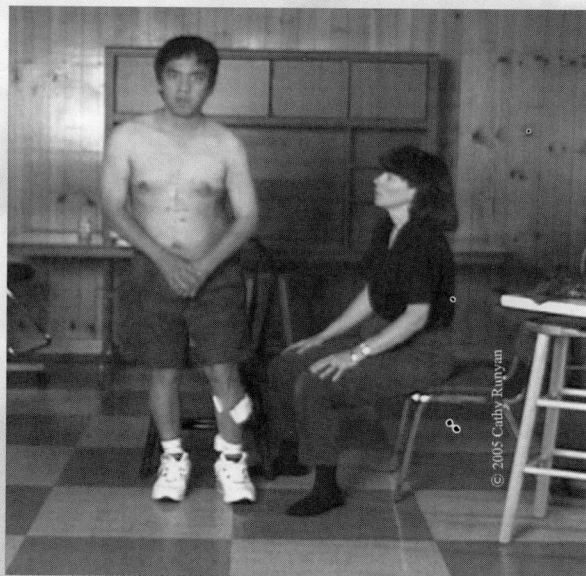

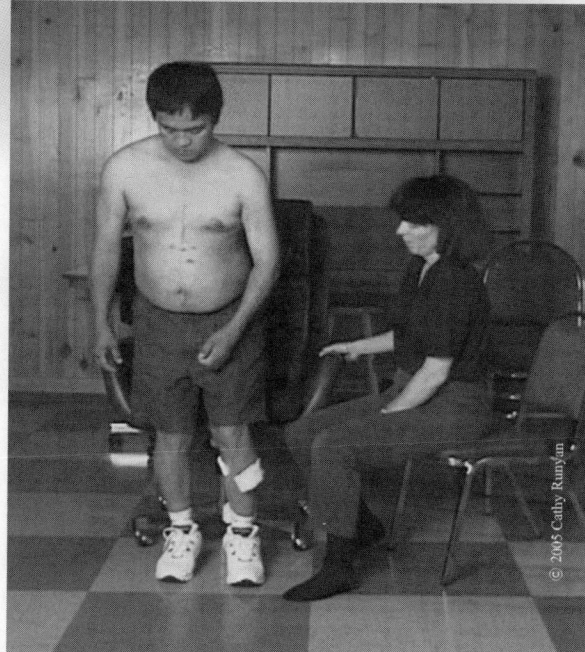

Figure 31-14 **A,** An appropriate individualized functional outcome for Joe is to sit to stand, or stand to sit from his dinette chair. **B,** An appropriate individualized functional outcome for Joe is to sit to stand, or stand to sit from his office chair. (Copyright © 2005 by Cathy Runyan OTR/L [www.RecoveringFunction.com].)

Life roles and environments	Joe expressed concern about requiring assistance from his wife when standing up from or sitting down on his dinette chair. He also expressed concern about standing up from or sitting down on his office chair.
Reimbursable	Increased access to various surfaces, including a dinette chair and an office chair
	Increased functional ability to stand, or sit without assistance from others
	Increased safety when standing up from, or sitting down on, a variety of surfaces as a result of the active use of his lower extremities

- Sit to stand, or stand to sit, with symmetrical use of his lower extremities while pushing a chair away from him or bringing a chair toward him, using his right, less involved upper extremity.

Life roles and environments	Joe expressed concern about requiring assistance from his wife to get up from the dinner table.
Reimbursable	Increased access to various life environments, including the dining room table
	Increased functional ability to pull his chair up to a table as well as push it back without assistance from others
	Increased independence when using his right, less involved hand to move a chair toward him or move a chair away while controlling his posture

- Sit to stand, or stand to sit, with symmetrical use of his lower extremities while carrying objects with his right, less involved upper extremity.

Life roles and environments	Joe expressed concern about not being able to hold his hymnal in church.
Reimbursable	Decreased requirement for others to hold objects for him while standing
	Increased functional ability to carry various objects (access to life environments) during the transitions of sit to stand, or stand to sit

Continued

THREADED CASE STUDY: JOE, PART 9–cont'd

- Stand, with symmetrical use of his lower extremities, from a standard-height chair in less time without using his right, less involved upper extremity in the lift off.

Life roles and environments	Joe expressed concern about the length of time his wife had to wait for him to stand up.
Reimbursable	Decreased requirement for assistance from others Increased productivity

- In standing, with symmetrical use of his lower extremities, safely pull up his pants with his right, less involved, upper extremity (Figure 31-15).

Life roles and environments	Joe expressed concern about requiring assistance from his wife to pull up his pants in the bathroom.
Reimbursable	Increased safety as a result of the active use of his lower extremities when standing

Increased functional ability to pull up his pants independently using his right, less involved hand for fastening his pants instead of holding onto his cane

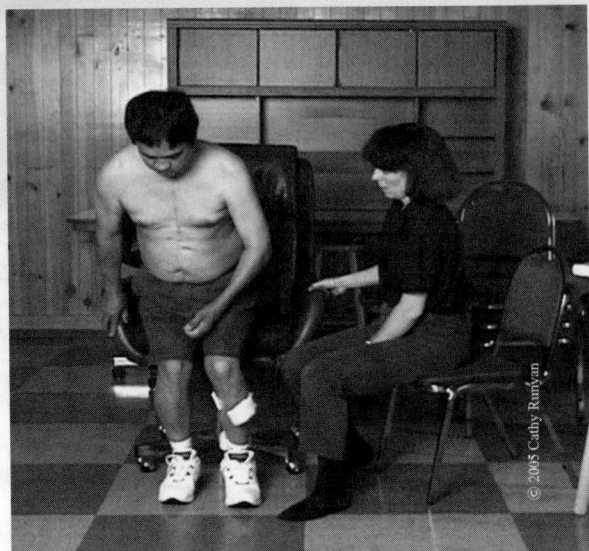

A

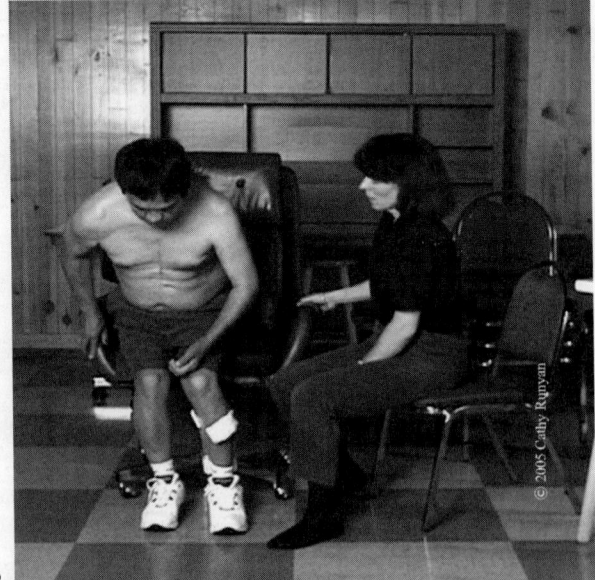

B

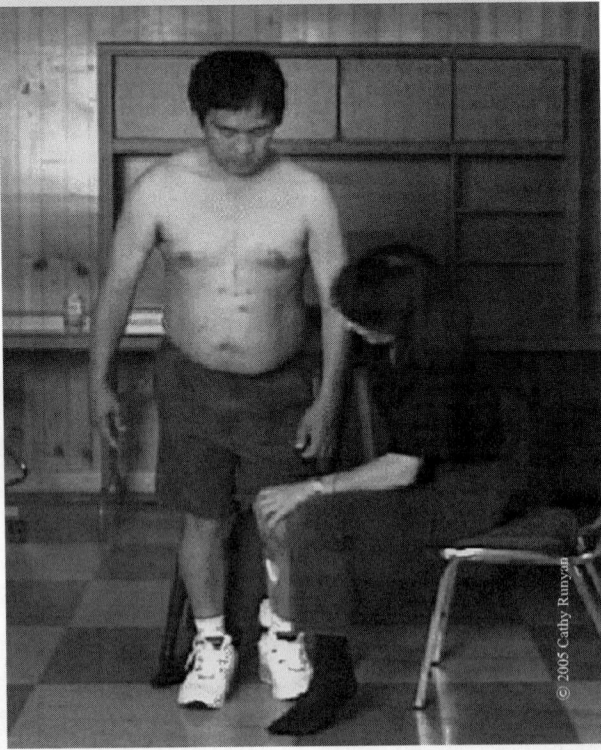

Figure 31-15 An appropriate individualized functional outcome for Joe is to safely pull up his pants with his right, less involved upper extremity when standing. (Copyright © 2005 by Cathy Runyan OTR/L [www.RecoveringFunction.com].)

Figure 31-16 **A,** An appropriate individualized functional outcome for Joe is to appropriately weight shift his hips backward and his shoulders forward to sit down on an unstable surface. **B,** This outcome requires Joe to actively use his lower extremities to control his posture during the descent. (Copyright © 2005 by Cathy Runyan OTR/L [www.RecoveringFunction.com].)

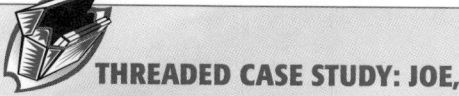

THREADED CASE STUDY: JOE, PART 9—cont'd

- In standing, with symmetrical use of his lower extremities, reach for an object placed high on a shelf and slightly to the left with his right, less-involved, upper extremity.

Life roles and environments	Joe expressed concern about being able to reach manuals in the bookcases at his real estate office.
Reimbursable	Increased functional ability to reach for objects placed high on a shelf

and slightly to his left (increased access to various life environments) Decreased assistance from others to reach for objects

- When sitting, appropriately weight shift his hips back and his shoulders forward to sit down on an unstable surface (Figure 31-16).

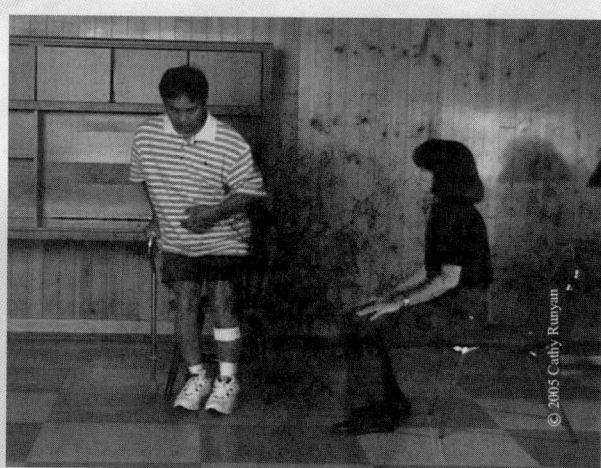
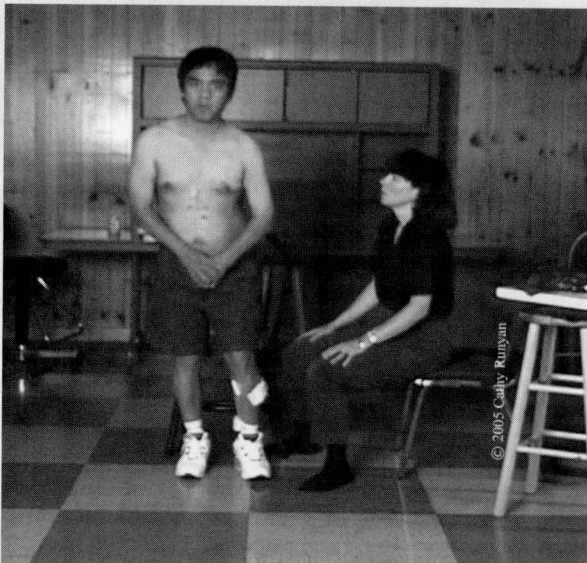
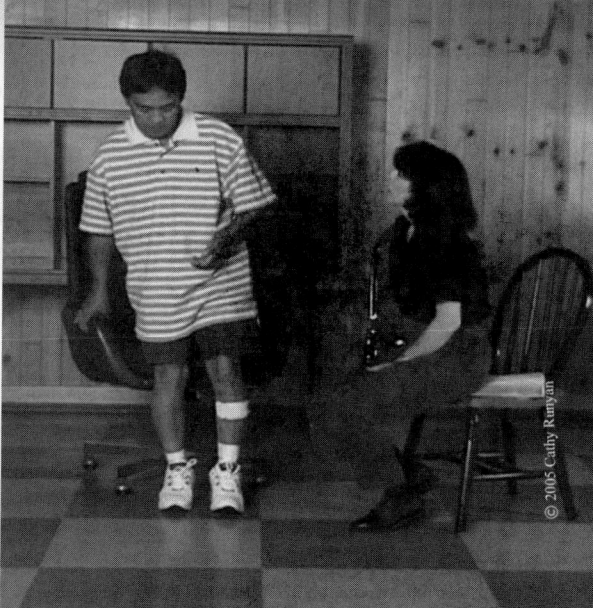
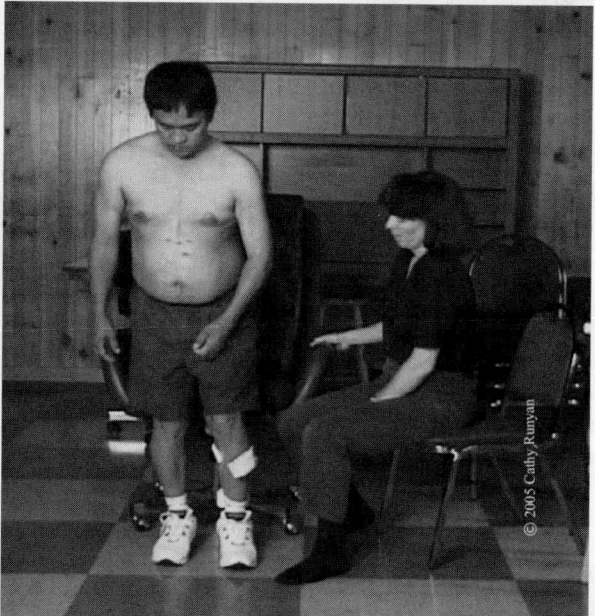

Figure 31-17 **A,** Joe standing from the dinette chair before intervention. **B,** Joe standing from the dinette chair after his 1-hour intervention session with Cathy. **C,** Joe standing from the office chair before intervention. **D,** Joe standing from the office chair after his 1-hour intervention session with Cathy. (Copyright © 2005 by Cathy Runyan OTR/L [www.RecoveringFunction.com].)

Continued

THREADED CASE STUDY: JOE, PART 9—cont'd

Life roles and environments	Joe expressed concern about being able to use his office chair at work because the chairs at his office have wheels
Reimbursable	Increased safety as a result of his ability to control eccentric use of his lower extremities with the appropriate weight shift to sit down on an unstable surface (an office chair on wheels)
	Decreased requirement for assistance from others to prevent him from falling
	Increased functional ability to change his direction of weight shift spontaneously

Figure 31-17, *A* and *C*, illustrates Joe's movement strategies before intervention. Figure 31-17, *B* and *D*, illustrates the changes in Joe's movement strategies after his 1-hour intervention session with Cathy. These changes in his movement strategies were required to achieve his functional outcomes.

Below are examples of individualized functional outcomes that are appropriate for Joe but for which he has limited potential for achievement because of his impairments:

- In standing, to bear weight equally on his lower extremities when reaching with his right, less involved upper extremity for an object on a high shelf (placed slightly to the left) while using his left, involved upper extremity to bear weight through his extended wrist and hand on a counter
- When standing from a table, bear weight on his left, involved upper extremity on the table while using his right, less involved upper extremity to move a chair toward him or away from him
- Using his left, involved upper extremity for active support in the lift off from or the descent to the office chair

SUMMARY

This chapter introduced the NDT approach. Application of the principle "Individualize Functional Outcomes" was described in detail because a thorough understanding of this principle is the first step toward becoming a skilled NDT therapist.

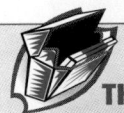

THREADED CASE STUDY: JOE, PART 10

The principle "Individualize Functional Outcomes" was illustrated through the case presentation of Joe by answering the critical thinking questions:

What factors influence the selection of outcomes for Joe?

Factors that influence the selection of outcomes for Joe (and all other adult clients with hemiplegia) are achievability, reimbursement, life roles, support systems, medical condition, life environments, and physical limitations resulting from his CVA.

What physical limitations resulting from the CVA are preventing Joe from participating in his occupation as a real estate agent?

The specific physical limitations preventing Joe from participating in his occupation are his underlying impairments. Joe's underlying impairments were determined via a progressive determination of his functional activity limitations, ineffective movement strategies, and missing components of movement. Examples of underlying impairments for Joe include the following:

- Neuromuscular system: Hypotonicity of left scapular adductors
- Neuromuscular system: Hypertonicity of left scapular abductors
- Neuromuscular system: Weakness of left scapular adductors
- Musculoskeletal system: Decreased ROM for left scapular adduction
- Sensory system: Diminished sensation of the left, involved upper extremity
- Proprioceptive system: Diminished position and kinesthetic sense of his left, involved upper extremity

What are examples of outcomes that are appropriate for Joe?

Examples of outcomes appropriate for Joe include the following:

- Sit to stand, or stand to sit, with symmetrical use of his lower extremities from a variety of surfaces without use of his right, less involved, upper extremity in the lift off or in the descent
- Sit to stand, or stand to sit, with symmetrical use of his lower extremities while pushing a chair away from him, or bringing a chair toward him, using his right, less involved upper extremity
- Sit to stand, or stand to sit, with symmetrical use of his lower extremities while carrying objects with his right, less involved upper extremity

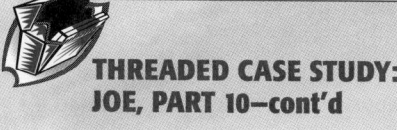

THREADED CASE STUDY:
JOE, PART 10—cont'd

- Stand with symmetrical use of his lower extremities from a standard-height chair in less time without using his right, less involved upper extremity in the lift off
- In standing, with symmetrical use of his lower extremities, safely pull up his pants with his right, less involved upper extremity
- In standing, with symmetrical use of his lower extremities, reach for an object placed high on a shelf and slightly to the left with his right, less involved upper extremity
- When sitting, appropriately weight shift his hips back and his shoulders forward to sit down on an unstable surface

Outcomes that are inconsistent with the potential for recovery of Joe's underlying impairments are not included, even though those outcomes might otherwise be appropriate.

The information in this chapter provides the foundation for the next steps in the development of your NDT skills: the use of problem-solving strategies and the use of appropriate manual cues.

It is essential that therapists use **problem-solving** strategies while managing the adult client with hemiplegia rather than adhere to strict protocols. Therapists skilled in the NDT approach use problem-solving strategies based on the core principles of the approach, which allow for dynamic decision making. For additional information on this topic, the reader is referred to the Runyan Problem Solving Framework™ (RPSF™), a set of problem-solving strategies built upon the core principles of NDT.[16] Examples of problems addressed by these strategies include the following:

- Use of static and dynamic features of the environment to facilitate movement for practice, challenge movement for learning, and investigate ineffective movement strategies
- Design of proper pretest and posttest environments
- Assessment of ineffective movement strategies, missing components of movement, and underlying impairments
- Application of movement analysis to identify individualized functional outcomes
- Creation of skilled intervention goals and design of progressive intervention activities leading to those goals

It is also essential that therapists wishing to become skilled in the NDT approach learn the appropriate use of manual cues. The NDT approach relies on the appropriate use of manual cues during examination, assessment, and treatment. Developing skills for the appropriate use of manual cues requires participation in hands-on NDT coursework that allows for self-movement experiences with feedback from the instructor. Examples of the use of manual cues include the following:

- Assessment of ineffective movement strategies, missing components of movement, and underlying impairments (and the potential for recovery)

- Access of missing components of movement via facilitation and inhibition
- Access of missing components of movement via preparation and challenge

By understanding the core principles of NDT, applying problem-solving strategies that adhere to those principles, and using appropriate manual cues during examination, assessment, and treatment, you will help adult clients with hemiplegia realize their potential for recovery and achieve individualized functional outcomes.

Review Questions

1. What is the purpose of the NDT approach?
2. Who began development of the NDT approach?
3. How does alignment of the trunk and limbs influence muscle activity?
4. List two important results provided by 24-hour management of adult clients with hemiplegia.
5. Why is the use of manual cues important when working with adult clients with hemiplegia?
6. What is meant by the "graded" use of manual cues?
7. What is the best way to promote acquisition of movement for a specific activity?
8. Describe a current model for describing functions of the CNS.
9. Define neuroplasticity, and explain its significance for adult clients with hemiplegia.
10. Describe how to promote neuroplasticity on the lesioned side of the cerebral cortex.
11. List six core principles of management of the NDT approach.
12. What is an individualized functional outcome?
13. List the factors that influence selection of individualized functional outcomes for adult clients with hemiplegia.
14. Write an example of an individualized functional outcome for Joe, the client featured in this chapter.
15. What is a functional activity limitation?
16. What is the role of functional activity limitations in the reimbursement process?
17. Write an example of a functional activity limitation for Joe, the client featured in this chapter.
18. Describe the progressive assessment process used when determining individualized functional outcomes for adult clients with hemiplegia.
19. What is an ineffective movement strategy?
20. Write an example of an ineffective movement strategy for Joe, the client featured in this chapter.
21. What is a missing component of movement?
22. What is one role of missing components of movement when determining intervention activities?
23. Write an example of a missing component of movement for Joe, the client featured in this chapter.
24. What is an underlying impairment?
25. What is the role of underlying impairments when individualizing functional outcomes?
26. Write an example of an underlying impairment for Joe, the client featured in this chapter.

27. List two unique aspects of the NDT approach, built upon the core principles, that are used routinely by therapists skilled in the NDT approach.

REFERENCES

1. Amaral DG: The anatomical organization of the central nervous system. In Kandel ER, Schwartz JH, Jessell TM, editors: *Principles of neural science*, ed 4, pp. 317, New York, 2000, McGraw Hill.
2. American Heart Association: *Heart disease and stroke statistics—2005 update*, Dallas, 2004, American Heart Association.
3. Bobath B: *Adult hemiplegia: evaluation and treatment*, ed 3, London, 1990, William Heinemann Medical Books, Ltd.
4. Bobath K: *A neurophysiological basis for the treatment of cerebral palsy*, Philadelphia, 1980, JB Lippincott.
5. Centers for Medicare and Medicaid Services: *Medicare coverage database*, Washington DC, 2005, Centers for Medicare and Medicaid Services. http://www.cms.hhs.gov/mcd/viewarticle.asp?article_id=27136&article_version=2&show=all
6. Engardt M et al: Dynamic muscle strength training in stoke patients: effects on knee extension torque, electromyographic activity and motor function, *Arch Phys Med Rehabil* 76(5):419, 1995.
7. Ferguson JM, Trombly CA: The effect on added-purpose and meaningful occupation on motor learning, *Am J Occup Ther* 51(7):508, 1998.
8. Fisher BE, Sullivan KJ: Activity-dependent factor affecting poststroke functional outcomes, *Stroke Rehabil* 8(3):42, 2001.
9. Howle JM: *Neuro-Developmental Treatment Approach: theoretical foundations and principles of practice*, Laguna Beach, CA, 2002, Neuro-Developmental Treatment Association.
10. Jenkins WM, Merzenich MM: Reorganization of neocortical representations after brain injury: a neurophysiological model of the bases of recovery after stroke, *Progress Brain Res* 71:249, 1987.
11. Library of Congress: *Project on the decade of the brain*, 2000. http://www.loc.gov/loc/brain
12. Loeb GE, Ghez C: The motor unit and muscle action. In Kandel ER, Schwartz JH, Jessell TM, editors: *Principles of neural science*, ed 4, pp. 674-693, New York, 2000, McGraw Hill.
13. Maquire EA et al: Navigation-related structural change in the hippocampi of cab drivers, *Proc Natl Acad Sci* 97:4398, 2000.
14. Nudo RJ: Role of cortical plasticity in motor recovery after stroke, neurology report, neurology section, *APTA* 22(2), 1998.
15. Nudo RJ et al: Neurophysiological correlates of hand preference in primary motor cortex of adult squirrel monkeys, *J Neuroscience* 12:1918, 1992.
16. Recovering Function: Recovering function for adults with hemiplegia using the principles of NDT, 2000, Recovering Function. http://www.recoveringfunction.com.
17. Rose DJ: *A multilevel approach to the study of motor control and learning*, Boston, 1997, Allyn & Bacon.
18. Sale D, MacDougall D: Specificity in strength training: a review for the coach and athlete, *Canad J Appl Sports Sci* 6:87, 1981.
19. Schleichkorn J: *The Bobaths: a biography of Berta and Karel Bobath*, Tucson, 1992, Therapy Skill Builders.
20. Schmidt RA: Motor learning principles for physical therapy. Contemporary management of motor control problems, Proceedings of the II Step Conference, Alexandria, VA, 1991, American Physical Therapy Association.
21. Sherrington CS: *The integrative action of the nervous system*, ed 2, New Haven, CN, 1947, Yale University Press.
22. Stein DG, Brailowsky S, Will B: *Brain repair*, New York, 1995, Oxford University Press.
23. Tangeman P, Banaitis D, Williams A: Rehabilitation of chronic stroke patients: changes in functional performance, *Arch Phys Med Rehabil* 71:876, 1990.
24. Vereijken B et al: Freezing degrees of freedom in skill acquisition, *J Motor Behav* 24:133, 1992.
25. Winstein CJ: Designing practice for motor learning: clinical implications. Contemporary management of motor control problems, Proceedings of the II Step Conference, Alexandria, VA, 1991, American Physical Therapy Association.

RESOURCES

Recovering Function
1582 Pam Lane
San Jose, CA 95120
www.RecoveringFunction.com

32

MOTOR LEARNING

SHAWN C. PHIPPS
PAMELA S. ROBERTS

KEY TERMS

Motor learning
Motor control
Brain plasticity
Dynamic systems theory

Heterarchical model
Hierarchical model
Task-oriented approach
Constraint-induced therapy

Learned nonuse
Shaping

LEARNING OBJECTIVES

After studying this chapter the student or practitioner will be able to do the following:

1. Describe the way that motor control affects occupational performance.
2. Describe dynamic systems theory and how it explains motor control.
3. Describe the task-oriented approach to motor learning.

4. Describe constraint-induced therapy as a method to increase functional use of a hemiparetic upper extremity following a neurological insult to the brain.
5. Develop client-centered and occupation-based treatment programs to facilitate motor learning.

CHAPTER OUTLINE

Theoretical foundations for motor learning
  Dynamic systems theory
  Task-oriented approach

Constraint-induced therapy
Summary

THREADED CASE STUDY: RICHARD, PART 1

Richard is a 66-year-old African-American man who was admitted to a rehabilitation hospital on July 11, 2005, secondary to an onset of left cerebral vascular accident (CVA) with resulting right-sided hemiparesis.

Before admission, the client lived with his wife in an apartment with four steps at the entrance. They have four grown children who do not live in the area. They also have three grandchildren. Richard is a retired electrician. He was independent in all activities of daily living before admission. He was responsible for cooking, household maintenance, and finances. He enjoys gardening, playing cards, and cooking. His social participation consisted of doing the weekly grocery shopping, attending church every Sunday, and going to the theater with his wife and family.

Richard's presenting symptoms include right-sided hemiparesis. He demonstrates selective motion at the shoulder, elbow, wrist, and hand. He is able to lift his affected arm above his head and to grasp and release objects of all sizes; however, he has difficulty with smaller objects.

Richard's daily routine consisted of getting up each morning at 6 AM and walking the dog for about a mile. He then cooked breakfast for himself and his wife. After breakfast, he was responsible for cleaning the kitchen and doing basic household maintenance.

Using the Canadian Occupational Performance Measure (COPM),[16] Richard identified the following occupational performance problems:

- Inability to perform cooking tasks using bilateral upper extremities
- Difficulty with fasteners and with manipulation of objects of different textures and sizes greater than 1 inch
- Inability to turn pages of prayer book while in church
- Difficulty with transition movements of sit to stand to kneel and kneel to stand to sit while in church
- Inability to perform transition movements during gardening activities
- Inability to manipulate cards with affected upper extremity

Critical Thinking Questions

1. How has Richard's motor control affected his ability to engage in meaningful occupation?
2. What motor control treatment strategies would enable Richard to engage more effectively in his daily occupations?

THEORETICAL FOUNDATIONS FOR MOTOR LEARNING

Motor learning is the acquisition and modification of learned movement patterns over time.[39] It involves cognitive and perceptual processes to code various motor programs. Motor learning involves practice and experience, which leads to permanent changes in the person's ability to produce movement sufficient to the demands of occupational performance. **Motor control** is the outcome of motor learning and involves the ability to produce purposeful movements of the extremities and postural adjustments in response to activity and environmental demands.[3]

The process of motor learning after cerebrovascular accident (CVA), traumatic brain injury, cerebral palsy, and other neurological insults to the brain has received a great deal of attention in research and occupational therapy (OT) practice. Researchers have found that 5 years after the onset of stroke, approximately 56% of clients have severe hemiparesis.[6] The explosion of new research on **brain plasticity,** or the ability of the brain to reorganize and develop new pathways, has paved the way for evolving approaches that target the ability of the individual to regain movement that enhances occupational performance, participation, and quality of life.[39] Recent studies support the theory that a form of brain plasticity, known as *cortical map reorganization*, plays a major role in regaining functional use of the hemiparetic upper extremity after CVA.[4,18]

DYNAMIC SYSTEMS THEORY

Modern motor control approaches are based on **dynamic systems theory,** which views motor behavior as a dynamic interaction between client factors (e.g., sensorimotor, cognitive, perceptual, and psychosocial), the context (e.g., physical, cultural, spiritual, social, temporal, personal, and virtual), and the occupations that must be performed to enact the client's roles.[21,22] Dynamic system theory is based on a **heterarchical model** that views each component (e.g., client, environment, and occupational performance) as critical in a dynamic interaction supporting the client's ability to engage in occupation.[3,39] Thus, movement and motor control are the result of a dynamic interaction between each of the subsystems. In addition, any change in the system has an effect on all the subsystems. For example, a CVA can lead to changes in the client's sensorimotor, cognitive, and perceptual skills, which affects motor control, engagement in occupation, and the person's ability to master their environment.

The heterarchical model is contrasted to the **hierarchical model,** which views higher centers in the central nervous system as having control over the subordinate lower centers.[22] The traditional sensorimotor approaches, such as neurodevelopmental treatment (NDT), proprioceptive neuromuscular facilitation (PNF), and the theories developed by Rood and Brunnstom are based on a hierarchical model. Recent research supports a dynamic systems approach in which motor learning and the development of motor control is a dynamic process that involves the interaction of the person, environment, and the occupations that the client needs to perform or wants to perform.

TASK-ORIENTED APPROACH

The **task-oriented approach** to motor recovery is based on dynamic systems principles, in which occupational performance and motor recovery occur from a dynamic interaction of the person, the environment, and the occupations that they are performing.[21,22] In OT, this approach is occupation based and client centered and focuses on enabling the client to obtain motor recovery through occupational performance using real objects, environments, and meaningful occupations.[35,37] Research shows that the use of real objects from the environment versus simulated objects produces better functional movement.[55] The client must also have the opportunity to attempt to solve motor problems in the context of multiple environments using a variety of strategies. For example, Richard must have the opportunity to turn the pages of a prayer book in the spiritual context of his place of worship using multiple strategies, such as various manipulation skills while kneeling, sitting, and standing. Research has shown that the environmental context plays a key role in the transfer of motor skill acquisition.[7,20]

Occupations that the client has identified as important through the Canadian Occupational Performance Measure[16] can be used to motivate the client to problem solve various motor strategies. An intervention plan that is developed collaboratively between the client and the therapist can aid the client in taking a more proactive role in making progress toward his or her outcomes and can facilitate more effective follow through. Research has shown that a client-centered and occupation-based approach can assist clients in attaining their personal goals.[47,48] Emerging research is also demonstrating that an occupation-based approach is more effective in remediating motor control impairments than rote exercise.[5,8,28,29,38,46,49,56] In addition, engaging in an occupation or activity from start to finish has been shown to elicit a more efficient, forceful, and coordinated motor response than performing only small portions of an activity.[19]

Activity analysis must be used to analyze the necessary movements that the client must perform to complete the task successfully. Effective upgrading and downgrading of the activity must be incorporated in order for clients to feel that they are successfully moving toward their goals. In addition, motor learning can take place only if the client has multiple practice opportunities in multiple real environments to transfer learning across multiple contexts.[7,17]

OT PRACTICE NOTE

Feedback and an analysis of factors that promote success or failure in a particular motor strategy must be a central problem-solving dialogue between the occupational therapist and the client.[10,11,23]

Qualitative (e.g., verbal encouragement) and quantitative (e.g., concrete measures of success or failure during a motor task) analyses have been shown to produce knowledge of results, which enables the client to cognitively reflect on the strengths and weaknesses of a particular motor strategy and implement a more effective strategy for completing an activity.[12,51,52] Through this dialogue, the client can learn to transfer various motor skills across multiple contexts.

CONSTRAINT-INDUCED THERAPY

Constraint-induced therapy, or forced use, is a technique designed to promote increased use of a weak or paralyzed arm and has been credited with speeding up the cortical map reorganization process in nonhuman primates[43] and in humans.[15] Constraint-induced therapy is also based on principles of dynamic systems theory and a task-oriented approach to motor control acquisition. In other methods of stroke rehabilitation, clients learn to use the stronger, or less involved, arm for daily activities. This type of treatment approach may foster learned nonuse of the stronger arm. **Learned nonuse** is proposed to be a phenomenon in which the individual effectively forgets to use the affected, or involved, extremity because of the extreme difficulty coordinating movement after the onset of a stroke.[15]

As an organism moves through its environment and manipulates objects, it receives sensory feedback from various sources simultaneously. Vision, audition, proprioception, and kinesthesia provide important sensory information for skilled movement. The importance of sensory information on motor action was demonstrated in the classic experiment carried out by Mott and Sherrington.[27] The afferent (sensory) input enters the spinal cord through the dorsal roots of the spinal nerves. By selectively severing the dorsal roots, sensory input was effectively eliminated while leaving motor innervation basically intact. Experiments conducted before 1955 demonstrated that deafferentation of a single forelimb in rhesus monkeys resulted in an essentially unused extremity when the animal is unrestricted.

Animal research has led to the discovery that cortical reorganization occurs after injury to the nervous system.[18] Research involving somatosensory deafferentation in monkeys has shown that if a single monkey forelimb is deafferented, the monkey will not use that extremity in the free situation.[13,14] In other words, the procedure left the monkeys with intact motor nerves but no feeling in the affected arm. The initial shock to the nervous system prevented arm movement. Even after the nervous system recovered, the monkeys failed to use their arms. Taub[40] theorized that use of the deafferented extremity can be regained if the intact extremity is restrained and the monkey is forced to use the extremity. If the restraint was used for a specific period of time, between 1 and 2 weeks, return of function could be permanent. These studies have shown that certain training procedures can be used to enable monkeys to regain use of their deafferented extremity.[13,14,41,42] Experimental evidence indicates that the persistent loss of motor function caused by deafferentation was due to learned behavioral suppression, a phenomenon called *learned nonuse.*[40] Conditioned response techniques did not show promise in returning the use of the extremity in daily life.

Another technique, **shaping,** did show substantial improvements in motor function in daily life situations. Shaping procedures are behavioral techniques that approach a desired motor outcome in small, successive increments.[25,32,44] Shaping techniques allow subjects to experience successful gains in performance with relatively small amounts of motor improvement. Explanations from these studies led to the development of a hypothesis that explained why the restraint and training procedures improved motor recovery after deafferentation.

The theory of learned nonuse was first described by Taub and is thought to extend to humans after central nervous system damage (Figure 32-1).[40,41,42,53] Animal research demonstrated that when the forelimb was not functional, the animal no longer used it in everyday tasks. This tendency led to the reinforcement and persistence of nonuse of the affected limb. Constraining the unaffected limb of the monkeys provided the first evidence of reversing learned nonuse.

To date, rehabilitation methods for those who have sustained a CVA have included but are not limited to biofeedback, neuromuscular facilitation, and operant conditioning. These various forms of rehabilitation are often used in conjunction with methods that teach clients to compensate by using their intact upper extremity to perform their day-to-day functional activities. This form of rehabilitation may improve the efficiency of the intact upper extremity, but at the same time, it encourages learned nonuse of the affected upper extremity. At present, there is minimal experimental evidence demonstrating the positive benefits of these forms of therapy.

An alternative therapy, constraint-induced therapy (CIT), has been used to rehabilitate individuals. Unlike more traditional therapies, CIT forces the client to use the affected upper extremity by immobilizing the unaffected upper extremity in a sling, mitt, or a combination of both (Figure 32-2). Clients then practice using their affected upper extremity on an intensive basis for several consecutive weeks by using shaping movements with the weaker arm. Taub[40] described this phenomenon as *learned nonuse;* thus, part of the theoretical framework of CIT is taken from the neurophysiological and behavioral studies of learned nonuse of the weaker limb seen in animal experiments. Constraining the intact forelimb of these monkeys provided the first evidence of changing the learned nonuse phenomenon. This success led to further studies incorporating humans with hemiparesis that developed after a stroke.

Wolf[40] and Miltner et al.[24] demonstrated positive effects of using CIT in individuals who had experienced a stroke. Liepert et al.[18] demonstrated cortical reorganization in humans undergoing CIT. In 1993, Taub et al.[45] found significant results when using CIT in a randomized clinical trial of nine individuals after stroke. These subjects had experienced strokes from 1 to 18 years after participation and were required to meet inclusion criteria similar to those used by Wolf et al.[53] (e.g., possessing some wrist and finger extension while still demonstrating significant disability). Additionally, subjects had to demonstrate good balance because they would be wearing a sling and would therefore be unable to use their stronger upper extremity to protect themselves in the event of a fall. Subjects were randomly assigned to either an experimental group or an attention-control group. The subjects assigned to the experimental group wore a sling on the less involved arm for a period of 12 days. During the 12 days, the sling was worn during all waking hours except when specific activities were being carried out, such as when it may be

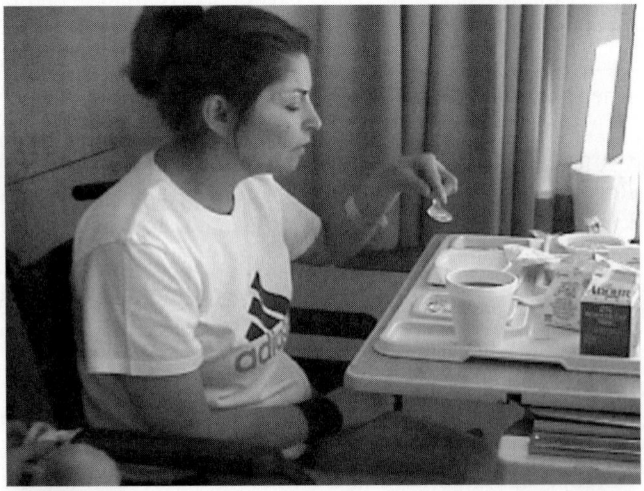

Figure 32-1 Client with left cerebrovascular accident and right hemiparesis before the initiation of the constraint-induced therapy (CIT) program. Client demonstrates learned nonuse by using her stronger, uninvolved left upper extremity during self-feeding. (Courtesy Remy Chu, OTR/L.)

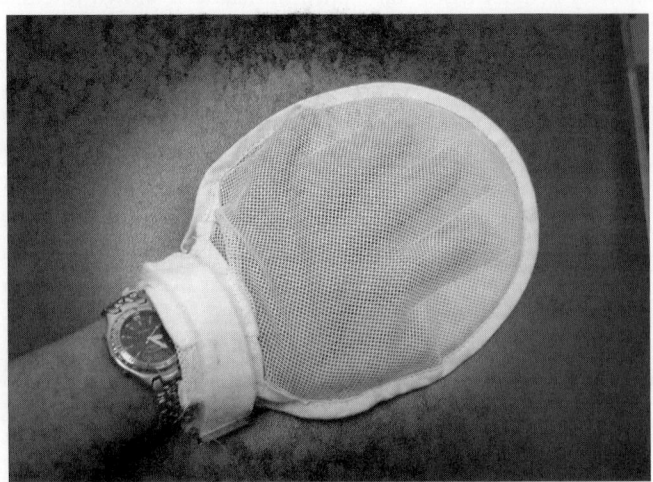

Figure 32-2 CIT forces the individual to use the affected upper extremity by immobilizing the unaffected upper extremity in a mitt.

unsafe or extremely difficult to use the weaker arm exclusively. The study also used a behavioral contract that included an agreement from subjects to wear the restraint device for at least 90% of their waking hours during the 12-day intervention period. The behavioral contract specifically identified activities during which the subject was to use the more involved arm exclusively, to use both arms, and to use the less involved arm (for safety reasons). Participants in the attention-control group were instructed to focus attention on the weaker arm and were encouraged to try using the weaker arm with as many new activities as possible at home. Activities were recorded throughout the 2-week period. Those in the attention-control group also received two sessions involving activities requiring either active movement or limbering of the weaker arm and were provided with an individualized range of motion exercise program. Effectiveness of treatment was measured using the Wolf Motor Function Test and the Motor Activity Log, a structured interview exploring functional use in the life setting. Speed, quality of movement, and functional use of the affected upper extremity were significantly improved for the research group versus the attention-control group and maintained over a 2-year period. In 1999, Kunkel et al.[15] showed a greater than 100% increase in the amount of use of the affected upper extremity in real-world environments. The effective factor in all forms of CIT appears to be inducing patients to repeatedly practice use of the weaker arm for many hours a day for a period of consecutive days.[54]

Over the past 30 years, numerous studies have further confirmed the effectiveness of CIT in improving clients' function after stroke compared with traditional therapy.[50] More recently, however, research involving CIT has used varied populations, altered the inclusion criteria, and modified the intensity of treatment and length of therapy program from the original research protocol. For example, Pierce et al.[34] found that the forced-use component of CIT in conjunction with a home program may be used in the traditional outpatient setting. Further, Page[31] found that repeated task-specific practice is more critical than intensity in improving function. These findings and others have broadened the scope and applicability of CIT to various populations.

Although recent CIT research has broadened its scope to include different diagnostic criteria, different treatment regimes, and different inclusion criteria, little of the current CIT research has addressed the participants' self-reported satisfaction in their life roles after completing a CIT program. After a person has a stroke, he or she experiences a disruption in his or her life roles. This disruption can lead to feelings of ineffectiveness, incompetence, and ultimately helplessness. To restore one's health, one must identify and alter one's lifestyle to improve the fit between oneself and the environment. CIT has already been proved effective in improving motor movement in individuals who have experienced a stroke. Functional carryover of CIT has been demonstrated from the clinic to the natural environment. Research has shown significant increases in the daily use of the impaired arm and an increase in the speed at which the individual carries out activities after participating in CIT. Increased satisfaction resulting from an increased ability to use their weaker arm has been noted in individuals who reported satisfaction with performance of meaningful daily activities and life roles.[30,36]

To determine whether a subject meets inclusion criteria, a telephone screening protocol is often administered.[26] Many research studies on CIT use a CIT protocol that contains typical inclusion criteria for use of this technique. These criteria include (1) a first-time CVA that occurred more than 1 year ago; (2) not currently receiving therapeutic intervention; (3) a score of ≥44 on the Berg Balance Test[1] or limited balance problems requiring an assistive device for mobility in clients who had a full-time caregiver to assist with any balance issues; (4) ability to move the affected arm in 45-degree shoulder flexion and abduction, 90-degree elbow flexion and extension, 20-degree wrist extension, and 10-degree extension at metacarpal phalanges and interphalanges as determined by active range of motion (Figure 32-3); (5) no significant cognitive deficits as demonstrated by a Mini Mental State Examination score of at least 22[9] or another type of cognitive test; (6) no preexisting co-morbidities that might interfere with mobility or function; (7) limited spasticity (score of 0 or 1) as measured by the Modified Ashworth Scale[2]; and (8) ability to identify an individual who could assist with the home program.[26,36] In summary, potential reasons for a person to be excluded may include motor ability that is too high or too low, cognitive deficits that prevent adequate participation, and an already high use of the weaker arm.

A battery of assessments[26] is usually performed with all clients included in CIT. Results from the tests are used to test certain research hypotheses, whereas other tests are used for

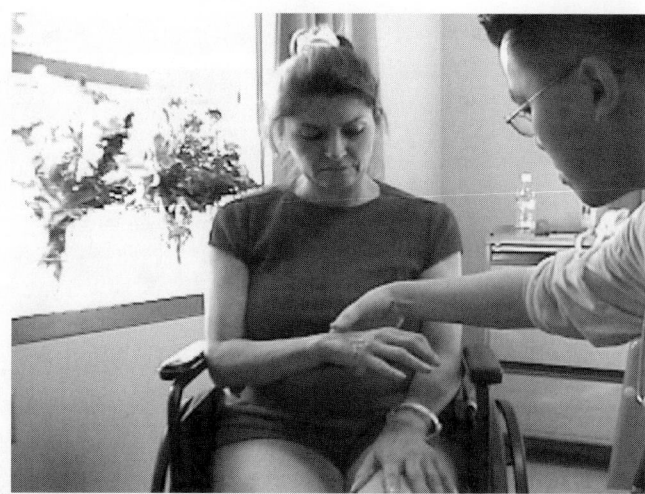

Figure 32-3 Client is asked to demonstrate active wrist and finger extension in her dominant right hand. Client is able to achieve 20 degrees of wrist extension and 10 degrees of finger extension (at the metacarpal phalanges) from a flexed position. (Courtesy Remy Chu, OTR/L.)

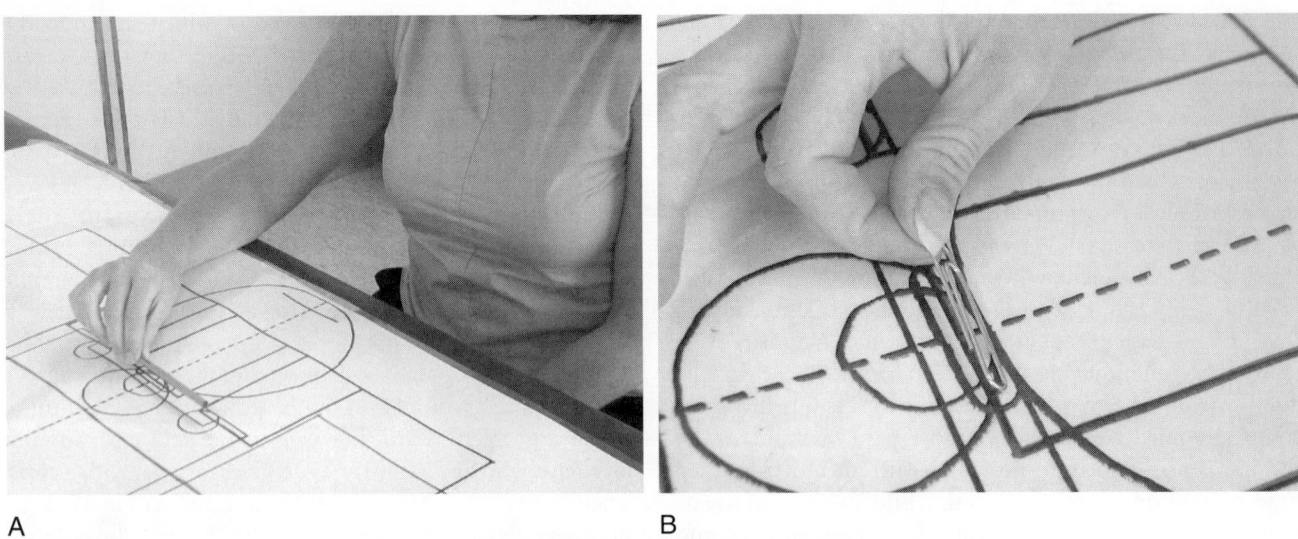

A   B

Figure 32-4   The Wolf Motor Function Test includes standard tasks such as lifting the forearm to the table and reaching for an object.

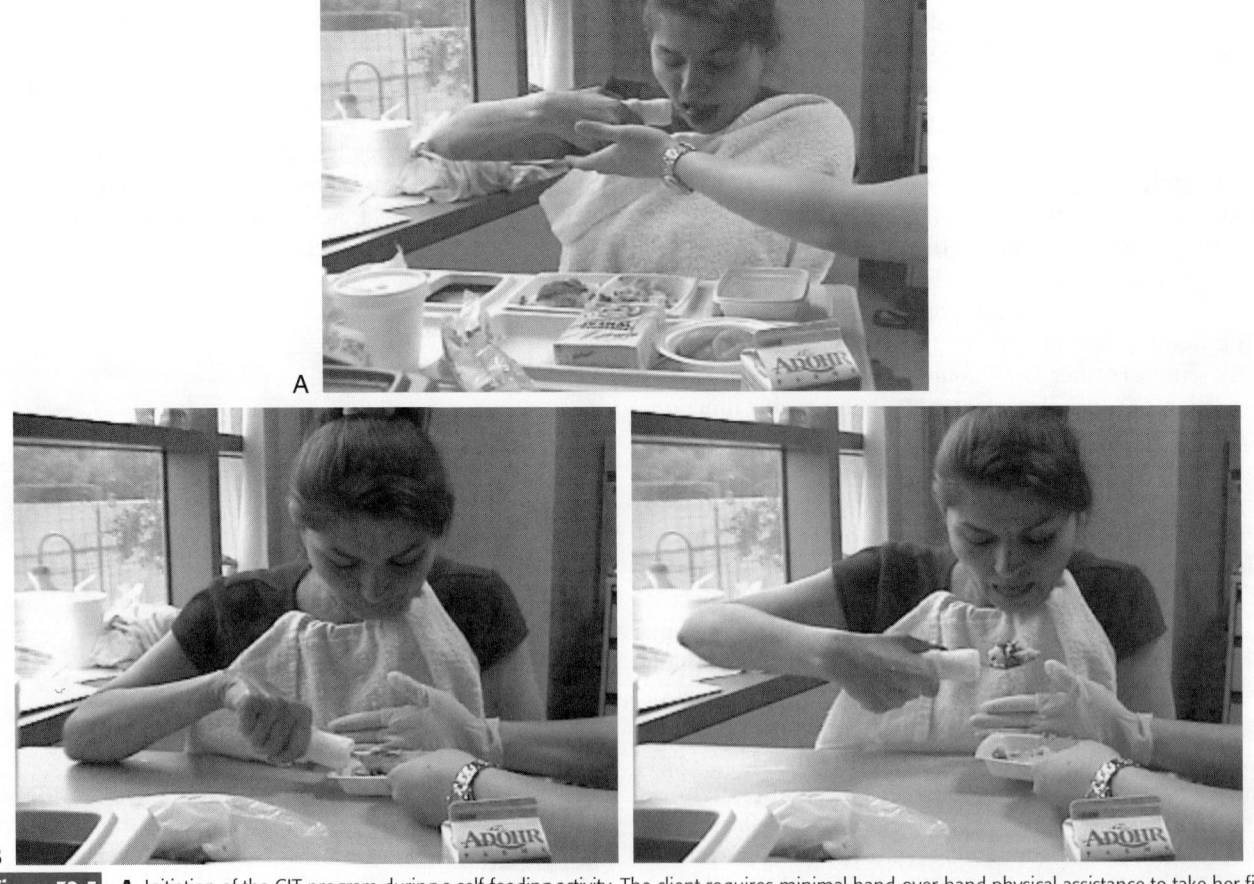

Figure 32-5   **A,** Initiation of the CIT program during a self-feeding activity. The client requires minimal hand-over-hand physical assistance to take her first bite with her weaker right hand. Hand-over-hand physical assistance focuses on eliminating gravity as the client brings the spoon to her mouth. **B** and **C,** After 10 CIT trials, the client is attempting to feed herself without physical assistance from the occupational therapist. (Courtesy Remy Chu, OTR/L.)

diagnostic purposes or to generate new hypotheses. Some typical tests include the Wolf Motor Function Test (WMFT) and the Motor Activity Log (MAL).

The WMFT consists of 15 motor items that examine contributions from the distal and proximal muscles of the arm. The tasks in the test are sequenced from proximal to distal and gross to fine motor. Most tasks are completed with the subject seated in a chair. Standard tasks such as lifting the forearm to the table, reaching for an object, or lifting a pencil are rated on a scale from 0 (does not attempt with weaker arm) to 5 (movement appears normal and time to complete the task is measured; Figure 32-4). The WMFT uses a diagrammed grid or template that is taped to the desk to specify standardized measurements. The WMFT is administered before the intervention, immediately after the intervention, and at a designated time following the intervention.

The MAL was developed for the purpose of exploring activities attempted outside the clinical setting. The MAL is a self-report, 30-item instrument administered in an interview format. Subjects are then asked to rate their performance on each activity, and emphasis is placed on performance at home. The test is administered about 10 times throughout the course of intervention. The instrument consists of specific activities, such as turning on a light switch or opening a drawer. The amount of use of the involved arm is rated by the participant from 0 (never used) to 5 (involved arm used the same as it was before the stroke). Quality of movement (how well) is also self-rated from 0 (not used) to 5 (normal movement).

Therapeutic procedures using CIT in the clinic are performed under supervision from the therapist (Figure 32-5). The procedures are effective only if the use of the weaker arm

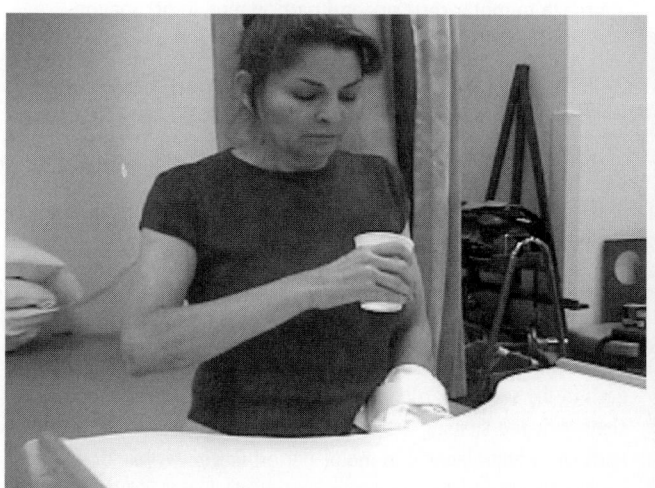
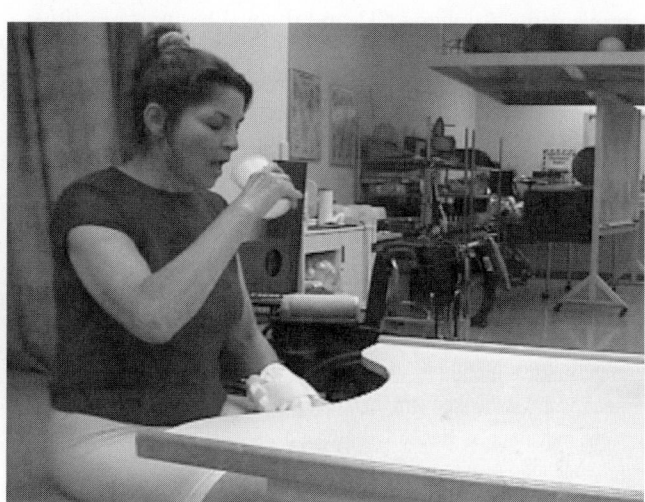

A   B

Figure 32-6   Client is performing a block trial (cup to mouth trial). The client demonstrates less strain in her neck and shoulder while bringing the cup to her mouth. (Courtesy Remy Chu, OTR/L.)

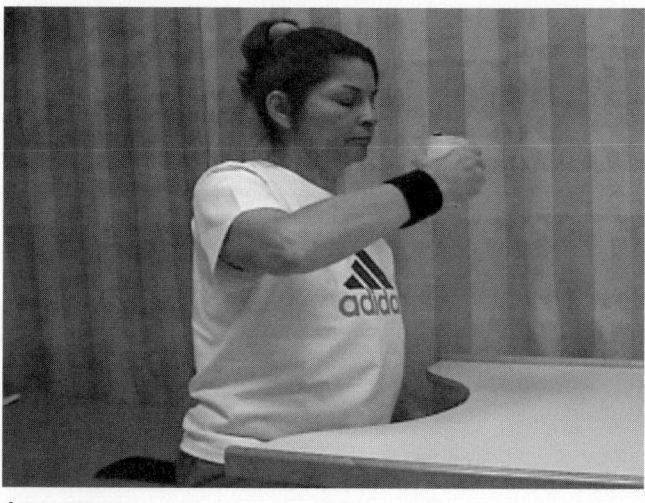
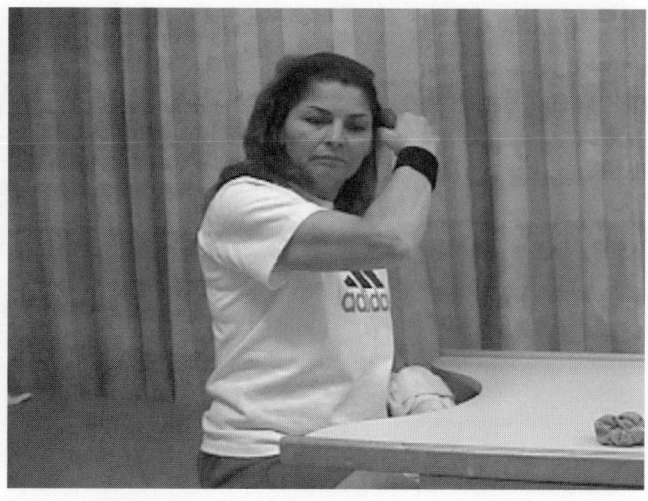

A   B

Figure 32-7   **A,** After 1.5 weeks of CIT, the client is able to bring a cup to her mouth independently using the weaker right upper extremity. **B,** She is also able to bring her right hand to her head to brush her hair. (Courtesy Remy Chu, OTR/L.)

is carried over in the home environment. Clients are asked about their compliance in filling out a daily entry in their home diaries. The home diary is used to outline the clients' activities from the time at which they are discharged from the clinic until they return for the daily sessions. A typical daily schedule is often used. The schedule includes time and length of rest periods. Further, specific shaping task practice is also listed on the daily schedule. Shaping is a behavioral training technique that is an effective form of CIT, especially when combined with the weaker arm. A desired motor or behavioral objective is approached in small steps with an individualized shaping plan. During shaping, explicit feedback is provided to identify small improvements in performance. Selection of shaping tasks depends on specific joint movements that exhibit the deficit, joint movements that have the greatest chance of improving, and the client's preference among tasks that have similar potential for producing specific improvements. Applying CIT and shaping requires repetitive,

supervised, constant practice. CIT study protocols call for 6 hours of continuous task practice per day (Figures 32-6 and 32-7).

SUMMARY

Dynamic systems theory supports a heterarchical model of motor control in which motor acquisition is influenced by the client, the environment, and the occupations that the client needs to perform or wants to perform. A task-oriented approach supports the use of occupation-based and client-centered interventions that assist the client in problem solving (e.g., learning how they will perform their desired occupations in a variety of contexts to support transfer of motor learning). CIT is a task-oriented approach that focuses on constraining the use of the unaffected upper extremity to facilitate motor recovery in the affected upper extremity during occupational performance. More research is needed in OT to support the use of a task-oriented and CIT approach to motor recovery and participation in occupation.

THREADED CASE STUDY: RICHARD, PART 2

At screening, Richard was determined eligible to meet the criteria to benefit from constraint-induced therapy (CIT) because his stroke occurred more than 1 year ago. He had residual right hemiparesis with selective motion in all joints. He was able to touch the top of his head with his weaker arm, bend his wrist, and grasp or release with slow movements. He had completed an inpatient and outpatient rehabilitation program. He has not had any major medical complications, has not had any falls within the past 6 months, and is able to walk without an assistive device. After screening, an upper extremity range of motion assessment and tone assessment using the Modified Ashworth Scale, Berg Balance Test, and the Folstein Mini-Mental State Examination were completed. Richard met all criteria and therefore was a good candidate for CIT.

Richard participated in the Motor Activity Log (MAL) throughout the intervention. Each task was modeled twice before the participant's performance, and the task was videotaped for scoring purposes. Specific tasks for grip strength and amount of weight added to the task of lifting a box with shoulder flexion were also scored separately. He also completed the WMFT. After completion of the pretraining assessment, Richard and his wife were taught how to don and doff the mitt and use the home diary, and they both signed a behavioral contract. Richard was then scheduled for 14 days of consecutive intervention, in which his less involved, or stronger, left arm was restrained by a mitt that required him to complete his daily activities using his more affected right arm. The behavioral contract stipulated that Richard would wear the mitt for 90% of waking hours. There was also a home program contract that included exceptions to wearing the mitt, such as while bathing and sleeping. Richard also kept a diary to record which arm was used for various daily activities and the time

that the mitt was worn. Richard recorded activities completed from the time he left the clinic until this return.

In addition to the activity-based home program, Richard's intervention was provided in both a group setting and individual sessions. Each of the sessions lasted for 6 hours. Tasks during the 6-hour sessions included shaping activities to ensure success in performance. Each small improvement in motor performance was reinforced with positive feedback. Tasks were progressively increased in difficulty as Richard's motor performance improved. To make sure that the activities were occupation based and client centered, activities were developed according to the information provided and identified by the COPM.

After Richard arrived in the clinic, the therapist reviewed his diary and performed the Motor Activity Log. The CIT activities were identified through information obtained from the COPM. For example, Richard participated in group activities such as playing cards, which required him to use his weaker hand to manipulate the cards while his stronger arm was constrained in the mitt. He further participated in activities such as cooking. He was responsible for set-up, preparation, and clean-up of the meal with his right upper extremity. His left upper extremity was constrained in the mitt, necessitating use of his weaker right hand to chop vegetables. Richard would often attempt to use his stronger arm in the mitt and would require prompting from the therapist. To focus on activities that were meaningful for Richard, all activities during the 6-hour intervention session were based on his goals from the COPM. CIT activities became progressively more challenging, with repetitions of task practice requiring range of motion, strength, endurance, and coordination. Verbal acknowledgments of daily achievements were provided.

THREADED CASE STUDY: RICHARD, PART 2—cont'd

After the 2-week intervention program, Richard had learned to incorporate his weaker upper extremity into meaningful daily occupations. It became routine for Richard to initiate activities with his right upper extremity, although he primarily used his left upper extremity before the intervention. Richard's level of participation grew to include gardening, attending church, and turning the pages of the prayer book with his right hand. He also resumed his roles in cooking and performing household maintenance.

How Has Richard's Motor Control Affected His Ability to Engage in Meaningful Occupation?

Because of his motor control impairments in the right upper extremity, Richard is unable to perform cooking tasks using bilateral upper extremities. He also has difficulty with fasteners and the manipulation of objects of different sizes and textures greater than 1 inch. Richard is unable to turn the pages of his prayer book while in church and has difficulty with transitional movements of sit to stand and stand to sit

while in church. He is also unable to perform transition movements during gardening activities and is unable to manipulate cards with the affected upper extremity.

What Motor Control Treatment Strategies Would Enable Richard to Engage More Effectively in His Daily Occupations?

Richard's CIT movement therapy program consisted of restriction of movement of the unaffected upper extremity by placing it in a splint, sling, or mitt for greater than 90% of his waking hours. He complied with this protocol for a period of 14 days and participated in training of the affected arm by a procedure termed *shaping* for approximately 7 hours per day during the 10 weekdays of that period. This approach enabled Richard to regain functional use of his right dominant upper extremity for occupations such as preparing meals, dressing, and opening the pages of a prayer book.

Review Questions

1. How does motor control affect occupational performance?
2. What is the task-oriented approach to motor learning?
3. What is dynamic systems theory, and how does it explain motor control?
4. What is constraint-induced therapy, and how does this approach increase functional use of the hemiparetic upper extremity after a neurological insult to the brain?
5. How would you develop a client-centered and occupation-based treatment program to facilitate motor learning?

REFERENCES

1. Berg K et al: Measuring balance in the elderly: validation of an instrument, *Can J Public Health* 83(Suppl 2):S7, 1992.
2. Bohannon RW, Smith MB: Interrater of a Modified Ashworth Scale of muscle spasticity, *Physician Ther* 67:206, 1986.
3. Carr JH, Shepherd RB: *Neurological rehabilitation: optimizing motor performance*, Oxford, 1998, Butterworth-Heinemann.
4. Cramer SC et al: A pilot study of somatotopic mapping after cortical infarct, *Stroke* 31:668, 2000.
5. Dearn CM, Shepherd RB: Task-related training improves performance of seated reaching tasks after stroke: a randomized controlled trial, *Stroke* 28:722, 1997.
6. Duncan PW et al: Measurement of motor recovery after stroke. Outcome assessment and sample size requirements, *Stroke* 23:1084, 1992.
7. Ferguson MC, Rice MS: The effect of contextual relevance on motor skills transfer, *Am J Occup Ther* 55:558, 2001.
8. Flinn NA: Clinical interpretation of effect of rehabilitation tasks on organization of movement after stroke, *Am J Occup Ther* 53(4):345, 1999.
9. Folstein MF, Folstein SE, McHugh PR: "Mini-mental state." A practical method for grading the cognitive state of patients for the clinician, *J Psychiatr Res* 12(3):189, 1975.
10. Jarus T: Is more always better? Optimal amounts of feedback in learning to calibrate sensory awareness, *Occup Ther J Res* 15:181, 1995.
11. Jarus T: Motor learning and occupational therapy: the organization of practice, *Am J Occup Ther* 48:810, 1994.
12. Kilduski NC, Rice MS: Qualitative and quantitative knowledge of results: effects on motor learning, *Am J Occup Ther* 57:329, 2003.
13. Knapp HD, Taub E, Berman AJ: Effect of deafferentation on a conditioned avoidance response, *Science* 128:842, 1958.
14. Knapp HD, Taub E, Berman AJ: Movement in monkeys with deafferented forelimbs, *Exp Neurology* 7:305, 1963.
15. Kunkel A et al: Constraint-induced movement therapy for motor recovery in chronic stroke patients, *Arch Phys Med Rehabil* 80:624, 1999.
16. Law M et al: *The Canadian Occupational Performance Measure*, ed 4, Ottawa, 2005, CAOT Publications.
17. Lee TD, Swanson LR, Hall AL: What is repeated in a repetition? Effects of practice conditions on motor skills acquisition, *Phys Ther* 71:150, 1991.
18. Liepert J et al: Treatment-induced cortical reorganization after stroke in humans, *Stroke* 31(6):1210, 2000.
19. Ma HI, Trombly CA: The comparison of motor performance between part and whole tasks in elderly persons, *Am J Occup Ther* 55(1):62, 2001.
20. Ma HI, Trombly CA, Robinson-Podolski C: The effect of context on skill acquisition and transfer, *Am J Occup Ther* 53:138, 1999.
21. Mathiowetz V: OT task-oriented approach to person post-stroke. In Gillen G, Burkhardt A, editors: *Stroke rehabilitation: a function-based approach*, ed 2, St Louis, 2004, Mosby.

22. Mathiowetz V, Bass Haugen J: Motor behavior research: Implications for therapeutic approaches to CNS dysfunction, *Am J Occup Ther* 47:733, 1994.

23. Merians A et al: Effects of feedback for motor skills learning in older healthy subjects and individuals post-stroke, *Neurology Report* 19:23, 1995.

24. Miltner W et al: Effects of constraint-induced movement therapy on patients with chronic motor deficits after stroke: a replication, *Stroke* 30(3):586, 1999.

25. Morgan GW: The shaping game: a technique, *Behav Ther* 5: 481, 1974.

26. Morris DM et al: Constraint-induced movement therapy for motor recovery after stroke, *Neurorehabil* 9:29, 1997.

27. Mott FW, Sherrington CS: Experiments upon the influence of sensory nerves upon movement and nutrition of the limbs, *Proc R Soc Lond* 57:481, 1895.

28. Nagel MJ, Rice MS: Cross-transfer effects in the upper extremity during an occupationally embedded exercise, *Am J Occup Ther* 55:317, 2001.

29. Neistadt M: The effects of different treatment activities on functional fine motor coordination in adults with brain injury, *Am J Occup Ther* 48:877, 1994.

30. Ostendorf CG, Wolf SL: Effect of forced use of the upper extremity of a hemiplegic patient on changes in function: a single-case design, *Phys Ther* 61:1022, 1981.

31. Page SJ et al: Efficacy of modified constraint-induced movement therapy in chronic stroke: a single-blinded randomized controlled trial, *Arch Phys Med Rehabil* 85(1):14, 2004.

32. Panyan MV: *How to use shaping*, Lawrence, KS, 1980, H and H Enterprises.

33. Phipps SC: *Outpatient occupational therapy outcomes for clients with brain injury and stroke using the Canadian Occupational Performance Measure*, unpublished master's thesis, San Jose State University, San Jose, California, 2002.

34. Pierce SR et al: Home forced use in an outpatient rehabilitation program for adults with hemiplegia: a pilot study, *Neurorehabil Neural Repair* 17(4):214, 2003.

35. Poole JL: Application of motor learning principles in occupational therapy, *Am J Occup Ther* 45:531, 1991.

36. Roberts P et al: Client-centered occupational therapy using constraint-induced therapy, *J Stroke Cerebrovascular Dis* 14(3): 115, 2005.

37. Sabari JS: Motor learning concepts applied to activity-based intervention with adults with hemiplegia, *Am J Occup Ther* 45:523, 1991.

38. Shepherd RB: Exercise and training to optimize functional motor performance in stroke: driving neural reorganization? *Neural Plasticity* 2:121, 2001.

39. Shumway-Cook A, Woollacott M: *Motor control: theory and practical applications*, ed 2, Philadelphia, 2001, Lippincott Williams & Wilkins.

40. Taub E: Movement in nonhuman primates deprived of somatosensory feedback, *Exer Sport Sci Rev* 4:335, 1977.

41. Taub E, Bacon R, Berman AJ: The acquisition of a trace-conditioned avoidance response after deafferentation of the responding limb, *J Comp Physiol Psychol* 58:275, 1965.

42. Taub E, Berman AJ: Avoidance conditioning in the absence of relevant proprioceptive and exteroceptive feedback, *J Comp Physiol Psychol* 56:1012, 1963.

43. Taub E et al: An operant approach to rehabilitation medicine: overcoming learned nonuse by shaping, *J Exp Anal Behav* 61: 281, 1994.

44. Taub E, Goldberg IA, Taub PB: Deafferentation in monkeys: pointing at a target without visual feedback, *Exper Neurol* 46:178, 1975.

45. Taub E et al: Technique to improve chronic motor deficit after stroke, *Arch Phys Med Rehabil* 74:347, 1993.

46. Thielman GT, Dean CM, Gentile AM: Rehabilitation of reaching after stroke: task-related training versus progressive resistive exercise, *Arch Phys Med Rehabil* 85:1613, 2004.

47. Trombly CA, Radomski MV, Davis ES: Achievement of self-identified goals by adults with traumatic brain injury: Phase I, *Am J Occup Ther* 52:810, 1998.

48. Trombly CA et al: Occupational therapy and achievement of self-identified goals by adults with acquired brain injury: Phase II, *Am J Occup Ther* 56:489, 2002.

49. Trombly C, Wu CY: Effect of rehabilitation tasks on organization of movement after stroke, *Am J Occup Ther* 53:333, 1998.

50. Van der Lee JH et al: Forced use of the upper extremity in chronic stroke patients: results from a single-blind randomized clinical trial, *Stroke* 30:2369, 1999.

51. Winstein CJ: Knowledge of results and motor learning: implications for physical therapy, *Phys Ther* 71:140, 1991.

52. Winstein CJ, Schmidt RA: Reduced frequency of knowledge of results enhances motor skills learning, *J Experiment Psychol Learning Memory Cognition* 16:677, 1990.

53. Wolf SL et al: Forced use in hemiplegic upper extremities to reverse the effect of learned non-use among chronic stroke and head injured patients, *Experiment Neurol* 104:125, 1989.

54. Wolfgang HR et al: Effects of constraint-induced movement therapy on patients with chronic motor deficits after stroke: a replication, *Stroke* 30(3):586, 1999.

55. Wu CY et al: A kinematic study of contextual effects on reaching performance in persons with and without stroke: influences of object availability, *Arch Phys Med Rehabil* 81:95, 2000.

56. Wu CY et al: Effects of task goal and personal preference on seated reaching kinematics after stroke, *Stroke* 32:70, 2001.

SUGGESTED READING

Donnelly M, Power M, Russell M, et al: Randomized control trial of an early discharge rehabilitation service: the Belfast stroke trial, *Stroke* 35:127, 2004.

Hanlon RF: Motor learning following unilateral stroke, *Arch Phys Med Rehabil* 77:811, 1996.

INTERVENTION
APPLICATIONS

33 CEREBROVASCULAR ACCIDENT/STROKE

GLEN GILLEN*

KEY TERMS

Ischemia
Transient ischemic attack
Dysarthria
Client-centered assessment

Top-down approach to
assessment
Postural control

Balance strategies
Aphasia
Neurobehavioral deficits

Motor control
Weight bearing
Subluxation

LEARNING OBJECTIVES

After studying this chapter the student or practitioner will be able to do the following:

1. List and describe evaluation procedures for survivors of a stroke.
2. Discuss the neuropathology of a stroke.
3. Identify risk factors associated with a stroke.
4. Identify multiple factors that impede task performance after a stroke.
5. Describe evaluation procedures for neurobehavioral deficits.
6. Identify balance strategies that support functional performance.
7. Describe motor control dysfunction associated with stroke.
8. Identify standardized stroke assessments for multiple areas of dysfunction.
9. Apply a client-centered approach to stroke rehabilitation.
10. Develop comprehensive occupation-based treatment plans to remediate or compensate for underlying deficits.

CHAPTER OUTLINE

Definition of cerebrovascular accident or stroke
Causes of cerebrovascular accident
  Ischemia
  Hemorrhage
  Related syndromes
  Transient ischemic attacks
Effects of cerebrovascular accident
  Internal carotid artery
  Middle cerebral artery
  Anterior cerebral artery
  Posterior cerebral artery
  Cerebellar artery system
  Vertebrobasilar system
Medical management
Evaluation and intervention procedures for clients who sustained a stroke

Client-centered assessments
Top-down approach to assessment
Effects of neurological deficits on performance in areas of occupation
Standardized tools
Adopting a philosophy for intervention
Functional limitations commonly observed after stroke
Inability to perform chosen occupations while seated
Inability to engage in chosen occupations in standing
Inability to communicate secondary to language dysfunction
Inability to perform chosen occupations secondary to neurobehavioral/cognitive-perceptual impairments
Inability to perform chosen tasks secondary to upper extremity dysfunction
Inability to perform chosen tasks secondary to visual impairment
Psychosocial adjustment
Summary

---

*The author would like to acknowledge the contribution of Michael P. Lawrence to this chapter.

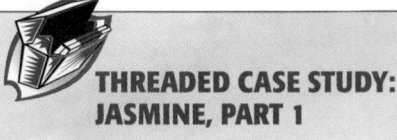

THREADED CASE STUDY: JASMINE, PART 1

Jasmine is a 39-year-old single mother of a 2-year-old boy. They live in a 2-bedroom rented apartment. She has converted her dining area into a home office, where she carries out her home-based business in desktop publishing. Jasmine drives her son to preschool each morning and shops on the way home before working for the rest of the day from home. While working on her computer, Jasmine experienced tingling and "clumsiness" in her left hand. She attributed this to long work hours. Still feeling "not quite right," she attempted to stand to go to the bathroom and collapsed on the floor. She was able to crawl to the phone to call 911.

Jasmine next remembers waking up in the emergency room, where she was told that she had just experienced a stroke. Her neuroimaging studies documented the presence of a right frontal-parietal infarct. Jasmine is unable to move or feel the left side of her body, has a left visual field cut, and tends to not respond to sensory stimuli on the left side of her body. Nurses and nurse's aides are lifting Jasmine out of bed and providing full assistance for self-care and mobility. Jasmine was told that by the end of the week she will be transferred to the local rehabilitation hospital and will require "aggressive" occupational and physical therapy. Her son is under the care of his aunt and uncle. Jasmine has been crying often and is concerned that she will not be able to work or take care of her son. She is also concerned about losing her apartment; she explains that she has been "just getting by" recently.

Critical Thinking Questions

1. How will Jasmine's impaired body functions and body structures (e.g., loss of motor control, sensory loss, visual dysfunction, and neglect) affect her ability to return to her previous lifestyle?
2. What three assessments are most critical to administer? Why?
3. Which interventions should be considered to address Jasmine's dependence in self-care (e.g., toileting, dressing), mobility (e.g., bed mobility, transfers), and instrumental activities of daily living (e.g., driving, child care) throughout her rehab stay?

Cerebrovascular accident (CVA), or stroke, continues to be a national health problem despite recent advances in medical technology. The American Heart Association[4] publishes stroke statistics that demonstrate the severity of this problem. Selected statistics include the following[4]:

- Stroke ranks as the third leading cause of death behind heart disease and cancer.
- On average, a United States citizen suffers a stroke every 45 seconds; every 3 minutes someone dies of a stroke.
- Each year, 700,000 people suffer a new or recurrent stroke. Approximately 500,000 strokes are first attacks, and 200,000 are recurrent.
- About 4,800,000 clients who sustained a stroke are alive today.

- The percentage of strokes that result in death within 1 year is about 29%, less if the stroke occurs before age 65.
- Of people who suffer a stroke, 28% are under age 65. For people over 55, the incidence of stroke more than doubles for each successive decade.
- The incidence of stroke is about 1.25 times higher for men than for women.

In addition, the aftermath of stroke is a substantial public health and economic problem:

- Stroke is a leading cause of serious, long-term disability in the United States.
- Stroke accounts for more than half of all clients hospitalized for acute neurological disease.
- Among long-term clients who sustained a stroke, 50% have hemiparesis, 30% cannot walk, 24% to 53% report complete or partial dependence on activities of daily living (ADL) scales, 12% to 19% are aphasic, 35% are clinically depressed, and 26% require nursing home care.

Obviously, stroke rehabilitation as a practice area for occupational therapists is a specialization that crosses multiple settings, from the intensive care unit to community-based programs.

DEFINITION OF CEREBROVASCULAR ACCIDENT OR STROKE

CVA is a complex dysfunction caused by a lesion in the brain. The World Health Organization[91] defines stroke as an "acute neurologic dysfunction of vascular origin ... with symptoms and signs corresponding to the involvement of focal areas of the brain." CVA results in upper motor neuron dysfunction that produces hemiplegia or paralysis of one side of the body, including limbs and trunk and sometimes the face and oral structures that are contralateral to the brain hemisphere that has the lesion. Thus a lesion in the left cerebral hemisphere (left CVA) produces right hemiplegia. Conversely, a lesion in the right cerebral hemisphere (right CVA) produces a left hemiplegia. When reference is made to the client's disability as right or left hemiplegia, the reference is to the paralyzed body side and not to the locus of the lesion.

Accompanying the motor paralysis may be a variety of dysfunctions other than the motor paralysis. Some of these are sensory disturbances, perceptual dysfunction, visual disturbances, personality and intellectual changes, and a complex range of speech and associated language disorders. The neurological deficits persist longer than 24 hours.

CAUSES OF CEREBROVASCULAR ACCIDENT

Bartels describes a stroke as "essentially a disease of the cerebral vasculature in which failure to supply oxygen to the brain cells, which are the most susceptible to ischemic damage, leads to their death. The syndromes that lead to stroke comprise two broad categories: ischemic and hemorrhagic stroke. Ischemic strokes account for approximately 80% of strokes, whereas hemorrhagic strokes account for the remaining 20%."[9]

ISCHEMIA

Ischemic strokes may be the result of embolisms to the brain from cardiac or arterial sources. Cardiac sources include atrial fibrillation (pooling of blood in the dysfunctional atrium leads to emboli production), sino-atrial disorders, acute myocardial infarction, endocarditis, cardiac tumors, and valvular (both native and artificial) disorders. Cerebral **ischemia** caused by perfusion failure occurs with severe stenosis of the carotid and basilar arteries, as well as when there is microstenosis of the small deep arteries.[4,9]

Age, gender, race, ethnicity, and heredity are considered nonmodifiable risk factors for ischemic strokes. In contrast, a major focus of stroke prevention and education programs is on the potentially modifiable risk factors discussed in the following list[4,46]:

1. *Hypertension* is considered the single most important modifiable risk factor for ischemic stroke; 40% of strokes have been attributed to systolic blood pressures greater than 140 mm Hg.[73]
2. Management of *cardiac diseases,* particularly atrial fibrillation (a-fib), mitral stenosis, and structural abnormalities (patent foramen ovale and atrial septal aneurysm), can reduce the risk of stroke.
3. Management of *diabetes and glucose metabolism* can also reduce the risk of stroke.
4. *Cigarette smoking* increases the relative risk of ischemic stroke nearly two times.
5. Although *excessive use of alcohol* is a risk factor for many other diseases, *moderate consumption of alcohol* may reduce incidence of cardiovascular disease, including stroke.
6. *Use of illegal drugs,* particularly cocaine, is commonly associated with stroke. Other drugs linked to stroke include heroin, amphetamines, LSD, PCP, and marijuana.
7. *Lifestyle factors* such as obesity, physical inactivity, diet, and emotional stress are associated with stroke risk.

"The realization that the probability of stroke is increased several fold by the presence of multiple risk factors may help the patient ... fully appreciate the need for serious risk factor management."[4] The responsibility for stroke prevention education (including the prevention of recurrence) falls on each member of the stroke rehabilitation team.

HEMORRHAGE

Hemorrhagic strokes include subarachnoid and intracerebral hemorrhage, which accounts for only 15% to 25% of total strokes.[4] This type of stroke has numerous causes. The four most common causes are deep hypertensive intracerebral hemorrhages, ruptured saccular aneurysms, bleeding from arteriovenous malformations, and spontaneous lobar hemorrhages.[53]

RELATED SYNDROMES

Cerebral anoxia and aneurysm can also result in hemiplegia. Some of the treatment approaches outlined in this chapter may be applicable to hemiplegia that results from causes other than CVA or stroke, such as head injuries, neoplasms, and infectious diseases of the brain.

TRANSIENT ISCHEMIC ATTACKS

Vascular disease of the brain can result in a completed CVA or cause **transient ischemic attacks** (TIAs). A TIA occurs as mild, isolated, or repetitive neurological symptoms that develop suddenly, last from a few minutes to several hours but not longer than 24 hours, and clear completely. The TIA is seen as a sign of impending CVA. Most TIAs occur in people with atherosclerotic disease. Of those who experience TIAs and do not seek treatment, an estimated one third will sustain a completed stroke, another third will continue to have additional TIAs without stroke, and one third will experience no further incidence.[71] If the TIA is caused by extracranial vascular disease, surgical intervention to restore vascular flow (carotid endarterectomy) may be effective in preventing the CVA and the resultant disability.

EFFECTS OF CEREBROVASCULAR ACCIDENT

The outcome of the CVA depends on which artery supplying the brain was involved (Figure 33-1). A client's inability to engage in areas of occupational performance depends on various pathological conditions resulting in CVA and the different anatomical structures involved. Stroke diagnostic workups help localize the lesion and find a cause of the stroke. Techniques include such cerebrovascular imaging techniques as computerized tomography (CT scanning), magnetic resonance imaging (MRI), and more recently, positron emission tomography (PET) and single photon emission computerized tomography (SPECT).[9] The information collected using these techniques (e.g., the extent of damage and location of the lesion) may help the occupational therapist identify neurological deficits that affect function. The information may also help the therapist develop hypotheses regarding recovery and plan appropriate treatment. Initial information may be collected during a medical record review that focuses on the chief complaint of the client on admission, previous medical and surgical history, results of diagnostics, and current pharmacological management. The following section and Tables 33-1 and 33-2 explain patterns of impairment resulting from CVA in both cortical and subcortical areas.

INTERNAL CAROTID ARTERY

In the absence of adequate collateral circulation, occlusion of the internal carotid artery results in contralateral hemiplegia, hemianesthesia, and homonymous hemianopsia.[7,9]

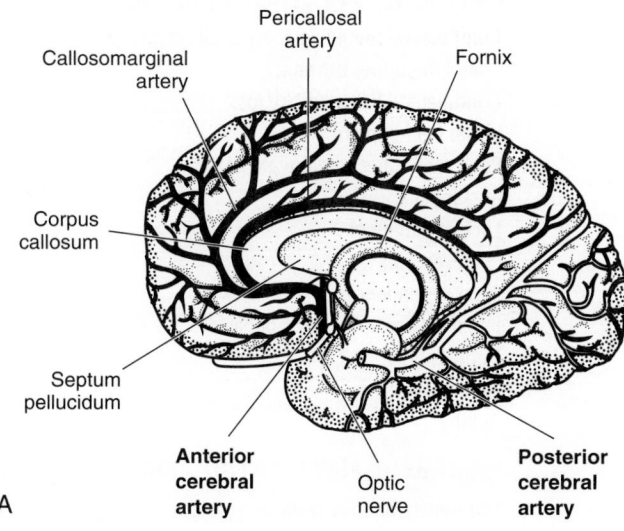

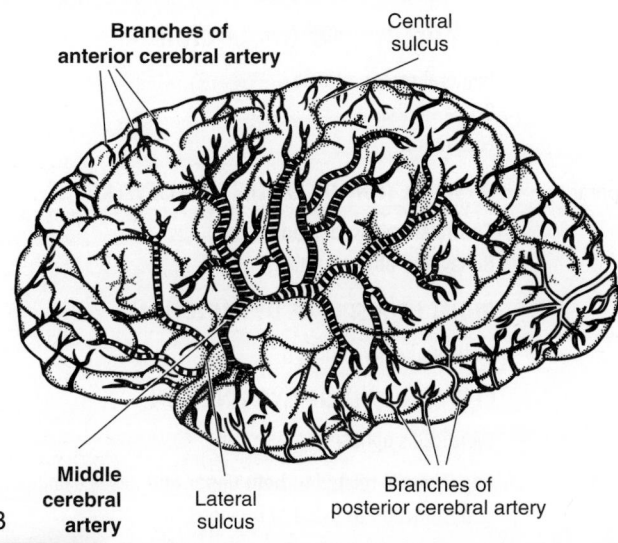

Figure 33-1 Blood supply to brain. Middle cerebral, anterior cerebral, and posterior cerebral arteries supply blood to cerebral hemispheres. **A,** Medial surface. **B,** Lateral surface. (From Nolte J: *The human brain,* ed 3, St Louis, 1993, Mosby.)

Additionally, involvement of the dominant hemisphere is associated with aphasia, agraphia or dysgraphia, acalculia or dyscalculia, right-left confusion, and finger agnosia. Involvement of the nondominant hemisphere is associated with visual perceptual dysfunction, unilateral neglect, anosognosia, constructional or dressing apraxia, attention deficits, and loss of topographic memory.

MIDDLE CEREBRAL ARTERY

Involvement of the middle cerebral artery (MCA) is the most common cause of CVA.[8,9,20] Ischemia in the area supplied by the MCA results in contralateral hemiplegia with greater involvement of the arm, face, and tongue; sensory deficits; contralateral homonymous hemianopsia; and aphasia if the lesion is in the dominant hemisphere. There is a pronounced deviation of the head and neck toward the side on which the lesion is located.[21,28] Perceptual deficits such as anosognosia, unilateral neglect, impaired vertical perception, visual spatial deficits, and perseveration are seen if the lesion is in the nondominant hemisphere.[7]

ANTERIOR CEREBRAL ARTERY

Occlusion of the anterior cerebral artery (ACA) produces contralateral lower extremity weakness that is more severe than that of the arm. Apraxia, mental changes, primitive reflexes, and bowel and bladder incontinence may be present. Total occlusion of the ACA results in contralateral hemiplegia with severe weakness of the face, tongue, and proximal arm muscles and marked spastic paralysis of the distal lower extremity. Cortical sensory loss is present in the lower extremity. Intellectual changes such as confusion, disorientation, abulia, whispering, slowness, distractibility, limited verbal output, perseveration, and amnesia may be seen.[7,9]

POSTERIOR CEREBRAL ARTERY

The scope of posterior cerebral artery (PCA) symptoms is potentially broad and varied because this artery supplies the upper brainstem region, as well as the temporal and occipital lobes. Possible results of PCA involvement depend on the arterial branches involved and the extent and area of cerebral compromise. Some possible outcomes are sensory and motor deficits, involuntary movement disorders (e.g., hemiballism, postural tremor, hemichorea, hemiataxia, and intention tremor), memory loss, alexia, astereognosis, dysesthesia, akinesthesia, contralateral homonymous hemianopsia or quadrantanopsia, anomia, topographic disorientation, and visual agnosia.[7,9,28]

CEREBELLAR ARTERY SYSTEM

Cerebellar artery occlusion results in ipsilateral ataxia, contralateral loss of pain and temperature sensitivity, ipsilateral facial analgesia, dysphagia and dysarthria caused by weakness of the ipsilateral muscles of the palate, nystagmus, and contralateral hemiparesis.[7,9,21,28]

VERTEBROBASILAR ARTERY SYSTEM

A CVA in the vertebrobasilar artery system affects brainstem functions. The outcome of the stroke is some combination of bilateral or crossed sensory and motor abnormalities, such as cerebellar dysfunction, loss of proprioception, hemiplegia, quadriplegia, and sensory disturbances, with unilateral or bilateral cranial nerve involvement of nerves III to XII.

TABLE 33-1 Cerebral Artery Dysfunction: Cortical Involvement and Patterns of Impairment

Artery	Location	Possible Impairments
Middle cerebral artery: upper trunk	Lateral aspect of frontal and parietal lobe	**DYSFUNCTION OF EITHER HEMISPHERE** Contralateral hemiplegia, especially of the face and the upper extremity Contralateral hemisensory loss Visual field impairment Poor contralateral conjugate gaze Ideational apraxia Lack of judgment Perseveration Field dependency Impaired organization of behavior Depression Lability Apathy **RIGHT HEMISPHERE DYSFUNCTION** Left unilateral body neglect Left unilateral visual neglect Anosognosia Visuospatial impairment Left unilateral motor apraxia **LEFT HEMISPHERE DYSFUNCTION** Bilateral motor apraxia Broca's aphasia Frustration
Middle cerebral artery: lower trunk	Lateral aspect of right temporal and occipital lobes	**DYSFUNCTION OF EITHER HEMISPHERE** Contralateral visual field defect Behavioral abnormalities **RIGHT HEMISPHERE DYSFUNCTION** Visuospatial dysfunction **LEFT HEMISPHERE DYSFUNCTION** Wernicke's aphasia
Middle cerebral artery: both upper and lower trunks	Lateral aspect of the involved hemisphere	Impairments related to both upper and lower trunk dysfunction as listed in previous two sections
Anterior cerebral artery	Medial and superior aspects of frontal and parietal lobes	Contralateral hemiparesis, greatest in foot Contralateral hemisensory loss, greatest in foot Left unilateral apraxia Inertia of speech or mutism Behavioral disturbances

From Arnadottir G: Impact of neurobehavioral deficits of activities of daily living. In Gillen G, Burkhardt A, editors: *Stroke rehabilitation: a function-based approach*, ed 2, St Louis, 2004, Elsevier.

TABLE **33-1** **Cerebral Artery Dysfunction: Cortical Involvement and Patterns of Impairment—cont'd**

Artery	Location	Possible Impairments
Internal carotid artery	Combination of middle cerebral artery distribution and anterior cerebral artery	Impairments related to dysfunction of middle and anterior cerebral arteries as listed in previous sections
Anterior choroidal artery, a branch of the internal carotid artery	Globus pallidus, lateral geniculate body, posterior limb of the internal capsule, medial temporal lobe	Hemiparesis of face, arm, and leg Hemisensory loss Hemianopsia
Posterior cerebral artery	Medial and inferior aspects of right temporal and occipital lobes, posterior corpus callosum and penetrating arteries to midbrain and thalamus	**DYSFUNCTION OF EITHER SIDE** Homonymous hemianopsia Visual agnosia (visual object agnosia, prosopagnosia, color agnosia) Memory impairment Occasional contralateral numbness **RIGHT SIDE DYSFUNCTION** Cortical blindness Visuospatial impairment Impaired left-right discrimination **LEFT SIDE DYSFUNCTION** Finger agnosia Anomia Agraphia Acalculia Alexia
Basilar artery proximal	Pons	Quadripareis Bilateral asymmetric weakness Bulbar or pseudobulbar paralysis (bilateral paralysis of face, palate, pharynx, neck, or tongue) Paralysis of eye abductors Nystagmus Ptosis Cranial nerve abnormalities Diplopia Dizziness Occipital headache Coma
Basilar artery distal	Midbrain, thalamus, and caudate nucleus	Papillary abnormalities Abnormal eye movements Altered level of alertness Coma Memory loss Agitation Hallucination
Vertebral artery	Lateral medulla and cerebellum	Dizziness Vomiting Nystagmus Pain in ipsilateral eye and face Numbness in face Clumsiness of ipsilateral limbs Hypotonia of ipsilateral limbs Tachycardia Gait ataxia

Continued

TABLE 33-1   Cerebral Artery Dysfunction: Cortical Involvement and Patterns of Impairment—cont'd

Artery	Location	Possible Impairments
Systemic hypoperfusion	Watershed region on lateral side of hemisphere, hippocampus, and surrounding structures in medial temporal lobe	Coma Dizziness Confusion Decreased concentration Agitation Memory impairment Visual abnormalities caused by disconnection from frontal eye fields Simultanognosia Impaired eye movements Weakness of shoulder and arm Gait ataxia

From Arnadottir G: Impact of neurobehavioral deficits of activities of daily living. In Gillen G, Burkhardt A, editors: *Stroke rehabilitation: a function-based approach*, ed 2, St Louis, 2004, Elsevier Mosby.

TABLE 33-2   Cerebrovascular Dysfunction in Noncortical Areas: Patterns of Impairment

Location	Possible Impairments	Location	Possible Impairments
Anterolateral thalamus, either side	Minor contralateral motor abnormalities Long latency period Slowness **RIGHT SIDE** Visual neglect **LEFT SIDE** Aphasia	Caudate	Good comprehension of speech Paraphasia Anomia Dysarthria Apathy Restlessness Agitation Confusion Delirium Lack of initiative Poor memory Contralateral hemiparesis Ipsilateral conjugate deviation of the eyes
Lateral thalamus	Contralateral hemisensory symptoms Contralateral limb ataxia		
Bilateral thalamus	Memory impairment Behavioral abnormalities Hypersomnolence		
Internal capsule or basis pontis	Pure motor stroke	Putamen	Contralateral hemiparesis Contralateral hemisensory loss Decreased consciousness Ipsilateral conjugate gaze Motor impersistence **RIGHT SIDE** Visuospatial impairment **LEFT SIDE** Aphasia
Posterior thalamus	Numbness or decreased sensibility of face and arm Choreic movements Impaired eye movements Hypersomnolence Decreased consciousness Decreased alertness **RIGHT SIDE** Visual neglect Anosognosia Visuospatial abnormalities **LEFT SIDE** Aphasia Jargon aphasia	Pons	Quadriplegia Coma Impaired eye movement
		Cerebellum	Ipsilateral limb ataxia Gait ataxia Vomiting Impaired eye movements

From Arnadottir G: Impact of neurobehavioral deficits of activities of daily living. In Gillen G, Burkhardt A, editors: *Stroke rehabilitation: a function-based approach*, ed 2, St Louis, 2004, Elsevier.

MEDICAL MANAGEMENT

Specific treatment of CVA depends on the type and location of the vascular lesion, the severity of the clinical deficit, concomitant medical and neurological problems, availability of technology and personnel to administer special types of treatment, and the cooperation and reliability of the client.

Early medical treatment involves maintenance of an open airway, hydration with intravenous fluids, and treatment of hypertension. Appropriate steps should be taken to evaluate and treat coexisting cardiac or other systemic diseases. Measures should be taken to prevent the development of deep venous thrombosis (DVT). DVT is the formation of emboli (blood clots) in the deep veins of the lower extremities, a common risk for clients who have prolonged periods of bed rest and immobility. The incidence of DVT in stroke ranges from 22% to 73%. Emboli that are released from deep veins and subsequently lodge in the lungs are referred to as *pulmonary emboli*. A pulmonary embolus is the most common cause of death in the first 30 days after a CVA.[9,19]

The physician oversees routine surveillance for thrombosis that includes daily evaluation of leg temperature, color, circumference, tenderness, and appearance. Preventive treatments for DVT may involve medication, the use of elastic stockings, the use of reciprocal compression devices, and early mobilization of the client.

Respiratory problems and pneumonia may complicate the early poststroke course. The National Survey of Stroke reported that one third of clients who had sustained strokes also had respiratory infections.[70]

Symptoms are a low-grade fever and increased lethargy. Medical management involves the administration of fluids and antibiotics, aggressive pulmonary hygiene, and mobilization of the client. Ventilatory insufficiency is a major factor contributing to the high frequency of pneumonia. The hemiparesis of stroke involves the muscles of respiration. Exercise programs that involve strengthening and endurance training of both inspiratory and expiratory muscles help improve breathing and cough effectiveness and reduce the frequency of pneumonia.[19]

Cardiac disease is another frequently occurring condition that complicates the poststroke course. The stroke itself may cause the cardiac abnormality, or the client may have had a preexisting cardiac condition. The former is treated in the same manner as any new cardiac diagnosis. A preexisting cardiac condition is reevaluated and the treatment regime modified as appropriate. Monitoring of heart rate, blood pressure, and an electrocardiogram (ECG) during self-care evaluations is frequently indicated to determine cardiac response to activity.

During the acute phase, bowel and bladder dysfunction is common. The physician is responsible for ordering a specific bowel program that includes a time schedule, adequate fluid intake, stool softeners, suppositories, oral laxatives, and medications or procedures to treat fecal impaction. A timed or scheduled toilet program is essential in treating urinary incontinence. Catheterization may be necessary in stroke rehabilitation.

EVALUATION AND INTERVENTION PROCEDURES FOR CLIENTS WHO SUSTAINED A STROKE

 OT PRACTICE NOTE

The evaluation of a client who sustained a stroke is a complicated process requiring the assessment of multiple client factors and performance in areas of occupation[5] that may be affected by the CVA. Therapists may have two or three clients who sustained a stroke assigned to their caseloads, each with completely different patterns of impairment and resulting functional deficits. Therefore, the most logical starting point in the evaluation process is the use of a client-centered approach to evaluation.

Tables 33-1 and 33-2 provide information related to patterns of impairments that are typically observed and that vary depending on the area of the brain that has been damaged. The location of the CVA is determined by CT (computerized axial tomography) scan or MRI (magnetic resonance imaging) and is typically documented in the medical record. Understanding this information is the first step of the evaluation process; it should take place before meeting the client and helps the therapist focus his or her evaluation procedures and begin to understand which client factors are impaired and affecting performance in areas of occupation.

For example, Jasmine has documented damage in her right frontal and parietal lobes (most likely secondary to a middle cerebral artery occlusion). Patterns of impairments that are typically observed for this type of stroke include contralateral motor loss, contralateral sensory loss, difficulty in the interpretation of spatial relationships (e.g., depth/distance, foreground from background), decreased attention or neglect of left-sided information (personal and extrapersonal), and left-limb motor-planning deficits. These impairments in turn may affect Jasmine's ability to engage in meaningful areas of occupation. Her sensory-motor loss may prevent her from fulfilling her role as a mother (e.g., assisting her child in the bath, lifting her son into the crib, preparing meals) and worker (e.g., typing, filing). Simultaneously, her attention deficits (left-sided neglect) will make driving unsafe, interfere with her self-care and her child's care, affect her computer use (e.g., finding information on the left side of the screen), and impede her ability to manage her household (e.g., read and write bills and checks, prepare meals.)

Typically, a client's clinical presentation immediately after the stroke (the acute stage) represents the worst case scenario. In other words, once the stroke is complete and the client who sustained the stroke is medically stabilized, the lesion is considered static or not progressive. At this point, the client who sustained the stroke may exhibit little to no contralateral motor function (hemiparesis or hemiplegia) because of severe weakness, no response to contralateral sensory stimuli, and a severe attention deficit; the client may also require assistance performing his or her job. Fortunately, barring another neurological insult, the client is usually expected to improve from both a neurological and functional perspective. Unfortunately, predicting the amount of improvement and the length of time necessary for improvement to take place is difficult. Clinicians generally agree that the first 3 to 6 months after the stroke is the most crucial time and that the greatest improvement takes place during this period. This time frame remains controversial and should be used only as a guideline. For example, more recent studies[80] have documented motor function improvements in clients who sustained a stroke many years earlier. It is important to note that some clients may recover only slightly and slowly, whereas others may recover fully.

Given this information, it is important to understand that neurological recovery and functional recovery are different aspects to consider. A motor control example will be used to illustrate this point. Clients A and B may share a similar presentation (no motor function on the left side of the body) immediately after experiencing the stroke. Client A may recover substantial motor function and resume engagement in previous occupations such as shopping and dressing with few residual impairments (perhaps a "limp or mild clumsiness) resulting from the stroke. Client B may not benefit from the same level of neurological motor recovery and yet still be able to resume engagement in previous occupations using adaptive methods. Dressing may require learning new one-handed techniques, wearing clothing with a looser fit, and using equipment such as a reacher. Shopping may be accomplished with the use of powered mobility (e.g., scooter or wheelchair), an ankle-foot orthotic and a cane, or the Internet. Despite these differences, both Client A and Client B are able to participate in occupations.

CLIENT-CENTERED ASSESSMENTS

"Client-centered practice is an approach to providing occupational therapy which embraces a philosophy of respect for, and partnership with, people receiving services. Client-centered practice recognizes the autonomy of individuals, the need for client choice in making decisions about occupational needs, the strengths clients bring to a therapy encounter, the benefits of client-therapist partnership, and the need to ensure that services are accessible and fit the context in which a client lives."[57]

Law, Baptiste, and Mills[56] and Pollack[67] suggest that the therapist implementing this approach to evaluation include the following concepts:

1. Recognizing that the recipients of occupational therapy (OT) are uniquely qualified to make decisions about their occupational functioning
2. Offering the client a more active role in defining goals and desired outcomes

3. Making the client-therapist relationship an *interdependent* one to enable the solution of performance dysfunction
4. Shifting to a model in which occupational therapists work with clients to enable them to meet their own goals
5. Evaluation (and intervention) focusing on the contexts in which clients live, their roles and interests, and their culture
6. Allowing the client to be the "problem-definer" so that the client will in turn become the "problem-solver"
7. Allowing the client to evaluate his or her own performance and set personal goals[56,67]

Through the use of these strategies, the evaluation process becomes more focused and defined, clients become immediately empowered, the goals of therapy are understood and agreed on, and a client-tailored treatment plan may be established. The Canadian Occupational Performance Measure[57] (COPM) is a standardized tool that uses a client-centered approach to allow the recipient of treatment to identify areas of difficulty, rate the importance of each area, and rate his or her satisfaction with current performance. It is a particularly useful tool to use with clients who sustained a stroke because of the multiple and extensive problems that this population experiences in performance of areas of occupation.

The COPM would be a good assessment to use with Jasmine. It would give the occupational therapist insight into the occupations that should be prioritized, assist in goal writing, and facilitate treatment planning. In addition, use of the COPM would empower Jasmine as an active participant in the rehabilitation process. If Jasmine completed the COPM, the results would identify toilet transfers, computer use, grooming, and feeding as the occupations that she wanted to pursue first—in other words, these occupations would be the focus of her initial occupational therapy.

TOP-DOWN APPROACH TO ASSESSMENT

A **top-down approach to assessment** process has been described in the literature[85] and is applicable to the evaluation of the client who sustained a stroke. Principles of this approach include the following:

1. Inquiry into role competency and meaningfulness is the starting point for evaluation.
2. Inquiry is focused on the roles that are important to the client who sustained a stroke, particularly those in which the client was engaged before the stroke.
3. Any discrepancy of roles in the past, present, or future is identified to help determine a treatment plan.
4. The tasks that define a person are identified, as well as whether those tasks can be performed and the reasons that the task is problematic.
5. A connection is determined between the components of function and occupational performance.

A top-down approach to evaluation is in contrast to a bottom-up approach that first focuses on dysfunction of client factors.[85]

EFFECTS OF NEUROLOGICAL DEFICITS ON PERFORMANCE IN AREAS OF OCCUPATION

Using activity analysis and keen observation allows therapists to identify errors during task performance and to analyze the errors and determine the underlying deficits blocking independent functioning. "A systematic evaluation of daily activities can be used as a structure for clinical reasoning that helps therapists detect neurobehavioral dysfunction or impaired neurologic performance components and assess functional independence in self-care activities. This method allows the therapist to analyze the nature or cause of a functional problem that requires occupational therapy intervention, so the analysis is made from the view of occupations" (Figure 33-2).[7]

Because the performance of a single functional task (e.g., donning a shirt) requires the use of multiple underlying client factors and performance skills that may have been affected by a stroke, multiple variables may be evaluated in the context of one client-chosen activity (Figure 33-3).[7,8]

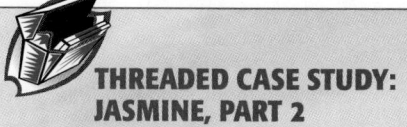

THREADED CASE STUDY: JASMINE, PART 2

Through standardized assessments and skilled observation made while Jasmine was performing her chosen occupations of feeding, grooming, toilet transfers, and computer use, it was determined that several impairments were affecting Jasmine's ability to perform independently:

- Feeding: Jasmine was unable to cut or open containers secondary to unilateral upper extremity weakness on the left, she had a tendency to eat only the food on the right side of her plate, and she was unable to locate utensils on the left side of the plate. In addition, food remained between her left gums and cheek ("pocketing") after meals, resulting in oral hygiene issues and putting Jasmine at risk for aspiration.
- Grooming: Jasmine had difficulty opening and applying toothpaste with one hand. She attended only to the right side of her body while grooming, leaving the left side of her mouth and hair not cared for during oral and hair care.
- Toilet transfers: Jasmine required moderate physical assistance to transfer to the toilet secondary to an inability to bear weight onto her left leg and an inability to control her trunk (she falls laterally when sitting on the toilet). The occupational therapist also noted that when Jasmine "completed" the transfer to the toilet, only the right side of her body was sitting on the toilet. She neglected to include the left side of her body into the transfer, leaving it in the wheelchair.
- Computer use: During attempts to use the computer, Jasmine became easily frustrated and made comments such as "I feel like a failure" and "I can't even provide for my child anymore." Jasmine agreed to attempt to write a letter to her friend on

the computer. Multiple mistakes were noted because Jasmine seemed to "not see" the left-sided keys, could not control the shift keys, and generally appeared disorganized in her approach to the task.
- Simulated child-care: A weighted doll was used to observe Jasmine's ability to care for her child. It was quickly decided that this area of occupation would be deferred until Jasmine's status improved. Jasmine and her occupational therapist made this decision collaboratively on the basis of safety concerns and Jasmine's emotional status. Jasmine was gravely concerned about her ability to care for her child. The occupational therapist wanted to focus on occupations that Jasmine could master, build her confidence, and upgrade her occupations systematically according to Jasmine's abilities.

STANDARDIZED TOOLS

The Clinical Practice Guidelines for Post-Stroke Rehabilitation[68] encourages the use of tools that are reliable, valid, and sensitive to change. In addition, the assessment tools focused on task performance should be used. Tools that are focused on evaluation of client factors in isolation from performance in areas of occupation, that use novel nonfunctional tasks, and that do not consider the effect of environmental context should be interpreted with caution. Tools are available to the occupational therapist that directly relate performance dysfunction observed during activities of daily living (ADLs) with the effect of underlying skills necessary for independent performance of activities.

The *Arnadottir Occupational Therapy Neurobehavioral Evaluation*[8] (A-ONE) objectively documents the way that dysfunction of client factors (e.g., left-sided neglect, apraxia, and spatial dysfunction) affects self-care and mobility tasks. The *Assessment of Motor and Process Skills*[36] (AMPS) uses predominantly instrumental activities of daily living (IADLs) to evaluate underlying performance skills related to the completion of various IADLs (e.g., reaching, grasping, and posture) and process skill dysfunction (e.g., using items and searching and locating). Table 33-3 provides a summary of standardized assessments used with clients who sustained a stroke. The A-ONE was used to objectively document the ways that Jasmine's various impairments (e.g., neglect, spatial relations dysfunction, loss of motor control, topographical disorientation) affected her ability to perform basic activities of daily living and mobility (e.g., bed mobility, transfers, wheelchair mobility, and walking when applicable).

ADOPTING A PHILOSOPHY FOR INTERVENTION

Therapists should consider overarching themes when deciding which interventions to use to address a client's inability to resume meaningful roles and successfully participate

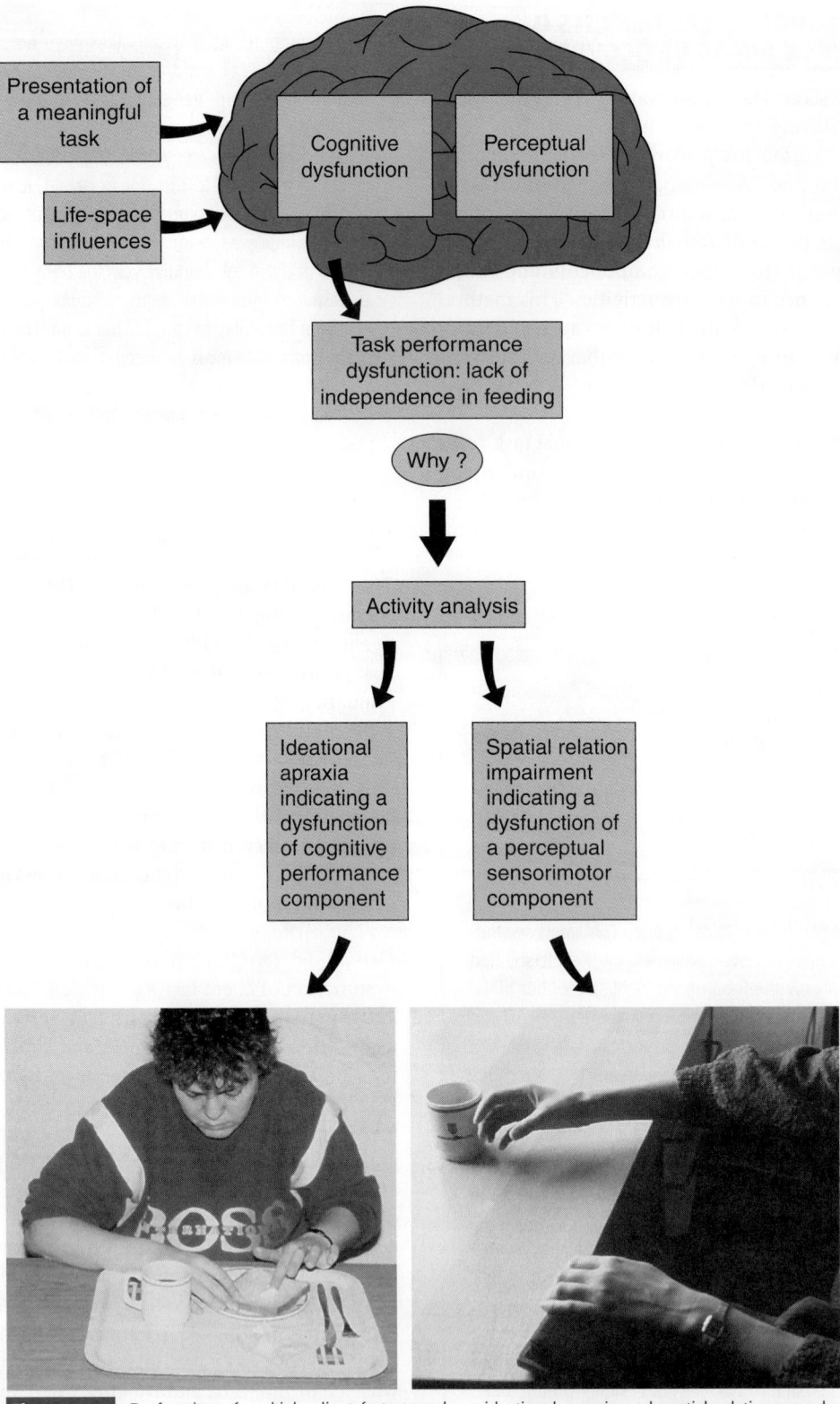

Figure 33-2 Dysfunction of multiple client factors such as ideational apraxia and spatial relations can be revealed by activity and error analysis during functional tasks such as feeding. (Modified from Arnadottir G: *The brain and behavior: assessing cortical dysfunction through activities of daily living,* St Louis, 1990, Mosby.)

Possible behavioral deficits interfering with function
Premotor perseveration: pulling up sleeve

Spatial-relation difficulties: differentiating front from back on shirt

Spatial-relation difficulties: getting an arm into the right armhole

Unilateral spatial neglect: not seeing shirt located on neglected side (or a part of the shirt)

Unilateral body neglect: not dressing the neglected side or not completing the dressing on that side

Comprehension problem: not understanding verbal information related to performance

Ideational apraxia: not knowing what to do to get shirt on or not knowing what the shirt is for

Ideomotor apraxia: having problems with the planning of finger movements in order to perform

Tactile agnosia (astereognosis): having trouble buttoning shirt without watching the performance

Organization and sequencing: dressing the unaffected arm first getting into trouble with dressing the affected arm; inability to continue the activity without being reminded

Lack of motivation to perform

Distraction: becomes interrupted by other things

Attention deficit: difficulty attending to task and quality of performance

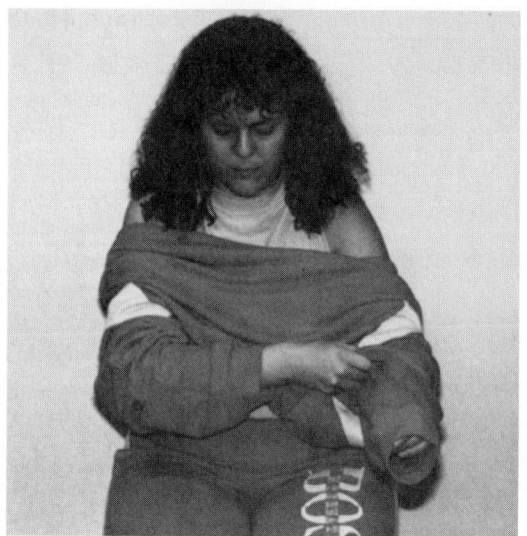

Irritated or frustrated when having trouble performing or when not getting the desired assistance

Aggressive when therapist touches patient in order to assist her (tactile defensiveness)

Difficulties recognizing foreground from background or a sleeve of a unicolor shirt from the rest of the shirt

Figure 33-3   Possible behavioral deficits interfering with function during donning a shirt. (From Arnadottir G: *The brain and behavior: assessing cortical dysfunction through activities of daily living,* St Louis, 1990, Mosby.)

TABLE **33-3** **Assessments Used with Clients Who Sustained a Stroke**

Instrument	Description and Usage
NIH Stroke Scale*[22]	Stroke deficit scale that scores 15 items (e.g., consciousness, vision, extraocular movement, facial control, limb strength, ataxia, sensation, and speech and language)
Canadian Neurological Scale*[27]	Stroke deficit scale that scores eight items (e.g., consciousness, orientation, speech, motor function, and facial weakness)
Rankin Scale*[18]	Global disability scale with six grades indicating degrees of disability
Canadian Occupational Performance Measure[57] (COPM)	Client-centered assessment tool based on clients' identification of problems in performance in areas of occupation (Clients rate importance of self-care, productivity, and leisure skills, as well as their perception of performance and satisfaction with performance.)
	Used as outcome measure, as well as client satisfaction survey
Barthel Index*[60]	Measure of BADL disability that ranges from 0 to 20 or 0 to 100 (by multiplying each item by 5); includes 10 items: bowels, bladder, feeding, grooming, dressing, transfer, toileting, mobility, stairs, and bathing
Kohlman Evaluation of Living Skills (KELS)[82]	Living skills evaluation that includes ratings of 17 tasks (e.g., safety awareness, money management, phone book use, and money and bill management)
Functional Independence Measure* (FIM)[50]	Measure of BADL disability that includes 18 items scored on a seven-point scale; includes subscores for motor and cognitive function; performance areas include self-care, sphincter control, mobility, locomotion, cognition, and socialization
Frenchay Activities Index*[47]	15-item IADL scale that evaluates domestic, leisure, work, and outdoor activities

*Recommended in AHCPR's Clinical Practice Guidelines #16, *Post-Stroke Rehabilitation,* 1995.

Continued

TABLE 33-3 **Assessments Used with Clients Who Sustained a Stroke—cont'd**

Instrument	Description and Usage
PCG Instrumental Activities of Daily Living*[58]	IADL evaluation of telephone use, walking, shopping, food preparation, housekeeping, laundry, public transportation, and medication management
Assessment of Motor and Process Skills[36]	16 motor skills (e.g., reach, manipulation, calibration, coordination, posture, and mobility) and 20 process skills (e.g., attends, organizes, searches and locates, initiates, and sequences) evaluated within context of client-chosen IADL skills; clients choose familiar and culturally relevant tasks from list of 50 standardized activities of various difficulties
Mini-Mental State Examination*[37]	Mental status screening test of orientation to time and place, registration of words, attention, calculation, recall, language, and visual construction
Glasgow Coma Scale*[81]	Level of consciousness scale that includes three sections scoring eye opening, motor, and verbal responses to voice commands or pain
Arnadottir Occupational Therapy Neurobehavioral Evaluation (A-ONE)[8]	Evaluates apraxias, neglect syndromes, body scheme disorders, organization/sequencing dysfunction, agnosias, and spatial dysfunction via BADL and mobility tasks; directly correlates impairment and disability levels of dysfunction
Neurobehavioral Cognitive Status Examination*[52]	Mental status screening test that includes the domains of orientation, attention, comprehension, naming, construction, memory, calculation, similarities, judgment, and repetition
Fugl-Meyer Test*[40]	Motor function evaluation that uses a three-point scale to score the domains of pain, range of motion, sensation, volitional movement, and balance
Functional Test for the Hemiparetic Upper Extremity[90]	Arm and hand function are assessed via 17 hierarchical functional tasks based on Brunnstrom's view of motor recovery; sample tasks are folding a sheet, screwing in a light bulb, stabilizing a jar, and zipping a zipper
Arm Motor Ability Test (AMAT)[54]	Arm function evaluated by functional ability and quality of movement; test involves performance of 28 tasks (e.g., eating with a spoon, opening jar, tying shoelace, and using telephone)
TEMPA[30,31]	Upper extremity performance test composed of nine standardized tasks (bilateral and unilateral) measured by three criteria: length of execution, functional rating, and task analysis; sample tasks are handling coins, picking up a pitcher and pouring water, writing and stamping an envelope, and unlocking a lock
Jebsen Test of Hand Function[49]	Hand function evaluation; includes seven test activities: writing a short sentence, turning over index cards, simulated eating, picking up small objects, moving empty and weighted cans, and stacking checkers during timed trials
Motor Assessment Scale*[24]	Motor function evaluation; includes disability and impairment measures; includes arm and hand movements, tone, and mobility (bed, upright, and ambulation)
Motricity Index*[29]	Measures impairments of limb strength with a weighted ordinal scale
Trunk Control Test[39]	Trunk control evaluated on a 0- to 100-point scale; tasks used: rolling, supine to sit, and balanced sitting
Berg Balance Scale*[13]	Balance assessment of 14 items scored on a 0- to 4-point ordinal scale
Tinetti Test[83]	Evaluates balance and gait in the older adult population
Rivermead Mobility Index*[26]	Measures bed mobility, sitting, standing, transfers, and walking on a pass or fail scale
Functional Reach Test[33]	Balance evaluation; objectively measures length of forward reach in the standing posture
Boston Diagnostic Aphasia Examination*[44]	Assesses sample speech and language behavior, including fluency, naming, word finding, repetition, serial speech, auditory comprehension, reading and writing
Western Aphasia Battery*[51]	Includes an "Aphasia Quotient" and "Cortical Quotient" scored on a 100-point scale: assesses spontaneous speech, repetition, comprehension, naming, reading, and writing
Beck Depression Inventory*[12]	21-item, self-rating scale with attitudinal, somatic, and behavioral components
Geriatric Depression Scale*[93]	Self-rated depression scale of 30 items with a yes-or-no format
Family Assessment Device*[34]	Family assessment of problem solving, communication, roles, affective responsiveness, affective involvement, behavioral control, and general functioning
Medical Outcomes Study/Short Form Health Survey (SF-36)*[89]	Quality of life measure that includes the domains of physical functioning, physical and emotional problems, social function, pain, mental health, vitality, and health perception
Sickness Impact Profile*[14]	Quality of life measure in the format of a 136-item scale with 12 subscales that measure ambulation mobility, body care, emotion, communication, alertness, sleep, eating, home management, recreation, social interactions, and employment

*Recommended in AHCPR's Clinical Practice Guidelines #16, *Post-Stroke Rehabilitation,* 1995.

TABLE **33-3** **Assessments Used with Clients Who Sustained a Stroke—cont'd**

Instrument	Description and Usage
Activity Card Sort[11]	Uses a Q-sort methodology to assess participation in 80 instrumental, social, and high and low physical demand leisure activities. Clients sort the cards into different piles to identify activities that were done before stroke, those activities they are doing less, and those they have given up since their stroke. The ACS uses cards with pictures of tasks that people do every day.
Stroke Impact Scale[55]	A stroke-specific measure that incorporates function and quality of life into one measure. It is a self-report measure including 59 items and forming 8 subgroups, including strength, hand function, basic and instrumental activities of daily living, mobility, communication, emotion, memory and thinking, and participation.

in chosen occupations. Embracing evidence-based practice should serve as the foundation for all OT interventions. To be successful in this endeavor, practitioners must remain abreast of new and emerging research in the OT literature as well as related fields. Review papers[59,77,88] and evidence-based libraries and search engines such as the Cochrane Library are sources of up-to-date information.

Mathiowetz[61] has outlined a series of intervention principles based on use of the Occupational Therapy Task Oriented Approach.[62] These include the following:

- Help clients adjust to role and task performance limitations by exploring new roles and tasks.
- Create an environment that includes the common challenges of everyday life.
- Practice functional tasks or close simulations that have been identified as important by participants to find effective and efficient strategies for performance.
- Provide opportunities for practice outside of therapy time (e.g., homework assignments).
- Minimize ineffective and inefficient movement patterns.

FUNCTIONAL LIMITATIONS COMMONLY OBSERVED AFTER STROKE

Multiple factors can impede effective and efficient performance of various tasks on which the client desires to focus in OT. The following section reviews problem areas that are typically observed during work with clients who sustained a stroke.

INABILITY TO PERFORM CHOSEN OCCUPATIONS WHILE SEATED

A commonly observed deficit after stroke is the loss of trunk and postural control.

Impairment in trunk control may lead to the following problems[42]:

1. Dysfunction of limb control
2. Increased risk for falls
3. Impaired ability to interact with the environment

4. Visual dysfunction secondary to resultant head and neck malalignment
5. Symptoms of dysphagia secondary to proximal malalignment
6. Decreased independence in ADLs

The loss of trunk control after a stroke may be manifested as an inability to sit in proper alignment, the loss of righting and equilibrium reactions, the inability to reach beyond the arm span because of lack of postural adjustments, and falling during attempts to function.

Clients who sustained a stroke who lose trunk control need to use the more functional upper extremity (UE) for postural support to remain upright and prevent falls. In these cases, the client effectively eliminates the ability to engage in ADL and mobility tasks because lifting the more functional arm from the supporting surface can result in a fall. "Trunk control appears to be an obvious prerequisite for the control of more complex limb activities that in turn constitute a prerequisite to complex behavioral skills."[39] Studies have found trunk control to be a predictor of gait recovery, sitting balance,[16] Functional Independence Measure scores,[39] and scores on the Barthel Index[75] after stroke.

Specific effects of a stroke on the trunk include the following:

1. Inability to perceive midline as a result of spatial relations dysfunction and resulting in sitting postures that are misaligned from the vertical
2. Assumption of static postures that do not support engagement in functional activities (e.g., posterior pelvic tilt, kyphosis, and lateral flexion)
3. Multidirectional trunk weakness[17]
4. Spinal contracture secondary to soft-tissue shortening
5. Inability to move the trunk segmentally (i.e., the trunk moves as unit; examples of this phenomenon are clients using "log rolling" patterns during bed mobility and an inability to rotate the trunk while reaching for an item across the midline.)
6. Inability to shift weight through the pelvis anteriorly, posteriorly, and laterally.

Specific deficits in trunk control are evaluated during observation of task performance (Box 33-1). Observing tasks allows the therapist to evaluate trunk control in many directions (i.e., isometric, eccentric, and concentric control of the trunk muscle groups [extensors, abdominal muscles, and lateral flexors]) and the client's limits of stability. The phrase *limits of stability* refers to "boundaries of an area of space in which the body can maintain its position without changing the base of support"[78] or "an area about which the center of mass may be moved over any given base of support without disrupting equilibrium."[34] The therapist must differentiate between the client's perceived limits of stability and the actual limits of stability. After a stroke, it is common to experience a disparity between the two because of body scheme disorder, fear of falling, or lack of insight into or awareness of disability. If the client's perceived limits are greater than his or her actual limits, there is a risk for falls. In other cases, the client's perceived limits are less than actual limits. In such instances, the client will not attempt more dynamic activities or will rely too greatly on adaptive equipment.

Treatment interventions aimed at increasing the client's ability to perform chosen tasks in seated postures include the following[42]:

1. *Establishing a neutral yet active starting alignment (i.e. a position of readiness to function).* This starting alignment (similar to a typist's posture) is a prerequisite to engaging the limbs in an activity. The desirable posture is as follows:
   - Feet flat on floor and bearing weight
   - Equal weight bearing through both ischial tuberosities
   - A neutral to slight anterior pelvic tilt
   - An erect spine
   - Head over the shoulders and shoulders over the hips
2. The client should attempt reaching activities from the above posture and do the same activities with a posterior pelvic tilt and flexed spine (a typical trunk pattern after stroke). The freedom of movement and the available range for each posture should be compared (Figure 33-4).
3. *Establishing the ability to maintain the trunk in midline using external cues.* Many clients have difficulty assuming and maintaining the correct posture. The therapist can provide verbal feedback (e.g., "Sit up nice and tall"). Visual feedback (e.g., using a mirror or the therapist assuming the same postural misalignment as the client) may be helpful. Environmental cues may be used to

---

Box 33-1   TRUNK CONTROL EVALUATION DURING TASK PERFORMANCE: EXAMPLES OF POSTURAL ADJUSTMENTS THAT SUPPORT PARTICIPATION IN CHOSEN ACTIVITIES

FEEDING

Anterior weight shift occurs to bring upper body toward table, to prevent spillage of food from utensils, and to support a hand-to-mouth pattern.

DRESSING

Lateral weight shift to one side of the pelvis occurs so that pants and underwear can be donned over hips.

ORAL CARE

Anterior weight shift occurs so that saliva and paste may be expectorated.

TRANSFER

Trunk extends with concurrent hip flexion to initiate a sit-to-stand transition.

MEAL PREPARATION

Trunk flexes into gravity in a controlled fashion to support a reach pattern to the lower shelf of the refrigerator.

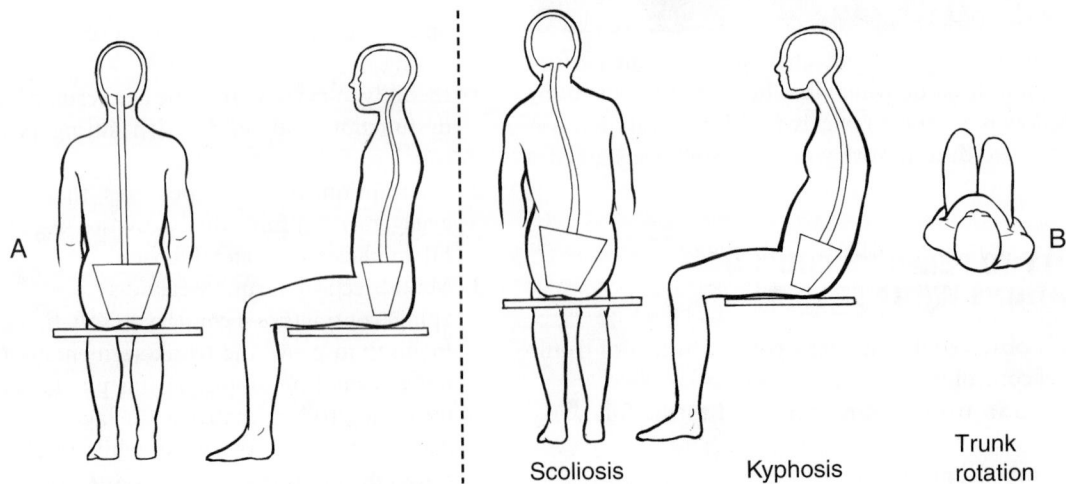

A   B

Scoliosis   Kyphosis   Trunk rotation

Figure 33-4   Normal and poststroke sitting alignment. (From Donato SM, Pulaski KH: Overview of balance impairments: functional implications. In Gillen G, Burkhardt A, editors: *Stroke rehabilitation: a function-based approach,* ed 2, St Louis, 2004, Elsevier Mosby.)

correct the posture. For example, the client may be instructed to maintain contact between the shoulder and an external target such as a bolster or wall, positioned so that the trunk is in the correct posture.

4. *Maintaining trunk range of motion (ROM) by wheelchair and armchair positioning that maintains the trunk in proper alignment.* The therapist can provide an exercise program focused on trunk range of motion and flexibility. Activities that elicit the desired movement patterns can be chosen, and hands-on mobilization of the trunk can be used if needed. Trunk ranges that should be addressed include flexion, extension, lateral flexion, and rotation.

5. *Prescribing dynamic weight-shifting activities to allow practice of weight shifts through the pelvis.* The most effective way to train the client in weight shifts is to coordinate the trunk and limbs. Successfully engaging in meaningful occupations that require reach beyond the span of either arm requires the client to adjust the posture. The client is encouraged to reach beyond arm span in all directions while seated (preferably while reaching for an object) and to analyze the corresponding postural adjustment of the pelvis and trunk. The position and goal of the task will dictate the required weight shift (Table 33-4).

6. *Strengthening the trunk, best achieved by using tasks that require the client to control the trunk against gravity.* Some examples are bridging the hips in the supine position to strengthen the back extensors and initiating a roll with the arm and upper trunk to strengthen the abdominal muscles. Strengthening occurs within the context of an activity.

7. *Using compensatory strategies and environmental adaptations when trunk control does not improve to a sufficient level and the client is at risk for injury.* Examples of interventions include wheelchair seating systems (e.g., lateral supports, lumbar rolls, chest straps, and tilt-in-space frames with head supports) and adaptive ADL equipment (e.g., reachers, long-handled equipment) to decrease the amount of required trunk displacements (see Chapter 10).

For Jasmine, therapy first focused on her ability to keep her trunk stable (i.e., not moving) while using her limbs to engage in occupations. Occupations that do not require substantial weight shifting in sitting (e.g., hair care, upper body washing, feeding, card playing) were chosen first, followed by those that required progressively more weight shifting in all directions (e.g., wiping after use of the toilet, lower body dressing, scooting, reaching to the floor to pick up shoes, washing her feet). As needed, the therapist provided external support at Jasmine's shoulders during these activities to increase her confidence, prevent falls, and provide necessary support to compensate for Jasmine's weakness. As Jasmine improved, more challenging seated activities were chosen and external support was diminished.

INABILITY TO ENGAGE IN CHOSEN OCCUPATIONS IN STANDING

The inability to assume and maintain a standing posture has a significant effect on the type of activities in which a person may engage; it may also play a significant role in the eventual discharge destination for the inpatient recovering from stroke. Impaired upright control has been correlated with an increased risk of falls,[92] as well as with less-than-optimal functional outcomes[60] on the Barthel Index. Because many basic and instrumental ADL, work, and leisure skills require control of standing postures, early training in upright control is a necessary component of stroke rehabilitation programs.

Similar to the deficits seen in sitting, upright standing postures are characterized by asymmetrical weight distribution; unlike deficits in sitting, the weight distribution in standing is seen through the lower extremities[92] in addition to the trunk. Clients who sustained a stroke often experience an inability to bear weight through the affected leg. Reasons for this disability include fear of falling or buckling of the knee, patterns of weakness that will not support the weight of the body, spasticity that impedes proper alignment (i.e., plantar flexion spasticity that effectively blocks weight bearing through the sole of the foot),[41] and perceptual dysfunction.

In addition to asymmetry and an inability to bear weight or shift weight through the affected leg, many clients who have sustained a stroke lose upright postural control and balance strategies. Effective upright control depends on the following automatic postural reactions[32,78]:

1. *Ankle strategies* are used to maintain the center of mass over the base of support when movement is centered on the ankles. These strategies control small, slow, swaying motions such as standing in a movie line, engaging in conversations while standing, and stirring a pot on a stovetop. They are most effective when the support surface (e.g., floor) is firm and longer than the foot. Ankle weakness, loss of the ankle's range of motion, and proprioceptive deficits may all contribute to ineffective ankle strategies and balance.

2. *Hip strategies* are used to maintain or restore equilibrium. These strategies are used specifically in response to larger, faster perturbations, when the support surface is compliant, or when the surface is smaller than the feet (e.g., walking on a beam).[48]

3. A *stepping strategy* is used when ankle and hip strategies are, or are perceived to be, ineffective. This strategy results in movement of the base of support toward the center of mass movement. A step is taken to widen the base of support. Tripping over an uneven sidewalk or standing on a bus that unexpectedly stops elicits this strategy.

Both the loss of postural reactions and the inability to bear and shift weight onto the affected leg will result in such functional limitations as gait deviations or dysfunction;

TABLE 33-4   **Effects of Object Positioning on Trunk Movements and Weight Shifts During Reaching Activities***

Position of Object	Trunk Response/Weight Shift
Straight ahead at forehead level, past arm's length	Trunk extension, anterior pelvic tilt Anterior weight shift
On floor, between feet	Trunk flexion Anterior weight shift
To side at shoulder level, past arm's length	Left trunk shortening, right trunk elongation, left hip hiking Weight shift to right

*These examples are for a patient with left hemiplegia. The left-hand column indicates where to position objects during a reaching task (using the right upper extremity). The right-hand column indicates the resultant trunk position and weight shift.
From Gillen G: Trunk control: a prerequisite to functional independence. In Gillen G, Burkhardt A, editors: *Stroke rehabilitation: a function-based approach,* ed 2, St Louis, 2004, Elsevier Science/Mosby.

Position of Object	Trunk Response/Weight Shift
On floor, below right hip	Right trunk shortening, left trunk elongation Weight shift to right

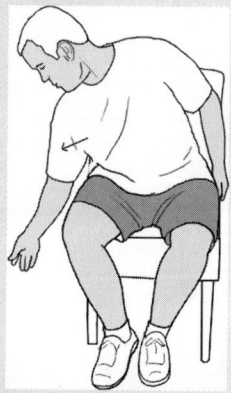

Behind right shoulder, at arm's length	Trunk extension and rotation (right side posteriorly) Weight shift to right

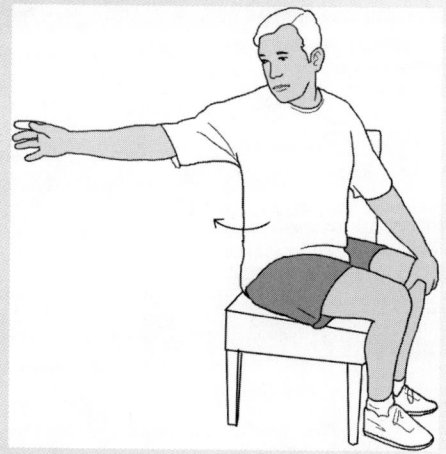

At shoulder level, to left of left shoulder	Trunk extension and rotation (left side posteriorly) Weight shift to left

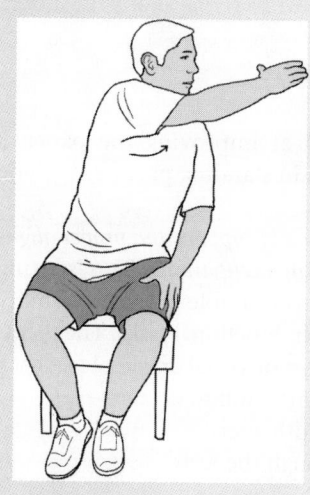

Continued

TABLE **33-4**   **Effects of Object Positioning on Trunk Movements and Weight Shifts During Reaching Activities*—cont'd**

Position of Object	Trunk Response/Weight Shift
On floor, to left of left foot	Trunk flexion and rotation (left side posteriorly) Weight shift to left
Above head, directly behind	Trunk extension, shoulders move behind hips Posterior weight shift

*These examples are for a client with left hemiplegia. The left-hand column indicates where to position objects during a reaching task (using the right upper extremity). The right-hand column indicates the resultant trunk position and weight shift.

an inability to climb stairs, transfer, and perform upright basic ADLs (BADLs) and IADLs; and an increased risk of falls. The assessment process provides the therapist with more specific information regarding the cause of dysfunction. "Specifically, therapists should observe what happens when patients have to move their center of mass over their base of support, move their head, stand on uneven surfaces, function in lower lighting, move from one type of surface to another, or function on a narrower base of support. Therapists should also observe patients' postural alignment, whether a bias in posture exists and in which direction that bias occurs, patients' limits of stability, the width between their feet during functional tasks, and what patients do after losing their balance."[32]

Treatment strategies aimed at improving the patient's ability to perform chosen tasks in standing postures include the following[32,78,92]:

1. *Establishing a symmetrical base of support and proper alignment to prepare to engage in occupations.* This starting alignment is assumed to provide ample proximal stability and to support engagement in functional tasks. The therapist may use hands-on support or visual or verbal feedback to establish proper alignment as follows:
   - Feet approximately hip width apart
   - Equal weight bearing through the feet
   - A neutral pelvis
   - Both knees *slightly* flexed
   - Aligned and symmetrical trunk

2. *Establishing the ability to bear weight and shift weight through the more affected lower extremity.*[27] The ability to bear weight may be graded at first. For example, if a client cannot assume a standing position because of postural insecurity or imbalance, sitting on a high surface (e.g., stool or raised therapy mat) allows the client to begin to bear weight but does not require bearing full body weight. As the client improves, full standing is encouraged, followed by graded weight shifts and progressing to full weight bearing on the affected leg. For example, a modified soccer activity requires the client to fully shift weight to kick the ball. The environment (e.g., work surface height and placement of objects) is manipulated in conjunction with the client's positioning to elicit the required weight shift.

3. *Encouraging dynamic reaching activities in multiple environments to develop task-specific weight-shifting abilities.* For example, kitchen activities that require retrieval of cleaning supplies under the sink, in a broom closet, and in overhead cabinets require mastery of multiple postural adjustments and balance strategies.

4. *Using the environment to grade task difficulty and provide external support.* Proper use of the environment can decrease the client's fear of falling and simultaneously improve confidence and challenge underlying balance skills. Examples include working in front of a high countertop, using one hand for weight bearing as a postural support, and using a walker for support. The client must not rely too much on external supports because balance strategies may not be fully challenged to reach optimal recovery.

5. *Training upright control within the context of functional tasks that are graded.* Tasks are graded in relation to length of required reach, speed, and progressively more challenging bases of support. Examples include making a bed,

changing a pet's food bowl, setting a table, stepping up on a curb, cleaning a wall mirror, playing horseshoes or shuffleboard, and doffing slippers in a standing posture. All of these activities require shifting of the body weight, balance strategies, and the ability to bear weight through both lower extremities. The activity choice is driven by the client's desires, and the therapist designs positioning and setup of the activity to elicit the desired postural strategies (Figure 33-5).

Jasmine was quickly engaged in activities that required standing despite persistent issues related to sitting balance. Standing was first attempted in front of stable work surfaces (e.g., kitchen counter, sink) to provide a balance point, increase Jasmine's feeling of security and safety, and highlight the functional relevance of standing. As needed, the therapist stabilized weak joints (e.g., hip and knee) with manual support, and Jasmine wore an ankle-foot orthotic to protect the integrity of her ankle. As Jasmine improved, she was asked to begin to use her upper body for function while controlling her standing. Examples include wiping the counter, organizing a shelf, and grooming while standing. Progressively more demanding occupations from a standing balance perspective were chosen (e.g., modified games such as volleyball, vacuuming, emptying a dishwasher, stand-pivot transfers), and external manual and environmental support were decreased as Jasmine improved. All occupations were chosen to improve Jasmine's ability to accept and shift weight through her left lower extremity.

INABILITY TO COMMUNICATE SECONDARY TO LANGUAGE DYSFUNCTION

CVA may result in a wide variety of speech or language disorders ranging from mild to severe. These deficits occur

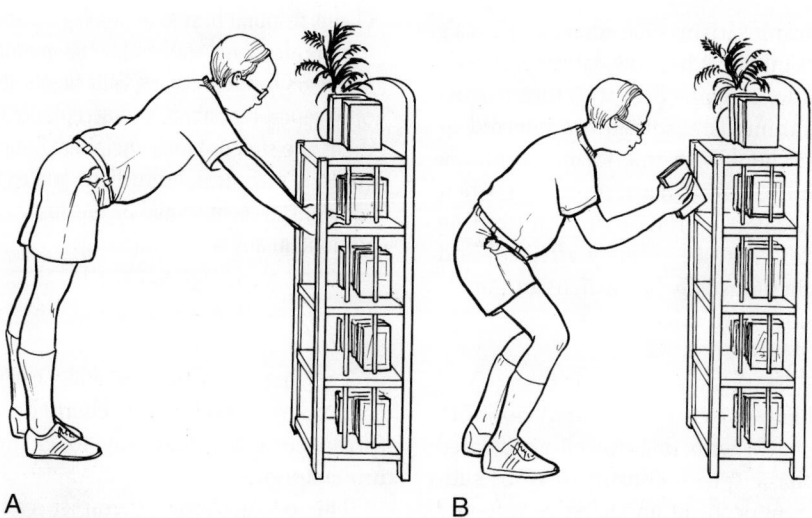

Figure 33-5 Activity is positioned to elicit the desired postural strategies. (From Donato SM, Pulaski KH: Overview of balance impairments: functional implications. In Gillen G, Burkhardt A, editors: *Stroke rehabilitation: a function-based approach*, ed. 2, St Louis, 2004, Elsevier Science/Mosby.)

most frequently in CVA resulting from damage to the left hemisphere of the brain. They can also occur less frequently after damage to the right hemisphere. All persons with CVA should be evaluated by a speech pathologist for the presence of speech and language disorders. The speech pathologist can provide valuable information to other members of the rehabilitation team and to the family regarding the best techniques for communicating with a particular client. The occupational therapist should continue the work of the speech therapist in the treatment sessions, as appropriate. Carryover may occur in reinforcing communication techniques the client is learning and in presenting instruction in ways that the client is able to understand and integrate.

The specific speech and language dysfunctions described in the following sections can exist in mild to severe forms and in combination with one another.

Aphasia

Aphasia is a language disorder that results from neurological impairment. It can affect auditory comprehension, reading comprehension (alexia), oral expression, written expression (agraphia), and the ability to interpret gestures. Mathematical deficits (acalculia) can also be present in aphasia. There are several different types of aphasia.

Global aphasia

Global aphasia is characterized by a loss of all language skills. Oral expression is lost, except for some persistent or recurrent utterance. Global aphasia is usually the result of involvement of the middle cerebral artery of the dominant cerebral hemisphere. The client with global aphasia may be sensitive to gestures, vocal inflections, and facial expression. Consequently, the client may appear to understand more than he or she actually does.[45]

Broca's aphasia

Speech apraxia and agrammatism characterize Broca's aphasia. The apraxia is manifested by slow, labored speech with frequent misarticulations. Syntactical structure is simplified because of the agrammatism, sometimes referred to as *telegraphic speech*. The client with this form of aphasia demonstrates good auditory comprehension, except when speech is rapid, grammatically complex, or lengthy. Reading comprehension and writing may be severely affected, and the client with Broca's aphasia usually has deficits in monetary concepts and the ability to do calculations.[45]

Wernicke's aphasia

Wernicke's aphasia is characterized by impaired auditory comprehension and feedback, with fluent, well-articulated paraphasic speech. Paraphasic speech consists of word substitution errors. Speech may occur at an excessive rate and may be hyperfluent. The client uses few substantive words and many function words. The client produces running speech composed of English words in a meaningless sequence.

English-speaking clients produce neologisms (non-English nonsense words) interspersed with real words. Reading and writing comprehension is often limited, and mathematical skills may be impaired.[45]

Anomic aphasia

Persons with anomic aphasia have difficulties with word retrieval. Anomia, or word-finding difficulty, occurs in all types of aphasia. However, clients in whom word-finding difficulty is the primary or only symptom may be said to have anomic aphasia. The speech of these clients is fluent, grammatically correct, and well articulated but reveals significant difficulty with word finding. This problem can result in hesitant or slow speech and the substitution of descriptive phrases for actual names of things. Mild to severe deficits in reading comprehension and written expression occur, and mild deficits in mathematical skills may be present.[2,45]

Dysarthria

Clients with dysarthria have an articulation disorder, in the absence of aphasia, because of a dysfunction of the central nervous system (CNS) mechanisms that control speech musculature. This disorder results in paralysis and incoordination of the organs of speech, causing the speech to sound thick, slurred, and sluggish.

Communication with Clients Who Have Aphasia

Although the speech pathologist is responsible for the treatment of speech and language disorders, the occupational therapist can facilitate communication and meaningful interaction with clients who have aphasia.

 OT PRACTICE NOTE

> Clients respond best to an intelligent and empathic approach from professional staff and family members. Staff and family members communicating with clients should adopt an attitude of patience, relaxation, and acceptance. When talking to the client, the staff or family member should use simple, short, concrete sentences. Instructions and explanations should be kept simple. The client should be encouraged, but not pressured, to respond in any way possible.

The use of gestures for communication should be encouraged. Having the client demonstrate through performance is the best way to ensure that instructions are understood.

The occupational therapist can use routine ADLs as opportunities to encourage speech. The client should be reassured that the language disorder is part of the disability, not a manifestation of mental illness. In addition, Rubio[72] has outlined strategies for the occupational therapist to use with clients and their caregivers:

- Understanding is facilitated when one person talks at a time. Extra noise creates confusion.
- Give the client time to respond.
- Carefully phrase questions to make it easier for the client to respond; for example, use "yes/no" and "either/or" questions.
- Use visual cues or gestures with speech to help the client understand.
- Never force a response.
- Use concise sentences.

Do not rush communication because this may increase frustration and decrease the effectiveness of communication.[72]

Given that Jasmine had a right hemispheric stroke, aphasia would not typically be expected. Jasmine did exhibit severe sensory motor loss related to her left oral structures. She presented with moderate dysarthria, occasional drooling, and difficulties in managing food in the left side of her mouth. Jasmine was encouraged to speak slowly and overenunciate. In addition, her occupational therapist taught her safe feeding strategies, including eating slowly, alternating solids and liquids, shifting food to the right side of her mouth, tilting her head to the right at a 45-degree angle, using her finger to sweep her mouth and clear out food pocketing on the left, and performing supervised oral care after each meal.

INABILITY TO PERFORM CHOSEN OCCUPATIONS SECONDARY TO NEUROBEHAVIORAL/COGNITIVE-PERCEPTUAL IMPAIRMENTS

Neurobehavioral deficit is defined as "a functional impairment of an individual manifested as defective skill performance resulting from a neurologic processing dysfunction that affects performance components such as affect, body scheme, cognition, emotion, gnosis, language, memory, motor movement, perception, personality, sensory awareness, spatial relations, and visuospatial skills."[7] A major responsibility of the occupational therapist treating a client who sustained a stroke is evaluating which neurobehavioral deficits are blocking independent performance of chosen occupations.

Arnadottir[7] has proposed a relationship among the ability to perform daily activities, neurobehavioral impairments, and the CNS origin of the neurobehavioral dysfunction (a CVA, for the purposes of this chapter). She supports this theory with the following relational statements:

1. Behaviors required for task performance are related to neuronal processing at the CNS level. Therefore, a relationship also exists between the defective behavioral responses of an individual with CNS damage during performance of ADLs and the dysfunction of neuronal processing and performance components resulting from CNS damage.
2. Performance of daily activities requires adequate function of specific parts of the nervous system. Consequently, CNS

impairment may result in dysfunction of specific aspects of ADL. For example, a CVA that causes a lesion of the posteroinferior parietal lobe of the left hemisphere commonly results in bilateral motor apraxia. "This neurobehavioral impairment may make manipulation of objects difficult during functional activities such as combing hair, brushing teeth, or holding a spoon while eating."[7]
3. Neurological impairment can be observed through the client's engagement in daily activities. Thus, through the analysis of ADL the integrity of the CNS can be evaluated (Box 33-2).

To properly evaluate the effect of neurobehavioral deficits on task performance, the therapist must develop activity analysis skills with the goal of analyzing which performance components are necessary to achieve an outcome that is satisfactory to the client. Even the simplest of BADL tasks challenges multiple underlying skills (Figure 33-3 and Boxes 33-3 and 33-4).[7,72]

Arnadottir[7,8] proposed a system of observing clients engaged in functional activities, allowing errors (as long as they are safe) to occur, analyzing the errors, and, finally, detecting the impairments that are interfering with task performance so that an appropriate treatment plan can be developed. She cautioned that when the therapist analyzes errors and observed behaviors, knowledge of neurobehavior, cortical function, activity analysis, and clinical reasoning must be considered in the results of the evaluation (Table 33-5).

Treatment aimed at counteracting the effects of neurobehavioral dysfunction may be based on an adaptive and compensatory approach or a restorative and remedial approach.[64,66,72] A combination of approaches has also been suggested (Table 33-6).[1]

Decisions regarding the selection of a particular treatment approach may be difficult. Neistadt[65,66] suggested evaluating a client's learning potential in the context of ADL evaluation and training, focusing on such issues as the number of repetitions needed to learn new approaches to tasks and the type of transfer of learning that is demonstrated.

Toglia[84] has suggested that the transfer of learning from one context to another (e.g., transferring skills learned from making a cup of tea in the OT clinic to meal preparation at home) may be facilitated by the therapist through the following methods:

1. Varying treatment environments
2. Varying the nature of the task
3. Helping clients become aware of how they process information
4. Teaching processing strategies
5. Relating new learning to previously learned skills

Toglia[84] has identified degrees of transfer of learning. The degree of transfer is defined by the number of task characteristics that differ from those of the original task. Examples of these characteristics are spatial orientation, mode of presentation (e.g., auditory or visual), movement requirements, and environmental context.

Box 33-2   Tooth Brushing Task: Treatment of Neurobehavioral Impairments

SPATIAL RELATIONS AND SPATIAL POSITIONING

Positioning of toothbrush and toothpaste while applying paste
   to brush
Placement of toothbrush in mouth
Positioning of bristles in mouth
Placement of brush under faucet

SPATIAL NEGLECT

Visual search for and use of brush, paste, and cup in affected
   hemisphere
Visual search for and use of faucet handle in affected
   hemisphere

BODY NEGLECT

Brushing of affected side of mouth

MOTOR APRAXIA

Manipulation of toothbrush during task performance
Manipulation of cap from toothpaste
Squeezing of toothpaste onto brush

IDEATIONAL APRAXIA

Appropriate use of objects (e.g., brush, paste, cup)
   during task.

ORGANIZATION AND SEQUENCING

Sequencing of task (e.g., removal of cap, application of paste to
   brush, turning on water, and putting brush in mouth)
Continuation of task to completion

ATTENTION

Attention to task (to increase difficulty, distractions such as
   conversation, flushing toilet, or running water may be added)
Refocusing on task after distraction

FIGURE-GROUND

Distinguishing white toothbrush and toothpaste from sink

INITIATION AND PERSEVERANCE

Initiation of task on command
Cleaning parts of mouth for appropriate period of time, then
   moving bristles to another part of mouth
Discontinuation of task when complete

VISUAL AGNOSIA

Use of touch to identify objects

PROBLEM SOLVING

Search for alternatives if toothpaste or toothbrush is missing

From Gillen G, Burkhardt A: *Stroke rehabilitation: a function-based approach*, ed 2, St Louis, 2004, Elsevier.

Box 33-3   Examples of Environmental and Task Manipulation to Challenge Component Skills During Meal Preparation

SPATIAL NEGLECT

Place ingredients in both visual fields.
Choose a task that requires use of right and left burners.

FIGURE-GROUND

Place necessary utensils in a cluttered drawer.
Use utensils that match the color of the counter.

SPATIAL DYSFUNCTION

Prepare items that require the client to pour ingredients from
   one container to another (e.g., pour pasta into a bowl or fill
   a pot with water).

MOTOR APRAXIA

Choose recipes that require manipulation of food items.
Choose recipes that require control of distal extremity adjustments
   (e.g., using a ladle, whisking, and stirring).

Box 33-4   Sample Compensatory Strategies for Neurobehavioral Deficits Affecting Dressing Skills

SPATIAL NEGLECT

Place necessary clothing on right side of closet and drawers.
Move dresser to right side of room.

MOTOR APRAXIA

Use loose-fitting clothing without fasteners.
Use Velcro closures.

SPATIAL DYSFUNCTION

Use shirts with a front emblem to identify proper orientation.
Lay out clothing in the proper orientation.

TABLE **33-5** **Evaluating the Effect of Neurobehavioral Dysfunction on Task Performance**

Performance Area	Observed Behavior	Possible Impairment
Grooming	Difficulty adjusting grasp on razor or toothbrush	Motor apraxia
	Using a comb to brush teeth	Ideational apraxia
	Repetitive brushing of one side of the mouth	Premotor perseveration
Feeding	Not eating food on the left side of the plate	Spatial neglect
	Overestimating or underestimating distance of glass, resulting in knocking over glass	Spatial relations dysfunction
	"Forgetting" that a glass of orange juice is in the hand, which results in spillage as the client attends to another aspect of the meal	Body neglect
	Hand placed in cereal bowl	
Dressing	Client attempting to put socks on after sneakers	Organization and sequencing dysfunction
	Client unable to locate armholes in an undershirt	Spatial relations dysfunction
	Dressing only the right side of the body	Body neglect
	Client attempting to dress the therapist's arms instead of his or her own	Somatoagnosia
Mobility	Client unable to locate the bathroom in his or her hospital room	Topographic disorientation
	Client neglecting to lock brakes or remove wheelchair footrests before attempting to transfer	Organization and sequencing dysfunction
	After a transfer, only the intact buttock in contact with the seat of the chair	Body neglect

From Arnadottir G: *The brain and behavior: assessing cortical dysfunction through activities of daily living,* St Louis, 1990, Mosby; Anadottir G: Impact of neurobehavioral deficits of activities of daily living. In Gillen G, Burkhardt A, editors: *Stroke rehabilitation: a function-based approach,* ed 2, St Louis, 2004, Elsevier Mosby.

TABLE **33-6** **Treatment Approaches for Neurobehavioral Deficits After Stroke**

Compensatory and Adaptive Approach	Restorative and Remedial Approach	Combination Approach
Repetitive practice of tasks	Restoration of component skills	Rejects dichotomy between compensatory and restorative approaches
Top-down approach	Bottom-up approach	
Emphasizes intact skill training	Deficit-specific	Uses optimally relevant occupations and environments as the treatment modality to challenge components
Emphasizes modification	Targets cause of symptoms and emphasizes components	
Uses environmental or task modifications to support optimal performance	Assumes transfer of training will occur	Treatment choice driven by tasks relevant to client needs; tasks presented so that the underlying deficits are challenged via the task
Activity choice driven by performance challenges, not component deficits	Assumes improved component performance will result in increased skill	
Treats symptoms, not the cause	Activity choice driven by component deficits	Rejects usage of contrived activities
Client-driven compensatory strategies	Research demonstrates short-term results with skills generalizable to very similar tasks	
Caregiver-therapist environmental adaptations		
Task-specific and not generalizable		

A near transfer of learning involves transfer between two tasks that have one or two differing characteristics. Intermediate transfer involves transfer of learning to a task that varies by three to six characteristics. A far transfer involves a task that is conceptually similar but has one or no characteristics in common. Finally, a very far transfer involves the "spontaneous application of what has been learned in treatment to everyday living."[84]

From her review of the literature, Neistadt[64] reached the following conclusions:
1. Near transfer from remedial tasks to similar tasks is possible for all clients with brain injury.
2. Intermediate, far, and very far transfer from remedial to functional tasks will occur only with localized brain lesions and good cognitive skills and after training with a variety of treatment tasks.

3. Far and very far transfer from remedial to functional tasks will not occur for clients with diffuse injury and severe cognitive deficits.

Using a functional and meaningful task as a treatment modality promotes acquisition of a desired skill, and the therapist may use this task to challenge multiple underlying performance components.[1,72] It is up to the therapist to present the task by manipulating the environment in a way that challenges the underlying skills (see Box 33-3). If a compensatory approach is chosen, adaptive techniques are used to counteract the effects of the underlying neurobehavioral deficits (see Box 33-4).

Jasmine's left-sided neglect had a substantial impact on her ability to perform relevant occupations independently and safely. A variety of strategies were used to improve her ability to attend to the left side. Organized visual scanning was taught during daily activities such as feeding and grooming. Occupations were chosen that required scanning to both the left and the right to be successful (e.g., finding ingredients in the refrigerator, locating the toothbrush on the left side of the sink and toothpaste on the right, reading, describing a room). Vanishing physical and verbal cues were used as Jasmine progressed. Another strategy that was helpful for Jasmine was the use of a left-sided anchor. A red strip of tape was placed to the left side (e.g., the left side of the computer monitor, placemat, sink, book), and Jasmine focused on scanning to the anchor to ensure that she was attending to all of the information required to be successful at performing each occupation. Because Jasmine's neglect persisted, driving was not an option. Other modes of transportation were considered, including supervised use of public transportation, assistance with transport by friends and neighbors, and local access-a-ride companies.

INABILITY TO PERFORM CHOSEN TASKS SECONDARY TO UPPER EXTREMITY DYSFUNCTION

The loss of UE control is common after stroke, with 88% of clients who sustained a stroke having some level of UE dysfunction.[68] The client's ability to integrate the affected arm into chosen tasks may be limited by multiple factors, including the following[43]:

1. Pain
2. Contracture and deformity
3. Loss of selective motor control
4. Weakness[20]
5. Superimposed orthopedic limitations
6. Loss of postural control to support UE control
7. Learned nonuse[80]
8. Loss of biomechanical alignment[23]
9. Inefficient and ineffective movement patterns

Integration into Function

UE evaluation procedures should focus primarily on assessing the client's ability to integrate the UE into performance

TABLE **33-7** **Suggestions for Categorizing Upper Extremity Tasks**

Category	Tasks
No functional use of arm	Teach shoulder protection
	Self range of motion
	Positioning
Postural support/weight bearing (forearm or extended arm)	Bed mobility assist
	Support upright function (e.g., work, leisure, activities of daily living)
	Support during reach with opposite hand
	Stabilize objects
Support reach (hand on work surface)	Wiping a table
	Ironing
	Polishing
	Sanding
	Smoothing out laundry
	Applying body lotion
	Washing body parts
	Vacuuming
	Locking wheelchair brakes
Reach	Multiple possibilities to engage upper extremity into activities of daily living, leisure, and mobility; grade tasks by height/distance reached, weight of object, speed, and accuracy

From Gillen G: Upper extremity function and management. In Gillen G, Burkhardt A, editors: *Stroke rehabilitation: a function-based approach*, ed 2, St Louis, 2004, Elsevier Mosby.

of functional tasks—in other words, to use the affected UE to support performance in areas of occupation. Standardized evaluations such as the TEMPA,[30,31] AMAT,[54] Jebsen,[49] and AMPS[36] (see Table 33-3) are available to objectively measure the client's ability to use the affected extremity during task performance.

The UE may be used during functional performance in different ways (Table 33-7), including but not limited to the following[39]:

1. *Weight bearing.* Weight bearing through the hand and forearm with an extended elbow is a pattern used during ADL and mobility tasks. The establishment of weight bearing is a goal of UE rehabilitation.[15] Effective control of weight bearing depends on the presence of sufficient trunk and scapula stability to accept partial body weight, control of *active* elbow extension, and ability of the hand to bear weight without losing the palmar arches. Once weight bearing is established, the client can effectively use the arm as a postural support (e.g., by supporting the upper body weight with the affected arm while wiping crumbs from the table with the more functional arm), as an aid during transitional movements (e.g., while pushing up from side-lying to sitting), and for fall prevention (increased postural support is provided).

2. *Moving objects across a work surface with a static grasp (Supported Reach)*. Activities such as ironing clothes, opening or closing a drawer, polishing furniture, and sliding a paper across the table are all examples of UE control of movement that does not occur with the arm in space. The hand is in contact with the objects involved in the task or is supported on the work surface; therefore, these types of tasks do not require the same control as, and may require less effort than, activities performed while the client is reaching in space, such as removing dishes from a cabinet or reaching for food in the refrigerator. This movement pattern can be used in multiple tasks and at the same time strengthens various muscle groups used to eventually support reach in space.

3. *Reach and manipulation*. Reviews of research on UE motor control[2,43] have identified two components of function during reaching activities. The first component is the transportation component, which is defined as the trajectory of the arm between the starting position and the object. The second component is the manipulation component, which is the formation of grip by combined movements of the thumb and the index finger during arm movement. Finger posturing anticipates the real grasp and occurs during transportation of the hand toward the object.[2] The shaping of the hand is independent of the manipulation itself. Trombly's[87] reaching studies of clients with left hemiparesis documented that the ability to reach smoothly and with coordination was significantly less on the affected than on the unaffected side. The continuous movement strategy was lost, movement time was longer, peak velocity occurred earlier, and weakness indicators were present.

Trombly[86] demonstrated that although muscular activity did not improve in the clients in her study, the discontinuity improved over time. She stated that the "level and pattern of muscle activity of these subjects depended on the biomechanical demands of the task rather than any stereotypical neurological linkages between the muscles."

Clients are commonly observed demonstrating the use of stereotypical movement patterns of the UE. These patterns are characterized by scapula elevation and fixation, humeral abduction, elbow flexion, and wrist flexion. Mathiowetz and Bass Haugen[62] suggested that the use of these movement patterns is evidence of attempts to use remaining systems to complete tasks. They gave an example of a client with weak shoulder flexors trying to lift an arm. The client flexes the elbow when trying to raise the arm because this movement strategy shortens the lever arm and eases shoulder flexion.

The following are examples of using treatment activities to improve the client's ability to integrate the UE into tasks[2,23,41,43,74,79]:

1. Using objects of different sizes and shapes to encourage control of the hand during reach and manipulation
2. Choosing activities that are appropriate to the client's level of available motor control

3. Using constraint-induced movement techniques (Box 33-5): a technique in which the *less* affected UE is constrained (e.g., with a sling and splint) to force use of the affected extremity, providing massed practice of graded activities for the affected side to increase functional use[77]
4. Specifically training the arm to be used in weight bearing, reach, and manipulation situations within the context of ADL and mobility
5. Presenting the client with graded tasks related to the number of degrees of freedom, the level of required antigravity control, and the resistance involved in the task (Figure 33-6)

Jasmine had very little motor activity throughout her left UE. Therapy focused on having Jasmine position her arm correctly (on the work surface and within her sightlines) during activities to prevent it from dangling all day, as well as use her arm as a stabilizer (e.g., using the weight of her arm to stabilize a paper while writing or hold a book open). As Jasmine improved, she was encouraged to use her arm in weight bearing as a postural support (e.g., pushing up when transitioning from the supine position to a seated position, pushing up to stand, reaching back to sit, and using the arm as support when standing at a sink or counter). Occupations were chosen that matched her available motor control and challenged her current level.

Upper Extremity Complications After Stroke

Subluxation

Subluxation, or malalignment caused by instability of the glenohumeral joint, is a common occurrence after stroke. The subluxation may be inferior (head of the humerus below the glenoid fossa), anterior (head of the humerus anterior to the fossa), or superior (head of the humerus lodged under the acromion-coracoid).[74] Cailliet[23] and Basmajian[10] have described the mechanism of inferior subluxation, in which the humeral head drifts inferior to the glenoid fossa. This common subluxation occurs as a result of malalignment of the scapula and the trunk. The normal position of the scapula is one of upward rotation, an orientation that cradles the head of the humerus and stabilizes it in alignment. The weight of the arm combined with instability and malalignment contributes to subluxation.

A common misunderstanding about subluxation is that it is associated with pain. The literature does not support this relationship.[94] Because the shoulder is unstable after a stroke, care must be taken to support the flail shoulder in bed (e.g., using pillows to maintain alignment), wheelchair (e.g., with lap boards or pillows), and in upright position (e.g., putting the hands in a pocket or taping the shoulder). Treatment to reduce a subluxation should focus on achieving trunk alignment and scapula stability in a position of upward rotation.[74]

Abnormal skeletal muscle activity

A change in the resting state of the limb and postural muscles is common after stroke.[15] Immediately after a stroke,

---

BOX 33-5   SUMMARY OF CONSTRAINT-INDUCED MOVEMENT THERAPY

- Use to counteract learned nonuse. Hypothesized causes of learned nonuse include therapeutic interventions implemented during the acute period of neurological suppression after stroke, an early focus on adaptations to meet functional goals, negative reinforcement experienced by the patients as they unsuccessfully attempt to use the affected limb, and positive reinforcement experienced by using the less involved hand and/or successful adaptations

- Motor inclusion criteria. Control of the wrist and digits is necessary to engage in this type of intervention. Current and past protocols have used the following inclusion criteria: 20 degrees of extension of the wrist and 10 degrees of extension of each finger; or 10 degrees extension of the wrist, 10 degrees abduction of the thumb, and 10 degrees extension of any two other digits; or ability to lift a wash rag from a table using any type of prehension and then release it.

- Main therapeutic factor. Massed practice and shaping of the affected limb during repetitive functional activities appear to be the therapeutic change agents. "There is thus nothing talismanic about use of a sling or other constraining device on the less-affected limb."

- Activity choices and therapist's interventions. Select tasks that address the motor deficits of the individual client, assist clients in carrying out parts of a movement sequence if they are incapable of completing the movement on their own at first, provide explicit verbal feedback and verbal reward for small improvements in task performance, use modeling and prompting of task performance, use tasks that are of interest and motivational to the patient, ignore regression of function, and use tasks that can be quantified related to improvements.

- Outcome measures. The Motor Activity Log (actual use outside of structured therapy or "real-world use"), Arm Motor Ability Test, Wolf Motor Function Test, and the Action Research Arm Test have been used to document outcomes.

- Cortical reorganization. Constraint-induced movement therapy is the first rehabilitation intervention that has been demonstrated to induce changes in the cortical representation of the affected upper limb.

- The continued rigorous research that has been and continues to be carried out to demonstrate the effectiveness or efficacy of constraint-induced movement therapy should be used as a gold standard for other rehabilitation interventions that are used traditionally (e.g., neurodevelopmental therapy) but have little or no research support.

- On the basis of available evidence, constraint-induced movement therapy appears to be an effective intervention for stroke survivors who have learned nonuse and who fit the motor inclusion criteria.

From Gillen G: Upper extremity function and management. In Gillen G, Burkhardt A, editors: *Stroke rehabilitation: a function-based approach*, ed 2, St Louis, 2004, Elsevier.)

---

a change in available, or resting, skeletal muscle activity occurs. Most commonly, the acute state is characterized by low tone ("low-tone stage"). During this low-tone stage, the limbs and trunk become increasingly influenced by the pull of gravity. Little or no available muscle activity is available at this stage, resulting in deviations from the normal resting alignment of the musculoskeletal system.

The inability to recruit and maintain muscle activity is generally the greatest limiting factor at this stage. Because of the generalized lack of muscle activity and the dependent nature of the trunk and limbs, secondary problems can occur.[41] These include the following:

1. Edema of the dorsal surface of the hand that pools under the extensor tendons, effectively blocking active or passive digit flexion

2. Overstretching of the joint capsule of the glenohumeral joint

3. Eventual shortening of muscles that are passively positioned, in an effort to support a weak limb (Commonly, flaccid upper extremities are positioned in the client's lap, on a pillow, on a lap tray, or in a sling. Although they support the arm, these static positions result in prolonged positioning of certain muscle groups [internal rotators, elbow flexors, and wrist flexors] in a shortened position, putting them at risk for mechanical shortening. Interestingly, these are the muscle groups that tend to become spastic as time progresses.)

4. Overstretching of the antagonists to the previously mentioned muscles

5. Risk of joint and soft-tissue injury during ADL and mobility tasks (Because of the lack of control associated with a low-tone stage, the arm dangles and is not positioned appropriately during dynamic activities. Common examples include an arm being caught in the wheel during wheelchair mobility, pinning of the arm during bed mobility or rest, sitting on the arm after a transfer, or weight bearing through a flexed wrist during engagement in self-care activities.)

The progression to a state of increased or excessive skeletal muscle activity (increased tone) with clonus, stereotypical posturing of the trunk and limbs, hyperactive stretch reflexes, and increased resistance to passive limb movements that are velocity dependent may occur within several days or months of the stroke.[41]

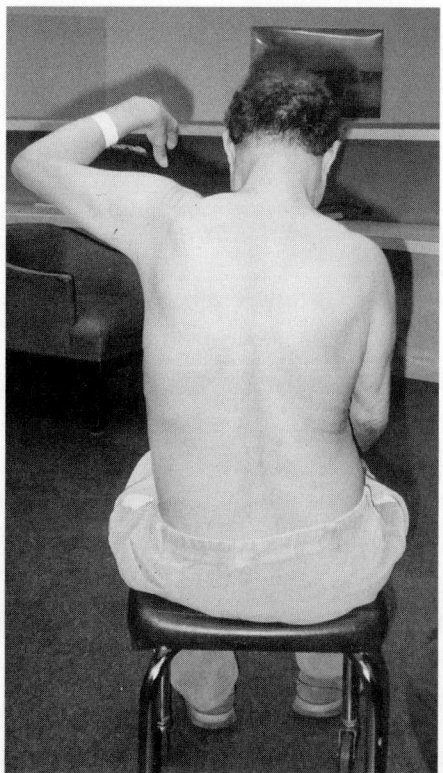

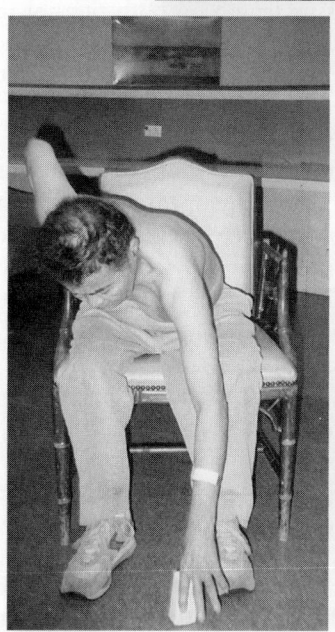 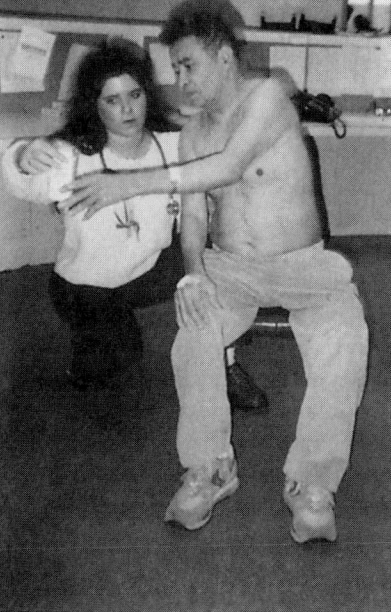

Figure 33-6   The task is designed to elicit the desired motor pattern; purpose of the activity drives the motor output. (From Gillen G: Upper extremity function and management. In Gillen G, Burkhardt A, editors: *Stroke rehabilitation: a function-based approach*, ed 2, St Louis, 2004, Elsevier.)

As spasticity increases, the risk for soft-tissue shortening is heightened. This factor may lead to a vicious circle of spasticity to soft-tissue shortening to overrecruitment of shortened muscles to increased stretch reflexes. Secondary problems that may occur if the spasticity is not managed in a therapy program include the following[41]:

1. Deformity of the limbs, specifically the distal upper limb (elbow to digits)
2. Maceration of the palm tissue
3. Possible masking of underlying selective motor control
4. Pain syndromes resulting from loss of normal joint kinematics (These syndromes are usually related to soft-tissue

contracture that blocks full joint excursion. A typical example is the loss of full passive external rotation of the glenohumeral joint. Attempts at forced abduction in these cases will result in a painful impingement syndrome of the tissues in the subacromial space.)

5. Impaired ability to manage BADL tasks, specifically UE dressing and bathing of the affected hand and axilla when flexor posturing is present

6. Loss of reciprocal arm swing during gait activities

In the past, the sensorimotor approaches were used to treat clients with abnormal skeletal muscle activity (see Chapters 30 and 31). These approaches were developed by Rood, Bobath, Knott, and Voss (PNF) and Brunnstrom and are based on an understanding of CNS dysfunction at the time these clinicians were doing their research (the mid-1900s). Although these interventions are commonly used, their effectiveness is being challenged as occupational therapists move toward models of evidence-based practice.[69] At present, there is limited research to support these neuro-facilitation approaches, whereas approaches that focus on the use of functional activities as the therapeutic change agent (e.g., task-oriented approaches) show promise from both a research and a clinical perspective. One final note on the subject: Approaches focused on the use of functional tasks are more consistent with traditional and current principles of occupational therapy.

Prevention of pain syndromes and contracture

Protection of unstable joints

During the low-tone stage, joints tend to become malaligned secondary to loss of muscular stabilization. In these cases, clients are at risk for injury to unstable joints (e.g., traction injuries and joint trauma) because of the joint instability. The glenohumeral and wrist joints are particularly at risk. The glenohumeral joint (usually already inferiorly subluxated at this stage) is at risk for a superimposed orthopedic injury if another individual unknowingly pulls on the affected arm during self-care and mobility or during unskilled passive range of motion (PROM) of the joint. The unstable glenohumeral joint is in a malaligned state, putting the client at risk for an impingement syndrome during PROM if normal joint mechanics is not addressed. Key joint motions of concern are upward rotation of the scapula and external (lateral) rotation of the shoulder. If these motions are not present and range of motion is forced, the client is at risk for the development of an impingement and pain syndrome.[41]

Clients with low tone also have an unstable wrist. Care should be taken to protect the wrist if the clients are not controlling the joint during ADL and mobility tasks. Clients commonly practice a bed mobility or lower extremity dressing sequence, then complete the task while bearing weight through a malaligned flexed wrist. These clients are at risk

for orthopedic injury (traumatic synovitis) and may be considered candidates for splinting to protect the wrist.[43]

Maintaining soft-tissue length

Clients who have both increased and decreased skeletal muscle activity are at risk for soft-tissue contracture secondary to the immobilization that occurs during both low-tone and increased-tone stages. The maintenance of tissue length is a 24-hour regimen. This regimen involves frequent variations in resting postures during waking hours, teaching the client and significant others *appropriate* ROM procedures, daytime and nighttime positioning programs, and staff and family education so that positioning and exercise programs may be carried out in the home environment.[41]

Prolonged static positioning (e.g., prolonged use of a sling) must be avoided. Rather, teaching clients to adjust their resting postures during the day will help prevent soft-tissue tightness.

Positioning programs

The same wheelchair and bed positioning programs should not be applied to every client. Instead, positioning should be individualized and focus on (1) promoting normal resting alignment of the trunk and limbs in an effort to maintain tissue length on both sides of the joints and (2) providing stretch to muscle groups that have been identified as contracture prone or already shortened.

Soft-tissue elongation

If soft-tissue shortening and length-associated changes have already developed, the treatment of choice is low-load prolonged stretch (LLPS). LLPS involves placing the soft tissues in question on submaximal stretch for prolonged periods. This technique is quite different from the common PROM with terminal stretch (high-load brief stretch) programs commonly used to treat this population.[63]

LLPS programs can be implemented in various ways, including splinting, casting, and positioning programs. For example, during a UE assessment, a client is noted to have tightness in the internal rotators, overactive internal rotation during attempts to move, and weakened external rotators. An effective LLPS would involve having the client rest in a supine position with both hands behind his or her head, allowing the elbows to drop toward the bed. This is a normal resting posture during recumbent leisure activities (e.g., watching television) and effectively elongates the muscle group identified as a contracture risk for a prolonged period.[41]

LLPS can also be achieved through splinting programs. A common example is that of a splint designed to elongate the long flexors of the hand during sleeping hours.

Splinting

Commonly a controversial subject in the management of stroke, splinting should be considered on a case-by-case basis and may be quite effective for many clients.[63] The most common uses for splints during the low-tone stage are maintaining joint alignment, protecting the tissues from shortening or overstretching, preventing injury to the extremity, and serving as an adjunctive treatment for edema control.[63] Specifically, splinting support may be needed to provide palmar arch support and maintain neutral wrist deviation and the neutral position of the wrist between flexion and extension. In most cases, the fingers do not require splinting in this stage of recovery.[63]

Splints may also be effective for clients developing spasticity. In these cases, the splints may be used to maintain soft-tissue length, provide LLPS, place muscles at their resting lengths on both sides of the joints, and attempt distal relaxation by promoting proximal alignment.[63]

Client Management

In addition to the interventions already described, it is helpful to train the client to manage his or her UE. For a client with low tone, the most important information to share with the client and significant others is the method for protecting the unstable joints and maintaining full range of motion. In the spastic stage, the treatment of choice is to teach positioning that will provide prolonged elongation to the overactive muscles and that will prevent contracture. Examples of positions that may be prescribed during leisure or self-care activities include the following[41]:

1. Weight bearing on the extended arm (elongates commonly shortened UE musculature)
2. In supine position, hands behind the head while allowing the elbows to drop toward the bed (provides stretch to the internal rotators)
3. In supine position, a pillow protracting the scapula and under the elbow to promote glenohumeral joint alignment
4. Lying on a protracted scapula to maintain stretch of the retractors and maintain scapulothoracic mobility
5. Supporting the involved wrist with the more functional hand and reaching down toward the floor with both hands (This pattern will elongate muscles that tend to contract during difficult activities, which is particularly helpful after gait activities or difficult self-care activities.)
6. Cradling the affected arm with the stronger arm, lifting to chest level, and gently raising and lowering (staying below 90 degrees) as well as gently abducting or adducting the arm (Figure 33-7). Cautionary note: Clasping the hands and lifting the affected arm overhead should be discouraged due to risk of increasing pain, causing an impingement syndrome, and stressing carpal ligaments (Figure 33-8).

The keys to prescribing a proper resting posture are to identify muscle groups in the trunk and upper limb that are shortening, overactive, or at risk to develop shortening and to select a comfortable posture that elongates the muscle group for a prolonged period.

Jasmine and her family were taught appropriate positioning when in bed and chairs and during upright activities. In addition, Jasmine learned how to safely perform self-range of motion exercises and was provided with a resting hand splint at night.

The Nonfunctional Upper Extremity

Although the restoration of UE control is a realistic goal for some clients, many clients will not regain enough control to integrate the affected UE into ADL and mobility tasks. Clients who will not regain sufficient control require extensive retraining in BADL and IADL[68] (see Chapter 13) using one-handed techniques and prescription of appropriate assistive devices (Box 33-6). Persons in this population are also candidates for dominance retraining. Deformity control to prevent body image issues is paramount for these clients.

INABILITY TO PERFORM CHOSEN TASKS SECONDARY TO VISUAL IMPAIRMENT

The processing of visual information is a complex act that requires intact functioning of multiple peripheral and CNS structures to support functional independence. The site of the lesion determines the visual dysfunction and the effect on task performance (Figure 33-9).[8]

Visual dysfunction and its treatment are detailed in Chapter 23. In general, treatment approaches may focus on remediation, such as eye calisthenics, fixations, scanning, visual motor techniques, and bilateral integration. Adaptive techniques are also used, including a change in working distance, the use of prisms, adaptations for driving and reading, changes in lighting, and enlarged print.[3,76]

PSYCHOSOCIAL ADJUSTMENT

The psychological consequences of a stroke are substantial. The incidence of depression in this population is 32%, according to statistics collected by the American Heart Association. Other studies suggest an incidence of depression after stroke that is as high as 61%. The highest levels of reported incidence are from acute and rehabilitation hospitals, and the lowest are from samples of community dwelling stroke survivors.[38] Other psychological manifestations that have been documented in survivors of stroke include anxiety, agoraphobia, substance abuse, sleep disorders, mania, aprosody (difficulty in expressing or recognizing emotion), behavioral problems (e.g., sexual inappropriateness, verbal outbursts, aggressiveness), lability (alteration between pathological laughing and crying), and personality changes (e.g., apathy, irritability, social withdrawal).[38]

A critical role of the occupational therapist is in helping the client adjust to hospitalization and, more important, to disability. Much patience and a supportive approach by the therapist are essential. The therapist must be sensitive

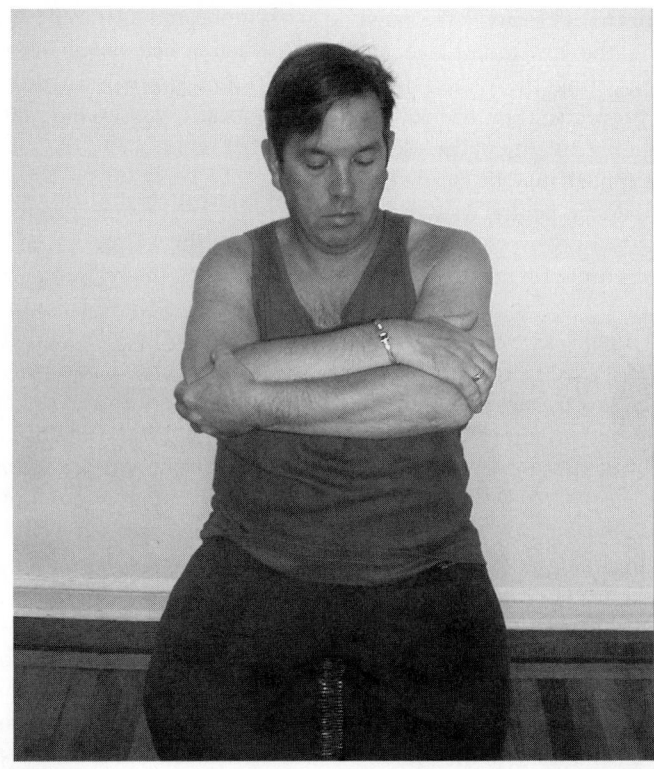

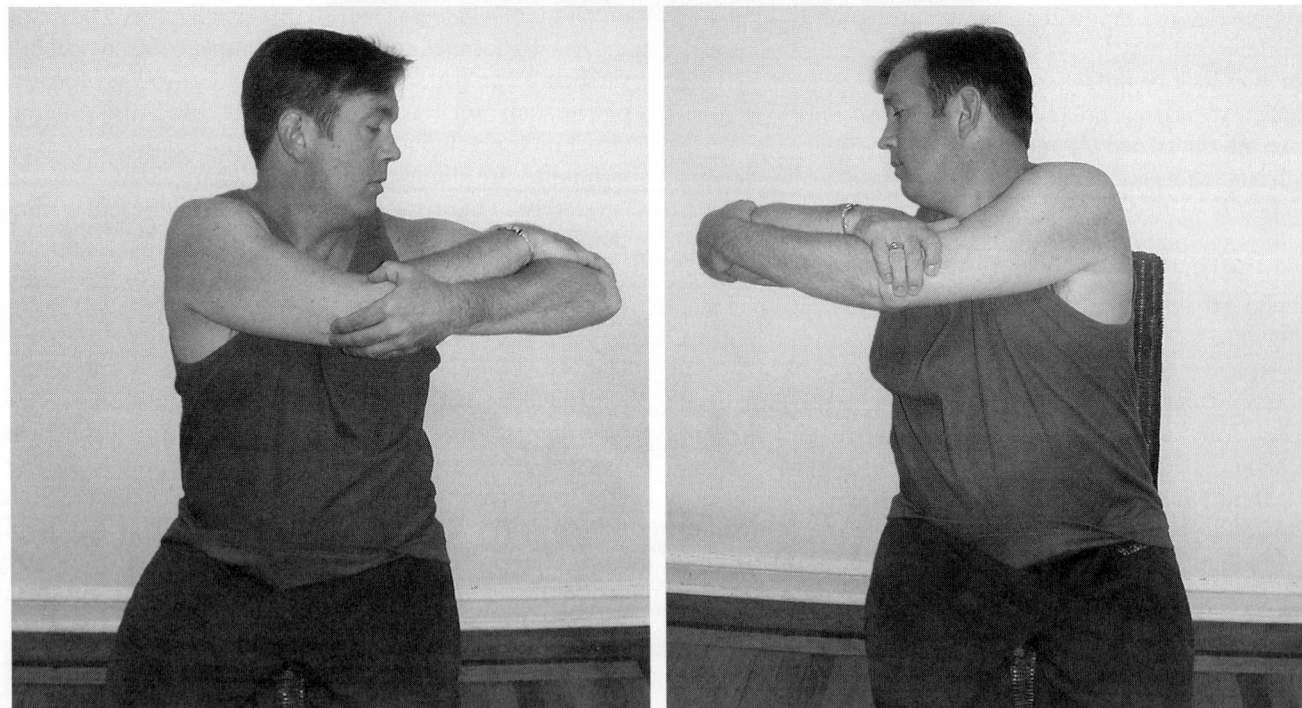

Figure 33-7   "Rock the baby." The client lifts the right upper extremity to chest level (**A**), adducts (**B**), and abducts (**C**), horizontally, allowing trunk rotation. (From Gillen G: Upper extremity function and management. In Gillen G, Burkhardt A, editors: *Stroke rehabilitation: a function-based approach*, ed 2, St Louis, 2004, Elsevier Mosby.)

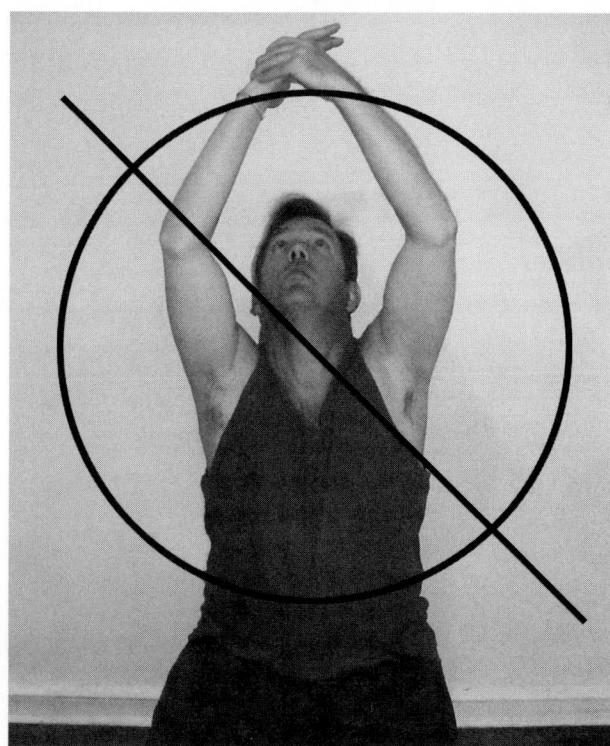

Figure 33-8 Because of multiple biomechanical concerns (e.g., impingement), self-overhead range of motion is discouraged. (From Gillen G: Upper extremity function and management. In Gillen G, Burkhardt A, editors: *Stroke rehabilitation: a function-based approach*, ed 2, St Louis, 2004, Elsevier Mosby.)

Box **33-6** EXAMPLES OF ASSISTIVE DEVICES USED AFTER STROKE TO IMPROVE TASK PERFORMANCE

Rocker knife
Elastic laces and lace locks
Adapted cutting board
Dycem
Plate guards
Pot stabilizer
Playing card holder
Suction devices to stabilize mixing bowls, cleaning brushes

---

to the fact that the client has experienced a devastating and life-threatening illness that has caused sudden and dramatic changes in the client's life roles and performance. The therapist must be cognizant of the normal adjustment process and must gear the approach and performance expectations to the client's level of adjustment. Frequently, the client is not ready to engage in rehabilitation measures with wholehearted effort until several months after onset of the disability.

Family education is extremely important throughout the treatment program. Family members are better equipped to assist their loved one with the adjustment to disability when they are knowledgeable about the disability and its implications.

Many clients dwell on the possibility of full recovery of function; they should gradually be made aware that some residual dysfunction is likely. The therapist may approach this probability by discussing in objective terms what is known about the prognosis for functional recovery after CVA. It may be necessary to review this information many times before the client begins to apply it to his or her recovery. This education should be done in a way that is honest and yet does not destroy all hope.

Falk-Kessler[35] provides occupational therapists with guidelines related to interventions for the psychological manifestations of stroke, including the following:
- Fostering an internal locus of control related to recovery
- Using therapeutic activities to improve self-efficacy or confidence in the performance of specific activities
- Promoting the use of adaptive coping strategies, such as seeking social support, information seeking, positive reframing, and acceptance
- Promoting success in chosen occupations to improve self-esteem
- Encouraging social support networks, such as families, friends, or support groups
- Using occupations to promote social participation

In addition to the aforementioned interventions, it is important to remember that pharmacological interventions have been shown to be effective for this population and should not be overlooked[35] as part of a team approach. These include, but are not limited to, antidepressants for depression or for those individuals with pathological affect, benzodiazepines for generalized anxiety disorder, and neuroleptic medications for those with poststroke psychosis.[25]

The OT program should focus on the skills and abilities of the patient. The patient's attention should be focused, through the performance of activity, on his or her remaining and newly learned skills. The OT program can also involve therapeutic group activities for socialization and sharing of common problems and their solutions. The discovery that there are residual abilities, and perhaps new abilities and success at performing many daily living skills and activities that were initially thought to be impossible, can improve the patient's mental health and outlook.

SUMMARY

CVA is a complex disability that challenges the skills of professional healthcare workers. Although the number and effectiveness of approaches for the remediation of affected motor, sensory, perceptual, cognitive, and performance dysfunctions have increased considerably, many limitations in treatment remain. The occupational therapist must bear in mind that the degree to which the patient achieves treatment goals depends on the CNS damage and recovery, psychoneurological residuals, psychosocial adjustment, and the skilled application of appropriate treatment by all concerned health professionals.

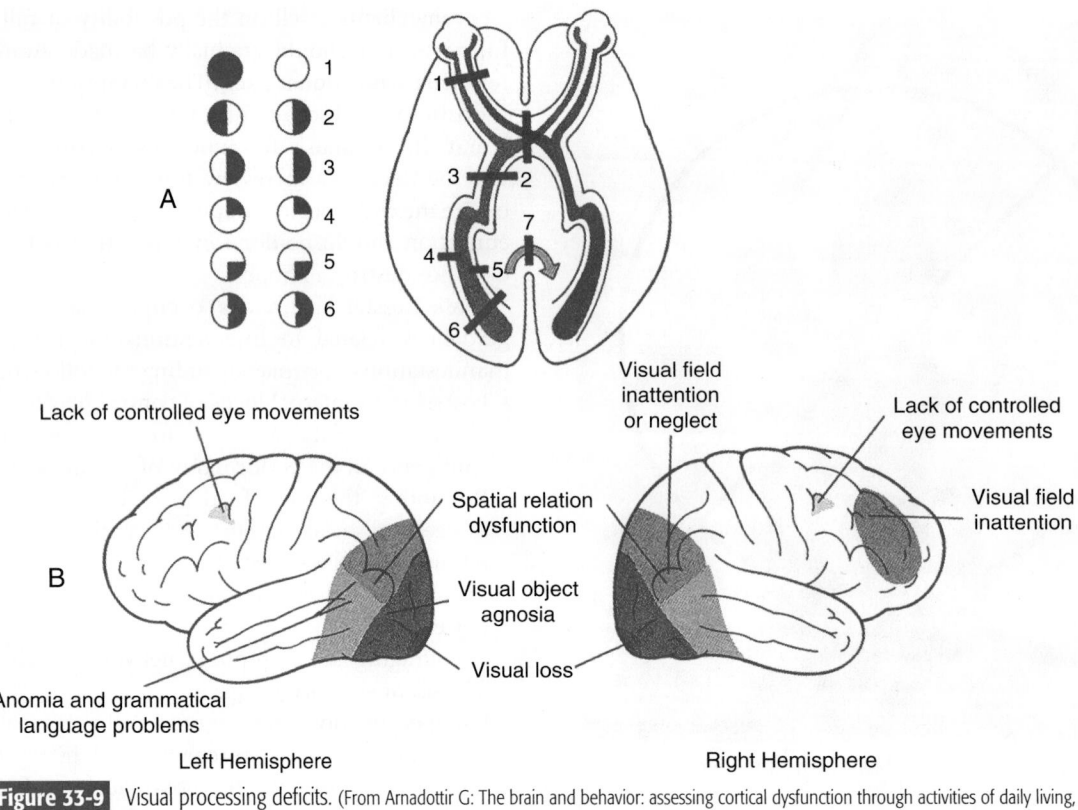

Left Hemisphere   Right Hemisphere

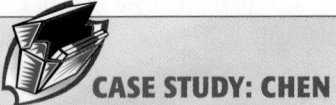 **Figure 33-9** Visual processing deficits. (From Arnadottir G: The brain and behavior: assessing cortical dysfunction through activities of daily living, St Louis, 1990, Mosby.)

Some patients remain severely disabled in spite of the noblest efforts of rehabilitation workers, whereas others recover quite spontaneously with minimal help in a short period. Most patients benefit from the professional skills of occupational therapists and other rehabilitation specialists and achieve improvement of performance skills and resumption of meaningful occupational roles.

CASE STUDY: CHEN

Chen is a 64-year-old man who lives alone in a building that has an elevator. He works as a manager for a garden center and was looking forward to retiring next year to enjoy his lifelong hobbies of furniture refinishing and antiquing.

Chen, who has a medical history of atrial fibrillation, awoke one morning with slurred speech and an inability to move his left side. His medical workup revealed a large right CVA of the middle cerebral artery. Chen was medically stabilized and admitted to the local rehabilitation center.

Chen was seen by personnel from OT, as well as physical therapy, speech-language pathology, and respiratory therapy. His OT evaluation revealed that he was cognitively intact except for mild, short-term memory loss that was attributed to his being overwhelmed with his situation. The evaluation also revealed the appearance of depression (poor eye contact, no initiation of conversation), 0/5 strength in his left upper extremity with an inferior subluxation, loss of trunk control characterized by falling to the left, and an impaired ability to stand secondary to knee buckling. He required moderate assistance for basic ADL (except being independent with oral care and shaving while seated) and maximal assistance for instrumental ADL requiring bilateral upper extremities.

Chen identified the desire to independently toilet, bathe, and dress in at least his undergarments in as the initial focus of OT intervention. Activities of interest, such as plant care and modified sports activities, were chosen with Chen's input. These activities were presented in such a manner as to remediate trunk control and standing balance. The activities were graded to promote increasing amounts of weight shifting and tolerance for sitting and standing postures.

Chen learned specific one-handed techniques for dressing and toileting. He was encouraged to practice these independently. Durable medical equipment (e.g., tub bench and commode) was prescribed to increase Chen's safety during bathroom activities and to compensate for his balance dysfunction. As he mastered his chosen tasks, Chen's affect brightened, he was able to continue his participation in treatment, and his outlook related to his future remained optimistic.

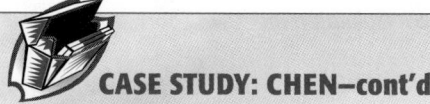

CASE STUDY: CHEN—cont'd

Although Chen did not regain use of his upper extremity, adaptive techniques and equipment allowed him to be independent in his chosen activities. He was provided with a home exercise program to maintain upper extremity flexibility and prevent pain. He continued to work on instrumental ADL and leisure task participation during his rehabilitation stay and with his home care occupational therapist.

Review Questions

1. Define *CVA*, and list three of its causes.
2. List the disturbances that can result from occlusion of the ACA, MCA, PCA, and cerebellar arteries.
3. Name three modifiable risk factors associated with stroke.
4. Define *transient ischemic attack.*
5. Name three functional deficits that occur as a result of loss of trunk control.
6. Besides the paralysis of limbs and trunk after CVA, what important motor disturbances can result?
7. Name two components of a "client-centered approach" to evaluation.
8. What are two frames of reference used to treat neurobehavioral impairments after stroke?
9. Name three postural reactions that support standing activities.
10. How does aphasia differ from dysarthria?
11. Describe four ways to aid effective communication with an aphasic client.
12. What is the importance of comprehensive occupational therapy evaluation of clients with hemiplegia?
13. Describe two methods used to maintain range of motion.
14. List four major elements of the occupational therapy program for hemiplegia. Describe the purposes of each.
15. How can occupational therapy assist with the psychosocial adjustment of the hemiplegic client?

REFERENCES

1. Abreu B et al: Occupational performance and the functional approach. In Royeen C: *AOTA self-study: cognitive rehabilitation,* Bethesda, MD, 1994, American Occupational Therapy Association.
2. Ada L et al: Task-specific training of reaching and manipulation. In Bennett KMB, Castiello U, editors: *Insights into the reach to grasp movements,* New York, 1994, Elsevier Science.
3. Aloisio L: Visual dysfunction. In Gillen G, Burkhardt A, editors: *Stroke rehabilitation: a function-based approach,* ed 2, St Louis, 2004, Elsevier Mosby.
4. American Heart Association: *Heart disease and stroke statistics 2004 Update,* Dallas, 2004, The Association.
5. American Occupational Therapy Association: Occupational therapy practice framework: domain and process, *Am J Occup Ther* 56(6):609, 2002.
7. Arnadottir G: Impact of neurobehavioral deficits of activities of daily living. In Gillen G, Burkhardt A, editors: *Stroke rehabilitation: a function-based approach,* ed 2, St Louis, 1998, Mosby.
8. Arnadottir G: *The brain and behavior: assessing cortical dysfunction through activities of daily living,* St Louis, 1990, Mosby.
9. Bartels MN: Pathophysiology and medical management of stroke. In Gillen G, Burkhardt A, editors: *Stroke rehabilitation: a function-based approach,* ed. 2, St Louis, 2004, Elsevier Mosby.
10. Basmajian JV: The surgical anatomy and function of the arm-trunk mechanism, *Surg Clin North Am* 43:1471, 1963.
11. Baum C, Edwards D: *The Activity Card Sort: Form C,* Unpublished Version, 2001.
12. Beck AT, Steer RA: *Beck Depression Inventory Manual,* rev ed, New York, 1987, Psychological Corp.
13. Berg K et al: Measuring balance in the elderly: preliminary development of an instrument, *Physiother Can* 41:304, 1989.
14. Bergner M et al: The sickness impact profile: development and final revision of a health status measure, *Med Care* 19(8): 787, 1981.
15. Bobath B: *Adult hemiplegia: evaluation and treatment,* ed 3, Oxford, 1990, Butterworth-Heinemann.
16. Bohannon RW: Recovery and correlates of trunk muscle strength after stroke, *Int J Rehabil Res* 18(4):162, 1995.
17. Bohannon RW, Cassidy D, Walsh S: Trunk muscle strength is impaired multidirectionally after stroke, *Clin Rehabil* 9(1):47, 1995.
18. Bonita R, Beaglehole R: Recovery of motor function after stroke, *Stroke* 19(12):1497, 1988.
19. Bounds JV, Wiebers DO, Whisnant JP: Mechanisms and timing of deaths from cerebral infarction, *Stroke* 12(4):414, 1981.
20. Bourbonnais D, Vanden Noven S: Weakness in patients with hemiparesis, *Am J Occup Ther* 43(5):313, 1989.
21. Branch EF: The neuropathology of stroke. In Duncan PW, Badke MB: *Stroke rehabilitation: the recovery of motor control,* Chicago, 1987, Year Book Medical.
22. Brott T et al: Measurements of acute cerebral infarction: a clinical examination scale, *Stroke* 20(7):864, 1989.
23. Cailliet R: *The shoulder in hemiplegia,* Philadelphia, 1980, FA Davis.
24. Carr JH et al: Investigation of a new motor assessment scale for stroke patients, *Phys Ther* 65(2):175, 1985.
25. Chemerinski E, Robinson RG: The neuropsychiatry of stroke, *Psychosomatics* 41(1):5, 2000.
26. Collen FM et al: The Rivermead mobility index: a further development of the Rivermead motor assessment, *Int Disabil Stud* 13(2): 50, 1991.
27. Cote R et al: The Canadian Neurological Scale: a preliminary study in acute stroke, *Stroke* 17(4):731, 1986.
28. Chusid J: *Correlative neuroanatomy and functional neurology,* ed 19, Los Altos, CA, 1985, Lange Medical Publications.
29. Demeurisse G, Demol O, Robaye E: Motor evaluation in vascular hemiplegia, *Eur Neurol* 19(6):382, 1980.
30. Desrosiers J et al: Development and reliability of an upper extremity function test for the elderly: the TEMPA, *Can J Occup Ther* 60(1):9, 1993.

31. Derosiers J et al: Upper extremity performance test for the elderly (TEMPA): normative data and correlates with sensorimotor parameters, *Arch Phys Med Rehabil* 76(12):1125, 1995.

32. Donato SM, Pulaski KH: Overview of balance impairments: functional implications. In Gillen G, Burkhardt A, editors: *Stroke rehabilitation: a function-based approach*, ed 2, St Louis, 2004, Elsevier.

33. Duncan P et al: Functional reach: a new clinical measure of balance, *J Gerontol* 45(6):M192, 1990.

34. Epstein NB et al: The McMaster family assessment device, *J Marital Fam Ther* 9(2):171, 1983.

35. Falk-Kessler J: Psychological aspects of stroke. In Gillen G, Burkhardt A, editors: *Stroke rehabilitation: a function-based approach*, ed 2, St Louis, 2004, Elsevier.

36. Fisher AG: *Assessment of motor and process skills*, ed 4, Fort Collins, CO, 2001, Three Star Press.

37. Folstein MF et al: Mini-mental state: a practical method for grading the cognitive state of patients for the clinician, *J Psychiatr Res* 12(3):189, 1975.

38. Fraley C: Psychosocial aspects of stroke rehabilitation. In Gillen G, Burkhardt A, editors: *Stroke rehabilitation: a function-based approach*, St Louis, 1998, Mosby.

39. Franchigoni FP et al: Trunk control test as an early predictor of stroke rehabilitation outcome, *Stroke* 28(7):1382, 1997.

40. Fugl-Meyer AR et al: The post-stroke hemiplegic patient: a method for evaluation of physical performance, *Scand J Rehabil Med* 7:13, 1975.

41. Gillen G: Managing abnormal tone after brain injury, *OT Practice* 3:8, 1998.

42. Gillen G: Trunk control: a prerequisite to functional independence. In Gillen G, Burkhardt A, editors: *Stroke rehabilitation: a function-based approach*, ed 2, St Louis, 2004, Elsevier.

43. Gillen G: Upper extremity function and management. In Gillen G, Burkhardt A, editors: *Stroke rehabilitation: a function-based approach*, ed 2, St Louis, 2004, Elsevier.

44. Goodglass H, Kaplan E: *Boston Diagnostic Aphasia Examination*, Philadelphia, 1983, Lea & Febiger.

45. Halper AS, Mogil SI: Communication disorders: diagnosis and treatment. In Kaplan PE, Cerullo LJ, editors: *Stroke rehabilitation*, Boston, 1986, Butterworth.

46. Helgason CM, Wolf PA: *American Heart Association prevention conference IV: prevention and rehabilitation of stroke*, Dallas, 1997, American Heart Association.

47. Holbrook M, Skilbeck CE: An activities index for use with stroke patients, *Age Ageing* 12(2):166, 1983.

48. Horak FB, Nashner L: Central programming of postural movements: adaptation to altered support surface configurations, *J Neurophysiol* 55(6):1369, 1986.

49. Jebsen RH et al: An objective and standardized test of hand function, *Arch Phys Med Rehabil* 50(6):311, 1969.

50. Keith RA et al: The functional independence measure: a new tool for rehabilitation. In Eisenberg MG, Grzesiak RC, editors: *Advances in clinical rehabilitation*, vol 1, New York, 1987, Springer-Verlag.

51. Kertesz A: *Western Aphasia Battery*, New York, 1982, Grune & Stratton.

52. Kiernan RJ: *The Neurobehavioral Cognitive Status Examination*, 1987, Northern California Neuro Group.

53. Kistler JP, Ropper AH, Martin JB: Cerebrovascular disease. In Isselbacher KJ et al, editors: *Harrison's principles of internal medicine*, New York, 1994, McGraw-Hill.

54. Kopp B et al: The arm motor ability test: reliability, validity, and sensitivity to change of an instrument for assessing disabilities in activities of daily living, *Arch Phys Med Rehabil* 78(6):615, 1997.

55. Lai S et al: Persisting consequences of stroke measured by the stroke impact scale, *Stroke* 33(7):1840, 2002.

56. Law M, Baptiste S, Mills J: Client-centered practice: what does it mean and does it make a difference? *Can J Occup Ther* 62(5): 250, 1995.

57. Law M et al: *The Canadian Occupational Performance Measure*, ed 2, Ottawa, 1994, CAOT Publications ACE.

58. Lawton MP: Instrumental activities of daily living scale: self-rated version, *Psychopharmacol Bull* 24(4):785, 1988.

59. Ma HI, Trombly CA: A synthesis of the effects of occupational therapy for persons with stroke. Part II: Remediation of impairments, *Am J Occup Ther* 56(3):260, 2002.

60. Mahoney FI, Barthel DW: Functional evaluation: the Barthel index, *Maryland State Med J* 14:61, 1965.

61. Mathiowetz, V: Task-oriented approach to stroke rehabilitaion. In Gillen G, Burkhardt A, editors: *Stroke rehabilitation: a function-based approach*, ed 2, St Louis, 2004, Elsevier.

62. Mathiowetz V, Bass Haugen J: Motor behavior research: implications for therapeutic approaches to central nervous system dysfunction, *Am J Occup Ther* 48(8):733, 1994.

63. Milazzo S, Gillen G: Splinting applications. In Gillen G, Burkhardt A, editors: *Stroke rehabilitation: a function-based approach*, ed 2, St Louis, 2004, Elsevier.

64. Neistadt ME: A critical analysis of occupational therapy approaches for perceptual deficits in adults with brain injury, *Am J Occup Ther* 44(4):299, 1990.

65. Neistadt ME: Occupational therapy treatments for constructional deficits, *Am J Occup Ther* 46(2):141, 1992.

66. Neistadt ME: Perceptual retraining for adults with diffuse brain injury, *Am J Occup Ther* 48(3):225, 1994.

67. Pollock N: Client-centered assessment, *Am J Occup Ther* 47(4): 298, 1993.

68. Post-Stroke Rehabilitation Guideline Panel: *Post-stroke rehabilitation: clinical practice guidelines # 16*, Rockville, MD, 1995, U.S. Department of Health and Human Services, Agency for Healthcare Policy and Research.

69. Rao A: Approaches to motor control dysfunction: an evidence-based review. In Gillen G, Burkhardt A, editors: *Stroke rehabilitation: a function-based approach*, ed 2, St Louis, 2004, Elsevier.

70. Roth EJ: Medical complications encountered in stroke rehabilitation, *Phys Med Rehabil Clin North Am* 2(3):563, 1991.

71. Rubenstein E, Federman D, editors: *Neurocerebrovascular diseases*, New York, 1994, Scientific American.

72. Rubio KB, Gillen G: Treatment of cognitive-perceptual deficits: a function-based approach. In Gillen G, Burkhardt A, editors: *Stroke rehabilitation: a function-based approach,* ed 2, St Louis, 2004, Elsevier Mosby.

73. Rutan GH et al: Mortality associated with diastolic hypertension and isolated systolic hypertension among men screened for the Multiple Risk Factor Intervention Trial, *Circulation* 77(3):504, 1988.

74. Ryerson S, Levit K: The shoulder in hemiplegia. In Donatelli RA, editor: *Physical therapy of the shoulder,* ed 2, Edinburgh, 1991, Churchill Livingstone.

75. Sandin KJ, Smith BS: The measure of balance in sitting in stroke rehabilitation prognosis, *Stroke* 21(1):82, 1990.

76. Scheiman M: *Understanding and managing vision deficits: a guide for occupational therapists,* Thorofare, NJ, 1997, Slack.

77. Steultjens EM, Dekker J, Bouter LM, et al: Occupational therapy for stroke patients: a systematic review, *Stroke* 34(3):676, 2003.

78. Shumway-Cook A, Horak FB: Balance rehabilitation in the neurological patient, *NERA,* 1992.

79. Shumway-Cook A, Woollacott M: *Motor control: theory and practical applications,* Baltimore, 1995, Williams & Wilkins.

80. Taub E et al: Technique to improve chronic motor deficit after stroke, *Arch Phys Med Rehabil* 74(4):347, 1993.

81. Teasdale G, Jennett B: Assessment of coma and impaired consciousness: a practical scale, *Lancet* 2(7872):81, 1974.

82. Thomson-Kohlman L: *The Kohlman Evaluation of Living Skills,* ed 3, Bethesda, MD, 1992, American Occupational Therapy Association.

83. Tinetti ME: Performance-oriented assessment of mobility problems in elderly patients, *J Am Geriatr Soc* 34(2):119, 1986.

84. Toglia J: Generalization of treatment: a multicontext approach to cognitive perceptual impairment in adults with brain injury, *Am J Occup Ther* 45(6):505, 1991.

85. Trombly CA: Anticipating the future: assessment of occupational function, *Am J Occup Ther* 47(3):253, 1993.

86. Trombly CA: Deficits in reaching in subjects with left hemiparesis: a pilot study, *Am J Occup Ther* 46(10):887, 1992.

87. Trombly CA: Observations of improvements in five subjects with left hemiparesis, *J Neurol Neurosurg Psychiatry* 56(1):40, 1993.

88. Trombly CA, Ma HI: A synthesis of the effects of occupational therapy for persons with stroke, Part I: Restoration of roles, tasks, and activities, *Am J Occup Ther* 56(3):250, 2002.

89. Ware JE, Sherbourne CD: The MOS 36-item short form health survey: conceptual framework and item selection, *Med Care* 30(6):473, 1992.

90. Wilson DJ, Baker LL, Craddock JA: Functional test for the hemiparetic upper extremity, *Am J Occup Ther* 38:159, 1984.

91. World Health Organization: *International classification of impairments, disabilities, and handicaps,* Geneva, 1980, The Organization.

92. Wu S et al: Effects of a program on symmetrical posture in patients with hemiplegia: a single-subject design, *Am J Occup Ther* 50(1): 17, 1996.

93. Yesavage JA et al: Development and validation of a geriatric depression screening scale: a preliminary report, *J Psychiatr Res* 17(1):37, 1982-1983.

94. Zorowitz RD et al: Shoulder pain and subluxation after stroke: correlation or coincidence? *Am J Occup Ther* 50(3):194, 1996.

34

TRAUMATIC BRAIN INJURY

MICHELLE TIPTON-BURTON
ROCHELLE McLAUGHLIN
JEFFREY ENGLANDER

KEY TERMS

Traumatic brain injury (TBI)
Diffuse axonal injury (DAI)
Post-traumatic amnesia (PTA)
Decorticate rigidity
Decerebrate rigidity

Postural deficits
Impaired initiation
Unilateral neglect
Sensory regulation
Neuromuscular re-education

Rehabilitative model
Neuroplasticity
Compensatory model
Environmental interventions
Interactive interventions

Tone normalization
Pelvic alignment

LEARNING OBJECTIVES

After studying this chapter the student or practitioner will be able to do the following:

1. Describe the pathology underlying traumatic brain injury (TBI).
2. State current medical, surgical, and pharmaceutical interventions for acute TBI.
3. Identify levels of consciousness in individuals with TBI using standard scales.
4. Describe the clinical picture of individuals with TBI, including common physical, cognitive, and psychosocial sequelae.
5. Identify occupational therapy evaluation methods for lower-, intermediate-, and higher-level individuals with TBI.
6. Identify several standard occupational therapy assessments for physical, cognitive, and psychosocial impairment after TBI.
7. Describe occupational therapy intervention methods for lower-, intermediate-, and higher-level individuals with TBI.
8. Describe the continuum of care services available for an individual with TBI in the acute, subacute, and postacute stages of rehabilitation.

CHAPTER OUTLINE

Introduction and epidemiology
Pathophysiology
  Focal brain injury
  Multifocal and diffuse brain injury
  Prevention of secondary brain injuries
Coma and levels of consciousness
Clinical picture
  Physical status
Dysphagia
  Self-feeding
  Cognitive status
  Visual status
  Perceptual skills
  Psychosocial factors
  Behavioral status
Evaluation of the lower-level individual
Intervention of the lower-level individual

Sensory stimulation
Wheelchair positioning
Bed positioning
Splinting and casting
Dysphagia
Behavior and cognition
Family and caregiver education
Evaluation of the intermediate- to higher-level individual
Physical status
Dysphagia
Cognition
Vision
Perceptual function
Activities of daily living
Driving
Vocational rehabilitation
Psychosocial skills

Intervention of the intermediate- to higher-level individual
  Neuromuscular impairments
  Ataxia
  Cognition
  Vision
  Perception
  Behavioral management
  Dysphagia and self-feeding

Functional mobility
Transfers
Home management
Community reintegration
Psychosocial skills
Substance use
Discharge planning
Summary

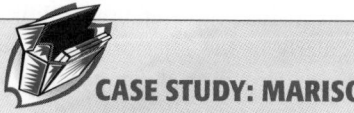

CASE STUDY: MARISOL

Marisol is an 18-year-old Hispanic female who sustained a severe brain injury as an unrestrained passenger in a sport utility motor vehicle accident. Marisol was a high school graduate who lived with her boyfriend and worked as a waitress. The computed tomography (CT) scan of her head showed a basilar skull fracture and a diffuse subdural hematoma. Approximately 2 weeks after injury, she was transferred to an acute rehabilitation unit to participate in a journey-to-recovery program, which is a program designed for patients whose progress is expected to be slower than that of typical acute care patients. This is determined by the extent of the injury; typically, these clients are determined to be at a Rancho Level II or III.

Results of the occupational therapy evaluation indicated that Marisol was dependent with all mobility and activities of daily living (ADLs) secondary to deficits in motor and process skills. She also displayed significant deficits in various client factors. Her right upper extremity (RUE) had full active and passive range of motion (A/PROM) with minimal ataxia in all joints. Her left upper extremity (LUE) had decreased ROM at her shoulder, elbow, and wrist. Severe spasticity was noted throughout her LUE. Marisol was alert and able to visually attend and track. She was nonverbal and was being fed through a gastrointestinal tube. When positioned at the edge of bed (EOB), she required total assistance to maintain a sitting position, including support to her head and trunk. She did not display sitting balance.

Occupational therapy was initiated to foster Marisol's ability to engage in self-care and some instrumental activities of daily living (IADLs) by accomplishing the following: (1) improve left upper extremity ROM, (2) decrease spasticity in her left UE, (3) improve functional use of RUE to facilitate participation in self-care tasks, (4) improve head and trunk control to allow her to sit upright in a wheelchair, (5) participate in bed mobility and transfers, and (6) improve cognition such that Marisol could participate in a self-care and self-feeding program as well as communicate with others.

Critical Thinking Questions

1. How should Marisol's injury be characterized?
2. What is her cognitive state?
3. How might Marisol's progress be measured?
4. How will her various problems be treated?

INTRODUCTION AND EPIDEMIOLOGY

Traumatic brain injury (TBI) is defined as damage to brain tissue caused by an external mechanical force with resultant loss of consciousness, post-traumatic amnesia (PTA), skull fracture, or objective neurological findings that can be attributed to the traumatic event on the basis of radiological findings or physical or mental status examination.[71] It is the most common cause of death and disability in young people.[24] More than 50,000 Americans die every year as a result of TBI, and 80,000 incur severe neurological disability.[66] The cost of TBI in the United States is estimated to be $48.3 billion annually. Approximately $31.7 billion of this figure is attributed to postacute hospitalization and supportive living arrangements because individuals with moderate to severe TBI often require lifelong rehabilitative assistance.[8]

The etiology of TBI is closely associated with age and gender. Children younger than 5 years tend to be injured in falls, in motor vehicle crashes, and by adults inflicting violence. Those between ages 5 and 15 are also injured on bicycles, skateboards, and horses; as pedestrians; and during sports activities. Between ages 15 and 40, high-speed motor vehicle and motorcycle crashes are the most common causes of TBI. After age 40, the incidence of violence-related injury approaches that of motor vehicles, particularly in metropolitan areas. Young and middle-aged adult males are 4 times more likely to be injured than their female counterparts. However, after the age of 65, the gender discrepancy narrows to 1.4 to 2 men for every woman; over the age of 80, injuries to women predominate by a ratio of 3 to 2. Elderly individuals are injured just as often by a fall or during a pedestrian mishap as they are in motor vehicles.[20,44]

Nontraumatic brain injuries include toxicity from drug overdose, chronic substance abuse, carbon monoxide poisoning, or environmental exposure; anoxia from cardiopulmonary arrest or near-drowning; brain abscess, meningitis, and encephalitis from bacteria, viruses, acquired immunodeficiency syndrome (AIDS), fungi, or parasites; nutritional deficiencies; genetic and congenital disorders; chronic epilepsy; and degenerative diseases such as dementia.[47]

Although the aforementioned conditions often have characteristics similar to those resulting from TBI (particularly with regard to rehabilitation approaches), this chapter's primary focus is assessment of and intervention for individuals with traumatic injury.

Substance abuse is strongly linked to TBI and many non-traumatic etiologies. Use of alcohol close to the time of injury is prevalent in more than half of adults with TBI.[45] An even greater number of individuals have a prior history of alcohol or other substance abuse in the year preceding the injury. As defined by the American Psychiatric Association's Diagnostic and Statistical Manual (DSM-IV), *substance abuse* is defined as follows: (1) failure to fulfill major role obligations at work, school, or home; (2) use in situations in which it is physically hazardous; (3) substance-related legal problems; or (4) continued use despite having persistent or recurrent social or interpersonal problems related to use.[2,16] Therefore, knowledge of the acute and chronic sequelae of substance abuse disorders is crucial in assessing and treating individuals with brain injuries.

Recovery from any type of brain injury depends on the patient's age and pre-injury capabilities, the severity of the injuries incurred, and the quality of intervention and support available during the patient's recovery. Recurrent brain injury is unfortunately all too common, occurring to those who have had previous trauma, developmental disabilities, or acquired disabilities associated with other etiologies.

Prevention of secondary complications is critical throughout all stages of the recovery process: at the time the person is resuscitated (i.e., at the site of injury), in acute medical care settings, during acute and post-acute rehabilitation programs, and when the individual is trying to reintegrate into his or her family and community. Many of the available medical and therapeutic interventions target these secondary complications. A well-coordinated team of knowledgeable professionals, family members, and supportive community caregivers can optimize the outcome for a given individual.[11]

PATHOPHYSIOLOGY

Neuropathologists and neurosurgeons currently categorize the early stages of TBI as *primary* (occurring at the moment of impact) and *secondary* (occuring in the days to several weeks after the injury). Prevention of primary injury includes the use of safety belts, protective helmets, air bags, and roadside barriers; these all can minimize the impact of the initial injury-causing agent. Prevention of secondary injury typically begins at the point of contact with those providing first aid at the scene of a trauma. It continues with emergency medical services, resuscitation and transport, and acute medical and surgical management, which carries over to rehabilitation settings. It is particularly the secondary interventions that will be discussed later, in the medical intervention section. An individual with TBI will typically have some combination of primary focal and diffuse brain injury depending on the etiology and mechanism of the initial injury; in best-case scenarios, there is a minimal amount of secondary brain damage and functional disability that occurs as a result of brain swelling, hypotension, hypoxia, and systemic injury. Prompt recognition of these complications improves survival and functional outcome when an appropriate intervention is implemented.[24]

FOCAL BRAIN INJURY

Focal brain injury is caused by a direct blow to the head after collision with an external object or fall, a penetrating injury resulting from a weapon, and the collision of the brain with the inner tables of the skull. The bones of the face or skull may or may not be fractured. Common findings of focal injury that results from falls include intracerebral and brain surface contusions, particularly in the inferior and dorsal-lateral frontal lobes, anterior and medial temporal lobes, and, less commonly, the inferior cerebellum. Assaults and missile wounds can occur anywhere in the brain depending on the direction of force. Other surface areas of the brain, including those not directly below the blow to the head, can also suffer contusions as a result of the collision of the brain with the inner tables of the skull. The directly injured area is referred as the *coup*, and the site of the indirect injury is known as the *contre coup*.[28,29]

If there are injuries to the coverings of the brain, especially the dura, pia, and arachnoid, then other focal hemorrhages occur. Epidural hematomas (EDH) are associated with skull fractures in adults with disruption of the integrity of the meningeal arteries; children may have arterial disruption with or without skull fracture. Individuals with EDH may be initially alert after the blow to the skull; as the hematoma develops between the skull and the dura, it can cause pressure on underlying brain tissue (secondary injury) with rapid deterioration in mental and physical status. Prompt recognition and neurosurgical treatment can save lives and limit morbidity.[34]

Subdural hematomas (SDH) occur between the dura and the brain surface through tearing of bridging veins. The rate of hemorrhage is often slower than that of an EDH because venous bleeding is more gradual than arterial. SDH may occur just as frequently on the side of the head opposite the direct blow; therefore, an EDH can occur on one side of the brain adjacent to the trauma with an SDH on the other. SDHs tend to spread around the entire surface of one hemisphere or less commonly in the posterior fossa. Acute SDH is diagnosed within 48 hours of injury; subacute SDH within 2 to 14 days after injury; and chronic SDH after 2 weeks. The fall or blow to the head in subacute or chronic SDH may have occurred days before the person arrives at the hospital, with symptoms typical of mental status changes. The urgency regarding SDH treatment depends on the clinical condition of the individual and the degree of mass of adjacent brain tissue observed on radiologic findings.[65]

MULTIFOCAL AND DIFFUSE BRAIN INJURY

With multifocal and diffuse brain injuries, there may be sudden deceleration of the body and head, with variable forces transmitted to the surface and deeper portions of the brain.

Motor vehicle, bicycle, and skateboard crashes are typical etiological factors, but falls from a high surface or off a horse or bull can also result in multifocal and diffuse injuries.

Intracerebral hemorrhage (ICH) is nearly always present with missile wounds as focal injury and is common after falls and assaults. Within the first week after the TBI, particularly in clients with blood-clotting abnormalities, ICH may appear on follow-up CT scans. With high-speed deceleration injury, multiple small, deep intracerebral hemorrhages occur throughout the neuraxis: on high-resolution CT or MRI scans, they are typically visible at the junction between the gray and white matter, basal ganglia, corpus callosum, midbrain, and/or cerebellum.

Subarachnoid (SAH) and intraventricular hemorrhages (IVH) occur when the pia or arachnoid are torn. SAH caused by trauma is less frequently associated with vasospasms than SAH caused by aneurysm rupture. A large IVH can block cerebral spinal fluid (CSF) flow, resulting in acute hydrocephalus. Thus, clinical evaluation of the possibility of a ruptured aneurysm that causes brain dysfunction, which may result from a fall or motor vehicle crash, is important with either of these entities.

Diffuse axonal injuries (DAI) are a prototypical lesion caused by rapid deceleration. The degree of injury may vary from primary axonotomy, with complete disruption of the nerve, to axonal dysfunction, wherein the structural integrity of the nerve remains but there is loss of ability to transmit normally along neuronal pathways. The clinical severity of DAI is measured by the depth and length of coma (i.e., the time from the onset of injury until the individual performs purposeful activity) and associated signs such as pupillary abnormalities.[45]

PREVENTION OF SECONDARY BRAIN INJURIES

The brain, like any body tissue, reacts to injury with swelling or edema, neurochemical injury cascades, changes in blood flow, and inflammation. Unlike other tissues, the brain is confined in a closed container, the skull, which protects it from outside injury but also confines the amount of swelling or blood accumulation that can occur. The brain is also the organ least able to tolerate loss of blood flow or oxygen. Secondary injury occurs as a result of the effects of brain swelling in a closed space, loss of perfusion, and decreased delivery of oxygen to healthy and damaged tissue. Recovery is related to the extent of the initial pathology and the secondary injury.[24]

Guidelines for the management of severe TBI have been developed over the last 10 years by the American Association of Neurological Surgeons and the Brain Trauma Foundation to minimize the impact of secondary injury. Some of these areas include resuscitation of blood pressure and oxygenation, management of elevated intracranial pressure (ICP) or hypertension, nutrition after acute trauma, and seizure prophylaxis.

These care recommendations are based on a critical review of the available literature on management of individuals with TBI and are categorized into the following groups: Standards, representing a high degree of clinical certainty; Guidelines, representing a moderate degree of clinical certainty; and Options, representing a low degree of clinical certainty.[10] Each of these terms, Standards, Guidelines, and Options, are used as labels for forms of intervention with the person who has sustained a TBI.

Those areas of intervention that are considered Standards are relatively few and relate to interventions that may be more harmful than helpful. They include the following:

- In the absence of increased ICP, chronic prolonged hyperventilation should be avoided.
- Steroids are not recommended to reduce ICP.
- Prophylactic anticonvulsants are not recommended for preventing late (i.e., after the first week) post-traumatic seizures.

Guidelines, which have a moderate degree of certainty in efficacy, include the following for individuals with severe TBI: (1) all regions should have an organized trauma care system; (2) hypotension (systolic blood pressure <90 mm Hg) or hypoxia (apnea, cyanosis, or oxygen saturation <90% in the field, or a PaO_2 of 60 mm Hg) must be monitored and corrected immediately; (3) ICP monitoring is appropriate for injuries in individuals younger than 40 years with systolic blood pressure (SBP) <90 mm Hg, Glasgow Coma scores between 3 and 8, or when CT scans show hematomas, contusions, edema, or compressed basal cisterns; (4) intervention should be initiated to lower ICP if it exceeds 20 to 25 mm Hg; (5) effective ICP treatments include mannitol, high-dose barbiturate therapy, ventriculostomy for drainage of CSF, and craniectomy (i.e., removal of portions of the skull to allow for external brain swelling); and (6) nutritional support at 140% basal rate in nonparalyzed and 100% in paralyzed individuals using enteral or parenteral formulas, with 15% calories as protein within 7 days of the TBI.

Post-traumatic seizures (PTS) are classified as immediate during the first 24 hours after injury, early during the first 7 days; and late after the first 7 days. Prophylactic treatment with phenytoin or carbamazepine during the first week after the TBI is an intervention option recognized by both the American Association of Neurological Surgeons and the American Academy of Physical Medicine and Rehabilitation. Both organizations recognize that the efficacy of prophylactic treatment diminishes greatly after the first week and thus recommend discontinuation of anticonvulsant medication as standard treatment after the first week.[9,10] If the patient develops late PTS, treatment is warranted because the reoccurrence rate is greater than 80%.[32] All patients and caregivers should learn recognition of and first aid for seizures as well as risk modification. Avoidance of alcohol, street drugs, and prescribed medications that lower seizure threshold is important for clients recovering from TBI. The groups at highest risk are those with metal and bone penetration into the brain substance, biparietal contusions, multiple intracranial operations, and any injury that causes more than a 5-mm lateral shift on CT scan.[19]

Implementation of the aforementioned standards and guidelines occurs more typically in designated trauma centers, where physicians, nurses, and allied health providers are accustomed to treating large numbers of individuals with TBI. Studies in both academic and community hospital settings have shown that morbidity and mortality can be reduced appreciably by following the AANS guidelines.[57]

After survival of the initial injury, ongoing optimal medical and health management can facilitate an individual's recovery and ability to participate in his or her own rehabilitation. Early detection and prompt management of sleep and mood disorders, pain, hydrocephalus, heterotopic ossification, and endocrinopathies, which are all common sequelae of TBI, must be addressed. Medical therapeutic interventions should be based on behavioral, cognitive, and functional performance factors that are observable and measurable by members of a rehabilitation team.

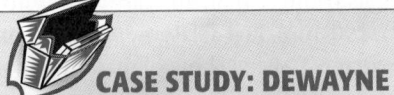

CASE STUDY: DEWAYNE

Dewayne, an 18-year-old with multiple cerebral contusions, has right arm and leg tremors with intentional movement and severe rigidity. He also has increased tone in the left arm and leg. He is dependent for all self-care and mobility.

After baseline evaluation over 2 days, both occupational and physical therapists note that tremors increase with any voluntary movement. Medication is introduced to reduce the tremors, and feedback is provided to the prescribing physician regarding Dewayne's performance of self-care activities and bed mobility. Over the next 2 weeks, Dewayne can wipe his face with minimal assistance using his right hand and taking 10 seconds; his medication is tapered, with no worsening of the tremor. Meanwhile the flexor tone on his left side is increasing, especially at the elbow; this prevents progress in upper body dressing. A temporary musculocutaneous nerve block with bupivacaine results in increased ability to extend the left arm so that dressing now requires only moderate assistance; the next day, a phenol nerve block is performed at the therapist's suggestion for longer-term relief of the elbow flexion tone.

This intervention is directed toward a focal area of difficulty for the patient, which is his ability to use his left arm for upper body self-care. Alternative interventions include systemic tone-reducing medications, which may have adverse side effects, or inhibitive casting of the elbow, which may help but makes the limb less useful while casted.

COMA AND LEVELS OF CONSCIOUSNESS

A TBI typically results in an altered level of consciousness. The continuum of consciousness includes coma at one end and conscious awareness at the opposite end. After a brain injury, an individual's progression along this continuum of consciousness depends on age; prior health status; severity of injury; and the methods of medical, therapeutic, and environmental management.

Consciousness is a state of environmental awareness and self-awareness. Coma involves the absence of awareness of self and the environment despite maximal external stimuli. No periods of wakefulness occur in the coma state.[58] When sedating and hypnotic medications are removed, the coma rarely lasts more than 4 weeks. When the coma resolves, the person becomes either partially aware of self and the environment ("minimally conscious") or, if no awareness is present, "vegetative."

The Glasgow Coma Scale (GCS) has been the traditional method used by healthcare professionals to assess levels of consciousness after a TBI (Table 34-1). The GCS has been used to quantify the severity of brain injury and predict outcome. Three behavioral areas assessed in the GCS are motor responses, verbal responses, and eye opening. The most reliable of these is the motor score; when it reaches 5, which signifies a purposeful response to pain, such as pushing away noxious stimuli, or 6, which represents an ability to follow simple commands, the injured individual is no longer in a coma or a vegetative state. This is an important landmark in recovery from TBI.[72]

The vegetative state is most succinctly described as wakefulness without awareness. A person in a vegetative state has the following characteristics: (1) no awareness of self or the environment and an inability to interact with others; (2) no sustained, reproducible, or voluntary behavioral responses to sensory stimuli; (3) no language comprehension or expression; (4) sleep-wake cycles of variable length; (5) ability to regulate temperature, breathing, and circulation to permit survival with routine medical and nursing care; (6) incontinence of bowel and bladder; and (7) variably preserved cranial-nerve and spinal reflexes. *Persistent vegetative state* refers to a condition of past and continuing disability with an uncertain future; the typical onset is within 1 month of a traumatic or nontraumatic brain injury or after a month-long metabolic or degenerative condition. The condition may improve, and the client may achieve a minimally conscious state over time. If the client does not improve, then the term *permanent vegetative state* is appropriate, signifying that the chance of regaining consciousness before death is exceedingly small.[69] Recovery of consciousness is rare for individuals in a persistent vegetative state 12 months after a traumatic brain injury or 3 months after a nontraumatic brain injury.[70]

Practice parameters regarding the care of individuals in a persistent vegetative state indicate that appropriate diagnosis of the condition is crucial; a physician with experience in

TABLE 34-1 **Glasgow Coma Scale**

Examiner's Test		Individual's Response	Assigned Score
Eye opening	Spontaneous	Opens eyes on own	4
	Speech	Opens eyes when asked to in a loud voice	3
	Pain	Opens eyes when pinched	2
	Pain	Does not open eyes	1
Best motor response	Commands	Follows simple commands	6
	Pain	Pulls examiner's hand away when pinched	5
	Pain	Pulls a part of body away when pinched by examiner	4
	Pain	Flexes body inappropriately to pain (decorticate posturing)	3
	Pain	Body becomes rigid in an extended position when examiner pinches victim (decerebrate posturing)	2
	Pain	Has no motor response to pinch	1
Verbal response (talking)	Speech	Carries on a conversation correctly and tells examiner where and who he or she is and the month and year	5
	Speech	Seems confused or disoriented	4
	Speech	Talks so examiner can understand but makes no sense	3
	Speech	Makes sounds that examiner can't understand	2
	Speech	Makes no noise	1

From Rosenthal M: *Rehabilitation of the head-injured adult*, Philadelphia, 1984, FA Davis.

this area should participate in the determination. Once the client is diagnosed, the prognosis should be explained in detail to the family, surrogates, and caregivers. Appropriate care respects the individual's comfort, hygiene, and dignity. Careful observation of any signs of emergence to a minimally conscious state is important in determining the intensity of therapeutic interventions. Positioning and other interventions to manage tone and prevent contractures should be included. The amount of extraordinary care will be guided by the advanced directives or presumed directives supplied by the patient's surrogate.[60]

Many individuals emerge from a persistent vegetative state to a minimally conscious state (MCS) in which there is definite behavioral evidence of awareness of self, environment, or both. Clearly discernible, reproducible behavior in one or more of the following areas must be demonstrated: (1) ability to follow commands; (2) gestural or verbal yes/no responses (regardless of accuracy); (3) intelligible verbalizations; and (4) purposeful movements or affective responses that are appropriate responses to environmental stimuli. Examples include reaching for objects; touching or holding objects that accommodate their size and shape; engaging in pursuit eye movements or sustained fixation in direct response to stimuli; and smiling, crying, vocalizing, or gesturing in response to relevant stimuli. Convenient ways to assess MCS are to test an individual with situational orientation questions (e.g., "Are you standing? Are you in a chair?") and giving the individual an object of common use, such as a washcloth or comb, and seeing whether the patient tries to use it. Testing for MCS should occur in a quiet environment when the patient is alert (i.e., not under sedating medication or in a physical position that encourages inattention). Requested commands should not exceed the patient's physical capabilities and not involve reflexive movements.[25] Serial assessment tools are available that can be useful for measuring the cognitive progress of individuals in MCS, such as the JFK Coma Recovery Scale, Wessex Head Injury Matrix, the Coma-Near Coma Scale, Sensory Stimulation Assessment Measure, and the Western Neuro Sensory Stimulation Profile.[13,55]

Another important landmark in recovery is **post-traumatic amnesia (PTA),** which is probably the single best measurable predictor of functional outcome in the research literature (Table 34-2). PTA is the length of time from the injury to the moment when the individual regains ongoing memory of daily events. Some evidence suggests that the duration of

TABLE 34-2 **Duration of Post-Traumatic Amnesia and Severity of Injury**

PTA Duration	Severity
Less than 5 min	Very mild
5 to 60 min	Mild
1 to 24 hr	Moderate
1 to 7 days	Severe
1 to 4 weeks	Very severe
More than 4 weeks	Extremely severe

From Rosenthal M: *Rehabilitation of the head-injured adult*, Philadelphia, 1984, FA Davis.
PTA, Post-traumatic amnesia.

PTA is highly correlated with individual outcomes. Longer PTAs are associated with poorer long-term cognitive and motor abilities and a decreased ability to return to work and school. A PTA of 4 weeks or greater is correlated with significant long-term disability.[51] Measurement of PTA is performed with the Galveston Orientation and Amnesia Test or the Orientation Log. The latter test is easier to administer in cases of moderate to severe TBI, in which the examiner may not know the details of circumstances that took place immediately before the injury and in which the injured individual has begun to remember events.[37,46]

The Rancho Los Amigos Scale of Cognitive Functioning is a descriptive measurement of the levels of awareness and cognitive function.[69] Progression through the various levels occurs most typically with traumatic injuries. However, the recovery curve of some individuals who are very severely injured may actually skip a level, typically Rancho 4, an agitated confused state. Others may never be as low as Rancho 1 or 2 but may be agitated and confused for several weeks (Rancho 4). These individuals may experience periods during which they also function at Rancho 5 or Rancho 6. Thus, it can be helpful to treating staff and family members in designing specific behavioral interventions for a given patient. Box 34-1 contains a complete description of the scale.

Although many studies have analyzed factors such as age, severity and etiology of the injury, substance abuse, and psychosocial status in predicting outcomes from TBI, they

---

| Box **34-1** | LEVELS OF COGNITIVE FUNCTIONING |

I. No response. Individual appears to be in a deep sleep and is completely unresponsive to any stimuli presented to him or her.

II. Generalized response. The individual reacts inconsistently and nonpurposefully to stimuli in a nonspecific manner. Responses are limited in nature and are often the same, regardless of the stimulus presented. Responses may be physiological changes, gross body movements, or vocalization. Often the earliest response is to deep pain. Responses are likely to be delayed.

III. Localized response. The individual reacts specifically but inconsistently to stimuli. Responses are directly related to the type of stimulus presented, as in turning the head toward a sound or focusing on an object presented. The individual may withdraw an extremity or vocalize when presented with a painful stimulus. He or she may follow simple commands in an inconsistent, delayed manner, such as in closing the eyes, squeezing, or extending an extremity. After the external stimulus is removed, the individual may lie quietly. He or she may also show a vague awareness of self and body by responding to discomfort by pulling at a nasogastric (NG) tube or catheter or resisting restraints. The individual may show bias by responding to some persons (especially family, friends) but not to others.

IV. Confused-agitated. The individual is in a heightened state of activity with a severely decreased ability to process information. He or she is detached from the present and responds primarily to his or her own internal confusion. Behavior is frequently bizarre and nonpurposeful relative to the immediate environment. The individual may cry out or scream out of proportion to stimuli even after removal and may show aggressive behavior, attempt to remove restraints or tubes, or crawl out of bed in a purposeful manner. The individual does not, however, discriminate among persons or objects and is unable to cooperate directly with treatment effort. Verbalization is frequently incoherent and inappropriate to the environment. Confabulation may be present; the individual may be euphoric or hostile. Thus, gross attention is very short and selective attention is often nonexistent. Being unaware of present events, the individual lacks short-term recall and may be reacting to past events. He or she is unable to perform self-care (e.g., feeding and dressing) without maximal assistance. If not disabled physically, the individual may perform motor activities as in sitting, reaching, and ambulating but as part of the agitated state and not as a purposeful act or on request.

V. Confused, inappropriate, nonagitated. The individual appears alert and is able to respond to simple commands fairly consistently. However, with increased complexity of commands or lack of any external structure, responses are nonpurposeful, random, or at best fragmented toward any desired goal. The individual may show agitated behavior, not on an internal basis (as in Level IV) but rather as a result of external stimuli and usually out of proportion to the stimulus. He or she has gross attention to the environment but is highly distractible and lacks the ability to focus attention to a specific task without frequent redirection back to it. With structure, the individual may be able to converse on a social, automatic level for short periods of time. Verbalization is often inappropriate; confabulation may be triggered by present events. Memory is severely impaired, with confusion of past and present in his or her reaction to ongoing activity. The individual lacks initiation with regard to functional tasks and often shows inappropriate use of objects without external direction. He or she may be able to perform previously learned tasks when they are structured for him or her, but the individual is unable to learn new information. He or she responds best to self, body, comfort—and often family members. The individual can usually perform self-care activities with assistance and may accomplish feeding with maximal supervision. Management on the ward is often a problem if the individual is physically mobile, because he or she may wander off either randomly or with the vague intention of going home.

VI. Confused-appropriate. The individual shows goal-directed behavior but is dependent on external input for direction. The response to discomfort is appropriate, and the individual is able to tolerate unpleasant stimuli (e.g., NG tube) when the need is explained. The individual follows simple directions consistently and shows carryover for tasks that have been relearned (such as self-care). He or she is at least supervised with old learning and is unable to maximally assist for new learning with little or no carryover. Responses may be incorrect because of memory problems, but they are appropriate to the situation. Responses may be delayed, and the individual shows a decreased ability to process information with little or no anticipation or prediction of events. Past memories show more depth and detail than recent memory. The individual may show beginning awareness of his or her situation by realizing he or she doesn't know an answer. The individual no longer wanders and is inconsistently oriented to time and place. Selective attention to tasks may be impaired, especially with difficult tasks and in unstructured settings, but the individual is now functional for common daily activities (30 min with structure). He or she shows at least vague recognition of some staff and has increased awareness of self, family, and basic needs (e.g., food), again in an appropriate manner, as in contrast to Level V.

VII. Automatic-appropriate. The individual appears appropriate and oriented within hospital and home settings and goes through the daily routine automatically but is frequently robot-like. The individual has minimal to absent confusion but has shallow recall of what he or she has been doing. He or she shows increased awareness of self, body, family, foods, people, and interaction in the environment. The individual has superficial awareness of, but lacks insight into, his or her condition; demonstrates decreased judgment and problem solving; and lacks realistic planning for the future. He or she shows carryover for new learning but at a decreased rate. He or she requires at least minimal supervision for learning and for safety purposes and is independent in self-care activities and supervised in home and community skills for safety. With structure the individual is able to initiate tasks in social and recreational activities in which he or she now has interest. Judgment remains impaired, such that the individual is unable to drive a car. Prevocational or avocational evaluation and counseling may be indicated.

VIII. Purposeful and appropriate. The individual is alert and oriented, is able to recall and integrate past and recent events, and is aware of and responsive to his or her culture. He or she shows carryover for new learning if it is acceptable to him or her and his or her life role. The individual needs no supervision after activities are learned within his or her physical capabilities. He or she is independent in home and community skills, including driving. Vocational rehabilitation, to determine ability to return as a contributor to society (perhaps in a new capacity), is indicated. The individual may continue to show a decreased ability, relative to premorbid abilities, in reasoning, tolerance for stress, judgment in emergencies, or unusual circumstances. His or her social, emotional, and intellectual capacities may continue to be at a decreased level but are functional for society.

From Rancho Los Amigos Medical Center, Downey, CA, Adult Brain Injury Service: Original Scale, Levels of Cognitive Functioning, 1980.

have definite limitations regarding the recovery of an individual patient.[7,11,16,21,33,76] Individuals with TBI improve over months to years especially once an individual becomes aware of his or her altered capabilities.[59] Following an individual's personal rate of recovery is probably more predictive of future recovery than any other factor.

CLINICAL PICTURE

PHYSICAL STATUS

An individual with TBI may exhibit a variety of symptoms, depending on the type, severity, and location of the injury. Individuals may have limitations in most of the areas listed in the following sections, or they may have subtle deficits evident only during more complex activities. Table 34-3 shows some of the most commonly diagnosed physical signs and symptoms of a client who has a TBI in a clinical setting.

Decorticate, Decerebrate, and Motor Rigidity

Rigidity is the presence of increased resistance to passive movement throughout most of the range that is independent of stretch velocity.[49] Comatose individuals often display one of two common positions: decorticate rigidity and decerebrate rigidity. In decorticate rigidity, the upper extremities (UEs) are in a spastic flexed position with internal rotation and adduction. The lower extremities (LEs) are in a spastic extended position but also internally rotated and adducted. **Decorticate rigidity** results from damage to the cerebral hemispheres (particularly the internal capsules), causing an interruption in the corticospinal tracts—those that emerge from the cortex and send voluntary motor messages to all extremities.

In **decerebrate rigidity,** both the UEs and LEs are in a position of spastic extension, adduction, and internal rotation. The wrist and fingers flex, the plantar portions of the feet flex and invert, the trunk extends, and the head retracts.

TABLE 34-3   **Motor Signs**

Motor Sign	Lesion Localization	Clinical Characteristics	Interventions
Decerebrate rigidity	Midbrain, pons, diencephalon	Extended internally rotated shoulders; extended elbows; flexed wrists, fingers; extended internally rotated hips, extended knees, ankle plantar flexion, inversion; increased rigidly when awake	Positioning, ROM, neuromuscular blocks and early casting
Decorticate rigidity	Cortical white matter, internal capsule, thalamus, cerebral peduncle, basal ganglia	Internally rotated shoulder; flexed elbow, wrists, fingers; extended internally rotated hips; knee flexion; ankle plantar flexion, inversion; increased rigidity when awake	Positioning; ROM, neuromuscular blocks and early casting
Bruxism		Persistent jaw clenching, teeth grinding +/− temporomandibular dislocation or subluxation	Neuromuscular blocks, oral orthotics
Spasticity	Upper motor neuron syndrome (UMN); cortical spinal pathways	Velocity-dependent resistance, hyper-reflexia/clonus, muscle shortening; present in face, neck, trunk, limbs; orse when awake and with effort	Bed/chair positioning, ROM, weight bearing, neuromuscular blocks, inhibitive casting, enteral and intrathecal medications, tendon releases, relaxation techniques
Rigidity and bradykinesia; "Parkinsonism"	Substantia nigra; extrapyramidal pathways; also with medications that block dopamine	Velocity-independent resistance; "lead-pipe," "cogwheeling" worse when awake	Positioning, ROM, functional activities, medications
Torticollis		Dystonic posture of neck; spasticity and or contracture of sternocleidomastoid, splenius muscles	Positioning, modalities and ROM, medications, neuromuscular blocks
Myoclonus	Variable	Abrupt, shocklike involuntary jerks in large (limb) or small muscles when sleep or awake	Medications, neuromuscular blocks
Tremor	Variable	Involuntary rhythmic oscillations while awake	Weighted devices, weight bearing, medications, neuromuscular blocks, appropriate assistive devices
Dystonia	Variable	Dynamic contraction/relaxation muscles with slow, writhing or repetitive twisting movements or sustained contortions; usually distal limb(s)	Positioning, ROM, neuromuscular blocks, medications appropriate assistive devices
Athetosis	Basal ganglia, medications with dopamine effect	Slow sinuous movements of face, tongue, or limbs	Relaxation techniques, taper offending medications
Chorea	Contralateral neostriatum thalamus	Involuntary dancelike or jerky movements without rhythmic pattern; distal	Medications
Hemiballismus/ Ballismus	Contralateral subthalamic nucleus, thalamus, cerebellum	Sudden irregular flinging movements starting hip or shoulder, occasionally facial or oral +/− rotatory component worse with arousal/excitement, absent in sleep	Medications
Tics	Variable	Sudden stereotypic coordinated automatic movements or vocalizations while awake	Medications, behavioral management, relaxation techniques
Pseudobulbar athetoid syndrome	Bilateral pyramidal tract	Postural dystonia with fragmentary athetosis, +/− bradykinesia; often preserved intellect/ personality	Positioning, appropriate assistive devices

Data from Mayer NH, Keenan MAE, Esquenzi A: Limbs with restricted or excessive motion after traumatic brain injury. In Rosenthal M: *Rehabilitation of the adult and child with traumatic brain injury*, ed 3, Philadelphia, 1999, FA Davis; Mayer NH: Choosing upper limb muscles for focal intervention after traumatic brain injury, *J Head Trauma Rehabil* 19(2):119, 2004; Zafonte R, Elovic E, Lombard L: Acute care management of post-TBI spasticity, *J Head Trauma Rehabil* 19(2):89, 2004.

Decerebrate rigidity occurs as a result of damage to the brainstem and extrapyramidal tracts—the tracts that send involuntary motor messages from the brainstem to the extremities. Individuals with decerebrate rigidity have a poorer prognosis than do those exhibiting decorticate rigidity.[14,29]

Cogwheel or lead-pipe rigidity resembling Parkinson's disease can occur, typically with severe TBI. It may respond to dopamine agonists such as L-dopa/carbidopa or amantadine. Dystonias in the neck (torticollis), jaw, or distal limbs can also occur. They may require treatment with motor point blocks.[49]

Abnormal Muscle Tone and Spasticity

Although decorticate rigidity and decerebrate rigidity manifest the most severe types of abnormal muscle tone and tend to occur in comatose individuals, hypertonicity may range from minimal to severe in any muscle group. Individuals who are functioning at a higher cognitive level than coma generally display a combination of both hypotonicity (i.e., decreased tone, or flaccidity) and hypertonicity (i.e., increased tone, or spasticity). Flaccidity, or hypotonicity, is a decrease of normal muscle tone. It is usually attributed to peripheral nerve injury resulting in a soft muscle feel, in which the muscles offer no resistance to passive movement. Spasticity, also known as *hypertonia*, is an involuntary increase in muscle resistance that is velocity dependent.[45] Because individuals with spasticity cannot voluntarily relax their limbs, voluntary movement of an affected limb may be impossible. Spasticity can be seen as early as a few days after a brain injury, or it may take between 3 and 6 months to develop. In as little as 2 weeks, spasticity may cause muscles to shorten permanently, which in turn can cause joints to lose motion. The condition of permanent shortening is called a *muscle contracture*.

 OT PRACTICE NOTE

It is important to instruct all members involved in the client's care that tone can fluctuate as a result of changes in position, volitional movement, medication, infection, illness, pain, environmental factors (i.e., ambient temperature), and emotional state.[6]

Primitive Reflexes

If damage has occurred to the midbrain, impaired righting reactions are commonly observed. Similarly, damage to the basal ganglia can result in the absence of equilibrium reactions and protective extension. The absence of righting reactions, equilibrium reactions, and protective extension puts the individual at a significant risk for further injury from falls during such activities as transfers, getting out of bed, toileting, bathing, and dressing.

Muscle Weakness

A decrease in muscle strength, without the presence of spasticity, can occur as a result of peripheral nerve or plexus injuries and lack of physical activity caused by secondary factors associated with the TBI (e.g., compromised respiration, fractures, and infection). A functional muscle and sensory test may be indicated when an individual exhibits decreased strength in the limbs. Additionally, impaired gross and fine motor coordination will be evident and should be assessed.

Decreased Functional Endurance

Decreased endurance and vital capacity usually accompany reduced muscle strength as a result of medical complications such as infections, poor nutrition, or prolonged bed rest. Increasing the individual's muscle strength and endurance are primary goals in the acute stage and in the initial stages of rehabilitation.

Ataxia

Ataxia results from impairment of the cerebellum itself or the motor pathways leading to and from the cerebellum; it can also occur with impaired proprioception. Ataxia is a movement abnormality characterized by incoordination, impaired sitting and standing balance, or both.[6] Ataxia can occur in the entire body, in the trunk, or in the UEs and LEs. The individual with ataxia has lost the ability to perform small adjustments in the distal and proximal extremities that are necessary for smooth, coordinated movement. The degree of ataxia ranges from mild to severe. The individual with ataxia in the trunk displays impaired postural stability when sitting and standing. He or she has difficulty maintaining the trunk in a stable position to free the upper or lower extremities for activities. The individual may compensate for this deficit by grasping a stable surface such as a tabletop. Ataxia in the UEs causes dysfunction in activities in which the individual attempts to perform a combination of gross and fine motor movements, such as bringing a glass of water to the mouth. The UE oscillates back and forth, causing the water to spill. Ataxia in the LEs results in an impaired ability to ambulate while maintaining balance; falls can easily occur with this condition.

Postural Deficits

Postural deficits develop as a result of an imbalance in muscle tone throughout the body. An individual may inadvertently accentuate postural deficits by using ineffective strategies to compensate for impaired motor control; delayed or absent righting reactions; or impaired vision, cognition, or perception. Therapists must possess a thorough knowledge of the postural deficits of their clients to position them properly in a wheelchair with the appropriate seating system, which is necessary to obtain an upright posture, maintain good postural alignment, and prevent further postural deformities. Frequently exhibited abnormal postures include the following:

1. *Pelvis.* Posterior pelvic tilt is often due to prolonged bed rest in the supine position, which causes loss of range of motion (ROM) in the lower back. Posterior pelvic tilt results in sacral sitting and facilitates kyphosis. Pelvic obliquity is observed when one side of the pelvis sits lower than the other side as a result of hypertonicity of the quadratus lumborum on the involved side.
2. *Trunk.* Kyphosis, scoliosis, and lordosis may all be present secondary to weak or spastic trunk muscles (e.g., pectoralis, abdominal, spinal, and paraspinal). It is also common to observe lateral flexion toward the involved side (trunk shortening) with elongation of muscle on the opposite side.
3. *Head and neck.* Forward flexion or hyperextension of the neck. Lateral flexion of the head often accompanies lateral flexion of the trunk.
4. *Scapula.* The scapula may be depressed, protracted or retracted, downwardly rotated, or all of these at once. This results from an imbalance in scapular muscle tone; some muscles are hypertonic, whereas others are hypotonic.
5. *Upper extremities.* UEs may be bilaterally or unilaterally involved. In unilateral involvement, it is common to see variations in ROM, tone, and strength in each muscle group and joint of the arm, forearm, wrist, and hand.
6. *Lower extremities.* Severe extension patterns are often observed in both LEs, which can pose a problem with wheelchair positioning; this is evident when the individual thrusts forward and slides out of the seating system. Hip adduction, internal rotation, knee flexion, plantar flexion, and inversion of the feet can all be observed.

Limitations of Joint Motion

Loss of ROM in the joints is a common problem. It is often difficult to distinguish between several possible causes of decreased ROM, such as the following: increased muscle tone, volitional resistance, contractures, heterotopic ossification (HO), fractures or dislocations, and pain. Because the intervention addressing decreased ROM depends on the cause, the therapist should consult a physician to determine the cause of the decreased ROM before initiating intervention. Fractures of distal limbs are often overlooked in acute trauma settings when patients are unable to communicate because of cognitive deficits. Therapists typically are the first to detect the hard end-feel of joints with limited ROM typical of HO, the formation of lamellar bone in soft tissue.[31]

Sensation

Clients with TBI may exhibit signs of absent or diminished sensation, including problems with light touch, differentiation between sharp and dull sensations, proprioception, temperature, pain, and kinesthesia. Additionally, impaired senses of taste and smell, caused by cranial nerve injury, may be observed.[6] Lost or diminished stereognosis, two-point discrimination, and graphesthesia (i.e., the ability to interpret letters written on the hand without visual input) may be present. Hypersensitivity, which can often interfere with postural alignment, may also occur.

Integration of Total Body Movements

Total body movements include the integration of head, neck, and trunk control, with dynamic sitting and standing balance while reaching, bending, stooping, and ambulating. To perform total body movements, the individual must coordinate and modulate gross and fine motor movements of the trunk, head, neck, and limbs while performing activities of daily living (ADLs). An individual with severe physical involvement often displays poor sitting and standing balance and is unable to maintain an upright position in order to free the UEs for activities. The individual functioning at a more advanced level may exhibit subtle deficits in total body movements, making it difficult to bend down, to reach overhead to retrieve items in a cabinet, or to stoop to retrieve an item that has fallen to the floor. Integrated total body movements are necessary for the performance of all ADLs.

DYSPHAGIA

Dysphagia, a difficulty in the four stages of chewing and swallowing, is caused by cranial nerve damage (see Chapter 26). There is a higher incidence of oral preparatory, oral, and pharyngeal stage dysphagia than esophageal stage dysphagia. Typically, more than one stage of chewing and swallowing is impaired.[4]

An individual may display oral muscular hypotonicity or hypertonicity; instability of the jaw; and abnormal oral reflexes, such as rooting, biting, sucking, gagging, and coughing, which prevent or impair the activity of speaking or eating. As a result of cognitive deficits, the individual may experience difficulty in sequencing chewing, swallowing, and breathing.

SELF-FEEDING

Clients with a TBI may be unable to sustain attention long enough to feed themselves. If impulsivity is apparent, these clients will have difficulty monitoring the amount and rate of food brought to the mouth, thus causing coughing and possible aspiration. Oral apraxia, the inability to perform an intended action or execute an act on command with the mouth or lips, may occur. If clients possess an ideational apraxia, they will have difficulty understanding the demands required of the self-feeding activity and will be unable to recognize utensils as tools for eating. Because they also may have lost the motor plan for self-feeding (ideomotor apraxia), they may be unable to gain access to the neurological motor pattern for bringing food to the mouth. A hemianopsia (visual field cut) or neglect may prevent them from seeing one half of the plate of food.

COGNITIVE STATUS

Cognitive deficits are always evident to varying degrees and can affect many aspects of the individual's quality of life, as mentioned in the previous sections. The most common include decreased attention and concentration, impaired memory, **impaired initiation** and termination of activities, decreased safety awareness and poor judgment, impulsivity, and difficulty with executive functions and abstract thinking (e.g., problem solving, planning, the integration of new learning, and generalization).

Attention and Concentration

Reduced attention and concentration impair the ability to maintain focus on an activity without becoming distracted and the ability to resume an activity when interrupted. Clients with TBI often lose the ability to concentrate for a length of time and the ability to filter out distractions from the surrounding environment. The inability to attend to and concentrate on activities severely impedes the ability to function at work and school and complete ADL activities. Although deficits in attention and concentration can diminish as neurological recovery progresses, such deficits can remain in varying degrees throughout an individual's life. Even those patients who experience mild TBI can demonstrate subtle deficits in attention and concentration that often linger for years after the injury and can affect their everyday functioning.

Memory

Impaired memory, the most frequently observed cognitive deficit in patients with TBI, can remain a lifelong problem. Memory impairment ranges from forgetting several words just heard (immediate memory), to forgetting which family members visited the night before (short-term memory), to forgetting events that occurred years before the injury (long-term memory). Despite neurological recovery, most of these patients continue to demonstrate difficulty in learning new information. Safety concerns include getting lost, leaving doors unlocked, and leaving stoves burning; patients with impaired memory typically require supervision if compensatory methods cannot be found. This loss of independence can be emotionally devastating because patients with TBI often have insight into who they were before the injury, as well as their accomplishments, goals, and plans for the future—many of which are severely disrupted and perhaps lost as a result of TBI.

Initiation and Termination of Activities

Impaired initiation and termination of activities affect the ability to start and end activities. The inability to initiate activities without assistance affects the individual's ability to live independently. In general, patients who exhibit deficits in initiation will demonstrate the greatest progress in a rehabilitation

setting that provides assistance and structure. After returning home, patients may regress and have difficulty completing basic daily activities if they have not set up the necessary structure. Similarly, patients may exhibit difficulty terminating an activity once it is started, which is a type of perseveration. For example, patients may initiate brushing their teeth and be unable to end the task because they feel compelled to continue. Perseveration sometimes involves a thought process. Clients may be unable to concentrate on one activity because they are perseverating on the idea that another activity (e.g., the laundry) must be completed.

Safety Awareness and Judgment

Frontal lobe damage often results in an impairment of insight regarding a person's limitations, as well as impulsivity, or the inability to consider consequences before acting. These results cause affected individuals to demonstrate poor safety awareness and judgment. For example, the client may attempt to rise out of a wheelchair without locking the brakes or moving the foot rests. A more mobile client who has been reintegrated into the community may attempt to cross streets without observing traffic signals or remove pots from the stove or oven without using protective oven mitts or pot holders. It is important for the occupational therapist to structure the client's environment to reduce accidents and increase the client's awareness of his or her limitations through repeated opportunities to practice and relearn safe and appropriate behaviors.

Processing of Information

Most people with TBI experience some degree of difficulty in processing external information from the environment. A delay in response time is often noted and can range from a few seconds to several minutes. It is important for the therapist to recognize the presence of delayed processing and distinguish the delay from the absence of function. For example, during a sensory evaluation a client may exhibit a delay in response to a dull stimulus. The therapist may mistakenly interpret the individual's delayed processing time as an absence seizure or impairment of sensory awareness. A delay in the processing of external information from the environment can involve visual, auditory, sensory, and perceptual processing.

Executive Functions and Abstract Thought

Executive function skills include the ability to plan, organize, set goals, understand the consequences of one's actions, and modify behaviors in accordance with environmental responses. Abstract thinking is the ability to hold and manipulate a concept in one's mind using critical reasoning and analytical skills. Many clients with TBI exhibit concrete thinking, in which they are able to interpret information only at the most literal level. For example, individuals with impaired executive and abstract functions may be able to complete a meal preparation activity accurately and safely only if step-by-step directions are provided. If the directions do not specifically direct the reader to modify the cooking temperatures, these individuals may burn the food because they are unable to foresee the consequences of maintaining the stove on a high setting.

Generalization

Generalization of new learning is the ability to learn a specific task and transfer the skills needed for that task to a similar activity. Deficits in executive functions, abstract thinking, and short-term memory significantly impair the generalization of new learning. For example, an individual who has learned in a day-treatment setting the skills for completing a laundry task may be unable to transfer the skills at home or at a different laundromat. Such deficits often occur as a result of concrete thinking and the inability to form abstractions. Although the cognitive pattern for completing laundry tasks using the laundry machine in the clinical setting is established, the individual cannot transfer that cognitive pattern to a similar but unfamiliar laundry machine in a different environment. Impaired generalization of new learning is one of the most significant problems impeding the individual's ability to resume independent functioning in a community setting.

VISUAL STATUS

Visual skills involve the ability to accurately see stimuli from the external environment (see Chapter 23). Visual skills do not involve the identification of objects, which is a function of perception. Among the many deficits in visual skills that may result from TBI are accommodative dysfunction (causing blurred vision), convergence insufficiency (the inability to maintain a single vision while fixating on an object), lateral or medial strabismus, nystagmus, hemianopsia, and impairment of scanning and pursuits. Saccades (fast, jerky movements of the eyes as they change from one position of gaze to another, as are needed to read a book) may also be compromised by TBI. Reduced blink rate, ptosis (drooping of the eyelid), and lagophthalmos (incomplete eyelid closure) are also common visual deficits resulting from oculomotor nerve damage.[6]

A dysfunction in any of these visual elements can profoundly affect daily life function. Individuals rely on vision indirectly in social and interpersonal interactions. Vision is used as a cueing and feedback system in motor skills such as ambulation and in eye-hand coordination activities. Deficits in vision can affect all daily life activities, including the areas of hygiene and grooming, meal preparation and eating, wheelchair mobility, reading and writing, and driving.

PERCEPTUAL SKILLS

Perception is the ability to interpret stimuli from the external environment (see Chapter 24). Perception is a function of the secondary cortical areas of the right hemisphere, including the secondary visual area, the secondary somatosensory area, the secondary auditory area, and the multimodal parietal-occipital-temporal area. Perceptual deficits are more often a result of right hemisphere damage but may occur with left hemisphere lesions. Perception can be grouped into the following categories: *visual* perception, *body schema* perception, *motor* perception, and *speech and language* perception. An individual with visual perceptual impairments may exhibit difficulty with right-left discrimination, figure-ground discrimination, form constancy, position in space, and topographical orientation. Visual perceptual deficits also include visual agnosia, in which the individual displays difficulty recognizing familiar objects and people. For example, prosopagnosia is the inability to connect faces with names. Prosopagnosia results from damage to the multimodal association area.[6]

Body schema perception is the awareness of the spatial characteristics of a person's own body. This awareness is derived from a neural synthesis of tactile, proprioceptive, and pressure sensory associations about the body and its individual parts. A common problem in persons with TBI is anosognosia, a failure to recognize deficits or limitations. This may lead to the body schema perceptual dysfunction of **unilateral neglect syndrome,** in which the individual has lost the ability to integrate perceptions from one side of the body or environment (usually the left). A unilateral neglect is commonly caused by a lesion to the right parietal lobe but also can occur as a result of frontal and occipital lobe damage. Patients with a left unilateral neglect may disown their left extremities, treating them as though they belonged to someone else. For example, these individuals may shave only the right side of their faces or dress only the right side of their bodies.[6]

Aphasia is a disturbance of comprehension or formulation of language (or both) caused by dysfunction in specific brain regions, typically the left hemisphere.[18] A few left-handed individuals have language dominance in the right hemisphere. Establishing reliable communication is crucial in treating anyone with aphasia. If auditory comprehension is compromised, gestural demonstration of instructions or activities will be more reliable. Common types of aphasia involving disorders of comprehension include Wernicke's and transcortical sensory types. Affected individuals will have longer periods of PTA because they do not understand orientation questions, and although their spoken language is fluent, it includes verbal paraphasias, or word substitutions. Clients with aphasia may also misinterpret speech and become suspicious and agitated. Insight into their communication deficit may be limited.

The nonfluent aphasias, Broca's aphasia, and transcortical motor aphasia are characterized by relatively preserved comprehension but effortful or explosive speech with phonemic paraphasias, (e.g., "bork" for "fork"). Conduction aphasia (i.e., intact comprehension, fluent speech, impaired repetition) and anomic aphasia are characterized by circumlocution and often paraphasias. Individuals with these types of aphasia typically are aware of their problems and often frustrated by their limitations. They should be encouraged to use gestures to express their immediate desires and needs.

Dyslexia (disturbance in reading), agraphia (disorder of writing), and dyscalculia (disturbance of calculation) often accompany the aphasias. However, with traumatic aphasias, these capabilities may be better preserved than with stroke; treating therapists should always attempt alternative modes of communication.

Dysprosody or aprosodia is the impaired production or comprehension of the tonal inflections or emotional tone of speech. Executive dysprosody is the inability to inflect one's voice to convey emotion. It can occur with cerebellar, basal ganglia, or right frontal lobe injury. Receptive dysprosody is the inability to perceive the emotional content of other people's spoken language. It occurs with right temporal or parietal injury and less often with left hemisphere injury. Individuals with this disorder may miss the point of a joke or story because they could not comprehend the subtle innuendoes and the implicit meanings conveyed through tonal qualities and inflections.[73] Even more disabling is the inability to interpret anger, humor, or sarcasm in communication with others.[17] Perceptual-motor dysfunction is impairment in motor planning, or an apraxia. It is a disorder of learned movement that cannot be explained by weakness, lack of sensation, inattention, or comprehension of the requested task.[17] The apraxias are usually a result of impairment to the premotor cortex, corpus callosum, or connections between the temporal/parietal lobes and frontal motor cortex.[35] It is in these cortical areas that established motor patterns for specific activities are stored and accessed for the execution of common movement patterns. Ideational apraxia is the inability to understand the demands of a task or the use of the wrong motor plan for a specific task. For example, individuals suffering from ideational apraxia may not understand that a shirt is an item of clothing to be placed on the torso and UEs. Not understanding the demands of the task, they may be unable to activate the motor plan for UE dressing or may activate the wrong plan and attempt to place their legs through the sleeve holes. This deficit is sometimes referred to as a *dressing apraxia*. Ideomotor apraxia is the loss of the kinetic memory of a movement pattern for a specific activity. Individuals with this disorder may understand that a shirt is an item of clothing to be placed on the torso and UEs but be unable to execute the appropriate movement plan because it is no longer accessible. Constructional apraxia is the inability to accurately assemble pieces of an object to form a three-dimensional whole. For example, a former carpenter who suffers from constructional apraxia may be unable to put together the wooden pieces of a basic birdhouse kit.

PSYCHOSOCIAL FACTORS

Researchers have found that the greatest concerns of clients 1 or more years after a TBI are the psychosocial deficits that prevent them from rebuilding a satisfactory quality of life.

As the time after the injury increases, clients and family members view such psychosocial factors as more detrimental than both the physical and the cognitive sequelae of TBI.

For example, in Marisol's case, it was initially difficult to assess her psychosocial status because she was nonvocal. The team was able to assess her mood on the basis of her level of participation and affect during therapy. Marisol would laugh appropriately and become visibly more interactive, with brighter affect, when her boyfriend arrived to visit.

Marisol continued to engage in positive interactions throughout her 4-month inpatient and day-treatment stay. Her discharge plan involved moving to Georgia with her mother. When the move was discussed with Marisol, it was evident that she was quite saddened by the knowledge that she would no longer be able to see her boyfriend. The team observed her closely to assess whether her sadness would eventually culminate in depressive symptoms.

Self-Concept

One of the most difficult psychosocial sequelae of TBI is the alteration in the individual's self-concept. Self-concept is the internal image a person holds regarding personal human identity; sexual and gender identity; body image; personal strengths and limitations; and position in the family, peer group, and community systems. An individual's self-concept changes drastically after TBI. One of the most difficult characteristics of TBI is that although short-term memory is often impaired, long-term memory commonly remains intact. Persons with TBI often have a clear memory of who they were before their injury and must now resolve the emotional conflict of having to replace their pre-injury self-concept with a post-injury self-concept that is both meaningful and satisfying. Affected individuals sometimes describe this process as an unwanted death and rebirth. They say that the person who lived before the injury is now gone, replaced by someone who is very different from the person they remember themselves to be.[56]

Social Roles

Self-concept is derived largely from the social roles that the person attains in the family, peer group, and larger community systems. Often, the individual with TBI loses most pre-injury roles and the activities that supported those roles. Family and peer group roles change. Family members and friends are often readily visible during the acute and subacute stages of TBI rehabilitation. However, as the time after the injury increases, family and friends become progressively less involved with the individual, often leading to feelings of isolation and abandonment. Many individuals with TBI report that the feeling of isolation and the inability to form and maintain social relationships are their most troubling post-injury concerns. The loss of the role of dating partner or spouse commonly leaves clients with TBI with a deep sense of loss and failure if they cannot rebuild a post-injury life that includes intimacy with another human being, partnership in a committed relationship, and parenting of children.

The loss of the work role and the inability to support oneself are intimately tied to feelings of dependence and lack of personal control.[42]

Independent Living Status

As a result of the physical, cognitive, and psychosocial sequelae of TBI, many affected individuals find that they require supportive living arrangements or must live with their parents. The loss of the ability to live independently in the community further reinforces feelings of dependence and decreased personal control. As a result of these role losses, adults who sustain a TBI commonly experience role strain and feel that they cannot re-enter their communities. The TBI, particularly if it occurred between the ages of 18 and 30, disrupts the developmental transition from adolescence to adulthood, leaving individuals feeling inadequate and unable to attain a post-injury adult status. Depression, withdrawal, and apathy are common psychosocial sequelae of the alterations in self-concept discussed earlier and of the loss of desired social roles.[50]

Dealing with Loss

Persons with TBI often experience a process that resembles the stages of death and dying experienced by the terminally ill.[43] These stages begin with denial, in which affected individuals deny that they are experiencing physical, cognitive, or psychosocial deficits. Denial can impede therapy because these clients may refuse to participate, believing that it is unnecessary. Denial gradually subsides as they continually confront their limitations in daily life activities. Anger follows denial. Clients grow increasingly aware of their deficits and become frustrated and angry because recovery is slower than desired. Bargaining is the next stage. Clients strike a deal with the Creator or the fates, offering to work as diligently as possible in therapy if only their pre-injury lifestyle could be restored. The bargaining stage is often marked by increased motivation and optimism. Depression tends to emerge next. Eventually, clients begin to realize the severity of the injury and its effect on the rest of their lives. Acceptance of the injury and resultant limitations, the next stage in the process, is necessary for clients to become sufficiently motivated to attempt to build a post-injury life that, although drastically different from their pre-injury goals and expectations, is nevertheless meaningful and personally valuable. These stages may require years of transition. Often denial, anger, and bargaining occur in the first few months to a year after the injury. Depression sets in as the individual is able to let go of some of the denial and becomes aware of the effect the injury will have on the future. It may take years before he or she can truly accept the injury and the alterations in personality, skill, and lifestyle and move on to rebuild a new life.

The process of denial, anger, depression, and acceptance does not generally proceed in a linear fashion. Clients with TBI commonly experience repeated periods of denial, anger, and depression throughout their years of rehabilitation. Renewed denial, anger, and depression may occur in response to a new environmental demand, such as a change in life condition (e.g., a need to move from the parental home to a community group home) or the development of further physical, cognitive, or psychosocial deterioration over time (e.g., the need for increased ambulatory assistance because of a deterioration in visual skills).

Affective Changes

Depression, increased emotional lability, and decreased affect can result from the neurological damage itself. Individuals with left hemisphere damage tend to exhibit increased depression and emotional lability. Lesions of the left orbitofrontal lobe often cause severe depression and heightened affect (including excitement, agitation, and tearfulness). Lesions of the left dorsolateral frontal lobe commonly result in a decreased or flat affect. Individuals with these lesions may appear depressed even though they feel fine. Neurological damage to the right hemisphere often causes a strange sense of euphoria or lack of emotional response to the severity of injury.[56]

BEHAVIORAL STATUS

Behavioral impairments are a natural part of the recovery process. The Rancho Los Amigos Scale cognitive level IV is typically described by the rehabilitation team as the agitated level "agitated, confused." During this stage of recovery, affected individuals can be described as restless and combative. They may be responding to internal bodily experiences, or some external environmental stimuli may be provoking the agitation. Commonly observed behaviors include yelling, swearing, grabbing, and biting. Behavioral problems can be disturbing for both the individual's family and the intervention team; therefore, behavioral management is an essential component in TBI rehabilitation.

 ## ETHICAL CONSIDERATIONS

Working with clients who have behavior problems can be frustrating and sometimes frightening. Untrained staff members can become injured and often reinforce the client's negative behaviors through their own actions and responses.

A comprehensive behavior management program should be established for anyone who exhibits behaviors that interfere with active participation in therapy and goal achievement. The goals and objectives of a comprehensive program include maintaining a safe environment for individuals and staff at all times, developing and consistently implementing behavior management techniques, minimizing the use of all restrictive modalities, and providing an environment that facilitates participation and appropriate behaviors in the hospital setting and after discharge.[63]

Interventions used in an effective behavior management program include one-on-one coaching, psychotropic medication intervention, a drug and alcohol abuse policy, and individually designed behavior management guidelines and interventions. One-on-one coaching, usually performed by a trained nursing assistant or rehabilitation technician, is especially necessary for clients who are at risk for harming themselves or others. In many cases, implementation of a behavior management program is necessary 24 hours a day, 7 days a week. A coach will help reinforce the client's behavior plan and redirect inappropriate or maladaptive behaviors. Medications are required to regulate sleep and minimize agitation and combative behaviors until clients can control the behaviors on their own. Medications must be chosen carefully to prevent side effects such as clouding of awareness and psychomotor slowing. Clients should have specific behavioral endpoints, such as establishing adequate sleep at night, facilitating attention during functional activities, and decreasing the frequency of verbal or physical outbursts.

Environmental modifications are a proactive approach to prevent and minimize undesirable behaviors. These may include use of a cubicle or net bed, an alarm system, a helmet, and walkie-talkies. The drug and alcohol policy is frequently necessary; it is well documented that many individuals with TBI have preexisting alcohol or drug problems (or both).[64]

The first step to become more comfortable when working with clients with behavior problems is to understand why they occur and how they manifest themselves.

Clients who are exhibiting agitation, combativeness, disinhibition, and refusal to cooperate and participate in activities typically have difficulty filtering distractions and can become agitated in noisy environments. Providing a quiet room during interventions and the use of a cubicle bed may help minimize noises and reduce outbursts.

A disinhibited individual may lack awareness of the external environment and may make indiscriminate sexual remarks or gestures to others. Ignoring comments, redirecting inappropriate behaviors, and modeling acceptable behaviors are typical therapeutic interventions.

Clients who refuse to cooperate and participate in intervention can be the most challenging because this attitude may affect their ability to remain in an acute rehabilitation program. The lack of participation is typically organically based and due to cognitive deficits such as impaired initiation and lack of insight into their disability. It is important to document these behaviors throughout the course of care; however, when clients refuse to participate, documenting progress can be challenging.

Interventions include providing consistent structure through daily schedules and goal sheets that provide visual cues of expectations, as well as visual and physical guidance through activities until clients are capable of completing tasks without assistance.

OT PRACTICE NOTES

Behavior management is essential to all TBI rehabilitation programs. It is important to develop and implement a behavioral program whether behaviors are passive (decreased initiation), active (agitation), or somewhere along the continuum.

An effective program includes comprehensive staff training, tools that track and monitor behaviors and techniques, and consistent multidisciplinary communication (behavior management meetings) to ensure that the individualized behavior plan is effective and goal oriented.[64]

EVALUATION OF THE LOWER-LEVEL INDIVIDUAL

Clients emerging from coma and at the beginning stages of the injury (Rancho Los Amigos level I to III) may exhibit minimal arousal and limited purposeful movements. It may be necessary to evaluate such individuals in short sessions and at different times of the day. A quiet environment with minimal distractions will enhance the client's ability to attend to and follow commands. Evaluation includes an assessment of the following:

1. *Level of arousal and cognition.* Can the client visually attend to the speaker and follow commands such as "Open your mouth" and "Squeeze your eyes closed"? Can he or she communicate through verbalizations, gestures, or eye movements? Does he or she demonstrate purposeful movements such as pulling at vital tubes? How easy/difficult is it to wake the client, and how long can the client stay awake?
2. *Vision.* Is the client able to visually scan or attend to a person, object, or activity? Can the client maintain eye contact?
3. *Sensation.* Does the client respond to external stimulation such as pain, temperature, and movement of the joints?
4. *Joint ROM.* Has the client lost ROM in certain joints as a result of decorticate or decerebrate posturing, increased tone or spasticity, contractures, or heterotopic ossification?
5. *Motor control.* Does the client exhibit decorticate or decerebrate posturing? Is there an increase of tone and spasticity? Is there deceased tone and hypotonicity? Are deep tendon responses present, diminished, or absent? Does the client exhibit the presence of primitive reflexes? Does the client engage in spontaneous motor movements, such as scratching the face?
6. *Dysphagia.* Does the client handle his or her own secretions, drool, or swallow spontaneously? Does the client demonstrate poor oral-motor control? Answers to these

questions provide valuable information as to whether a swallowing evaluation is indicated.

7. *Emotional and behavioral factors.* Is the client's affect flat or expressive? Are responses such as crying or laughing observed in response to interactions with the rehab team or family members?

Evaluation of the lower-level individual with TBI is generally accomplished with tools such as a goniometer, clinical muscle and tone testing, traditional neurological screening, and clinical observations. Many acute TBI rehabilitation facilities have developed their own initial evaluation forms. There are a variety of scales that can be utilized to establish a baseline and predict recovery. The Glasgow Coma Scale and Rancho Los Amigos Scale are common; however, newer cognitive scales, such as the JFK Coma Recovery Scale (JFK)[60] and the Wessex Head Injury Matrix (WHIM), are also being used.[60] Some clients tend to emerge quickly and move expeditiously through the Rancho levels, whereas others (e.g., those with anoxia) may demonstrate limited or slow recovery. A subacute program or a rehabilitation center that specializes in slow-to-recover clients may be necessary. In either case, a rehabilitation program with active therapeutic intervention is necessary to prevent contractures, encourage activity, and facilitate the client's progress through the rehabilitative process.

In the case of Marisol, the team decided to address her spasticity and joint contractures first by providing appropriate medical interventions, including a block to her musculocutaneous nerve to decrease her spasticity. This was followed by casting to reduce her elbow contracture. The team also gave Marisol a comprehensive activity schedule in a multistimulus environment. This schedule involved transferring her out of bed and into a customized wheelchair, in which she would remain between 6 and 8 hours a day, and requiring active participation in all therapies 4 hours per day. Her cognitive level was assessed weekly by using the JFK Coma Recovery Scale and assessing her ability to follow through with basic mobility and self-care tasks.

INTERVENTION OF THE LOWER-LEVEL INDIVIDUAL

The general aim of intervention for those at Rancho Levels I through III is to increase the individual's level of response and overall awareness of self and environment. All stimulation should be well structured and broken down into simple steps and commands. Sufficient time is necessary for an individual's response because cognitive processing is often significantly delayed during this phase of recovery. Intervention at this stage can be grouped into six areas: sensory stimulation, bed positioning, casting or splinting, wheelchair positioning, dysphasia management, and emotional and behavioral management, as well as family and caregiver education. Interventions may occur simultaneously to optimize progress. Each intervention affects and enhances the next.

Because clients often respond more to the familiar and routine, it is important to incorporate close family members and friends into sessions.

SENSORY STIMULATION

Intervention for clients emerging from coma should start as soon as they are medically stable. Intervention generally begins in the intensive care unit. At this stage, clients often lack responsiveness to pain, touch, sound, or sight. They may exhibit a generalized response to pain that appears reflexive (e.g., attempting to pull away from painful stimulus). The goal of intervention is to increase the client's level of awareness by trying to increase arousal with controlled sensory input. **Sensory regulation** increases neurological signals to the reticular activation system, the structure of the brainstem that alerts the brain to important sensory input from the external environment.

Sensory stimulation can be introduced in a variety of ways and methods. Introducing isolated visual, auditory, tactile, olfactory, and gustatory stimulants to the individual may heighten arousal. For example, a flashlight may be used to elicit eye opening and visual tracking. Playing familiar music may facilitate autonomic responses, such as a change in respiratory rate or blood pressure changes. Introducing olfactory stimulation through a variety of scents may elicit eye opening or head turning. Gustatory stimulation involves the controlled presentation of taste to the client's lips and tongue through use of a cotton swab. Such stimulants may include salty, sweet, bitter, and sour tastes. Any response from the client is noted.

 OT PRACTICE NOTE

The most effective types of sensory stimulants are those that have personal meaning to the client, such as favorite songs or stories. Family members often bring in familiar objects and pictures that can facilitate responses from the client. It is helpful to learn about the client's pre-injury history in order to incorporate familiar items and routines into his or her intervention plan.

Kinesthetic input is incorporated early in the intervention. One of the most effective ways to facilitate volitional movement is by actively guiding movements in a normalized fashion while performing functional activities. The therapist actively helps the client to perform simple movements, such as rolling from side to side, and simple functional activities, such as wiping the mouth with a washcloth, combing hair, and applying lotion to the skin. The theoretical aim of functional sensory stimulation is to reactivate highly processed neural pathways that had been established before the injury. Other activities related to functional sensory stimulation include sitting the individual up at the edge of the bed and having the client stand by using a tilt table or a hydraulic standing frame. During all these activities, the therapist observes the client for any changes such as the following: visual tracking, turning of the head, physical responses, vocalizations, and ability to follow verbal commands.

WHEELCHAIR POSITIONING

Seating and positioning are important components of treatment for lower-level patients. Being properly positioned in a wheelchair allows these patients to interact with their immediate environment in an upright, midline posture. Proper positioning aims to facilitate head and trunk control so that clients can see and interact with people and objects in the environment. A proper wheelchair seating position helps prevent skin breakdown and joint contractures, facilitate normal muscle tone, inhibit primitive reflexes, increase sitting tolerance, enhance respiration and swallowing function, and promote function (Figure 34-1).

Effective seating and positioning require a stable base of support at the pelvis, maintenance of the trunk in midline, and facilitation of the head in an upright, midline position. This position frees the upper extremities for use and allows the client to visually scan the environment. Once the client has a seating system that encourages and promotes function, therapy sessions can be more effective and beneficial. For example, clients generally find it easier to handle their

secretions in this position, so swallowing trials may be safer and more effective.

Marisol required a wheelchair and specific positioning devices when she entered the acute rehabilitation program. Given her motor abilities and deficits, what type of wheelchair set-up would you prescribe?

Pelvis

Wheelchair positioning should begin at the pelvis. Poor hip placement adversely alters the trunk and head alignment and influences tone in the extremities. Because sling-seat wheelchairs contribute to internal rotation and adduction of the hips, it is important to insert a firm, solid seat (padded with foam and covered by vinyl) to facilitate a neutral to slightly anterior pelvic tilt. A lumbar support will also help maintain the natural curve in the lumbar spine. A wedged seat insert (with the downward slope pointing toward the back of the chair) can be used to facilitate hip flexion and inhibit extensor tone in the hips and LEs. The individual's buttocks should bear weight evenly, with both ischial tuberosities firmly resting on the wheelchair seat. A seatbelt angled across the pelvis helps maintain this desired position.

Trunk

The trunk should be positioned after the pelvis because it is the next most proximal body structure. A solid back insert or firm contoured back should be placed behind the client's

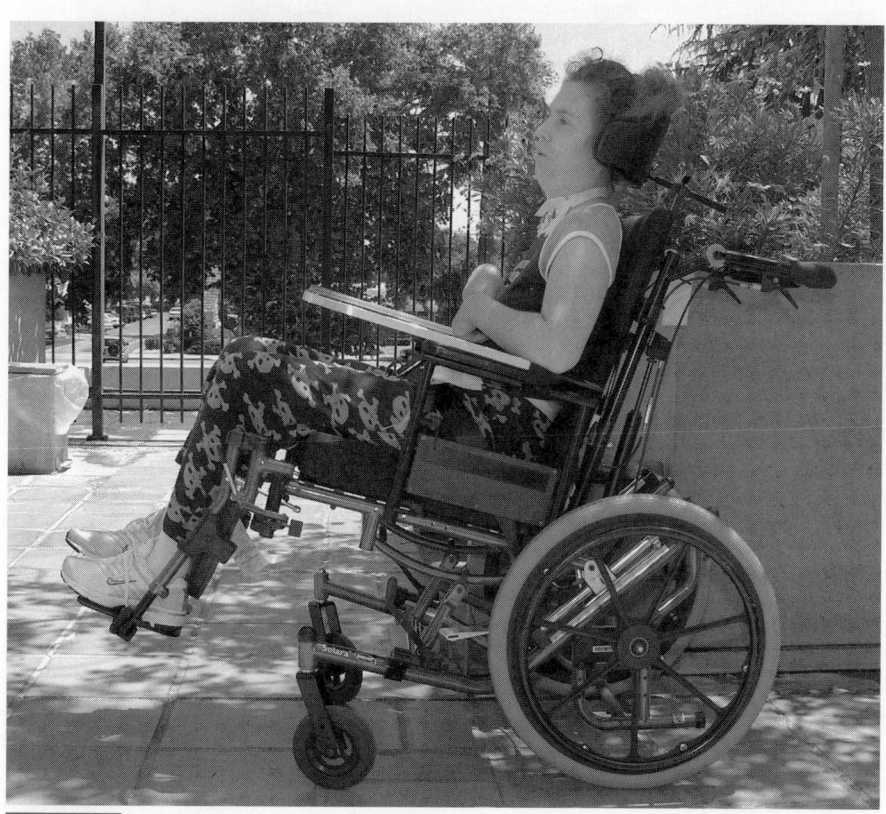

Figure 34-1 Proper wheelchair seating position.

back to maintain the spine in an erect posture. A back insert that is contoured to the curves in the spine will maintain the lumbar and thoracic curves. Lateral trunk supports can be used to reduce scoliosis and lateral trunk flexion caused by imbalanced tone of the intrinsic muscles of the back. A chest strap (with easily opened Velcro fasteners) can be used to decrease kyphosis, facilitate shoulder retraction and abduction, and expand the upper chest for proper diaphragmatic breathing and UE use.

Lower Extremities

An abductor wedge placed between the LEs just proximal to the knees may be used to decrease hip adduction and internal rotation. If hip abduction is present, padded abductor wedge can be placed along the lateral aspect of the thigh to reduce LE abduction. Ideally, the knees should be positioned at 90 degrees, with the heels slightly behind the knees in sitting. It is desirable to maintain both feet securely on the foot plates to provide proprioceptive input and facilitate weight bearing in both heels to normalize tone.

Upper Extremities

The UEs should be positioned with the scapulae in a neutral position (neither elevated nor depressed), the shoulders slightly externally rotated and abducted, the elbows in a neutral position of slight flexion with forearm pronation, and the wrists and digits in a functional position. This position is often difficult to achieve because of severe spasticity and soft-tissue contractures of the UEs. A splint or cast may be applied to decrease spasticity and facilitate a functional position of the UEs. Frequently, a lap tray is used to provide support for the UEs and encourage bilateral UE weight bearing and use.

Head

Clients with TBI at a lower functioning level often have little or no active head control. Attaining a neutral-midline head position, which allows optimal visual contact with the environment, is difficult. A dynamic head-positioning device (Figure 34-2) can be used to maintain neutral head alignment and facilitate head control. A contoured head rest that

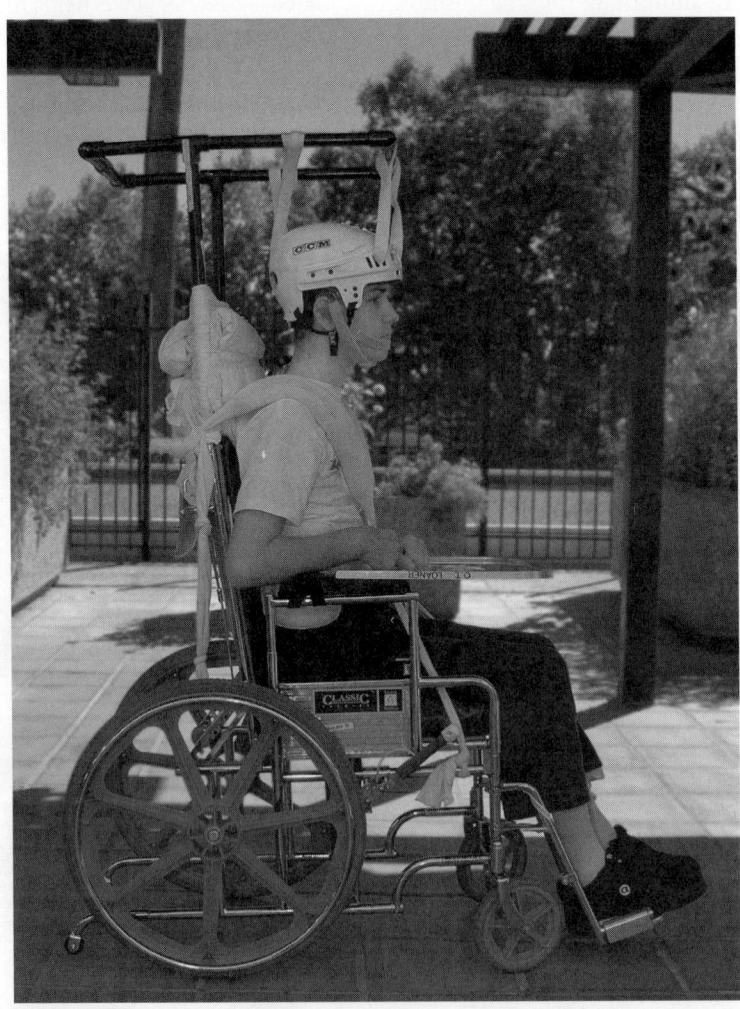

Figure 34-2 A dynamic head positioning device maintains neutral head alignment and facilitates head control.

cradles the head posteriorly and laterally may be used to support the head in a midline position. A forehead strap (fabricated from soft, padded material) may be used to prevent the head from falling forward. Slightly reclining the wheelchair also prevents the client's head from falling forward and facilitates visual interaction with the environment. The client should be reclined between 10 and 15 degrees; reclining the client beyond this point reduces weight bearing through the trunk and pelvis and tends to encourage extensor tone, a posterior pelvic tilt, and sacral sitting.

As the client progresses in rehabilitation, wheelchair seating and positioning should be reevaluated continually to better meet his or her specific needs. Devices should be modified gradually or removed as the client begins to control his or her body actively and manipulate more items in the environment. A schedule is necessary to indicate the length of time that the client can tolerate being seated in the wheelchair. Keeping the client in a wheelchair longer than can be tolerated may result in fatigue, which can subsequently interfere with active participation in therapy.

BED POSITIONING

Proper bed positioning is critical in the early stages of TBI. Because the client tends to spend a lot of time in bed, proper bed positioning is crucial to prevent pressure sores and facilitate normal muscle tone. It is often difficult to maintain optimal positioning because of spasticity and abnormal posturing. Other complications that may interfere with proper positioning are casts or splints, intravenous tubes, nasogastric tubes, fractures, or any other medical precautions that must be maintained while in bed.

If the client exhibits abnormal tone or posturing, a side-lying or semi-prone position is preferable. This position assists in normalizing tone and providing sensory input. A supine position may elicit tonic labyrinthine reflex and extensor tone. A supine position with the head in a lateral position could elicit the asymmetrical tonic neck reflex. Clients with TBI generally have bilateral involvement requiring a program for side-lying on both sides. The traditional bed positioning techniques used with patients who have had a cerebral vascular accident (CVA) may require modification depending on the extent of bilateral involvement. Pillows, foam wedges, and splints may be incorporated into the bed-positioning program to facilitate normal positions and prevent abnormal postures such as extreme elbow flexion, head and neck extension, and foot drop deformity.

 OT PRACTICE NOTE

Because all clients have unique needs, each should be assessed and set up with an ideal positioning program. It often helps to take a photo of the client once positioned and post it to ensure that it may be easily duplicated and carried out by staff and family members.

SPLINTING AND CASTING

Splinting or casting may be indicated when (1) spasticity interferes with functional movement and ADL independence, (2) joint ROM limitations are present, and (3) soft-tissue contractures are possible. Splints have been thought to provide elongation and inhibition by positioning the joint in a static position with the muscles and soft tissues on stretch. Splinting of the elbows, wrists, and hands is often implemented to maintain a functional position at rest and to reduce tone. Serial casting is a more aggressive intervention to increase ROM in the joints when contractures have formed or spasticity is present (or both). Splinting and casting not only reduce contractures and increase ROM but also prevent skin breakdown. Because clients with TBI often have limited active ROM, the UE joints often assume a position of flexion (particularly when severe finger flexor spasticity has caused the fingers and nails to embed in the palmar surface of the hand), and this may cause moisture, redness, and breakdown of the skin.

The resting or functional position splint (Figure 34-3) is one that is worn when the client is not involved in active movements or functional tasks. Once the splint has been fitted, a wearing schedule must be established for the rehabilitation team and caregivers to follow. A typical splint schedule during the day requires the client to wear the splint for repeated, alternating 2-hour periods (2 hours on, followed by 2 hours off). The client must be monitored frequently for skin breakdown or tonal changes that may change the initial fit of the splint. The team and caregivers should be trained in proper application and removal of each splint.

Other common splints worn at this stage of recovery are cone splints, used in the palm of the hand to keep the fingers from digging into the palmar surface. Often, rolled cloths are put into the clenched hand; however, because this may facilitate increased spasticity, a hard cone splint is more appropriate. An antispasticity splint (Figure 34-4) not only positions the hand and wrist in a functional position but also abducts the fingers to further decrease spasticity. Splints are modified as needed and may eventually be discontinued if the individual's motor control and tone improve.

A serial casting program is indicated when moderate to severe spasticity cannot be managed by splints. The goal of casting is to increase ROM and decrease tone gradually by

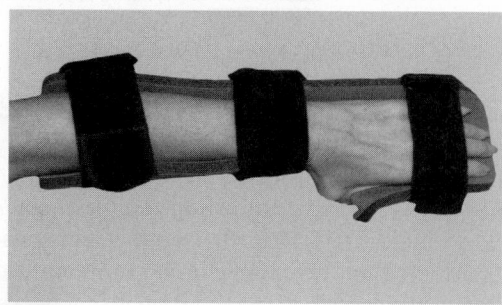

Figure 34-3 A resting splint.

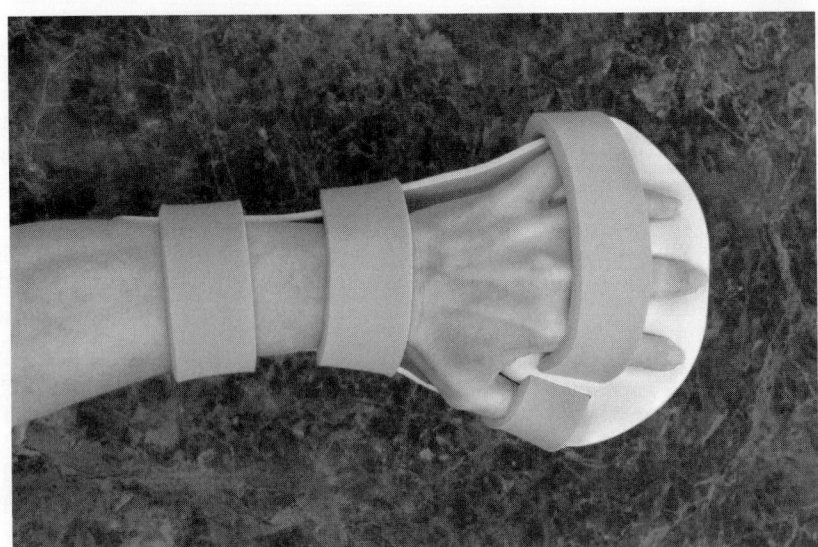

Figure 34-4 Antispasticity splint.

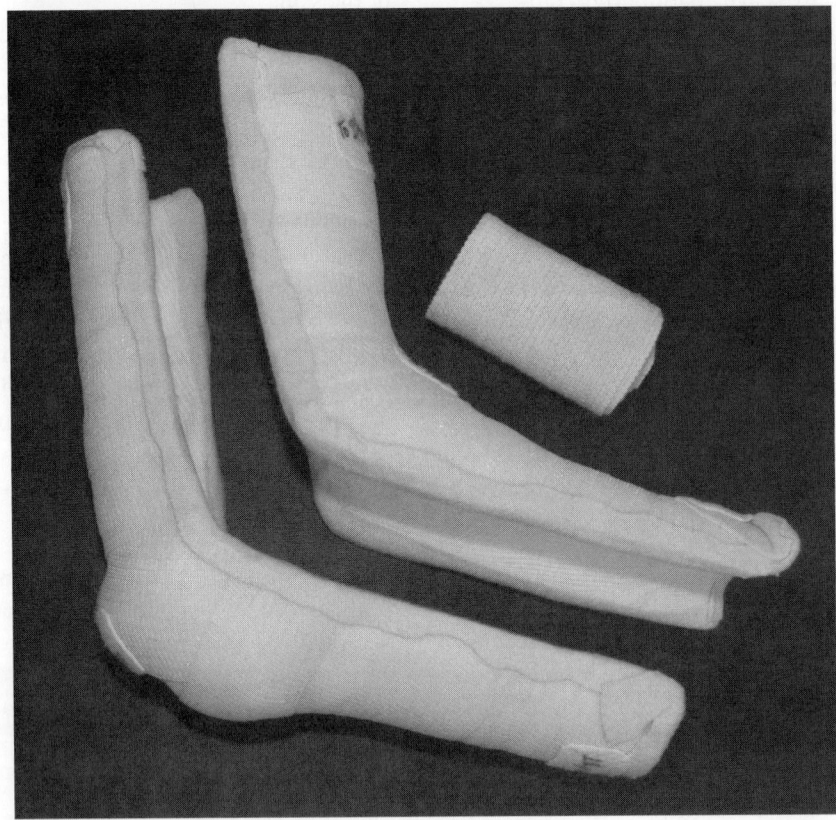

Figure 34-5 Spasticity splint.

using a progressive succession of separately fabricated casts, each worn continuously for a period of weeks. Casts are often left on for 5 to 7 days, which puts the muscle and tendons on a prolonged stretch and reduces tone. Successive casts are designed to increase ROM further until a functional joint range is achieved and maintained. The common difficulty that prevents the success of serial casting is skin breakdown.

If skin breakdown occurs because of a cast that is worn for several days, the cast must be removed until the skin has healed. While wound healing is occurring, spasticity again increases and any gain in joint ROM is often lost.

The most common UE casts are the elbow cast, which is used for loss of passive range of motion (PROM) in the elbow flexors, and the wrist-hand cast, which is used for loss of

PROM in the wrist and finger flexors. Other variations of these casts include elbow drop-out, wrist, thumb, hand, and individual finger casts. However, the casting of more than one joint at a time often leads to skin breakdown as a result of multiple pressure points. It is thus recommended that casting be applied to one joint at a time.[27]

Casting is frequently used in conjunction with motor point, nerve blocks or *Botulinum* toxin injections. Blocks involve the injection of a chemical substance (e.g., Lidocaine, marcaine, phenol) into the nerve or motor point to inhibit the innervation of spastic muscles temporarily. *Botulinum* toxin is injected directly into the target muscle and works by causing presynaptic blockade of acetylcholine release.

Indications for the completion of a casting program include obtaining a functional ROM or plateauing (e.g., the individual has not gained significant improvement in ROM after two consecutive casts). When improvement in ROM has been made and the goal has been achieved, the final cast is cut in half lengthwise, the edges are finished, and the cast is used as a bivalve splint to maintain the functional position. Velcro straps or elastic wrap bandages are used to secure them in place (Figure 34-5). A wearing schedule is then established.

Casting is an advanced intervention technique that carries some risk. Competent use of the technique requires knowledge and advanced clinical training. Marisol presented with increased spasticity and reduced function in her UEs. What splint or cast (or both) would best suit her needs initially?

DYSPHAGIA

Patients emerging from coma are fed through a nasogastric (NG) tube or gastrointestinal (G) tube. Once the patient is alert and more oriented, the physician decides when a dysphagia evaluation is indicated. Dysphagia programs usually begin in the intermediate- to advanced-level stages of rehabilitation (see Chapter 26).

BEHAVIORAL AND COGNITION

As clients emerge from coma and become more alert and aware of their surroundings, it is important to track their improvement and attempts to establish a form of communication. In acute rehabilitation, tracking the level of arousal and awareness is important because it demonstrates progress. Several scales and assessments are available, including the Wessex Head Injury Matrix (WHIM), JFK Coma Recovery Scale (JFK), and the Orientation-Log (O-Log). These measurement tools will document improvements in visual attention, visual tracking, and ability to follow commands.

Establishing a way for the client to communicate wants and needs is of the utmost importance because it helps guide intervention. It also allows the team to more accurately assess the client's cognitive level. A reliable yes/no system should typically be implemented. Examples include eye blinks, eye gaze, head nods, and motor movements such as thumb up

and down. Once a system is established, communication is possible.

FAMILY AND CAREGIVER EDUCATION

Education of family members and caregivers starts immediately because they are an integral part of the intervention team. Family members often play an essential role in eliciting the client's responses and in implementing the sensory regulation program, positioning the client in bed, and contributing to the ROM program. At the earliest stage after the injury, therapy may be limited; therefore, setting up a simple intervention plan for the family to implement is important in fostering the client's recovery and in maintaining passive joint motion. Family members often feel helpless, and allowing them to be actively involved helps alleviate their feelings of helplessness and focus their array of emotions. Later, when the individual is more alert and mobile, family members can be involved in transfers, wheelchair positioning, feeding programs, and ADL retraining.

EVALUATION OF THE INTERMEDIATE- TO HIGHER-LEVEL INDIVIDUAL

During the intermediate to advanced level of recovery (Rancho Los Amigos Scale score of IV to VIII), the client is alert but often displays confused, agitated, and inappropriate responses. The client may be able to follow simple two- to three-step verbal commands but is easily distracted. Minimal or moderate cues are often necessary to assist intermediate- to higher-level clients in the performance of ADLs. In general, they can complete most components of the occupational therapy evaluation; however, they may require several breaks during the evaluation process on account of distractibility or agitation. The evaluation is similar to that for the beginning-level client, in that physical status, dysphagia, psychosocial and behavioral factors, vision, sensation, and perception are assessed. Additionally, these patients require more extensive evaluation of ADL (including driving), work readiness, and ability to reintegrate into the community.

PHYSICAL STATUS

The physical status evaluation includes an assessment of joint ROM, muscular strength, sensation, proprioception, kinesthesia, fine and gross motor control, and total body control (i.e., dynamic sitting or standing balance). Limitations in physical status are usually the result of abnormal tone, spasticity, and muscle weakness without abnormal tone, heterotopic ossification, fractures, soft-tissue contractures, and peripheral nerve compression. Tools to assess physical status include goniometers, dynamometers, manual muscle testing, and clinical observation. Standard assessments may include the Jebsen Hand Function Test,[38] the

Minnesota Rate of Manipulation Tests,[52] the Minnesota Manual Dexterity test,[52] and the Purdue Pegboard.[68]

DYSPHAGIA

Dysphagia assessment may include both a clinical (bedside) assessment and videofluoroscopy. The bedside examination provides the therapist with a variety of information. For example, aspiration can be caused by impulsivity because the client may gulp large portions of food quickly. Pocketing food and drooling may be apparent; these are a result of impaired oral motor control. The dysphagia examination can also provide the therapist with information regarding cognitive status. Does the client appear to understand what to do with the utensils and food items? Is neglect present, causing the client to leave one side of the plate untouched? Does the client know the names of the utensils and food items, or is aphasia suspected?

Performed by a speech pathologist or a trained occupational therapist, the videofluoroscopy provides information regarding the anatomy and physiology of the oral, pharyngeal, and esophageal stages of swallowing. Videofluoroscopy is the only dysphagia assessment tool that can provide information regarding the individual's ability to manage liquids and solid foods. This information will be used to design a feeding program that may require a diet of thick liquids and puréed foods. Reevaluation of swallowing status should be made as the individual improves in rehabilitation and can progress to thin liquids and solid foods. (See Chapter 26 for more information on dysphagia.)

Improper positioning, behavioral disorders, and cognitive-perceptual impairment have all been implicated as factors contributing to swallowing disorders. Dysphagia intervention must address seating and positioning and cognitive-perceptual distortions. Formal assessments to evaluate dysphagia include the Dysphagia Evaluation Protocol 4 and the Evaluation of Oral Function in Feeding.[67]

COGNITION

Cognitive skills will be assessed within functional tasks (e.g., ADLs, meal preparation, money management, and community skills). Tasks that involve paper and a pencil can also provide valuable information, although they are only part of the equation. Assessment of a client's cognitive skills during preparation of a cold meal may include the following skills: (1) following two- to three-step written or spoken directions, (2) correctly sequencing the order of steps, (3) attending to the task with minimal distraction, and (4) displaying good safety and judgment. The therapist may evaluate the client's cognitive status by measuring any of the following: (1) counting the number of errors and correct responses, (2) assessing the amount of assistance or cueing required (minimal, moderate, or maximal), and (3) determining the percentage of the task that was completed correctly.

Assessment of the complexity of the activity (simple versus multistep or basic to complex) and the conditions of the environment (isolated versus multistimulus or quiet to distracting) is also important.

When assessing an individual's cognitive skills, the therapist must consider and document other factors that may affect performance. These include language barriers (e.g., the presence of aphasia, a primary language other than English), visual-perceptual deficits, the effects of medication on cognitive level, educational and cultural background, and previous experience with the task. Formal cognitive assessments that may be used with a TBI population include the Allen Cognitive Level Test,[1] the Loewenstein Occupational Therapy Cognitive Assessment,[48] the Rivermead Behavioral Memory Test,[75] Kohlman Evaluation of Living Skills,[41] and the Cognitive Assessment of Minnesota.[62]

VISION

Clients with TBI should undergo a vision screening. The vision screening should be completed as early as possible in the rehabilitation process because early detection of vision deficits will allow the intervention team to obtain more reliable information regarding the client's overall health status. For example, diplopia (double vision) or accommodative dysfunction (inability to adjust focus for changes in distance) will probably influence the results of the neuropsychology or speech-language pathology assessments.

A vision screening is a tool that allows therapists to identify potential vision deficits. Although therapists cannot diagnose conditions of vision dysfunction, they can determine whether an individual passes or fails a visual screening based on standard criteria. The screening is a means to determine which clients require a referral to an optometrist or ophthalmologist for a complete evaluation and intervention. A comprehensive vision intervention program is designed by an optometrist and implemented by an occupational therapist or vision therapist. A vision history questionnaire should be completed as well. The vision history questionnaire should contain an ophthalmological history, questions regarding the use of glasses and contact lenses, and questions regarding the presence of blurred vision, dizziness, headaches, eyestrain, diplopia, and visual field loss.

Common areas evaluated in a vision screening include visual attention, near and distant acuities, ocular movement (e.g., pursuits and saccades), convergence, accommodation, ocular alignment, depth perception (stereopsis), and visual field function. Vision dysfunction can also be identified during the clinical observation of the individual's performance in functional activities. Tilting the head as a result of a field deficit, closing or covering one eye to decrease blurred vision, and bumping into walls or objects in the environment because of a field deficit or unilateral neglect are all easily observed behaviors indicative of vision dysfunction.

PERCEPTUAL FUNCTION

The perceptual evaluation should be administered when the therapist has obtained a clear understanding of the individual's cognitive, sensory, motor, and language status because deficits in these areas may skew the client's performance on a perceptual evaluation. Evaluation of visual perception should include right-left discrimination, form constancy, position in space, topographical orientation, and naming of objects. Evaluation of perceptual-speech and language function should assess for aphasia, agrommation, and anomia. Evaluation of perceptual motor function should include the functions of ideational praxis, ideomotor praxis, three-dimensional constructional praxis, and body schema perception (including the identification of unilateral neglect). Formal perceptual assessments that can be used with a population of adults with TBI include the Hooper Visual Organization Test,[36] Motor-Free Visual Perception Test—Revised,[16] Rivermead Perceptual Assessment Battery,[74] and Loewenstein Occupational Therapy Cognitive Assessment.[48]

ACTIVITIES OF DAILY LIVING

The intermediate-level client should be assessed in all basic ADLs (e.g., grooming, oral hygiene, bathing, toileting, dressing, functional mobility, and emergency response). The advanced-level client should also be assessed with regard to instrumental activities of daily living (IADLs), such as hot and cold meal preparation, money management, community shopping, (Figure 34-6) household maintenance, cleaning and clothing care, safety procedures, medication routine, and work readiness. The therapist will have ample opportunity during assessment to observe cognitive skills, perceptual skills, and behavioral appropriateness. Formal assessments that can be used with a population with TBI to assess ADL skills include the Arnadottir OT-ADL Neurobehavioral Evaluation,[3] Assessment of Motor and Process Skills,[24] Functional Independence Measure,[33] and Klein-Bell Activities of Daily Living Scale.[40]

Clients with a history of alcohol abuse require assessment of leisure patterns. An interest history and interest checklist may reveal healthful leisure interests that can replace alcohol use. The combination of leisure skills development and substance abuse rehabilitation will help clients manage time more effectively and thereby refrain from using alcohol after discharge.

Driving

Many states require physicians to report to the Department of Motor Vehicles anyone who has lapses of consciousness;

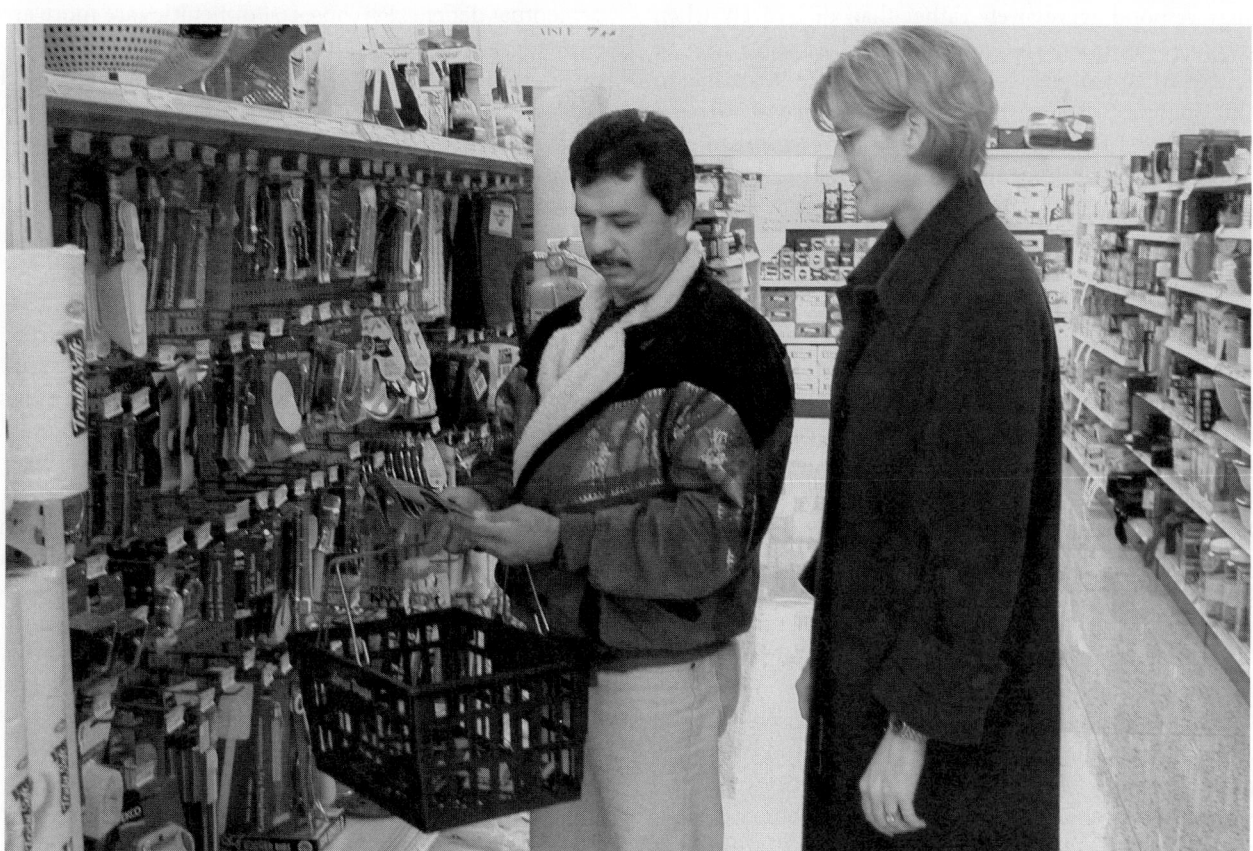

Figure 34-6 Community shopping.

seizure disorders; and cognitive, visual, and perceptual dysfunction caused by TBI. Regulations regarding such disorders often mandate that the driver's license be revoked until further assessment confirms that the person can drive without posing a safety risk to self or others.

Advanced-level clients with TBI who do not have seizure disorders or severe cognitive deficits must undergo a comprehensive driving evaluation to assess their ability to resume driving. Two types of driving evaluations can be completed: a clinical assessment (evaluation of the individual's visual, cognitive, perceptual, and physical status as it relates to driving) and an on-road assessment. Both types of evaluation are necessary because the client may fail the clinical assessment but pass the on-road assessment using compensatory strategies. Conversely, the client may perform successfully on the clinical assessment but fail the on-road assessment (see Chapter 11).

Clients with TBI frequently exhibit deficits (e.g., visual processing disorders, figure-ground discrimination dysfunction, and impulsivity) that significantly affect their ability to drive safely. When visual processing is delayed, affected persons hesitate during driving maneuvers and stop in an unsafe manner (e.g., in the middle of the road or at a corner) to allow themselves adequate time to process visual information. Those with figure-ground impairments may be unable to identify stop signs and traffic signals at intersections or locate the gearshift near the dashboard. Impulsive individuals may respond aggressively rather than defensively when driving, increasing the risk of accidents. They may use poor judgment when making driving decisions and be unable to inhibit inappropriate responses. The Elemental Driving Simulator[26] and Driving Assessment System[26] constitute an off-the-road clinical driving assessment that can be used, with an on-road assessment, to determine a client's ability to resume driving after brain injury.

VOCATIONAL REHABILITATION

Advanced-level clients may be evaluated to determine whether they are ready to return to work. It has been well documented that the return to work after a moderate to severe TBI is generally unsuccessful. High unemployment rates have been attributed to the adverse emotional, behavioral, and neuropsychological changes arising from TBI. Substance abuse in the TBI population is also a major factor inhibiting the ability to return to and maintain employment.[25]

The vocational assessment for the advanced-level client must involve assessment in the actual work setting because psychometric tests and job simulations in themselves do not accurately determine work potential. The client is often able to compensate in a familiar work setting for deficits that may appear as significant impairments on a psychometric test. The therapist's vocational evaluation should summarize the individual's interests, strengths, and areas of deficit.

The report should conclude with recommendations stating modifications required, realistic job goals, and a plan for achieving those goals with professional assistance as needed.

PSYCHOSOCIAL SKILLS

Advanced-level clients who will be discharged to home or a community-supported living residence should also receive a psychosocial skill evaluation. Such an evaluation should assess role loss, social conduct, interpersonal skills, self-expression, time management, and self-control. The therapist should also assess the client's social support system, ability to form and maintain friendships, and resources to decrease feelings of isolation (such as TBI support groups). The ability to form and maintain intimate and sexual relationships after TBI will be of paramount concern to single clients who sustained their TBI between the ages of 18 and 30. Child rearing and care of family members will be of concern for clients who are responsible for children and other family members.

The assessment of psychosocial skills in clients with TBI is critical. For 1 or more years after injury, clients with TBI report that their psychosocial deficits significantly diminish life satisfaction and are a greater problem than physical and cognitive deficits combined. Psychosocial impairment is often neglected in the rehabilitation setting, which prioritizes the intervention of acute physical, cognitive, and perceptual deficits. Psychosocial difficulties are more apparent after discharge, when the individual has left the structured and safe setting of the rehabilitation hospital to reenter the community. It is important to address psychosocial difficulties before the individual is discharged. Psychosocial assessment tools that can be used for this population include the Assessment of Communication and Interaction Skills,[63] the Occupational Role History,[23] and the Role Checklist.[54]

Marisol received skilled occupational therapy intervention throughout a 3-month inpatient rehabilitation stay followed by 6 weeks in a day treatment program. Marisol participated in a multifaceted spasticity reduction program and **neuromuscular re-education,** thus improving ROM and functional use of her right UE. As ROM and selective movement improved, Marisol learned how to feed, dress, and bathe herself with minimal assistance. As Marisol's head and trunk control improved, she was able to participate in all aspects of bed mobility and transfers. Daily guided self-care tasks were a critical part of her morning schedule. Performing meaningful, routine tasks allowed Marisol to work on her basic cognitive abilities. Spontaneous neurological recovery, cognitive re-education, and memory strategies improved Marisol's ability to plan, organize, and sequence her ADLs and recall her daily therapy schedule with occasional verbal cues. Marisol was referred to an outpatient occupational therapy program after discharge from the day treatment program.

INTERVENTION OF THE INTERMEDIATE- TO HIGHER-LEVEL INDIVIDUAL

Intervention of the intermediate- to higher-level individual involves two primary approaches: the *rehabilitative* model and the *compensatory* model. The **rehabilitative model** is supported by the theory of **neuroplasticity,** which holds that the brain can repair itself or reorganize its neural pathways to allow the relearning of functions that had been lost as a result of neural damage sustained in the accident. The **compensatory model** holds that the repair of damaged brain tissue either has occurred to its full extent or cannot occur, leaving the individual unable to perform lost functions without external assistance. Tools used in the compensatory model are adaptive equipment, environmental modification, and compensatory strategies that allow the client to perform ADLs. It is valuable to approach intervention using both the rehabilitative and compensatory approaches through addressing neuromuscular impairment, cognitive deficits, perceptual deficits, vision dysfunction, and behavioral disorders. In general, a rehabilitative approach is used in the acute stage of TBI recovery until the client has plateaued or progress has slowed, at which time a compensatory approach is attempted.

NEUROMUSCULAR IMPAIRMENTS

As with a beginning-level individual with TBI, numerous types of neuromuscular impairment can be present in the intermediate- to advanced-level individual. Spasticity, rigidity, soft-tissue contractures, the presence of primitive reflexes, diminished or lost postural reactions, muscular weakness, and impaired sensation affect the ability to perform activities independently and with normal control (see Table 34-3). The prerequisites for normal movement include normal postural tone, a balanced integration of flexor control (reciprocal innervation), normal proximal stability, and the ability to implement selective movement patterns.

The common principles of intervention for neuromuscular impairment are to facilitate control of muscle groups, progressing proximally to distally; encourage symmetrical posture; facilitate integration of both sides of the body into activities; encourage bilateral weight bearing; and introduce a normal sensory experience. The variety of effective rehabilitation techniques for this individual include neurodevelopmental intervention (NDT), proprioceptive neuromuscular facilitation (PNF), myofascial release, Rood techniques, and some physical agent modalities (see Chapters 28 and 30 through 32). These clinical interventions require education beyond the entry level and must be either incorporated into or followed by a meaningful functional activity that requires the same movement. The following brief overview of principles is merely an introduction and cannot substitute for training in the specific techniques.

The intervention of impaired neuromuscular control should begin at the pelvis because positioning of the pelvis affects motor control of all other body parts. A variety of approaches may be used to normalize pelvic positioning. For example, clients with TBI commonly have a posterior pelvic tilt. To move the client to a more functional erect pelvic position, a therapist trained in NDT might use an anterior pelvic tilt mobilization. A therapist with a different approach might use a bedsheet behind the pelvis to lift and rotate the pelvis forward over the heads of the femurs. In either case, the individual would be directed to raise the head, and sit up tall.

The trunk is positioned after the pelvis. Proper positioning of the trunk frees the UEs for functional activities. Major principles include the following: (1) facilitating trunk alignment, (2) stimulating reciprocal trunk muscle activity, (3) encouraging the individual to shift weight out of a stable posture into all directions (bending forward, bending backward, reaching to each side while laterally flexing the trunk), and (4) helping the individual move the lower trunk on a stable upper trunk or to move the upper trunk on a stable lower trunk. Once trunk control improves, intervention should progress to the UEs.

The competent practitioner may apply rehabilitative techniques in a variety of ways. The client with soft-tissue contractures or spasticity in a particular muscle group may benefit from NDT mobilizations and inhibitory techniques of the agonistic muscle group. The client with low tone or weak muscles (without the presence of spasticity) may benefit from NDT, PNF, Rood, and physical agent modalities. Kineseo-taping can assist with providing stability to weak muscle groups. Neuromuscular electrical stimulation can effectively stimulate UE muscle groups, including the triceps, pronators, supinators, wrist and finger extensors, to enhance muscle strength, increase sensory awareness, and assist in motor learning and coordination.[12]

Many advanced-level clients have fairly intact motor control and are able to ambulate independently and use both UEs in functional activities. However, close observation reveals subtle trunk and extremity deficits related to coordination and speed of movement. The intervention for trunk control focuses on developing full isolated movements of the trunk and extremities, good dynamic standing balance for all activities (including reaching and bending to high and low surfaces), and the ability to shift weight naturally from one LE to the other during activities. UE intervention programs are designed to increase scapular stability and improve fine motor control. A goal of intervention is to improve the client's speed while maintaining good coordination and minimizing compensatory strategies (Figure 34-7).

ATAXIA

Ataxia is a common motor dysfunction that occurs primarily as a result of damage to the cerebellum or to the neural pathways leading to and from the cerebellum. Ataxia develops early in the acute stage of recovery and may remain permanently. Ataxia is a clinical problem for which

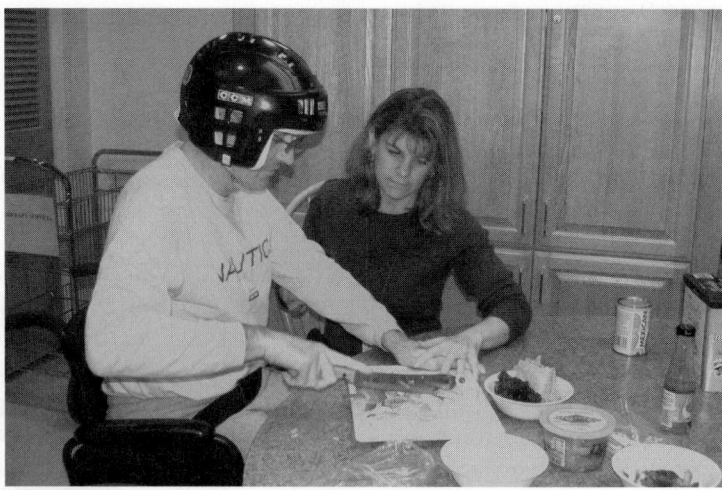

Figure 34-7 Use of both hands during meal preparation.

rehabilitation methods are generally ineffective. More often, therapists train the client in the use of compensatory strategies to control the effects of ataxia. For example, weighting of body parts and the use of resistive activities often improve control during the performance of tasks but show inconsistent carryover of muscular control when the resistance is removed. When applying weights to the client, the therapist must identify at which joint (or joints) the tremor originates. Applying weights to the client's wrists when the tremor emerges from the trunk and shoulders is ineffective. Weighted eating utensils and cups are also used as compensatory aids to reduce effects of ataxia in the UEs; however, these assistive devices are limited in their effectiveness.

COGNITION

Intervention designed to enhance cognitive skills should be implemented through functional ADLs and instrumental ADLs (IADLs). A common impairment of cognition is concrete thinking, in which the individual is likely to have difficulty with abstract concepts. Activities that require the generalization of skills from one task to another will be difficult for clients with TBI. It is best to engage these clients in activities that they need to participate in everyday life. For example, if the client will return to a community environment in which it is necessary to use public transportation, interpreting bus schedules is a meaningful and relevant activity that addresses many critical cognitive skills, including problem solving, planning, organization, concentration, frustration tolerance, sequencing, money management, and categorization. Another way to address the aforementioned cognitive skills is by planning a trip to the hardware store to purchase supplies necessary to install a hand-held showerhead.

Clients at an advanced level of recovery who demonstrate high-level cognitive skills often display subtle cognitive

deficits in the areas of organization, planning, sequencing, and short-term memory.

 OT PRACTICE NOTE

Activities such as establishing a monthly budget to live independently and negotiating the community public transportation system to pay a utility bill provide a context for cognitive retraining to address subtle cognitive deficits. Activities should be challenging, age appropriate, and relevant to the individual's real-life needs. Compensatory strategies may include the use of a schedule, memory book, electronic hand-held device, monthly budget chart, and the use of simplified maps of the client's community. For optimal success, the system chosen must take into account the client's familiarity with and motivation to use the given strategy. For example, a client may have used a high-tech cell phone as a day planner before the injury and may prefer to use this system after the injury as well.

Generally, neuropsychologists and cognitive educators have implemented the use of computers in cognitive retraining. Use of computer programs has not been shown to generalize to the cognitive skills needed to improve performance in IADLs.[53] Computers can be used in therapy if they are meaningful in the client's daily life; the therapist should address the client's specific computer needs. For example, by simplifying tool bars and menus and programming step-by-step written directions that appear on screen, therapists may reprogram a client's home computer to make it less complicated to use. Software programs that do not represent functional activities should be avoided.

VISION

Intervention alternatives for clients with TBI and vision dysfunction include the use of corrective lenses, occlusion (e.g., patching one eye), prism lenses, vision exercises, environmental adaptations, and corrective surgery. An optometrist or ophthalmologist can evaluate the client's vision and prescribe glasses to address accommodative dysfunction caused by brain injury. However, the glasses should not be prescribed until the client has passed the subacute phase of rehabilitation because an accommodative dysfunction that appears in the acute stage of brain injury may improve during the recovery process.

A common technique to eliminate double vision (diplopia) is patching, or occlusion. The client wears a patch over one eye, blocking the image seen by that eye and eliminating diplopia. Patching is a temporary compensatory strategy. An optometrist may prescribe prism glasses or binasal occluders for clients with consistent diplopia resulting from permanent oculomotor nerve damage. The prisms assist the eyes in fusing images. Prism glasses are not effective for those with a significant lateral strabismus or exotropia (outward eye turn). Binasal occluders encourage the malaligned eye to fixate centrally. Prism glasses and binasal occluders are used conjointly with vision exercises. The goal of this intervention is to decrease the diplopia and eventually eliminate the need for prisms or occluders.

Vision exercises consist of a series of activities that (1) maximize residual vision, (2) enhance impaired vision skills (the rehabilitative approach), (3) increase the client's awareness of his or her vision deficits, and (4) help the client learn compensatory strategies. Intervention progresses from monocular to binocular vision and follows a developmental progression (supine to sitting to standing). Exercises initially address basic skills such as visual attention, pursuits, and saccades and may progress to more difficult skills such as fusion and stereopsis. These vision exercises are based on the rehabilitative model that holds that impaired vision skills can improve with training.

Environmental adaptations for vision deficits are based on the compensatory model. Compensatory strategies for vision deficits include using a colored border along one side of a page to facilitate reading. A colored strip of tape along one side of a plate or meal tray to promote self-feeding is one option. Use of large objects, such as a clock with bold numbers or a telephone with enlarged buttons, is another compensatory technique. Contrasting colors to highlight controls and knobs (e.g., marking a TV/VCR remote control buttons with fluorescent paint) may be helpful. Increasing lighting in an environment and using textures as cues (e.g., placing textured tape on a banister by the bottom step to alert the individual that the bottom step is coming and thereby reduce falls) may be used for clients with low vision. The latter compensatory strategy is also valuable for clients with vertical gaze paralysis who can look neither up nor down.

Those who have lost pupil constriction should wear sunglasses whenever they are in bright light.

Corrective surgery performed by an ophthalmologist may be indicated to align the eyes and eliminate double vision; however, the individual must wait at least a year after the injury to allow for any improvement that may occur naturally in the course of recovery.

PERCEPTION

Treatment of perceptual deficits involves both rehabilitative and compensatory intervention. For example, impairment of figure-ground perception might be treated using a rehabilitative approach through the repeated practice of locating objects against a similar background (e.g., finding a white shirt on a bed with white sheets or finding a spoon in a drawer of similar stainless-steel utensils). Using a compensatory approach, the therapist would help the client to arrange the kitchen drawers so that utensils were categorized (perhaps color-coded) and distinctly divided to facilitate identification.

Aphasia (a perceptual-speech disorder) can also be treated using both rehabilitative and compensatory approaches. An expressive aphasia may be treated rehabilitatively through repeated conversation exercises in which clients are given feedback regarding their incorrect spoken words and challenged to express the words that they meant to verbalize. If the client has not made significant gains in expressive speech through the use of the rehabilitative approach, the compensatory approach should be used to help the client articulate his or her needs to caregivers. For example, a chart with letters, words, or pictures (or a combination of the three) of important items in the client's environment can be used to help the client identify needs such as eating, toileting, and medications. Such a chart may be used concomitantly with rehabilitative approaches.

Through a rehabilitative approach, apraxia can be treated by helping the client to perform specific tasks (e.g., hair combing) hand over hand (i.e., the therapist's hands guide the client's hands during hair combing). The rehabilitative approach holds that through repeated hand-over-hand exercise, the client's brain can repair the neural pathways that mediate specific motor patterns, such as those needed in hair combing, or can reorganize pathways so that different, undamaged areas of the brain can establish new pathways for specific motor patterns. Using a compensatory approach, the client may comb his or her hair by following the steps through the visual interpretation of pictures sequentially depicted (pictures) or listed (words) on a poster or note card.

Neglect syndrome (a disorder of body schema) can also be addressed using rehabilitation and compensatory strategies. Severe neglect syndromes tend to decrease as a natural part of the recovery process. However, some neglect syndromes may continue into the post-acute rehabilitation stage. With a rehabilitative approach, the client is encouraged to use the neglected extremity in all ADLs. The client's room may be rearranged to encourage interaction with the neglected part of the environment (e.g., placing the television or standing-bed tray in the left side of the room if the client has a left-sided neglect). A compensatory model is used when the client has not demonstrated significant improvement in attending to the neglected side of the body or environment. The meal tray may be placed within the client's field of vision to maximize success. A colored border may be placed on the left side of book pages to cue the individual to scan the entire line while reading.

BEHAVIORAL MANAGEMENT

The types of intervention strategies used to decrease and eliminate problem behaviors may be divided into two categories: *environmental* and *interactive*. **Environmental interventions** alter objects or other environmental features to facilitate appropriate behaviors, inhibit unwanted behaviors, and maintain individual safety. Agitated clients should be placed in a quiet, isolated room without a roommate. All extraneous stimuli (e.g., radios and televisions) should be removed. Similarly, therapy is provided in a private, quiet room away from other people and extraneous stimuli.

An agitated client who demonstrates severe behavioral problems may require one-to-one care. The client is assigned a rehabilitation aide who remains with the client throughout the day (including during therapy) to monitor and regulate his or her behavior. The rehabilitation aide may wear an alarm bracelet that signals staff when the client attempts to wander away from the appropriate floor or out of the building. Walkie-talkies and pagers may be used with those who are at risk of eloping. One walkie-talkie or pager remains in the nursing station; the other is held by the therapist or staff member who is providing one-to-one care to the client. If the client begins to act aggressively or attempts to elope, the rehabilitation aide can alert the staff that assistance is needed.

Interactive interventions are the approaches that the staff and caregivers use to interact with the client. The entire team should implement these interventions in a consistent way. Consistent implementation includes speaking in a calm and concise manner, deliberately refraining from detailed explanations that will only increase the client's confusion and frustration. For safety's sake, therapists should also keep the door open when working with the client at bedside and should always maintain an awareness of the individual in relation to self.

The client who is in the post-acute stages of rehabilitation and who continues to exhibit behavioral problems should be placed on a behavioral management program. Such a program should allow the client to experience the natural consequences of inappropriate behavior (e.g., losing community recreational privileges) in an effort to encourage more appropriate responses. Drug therapy may be used for those who do not make significant improvements in their behaviors and who present a safety risk to themselves and others.

DYSPHAGIA AND SELF-FEEDING

Intervention strategies for dysphagia follow the same guidelines as for other neurological impairments; intervention, however, may be more complex in this population as a result of bilateral neurological involvement, cognitive and behavioral issues, and severe neuromuscular impairments. A self-feeding program may begin in a quiet area, such as the client's room. Eating is graded to more social situations, such as the hospital dining room. Common pieces of adaptive equipment, such as a rocker knife, plate guard, and nonspill mug, may be used if the client demonstrates diminished strength, coordination, or perceptual deficits. If the client displays decreased attention, introducing one piece of adaptive equipment at a time may help. Clients who display heightened impulsivity may benefit from the strategy of placing the fork down after each bite to ensure that they completely chew and swallow before initiating the next bite. Depending on the client's level of dysphagia (i.e., pre-oral, oral, pharyngeal, and esophageal), a diet of thick liquids or puréed foods may be indicated until the client makes progress toward recovery.

FUNCTIONAL MOBILITY

Mobility training can be subdivided into bed mobility, transfer training, wheelchair mobility, functional ambulation in ADL, and community mobility. The NDT principles of bilateral extremity use, equal weight bearing, and **tone normalization** are used in intervention strategies that address functional mobility. The rehabilitation model, based on the principles of NDT and PNF, should be used with the intermediate-level client with TBI in the acute and subacute stages of rehabilitation. Allowing the client with loss of function to use compensatory strategies, such as grabbing a bed rail with one hand and rolling or standing on one leg to transfer, may appear to enable the client to function more independently earlier. However, the use of such strategies diminishes the client's ability to perform activities using a bilateral UE pattern at a later point. In time, the unilateral performance of activities results in hemiplegic postures, contractures, and abnormal gait deviations. Compensatory strategies should be used only in the later stages of recovery and when the client has not been able to demonstrate significant improvement in functional mobility skills and so must learn compensatory strategies to enhance the ability to live independently in the community.

Bed Mobility

An intermediate-level client with TBI may require training in bed mobility skills. These include (1) scooting up and down in bed, (2) rolling, (3) bridging, and (4) moving from a supine position to and from sitting and standing positions.

Wheelchair Management

Wheelchair management includes the ability to manage wheelchair parts (e.g., removing footrests and locking brakes) and propelling the wheelchair both indoors and outdoors on a variety of surfaces (e.g., low-pile carpeting, sidewalks, and ramps). Customized wheelchairs may be ordered for the client who is in the post-acute stage of rehabilitation and continues to exhibit neuromuscular impairment that requires use of a wheelchair for long-term mobility needs. A custom wheelchair provides a seating and positioning system that contours the client's body for comfort and skin protection, includes adaptive supports for proper **pelvic and trunk alignment,** and offers a seating position that enhances the client's ability to interact with the environment. Clients who cannot propel or control a manual wheelchair may require an electric wheelchair for independent home or community mobility.

Functional Ambulation

Functional ambulation refers to the ability to walk during functional activities. Whereas physical therapists address gait training, occupational therapists facilitate the carryover of ambulation skills into ADLs. Ambulation during ADL performance often requires the integrated use of UEs and LEs to carry and manipulate objects (e.g., carrying a plate to a table, holding a book bag or purse, sweeping with a broom or vacuum cleaner, carrying an infant). Functional ambulation also requires the ability to negotiate an ambulatory device (e.g., straight or quad cane and walker) with one or both UEs during ADL performance. This is a high-level activity that requires eye-hand coordination and the integration of total body movements. Compensatory aids to improve the client's ability to negotiate an ambulatory device while performing ADLs include walker bags and baskets, wheeled carts (to provide balance and support while transporting items such as plates to a table), canes with built-in reachers, pouch belts (to hold keys, wallet, and memory books), and apron during meal preparation (see also Chapter 10).

Community Travel

For clients who will be discharged to home or a community supportive living arrangement, the ability to negotiate their environment must be considered. Negotiating uneven sidewalks and curb cut-outs and correctly interpreting traffic light signals, as well as the direction and speed of oncoming traffic, are important skills to practice for safe and independent community mobility. Functional ambulation in the community requires the client to respond and initiate actions quickly—for example, to cross the street after the light turns green and before it turns red. Clients must perceive depth and spatial relations (to correctly judge the distance and speed of oncoming and turning traffic) and visually identify and avoid environmental hazards that could cause falls (e.g., potholes and cracks in the sidewalk). Electric mobile scooters or electric wheelchairs are often recommended for clients who must perform long-distance mobility in the community but who fatigue easily or are unable to walk independently. The use of an electric mobile scooter or electric wheelchair requires good static sitting balance and the ability to quickly integrate UE hand control and cognitive decisions regarding the environment. Practicing with clients during the wheelchair evaluation is crucial to determine whether they are able to safely propel an electric system within the community.

TRANSFERS

Because individuals with TBI commonly have memory deficits and limited carryover of information, transfer training should be consistent (in technique and sequence) among all staff members treating the client. It is preferable that transfers for intermediate- and advanced-level clients be practiced moving to both the right and left sides. Without this practice, clients who become proficient in a transfer toward the uninvolved side (in the hospital) may be dismayed to find that the home setting or public restroom requires transfers toward the opposite side. Additionally, teaching them to transfer to both sides provides weight bearing on both LEs, the use of bilateral trunk muscles, and bilateral sensory input.

Family members and caregivers should be trained in proper transferring techniques (including proper body mechanics) and cleared by a therapist before transferring the individual alone. The decision about when to begin caregiver training depends on the client's functional level and ability to cooperate, the discharge date, and the caregiver's physical and cognitive abilities.

HOME MANAGEMENT

As the client's skills and independence in self-care, dressing, self-feeding, and functional mobility increase, intervention is expanded to include home management skills in preparation for discharge to the community. Home management skills include meal preparation, laundry, cleaning, money management (e.g., balancing a checkbook, paying bills, and budgeting), home repairs (e.g., changing a washer in a leaking faucet), and community shopping (which includes planning a shopping list, locating the correct items in the store, and paying the correct amount of money at the cash register). Examples of high-level activities include planning a monthly budget, organizing a file cabinet, ordering from a catalog or the Internet, and filing income taxes. These are skills that adults need to live independently in the community and are thus relevant for most clients with TBI.

The degree to which clients participate in home management activities varies. For example, some prepare only simple meals, using a microwave oven. For those who must prepare meals to live independently in the community but who are not interested in cooking, the goal is to help them safely prepare simple hot and cold meals at home. Some clients perform no household cleaning activities other than making their bed and doing the laundry. Common sense dictates that therapeutic interventions first address the activities that the client performed before the injury.

As in all other areas of intervention, home management skills are graded to accommodate the client's functional level. Beginning meal preparation tasks may involve making a cold sandwich, whereas beginning money management skills may involve learning to perform basic cash transactions. As clients progress in home management skills, the meal preparation task may be graded to preparing a two-item hot meal using a stovetop, oven, or microwave oven. Money management skills may be graded to writing checks and balancing a checkbook. As the client continues to gain skills, activities requiring higher-level demands are made until the client reaches desired goals.

Childcare, if appropriate, must not be overlooked as an area of intervention. Family involvement is critical if a mother or father is to return effectively to his or her role as a spouse and parent. Sensory overload and its resultant agitation in the parent with a TBI are a commonly reported problem for families. Occupational therapy sessions should gradually reintroduce parents to their role of caring for their children. Some hospitals have a family suite in which family members can practice ADLs and interpersonal skills with the client on weekends, in preparation for discharge. This allows family members to gain a greater awareness of their loved one's impairments and need for assistance. It also makes the transition from hospital to home less stressful for both clients and family members.

The occupational therapist can also assist parents with TBI in the adaptation of strollers, cribs, and childcare equipment to make the handling of such items easier. Safely bathing or carrying a baby, preparing a meal while simultaneously caring for children, and one-handed diapering and dressing techniques are all examples of areas that could be addressed by occupational therapy services.

COMMUNITY REINTEGRATION

Clients who will be discharged from the subacute rehabilitation hospital to home or to a post-acute, residential supportive-living arrangement should receive training to facilitate the transition from the hospital to the community. Clients who achieve a maximal level of independence in the protected and structured environment of the rehabilitation hospital may find that community reintegration holds even greater challenges. Community trips—in which the advanced-level client with TBI is accompanied in the community by the occupational therapist (and perhaps a family member) to practice IADLs in the natural environment—should be implemented to provide the client with the opportunity to rebuild daily life skills. Depositing or withdrawing money from the bank or ATM, using the public transportation

system, planning a shopping list, and purchasing items at the grocery or hardware store are activities that will facilitate the beginning of the client's re-entry into the community. Having the client perform ADLs within the community setting will also allow the therapist to observe the client's ability to interact successfully or otherwise with the environment. The client will be provided with a chance to receive valuable feedback from others in the community regarding his or her behaviors.

Some clients are discharged from the subacute rehabilitation center to a transitional living center. Transitional living centers are designed to develop daily life skills by providing the client with an opportunity to live temporarily in a community group setting with 24-hour staff supervision and assistance. The goal of transitional living centers is to facilitate progression from supervised living to greater independence in community living. The client is usually discharged from the transitional living center to a relative's home or to a residential supportive-living facility that provides various levels of living arrangements (e.g., community apartments and shared community group homes). Because long-term residential community facilities for people with TBI are expensive for insurance companies, many are discharged home, where they receive continued intervention in outpatient rehabilitation or in day treatment programs that provide community, work, and school re-entry training.

PSYCHOSOCIAL SKILLS

Individuals with TBI commonly report one or more years after the injury that psychosocial impairment is the greatest obstacle to rebuilding a meaningful lifestyle. Many report feeling a deep sense of isolation and loneliness. Loss of roles such as partner or spouse, worker or student, independent home maintainer, friend, and community member often leaves individuals feeling as though they have lost their identity. The goal of the occupational therapist, particularly in post-acute TBI centers (e.g., day treatment programs, outpatient rehabilitation, transitional living sites, and long-term community supportive living arrangements), is to help rebuild desired occupational and social roles. This involves a three-step process: (1) identifying the desired roles that were lost secondary to TBI; (2) identifying the activities that would support desired roles; and (3) identifying rites of passage that were either lost or never transitioned through as a result of TBI. Rites of passage are socially recognized events that mark the transition from one life stage to another. Common rites of passage in Western society include obtaining a driver's license, graduating from secondary school or obtaining a higher education degree, securing full-time employment, living independently in the community, dating, marrying, and parenting.

Once desired occupational and social roles, activities, and rites of passage have been identified, the therapist facilitates the client's use of adaptation, compensatory strategies, and the integration of new learning. The therapist will also help the client enhance or regain interpersonal skills, self-expression, social appropriateness, time management, and self-control. Such psychosocial skills will be critical if the client is to re-enter the community—to live in a neighborhood setting, hold a job, perform volunteer work in the community, and participate in desired recreational opportunities along with other adult community members.

Group intervention is beneficial because it enables the client to meet others experiencing the same life concerns (thereby decreasing feelings of isolation). Groups can offer exposure to peer reactions, which is particularly helpful if the client exhibits socially inappropriate behaviors. Groups may also facilitate problem solving by providing the opportunity to speak with others who have successfully dealt with the same or similar problems. Participants who have been in the group longer can become peer mentors to new group members. The opportunity to help others—to share one's experience of having a brain injury with others who can benefit from that knowledge—has been shown to enhance an individual's life satisfaction, feelings of competence, and sense of usefulness. Many states have support groups for individuals with TBI, run by state associations for brain injury.

SUBSTANCE USE

If the client's pre-injury history includes substance use, the client should receive drug and rehabilitation services specifically designed for individuals with TBI. Clients with a history of substance use may not display any signs of a desire to return to substance use while in the structured and protective environment of the subacute rehabilitation facility. Substance use may become a problem only after the client is discharged to home, a community supported-living arrangement, or any residential situation in which long periods of time may be spent alone and unsupervised. Drug rehabilitation services are critical for clients with a substance abuse history because a return to substance use after brain injury has been closely implicated in the occurrence of a second TBI.

DISCHARGE PLANNING

Planning for discharge from occupational therapy services begins at the initial evaluation and continues until the last day of intervention. Components of discharge planning include a home safety evaluation (if the client will be discharged home), equipment evaluation and ordering, family and caregiver education, recommendations for a driver's training program (if indicated), and recommendations for successful return to school or vocational retraining and work skills.

Home Safety

If the client is to be discharged home, the therapist should visit the home (or transitional living setting) to recommend modifications for increased safety. For example, clients with balance difficulties should have grab bars in the shower stall. Increased lighting should be provided as necessary for clients with vision deficits because low lighting has been linked to falls. Recommendations should also be made regarding the client's ability to handle sharp items (e.g., knives or glass items that could shatter easily), use the stove, and remember to turn off the faucet and other appliances. The temperature setting on the hot water system should be set at or below 120° F to prevent scalding. Anything that could be tripped over (e.g., throw rugs, appliance cords, furniture legs, objects placed on steps) should be removed. If feasible, non-slip flooring should be added to slippery surfaces (e.g., bathroom and kitchen tiles). If a wheelchair is indicated, the therapist should recommend modifications to doorways and bathroom spaces and should suggest the replacement of high-pile carpeting with tiles, wood, or other surfaces that can be easily traversed by a wheelchair. Additionally, family members and caregivers should be educated in the appropriate steps to follow during a seizure, should understand how to evacuate the individual in case of emergency, and should practice methods by which to transfer the individual safely. Caregivers should be able to identify unsafe activities in which their loved one should not participate and should know the length of time that he or she can be left alone safely (if this is possible at all).

Equipment Evaluation and Ordering

Clients who will be discharged from the subacute rehabilitation facility will require an evaluation for equipment needed in the next setting. This may necessitate a reevaluation of the client's equipment needs because many of the adaptive devices that were valuable in the beginning and intermediate stages of rehabilitation may be discarded as the client improves. For example, a tub bench or shower chair may have been needed initially because of dynamic standing balance difficulties. This client may have progressed sufficiently during the course of rehabilitation to stand in the shower while using only a grab bar.

Family and Caregiver Education

Family members and caregivers should be involved in the client's rehabilitation from the beginning of treatment and should be considered members of the intervention team. Education of the caregivers in such activities as transfers, wheelchair mobility, ADLs, bed positioning, splint schedules, equipment usage, ROM exercises, and self-feeding techniques will facilitate follow-through with the skills that have been learned in the rehabilitation hospital. Individual safety is of primary importance for caregiver education. The caregiver should be trained in the implementation of the home program (in either written or videotape form). Home programs may include the areas listed previously, as well as specific activities for the improvement of cognition, vision, perception, and motor control.

Recommendations for Driver's Training

If the client passes the clinical driver's evaluation, the occupational therapist may recommend a specific number of hours of driver's training. An occupational therapist or a driving instructor who has experience working with individuals with TBI (see Chapter 14) should implement driver's training.

Recommendations for Vocational Training and Work Skills

If indicated, an occupational therapist may make recommendations for vocational training if the client is discharged to a day treatment program, outpatient rehabilitation center, or a transitional living site. Vocational training is an extended process requiring the involvement of an occupational therapist and possibly a vocational counselor. The client's eventual return to work may require the assistance of a job coach. The success of a client's return to work depends highly on the environment to which he or she is returning and the supportiveness of the environment. These are all aspects that must be considered when evaluating a client's potential.

SUMMARY

Treatment of the adult with TBI is challenging and requires flexibility, stamina, and creativity. Behavioral and psychosocial deficits greatly influence recovery. Substance abuse, a possible contributing factor, must be assessed and addressed. Most clients have a multitude of problems requiring intervention. Coordination of evaluation and goal setting with the interdisciplinary team (including the client and family) is assumed. Intervention should be individualized and oriented toward functional outcomes that are meaningful to the client. An effective transition from acute care to intermediate-level care and then to the community requires the therapist to plan thoughtfully and communicate clearly. For the person with TBI, recovery and adjustment may be a lifelong challenge.

Review Questions

1. What are two important measurable landmarks of recovery from TBI?
2. Name five types of neuromuscular impairment that may be present in the client with TBI.
3. Describe the types of care settings available for clients with TBI in the acute, subacute, and post-acute stages of rehabilitation.
4. Describe the psychosocial deficits that may be present in a client with TBI.
5. List two components of a behavioral management program.
6. Name three standard assessments for a population with TBI, and describe what performance components and areas they assess.
7. List four vision skills that are evaluated in a vision screening.
8. Why is it important for the client with TBI to complete an on-road driving assessment?
9. What are the goals of a proper wheelchair-positioning program?
10. What are the indications for splinting? Casting?
11. Describe three areas that should be addressed during discharge planning.
12. Why is it important to address substance use with a population with TBI?

REFERENCES

1. Allen CK: Occupational therapy for psychiatric diseases: measurement and management of cognition disabilities, Boston, 1985, Little, Brown.
2. American Psychiatric Association: *Diagnostic and statistical manual of mental disorders*, ed 4, Washington, DC, 1994, The Association.
3. Arnadottir G: *The brain and behavior*, Philadelphia, 1990, Mosby.
4. Avery-Smith W, Dellarosa DM: Approaches to treating dysphagia in individuals with brain injury, *Am J Occup Ther* 48(3):235, 1994.
5. Avery-Smith W, Dellarosa DM, Brod Rosen A: *Dysphagia evaluation protocol*, San Antonio, 1996, Therapy Skill Builders.
6. Bennett SE, Karnes JL: *Neurological disabilities*, Philadelphia, 1998, JB Lippincott.
7. Bombardier CH et al: The natural history of drinking and alcohol-related problems after traumatic brain injury, *Arch Phys Med Rehabil* 84(2):185, 2003.
8. Brain Injury Association: *Fact sheets*, Washington, DC, 1997, The Association.
9. Brain Injury Special Interest Group of the American Academy of Physical Medicine and Rehabilitation: Practice parameter: antiepileptic drug treatment of posttraumatic seizures, *Arch Phys Med Rehabil* 79(5):594, 1998.
10. Brain Trauma Foundation and American Association of Neurological Surgeons: *Management and prognosis of severe traumatic brain injury*, 2000, Brain Trauma Foundation, Inc.
11. Brain Trauma Foundation and American Association of Neurological Surgeons: *Management and prognosis of severe traumatic brain injury. Part II: Early indicators of prognosis in severe brain injury*, 2000, Brain Trauma Foundation, Inc.
12. Carmick J: Clinical use of neuromuscular electric stimulation for children with cerebral palsy. Part 2: Upper extremity, *Phys Ther* 73(8):514, 1993.
13. Center for Outcome Measures in Brain Injury, Santa Clara Valley Medical Center. www.tbi-sci.org.
14. Chestnut RM: The management of severe traumatic brain injury, *Emerg Med Clin North Am* 15(3):581, 1997.
15. Colarusso RP, Hammill DD, Mercier L: *Motor-Free Visual Perception Test—Revised*, Novato, CA, 1995, Academic Therapy Publications.
16. Corrigan JD et al: Systemic bias in outcome studies of persons with traumatic brain injury, *Arch Phys Med Rehabil* 78(2):132, 1997.
17. Cummings JL, Mega MS: *Neuropsychiatry and behavioral neuroscience*, 2003, Oxford University Press, Oxford, England.
18. Damasio AR: Aphasia, *N Engl J Med* 326(8):531, 1992.

19. Englander J et al: Analyzing risk factors for late posttraumatic seizures: a prospective, multicenter investigation, *Arch Phys Rehabil* 84(3):365, 2003.

20. Englander J, Cifu DX: The older adult with traumatic brain injury. In Rosenthal M et al: *Rehabilitation of the adult and child with traumatic brain injury*, ed 3, Philadelphia, 1999, FA Davis.

21. Englander J et al: The association of early computed tomography scan findings and ambulation, self-care and supervision needs at rehabilitation discharge and at 1 year after traumatic brain injury, *Arch Phys Med Rehabil* 84(2):214, 2003.

22. Fisher AG: *Assessment of motor and process skills*, Fort Collins, CO, 1994, Colorado State University.

23. Florey LL, Michelman SM: Occupational role history: a screening tool for psychiatric occupational therapy, *Am J Occup Ther* 36(5):301, 1982.

24. Ghajar J: Traumatic brain injury, *Lancet* 356:923, 2000.

25. Giacino JT et al: The minimally conscious state: definition and diagnostic criteria, *Neurology* 58(3):349, 2002.

26. Giatnutsos R: *Elemental driving simulator and driving assessment system*, Bayport, NY, 1994, Life Sciences Associates.

27. Goga-Eppenstein P et al: *Casting protocols for the upper and lower extremities*, Gaithersburg, MD, 1999, Aspen.

28. Graham DI et al: The nature, distribution and causes of traumatic brain injury, *Brain Pathol* 5(4):397, 1995.

29. Graham DI: Pathophysiological aspects of injury and mechanisms of recovery. In Rosenthal M et al: *Rehabilitation of the adult and child with traumatic brain injury*, ed 3, Philadelphia, 1999, FA Davis.

30. Granger CV et al: Functional assessment scales, *Arch Phys Med Rehabil* 74(2):133, 1993.

31. Hammond FM, McDeavitt JT: Medical and orthopedic complications. In Rosenthal M et al: *Rehabilitation of the adult and child with traumatic brain injury*, ed 3, Philadelphia, 1999, FA Davis.

32. Haltiner AM, Temkin NR, Dikmen SS: Risk of seizure recurrence after the first late posttraumatic seizure, *Arch Phys Med Rehabil* 78(8): 835, 1997.

33. Hart T et al: The relationship between neuropsychological function and level of caregiver supervision at 1 year after traumatic brain injury, *Arch Phys Med Rehabil* 84(2):221, 2003.

34. Haselberger K, Pucher R, Auer LM: Prognosis after acute subdural or epidural hemorrhage, *Acta Neurochir* 90(3-4):111, 1988.

35. Heilman KM, Gonzales Rothi LJ: Apraxia. In Heilman KM, Valenstein E: *Clinical neuropsychology*, ed 4, New York, 2003, Oxford University Press.

36. Hooper HE: *Hooper Visual Organization Test*, Los Angeles, 1983, Western Psychological Services.

37. Jackson WT, Novack TA, Dowler RN: Effective serial management of cognitive orientation in rehabilitation: The Orientation Log, *Arch Phys Med Rehabil* 79(6):718, 1998.

38. Jebsen RH et al: An objective and standardized test of hand function, *Arch Phys Med Rehabil* 50(6):311, 1969.

39. Kraus JF et al: Blood alcohol tests, prevalence of involvement, and outcomes following brain injury, *J Public Health*, 79(3):294, 1989.

40. Klein RM, Bell BJ: *Klein-Bell Activities of Daily Living Scale*, Seattle, 1982, Health Science Center for Educational Resources.

41. Kohlman Thomson L: *The Kohlman Evaluation of Living Skills*, ed 3, Bethesda, MD, 1992, AOTA.

42. Kreuter M et al: Partner relationships, functioning, mood and global quality of life in persons with spinal cord injury and traumatic brain injury, *Spinal Cord* 36(4):252, 1998.

43. Kubler-Ross E: *On death and dying*, New York, 1969, Macmillan.

44. Langlois JA et al: Traumatic brain injury–related hospital discharges: results from a 14-state surveillance system, 1997, *MMWR Surveill Summ* 52(4):1, 2003.

45. Levi L et al: Diffuse axonal injury: analysis of 100 individuals with radiological signs, *Neurosurgery* 27(3):429, 1990.

46. Levin HS, O'Donnell VM, Grossman RG: The Galveston Orientation and Amnesia Test: a practical scale to assess cognition after head injury, *J Nerv Ment Dis* 167(11):675, 1979.

47. Levy DE et al: Prognosis in nontraumatic coma, *Ann Intern Med* 94(3):293, 1981.

48. Loewenstein Rehabilitation Hospital, Israel: *Loewenstein Occupational Therapy Cognitive Assessment*, Pequannock, NJ, 1990, Maddak.

49. Mayer NH, Keenan ME, Esquenazi A: Limbs with restricted or excessive motion after traumatic brain injury. In Rosenthal M et al: *Rehabilitation of the adult and child with traumatic brain injury*, ed 3, Philadelphia, 1999, FA Davis.

50. Mazaux JM et al: Long-term neuropsychological outcome and loss of social autonomy after traumatic brain injury, *Arch Phys Med Rehabil* 78(12):1316, 1997.

51. McKinlay WM, Watkiss AJ: Cognitive and behavioral effects of brain injury. In Rosenthal M et al: *Rehabilitation of the adult and child with traumatic brain injury*, ed 3, Philadelphia, 1999, FA Davis.

52. *Minnesota rate of manipulation tests*, Circle Pines, MN, 1969, American Guidance Service.

53. Novak TA et al: Focused versus unstructured intervention for attentional deficits after traumatic brain injury, *J Head Trauma Rehabil* 11(3):52, 1996.

54. Oakley FM: The role checklist, *Occup Ther J Res* 6(3):157, 1986.

55. O'Dell MW et al: Standardized assessment instruments for minimally-responsive, brain-injured patients, *Neuro Rehab* 6(1):45, 1996.

56. Ownsworth TL, Oei TP: Depression after traumatic brain injury: conceptualization and treatment considerations, *Brain Inj* 12(9):735, 1998.

57. Palmer S et al: The impact on outcomes in a community hospital setting of using the AANS traumatic brain injury guidelines, *J Trauma* 50(4):657, 2001.

58. Plum F, Posner JB: *The diagnosis of stupor and coma*, ed 3, Philadelphia, 1980, FA Davis.

59. Prigitano GP, Schacter DL: *Awareness of deficit after brain injury: clinical and theoretical issues*, New York, 1991, Oxford University Press.

60. Quality Standards Subcommittee of the American Academy of Neurology: Practice parameters: Assessment and management

of patients in the persistent vegetative state (Summary statement), *Neurology* 45:1015-1018, 1995.

61. Ranchos Los Amigos Medical Center: *Levels of cognitive functioning*, Downey, CA, 1980, The Center.

62. Rustad RA et al: *Cognitive assessment of Minnesota*, San Antonio, 1999, Therapy Skill Builders.

63. Salamy M et al: *Assessment of communication and interaction skills*, Chicago, 1993, Department of Occupational Therapy, University of Illinois at Chicago.

64. Santa Clara Valley Medical Center: *Behavior Management Program Policy and Procedure Manual*, San Jose, CA, 2003, Santa Clara Valley Medical Center.

65. Seelig JM, Becker DP, Miller JD et al: Traumatic acute subdural hematoma: Major mortality reduction in comatose patients treated within four hours, *N Engl J Med* 304(25):1511, 1981.

66. Sosin DM, Sniezek JE, Thurman DJ: Incidence of mild and moderate brain injury in the United States, 1991, *Brain Inj* 10(1): 47, 1996.

67. Stratton M: Behavioral assessment scale of oral functions in feeding, *Am J Occup Ther* 35(11):719, 1981.

68. Tiffan J: *Purdue pegboard*, Lafayette, IN, 1960, Lafayette Instruments.

69. The Multi-Society Task Force Report on PVS: Medical aspects of the persistent vegetative state (first of two parts), *N Engl J Med* 330(21):1499, 1994.

70. The Multi-Society Task Force Report on PVS: Medical aspects of the persistent vegetative state (second of two parts), *N Engl J Med* 330(22):1572, 1994.

71. Thurman DJ, Jeppson L, Burnett CL, et al: *Guidelines for surveillance of central nervous system injury*, Atlanta, 1995, U.S. Department of Health and Human Services, Public Health Service, CDC, National Center for Injury Prevention and Control.

72. Traumatic Brain Injury Model Systems National Data Base Syllabus, 2003.

73. Tucker FM, Hanlon RE: Effects of mild traumatic brain injury on narrative discourse production, *Brain Inj* 12(9):783, 1998.

74. Whiting S et al: *Rivermead Perceptual Assessment Battery*, Los Angeles, 1985, NFER-Nelson.

75. Wilson B, Cockburn J, Baddeley A: *The Rivermead Behavioural Memory Test*, Gaylord, MI, 1991, National Rehabilitation Services.

76. Zasler ND: Prognostic indicators in medical rehabilitation of traumatic brain injury: a commentary and review, *Arch Phys Med Rehabil* 78(8 Suppl 4):12, 1997.

35

Degenerative Diseases of the Central Nervous System

WINIFRED SCHULTZ-KROHN

DIANE FOTI

CAROLYN GLOGOSKI

KEY TERMS

Amyotrophic lateral sclerosis (ALS)

Fasciculations

Alzheimer's disease

Huntington's disease (HD)

Chorea

Multiple sclerosis (MS)

Exacerbation

Remission

Parkinson's disease (PD)

Rigidity

Stereotactic surgery

LEARNING OBJECTIVES

After studying this chapter the student or practitioner will be able to do the following:

1. Describe the course of ALS.
2. Describe the differences between familial ALS (FALS) and sporadic ALS (SALS).
3. Describe the role of the occupational therapist for a client with ALS.
4. Describe the three subtypes of ALS.
5. Identify the symptoms and incidence of Alzheimer's disease.
6. Describe the pathophysiology of Alzheimer's disease.
7. Describe the overall model of medical management used by primary care providers and other health professionals.
8. Describe an approach to evaluation used by occupational therapists.
9. Identify stages of disease progression and general methods of treatment interventions associated with stages of dementia.
10. Describe the course and stages of HD.
11. Identify current research regarding the etiology of the disease.
12. Describe the medical management of HD.
13. Describe the purpose of occupational therapy for a client with HD.
14. Describe the three typical forms of multiple sclerosis.
15. Describe current research regarding the etiology of the disease.
16. Describe the symptoms of multiple sclerosis.
17. Describe complications that may occur as a result of the disease.
18. Describe the role of the occupational therapist for the person with multiple sclerosis.
19. Describe the course and stages of PD.
20. Identify current research regarding the etiology of the disease.
21. Describe the medical management of PD.
22. Describe the role of the occupational therapist for a client with PD.

CHAPTER OUTLINE

Section 1: Amyotrophic Lateral Sclerosis
  Pathophysiology
  Clinical picture
  Medical management
  Role of the occupational therapist
  Summary
Section 2: Alzheimer's Disease
  Incidence
  Pathophysiology
  Clinical picture
  Medical management

  Role of the occupational therapist
  Evaluation
  Intervention methods
  Summary
Section 3: Huntington's Disease
  Incidence
  Pathophysiology
  Clinical picture
  Medical management
  Role of the occupational therapist
  Summary

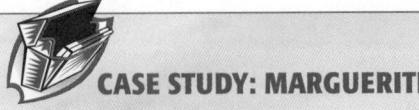

CASE STUDY: MARGUERITE

Marguerite is a 35-year-old woman who was diagnosed with multiple sclerosis (MS) when she was 26. Although Marguerite was initially identified as having the relapsing-remitting form of MS, her neurologist recently diagnosed her with the secondary progressive form of MS and referred Marguerite to OT. Marguerite now uses an AFO on her RLE when walking and has diminished sensation and dexterity in her nondominant left hand.

An occupational profile revealed the following background information about Marguerite. She is married and has two boys, ages 8 and 6. Both children are involved with soccer and swimming on a weekly basis. Her husband travels every month for his job as a sales manager at an insurance company. Marguerite is a special education teacher in an elementary school and works full time, although she was unable to work during relapses. She cares for her 69-year-old mother, who has been diagnosed with Alzheimer's disease. Her mother lives alone in her own apartment in the same city. Although Marguerite has two sisters, neither lives within driving distance; Marguerite has the primary responsibility of caring for her mother and her children.

Marguerite was asked to identify what areas of occupational performance were problematic or successful. She quickly replied that being a chauffeur for her children, a manager of her mother's medical care, and a housekeeper for her family were problematic. She felt as though she was constantly juggling schedules; recently, her children's swimming class changed to a different day, causing a big change in the schedule. Although she wants her children to have the opportunity to pursue sports, Marguerite finds it difficult to supply snacks every month for these extracurricular activities, an obligation that each participant's mother is expected to fulfill. Her husband does try to help with household chores when he is home, but he works long hours and does not have time to shop for the family's groceries. Marguerite is also responsible for arranging all of her mother's medical appointments; shopping for her mother, who no longer drives; and visiting her mother daily. Marguerite reports that she often feels so tired after teaching all day and running all of her errands that she has trouble making dinner when she returns home.

Marguerite was most comfortable with her work situation and reported that many of her colleagues had offered to help with various tasks such as playground duty or monitoring the students during lunchtime. This allowed Marguerite to have a brief break during the day to rest.

Critical Thinking Questions

1. What evaluations would you perform to collect additional data to develop an intervention plan?
2. Where would you start your intervention plan, considering Marguerite's report of her occupational profile?
3. How would the change in Marguerite's diagnosis from the relapsing-remitting form to the secondary progressive form of MS affect her current occupational roles?
4. How would the strategies you select for Marguerite be applied to other clients who have degenerative neurological disorders?

This chapter addresses the impact of degenerative neurological disorders on a person's occupational performance and outlines the role of occupational therapy (OT) in providing services to clients with these disorders. The specific disorders discussed in this chapter are amyotrophic lateral sclerosis (ALS), Alzheimer's disease (AD), Huntington's disease (HD), multiple sclerosis (MS), and Parkinson's disease (PD).

In degenerative neurological disorders, the disease progresses and an individual's occupational performance is often increasingly compromised. Occupational therapy aims to help the client compensate and adapt as function declines secondary to the disease process. Environmental adaptations and modifications are often necessary to maintain functional skills for as long as possible.

Degenerative neurological diseases may occur because of structural or neurochemical changes within the central nervous system (CNS).[55] In the disorders discussed in this section, the client's CNS usually functions normally during childhood and adolescence. After these years, the client experiences signs and symptoms indicating that CNS functions are deteriorating. The progressive nature of the disorder varies from person to person. Some clients have a rapid decline in function, whereas others maintain functional skills for many years.

The decline in function may compromise the individual's sense of self-efficacy in performing various tasks.[143] No longer is the individual able to perform personal or instrumental activities of daily life at the same level of independence. Dependence on others can alter the client's concept of self-worth and self-control. The OT practitioner serves an important role in reframing the client's sense of self even though functional independence may be deteriorating. A man with PD who is unable to dress independently may now direct a personal care attendant (PCA) or home health aide (HHA) to perform these tasks. A woman with MS who was previously responsible for household finances may need to instruct a member of the family to complete these activities.

The disorders discussed in this chapter are most often diagnosed during adult or later adult life, after habits and patterns of independent behavior are well established. A client may encounter a significant change in social relationships and interactions secondary to a decline in functional abilities. The OT practitioner must consider the ways in which progressive loss of function affects the client's social and occupational roles, whether those roles are as husband, wife, parent, adult child, worker, sibling, or friend. OT must address the needs of the client within the context of his or her social, physical, and cultural environment.

OT intervention aims to support the client's ability to function within his or her environment. The rate at which the client's symptoms progress influences the intervention plan. A client who displays a progressive loss of fine motor skills over 20 years has a much different profile than a client who loses all upper extremity function within 2 years. Use of adaptive equipment must be carefully weighed against the rate of deteriorating skills.

The OT practitioner must be knowledgeable about support services and respite care available to clients with a degenerative neurological disorder. A PD support group may provide the necessary social support for both a man with this disorder and his family. MS support groups may offer clients information regarding new intervention methods available, along with the opportunity to share life experiences.

An OT intervention plan should address not only the physical limitations associated with various disorders but also their cognitive, social, and emotional implications. Many individuals with neurodegenerative disorders have concomitant depression. Depression can be a reaction to the loss of function associated with some disorders or the primary symptom of other disorders. Occupational therapists should regularly screen for depressive features. An instrument such as the Beck Depression Inventory can effectively evaluate this component.[18,19] In addition to the evaluation of depression in clients with neurodegenerative disorders, cognitive abilities should be evaluated. Clients may have concomitant cognitive problems because of the destruction of neurological structures, and these deficits can have a dramatic effect on intervention. Brief assessments such as the Mini Mental State Examination (MMSE)[51] or the Cognistat[110] can be used to determine cognitive abilities and establish a baseline of performance.

In most cases, the occupational therapist is a member of a team providing services to the individual with a degenerative neurological disorder.[73] As a team member, the occupational therapist must consider the roles other professionals and family members play in the client's life and incorporate this knowledge into the intervention plan. OT practitioners provide a unique and needed service to individuals with degenerative neurological disorders. A client who is able to engage in meaningful occupations despite deteriorating skills reflects the significant contribution of OT.

Two case studies are presented to illustrate the similarities and differences among clients faced with degenerative neurological disorders. The first case concerns a woman who has MS. That case is presented at the beginning of the chapter. The second case concerns a man with PD and is presented at the end of the chapter to serve as a review. The cases should serve to prompt clinical reasoning and decision making as you read this chapter.

SECTION 1: AMYOTROPHIC LATERAL SCLEROSIS

Diane Foti

The term **amyotrophic lateral sclerosis (ALS)** is used to identify a group of progressive, degenerative neuromuscular diseases. The underlying neurological process involves destruction of the motor neurons within the spinal cord, brainstem, and motor cortex.[21,63] There is a combination of both upper motor neuron (UMN) and lower motor neuron (LMN) deficits at some point in the progression of the disease.

The term *motor neuron disease* is used interchangeably with ALS. In the United States, ALS is also known as *Lou Gehrig's disease*; in France, it is referred to as *Charcot's disease.*[20] As mentioned initially, the term *ALS* refers to a group of diseases. This group of diseases consists of progressive bulbar palsy (PBP), progressive spinal muscular atrophy (PSMA), and primary lateral sclerosis (PLS). Table 35-1 provides a description of each of these distinct subtypes of ALS. The classic forms of ALS are presented in this section.

The incidence of ALS is about 2.0 per 100,000 people. Approximately 5600 people in the United States are diagnosed with ALS each year. There are two forms of ALS: sporadic (SALS) and familial (FALS). SALS makes up about 90% to 95% of the ALS population. Between 5% and 10% of individuals with ALS are found to have a family history of the disease. Families with FALS have been found to have an autosomal

TABLE 35-1   **Clinical Subtypes of ALS**

Name	Area of Destruction	Symptoms
Progressive bulbar palsy (PBP; bulbar form)	Corticobulbar tracts and brainstem motor nuclei involved	Dysarthria, dysphagia, facial and tongue weakness, and wasting
Progressive spinal muscular atrophy (PMA or PSMA) (LMN form)	Lower motor neurons in the spinal cord and sometimes the brainstem	Marked muscle wasting of the limbs, trunk, and sometimes the bulbar muscles
Primary lateral sclerosis (PLS; UMN form)*	Destruction of the cortical motor neurons; may involve both corticospinal and corticobulbar regions	Progressive spastic paraparesis

From Belsh JM, Schiffman PL, editors: *ALS diagnosis and management for the clinician*, Armonk, NY, 1996, Futura Publishing; Guberman A: *An introduction to clinical neurology, pathophysiology, diagnosis, and treatment*, Boston, 1994, Little, Brown.
*The World Federation of Neurology Classification of SMAs and other disorders of the motor neurons does not identify PLS as a subtype of ALS.[20] This author is including PLS in the list in recognition of the many other articles and books that recognize it as a subtype of ALS.

dominant transmission pattern.[21] There is no difference in symptoms of clients with FALS and those with SALS. Differences between FALS and SALS pertain to age of onset and incidence. Onset for FALS is between 45 and 52 years of age, and onset for SALS is between 55 and 65 years of age. The ratio of male to female incidence for FALS is 1:1, but with SALS the ratio is between 1.5:1 and 2:1.[21]

As with other neurological diagnoses, multiple tests and a thorough neurological examination provide a differential diagnosis. Tests include electromyography (EMG) and nerve conduction velocity (NCV); blood and urine studies including high-resolution serum protein electrophoresis, thyroid, and parathyroid hormone levels, and 24-hour urine collection to assess for heavy metals; spinal tap; X-rays; magnetic resonance imaging (MRI); myelogram of cervical spine; and muscle and/or nerve biopsy.

PATHOPHYSIOLOGY

The etiology of ALS has not been established. There are multiple theories regarding the cause of the motor neuron destruction, including metabolic disorders of glutamate insufficiency, metal toxicity, autoimmune factors, genetic factors, and viral infection.[137]

CLINICAL PICTURE

The symptoms of ALS are variable, depending on the initial area of motor neuron destruction. The individual with ALS typically has a focal weakness beginning in the arm, leg, or bulbar muscles. The individual may trip or drop things and may have slurred speech, abnormal fatigue, and uncontrollable periods of laughing or crying (i.e., emotional lability). As the disease progresses, there is marked muscle atrophy, weight loss, spasticity, muscle cramping, and **fasciculations** (i.e., twitching of the muscle fascicles at rest). The individual may have greater difficulty with walking, dressing, fine motor activities, swallowing, and breathing. In the end stages

the individual may require tube feedings and the support of a ventilator for respiration. Half of all people diagnosed with ALS live at least 3 or more years after diagnosis. Approximately 20% live 5 years or more; close to 10% will live more than 10 years.

As ALS progresses, the disorder does not affect a person's eye function, cognition, bowel and bladder function, or sensory function.

Prognosis is difficult to predict. Generally, individuals with early bulbar involvement have a poorer prognosis. A more positive prognosis is usually associated with the following factors: younger age of onset; onset involving the LMN located in the spinal cord; deficits of either UMN or LMN, not a combination of both areas; absent or slow changes in respiratory function; fewer fasciculations; and a longer time from onset of symptoms to diagnosis. In some cases, the client's condition stabilizes, with little progression of the disease.[63]

A person with ALS differs from a person, such as Marguerite, with MS; with ALS the loss of function is more rapid, without episodes of remission. The person with ALS must cope with a fatal disease, whereas a person with MS must cope with a chronically disabling condition.

MEDICAL MANAGEMENT

The American Academy of Neurology has established practice parameters and standards to address major management issues for the person with ALS. An OT practitioner working with this population should be familiar with the standards to better understand the approaches and rationale for intervention. The parameters cover the following topics: how to inform the client of the diagnosis, when to consider noninvasive and invasive ventilator support, evaluating dysphagia and intervention with a feeding tube, management of saliva and pain, and use of hospice services.[89]

Symptoms such as muscle cramping, excessive saliva, depression, and pain are managed with medication. The patient's respiratory status should be reevaluated frequently to determine when noninvasive and invasive ventilator support is necessary. Swallow function should also be evaluated frequently to prevent aspiration and to determine when and if a feeding tube should be placed.

The Federal Drug Administration approved the drug riluzole (Rilutek) in 1995. Riluzole, an antiglutamate, is the first drug used specifically to alter the course of the disease by prolonging survival. In addition to inhibiting the release of glutamate from nerve endings, it blocks the amino acid receptors on the cell bodies.[137] Researchers believe that the success of riluzole indicates that an excess of glutamate leads to the death of the motor neuron. Research has shown that riluzole prolongs the life of patients with ALS by at least a few months.[106]

Other medications for the treatment of ALS are currently in clinical trial. These medications are ciliary neurotrophic factor (CNTF), insulin-like growth factor-1 (IGH-1), brain-derived neurotrophic factor (BDNF), and Sanofi Recherche (SR57746A). Exactly how these factors act on the motor neuron is unclear.[21,160] Stem cell research also offers potential treatment options for those with ALS.[151] The clinical trials are focused on extending survival and slowing decline of the disease.

It is essential to work with the client and family throughout the progression of the disease as needs change. The client and family members must regularly update decisions about care. Decisions range from when or if a wheelchair or adaptive eating device should be used to whether the client should undergo a tracheostomy, choose tube feeding, or use a ventilator.[32] Psychosocial support regarding decisions about the extent of life support and medical intervention should be provided by the entire healthcare team, with the physician and client having primary responsibility. The family's and client's cultural, social, and spiritual values must be understood because these factors will influence ongoing decisions about personal care and life support.

Cobb and associates[32] found that physicians frequently tell clients "nothing can be done" and that families often are not informed of services that can be provided by occupational, physical, and speech therapy. Education is needed for nursing staff and physicians to understand the occupational therapist's role in the treatment of clients with ALS. Ongoing OT assessment is essential to educate the client regarding ways to adapt functional activities as the disease progresses.

ROLE OF THE OCCUPATIONAL THERAPIST

ALS progresses rapidly, with ongoing deterioration of physical status. The intervention plan should focus on the client's participation in occupational performance because the client's functional status changes frequently and intervention focused on physical performance is limited. As the client's physical status declines, there is a greater need for environmental support through providing durable medical equipment,

modifying the home, and providing adaptive equipment. Depending on the client's level of understanding, life support choices, and acceptance of the disease, the OT intervention may focus on structuring the client's environment to support independence. Some clients with ALS may choose to have the maximum environmental and life support available to extend life. In this case, the occupational therapist may provide periodic reevaluations to determine the client's need for adapting self-care, work, and leisure activities. Other clients may request that no extraordinary life support be used, in which case the occupational therapist would assume a supportive role, perhaps helping these clients to create a memory book to give to their loved ones. Table 35-2 provides a list of the functional deficits at various stages of the disease and interventions that may be required. When referring to this table, the OT practitioner must remember that each client's clinical picture is unique and symptoms may appear in a different sequence than the table indicates. For example, a client with early onset bulbar signs may require earlier intervention regarding swallowing assessment and communication devices; another client may not need a wheelchair until the very late stages.

Individuals and their families require an interdisciplinary approach to the rapid functional changes, complex psychosocial factors, and quality-of-life issues associated with ALS. The impact of the disease on the client's quality of life is frequently examined. One study indicated that those who were less distressed and less depressed[96] and had a more positive attitude lived longer.[67] Fatigue and depression have been associated with a poor quality of life for the individual with ALS.[91] The same study found that disease progression was not necessarily associated with a poor quality of life. Hecht et al.[67] found that social withdrawal correlated with levels of disability; based on the results of this investigation, the authors recommended that mobility be improved with power wheelchairs and public transportation to prevent social withdrawal. Studies have also examined the impact of hope, spirituality, and religion as a means of coping with the disease.

OT PRACTICE NOTE

The formulation of the occupational profile during the OT evaluation can promote better understanding of the client's outlook and determine the most appropriate interventions to improve quality of life with this rapidly progressing disease.

SUMMARY

ALS is a rapidly progressing, fatal condition of unknown etiology. OT aims to maximize the client's function by providing interventions to compensate for declining motor function and by helping the client to achieve self-identified goals.

TABLE 35-2 **ALS Interventions**

Patient Characteristics	Interventions with Focus on Performance Areas of Occupation	Interventions with Focus on Client Factors
PHASE I (INDEPENDENT)		
Stage I Mild weakness Clumsiness Ambulatory Independent with ADLs	Continue normal activities or increase activities if client is sedentary to prevent disuse atrophy and prevent depression. Integrate energy conservation into daily activities, work, and leisure. Provide opportunity for individual to voice concerns (provide psychological support as needed).	Begin range-of-motion program (e.g., stretching, yoga, tai chi). Add strengthening program of gentle resistance exercise to all musculature, using caution to prevent overwork fatigue.
Stage II Moderate, selective weakness Slightly decreased independence in ADLs; for example, difficulty climbing stairs, difficulty raising arms, difficulty buttoning clothing	Assess self-care, work, and leisure skills impaired by loss of function; if patient continues to work, focus on how to adapt tasks with current deficits; assist with balance between work, home, and leisure activities; include significant others in treatment. Use adaptive equipment to facilitate ADLs (e.g., button hook, reacher, built-up utensils, shower seat, grab bar). Integrate hand orthotic use into daily activities. Perform baseline dysphagia evaluation; reevaluate throughout each stage of the disease.	Continue stretching to avoid contractures. Continue cautious strengthening of muscles with MMT grades above F+ (3+). Monitor for overwork fatigue. Consider orthotic support (e.g., AFOs, wrist or thumb splints—short opponens splint).
Stage III Severe, selective weakness in ankles, wrists, and hands Moderately decreased independence in ADLs Tendency to become easily fatigued with long-distance ambulation Slightly increased respiratory effort	Prescribe manual or power wheelchair with modifications to eventually allow recline or tilt posture with headrest, elevating leg rests, adequate trunk and arm support. Help patient prioritize activities and provide work simplification. Reassess for adaptive equipment needs (universal cuff to eat). Assess and adapt use of communication devices (e.g., regular phone to cordless or speaker phone; pen and paper to computer with adapted typing aid). Provide support if there is loss of employment or other activities; explore alternative activities. Begin discussing need for home modification, such as installing ramps or moving the bedroom to the lowest floor. Provide education regarding the types of bathroom equipment available for energy conservation and safety.	Keep patient physically independent as long as possible through pleasurable activities and walking. Encourage deep breathing exercises, chest stretching, and postural draining if needed.

Modified from Yase Y, Tsubaki T, editors: *Amyotrophic lateral sclerosis: recent advances in research and treatment,* Amsterdam, 1988, Elsevier Science. In Umphred DA, editor: *Neurological rehabilitation,* ed 3, St Louis, 1995, Mosby.

TABLE 35-2   **ALS Interventions—cont'd**

Patient Characteristics	Interventions with Focus on Performance Areas of Occupation	Interventions with Focus on Client Factors
PHASE II (PARTIALLY INDEPENDENT)		
Stage IV Hanging-arm syndrome with shoulder pain and sometimes edema in the hand Wheelchair dependent Severe lower extremity weakness (with or without spasticity) Able to perform some ADLs, but fatigues easily	Evaluate need for arm slings, overhead slings, mobile arm supports for eating, typing, page turning. Prescribe power wheelchair if the patient wants to be independent with mobility; controls must be adaptable from hand to other mode of control. Evaluate need for assistive technology such as environmental control systems, voice-activated computer; augmentative communication device. Help the patient prioritize activities, and consider negotiating roles with significant others. Reinforce the need for home modifications. Reinforce the need for shower seat or transfer tub bench and shower hose. Assist with patient's ability to participate in closure activities, such as writing letters or making tapes for children, completing a life history, and writing a log on household management for family.	If arm supports are not used, provide arm troughs or wheelchair lap tray for wheelchair positioning; wrist cock-up splints for full resting; hand splints may be needed for positioning. Provide pain and spasm management through the following: Heat, massage as indicated to control spasm and pain Anti-edema measures Active assisted or passive range-of-motion exercises to the weak joints; caution to support and rotate shoulder during abduction and joint accessory motions Isometric contractions of all musculature to tolerance
Stage V Severe lower extremity weakness Moderate to severe upper extremity weakness Wheelchair dependent Increasingly dependent in ADLs At risk for skin breakdown caused by poor mobility	Instruct family in methods to assist patient with self-care, especially bathing, dressing, and toileting; aim to minimize caregiver's burden and stress. Family training to learn proper transfer, positioning principles, and turning techniques. Instruct in use of mechanical lift if needed for transfers out of bed (patients in slings require head support). Adapt and select essential control devices for telephone, stereo, television, electric hospital bed controls for independent use. Adapt wheelchair for respiratory unit if needed to allow for continued community access.	Instruct family and patient in skin inspection techniques. Instruct in use of electric hospital bed and antipressure device. Adapt wheelchair for respiratory unit if needed; reassess adequacy of wheelchair cushion for pressure relief.
PHASE III (DEPENDENT)		
Stage VI Dependent, with all positioning in bed or wheelchair Completely dependent in ADLs Extreme fatigue	Eating: Evaluate dysphagia, and recommend appropriate diet; therapist may recommend tube feedings if patient is at high risk for aspiration; recommend suction machine for handling secretions and preventing aspiration. Augmentative speech devices may be recommended, in addition to speech therapy.	Continue with passive-range-of-motion exercises for all joints Provide sensory stimulation with massage and skin care.

SECTION 2: ALZHEIMER'S DISEASE

Carolyn Glogoski

Alzheimer's disease (AD), the most common form of dementia, is an insidious and progressive neurological disorder. AD is classified as a mental disorder by the American Psychiatric Association.[7] The exact etiology of AD is unknown. Because of the disease's damaging effects on the brain, higher mental processes are impaired, behavior is altered, and mood is disturbed. The onset of the disorder is gradual, with multiple cognitive deficits, a significant decline from previous levels of functioning, and noticeable impairment in social and occupational functioning. Effects on the motor and sensory systems are not apparent until later in the disease process. Dementia is a significant healthcare problem because of the increasing number of individuals who are living longer, the higher incidence of dementia among older persons, the very high cost of supervised care, and the extensive use of medical resources.[68] Early recognition of cognitive decline by physicians, occupational therapists, and all other healthcare professionals is critical. The AD diagnosis is often overlooked or mistaken for other disorders, especially in the early stages.

 OT PRACTICE NOTE

Occupational therapists have an essential role in helping the client with AD enjoy life and remain as self-sufficient as possible and in supporting families and caregivers over the course of this difficult disease.

INCIDENCE

Alzheimer's disease accounts for almost two thirds of the cases of dementia, and the incidence increases dramatically as people age.[46,152] Approximately 6% to 8% of adults 65 years of age and older have AD. The disease affects approximately 4 million people in the United States. Age is a primary risk factor. The incidence of AD doubles every 5 years after age 65, and AD is expected to occur in 20% to 40% of the population of old-old (85+ years) adults.[152] Family history is another primary risk factor for AD. Early-onset, familial forms of AD are linked to genetic mutations on chromosomes 1, 14, and 21.[60,89,147] Late-onset AD has been linked to the apolipoprotein E-4 (APOE-4) allele on chromosome 19, but it should be noted that this allele has also been found in older persons who do not have AD.[38,152] Previous head trauma, lower educational levels, Down's syndrome, and female sex are other potential risk factors.

Although the incidence of dementia is growing rapidly, it does not occur in all older adults. Many older adults experience a normal slowing of information processing but do not develop clinically significant cognitive deficits. *Senility* is a misleading and nonspecific term that has been used in conjunction with older persons and aging. Early signs of what could really be a dementing illness have been erroneously attributed to the normal aging process[152] and identified as senility. The use of the term *senility* perpetuates stereotypical impressions that progressive cognitive decline occurs in normal aging. Such ideas prevent early recognition and accurate diagnosis of dementia.

PATHOPHYSIOLOGY

AD is the result of degenerative changes in the CNS. Neuroanatomical (structural) and neurochemical changes occur in genetically or environmentally susceptible brains. The result of these changes is progressive and diffuse neuronal loss in the cerebral cortex and the hippocampus.[100,142] Pathological changes have been found through microscopic examination of brain tissue after death. These changes include increased neuritic plaques and neurofibrillary tangles, with loss of neurons and synapses. Early AD is associated with decreased cholinergic markers in areas of the brain where there is also increased distribution of plaques and tangles. Many of the changes in the brains of persons with AD can be seen only at autopsy, although neuroimaging techniques (e.g., CT, MRI, and PET) provide further diagnostic information such as enlarged ventricles.

Degenerative changes in the brain involve several processes that affect neurotransmission and result in neuronal death.[142] An inflammatory process causes the tau proteins in the cortical and limbic neurons to undergo microtubular dysfunction, preventing the neurons from sending nutrients and hormones along the axons. The paired filaments of these intracellular proteins actually become cross-linked in an abnormal metabolic process. These filaments form neurofibrillary tangles that eventually lead to neuron death. Neurofibrillary tangles are also seen in the temporal areas and to a lesser degree in the parietal association areas.

Neuritic plaques are large, extraneuronal bodies consisting of accumulated β-amyloid and neuronal debris—small axons and dendrites. This material degenerates, taking up cellular space. Extracellular accumulation of too much insoluble β-amyloid into neuritic plaques contributes to neuron degeneration. Distribution of neuronal plaques predominates in the temporal and parietal areas in early AD. The production of high levels of insoluble β-amyloid, associated with familial AD, has been linked to genetic markers on chromosomes 1, 14, and 21.[60,89,147] The accumulation of amyloid deposits may be affected by APOE-4 on chromosome 19 and can also affect the development of neurofibrillary tangles.[145]

The ongoing neurodegenerative process itself may lead to further damage to cell membranes, enzymes, DNA, and proteins through the excess production of oxygen-based free radicals.[142] The metabolic processes triggering excess free radicals may further be associated with activation of the amyloid precursor protein (APP) gene and the formation of insoluble β-amyloid.

Cholinergic dysfunction is the process responsible for the expression of clinical symptoms, such as memory deficits and word-finding problems, in early AD. Specifically, cholinergic deficits, thought to be linked to APOE-E4, include less choline acetyltransferase (ChAT) activity in the frontal cortex and less ChAT activity in the hippocampus and temporal cortex.[122,123,142] These areas of the brain are associated with the symptoms of AD, such as recent memory impairment and problems with executive functions.

CLINICAL PICTURE

Symptoms and patterns of behavior in AD are most often described in terms of stages. The simplest description of staging, useful for caregivers and consumers, defines the progression of AD either in terms of a three-point scale using early, middle, and late stages or in terms of a four-point scale (Table 35-3).[59,64,102] More clinically and diagnostically complex scales, such as the seven-point Global Deterioration Scale,[133,134] are used in research or modified for diagnostic purposes and used as part of an assessment battery.

The primary symptom of AD is impairment in recent memory that worsens with time, followed by at least one other cognitive deficit such as apraxia, aphasia, agnosia, or impaired executive function, according to the American Psychiatric Association.[7] Memory impairment involves increased difficulty learning new information and recalling information after more than a few minutes.[152] Over time, the ability to learn deteriorates further and the ability to recall old memories also declines. Symptoms such as speech and language problems, impaired recognition of previously familiar objects, and impaired ability to perform planned motor movement are more variable and may not be seen in all persons with AD. The expression of symptoms depends on the areas of the brain most affected by the disease. Executive function (the ability to initiate, plan, organize, safely implement, and judge and monitor performance) inevitably deteriorates as AD progresses. Visuospatial dysfunction is common. Mood and behavioral changes are often observed in the early stages of AD, with personality shifts and the development of depression, anxiety, and increased irritability. Later in the course of the disease, troubling behavioral problems such as agitation, psychosis (i.e., delusions and hallucinations), aggression, and wandering can emerge.[97,141,154] Motor performance areas such as gait and balance may become impaired, and sensory changes usually arise in the middle to later stages in the course of AD (see Table 35-3). Frequently, delirium and depression complicate the clinical picture. The life expectancy following the diagnosis of AD is typically from 8 to 10 years but can range from 3 to 20 years, with a variable rate of progression.

Deterioration in the individual's functional performance usually occurs in a hierarchical pattern. This pattern of decline consists of initially a gradual progression from mild impairments in work and leisure performance to more moderate difficulties in performing instrumental activities of daily living (IADLs) to a progressive loss of the ability to perform even basic self-care tasks in activities of daily living (ADLs). The trend is for cognitive deficits to increase and executive function to become more impaired (see Table 35-3).[28,53,56,144] Motivation and perception can influence functional performance but may not be routinely considered in individuals with AD.[56]

MEDICAL MANAGEMENT

According to Larson,[81] medical management of the individual with AD in primary care settings generally includes several areas. Many aspects of what is termed *medical management* may also be performed by certain other members of an interdisciplinary healthcare team, including the nurse, social worker, physical therapist, or occupational therapist. First, there is a need for early recognition and diagnosis of AD.[81] Second, there is the issue of how to intervene on behalf of the person with AD who is living in the community, before institutionalization or more restrictive care becomes necessary. The third area concerns intervention issues as the disease progresses. Last is the role of healthcare providers in recognizing and addressing treatment of other conditions that lead to excess disability in the person with AD.

Although dementia is relatively common in persons who are more than 80 years of age, such individuals often are not diagnosed until approximately 2 to 4 years after the onset of dementia symptoms.[80,81,83,95] A comprehensive physical examination, laboratory evaluation, mental status examination, brief neurological examination, and informant interview are essential in diagnosing AD. It is important to identify and treat medical conditions (e.g., metabolic disturbances, infections, alcohol use, vitamin deficiencies, chronic obstructive pulmonary disease, heart disease, and drug toxicity) that can contribute to comorbidity. MRI, PET, and CT scan results can be useful, but overreliance on these techniques should be avoided because their value is in identifying relatively uncommon, treatable causes of cognitive impairment. A comprehensive and skillful interview with a reliable informant is essential to the evaluation and diagnostic process in order to recognize decline by comparing current changes with past performance. Informant questionnaires, interviews, and screening measures may be performed by many healthcare professionals other than physicians and are important to the diagnostic process.

The goal of healthcare providers in the successful management of an individual with dementia, whether in the community or in a semi-institutional or institutional setting, is to "minimize behavior disturbances, maximize function and independence, and foster a safe and secure environment"[152] (p. 1367). Increased mortality is associated with dementia.[25] Regular health maintenance visits in primary

TABLE 35-3 **Progression of Alzheimer's Disease and Intervention Considerations**

Client Characteristics	Intervention Using Occupational Performance	Intervention Using Performance Patterns and Client Factors
STAGE I: VERY MILD TO MILD COGNITIVE DECLINE		
Feels loss of control, less spontaneous; may become more anxious and hostile if confronted with losses	Listen to client concerns; collaborate with client in identifying areas that are challenging, and identify associated feelings (depression or anxiety).	Encourage physical exercise and wellness behavior.
Mild problems with memory and less initiative; difficulty with word choice, attention, and comprehension; repetition sometimes necessary; conversation more superficial; mild problems with gnosis or praxis	Begin training the caregiver to serve as a case manager.[15]	Help client and caregiver establish a daily routine, and post it in a central place.
Seems socially and physically intact except to intimates; decline in job performance	Provide educational and other resources for disease information, support and relaxation, support groups, or activities for both client and caregiver.	Use environmental aids such as calendars, appointment books, adhesive notes, and notebooks to enhance memory and reinforce engagement in occupation.
	Identify roles, activity frequency, and configuration; encourage continuation of or increase in enjoyable activities by keeping a log and planning enjoyable activity daily or weekly[156]; use activity or task as a focus in socialization.	Identify appropriate environments, or adapt for activities that are currently challenging.
	Explore meaning of occupations and occupational role changes with client and caregiver.	In teaching new tasks, use auditory, visual, and kinesthetic input, and provide supportive or positive feedback; grade activity for success to decrease anxiety.
	Identify needs, preferences, and goals of the caregiver.	During communication training, rehearse with client how to use "I" statements and assertively express self and needs in response to changed ability and the feelings aroused.
	Discuss driving skills, and plan for future evaluation and restrictions.	Educate and train caregiver in how to empower client to keep active and facilitate initiation of tasks.
STAGE II: MILD TO MODERATE DECLINE (PROBLEMS FROM STAGE I ARE EXACERBATED)		
Use of denial, labile moods, anxious or hostile at times; excessive passivity and withdrawal in challenging situations; possible development of paranoia	Emphasize to caregiver the importance of environment in managing dementia at home.[36]	Maintain routines and design environmental support (e.g., lists, posters, and pictures) and level of assistance for cues to remember daily routine and important events
Moderate memory loss, with some gaps in personal history and recent or current events; decreased concentration; possible tendency to lose valued objects; difficulty with complex information and problem solving; difficulty learning new tasks; visuospatial deficits more apparent	Analyze and adapt meaningful leisure, home management, and other productive activities so as to allow the client to safely participate and exert initiation, independence, and control.	Avoid tasks involving new learning; help to simplify surroundings and tasks; make objects accessible, establish expectations for object use, simplify instructions, and clarify the meaning of "success."
Need for supervision slowly increases; decreased sociability; moderate impairment in IADLs that are complicated and mild impairment in some ADLs (e.g., finances, shopping, medications, community mobility, cooking complex meals); no longer employed; complicated hobbies dropped	Identify needs, and design ways to adapt and grade activity by simplifying complex tasks; train the caregiver to provide cognitive support (verbally) with the client on IADLs and some ADLs.[15]	Help caregiver interpret behavioral problems by understanding source of frustration and the effects of memory loss on behavior.
	Encourage scrutiny of family structure and resources to respond to increasing need for supervision; consider outside resource (e.g., day care, legal planning, friendly visitor volunteer, public transportation for the disabled).	Maintain socialization, and structure opportunities in which others initiate socialization to ensure satisfying relationships in group activity and other social activities.
		Use reality orientation activities, photo albums, and pictures around the home as a reminder of the past, past competence, and opportunities for socializing.
		Encourage stretching, walking, and other balance activities.

TABLE 35-3 **Progression of Alzheimer's Disease and Intervention Considerations—cont'd**

Client Characteristics	Intervention Using Occupational Performance	Intervention Using Performance Patterns and Client Factors
STAGE III: MODERATE TO MODERATELY SEVERE DECLINE IN COGNITION (PROBLEMS FROM STAGE II ARE EXACERBATED—DIFFICULTIES INVOLVING PHYSICAL STATUS MORE)		
Reduced affect, increased apathy; sleep disturbances; repetitive behaviors; hostile behavior, paranoia, delusions, agitation and violence possible if client becomes overwhelmed	Maintain involvement in meaningful activity and reactivate alternative roles; identify and design tasks in home management activity; client can assist caregiver with design of productive activity related to former work role.[86,87,159]	In managing problem behaviors (e.g., assaultive behavior), teach caregivers to identify problem, understand and consider possible precipitants for the behavior (e.g., feelings; antecedent events; who, where, when; medical problem or task; environment; or communication problem), and adapt own behavior or change the environment.[29,41,167]
Progressive memory loss of well-known material; some past history retained; client unaware of most recent events; disorientation to time and place and sometimes extended family; progressively impaired concentration; deficits in communication severe; apraxia and agnosia more evident	Help caregiver problem solve and recognize degree of need for initiation, verbal cues, physical assistance, and ADLs; provide time orientation; simplify environment. Support socialization at home and with family or in structured settings outside of the home.	It is essential to maintain consistent daily routines as means of facilitating participation in overlearned tasks, maintain function, and continue to define the self.[29] Teach family that overlearned tasks are possible but require safe environment; overall, tasks take longer, need to be simplified, and require setup and grading to comprise two steps or less.
Slowed response, impaired visual and functional spatial orientation Unable to perform most IADLs; in ADLs, assistance eventually needed with toileting, hygiene, eating, and dressing; beginning signs of urinary and fecal incontinence; wandering behavior	Ensure safety in the home and other environments by making adaptations suited to level of client functioning (e.g., alarms, restricted use of heating devices and sharps, cabinet latches, ID bracelet, visual cues for item location, and visual camouflaging).[30,52,72,146]	Make further environmental adaptations to compensate for perceptual deficits and ensure safe mobility. Rehearse and review names of family and others, using pictures. Encourage standby or assisted ambulation, stretching, and exercise on a regular basis. In new environments, cue and assist client in navigation, and provide more light and pictorial representations to cue.
STAGE IV: SEVERE COGNITIVE DECLINE AND MODERATE TO SEVERE PHYSICAL DECLINE		
Memory impairment severe; may forget family member's name but still recognize familiar people; can become confused even in familiar surroundings Gait and balance disturbances; difficulty negotiating environmental barriers; generalized motoric slowing Often unable to communicate except by grunting or saying single word; psychomotor skills deteriorate until unable to walk; incontinent of both urine and feces; unable to eat; often becomes necessary to place client in nursing home at this time	For ADLs (hygiene, feeding), instruct caregivers (family or nursing assistants) regarding need for simple communication, one-step commands, step-by-step verbal cues, and physical guidance. Encourage continued socialization by family; socialization depends on initiation of conversation by others and may not consistently include a response from the client. Use dysphagia techniques to promote swallowing, prevent choking, and encourage eating. Instruct family in transfer techniques.	Encourage caregiver to use respite programs and maintain recreation and leisure activity for himself or herself. Encourage assisted ambulation methods until client is no longer able to use them. Maintain proper positioning in bed and wheelchair; instruct family in skin inspection. Provide controlled sensory stimulation involving sound, touch, vision, and olfaction to maintain contact with reality. Begin program of active and assisted and passive ROM exercises.

Adapted from Baum C: Addressing the needs of the cognitively impaired elderly from a family policy perspective, *Am J Occup Ther* 45:594, 1991; Morscheck P: An overview of Alzheimer's disease and long term care, *Pride J Long-Term Health Care* 3:4, 1984; Glickstein J: *Therapeutic interventions in Alzheimer's disease*, Gaithersburg, MD, 1997, Aspen; Gwyther L, Matteson M: Care for the caregivers, *J Gerontol Nurs* 9, 1983.

care settings to identify treatable illnesses such as depression, Parkinson's disease, low folate levels, arthritic conditions, urinary tract infections, and other conditions that may exacerbate dementia are important for all older adults, but especially those with AD.[85,142]

Depression and dementia easily may be mistaken for each other, or they may coexist.[152] Careful attention to whether the onset of symptoms has been gradual (dementia) or more recent (depression) is an important diagnostic issue because affective and cognitive symptoms frequently occur together.[132] Cognitive impairments and especially functional performance may improve in individuals with both dementia and depression after they are treated for depression. Delirium (i.e., impairment in attention, alertness, and perception) and dementia frequently coexist as well, especially in hospital settings.[152] Both conditions involve global cognitive impairment, but delirium is usually acute in onset, shows fluctuating symptoms, disrupts consciousness and attention, and interferes with sleep. Adverse drug reactions are more common in AD because of the vulnerable, impaired brain.[82] Often, a cause of delirium, such as drug toxicity, is treatable.

Hearing, vision, and other sensory impairments are known to make dementia worse and cause greater strain on the caregiver.[161,162] Falls with hip fractures are 5 to 10 times more common in persons with AD than in normal persons of the same age and often result in earlier institutionalization for the individual and the need for higher levels of care.[26] Unsafe mobility quickly becomes an overwhelming burden for caregivers, especially those who are aged.

According to Small and colleagues,[152] pharmacotherapy for the treatment of individuals with AD should be assessed carefully and justified at regular intervals. Although OT practitioners do not prescribe medications, knowledge of pharmacotherapy is useful. Cholinesterase inhibitors such as tacrine and donepezil may improve cognition and functional performance, at least in the short term. Promising research is under way in this area. Other agents that may improve cognitive function include estrogen, nonsteroidal antiinflammatory agents, gingko biloba, and vitamin E.[141] Evidence about the benefits of these agents is inconclusive. Antidepressant medications, especially selective serotonin reuptake inhibitors (SSRIs), are often prescribed.[152] However, some of the tricyclic antidepressants (e.g., amitriptyline, imipramine, and clomipramine) and monoamine oxidase inhibitors (MAOIs) can have troublesome side effects in older adults. Atypical antipsychotics such as clozapine, risperidone, and olanzapine may be used to reduce agitation and psychosis.[93,152] Benzodiazepines are prescribed for treating anxiety and infrequent agitation but have been found to be less effective than antipsychotics when the symptoms are severe.[152]

ROLE OF THE OCCUPATIONAL THERAPIST

In the early stages of AD, most individuals with the disorder live alone or with family and friends, rather than in institutions. A predominant feature of AD is significant and progressive deterioration of function from previous levels of performance because of advancing brain atrophy and pathological tissue changes. These changes cause deficits in client factors, which in turn lead to deterioration in occupational performance and major changes in occupational roles. Over time, more structured and supervised living environments are needed. Increased difficulties in performing everyday functions create challenges for the individual with AD and have an impact on the quality of life for the client, family, and caregivers as the disease progresses. Effective OT interventions must be directed at supporting occupational performance for the individual. Intervention should focus on maintaining capabilities and adapting tasks and environments or otherwise compensating for declining function in individuals with AD while trying to help them retain as much control as possible over their lives in the least restrictive environment.[6]

ETHICAL CONSIDERATIONS

Support for the caregiver is a must. Collaboration with and training of the caregiver is essential in the management of clients with dementia. Family members should encounter an open and encouraging environment in which to discuss safety, security, and dependence issues. Legal, financial, and health concerns that require advance directives (e.g., medical and legal), trusts, activity restrictions (e.g., driving, financial matters, and medication management), and contingency and transitional care plans (e.g., day care, residential care, and long-term care) are important in preparation for the inevitable progression of the disease.[81,151]

Behavioral problems can be expected in the client with AD until the terminal or bed-bound stage. Encouragement to use respite care, in-home support services, and support groups is important. Caregivers also need effective strategies for dealing with behavioral disturbances and disruptions in mood. The use of environmental adaptations, therapeutic interpersonal approaches, referral to other disciplines, and resource sharing helps in collaborating with the client's family and handling these problems. Health professionals use education, training, counseling, and support to help caregivers deal with their feelings, manage behaviors, and maintain quality of life for themselves and for the client with AD. Awareness of the multidimensional effects of this illness on the individual, the family, and the society at large is important to promote more effective and efficient care.[129]

EVALUATION

An OT screening is often performed before the evaluation. OT services are indicated for individuals who have demonstrated a recent decline in function; whose behaviors pose a safety hazard to family, staff, other residents, or self; or who may experience improved quality of life.[23] Much of the therapist's time in community settings and in long-term care is spent helping families and caregivers develop strategies and environmental adaptations to cope with the overwhelming stresses of safely managing a cognitively impaired individual.[15]

The type of assessment and the depth of the evaluation process used are influenced by the setting, the stage of progression of AD, the reimbursement process, the presence of other medical and mental health disorders, and the cooperation and interest of the caregiver or care staff. The consequences of caregiving and the needs of the caregiver can vary greatly, depending on gender, family relationships, culture, and ethnicity. The caregiver's understanding of dementia, reaction to dementia-related behaviors, use of problem-solving skills, use of the environment, use of formal and informal support systems, and decision-making style greatly affect the caregiver's ability to participate in the care plan and treatment of persons with dementia.[13,37,45,90,165]

Evaluation should be comprehensive despite changing reimbursement. Much information can be gathered before an interview and intervention session by asking caregivers, family members, and staff informants to complete questionnaires and rating scales. These scales assess occupational performance, functional abilities, and skills using measures such as the Functional Behavior Profile,[17] the Activity Profile,[15] the Caregiver's Strain Questionnaire,[138] the Katz Activities of Daily Living Scale (KADL),[77] and the Instrumental Activities of Daily Living Scale (IADL).[84] Informant rating measures should routinely be followed by an interview either before or during the first visit. The use of a few brief screening instruments for mental status (e.g., the MMSE),[51] depression,[19,166] and anxiety[85] provides baseline data and a wealth of information about factors that are likely to influence performance.

The functional evaluation of an individual with AD depends on the stage of cognitive decline.[6] The American Occupational Therapy Association's statement on services for persons with AD suggests that tasks involving work, home management, driving skills, and safety should be targeted in the early stages of the disease. In the later stages, the focus shifts to self-care, mobility, communication, and leisure skills.

The concerns and observations of the caregiver are important, but the therapist's observation of task performance is also necessary. Unfortunately, many of the functional ADL scales developed for use with older adults have targeted physical performance and are not appropriate for persons experiencing cognitive decline.[56] Fortunately, several excellent, standardized measures that determine whether individuals are able to use their cognitive skills to perform tasks in ADLs and IADLs have been developed over the last 15 years. The Kitchen Task Assessment (KTA) determines the level of cognitive support a person with AD needs to complete a cooking task successfully.[16] The Allen Cognitive Level (ACL)[1] test determines the quality of problem solving an individual

uses while engaged in perceptual motor tasks. Levy[87,88] has written at great length about the use of the ACL for clients with cognitive impairments. Consistent with the Allen theoretical approach, the Cognitive Performance Test (CPT)[2,27] was developed to identify cognitive deficits that are predictive of functional capacity using several ADL and IADL tasks. Another measure, the Assessment of Motor and Process Skills (AMPS),[48] has been used with individuals who have dementia.[48,113] The AMPS measures motor (e.g., posture, mobility, and strength) and process (e.g., attentional, organizational, and adaptive) skills by using task performance in IADLs. The Disability Assessment for Dementia (DAD)[56] uses informant ratings to determine the ability of the individual with AD to complete tasks in both ADLs and IADLs. The DAD also provides information relevant to executive functioning, such as the person's ability to initiate, plan, and execute the activity. Further information regarding the evaluation of cognitive function and ADL performance is given in Chapters 10 and 25. After obtaining through evaluation a good understanding of the disease process and the functional level of the person with AD, the therapist can begin to look at the all-important question of what aspects of the occupational performance context, especially the environment and care provider interactions, must be modified to optimize function of the person with AD.[113]

INTERVENTION METHODS

The goals of OT services are to provide services to persons with dementia and their families and caregivers so as to emphasize remaining strengths, maintain physical and mental activity for as long as possible, decrease caregiver stress, and keep the person in the least restrictive setting possible.[7,9,65,76] Intervention planning takes into account the progressive nature of the disorder, the expected decline in function, and the care setting itself. OT interventions for clients with dementia are directed toward maintaining, restoring, or improving functional capacity; promoting participation in occupations that are satisfying and that optimize health and well-being; and easing the burdens of caregiving.[15] The methods therapists use in the intervention process include activity analysis, caregiver training, behavior management techniques, environmental modification, use of purposeful activity, and the provision of resources and referrals. Services are provided in many different settings, such as home care, adult daycare, and semi-institutional or institutional long-term care. The intervention setting and the stage of the illness help frame the focus of intervention, determine the recipients of service, and prescribe the methods used (see Table 35-3).

SUMMARY

AD is a neurological condition characterized by the development of multiple cognitive impairments with a gradual onset. The effect of these impairments is a significant and progressive decline from previous levels of functioning. The course of the disorder is variable, but loss of function generally occurs in a hierarchical pattern, beginning with work and progressing to difficulties with home management, driving, and safety until even basic self-care skills such as dressing, functional mobility, toileting, communication, and feeding are affected.

OT interventions should be directed at enhancing the abilities of the client with AD by continually adapting tasks of daily living and modifying the physical and social environment as the client experiences progressive loss of function. Given many of the current limitations in treatment time imposed by third-party payment, therapists may find it useful to employ some of the self-report and informant report measures identified in this chapter as a means of gathering information more efficiently during the evaluation process. Several standardized measures also have been identified to assist with the assessment of functional performance and the establishment of a baseline of performance. Recommendations for OT treatment of AD have been identified. The focus of intervention must be flexible and depends on an understanding of the particular expression of the disease process in the client, the specific treatment setting, and the needs of the caregiver. Generally, the goals of OT services for persons with dementia are to maintain or enhance function, promote continued participation in meaningful occupation, optimize health and quality of life, and work collaboratively with the caregiver to ease the burden of caregiving.

SECTION 3: HUNTINGTON'S DISEASE

Winifred Schultz-Krohn

INCIDENCE

Huntington's disease (HD) is a fatal, degenerative neurological disorder that affects 5 to 10 of every 100,000 individuals.[58,120] The disorder is transmitted in an autosomal dominant pattern. Each offspring of an affected parent has a 50% chance of having HD. Genetic studies have identified a mutation on chromosome 4 as the cause of this disease.[107,120,128,131] Presymptomatic diagnosis of HD is possible with genetic testing when the family history shows this disease.[118,120] Diagnosis is also made through clinical examination when the family history is unavailable or unknown.

PATHOPHYSIOLOGY

The neurological structure associated with HD is the corpus striatum. Deterioration of the caudate nucleus is more severe and occurs earlier than atrophy of the putamen.[31,116] The corpus striatum plays an important role in motor control, and deterioration in this area contributes to the chorea associated with HD. The caudate nucleus is also linked to cognitive and emotional function through connections with the cerebral cortex. A progressive loss of tissue occurs in the frontal cortex, globus pallidus, and thalamus as the disease

advances.[120] The degeneration of the corpus striatum results in a decrease in the neurotransmitter gamma-aminobutyric acid (GABA). Additional deficiencies in acetylcholine and substance P, both neurotransmitters, are noted in clients with HD. The triggering mechanism for the neuronal degeneration has not been clearly identified, but it is linked to genetic coding on chromosome 4.[131]

CLINICAL PICTURE

HD is characterized by progressive disorders of both voluntary and involuntary movement, in addition to a significant deterioration of cognitive and behavioral abilities.[120,148] A client usually experiences an insidious onset of symptoms in the third to fourth decade of life, but cases have been reported in teenage and younger clients.[164] Clients who are positively identified by genetic testing should be carefully monitored for the first indications of HD symptoms. Not all individuals who have the potential to develop HD because of family history elected to undergo genetic testing, a fact that may affect determination of the time at which first symptoms emerged. The symptoms progress over a 15- to 20-year period, ultimately necessitating long-term care or hospitalization for the client.[120] Death is often the result of secondary causes, such as pneumonia.[118]

The initial symptoms vary but are most often reported as alterations in behavior, changes in cognitive function, and choreiform movements of the hands.[164] The early symptoms of cognitive disturbances are probably related to the degeneration of the caudate nucleus. The client may appear forgetful or display difficulty in concentrating. During the initial stages of HD, a client may have difficulty maintaining adequate work performance. Family members often identify the initial behavioral changes seen in the person with HD as increased irritability or depression. Irritability and depression may be attributed inappropriately to the decline in work performance rather than to the disease process. Emotional and behavioral changes are often the earliest symptoms of HD.[50] **Chorea,** seen in clients with HD, consists of rapid, involuntary, irregular movements.[119] During the early stages of HD, chorea is often limited to the hands. A client may mask the initial chorea by engaging in behaviors such as manipulating small objects within the hands. These irregular movements are exacerbated during stressful conditions and decrease during voluntary motor activities. Chorea is absent when the client is sleeping. Onset of HD in teenage years is associated more often with early symptoms of **rigidity** than with chorea.[164]

Cognitive and emotional abilities progressively deteriorate over the course of the disease.[164] Disturbances in memory and in decision-making skills become more apparent during the middle stages of HD. Establishing and maintaining meaningful habits and routines for the individual who has HD are important ways to support continued participation in occupational pursuits. A client may be able to complete familiar tasks at work or in the home, but if the environment is changed or if additional demands are placed on the individual, task performance is significantly compromised. Further deterioration of cognitive abilities in the person with HD may result in dismissal from employment. The cognitive deficits most frequently associated with HD are problems with mental calculations, the performance of sequential tasks, and memory.[50] Verbal comprehension often is spared until the later stages of the disease and even then appears to be more compromised by dysarthria than by difficulty in comprehension.

As HD progresses, depression often worsens and suicide is not uncommon.[164] Clients with HD are often hospitalized because of various psychiatric problems, including depression, emotional lability, and behavioral outbursts. Although the loss of function may contribute to the client's level of depression, depression is clearly identified as a specific characteristic of HD.[50] This affective disorder frequently is treated with various antidepressants. Periods of mania have also been reported in approximately 10% of individuals diagnosed with HD.

As the disease progresses, the chorea becomes more severe and may be observed throughout the entire body, including the face.[120] Disturbances in gait are often observed during the middle stages of the disease, and balance is frequently compromised.[50] The individual with HD may display a wide-based gait pattern and have difficulties walking on uneven terrain. This staggering gait is at times misinterpreted by others in the client's life as evidence of alcoholism.[119] The client also has progressive difficulty with voluntary movements.[120] The performance of voluntary motor tasks is slowed (bradykinesia), and the initiation of movement is compromised (akinesia). Although handwriting ability may be spared initially, the client displays increasing difficulties with this task as the disease progresses. Letter size is enlarged, and letter formation, such as slant and shape, is distorted. Saccadic eye movements and ocular pursuits may be slowed at this stage of HD.[118] Slight dysarthria may be noted, which compromises communication.[50] Dysphagia is seen, and the client may choke on various foods. Difficulties may be noted with the coordination of both chewing and breathing while eating.

In the later stages of HD, choreiform movements may be reduced because of the further deterioration of the corpus striatum and globus pallidus.[120] Hypertonicity often replaces the chorea, and the client experiences a severe reduction in voluntary movements. Severe difficulties in eye movement are common during the final stage of the disease.[118] At this stage, the client often needs significant support from others or resides in a long-term care facility. The client is usually unable to talk, walk, or perform basic ADLs without significant assistance.[107]

MEDICAL MANAGEMENT

Medical management of clients with HD can address symptoms, but no effective course of treatment has been identified to arrest the progression of this disease.[130] Intervention based on replacing the deficient neurotransmitters has not been effective in changing the course or rate of progression of HD. Tricyclic antidepressants are often used to treat the depression seen in clients with HD, but MAOIs are contraindicated because of possible exacerbation of chorea.[164] Haloperidol may be used to decrease the negative effects of chorea on the performance of functional activities.[120] Haloperidol is prescribed cautiously and only when the chorea significantly compromises a person's daily activities.

Systematic evaluation of a client with HD must be performed at regular intervals to identify the rate of symptom progression and modify intervention strategies. Standardized instruments are available for determining the presence and severity of various symptoms.[71,148] One evaluation tool, known as the Unified Huntington's Disease Rating Scale (UHDRS), combines aspects from several instruments into a scale that can be administered within 30 minutes. The UHDRS is often administered by a team. This tool provides an accurate means of determining a change in the areas of "motor function, cognitive function, behavioral abnormalities, and functional capacity."[71] The occupational therapist should complete additional assessments before an intervention plan is developed. An evaluation would address functional daily living skills; cognitive abilities such as problem solving, motor performance, and strength; and personal interests and values. The occupational therapist must consider the client's role within the family and community and incorporate these data into the intervention plan. An evaluation at both the home and work site would provide needed information that could be modified if necessary.

ROLE OF THE OCCUPATIONAL THERAPIST

The role of the OT practitioner varies depending on the stage of the disease.[73] During the early stages of HD, an occupational therapist should address the cognitive components of memory and concentration. A client may still be employed at this stage. Strategies such as establishment of a daily routine, the use of checklists, and task analysis to break down tasks into manageable steps can be very helpful. These strategies provide the external structure and support to help the person with HD maintain functional abilities at both the workplace and home. A work-site evaluation can identify changes that would allow the person with HD to continue working. Modification may include tools such as organizers. The use of a kitchen timer or a watch with a beeper can remind the client to perform a specific task. Family members should also be instructed in the use of these techniques. Environmental modifications such as providing a quiet workplace and reducing extraneous stimuli will decrease the impact of compromised memory and concentration on performing functional tasks.

Psychological issues during this stage of the disease often include anxiety, depression, and irritability.[50,66] A client may express guilt that any of his or her children have a 50%

chance of having HD.[119] The diagnosis of HD often is not confirmed until a person is 30 to 40 years old. The client may already be married and have children by that time. Decisions as to whether to complete predictive genetic testing on children may be a significant stressor for the client with HD and for his or her family members. Although genetic testing can confirm HD, it does not predict when the first symptoms will appear. As mentioned previously, not all individuals elect to be tested.

Maintaining social contacts and engaging in purposeful activities are important in designing interventions for clients with HD.[119] Changes in cognitive abilities and emotional responses may result in the loss of a job and decreased income for the family, even during this early stage of the disease.[50] This additional stress should also be considered when developing an intervention plan. The OT intervention plan must include community support services for the client with HD. OT services should include providing clients with information regarding support groups, opportunities to engage in community activities, and connecting with virtual resources through the Internet.

The motor disturbances during the early stages of HD are usually limited to fine motor coordination problems.[50] The characteristic chorea may be noticed only as a twitching of hands when the client is anxious. OT should provide modifications to diminish the effect of chorea and fine motor incoordination on performance of functional activities.[73] This would include modifications to clothing and selection of clothing that does not require small fasteners such as small buttons, snaps, or hooks. Shoes with Velcro closures or elastic closures are recommended to compensate for diminished fine motor skills. Home modifications should be instituted at this stage to allow the client with HD to become familiar with the changes. Developing the skills of using adaptive equipment or modifications and then converting these skills into habits are critical during the early stage of HD. Typical modifications are the use of cooking and eating utensils with built-up handles, unbreakable dishes, a shower bench or seat with tub safety bars, and sturdy chairs with high backs and armrests. Throw or scatter rugs should be eliminated wherever possible in the home, and walkways should be kept free of clutter. The occupational therapist should establish a home exercise program with the client to address the flexibility and endurance of the entire body. These exercises will be incorporated into the client's daily routine. As the movement disorder progresses, the client will have to stop driving a car. These further losses of independent function and control must be considered within the OT intervention plan. Alternative methods of community mobility must be explored.

As HD progresses, the role of OT changes to meet the client's needs.[73] During the middle stages of HD, further deterioration of cognitive abilities often requires the person to resign from a job. Engagement in purposeful activities is greatly needed at this stage and should be a focus of the OT intervention plan.[66,119] Decision-making and arithmetic skills show further deterioration, and family members may need to arrange for others to handle the client's financial matters.[50,108] Generally, comprehension of verbal information is better preserved than ability to complete sequential tasks during this stage. The occupational therapist should encourage the family to use simple written cues or words to help the family member with HD complete self-care and simple household activities. For example, selecting clothing items for the person with HD and placing the clothes in a highly visible area can provide the prompt to change from pajamas to clothes in the morning. Arranging the bathroom with visual cues, such as putting the toothpaste and toothbrush by the sink, can remind the client to brush his or her teeth in the morning and evening.

During the middle stage of HD, the client may display increasing levels of irritability and depression.[164] Clients with HD may attempt suicide. The OT intervention plan should focus on the client's engagement in purposeful activities, particularly leisure activities. When selecting craft activities, the therapist should always consider the client's interests but should also strive to ensure that no sharp instruments are required.[66,108] Modification of craft activities allows the client with HD to successfully complete a task with minimal support. Materials often require additional stabilization to compensate for the client's movement disorders, and any tools used in the leisure activity, such as a wood sander and paintbrushes, should have enlarged or built-up handles.

Motor problems become more apparent during the middle stage of HD, necessitating further modifications in daily living tasks.[73,148] The client's compromised balance may require that tasks such as dressing, brushing teeth, shaving, and combing hair be performed while the client is seated. The client may require the use of a walker or wheelchair at this stage. A rollator walker is preferred to a standard walker without wheels. The walker may need to be fitted with forearm supports to provide additional support when the client is ambulating. When a wheelchair becomes necessary, it should have a firm back and seat; however, additional padding is often required on the armrests because of the client's chorea. Many clients with HD are better able to move the wheelchair with their feet than with their hands. The seat height of the wheelchair should be fitted to allow the client to use his or her feet to move the chair, if possible.

Fatigue is a common issue during the middle stage of HD and can be addressed by taking frequent breaks during the day. Breaks must be scheduled because the person with HD may not readily recognize fatigue. Clothing should have few or no fasteners, and shoes should be sturdy with low heels.[108] Additional adapted equipment that may prove helpful for the client with HD includes shower mitts, electric razor or chemical hair removal method, covered mugs, and non-slip placemats.[73] The choreic movements may become so severe as to necessitate the use of a bed with railings.

Padding should be used on the railings, and additional cushions should be used in the bed.

Because of excessive movements associated with chorea, the client with HD often needs to consume 3000 to 5000 calories per day to maintain weight.[108] Smaller, high-calorie meals should be provided five times a day. This schedule may require additional support from family members or a personal care attendant. Dysphagia, poor postural control, and deficient fine motor coordination compromise the client's ability to eat.[73] Positioning during feeding is crucial, and the trunk should be well supported during mealtime. The client with HD should be able to support his or her arms on the table while the feet are stabilized. Feet may be supported on the floor, or the client may wrap the feet around the legs of the chair for additional support. Problems with dysphagia can be addressed with positioning, oral motor exercises, and changes in diet consistency. Soft foods and thickened fluids are preferable to chewy foods, foods with mixed textures, and thin liquids.

During the final stages of HD, the client often depends on others for all self-care tasks because of the lack of voluntary motor control.[73,107] In some clients, the chorea may diminish, leading to rigidity. The occupational therapist provides important input on positioning and the use of splints to prevent contractures at this stage. Because of the risk of aspiration, oral feedings are provided by trained personnel; alternatively, the client may receive nutrition through a feeding tube.[108] A combination of oral feedings and tube feedings may be used during this stage.

Although cognitive abilities continue to deteriorate, the level of functional decline is difficult to assess because of dysarthria and the loss of motor control.[50] Dementia is part of the HD profile and must be considered in development of the intervention plan. For example, a person in the late stage of HD may still recognize family members and enjoy watching television. The occupational therapist should explore the use of various environmental controls to allow the client control of and access to the immediate environment.[11] Providing a touch pad or switch for selecting television channels may prove beneficial for the client.

Behavioral outbursts have been reported in approximately one third of clients with HD living in long-term care facilities.[107] OT can decrease the frequency of these outbursts by organizing consistent daily schedules and routines for the client with HD.

SUMMARY

Although HD is a progressive, degenerative process, OT has much to offer clients with this disease.[66,73,108,119] The diminishing ability to control the environment has been identified as one of the variables contributing to the deterioration of function in clients with HD. Throughout the course of the disease, OT addresses the client's ability to exercise a degree of control over the environment and engage in purposeful activity.

SECTION 4: MULTIPLE SCLEROSIS

Diane Foti

INCIDENCE

Multiple sclerosis (MS) is a progressive neurological disease that damages the myelin sheath in the CNS. Onset usually occurs between the ages of 20 and 40 years.[94] The disease affects 60 to 100 people per 100,000.[63] It is more prevalent in women than in men.[35] The highest prevalence of the disease is in Caucasians of northern European ancestry. Recent studies show that MS also occurs in people younger than 20, with 3% to 5% diagnosed before age 15 and 17% before the age of 21.[94,111,121]

The myelin is typically damaged in discrete regions of the white matter, with the axon remaining preserved. Disruption of the myelin sheath has differing effects on the axonal conduction, depending on the degree of breakdown and the length of the damaged segment.[63] When axons are conducting in a slower manner because of inflammation of the myelin sheath, the person with MS may have intermittent symptoms of sensory distortions, incoordination, or weakness. This inflammatory process accounts for the unpredictability of the disease.

In advanced cases of MS, acute and chronic plaques develop throughout the white matter, especially in the spinal cord, optic nerve, and periventricular white matter, including the corpus callosum.[63] Axons may be damaged and severed in advanced cases, resulting in extensive loss of function. MRI results may show lesions and changes in the brain volume.[22,75]

ETIOLOGY

The specific cause of MS is unknown, although it is suspected to be the result of a combination of environmental and genetic factors. The most current theory is that MS is an immune system reaction that acts on the nervous system. Recent studies have shown that 30% to 60% of the new clinical attacks of the disease occur after a cold, flu, or common viral illness. Some researchers theorize that the immune system mistakes a portion of the myelin protein for a virus and destroys it. Other researchers believe that the viral infection damages the myelin and releases small amounts into the body, resulting in an autoimmune reaction.[149]

CLINICAL PICTURE

The symptoms that occur with MS are related to the area of the CNS affected.[5] Early symptoms may be paresthesias, diplopia, or visual loss in one eye; fatigability, emotional lability; and sensory loss in the extremities. Cognitive deficits have also been documented in individuals with a disease duration of less than 2 years and with few neurological signs.[4] Other initial symptoms are trigeminal neuralgia and a worsening of symptoms when the body temperature is elevated. Symptoms that occur with elevated body temperature are generally temporary and resolve in time.

Persons with MS and other chronic conditions experience a higher rate of depression than the general population.[109] Depression may have different causes and should be assessed by the team. Depression may be caused by a physiological response to the disease process, may be a psychological response to the diagnosis, or may be a side effect of one of the disease-modifying medications. Depression may occur at any stage of the disease process. It should be addressed promptly because it may contribute to fatigue and an inability to cope with challenges and make adaptations as needed.[109]

In advanced stages of the disease process, the individual may have varying degrees of paralysis, from total lower extremity paralysis to involvement of the upper extremities, dysarthria, dysphagia, severe visual impairment, ataxia, spasticity, nystagmus, neurogenic bladder, and impaired cognition. Cognitive deficits are reported to occur in 30% to 70% of persons with MS but do not necessarily correlate with a physical decline.[3,4,62] Emotional changes such as depression may also be present; less commonly seen are euphoria and a sense of indifference. Dementia may develop in individuals who exhibit euphoria and indifference. Dementia occurs in less than 5% of the population with MS.[63]

The course of MS is unpredictable. It is marked by episodes of exacerbation and remission. An **exacerbation** may be an episode as minor as fatigue and sensory loss or as extensive as total paralysis in all extremities and loss of bladder control. **Remission** may involve a total resolution of the symptoms, result in a short plateau, or lead to some loss of function.

The three typical patterns seen in MS are (1) relapsing and remitting, (2) secondary-progressive, and (3) primary-progressive.[5] The relapsing and remitting form of MS involves 85% of the MS population and leads to episodes of exacerbation and remission, resulting in a slow, stepwise progression as the deficits accumulate. The secondary-progressive course begins with a pattern of relapses and remissions but evolves into the progressive form of the disease. Before the introduction of disease-modifying drugs, approximately 50% of clients with relapsing and remitting MS progressed to the secondary-progressive form of the disease. Long-term studies regarding the impact of the disease-modifying drugs on this progression have not been completed. Marguerite was first diagnosed with the relapsing-remitting form of MS and was recently diagnosed with the secondary-progressive course of the disease. She is now experiencing sustained diminished fine motor abilities and sensation in her left hand.

The primary-progressive form of MS (10% of the MS population) is distinguished by a downward course and little recovery after exacerbations. Individuals with this form eventually become nonambulatory and incontinent of urine and may have dysphagia and dysarthria, severely compromised lower extremity function, and varying limitations in upper extremity function. For individuals with the primary-progressive form of MS, the average time to reach the stage of severe disability is 10 to 25 years. Overall, life expectancy is near normal for those with MS.[149]

The two atypical patterns of MS are the benign course and the progressive-relapsing form. The clinical signs of a benign course are a younger age at onset, female sex, and onset with sensory symptoms. The symptoms usually resolve within 6 weeks, and there may be only a few residual deficits. If the disability is minimal after 5 years, the course is considered benign.[63] The progressive-relapsing form of MS is rare (5% of the MS population). It is identified as steadily progressive but has specific relapses.[5]

MEDICAL MANAGEMENT

In recent years new interventions have been introduced to limit inflammation during periods of exacerbation and to slow the immune system response. Medical management is primarily focused on treating the symptoms of the disease.

Antiinflammatory medications such as prednisone or methylprednisolone are used during an exacerbation. These medications are usually given in high doses for short periods because of their extensive side effects. In lower doses that can be tolerated for long periods, these medications have not demonstrated the ability to prevent further exacerbations or change the long-term course of the disease but are effective primarily for shortening the duration of an exacerbation.[149]

In the relapsing and remitting form of MS, several new medications are being used to modify the disease process and are thought to have an effect in slowing the progression of the disease. Four different medications for this group have recently been introduced: interferon β-1 b (Betaseron), interferon β-1 a (Avonex), glatiramer (Copaxone). and Rebif.[70] Patients treated with these medications, administered by subcutaneous self-injection, showed a one-third reduction in frequency of exacerbations. Studies regarding the effects of these medications on individuals with the progressive form of the disease are ongoing.

A new medication, mitoxantrone (Novatrone), is the first drug approved in the United States for secondary-progressive MS. It is a form of chemotherapy that can also be offered as a treatment option for those with secondary-progressive, progressive-relapsing, or worsening relapsing-remitting MS. Novatrone is reported to help in reducing neurological disability and the frequency of clinical relapses.

Use of the disease-modifying medications requires the client or caregiver to learn to give the injections and evaluate the impact of the medication regime on habits and routines. Integrating use of the medication and managing the side effects may require consideration of how activity is managed, how it fits into the client's daily or weekly routines, and how management of the side effects may affect activities.

Symptom management includes treatment of spasticity, bladder management, prevention of bladder infection, and management of pain and fatigue. Spasticity is often managed with medication; unfortunately, this may also worsen muscle weakness. Bladder management may involve the use of incontinence pads or catheters, along with the prevention of bladder infections. Fatigue should be managed with good nutrition, the prevention of overfatigue with energy conservation methods, regular exercise, establishing routines for rest and sleep, and control of stress.[104] Bowel incontinence is rarely a problem related to a neurological deficit but is usually a functional impairment resulting from immobility.

ROLE OF THE OCCUPATIONAL THERAPIST

The OT practitioner may provide services for the person with MS in a number of settings. The type and degree of intervention provided will be determined by the setting, the type of reimbursement, and the client's and caregiver's responses to intervention.

The evaluation should include the gathering of information about all performance areas: ADLs, IADLs, education, work, leisure, and social participation. During the performance of various occupations, the following performance skills should be evaluated: motor, process, and communication skills. Optimally, a home evaluation should be completed. Because not all settings allow a home evaluation, the occupational therapist should interview the client and caregiver regarding the home environment and potential barriers. Because MS has an unpredictable course, the client may need a referral for other resources and periodic reevaluation by an occupational therapist.

The evaluation includes an occupational profile to guide the evaluation process. The occupational therapist then selects the necessary instruments to assess occupational performance, performance skills, and client factors. This is generally accomplished with a combination of standardized and nonstandardized assessments, through the use of interviews with the family and client, and through observation. If the client has a cognitive deficit, a family member or significant other should be included in the evaluation process to provide accurate information. Having an understanding of the client's cultural, social, and spiritual perspective will provide insight into available support systems and their mpact on the client's adaptation to the disability.

Assessment of the sensorimotor skills is discussed thoroughly in previous chapters. Because endurance and fatigue are such significant factors, it is important not to rely solely on the results of an assessment of a specific client factor. For example, a manual muscle test is not likely to accurately reflect the degree of weakness experienced throughout the day. Observing a client performing a functional activity over a period of time or gathering information about the client's daily activity patterns will provide the clinician with a more accurate evaluation of fatigue.[70] The National MS Society recommends use of the Modified Fatigue Scale (MFS) or the Fatigue Questionnaire to understand specific problems resulting from fatigue.[104] In the case of Marguerite, the MFS assessment may help determine the impact of fatigue on her daily activities.

When evaluating a client's activity patterns, the OT practitioner should also ask about sleep patterns. Disrupted sleep patterns sometimes contribute to fatigue in the MS population. The information can be shared with the client's physician so that appropriate intervention can be made either medically or with counseling that addresses the habits and routines that may contribute to the client's disrupted sleep.[10]

MS may also affect visual abilities, and compromises may be noted in visual tracking, scanning, and acuity. An objective evaluation will help determine the type of deficits, when the deficits occur, and more specifically how it affects ADLs and IADLs.

Perceptual processing and cognitive status should be reassessed periodically. The data gathered will help identify specific deficits and their potential impact on functional activities, allowing the OT practitioner to incorporate this information into family training. Cognitive deficits vary from a slight decrease in short-term memory and attention span to poor orientation and severely impaired short-term memory. Cognitive deficits are not necessarily correlated with the degree of physical deficits. The volume of lesions on the MRI correlates with cognitive decline in complex attention, processing speed, and verbal memory.[153] One investigation evaluated overall brain atrophy and size of ventricles in relation to cognitive abilities. The results suggested a relationship between an increase in the size of the third ventricle and a decrease in cognition.[22] The client's perceptual and cognitive deficits are factors that must be considered when deciding whether the client needs close, constant supervision or can stay home alone. Various standardized cognitive and perceptual assessments are included in previous chapters of the text. Basso developed a screening tool for cognitive dysfunction for individuals with MS. Basso's tool was found to be both sensitive to functional impairment and cost effective.[14] This tool can be used by an occupational therapist or practitioners in other disciplines when evaluating the person with MS for cognitive deficits.

ADLs may be evaluated with a check-off list, a standardized assessment such as the Assessment of Motor and Process Skills,[42] or other standardized assessments for ADLs.[8] The most widely accepted tool to measure clinical impairment for the person with MS is the Expanded Disability Status Scale (EDSS).[117] The scale should be completed by a physician because it includes a detailed neurological examination. The EDSS combines an assessment of neurological function and a scale to measure a client's ambulatory and functional mobility status. There are limitations with this tool; it does not allow for specific assessment of all ADLs and is not sensitive to potential cognitive and sexual deficits in MS.[117] The OT practitioner should be familiar with the EDSS because it is often mentioned in the literature as a baseline for evaluating disability and has been adopted by the International Federation of MS Societies.[74,163] The MS Functional Composite (MSFC) was developed to measure leg function and ambulation, arm and hand function, and cognition.[33,105] It can be used for periodic baseline function. It may be more sensitive for use as baseline cognitive evaluation than the EDSS.

Evaluation of the social environment is important to consider with each client. MS is usually identified during the phase of life in which a person is raising a family and developing a career, as in the case study example of Marguerite. She is in the "sandwich," generation, simultaneously caring for her children and her mother. Because the disease is unpredictable and fluctuating, it leads to disruptions in normal daily activities and in family life. These disruptions create stress for the spouse or partner, children, and other family members. The occupational therapist must determine the type of support that the client can expect from family members.

Behavioral issues vary depending on the premorbid personality, progression of the disease, coping skills, and social environment of the person with MS. Cognitive deficits and denial of the progressive nature of the disease may lead to behavior that puts the client at risk and makes management difficult. If family members do not understand or recognize the client's behavioral problems, further complications may arise when the behavior is not restricted or modified by the family.

Ethical Considerations

A client with MS is able to ambulate to the car but has cognitive deficits that are exacerbated by fatigue in the afternoon. Because the client has discontinued work, the family members do not want to take away driving privileges as well. However, by continuing to drive, the client places himself and others at risk of injury. The occupational therapist may need to educate his family about the deficits by providing examples of the ways in which cognition is evaluated and by discussing the ways in which cognitive deficits affect driving and other daily activities. The occupational therapist is responsible for reporting the driving risk to the client's physician.

Other behavioral examples include the client who is depressed or labile, has poor memory, refuses assistance from outside caregivers, or uses poor judgment regarding safety with medications and transfers. Each client demonstrates a unique set of behavioral issues and requires individual evaluation and an intervention approach that encompasses the family, client, and caregivers.

GOAL SETTING

For the client with a progressive disease such as MS, goal setting focuses on the client's need to adapt as the disability progresses. Families often need to negotiate role changes to accommodate the person with MS, who may not be able to participate consistently in a previously established family role. The client's ability to adapt depends on the family and client's acknowledgment of deficits and willingness to consider alternatives. OT intervention may include: (1) problem-solving compensatory strategies; (2) time management; (3) role delegation; and (4) use of adaptive equipment to compensate for motor, sensory, endurance, cognitive, and visual deficits. Marguerite's intervention may involve analyzing her daily and weekly routine to identify activities that can be eliminated, modified, or delegated. She may consider grocery shopping on-line or delegating this task to her husband. Marguerite will need to evaluate the number of activities in which her children participate and the possibility of carpooling. She may need adaptive equipment for activities that require bilateral strength and dexterity because of the loss of sensation and dexterity in her left hand.

A client may initially be capable of working outside the home and completing household management tasks. Clients with the progressive form of MS may experience such a significant decline that employment outside of the home is eventually no longer feasible. These clients also may need to delegate household management tasks to others, until finally only basic self-care activities remain. These clients eventually may become totally dependent on others for basic self-care. The adaptation of roles requires working not only with the client but also with family members and significant others. The occupational therapist may identify areas of difficulty for the family and client and provide training in methods to better handle those situations. The therapist also may refer the client and family to a social worker or psychologist for further support.

SUMMARY

MS affects each patient in a unique way, necessitating individual evaluation to determine the patient's deficits and strengths. Working with patients who have MS requires the practitioner to use expertise in the evaluation and intervention of all areas of OT. Because of relapses and remissions over the course of the disease process, developing an intervention plan is particularly challenging. Because the client may expect the return of function, he or she may deny deficits, refusing to adapt to a change in status; this attitude can create safety problems. The OT practitioner focuses on assessing the current level of functioning and the best methods for the client to adapt to current changes in status. The occupational therapist may also assist the family with making long-range, realistic plans. For example, if the family is planning to remodel the bathroom, the therapist may encourage consideration of a roll-in shower and not just a standard shower stall with a shower seat.

Quality of life is assessed more often when considering the impact of the disease on the individual. One type of assessment, the MS Quality of Life Inventory, measures 36 areas of functioning.[112] Study results vary regarding the impact of quality of life for the person diagnosed with MS. Some studies show that individuals with MS experience a lower quality of life; other studies report no difference in this area between individuals with MS and the general population.[75,99,122] These studies are based on the perceptions of the person with MS and do not consider the impact of quality-of-life issues on the family.

Working with clients with MS requires a multidisciplinary approach. In addition to the occupational therapist, the physician, physical therapist, registered nurse, social worker, and psychologist may be involved as team members. Because the social environment may create complex and difficult problems, good communication among all team members is needed to ensure that the team goals are congruous. The occupational therapist has a unique perspective to offer to the team as cognition, perception, psychosocial, and motor abilities are assessed and treated in a functional context.

SECTION 5: PARKINSON'S DISEASE

Winifred Schultz-Krohn

INCIDENCE

Parkinson's disease (PD) is one of the most common adult-onset, degenerative neurological disorders.[43] Three classic symptoms are associated with PD: tremor, rigidity, and bradykinesia. The prevalence rate for PD varies greatly, from 10 to over 400 per 100,000.[168] Incidence increases with age, and the disease affects 1.4% of the population over the age of 55.[136] Gender differences have been noted; the prevalence of PD in men between the ages of 55 and 74 is slightly higher than in women of the same age. After the age of 74, women show a slightly greater prevalence of PD than do men. Diagnosis is most often made after the age of 60.

The etiology for PD has not been definitively established.[12,61] Although a positive family history has been established as a risk factor for PD, a clear genetic marker has not been identified. Twin studies have not conclusively identified a genetic factor as the cause of PD. Current genetic work is looking at a specific gene mutation on chromosome 4 in familial PD, but whether this genetic mutation will also be identified as the causal factor in sporadic occurrences of PD is unknown. A mutation on the gene that encodes a specific protein has also been linked to PD.[12]

Environmental factors have been considered as a possible cause of PD.[61] The possibility of an exogenous agent's producing PD gained considerable recognition when narcotic addicts began using 1-methyl-4-phenyl-1,2,3,6-tetrahydropyridine (MPTP). After using MPTP, many addicts quickly exhibited parkinsonism that "strictly mimics the clinical and anatomical features of Parkinson's disease"[61] (p. 143). Other toxins, such as manganese and hydrocarbon solvents, produced more widespread neurological damage and lacked the selective deterioration in the basal ganglia.

Researchers have also considered dietary habits as a potential risk factor for PD. The incidence of PD was higher among persons with a diet high in animal fat. The incidence of PD was inversely related to a diet high in nuts, legumes, and potatoes. Many researchers are now investigating a possible interactional effect between a genetic predisposition and environmental agents as the possible cause of PD. Although many possible etiologies are being considered, most individuals with diagnosed PD are identified as having idiopathic parkinsonism.[44]

PATHOPHYSIOLOGY

The neurological structure associated with PD is the substantia nigra, specifically the pars compacta portion.[115] The pars compacta receives input from other basal ganglia nuclei and appears to serve as a modulator of striatal activity.[120] The substantia nigra nuclei undergo significant deterioration as the disease progresses. The significant reduction in the dopaminergic neurons in the substantia nigra pars compacta produces a decrease in activity within the basal ganglia and an overall "reduction in spontaneous movement"[120] (p. 426). The substantia nigra serves as one of the major output nuclei for the basal ganglia to other structures.[116] In addition to the loss of dopaminergic neurons, intracytoplasmic inclusions are found on postmortem examination within the substantia nigra.[115] These intracytoplasmic inclusions are also known as *Lewy bodies*.[44] Although the greatest amount of neurodegeneration is found in the pars compacta substantia nigra, destruction of other neurological structures has been reported.[115] Deterioration is also seen in the remainder of the substantia nigra, locus ceruleus, nucleus basilis, and hypothalamus.

CLINICAL PICTURE

PD is characterized as a slowly progressive, degenerative movement disorder.[120] The diagnosis of PD is usually made after the age of 55. Although PD is not considered fatal, the degeneration of various neurological structures severely compromises performance of functional tasks. A person diagnosed with PD may live an additional 20 to 30 years, with a progressive loss of motor function that eventually requires specialized care.[44] A person with MS has an increased risk for developing pneumonia, which may be fatal.

PD is characterized by dysfunction in both voluntary and involuntary movements.[120] A classic triad of symptoms includes tremor, rigidity, and a voluntary movement disorder. The disturbances in voluntary movement are identified as difficulty initiating movement (akinesia) and slowness in maintaining movement (bradykinesia). The bradykinesia and akinesia are often the most disabling motor symptoms for the client with PD.[40] The delay in initiating movement patterns and the slowness in executing the motion compromise functional tasks such as driving, dressing, and eating.

In addition to the slowness of movement, rigidity is a characteristic of PD. **Rigidity** is the stiffness within a muscle that impedes smooth movement. This stiffness occurs in both directions for each plane of motion at a specific joint.[127] The characteristic resting tremor with a rate between 4 and 5 Hz is a disturbance of involuntary movement.[101] This tremor often diminishes with activity, but in some clients the tremor persists during performance of functional activities.

Additional symptoms of PD are disturbances in gait and postural reactions and masked face with decreased facial expressions and depression.[120] Deterioration in gait is seen throughout the course of the disease.[139] Initially, gait may be fairly normal, but as the disease progresses, changes in stride length and speed of gait are apparent. The characteristic festinating gait is often seen; as the client walks, the stride length decreases in length and the speed slightly increases, creating a shuffling effect. A reduced arm swing during ambulation is evident, and trunk rotation is markedly decreased during walking. Another motor disturbance associated with gait is the phenomenon of "freezing."[57] Freezing occurs when the person ceases to move, often after attempting to initiate, maintain, or alter a movement pattern. During gait, freezing may be seen as the client attempts to change directions or approach a narrow hallway or stairs. As the client attempts to alter the trajectory of walking to turn to enter another room, he or she may cease moving. Freezing can also be seen during other motor tasks, such as writing, brushing teeth, and speaking.

Postural abnormalities associated with PD include a flexed, stooped posture with the head positioned forward.[103] The client tends to stand with flexion at the knees and hips. In addition to the stooped posture, balance reactions are compromised.[126] Righting and equilibrium reactions are markedly reduced in effectiveness, and the person with PD may experience frequent falls.

Approximately 50% of individuals with diagnosed PD exhibit depression,[126] which is not merely reactive to the severity of symptoms or the chronic nature of the disease.[44] The depression seen in individuals with PD appears to be related to a serotonergic deficit, which is similar to that in clients without PD who have depression. Complicating the feature of depression is a decrease in facial expressiveness caused by akinesia.[126] This decrease in spontaneous facial expressions, or so-called masked face, is characteristic of clients with PD. Initially, decreased facial expressions are seen unilaterally, but as the disease progresses, spontaneous expression decreases on both sides of the face.[44] Individuals with PD may also self-limit social interaction because they are embarrassed by their decreased facial expressions and movement disorders.

Mental status is fairly normal throughout the early stages of PD, but visual-spatial perception is often compromised.[126]

Higher-order cognitive disorders are common in clients with PD. Clients with PD often have difficulty shifting attention among various stimuli. Processing simultaneous information is often difficult for the individual with PD, and tasks that require a sequential process are somewhat easier to perform. Driving a car presents a particular challenge because it necessitates the processing of multiple forms of information in a simultaneous manner. Some self-care tasks, such as brushing teeth, have a clear sequence that can be followed; these activities can be performed with less demand on cognitive functioning. Although dementia is seldom seen in clients with an earlier-onset form of PD, approximately one third of people over 70 years old who have PD display dementia.

Additional symptoms associated with PD include autonomic dysfunction, dysphagia, and dysarthria.[126] A client with PD may have bowel and bladder problems, with reduced intestinal motility producing constipation. Clients often report an increase in the frequency and urgency of urination. Clients also frequently complain of orthostatic hypotension, but syncope is rare.[44] Clients with PD occasionally report periods of sweating and abnormal tolerance of heat and cold.[126] Because speech volume is often decreased, persons with PD often seem to whisper. Articulation is imprecise, and speech is monotone. Dysphagia tends to occur in the later stages of PD, and afflicted clients may be at risk for choking and aspiration pneumonia resulting from the dysphagia.

The course of the disease varies from person to person, but the first clinical symptom identified is typically a unilateral resting tremor in the hand.[101] Hoehn and Yahr[69] established a scale identifying the progression of symptoms in PD. A client at stage I exhibits unilateral involvement, typically a hand tremor, but no impairment of functional abilities is reported. A client is able to complete personal ADLs and IADLs, but performance often requires additional effort and energy. Depending on job demands, a client with PD at stage I is often employed but may require modifications to the work site. During this stage the client's handwriting may become very small, with letters that are cramped together.[44] This change in handwriting is referred to as *micrographia*. The client may also complain of muscle cramping when required to write for extended periods. Slight rigidity may be seen when the client is asked to rapidly open and close the involved hand.

Stage II denotes a progression of symptoms and the development of bilateral motor disturbances.[69] Although the course of PD is variable, this stage is usually seen 1 to 2 years after initial diagnosis. Even though tremors or rigidity may be noted bilaterally, the client can still perform ADL skills. Performance of IADL skills may require modification because of motor difficulties. Work, depending on the job requirements, often requires additional modifications, and the client may require several rest breaks during the day. The client should make decisions at this point regarding the benefits of remaining employed relative to the energy expenditures. Posture becomes slightly stooped, with flexion at the knees and hips. The person with stage II PD is still able to ambulate independently. As PD progresses to stage III, the client experiences delayed righting and equilibrium reactions. Balance is impaired; the client has difficulty performing daily tasks that require standing, such as showering and meal preparation. Employment may be difficult because of its energy demands. Safety in walking is a concern because of the client's reduced balance, and home modifications are necessary at this stage. A person with stage IV PD has significant deficits in completing daily living tasks. The client is still able to ambulate at this stage, but motor control is severely compromised and negatively affects dressing, feeding, and hygiene skills. Stage V is the final stage of PD. The client is typically confined to a wheelchair or bed and depends on others for most self-care activities. The rate of progression through these stages varies from person to person, but PD is a slowly progressive disorder.

The extent of PD symptoms in individual clients has been measured using the Unified Parkinson's Disease Rating Scale.[47] This scale evaluates a client's motor skills, functional status, and extent of disability. Motor skills are evaluated by a trained observer.[135] The functional status and extent of disability are measured through a client interview that includes items addressing ADL skills and cognitive and emotional factors.[92] This instrument has been used for research and clinical practice to measure the effectiveness of various interventions in reducing PD symptoms.

MEDICAL MANAGEMENT

The most frequently used medical management strategy for PD is the provision of a dopamine agonist to make up for the depletion of dopamine caused by the destruction of the substantia nigra.[43,140] Levodopa is the medication most commonly used in the treatment of PD.[125] This oral medication is actually a precursor to dopamine because dopamine is too large to cross the blood-brain barrier. Levodopa provides substantial relief from tremors and rigidity during the initial stages of PD. After approximately 5 to 10 years of chronic use of levodopa, motor side effects are reported.[126] Those most often reported are dyskinesias and motor fluctuations. This so-called on-off phenomenon is related to the levodopa dosage. A decrease in tremors and rigidity occurs during the "on" period after administration of levodopa, but the client also has various dyskinesias, such as abnormal movements of the limbs. As the dosage of levodopa wears off, the motor symptoms associated with PD return. Timing of the medication and the periods of "on-off" are important considerations in planning the client's daily activities. Even though abnormal movements are observed during the "on" period, the client has greater freedom of movement to complete functional activities.

As PD progresses, control of various motor symptoms through the use of levodopa becomes less effective.[126] Surgical intervention, known as **stereotactic surgery,** has been used.

In this surgery, specific lesions are made in neurological structures to decrease the severity of PD symptoms. Stereotactic surgery of the globus pallidus internus has been used to decrease the severity of motor symptoms associated with PD and thus reduce the needed dosage of levodopa.[78,114] This surgical procedure is known as a *pallidotomy*. Pallidotomies have also been shown to reduce the dyskinesias associated with long-term use of levodopa.[126] Stereotactic surgery has also been used to create lesions in portions of the thalamus to reduce tremor and rigidity associated with PD.[79]

Neural transplantation has been used selectively for clients with PD.[24] This process involves harvesting fetal mesencephalic neural tissue and then transplanting this tissue into the basal ganglia of clients with PD.[34] The results of fetal brain transplants have been varied. The best success for this procedure has been reported when bilateral implants are placed in the putamen from multiple fetuses. The transplanted fetal tissue produces dopamine and thereby reduces the debilitating symptoms of progressive PD. Clients must continue to use levodopa but at a reduced dosage.

ROLE OF THE OCCUPATIONAL THERAPIST

Occupational therapy services vary depending on the client's stage of PD. Typically, an OT program would provide compensatory strategies, client and family education, environmental and task modifications, and community involvement.

During the initial stages of the disease, the occupational therapist should develop an occupational profile with the client and significant others to establish intervention priorities. The focus of intervention is developing the habits and routines to foster participation in desired occupations as the disease process progresses. Educating the client and significant others regarding the course of the disease is an important step in this process, one that aids in selection of occupations. For example, the case study at the end of this chapter introduces Carl. He identified traveling and painting as important occupations, and interventions were designed to help him continue participating in these occupations as the disease progressed.

During the early stages of the disease, the client and family should be informed of community resources and support groups. In one study, clients with PD were found to be far more dependent on others for personal care and household activities than were same-age peers without PD.[158] This dependence can place additional stress on the family. Involvement in a community-based group may provide the support needed to accommodate the changes in family roles and interaction.

Modification of household items may decrease the impact of tremors during the initial stage of the disease process. The use of built-up handles for eating and writing utensils should be introduced during the initial stages of PD. Handwriting often becomes small and difficult to read during the initial stage of PD. Time management techniques should be introduced at this stage. Paying bills, signing forms, or doing other written work should be completed soon after taking levodopa, using utensils with built-up handles. Even though tremors are not severe during the early stages of PD, clothing fasteners should be modified. The use of slip-on shoes or Velcro closures for clothing should be considered at this time. Although a client may be able to complete the fastening of clothing during this stage of PD, the occupational therapist must consider the amount of energy and time needed to perform such a task. In addition to the modification of specific tasks, household changes should be made at this time. Loose rugs should be removed from floors and furniture placed close to the wall to decrease obstacles. Chairs should have armrests to allow the client to push up from the chair to stand. Although balance is not significantly compromised during the early stages of PD, the family and client should become familiar with the new arrangement of furniture before this becomes a necessity. Bath and toilet railings and a raised toilet seat should be provided within the home. Because fatigue is a common complaint, clients should develop the habit of taking frequent breaks during the day. Modifying the household setting early in the course of PD allows the client and family members to adjust to changes and incorporate these changes into daily routines before they become a necessity.

A work evaluation should be performed during the early stage of the disease process to assess safety risks, potential hazards, and work simplification techniques that could be used. An ergonomic assessment of the work site and modifications to the tools would be appropriate. In the case of Carl, computer modifications were considered. A client may have the option of reducing the number of work hours, but that decision may result in reduced medical benefits. These decisions and available options are part of the OT intervention process during the early stage of the disease.

During the initial stage of PD, the occupational therapist should establish a daily exercise program addressing full range of motion.[155] It is preferable to have a client with PD perform a short exercise program for 5 to 10 minutes daily rather than a longer program three times a week. Postural flexibility exercises should be included in the program, with specific attention given to trunk extension. The most common postural change noted with the progression of PD is a stooped posture. In addition to the flexibility exercises, occupational therapists should instruct clients in the use of relaxation techniques and controlled breathing. Inhaling slowly through the nose and exhaling through pursed lips two or three times in succession, combined with improved postural alignment, can promote relaxation.

As the disease progresses, additional exercises can improve gait.[157] Rhythmic auditory stimulation in the form of music with an accentuated initial beat has been found to significantly improve stride length and speed in clients with PD. Dancing can also enhance gait patterns, in addition to providing a social environment for the client with PD. As akinesia becomes more apparent, the client with PD should be instructed to use a rocking motion to begin movement activities. Rocking forward and backward a few times while seated can produce the momentum needed to rise from a chair.

As a person with PD progresses to the middle stages of the disease, the client experiences further deterioration of motor skills, particularly the execution of skilled sequential movements.[39] These types of movements are needed to complete personal care and household tasks. Curra and associates[39] found that external cues improved the speed and sequential performance of novel motor tasks. The occupational therapist should suggest modifying activities to include visual cues, verbal prompts, and rehearsal of movements. These strategies increase a client's ability to perform personal care and household activities.

During the middle stages of PD, clients may have decreased oral motor control.[126] Dysphagia and drooling may embarrass them and further restrict social engagements. The occupational therapist should encourage oral motor exercises and provide education regarding food selection. Food consistencies can be altered to improve the client's ability to eat.

The ability to complete personal care tasks has been identified as a critical variable in a client's perception of quality of life.[49] Although progressive movement problems are characteristic of PD, the occupational therapist can minimize the impact the movement disorder has on functional activities. Tremors have less effect on the completion of personal care tasks than compensations for postural instability.[54] The use of group OT sessions has been demonstrated to be effective in reducing the impact of postural instability in clients with PD. An additional benefit of these group sessions is the reported improvement in the perception of quality of life in clients attending the sessions.

Access to community mobility and support programs should be included in the OT intervention plan during the middle stages of PD. A client with PD is often dependent on others for transportation. The use of community mobility services can decrease the client's dependence on family members for shopping and errands.

During the last stages of PD, movement disorders and rigidity may eliminate the client's ability to perform personal care tasks such as dressing and grooming.[69] Depression caused by the decreased ability to perform these tasks can significantly compromise a person's quality of life.[49] OT services should be provided to further modify the home environment for access and control. The use of environmental control units, such as a switch-operated television or radio, can be helpful. The switch plate should be activated with only light touch. Voice- or sound-activated environmental control units may not be as useful because of decreased vocal volume and poor articulation control during speech production. The client's ability to control the immediate environment can compensate for the losses experienced during the final stages of PD. The client may no longer be able to dress himself or herself, but through the use of various switches the client can select preferred television or radio programs, control room lighting, and operate a computer by using minimal motor action.

SUMMARY

Although PD is a progressive, neurodegenerative disorder, OT has much to offer the client with this disease.[49,54] The diminishing ability to perform personal care activities and engage in self-selected tasks has been identified as one of the variables contributing to depression and the decreased quality of life in clients with PD. Throughout the progressive course of PD, OT addresses the ability of the client to engage in meaningful activities. The client's wishes and family circumstances are incorporated into the OT intervention plan at every stage of the disease process.

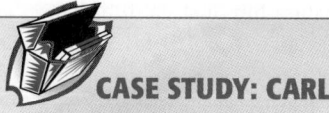

CASE STUDY: CARL

Carl is a 62-year-old college professor diagnosed with PD at the age of 57. He is married and lives in a small one-story home with his wife. He has two adult children, who live in another state. Carl reports that he enjoys traveling, reading, painting, and attending concerts.

Carl recently considered taking early retirement because of the increase in tremors in both of his hands, which made correcting papers difficult. He also reports some problems with endurance as a result of stiffness. Carl indicates that he is no longer able to paint because of the tremors in his hands. He also reports that he is unsure whether he should continue driving because of these tremors.

Results of the OT evaluation indicate that Carl is cooperative and motivated for therapy. Although he does not indicate that he is depressed, his wife reports features of depression, such as a decreased interest in going to concerts and planning summer vacations to see their adult children and grandchildren. His wife also reports that Carl seems depressed about his possible early retirement and loss of status as a college professor.

Carl is able to complete most personal ADLs independently but has difficulties stepping into and out of the tub and shower. His wife reports that she is afraid he will fall and that she often assists him in getting into and out of the shower. Carl also has difficulty tying his tie and buttoning his shirt. Tremors are noted bilaterally in his hands, and slight rigidity is present during PROM. Dynamic balance is slightly compromised on uneven surfaces and stairs.

Carl has been taking Sinemet (levodopa and carbidopa medication) for the past 3 years to decrease the rigidity and tremors. He does not report any dyskinesias.

When asked about his personal goals, Carl replies, "I guess I'll have more time to read now."

OT was initiated to accomplish the following:

1. Improve ADL performance
   a. Instruct in use of a buttonhook
   b. Make suggestions regarding clothing modifications such as clip-on ties and slip-on shoes
   c. Instruct in use of momentum to initiate movement, such as rocking back and forth to rise from a chair
2. Modify home environment
   a. Remove throw rugs and obstacles in walkways
   b. Provide a tub seat and shower extension hose
   c. Provide a raised toilet seat
   d. Provide a cushion on dining room chairs
3. Assess work setting for modifications
   a. Assess for computer access
   b. Instruct in energy conservation, urging him to take frequent breaks and schedule activities during "on" phase of medications
4. Investigate leisure pursuits
   a. Provide modifications to his easel, using forearm supports to allow him to continue to paint
   b. Provide information regarding community-based Parkinson's disease support groups
5. Instruct in daily active ROM exercise program
   a. Trunk extension and rotation exercises
   b. Bilateral upper extremity exercise
   c. Use of music during exercise program

Carl responded well to OT intervention. Although he was able to complete the academic school year, he decided to retire afterwards. He stopped driving, but his wife began to drive them to concerts and art exhibits. He was able to complete personal ADLs safely with the use of adapted equipment and home modifications. He resumed painting during the "on" periods of his medications schedule, using the forearm supports attached to an angled table. He attended a Parkinson's support group two times a week and began to socialize with members from that group. Carl reported that the daily exercises seemed to decrease his stiffness, and he and his wife took frequent strolls in the park when weather permitted. He and his wife also joined a book club.

Review Questions

1. What are the symptoms of ALS at onset?
2. What is the underlying neurological process in ALS?
3. What bodily functions remain intact throughout the disease process?
4. What is the prognosis for ALS? Given this prognosis, what is the goal of the occupational therapist?
5. What are the symptoms of ALS at each stage of the disease?
6. What interventions are appropriate at each stage of ALS?
7. What are the initial symptoms of AD?
8. What is the underlying degenerative neurological process associated with AD?
9. What changes in symptoms occur over the course of AD?
10. How do the changes in symptoms affect occupational performance in clients with AD?
11. What is the prognosis for a client with AD?

12. What OT interventions are appropriate for the client at each stage of AD?
13. What environmental modifications should be made to accommodate the client with AD?
14. What are the symptoms of MS at onset?
15. What is the underlying neurological process in MS?
16. What are the three typical patterns of MS? How do they differ?
17. What symptoms of MS are managed with medication? What are the side effects of medication management?
18. How is medication management in the relapsing and remitting form of MS different than in the other forms of MS?
19. What does the OT evaluation include for the person with MS?
20. Why is it important to include the family in the evaluation and treatment process for the client with MS?
21. What are the initial symptoms of HD?
22. What is the underlying degenerative neurological process associated with HD?
23. What changes in symptoms occur over the course of the disease?
24. How do the changes in symptoms affect occupational performance?
25. What is the prognosis for a client with HD?
26. What OT interventions are appropriate for the client with HD at the various stages of the disease?
27. What environmental modifications should be made to accommodate the client with HD?
28. What are the initial symptoms of PD?
29. What is the underlying degenerative neurological process associated with PD?
30. What changes in symptoms occur over the course of the disease?
31. How do the changes in symptoms affect occupational performance?
32. What is the prognosis for a client with PD?
33. What OT interventions are appropriate for the client with PD?
34. How does the medication schedule of levodopa affect a client's daily routine?
35. What environmental modifications should be made to accommodate the client with PD?

REFERENCES

1. Allen C: *Allen Cognitive Level (ACL) test*, Rockville, MD, 1991, American Occupational Therapy Foundation.
2. Allen CK, Earhart CA, Blue T: *Occupational therapy treatment goals for the physically and cognitively disabled*, Rockville, MD, 1992, American Occupational Therapy Association.
3. Amato MP, Ponziani G, Guiseppina MD, Siracus G, Sorbi, S: Cognitive impairment in early-onset multiple sclerosis: a reappraisal after 10 years, *Arch Neurol* 58(10):1602, 2001.
4. Amato MP et al: Cognitive impairment in early-onset multiple sclerosis, *Arch Neurol* 52(2): 168, 1995.
5. American Occupational Therapy Association: *Occupational therapy practice guidelines for adults with neurodegenerative diseases: multiple sclerosis, transverse myelitis, and amyotrophic lateral sclerosis*, Bethesda, MD, 1999, The Association.
6. American Occupational Therapy Association: Statement: occupational therapy services for persons with Alzheimer's disease and other dementias, *Am J Occup Ther* 48(11):1029, 1994.
7. American Psychiatric Association: *DSM IV: Diagnostic and statistical manual of mental disorders*, ed 4, Washington, DC, 1994, The Association.
8. Asher IE: *Occupational therapy assessment tools: an annotated index*, ed 2, Bethesda, MD, 1996, American Occupational Therapy Association.
9. Atchison P: Helping people with Alzheimer's and their families preserve independence, *OT Week* 8:16, 1994.
10. Attarian HP et al: The relationship of sleep disturbances and fatigue in multiple sclerosis, *Arch Neurol* 61 (4):525, 2004.
11. Bain BK: Switches, control interfaces, and access methods. In Bain BK, Leger D, editors: *Assistive technology*, New York, 1997, Churchill Livingstone.
12. Bandmann O, Marsden CD, Wood NW: Genetic aspects of Parkinson's disease, *Mov Disord* 13(2):203, 1998.
13. Barusch A, Spaid W: Gender differences in caregiving: why do wives report greater burden? *Gerontologist* 29(5):667, 1989.
14. Basso MR et al: Screening for cognitive dysfunction in multiple sclerosis, *Arch Neurol* 53(10): 980, 1996.
15. Baum C: Addressing the needs of the cognitively impaired elderly from a family policy perspective, *Am J Occup Ther* 45(7):594, 1991.
16. Baum C, Edwards D: Cognitive performance in senile dementia of the Alzheimer's type: the kitchen task assessment, *Am J Occup Ther* 47(5):431, 1993.
17. Baum C, Edwards D: Identification and measurement of productive behaviors in senile dementia of the Alzheimer's type, *Gerontologist* 33(3):403, 1993.
18. Beck AT, Steer RA: *Beck Depression Inventory*, rev ed, San Antonio, TX, 1987, Psychological Corporation.
19. Beck AT et al: An inventory for measuring depression, *Arch Gen Psychiatry* 4:561, 1961.
20. Belsh JM: Definitions of terms, classifications, and diagnostic criteria of ALS. In Belsh JM, Schiffman PL, editors: *ALS diagnosis and management for the clinician*, Armonk, NY, 1996, Futura Publishing.
21. Belsh JM, Schiffman PL, editors: *ALS diagnosis and management for the clinician*, Armonk, NY, 1996, Futura Publishing.
22. Berg D et al: The correlation between ventricular diameter measured by transcranial sonography and clinical disability and cognitive dysfunction in patients with multiple sclerosis, *Arch Neurol* 57(9):1289, 2000.
23. Birnesser L: Treating dementia: practical strategies for long-term care, *OT Practice* 2(6):16, June 1997.
24. Borlongan CV, Sanberg PR, Freman TB: Neural transplantation for neurodegenerative disorders, *Lancet* 353(suppl 1):29, 1999.
25. Bowen J et al: Predictors of mortality in patients diagnosed with probable Alzheimer's disease, *Neurology* 47(2):433, 1996.
26. Buchner D, Larsen E: Falls and fractures in patients with Alzheimer's-type dementia, *JAMA* 257(11):1492, 1987.
27. Burns T, Mortimer JA, Merchak P: Cognitive performance test: a new approach to functional assessment in Alzheimer's disease, *J Geriatr Psychiatry Neurol* 7(1):46, 1994.

28. Carswell A, Eastwood R: Activities of daily living, cognitive impairment and social function in community residents with Alzheimer disease, *Can J Occup Ther* 60:130, 1993.

29. Cherry D: Teaching others how to manage the challenging behaviors of dementia. In *Summer series on aging*, San Francisco, CA, 1997, American Society on Aging.

30. Christenson M: Environmental design, modification and adaptation. In Larson O et al, editors: *Role of occupational therapy and the elderly*, Rockville, MD, 1996, American Occupational Therapy Association.

31. Cicchetti F, Parent A: Striatal interneurons in Huntington's disease: selective increase in the density of calretinin-immunoreactive medium-sized neurons, *Mov Disord* 11(6):619, 1996.

32. Cobb AK, Hamera E, Festoff BW: The decision-making process in amyotrophic lateral sclerosis. In Charash L et al, editors: *Coping with progressive neuromuscular diseases*, Philadelphia, 1987, Charles Press.

33. Cohen JA et al: Intrarater and interrater reliability of the MS functional composite outcome measure, *Neurology* 54(4):802, 2000.

34. Collier TJ, Kordower JH: Neural transplantation for the treatment of Parkinson's disease: present-day optimism and future challenges. In Jankovic J, Tolosa E, editors: *Parkinson's disease and movement disorders*, ed 3, Baltimore, 1998, Williams & Wilkins.

35. Comptson A, editor: *McAlpine's multiple sclerosis*, ed 3, New York, 1998, Churchill.

36. Corcoran M, Gitlin L: Family acceptance and use of environmental strategies provided in an occupational therapy intervention, *Occup Phys Ther Geriatr* 19(1):1-20, 2001.

37. Corcoran M, Gitlin L: Dementia management: an occupational therapy home based intervention for caregivers, *Am J Occup Ther* 46(9):801, 1992.

38. Corder E et al: Gene dose of apolipoprotein E type allele and the risk of Alzheimer's disease in late onset families, *Science* 261(5123):921, 1993.

39. Curra A, Berardelli A, Agostino R: Performance of sequential arm movements with and without advanced knowledge of motor pathways in Parkinson's disease, *Mov Disord* 12(5):646, 1997.

40. Delwaide PJ, Gonce M: Pathophysiology of Parkinson's signs. In Jankovic J, Tolosa E, editors: *Parkinson's disease and movement disorders*, ed 3, Baltimore, 1998, Williams & Wilkins.

41. Dixon C: Preventing striking out behavior by a geriatric resident, *OT Practice* 1(2):39, 1996.

42. Doble SE et al: Functional competence of community-dwelling persons with multiple sclerosis using the Assessment of Motor Process Skills, *Arch Phys Med Rehabil* 75(8):843, 1994.

43. Dodel RC et al: Cost of drug treatment in Parkinson's disease, *Mov Disord* 13(2):249, 1998.

44. Duvoisin RC, Sage JI: The spectrum of parkinsonism. In Chokroverty S, editor: *Movement disorders*, New Brunswick, NJ, 1990, PMA Publishing.

45. Edwards D, Baum C: Caregiver burden across stages of dementia, *OT Practice* 2:17, 1990.

46. Evans D: Estimated prevalence of Alzheimer's disease in the U.S., *Milbank Quarterly* 68:267, 1990.

47. Fahn S, Elton RL: The Unified Parkinson's Disease Rating Scale. In Fahn S et al, editors: *Recent developments in Parkinson's disease*, vol 2, Florham Park, NJ, 1987, Macmillian Healthcare Information.

48. Fisher A: The assessment of motor and process skill (AMPS) in assessing adults: functional measures and successful outcomes, Rockville, MD, 1991, American Occupational Therapy Foundation.

49. Fitzpatrick R, Peto V, Jenkinson C: Health-related quality of life in Parkinson's disease: a study of outpatient clinic attenders, *Mov Disord* 12(6):916, 1997.

50. Folstein SE: *Huntington's disease: a disorder of families*, Baltimore, 1989, Johns Hopkins University Press.

51. Folstein MF, Folstein SE, McHugh PR: Mini-Mental State: a practical method for grading the cognitive state of patients for the clinician, *J Psychiatr Res* 12(3):189, 1975.

52. Foti D: Gerontic occupational therapy: specialized intervention for the older adult. In Larson O et al, editors: *Role of occupational therapy and the elderly*, Rockville, MD, 1996, American Occupational Therapy Association.

53. Galasko D et al: The consortium to establish a registry for Alzheimer's disease (CERAD). XI: Clinical milestones in your patients with Alzheimer's disease followed over 3 years, *Neurology* 45(8):1451, 1995.

54. Gauthier L, Dalziel S, Gauthier S: The benefits of group occupational therapy for patients with Parkinson's disease, *Am J Occup Ther* 41(6):360, 1987.

55. Gelb DJ: *Introduction to clinical neurology*, Boston, 1995, Butterworth-Heinemann.

56. Gelinas I et al: Development of a functional measure for persons with Alzheimer's disease: the disability assessment for dementia, *Am J Occup Ther* 53(5):471, 1999.

57. Giladi N, Kao R, Fahn S: Freezing phenomenon in patients with parkinsonian syndromes, *Mov Disord* 12(3):302, 1997.

58. Gilliam TC, Kandel ER, Jessell TM: Genes and behavior. In Kandel ER, Schwartz JH, Jessell TM, editors: *Principles of neural science*, ed 4, New York, 2000, McGraw-Hill.

59. Glickstein J: *Therapeutic interventions in Alzheimer's disease*, Gaithersburg, MD, 1997, Aspen Publishers.

60. Goate A, Chartier-Harlin MC, Mullan M: Segregation of a missense mutation in the amyloid precursor protein gene with familial Alzheimer's disease, *Nature* 349(6311):973, 1991.

61. Goldman SM, Tanner C: Etiology of Parkinson's disease. In Jankovic J, Tolosa E, editors: *Parkinson's disease and movement disorders*, ed 3, Baltimore, 1998, Williams & Wilkins.

62. Grigsby J et al: Prediction of deficits in behavioral self-regulation among persons with multiple sclerosis, *Arch Phys Med Rehabil* 74(12): 1350, 1993.

63. Guberman A: *An introduction to clinical neurology, pathophysiology, diagnosis, and treatment*, Boston, 1994, Little, Brown.

64. Gwyther L, Matteson M: Care for the caregivers, *J Gerontol Nurs* 9(2):93, 1983.

65. Hasselkus B: Occupation and well being in dementia: the experience of day-care staff, *Am J Occup Ther* 52(6):423, 1998.

66. Hayden MR: *Huntington's chorea*, New York, 1996, Springer-Verlag.

67. Hecht M et al: Subjective experience and coping in ALS, *ALS Other Motor Neuron Disorders* 3:225, 2002.

68. Hendrie H: Epidemiology of dementia and Alzheimer's disease, *Am J Geriatric Psychiatry* 6(2):S3, 1998.

69. Hoehn MM, Yahr MD: Parkinsonism: onset, progression and mortality, *Neurology* 17(5):427, 1967.

70. Hugos C, Copperman L: Workshop: the new multiple sclerosis guidelines, delivering effective comprehensive therapy services, Monterey, CA, 1999.

71. Huntington Study Group: Unified Huntington's Disease Rating Scale: reliability and consistency, *Mov Disord* 11(2):136, 1996.

72. Hussian R: Modification of behaviors in dementia via stimulus manipulation, *Clin Gerontol* 8:37, 1988.

73. Imbriglio S: *Physical and occupational therapy for Huntington's disease*, New York, 1997, Huntington's Disease Society of America.

74. International Federation of Multiple Sclerosis Societies: Symposium on a minimal record of disability for multiple sclerosis, *Acta Neurol Scand* 70:169, 1984.

75. Janardhan V, Bakshi R: Quality of life and its relationship to brain lesions and atrophy on magnetic resonance images in 60 patients with Multiple Sclerosis, *Arch Neurol* 57(10):1485, 2000.

76. Joiner C, Hansel M: Empowering the geriatric client, *OT Practice* 1:34-39, 1996.

77. Katz S et al: Studies of illness in the aged. The index of ADL: a standardized measure of biological and psychological function, *JAMA* 135:75, 1963.

78. Kelly PJ: Pallidotomy in Parkinson's disease, *Neurosurgery* 36(6):1154, 1995.

79. Krauss JK, Grossman RG: Surgery for hyperkinetic movement disorders. In Jankovic J, Tolosa E, editors: *Parkinson's disease and movement disorders*, ed 3, Baltimore, 1998, Williams & Wilkins.

80. Kukull W et al: The Mini-Mental Status Examination and the diagnosis of dementia, *J Clin Epidemiol* 47(9):1061, 1994.

81. Larson E: Management of Alzheimer's disease in primary care settings, *Am J Geriatr Psychiatry* 6(2):S34, 1998.

82. Larson E et al: Adverse drug reactions associated with global cognitive impairment in elderly persons, *Ann Intern Med* 107(2):169, 1987.

83. Larson E et al: Dementia in elderly outpatients: a prospective study, *Ann Intern Med* 100(3):417, 1984.

84. Lawton M, Brody E: Assessment of older people: self-maintaining and IADL, *Gerontologist* 9(3):179, 1969.

85. LeBarge E: A preliminary scale to measure degree of worry among mildly demented Alzheimer disease patients, *Phys Occup Ther in Geriatrics* 11:43, 1993.

86. Levy LL: Activity, social role retention and the multiply disabled aged: strategies for intervention, *Occup Ther in Mental Health* 10:1, 1990.

87. Levy LL: Cognitive integration and cognitive components. In Larson KO et al, editors: *The role of occupational therapy with the elderly*, Bethesda, MD, 1996, American Occupational Therapy Association.

88. Levy LL: Cognitive treatment. In Davis LJ, Kirkland M, editors: *The role of occupational therapy with the elderly*, Rockville, MD, 1988, American Occupational Therapy Association.

89. Levy-Lahad E et al: Candidate gene for chromosome 1 familial Alzheimer's disease locus, *Science* 269(5226):973, 1995.

90. Lewis I, Kirchen S, editors: *Dealing with ethnic diversity in nursing homes*, Washington, DC, 1996, Taylor & Francis.

91. Lou JS et al: Fatigue and depression are associated with poor quality of life in ALS, *Neurology* 60:122, 2003.

92. Louis ED et al: Reliability of patient completion of the historical section of the Unified Parkinson's Disease Rating Scale, *Mov Disord* 11(2):185, 1996.

93. Madhusoodanan S et al: Efficacy of risperidone treatment for psychoses associated with schizophrenia, bipolar disorder or senile dementia in 11 geriatric patients: a case series, *J Clin Psychiatry* 56(11):514, 1995.

94. Matthews WB et al, editors: *McAlpine's multiple sclerosis*, New York, 1985, Churchill Livingstone.

95. McCormick W et al: Symptom patterns and co-morbidity in the early stages of Alzheimer's disease, *J Am Geriatr Soc* 42:517, 1994.

96. McDonald ER et al: Survival in amyotrophic lateral sclerosis, *Arch Neurol* 51:17, 1994.

97. Mega M et al: The spectrum of behavioral changes in Alzheimer's disease, *Neurology* 46(1):130, 1996.

98. Miller RG et al: Practice parameter: the care of the patient with amyotrophic lateral sclerosis (an evidence-based review): Report of the Quality Standards Subcommittee of the American Academy of Neurology, *Neurol* 52:1311, 1999.

99. Miller DM et al: Clinical significance of the Multiple Sclerosis Functional Composite: relationship to patient-reported quality of life. *Arch Neurol* 57(9):1319, 2000.

100. Mirra S et al: The consortium to establish a registry for Alzheimer's disease (CERAD). II: Standardization of the neuropathologic assessment of Alzheimer's disease, *Neurology* 41(4):479, 1991.

101. Misulis KE: *Neurologic localization and diagnosis*, Boston, 1996, Butterworth-Heinemann.

102. Morscheck P: An overview of Alzheimer's disease and long term care, *Pride J Long-Term Health Care* 3:4, 1984.

103. Muller V et al: Short-term effects of behavioral treatment on movement initiation and postural control in Parkinson's disease: a controlled clinical study, *Mov Disord* 12(3):306, 1997.

104. Multiple Sclerosis Council: *Fatigue and multiple sclerosis*, Washington, DC, 1998, Paralyzed Veterans of America.

105. Multiple Sclerosis Council: *MS Functional Composite*, Oct 2001, National MS Society. www.nationalmssociety.org

106. Munsat TL: Slowing down ALS—is this good or bad? *ALS Other Motor Neuron Disorders* 2(Suppl 1):S19, 2001.

107. Nance MA, Sander G: Characteristics of individuals with Huntington's disease in long-term care, *Mov Disord* 11(5):542, 1996.

108. National Institutes of Health: *Huntington's disease: hope through research*, NIH Publication No. 98-19, Bethesda, MD, 1998, The Institutes.

109. National Multiple Sclerosis Society, *Depression and Multiple Sclerosis*. http://www.nationalmssociety.or/brochures, 2004.

110. Northern California Neurobehavioral Group: *Cognistat: the neurobehavioral cognitive status examination*, Fairfax, CA, 1995, The Group.

111. Noseworthy JH et al: Multiple sclerosis, *New Engl J Med* 343(13):938, 2000.

112. Nuyens G et al: Predictive value of SF-36 for MS-specific scales of the MS Quality of Life Inventory, *Internat J MS Care* 5(1):8, 2003.

113. Nygard L et al: Comparing motor and process ability of persons with suspected dementia in home and clinic settings, *Am J Occup Ther* 48(8):689, 1994.

114. Olanow CW: Gpi pallidotomy—have we made a dent in Parkinson's disease? *Ann Neurol* 40(3):341, 1996.

115. Olanow CW et al: Neurodegeneration and Parkinson's disease. In Jankovic J, Tolosa E, editors: *Parkinson's disease and movement disorders*, ed 3, Baltimore, 1998, Williams & Wilkins.

116. Parent A, Cicchetti F: The current model of basal ganglia organization under scrutiny, *Mov Disord* 13(2):199, 1998.

117. Paty D, Willoughby E, Whitaker J: Assessing the outcome of experimental therapies in multiple sclerosis patients. In Rudick RA, Goodkin DE, editors: *Treatment of multiple sclerosis: trial design, results, and future perspectives*, London, 1992, Springer-Verlag.

118. Penney JB, Young AB: Huntington's disease. In Jankovic J, Tolosa E, editors: *Parkinson's disease and movement disorders*, ed 3, Baltimore, 1998, Williams & Wilkins.

119. Phillips DH: *Living with Huntington's disease*, Madison, WI, 1982, University of Wisconsin Press.

120. Phillips JG, Stelmach GE: Parkinson's disease and other involuntary movement disorders of the basal ganglia. In Fredericks CM, Saladin LK, editors: *Pathophysiology of the motor systems*, Philadelphia, 1996, FA Davis.

121. Pinhas-Hamiel O, Sarova-Pinhas I, Achiron A: Multiple sclerosis in childhood and adolescence: clinical features and management, *Paediatr Drugs* 3(5):329, 2001.

122. Pittock SJ et al: Quality of life is favorable for most patients with multiple sclerosis: a population-based cohort study, *Arch Neurol* 61(5):679, 2004.

123. Poirier J: Apolipoprotein E in animal models of CNS injury and in Alzheimer's disease, *Trends Neurosci* 17(12):525, 1994.

124. Poirier J et al: Apolipoprotein E4 allele as a predictor of cholinergic deficits and treatment outcome in Alzheimer's disease. In *Proceedings of the National Academy of Science* 92:12260, Washington, DC, The Academy.

125. Poewe W, Wenning G: Levodopa in Parkinson's disease: mechanisms of action and pathophysiology of late failure. In Jankovic J, Tolosa E, editors: *Parkinson's disease and movement disorders*, ed 3, Baltimore, 1998, Williams & Wilkins.

126. Pollak P: Parkinson's disease and related movement disorders. In Bogousslasky J, Fisher M, editors: *Textbook of neurology*, Boston, 1998, Butterworth Heinemann.

127. Prochazka A et al: Measurement of rigidity in Parkinson's disease, *Mov Disord* 12(1):24, 1997.

128. Quinn N et al: Core assessment program for intracerebral transplantation in Huntington's disease, *Mov Disord* 11(2):143, 1996.

129. Rabins P, Cummings J: Introduction, *Am J Geriatr Psychiatry* 6(2):S1, 1998.

130. Ranen NG et al: A controlled trial of idebenone in Huntington's disease, *Mov Disord* 11(5):549, 1996.

131. Reddy PH, Williams M, Tagle DA: Recent advances in understanding the pathogenesis of Huntington's disease, *Trends Neurosci* 22(6):248, 1999.

132. Reifler B: Detection and treatment of mixed cognitive and affective symptoms in the elderly: is it dementia, depression or both? *Clin Geriatrics* 6:17, 1998.

133. Reisberg B, Ferris S, Anand R: Functional staging of dementia of the Alzheimer's type, *Ann New York Acad Sci* 435:481, 1984.

134. Reisberg B et al: The Global Deterioration Scale for assessment of primary degenerative dementia, *Am J Psychiatry* 139(9):1136, 1982.

135. Richards M et al: Interrater reliability of the Unified Parkinson's Disease Rating Scale Motor Examination, *Mov Disord* 9(1):89, 1994.

136. de Rijk MC et al: Prevalence of Parkinson's disease in the elderly: the Rotterdam study, *Neurology* 45(12):2143, 1995.

137. Robberecht W, Brown RH: Etiology and pathogenesis of ALS: biochemical, genetic, and other theories. In Belsh JM, Schiffman PL, editors: *ALS diagnosis and management for the clinician*, Armonk, NY, 1996, Futura Publishing.

138. Robinson B: Validation of caregiver strain index, *J Gerontol* 38(3):99, 1983.

139. Rosin R, Topka H, Dichgans J: Gait initiation in Parkinson's disease, *Mov Disord* 12(5):682, 1997.

140. Sage JI, Duvoisin RC: The modern management of Parkinson's disease. In Chokroverty S, editor: *Movement disorders*, New Brunswick, NJ, 1990, PMA Publishing.

141. Sano M et al: A controlled trial of selegiline, alpha-tocopherol or both as treatment for Alzheimer's disease, *New Engl J Med* 336(17):1216, 1997.

142. Schneider LS: Cholinergic deficiency in Alzheimer's disease: pathogenic model, *Am J Geriatr Psychiatry* 6(2):S49, 1998.

143. Schwartz CE et al: Measuring self-efficacy in people with multiple sclerosis: a validation study, *Arch Phys Med Rehabil* 77(4):394, 1996.

144. Sclan S, Reisberg B: Functional assessment staging (FAST) in Alzheimer's disease: reliability, validity, and ordinality, *Int Psychogeriatrics* 4(Suppl 1):55, 1992.

145. Seshadri S, Drachman D, Lippa C: Apolipoprotein E epsilon 4 allele and lifetime risk of Alzheimer's disease: what physicians know and what they should know, *Arch Neurol* 52(11):1074, 1995.

146. Shamberg S, Shamberg A: Blueprints for independence, *OT Week* June: 24, 1996.

147. Sherrington R et al: Cloning of a gene bearing missense mutations in early-onset familial Alzheimer's disease, *Nature* 375(6534):754, 1995.

148. Shoulson I, Fahn S: Huntington's disease: clinical care and evaluation, *Neurology* 29(1):1, 1979.

149. Sibley W: *Therapeutic claims in multiple sclerosis: a guide to treatments*, ed 4, New York, 1996, Demos Medical Publishing.

150. Siesling S, Zwinderman AH, van Vugt JP, et al: A shortened version of the motor section of the Unified Huntington's Disease Rating Scale, *Mov Disord* 12(2):229, 1997.

151. Silani V et al: Stem cells in the treatment of amyotrophic lateral sclerosis (ALS), *ALS Other Motor Neuron Disorders* 3:173, 2002.

152. Small GW et al: Diagnosis and treatment of Alzheimer's disease and related disorders. Consensus statement of the American Association of Geriatric Psychiatry, the Alzheimer's Association, and the American Geriatrics Society, *JAMA* 278(16):1363, 1997.

153. Sperling RA et al: Regional magnetic resonance imaging lesion burden and cognitive function in multiple sclerosis: a longitudinal study, *Arch Neurol* 58(1):115, 2001.

154. Stern Y et al: Measurement and prediction of functional capacity in Alzheimer's disease, *Neurology* 40(1):8, 1990.

155. Stern G, Lees A: *Parkinson's disease*, Oxford, 1990, Oxford University Press.

156. Teri L, Logsdon R: Identifying pleasant activities for Alzheimer's disease patients: the pleasant events schedule, *Gerontologist* 31:124, 1990.

157. Thaut MH et al: Rhythmic auditory stimulation in gait training for Parkinson's disease patients, *Mov Disord* 11(2):193, 1996.

158. Tison F et al: Dependency in Parkinson's disease: a population-based survey in nondemented elderly subjects, *Mov Disord* 12(6):1073, 1997.

159. Trace S, Howell T: Occupational therapy in geriatric mental health, *Am J Occup Ther* 45(9):833, 1991.

160. Turner MR, Parton MJ, Leigh PN: Clinical trials in ALS: an overview, *Semin Neurol* 21(2):167, 2001.

161. Uhlmann R, Larson E, Koepsell T: Visual impairment and cognitive dysfunction in Alzheimer's disease, *J Gen Intern Med* 6(2):126, 1991.

162. Uhlmann R, Larson E, Rees T: Relationship of hearing impairment to dementia and cognitive dysfunction in older adults, *JAMA* 261(13):1916, 1989.

163. Weinshenker BG, Issa M, Baskerville J: Long-term and short-term outcome of multiple sclerosis, *Arch Neurol* 53(4): 353, 1996.

164. Wiederholt W: Parkinson's disease and other movement disorders. In *Neurology for non-neurologists*, ed 4, Philadelphia, 2000, WB Saunders.

165. Yeo G, editor: *Background*, Washington, DC, 1996, Taylor & Francis.

166. Yesavage JA et al: Development and validation of a geriatric depression scale: a preliminary report, *J Psychiatr Res* 17(1):37, 1982-1983.

167. Zarit S, Orr N, Zarit J: *The hidden victims of Alzheimer's disease*, New York, 1985, NYU Press.

168. Zhang Z, Roman GC: Worldwide occurrence of Parkinson's disease: an updated review, *Neuroepidemiology* 12(4):195-208, 1993.

SUGGESTED READING

Bello-Haas VD, Kloos AD, Mitsumoto H: Physical therapy for a patient through six stages of amyotrophic lateral sclerosis, *Phys Ther* 78(12):1312, 1998.

Borasio, GD, Votz, R, Miller RG: Palliative care in amyotrophic lateral sclerosis, *Palliative Care* 19(4): 829, 2001.

Frankel D: Multiple sclerosis. In Umphred DA, editor: *Neurological rehabilitation*, ed 3, St Louis, 1995, Mosby.

Kraft GH, Freal JE, Coryell JK: Disability, disease duration, and rehabilitation service needs in multiple sclerosis: patient perspectives, *Arch Phys Med Rehabil* 67(3):353, 1986.

LaBan MM et al: Physical and occupational therapy in the treatment of patients with multiple sclerosis, *Phys Med Rehabil Clin North Am* 9(3):603, 1998.

Lechtzin N et al: Amyotrophic lateral sclerosis: evaluation and treatment of respiratory impairment, *ALS Other Motor Neuron Disorders* 3:5, 2002.

Newman EM, Echevarria ME, Digman G: Degenerative diseases. In Trombly CA, editor: *Occupational therapy for physical dysfunction*, ed 4, Boston, 1995, Williams & Wilkins.

Pulaski KH: Adult neurological dysfunction. In Neistadt ME, Crepeau EB, editors: *Willard & Spackman's occupational therapy*, ed 9, Philadelphia, 1998, Lippincott.

Struifbergen AK, Rogers S: Health promotion: an essential component of rehabilitation for persons with chronic disabling conditions, *Adv Nurs Sci* 19(4):1, 1997.

Verma A, Bradley WG: Atypical motor neuron disease and related motor syndromes, *Semin Neurol* 21(2):177, 2001.

Walling AD: Amyotrophic lateral sclerosis: Lou Gehrig's disease, *Am Fam Physician* 59(6):1489, 1999.

RESOURCES

Amyotrophic Lateral Sclerosis Association
http://www.alsa.org

Brunel University, Centre for the Study of Health and Illness
www.brunel.ac.uk/about/acad/sssl/ssslresearch/centres/cshi/

International Journal of MS Care
www.mscare.org/journal/

MS Watch
www.mswatch.com

National Multiple Sclerosis Society
www.nmssociety.org.

36

SPINAL CORD INJURY

CAROLE ADLER

KEY TERMS

Tetraplegia/quadriplegia
Paraplegia
Autonomic dysreflexia

Spasticity
Heterotopic ossification
Decubitus ulcer

Rehabilitation technology
supplier

LEARNING OBJECTIVES

After studying this chapter the student or practitioner will be able to do the following:

1. Understand the difference between complete and incomplete spinal cord injury and the classification system used to describe such levels of injury.
2. Recognize and identify the various spinal cord injury syndromes.
3. Briefly describe the medical and surgical management of the individual who has experienced a traumatic spinal cord injury.
4. Identify some of the complications that can limit optimal functional potential.
5. Describe the changes in sexual functioning in males and females after spinal cord injury.
6. Identify the specific assessment tools that must be considered before developing intervention objectives.

7. Analyze the critical issues in factors to consider when developing intervention objectives during the acute, active, and discharge phases of the rehabilitation process.
8. Identify in detail the functional outcomes, including equipment considerations and personal and home care needs, that can be reached at each level of complete injury under optimal circumstances.
9. Analyze how the normal aging process is accelerated by the effects of spinal cord injury, and explain how functional status may change.

CHAPTER OUTLINE

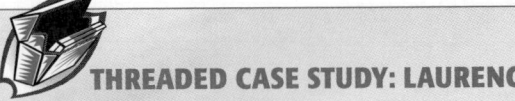

THREADED CASE STUDY: LAURENCE, PART 1

Laurence is a 44-year-old Caucasian man who sustained a C7 complete (ASIA A) spinal cord injury (SCI) as a result of a fall. He also sustained facial lacerations and bilateral radial wrist fractures, which necessitated casting without internal fixation. Laurence is divorced with no biological children. He has a 21-year-old stepdaughter with whom he is very close. He is a firefighter and has a background in auto mechanics. Laurence is very athletic, a triathlete and marathon runner. Just before his accident, Laurence had moved into a second-story apartment.

Laurence was referred to occupational therapy (OT) on the day of his injury and was initially evaluated in the intensive care unit (ICU) within 24 hours of the injury. Because of the acute nature of his injury and the immediacy of his needs related to client factors, the occupational profile and history, which are normally the first priority in the OT evaluation, were temporarily postponed until his physical and environmental control needs could be addressed. He was immobilized in cervical traction and bilateral wrist casts on a kinetic bed. His specific manual muscle test revealed 3+ (Fair +) to 4 (Good) strength in deltoids, biceps, and triceps. Wrists could not be tested secondary to bilateral wrist casts, and finger and thumb flexion and extension were noted to be at least 2− (Poor −) bilaterally. Sensory examination was intact to the C7 dermatome. Vital capacity was low secondary to the absence of innervation of intercostals and abdominal musculature, and Laurence required respiratory treatments four times per day to mobilize lung secretions. Because of his immobilization, he required assistance for all aspects of his activities of daily living (ADLs), including bed and wheelchair mobility.

OT intervention objectives included (1) maintaining optimal range of motion (ROM) in all joints for maximal upper extremity function and seated positioning; (2) achieving optimal strength and endurance in available musculature; (3) achieving optimal independence in all ADLs, including bathing, toileting, and skin care; (4) achieving independent wheelchair mobility on all indoor and outdoor surfaces; (5) receiving appropriate durable medical equipment (DME) to meet both short- and long-term needs (e.g., manual and power wheelchairs, cushion, and bathing and toileting equipment); (6) achieving optimal independence in the instrumental activities of daily living (IADLs), such as returning to safe and accessible housing; and (7) being educated in all aspects of care and independently instructing caregivers in assistance needed.

Laurence has had a very difficult time accepting the fact that he had a complete SCI. He could not imagine how he could function at work and in his community as a person with quadriplegia. The occupations of most importance to him were to resume his work as a firefighter and to continue in his previous athletic activities. Clearly, the severity of his injury makes him unable to return to those occupations as he knew them. His work and church community offered a tremendous amount of support, yet he continued to be depressed and angry over his loss of mobility and independence. He received regular psychological counseling and attended a weekly peer support group.

Throughout this chapter, consider the long-term consequences of Laurence's injuries to his ability to engage in occupation to support participation in his life contexts. Keep in mind the effects of SCI on client factors, performance skills and patterns, and the relationship of activity demands to selection of the optimal equipment to enhance mobility and other areas of occupation.

Critical Thinking Questions

1. Considering Laurence's level of SCI, what expectations would there be for functional recovery and what interventions would the therapist provide to maximize his independence in performance of ADLs and IADLs?
2. What durable medical equipment (DME) and adaptive equipment will maximize efficiency in his mobility and ADLs?
3. How will the therapist approach OT interventions and realistic expectations regarding work, social participation, leisure, and other important lifestyle options considering Laurence's depression and anger over his situation?

Rehabilitation of the client with a spinal cord injury (SCI) is a lifelong process that requires readjustment to nearly every aspect of life. Occupational therapists and occupational therapy (OT) assistants play a significant role in physical and psychosocial restoration and help the client achieve maximal independence. Through accurate evaluation, retraining, and adaptive techniques and equipment, occupational therapists provide their clients with the tools and resources needed to resume engagement in occupation to support participation in life situations to their maximal physical and functional potential.

SCIs have many causes, trauma being the most common. Trauma can result from motor vehicle accidents, violent injuries such as gunshot and stab wounds, falls, sports accidents, and diving accidents.[5,12] Normal spinal cord function may also be disturbed by diseases such as tumors, myelomeningocele, syringomyelia, multiple sclerosis, cancer, and amyotrophic lateral sclerosis. Some of the intervention principles outlined in this chapter may apply to these conditions; however, the emphasis is on rehabilitation of the individual with a traumatic SCI.

RESULTS OF SPINAL CORD INJURY

SCI results in quadriplegia (labeled *tetraplegia* by the American Spinal Cord Injury Association) or paraplegia. **Tetraplegia,** which will be referred to as *quadriplegia* throughout the remainder of the chapter, is any degree of paralysis of the four limbs and trunk musculature. There may be partial upper extremity (UE) function, depending on the level of the cervical lesion. **Paraplegia** is paralysis of the lower extremities (LEs) with some involvement of the trunk, depending on the level of the lesion.[5,12]

SCIs are referred to in terms of the regions (cervical, thoracic, and lumbar) of the spinal cord in which they occur and the numerical order of the neurological segments. The level of SCI designates the last fully functioning neurological segment of the cord. For example, *C6* refers to the sixth neurological segment of the cervical region of the spinal cord as the last fully intact neurological segment.[3,5] Complete lesions result in the absence of motor or sensory function of the spinal cord below the level of the injury.

Incomplete lesions may involve several neurological segments, and some spinal cord function may be partially or completely intact.[2,3]

COMPLETE VERSUS INCOMPLETE NEUROLOGICAL CLASSIFICATIONS

The extent of neurological damage depends on the location and severity of the injury (Figure 36-1). In a complete injury, total paralysis and loss of sensation result from a complete interruption of the ascending and descending nerve tracts below the level of the lesion. In an incomplete injury, there is some degree of preservation of the sensory or motor nerve pathways below the level of the lesion. Segments at which normal function is found often differ in the side of the body and in terms of sensory versus motor testing.

It is essential that a very careful neurological examination be done before determining whether an injury is complete or incomplete.

The American Spinal Injury Association (ASIA) uses the findings from the neurological examination to classify injury types to further objectify specific clinical findings:

- *ASIA impairment scale classification A* indicates a complete lesion; there is no motor or sensory function preserved in the sacral segments S4 through S5. Any preservation of strength without sensory sparing in the sacral segments of S4 through S5 is considered a zone of partial preservation (ZPP) and still considered a complete (ASIA A) neurological classification.
- *ASIA classification B* indicates an incomplete lesion in which sensory but not motor function is preserved below the neurological level and must include the sacral segments S4 through S5.
- *ASIA classification C* indicates an incomplete lesion in which motor function is preserved below the neurological level and more than half of the key muscles below the neurological level have a muscle grade of less than 3 (Fair).
- *ASIA classification D* indicates an incomplete lesion in which motor function is preserved below the neurological level and at least half of the key muscles below the neurological level have a muscle grade of 3 or more.
- *ASIA classification E* indicates that motor and sensory functions are normal.[1]

Incomplete injuries are categorized according to the area of damage: central, lateral, anterior, or peripheral.

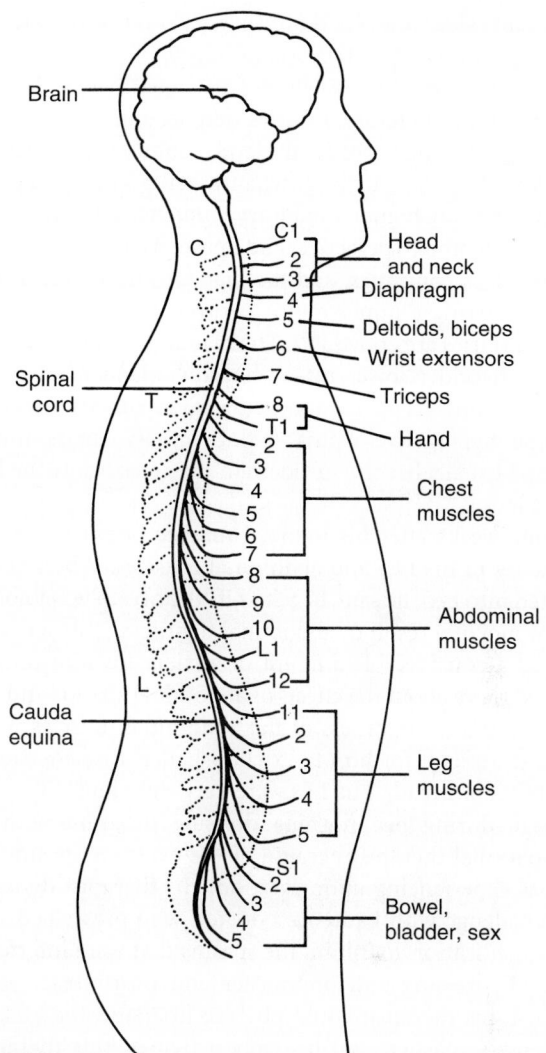

Figure 36-1 Spinal nerves and major areas of body they supply. (From Paulson S, editor: *Santa Clara Valley Medical Center spinal cord injury home care manual,* ed 2, San Jose, CA, 1994, Santa Clara Valley Medical Center.)

After thorough muscle and sensory testing, Laurence's neurological diagnosis was C7 ASIA A. Key musculature innervated by the C7 nerve root (triceps) was graded at 4 (good). He had 2– (Poor –) strength in his finger flexors, extensors, and thumb flexors. Because sensation was intact to the C7 dermatome level and completely absent below and in the sacral segments, his diagnosis was clearly ASIA A with a ZPP (zone of partial preservation) at C8.

CLINICAL SYNDROMES

After SCI the individual enters a stage of spinal shock that may last from 24 hours to 6 weeks. This period is one of areflexia, in which reflex activity ceases below the level of the injury.[3] The bladder and bowel are atonic or flaccid. Deep tendon reflexes are decreased, and sympathetic functions are disturbed. This disturbance results in decreased constriction of blood vessels, low blood pressure, a slower heart rate, and no perspiration below the level of injury.[10,16]

The spinal cord is usually not damaged below the level of the lesion. Therefore, muscles that are innervated by the neurological segments below the level of injury usually develop spasticity, because the monosynaptic reflex arc is intact but separated from higher inhibitory influences. Deep tendon reflexes become hyperactive, and spasticity may be evident. Sensory loss continues, and the bladder and bowel usually become spastic ("upper motor neuron" bladder) in clients whose injuries are above T12. The bladder and bowel usually remain flaccid ("lower motor neuron" bladder) in clients whose lesions are at L1 and below. Sympathetic functions become hyperactive. Spinal reflex activity (mass muscle spasms) usually becomes evident in the areas below the level of the lesion.[2,12,14]

Four weeks after his injury, Laurence began to develop spasticity in his LEs and abdominal muscles. When he was assisted into bed, he said, he felt as if "the breath was knocked out of me" as a result of abdominal tightness. This sensation created a considerable amount of anxiety for him until he learned more about the effects of abdominal spasms and how the involuntary tightness of the abdominal muscles would make it difficult for him to exhale—hence, the sensation of shortness of breath. His LEs were very tight and difficult to manage during his morning dressing program with the occupational therapist because of the extensor spasms that he was experiencing upon exertion. His therapist discussed this challenge with Laurence's doctor, who prescribed spasticity medication to inhibit the spasms that were interfering with LE dressing and pretransfer and posttransfer setup. Because his therapist could observe firsthand the effect of Laurence's spasticity on his daily activities, this therapist's feedback to Laurence's physician considerably influenced the dosage of his spasticity medications.

CENTRAL CORD SYNDROME

Central cord syndrome occurs when there is more cellular destruction in the center of the cord than in the periphery. Paralysis and sensory loss are greater in the UEs because these nerve tracts are more centrally located than those of the LEs. Central cord syndrome is often seen in older people in whom arthritic changes have caused a narrowing of the spinal canal; in such cases, cervical hyperextension without vertebral fracture may precipitate central cord damage.

BROWN-SEQUARD SYNDROME (LATERAL DAMAGE)

Brown-Sequard syndrome results when only one side of the cord is damaged, as in a stabbing or gunshot injury. Below the level of injury, there is motor paralysis and loss of proprioception on the ipsilateral side and loss of pain, temperature, and touch sensation on the contralateral side.

ANTERIOR SPINAL CORD SYNDROME

Anterior spinal cord syndrome results from injury that damages the anterior spinal artery or the anterior aspect of the cord. This syndrome involves paralysis and loss of pain, temperature, and touch sensation. Proprioception is preserved.

CAUDA EQUINA (PERIPHERAL)

Cauda equina injuries involve peripheral nerves rather than directly involving the spinal cord. This type of injury usually occurs with fractures below the L2 level and results in a flaccid-type paralysis. Because peripheral nerves possess a regenerating capacity that the cord does not, this injury is associated with a better prognosis for recovery. Patterns of sensory and motor deficits are highly variable and asymmetrical.

CONUS MEDULLARIS SYNDROME

Conus medullaris syndrome involves injury of the sacral cord (conus) and lumbar nerve roots within the neural canal, which usually results in an areflexic bladder, bowel, and LEs.

PROGNOSIS FOR RECOVERY

The prognosis for substantial recovery of neuromuscular function after SCI depends on whether the lesion is complete or incomplete. If there is no sensation or return of motor function below the level of lesion 24 to 48 hours after the injury in carefully assessed complete lesions, motor function is less likely to return. However, partial to full return of function to one spinal nerve root level below the fracture can be gained and may occur in the first 6 months after injury. In incomplete lesions, progressive return of motor function is possible, yet it is difficult to determine exactly how much and how quickly return will occur.[14] Frequently, the longer it takes for recovery to begin, the less likely it is that it will occur.

The following statements can be used as guidelines to predict and assist the therapist and their clients in understanding the recovery process after a new SCI[11]:

- The severity of the original injury determines whether recovery will occur. Unfortunately, no test to measure this severity exists at this time, and predictions must be based on what has happened to others in the past with similar neurological findings.
- Incomplete injuries are associated with a better chance of further recovery than are complete injuries, but even with incomplete injuries there is no guarantee that further recovery will occur.
- Most of the recovery that will occur starts within the first few weeks. Therefore, each day that goes by without any return of function means that the likelihood of recovery is reduced.

- No amount of hard work will cause nerve function to return. If hard work were all it took, very few people would end up with permanent paralysis.
- Rehabilitation will not affect the degree of recovery. The purpose of rehabilitation is to prevent further medical complications through education, to maintain and improve the strength and skills that are present, to maximize function in self-care activities, to facilitate mobility, and to optimize lifestyle options for the patient and their family.

MEDICAL AND SURGICAL MANAGEMENT OF THE PERSON WITH SPINAL CORD INJURY

After a traumatic event in which SCI is likely, the conscious client should be carefully questioned about cutaneous numbness and skeletal muscle paralysis before being moved. Emergency medical technicians, paramedics, and air transport personnel are trained in SCI precautions and extrication techniques for moving a person who has sustained a possible SCI from an accident site. Movement of the spine must be prevented during the transfer procedures. A firm stretcher or board to which the person's head and back can be strapped should be procured before moving the person. After the patient is transferred to the stretcher or board, he or she should be strapped to the board or stretcher and carefully transferred via air or ground transport to the nearest hospital emergency room. Axial traction on the neck should be maintained, and any movement of the spine and neck prevented during this process. Careful examination, stabilization, and transportation of the patient may keep a temporary or minimal SCI from becoming more severe or permanent. Initial care is directed toward preventing further damage to the spinal cord and reversing neurological damage, if possible, by stabilization or decompression of the injured neurological structures.[5,10,12] Antiinflammatory and steroidal drugs are administered immediately after injury in an effort to minimize swelling to the specific lesion and therefore minimize neurological damage, although the significance of their effect on neurological recovery remains unclear.

A careful neurological examination is carried out by the examining physician to aid in determining the site and type of injury. The client is in a supine position for this procedure, with the neck and spine immobilized. A catheter is usually placed in the client's bladder for drainage of urine. Anteroposterior and lateral X-ray films may be taken, with the individual's head, neck, or spine immobilized, to help determine the type of injury. A computed tomography (CT) scan or magnetic resonance imaging (MRI) may be needed for further evaluation. In early medical treatment the goals are to restore normal alignment of the spine, maintain stabilization of the injured area, and decompress neurological structures that are under pressure.

Bony realignment and stabilization are usually achieved by placing the client on a rotating kinetic bed (Figure 36-2)

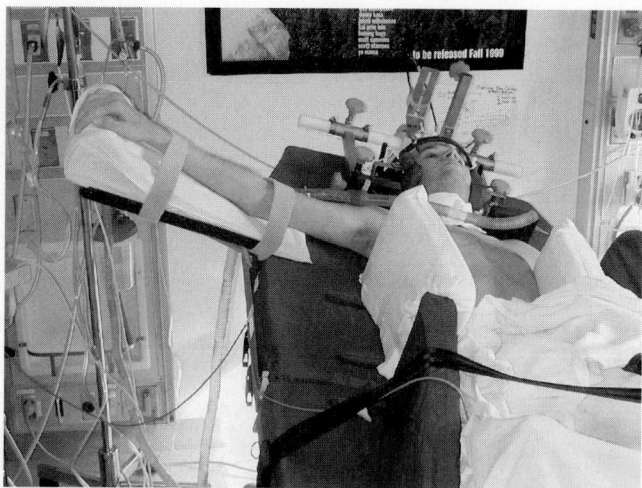

Figure 36-2 Kinetic bed with custom arm positioner. Designed and fabricated by the Occupational Therapy Department, Santa Clara Valley Medical Center, San Jose, CA. (Courtesy of Luis Gonzalez, Media Resource Department, Santa Clara Valley Medical Center.)

that allows skeletal traction and immobilization. The bed's constant rotation allows continuous pressure relief, mobilization of respiratory secretions, and easy access to the client's entire body for bowel, bladder, and hygiene care. Open surgical reduction with internal fixation and spinal fusion may be indicated.

The goals of surgery are to decompress the spinal cord and achieve spinal stability and normal bony alignment.[5,12] Surgery is not always necessary, and adequate immobilization may allow the individual to heal. As soon as possible, a means of portable immobilization is provided—usually a halo vest for cervical injuries (Figure 36-3, *A*) and a thoracic brace or body jacket for thoracic injuries (Figure 36-3, *B*). This approach enables the client to be transferred to a standard hospital bed and, subsequently, to be upright in a wheelchair and involved in an active therapy program in as little as 1 to 2 weeks after injury. Initiating an upright sitting tolerance program shortly after injury can substantially reduce the incidence and severity of further medical complications, such as deep vein thrombosis, joint contractures, and the general deconditioning that can result from prolonged bed rest.

The benefits of early transport to an SCI center have been documented.[7] Clients treated initially in a spinal cord acute-care unit rather than a general hospital had shorter acute-care lengths of stay. Clients treated in general hospitals tended to have a higher incidence of skin problems and spinal instability. It has been found that individuals sent to rehabilitation centers specializing in the treatment of SCI made functional gains with greater efficiency.[16] Spinal cord centers are equipped to offer a complete, multidisciplinary program executed by an experienced team of professionals who specialize in this unique and demanding disability.

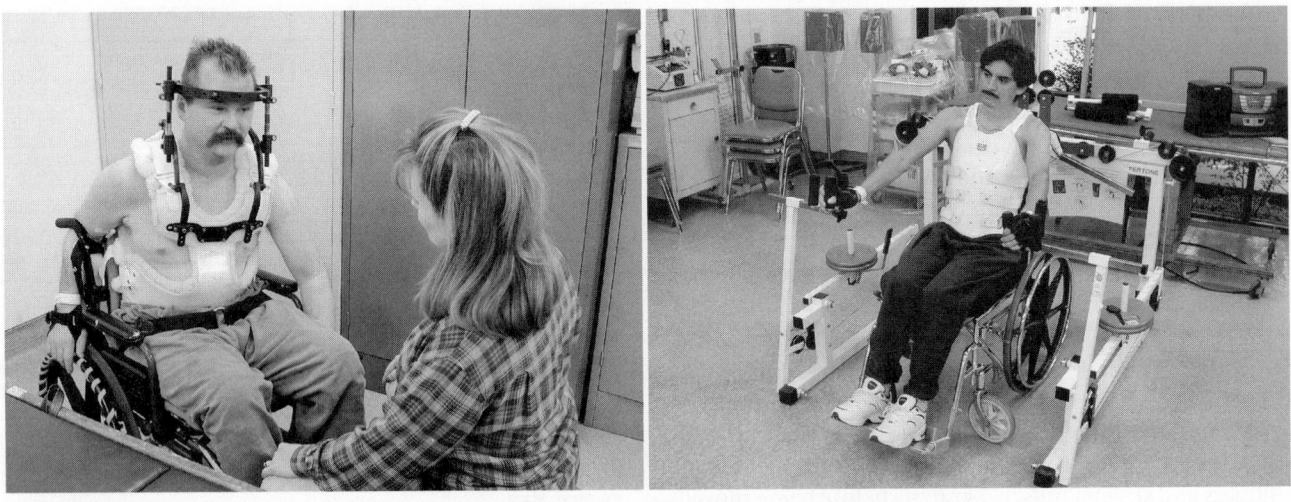

A   B

Figure 36-3 **A,** Halo vest: neck immobilization device for individuals with quadriplegia and high-level paraplegia (T1 to T4). **B,** Body jacket: one type of immobilization device for paraplegia. (Courtesy of Luis Gonzalez, Media Resource Department, Santa Clara Valley Medical Center.)

Laurence was injured at his work site, which happened to be very close to a hospital in which a designated SCI center was located. In addition to his cervical spine injury, he sustained bilateral wrist fractures and facial lacerations as a result of the nature of the fall from the equipment on which he had been standing. Standard practice at this particular hospital is to contact the physiatrist on call for an immediate opinion regarding trauma care.

COMPLICATIONS OF SPINAL CORD INJURY

SKIN BREAKDOWN, PRESSURE SORES, OR DECUBITUS ULCERS

Sensory loss increases the risk of skin breakdown. Persons with sensory loss cannot feel the pressure and shearing of prolonged sitting or lying in one position or the presence of pain or heat against the body. Pressure causes the loss of blood supply to the area, which can ultimately result in necrosis. Heat can quickly burn and destroy tissues. Shearing can destroy underlying tissue. Any combination of the aforementioned factors will hasten skin breakdown. The areas most likely to develop skin breakdown are bony prominences over the sacrum, ischium, trochanters, elbows, and heels; however, other bony prominences, such as the iliac crest, scapula, knees, toes, and rib cage, are also at risk.

All rehabilitation personnel must be aware of the signs of developing skin problems. At first the area reddens and then blanches when pressed. Later, the reddened or abraded area does not blanch, which indicates that necrosis has begun. Finally, a blister or ulceration appears in the area. The problem is often more severe below the level of the skin surface. The visible sore may be only the tip of the iceberg. If allowed to progress, a sore can become severe, destroying underlying tissues even as deep as the bone.

Skin breakdown can be prevented by relieving and eliminating pressure points and protecting vulnerable areas from excessive shearing, moisture, and heat. Routine turning of clients in bed, specialized mattresses and wheelchair seat cushions, protection of bony prominences with various types of padding, and the performance of weight shifts are some of the methods used to prevent pressure sores.

The use of hand splints, body jackets, and other orthoses can also cause skin breakdown, particularly when protective sensation in those areas is impaired. The therapist must inspect the skin, and the client must be taught to examine his or her skin on a consistent, daily basis, using a mirror or caregiver assistance to watch for signs of developing problems. Skin damage can develop within 30 minutes; therefore, frequent weight shifting, repositioning, and vigilance are essential if skin breakdown is to be prevented.[12,14]

DECREASED VITAL CAPACITY

Decreased vital capacity is a problem among people who have sustained cervical and high thoracic lesions. Such individuals have markedly limited chest expansion and a decreased ability to cough because of weakness or paralysis of the diaphragm and the intercostal and latissimus dorsi muscles. This scenario can result in a tendency toward respiratory tract infections. Reduced vital capacity affects the overall endurance level for activity. Endurance can be improved by assisted breathing and by vigorous respiratory and physical therapy. Strengthening of the sternocleidomastoids and the diaphragm, manually assisted cough, and deep breathing exercises are essential to maintain optimal vital capacity.[12,14]

Laurence's vital capacity was 50% of normal capacity for a man of his size. He required assistance to cough because he did not have the force to clear his secretions upon exhaling.

His endurance was low during his 4- to 5-hour therapy program. He required much education in this area because he was previously a triathlete and in exceptional cardiovascular shape.

OSTEOPOROSIS

Osteoporosis is likely to develop in individuals with SCIs because of disuse of long bones, particularly of the LEs. Osteoporosis may be sufficiently advanced for pathological fractures to occur a year after the injury. Pathological fractures are most common in the supracondylar area of the femur, proximal tibia, and distal tibia, the intertrochanteric area of the femur, and the neck of the femur. Pathological fractures are usually not seen in UEs. Daily standing with a standing frame may slow the onset of osteoporosis[12,14]; however, this is a controversial method and not embraced in all rehabilitation programs. A standing program must fit into the patient's activities of daily living (ADLs) after discharge to be effective on an ongoing basis. Not all reimbursement sources will cover the cost of standing equipment.

ORTHOSTATIC HYPOTENSION

A lack of muscle tone in the abdomen and LEs leads to pooling of blood in these areas, with a resultant decrease in blood pressure (hypotension). This problem occurs when the patient moves from a supine to upright position or changes body position too quickly. Symptoms are dizziness, nausea, and loss of consciousness.[4] The client must be reclined quickly and, if sitting in a wheelchair, should be tipped back with legs elevated until symptoms subside. With time, this problem can diminish as sitting tolerance and level of activity increase; however, some people continue to have hypotensive episodes. Abdominal binders, leg wraps, antiembolism stockings, and medications can help reduce symptoms.

AUTONOMIC DYSREFLEXIA

Autonomic dysreflexia is a phenomenon seen in persons whose injuries are above the T4 to T6 level. It is caused by reflex action of the autonomic nervous system in response to some stimulus, such as a distended bladder, fecal mass, bladder irritation, rectal manipulation, thermal or pain stimuli, or visceral distention. The symptoms are immediate pounding headache, anxiety, perspiration, flushing, chills, nasal congestion, paroxysmal hypertension, and bradycardia.

Autonomic dysreflexia is a medical emergency and life threatening. The client should not be left alone.[5,12,14] The condition is treated by placing the client in an upright position and removing anything restrictive, such as abdominal binders or elastic stockings, to reduce blood pressure. The bladder should be drained or leg bag tubing checked for obstruction. Blood pressure and other symptoms should be monitored until they return to normal. The occupational therapist must be aware of symptoms and treatment because autonomic dysreflexia can occur at any time after the injury.

Individuals who are susceptible to this condition are encouraged to carry an emergency card describing the condition and treatment because many emergency rooms and medical personnel may be unfamiliar with it.

SPASTICITY

Spasticity is a nearly universal complication of SCI.[14] It is an involuntary muscle contraction below the level of injury that results from lack of inhibition from the brain. Patterns of spasticity change over the first year, gradually increasing in the first 6 months and reaching a plateau about 1 year after the injury. A moderate amount of spasticity can be helpful in the overall rehabilitation of the patient with an SCI. It helps to maintain muscle mass, assists in the prevention of pressure sores by facilitating blood circulation, and can be used to assist in range of motion (ROM) and bed mobility. A sudden increase in spasticity can alert the individual to other medical problems, such as bladder infections, skin breakdown, and fever.

Because it can interfere with function, severe spasticity can be quite frustrating to both the client and the therapist. It may be treated more aggressively with a variety of medications. In select instances, local injections of nerve blocks or Botox may benefit some individuals. In severe cases, neurosurgical procedures can be performed.[5,12,14]

HETEROTOPIC OSSIFICATION

Heterotopic ossification (HO), also called *ectopic bone*, is bone that develops in abnormal anatomical locations.[16] It most often occurs in the muscles around the hip and knee, but occasionally it can also be noted at the elbow and shoulder. The first symptoms are swelling, warmth, and decreased joint ROM. The onset of HO is usually 1 to 4 months after injury. Early diagnosis and initiation of treatment can minimize complications. Treatment consists of medication and the maintenance of joint ROM during the early stage of active bone formation to preserve the functional ROM necessary for good wheelchair positioning, symmetrical position of the pelvis, and maximal functional mobility. If HO progresses to the phase of substantially limiting hip flexion, pelvic obliquity while in the sitting position is likely to occur. This problem contributes to trunk deformities such as scoliosis and kyphosis, with subsequent skin breakdown at the ischial tuberosities, trochanters, and sacrum.[5,12]

SEXUAL FUNCTION

The sexual drive and the need for physical and emotional intimacy are not altered by SCI. However, problems of mobility, functional dependency, and altered body image, as well as complicating medical problems and the attitudes of partners and society, affect social and sexual roles, access, and interest and satisfaction. Education is essential for the individual with an SCI and, as an important area of occupation (both in ADLs and social participation), is a critical part of the rehabilitation process. Lack of sensation over one part of the body is accompanied by increased or altered sensation over other parts of the body. The sexual response of the body after SCI needs to be explored in the same way a person learns what muscles are working and where he or she can feel.

In males, erections and ejaculations are often affected by SCI. However, because this problem is variable, it should be evaluated individually. The viability of sperm in men with SCI is frequently decreased, even when other function is near normal.[1] Research is under way to investigate the possible sources of infertility caused by SCI and to reverse the problem.

In women, menstruation usually ceases for an interval of weeks to months after injury. It will usually start again and return to normal in time. There may also be changes in lubrication of the vagina during sexual activity. In contrast to males, however, there is no change in female fertility. Females with SCI can conceive and give birth. Special attention must be given to the interaction of pregnancy and childbirth with SCI, especially with regard to blood clots, respiratory function, bladder infections, autonomic dysreflexia, and the use of medications during pregnancy and breast-feeding.

To avoid pregnancy, women with SCI must take precautions, and the type of birth control used must be considered carefully. Birth control pills are associated with blood clots, especially when combined with smoking, and probably should not be used. The intrauterine device (IUD) is not recommended, even for able-bodied females. Diaphragms may be difficult to position properly when there is loss of sensation in the vagina or decreased hand function. Foams and suppositories are not very effective. The use of condoms by the male partner is probably the safest method.

Disabled individuals quickly sense the attitudes of professionals and caregivers toward their sexuality. Awareness and acceptance by professionals is increasing, and sexual counseling and education are a regular part of many rehabilitation programs for all types of physical disabilities. Some clients lack basic sex education. Others feel asexual because of their disability and altered self-esteem and are isolated from peers; thus, they may feel uncomfortable with any type of sexual interaction. For these reasons, sexual education and counseling must be geared to the needs of the individual client and his or her significant other. In some instances, social interaction skills require improvement before sexual activity can be considered, and occupational therapists play an important role in providing information and a forum to deal with these issues. (See Chapter 12 for more information on sexuality with physical dysfunction.)

Laurence was divorced at the time of his accident. He was very close to his stepdaughter and was having a difficult time dealing with the dissolution of his family. While in the hospital, his ex-wife and stepdaughter resumed their relationship with Laurence in hopes of resolving their conflicts. After acknowledging the permanency of his disability, Laurence felt considerable depression, anger, and low self-esteem. Even with the resumption of family support and the large professional community of support he was given, he could not imagine himself as a sexual person who could offer his family and friends the love and relationships he had known in the past.

OCCUPATIONAL THERAPY INTERVENTION

EVALUATION

Evaluation of the client is an ongoing process that begins on the day of admission and continues long after discharge on an outpatient follow-up basis. Depending on whether the patient is in an acute inpatient rehabilitation, outpatient, or home setting, the occupational therapist should continually evaluate the client's functional progress and the appropriateness of intervention and equipment. An accurate and comprehensive formal initial evaluation is essential. Initial data gathered from the medical chart will provide personal information, a medical diagnosis, and a history of other pertinent medical information. Input from the multidisciplinary team will enhance the occupational therapist's ability to predict realistic optimal outcomes accurately.

Discharge planning begins during the initial evaluation. Therefore, the individual's social and vocational histories, as well as personal contexts such as past and expected living situations, are necessary for planning an intervention program that meets the client's ongoing needs. Intervention should begin as soon as possible. It is possible to quickly gather enough information to begin addressing high-priority areas such as splinting, positioning, and family training without having to wait for the evaluation to be completed.

OCCUPATIONAL AND PSYCHOSOCIAL STATUS

The top-down and client-centered approaches recommended in the Occupational Therapy Practice Framework (OTPF) suggest that the evaluation process begin with an occupational profile, which includes obtaining an occupational history and ascertaining the goals of the client as they pertain to resuming performance of favored occupations. Frequently, given the acute nature and overwhelming impact of an SCI, some of the physical problems associated with client factors crucial to survival must initially be given priority for evaluation. Efforts may be directed toward determining baseline neurological, clinical, and functional status from which to formulate an early intervention program. However, while the occupational therapist is initially addressing these critical client factors, he or she can be simultaneously engaging the client in an occupational profile, learning the areas of occupation that comprise and give meaning to the client's life. By involving the client as central to the intervention plan and identifying occupational goals as primary, the more physical aspects and client factors (body structure and body functions) are put into perspective as underlying and supportive to these occupational goals.

Through conducting the occupational profile and occupational history and beginning interventions, the occupational therapist has the opportunity to learn about and observe the client's psychosocial adjustment to the disability and life in general through the nature of the activities and occupations in which the patient participates.[12] The evaluation phase is important for establishing rapport and mutual trust, which will facilitate participation and progress in later and more difficult phases of rehabilitation. The client's motivation, determination, and contexts—including socioeconomic background, education, family support, personal attitudes toward disability, problem-solving abilities, and financial resources—can prove to be invaluable assets or limiting factors in determining the outcome of rehabilitation. A therapist must carefully observe the client's status in each of these areas before recommending the course of intervention.

PHYSICAL STATUS

Before evaluation of the client's physical status (or "client factors: body functions and body structures"), specific medical precautions should be obtained from the primary and consulting physicians. Skeletal instability and related injuries or medical complications will affect the way in which the client is moved and the active or resistive movements allowed.

Passive range of motion (PROM) should be measured before specific manual muscle testing to determine available pain-free movement. This evaluation also identifies the presence of or potential for joint contractures, which could suggest the need for preventive or corrective splinting and positioning.

Shoulder pain, which ultimately causes decreased shoulder and scapular ROM, is extremely common in those individuals with C4 through C7 quadriplegia. Among the possible causes is scapular immobilization resulting from prolonged bed rest and nerve root compression subsequent to the injury. Shoulder pain should be thoroughly assessed and diagnosed so that proper intervention can be provided before the onset of chronic discomfort and functional loss.

Accurate assessment of the client's muscle strength is critical in determining a precise diagnosis of neurological level and establishing a baseline for physical recovery and functional progress. Because the occupational therapist's skills with activity analysis greatly enhance his or her effectiveness in treating the client with SCI, a precise working knowledge of musculoskeletal anatomy and specific manual muscle testing techniques is essential. Use of accepted muscle testing protocols ensures accurate technique during performance of this complex evaluation. The muscle test should be repeated

as often as is necessary to provide an ongoing picture of the client's strength and progress.

Sensation is evaluated for light touch, superficial pain (pin prick), and kinesthesia, which determines areas of absent, impaired, and intact sensation. These findings are useful in establishing the level of injury and determining functional limitations (Figure 36-4).[1]

If the client is evaluated in the acute stage, spasticity is rarely noted because the client is still in spinal shock. When spinal shock subsides, increased muscle tone may be present in response to stimuli. The therapist should then determine whether the spasticity interferes with or enhances function.

An evaluation of wrist and hand function determines the degree to which a client can manipulate objects. This information is used to suggest the need for equipment such as positioning splints or universal cuffs or, later, consideration of a tenodesis orthosis (wrist-driven flexor hinge splint). Gross grasp and pinch measurements indicate functional abilities and may be used as an adjunct to manual muscle testing to provide objective measurements of baseline status and progress for clients who have active hand musculature.[8]

Clinical observation is used to assess endurance, oral motor control, head and trunk control, LE functional muscle strength, and total body function. More specific assessment in any of these areas may be required, depending on the client's specific needs.

An increased number of combined SCI and head-injury diagnoses suggests that a specific cognitive and perceptual evaluation may be necessary.[9] Assessing a client's ability to initiate tasks, follow directions, carry over learning day to day, and handle problem-solving tasks contributes to the information base necessary for appropriate and realistic goal setting. Understanding the client's learning style, coping skills, and communication style is also essential.

In Laurence's case, he had no memory of his fall and several hours of the time that elapsed after his accident. He also exhibited a slight memory deficit, as shown by his poor carryover of tasks from day to day during the first 2 weeks of his rehabilitation. He received a full cognitive assessment and was determined to be below his baseline for cognition and memory. His therapists helped him complete a memory book of his daily activities to assist in carryover. Because his therapists believed that his extreme depression contributed to his poor memory, he was seen daily for individual counseling. His memory and affect significantly improved over the next several weeks.

FUNCTIONAL STATUS

Observing as the client performs ADLs is an important part of the OT evaluation. The purpose of this observation is to determine present and potential levels of functional ability. If the client is cleared of bed-rest precautions, evaluation and simultaneous intervention should begin as soon as possible after injury. Light activities such as feeding, light

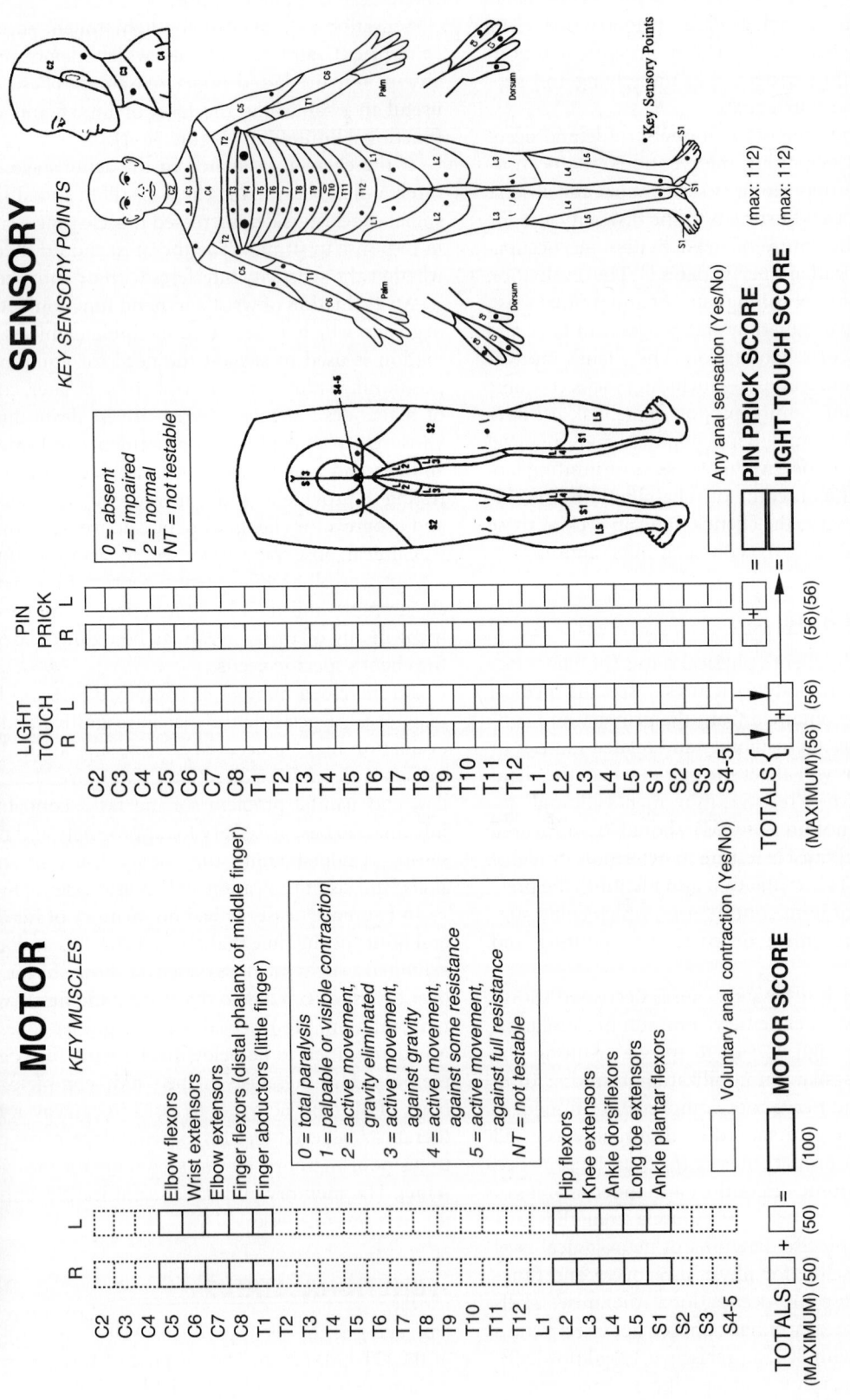

Figure 36-4 Standard neurological classification of spinal cord injury. (Courtesy of American Spinal Injury Association, 2000.)

hygiene at the sink, and object manipulation may be appropriate, depending on the level of injury.

Direct interaction with the client's family and friends provides valuable information regarding the client's support systems while in the hospital and, more important, after discharge. This information is relevant to later caregiver training in areas in which the client may require the assistance of others to accomplish self-care and mobility tasks.

ESTABLISHING INTERVENTION OBJECTIVES

Establishing intervention objectives in concert with the client and with the rehabilitation team is important. The primary objectives of the rehabilitation team may not be those of the client. Psychosocial factors, cultural factors, cognitive deficits, environmental limitations, and individual financial considerations must be identified and integrated into a comprehensive intervention program that will meet the unique needs of each individual. Every client is different; therefore, a variety of intervention approaches and alternatives may be necessary to address each factor that may affect goal achievement.[7] Increased participation can be expected if the client's priorities are respected to the extent that they are achievable and realistic.

The occupational therapist's general objectives for intervention with the person with SCI are as follows:

1. To maintain or increase joint ROM and prevent problems associated with body functions and other body structures (skin) via preparatory activities such as active and passive ROM, splinting, positioning, and client education
2. To increase the strength of all innervated and partially innervated muscles and address problems associated with other body functions (e.g., sensation, higher level cognitive functions, emotional functions) through preparatory activities and engagement in purposeful activities and occupations
3. To increase physical endurance and other performance skills and performance patterns through engagement in purposeful activities and occupations
4. To maximize independence in performance in all areas of occupation, including ADLs, IADLs, education, work, play, leisure, and social participation
5. To aid in the psychosocial adjustment to disability
6. To evaluate, recommend, and educate the client in the use and care of necessary durable medical and adaptive equipment
7. To ensure safe and independent home and environmental accessibility through consultation and safety and accessibility recommendations
8. To assist the client in developing the communication skills necessary for training caregivers to provide safe assistance
9. To educate the client and his or her family regarding the benefits and consequences of maintaining healthy and responsible lifestyle habits in relation to long-term function and the aging process

The client's length of stay in the inpatient rehabilitation program and the ability to participate in outpatient therapy determine the appropriateness and priority of the aforementioned activities.

INTERVENTION METHODS

ACUTE PHASE

During the acute, or immobilized, phase of the rehabilitation program, the client may be in traction or wearing a stabilization device such as a halo brace or body jacket. Medical precautions must be in force during this period. Flexion, extension, and rotary movements of the spine and neck are contraindicated.

Evaluation of total body positioning and hand splinting needs should be initiated at this time. In clients with quadriplegia, scapular elevation and elbow flexion (as well as limited shoulder flexion and abduction while on bed rest) can cause pain in the shoulders and ROM limitations. UEs should be intermittently positioned in 80 degrees of shoulder abduction, external rotation with scapular depression, and full elbow extension to assist in alleviating this common problem. The forearm should be positioned in forearm pronation because the client is at risk for supination contractures, such as at the C5 level. At Santa Clara Valley Medical Center, a device has been designed and fabricated by the OT department to maintain the arm in an appropriate position while the patient is immobilized on a kinetic bed (see Figure 36-2).

Selection of appropriate splint style and accurate fabrication and fit of the splint by the occupational therapist enhance client acceptance and optimal functional gain. If musculature is not adequate to support the wrist and hands properly (radial wrist extensors—extensor carpi radialis longus [ECRL] and extensor carpi radialis brevis [ECRB]) below 3+ (F+) for functional or cosmetic reasons—splints should be fabricated to support the wrist properly in extension and the thumb in opposition and to maintain the thumb web space while allowing the fingers to flex naturally at the metacarpophalangeal (MP) and proximal interphalangeal (PIP) joints. Splints should be dorsal rather than volar in design to allow maximal sensory feedback while the patient's hand is resting on any surface. If at least 3+ (F+) strength of wrist extension is present, a short opponens splint should be considered to maintain the web space and support the thumb in opposition. This splint can be used functionally while the client is trained to use a tenodesis grasp.

Active and active-assisted ROM of all joints should be performed within strength, ability, and tolerance levels. Muscle reeducation techniques for wrists and elbows should be employed when indicated. Progressive resistive exercises for wrists may be carried out. The client should be encouraged to engage in self-care activities such as feeding, hygiene, and keyboard and writing activities if possible, using simple devices such as a universal cuff or a custom writing splint.

Even though the client may be immobilized in bed, discussion of anticipated durable medical equipment (DME), home modifications, and caregiver training should be initiated to allow sufficient time to prepare for discharge. When indicated, bedside activities that might be of interest to the client, such as modified call systems, laptop computer setup on bed tables, and avocational activities, can be explored.

During the immobilization phase of Laurence's rehabilitation, he was given a U-cuff for self-feeding, which was fitted over his wrist cast. A typing splint was fabricated for him for page turning and computer use while he was lying on his side in bed.

ACTIVE PHASE

During the active, or mobilization, phase of the rehabilitation program, the client can sit in a wheelchair and should begin developing upright tolerance. A high priority at this time is determining a method of relieving sitting pressure for the purpose of preventing **decubitus ulcers**, or pressure sores, on the ischial, trochanteric, and sacral bony prominences. If the client has quadriplegia yet has at least F+ (3+) shoulder and elbow strength bilaterally, pressure can be relieved on the buttocks by leaning the client forward over the feet. Simple cotton webbing loops are secured to the back frame of the wheelchair (Figure 36-5). A person with low quadriplegia (C7 with F+ or better triceps) or a person with paraplegia with intact UE musculature can perform a full depression weight shift off the arms or wheels of the wheelchair. Some clients with C6 quadriplegia can also perform this type of weight shift by mechanically locking the elbows in extension while simultaneously externally rotating the shoulders and using their strong shoulder muscles to support their weight. Weight shifts should be performed every 30 to 60 minutes until skin tolerance is determined.

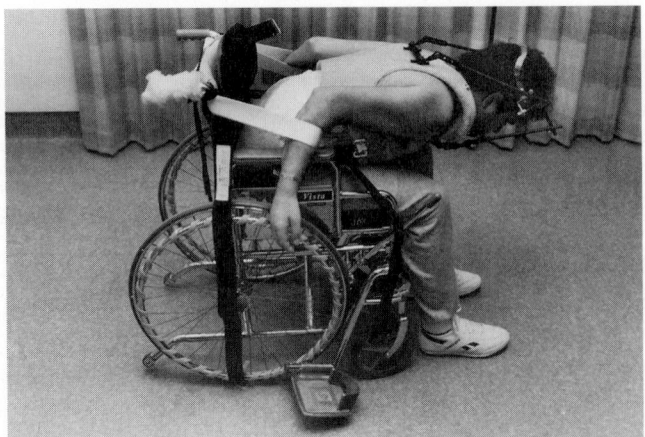

Figure 36-5 Forward weight shift using loops attached to wheelchair frame. A client with C6-level quadriplegia with symmetrical grade 4 deltoids and biceps and wrist extensors.

Active and passive ROM exercises should be continued regularly to prevent undesirable contractures. Splinting or casting of the elbows may be indicated to correct contractures that are developing. Some clients will have active wrist extension, which will be used to substitute for absent grasp through tenodesis action of the long finger flexors. With these clients, it is desirable to develop some tightness in these tendons to give some additional tension to the tenodesis grasp. The desirable contracture is developed by ranging finger flexion with the wrist fully extended and finger extension with the wrist flexed, thus never allowing the flexors or extensors to be in full stretch over all of the joints that they cross (Figure 36-6).[14]

Elbow contractures should never be allowed to develop. Full elbow extension is essential for allowing propping to maintain balance during static sitting and for assisting in transfers. With zero triceps strength, a person with C6-level quadriplegia can maintain forward sitting balance by shoulder depression and protraction, external rotation, full elbow extension, and full wrist extension (Figure 36-7).

Progressive resistive exercise and resistive activities can be applied to innervated and partially innervated muscles. Shoulder musculature should be exercised so as to promote proximal stability, with emphasis on the latissimus dorsi (shoulder depressors), deltoids (shoulder flexors, abductors, and extensors), and the remainder of the shoulder girdle and scapular muscles. The triceps, pectoralis, and latissimus dorsi muscles are needed for transfers and for shifting weight when in the wheelchair. Wrist extensors should be strengthened to maximize natural tenodesis function, thereby maximizing the necessary prehension pattern in the hand for functional grasp and release. Strengthening wrist extensors also increases the client's ability to use the tenodesis splint more effectively, mechanically transferring the strength of the wrist extensors to the finger pieces of the splint for a stronger pinch.

The intervention program should be graded to increase the amount of resistance that can be tolerated during activity. As muscle power and endurance improve, increasing the amount of time in wheelchair activities will help the patient participate in activities and occupation throughout the day.

Many assistive devices and equipment items can be useful to the person with SCI. However, every attempt should be made to have the client perform the task with no equipment or with as little as possible. Modified techniques are available that enable an individual to perform efficiently without the need for expensive or bulky equipment.

When appropriate, the universal cuff for holding eating utensils, toothbrushes, pens, and typing sticks is a simple and versatile device that offers increased independence. A wrist cock-up splint to stabilize the wrist with attachment of the universal cuff may be useful for clients with little or no wrist extension. A plate guard, cup holder, extended straw with straw clip, and non-skid table mat can facilitate independent feeding. A wash mitt, soap holder, or

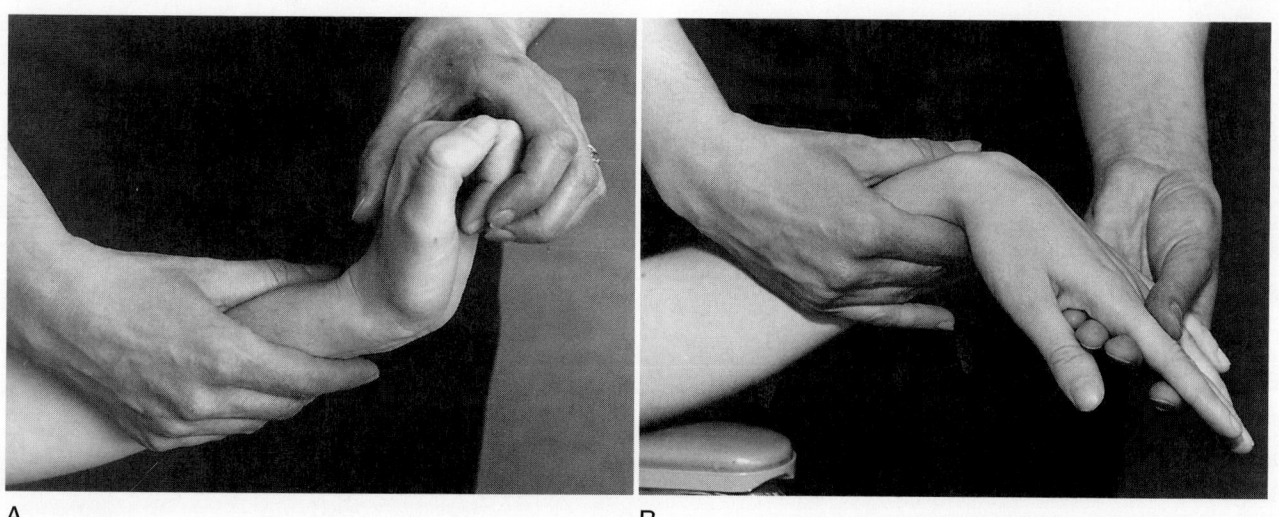

Figure 36-6 Tenodesis action. **A,** Wrist is extended when fingers are passively flexed. **B,** Wrist is flexed when fingers are passively extended.

soap-on-a-rope appears to make bathing easier; however, the added difficulty of donning and doffing such equipment must be considered. A sliding board is a valuable option for safe transfers. Through intervention, optimal muscle strength and coordination can occur, enabling the client to outgrow the use of initially necessary equipment.

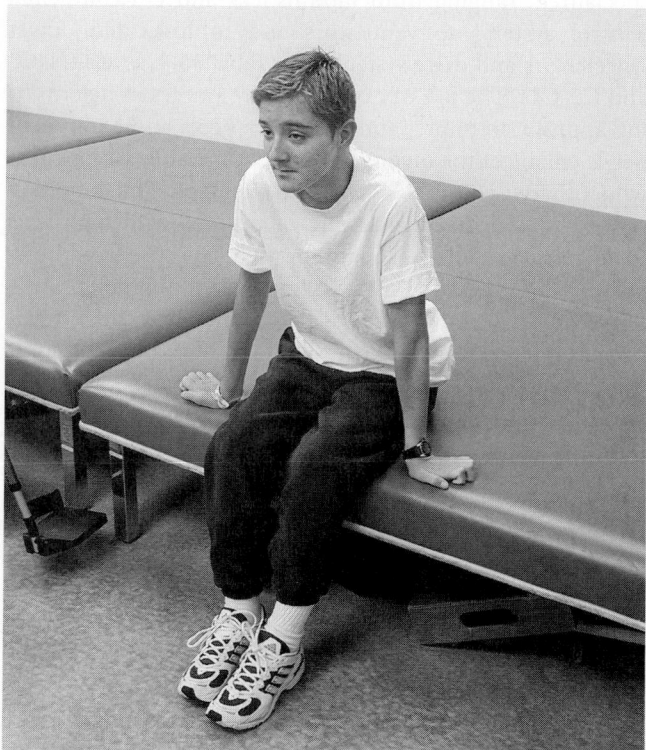

Figure 36-7 A client with C6-level quadriplegia; forward sitting balance is maintained (without triceps) by locking elbows. This is a valuable skill for maintaining sitting balance, bed mobility, and transfers. (Courtesy of Luis Gonzalez, Media Resource Department, Santa Clara Valley Medical Center.)

During the active phase, the ADL program may be expanded to include independent feeding with devices, oral and facial hygiene, upper-body bathing, bowel and bladder care (e.g., digital stimulation and intermittent catheterization), UE dressing, and transfers using the sliding board. Communication skills in writing and using the telephone, tape recorder, stereo equipment, computer, and calculator keyboard should be an important part of the intervention program (Figure 36-8). Training in the use of the mobile arm support and overhead slings (see Chapter 29, Section 1), wrist-hand orthosis (flexor hinge or tenodesis splint), and assistive devices is also part of the OT program.

The occupational therapist should continue to provide psychological support by allowing and encouraging the client to express frustration, anger, fears, and concerns.[12] The OT clinic in an SCI center can provide an atmosphere where clients can establish support groups with other inpatients and outpatients who can share their experiences and problem-solving advice with those in earlier phases of their rehabilitation. Direct OT intervention to address psychosocial issues of SCI can include training in stress management; coping-skills training; and education regarding social connectedness, sexuality, and relationship-building strategies; and the connection between occupation and emotional health. Such intervention is particularly helpful when conducted by the occupational therapist in the supportive clinic atmosphere described previously. Occupational therapists have also found it beneficial to involve successful former clients as expert peer participants or co-leaders during such psychosocial intervention groups and individual sessions.[13]

The assessment, ordering, and fitting of DME such as wheelchairs, seating and positioning equipment, mechanical lifts, beds, and bathing equipment are extremely important parts of the rehabilitation program. Such equipment should be specifically evaluated, however, and ordered only when

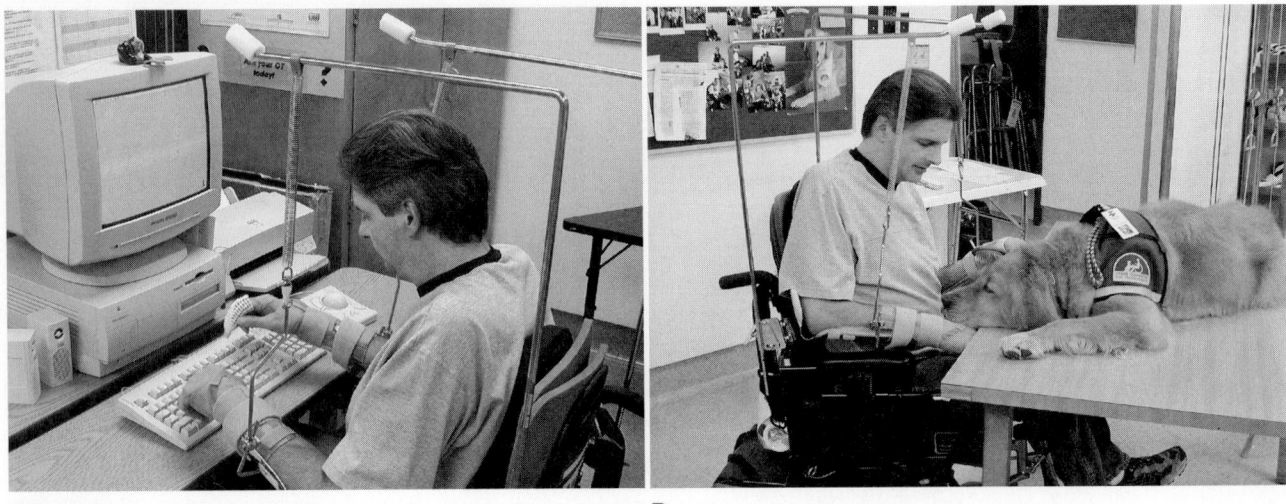

A   B

Figure 36-8   **A,** Individual with injury at C4 to C5 typing at keyboard with bilateral overhead slings, bilateral wrist splints, and typing splints. **B,** Use of a service dog as a treatment option to facilitate bilateral upper extremity use. (Courtesy of Luis Gonzalez, Media Resource Department, Santa Clara Valley Medical Center.)

definite goals and expectations are known. Inappropriate equipment can impair function and cause further medical problems, such as skin breakdown or trunk deformity; the therapist must take into account all functional, positioning, environmental, psychological, and financial considerations in evaluating the client's equipment needs. The desired equipment—especially wheelchairs, seat cushions, back supports, positioning devices, and bathing equipment—should be available for demonstration and trial by the client before final ordering. It is imperative that the therapist involved in the evaluation and ordering of this costly and highly individualized equipment be familiar with currently available products and be knowledgeable in ordering equipment that will provide the client with optimal function and body positioning on a short- and long-term basis. A good working relationship with an experienced **rehabilitation technology supplier** (RTS), an equipment supplier specializing in custom rehabilitation equipment, is crucial. Advancements in technology and design have provided a wide variety of equipment from which to choose, and working with another professional specializing in such equipment will help ensure correct selection and fit. (See Chapter 11, Section 2 for a more detailed discussion of wheelchairs, seating, and positioning equipment.)

In addition to enhancing respiratory function by supporting the client in an erect, well-aligned position that maximizes sitting tolerance and optimizes UE function, wheelchair seating must assist in the prevention of deformity and pressure sores. An appropriate and adequate wheelchair cushion helps distribute sitting pressure, assists in the prevention of pressure sores, stabilizes the pelvis as necessary for proper trunk alignment, and provides comfort. Whether it is the occupational therapist's or the physical

therapist's role to evaluate and order the wheelchair and cushion, both should work closely together to ensure consistent training and use for the individual needs of each client.

The intervention and equipment needs of clients with high-level SCI (C4 and above) are unique and extremely specialized, ranging from mouthsticks and environmental control systems to ventilators and sophisticated power wheelchairs and drive systems (see Table 36-1, levels C1-C3 and C3-C4). The use of experienced resources in determining appropriate short- and long-term goals and equipment needs enhances the quality and functional ability of a client who otherwise would be quite dependent. Rehabilitation centers specializing in the care of persons with high-level quadriplegia should be sought for their expertise in addressing all aspects of care for this unique client population.

When discharge location is determined and the individual can tolerate leaving the hospital for a few hours, a home evaluation should be performed. The therapist, client, and family members can then view and attempt activities in the home in anticipation of return to a safe and accessible environment.

OT PRACTICE NOTE

The therapist must be knowledgeable about safety and accessibility options for a variety of environments and often must advise architects or contractors to ensure that appropriate modifications are made. The therapist must be aware of accessibility requirements in the home, as well as those required in the workplace by the Americans with Disabilities Act of 1990 (ADA; see Chapter 14).

Table 36-1   **Expected Functional Outcomes**

Level	Functionally Relevant Muscles Innervated	Movement Possible	Patterns of Weakness	NSCISC sample size
C1-C3	Sternocleidomastoid: cervical paraspinal; neck accessories	Neck flexion, extension, rotation	Total paralysis of trunk, upper extremities, lower extremities; dependent on ventilator	FIM = 15/ assist = 12
C4	Upper trapezius; diaphragm; cervical paraspinal muscles	Neck flexion, extension, rotation; scapular elevation; inspiration	Paralysis of trunk, upper extremities, lower extremities; inability to cough, endurance and respiratory reserve low secondary to paralysis of intercostals	FIM = 28/ assist = 12
C5	Deltoid, biceps, brachialis, brachioradialis, rhomboids, serratus anterior (partially innervated)	Shoulder flexion, abduction, and extension; elbow flexion and supination; scapular adduction and abduction	Absence of elbow extension, pronation, all wrist and hand movement; total paralysis of trunk and lower extremities	FIM = 36/ assist = 35
C6	Clavicular pectoralis; supinator; extensor carpi radialis longus and brevis; serratus anterior; latissimus dorsi	Scapular protractor; some horizontal adduction, forearm supination, radial wrist extension	Absence of wrist flexion, elbow extension, hand movement; total paralysis of trunk and lower extremities	FIM = 43/ assist = 35
C7-8	Latissimus dorsi; sternal pectoralis; triceps; pronator quadratus; extensor carpi ulnaris; flexor carpi radialis; flexor digitorum profundus and superficialis; extensor communis; pronator/flexor/extensor/abductor pollicis; lumbricals (partially innervated)	Elbow extension; ulnar/wrist extension; wrist flexion; finger flexions and extensions; thumb flexion/extension/abduction	Paralysis of trunk and lower extremities; limited grasp and dexterity secondary to partial intrinsic muscles of the hand	FIM = 43/ assist = 35
T1-9	Intrinsics of the hand including thumbs; internal and external intercostals; erector spinae; lumbricals; flexor/extensor/abductor pollicis	Upper extremities fully intact; limited upper trunk stability; endurance increased secondary to innervation of intercostals	Lower trunk paralysis; total paralysis of lower extremities	FIM = 144/ assist = 122
T10-L1	Fully intact intercostals; external obliques; rectus abdominis	Food trunk stability	Paralysis of lower extremities	FIM = 71/ assist = 57
L2-S5	Fully intact abdominals and all other trunk muscles; depending on level, some degree of hip flexors, extensor, abductors; knee flexors, extensors; ankle dorsiflexors, plantar flexors	Good trunk stability; partial to full control of lower extremities	Partial paralysis of lower extremities, hips, knees, ankle, foot	FIM = 20/ assist = 16

FIM/assistance data: *Exp*, expected FIM score; *Med*, NSCISC median; *IR*, NSCISC Interquartile Range.

Table 36-1 **Expected Functional Outcomes—cont'd**

	Expected Functional Outcomes	Equipment	FIM/Assistance Data		
			Exp	Med	IR
BASIC BODY FUNCTIONS					
Level C1-C3					
Respiratory	Ventilator dependent	Two ventilators (bedside, portable)			
	Inability to clear secretions	Suction equipment or other suction management device			
		Generator/battery backup			
Bowel	Total assist	Padded reclining shower/commode chair (if roll-in shower available)	1	1	1
Bladder	Total assist		1	1	1
Level C4					
Respiratory	May be able to breathe without a ventilator	If not ventilator free, see C1-C3 for equipment requirements			
Bowel	Total assist	Reclining shower/commode chair (if roll-in shower available)	1	1	1
Bladder	Total assist		1	1	1
Level C5					
Respiratory	Low endurance and vital capacity caused by paralysis of intercostals; may require assist to clear secretions				
Bowel	Total assist	Padded shower/commode chair or padded transfer tub bench with commode cutout	1	1	1
Bladder	Total assist	Adaptive devices may be indicated (electric leg bag emptier)	1	1	1
Level C6					
Respiratory	Low endurance and vital capacity secondary to paralysis of intercostals; may require assist to clear secretions				
Bowel	Some total assist	Padded tub bench with commode cutout or padded shower/commode chair	1-2	1	1
		Other adaptive devices as indicated			
Bladder	Some total assist with equipment; may be independent with leg bag emptying	Adaptive devices as indicated	1-2	1	1
Level C7-8					
Respiratory	Low endurance and vital capacity secondary to paralysis of intercostals; may require assist to clear secretions				
Bowel	Some to total assist	Padded tub bench with commode cutout or shower/commode chair	1-4	1	1-4
		Adaptive devices as indicated			
Bladder	Independent to some assist	Adaptive devices as indicated	2-6	3	1-6

Level / Function	Pattern of ability	Equipment	Exp	Med	IR
Level T1-T9					
Respiratory	Compromised vital capacity and endurance				
Bowel	Independent	Elevated padded toilet seat or padded tub bench with commode cutout	6-7	6	4-6
Bladder	Independent		6	6	5-6
Level T10-L1					
Respiratory	Intact respiratory function				
Bowel	Independent	Padded standard or raised padded toilet seat	6-7	6	6
Bladder	Independent		6	6	6
Level L2-S5					
Respiratory	Intact function				
Bowel	Independent	Padded toilet seat	6-7	6	6-7
Bladder	Independent		6	6	6-7
MOBILITY, LOCOMOTION, AND SAFETY					
Level C1-C3					
Bed mobility	Total assist	Full electric hospital bed with Trendelenburg feature and side rails	1	1	1
Bed/wheelchair transfers	Total assist	Transfer board; Power or mechanical lift with sling	1	1	1
Wheelchair propulsion	Manual: total assist; Power: independent with equipment	Power recline and/or tilt wheelchair with head, chin, or breath control and manual recliner; Vent tray	6	1	1-6
Pressure relief/positioning	Total assist; may be independent with equipment	Power recline and/or tilt wheelchair; Wheelchair pressure-relief cushion; Postural support and head control devices as indicated; Hand splints may be indicated; Specialty bed or pressure-relief mattress may be indicated			
Level C4					
Bed mobility	Total assist	Full electric hospital bed with Trendelenburg feature and side rails	1	1	1
Bed/wheelchair transfers	Total assist	Transfer board; Power or mechanical lift with sling	1	1	1
Wheelchair propulsion	Power: independent; Manual: total assist	Power recline and/or tilt wheelchair with head, chin, or breath control and manual recliner; Vent tray	6	1	1-6
Pressure relief/positioning	Total assist; may be independent with equipment	Power recline and/or tilt wheelchair; Wheelchair pressure-relief cushion; Postural support and head control devices as indicated; Hand splints may be indicated; Specialty bed or pressure-relief mattress may be indicated			

FIM/assistance data: *Exp*, expected FIM score; *Med*, NSCISC median; *IR*, NSCISC Interquartile Range.

Continued

Table 36-1 Expected Functional Outcomes—cont'd

	Expected Functional Outcomes	Equipment	FIM/Assistance Data		
			Exp	Med	IR
Level C5					
Bed mobility	Some assist	Full electric hospital bed with Trendelenburg feature with client control; Side rails	1	1	1
Bed/wheelchair transfers	Total assist	Transfer board; Power or mechanical lift			
Wheelchair propulsion	Power: independent; Manual: independent to some assist indoors on noncarpeted, level surface; some to total assist outdoors	Power recline and/or tilt with arm drive control; Manual: lightweight rigid or folding frame with handrim modifications	6	6	5-6
Pressure relief/positioning	Independent with equipment	Power recline and/or tilt wheelchair; Wheelchair pressure-relief cushion; Hand splints; Specialty bed or pressure-relief mattress may be indicated; Postural support devices			
Level C6					
Bed mobility	Some assist	Full electric hospital bed; Side rails; Full to king standard bed may be indicated			
Bed/wheelchair transfers	Level: some assist to independent; Uneven: some to total assist	Transfer board; Mechanical lift	3	1	1-3
Wheelchair propulsion	Power: independent with standard arm drive on all surfaces; Manual: independent indoors; some total assist outdoors	Manual: lightweight rigid or folding frame with modified rims; Power: may require power recline or standard upright power wheelchair	6	6	4-6
Pressure relief/positioning	Independent with equipment and/or adapted techniques	Power recline wheelchair; Wheelchair pressure-relief cushion; Postural support devices; Pressure-relief mattress or overlay may be indicated			
Level C7-C8					
Bed mobility	Independent to some assist	Full electric hospital bed or full to king standard bed			
Bed/wheelchair transfers	Level: independent; Uneven: independent to some assist	With or without transfer board	3-7	4	2-6
Wheelchair propulsion	Manual: independent on all indoor surfaces and level outdoor terrain; some assist with uneven terrain	Manual: rigid or folding lightweight or folding wheelchair with modified rims	6	6	6

				Med	IR
Pressure relief/positioning	Independent	Wheelchair pressure-relief cushion			
		Postural support devices as indicated			
		Pressure-relief mattress or overlay may be indicated			
Level T1-T9					
Bed mobility	Independent	Full to king standard bed			
Bed/wheelchair transfers	Independent	May or may not require transfer board		6-7	6-7
Wheelchair propulsion	Independent	Manual rigid or folding lightweight wheelchair		6	6
Pressure relief/positioning	Independent	Wheelchair pressure-relief cushion			
		Postural support devices as indicated			
		Pressure-relief mattress or overlay may be indicated			
Level T10-L1					
Bed mobility	Independent	Full to king standard bed			
Bed/wheelchair transfers	Independent			7	7
Wheelchair propulsion	Independent all indoor and outdoor surfaces	Manual rigid or folding lightweight wheelchair		6	6
Pressure relief/positioning	Independent	Wheelchair pressure-relief cushion			
		Postural support devices as indicated			
		Pressure-relief mattress or overlay may be indicated			
Level L2-S5					
Bed mobility	Independent	Full to king standard bed			
Bed/wheelchair transfers	Independent			7	7
Wheelchair propulsion	Independent all indoor and outdoor surfaces	Manual rigid or folding lightweight wheelchair		6	6
Pressure relief/positioning	Independent	Wheelchair pressure-relief cushion			
		Postural support devices as indicated			

STANDING AND AMBULATION

Level C1-C3	Standing: total assist	Tilt table
	Ambulation: not indicated	
Level C4	Standing: total assist	Hydraulic standing table
	Ambulation: not usually indicated	
Level C5	Total assist	Hydraulic standing table
Level C6	Standing: total assist	Hydraulic standing frame
	Ambulation: not indicated	
Level C7-C8	Standing: independent to some assist	Hydraulic or standard standing frame
	Ambulation: not indicated	
Level T1-9	Standing: independent	Standing frame
	Ambulation: typically not functional	

FIM/assistance data: *Exp*, expected FIM score; *Med*, NSCISC median; *IR*, NSCISC Interquartile Range.

Continued

Table 36-1 **Expected Functional Outcomes—cont'd**

	Expected Functional Outcomes	Equipment	FIM/Assistance Data		
			Exp	Med	IR
STANDING AND AMBULATION—cont'd					
Level T10-L1	Standing: independent	Standing frame			
	Ambulation: functional, some assist to independent	Forearm crutches or walker			
		Knee, ankle, foot orthosis (KAFO)			
Level L2-S5	Standing: independent	Standing frame			
	Ambulation: functional, independent to some assist	Knee-ankle-foot orthosis (KAFO) or ankle-foot orthosis (AFO)			
		Forearm crutches or cane as indicated			
ACTIVITIES OF DAILY LIVING					
Level C1-C3					
Eating	Total assist		1	1	1
Grooming	Total assist		1	1	1
Dressing	Total assist	Handheld shower	1	1	1
Bathing	Total assist	Shampoo tray	1	1	1
		Padded reclining shower/commode chair (if roll-in shower available)			
Level C4					
Eating	Total assist		1	1	1
Grooming	Total assist		1	1	1
Dressing	Total assist	Shampoo tray	1	1	1
Bathing	Total assist	Handheld shower	1	1	1
		Padded reclining shower/commode chair (if roll-in shower available)			
Level C5					
Eating	Total assist for setup, then independent eating with equipment	Long opponens splint	5	5	2.5-5.5
		Adaptive devices as indicated			
Grooming	Some to total assist	Long opponens splint	1-3	1	1-5
		Adaptive devices as indicated			
Dressing	Lower extremity: total assist	Long opponens splint	1	1	1-4
	Upper extremity: some assist	Adaptive devices as indicated			
Bathing	Total assist	Padded tub transfer bench or shower/commode chair	1	1	1-3
		Handheld shower			

	Description	Equipment	Exp	Med	IR
Level C6					
Eating	Independent with or without equipment; except cutting, which is total assist	Adaptive devices as indicated (e.g., U-cuff, tenodesis splint, adapted utensils, plate guard)	5-6	5	4-6
Grooming	Some assist to independent with equipment	Adaptive devices as indicated (e.g., U-cuff, adapted handles)	3-6	4	2-6
Dressing	Independent upper extremity; some assist to total assist for lower extremities	Adaptive devices as indicated (e.g., button-hook; loops on zippers, pants; socks, velcro on shoes)	1-3	2	1-5
Bathing	Upper body: independent / Lower body: some to total assist	Padded tub transfer bench or shower/commode chair / Adaptive devices as needed / Handheld shower	1-3	1	1-3
Level C7-C8					
Eating	Independent	Adaptive devices as indicated	6-7	6	5-7
Grooming	Independent	Adaptive devices as indicated	6-7	6	4-7
Dressing	Independent in upper extremities; independent to some assist in lower extremities	Adaptive devices as indicated	4-7	6	4-7
Bathing	Upper body: independent / Lower body: some assist to independent	Padded tub transfer tub bench or shower/commode chair / Handheld shower / Adaptive devices as needed	3-6	4	2-6
Level T1-T9					
Eating	Independent		7	7	7
Grooming	Independent		7	7	7
Dressing	Independent		7	7	7
Bathing	Independent	Padded tub transfer bench or shower/commode chair / Handheld shower	6-7	6	5-7
Level T10-L1					
Eating	Independent		7	7	7
Grooming	Independent		7	7	7
Dressing	Independent		7	7	7
Bathing	Independent	Padded transfer tub bench / Handheld shower	6-7	6	6-7
Level L2-S5					
Eating	Independent		7	7	7
Grooming	Independent		7	7	7
Dressing	Independent		7	7	7
Bathing	Independent	Padded tub bench / Handheld shower	7	7	6-7

FIM/assistance data: *Exp*, expected FIM score; *Med*, NSCISC median; *IR*, NSCISC Interquartile Range.

Continued

Table **36-1** **Expected Functional Outcomes—cont'd**

	Expected Functional Outcomes	Equipment	FIM/Assistance Data		
			Exp	Med	IR
COMMUNICATION					
Level C1-C3	Total assist to independent, depending on work station setup and equipment availability	Mouth stick, high-tech computer access, environmental control unit			
		Adaptive devices everywhere as indicated			
Level C4	Total assist to independent, depending on work station setup and equipment availability	Mouth stick, high-tech computer access, environmental control unit			
Level C5	Independent to some assist after setup with equipment	Long opponens splint			
		Adaptive devices as needed for page turning, writing, button pushing			
Level C6	Independent with or without equipment	Adaptive devices as indicated (e.g., tenodesis splint; writing splint for keyboard use, button pushing, page turning, object manipulation)			
Level C7-8	Independent	Adaptive devices as indicated			
Level T1-9	Independent				
Level T10-L1	Independent				
Level L2-S5	Independent				
TRANSPORTATION					
Level C1-C3	Total assist	Attendant-operated van (e.g., lift, tie downs) or accessible public transportation			
Level C4	Total assist	Attendant-operated van (e.g., lift, tie-downs) or accessible public transportation			
Level C5	Independent with highly specialized equipment; some assist with accessible public transportation; total assist for attendant-operated vehicle	Highly specialized modified van with lift			
Level C6	Independent driving from wheelchair	Modified van with lift			
		Sensitized hand controls			
		Tie-downs			
Level C7-C8	Independent in car if independent with transfer and wheelchair loading/unloading; independent in driving modified van from captain's seat	Modified vehicle			
		Transfer board			
Level T1-9	Independent in car, including loading and unloading wheelchair	Hand controls			
Level T10-L1	Independent in car, including loading and unloading wheelchair	Hand controls			

Level	Description	Equipment	Exp	Med	IR
Level L2-S5	Independent in car, including loading and unloading wheelchair	Hand controls			

HOMEMAKING

Level	Description	Equipment
Level C1-C3	Total assist	
Level C4	Total assist	
Level C5	Total assist	
Level C6	Some assist with light meal preparation; total assist for all other homemaking	Adaptive devices as indicated
Level C7-C8	Independent light meal preparation and homemaking; some to total assist for complex meal preparation and heavy housecleaning	Adaptive devices as indicated
Level T1-T9	Independent with complex meal preparation and light housecleaning; total to some assist with heavy housecleaning	
Level T10-L1	Independent with complex meal prep and light housecleaning; some assist with heavy housecleaning	
Level L2-S5	Independent with complex meal preparation and light housecleaning; some assist with heavy housecleaning	

ASSISTANCE REQUIRED

Level	Description	Exp	Med	IR
Level C1-C3	24-hour attendant care to include homemaking / Able to instruct in all aspects of care	24*	24*	12-24*
Level C4	24-hour attendant care to include homemaking / Able to instruct in all aspects of care	24*	24*	16-24*
Level C5	Personal care: 10 hours/day / Homecare: 6 hours/day / Able to instruct in all aspects of care	16*	23*	10-24*
Level C6	Personal care: 6 hours/day / Homecare: 4 hours/day	10*	17*	8-24*
Level C7-C8	Personal care: 6 hours/day / Homecare: 2 hours/day	8*	12*	2-24*
Level T1-T9	Homemaking: 3 hours/day	2*	3*	0-15*
Level T10-L1	Homemaking: 2 hours/day	2*	2*	0-8*
Level L2-S5	Homemaking: 0-1 hour/day	0-1*	0*	0*

FIM/assistance data: *Exp*, expected FIM score; *Med*, NSCISC median; *IR*, NSCISC Interquartile Range.
*Hours per day

Accompanied by his occupational therapist, Laurence went to his new rental home to determine its safety and accessibility in light of his mobility and ADL needs. Modifications to both the front and rear entrances, as well as bathroom modifications, were recommended. He and his therapist discussed the recommendations with the contractor who would be performing the work on the house to determine the feasibility of door widening and ramping in terms of the house's structural stability. It was important that Laurence participate in the plans not only because he needed to manage this part of his life but also because he needed to learn about regulations related to the Americans with Disabilities Act (ADA) and his rights as a renter. Laurence took control of managing his housing needs, as well as his discharge supplies and follow-up services. His sense of helplessness was subsiding as he began to assume control of his life again.

AFTER DISCHARGE FROM ACUTE REHABILITATION

Decreases in the amount of time devoted to inpatient rehabilitation have moved the extended phase of intervention to an outpatient basis or home therapy context. Adaptive driving, home management, leisure activities, and work skill assessments using hand- or power-based tools are feasible and appropriate intervention modalities for evaluating and increasing UE strength, coordination, and trunk balance; however, they may not be a priority during inpatient hospitalization. OT training in such activities can improve the client's socialization skills and can also assess and improve problem-solving skills and potential work habits.

OT services can offer valuable evaluation and exploration of the vocational potential of persons with SCI. Because of the sheer magnitude of the physical disability, vocational possibilities for clients with high levels of SCI are limited. Many clients must change their vocation or alter former vocational goals. Decreased motivation, threat of loss of health benefits, and lack of perseverance on the part of many patients make vocational rehabilitation challenging.

The occupational therapist can assess the client's level of motivation, functional aptitudes, attitudes, interests, and personal vocational aspirations during the process of the intervention program and through the use of ADL, mobility, and work simulation activities. The therapist can observe the client's attention span, concentration, problem-solving ability, judgment, and other high-level cognitive functions, as well as his or her manual ability with splints and devices, accuracy, speed, perseverance, work habits, and work tolerance level. The therapist can serve as a liaison between the client and the vocational rehabilitation counselor by offering valuable information gleaned from observation during the client's performance of activities and occupations. When suitable vocational objectives have been selected, they may be pursued in an educational setting or in a work setting, usually out of the realm of OT.

AGING WITH SPINAL CORD INJURY

Following survival of acute SCI, the primary goal of rehabilitation is independence. Independence as the measure of quality of life for people with disabilities is a concept accepted and often perpetuated by professionals and survivors alike.[15]

Occupational therapists work in concert with these clients to identify and prioritize their favored and meaningful occupations and provide intervention to enable them to resume their engagement in these occupations for participation in a satisfying life. Occupational therapists treating clients with SCI have considerable responsibility in influencing the level of independence, whether in the acute setting, during active rehabilitation, or in follow-up care throughout the life of the client. Understanding the aging process in both able-bodied and individuals with disabilities is necessary for providing appropriate options and fostering attitudes that enhance the quality of the client's life at any age.

Physical aging is a natural, inevitable process. The signs of the process can occur at varying rates for each individual, and aging affects most systems of the body (see Chapter 46). In individuals with SCI, aging is usually accelerated by the secondary effects of the disability, such as the presence of muscle imbalance, infections (urinary and respiratory), deconditioning, pain, and joint degeneration secondary to overuse.[12] Issues to be considered at an age much earlier than normal are urinary problems brought on by years of catheterization, bladder infections, and urinary retention. Also to be considered are osteoporosis, arthritis and joint degeneration, constipation, weakening of already precarious skin, substance abuse, and the need for an increasing amount of personal care over time.

Approximately 20 years after injury appears to be a point at which some of the aging problems begin to increase. Because at least one of four SCI survivors experienced an SCI more than 20 years ago,[15] a significant portion of SCI survivors are prematurely experiencing the problems of aging. Individuals with SCI onset in their later years have very different patterns of functional outcomes, program needs, and financial resources than do those with onset in their earlier years. For someone who acquired quadriplegia in his or her 20s, when the majority of SCIs occur, the degenerating conditions of normal aging become evident prematurely, usually before the 40s.[4] Thus, someone who was independent during transfers at home and the loading of a wheelchair in and out of the car may now require assistance getting in and out of bed; because his or her shoulders have deteriorated, this person may have to trade the car for a van that requires costly modifications. Similarly, someone who is at a level normally associated with functional independence (e.g., T10-level paraplegia) may, in fact, need personal care assistance and possibly a power wheelchair because of degenerative changes in shoulders, elbows, and wrists. The occupational therapist should make good trunk alignment and seating a priority from the onset to prevent fixed trunk and pelvic deformities such as kyphosis and scoliosis, which can lead to considerable skin problems and uncorrectable cosmetic deformities years later. In addition, it is necessary to be aware of how the lightest possible weight of a manual wheelchair and the optimal distance from shoulder to push rim when propelling a chair can positively affect a weak or imbalanced shoulder complex. Also to be considered is the advantage of the cardiopulmonary conditioning that such an activity can provide. The occupational therapist must simultaneously consider those benefits while weighing the benefit of a power wheelchair for joint and energy conservation.

When SCI is compounded by the increased fatigue and weakness often associated with normal aging, the functional status of the individual with SCI may decline. Occupational therapists may cite this change to justify additional services or equipment. Many considerations must be weighed to make appropriate short- and long-term decisions. Consulting experienced experts, who have a perspective on both acute and long-term injuries and issues, can provide valuable insight into intervention decisions.

RESEARCH

Current research conducted in clinical settings and scientific laboratories around the world focuses on understanding the nature of SCI and defining the nervous system's response to this injury. There is now a sense of optimism in the scientific community that it will be possible someday to restore function after SCI. This optimism is based on the combined research efforts of scientists in many different disciplines. It is important for occupational therapists treating SCI to be aware of the scientific and technologicaladvances so as to better educate clients, while at the same time providing them with the most realistic and comprehensive rehabilitation interventions for their immediate and long-term needs.

SUMMARY

SCI can result in substantial paralysis of the limbs and trunk. The degree of residual motor and sensory dysfunction depends on the level of the lesion, whether the lesion was complete or incomplete, and the area of the spinal cord that was damaged.

After an SCI, bony realignment and stabilization are established surgically, by way of an external immobilization device, or through a combination of both methods. The many possible complications of SCI include skin breakdown, rapid loss of bone density, and spasticity.

The goal of OT is to facilitate the client's achievement of optimal independence and functioning. Areas of focus are physical restoration of available musculature; self-care; independent living skills; short- and long-term equipment needs; environmental accessibility; and educational, work, and leisure activities. The psychosocial adjustment of the client is instrumental, and the occupational therapist offers emotional support and intervention toward this end in every phase of the rehabilitation program.

THREADED CASE STUDY: LAURENCE, PART 2

The case of Laurence, presented in the beginning of this chapter, discussed a very common occurrence of a client who believed he would recover from his SCI and return to his previous lifestyle and occupations. Clearly, because he had a complete, C7, 8 Asia A injury, he did not recover motor or sensory function below his level of injury. Although his occupational therapist offered him hope for recovery, it was also essential for his therapist to provide positive but realistic expectations and options. Upon discharge from acute rehabilitation, Laurence returned to a newly rented single-story home that required ramps at the front and back entrances and bathroom modifications. Laurence initially received 4 hours of attendant care daily. He required assistance only for completion of his daily bath and bowel program, as well as for homemaking tasks. He required a transfer tub bench with a commode cutout for his bath and bowel program that was performed for him by his caregiver.

He was evaluated for the lightest-possible weight, customizable manual wheelchair to offer him independent manual wheelchair mobility at home and in his community. He does not require a power wheelchair at this time; however, he is aware that he may require one in the future. He has been educated on the premature degenerative changes that will likely occur in his shoulders from pushing a manual wheelchair and transferring himself to many necessary surfaces. He has been educated on skin care and the need for a maximal pressure-relieving wheelchair cushion. He was specifically evaluated for the optimal wheelchair sitting position that will offer him good trunk and pelvic alignment and pressure relief.

After Laurence received in-home OT services for home setup and community transition issues, his need for personal care diminished; he now requires only homemaking assistance. He regularly visits a neighborhood gym to maintain upper extremity strength and endurance, and he will soon be driving a modified van. He and his occupational therapist had many discussions regarding how he could pursue a teaching position within the fire department, given that he could not return to his previous assignment. His department is very willing to work with him in modifying his responsibilities to accommodate his limitations. His vocational plans are on hold until his van and driving training are completed.

Laurence continues with psychotherapy to deal with his change in function and lifestyle. He has had a very difficult time maintaining his friendships and personal relationships with his family. As time passes, he has begun to adapt to his lifestyle, if not necessarily accept it, and is still hoping that researchers will discover a cure for spinal cord injury in his lifetime.

Table 36-1 presents expectations of functional performance of SCI at 1 year after injury and at each of the eight levels of injury (C1-C3, C4, C5, C6, C7-C8, T1-T9, T10-L1, L2-S5). The outcomes reflect a level of independence that can be expected of a person with motor-complete SCI, given optimal circumstances.

The categories presented reflect expected functional outcomes in the areas of mobility, ADLs, instrumental activities of daily living (IADLs), and communication skills. The guidelines are based on the consensus of clinical experts, available literature on functional outcomes, and data compiled from Uniform Data Systems (UDS) and the National Spinal Cord Injury Statistical Center (NSCISC).

Within the functional outcomes for people with SCI listed in Table 36-1, a series of essential ADLs and IADLs, including the attendant care likely to be needed to support the predicted level of independence at 1 year after injury, have been identified. These outcome areas include the following categories of ADLs and IADLs:

- *Respiratory, bowel, and bladder function.* The neurological effects of SCI may result in deficits in the ability to perform basic body functions. Respiratory function includes the ability to breathe with or without mechanical assistance and to adequately clear secretions. Bowel and bladder function includes the ability to manage elimination, maintain perineal hygiene, and adjust clothing before and after elimination. Adapted or facilitated methods of managing these bodily functions may be required to attain expected functional outcomes.
- *Bed mobility, bed/wheelchair transfers, wheelchair propulsion, and positioning/pressure relief.* The neurological effects of SCI may result in deficits in the ability of the individual to perform the activities required for mobility, locomotion, and safety. Adapted or facilitated methods of managing these activities may be required to attain expected functional outcomes in standing and ambulation.
- *Standing and ambulation.* SCI may result in deficits in the ability to stand for exercise or psychological benefit or to ambulate for functional activities. Adapted or facilitated methods of management may be outcomes in standing and ambulation.
- *Eating, grooming, dressing, and bathing.* The neurological effects of SCI may result in deficits in the ability of the individual to perform these ADLs. Adapted or facilitated methods of managing ADLs may be necessary to attain expected functional outcomes.
- *Communication (keyboard use, handwriting, and telephone use).* The neurological effects of SCI may result in deficits in the ability to communicate. Adapted or facilitated methods of communication may be required to attain expected functional outcomes.
- *Transportation (driving, attendant-operated vehicle, and public transportation).* Transportation activities are critical for individuals with SCI to become maximally independent in their community. Adaptations may be required

to help the individual meet the expected functional outcomes.
- *Homemaking (meal planning and preparations and home management).* Adapted or facilitated methods of managing homemaking skills may be required to attain expected functional outcomes. Individuals with complete SCI at any level will require some level of assistance with some homemaking activities. The hours of assistance required for homemaking activities are presented in Table 36-1.
- *Assistance required.* Table 36-1 lists the number of hours that may be required from a caregiver to assist with personal care and homemaking activities. Personal care includes hands-on delivery of all aspects of self-care and mobility, as well as safety interventions. Homemaking assistance is also included in the recommendation for hours of assistance and includes activities previously presented. The number of hours presented in both the panel recommendations and the self-reported CHART data is representative of skilled and unskilled and paid and unpaid hours of assistance. The 24-hour-a-day requirement noted for the C1 through C3 and C4 levels includes the expected need for unpaid attendant care to provide safety monitoring.

Adequate assistance is required to ensure that the individual with SCI can achieve the outcomes set forth in Table 36-1. The hours of assistance recommended do not reflect changes in assistance required over time, as reported by long-term survivors of SCI,[6] nor do they take into account the wide range of individual variables that may affect the required hours of assistance. The Functional Independence Measure (FIM) estimates are widely variable in several of the categories. Whether the representative individuals with SCI in the individual categories attained the expected functional outcomes for their specific level of injury is unclear, as is whether there were mitigating circumstances, such as age, obesity, or concomitant injuries, that would account for variability in assistance reported. An individualized assessment of needs is required in all cases.
- *Equipment requirements.* Minimum recommendations for DME and adaptive devices are identified in each of the functional categories. The most commonly used equipment is listed, with the understanding that variations exist among SCI rehabilitation programs and that use of such equipment may be necessary to achieve the identified functional outcomes. Additional equipment and devices that are not critical for the majority of individuals at a specific level of injury may nonetheless be required for some individuals. The equipment descriptions are generic to allow for variances in program philosophy and financial resources. Rapid changes and advances in equipment and technology will be made and therefore must be considered.

Healthcare professionals should remember that the recommendations set forth in Table 36-1 are not intended to be prescriptive; rather, they should serve as a guideline. The importance of completing an individual functional assessment of people with SCI before making equipment recommendations cannot be overemphasized. All DME and adaptive devices must be thoroughly assessed and tested to determine medical necessity, to prevent medical complications (e.g., postural deviations, skin breakdown, pain), and to foster optimal functional performance. Environmental control units and telephone modifications may be needed for safety and maximal independence, and each person must be individually evaluated to determine the need for this equipment. Recommendations for disposable medical products are not included in this document.

- *FIM.* Evidence for the specific levels of independence provided in Table 36-1 relies both on expert consensus and on data from FIM in large-scale, prospective, and longitudinal research conducted by NSCISC. FIM is the most widely used disability measure in rehabilitation medicine, and although it may not incorporate all of the characteristics of disability in individuals recovering from SCI, it captures many basic disability areas.

FIM consists of 13 motor and five cognitive items that are individually scored from 1 to 7. A score of 1 indicates complete dependence, and a score of 7 indicates complete independence (Box 36-1). The sum of the 13 FIM motor score items can range from 13, indicating complete dependence for all items, to 91, indicating complete independence for all items. FIM is a measure usually completed by healthcare professionals; different observers, including the client, family members, and caregivers, can contribute information to the ratings. Each of these reporters may represent a different type of potential bias.

Although the sample sizes of FIM data for certain neurological level groups are quite small, the consistency of the data suggests that the interpretation is reliable. Other pertinent data regarding functional independence must be factored into outcome analyses, including medical information, patient factors, social role participation, quality of life, and environmental factors and supports.

In Table 36-1, FIM data, when available, are reported in three areas. First, the expected FIM outcomes are documented on the basis of expert clinical consensus. The second number reported is the median FIM score, as compiled by NSCISC. The interquartile range for NSCISC FIM data is the third set of numbers. In total, the FIM data represent 1-year postinjury FIM assessments of 405 survivors with complete SCI and a median age of 27 years. The NSCISC sample size for FIM and Assistance Data is provided for each level of injury. Different outcome expectations should clearly apply to different client subgroups and populations. Some populations are likely to be significantly older than the referenced one. Functional abilities may be limited by advancing age.[14,17]

- *Home modifications.* To provide the best opportunity for individuals with SCI to achieve the identified functional outcomes, a safe and architecturally accessible environment is necessary. An accessible environment must take into consideration, but not be limited to, entrance and egress, mobility in the home, and adequate setup to perform personal care and homemaking tasks.

Review Questions

1. List three causes of SCI. Which is most common?
2. Describe the patterns of weakness in quadriplegia and paraplegia.
3. Describe the functional and prognostic differences between complete and incomplete lesions.
4. When reference is made to C5 in quadriplegia, what is meant in terms of level of injury and functioning muscle groups?
5. What are the characteristics of spinal shock?
6. What physical changes occur after the spinal shock phase?
7. What is the prognosis for recovery of motor function in complete lesions and incomplete lesions?
8. What are the purposes of surgery in management of SCI?
9. What are some medical complications common among clients with SCI that can limit achievement of functional potential?
10. How should postural hypotension be treated?
11. How should autonomic dysreflexia be treated?
12. What is the role of the occupational therapist in the prevention of pressure sores?
13. Why is vital capacity affected in individuals with SCI?
14. What effect does reduced vital capacity have on the rehabilitation program?
15. Which level of injury features full innervation of the rotator cuff musculature, biceps, and extensor carpi radialis and partial innervation of the serratus anterior, latissimus dorsi, and pectoralis major?
16. What additional muscle power does the client with C6-level quadriplegia have over the client with C5-level quadriplegia? What is the major functional advantage of this additional muscle power?
17. What are the additional critical muscles that the client with C7-level quadriplegia has, as compared with the client with C6-level quadriplegia?
18. What additional functional independence can be achieved because of this additional muscle power?

Box **36-1**	FUNCTIONAL INDEPENDENCE MEASURE LEVELS

(7) Complete independence (timely, safely)	No helper
(6) Modified independence (device)	
MODIFIED DEPENDENCE	Helper
(5) Supervision	
(4) Minimal assist (subject = 75% or more)	
(3) Moderate assist (subject = 50% to 74%)	
COMPLETE DEPENDENCE	
(2) Maximal assist (subject = 25%-49%)	
(1) Total assist (subject = 0%-24%)	

From *Guide for the uniform data set for medical rehabilitation* (including the FIM instrument), Version 5.0, Buffalo, NY, State University of New York at Buffalo.

19. What is the first spinal cord lesion level that features full innervation of the UE musculature?

20. Which assessments do occupational therapists use to evaluate the client with SCI? What is the purpose of each?

21. List five goals of OT for the client with SCI.

22. How is wrist extension used to affect grasp by the individual with quadriplegia?

23. How does the individual with C6-level quadriplegia substitute for the absence of elbow extensors?

24. What is the contracture that is encouraged in clients with SCI? Why? How is it developed?

25. What is the splint that allows the client with C6-level quadriplegia to achieve functional prehension?

26. What are some of the first self-care activities that the client with a C6-level SCI should be expected to accomplish?

27. List four assistive devices commonly used by persons with quadriplegia, and tell the purpose of each.

28. How can ordering an ill-fitting wheelchair affect the UE function and skin care of someone with C6-level quadriplegia?

29. Describe the role of OT in the vocational evaluation of a client with SCI.

30. What are two considerations when predicting the future functional outcomes for a 25-year-old client with T4-level paraplegia?

31. Why would a person with paraplegia require homemaking assistance if he is independent in all self-care and mobility activities?

REFERENCES

1. Amador J: Contemporary information regarding male infertility following spinal cord injury, *SCI Nursing* 15(3):61, 1998.

2. Bromley I: *Tetraplegia and paraplegia: a guide for physiotherapists*, ed 5, New York, 1998, Churchill Livingstone.

3. Consortium for Spinal Cord Medicine, Paralyzed Veterans of America: *Outcomes following traumatic spinal cord injury: clinical practice guidelines for health-care professionals*, Washington, D.C., 1999, The Consortium.

4. Frankel H et al: The value of postural reduction in the initial management of closed injuries to the spine with paraplegia and tetraplegia, *Paraplegia* 7:179, 1969.

5. Freed MM: Traumatic and congenital lesions of the spinal cord. In Kottke FJ, Lehmann JF, editors: *Krusen's handbook of physical medicine and rehabilitation*, Philadelphia, 1990, WB Saunders.

6. Gerhart KA et al: Quality of life following spinal cord injury: knowledge and attitudes of emergency care providers, *Ann Emerg Med* 23(4):807, 1994.

7. Hanak M, Scott A: *An illustrated guide for health care professionals*, ed 2, New York, 1993, Springer-Verlag.

8. Heinemann AW et al: Mobility for persons with spinal cord injury: an evaluation of two systems, *Arch Phys Med Rehabil* 68(2):90, 1987.

9. Hill JP, editor: *Spinal cord injury: a guide to functional outcomes in occupational therapy*, Rockville, MD, 1987, Aspen.

10. Institute for Medical Research, Santa Clara Valley Medical Center: *Severe head trauma, a comprehensive medical approach*, Project 13-9-59156/9 (Report to National Institute for Handicapped Research), Nov., 1982.

11. Lammertse D: Why some injured people get better and others don't. In Maddox S: *Spinal network*, Boulder, CO, 1987, Spinal Network.

12. Paulson S, editor: *Santa Clara Valley Medical Center spinal cord injury home care manual*, ed 3, San Jose, CA, 1994, Santa Clara Valley Medical Center.

13. Pendleton HMcH, Schultz-Krohn W: Psycho-social issues of physical disability. In Cara EM, MacRae A, editors: *Psychosocial occupational therapy in clinical practice*, New York, 2005, Delmar.

14. Penrod LE, Hegde SK, Ditunno JF Jr: Age effect on prognosis for functional recovery in acute traumatic central cord syndrome (CCS), *Arch Phys Med Rehabil* 71(12):963, 1990.

15. Pierce DS, Nickel VH: *The total care of spinal cord injuries*, Boston, 1977, Little, Brown.

16. Spencer EA: Functional restoration. In Hopkins HL, Smith HD, editors: *Willard and Spackman's occupational therapy*, ed 8, Philadelphia, 1993, JB Lippincott.

17. Yarkony GM et al: Spinal cord injury rehabilitation outcomes: the impact of age, *J Clin Epidemiol* 41(2):173, 1988.

37

DISORDERS OF THE MOTOR UNIT

MARTI SOUTHAM
AMY SCHMIDT
(contributing author for Guillain Barré syndrome)

KEY TERMS

Motor unit	Guillain-Barré syndrome	Postpolio syndrome	Myasthenia gravis
Lower motor neuron system	Poliomyelitis	Brachial plexus	Muscular dystrophy
Peripheral neuropathies	Peripheral nerve injuries		

LEARNING OBJECTIVES

After studying this chapter the student or practitioner will be able to do the following:

1. Describe the characteristics of motor unit disorders.
2. Discuss the clinical manifestations of motor unit disorders.
3. Discuss the impact of motor unit disorders on occupational performance.

4. Identify assessments and interventions for an occupational therapy program for the various motor unit disorders discussed in this chapter.

CHAPTER OUTLINE

Neurogenic disorders
  Peripheral neuropathies
  Peripheral nerve injuries
Neuromuscular disorders

Neuromuscular junction: myasthenia gravis
Myopathic disorders
  Muscular dystrophies
Summary

THREADED CASE STUDY: EDITH, PART 1

Although this case study is specific to Guillain-Barré syndrome, many of the aspects of Edith's occupational profile and occupational performance needs apply to the other diagnoses in this chapter.

At age 67, Edith had been enjoying her retirement, primarily spending time with her husband, three children, and five grandchildren. She had recently recovered from the flu and was looking forward to a day at the park with her family. While showering, she suddenly lost strength in her legs and collapsed. While lying on the shower floor, she noticed that her arms also felt weak. Her cognition was intact, but she was physically helpless. Her husband called 911. It was fortunate that she received immediate medical care because she later required mechanical assistance to breathe. After extensive neurological testing, Edith was diagnosed with Guillain-Barré syndrome (GBS). Neither she nor her family had ever heard of GBS.

Edith suddenly found herself dependent in all of her life roles and occupations. She was hospitalized in the intensive care unit (ICU) for several weeks, was dependent on a ventilator to breathe, and needed physical assistance because of her total body paralysis. Her muscles were painful, sore, and tender, and pain medications helped to manage the discomfort.

Jen, the occupational therapist assigned to the ICU, interviewed Edith, and together they identified the occupational needs and client factors that should be addressed. Jen performed passive range of motion (ROM) exercises, fabricated static hand splints to maintain a functional resting position and to prevent contractures, provided proper bed positioning, and taught the family about GBS. Jen also provided support, encouragement, and active listening, employing therapeutic use of self during the intervention. Edith often spoke about her spiritual beliefs and reported that she found hope and strength with prayer and meditation. She spoke of her favorite previous performance pattern of reading her Bible every morning and said she felt depressed because she was now unable to physically hold a book or turn pages. After receiving training and modifications from Jen, Edith was able to listen to the Bible on CD, using a mouth switch to turn it on and off; this modification allowed her to resume her previous morning routine.

Edith made slow but steady gains in physical abilities and was transferred to an acute rehabilitation hospital to actively participate in an intensive interdisciplinary therapy program. Lara, the occupational therapist on the rehabilitation unit, evaluated Edith's specific functions as they related to supporting performance and engagement in occupations and activities targeted for intervention. The goals from the Canadian Occupational Performance Measure[26] included the following: (1) to be able to feed herself, brush her teeth, and shower; (2) to cook for her family; (3) to be able to go shopping at the mall with her granddaughter; and (4) to be able to drive to her friend's house to play cards. Detailed upper extremity manual muscle testing, muscle belly tenderness screening, ROM measurements, and sensation testing were completed during the evaluation phase.

Intervention strategies focused on using compensatory methods and improving strength and endurance. Lara taught Edith adaptive strategies to eat, groom, and bathe. The use of adaptive equipment, work simplification, and energy conservation techniques were encouraged while Edith engaged in activities such as cooking and light cleaning. Lara supported Edith's community mobility and accompanied Edith to the mall with her granddaughter. After the brief outing, Edith expressed a sense of increased self-confidence and accomplishment. She practiced card playing with other clients in a group environment. She also participated in a daily individualized strengthening program.

Lara provided Edith with community resources to aid in her independence. For example, the Guillain-Barré Syndrome Foundation International (GBSFI) offers local support groups, literature, and conferences to GBS survivors and caregivers. In addition, her family received extensive training from the interdisciplinary team members to assist with application of learned strategies and equipment in the home and community. Driving was not addressed at an inpatient level, but Edith was referred to an outpatient training program.

Critical Thinking Questions

1. What are the phases of Guillain-Barré, and what occupational therapy interventions might be used in each phase?
3. In what ways were the client's psychosocial needs addressed during recovery?
4. Describe energy conservation techniques that you think would be appropriate for Edith while engaging in her valued occupation of cooking.

The symptoms, course, medical treatment, and occupational therapy (OT) assessment and intervention for clients who have motor unit disorders most commonly seen in OT practice are presented in this chapter. The **motor unit** is the basic functional unit of the peripheral nervous system and consists of four elements: the cell body of the motor neuron in the anterior horn of the spinal cord; the axon of the motor neuron, which travels via spinal nerves and peripheral nerves to muscle; the neuromuscular junction; and the muscle fibers innervated by the neuron (Figure 37-1). Disorders of the motor unit generally cause muscle weakness and atrophy of skeletal muscle that may be of neurogenic, neuromuscular, or myopathic origin. Those with a neurogenic basis are the lower motor neuron disorders, affecting the cell bodies and peripheral nerves. Those with a neuromuscular or myopathic basis affect the neuromuscular junction or the muscle itself.[43]

This chapter will discuss the physical, psychosocial, and emotional factors that occupational therapists address when

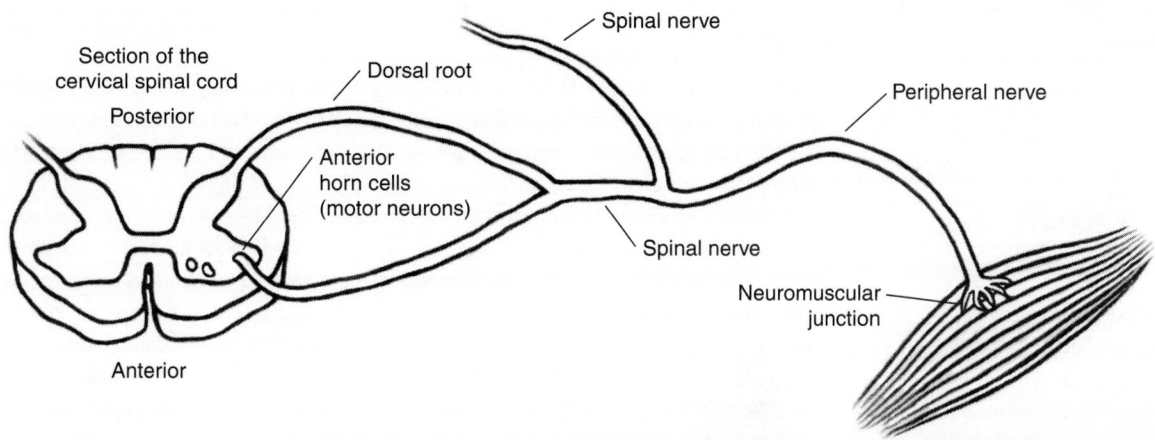

Figure 37-1   Motor unit consisting of motor neuron cell body in the anterior horn of the spinal cord, the axon of the motor neuron (which travels via spinal nerves and peripheral nerves to muscle), the neuromuscular junction, and the muscle fibers innervated by the neuron.

assessing and providing interventions for people with motor unit disorders.

Occupational therapists, with their holistic view of persons with physical disabilities, are uniquely positioned to recognize and include interventions that address mental health concerns for persons with disorders of the motor unit. The sudden onset of severely disabling peripheral neuropathies, such as Guillain-Barré, or the chronic aspects of living with fatigue and experiencing role alterations will have ramifications on the client, the family, and their social network as described in the case study of Edith.

NEUROGENIC DISORDERS

PERIPHERAL NEUROPATHIES

The motor neurons in the anterior horn of the spinal cord mediate voluntary movement and reflexes that produce motor behavior. Muscle strength and endurance contribute to coordinated and skilled movement and the ability to move through available range of motion. The characteristics of movement are determined by the pattern and firing frequency of specific motor units. Muscle contraction is the output of the motor system.[43]

The **lower motor neuron system** includes the cell bodies in the anterior horn of the spinal cord and their axons (which pass by way of the spinal nerves and peripheral nerves to the neuromuscular junction) and the nuclei of cranial nerves III through X (located in the brainstem) and their axons. The motor fibers of the lower motor neurons contain somatic motor components, including the alpha motor neurons, which innervate skeletal muscles (extrafusal fibers), and gamma motor neurons, which innervate muscle spindles (intrafusal fibers). A lesion in any of these neurological structures results in peripheral neuropathy or a lower motor neuron dysfunction.[43]

Peripheral neuropathies involve lesions of the lower motor neuron system and may be located in the anterior horn cells of the spinal cord, spinal nerves, peripheral nerves, and cranial nerves or their nuclei in the brainstem. Lesions can result from nerve root compression, trauma (e.g., bone fractures and dislocations, lacerations, traction, or penetrating wounds and friction), toxins (e.g., lead, phosphorus, alcohol, benzene, or sulfonamides), infections (e.g., poliomyelitis or Guillain-Barré syndrome), neoplasms (e.g., neuromas and multiple neurofibromatosis), vascular disorders (e.g., arteriosclerosis, diabetes mellitus, peripheral vascular anomalies, and polyarteritis nodosa), degenerative diseases of the central nervous systems (e.g., amyotrophic lateral sclerosis), and congenital malformations.[50] "Like static on a telephone line, peripheral neuropathy distorts and sometimes interrupts messages between the brain and the rest of the body." [35]

OT assessments for motor unit disorders follow a similar sequence and are described in Table 37-1. An occupational profile is developed during an interview with the client and caregivers. The Canadian Occupational Performance Measure[26] is an excellent instrument to establish goals and measure intervention outcomes. Performance skills, performance patterns, client factors, and activity demands in context must also be clinically assessed. Specific assessments such as range of motion, manual muscle testing, scales designed to measure coping and depression, and activities of daily living assessments are appropriate for each of the motor unit disorders described in this chapter.

A description of two complex syndromes, Guillain-Barré and postpolio, will be discussed in detail in the following section. The concepts are applicable to the other motor unit disorders described later in the chapter.

TABLE 37-1 **Occupational Therapy Assessments and Descriptions**

Assessments	Descriptions
Occupational profile	Interview client (and family members and caregivers, if appropriate) to gain information about problems and concerns, successful and unsuccessful strategies when engaging in occupations, ways in which contexts influence functional abilities, activity demands, and priorities of meaningful occupations.
Canadian Occupational Performance Measure[26]	The interview is conducted before and after intervention to describe problems, level of satisfaction with performing activities, and level of perceived performance abilities in areas of self-care, productivity, and leisure. Testing methods must be measurable to assess intervention results.
Performance skills in areas of occupation: activities of daily living, instrumental activities of daily living, education, work, play, leisure, social participation	Following the occupations that the client prioritizes in the occupational profile, the therapist can perform formal assessments and observation of the client's performance during activity engagement in the appropriate context, with attention paid to motor, process, and communication/interaction skills. (See Chapter 17 for additional assessment details and Chapter 18 for a description of specific leisure assessments.)
Performance patterns	Client (independently or with assistance from caregivers or occupational therapist) maintains a log of activities and symptoms to analyze in collaboration with the occupational therapist to discover habits and routines that are detrimental or helpful to occupational performance. Reestablishment or adjustment of roles should be discussed and implemented.
Client factors: manual muscle testing, range of motion testing, eating and swallowing assessments, pain scale, sensory testing, depression scale, Ways of Coping Scale, clinical observations during activities of daily living.	The therapist should perform specific assessments of the client's bodily function, including systems that support participation in meaningful occupations (e.g., neuromusculoskeletal, pain, joint range of motion, sensation, cardiovascular, respiratory, swallowing, pain, skin). Because fatigability is so prevalent in these disorders, assessments should be adequately spaced and preferably performed when clients are feeling their best (often in the morning). Assessment of emotional stability, motivation, sexual activity, depression, ways of coping, and so forth is critical to forming an overall picture of the client's strengths and weaknesses.
Activity demands	Analysis of the required sequence, body functions, and body structures is necessary to complete the activity. Analysis must include assessment of the tools or equipment used to perform the activity and any adaptations that could be made to ensure success.
Contexts	The therapist should always consider the client's culture, physical environment, socioeconomic status, personal and spiritual beliefs, temporal aspects, and virtual contexts.

Data from American Occupational Therapy Association: Occupational therapy practice framework: domain and process, *Am J Occup Ther* 56:609, 2002.

Guillain-Barré Syndrome

Guillain-Barré (ghee-YAN bah-RAY) **syndrome** (also known as *acute idiopathic neuropathy, infectious polyneuritis,* and *Landry's syndrome*) is an acute, inflammatory condition involving the spinal nerve roots, peripheral nerves, and, in some cases, selected cranial nerves. Guillain-Barré syndrome (GBS) is an autoimmune disease with no known cause or cure.[33] The immune system destroys the myelin sheath that surrounds the axons of many peripheral nerves or even the axons themselves. It often follows a viral illness, immunization, or surgery. Upper respiratory infection, gastrointestinal infection, or a nonspecific febrile illness precedes the onset of weakness in 40% to 60% of individuals, usually within 1 to 2 weeks.[4]

This acute and complex disorder came to public attention when it struck a number of people who received the 1976 swine flu vaccine. It continues to claim thousands of new victims each year, striking any person, at any age, regardless of gender or ethnic background.[16] The worldwide incidence of GBS ranges from 0.6 to 1.4 people per 100,000 annually.[10]

It is the most common cause of acute neuromuscular paralysis in developed countries; about 5000 people are diagnosed annually in the United States, and GBS occurs almost twice as often in males as in females.[31]

The initial symptoms of Guillain-Barré syndrome most often include varying degrees of weakness and sensory changes in the legs. GBS is characterized by rapidly progressive ascending weakness of bilateral extremities, usually proceeding from distal to proximal (feet to trunk). Descending paralysis with predominant proximal muscle weakness rarely appears.[4,33] Because the myelin sheath of the peripheral nerves are injured or degraded, the nerves cannot transmit signals efficiently. The muscles begin to lose their ability to respond to the brain's commands. The brain also receives fewer sensory signals from the rest of the body, resulting in an inability to feel textures, heat, pain, and other sensations. Clients often report initial sensations such as tingling, "crawling-skin," or painful sensations. Because the signals to and from the arms and legs must travel the longest distances, they are most vulnerable to interruption. Therefore, muscle weakness and tingling sensations usually first appear distally in the hands and feet and progress proximally.[33]

Typically, the weakness and abnormal sensations first noticed in the legs progress to the arms and upper body, and some muscles are almost totally paralyzed. As the demyelination continues, the client may experience problems with breathing, speaking, swallowing, blood pressure, or heart rate. The client may require use of a respirator to assist with breathing and is monitored closely for an abnormal heart rhythm, infections, blood clots, and high or low blood pressure. After the first clinical manifestations of the disease, the symptoms can progress over the course of hours, days, or weeks. By the third week of the illness, 90% of all clients are at their weakest. Some may be completely paralyzed and dependent on the respirator.[33]

Cooke and Orb[10] define three phases of Guillain-Barré syndrome. The initial, or acute, phase begins with the client's first conclusive symptoms and lasts until there is no further decline in physical status. This phase may last from 1 to 3 weeks.[18] The plateau phase begins when the client's physical state is stable, with no further deterioration of physical status and no evidence of physical recovery. The plateau phase generally lasts a few weeks, during which the physical status of the client remains unchanged. The recovery phase is that period when the client slowly begins to recover physical abilities and symptoms gradually decrease. This phase can last up to 2 years, depending on the extent of paralysis.

Being paralyzed is a frightening experience for people with GBS and their family members and friends. Clients can be expected to proceed through varying stages of adapting to the acute and residual effects of this physical disability.[38] However, the prognosis is generally good for the majority of clients; therefore, it is appropriate to be optimistic during intervention sessions and encourage clients and families to look forward to recovery (Table 37-2).

There is no known cure for GBS. However, there are interventions that lessen the severity of the illness and accelerate the recovery in most individuals. There are also a number of ways to treat the complications of the disease.[33] Immunomodulatory therapy (plasmapheresis or intravenous immunoglobulin IVIg) is the recommended medical treatment at the onset of GBS. Plasmapheresis has shown clinical improvements, reducing the time required for ventilation and critical care, time to achieve ambulation, and hospital length of stay.[4,29] This process is used to separate the whole blood from the plasma and then return the whole blood to the client without the plasma to reduce the length of the acute phase.

Role of the occupational therapist

The client with GBS may be referred to OT when medically stable. An occupational profile of the client will be developed through OT assessments related to the level of dysfunction that the client is experiencing. For example, physical abilities

TABLE 37-2 Guillain-Barré Syndrome: Prognosis and Outcomes

Recovery Status	Percentage of Clients	Description
Recover well spontaneously	85%	70% of those who recover well have some residual deficits such as distal numbness, weakness, fatigue; these may interfere with some daily functions but usually are not severe.
Significant impairments	10%	Fatigue and severe weakness in specific muscle groups significantly impair daily function
Death	5%	Death is usually the result of pneumonia, sepsis, adult respiratory distress syndrome, autonomic dysfunction, or pulmonary embolism.

Data from Lawn N, Wijdicks E: Fatal Guillain-Barré syndrome, *Neurology* 52: 635, 1999;
Nicholas R, Playford ED, Thompson AJ: A retrospective analysis of outcome in severe Guillain-Barré syndrome following combined neurological and rehabilitation management, *Disabil Rehabil* 22(10):451, 2000.

are assessed using range of motion (ROM) and manual muscle testing (MMT), sensation testing, and swallowing assessment. Functional assessments of quality of movement, coordination, and self-care may also be performed. It is critical to assess emotional and psychosocial factors of the client and family. See Table 37-1 for OT assessments.

After the initial OT evaluation, an intervention plan is developed. Frequent revisions may be necessary, depending on the client's recovery status. During the initial phase of intervention, problematic client factors are immediately addressed in conjunction with the healthcare team. These may include providing daily passive ROM, positioning, and splinting to prevent contracture and deformity and to protect weak muscles. Passive ROM should begin with gentle movement of the joints and should not exceed the point of pain. Particular attention should be paid to determining residual weakness in the intrinsic muscles of the hands. Passive activities (e.g., watching television) and nonstrenuous social visits from family and friends are encouraged. Muscle belly tenderness (a flu-type muscle soreness) is closely monitored, and activities are modified as needed.[6] Many clients may benefit from the use of electronic aids for daily living (EADLs). EADLs increase the level of independence in the client's control of the environment through the use of technology. For example, a client with GBS might lack the strength and motor skills to operate the television, lights, telephone, and radio in the environment. With the use of EADLs, the client may be able to use the head, mouth, or other parts of the body to operate control switches and successfully control the environment.

An intensive interdisciplinary rehabilitation program is typically implemented during the recovery phase as the client begins to regain physical movement. After the evaluation process, the OT intervention plan, developed in collaboration with the client, must be carefully designed to respect muscle belly tenderness and to prevent fatigue and further damage to the nerves. Because muscle belly tenderness usually decreases in the proximal musculature before it decreases distally, proximal musculature movements can be facilitated first while distal joints continue to be supported (e.g., using mobile arm supports).[6] Activity is gradually increased with close monitoring of pain or fatigue after each intervention session. The therapist should continue to monitor for increased muscle belly tenderness, muscle imbalance, and substitution patterns. Progressive resistive exercises should be used conservatively, with attention to joint protection and fatigue. Throughout the course of recovery, the therapist should guard against fatigue and irritation of the inflamed nerves. Instruction to client and family in key concepts such as energy conservation, work simplification, avoidance of over-stretching, and overuse of muscles is critical to recovery.[44]

As the client's strength increases, activities promoting more resistance can be incorporated into the intervention program. Self-care (grooming, eating, dressing, bathing, and toileting) and other activities of daily living (ADLs), instrumental activities of daily living (IADLs), and leisure occupations should be included as soon as the client is capable of participating in them. Activities should be graded for success as strength and endurance improve. Adaptive equipment, frequent rest breaks, and creative strategies are typically necessary during this phase. Mobile arm supports may be used to alleviate muscle fatigue, promote active assistive use of upper extremities, and encourage independence with occupations. Activities and occupations should be varied among gross motor, fine motor, resistive, and non-resistive exercises to prevent undue fatigue.[44]

 OT PRACTICE NOTE

Engagement in light occupations that are meaningful to the client is essential for building the self-confidence necessary to resume previous life roles and interests. For example, a client may be able to participate in enjoyable leisure occupations such as scrapbooking, surfing the web, planning a family gathering, and reading books to grandchildren (see Chapter 18).

People with GBS face not only physical difficulties but emotionally painful periods as well. It is often extremely difficult for clients to adjust to sudden paralysis and dependence on others for help with routine daily activities.[38]

Eisendrath, Matthay, and Dunkel found severe anxiety, fear, and panic in the acute progressive phase.[13] When clients reached the plateau phase, they often expressed anger and depression. When improvement began during the recovery phase, severe depression occurred as clients contemplated the long, slow convalescence and the possibility of permanent neurological deficits. An occupational therapist can support the client by facilitating feelings of self-worth, a positive attitude, and encouragement through the engagement in occupations (see Chapter 18).[38,46] A psychologist or physician should also closely monitor the mood of the client and provide necessary interventions as a member of the intervention team.

After becoming medically stable and being discharged from the hospital, many GBS survivors find themselves living at home without proper medical follow-up and therapy. Families are left to their own devices to successfully create real-life solutions to functional limitations and to locate and use resources. Schmidt conducted a survey of 90 voluntary participants from the Guillain-Barré Syndrome Foundation International to explore the extent of functional limitations within home, work, community, and leisure roles after hospitalization.[44] The majority of the participants stated that they had to independently research information about GBS because their doctors and team members either lacked the knowledge or did not provide them with any verbal or written information. One participant noted, "My family had to learn everything about GBS on the Internet. My doctors and nurses didn't know anything about it. *We* had to educate *them* (doctors, nurses, therapists, etc.)." These families reported feeling most frustrated about the fact that significant psychosocial issues such as depression, anxiety, fear, and hopelessness were not addressed by healthcare professionals. Physically demanding tasks that required fair to good strength and endurance were scored the lowest in satisfaction and ability by participants. The great majority of respondents (98%) reported that they were living with limiting factors affecting their ability to participate in life, such as fatigue, weakness, pain, sensation disturbances, coordination problems, and psychosocial changes. Nearly half of the participants agreed that they would benefit from OT services to improve the use of their upper extremities and to learn ways to manage daily fatigue and maintain their current health status. This study indicates the need for continued OT to optimize occupational performance and occupational roles many years after the onset of the syndrome and apparent recovery.

The complex process of adjusting to the disabling condition, problem solving, learning, and redesigning a life for a GBS survivor is a long-term, therapeutic experience. The lifestyle redesign process can be initiated by the occupational therapist at the inpatient rehabilitation phase; however, there must be a continuum of care established for follow-up treatment. An occupational therapist working in an outpatient or home setting can skillfully guide clients back to the resumption of their previous life roles, assist clients in returning to productive community involvement and leisure occupations (see Chapter 18), and teach engagement and participation in meaningful occupations.[28,44]

Poliomyelitis and Postpolio Syndrome

Transmission of the poliomyelitis virus has been severely curtailed throughout the world as a result of the Global Polio Eradication Program; only 784 confirmed cases of polio were reported globally in 2003.[8] The peak of polio cases in the United States was in 1952, with over 21,000 persons paralyzed. A great number of children were infected during the summer and fall months. According to the Centers for Disease Control and Prevention (CDC), the last case of indigenous polio acquired in the United States was in 1979. A program to eradicate polio in the Western hemisphere, led by the Pan American Health Organization, eliminated polio in this region of the world in 1991.

Poliomyelitis is a highly contagious viral disease that enters through the mouth via the fecal-oral route (i.e., it is spread in unsanitary conditions with poor hand-washing techniques). The virus moves from the throat into the digestive tract and is shed through fecal material for several weeks. The polio virus enters the bloodstream and, in some cases, infects the motor neurons of the anterior horn and brainstem. Generally, people who contract the disease are asymptomatic but can still spread the disease. According to the CDC, flaccid paralysis results in less than 1% of all polio infections, and most people recover completely. If weakness or paralysis lasts more than 12 months, it is usually permanent.

The CDC recognizes three types of paralytic polio: spinal polio, bulbar polio, and bulbospinal polio. Spinal polio was the most commonly diagnosed type between 1969 and 1979, involving 79% of the reported cases. This type produced asymmetric flaccid paralysis predominantly in the legs. Bulbar polio (2% of cases) infected the cranial nerves, leading to muscle weakness in oral and facial musculature, and a combination of the two types resulted in bulbospinal polio (19% of cases). Marked atrophy could be seen in the involved extremities, and deep tendon reflexes were often absent. Sensation and cognition remained intact. The asymmetry of muscles pulling on various joints sometimes produced deformities, such as subluxation, scoliosis, and contractures.[45,53]

Even though substantial efforts have dramatically reduced the presence of poliomyelitis, the effects of polio still exist. Between 12 and 20 million people in the world who had polio are still alive (approximately two million of these people live in the United States). These adults are currently dealing with new muscle pain and increasing weakness or are developing new weakness or paralysis that is diagnosed as **postpolio syndrome** (PPS). In fact, between 25% and 40% of persons who had paralytic and nonparalytic polio in childhood are experiencing these symptoms.[8,39] According to the CDC, "the pathogenesis of postpolio syndrome is thought to involve the failure of oversized motor units created during

the recovery process of paralytic poliomyelitis".[8] Fortunately, postpolio syndrome is not contagious.

According to Postpolio Health International,[39] six criteria should be considered for this diagnosis: period of partial or complete recovery, gradual or sudden onset of progressive new muscle weakness or muscle fatigue, new difficulties with breathing and swallowing, a year or more of these symptoms, and other causes of symptoms ruled out (Table 37-3). PPS progresses slowly with intermittent periods of stability. People who had severe cases of acute polio experience a greater degree of disability resulting from PPS than do those whose initial response to the polio virus was mild. Fatigue is the most debilitating symptom because it limits activity. The fatigue may be severe and out of proportion to the apparent physical demands of the activity and can be overwhelming. People with PPS risk additional disabling problems such as muscle atrophy, scoliosis, osteoporosis, fractures, contractures, and depression.[19,56,57] An increase in difficulty with ADLs and IADLs accompanies the symptoms. Problems with ambulation, transfers, stairs, home management, driving, dressing, eating and swallowing, and bladder and bowel control may occur, and people report a poorer functional status

TABLE **37-3** **Six Criteria for Postpolio Syndrome**

Criteria	Description
Prior paralytic poliomyelitis	Documented polio diagnosis, motor neuron loss, residual weakness, muscle atrophy, and electromyography (EMG) showing denervation of muscles
Period of partial or complete recovery	Evidence of acute paralytic polio with recovery and stable neurological functions for an interval of about 15 years or more
Gradual or sudden onset of progressive and persistent new muscle weakness or abnormal muscle fatigability	Decreased endurance, muscle and joint pain; onset possibly occurring after surgery, trauma, or periods of inactivity
New difficulties with breathing and swallowing	Unlikely but possible development of problems with breathing and swallowing
Symptoms as listed above that may persist for at least a year	Length of time that client reports having symptoms sometime relevant in the diagnosis of postpolio syndrome
Other causes of above symptoms ruled out	Exclusion of other neurological, medical, and orthopedic problems

Data from Jubelt B, Agre JC: Characteristics and management of postpolio syndrome, *J Am Med Assoc* 284:412, 2000; Postpolio Health International: *Information about the late effects of polio.* Retrieved on July 14, 2005, from www.post-polio.org/ipn/aboutlep.html.

and health-related quality of life.[25,56] Unless there is severe pulmonary or swallowing involvement in postpolio syndrome, the symptoms are rarely life threatening.

Role of the occupational therapist

Occupational therapists should consider that the psychological and emotional aspects of PPS may be as disabling as the physical symptoms. Persons who originally had polio most likely assumed that the disease was over, that disability was in the past, and that any residual weakness was static. Therefore, the onset of new symptoms and accompanying disruption of occupational performance and lifestyle may be devastating as the client, family, and friends are confronted for a second time with the notion of being disabled. A supportive and realistic approach by the healthcare team, along with client and family education, is the key to lifestyle modification.[56,57]

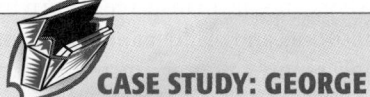

CASE STUDY: GEORGE

During his ninth birthday party, in February of 1955, George fell after another child kicked a ball, which hit George's legs. By the next morning, he could not get out of bed or stand on his own. He was admitted to a hospital and diagnosed with polio. George was placed in an iron lung that did the breathing for him. This was at the height of the polio epidemic, and the hospital wards and even the halls were filled with children in iron lungs. The complete confinement was terrifying, as was the constant presence of medical staff and equipment.

Over the years, George gradually recovered and was able to walk unassisted and participate fully in life. Recently, however, at the age of 60, George has begun experiencing new weakness in his legs, muscle pain, disproportionate fatigue related to activities, and an unstable gait. He is afraid that he is getting polio again. George quit his full-time job, stopped playing tennis, and became disengaged from his social life because he feared the full re-emergence of polio and did not want anyone to know. His wife was very concerned and scheduled an appointment for George with their doctor, who prescribed occupational therapy, physical therapy, and counseling.

Analysis

George is among the many people worldwide who are affected by postpolio syndrome. Through occupational and physical therapy and counseling, he will be able to resume a near-normal life. His fears must be addressed because they will hamper whatever remaining function he has. Through occupational therapy, George can learn to pace his activities, protect his joints, recognize fatigue before it becomes severe, and modify his leisure occupations so that he can lead an enjoyable life.

Occupational therapy has an important role to play in helping the client to stabilize function. Goals to adjust lifestyle may be accomplished by collaborating with the client and family to use work simplification, energy conservation, and adaptive equipment as needed. These measures, along with a healthy diet and enjoyment of remaining abilities, may provide improved engagement in meaningful occupations and participation in the various contexts of the client's life.[36,57]

When assessing a client with the diagnosis of PPS, the occupational therapist collaborates with the client and caregivers (if appropriate) to develop the occupational profile. After discussing the client's problems and concerns, the therapist can explore what strategies have been used by the client and the client's report of the usefulness of those strategies. The occupational therapist selects specific assessments, such as ROM, MMT, and assessment of client's equipment for proper fit and function, to provide additional needed information (see Table 37-1).

Information gained from the evaluation process is used to prioritize and select valued, relevant activities for the client with PPS. The Knowledge of Polio Test can reveal what the client and family understands about polio and its sequelae.[55] Education about the effects of polio when the client was a child, combined with information about current symptoms, is important. In most cases, little family education was available in the 1950s and 1960s, when the client first contracted polio.[45]

Fatigue and pain are the two symptoms most frequently mentioned by clients with PPS. Scoliosis is found in nearly all survivors of polio. Even though scoliosis itself generally does not produce pain, the strain it puts on joints and muscles through abnormal biomechanics can produce degenerative disk disease, as well as pain in the shoulders, knees, and other joints and muscles.[53] Decreased vital capacity and difficulty breathing with deventilation during sleep is seen frequently in these clients. If the client complains of frequent awakening during the night or breathing problems, the therapist should refer the client to a pulmonologist immediately.[53,57]

A client-centered intervention plan is designed to help the client and caregiver improve functional outcomes. Adaptive strategies and preventative measures are key factors to include in the OT intervention plan. Prognosis and selection of intervention methods depend on the progression of the disorder. Functional and leisure activities that are meaningful to the client are used in combination with work simplification, pacing the activity for energy conservation, passive and active ROM exercises, muscle reeducation, proper posture and body mechanics, joint protection, and training in the use of assistive and adaptive devices and mobility aids, as needed. In all cases, the therapist must teach the client to carefully monitor fatigue level and to modify or stop the activity when necessary.[57] Establishing priorities of goals is critical to reach the desired outcome, and intervention goals should be coordinated with the client and members of the interdisciplinary team for a comprehensive rehabilitation program. Psychosocial aspects of the disorders must be addressed in the intervention plan.[22,38]

Understanding the client's psychosocial reactions to the various disabilities associated with PPS will help the therapist and client select interventions that will facilitate rehabilitation efforts and the patient's adjustment to new limitations. Changes in physical capacities, abnormal fatigue, and curtailment of valued life skills confront the client with psychological issues of coping, adjustment, and adaptation. These changes may be as traumatic as they were at the time of the original illness. It is important to be aware of the stages of adapting to a chronic disabling condition.[38,39] Feelings of denial, anger, and hopelessness and the sense of being a burden should be identified and addressed as a part of the OT intervention. Helping clients and families connect with support groups can make a difference in psychosocial acceptance and motivation.[57] If the client's psychological needs are beyond the scope of the OT practice, referral to a psychologist is appropriate.

Because the client with PPS may be psychologically fragile when facing renewed disabilities, the occupational therapist should introduce lifestyle changes gradually because modifying performance patterns and introducing adaptive equipment could threaten the client's self image. Small changes may be more acceptable than major ones, even if the latter are obviously necessary. The client's spiritual beliefs must be considered when developing an intervention plan, and "activities of the spirit" may be helpful to foster a sense of hope.[9]

The benefits of exercise are controversial. Muscles affected by PPS may actually function at levels of strength lower than estimated from the results obtained on the MMT, and upper extremity strength varies markedly throughout the ROM. Thus, careful observation is essential during engagement in occupations. Exercise must be carefully supervised because it may aggravate pain and overwork of muscles innervated by a limited number of motor units.[14,57] Signs of excessive activity are further weakness, discomfort, pain, muscle spasm, and chronic fatigue.[36,45,56,57]

Chronic pain can be managed or alleviated by prescribed pharmaceuticals, improving body mechanics during occupations, supporting weakened muscles through splinting and adaptive equipment, and promoting lifestyle and role modifications through a multidisciplinary treatment approach that is based on cognitive-behavioral therapy (CBT), a method that is frequently used by chronic pain management programs and may be employed by occupational therapists. CBT teaches clients about the dynamics of pain and coping strategies such as stress management, relaxation and visualization, appropriate use of play and humor, recognition of fatigue and implementation of activity pacing, monitoring of self-talk, and family training.[7,12,24,46,47,53] Strategies can be taught to reduce or eliminate nonessential activities, thus reducing overuse of muscles and resultant pain. Energy conservation

for the most valued activities may mean delegating less valued ones to others or performing them with the assistance of equipment, such as orthoses, assistive devices, or ambulation aids.[40,45,56,57] Body weight reduction may be medically recommended for some clients to reduce pain, and occupational therapists can work in conjunction with dietitians to address weight loss through cooking groups that create the recommended high-protein diet.[40]

It is important to make referrals to appropriate healthcare professionals depending on the needs of the client and family. These healthcare professionals may include an orthotist, physical therapist, pulmonologist, and psychologist.[57]

GBS and PPS are two disorders requiring OT services; they have been presented in detail to outline the process used for individuals with these disorders. The remaining portion of this chapter describes other disorders related to the motor unit that result in compromised occupational performance. The principles behind the interventions described for both GBS and PPS have application to the following disorders.

PERIPHERAL NERVE INJURIES

Thus far, this chapter has described diseases affecting the anterior horn cell and peripheral nerves. This section of the chapter will cover three specific upper extremity **peripheral nerve injuries**: axillary nerve, brachial plexus, and long thoracic nerve injury. The **brachial plexus** includes the nerves from C5 through T1.[37] These nerve fibers, both sensory and motor, intertwine very closely to the vertebral column. The fibers join together to form trunks of the brachial plexus, and from the trunks arise the divisions at which further interweaving of fibers occurs. The divisions give rise to the cords of the brachial plexus, and from the cords the terminal branches or named peripheral nerves arise. From an anatomical presentation, this complexity has the potential to preserve function if one root is compressed. For example, the radial nerve is composed of fibers originating from C6, C7, C8, and T1. For a list of nerves, muscles innervated, and actions performed, see Table 37-4. (See Chapter 39 for additional information on peripheral nerve injuries, peripheral pain syndromes, and the management of these disorders.)

Many people are injured every year by car accidents, falls, sports mishaps, gunshots, and violent acts (e.g., blunt and sharp wounds) that result in severed, crushed, compressed, or stretched peripheral nerves.[35] The most obvious manifestation of peripheral nerve injury is muscle weakness or flaccid paralysis, with symptoms depending on the extent of the nerve damage. Deep tendon reflexes are depressed or absent. Sensation along the cutaneous distribution of the nerve is also altered or lost. Trophic changes, such as dry skin, hair loss, cyanosis, brittle fingernails, painless skin ulcerations, and slow wound healing in the area of involvement, may be present.

TABLE **37-4** **Clinical Manifestations of Peripheral Nerve Lesions of the Brachial Plexus**

Spinal Nerves	Nerve	Motor Distribution	Clinical Manifestations
C5	Dorsal scapular	Rhomboid major and minor, levator scapulae	Loss of scapular elevation, adduction, downward rotation
C5-6	Suprascapular	Supraspinatus, infraspinatus	Weakened lateral rotation of humerus
C5-6	Subscapular	Subscapularis, teres major	Weakened internal rotation of humerus
C5-6	Axillary	Deltoid, teres minor	Loss of shoulder abduction, flexion and external rotation and extension
C5-7	Musculocutaneous	Biceps brachii, brachialis, coracobrachialis	Loss of forearm flexion and supination
C5-7	Long thoracic	Serratus anterior	Winging of the scapula
C6-8	Thoracodorsal	Latissimus dorsi	Loss of arm adduction and shoulder extension
C6-8, T1	Radial	All extensors of arm, wrist, fingers, thumb, abductor pollicis longus, supinator, brachioradialis	Wrist drop, extensor paralysis, inability to supinate
C6-8, T1	Median	Flexors of wrist, hand, and digits; forearm pronators; opponens pollicis; abductor pollicis brevis; flexor pollicis brevis; first and second lumbricales	"Ape-hand" deformity, weakened grip, thenar atrophy, unopposed thumb
C8-T1	Ulnar	Supplies muscles on ulnar side of forearm and hand; adductor pollicis, abductor digiti minimi, opponens digiti minimi, flexor digiti minimi brevis, flexor digitorum profundus (digits 4, 5), third and fourth lumbricales, flexor carpi ulnaris, palmaris brevis, dorsal and palmar interossei, flexor pollicis brevis (deep head)	"Claw-hand" deformity, also known as an *intrinsic minus hand deformity*, interosseus atrophy, loss of thumb adduction

From Hislop HJ, Montgomery J: *Daniels and Worthingham's muscle testing: techniques of manual examination*, ed 6, Philadelphia, 1995, WB Saunders.

Extensive peripheral nerve damage may produce deformity if contractures, joint stiffness, and poor positioning are allowed to occur. Disfigurement of the hands is particularly noticeable and may produce psychological distress. Other complications may include osteoporosis of bone and epidermal fibrosis of the joints. See Table 37-4 for descriptions of clinical manifestations of peripheral nerve lesions of the brachial plexus.

Axillary Nerve Injury

The axillary nerve is composed of the C5-C6 spinal nerves and arises from the upper trunk of the brachial plexus. The motor branches of the axillary nerve innervate the deltoid muscle and the teres minor muscle (see Table 37-4).[21] The axillary nerve is "the most commonly injured nerve in the shoulder, and the most common cause of injury is anterior dislocation of the shoulder or fracture of the neck of the humerus."[27] Nerve damage may occur as a result of the actual dislocation or of the reduction; other causes include compression (e.g., crutches) or trauma (e.g., blunt or lacerating wounds). As a result, the client has weakness or paralysis of the deltoid muscle, which causes limitations in shoulder flexion, abduction, extension, and weakness in lateral rotation of the arm. In addition to the loss of muscle power, atrophy of the deltoid muscle produces asymmetry of the shoulders, which may cause issues with body image.[27]

See Table 37-1 for OT assessments. ROM assessment and MMT, as well as clinical observation of the client's ability to use the arm functionally, are critical.

Interventions for axillary nerve injury require that the shoulder dislocation be reduced and that the arm be supported for a brief time in a sling. When the physician prescribes OT for rehabilitation of shoulder function, interventions include passive and active ROM of shoulder flexion and extension and shoulder abduction and adduction exercises while the client is supine or lying on the noninjured side to minimize gravity (Table 37-5). Functional movements are graded as the muscles become stronger.

Brachial Plexus Injuries

The nerve roots that innervate the upper extremity originate in the anterior rami between the C5, C6, C7, C8, and T1

TABLE 37-5 **Occupational Therapy Interventions for Peripheral Nerve Injuries**

Nerve Injury	Intervention	Example of Activities
Axillary nerve	Passive ROM to prevent deformity and improve circulation; necessary to protect teres minor and deltoid muscles from stretch during the passive ROM activities	Passive ROM performed two or three times daily while client is supine or lying on uninjured side to minimize effects of gravity; family or caregiver instructed in techniques; client instructed in self-ranging techniques performed on a daily basis
	Adaptive equipment	Instruction in use of long-handled assistive devices to compensate for upper extremity abduction deficit
	Joint protection	Instruction in joint protection to allow nerve time to heal and to prevent further injury; instruction in adaptive equipment, as needed for activities of daily living and leisure, work and play occupations
	EMG biofeedback	Biofeedback potentially beneficial in providing the client with visual and auditory incentives during muscle reeducation sessions
	Retrograde massage	Use of retrograde massage if edema occurs in hand or arm; client, family, or caregivers instructed in technique to be performed several times per day
	Graded activities	Shoulder movement critical to recovery; incorporation of long, sweeping shoulder movements in the client's meaningful activities; graded from horizontal to vertical.
Brachial plexus	Passive ROM to maintain joint flexibility	Passive ROM performed while supine twice daily, with emphasis on shoulder flexion, abduction, and external rotation; family or caregiver instructed in techniques
	Tactile stimulation to upper extremity to increase awareness	Massage, vibration, application of various textures to the arm
	Proprioceptive stimulation to upper extremity	Joint approximation through progressive weight bearing to increase awareness; always necessary to ensure proper alignment of joints
	Bilateral integration to improve body scheme	Use of developmentally appropriate bilateral activities (e.g., toys, crafts, or activity that requires two hands)
	Pool therapy	Therapeutic exercises with gravity minimized in water; swimming or weight lifting possible as client's strength improves
	Electrical stimulation	As prescribed by physician after EMG
	Slings	For damage to C5 and C6, sling fabricated to fit around humerus to support arm and allow hand to engage in occupations; especially important if arm is flaccid and the individual is able to walk—prevents further traction injury to nerves
	Splints	Resting splint for flaccid hand/wrist seen with damage to C8 and T1 to maintain part in functional position and prevent contractures; other splints available or fabricated for specific joints; air splints sometimes used to provide stability in elbow extension to bear weight with damage to C7
	Retrograde massage	For edema in hand or arm; client, family, or caregivers instructed in technique to be performed several times per day
Long thoracic nerve	Shoulder stabilized to limit scapular motion while nerve heals	After medical treatment, encouragement of maximal functional independence during activities and education in use of long-handled devices to compensate for shoulder limitations
	If nerve regeneration is not complete, possible consideration of surgery to relieve the excessive mobility of the scapula	
	Retrograde massage	For edema in hand or arm; client, family, or caregivers instructed in technique to be performed several times per day

ROM: Range of motion.
Data from Storment M: *Margaret Storment's guidelines for therapists: treating children with brachial plexus injuries.* Retrieved on August 25, 2005, from www.ubpn.org/awareness/A2002storment.

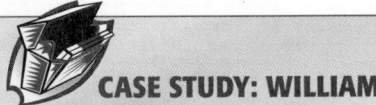

CASE STUDY: WILLIAM

William, a 60-year-old husband and teacher, was in a car accident that dislocated his right dominant shoulder. He was taken to the emergency room, given a sling, and sent home. Over the next few days, he noticed that he could neither flex nor abduct his humerus more than approximately 45 degrees. His physician reviewed his X-rays, repositioned the humerus, and diagnosed axillary nerve injury. Once the glenohumeral joint was stable, she prescribed occupational therapy to recover arm function.

During his therapy sessions, Marla, his occupational therapist, instructed William and his wife about joint protection, range of motion (ROM) exercises, and use of a reacher. As William's strength improved, Marla explored meaningful activities with him. After he enthusiastically mentioned a map project illustrating the places where he and his family had traveled, the two of them worked together to mount the map on poster board. Marla graded the activity and encouraged William to use long, sweeping movements of his right shoulder in flexion/extension and abduction/adduction when spreading the glue. William then sanded the frame and painted it, again using gliding shoulder movements. His home program also included smooth, gliding shoulder movements (e.g., wiping the counters, which his wife happily endorsed).

Analysis

Injury to the axillary nerve is one of the most common peripheral nerve injuries. Once the dislocation of the humerus has been reduced and the nerve begins to regenerate, rehabilitation of function may be possible. In this case, the occupational therapist was able to identify an activity that related to William's role as husband and home project enthusiast. This meaningful occupation caught his attention and engaged him in participation to accomplish the task.

spinal segments. This network of peripheral nerves is collectively called the **brachial plexus.** This important nerve complex can be palpated just behind the posterior border of the sternocleidomastoid as the head and neck are tilted to the opposite side.[17]

Most brachial plexus injuries are typically unilateral and occur during birth.[32] Obstetrical brachial plexus injury occurs if the baby's shoulders become impacted, which causes the brachial plexus nerves to stretch or tear. For example, if the infant's shoulder is stuck in the birth canal and the head is pulled, the neck is stretched, which can subsequently stretch or tear the brachial plexus. In adults, traumatic brachial plexus injuries are caused by damage to the nerve roots through a variety of causes (e.g., car or motorcycle accidents, sports misadventures, falls, blows to the neck with blunt or sharp objects, radiotherapy). The two types of brachial plexus lesions are Erb-Duchenne syndrome and

Klumpke's (Dejerine-Klumpke) syndrome.[17,27,41] These disorders are also referred to as *Erb's palsy* and *Klumpke's palsy*.

Erb-Duchenne syndrome is seen with lesions to the upper trunk of the brachial plexus, which consists of C5 and C6 nerve fibers. The incidence among newborns is 2 to 5 per 1000 births with 80% to 90% full recovery within 3 to 24 months.[48] The incidence among adults is not known. Typically, the muscles of the shoulder and elbow are affected and hand movement is retained. Paralysis and atrophy occur in the deltoid, brachialis, biceps, and brachioradialis muscles (see Table 37-4). Upon observation, the arm hangs limp in internal rotation and adduction. The elbow is extended, the forearm pronated, and the wrist flexed, resulting in the "waiter's tip position." Even though hand muscles are unaffected, functional movement of the upper extremity is extremely limited.[17,27,48]

Klumpke's syndrome results from compression or traction to the lower trunk of the brachial plexus (comprising nerves arising from C8 and T1) and is seen less often than Erb-Duchenne syndrome. Traction during birth or later in life that is caused by a strong upward pull on the upper extremity when it is in an abducted position can result in this disorder. The involved nerves innervate muscles whose actions are wrist and finger flexion and abduction and adduction of the fingers (see Table 37-4). Consequently, paralysis to the distal musculature of the wrist flexors and the intrinsic muscles of the hand results in a "claw-hand deformity," also referred to as an *intrinsic minus hand deformity* (Figure 37-2).[17,27,48]

See Table 37-1 for OT assessments.

OT interventions initially involve partial immobilization and positioning. Passive ROM is critical in maintaining joint flexibility, and the client's family or caregiver should be taught to perform these exercises with the client two or three times daily. Intervention includes a variety of tactile and proprioceptive sensory input to increase sensory awareness. Preventing contractures is critical to a functional outcome. For individuals with Erb-Duchenne syndrome, performance

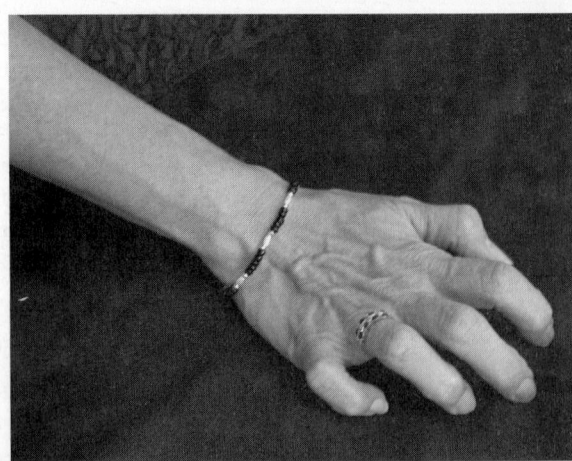

Figure 37-2   Klumpke's syndrome: paralysis to the distal musculature of the wrist flexors and the intrinsic muscles of the hand that results in a "claw-hand deformity" or intrinsic minus hand.

of passive and active assistive exercises and fabrication of a sling that fits around the humerus to support the arm are important. If strength improves, resistive exercises and activities can be implemented and the sling may be removed or used intermittently when walking to support the shoulder.[41,48] For those with Klumpke's syndrome, a short opponens hand splint that supports the thumb in opposition is often used. It is important to provide occupations that are appropriate to developmental ages and stages and that appeal to the client and encourage active use of the extremity in bilateral activities. Surgery to improve nerve growth and upper extremity function may be recommended if improvement is not spontaneously observed within a few months.[41,48] Other interventions are described in Table 37-5.

Long Thoracic Nerve Injury

The long thoracic nerve, arising from C5-C7 nerve roots, innervates the serratus anterior muscle, which anchors the apex of the scapula to the posterior of the rib cage. The serratus anterior's action is scapular abduction and upward rotation (see Table 37-4).[21] Although injury to this nerve is not common, the nerve can be injured in a number of ways: carrying heavy weights on the shoulder (e.g., backpacks), blows to the neck, compression caused by prolonged lying on the lateral trunk, and wounds. The resulting clinical picture involves winging of the scapula, difficulty flexing the outstretched arm above shoulder level, and difficulty protracting the shoulder or performing scapula abduction and adduction.[17,27] Asking the client to perform a wall pushup is commonly used as a screening assessment technique. If the long thoracic nerve is impaired, the scapula on that side will elevate and move medially, with the inferior angle rotating medially to produce a winging of the scapula.[27] Other OT assessments are described in Table 37-1.

Lesions of the radial, median, and ulnar nerves and cumulative trauma disorders affecting the hand are discussed in Chapter 39.

Psychosocial Interventions for Peripheral Nerve Injuries

Brachial plexus, thoracic, and axillary nerve injuries are life changing, affecting the psychological and emotional states of clients and their families and friends. Clients often experience depression, which may be a reaction to the traumatic event that caused the injury or may become chronic and serious. Occupational therapists can be helpful in this regard by discovering activities that are meaningful to the client and adapting them for success. The client's self-image is challenged and may require revision to accommodate the client's changed health status. For example, if the deltoid muscle has atrophied, a foam or thermoplastic pad can be worn under clothing to round out the shoulders. Use of these aesthetic pads may increase the client's willingness to venture out into society. Referrals to support groups or a psychologist also may help clients adjust to a changed appearance.[38,51]

Participation in leisure occupations has been found to help people with physical disabilities redefine themselves (see Chapter 18), and occupational therapists should consider leisure as an important area of occupation to include in an intervention plan.[2]

NUEROMUSCULAR DISORDERS

NEUROMUSCULAR JUNCTION: MYASTHENIA GRAVIS

Myasthenia gravis (MG) is the most common chronic disease involving a disorder of chemical transmission at the nerve-muscle synapse, or neuromuscular junction. The term *myasthenia gravis* is derived from Greek and Latin and means "grave muscle weakness."[54] It is caused by an autoimmune response in which antibodies are produced that block, alter, or destroy the nicotinic acetylcholine receptors on the postsynaptic membrane and interfere with synaptic transmission at the nerve-muscle junction. Because neurotransmission is defective, skeletal (voluntary) muscles, typically the cranial muscles, become weak and easily fatigued. The incidence of MG in the United States is approximately 14 in a population of 100,000, but it may be underdiagnosed, especially among very old persons. The latest statistics show that with the aging of the population, males are diagnosed more often than women, with symptoms beginning after 50 years of age.[3,23,42,49,50]

Most clients diagnosed with MG initially experience symptoms in the oculomotor muscles that cause eyelid drooping, referred to as *ptosis*, and double vision, referred to as *diplopia*. Oropharyngeal muscle weakness, which results in difficulty in chewing, swallowing, and speaking, is seen in some clients. Weakness of limb musculature is not typically an initial symptom. People with MG tend to be stronger in the morning, but their strength and endurance decrease as the day progresses and muscles fatigue. Therefore, the client may experience increased double vision, severe drooping of the eyelids, difficulty with speech or swallowing, and fatigue with repetitive activity as muscles tire (Table 37-6).

Most clients with MG have abnormalities of the thymus glands, and some have thymic tumors. Removal of the thymus gland (thymectomy) is standard therapy for most clients, but response time for symptom reduction varies with individuals and may take between 2 and 5 years after surgery. Clients without thymomas have a better response to surgery than those with a tumor. Clients are also treated with corticosteroids (prednisone) and immunosuppressive and cholinesterase-inhibiting drugs.[42] High-dose intravenous immune globulin has been reported to decrease symptoms in 50% to 100% of clients for a period of weeks to months. For clients with symptoms that suddenly worsen, those about to have surgery, or those who have not responded well to other interventions, plasma exchange is used as a short-term treatment. Nearly all people with MG improve for weeks to months after plasma exchange.[23,50]

TABLE **37-6** **Myasthenia Gravis: Initial Symptoms, Description, and Percentage of Clients with Symptoms**

Initial Symptoms	Description	Approximate Percentage of Clients with Initial Symptoms
Oculomotor dysfunction	Severe drooping of eyelids (ptosis), double vision (diplopia), inability to move eyes in certain directions	70%
Otopharyngeal muscle weakness	Difficulty in chewing, swallowing, speaking; in severe cases, problems breathing and coughing resulting in aspiration	20%
Limb weakness	May be limited to specific muscles or may progess to generalized fatigue	10%

Data from Cabrera CS et al: Myasthenia gravis: the otolaryngologist's perspective, *Am J Otolaryngology* 23(3):169, 2002; Howard JF. *Myasthenia gravis: a summary.* Retrieved on July 22, 2005, from www.myasthenia.org/information/summary; Rowland LP: Diseases of chemical transmission at the nerve-muscle synapse: myasthenia gravis. In Kandel ER, Schwartz JH, Jessell TM, editors: *Principles of neural science*, ed 4, New York, 2000, McGraw-Hill; Kernich CA, Kaminski HJ: Myasthenia gravis: pathophysiology, diagnosis and collaborative care, *J Neuroscience Nurs* 27(4):207, 1995; Yee CA: Getting a grip on myasthenia gravis, *Nursing 2002* 32(1):1, 2002.

Most people with MG usually experience maximal weakness during the first year after diagnosis. The course of the disease fluctuates but is usually progressive. However, according to the Myasthenia Gravis Foundation of America (www.myasthenia.org), the current prognosis for most patients with this disease is good; most live normal or nearly normal lives. Remissions or a decrease in symptoms and an improvement in strength and function can last for years. However, emotional upset, extended exertion, infections, medications, thyroid conditions, elevated body temperature, or childbirth may induce exacerbations of unpredictable severity.[23] With modern diagnosis and treatment effectiveness, the mortality rate of MG is nearly zero.[49]

Role of the Occupational Therapist

Because similarities exist among the diagnoses of motor unit disorders, OT evaluation follows the same pattern with specific assessments selected according to the disorder (see Table 37-1). A significant area for assessment in MG is eating and swallowing because of the dangers of aspiration. Because some clients may experience difficulty with diaphragmatic and intercostal muscle strength, they may have trouble coughing to clear secretions. An occupational therapist with advanced training in dysphagia should assess and treat clients with severe eating and swallowing dysfunction (see Chapter 26).

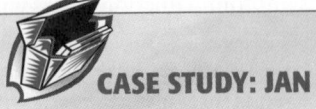

CASE STUDY: JAN

For several months, Jan, a 45-year-old photographer, had noticed unusual changes in her body. Her eyelids felt heavy, and her vision would blur when she was reading; it felt as if she was cross-eyed. Jan's speech became slurred if she was in a lengthy conversation. More recently, she had become aware that when she was drinking thin liquids, such as coffee, she would frequently choke. When she visited her doctor and received the results of medical tests, she was shocked to hear that she had an autoimmune disorder called *myasthenia gravis*. Jan's physician referred her to a surgeon for removal of her thymus gland, and she was given a prescription for prednisone.

Jeri, an occupational therapist trained in dysphagia, assessed Jan's swallowing abilities and recommended that thickening agents be added to liquids to decrease choking. As Jan improved, Jeri performed ongoing swallowing assessments and was able to gradually add thinner liquids so that Jan could again enjoy coffee. Jan reports that the most important thing that anyone did for her was when Jeri helped her enroll in a myasthenia gravis support group, where she experienced empathy, was given resources, and, to her surprise, found herself laughing again.

Analysis

People with myasthenia gravis can be helped through a variety of therapies to lead a near normal life. When a swallowing disorder is present, an occupational therapist with advanced training must perform a dysphagia assessment and make recommendations to prevent aspiration and pneumonia. A social support system is critical to the well-being and recovery of people with this disease.

Interventions for clients with MG depend on the results of the OT evaluation, which includes client and caregiver goals. The therapeutic program should not cause fatigue; therefore, the therapist must be aware of the client's medication regimen and ability to tolerate activity and the time of day that the client has the most energy. The client's muscle strength must be monitored on a regular basis, and the occupational therapist keeps a running record to document any important changes that must be reported to the medical team. Specific intervention protocols for MG are scarce, but a recent study described the ways in which subjects with MG self-managed fatigue. "Effective self-care actions include stress reduction techniques, pacing all activities, and increased rest and sleep."[15]

An important aspect of treatment is to educate the client and family members to use energy conservation and work simplification strategies when engaging in ADLs, IADLs, and leisure occupations (see Chapter 18). Adaptive and assistive devices may be introduced to decrease effort during daily activities. Because vision may be impaired, the occupational therapist should visit the client's home to assess architectural barriers, bathroom safety, and furniture arrangements; otherwise, the client might fall. If chewing and swallowing are problems, an eating program should be designed and monitored by an experienced occupational therapist (see Chapter 26).

Because of the client's facial appearance (e.g., drooping eyelids), fear of choking, or steroid-related changes in appearance, the psychosocial effects of MG may be distressing to clients and their family and friends. The therapist should always treat the client with empathy and encourage honest discussion. For general well-being, the client must be able to express his or her feelings about these physical changes.[38] The client and family members may also be referred to an MG support group, a psychologist, or both.

MYOPATHIC DISORDERS

MUSCULAR DYSTROPHIES

The muscular dystrophies are a group of genetic diseases. There are three major types of **muscular dystrophy** (MD): Duchenne, facioscapulohumeral, and myotonic (Table 37-7). A fourth group, limb-girdle MD, includes forms of inherited MD that do not fit into the three major types. The dystrophies have in common the progressive degenerations of muscle fibers while the neuronal innervation to muscle and sensation remains intact. As the number of muscle fibers declines, each axon innervates fewer and fewer of them, resulting in progressive weakness.[34]

Because this group of diseases is degenerative, the decline of muscle function cannot be prevented. As yet, there is no cure. Medical management is largely supportive, and rehabilitation measures are vital in delaying deformity and achieving maximal function within the limits of the disease and its debilitating effects. Gene therapy is being investigated but is not yet available.[41]

Role of the Occupational Therapist

The primary goal of OT is to help the client with MD maintain maximal independence as long as possible. Self-care activities and assistive devices that promote independence during home, school, leisure, and work activities are a vital part of the treatment program.[41] Leisure occupations need to be considered in a comprehensive OT intervention plan to ensure balance in all areas of the client's life. Play and laughter are particularly important to the health, well-being, and social adjustment of the growing youth (see Chapter 18).

A comprehensive team evaluation of the client's abilities and disabilities should be administered. The team includes the physician, occupational therapist, physical therapist, and psychologist. A social worker may advise the family on community resources. The occupational therapist assesses the client's functional status in ADLs and IADLs, ROM exercises, and muscle strength, as well as the fit and proper use of adaptive equipment, engagement in leisure activities, and emotional status. (See Table 37-1 for assessments.)

After the evaluation process is complete, an OT intervention plan is developed to address specific concerns. Active exercise

Table **37-7** **Major Types of Muscular Dystrophy**

Type	Description	Age of Onset and Progression
Duchenne	Affects boys only because it is inherited as an X-linked recessive trait Results from gene mutation that regulates the protein involved in maintenance of muscle integrity.	Onset age: 3-5 years—begins in muscles of pelvic girdle and legs. By 12 years unable to walk; uses wheelchair. Weakness spreads upwards to shoulder girdle and trunk. By 20 most need respirator to breathe with death usually occurring by age 30.
Fascioscapulohumeral	Affects both genders Autosomal dominant Affects primarily the muscles of the face and shoulder girdle (hence its name).	Onset age: Adolesence Slow progression of weakness resulting in a near normal life span
Myotonic	Affects both genders Causes weakness but also myotonia—prolonged muscle spasm or delayed muscle relaxation after vigorous contraction—especially in fingers and face. Floppy, high-stepping gait. Appearance of long face and drooping eyelids.	Onset age: Varies, often adult Involves cranial muscle and distal limb weakness rather than proximal May be mild or severe Associated symptoms progress to involve cardiac abnormalities, endocrine disturbances, cataracts, and in men, testicular atrophy and baldness
Limb-girdle (dystrophies that do not fit into the other types)	Affects both genders Families differ in extent of limb weakness and patterns of inheritance	Onset age: Varies

Source: National Institute of Neurological Disorder and Stroke: Muscular Dystrophy Information Page, 7/22/05; Rowland, Diseases of the motor unit, 2000.

may be helpful in maintaining strength, but overexertion and fatigue must be prevented. Because people with MD may experience cardiac complications, occupational therapists must be aware of the client's medical history and use exercise judiciously, observing cardiac precautions when necessary. Incorporating exercise into meaningful, age-related activities that are monitored by a therapist can promote engagement in participation. Parachute games, obstacle courses, and swimming may be implemented with frequent built-in rest breaks.[18]

Two recent pilot studies involving clients with MD and exercise show that improvements are possible; investigators recommend further research. Clients with myotonic dystrophy showed significant improvement in hand function and in self-rated occupational performance on the Canadian Occupational Performance Measure after a 3-month hand training OT intervention.[1] An experimental pilot study quantitatively evaluated that *qigong* may be used as an adjunct therapy program. Subjects with MD reported perceived maintenance of general health and positive coping when compared to the control group. The treatment group tended to "maintain balance function during training and performance of *qigong* whilst there was a decline when not training." The researchers concluded that *qigong* brought about a decreased rate of decline and is worthy of further study.[52]

Adaptive equipment and environmental modifications are often used as OT interventions. Instruction in work simplification and energy conservation, as well as in creative and effective strategies to perform ADLs, IADLs, and various other occupations, are important in the OT program.[18,41] A powered wheelchair, a wheelchair lap board, suspension slings, or mobile arms supports may be indicated to facilitate self-feeding, writing, reading, use of a computer, and table-top leisure activities when there is substantial shoulder girdle and upper limb weakness. Built-up utensils are helpful when grip strength declines. Home and workplace modifications will be necessary for most clients. Client and family education is an important part of a team rehabilitation program.[41] A supportive approach to the client and family is helpful as function declines and new mobility aids, assistive devices, and community resources become necessary.[18]

Wheelchair prescription and mobility training in either a manual or powered wheelchair are included in the OT intervention program. The wheelchair may require a special seating system or supports to minimize the development of scoliosis, hip and knee flexion contractures, and ankle plantar flexion deformity.[18,41] Powered wheelchairs are often recommended to conserve energy and decrease strain on shoulders and trunk. Instruction in methods to maneuver power chairs can cause overexertion, and this activity, like any other, must be graded for difficulty. A recent study found that young people (i.e., those between 7 and 22 years of age) diagnosed with either MD or cerebral palsy who were inexperienced powered wheelchair drivers significantly improved their wheelchair driving performance through the use of simulator training. The researchers concluded that this method of instruction conserved energy and was effective.[20]

Chronic pain in children, adolescents, and young adults (i.e., persons between 8 and 20 years of age) with physical disabilities has not been widely studied, but recent research indicates that chronic pain interferes with ADLs and IADLs in young people with MD, cerebral palsy, spinal cord injury, acquired and congenital limb deficiency, and spina bifida.[30] Pain appears to be more prevalent in female subjects than male subjects during the performance of daily routines, and it interfered most often with physical activities, as well as negatively affecting mood. McKearnan (2004) reports that the young people in this study frequently reported pain associated with physical therapy, OT, and therapeutic home programs. They also complained that the use of splints, orthotics, and prosthetics was sometimes painful. Therapists must be aware of their client's pain levels and modify activities, splints, and orthotics as needed. Helping clients with MD to manage pain will most likely lead to improved quality of life.

The sense of self is challenged as clients with MD realize that they will experience a progressive loss of bodily function. Occupational therapists must realize that these clients are constantly forced to redefine themselves as they go through life, making "continuous trade-offs as function is lost."[38] A critical element in OT intervention is to help client and family members find meaningful activities in which to participate either as individuals or as a family. For example, connecting with spiritual activities that engage clients and families on the deepest level could be critical to a sense of hope and well-being.[9] Alternatively, encouraging families to use humor and to play and laugh together can promote bonding, reduce fear and anxiety, and produce positive physical and emotional feelings (see Chapter 18).[5,11]

Psychosocial issues related to MD involve the whole family. Parents go through phases of shock, fear, and despair when the diagnosis is made and as the child ages and function decreases (e.g., when the wheelchair is prescribed). Encouraging parents not to be overprotective and to continue to promote their child's independence is an important aspect of therapy. Further, therapists can anticipate times in the growing child's life when psychosocial support will be most essential and can offer education and support during intervention sessions. Some potentially disturbing developmental milestones for the client and family occur when the child starts school (at approximately age 5), when the child loses the capacity for independent ambulation (at 8-12 years), when adolescent social life is limited, and, of course, when young adulthood arrives with the expectation that death is imminent.[18,41] Referral to a psychologist or family counselor, or spiritual advisor, during these times should be considered.

SUMMARY

The motor unit consists of the lower motor neuron, neuromuscular junction, and muscle. Some motor unit dysfunctions are reversible, and others are degenerative. The role of the occupational therapist is to assess functional capabilities in all occupational performance areas and contexts. ADLs and IADLs (including self-care, home management, mobility, and work-related tasks), energy conservation, work simplification, joint protection, spiritual approaches, and appropriate humor may be used to restore or maintain function. Proper positioning, exercise programs, and pain management techniques are used as indicated to facilitate recovery and increase functional capacity. Orthoses, assistive devices, communication aids, and mobility equipment and training in their use may be necessary. Psychosocial considerations and client and family education are important aspects of the OT program.

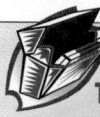

THREADED CASE STUDY: EDITH, PART 2

Return to the case study presented at the beginning of this chapter, and compare your answers with the ones given here.

What are the Phases of Guillain-Barré, and What Occupational Therapy Interventions Might be Used in Each Phase?

Cooke and Orb[10] define three phases of Guillain-Barré syndrome. The initial, or acute, phase begins with the client's first conclusive symptoms and lasts until there is no further decline in physical status. This phase may last from 1 to 3 weeks.[18] During this phase, Edith's condition progressed from generalized weakness to paralysis of her extremities and muscles of the trunk and diaphragm. She was completely dependent in activities of daily living and required a ventilator to breathe. Jen, the occupational therapist assigned to the intensive care unit, established four goals with Edith and her family.

Goal	Intervention
1. Maintain full range of motion (ROM) in all joints.	1. Perform passive ROM two times per day to all joints.
2. Prevent contractures.	2. Fabricate resting hand splints, and educate client, family, and nursing aides in proper ways to position Edith in bed.
3. Teach client and family about Guillain-Barré syndrome (GBS).	3. Provide and discuss with clients handouts, reading materials, and GBS Web sites.
4. Provide a strategy for Edith to listen to the Bible.	4. Instruct Edith in ways to use control switch with her tongue to turn CD player on and off.

Phase two, the plateau phase, began when Edith's physical status stabilized, with no further deterioration. She was transferred to a regular hospital unit. She was able to breathe on her own, speak softly, and sit up in bed in a semireclining position with pillows positioned for support. Some strength had returned to her proximal musculature, but her hands remained paralyzed and she fatigued easily. The plateau phase lasted a few weeks during which Edith's physical status remained unchanged. The goals for this phase were essentially the same as for the acute phase except that now Edith could choose to either read the Bible by turning the pages with a mouth stick or listen to the CD using the mouth stick to turn the player on and off. She could also control the television set with the mouth stick and was able to view her favorite shows. Family and friends were encouraged to visit but cautioned not to fatigue her.

The recovery phase began when Edith's strength and sensation began to return to her distal extremities. She was transferred to the rehabilitation unit. The occupational therapist, Lara, and Edith came up with four goals during the recovery phase. The use of adaptive equipment such as built-up handles, work simplification and energy conservation techniques (e.g., breaking the task down into steps and resting between steps), and the use of electric appliances were encouraged during activities. Edith practiced playing cards with other clients in a group environment. Lara set her up with a card holder and a battery-powered card shuffler when her hands were too weak to hold the cards, but Edith eventually was able to play independently. Edith went to the mall with her granddaughter and Lara. During the outing, Lara taught them, in the context of shopping, how to gauge fatigue and to rest for 5 or 10 minutes when feeling tired. She also served as a role model, pacing the activity by limiting the initial shopping trip to 30 minutes and encouraging gradual lengthening of the experience over time. Lara provided Edith with community resources to aid in her independence. For example, the Guillain-Barré Syndrome Foundation International (GBSFI) offers local support groups, literature, and conferences to all GBS survivors and caregivers. In addition, Edith's family received extensive training from the interdisciplinary team members to assist with carryover of learned strategies and equipment in the home and community. Driving was not addressed at an inpatient level, but Edith was referred to the OT driver training program, where she would be assessed when her strength returned.

In What Ways Were the Client's Psychosocial Needs Addressed During Recovery?

Edith's fears about being paralyzed were addressed in several ways. Edith and her family were taught about the disease and encouraged to have hope because most people with GBS recover well. Edith's spiritual needs were met by making it possible for her to continue her morning Bible routine; she initially used a tongue switch to turn a Bible CD on and off and then was able to use a mouth stick to

THREADED CASE STUDY: EDITH, PART 2–cont'd

turn pages until her hands recovered strength. Edith expressed a desire to be as independent as possible in activities of daily living, to cook for her family, and to enjoy family outings and card playing. These activities were all made possible through occupational therapy adaptive interventions. Her family members and friends were encouraged to visit, gradually increasing the length of time that they stayed.

Describe Energy Conservation Techniques that You Think Would Be Appropriate for Edith While Engaging in Her Valued Occupation of Cooking During the Recovery Phase.

First, Edith and Lara reviewed the recipe and listed the necessary items while seated at the kitchen table. Edith used a wheeled kitchen cart to gather items and carry them to the counter. Lara provided her with a reacher to obtain items on high shelves. When the items were assembled, Edith sat and rested on a bar stool near the counter while she and Lara reviewed the next step. Electric appliances were used to chop and stir the ingredients. Edith rested after this step. Lara showed Edith how to slide containers along the counter to the stove without lifting. They walked back to the table to play a game of cards while the meal cooked. When the food was cooked, Edith placed plates and utensils on the kitchen cart with the one-dish meal and wheeled the cart to the table to enjoy her meal.

Review Questions

1. Name the components of the motor unit and one disorder that may result in dysfunction for each component.
2. Describe Guillain-Barré syndrome and the occupational therapy interventions used for clients with this disorder.
3. Describe the symptoms of postpolio syndrome.
4. What are the elements of the occupational therapy program for the client with postpolio syndrome?
5. List at least six clinical manifestations of peripheral nerve injury.
6. Describe the occupational therapy treatment strategies, including any contraindications, for peripheral nerve injuries.
7. Describe a method of managing pain that may be used by an occupational therapist.
8. Discuss the clinical signs of myasthenia gravis.
9. Describe the role of occupational therapy for clients who have myasthenia gravis.
10. What is the primary treatment precaution in myasthenia gravis?
11. Name and differentiate the four types of muscular dystrophy.
12. What are the treatment goals for muscular dystrophy?
13. Discuss ways that occupational therapists address the psychosocial needs of clients with each of the motor unit disorders.

REFERENCES

1. Aldehag AS, Jonsson H, Ansved T: Effects of a hand training programme in five patients with myotonic dystrophy type 1, *Occup Ther International* 12(1):14, 2005.
2. American Occupational Therapy Association: Occupational therapy practice framework: domain and process, *Am J Occup Ther* 56:609, 2002.
3. Aragones JM et al: Myasthenis gravis: a higher than expected incidence in the elderly, *Neurology* 60(6):1024, 2003.
4. Barohn R, Gooch C: Guillain-Barré syndrome: clinical features, diagnosis, and therapeutic strategies, *Advances Immunotherapy* 11:3, 2004.
5. Berk L, Tan S, Fry W: Eustress of humor associated laughter modulates specific immune system components, *Annals Behavioral Med* 15:111, 1993.
6. Blaskey J et al: *Therapeutic management of patients with Guillain-Barré syndrome*, Downey, CA, 1989, Rancho Los Amigos National Rehabilitation Center.
7. Bradshaw DC, Keane GP: Management of chronic pain. In Sine R et al: *Basic rehabilitation techniques: a self-instructional guide*, ed 4, New York, 2000, Aspen.
8. Centers for Disease Control and Prevention: *Poliomyelitis*. Retrieved on July 22, 2005, from www.cdc.gov/doc.do/id/9099f3ec802286ba.
9. Christiansen C: Acknowledging a spiritual dimension in occupational therapy practice, *Am J Occup Ther* 3:169, 1997.
10. Cooke J, Orb A: The recovery phase in Guillain-Barré syndrome: moving from dependency to independence, *Rehabil Nursing* 28:105, 2003.
11. Cousins N: *Head first: the biology of hope*, New York, 1989, Penguin.
12. Dillard JN: *The chronic pain solution: your personal path to pain relief*, New York, 2002, Bantam.
13. Eisendrath S, Matthay M, Dunkel J: Guillain-Barré syndrome: psychosocial aspects of management, *Psychosomatics* 24:465, 1983.
14. Gawne A: Strategies for exercise prescription in post-polio patients. In Halstead L, Grimby G, editors: *Post-polio syndrome*, Philadelphia, 1995, Hanley & Belfus.
15. Grohar-Murray ME et al: Self-care actions to manage fatigue among myasthenia gravis clients, *J Neuroscience Nursing* 30(3):191, 1998.
16. Guillain-Barré Syndrome/Chronic Inflammatory Demyelinating Polyneuropathy Foundation International: *GBS: an overview*. Retrieved on August 6, 2005, from www.gbsfi.com/overview.html.
17. Gutman SA, Schonfeld AB: *Screening adult neurologic populations: a step-by-step instruction manual*, Bethesda, MD, 2003, American Occupational Therapy Association.
18. Hallum A: Neuromuscular diseases. In Umphred D, editor: *Neurological rehabilitation*, ed 4, St Louis, 2001, Mosby.
19. Halstead LS: Late complications of poliomyelitis. In Goodgold J, editor: *Rehabilitation medicine*, St Louis, 1988, Mosby.
20. Hasdai A, Jessel AS, Weiss PL: Use of a computer simulator for training children with disabilities in the operation of a powered wheelchair, *Am J Occup Ther* 52(3):215, 1998.

21. Hislop HJ, Montgomery J: *Daniels and Worthingham's muscle testing: techniques of manual examination*, ed 6, Philadelphia, 1995, WB Saunders.

22. Hollingsworth L, Didelot MJ, Levington C: Post-polio syndrome: psychological adjustment to disability, *Issues Ment Health Nurs* 23(2):135, 2002.

23. Howard JF: *Myasthenia gravis: a summary*. Retrieved on July 22, 2005, from www.myasthenia.org/information/summary.htm.

24. Keefe FJ: Cognitive behavioral therapy for managing pain, *Clin Psychologist* 49(3):4, 1996.

25. Kling C, Persson A, Gardulf A: The health-related quality of life of patients suffering from the late effects of polio (post-polio), *J Adv Nurs* 32(10):164, 2000.

26. Law M et al: *Canadian occupational performance measure*, ed 3, Toronto, 1999, Canadian Association of Occupational Therapy.

27. Magee DJ: *Orthopedic physical assessment*, ed 3, Philadelphia, 1997, WB Saunders.

28. Mandel DR et al: *Lifestyle redesign: implementing the well elderly program*, Bethesda, MD, 1999, American Occupational Therapy Association.

29. Mayo Clinic Medical Services, Brain and Nervous System Center: *Guillain-Barré syndrome*. Retrieved on August 6, 2005, from www.mayoclinic.com/health/guillain-barre-syndrome/DS00413.

30. McKearnan KA: *Chronic pain in youths with physical disabilities* (unpublished doctoral dissertation), University of Washington, 2004.

31. Meythaler J, DeVivo M, Braswell W: Rehabilitation outcomes of patients who have developed Guillain-Barré syndrome, *Am J Phys Med Rehabili* 14:411, 1997.

32. National Institute of Neurological Disorders and Stroke: *Brachial plexus injuries information page*, p. 1. Retrieved on August 28, 2005, from www.ninds.nih.gov/disorders/brachial_plexus/brachial_plexus.htm.

33. National Institute of Neurological Disorders and Stroke: *Guillain-Barré syndrome fact sheet*. Retrieved on August 6, 2005, from www.ninds.nih.gov/disorders/gbs/gbs.htm.

34. National Institute of Neurological Disorders and Stroke: *Muscular dystrophy information page*. Retrieved on July 22, 2005, from www.ninds.nih.gov/disorders/md/md.htm.

35. National Institute of Neurological Disorders and Stroke: *Peripheral neuropathy fact sheet*. Retrieved on August 14, 2005, from www.ninds.nih.gov/disorders/peripheralneuropathy/peripheralneuropathy.htm.

36. National Institute of Neurological Disorders and Stroke: *Post-polio syndrome information page*, p. 1. Retrieved on July 14, 2005, from www.ninds.nih.gov/disorders/post_polio/post_polio.htm.

37. Netter FH: *The CIBA collection of medical illustrations*. Vol 1: *Nervous system*, West Caldwell, NJ, 1986, CIBA.

38. Pendleton HM, Schultz-Krohn W: Psychosocial issues in physical disability. In Cara E, MacRae A, editors: *Psychosocial occupational therapy: a clinical practice*, ed 2, Clifton Park, NY, 2005, Thomson Delmar Learning.

39. Postpolio Health International: *Information about the late effects of polio*. Retrieved on July 14, 2005, from www.post-polio.org/ipn/aboutlep.html.

40. Postpolio Institute. Retrieved on July 14, 2005, from www.englewoodhospital.com/PostPolio_old/PostPolio_at_EHMC3.

41. Rogers SL: Common conditions that influence children's participation. In Case-Smith J, editor: *Occupational therapy for children*, ed 5, St Louis, 2005, Mosby.

42. Rowland LP: Diseases of chemical transmission at the nerve-muscle synapse: myasthenia gravis. In Kandel ER, Schwartz JH, Jessell TM, editors: *Principles of neural science*, ed 4, New York, 2000, McGraw-Hill.

43. Rowland LP: Diseases of the motor unit. In Kandel ER, Schwartz JH, Jessell TM, editors: *Principles of neural science*, ed 4, New York, 2000, McGraw-Hill.

44. Schmidt A: *How do people with Guillain-Barré syndrome (GBS) participate in daily life: a pilot study* (unpublished master's thesis project), San Jose State University, San Jose, CA, 2004.

45. Smith LK, Kelly C: The postpolio syndrome. In Umphred D, editor: *Neurological rehabilitation*, ed 4, St Louis, 2001, Mosby.

46. Southam M: Psychosocial aspects of chronic pain. In Cara E, MacRae A, editors: *Psychosocial occupational therapy: a clinical practice*, ed 2, Clifton Park, NY, 2005, Thomson Delmar Learning.

47. Stewart D et al: The effectiveness of cognitive-behavioral interventions with people with chronic pain: an example of a critical review of the literature. In Law M, editor: *Evidence-based rehabilitation: a guide to practice*, Thorofare, NJ, 2002, Slack.

48. Storment M: *Margaret Storment's guidelines for therapists: treating children with brachial plexus injuries*. Retrieved on August 25, 2005, from www.ubpn.org/awareness/A2002storment.html.

49. Thanvi BR, Lo TC: Update on myasthenia gravis, *Postgrad Med J* 80(950):690, 2004.

50. Tierney LM, McPhee SJ, Papadakis MA: *Current medical diagnosis and treatment*, ed 33, Norwalk, CN, 1994, Appleton & Lange.

51. United Brachial Plexus Network: Brachial plexus injury awareness: information for adults with brachial plexus injuries. Retrieved on August 27, 2005, from http://www.ubpn.org/awareness/A2002adultinfo.html.

52. Wenneberg S, Gunnarsson LG, Ahlstrom G: Using a novel exercise programme for patients with muscular dystrophy. Part II: A quantitative study. *Disabil Rehabil* 26(10):595, 2004.

53. Yarnell SK: The late effects of polio. In Sine R et al, editors: *Basic rehabilitation techniques: a self-instructional guide*, ed 4, New York, 2000, Aspen.

54. Yee CA: Getting a grip on myasthenia gravis, *Nursing 2002* 32(1):1, 2002.

55. Young G: Energy conservation, occupational therapy, and the treatment of postpolio sequelae, *Orthopedics* 14:1233, 1991.

56. Young G: Occupational therapy and the postpolio syndrome, *Am J Occup Ther* 43(2):97, 1989.

57. Young G: Treating post-polio syndrome, *OT Practice* 6(21):10, 2001.

RESOURCES

Ways of Coping Scale
Available at Mind Garden Inc.
1690 Woodside Rd., Suite 202
Redwood City, CA 94961
www.mindgarden.com

38 ARTHRITIS

LISA DESHAIES

KEY TERMS

Arthritis
Osteoarthritis
Systemic
Crepitus

Gelling
Rheumatoid arthritis
Synovitis

Flare
Nodules
Tenosynovitis

Joint laxity
Nodes
Subluxation

LEARNING OBJECTIVES

After studying this chapter the student or practitioner will be able to do the following:

1. Understand the distinct disease processes of osteoarthritis and rheumatoid arthritis.
2. Describe common symptom similarities and differences of osteoarthritis and rheumatoid arthritis.
3. Identify joint changes and hand deformities commonly seen in osteoarthritis and rheumatoid arthritis.
4. Recognize medications commonly used in the treatment of arthritis and their side effects.
5. Understand the physical and psychosocial effects of arthritis and their impact on occupational functioning.

6. Identify important areas to evaluate in clients with arthritis.
7. Identify intervention objectives of occupational therapy for clients with arthritis.
8. Design an appropriate individualized intervention plan based on diagnosis, stage of disease, functional activity limitations, and client goals and lifestyle.
9. Identify key resources helpful to persons with arthritis and to healthcare providers.
10. Identify evaluation and treatment precautions related to arthritis.

CHAPTER OUTLINE

Overview of rheumatic diseases
Osteoarthritis
  Clinical features
  Diagnostic criteria
  Medical management
  Surgical management
Rheumatoid arthritis
  Clinical features
  Diagnostic criteria
  Medical management
  Surgical management
Occupational therapy evaluation
  Client history
  Occupational profile
  Occupational performance status

Cognitive, psychological, and social status
  Clinical status
Goal setting
Intervention objectives and planning
Occupational therapy intervention
  Rest
  Physical agent modalities
  Therapeutic exercise
  Therapeutic activity
  Splinting
Occupational performance training
  Assistive devices
  Client and family education
Summary

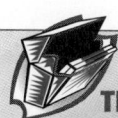

THREADED CASE STUDY: NINA, PART 1

Nina is a 52-year-old woman with a 4-year history of rheumatoid arthritis. She lives with her husband in a large two-story home. Her primary roles are managing her household and caring for her two grandchildren (ages 7 and 9) after school. Additionally, she is self-employed as an accountant who contracts her services to three small companies in nearby cities. Nina values being active and productive. Her part-time job serves as both a source of enjoyment and needed household income. In her leisure time, she participates in church activities and attends her grandchildren's school and sporting events.

Nina was referred to outpatient occupational therapy after an exacerbation of her arthritis that resulted in increased pain, fatigue, and difficulty engaging in many important daily occupations. On initial evaluation, Nina identifies her primary concerns as maximizing her functional level and reducing her pain so that she can resume her full participation in work, house cleaning, and child care. Clinical examination reveals pain and active range of motion limitations in all upper extremity joints, especially her wrists and fingers. Mild synovitis is present at her wrist and metacarpophalangeal joints, but no other joint changes are noted. Pain and stiffness are interfering with daytime activities and are also making sleep difficult. Her energy level is significantly decreased, and she reports feeling tired all the time. Although she still manages to watch her grandchildren for 2 hours each afternoon, she is unable to care for her house to her liking and is able to work only half of her usual 20 hours a week; she is fearful of losing her contracts.

Critical Thinking Questions

1. What evaluation components would you choose to assess regarding Nina's prior and current clinical and functional status?
2. Which aspects of the disease process are most problematic, and what are the major performance skills, performance patterns, contexts, activity demands, and client factors influencing Nina's ability to engage in her employment and other areas of occupation?
3. What interventions would you use to help Nina reach her goal of being able to continue working?

OVERVIEW OF RHEUMATIC DISEASES

The term **arthritis** is of Greek derivation and literally means "joint inflammation." It is used to describe many different conditions that fall under the larger umbrella of rheumatic diseases. Rheumatic diseases encompass more than 100 conditions characterized by chronic pain and progressive physical impairment of joints and soft tissues (e.g., skin, muscles, ligaments, tendons). These include osteoarthritis, rheumatoid arthritis, systemic lupus erythematosus, ankylosing spondylitis, scleroderma, gout, and fibromyalgia.[17,40] Almost one third of adults in the United States have signs and symptoms of arthritis, and these have been reported to be the main reason that adults over the age of 65 visit a physician.[40,53] Rheumatic diseases are a leading cause of disability, with significant economic, social, and psychological impacts.[17,21] In the late 1990s, approximately 43 million Americans were affected by arthritis and other rheumatic conditions, with 7 million experiencing limitations in their ability to participate in daily activities such as work, school, and housekeeping. As the population continues to age, the prevalence of arthritis-related conditions is expected to increase to an estimated 60 million by the year 2020, causing disability for 11.6 million.[17,20]

Occupational therapists are likely to encounter clients with rheumatic diseases in their practice settings, whether the condition manifests as a primary or a secondary type. To recognize problem areas and plan effective intervention strategies, the occupational therapist should know the unique features of each disease, its underlying pathology, and its typical clinical presentations; the therapist should also be familiar with commonly prescribed medications and their adverse reactions. Given the scope and intended purpose of this book, it is neither appropriate nor possible to adequately describe every rheumatic disease. Therefore, this chapter focuses on two of the most prevalent diseases: osteoarthritis and rheumatoid arthritis. With an understanding of the noninflammatory and inflammatory disease processes that they represent, the therapist can apply many of the evaluation and intervention principles to other rheumatic conditions. Table 38-1 provides a quick summary of the contrasting features of osteoarthritis and rheumatoid arthritis.[2,3,4,8,35,36,58]

OSTEOARTHRITIS

Osteoarthritis (OA), also referred to as *degenerative joint disease (DJD)*, is the most common rheumatic disease, affecting approximately 21 million people in the United States.[3,17,53] It ranks third among health problems in the developed world.[13,51] Its prevalence strongly correlates with age. In fact, evidence of characteristic cartilage damage is almost universal in persons over 65 years of age.[13] Before the age of 50, men are more likely to have OA; over the age of 50, women predominate.[8] In addition to age and gender, risk factors include heredity, obesity, anatomical joint abnormality, injury, and occupation leading to overuse of joints.[8] It is interesting to note that because rheumatoid arthritis may cause malalignment or instability of joints, it often results in premature OA.[22]

OA is classified as primary or secondary. Primary OA has no known cause and may be localized (i.e., involvement of one or two joints) or generalized (i.e., diffuse involvement generally including three or more joints). Secondary OA can

TABLE 38-1   **Primary Features of Osteoarthritis and Rheumatoid Arthritis**

	Osteoarthritis	Rheumatoid Arthritis
Prevalence	Affects 21 million Americans	Affects 2.1 million Americans
Peak incidence	Increases with age, <50 years old more common in males and >50 years old more common in females	Ages 40-60, 3:1 female-to-male ratio
Onset	Usually develops slowly, over years	Usually develops suddenly, within weeks or months
Systemic features	None	Fever, fatigue, malaise, extraarticular manifestations
Disease process	Noninflammatory, characterized by cartilage destruction	Inflammatory, characterized by synovitis
Joint involvement	Individual	Polyarticular, symmetrical
Joints commonly affected	Neck, spine, hips, knees, MTPs, DIPs, PIPs, thumb CMCs	Neck, jaw, hips, knees, ankles, MTPs, shoulders, elbows, wrists, PIPs, MPs, thumb joints
Morning stiffness	<30 minutes	At least 1 hour, often >2 hours

MTP = metatarsophalangeal, DIP = distal interphalangeal, PIP = proximal interphalangeal, CMC = carpometacarpal

be related to an identifiable cause, such as trauma, anatomical abnormalities, infection, or aseptic necrosis.[13]

OA is a disease that causes the breakdown of cartilage in joints, leading to joint pain and stiffness. Unlike rheumatoid arthritis, which is **systemic** (affecting the entire body), OA limits its attack to individual joints. Also in contrast to rheumatoid arthritis, the basic process of OA is noninflammatory, although secondary inflammation caused by joint damage is quite common. Once considered simply "wear and tear" arthritis, OA is now considered to involve more than just the passive deterioration of cartilage. The agent that initiates OA is not well understood, but it is known to involve a complex dynamic process of biomechanical, biochemical, and cellular events.[58] These are affected by local, systemic, genetic, environmental, and mechanical factors, which directly or indirectly influence cartilage vulnerability.[8] It is, in essence, the "final common pathway" for a variety of conditions.[13]

A healthy joint is lined by articular cartilage that is relatively thin, highly durable, and designed to distribute loads and limit stress on subchondral bone (Figure 38-1).[13] OA destabilizes the normal balance of degradation and synthesis of articular cartilage and subchondral bone and involves all of the tissues of a diarthrodial (i.e., synovial-lined) joint.[8,13] OA is basically a two-part process: deterioration of articular cartilage and reactive new bone formation.[66] This breakdown of joint tissue occurs in several stages. First, the smooth cartilage softens and loses its elasticity, which makes it more susceptible to further damage. Eventually, large sections of the cartilage wear away completely, causing reduced joint space and painful bone-on-bone contact. The ends of the bone thicken, osteophytes (bony growths) are formed where the ligaments and capsule attach to the bone, and the joint may lose its normal shape (Figure 38-2). Fluid-filled cysts may form in the bone near the joint, and bone or cartilage particles may float loose in the joint space.[3,65]

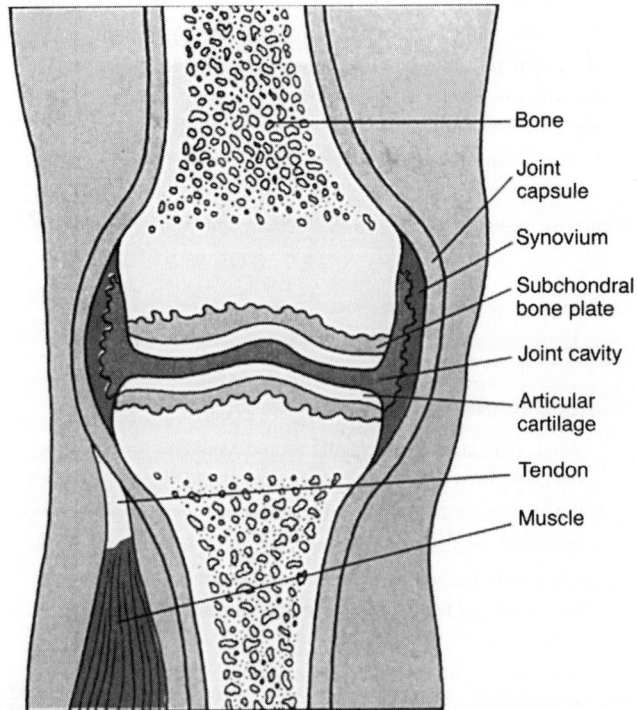

— Bone

Joint capsule

Synovium

Subchondral bone plate

Joint cavity

Articular cartilage

Tendon

Muscle

Figure 38-1   Normal joint structures. (From Ignatavicius DD, Bayne MV: *Medical-surgical nursing: a nursing process approach*, p. 720, Philadelphia, 1991, WB Saunders.)

CLINICAL FEATURES

OA is characterized by joint pain, stiffness, tenderness, limited movement, variable degrees of local inflammation, and **crepitus** (an audible or palpable crunching or popping in the joint caused by the irregularity of opposing cartilage surfaces).[47] It can affect axial and peripheral joints. The most common joints are distal interphalangeal (DIP), proximal interphalangeal (PIP), and first carpometacarpal (CMC) joints

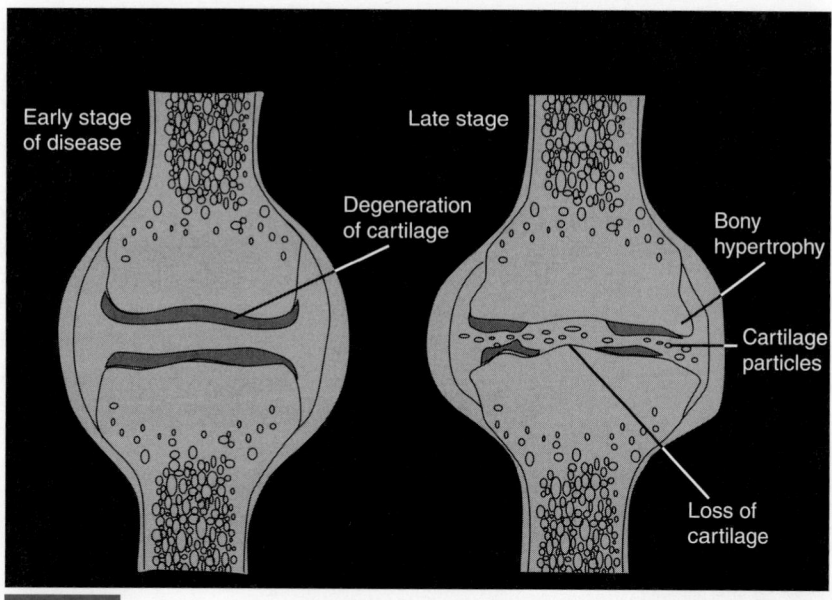

Figure 38-2   Joint changes in osteoarthritis. (From ARHP Arthritis Teaching Slide Collection, American College of Rheumatology.)

of the hand; cervical and lumbar apophyseal joints; first metatarsophalangeal (MTP) joints of the feet; and knees and hips.[4] Symptoms are usually gradual and may begin as a minor ache with motion. Pain and stiffness typically occur with activity and are relieved by rest but eventually become present at rest and at night. Morning stiffness (lasting less than 30 minutes) and stiffness after periods of inactivity (known as **gelling**) may develop. With advanced disease, patients may complain of the "bony" appearance of their joint, which is a result of osteophyte formation and possibly muscle atrophy.[58]

DIAGNOSTIC CRITERIA

The diagnosis of OA is initially made on the basis of patient history and physical examination, with a lack of systemic symptoms ruling out inflammatory disorders such as rheumatoid arthritis. The clinical diagnosis is typically confirmed with radiographs of the affected joint, which will show osteophyte formation at the joint margin, asymmetrical joint space narrowing, and subchondral bone sclerosis.[47] Magnetic resonance imaging (MRI) may be used to improve diagnostic imaging; MRI is able to more sensitively detect cartilage loss, osteophytes, and subchondral cysts.[19] The American College of Rheumatology Classification Criteria for Osteoarthritis of the Hand are listed in Box 38-1.

MEDICAL MANAGEMENT

OA currently has no cure. The goals in the treatment of OA are to relieve symptoms, improve function, limit disability, and avoid drug toxicity.[19,58] Pharmacological treatment

---

Box 38-1 | AMERICAN COLLEGE OF RHEUMATOLOGY CLASSIFICATION CRITERIA FOR OSTEOARTHRITIS OF THE HAND

Hand pain, aching, or stiffness and three or four of the following features:
- Hard tissue enlargement of two or more of 10 selected joints*
- Hard tissue enlargement of two or more DIP joints
- Fewer than three swollen MP joints
- Deformity of at least one of 10 selected joints

*The 10 selected joints are the second and third DIP, the second and third PIP, and the first CPC joints of both hands. This classification method yields a sensitivity of 94% and a specificity of 87%.
From Altman R, et al: The American College of Rheumatology criteria for the classification and reporting of osteoarthritis of the hand, *Arthritis Rheum* 33:1601, 1990.

may be systemic or local. Commonly prescribed systemic medications include analgesic agents and anti-inflammatory agents (Table 38-2).[29] Analgesic agents provide relief to painful joints and may be non-narcotic or narcotic for advanced and severe OA that fails to respond to other measures. Anti-inflammatory agents provide pain relief, with the added benefit of decreasing local joint inflammation. Because of the risk of gastrointestinal and renal toxicity, these drugs are typically used when analgesics are ineffective. Nonsteroidal anti-inflammatory drugs (NSAIDs) and Cox-2 inhibitors fall into this category. Although proven effective in treating OA, NSAIDs must be chosen and monitored carefully to minimize potentially serious side effects. Newer Cox-2 inhibitors are thought to provide clinical benefits similar

TABLE 38-2 Common Arthritis Medications and Side Effects

Class	Medication	Possible Side Effects
ANALGESICS		
Non-narcotic	Excedrin, Tylenol	Usually none if taken as prescribed
Narcotic	Darvon, Tylenol with codeine, Vicodin	Dizziness or lightheadedness, drowsiness, nausea, vomiting, drug tolerance, and physical dependence with long-term use
NONSTEROIDAL ANTI-INFLAMMATORY DRUGS (NSAIDs)		
Traditional	Advil, Aleve, Motrin, Naprosyn	Abdominal pain, dizziness, drowsiness, gastric ulcers and bleeding, greater susceptibility to bruising or bleeding, heartburn, indigestion, lightheadedness, nausea, tinnitus, kidney and liver effects
Cox-2 inhibitors	Celebrex	Same as traditional NSAIDs except less likely to cause gastric ulcers and susceptibility to bruising or bleeding; increased risk of heart attack and stroke
Salicylates	Anacin, Bayer, Bufferin	Abdominal cramps, gastric ulcers, increased bleeding tendency, confusion, dizziness, tinnitus, nausea, vomiting, deafness
CORTICOSTEROIDS		
	Cortisone, methylprednisone, prednisone	Cushing's syndrome (weight gain, moon-face, thin skin, muscle weakness, osteoporosis), cataracts, hypertension, elevated blood sugar, insomnia, mood changes, nervousness or restlessness
DISEASE-MODIFYING ANTIRHEUMATIC DRUGS (DMARDs)		
	Gold salts	Sun sensitivity, blood and kidney effects
	Imuran	Immunosuppression
	Methotrexate	Liver and blood effects, decreased fertility
	Penicillamine	Blood and kidney effects
	Plaquenil	Vision damage with long-term use
	Enbrel	Injection site irritation
BIOLOGICAL RESPONSE MODIFIERS		
	Remicade	Upper respiratory infection, headache, cough

to NSAIDs but with fewer incidences of gastric problems; however, more experience among prescribing physicians and longer-term use will help better define their role. The withdrawal of two popular Cox-2 drugs from the market (Vioxx in 2004 and Bextra in 2005) because of links with an increased risk of heart attack and stroke points to the need for further study.[29] Local pharmacological treatment of OA includes topical agents (e.g., aspirin and capsaicin creams) and intraarticular corticosteroid injections. These may be used alone or as an adjunct to systemic medications. Repeated injections in a joint are often limited to fewer than three per year because of the possible risk of progressive cartilage damage.[19]

Nonpharmacological agents, also known as *neutraceuticals*, are used by an estimated 23% of persons with OA as alternative or complementary treatments and seem to be gaining favor in the general public.[19,58,74] These include nutritional supplements such as glucosamine sulfate and chondroitin sulfate. Although they may have some effect on improving symptoms or slowing the progression of OA, studies citing their efficacy have not yet been of optimal quality.[50] However, even if their benefits have not been convincingly proved, the use of neutraceuticals carries little risk. Only minimal adverse effects related to their use have been described.[19,50]

SURGICAL MANAGEMENT

Operative intervention may be performed to improve joint integrity, restore joint stability, or reduce pain, with the overarching goal of improving the patient's overall function. Common surgical procedures in OA include arthroscopic joint debridement, use of grafts to replace damaged cartilage, joint fusion, and joint replacement.[16]

RHEUMATOID ARTHRITIS

Rheumatoid arthritis (RA) is a chronic, systemic inflammatory condition that affects approximately 2.1 million Americans.[4] The etiology of RA is not well understood, other than that a yet-unknown trigger causes an autoimmune inflammatory response in the joint lining of a genetically predisposed host.[36] Onset can happen at any age, but prevalence does increase with age. Peak incidence occurs between 40 and 60 years of age, with a rate of disease two to three times higher for females.[4,36] Onset is commonly insidious, with symptoms developing over several weeks to several months.

The disease manifests itself as **synovitis**, which is inflammation of the synovial membrane that lines the joint capsule of diarthrodial joints. The function of normal synovial tissue is to secrete a clear fluid into the joint for the purpose of lubrication.[1,22] In RA, synovial cells produce matrix-degrading enzymes that destroy cartilage and bone. Joint swelling results from excessive production of synovial fluid, enlargement of the synovium, and thickening of the joint capsule. This weakens the joint capsule and distends tendons and ligaments. As the inflammatory process continues, the diseased synovial membrane forms a pannus that actively invades and destroys cartilage, bone, tendon, and ligament (Figure 38-3). Scar tissue can form between the bone ends and cause the joint to become permanently rigid and immovable.

Articular manifestations of RA fall into two categories: (1) reversible signs and symptoms related to acute inflammatory synovitis and (2) irreversible cumulative structural damage caused by recurrent synovitis over the course of disease. Structural damage typically begins between the first and second years of disease and progresses as a linear function of the amount of prior synovitis.[2,33] Almost 90% of joints ultimately affected by RA become involved during the first year.[2,78] Progressive joint damage in the majority of patients results in significant disability within 10 to 20 years.[35]

The course of RA is variable from person to person. Approximately 20% of those affected have a single episode of inflammation with a long-lasting remission. The majority of people with RA experience a series of exacerbations and remissions, with periodic flare-ups of inflammation followed by complete or incomplete remissions.[63] Outcomes are similarly variable. Patients' functional abilities vary according to the course of the disease, the severity of the symptoms, and the amount of joint damage. Because RA is a systemic disease, certain extraarticular features occur in most patients. These features include fatigue, rheumatoid nodules, and vasculitis. Ocular, respiratory, cardiac, gastrointestinal, renal, and neurological manifestations are also seen as secondary complications. Patients with severe forms of RA may die between 10 and 15 years earlier than expected as a result of accompanying infection, pulmonary and renal disease, gastrointestinal bleeding, and possibly cardiac disease.[35]

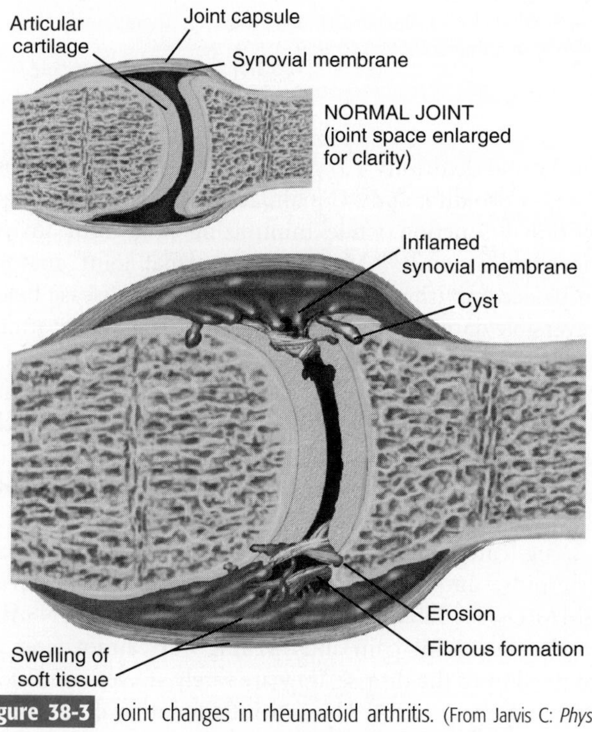

CLINICAL FEATURES

RA is characterized by symmetrical polyarticular pain and swelling, prolonged morning stiffness, malaise, fatigue, and low-grade fever. Joints most commonly affected are the PIP, MCP, and thumb joints of the hands, wrists, elbows, ankles, MTPs, and temporomandibular (TMJ) joints, with hips, knees, ankles, shoulders, and cervical spine also frequently involved.[2,35] Even though joint involvement is bilateral, the disease progression may not be equal on both sides. For instance, a patient's dominant hand may show more severe involvement and different joint changes or deformities than the other hand. Clinical features vary from patient to patient and also in individual patients over the course of their disease. Pain can be acute or chronic. Acute pain occurs during a disease exacerbation, or **flare.** Chronic pain is experienced from progressive joint damage. Synovial inflammation manifests as warm, spongy, and sometimes erythematous, or red, joints. This is seen in active phases of the disease process. Rheumatoid **nodules,** a cutaneous manifestation of RA, develop in up to 50% of afflicted persons during periods of increased disease activity. These soft tissue masses are commonly found over the extensor surface of the proximal ulna or at the olecranon.[2] Morning stiffness is an almost universal feature of RA. Unlike the shorter-duration stiffness seen in OA, RA morning stiffness can last one or two hours. It frequently disappears during periods of disease remission. Duration of morning stiffness tends to correlate with the degree of synovial inflammation, and its presence and length are useful measures of following the patient's course of RA.[36] Feelings of malaise, fatigue, and depression also fluctuate, with many patients experiencing worse symptoms in the afternoon. These non-specific symptoms may precede other typical signs of RA by weeks or months.[35]

The inflammatory process has been described as having four stages: acute, subacute, chronic active, and chronic inactive.[65] Stages may overlap, and patients may move back or forward through them depending on the course of their disease. Clinical symptoms seen in the acute stage include limited movement; pain and tenderness at rest that increases with movement; overall stiffness, weakness, tingling, or numbness; and hot, red joints. In the subacute stage, limited movement and tingling remain. A decrease in pain and tenderness indicates that inflammation is subsiding. Stiffness is limited to morning stiffness, and the joints appear pink and warm.

Articular cartilage
Joint capsule
Synovial membrane

NORMAL JOINT
(joint space enlarged for clarity)

Inflamed synovial membrane
Cyst

Erosion
Fibrous formation
Swelling of soft tissue

Figure 38-3   Joint changes in rheumatoid arthritis. (From Jarvis C: *Physical examination and health assessment,* ed 4, Philadelphia, 2004, WB Saunders.)

The chronic-active stage is characterized by less tingling, pain, and tenderness and increased activity tolerance, although endurance remains low. No signs of inflammation are present in the chronic-inactive stage. The patient's low endurance and pain and stiffness at this stage result from disuse. Overall functioning may be decreased as a result of fear of pain, limited range of motion (ROM), muscle atrophy, and contractures.[65]

More than 33% of patients with RA will develop characteristic joint deformities that are late manifestations of the disease. More than 10% will develop deformity of the small joints of the hand within the first 2 years.[35] Wrist radial deviation, MP ulnar deviation, and swan-neck and boutonnière deformities of digits are the joint changes most often seen. Joint changes, or deformities, can result from a variety of mechanisms, including joint immobility; destruction of cartilage and bone; and alterations in muscles, tendons, and ligaments.[36] **Tenosynovitis** (inflammation of the tendon sheath) and the presence of nodules within the flexor tendon sheaths can cause trigger finger. Patients may also exhibit symptoms of nerve compression of the median or ulnar nerves at the wrist. Tendon rupture may also be seen, usually in the extensor tendons of the fifth, fourth, and third digits. Stages of the disease based on joint deformity and radiographic changes are defined in Box 38-2.

DIAGNOSTIC CRITERIA

There is no single test leading to a definitive diagnosis of RA. Diagnosis is based on clinical evaluation of characteristic signs and symptoms, laboratory findings, and radiological findings.[35] The American College of Rheumatology Criteria for the Classification of Rheumatoid Arthritis require that the patient demonstrate at least four of seven criteria for a diagnosis of RA to be made (Table 38-3). A positive laboratory test is not necessary to establish a diagnosis of RA, but such tests may help confirm the clinical impression. Rheumatoid factor is an antibody found in the blood serum of approximately 85% of persons with RA, but it can also be found in other inflammatory diseases associated with synovitis. The presence of rheumatoid factor correlates with increased severity of symptoms and increased systemic manifestations. Erythrocyte sedimentation rate (ESR) correlates with degree of synovial inflammation and is useful in ruling out non-inflammatory conditions such as OA and tracking the course of inflammatory activity.[2,35] Radiographs may show nothing other than soft tissue swelling early in RA, but more than half of patients will develop radiographic changes within the first 2 years of developing the disease.[35]

MEDICAL MANAGEMENT

RA currently has no known cure. The major goals in the treatment of RA include (1) reducing pain, swelling, and fatigue; (2) improving joint function and minimizing joint damage and deformity; (3) preventing disability and disease-related morbidity; and (4) maintaining physical, social, and emotional function while minimizing long-term toxicity from medication.[35,63] Maintaining normal joint anatomy can be accomplished only by controlling the disease before irreversible damage occurs. Major advances in the treatment of RA have occurred over the past several years because of an improved understanding of the pathenogenic mechanisms of the disease, development of therapies that more specifically target pathophysiological processes, and recognition that early use of aggressive drug therapies can alter the outcome and reduce RA severity and disability.[63,97]

Drug categories used in RA include NSAIDs, corticosteroids, and disease-modifying antirheumatic drugs (DMARDs; see Table 38-2).[29] Because the fast-acting NSAIDs can decrease joint pain and swelling but cannot alter the progression of the disease, they are rarely, if ever, used alone in the treatment of RA. The anti-inflammatory effects of the

---

> ### Box 38-2 AMERICAN COLLEGE OF RHEUMATOLOGY CRITERIA FOR THE CLASSIFICATION OF RHEUMATOID ARTHRITIS
>
> **STAGE I: EARLY**
>
> 1. No destructive changes on roentgenographic examination*
> 2. Possible presence of radiographic evidence of osteoporosis
>
> **STAGE II: MODERATE**
>
> 1. Radiographic evidence of osteoporosis, with or without slight subchondral bone destruction; possible presence of slight cartilage destruction*
> 2. No joint deformities, although possible limitation of joint mobility*
> 3. Adjacent muscle atrophy
> 4. Possible presence of extraarticular soft tissue lesions, such as nodules and tenosynovitis
>
> **STAGE III: SEVERE**
>
> 1. Radiographic evidence of cartilage and bone destruction, in addition to osteoporosis*
> 2. Joint deformity, such as subluxation, ulnar deviation, or hyperextension, without fibrous or bony ankylosis*
> 3. Extensive muscle atrophy
> 4. Possible presence of extraarticular soft tissue lesions, such as nodules and tenosynovitis
>
> **STAGE IV: TERMINAL**
>
> 1. Fibrous or bony ankylosis*
> 2. Criteria of stage III

*These criteria must be present to permit classification in any particular stage or grade.
From Steinbrocker O, Traeger CH, Batterman RC: Therapeutic criteria in rheumatoid arthritis, *JAMA* 140:659, 1949.

TABLE **38-3** **American College of Rheumatology Classification of Rheumatoid Arthritis**

Criterion	Definition
Morning stiffness	Morning stiffness occurs in and around the joints, lasting at least 1 hour before maximal improvement.
Arthritis of three or more joint areas	At least three joint areas simultaneously have had soft tissue swelling or fluid (not bony overgrowth alone) observed by a physician. The 14 possible areas are right or left PIP, MP, wrist, elbow, knee, ankle, and MTP joints.
Arthritis of hand joints	At least one area is swollen (as defined above) in a wrist, MCP, or PIP joint.
Symmetrical arthritis	Simultaneous involvement of the same joint areas (as defined in the second example) occurs on both sides of the body (bilateral involvement of PIPs, MPs, or MTPs is acceptable without absolute symmetry).
Rheumatoid nodules	Subcutaneous nodules, over bony prominences, or extensor surfaces, or in juxtaarticular regions, are observed by a physician.
Serum rheumatoid factor	Abnormal amounts of serum rheumatoid factor are demonstrated by any method for which the result has been positive in <5% of normal control subjects.
Radiographic changes	Radiographic changes are typical of rheumatoid arthritis on posteroanterior hand and wrist radiographs, which must include erosions or unequivocal bony decalcification localized in or most marked adjacent to the involved joints (osteoarthritic changes alone do not qualify).

For classification purposes, a client shall be said to have rheumatoid arthritis if he or she has satisfied at least four of these criteria. The first four criteria must have been present for at least 6 weeks. Patients with two clinical diagnoses are not excluded. Designation as classic, definite, or probable rheumatoid arthritis is *not* to be made.

From Arnett FC, et al: The American Rheumatism Association 1987 revised criteria for the classification of rheumatoid arthritis, *Arthritis Rheum* 31:315, 1988.

large number of medications in this category are about equal. Cox-2 inhibitors, a newer type of medication, show no evidence of greater efficacy than other NSAIDs but are thought to pose a lower risk of serious gastrointestinal side effects.[2] Corticosteroids have a long history in the medical management of RA and still remain a key element. They produce rapid and potent suppression of inflammation with improvement in joint pain and fatigue. Because of the significant adverse effects of corticosteroids, they are frequently used on a temporary basis in patients with active disease and significant functional decline while awaiting the full therapeutic effect of DMARDs. DMARDs lack a pain-relief effect, but they may actually affect the course of the disease. Because of their slow-acting nature, weeks or months of drug therapy may be necessary before a clinical benefit is recognized. The potency of these drugs requires that patients must be closely monitored for side effects.

Traditionally, the approach for RA began with less toxic medications such as NSAIDs and progressed to the stronger drugs needed later in the disease course. The approach is becoming more aggressive, with early use of DMARDs to control the disease process as soon as possible, as completely as possible, and for as long as possible.[2,97] Drug therapy constantly changes, depending on the patient's needs and response to treatment as well as the physician's treatment philosophy. This uncertainty can be frustrating for the patient, who may have to experiment with myriad new medications when current drugs become ineffective or side effects too severe. It is important for the occupational therapist and other team members to know the specific medications that the patient is taking and what adverse reactions may arise.

SURGICAL MANAGEMENT

Because of the extensive joint damage caused by RA, surgical intervention is frequently indicated to relieve pain and improve function. Several surgical procedures may be of benefit to patients with RA. Synovectomy (excision of diseased synovium) and tenosynovectomy (removal of diseased tendon sheaths) are performed to relieve symptoms and slow the process of joint destruction, but they do not prevent progression of the disease. These procedures are most commonly performed in the wrist and hand. Tendon surgery, including relocation of displaced tendons, repair of ruptured tendons, and release of shortened tendons, may be performed to correct hand impairments. Tendon surgery occurs most frequently on the extensor tendons of the wrist and hand. Tendon transfers and peripheral nerve decompressions (such as carpal tunnel releases) are also performed to optimize function. Arthroplasty (joint reconstruction) and arthrodesis (joint fusion) are options when joint restoration is not possible. These may be performed to relieve pain, provide stability, correct deformity, and improve function. Common sites for arthroplasty include hips, knees, and MCPs. Common sites for arthrodesis include wrists, thumb MPs and IPs, and the cervical spine.[63,65]

OCCUPATIONAL THERAPY EVALUATION

It is important to recognize that every client with arthritis has a unique presentation of clinical problems and functional impairment. A strong client-centered and occupation-based approach is helpful in determining each client's specific needs. The evaluation process for clients with arthritis includes many of the same elements as for any physical disability. Special considerations related to arthritis include closer attention to pain, joint stiffness, joint deformity, fatigue, and coping strategies, especially as they relate to activity limitations.

Because clients with arthritis typically experience good days and bad days, many symptoms and problems are fluctuant. A thorough systematic assessment of the client's functional, clinical, and psychosocial status is key to prioritizing problems and planning effective intervention.

The extent of specific evaluation components will often be driven by the main reason for referral. Clients seen for preoperative hand assessment, postoperative hip replacement, education after diagnosis, splinting while in a flare, or a decline in functional status will all require the therapist to customize evaluation priorities.

Because of the chronic nature of rheumatic diseases, some clients are able to clearly state their specific needs and should be afforded the opportunity to do so. Other clients may be overwhelmed by multiple problems or a newly made diagnosis and will look to the therapist to guide the intervention process. Regardless of the client's status, a close collaboration and partnership among the client, family, therapist, and other team members is crucial in helping deliver the best treatment possible.

The occupational therapy (OT) evaluation process consists of (1) a client history, (2) occupational profile, (3) occupational performance status, (4) cognitive, psychological, and social status, and (5) clinical status.

CLIENT HISTORY

A thorough history should be obtained through review of the client report and medical record. Important details include diagnosis, dates of onset and diagnosis, secondary medical conditions, current medications and medication schedule, alternative or complementary therapies, and surgical history.[83] Asking the client questions such as "What type of arthritis do you have?," "How long have you had it?," "What medications are you currently taking?," and "What other things are you doing to manage your arthritis?" can provide helpful insights regarding the client's level of understanding about his or her condition, medical treatment, and health habits. Prior experiences with OT and physical therapy should also be ascertained in order to build on them. The therapist must ask and actively listen to the client's current primary complaints through questions such as "What is bothering you most about your arthritis?," "How is your arthritis limiting your ability to do things right now?," and "What are you hoping therapy can help you with?"

This was Nina's first referral to OT. She was knowledgeable about her diagnosis and medications but uncertain about the potential benefits of therapy. Through her responses to key questions, Nina was able to clearly state that her pain and her difficulty with performing household and work activities were her main priorities.

OCCUPATIONAL PROFILE

It is helpful to begin the process of assessing occupational performance with an occupational profile. Obtained through an open-ended interview, the profile yields important details about the client's prior and current roles, occupations, overall activity level, and ability to participate in meaningful activities. It can also provide insight into the client's sense of self-efficacy, adjustment to disability, and themes of meaning in his or her life.[54,62] An effective method to obtain a client's occupational profile is to have the client describe how he or she spends a typical day. This typical-day assessment allows the therapist to become familiar with the client's routines, use of time, sleep/wake habits, energy and fatigue patterns, important people and environments, activity contexts, and other details that otherwise may not come up in conversation. Because arthritis involves fluctuant symptoms, the client should be asked to describe how time is spent on a good day and a bad day so that the therapist can compare the two and understand how arthritis affects the client's daily life and how effectively the client is able to balance activity and rest. It is helpful to ask the client to estimate the percentage of good versus bad days per week or month. It also may be advantageous to explore time spent on weekend days versus weekdays; the client may reveal other occupations, such as those involving spirituality, social participation, and leisure. This fluid dialog also serves to develop rapport, establish the client as the valued expert in his or her occupations and lifestyle, and frame the role of OT in the client's rehabilitation.

OCCUPATIONAL PERFORMANCE STATUS

Once the client's typical and preferred occupations are identified, his or her level of independence engaging in these functional activities can be assessed by interview or by observation. If observation is used, the activity should occur as closely as possible to the time it is normally performed because the client's abilities may fluctuate at different times of the day. For instance, stiffness and pain may make dressing very difficult in the early morning, but if this task is assessed in the afternoon, the client's status may appear much better. Ideally, the activity should also be done in the client's own home, community, or work contexts.[6] In addition to assessing the client's level of independence during activities of daily living (ADLs), instrumental activities of daily living (IADLs), school, work, play, leisure, and social engagements, it is important to note any assistive devices (e.g., mobility aids or adaptive equipment) and compensatory techniques that the client may use. The activity demands of the occupation performed (e.g., tools, equipment, and skills required) as well as the specific contexts in which it is performed (e.g., the client's living situation, others in the home, and architectural setup relative to occupational performance) should be detailed in tandem with existing physical, environmental, or social barriers. Finally, the amount of time required to complete certain activities should be explored. A client who experiences significant morning stiffness or limited endurance often chooses to accept assistance with an activity such as dressing to save time or conserve energy to participate in

TABLE 38-4 **American College of Rheumatology Classification of Global Functional Status in Rheumatoid Arthritis**

Classification	Description
Class I	Completely able to perform usual activities of daily living (self-care,* vocational, and avocational)
Class II	Able to perform usual self-care and vocational activities, but limited in avocational activities
Class III	Able to perform usual self-care and vocational activities, but limited in vocational and avocational activities
Class IV	Limited in ability to perform usual self-care, vocational, and avocational activities

*Usual self-care activites include dressing, feeding, bathing, grooming, and toileting. Avocational (recreational or leisure) and vocational (work, school, homemaking) activities are client-desired and age- and sex-specific.
Courtesy of American College of Rheumatology © 2004.

a more meaningful occupation later in the day. This strategy may contribute to the client's overall satisfaction with and participation in life, and it should be respected as such.

In RA, functional status may be classified according to the American College of Rheumatology Revised Criteria for Classification of Functional Status in Rheumatoid Arthritis (Table 38-4). This system was devised for rapid, global assessment of functional status by health professionals.[47] The therapist should be familiar with this system because it is often used in clinical research and can provide a general framework for defining advancing disability.[44,100] Nina would be considered Class III because of her limitations in her work activities.

A decrease in occupational functioning in clients with arthritis may be due to pain, joint changes or instability, loss of motion, weakness, fatigue, change in living environment, or change in social support, among other contributing circumstances. Effects of medication can also limit performance. The challenge for the therapist is not only to identify occupational performance deficits but also to determine the factors that are causing them. Asking the client why an activity cannot be done yields the important client perspective.[6] Nina was having difficulty with many occupations, including sleeping, playing actively with her grandchildren, managing her home, and performing her job to her level of satisfaction. She reported having to give up or cut back on activities because of increased pain, stiffness, and fatigue from her recent flare.

COGNITIVE, PSYCHOLOGICAL, AND SOCIAL STATUS

The effects of arthritis are not merely physical and functional. Clients with arthritis should be screened for cognitive and psychosocial deficits. Although arthritis does not directly affect cognition, pain, sleep disturbances, depression,

and medication can all have profound effects on attention span, short-term memory, and problem-solving skills.[65] People with a chronic illness must develop coping strategies to deal with the disability. Coping strategies are particularly crucial for the person with arthritis, who may face serious changes in physical function, life roles, and appearance because of deformity and pharmacological side effects. Because arthritis is both unpredictable and painful, normal responses to the disability include depression, denial, a need to control the environment, and dependence. Psychosocial adaptation is affected by the complex interplay of physical, psychological, and situational factors.[38,54] Approximately 20% of persons with RA are estimated to suffer from major depression.[27] About one half of individuals with RA or OA may experience loss in social relationships.[99] Constant pain and fear of pain, changed body image, perception of self as a sick person, continuous uncertainty about the course and progression of the disease, sexual dysfunction, altered roles, and loss of income resulting from the inability to work can lead to significant psychological stressors.[54,72] Evidence has shown that disability from RA relates to psychosocial factors almost to the same extent as biomedical factors.[30] Occupational therapists must understand the ways in which their clients manage stress in their lives because these stressors may exacerbate the disease.[54] Family relationships and cultural backgrounds also affect the client's healthcare behaviors and response to disability.[77] The therapist should be sensitive to all factors that will influence rehabilitation. Referrals to other health professionals (such as psychiatrists, psychologists, and social workers) should be made if needed.[72]

Nina reported that she had increasing difficulty in concentrating on tasks because she was unable to get adequate restful sleep. She expressed frustration about her inability to keep her house in order and anxiety about losing income because she was unable to work her customary hours. She was also fearful about her health because her arthritis had been adequately controlled for the past few years, and she had not experienced any flares.

CLINICAL STATUS

For clients with arthritis, the elements of inflammation, ROM, strength, hand function, stiffness, pain, sensation, joint instability and deformity, physical endurance, and functional mobility should be included through either brief screening or detailed evaluation. As with assessment of function, the time of day and anti-inflammatory or analgesic medication taken should be noted because these may influence results. In addition, future reevaluations should be performed under the same conditions.[65] When the client's functional deficits are identified first, the assessment of client factors can be much more focused. Additionally, asking the client a question such as "What joints are you having the most problems with?" can help prioritize assessment needs. Given Nina's initial presentation, the detailed evaluation focused primarily on synovitis, pain, stiffness, ROM, strength, physical endurance, and functional mobility. Even though joint deformities were not immediately evident, the therapist was careful to search for signs of instability that would place Nina's joints at risk for deformity.

The clinical evaluation may take considerable time. It should be approached in a systematic manner, with results clearly documented. The occupational therapist may need to perform assessments over several sessions, especially if the client is experiencing significant pain or fatigue. Intervention can begin immediately and does not necessarily depend on completion of the evaluation. The evaluation actually begins with a general observation of the client's posture, willingness to move, and pain behaviors during the initial interview.

The presence and location of inflammation or synovitis should be noted because these indicate an active disease process. Several types of swelling may be present and should be described. An effusion (excess fluid in the joint capsule) is seen as fusiform swelling that is spindle-shaped and conforms to the shape of the joint. Boggy swelling is thin and full of fluid. Puffy, spongy, and soft to the touch, boggy swelling is seen in the early active stages of synovitis. Chronic synovitis feels firm because the joint fills with synovial tissue.[65]

Active and passive ROM can be measured. Depending on the reason for referral and the client's complaints, the therapist may not find it necessary to obtain goniometric measurements of all joints, instead focusing only on those joints of most concern. Active motion will allow the therapist to see the amount of mobility the client has available for function, whereas passive motion will elicit the joint's capacity to move. The client's range of active motion may be significantly less than that of passive ROM; this is known as a lag and is caused by pain, weakness, or the mechanical inefficiencies caused by joint damage. Goniometric measurement of hand joints may be difficult in the presence of deformity. Assessing composite (combined motion of all joints) flexion, composite extension, and thumb opposition can provide more functional information.[9] Active opening and closing of the hand can be measured by the distance from the fingertips to the table top in maximal extension (opening) when the dorsal side of the hand is resting on the table and the distance from the fingertips to the distal palmar crease (closing). While performing the ROM assessment, the therapist should note whether the client's joints feel stiff or unstable. A hard end-feel in the presence of contracture indicates bony blockage.[66] A firm end-feel that still has some give indicates that the joint capsule or ligaments are limiting motion.[46] The presence and location of crepitus, along with the motions that cause it, should also be noted because crepitus often indicates extensive joint damage. The source of crepitation may be bony, synovial, bursal, or tendinous (see Chapters 19 through 21 for additional information).[9,65]

Gross strength should be assessed with more specific manual muscle testing as indicated. One important detail to understand is that strength testing in clients with arthritis differs from normal testing procedures. Resistance is applied at the end range of pain-free motion rather than at the true end of the ROM. It is not unusual for clients with arthritis to have pain in the last 30 to 40 degrees of joint motion. When resistance is applied within the pain-free range, the inhibition of muscle strength by pain will be avoided. It is also important to consider joint protection principles when applying resistance and to discontinue resistance if the client experiences pain. If use of resistance is contraindicated (as may be the case in an acute or active phase of arthritis, in which resistance may be harmful to inflamed tissue and joints), functional muscle or motion testing may be substituted.[65]

Hand strength and function are important to test, but care must be taken not to stress painful or vulnerable joints during assessment. Grip and pinch may be measured by standard meters, but in the presence of severe weakness or hand deformity, adapted methods, such as use of a blood pressure cuff to measure force in millimeters of mercury, may be indicated.[9,65] Although it is more comfortable for the client, results of testing strength in this manner are less reliable, with no established norms. Other specific devices for measuring grip strength in hands with arthritis, including pneumatic bulb dynamometers, are commercially available. As a result of joint deformity, the client may not be able to assume the standard testing positions for lateral and palmar pinch. Because it is important to assess pinch strength relative to function, pinch should still be tested, with a notation made of the client's prehensile pattern (e.g., "4 pounds of pinch with meter placed in web space between thumb and second metacarpal"). The presence and location of muscle atrophy should be recorded because it indicates severe weakness and possible nerve compression that may require further investigation. Intrinsic atrophy can be seen as flattening of thenar and hypothenar eminences and as hollowing between metacarpals on the dorsal aspect of the hand.

Hand function can be assessed through standardized tests (e.g., the Jebsen Taylor Hand Function Test)[49] or observation of the client performing common functional tasks that involve various grasp and prehensile patterns. These tasks can include opening a medication bottle, writing, holding a glass, picking up small pins, turning a doorknob and key, cutting with a knife, and fastening buttons. In addition to noting whether the client is able to perform each task, the value of this testing lies in the observation of how the client uses his or her hands and the determination of which factors interfere most with activity: instability, lack of motion, deformity, pain, weakness, or something else. The therapist cannot predict function solely on the basis of the hand's appearance. Deformities caused by arthritis often develop slowly, and many clients learn how to adapt their hand function gradually over time. It may be surprising to see significantly deformed hands performing tasks with relatively good function. The therapist should remember this when planning an intervention because it might eliminate a problem that is actually functional for the client.

Joint stiffness is a distinct feeling of excessive stiffness that eventually wears off.[65] It can occur from low-grade inflammation, effusion, synovial thickening, muscle shortening, or spasm.[10,66] The therapist can determine the extent of joint stiffness by asking the client which joints experience stiffness, under what conditions, and for how long. Morning stiffness and gelling should be considered separately and can be measured in hours or minutes. The duration of morning stiffness is often used as an objective indicator of the degree of disease activity present. The gelling phenomenon, stiffness after prolonged periods of inactivity, is so named because fluid in the joint and surrounding tissues sets up like gelatin.[66]

Because pain is often the primary clinical manifestation of arthritis, it should be closely evaluated. Pain that interferes with the client's ability to engage in occupations should be of primary concern. The presence and location of joint pain should be noted. To elicit important details, the therapist should ask questions such as "When does the pain occur?," "What tends to make the pain worse?," and "What seems to make the pain better?" An attempt should be made to distinguish between articular (joint) pain and periarticular (soft tissues surrounding the joint) pain. Secondary conditions such as tendonitis and bursitis are frequent causes of pain. Pain has different meanings for individuals and is often difficult to describe.[85] The therapist can obtain measurements of pain intensity by asking the client to rate the pain on a numerical scale of "1" (no pain) to "10" (greatest pain) or on a visual analog scale in which the client places a mark along a 10-cm line.[48] These scales can also be used to measure other subjective symptoms, including fatigue and degree of stiffness.[43] Because pain related to arthritis is fluctuant, the client may be asked to rate pain at its current level, at its best, at its worst, and at various times of the day or to compare pain at rest versus pain upon motion or activity. Interestingly, pain caused by acute inflammation in early stages of RA tends to be greater than pain at end stages, when severe deformities are present.[9] The presence and location of joint tenderness should also be noted. Tenderness is assessed by applying manual compression to the medial/lateral aspects of the joint (see Chapter 27 for additional information).[65]

Sensation should be evaluated if the potential for peripheral nerve damage or compression caused by swelling exists. The therapist should obtain a subjective report from the client with regard to the presence of numbness or tingling. This report can be followed by a screening of touch/pressure threshold of the fingertips using monofilaments.[7] If sensory impairment is noted, further assessment may be indicated. This may include provocative tests to replicate or aggravate symptoms in order to localize areas of compression. Examples of these tests are Phalen's test and Tinel's test in the case of suspected median nerve compression at the carpal tunnel.[5] When cervical spine involvement is known or suspected, dermatomal light touch, sharp-dull, and proprioception should be evaluated (see Chapters 22 and 39 for additional information).

The examiner assesses **joint laxity** (instability) by applying stress to individual joints in medial/lateral and anterior/posterior directions. When testing medial/lateral stability of the MP joints, the examiner must first place the MPs in flexion to tighten the collateral ligaments, which are naturally loose in MP extension. Unstable joints should be noted. Ligamentous laxity can be described as slight (5-10 degrees in excess of normal), moderate (10-20 degrees in excess), or severe (20 or more degrees in excess).[65] In the hand joints, instability with medial/lateral motion indicates laxity of collateral ligaments whereas excessive anterior/posterior motion is caused by laxity of the joint capsule and volar plate. Normal joint stability is highly variable, and whenever possible, it is helpful to compare it to the client's uninvolved joints.[65]

The evaluation of joint deformities is done primarily through observation and palpation. The location and type of deformity should be noted. Comparison with previous evaluations, if available, allows the therapist to see how deformities have progressed over the course of the disease. If a deformity is correctable, either actively or passively, it is considered *flexible*; if the deformity cannot be reduced, it is considered *fixed*. Patterns of deformity can be different in a client's two hands, and a person with RA can also exhibit deformities caused by osteoarthritic joint damage.

Common hand deformities in arthritis include the following:
- A *boutonnière deformity* is characterized by flexion of the PIP joint and hyperextension of the DIP joint (Figure 38-4). This zigzag collapse represents an alteration in muscle-tendon balance. Pathology begins at the

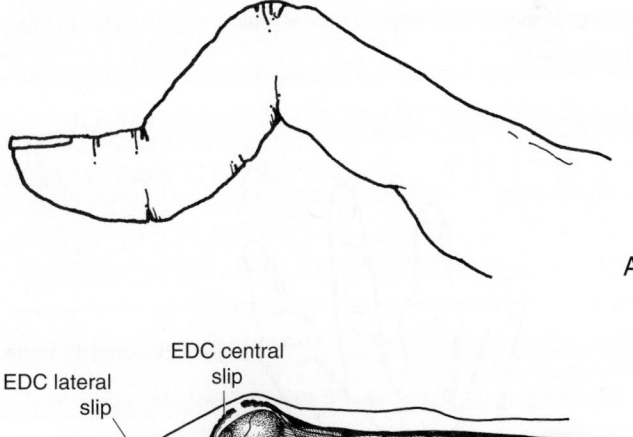

Figure 38-4   **A,** Boutonnière deformity results in distal interphalangeal hyperextension and proximal interphalangeal flexion. **B,** Boutonnière deformity caused by rupture or lengthening of central slip of extensor digitorum communis tendon.

PIP joint with secondary changes in the DIP. It occurs when synovitis weakens, lengthens, or disrupts the dorsal capsule and central slip of the extensor mechanism, causing incomplete or weak-to-absent extension at the PIP joint. The lateral bands of the extensor mechanism displace

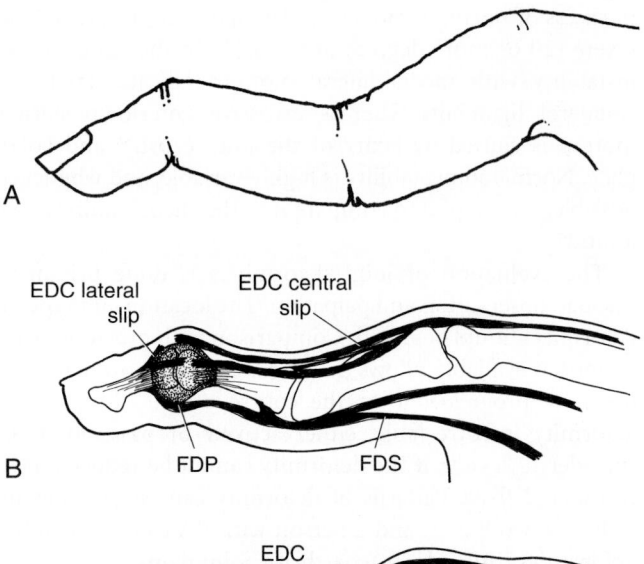

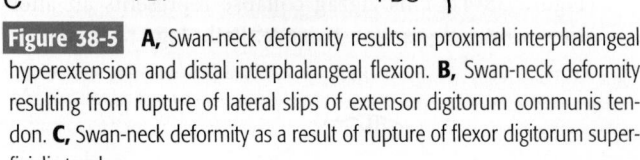

Figure 38-5   **A,** Swan-neck deformity results in proximal interphalangeal hyperextension and distal interphalangeal flexion. **B,** Swan-neck deformity resulting from rupture of lateral slips of extensor digitorum communis tendon. **C,** Swan-neck deformity as a result of rupture of flexor digitorum superficialis tendon.

volarly below the axis of the PIP joint, becoming flexors of that joint. Increased force on the lateral bands at the DIP, where they insert, causes hyperextension. Function of the finger is compromised by the inability to straighten the finger and the loss of flexion at the fingertip for pinching.[1,9,65]

- A *swan-neck deformity* is characterized by hyperextension of the PIP joint and flexion of the DIP joint, with possible flexion of the MP joint (Figure 38-5). This zigzag collapse is also a result of muscle-tendon imbalance and joint laxity. It can originate from abnormalities at any finger joint. Causes of this deformity include intrinsic muscle tightness, stretching or rupture of the terminal extensor tendon at the DIP, and chronic synovitis that leads to stretching of the volar capsular supporting structures at the PIP. Here the lateral bands of the extensor mechanism slip above the axis of the PIP joint, hyperextending the PIP joint and flexing the DIP joint. Function of the finger is compromised by inability to flex the PIP, with loss of the ability to make a fist or hold small objects.[1]

- A *mallet finger* is characterized by flexion of the DIP joint. This is caused by rupture of the terminal extensor tendon as it crosses the DIP. The finger loses the ability to extend the distal phalanx.

- ***Nodes*** are bony enlargements that indicate cartilage damage caused by OA. Joints affected by RA can also have degenerative joint disease, so nodes may be seen in clients with RA as well. These osteophytes are hard to the touch and are typically not painful. They are most commonly seen at the DIP joint (Heberden's nodes) and the PIP joint (Bouchard's nodes; Figure 38-6).[9,13,65,66]

- ***Nodules*** are granulomatous and fibrous soft tissue masses that are sometimes painful. These usually occur along weight-bearing surfaces such as the ulna or at the olecranon (Figure 38-7) and can be prognostic of rheumatoid arthritis disease severity.[9]

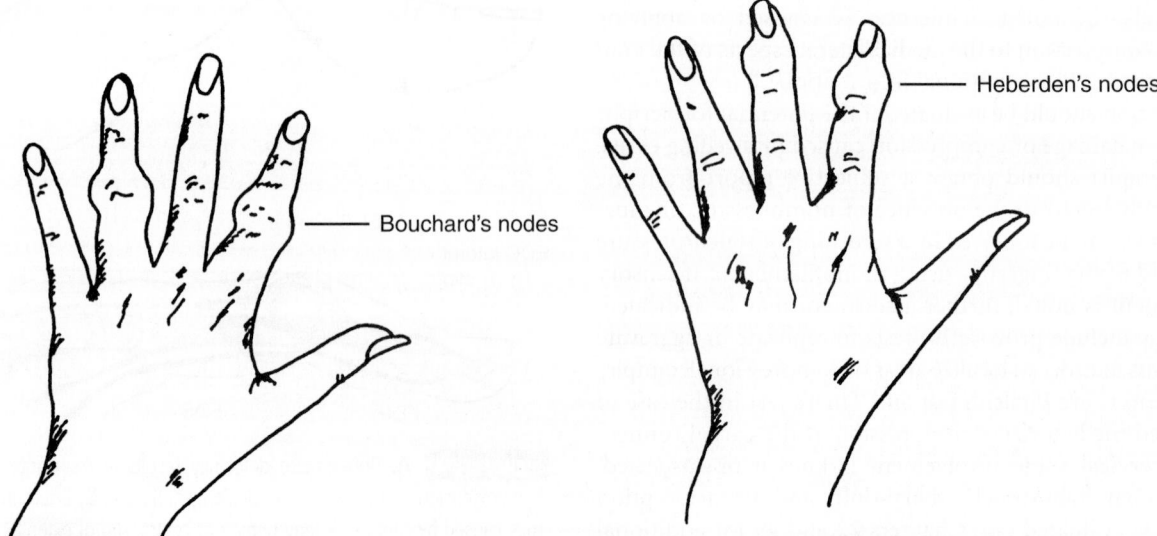

Figure 38-6   Osteophyte formation of the proximal interphalangeal joints (Bouchard's nodes) and the distal interphalangeal joints (Heberden's nodes) are common findings in osteoarthritis.

- *Deviation* is characterized by a change in normal joint position. It is typically described as radial or ulnar. In RA the most common pattern of deviation is radial deviation of the wrist and ulnar deviation (commonly referred to as *ulnar drift*) of the MPs (Figure 38-8). Deviation is caused by ligament weakening or disruption. Small joints are especially vulnerable because daily activities involving gripping and pinching apply strong forces to them.[1,9,65]
- *Subluxation* is characterized by volar or dorsal displacement of joints. It is any degree of malalignment in which

articular structures are only in partial contact. In RA the most common sites of subluxation are the wrist and MP joints.[65] Volar subluxation of the wrist occurs as the carpal bones slip relative to the distal radius as a result of chronic synovitis that weakens the supporting ligaments. Because of the condyloid nature of their joints, MPs have more planes of movement and are inherently less stable than IP joints. Volar subluxation of the MPs is frequent and often accompanied by ulnar drift and lateral displacement of the extensor tendons into the ulnar valleys between the metacarpal heads (Figure 38-9).[1,9,65]
- *Dislocation* is characterized by joints whose articulating surfaces are no longer in contact. In cases of severe RA, volar dislocation of the carpals on the radius or dislocation of other joints can occur from complete destruction of ligamentous integrity.[9,65]
- *Ankylosis* is characterized by lack of joint mobility. This spontaneous joint fusion can be bony (caused by ossification within or around the joint) or fibrous (caused by growth of fibrous tissue around the joint).[65]

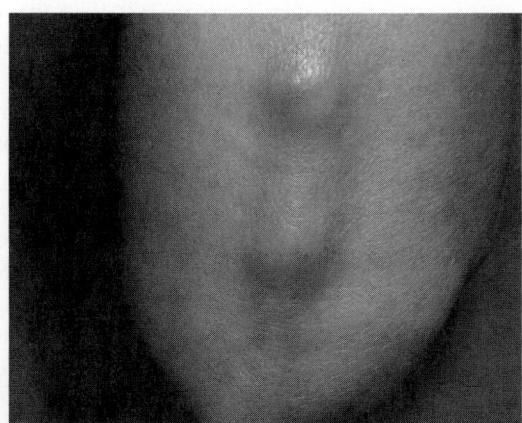

Figure 38-7 Rheumatoid nodules present on the extensor surface of the elbow. (From Jarvis C: *Physical examination and health assessment*, ed 4, Philadelphia, 2004, WB Saunders.)

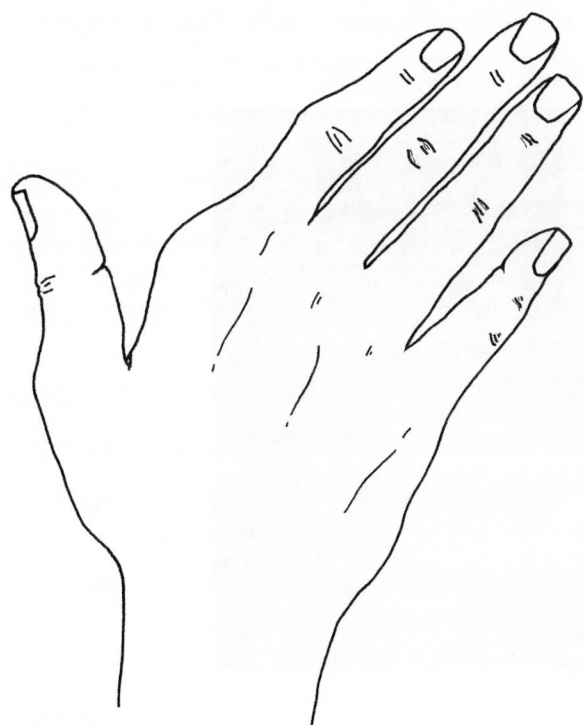

Figure 38-8 Metacarpophalangeal joint ulnar drift.

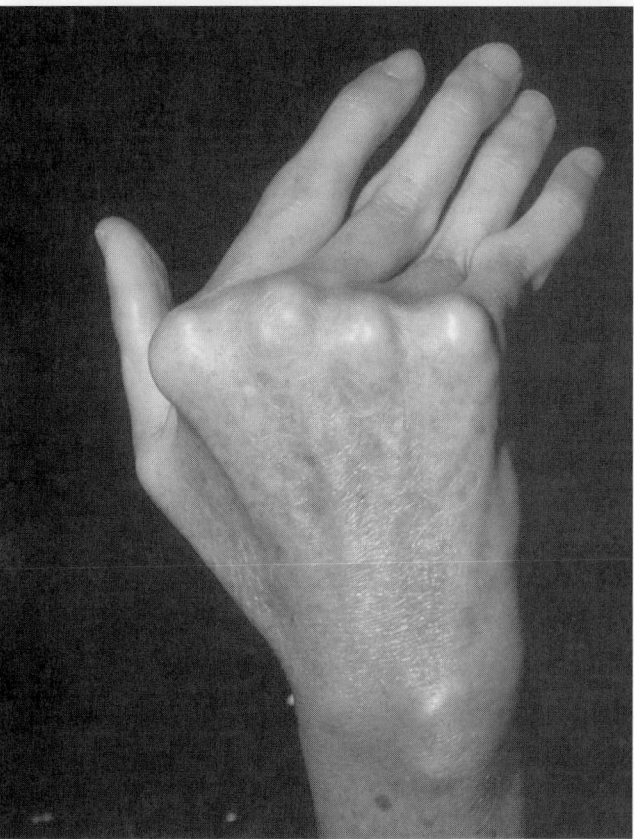

Figure 38-9 Volar subluxation and ulnar deviation of the metacarpophalangeal joints with lateral displacement of extensor tendons characteristic of rheumatoid arthritis. (From Alter S, Feldon T, Terrono AL: Pathomechanics of deformities in the arthritic hand and wrist. In Mackin EJ et al, editors: *Rehabilitation of the hand and upper extremity*, ed 5, pg. 1550, St Louis, 2002, Mosby.)

- *Extensor tendon rupture* is characterized by the inability to actively extend a joint in the absence of muscle weakness (Figure 38-10). The extensor digiti minimi is often the first to rupture. The extensor pollicis longus and extensor digitorum communis of the third, fourth, and fifth digits are also vulnerable.[9] Tendon rupture can occur from rubbing of the tendon over rough bony surfaces or tendon damage caused by direct synovial invasion or increased pressure that decreases blood supply to the tendon.

- *Trigger finger* is characterized by inconsistent limitation of finger flexion or extension. It is often caused by a nodule on a flexor tendon or stenosis of a tendon sheath, which impedes the tendon's ability to glide.[65] The client often experiences "catching" or "locking" of a finger into flexion and has to passively extend the finger out of the flexed position.

- *Mutilans deformity* is characterized by very floppy joints with redundant skin (Figure 38-11). The cause is unknown, but the result is resorption of the bone ends, which shortens the bones and renders the joints completely unstable. This is most commonly seen at the MP and PIP joints of the hands and the radiocarpal and radioulnar joints of the wrist.[65]

- *Thumb deformities* can manifest as any of the deformities previously described. Six patterns of thumb deformity have been classified by Nalebuff (Table 38-5).[92] Type I is the most common in RA, followed by type III, seen in both OA and RA.[65,92] Boutonnière (type I) is characterized by MP joint flexion and IP joint hyperextension. Swanneck (type III) is characterized by CMC joint subluxation, adduction, and flexion; MP joint hyperextension; and IP joint flexion. Also common in RA and OA is an adduction contracture of the thumb CMC joint caused by subluxation of the first metacarpal, radial deviation of the MP joint, or shortening or weakness of intrinsic muscles.[66,92] Subluxation causes a characteristic squared appearance of the CMC (Figure 38-12). Disruption of the thumb biomechanics often leads to significant loss of hand function, especially given the fact that the thumb is thought to account for as much as 60% of hand function.[41]

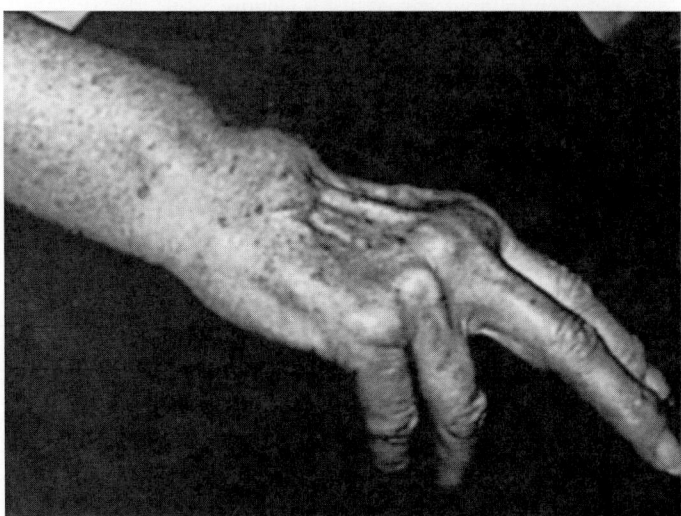

Figure 38-10 Extensor tendon rupture of the fourth and fifth digits resulting in loss of active extension. Tenosynovitis of the extensor tendons and volar subluxation of the wrist caused by rheumatoid arthritis are contributing factors. (From Harris ED, et al: *Kelley's textbook of rheumatology*, ed 7, Philadelphia, 2005, WB Saunders.)

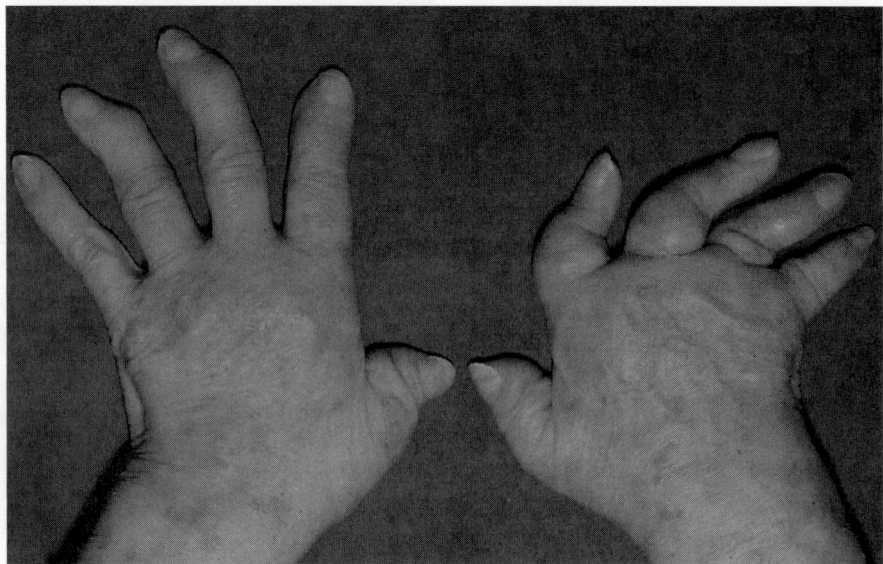

Figure 38-11 Mutilans deformity. (From Klippel JH, Dieppe P, Ferri FF: *Primary care rheumatology*, St Louis, 1999, Mosby.)

TABLE **38-5** **Rheumatoid Thumb Deformities**

Type	CMC Joint	MP Joint	IP Joint
I (boutonnière)	Not involved	Flexed	Hyperextended
II (uncommon)	CMC flexed and adducted	Flexed	Hyperextended
III (swan neck)	CMC subluxed, flexed, and adducted	Hyperextended	Flexed
IV (gamekeepers)	CMC not subluxed; flexed and adducted	1 degree, hyperextended, ulnar collateral ligament unstable	Not involved
V	May or may not be involved	1 degree, volar plate unstable	Not involved
VI (arthritis mutilans)	Bone loss at any level	Bone loss at any level	Bone loss at any level

From Terrono AL, Nalebuff EA, Philips CA: The rheumatoid thumb. In Mackin EJ et al: *Rehabilitation of the hand and upper extremity*, ed 5, p. 1556, St Louis, 2002, Mosby.

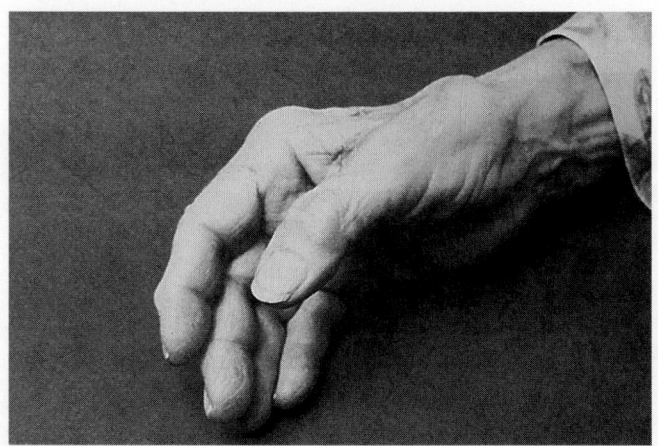

Figure 38-12   Osteoarthritis of the thumb carpometacarpal joint resulting in squaring and subluxation of the base of the thumb. (From ARHP Arthritis Teaching Slide Collection, American College of Rheumatology.)

Physical endurance can be evaluated by observation during the assessment process and by client report. Pain, weakness, deconditioning, lack of sleep, and emotional stress can all lead to decreased stamina. The pattern and severity of fatigue should be noted.[83] Functional mobility, including ambulation, sitting, and standing tolerances, and ability to transfer, should be assessed relative to occupational performance.

GOAL SETTING

Therapy goals should be determined by careful consideration of the client's stated goals, the client's individual needs, and the stage of the disease process. The Canadian Occupational Performance Measure (COPM) is a useful client-centered tool that can be used for goal setting, treatment planning, and outcomes measurement.[52] It is designed to detect change in a client's self-perception of occupational performance over time. It engages the client in defining activity problems and helps the client to more clearly understand

the purpose of OT. The COPM involves a semi-structured interview in which the client is asked to identify occupations that the client needs to, wants to, or is expected to perform but that are not done satisfactorily. Occupational goals in the areas of self-care, productivity, and leisure (based on the Canadian Model of Occupational Performance [CMOP]) are listed, and the client is then asked to rate his or her self-perception of importance of, current performance of, and satisfaction with performance of each occupation. Through this process of collaboration with the client, occupation-based therapy goals can be identified, priorities determined, and a treatment plan designed to facilitate optimal outcome. The rating process is repeated at time of discharge for outcome purposes. The COPM has been used with people who have arthritis in both inpatient and outpatient settings.[6] COPM goals for Nina were to return to work 20 hours a week, to clean her house independently, and to be able to take her grandchildren to the park after school.

INTERVENTION OBJECTIVES AND PLANNING

Treatment of the client with arthritis must take into account the progressive nature of the disease.[22] The overarching goal of therapy is to decrease pain, protect joints, and increase function. General objectives of OT are to (1) maintain or increase the ability to engage in meaningful occupations; (2) maintain or increase joint mobility and strength; (3) maximize physical endurance; (4) protect against or minimize the effect of deformities; (5) increase understanding of the disease and the best methods of dealing with physical, functional, and psychosocial effects; and (6) assist with adjustment to disability.[65]

The intervention plan should be designed for the individual client and based on the stage of disease, the severity of symptoms, general health status, lifestyle, and mutually agreed-upon goals. Given the limited time for therapy, prioritizing treatment is essential. The therapist should focus on addressing the most important factors by answering the following question: "What are the essential interventions necessary to enable the client to function at an optimal level?" It is important to have the client and significant others be active participants throughout therapy. Everyone involved must understand the disease process and the rationale for intervention methods. Because therapy intervention will most likely be intermittent throughout the client's course of disease, the client's ability to follow through with and self-manage interventions at home will greatly influence the ultimate success of treatment.

Table 38-6 outlines some common symptoms, general objectives, and OT interventions typically appropriate for each stage of inflammatory disease; it can be used as a starting point for treatment planning.[9,65] Nina was in the subacute stage of her RA flare. All six general objectives listed previously were important to address in her OT program.

 OT PRACTICE NOTE

As always, the occupational therapist's clinical judgment of each client's unique status is crucial for tailoring programs appropriately.

OCCUPATIONAL THERAPY INTERVENTION

Treatment methods useful in the remediation of clinical or functional problems include rest, physical agent modalities, therapeutic exercise and activity, splinting, occupational performance training, and client education. It is important to foster the client's self-efficacy in his or her ability to follow through with treatment at home given the influences of the home contexts because building the client's confidence will likely lead to the desired behavior. Asking the client a question such as "How certain are you that you can perform this activity at home as well as you did in the clinic?" can provide feedback on the need for further training and practice.[57] Chosen interventions should reflect the individual client's needs and choices whenever appropriate. General treatment precautions related to arthritis are listed in Box 38-3.

REST

Rest should be considered an active way of reducing inflammation and pain. Rest and relaxation can effectively break

TABLE 38-6 **Treatment Objectives by Stage of Inflammatory Disease**

Stage	Symptoms	Objectives	Treatment Considerations
I. Acute	Pain; inflammation; hot, red joints; tenderness; overall stiffness; limited motion	Decrease pain and inflammation. Maintain ROM. Maintain strength and endurance.	Splinting for localized rest day and night, increased bed rest, joint protection, assistive devices, physical agent modalities Gentle active ROM and/or passive ROM to point of pain (no stretch), proper positioning Functional activities to tolerance, isometric exercises
II. Subacute	Inflammation subsiding; warm, pink joints; decreased pain and tenderness; stiffness limited to morning	Decrease pain and inflammation. Maintain ROM. Maintain strength and endurance.	Less restrictive splinting for day, splinting continued at night, joint protection, assistive devices, physical agent modalities Active ROM and/or passive ROM with gentle stretch, proper positioning Increased functional activities to tolerance, isometric exercises
III. Chronic Active	Minimal inflammation, less pain and tenderness, increased activity tolerance, low endurance	Decrease pain and inflammation. Increase ROM. Increase strength and endurance.	Joint protection, splinting as needed, assistive devices as needed, physical agent modalities as needed Active ROM and/or passive ROM with stretch at end range Resistive exercises (isometric or isotonic if no risk of overstressing joints), cardiovascular exercises, increased functional activities
IV. Chronic Inactive	No inflammation, pain and stiffness from disuse, low endurance	Decrease pain. Increase or maintain ROM. Increase strength and endurance.	Joint protection, splinting as needed, assistive devices as needed, physical agent modalities as needed Active ROM and/or passive ROM with stretch at end range Resistive exercises (isometric or isotonic if no risk of overstressing joints), cardiovascular exercises, increased functional activities

Box **38-3** TREATMENT PRECAUTIONS RELATED TO ARTHRITIS
Respect pain.
Avoid fatigue.
Avoid placing stress on inflamed or unstable joints.
Use resistive exercise or activity with caution.
Be aware of sensory impairments.
Be cautious with fragile skin resulting from systemic disease or pharmacological side effects.

the vicious cycle of pain, stress, and depression by allowing the body time to heal itself. Rest can be either systemic or local. Whole body general rest, including recuperative sleep, is necessary for health. During periods of active systemic inflammatory disease, at least eight to ten hours of sleep at night and one-half to one hour morning and afternoon rest periods are recommended.[68] The amount of systemic rest needed varies by individual, from complete bed rest to an extra nap during the day. Localized rest of symptomatic joints in RA and OA may include wearing a splint, avoiding or modifying activity, or positioning during the day or at night to prevent joint stress.[22] Repetitive joint loading or motion from activity should be alternated with rest. The effectiveness of rest will be seen as improved energy level with less joint swelling, pain, and fatigue.[68]

Nina required both general rest for her body and localized rest for her inflamed wrists and hands. It was important to help her realize the physiological need for rest in the recovery from her flare. This assurance permitted her to feel less guilty about tasks left undone and enabled her to understand that taking care of herself in the short term would allow her to return to activity in the long term.

PHYSICAL AGENT MODALITIES

Physical agent modalities (PAMs) may be helpful in relieving pain or in maintaining or improving ROM. Although modality use alone has not been shown to provide sustained benefits in rheumatic disease, clients do report less pain and stiffness from a clinical standpoint.[9,84] The most commonly used PAMs are superficial heat and cold agents. Benefits of heat in arthritis include increased blood flow, pain relief, and increased tissue elasticity, with a negative effect of increasing inflammation also possible.[75] Benefits of cold include reduced inflammation and decreased pain threshold, with possible negative effects of increased tissue viscosity and decreased tissue elasticity causing more joint stiffness.[93] Heat can be delivered through hot packs, paraffin, fluidotherapy, hydrotherapy in a heated pool, and even a warm shower or bath; cold can be delivered through ice packs or gel packs. When selecting the proper modality, the therapist must consider the activity and stage of disease process. Acutely inflamed joints may be exacerbated by heat, whereas ice may be more helpful in reducing pain and inflammation. In subacute or chronic stages, heat or cold may be equally effective.[84] Nina preferred the use of heat and found it helpful in loosening her joints and lessening her pain. Even though she was in the subacute phase, some inflammation was still present; therefore, her response to heat was closely monitored so as not to worsen her inflammation. She was educated in the safe use of warm baths and microwave packs at home.

There are some medical conditions associated with rheumatic disease that contraindicate the use of thermal agents. For example, use of cold is contraindicated in clients with Raynaud's phenomenon, a vasospastic disorder of digits.[84] Clients with RA often have unstable vascular reactions to heat and cold, causing greater than normal heat retention with heat agents or increased coldness and stiffness with cold exposure.[45] Careful monitoring of client responses to PAMs is crucial. Client preference and ease of home application should also be considered before choosing an agent to use. Home paraffin units, microwave packs, and continuous low-level heat wraps are increasingly accessible and affordable in community stores, providing clients with more options.[67] Safety should always be a primary concern. Clients and significant others should be carefully instructed in proper application techniques to prevent burns or other tissue damage. Before using any modality, the therapist must fully understand tissue responses and related precautions and be competent in the safe delivery of the agent. This typically requires specific education beyond entry-level preparation. Therapists must also adhere to any state licensure or training requirements.

THERAPEUTIC EXERCISE

The purpose of exercise in the treatment of arthritis is to keep muscles and joints functioning as normally as possible by maintaining muscle strength, preventing disuse atrophy, and maintaining or improving ROM.[96] It is helpful to find out what exercises the client may already be performing and whether these exercises were suggested by a professional or a well-meaning family member or friend; many self-initiated exercises can be harmful to a person with arthritis. There is no universal exercise program suitable for all clients with arthritis. Exercise programs should be designed with regard to individual client needs and tolerances. As a good rule of thumb, pain lasting greater than 1 or 2 hours after completion of exercise signals a need to modify or decrease an exercise.[65,96] General guidelines for exercise in arthritis are to avoid undue joint stress, avoid pain and joint swelling, and work within the client's comfortable ROM.[9,55,96] The client should be taught to perform exercises slowly, smoothly, and with proper technique. The client must also understand the rationale behind the prescribed exercises.[96] Exercises to maintain ROM should be performed at least once daily, even during a flare. For RA each major joint should be taken through its full comfortable ROM. This includes the neck and possibly the jaw if symptomatic. The stiffest joints require the most attention. The type of ROM exercise selected depends on the disease activity and the joint location. Active ROM is typically preferred, with assisted or passive ROM if pain or weakness precludes it. In cases of active synovitis, AROM can exert more stress on a joint than gentle passive ROM, so passive ROM exercises may be safer.[65] Performing shoulder exercises is often easier in a supine position, which eliminates the effects of gravity. The number of repetitions should be weighed against the potential inflammatory response.[96] On good days, ten repetitions may be appropriate; on bad days, three or four repetitions within a smaller arc of motion may be indicated.[96] If the goal of exercise is to increase joint mobility, active or passive stretch can be incorporated. This is appropriate for subacute or chronic phases of disease but never for the acute phase.[65] Box 38-4 shows general active ROM exercises for rheumatoid arthritis.

Exercises for strengthening can be dynamic (isotonic) or static (isometric) and should be aimed toward recovery of function.[25,65] Strengthening must be approached cautiously so as not to increase pain, create deforming forces, and compromise joint stability. Grip-strengthening exercises, even those using light putty, can impart large forces to unstable

hand joints.[14] Additionally, this type of dynamic exercise may aggravate joints or pose a risk for potential deformity and in general should be avoided for clients with rheumatoid hand involvement.[9] Resistive exercise of any kind should never be performed during periods of acute flare or inflammation but may be used at other stages. Isometric exercises are usually the least painful for clients with RA because they eliminate joint motion and can be as effective or more effective in improving muscle strength and endurance.[65] Isometric contractions are generally held for 6 to 12 seconds.[25] Programs to maintain strength vary depending on the client's overall activity level. Clients who are sedentary may require a daily program, whereas clients who are active may need to perform only specific exercises once a week.[65] A gradual progression of repetitions or resistance is recommended.[68]

Exercises to promote general health and fitness are recommended for all adults as part of a healthy lifestyle and should be encouraged in clients with arthritis. Stationary bicycling, walking, and low-impact aerobic dancing, once thought to cause joint damage, have been found to increase flexibility, strength, endurance, and cardiovascular fitness without aggravation of symptoms.[68] T'ai Chi has been reported to have positive effects on self-efficacy, quality of life, general

---

Box **38-4** RANGE OF MOTION EXERCISES FOR RHEUMATOID ARTHRITIS

INSTRUCTIONS

1. Start with five of each exercise, one or two times each day.
2. Progress to 10 of each exercise, one or two times each day.
3. Do all exercises slowly and smoothly.
4. If in a flare, cut down on exercises but do not discontinue them entirely.

JAW

1. Open your mouth wide, then close it.
2. With your mouth open, move your jaw from side to side.
3. Bring your lower jaw forward, then relax.

NECK

4. Look up toward ceiling, then look down to the floor.
5. Bend your head toward one shoulder, then bend your head toward the other shoulder.
6. Slide your chin forward, then relax.
7. Slide your chin toward the back of your neck, then relax.

SHOULDERS AND ELBOWS

8. Shrug your shoulders up and down.
9. With your hands on your shoulders, make circles clockwise then counter-clockwise.

10. With your hands behind your head (or, if unable, on your shoulders), bring your elbows together in front of you and then spread your elbows apart.
11. Touch your shoulders with your hands, then straighten your elbows.

FOREARMS AND WRISTS

12. With your elbows partially bent and kept at your sides, turn your palms up and then down.
13. Lift your hands backward, letting your fingers curl, then bend your hands down, letting your fingers straighten.

FINGERS

14. Make fists, then open your hands and straighten your fingers.
15. Touch your thumb tips to the tips of each finger.
16. With your palms on your thigh or a table, move your thumbs away from your fingers and then slide each finger toward your thumbs.

Courtesy Occupational Therapy Department, Rancho Los Amigos National Rehabilitation Center, Downey, CA.

health status, pain, stiffness, and physical functioning in older adults with lower extremity OA[42,82] and is being used for clients with RA as well.

Whether for ROM, strengthening, or overall conditioning, the occupational therapist should work closely with the client to help ensure that any exercise program can be successfully integrated into the client's typical daily routine with a proper balance of rest and activity. Exercises ideally should be done when the client feels most limber and has the least pain. Community land- and water-based exercise classes specifically designed for people with arthritis are available through the Arthritis Foundation. They offer the added benefits of social interaction and peer support and have been shown to be safe and effective for increasing fitness and strength and decreasing pain and difficulty in daily functioning.[11,86,90] Daily upper body active ROM exercises with gentle stretch and isometric exercises for shoulders and elbows were prescribed to improve Nina's motion and strength. It was decided that the best time to perform these exercises was after her morning shower, when she felt less stiff and least fatigued. The therapist recommended that Nina become involved with an Arthritis Foundation exercise class, once her flare subsided, to build her endurance and cardiovascular conditioning. She was interested in joining and planned to attend classes on the days she worked fewer hours.

THERAPEUTIC ACTIVITY

Performance of therapeutic activities offers many benefits, both physical and psychological. Discussing current and past hobbies or having the client complete an interest survey can help the therapist determine activities that may be most appropriate for the client. New activities may be suggested or previously enjoyed activities re-introduced. A carefully chosen and graded activity can be an effective means of encouraging ROM and strength. When selecting therapeutic activities, the therapist should apply the same principles as with exercise.[65] Activities should be nonresistive, avoid patterns of deformity, and not overstress joints; instead, they should offer enough repetition of movement to help improve ROM and strength. The effect of the activity on all joints should be considered.

It is typically recommended that clients with RA not engage in activities that require the use of the hand in prolonged static positions. However, sometimes the psychological benefits of doing activities that one enjoys outweigh the risks involved, especially if the risks can be minimized. Examples of activities that are often frowned upon include knitting and crocheting. These activities are truly contraindicated only if there is active MP synovitis, developing swan-neck deformity, or thumb CMC joint involvement.[65] Potential problems may be averted by having the client wear a hand or thumb splint to support vulnerable joints while performing the activity. Additionally, educating the client to incorporate frequent rest breaks and stretching exercises for the intrinsic muscles will help to limit risks (see Chapter 28 for additional information regarding therapeutic exercise and activity).[26,65]

SPLINTING

Indications

Splinting is often an integral component in the treatment of arthritis. Splints can be used for numerous reasons, with the fundamental goal of maximizing function. It is important for the therapist to understand the pathomechanics of the disease process in order to prescribe an appropriate and feasible splinting plan. The inappropriate use of splints can be harmful. Indications for splinting in arthritis include reducing inflammation, decreasing pain, supporting unstable joints, properly positioning joints, limiting undesired motion, and increasing ROM. Although it is generally agreed that splinting has a place in the acute phase of RA, there are few documented or well-established protocols for splinting in later stages.[32] Table 38-7 summarizes potential splinting indications on the basis of the progression of joint destruction in RA.[9,65]

Ultimately, the individual needs of each client must be carefully measured. What are the primary goals for splinting? What benefits will a splint provide? What limitations will a splint impose? Which joints are involved and should be incorporated into a splint design? What effect will splinting have on unsplinted joints? Is the client receptive to splinting? What splints has the client tried or worn before? When should the splint be worn? These factors should be considered when deciding on an appropriate splinting plan.

Considerations

There are some special considerations for splinting clients with rheumatoid arthritis. Because the added weight of a splint puts additional stress on the upper extremity and may cause problems with pain and fatigue, a splint should be as lightweight as possible. Forces are also transferred from splinted to adjacent unsplinted joints. For example, a thumb splint leaving the wrist and IP joints free may cause these joints to become more symptomatic. Skin tolerance can be an issue because skin is often more fragile as a result of the RA disease process and medication effects. The presence of sensory impairments may also require closer monitoring for signs of pressure. Lastly, splint straps may need to be modified to allow for increased ease and decreased joint stress during donning and doffing of splints.

Options

If splinting is indicated, the therapist must then determine which type of splint will work best. The growing array of commercial products has led to a greater number of choices. Should the splint be rigid, semi-rigid, or soft? This will often

TABLE 38-7 **Splinting Indications by Classification of Progression of Rheumatoid Arthritis**

Stage	Symptoms/Radiographic Changes	Splinting Indications
Stage I: Early	No destructive changes; possible osteoporosis	Resting splints to decrease acute inflammation, decrease pain, protect joints
Stage II: Moderate	Osteoporosis with or without slight subchondral bone destruction, slight cartilage destruction, no joint deformities, limited joint mobility possible, muscle atrophy, extraarticular soft tissue lesions possible	Day splints to provide comfort Night splints to relieve pain and/or protect joints against potential deformity Splints to increase ROM
Stage III: Severe	Cartilage and bone destruction, joint deformity, extensive muscle atrophy, extraarticular soft tissue lesions possible	Day splints to improve function (decrease pain, provide stability, limit undesired motion, properly position joints) Night splints to provide positioning and comfort
Stage IV: Terminal	Criteria of Stage III, with fibrous and bony ankylosis	Day splints to improve function (decrease pain, provide stability, limit undesired motion, properly position joints) Night splints to provide positioning and comfort

be decided by the splint's proposed purpose and the client's preference. Rigid splints provide maximal immobilization or stability; soft splints allow for more freedom of motion; semi-rigid splints combine elements of both. Should the splint be prefabricated or custom-made? This decision is based on many splint- and client-related factors, including splint availability, cost to purchase or fabricate, durability, weight, ease of care, ease of donning and doffing, cosmetic appearance, and extent of the client's existing deformity.

Providing the client with choices will enhance splint use and client satisfaction. Studies have shown that these additional factors may encourage splint wear: flexibility of the splinting regimen and vigorous client education regarding the splint's purpose and wearing schedule, individualized splint prescriptions based on the client's comfort and preference, strong family support, positive attitudes and behaviors exhibited by healthcare providers, and benefits that are immediately obvious to the client.[18,31,37,70,71,88] Rapport, trust, sensitivity to clients' learning styles, splint trial evaluations, and providing clients with the opportunity to voice their concerns and frustrations can also enhance the collaborative process and splinting outcome.[23] The therapist can recommend splinting, but ultimately the client will decide whether the splint's benefits outweigh the limitations it imposes.

Commonly Used Splints in Arthritis

A resting hand splint is useful for the treatment of acute synovitis of the wrist and hand. Its primary function is to provide localized rest to the involved joints. It can also serve to relieve pain, decrease muscle spasm, and protect joints vulnerable to contracture or deformity from synovitis. Joints are rested in positions that place the least internal pressure on them and that are opposite that of potential deformity.[9] The recommended joint positions of rest are slight wrist

extension (0-20 degrees) and ulnar deviation (10-20 degrees), MP flexion (20-30 degrees), slight PIP and DIP flexion (10-30 degrees), and slight thumb extension and abduction at the CMC with slight flexion of the MP and IP.[32,65,98] However, the client's comfort should always take precedence, and joints should never be forced into the ideal position. The splint is worn continually for the duration of the flare and removed at least once a day for skin hygiene and gentle ROM exercises. Splint use should continue full-time for at least 2 weeks after the flare subsides, with a gradual decrease in wearing time to allow the joints to recover.[32,65] In later stages of disease, the splint is often used at night only to increase comfort and protect against deforming positions. If bilateral splints are needed, clients may alternate splints or wear the splint on the most symptomatic hand.

Commercial splints, such as those made from wire-foam or a malleable metal frame covered by soft padding (Figure 38-13), may be used if the limited adjustments they allow for can provide the client with a proper fit. This is often not possible in the presence of established joint deformities. A custom-fabricated thermoplastic splint will allow for a precise individualized fit. Joints that are asymptomatic may not need to be included in the splint. Modified resting splints with uninvolved joints left free may lessen joint stiffness related to splint wear, allow some degree of hand function while the splint is worn, and improve splint wear and comfort.

Although the benefits of resting hand splints are recognized by healthcare professionals, studies have shown that client compliance is less than optimal, at approximately 47%.[31] In a study comparing the use of soft and hard resting splints in clients with RA, pain was significantly decreased with splint wear, 57% preferred the soft splint, 33% the hard splint, and 10% no splint at all. The rate of compliance was greater for the soft splint than for the hard splint.[18]

A wrist splint is often used to provide wrist stability, decrease pain, and improve function. Supports may be custom-fabricated (Figure 38-14) or prefabricated. Because they are intended to provide support while allowing functional use of the hand, fit and comfort are crucial. A variety of commercial splints made from many materials is available, offering a full range of soft to rigid support. Aside from support, clients with arthritis frequently report a benefit from the neutral warmth that many fabrics provide. Studies have shown conflicting results across different splint styles in grip strength, dexterity, pain reduction, hand function, comfort, security during task performance, effects of stiffness, or muscle atrophy related to wrist splint wear in clients with RA.[71,88] In a study of splint preference, most clients were able to identify their preferred splint within only a few minutes of wear when given three styles to try.[87] These studies illustrate the importance of offering a wide variety of splints for each client to try. When MPs are symptomatic, a splint can be used to support them along with the wrist (Figure 38-15).

MP ulnar deviation splints may be beneficial in providing pain relief, stability, alignment, and reduced joint stress to painful, subluxed, or deviated joints. They may slow the progression of deformity, but they will not prevent or correct it.[64,73] Splints can be fabricated or obtained commercially, with support ranging from soft to rigid (Figure 38-16). Despite the variety of splint designs and materials, MP ulnar deviation splints are reported to be infrequently prescribed and used by clients.[76] Immobilization of the MPs can impede functional use of the hand or increase pain and stress on adjacent PIP joints.[64,73] Bulky or volar-based splints can also interfere with palmar sensation or impair the ability to grasp objects. However, some clients benefit from pain relief and improved digital alignment. High client satisfaction rates have been reported for a custom dorsal-based design.[76] Soft splints are commercially available or can be custom-fabricated.[34] The client's preference for use and selection of an MP ulnar deviation support should be the primary factor in decision making.[41,64]

A swan-neck splint, also known as a *PIP hyperextension block*, is used to restrict unwanted PIP hyperextension motion. Swan-neck deformities often cause difficulty with hand closure because PIP tendons and ligaments can catch during motion and the finger flexors have less of a mechanical advantage to initiate flexion when the PIP is in a hyperextended position. By blocking the PIP in slight flexion, the client can flex the PIP more efficiently, thus improving

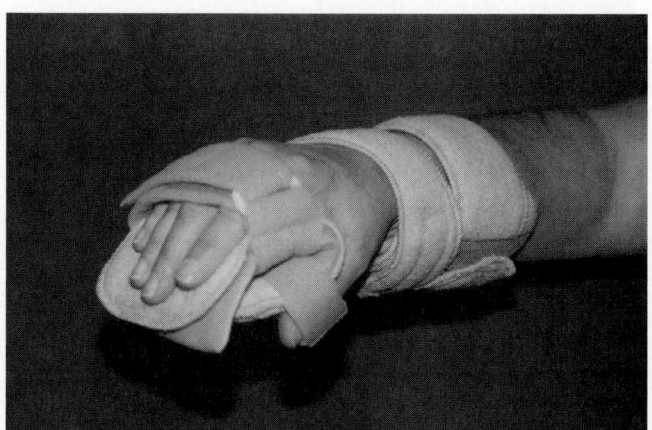

Figure 38-13 Prefabricated resting hand splint. (Courtesy Occupational Therapy Department, Rancho Los Amigos National Rehabilitation Center, Downey, CA.)

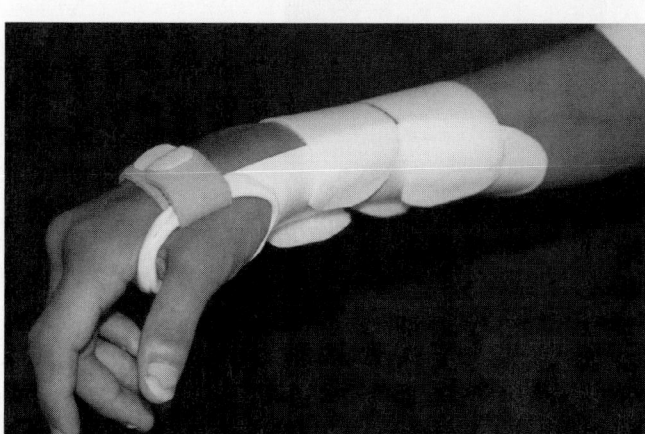

Figure 38-14 Custom-fabricated thermoplastic wrist splint. (Courtesy Occupational Therapy Department, Rancho Los Amigos National Rehabilitation Center, Downey, CA.)

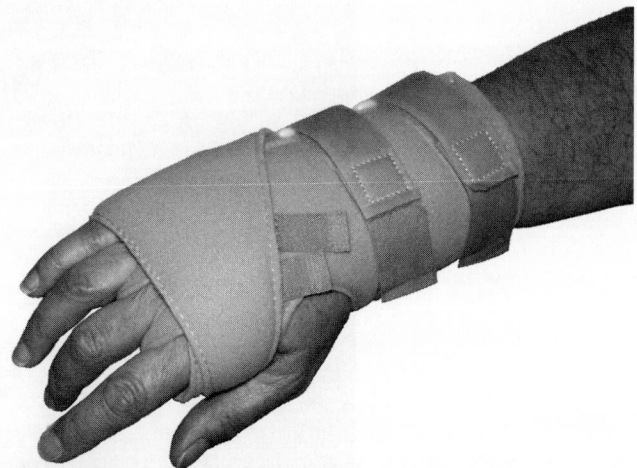

Figure 38-15 Prefabricated wrist and metacarpophalangeal joint soft support. (Courtesy Occupational Therapy Department, Rancho Los Amigos National Rehabilitation Center, Downey, CA.)

hand function. Swan-neck splints can be custom-fabricated from thermoplastics for short-term or trial use. For long-term use or for use on adjacent fingers, commercial products made from metal or polypropylene are often recommended because they are more durable, less bulky, more easily cleaned, and more cosmetically appealing (Figure 38-17). Swan-neck splints

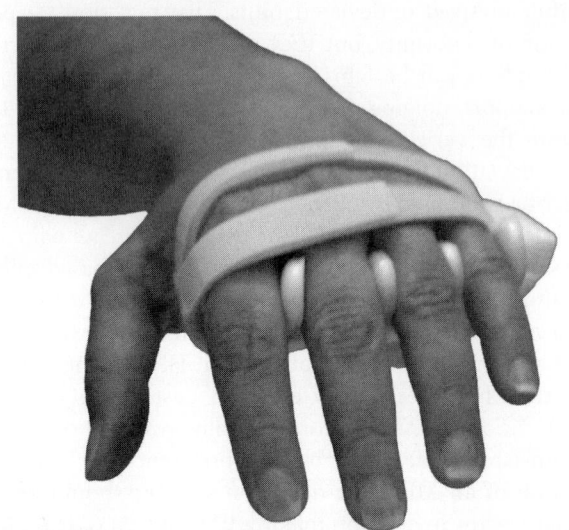

Figure 38-16 Rigid prefabricated wire-foam metacarpophalangeal joint ulnar deviation splint. (Courtesy Occupational Therapy Department, Rancho Los Amigos National Rehabilitation Center, Downey, CA.)

or splints of similar design can also be used to provide lateral stability to unstable IP joints of the fingers or thumb.[9,41]

Flexible boutonnière deformities may benefit from boutonnière splints to block the PIP in extension and leave the DIP free to flex. These can be fabricated by the therapist or custom-ordered from the same companies that manufacture swan-neck splints. As a result of the direct pressure that they exert over the dorsum of the PIP, the skin must be monitored closely. Clients may reject wearing these splints during the day if limiting PIP flexion impedes function. Night splinting with the PIP in maximal extension can be used in an attempt to maintain ROM.[9]

Thumb splinting can provide positioning opposite that of developing deformity in early stages of disease and a more stable and pain-free pinch for function in later stages.[9] Hand-based short thumb spica splints or opponens splints leave the wrist and IP free and can be used for problems at the MP or CMC. Splinting for the CMC joint may sometimes necessitate inclusion of the wrist or MP joints, but both hand-based and forearm-based (long thumb spica) types have been found to be effective.[41,91,94] Several thermoplastic splint designs exist, as do numerous prefabricated splints made from a variety of materials. Depending on the client's symptoms and stage of disease, a soft support (Figure 38-18, *A*) may suffice or the client may require a rigid support (see Fig. 38-18, *B*) to counteract the stressors applied to joints during functional use. In a recent study comparing a short neoprene thumb spica and a custom

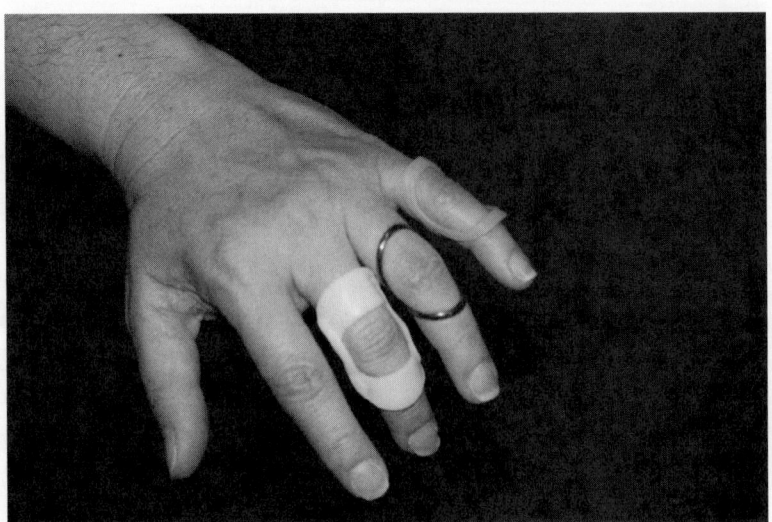

Figure 38-17 Splints for swan-neck deformity: custom-fabricated thermoplastic, commercial custom-sized metal, and prefabricated polypropylene. (Courtesy Occupational Therapy Department, Rancho Los Amigos National Rehabilitation Center, Downey, CA.)

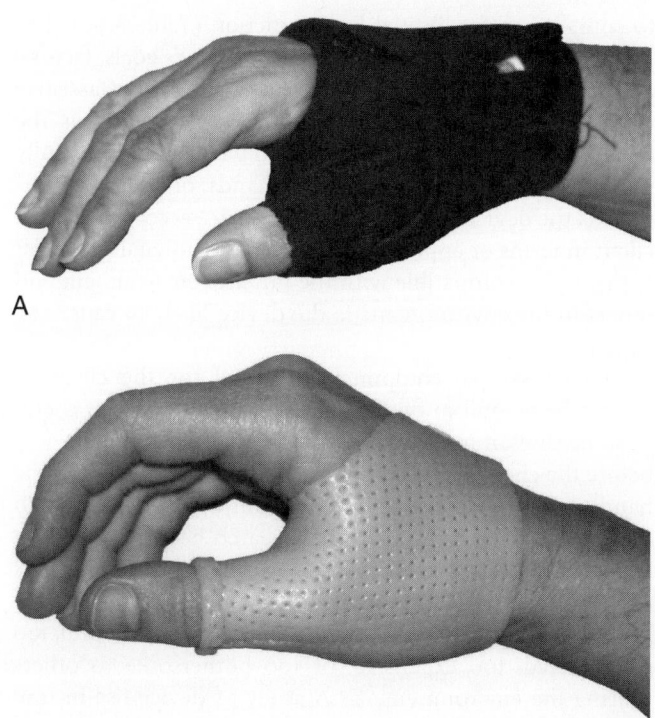

A

B

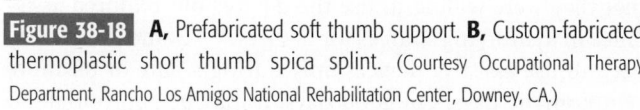
Figure 38-18 **A,** Prefabricated soft thumb support. **B,** Custom-fabricated thermoplastic short thumb spica splint. (Courtesy Occupational Therapy Department, Rancho Los Amigos National Rehabilitation Center, Downey, CA.)

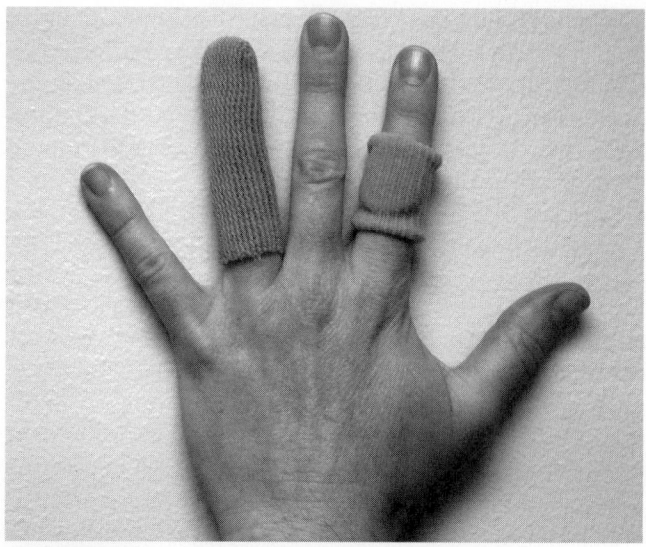
Figure 38-19 Silicone-lined digital sleeve and pad. (Courtesy Occupational Therapy Department, Rancho Los Amigos National Rehabilitation Center, Downey, CA.)

thermoplastic hand-based splint in OA of the CMC, both splints improved pain and function and reduced subluxation. The thermoplastic splint reduced subluxation more, but the neoprene splint provided better pain relief and was preferred by clients.[95]

Dynamic splints and serial static splints may be used to regain ROM lost by shortening of periarticular structures or to maximize motion after surgical procedures such as joint arthroplasty. If the joint space is preserved (as determined by radiographs), there is a soft end-feel, and there is no more than minimal inflammation, gentle splinting may be indicated. The program should be monitored closely for adverse signs of increased pain and swelling. Static splints are often better tolerated than dynamic ones because they apply lesser amounts of force to the joint.[41]

Finally, silicone-lined digital sleeves and pads (Figure 38-19) may be helpful in protecting painful nodes or nodules from external trauma.

The splinting program for Nina focused on decreasing her inflammation and pain and protecting vulnerable joints. Because she had no established deformity, prefabricated splints were a viable option, one that she preferred. Bilateral lightweight resting hand splints were selected for use at night. To afford her some ability to function,

semi-rigid wrist splints were prescribed for use during the day. She was taught to monitor her symptoms and intermittently use the resting hand splints as needed if daytime activity led to increased pain or inflammation. Splint straps were modified by attaching loops to one end so that she could more easily manage them (see Chapter 29 for additional information).

OCCUPATIONAL PERFORMANCE TRAINING

An effective means of maintaining functional motion and strength with arthritis is to have clients perform daily occupations.[65] During active stages of disease, these may be limited to just a few, such as feeding and hygiene. As the client's condition improves, usual life activities should be resumed because this will help promote physical status and psychological well-being. An important but sometimes neglected aspect of ADL training is sexual counseling. Given pain and ROM limitations resulting from arthritis or movement restrictions imposed postoperatively after joint replacement, an open discussion of issues and illustrations of more comfortable and safe positions for intercourse may prove helpful for clients and their partners. Excellent resources for sexual functioning with disabilities are available (see Chapter 12 for additional information).[24,81]

Analysis of activity demands and activity contexts is a critical component in helping clients maintain, restore, or enhance their engagement in desired activities and occupations. Environmental modifications, alternative methods, or assistive devices often make a difference by increasing clients' independence, ease, and safety in completing meaningful occupations with less pain and stress to their joints. Creative problem solving with the client as an active participant can lead to solutions for unique challenges. Understanding the client's perspective, the meaning of roles, and the cultural and physical environment will allow the therapist to propose more effective intervention.[6]

ASSISTIVE DEVICES

Numerous assistive devices can be fabricated or purchased commercially. The therapist should be familiar with types of available devices and sources where they can be obtained at minimal expense. Many devices that were previously available exclusively from medical suppliers can now be found in retail stores at much less cost. Commonly used in arthritis interventions are extended handle devices (e.g., dressing sticks, sock aids, shoe horns, bath sponges, hair brushes, toilet aids; Figure 38-20, A) to compensate for loss of proximal ROM and strength, and built-up handle devices (e.g., eating utensils, button aids, writing implements; see Figure 38-20, B)

to compensate for limited hand function (Table 38-8). The therapist should carefully consider the client's goals, factors, activity demands, and contexts when suggesting assistive devices.[59,65] Most relevant to clients with arthritis: Is the client receptive to using a device? Will the device successfully reduce pain, joint stress, energy demands, or time expenditure? Is the device easy to use? Is the device acceptable to the client in terms of appearance, cost, and maintenance needs? Is the device compatible with the physical environment and others in the environment? Is the device likely to cause any negative effects?

Having sample equipment on hand for the client to try can be helpful in finding the best device for each client. In some cases, it may be necessary to modify existing devices before the client can use them successfully. For example, the handle of a dressing stick may be built up for a client with limited grasp. Surprisingly little research has been done on assistive devices in arthritis and characteristics of device users and non-users, but clinical experience shows that clients are less likely to use devices that they perceive as not helpful, too complicated, too expensive, or too bothersome to others sharing the environment.[79,89] A study of device use in frail elderly clients, including some with arthritis, demonstrated that they were willing to use the devices but required assistance in identifying sources for devices.[60,61] Some clients may need to use assistive devices only during a flare or on more symptomatic days. On good days, it may be appropriate to encourage clients to perform tasks without them to promote strength and mobility.

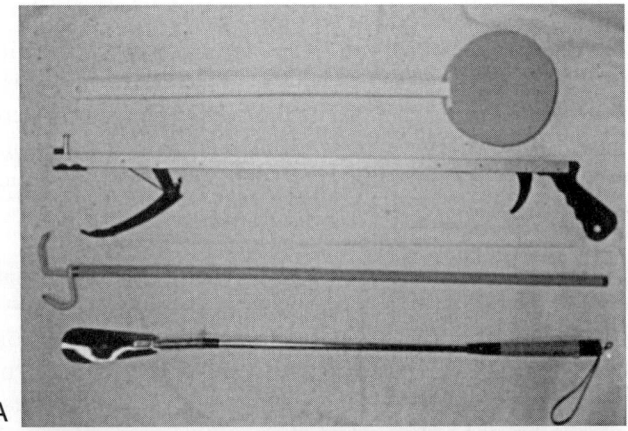

A

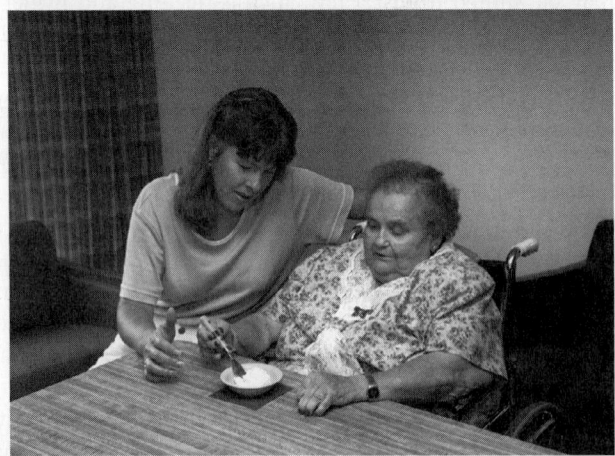

B

Figure 38-20 **A,** Extended-handle devices. (From Harris ED, et al: *Kelley's textbook of rheumatology*, ed 7, Philadelphia, 2005, WB Saunders.) **B,** Built-up handle. (From Byers-Connon S, Lohman H, Padilla RL: *Occupational therapy for elders: strategies for the COTA*, ed 2, St Louis, 2004, Mosby.)

TABLE 38-8 **Commonly Used Assistive Devices for Arthritis**

Activity	Assistive Devices
Dressing	Dressing stick, shoe horn, sock aid, button hook, zipper pull, elastic shoe laces
Bathing	Hand-held shower hose, bath bench, grab bars, long-handled sponge
Toileting	Raised toilet seat, grab bars, extended perineal hygiene aid
Hygiene and grooming	Built-up or extended-handle toothbrush, suction denture brush, extended-handle hair brush or comb, suction nail brush, mounted nail clipper
Feeding	Built-up or extended-handle utensils, lightweight T-handle mug
Meal preparation	Electric can and jar openers, adapted cutting board, built-up handle utensils, ergonomic right-angled knives, rolling utility cart, knob turner for stove, reacher
Miscellaneous	Door knob levers, built-up or extended key holder, extended-handle dust pan, built-up pen, loop or spring-loaded scissors, speaker phone

CLIENT AND FAMILY EDUCATION

Providing clients with as much information as possible regarding their conditions and treatment is a crucial component of OT and should be integrated throughout all phases of the program. Whether it is the client's first visit or one of many therapy encounters, educational needs should always be explored. The client's estimation of the therapist's credibility, the quality of the therapeutic relationship, and whether the client's experience confirms the therapist's statements are important factors tied to success in changing the client's knowledge and beliefs.[57] Client education has been shown to empower clients and lead to changes in disease management behaviors and self-efficacy.[15,56,62]

 ETHICAL CONSIDERATIONS

Information should be presented at a level appropriate for each client and significant other, with sensitivity to learning styles; socioeconomic status; educational level; cultural implications; and personal values, beliefs, and feelings.

Rather than focusing exclusively on providing basic information and generic skills, encouraging client self-reflection and transformation of client perspectives has been suggested as a helpful part of rehabilitation.[28] Repetition, reinforcement, and real-life application to the client's situation are other keys to education. By focusing on the client's symptoms and concerns, the therapist can capitalize on "teachable moments" to provide present-oriented and problem-focused learning activities.[12] It may be helpful to provide both verbal and written instructions. The following are some important educational aspects to cover: disease process, symptom management, joint protection and fatigue management, and community resources.

Disease Process

Does the client understand the type of arthritis, basic underlying pathology, medications, and medication side effects? Does the client understand that prolonged synovitis in RA can lead to irreversible joint damage and potential disability? Does the client feel comfortable in discussing questions with the physician, nurse, or other treating clinicians? Does the client know of available resources to learn more?

Symptom Management

Does the client know how to monitor for signs and symptoms of inflammation? Does the client understand that pain lasting for more than 1 or 2 hours after an activity signals a need to modify or cease doing that task? Does the client

understand the rationale behind, demonstrate appropriate use of, and appropriately integrate rest, exercise, splinting, and physical agent modalities into a daily routine? Do family members understand the client's abilities and when they should or should not assist the client with activities? Does the client know to take a cautious approach to nontraditional arthritis remedies so as not to fall prey to medical quackery?

Joint Protection and Fatigue Management

Does the client understand the rationale and general principles of joint protection and fatigue management? More important, does the client successfully integrate them into daily activities? It can be challenging not just to help the client understand the potential implications but to translate learning into action. The purpose of joint protection is to reduce internal and external joint stress, pain, and inflammation in involved joints and preserve the integrity of joint structures during performance of daily activities.[65] Although it has not been proved that use of joint protection techniques prevents deterioration, knowledge of the disease process, pathomechanics of deformity, and clinical experience suggest that joint protection is a sound idea.[26] Studies have shown that clients who experience pain relief or improved function may be more receptive to changing behaviors.[26,39,69] Fatigue management, a more contemporary term for energy conservation, is aimed toward saving and expending energy wisely (Box 38-5). Organizing the environment, pacing activity, and resting can successfully moderate fatigue.[26] Instruction of principles should be based on teaching key concepts rather than general rules and should be specifically applied to each client's lifestyle and pattern of occupation.[65,80] Practice in the therapy setting can help with carryover because following these principles often necessitates a change in lifelong habits. General principles of joint protection and fatigue management are especially helpful for clients with RA or clients with OA involving the hands, hips, or knees.[22,26,65] A summary of principles follows; more detailed information can be found in the sources cited.

Joint protection and fatigue management principles are as follows:

- *Respect pain.* Pain is a signal from the body that something is wrong. Clients often feel that they can ignore and work through pain, but the result is often more pain. If pain is present from an acute episode of inflammation, rest and avoidance of activity are indicated so as not to worsen pain and inflammation. In chronic stages, pain that lasts for more than 1 or 2 hours after completion of an activity indicates that the activity should be modified or avoided. Clients should be encouraged to be aware of their limits and stop activities *before* pain occurs. Disregard of pain can lead to joint damage.
- *Maintain muscle strength and joint ROM.* Joints that are less stiff and have balanced strength will be less susceptible to further injury. Limited motion at one joint transmits force to another and may require exaggerated motions

BOX **38-5** PRINCIPLES OF FATIGUE MANAGEMENT

ATTITUDES AND EMOTIONS

Remove yourself from stressful situations.
Refrain from concentrating on things that make you tense.
Close your eyes, and visualize pleasant places and thoughts.

BODY MECHANICS

When lifting something that is low, bend your knees and lift by straightening your legs. Try to keep your back straight.
Avoid reaching (use reachers). Avoid stretching, bending, carrying, and climbing. If you have to bend, keep your back straight.
Incorporate good posture into your activities.
Whenever possible, sit when working.
To get up from a chair, slide forward to the edge of the chair. With your feet flat on the floor, lean forward and push with your *palms* on the arms or seat of the chair. Stand by straightening your legs.
Before you get tired, stop and rest.

WORK PACE

Plan on getting 10 to 12 hours of rest daily (naps and nights).
Work at your own pace.
Spread tedious tasks throughout the week.
Do the tasks that require the most energy at the times when you have the most energy.
Alternate easy and difficult activities, and take a 10- to 15-minute rest break each hour.

LEISURE TIME

Devote a portion of your day to an activity that you enjoy and find relaxing.
Check out what's available in the community.

WORK METHODS

Keep items within easy reach.
Use good light and proper ventilation and room temperature.
Use joint protection techniques.
Work surfaces should be at a correct height.

ORGANIZATION

Plan ahead; don't rush or push yourself.
Decide which jobs are absolutely necessary.
Share the workload with family and friends.

HOW TO BEGIN

Plan ahead by charting your daily routine.
Make a list of tasks, and spread them out in your schedule.
Include daily rest periods and rest breaks during energy-consuming times.

WEEKLY SCHEDULE

TIME.	SUN.	MON.	TUES.	WED.	THUR.	FRI.	SAT.
7:00							
8:00							
9:00							
10:00							
11:00							
12:00							
1:00							
2:00							
3:00							
4:00							
5:00							
6:00							
7:00							
8:00							
9:00							
10:00							

Check your schedule for the following factors:
- Is there one day in the week that is longer than the others?
- Are heavier tasks distributed through the week?
- Is there a long task that could be done in several steps?
- Will your plan allow for flexibility?
- Have you devoted part of your day to a relaxing activity?
- Does your plan use the principles of energy conservation?

---

at other joints to accomplish a task. For example, loss of MP motion will affect the PIP. Daily functioning and exercise programs should be done with all joint protection principles in mind to ensure that they are as least stressful as possible.
- *Use each joint in its most stable anatomical and functional plane.* This plane is the point at which the resistance to motion is provided by muscle rather than ligament. Following this principle will minimize excessive stress on ligaments and allow muscle power to be used with the greatest mechanical advantage. Examples include not leaning to

either side when rising from a seated position to lessen rotational forces on the knees and pinching with the pad of the thumb and the IP in a flexed position to minimize force on the ulnar collateral ligament.
- *Avoid positions of deformity.* The customary way of performing tasks may cause forces to be applied in directions of deformity. Tasks involving tight squeezing, pinching, or twisting motions are especially stressful. Opening a jar lid, turning a doorknob, cutting food with a knife, and lifting a coffee cup are all activities promoting MP ulnar deviation. Instead, the client with hand involvement can be encouraged

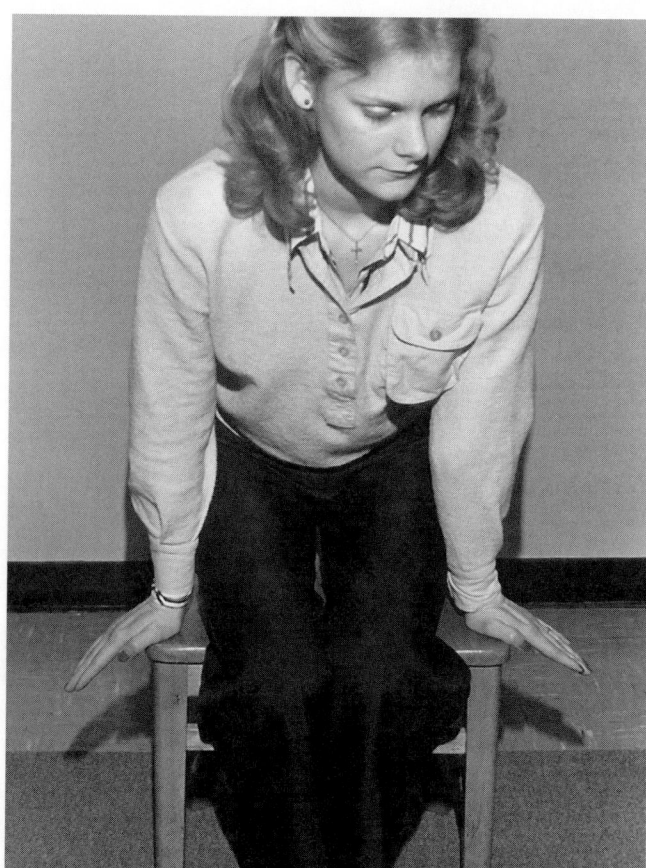

Figure 38-21 Use of palms to push off chair helps to prevent dislocation of finger joints.

to open lids using the palm of the hand and shoulder motion or a jar opener; to turn a doorknob with an adapted lever; to cut food using a dagger-type grip, rolling pizza cutter, or adapted knife; and to lift coffee mugs using two hands. Static positioning should also be considered. For example, the client should be discouraged from leaning his or her chin on the back of the fingers because this applies considerable force to the flexed MPs.

- *Use the strongest joints available.* Using larger, inherently stronger joints reduces the stress on smaller joints. Carrying bags and purses on the shoulder or elbow lessens strain on the wrist and hand. Properly fitting backpacks or waist packs are other good alternatives, as is pushing or pulling a rolling cart instead of carrying items on the body. The palms rather than the fingers should be used to lift, push, or take weight to better distribute the forces.

- *Ensure correct patterns of movement.* The client may adopt incorrect patterns because of pain, deformity, muscle imbalance, or habit. For example, the client may use the dorsum of the fingers to push up from a seated position. This movement places deforming forces toward MP flexion. A more suitable pattern is to use the flat surface of the palm (Figure 38-21). In the hand, use of the long extensors

during finger movement should be maintained. Finger flexion should be initiated at the DIPs while maintaining extension at the MPs versus leading motion with the intrinsic muscles.

- *Avoid staying in one position for long periods.* Prolonged static positions can lead to joint stiffness and muscle fatigue. Positional stress is then transmitted to the joint ligaments, which may already be in a weakened state. Changing body positions and gripping postures, taking frequent breaks, and integrating active motion exercises during activities such as computer keyboarding, writing, gardening, and knitting can prevent fatigue, soreness, stiffness, and resulting poor movement patterns.

- *Avoid starting an activity that cannot be stopped immediately if it becomes too stressful.* This will prevent the load from going to the joint capsule and ligaments if muscles tire. Continuing a task that causes sudden or severe pain is likely to cause joint damage, and severe fatigue can cause poor movement patterns and safety risks. Realistic planning of options can help prevent these situations. For example, clients can keep a bath bench available in case they need to rest while standing in the shower. Clients can also can note the location of benches in a mall in relation to the stores where they plan to shop.

- *Balance rest and activity.* Chronic pain and a systemic disease such as RA can drain both physical and psychological resources. Helping the client understand the physiological need for proper rest can facilitate this often difficult lifestyle change. The key to increasing functional endurance is to rest *before* becoming overfatigued, which could mean napping or taking breaks during or between activities. Clients with arthritis often relate similar stories of feeling the need to take advantage of good days by trying to complete as many tasks as possible. These good days are more than likely followed by several bad days as their bodies try to recover. Balancing activities during the day and longer-term across the week or month can be accomplished through planning and establishing priorities.

- *Reduce the force and effort.* Less force and effort equates to less joint stress, less pain, and less fatigue. Using built-up handles, levers, more even distribution of loads, alternative methods, and other aforementioned joint protection and fatigue management techniques can help toward this end. For example, rearranging the kitchen environment to have everything within easy reach, planning tasks and gathering all needed items, sitting down while at the sink or stove, and using assistive devices all contribute to easier meal preparation.

Community Resources

Does the client know of and use available resources? Clients should be made aware, and encouraged to take advantage, of them. Reading materials, exercise and educational programs, and support groups can supplement medical and therapy intervention and promote lasting positive

---

Box **38-6** SELECT ARTHRITIS FOUNDATION PROGRAMS AND MATERIALS

EXERCISE PROGRAMS

Arthritis Foundation Aquatic Program (community water exercise)

People with Arthritis Can Exercise (community exercise, basic and advanced levels)

Arthritis Today Walking Guide (tips, 12-week home walking plan)

Walk with Ease (audiotape and book)

EDUCATIONAL PROGRAMS

Arthritis Basics for Change (self-help home study)

Arthritis Self-Help Course (group education)

WRITTEN MATERIALS

Alternative and Complementary Therapies

Arthritis Answers

Arthritis and Pregnancy

Arthritis in the Workplace

Arthritis Today magazine

Arthritis Today Drug Guide

Arthritis Today Supplement Guide

Diet and Your Arthritis

Exercise and Your Arthritis

Gardening with Arthritis

Golf and Arthritis

Guide to Intimacy and Arthritis

Living With Osteoarthritis

Living With Rheumatoid Arthritis

Managing Your Activities

Managing Your Pain

Managing Your Stress

Protect Your Joints

Range of Motion Exercises

Surgery and Arthritis

RESOURCES

RA Connect Online Community

---

self-management behaviors. The Internet, libraries, YMCAs, and senior centers are sources of information and activity or exercise programs. The Arthritis Foundation, a national organization with many local chapters throughout the country, is an excellent resource for clients, families, and clinicians. Among other services, the Foundation offers educational pamphlets, pool- and land-based exercise programs, self-help groups, and support groups designed exclusively for persons with arthritis. Box 38-6 highlights some programs and materials of special relevance to persons with RA and OA.

Occupational performance training was an important component of Nina's OT intervention. Her ability to continue working was addressed through a combination of activity modification, assistive devices, and client education. Client education focused on her ability to better understand her disease process, manage her symptoms, and integrate joint protection and fatigue management principles into her life. Nina and the therapist reviewed her typical weekly schedule and together planned one that allowed for a more suitable balance of rest and activity given her patterns of fatigue and peak energy. The therapist recommended ways to improve Nina's computer work station at home, including moving the keyboard and monitor to more appropriate heights, adjusting her chair for optimal body positioning, using a pad to support her wrists, and switching from a standard mouse to a track-ball device. Assistive devices were recommended for other occupations, such as cooking and managing her home. Mutual problem solving identified solutions that allowed Nina to gradually return to her previous level of work hours. Among these solutions were having Nina do

much more work from her home, where she could rest as needed, and to spread out visits to her contracted businesses over several weeks and only when needed. Planning and taking an afternoon rest before picking up her grandchildren from school gave her the energy to take them to the park more frequently.

SUMMARY

Arthritis is a chronic condition that can impose devastating limitations on a person's ability to engage in meaningful occupations. It is important for the therapist to understand the different disease processes and pathomechanics of joint destruction found in OA and RA. Through a carefully crafted program based on a thorough evaluation of physical, psychosocial, and functional barriers, OT can decrease pain, protect joints, and enable increased participation in life skills.

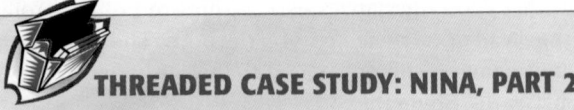

THREADED CASE STUDY: NINA, PART 2

Critical evaluation components in assessing Nina's prior and current functional status were the occupational profile and typical day assessment; assessment of clinical status included pain, inflammation, stiffness, range of motion, strength, endurance, and functional mobility. The aspects of the disease process most problematic to Nina were inflammation, pain, and fatigue from a flare

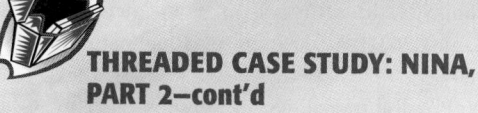

THREADED CASE STUDY: NINA, PART 2—cont'd

of her rheumatoid arthritis. Her ability to engage in her employment was affected by her motor and process performance skills; roles and routines performance patterns; physical, social, personal, temporal, and virtual contexts; object, space, body functions, and body structures activity demands; sleep, energy, attention, joints, and muscle function client factors.

Nina benefited from splinting, exercise, heat, and occupational performance training with activity modification, assistive devices, and client education in symptom management, joint protection, fatigue management, and available resources. A collaborative approach throughout the entire therapy process was essential to promoting lasting benefits and engagement in meaningful occupations.

Review Questions

1. What are the major differences between osteoarthritis and rheumatoid arthritis?
2. What are three systemic signs of rheumatoid arthritis?
3. What are clinical signs of joint inflammation?
4. When is resistive exercise appropriate for persons with rheumatoid arthritis?
5. What are typical indications for splinting in arthritis?
6. What are the purposes and major principles of joint protection and fatigue management?
7. What assistive devices are commonly helpful for clients with arthritis?
8. What are general treatment precautions related to arthritis?

REFERENCES

1. Alter S, Feldon T, Terrono AL: Pathomechanics of deformities in the arthritic hand and wrist. In Mackin EJ, et al: *Rehabilitation of the hand and upper extremity*, ed 5, St Louis, 2002, Mosby.
2. Anderson RJ: Rheumatoid arthritis clinical and laboratory features. In Klippel JH, editor: *Primer of the rheumatic diseases*, ed 12, Atlanta, 2001, Arthritis Foundation.
3. Arthritis Foundation: *Osteoarthritis*, Atlanta, 2003, Arthritis Foundation.
4. Arthritis Foundation: *Rheumatoid arthritis*, Atlanta, 2003, Arthritis Foundation.
5. Aulicino PL: Clinical examination of the hand. In Mackin EJ, et al: *Rehabilitation of the hand and upper extremity*, ed 5, St Louis, 2002, Mosby.
6. Backman C: Functional assessment. In Melvin J, Jensen G, editors: *Rheumatologic rehabilitation series, volume 1: assessment and management*, Bethesda, MD, 1998, American Occupational Therapy Association.
7. Bell-Krotoski JA: Sensibility testing with the Semmes-Weinstein monofilaments. In Mackin EJ, et al: *Rehabilitation of the hand and upper extremity*, ed 5, St Louis, 2002, Mosby.
8. Berenbaum F: Osteoarthritis epidemiology, pathology, and pathogenesis. In Klippel JH, editor: *Primer of the rheumatic diseases*, ed 12, Atlanta, 2001, Arthritis Foundation.
9. Biese J: Therapist's evaluation and conservative management of rheumatoid arthritis in the hand and wrist. In Mackin EJ, et al: *Rehabilitation of the hand and upper extremity*, ed 5, St Louis, 2002, Mosby.
10. Bland JH, Melvin JL, Hasson S: Osteoarthritis. In Melvin J, Jensen G, editors: *Rheumatologic rehabilitation series, volume 1: assessment and management*, Bethesda, MD, 1998, American Occupational Therapy Association.
11. Boutaugh ML: Arthritis Foundation community-based physical activity programs: effectiveness and implementation issues, *Arthritis Rheum* 49:463, 2003.
12. Boutaugh ML, Brady TJ: Patient education for self-management. In Melvin J, Jensen G, editors: *Rheumatologic rehabilitation series, volume 1: assessment and management*, Bethesda, MD, 1998, American Occupational Therapy Association.
13. Bozentka DJ: Pathogenesis of osteoarthritis. In Mackin EJ, et al: *Rehabilitation of the hand and upper extremity*, ed 5, St Louis, 2002, Mosby.
14. Brand PW, Hollister A: *Clinical mechanics of the hand*, ed 2, St Louis, 1993, Mosby.
15. Brekke M, Hjortdahl P, Kvien TK: Changes in self-efficacy and health status over five years: a longitudinal observational study of 306 patients with rheumatoid arthritis, *Arthritis Rheum* 49: 342, 2003.
16. Buckwalter JA, Ballard WT: Operative treatment of arthritis. In Klippel JH, editor: *Primer of the rheumatic diseases*, ed 12, Atlanta, 2001, Arthritis Foundation.
17. Callahan LF, Yelin EH: The social and economic consequences of rheumatic disease. In Arthritis Foundation: *Osteoarthritis*, Atlanta, 2003, Arthritis Foundation.
18. Callinan NJ, Mathiowetz V: Soft versus hard resting splints in rheumatoid arthritis: pain relief, preference, and compliance, *Am J Occup Ther* 50:347, 1996.
19. Cannon GW: Osteoarthritis treatment. In Klippel JH, editor: *Primer of the rheumatic diseases*, ed 12, Atlanta, 2001, Arthritis Foundation.
20. Centers for Disease Control and Prevention: Arthritis prevalence and activity limitations, U.S., 1990, *Morb Mortal Weekly Rep* 43:433, 1994.
21. Centers for Disease Control and Prevention: Prevalence of disabilities and associated health conditions among adults, U.S., 1999, *Morb Mortal Weekly Rep* 50:120, 2000.
22. Chang RW: *Rehabilitation of persons with rheumatoid arthritis*, Gaithersburg, MD, 1996, Aspen.
23. Collins L: Helping patients help themselves: improving orthotic use, *OT Practice* 4:30, 1999.
24. Comfort A: *Sexual consequences of disability*, Philadelphia, 1978, George F Stickley.

25. Coppard BM, Gale JR: Therapeutic exercise. In Melvin J, Jensen G, editors: *Rheumatologic rehabilitation series, volume 1: assessment and management*, Bethesda, MD, 1998, American Occupational Therapy Association.

26. Cordery J, Rocchi M: Joint protection and fatigue management. In Melvin J, Jensen G, editors: *Rheumatologic rehabilitation series, volume 1: assessment and management*, Bethesda, MD, 1998, American Occupational Therapy Association.

27. Creed F, Ash G: Depression in rheumatoid arthritis: aetiology and treatment, *Int Rev Psychiatry* 4:23, 1992.

28. Dubouloz CJ, et al: Transformation of meaning perspectives in clients with rheumatoid arthritis, *Am J Occup Ther* 58(4): 398, 2004.

29. Duncan MA, Siegfried DR: *Arthritis today 2005 drug guide*, Atlanta, 2005, Arthritis Foundation.

30. Escalante A, Rincon I: The disablement process in rheumatoid arthritis, *Arthritis Rheum* 47:333, 2002.

31. Feinberg J: Effects of the arthritis health professional on compliance with use of resting hand splints by patients with rheumatoid arthritis, *Arthritis Care Res* 5:17, 1992.

32. Fess EE, et al: *Hand and upper extremity splinting: principles and methods*, ed 3, St Louis, 2005, Mosby.

33. Fleming A, et al: Early rheumatoid disease. II. Patterns of joint involvement, *Ann Rheum Dis* 35(4):361, 1976.

34. Gilbert-Lenef L: Soft ulnar deviation splint, *J Hand Ther* 7: 29, 1994.

35. Gornisiewicz M, Moreland LW: Rheumatoid arthritis. In Robbins L, editor: *Clinical care in the rheumatic diseases*, ed 2, Atlanta, 2001, Association of Rheumatology Health Professionals.

36. Goronzy JJ, Weyand CM: Rheumatoid arthritis epidemiology, pathology, and pathogenesis. In Klippel JH, editor: *Primer of the rheumatic diseases*, ed 12, Atlanta, 2001, Arthritis Foundation.

37. Groth GN, Wulf MB: Compliance with hand rehabilitation: health beliefs and strategies, *J Hand Ther* 8:18, 1995.

38. Hagglund KJ, Frank RG: Mood disorders. In Robbins L, editor: *Clinical care in the rheumatic diseases*, ed 2, Atlanta, 2001, Association of Rheumatology Health Professionals.

39. Hammond A: Joint protection behavior in patients with rheumatoid arthritis following an education program, *Arthritis Care Res* 7:5, 1994.

40. Hannan MT: Epidemiology of rheumatic diseases. In Robbins L, editor: *Clinical care in the rheumatic diseases*, ed 2, Atlanta, 2001, Association of Rheumatology Health Professionals.

41. Harrell PB: Splinting of the hand. In Robbins L, editor: *Clinical care in the rheumatic diseases*, ed 2, Atlanta, 2001, Association of Rheumatology Health Professionals.

42. Hartman CA, Manos TM, Winter C, et al: Effects of T'ai Chi training on function and quality of life indicators in older adults with osteoarthritis, *J Am Geriatr Soc* 48(12):1553, 2000.

43. Hawley DJ: Clinical outcomes: issues and measurement. In Melvin J, Jensen G, editors: *Rheumatologic rehabilitation series, volume 1: assessment and management*, Bethesda, MD, 1998, American Occupational Therapy Association.

44. Hawley DJ: Functional ability, health status, and quality of life. In Robbins L, editor: *Clinical care in the rheumatic diseases*, ed 2, Atlanta, 2001, Association of Rheumatology Health Professionals.

45. Hayes KW: Physical modalities. In Robbins L, editor: *Clinical care in the rheumatic diseases*, ed 2, Atlanta, 2001, Association of Rheumatology Health Professionals.

46. Hayes KW, Petersen CM: Joint and soft tissue pain. In Melvin J, Jensen G, editors: *Rheumatologic rehabilitation series, volume 1: assessment and management*, Bethesda, MD, 1998, American Occupational Therapy Association.

47. Hochberg MC: Osteoarthritis clinical features. In Klippel JH, editor: *Primer of the rheumatic diseases*, ed 12, Atlanta, 2001, Arthritis Foundation.

48. Huskisson EC: Measurement of pain, *Lancet* 2:1127, 1974.

49. Jebsen RH, et al: An objective and standardized test of hand function, *Arch Phys Med Rehabil* 50(6):311, 1969.

50. Kolasinski SL: Complementary and alternative treatments. In Robbins L, editor: *Clinical care in the rheumatic diseases*, ed 2, Atlanta, 2001, Association of Rheumatology Health Professionals.

51. Kraus V: Pathogenesis and treatment of osteoarthritis, *Med Clin North Am* 81:85, 1997.

52. Law M, et al: *The Canadian Occupational Performance Measure manual*, ed. 3, Ottawa, 1998, CAOT Publications ACE.

53. Lawrence RC, et al: Estimates of the prevalence of arthritis and selected musculoskeletal disorders in the United States, *Arthritis Rheum* 41(5):778, 1998.

54. Livneh H, Antonak RF: *Psychosocial adaptation to chronic illness and disability*, Gaithersburg, MD, 1997, Aspen.

55. Lockard MA: Exercise for the patient with upper quadrant osteoarthritis, *J Hand Ther* 13:175, 2000.

56. Lorig KR, Holman HR: Arthritis self-management studies: a twelve-year review, *Health Edu Q* 20:17, 1993.

57. Lorish C: Psychological factors related to treatment and adherence. In Melvin J, Jensen G, editors: *Rheumatologic rehabilitation series, volume 1: assessment and management*, Bethesda, MD, 1998, American Occupational Therapy Association.

58. Lozada CJ, Altman RD: Osteoarthritis. In Robbins L, editor: *Clinical care in the rheumatic diseases*, ed 2, Atlanta, 2001, Association of Rheumatology Health Professionals.

59. Luck JN: Enhancing functional ability. In Robbins L, editor: *Clinical care in the rheumatic diseases*, ed 2, Atlanta, 2001, Association of Rheumatology Health Professionals.

60. Mann W: Assistive technology for persons with arthritis. In Melvin J, Jensen G, editors: *Rheumatologic rehabilitation series, volume 1: assessment and management*, Bethesda, MD, 1998, American Occupational Therapy Association.

61. Mann WC, et al: The need for information on assistive devices by older persons, *Assist Technol* 6(2):134, 1994.

62. Marks R: Efficacy theory and its utility in arthritis rehabilitation: review and recommendations, *Disabil Rehabil* 23:271, 2001.

63. Matteson EL: Rheumatoid arthritis treatment. In Klippel JH, editor: *Primer of the rheumatic diseases*, ed 12, Atlanta, 2001, Arthritis Foundation.

64. Melvin JL: Orthotic treatment of the hand: what's new? *Bull Rheum Dis* 44:5, 1995.

65. Melvin JL: *Rheumatic disease in the adult and child: occupational therapy and rehabilitation*, ed 3, Philadelphia, 1989, FA Davis.

66. Melvin JL: Therapist's management of osteoarthritis in the hand. In Mackin EJ, et al: *Rehabilitation of the hand and upper extremity*, ed 5, St Louis, 2002, Mosby.

67. Michlovitz SM, Hun L, Erasala GN, et al: Continuous low-level heat wrap therapy is effective for treating wrist pain, *Arch Phys Med Rehabil* 85(9):1409, 2004.

68. Minor MA, Westby MD: Rest and exercise. In Robbins L, editor: *Clinical care in the rheumatic diseases*, ed 2, Atlanta, 2001, Association of Rheumatology Health Professionals.

69. Nordenskiöld U: Evaluation of assistive devices after a course in joint protection, *Internat J Technol Assess Heath Care* 10:283, 1994.

70. Oakes TW, et al: Family expectations and arthritis patients' compliance to a resting hand splint regimen, *J Chronic Dis* 22:757, 1970.

71. Pagnotta A, Baron M, Korner-Bitensky N: The effect of a static wrist orthosis on hand function in individuals with rheumatoid arthritis, *J Rheumatol* 25:879, 1998.

72. Parker JC, Wright GE, Smarr KL: Psychological assessment. In Robbins L, editor: *Clinical care in the rheumatic diseases*, ed 2, Atlanta, 2001, Association of Rheumatology Health Professionals.

73. Philips CA: Management of the patient with rheumatoid arthritis: the role of the hand therapist, *Hand Clin* 5:291, 1989.

74. Rao JK, et al: Use of complementary therapies for arthritis among patients of rheumatologists, *Ann Intern Med* 131(6):409, 1999.

75. Rennie GA, Michlovitz SL: Biophysical principles of heating and superficial heating agents. In Michlovitz SL, editor: *Thermal agents in rehabilitation*, ed 3, Philadelphia, 1996, FA Davis.

76. Rennie HJ: Evaluation of the effectiveness of a metacarpophalangeal ulnar deviation orthosis, *J Hand Ther* 9:371, 1996.

77. Robbins L: Social and cultural assessment. In Robbins L, editor: *Clinical care in the rheumatic diseases*, ed 2, Atlanta, 2001, Association of Rheumatology Health Professionals.

78. Roberts WN, Daltroy LH, Anderson RJ: Stability of normal joint findings in persistent classical rheumatoid arthritis, *Arthritis Rheum* 31:267, 1988.

79. Rogers JC, Holm MB, Perkins L: Trajectory of assistive device usage and user and non-user characteristics: long-handled bath sponge, *Arthritis Rheum* 47:645, 2002.

80. Shapiro-Slonaker DM: Joint protection and energy conservation. In Riggs MA, Gall EP, editors: *Rheumatic diseases: rehabilitation and management*, Boston, 1984, Butterworth.

81. Sidman JM: Sexual functioning and the physically disabled adult, *Am J Occup Ther* 31:81, 1977.

82. Song R, et al: Effects of tai chi exercise on pain, balance, muscle strength, and perceived difficulties in physical functioning in older women with osteoarthritis: a randomized clinical trail, *J Rheumatol* 30(9):2039, 2003.

83. Sotosky JR, Melvin JM: Initial interview: a client-centered approach. In Melvin J, Jensen G, editors: *Rheumatologic rehabilitation series, volume 1: assessment and management*, Bethesda, MD, 1998, American Occupational Therapy Association.

84. Sotosky JR, Michlovitz SL: Use of heat and cold in the management of rheumatic diseases. In Michlovitz SL, editor: *Thermal agents in rehabilitation*, ed 3, Philadelphia, 1996, FA Davis.

85. Spiegel TM, Forouzesh SN: Musculoskeletal examination. In Riggs MA, Gall EP, editors: *Rheumatic diseases: rehabilitation and management*, Boston, 1984, Butterworth.

86. Stenstrom CH, Minor MA: Evidence for the benefit of aerobic and strengthening exercise in rheumatoid arthritis, *Arthritis Rheum* 49:428, 2003.

87. Stern EB, et al: Commercial wrist extensor orthoses: a descriptive study of use and preference in patients with rheumatoid arthritis, *Arthritis Care Res* 10:27, 1997.

88. Stern EB, et al: Finger dexterity and hand function: effect of three commercial wrist extensor orthoses on patients with rheumatoid arthritis, *Arthritis Care Res* 9:197, 1996.

89. Steultjens EM, et al: Occupational therapy for rheumatoid arthritis: a systematic review, *Arthritis Rheum* 47(6):672, 2002.

90. Suomi R, Collier D: Effects of arthritis exercise programs on functional fitness and perceived activities of daily living measures in older adults with arthritis, *Arch Phys Med Rehabil* 84:1589, 2003.

91. Swigart CR, et al: Splinting in the treatment of arthritis of the first carpometacarpal joint, *J Hand Surg* 24(1):86, 1999.

92. Terrono AL, Nalebuff EA, Philips CA: The rheumatoid thumb. In Mackin EJ et al: *Rehabilitation of the hand and upper extremity*, ed 5, St Louis, 2002, Mosby.

93. Von Nieda K, Michlovitz SL: Cryotherapy. In Michlovitz SL, editor: *Thermal agents in rehabilitation*, ed 3, Philadelphia, 1996, FA Davis.

94. Weiss S, et al: Prospective analysis of splinting the carpometacarpal joint: an objective, subjective, and radiographic assessment, *J Hand Ther* 13:218, 2000.

95. Weiss S, et al: Splinting the degenerative basal joint: custom-made or prefabricated neoprene? *J Hand Ther* 17:401, 2004.

96. Wickersham BA: The exercise program. In Riggs MA, Gall EP, editors: *Rheumatic diseases: rehabilitation and management*, Boston, 1984, Butterworth.

97. Wilske KK, Healey LA: Remodeling the pyramid: a concept whose time has come, *J Rheumatol* 16:565, 1989.

98. Wilton JC: *Hand splinting: principles of design and fabrication*, Philadelphia, 1997, WB Saunders.

99. Wright GE, et al: Risk factors for depression in rheumatoid arthritis, *Arthritis Care Res* 9(4):264, 1996.

100. Yasuda YL: *Occupational therapy practice guidelines for adults with rheumatoid arthritis*, ed 2, Bethesda, MD, 2001, American Occupational Therapy Association.

SUGGESTED READING

Lorig K, Fries JF, editors: *The arthritis helpbook*, ed 3, Reading, MA, 1990, Addison-Wesley.

Melvin JL: *Osteoarthritis: caring for your hands*, Bethesda, MD, 1995, American Occupational Therapy Association.

Melvin JL: *Rheumatoid arthritis: caring for your hands*, Bethesda, MD, 1995, American Occupational Therapy Association.

RESOURCES

American College of Rheumatology and Association of Rheumatology Health Professionals
www.rheumatology.org
Arthritis Foundation
www.arthritis.org
National Institute of Arthritis and Musculoskeletal and Skin Diseases
www.nih.gov/niams

39

HAND AND UPPER EXTREMITY INJURIES

MARY C. KASCH

J. MARTIN WALSH

KEY TERMS

Upper quadrant	Splinting	Complex regional pain	Functional capacity evaluation
Edema	Peripheral nerve injuries	syndrome	Ergonomic
Provocative tests	Tendon injuries	Cumulative trauma disorders	

LEARNING OBJECTIVES

After studying this chapter the student or practitioner will be able to do the following:

1. Discuss the incidence and effect of upper extremity (UE) injuries in the United States and their effects on occupational performance.
2. Identify three upper quarter screening tests, and explain their significance in developing an intervention plan.
3. Discuss the importance of joint mobility in regaining the motor performance skill of hand function.
4. Describe the four categories of tests used to evaluate peripheral nerve function, and explain how the results would be used in developing an intervention plan.
5. Compare the standardized tests used to assess the motor performance skill of hand function.
6. Describe the sensory and motor innervation patterns of the three major nerves, and differentiate between the effects of proximal and distal lesions in each of the nerves and how they might affect occupational performance.
7. Discuss complex regional pain syndrome and the intervention approaches that should be included in the occupational therapy (OT) intervention plan for that disorder.
8. Compare techniques used in the rehabilitation of tendon injuries.
9. Describe the significance of edema with regard to wound healing and joint mobility.
10. Discuss the role of the occupational therapist in evaluation and rehabilitation of injured workers.

CHAPTER OUTLINE

Examination and evaluation
  Observation and topographical assessment
  Assessment of performance skills and client factors
  Grip and pinch strength
  Functional assessment
Intervention
  Fractures
  Nerve injuries
  Tendon injuries
  Complex injuries
  Edema

Wound healing and scar remodeling
Pain syndromes
Joint stiffness
Cumulative trauma disorders
Strengthening activities
Purposeful and occupation-based activity
Functional capacity evaluation
  Work hardening
Consultation with industry
Psychosocial effects of hand injuries
Summary

THREADED CASE STUDY: GERRY, PART 1

Gerry is a 32-year-old man who is self-employed as a cabinetmaker. He sustained a table saw injury to his nondominant left hand while working. The thumb, index, and middle fingers of Gerry's left hand were amputated as a result of the saw injury at the level of the proximal phalanges and were subsequently replanted by a hand surgeon using microsurgical techniques. Gerry is single, lives with a roommate, and is in business with his father in a small but busy cabinet shop. Gerry is extremely active at work and during his free time. He is very social and has an extensive network of supportive friends and family.

Gerry was referred to hand therapy as an inpatient 5 days after the replantation surgeries, as soon as he was discontinued from the anticoagulation medications. The initial interview with Gerry was performed at bedside. He was to be discharged from the hospital the following day with instructions to return for outpatient hand therapy. A protective splint was fabricated on the first therapy session, and Gerry was taught about post-surgical precautions, wound care, and dressing changes. During the initial evaluation, Gerry said that he was very distressed about the potential loss of function of his left hand and that he wanted to accomplish three of his most valued occupations in the months to come. The first occupation was to return to work with his father making cabinets in the family business, the second was to resume playing softball with his league, and the third was to play golf again. The first occupation was one he valued not only

as a source of livelihood but also as a profession in which he demonstrated great skill and derived joy. The second two occupations were important to him not only as a source of relaxation but, more important, as a primary venue for social interaction with friends and family.

Gerry initiated hand therapy in the hospital during the acute phase of his recovery. He was followed in hand therapy for 15 months from the date of his injury and through several additional surgeries and throughout all phases of his rehabilitative process: the acute or immobilization phase, the intermediate or mobilization phase, and the late or strengthening phase.[21] During the initial evaluation, Gerry clearly expressed a desire to return to three specific occupations of value to him: working as a cabinetmaker, playing golf, and playing softball.

Critical Thinking Questions

1. How will the intervention plan change over the course of Gerry's recovery? What specific intervention approaches will be used during the three phases of his recovery?
2. What specific tools or instruments will be used to assess Gerry's performance skills during the different phases of his recovery?
3. What are some of the specific preparatory methods and purposeful activities that may be used in preparation for Gerry's occupation-based performance activity of golf?

Treatment of the upper extremity (UE) is important to all occupational therapists who work with persons with physical disabilities. The incidence of UE injuries is significant and accounts for about one third of all acute injuries. About 63% of the 90,000 work-related repetitive motion injuries per year in the United States involve the wrist, hand, and shoulder. Combined, these injuries account for 98 million days of restricted activity. The UEs are involved in about one third of work-related farm injuries and one quarter of all disabling injuries. In addition, disease and congenital anomalies contribute to UE dysfunction, and it is estimated that only about 15% of those who experience severe cerebrovascular accident recover hand function.[53]

The hand is vital to human function and appearance. It flexes, extends, opposes, and grasps thousands of times daily, allowing the performance of necessary daily activities. The hand's sensibility allows feeling without looking and provides protection from injury. The hand touches, gives comfort, and expresses emotions. Loss of hand function through injury or disease thus affects much more than the mechanical tasks that the hand performs. Hand injury may jeopardize a family's livelihood and, at the least, affects every daily activity. The occupational therapist with training in

physical and psychological assessment, prosthetic evaluation, fabrication of orthoses, assessment and training in the activities of daily living (ADLs), and functional restoration is uniquely qualified to treat UE disorders.

Hand rehabilitation, or hand therapy, has grown as a specialty area of occupational therapy (OT) and physical therapy (PT). Many of the intervention techniques used with hand-injured clients have evolved from the application of therapy and knowledge of both specialties to be used by the hand therapist. It is not the purpose of this chapter to instruct the OT student in physical agent modalities. Rather, intervention techniques that have been found to be beneficial to clients with hand injuries are presented. It is assumed that therapists best trained to provide them will provide these techniques.

As used in this chapter, *hand therapy* is a term that includes intervention of the entire **upper quadrant,** which includes the scapula, shoulder, and arm. Upper quadrant and UE are used interchangeably. UE rehabilitation requires advanced and specialized training by both occupational and physical therapists. A practice analysis study of the theory and knowledge that serves as the underpinning for hand therapy has been reported.[75] Intervention techniques, whether thermal modalities or specifically designed exercises, are used as a bridge to reach a further goal of restoring functional performance. Thus, some modalities may be used as adjunctive or enabling modalities in preparation for functional use. It is within this context that intervention techniques will be presented in this chapter.

Intervention for the injured UE is a matter of timing and judgment. After trauma or surgery, a healing phase must occur in which the body performs its physiological function of wound healing. After the initial healing phase, when cellular restoration has been accomplished, the wound enters its restorative phase. It is in this phase that hand therapy is most beneficial. Early intervention that occurs in this restorative phase is ideal and in some cases essential for optimal results.

Although sample timetables may be presented, the therapist should always coordinate the application of any intervention with the referring physician. Surgical techniques may vary, and inappropriate treatment of the client with hand injury can result in failure of a surgical procedure.

Communication among the surgeon, therapist, and client is especially vital in this setting. A comfortable environment that allows group interaction may increase client motivation and cooperation. The presence of the therapist as an instructor and evaluator is essential, but without the client's cooperation limited gains will be achieved. Treating the psychological loss suffered by the client with a hand injury is also an integral part of the rehabilitative therapy.

 OT PRACTICE NOTE

> Hand therapy is provided in a number of intervention settings, ranging from private therapy offices to outpatient rehabilitation clinics and hospitals. Reimbursement for services may come directly from the client or through private medical insurance, workers' compensation insurance, or a variety of managed care programs. Changes in reimbursement have driven changes in the marketplace and employment patterns. In the future, OT will be provided in a variety of new settings and OT intervention will continue to evolve.

In UE rehabilitation, changes have been manifested as changes in delivery of services. In some cases, therapists are not members of the approved provider panel and are no longer able to treat clients who are members of a health maintenance organization. Reimbursement patterns have altered the provision of services by limiting the number of visits authorized. Therapists are also being asked to provide outcome data that support the need for services. It is likely that outcome-based intervention plans with functional goals and analysis of goal achievement will become the standard for the reimbursement of OT services. In addition, client satisfaction and perception of health status have become

crucial in the delivery of medical care in a consumer-based economy. Continuous quality improvement documentation is often required for participation in managed care programs. With fewer authorized visits, the therapist must be more adept in instructing the client in self-management of the condition being treated. In the future, occupational therapists should anticipate a greater need to justify intervention as part of the national challenge to control medical costs. Aides, certified assistants, and other support personnel will be used increasingly, but the quality of services provided must continue to meet all professional and ethical standards. This climate of change will present unique opportunities for the occupational therapist. Clinical specialists may find new roles as consultants and trainers. Just as OT teaches the client to adapt to changes in health status, the profession of OT will need to adapt to social and economic changes to remain a leader in health management.

EXAMINATION AND EVALUATION

When approaching a client who has a hand injury, the occupational therapist must gather information about the client's occupational history, including a detailed description, from the client's perspective, regarding how the hand injury may interfere with resumption of daily rounds of meaningful occupation. Armed with this occupational profile, the therapist and client continue the evaluation process. The therapist must be able to evaluate the nature of the injury and the limitations it has produced. First, the injured structures must be identified by consulting with the hand surgeon, reviewing operative reports and X-ray films, and discussing the injury with the client. Assessment of bone, tendon, and nerve function must be ascertained, using standardized assessment techniques whenever possible.

The client's age, occupation, and hand dominance should be taken into account in the initial evaluation. The type and extent of medical and surgical treatment that has been received and the length of time since such intervention are important in determining a intervention plan. Any further surgery or conservative intervention that is planned should also be noted. A written intervention plan should have the approval of the referring physician. Most physicians welcome observations and evaluation-based recommendations from the therapist regarding the client's care.

The purposes of hand evaluation are to identify physical limitations, such as loss of range of motion (ROM); functional limitations, such as an inability to perform daily tasks;[3] substitution patterns to compensate for loss of sensibility or motor function;[4] and abnormalities, such as joint contracture.

The movement of the arm and hand must be coordinated for maximal function. Shoulder motion is essential for positioning the hand and elbow for daily activities.[20] The wrist is the key joint in the position of function.[12] Skilled hand performance depends on wrist stability. Although a mobile wrist is preferable, function is possible as long as the wrist is positioned to maximize movement of the fingers. Function also depends on arm and shoulder stability and mobility for fixing or positioning the hand for activity. The thumb is of greater importance than any other digit. Effective pinch is almost impossible without a thumb, and attempts will be made to salvage or reconstruct an injured thumb whenever possible. Within the hand the proximal interphalangeal (PIP) joint is critical for grasp and is considered to be the most important small joint.[12] Limitations in flexion or extension will result in significant functional impairment.

The hand therapy evaluation should, therefore, consist of two concurrent stages. One stage consists of assessing the client's occupational profile to help the therapist select an effective intervention that addresses the client's occupational priorities. The other stage of the hand therapy evaluation consists of assessing specific performance skills, such as coordination and strength, and client factors, such as sensory functions, neuromusculoskeletal and movement-related functions, and the functions of the hand and related structures. Evaluating both the client's occupational profile and the client's performance skills ensures that the client's priorities are addressed and makes the intervention more meaningful.

OBSERVATION AND TOPOGRAPHICAL ASSESSMENT

The occupational therapist should observe the appearance of the entire UE. The position of the hand and arm at rest and the carrying posture can yield valuable information about the dysfunction. The therapist should observe the way that the client treats the disease or injury. The therapist should note if the hand and arm are overprotected and carefully guarded or ignored and if the client carries the arm close to the body, in an awkward posture, or even covered.

The cervical and shoulder area posture should be observed for evidence of abnormalities in cervical and thoracic curvature that may reduce the potential for shoulder movement. Muscle atrophy may be evident in the scapular area if there has been significant long-term weakness or if the rotator cuff is torn. The scapula may appear asymmetrical or altered if muscle imbalances of length or strength are present.

The skin condition of the hand and arm should be noted. In particular, the therapist should note any lacerations, sutures, or evidence of recent surgery; whether the skin is dry or moist; whether scales or crusts are present; and whether the hand appears swollen or has an odor. Palmar skin is less mobile than dorsal skin normally. The therapist should determine the degree of mobility and elasticity and the adherence of scars. The therapist should also observe trophic changes in the skin. The vascular system is assessed by observing the skin color and temperature of the hand and evaluating for presence of edema (swelling). Any contractures of the web spaces should be noted. The therapist should

observe the relationship between hand and arm function as the client moves about and performs test items or tasks.

The therapist should ask the client to perform some simple bilateral ADLs, such as buttoning a button, putting on a shirt, opening a jar, and threading a needle, and observe the amount of spontaneous movement and use of the affected hand and arm. Similar screening tests can be used to determine shoulder mobility, such as reaching overhead, as well as placing the hand behind the back and behind the head.

ASSESSMENT OF PERFORMANCE SKILLS AND CLIENT FACTORS

A number of standardized tests can be used to determine physical limitations in the UE. Joint measurement and manual muscle testing are crucial and are described in other chapters. Special tests used by the hand therapist are described here in a general sense, but the student should consult other textbooks for detailed instructions in such areas as assessment of adverse neural tension.[16]

Screening the Cervical Neck and Shoulder

Screening examination of the cervical neck and shoulder regions should be included in evaluation of hand conditions to determine whether these areas are contributing to the client's symptoms or limitations in function.

Active movements of the neck should be conducted, with attention paid to complaints of UE symptoms during cervical extension or lateral flexion to the same side. Complaints during these movements may suggest nerve root irritation. Hand symptoms with opposite side bending may be a sign of adverse neural tension. Few occupational therapists are knowledgeable in the intervention of cervical conditions, and care must be taken not to aggravate an existing condition. The therapist should return the client to the referring physician with recommendations for referral to an appropriate practitioner if the results of this testing are positive.

Assessment of Movement

The effect of trauma or dysfunction on anatomical structures is the first consideration in evaluating hand function. The joints must be assessed for active and passive mobility, fixed deformities, and any tendency to assume a position of deformity. The ligaments must be assessed for laxity or contracture and their ability to maintain joint stability. Tendons must be examined for integrity, contracture, or overstretching; muscles are tested for strength and function.

Limited Movement in the Shoulder

Examples of conditions in the shoulder region leading to reduced strength, reduced ROM, or pain in the shoulder are outlined in Table 39-1. Comparing initial responses with the results of follow-up evaluation will help document a positive response to intervention. Patterns of impairments in UE ROM and strength, as well as a positive response to

TABLE 39-1 **Clinical Tests for Specific Dysfunction in the Shoulder**

Condition	Pattern of Impairment	Characteristic Findings/Special Tests
Adhesive capsulitis	Loss of active and passive shoulder motion with the most pronounced loss in external rotation and, to a lesser degree, abduction and internal rotation	Capsular end feel to passive motions in restricted planes of movement
Subacromial impingement	Painful arc of motion between approximately 80 and 100 degrees elevation or at end range of active elevation	In early stages, muscle tests may be strong and painless despite positive impingement test
Rotator cuff tendinitis	Painful active or resistive rotator cuff muscle use	Painful manual muscle test of scapular plane abduction or external rotation Nonpainful passive motion end ranges Tenderness at tendons of supraspinatus or infraspinatus.
Rotator cuff tear	Significant substitution of scapula with attempted arm elevation	Positive drop arm test Very weak, less than $^3/_5$ abduction or external rotation

provocative testing, should be reported to the referring physician if they would affect the client's planned intervention or outcome. Therapists must not attempt to treat conditions that are beyond their scope of knowledge. Referral to an appropriate practitioner should be discussed with the physician if indicated.

Impingement tests

The examiner passively overpressures the client's arm into end-range elevation. This movement causes a jamming of the greater tuberosity against the anterior inferior acromial surface.[76] The test is positive if the client's facial expression shows pain. An alternative test is described by Hawkins and Kennedy.[44] The examiner forward flexes the arm to 90 degrees, then forcibly internally rotates the arm. Pain indicates a positive test result.

Drop arm test

The client's arm is passively abducted by the examiner to 90 degrees with the client's palm down. The client is then asked to lower the arm actively. Pain or inability to lower the arm smoothly with good motor control is considered a positive test result.[62, 82]

Soft-Tissue Tightness

Joints may develop dysfunction after trauma, immobilization, or disuse. Mennell emphasizes the importance of the small, involuntary motions of the joint, which he refers to as "joint play."[70] Others[63] describe these as "accessory motions." Both terms describe those movements that are involuntary and physiological and can be performed only by someone else.[54] Examples of accessory motions are joint rotation and joint distraction. If accessory motions are limited and painful, the active motions of that joint cannot be normal.

Therefore, it is necessary to restore joint play through the use of joint mobilization techniques before attempting passive or active ROM.[71]

Joint mobilization may date back to the fourth century BC, when Hippocrates first described the use of spinal traction.[54] In the 1930s, an English physician, James Mennell, encouraged physicians to perform manipulation without anesthesia, a practice that is advocated today by James Cyriax,[28] who explored the use of manipulation of the intervertebral disks. Current theorists include Cyriax, Robert Maigne, F.M. Kaltenborn, G.D. Maitland, Stanley Paris, and John Mennell, son of the late James Mennell. Although physicians originally practiced manipulation, therapists have adapted the techniques, which are now called *joint mobilization.*

The techniques used to assess joint play are also used in the treatment of joint dysfunction. During assessment the evaluator determines the range of accessory motion and the presence of pain by taking up the slack only in the joint. Some practitioners advocate use of a high-velocity, low-amplitude thrust or graded oscillation to regain motion and relieve pain.[63]

Guidelines must be followed in applying joint mobilization techniques, and the untrained or inexperienced practitioner should not attempt to use the techniques. Postgraduate courses are offered in joint mobilization of the extremities, and the therapist must be familiar with the orthokinematics of each joint, as well as with the techniques used.

Joint mobilization is generally indicated with restriction of accessory motions or the presence of pain caused by tightness of the joint capsule, meniscus displacement, muscle guarding, ligamentous tightness, or adherence. It is contraindicated in the presence of infection, recent fracture, neoplasm, joint inflammation, rheumatoid arthritis, osteoporosis, degenerative joint disease, and many chronic diseases.[54]

TABLE 39-2 **Clinical Tests for Specific Dysfunction in the Wrist**

Condition	Pattern of Impairment	Special Tests
Thumb ulnar collateral ligament instability (gamekeeper's or skier's thumb)	Pain and instability of the thumb MP joint	Movement greater than 35 degrees when valgus stress is applied to the thumb MP joint
Instability of the scaphoid	Pain in the area of the scaphoid bone (anatomical snuffbox) or "clunking" with movement of the wrist	Watson test Pain or sound associated with subluxation of the dorsal pole of the scaphoid while performing test
Instability of the distal radioulnar joint	Pain and tenderness in the wrist	"Piano keys" test Hypermobility and pain associated with pressure on the distal ulna
Lunate dislocation	Pain or instability in the central wrist	Murphy's sign Head of the third metacarpal level with the second and fourth metacarpals while making a fist
Lunotriquetral instability	Pain or instability in the central or ulnar wrist	Lunotriquetral ballottement test Crepitus; laxity or pain with isolated movement of the lunate
TFCC tear	Pain and instability in the ulnar wrist	Wrist arthrogram or MRI

Limitations in joint motion may also be caused by tightness of the extrinsic or intrinsic muscles and tendons. If the joint capsule is not tight and accessory motions are normal, the therapist should test for extrinsic and intrinsic tightness.

To test for extrinsic extensor tightness, the metacarpophalangeal (MP) joint is passively held in extension and the PIP joint is moved passively into flexion. Then the MP joint is flexed, and the PIP joint is again passively flexed. If the PIP joint can be flexed easily when the MP joint is extended but not when the MP joint is flexed, the extrinsic extensors are adherent.[4]

If there is extrinsic flexor tightness, the PIP and distal interphalangeal (DIP) joints will be positioned in flexion, with the MP joints held in extension. It will not be possible to pull the fingers into complete extension. If the wrist is then held in flexion, the IP joints will extend more easily because slack is placed on the flexor tendons.

Tightness of the intrinsic musculature is tested by passively holding the MP joint in extension and applying pressure just distal to the PIP joint. This action is repeated with the MP joint in flexion. If there is more resistance when the MP joint is extended, intrinsic tightness is indicated.[4]

If passive motion of the PIP joint remains the same whether the MP joint is held in extension or flexion and there is limitation of PIP joint flexion in any position, tightness of the joint capsule is indicated. The therapist should assess the joint for capsular tightness if this has not already been done.

Provocative tests that are used to assess ligament, capsule, and joint instability are summarized in Table 39-2. For more detailed and comprehensive information regarding administration of these tests, the reader is referred to textbooks dedicated solely to hand therapy or to the specific topic.[62,82]

Assessment of Peripheral Nerve Status

Nerve dysfunction can occur at any point from the nerve roots through the digital nerves in the fingers. A good understanding of the peripheral nervous system is essential for appropriate treatment of the UE. Determining the approximate location of nerve dysfunction can assist in intervention planning.

Categories of tests

A variety of tests may be required to assess nerve function adequately. These tests can be divided into four categories: (1) modality tests for pain, heat, cold, and touch pressure; (2) functional tests to assess the quality of sensibility, or what Moberg[74] described as "tactile gnosis"; (3) objective tests that do not require active participation by the client; (4) and provocative tests that reproduce symptoms.

Examples of functional tests are stationary and moving two-point discrimination and the Moberg pick-up test; objective tests include the wrinkle test, the Ninhydrin sweat test, and nerve-conduction studies.[18] Electrodiagnostic testing is the most conclusive and widely accepted method of determining nerve dysfunction.

Provocative tests are highly suggestive of a nerve lesion if results are positive but do not rule out a problem if results are negative. Tests of nerve dysfunction are summarized in Table 39-3. Instructions for administration of the most common tests are described in the following paragraphs.

Adson maneuver

The examiner palpates the radial pulse on the arm to be tested. The client then rotates the head toward the arm

TABLE **39-3** **Clinical Tests for Specific Nerve Dysfunction in the Upper Extremity**

Condition	Pattern of Impairment	Characteristic Findings/Special Tests
Thoracic outlet syndrome	Nonspecific paresthesias or heaviness with sustained positioning or activity above shoulder level or behind the plane of the body	Adson test Roos test
Adverse neural tension	Nonspecific pain or paresthesias with reaching in positions that place tension on brachial plexus nerves	Positive upper limb screening test
Carpal tunnel syndrome	Pain and numbness, primarily in the thumb, index, and middle fingers Usually worse at night and may be associated with activity	Tinel's sign at the wrist Phalen's test Reverse Phalen's test Carpal compression test
Cubital tunnel syndrome	Compression of ulnar nerve at elbow	Elbow flexion test
Ulnar nerve paralysis	Paralysis of the adductor pollicis muscle	Froment's sign Jeanne's sign Wartenberg's sign

being tested. The client then extends the head and holds a deep breath while the arm is being laterally rotated and extended. Disappearance or slowing of pulse rate is considered a positive test result suggesting presence of thoracic outlet syndrome.[1,62]

Roos test

In this test the client maintains a position of bilateral arm abduction to 90 degrees, shoulder external rotation, and elbow flexion to 90 degrees for 3 minutes while slowly alternating between an open hand and a clenched fist. Inability to maintain this position for the full 3 minutes or onset of symptoms is considered a positive test result for thoracic outlet syndrome.[62,84]

Upper limb tension test (brachial plexus tension test)

This test is designed to screen for symptoms that are produced when tension stress is placed on the brachial plexus. The maneuver described primarily stresses the median nerve and C5-C7 nerve roots. Adverse neural tension in the ulnar or radial nerves may also be tested. However, we have found that using the median nerve test as a screening device establishes a marker against which to gauge the success of intervention. Although some authors recommend using the neural tension tests for intervention as well as assessment, this has not been the practice of the authors. The occupational therapist should use this screening process to rule out or confirm the involvement of more proximal structures.

The client is positioned supine, and the examiner takes the client's arm into abduction and external rotation behind the coronal plane at the shoulder. The shoulder girdle is fixed in depression. The elbow is then passively extended with the wrist in extension and the forearm in supination. Symptoms of stretch or ache in the cubital fossa or tingling in the thumb and first three fingers indicate tension on the median nerve. Lateral flexion of the neck to the opposite side will amplify

symptoms by increasing tension on the dura mater. Elbow extension ROM should be compared with the uninvolved side to indicate the degree of restriction.[62]

Tinel's sign

The test is performed by tapping gently along the course of a peripheral nerve, starting distally and moving proximally to elicit a tingling sensation in the fingertip. The point at which tapping begins to elicit a tingling sensation is noted and indicates the approximate location of nerve compression. This test is also used after nerve repair to determine the extent of sensory axon growth.[89]

Phalen's test and reverse Phalen's test

Phalen's test is performed by fully flexing the wrists with the dorsum of the hands pressing against each other. Reverse Phalen's is performed by holding the hands in the "prayer" position for 1 minute. The test results are positive if the client reports tingling in the median nerve distribution (thumb, index, middle and radial aspect of ring finger) within 1 minute.

Carpal compression test

The examiner places pressure over the median nerve in the carpal tunnel for up to 30 seconds. The test result is positive if tingling occurs in the median nerve distribution. The combination of wrist flexion and compression of the median nerve for 20 seconds has been found to be more sensitive than other provocative tests used alone.[93]

Elbow flexion test

The elbow flexion test is used to screen for cubital tunnel syndrome (compression of the ulnar nerve in the cubital tunnel). The client is asked to fully flex the elbows with the wrists fully extended for a period of 3 to 5 minutes. The test result is positive if tingling is reported in the ulnar nerve distribution of the forearm and hand (ulnar ring finger and small finger).[62]

Quick tests for motor function in the peripheral nerves

The ulnar nerve may be tested by asking the client to pinch with the thumb and index finger and palpating the first dorsal interosseous muscle. Another test for ulnar nerve paralysis involves asking a client to grasp a piece of paper between the thumb and index finger. When the examiner pulls away the paper, the tip of the thumb flexes because of absence of the adductor pollicis muscle (Froment's sign). If the MP joint of the thumb also extends at the same time, it is known as *Jeanne's sign*. Wartenberg's sign for ulnar nerve compression is positive if the client is unable to adduct the small finger when the hand is placed palm down on the table with the fingers passively abducted.

The radial nerve may be tested by asking the client to extend the wrist and fingers. Median nerve function is tested by asking the client to oppose the thumb to the fingers and flex the fingers.[62]

Sensory mapping

Detailed sensibility testing can begin with sensory mapping of the entire volar surface of the hand.[18] The hand must be supported by the examiner's hand or be resting in a medium such as therapy putty to stabilize the hand during testing. The examiner draws a probe, usually the eraser end of a pencil, lightly over the skin from the area of normal sensibility to the area of abnormal sensibility. The client must immediately report the exact location where the sensation changes. This is done from proximal to distal and radial and ulnar to medial directions. The areas are carefully marked and transferred to a permanent record. Mapping should be repeated at monthly intervals during nerve regeneration.

Sympathetic function

Recovery of sympathetic response such as sudomotor (sweating), vasomotor (temperature discrimination), pilomotor (gooseflesh), and trophic (skin texture, nail, and hair growth) may occur early but does not correlate with functional recovery.[30] O'Rain[78] observed that denervated skin does not wrinkle. Therefore, nerve function may be tested by immersing the hand in water for 5 minutes and noting the presence or absence of skin wrinkling. This test may be especially helpful in diagnosing a nerve lesion in young children. The ability to sweat is also lost with a nerve lesion. A Ninhydrin test[74] evaluates sweating of the finger.

The wrinkle test and the Ninhydrin test are objective tests of sympathetic function. Recovery of sweating has not been shown to correlate with the recovery of sensation, but the absence of sweating correlates with the lack of discriminatory sensation. Other signs of sympathetic dysfunction are smooth, shiny skin; nail changes; and "pencil-pointing" or tapering of the fingers.[100]

Nerve compression and nerve regeneration

Sensibility testing is performed to assess the recovery of a nerve following laceration and repair, as well as to determine the presence of a nerve compression syndrome and the return of nerve function after surgical decompression, or the efficacy of conservative intervention to reduce compression. Therefore, tests such as vibratory tests may be interpreted differently, depending on the mechanism of nerve dysfunction. In the following section, tests will be described and differences drawn as appropriate to assist the therapist in selecting the correct assessment technique, as well as in planning treatment based on the evaluative measures.

During the first 2 to 4 months after nerve suture, axons regenerate and travel through the hand at a rate of about 1 mm per day, or 1 inch (2.54 cm) per month. Tinel's sign may be used to follow this regeneration. As regeneration occurs, hypesthesias develop. Although this hypersensitivity may be uncomfortable for the client, it is a positive sign of nerve growth. An intervention program for desensitization of hypersensitive areas can be initiated as soon as the skin is healed and can tolerate gentle rubbing and immersion in textures. Desensitization is discussed further in the intervention section.

Vibration

Dellon was an early advocate of the use of 30-cycles-per-second (30-cps) and 256-cps tuning forks for assessing the return of vibratory sensation after nerve repair, as regeneration occurs and as a guideline for initiating a sensory reeducation program.[31,32] However, many clinicians found that use of a tuning fork was not discrete enough to detect sensory abnormalities.

Lundborg[60] has described the use of commercial vibrometers to detect abnormal sensation. This method was less subjective and thought to be more reliable. In a study of induced median nerve compression, Gelberman[41] found that vibration and touch perception as measured by the Semmes-Weinstein monofilaments are altered before two-point discrimination because they measure a single nerve fiber innervating a group of receptor cells. Two-point discrimination is a test of innervation density that requires overlapping sensory units and cortical integration. Thus, two-point discrimination is altered after nerve laceration and repair but remains normal if the nerve is compressed, as long as there are links to the cortex. Bell-Krotoski[10] has also found normal two-point values in the presence of decreased sensory function.

Vibration and the Semmes-Weinstein test are more sensitive in picking up a gradual decrease in nerve function in the presence of nerve compression where the nerve circuitry is intact. They also correlate with decreases in the potential amplitude of sensory nerve action as measured by nerve conduction studies.[92] Therefore, vibration, Semmes-Weinstein, and electrical testing are reliable and sensitive tests for early detection of carpal tunnel syndrome and other nerve compression syndromes. Vibration and Semmes-Weinstein can be performed in the clinic with no discomfort to the client and are excellent screening tools when nerve compression is suspected.

Touch pressure

Moving touch is tested using the eraser end of a pencil. The eraser is placed in an area of normal sensibility and, with application of light pressure, is moved to the distal fingertip. The client notes when the perception of the stimulus changes. Light and heavy stimuli may be applied and noted.[30] Constant touch is tested by pressing with the eraser end of a pencil, first in an area with normal sensibility and then placing the eraser distally by lifting up the pencil before placement. The client responds when the stimulus is altered; again, light and heavy stimuli may be applied.[30]

The Semmes-Weinstein monofilaments are the most accurate instruments for assessing cutaneous pressure thresholds.[10] The original testing equipment consisted of 20 nylon monofilaments housed in plastic hand-held rods. Many therapists today use the smaller five-pack filaments. These five monofilaments correspond to the categories of light touch sensation described later. The diameter of the monofilaments increases, and when applied correctly, they exert a force ranging from 4.5 mg to 447 g. Markings on the probes range from 1.65 to 6.65 but do not correspond to the grams of force of each rod. Normal fingertip sensibility has been found to correspond to the 2.44 and 2.83 probes.

The monofilaments must be applied perpendicularly to the skin and are applied just until the monofilament bends. The skin should not blanch when the monofilament is applied. Probes 1.65 through 2.83 are bounced three times. Probes marked 3.22 to 4.08 are applied three times with a bend in the filament, and probes marked 4.17 to 6.65 are applied once. The larger monofilaments do not bend; therefore, skin color must be observed to determine how firmly to apply the probe.

The examiner should begin with a probe in the normal range and progress through the rods in increasing diameters to find the client's threshold for touch throughout the volar surface.[10] A grid should be used to record the responses so that varying areas of touch perception can be demonstrated. Two correct responses out of three applications are necessary for an area to be considered as having intact sensibility. It is preferable to place the monofilaments randomly rather than to concentrate on an area, to allow the nerves recovery time. When a filament is placed three times, it should be held for a second, rested for a second, and reapplied. Results can be graded from normal light touch (probes 2.83 and above) to loss of protective sensation (probes 4.56 and below). Diminished light touch and diminished protective sensation are in the range reflected by the central probes (probes 3.22 to 4.31).[10]

Two-point and moving two-point discrimination

Discrimination, the second level of sensibility assessment, requires the subject to distinguish between two direct stimuli. Static or stationary two-point discrimination measures the slowly adapting fibers. The two-point discrimination test, first described by Weber in 1853, was modified and popularized by Moberg,[74] who was interested in a tool that would assess the functional level of sensation. A variety of devices have been proposed to use in measuring two-point discrimination. The bent paper clip is inexpensive but often has burrs on the metal tip. Other devices include industrial calipers* and the Disk-Criminator.[61][†] A device with parallel prongs of variable distance and blunted ends should produce replicable results.

The test is performed as follows[89]:
1. The client's vision is occluded.
2. An area of normal sensation is tested as a reference, using blunt calipers or a bent paper clip.
3. The calipers are set 10 mm apart and are randomly applied, starting at the fingertip and moving proximally and longitudinally in line with the digital nerves, with one or two points touching. The skin should not be blanched by the caliper.
4. The distance is decreased until the client no longer feels two distinct points, and that distance is measured.

Between 3 and 4 seconds should be allowed between applications, and the client should have four correct responses out of five administrations. Because this test indicates sensory function, it is usually administered at the tips of the fingers. It may be used proximally to test nerve regeneration. Normal two-point discrimination at the fingertip is 6 mm or less.

Moving two-point discrimination measures the innervation density of the quickly adapting nerve fibers for touch. It is slightly more sensitive than stationary two-point discrimination. The test is performed as follows[30]:
1. The client's vision is occluded.
2. An area of normal sensation is tested as a reference, using blunt calipers or a bent paper clip.
3. The fingertip is supported by the examining table or the examiner's hand.
4. The caliper, separated 5 mm to 8 mm, is moved longitudinally from proximal to distal in a linear fashion along the surface of the fingertip. One and two points are randomly alternated. The client must correctly identify the stimulus in seven out of eight responses before proceeding to a smaller value. The test is repeated down to a separation of 2 mm.

Two-point values increase with age in both sexes, with the smallest values occurring between the ages of 10 and 30 years.

---

*Central Tool Company of Germany (available from Anthony Products, Indianapolis, IN).

†Disk-Criminator (available from Smith & Nephew, Germantown, WI).

Women tend to have smaller values than men, and there is no significant difference between dominant and nondominant hands.[58]

Modified Moberg pick-up test

Recognition of common objects is the final level of sensory function. Moberg used the phrase *tactile gnosis* to describe the ability of the hand to perform complex functions by feel. Moberg described the pick-up test in 1958,[74] and it was later modified by Dellon.[30] This test is used with either a median nerve injury or an injury to a combination of median and ulnar nerves. It takes twice as long to perform the tests with vision occluded as with vision unimpaired. The test is performed as follows:

1. Nine or 10 small objects (e.g., coins or paper clips) are placed on a table, and the client is asked to place them, one at a time, in a small container as quickly as possible, while looking at them. The client is timed.
2. The test is repeated for the opposite hand with vision.
3. The test is repeated for each hand with vision occluded.
4. The client is asked to identify each object one at a time, with and then without vision.

It is important to observe any substitution patterns that may be used when the client cannot see the objects.

Edema Assessment

Hand volume is measured to assess the presence of extracellular or intracellular edema. Volume measurement is generally used to determine the effect of intervention and activities. By measuring volume at different times of the day, the therapist can measure the effects of rest versus activity, as well as the effects of **splinting** or intervention designed to reduce edema.

A commercial volumeter[26] may be used to assess hand edema. The volumeter has been shown to be accurate to 10 ml[101] when used in the prescribed manner. Variables that have been shown to decrease the accuracy of the volumeter include the use of a faucet or hose that introduces air into the tank during filling, movement of the arm within the tank, inconsistent pressure on the stop rod, and the use of a volumeter in a variety of places. The same level surface should always be used.[101] The evaluation is performed as follows (Figure 39-1):

1. A plastic volumeter is filled and allowed to empty into a large beaker until the water reaches spout level. The beaker is then emptied and dried thoroughly.
2. The client is instructed to immerse the hand in the plastic volumeter, being careful to keep the hand in the midposition.
3. The hand is lowered until it rests gently between the middle and ring fingers on the dowel rod. It is important that the hand not press onto the rod.
4. The hand remains still until no more water drips into the beaker.
5. The water is poured into a graduated cylinder. The cylinder is placed on a level surface, and a reading is made.

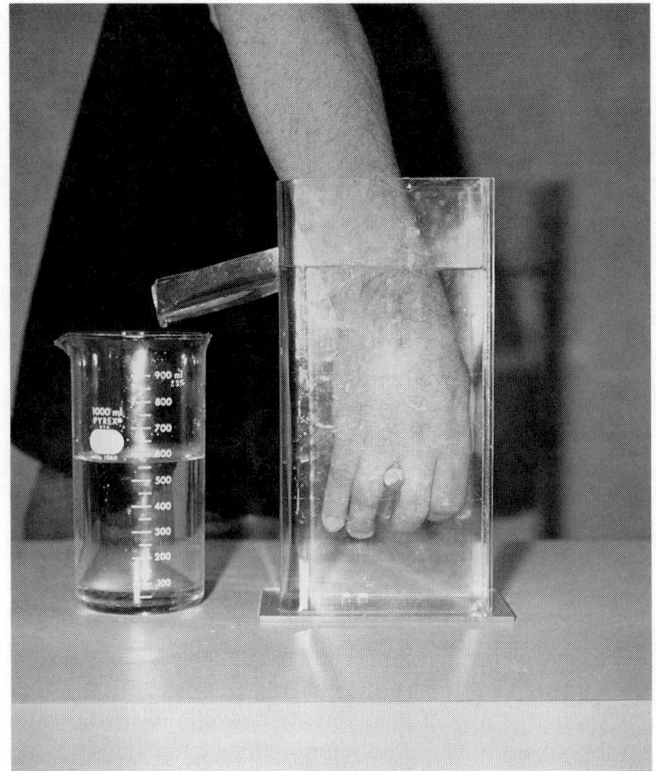

Figure 39-1 Volumeter is used to measure volume of both hands for comparison. Increased volume indicates presence of edema.

A method of assessing edema of an individual finger or joint is circumferential measurement using either a circumference tape* or jeweler's ring-size standards. Measurements should be made before and after intervention and especially after the application of thermal modalities or splinting. Although clients often have subjective complaints relating to swelling, objective data of circumference or volume will help the therapist to assess the response of the tissues to intervention and activity. Edema control techniques are discussed later in this chapter.

GRIP AND PINCH STRENGTH

UE strength is usually assessed after the healing phase of trauma. Strength testing is not indicated after recent trauma or surgery. Testing should not be performed until the client has been cleared for full-resistive activities, usually 8 to 12 weeks after injury.

A standard adjustable-handle dynamometer is recommended for assessing grip strength (Figure 39-2). The subject should be seated with the shoulder adducted and neutrally rotated, the elbow flexed at 90 degrees,[65] forearm in the neutral position, and wrist between 0 and 30 degrees extension and between 0 and 15 degrees of ulnar deviation.

---

*DeRoyal/LMB, DeRoyal Industries, Powell, TN.

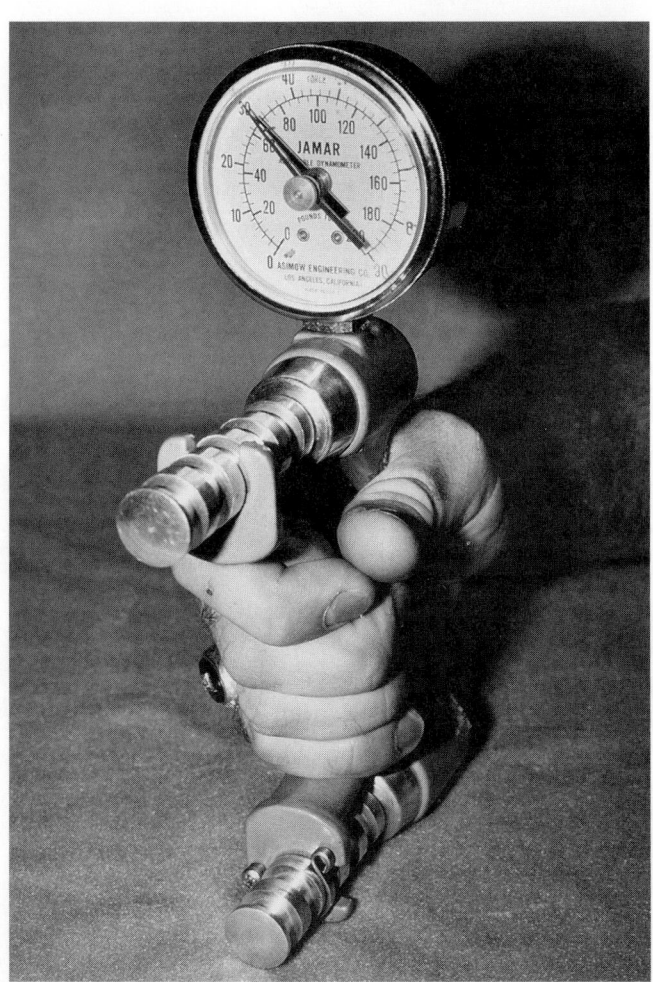

Figure 39-2   Jamar dynamometer is used to evaluate grip strength in both hands.

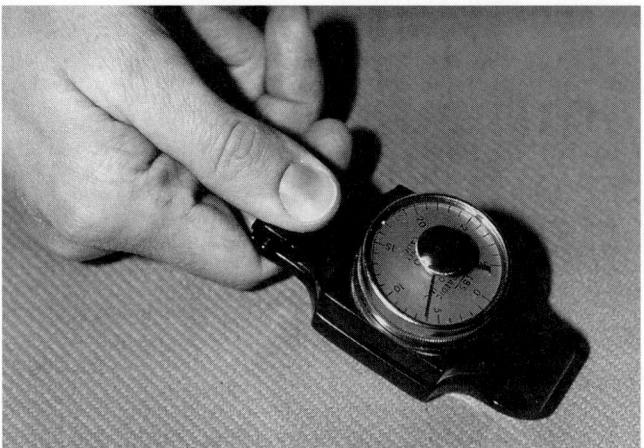

Figure 39-3   Pinch gauge is used to evaluate pinch strength to variety of prehension patterns of pinch.

Three trials are taken of each hand, with the dynamometer handle set at the second position.[68] The examiner should hold the dynamometer lightly to prevent accidental dropping of the instrument. A mean of the three trials should be reported. The noninjured hand is used for comparison. Normative data may be used to compare strength scores.[52, 67] Variables such as age will affect the strength measurements.

Pinch strength should also be tested, using a pinch gauge. The pinch gauge has been found to be the most accurate.[68] Two-point pinch (thumb tip to index fingertip), lateral or key pinch (thumb pulp to lateral aspect of the middle phalanx of the index finger), and three-point pinch (thumb tip to tips of index and middle fingers) should be evaluated. As with the grip dynamometer, three successive trials should be obtained and compared bilaterally (Figure 39-3).[39]

Manual muscle testing is also used to test UE strength. Accurate assessment is especially important when the client is being prepared for tendon transfers or other reconstructive surgery. The student who wishes to study kinesiology of the UE is referred especially to Brand's work.[14] Additionally, muscle testing is addressed in Chapter 21.

Maximal voluntary effort during grip, pinch, or muscle testing will be affected by pain in the hand or extremity, and the therapist should note if the client's ability to exert full force is limited by subjective complaints. Localization of the pain symptoms and consistency in noting pain will help the therapist evaluate the role that pain is playing in the recovery from injury. Pain problems are discussed in more detail later in this chapter.

FUNCTIONAL ASSESSMENT

Assessment of hand function or performance is important because the physical assessment does not measure the client's ingenuity and ability to compensate for loss of strength, ROM, or sensation or the presence of abnormalities.[20]

The physical assessment should precede the functional assessment because awareness of physical dysfunction can result in a critical analysis of functional impairment and an understanding of the reasons that the client functions as he or she does.[69]

The occupational therapist should observe the effect of the hand dysfunction on the use of the hand during ADLs. In addition, some type of a standardized performance test, such as the Jebsen Test of Hand Function[46] or the Carroll Quantitative Test of Upper Extremity Function,[20] should be administered.

The Jebsen Test of Hand Function[46] was developed to provide objective measurements of standardized tasks with norms for client comparison. It is a short test that is assembled by the administrator. It is easy to administer and inexpensive. The test consists of seven subtests, which test writing a short sentence, turning over 3- × 5-inch cards, picking up small objects and placing them in a container, stacking checkers, simulated eating, moving empty large cans, and moving weighted large cans. Norms are provided for dominant and nondominant hands for each subtest and further categorized by gender and age. Instructions for assembling the test, as well as specific instructions for administering it, are provided by the authors.[46] This has been found to be a good test for overall hand function.

The Quantitative Test of Upper Extremity Function described by Carroll[20] was designed to measure ability to perform general arm and hand activities used in daily living. It is based on the assumption that complex UE movements used to perform ordinary ADLs can be reduced to specific patterns of grasp and prehension of the hand, supination and pronation of the forearm, flexion and extension of the elbow, and elevation of the arm.

The test consists of six parts: grasping and lifting four blocks of graduated sizes to assess grasp; grasping and lifting two pipes of graduated sizes to test cylindrical grip; grasping and placing a ball to test spherical grasp; picking up and placing four marbles of graduated sizes to test fingertip prehension or pinch; putting a small washer over a nail and putting an iron on a shelf to test placing; and pouring water from pitcher to glass and glass to glass. In addition, to assess pronation, supination, and elevation of the arm, the therapist instructs the subject to place his or her hand on top of the head, behind the head, and to the mouth and write his or her name. The test uses simple, inexpensive, and easily acquired materials. Details of materials and their arrangement, test procedures, and scoring can be found in the original source.[20]

Other tests that are useful in the assessment of hand dexterity are the Crawford Small Parts Dexterity Test,[25] the Bennett Hand Tool Dexterity Test,[11] the Purdue Pegboard Test,[95] and the Minnesota Manual Dexterity Test.[73] The VALPAR Corporation* has developed a number of standardized tests that measure an individual's ability to perform work-related tasks. They provide information about the test taker's results, compared with industry performance standards. All of these tests include comparison with normal subjects working in a variety of industrial settings. This information can be used in predicting the likelihood of successful return to a specific job. The tests are especially useful when administering a work capacity evaluation. Tests may be purchased and come with instructions for administration of the test and the standardized norms. Melvin[69] lists a variety of additional hand function tests. Further discussion of vocational evaluation can be found in Chapter 13.

INTERVENTION

FRACTURES

In treating a hand or wrist fracture, the surgeon attempts to achieve good anatomical position through either a closed (nonoperative) or open (operative) reduction. Internal fixation

with Kirschner wires, metallic plates, or screws may be used to maintain the desired position. External fixation may also be used with internal fixation. The hand is usually immobilized in wrist extension and MP joint flexion, with extension of the distal joints whenever the injury allows this position. Trauma to bone may also involve trauma to tendons and nerves in the adjacent area. Intervention must be geared toward the recovery of all injured structures, and this fact may influence treatment of the fracture.

OT may be initiated during the period of immobilization, which is usually 3 to 5 weeks. Uninvolved fingers of the hand must be kept mobile through the use of active motion. Edema should be carefully monitored, and elevation is required whenever edema is present.

As soon as there is sufficient bone stability, the surgeon allows mobilization of the injured part. The surgeon should provide guidelines for the amount of resistance or force that may be applied to the fracture site. Activities that correct poor motor patterns and encourage use of the injured hand should be started as soon as the hand is pain free. Early motion will prevent the adherence of tendons and reduce edema through stimulation of the lymphatic and blood vessels.

As soon as the brace or cast is removed, the client's hand must be evaluated. If edema remains present, edema control techniques can be initiated using techniques described later in this chapter. A baseline ROM should be established, and the application of appropriate splints may begin. A splint may be used to correct abnormal joint changes that have resulted from immobilization, or it may be used to protect the finger from additional trauma to the fracture site. An example of this type of splinting would be the application of a Velcro "buddy" splint (Figure 39-4). A dorsal block splint that limits full extension of the finger may be used after a fracture or dislocation of the PIP joint. A dynamic splint may be used to

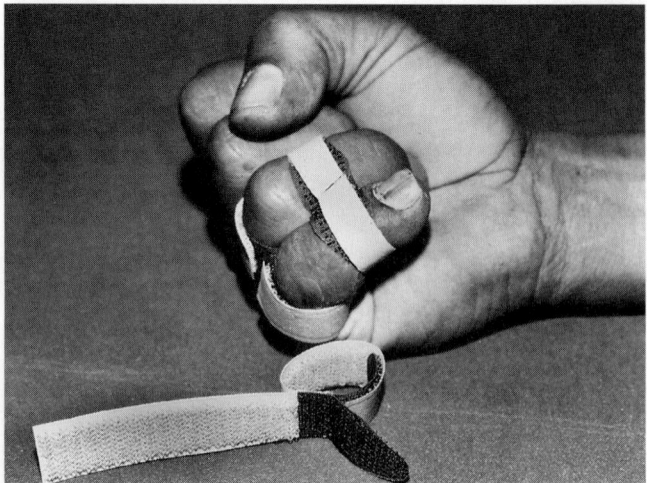

Figure 39-4 Velcro "buddy" splint may be used to protect finger following fracture or to encourage movement of stiff finger. (Splint available from Smalley and Bates, Inc.)

---

*VALPAR Assessment Systems (available from VALPAR International, Tuscon, AZ, http://www.valparint.com)

achieve full ROM or to prevent the development of further abnormal joint changes at 6 to 8 weeks after fracture.

Intraarticular fractures may result in injury to the cartilage of the joint, causing additional pain and stiffness. An X-ray examination will indicate whether the joint surface has been damaged, which might limit the treatment of the joint. Joint pain and stiffness after fracture without the presence of joint damage should be alleviated by a combination of thermal modalities, restoration of joint play, or joint mobilization and corrective and dynamic splinting followed by active use. Resistive exercise can be started when bony healing has been achieved.

Wrist fractures are common and may present special problems for the surgeon and therapist. Colles fractures of the distal radius are the most common injury to the wrist[12] and may result in limitations in wrist flexion and extension, as well as pronation and supination resulting from the involvement of the distal radioulnar joint. External fixators, which may be used with or without internal fixation, are now common in the reduction of distal radius fractures. The external fixator maintains the anatomical relationship

between the radius and ulna by maintaining the length of the radius, often with excellent results. The therapist must carefully instruct the client in active ROM of the fingers and proper care of the pin sites while the fixator is in place. Use of splints, active motion that emphasizes wrist movement, and joint mobilization may be beneficial after removal of the fixator or cast. The Weight Well may be used to provide resistance to wrist motions (Figure 39-5).

The scaphoid is the second most commonly injured bone in the wrist[12] and is often fractured when the hand is dorsiflexed at the time of injury. Fractures to the proximal pole of the scaphoid may result in nonunion because of poor blood supply to this area. Scaphoid fractures require a prolonged period of immobilization, sometimes up to several months in a cast, with resulting stiffness and pain. Care should be taken to mobilize uninvolved joints early.

Trauma to the lunate bone of the wrist may result in avascular necrosis of the lunate or Kienböck's disease,[12] which may result from a one-time accident or repetitive trauma. Lunate fractures are usually immobilized for 6 weeks. Kienböck's disease may be treated with a bone graft, removal of the proximal carpal row, or partial wrist fusion.

Stiffness and pain are common complications of fractures. The control of edema coupled with early motion and good client instruction and support will minimize these complications, however.

NERVE INJURIES

Nerve injury may be classified into the following three categories:

1. Neurapraxia is contusion of the nerve without wallerian degeneration. The nerve recovers function without intervention within a few days or weeks.
2. Axonotmesis is an injury in which nerve fibers distal to the site of injury degenerate, but the internal organization of the nerve remains intact. No surgical intervention is necessary, and recovery usually occurs within 6 months. The length of time may vary, depending on the level of injury.
3. Neurotmesis is a complete laceration of both nerve and fibrous tissues. Surgical intervention is required. Microsurgical repair of the fascicles is common. Nerve grafting may be necessary in situations in which there is a gap between nerve endings.[89]

Peripheral nerve injuries may occur as a result of disruption of the nerve by a fractured bone, laceration, or crush injury. Symptoms of nerve injuries include weakness or paralysis of muscles that are innervated by motor branches of the injured nerve and sensory loss to areas that are innervated by sensory branches of the injured nerve. Before evaluating the client for nerve loss, the therapist must be familiar with the muscles and areas that are innervated by the three major forearm nerves. A summary of UE peripheral neuropathic conditions can be found in Table 39-4.

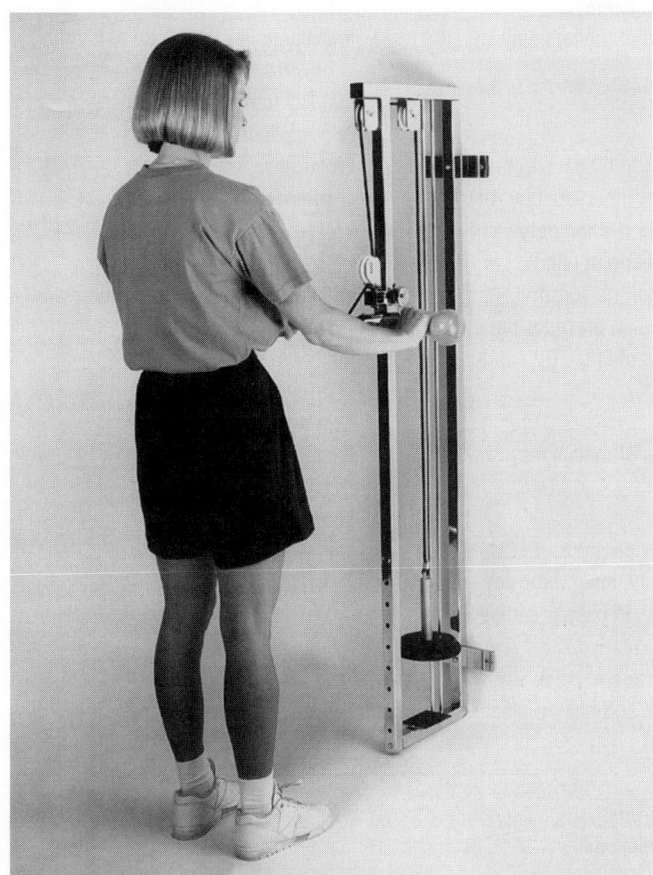

Figure 39-5 Weight Well is used for strengthening upper extremity with progressive resistance applied to weakened musculature and is also useful in retraining prehension of pinch and grip. (Photo courtesy of Karen Schultz Johnson.)

TABLE 39-4 **Nerve Injuries of the Upper Extremity**

Nerve	Location	Affected	Test
Radial nerve (posterior cord, fibers from C5, C6, C7, C8)	Upper arm	Triceps and all distal motors Sensory to SRN	MMT Sensory test
Radial nerve	Above elbow	Brachioradialis and all distal motors Sensory to SRN	MMT Sensory
Radial nerve	At elbow	Supinator, ECRL, ECRB, and all distal motors Sensory to SRN	MMT Sensory
Posterior interosseous nerve	Forearm	ECU, ED, EDM, APL, EPL, EPB, EIP No sensory	Wrist extension—if present, indicates PIN rather than high radial nerve
Radial nerve at ECRB, radial artery, arcade of Frohse, origin of supinator	Radial tunnel syndrome	Weakness of muscles innervated by PIN No sensory loss	Palpate for pain over extensor mass Pain with wrist flexion and pronation Pain with wrist extension and supination Pain with resisted middle finger extension
Median nerve (lateral from C5, C6, C7, medial cord from C8, T1)	High lesions (elbow and above)	Paralysis/weakness of FCR, PL, all FDS, FDP I and II FPL, pronator teres and quad., opponens pollicis, APB, FPB (radial head), lumbricals I and II Sensory cutaneous branch of median nerve	MMT Sensory
Median nerve	Low (at wrist)	Weakness of thenars only	Inability to flex thumb tip and index fingertip to palm Inability to oppose thumb Poor dexterity
Median nerve under fibrous band in PT, beneath heads of pronator, arch of FDS, origin of FCR	Pronator syndrome	Weakness in thenars, but not muscles innervated by AIN Sensory in median nerve distribution in hand	Provocative tests to isolate compression site
Median nerve under origin of PT, FDS to middle	Anterior interosseous nerve syndrome	Pure motor, no sensory Forearm pain precedes paralysis Weakness of FPL, FDP I and II, PQ	Inability to flex IP joint of thumb and DIP of index Increased pain with resisted pronation Pain with forearm pressure
Median nerve at wrist	Carpal tunnel syndrome	Weakness of medial intrinsics Sensory	Provocative tests Tinel's Sensory
Ulnar nerve at elbow (branch of medial cord from C7, C8, T1)	Cubital tunnel syndrome	Weakness/paralysis of FCU, FDP III and IV, ulnar intrinsics Numbness in palmar cutaneous and dorsal cutaneous distribution Loss of grip and pinch strength	Pain with elbow flexion and extension
Ulnar nerve at wrist	Compression at canal of Guyon	Weakness and pain in ulnar intrinsics	Reproduced by pressure at site

AIN, Anterior interosseus nerve; *APB*, abductor pollicis brevis; *APL*, abductor pollicis longus; *ECRB*, extensor carpi radialis brevis; *ECRL*, extensor carpi radialis longus; *ECU*, extensor carpi ulnaris; *ED*, extensor digitorum; *EDM*, extensor digitorum minimus; *EIP*, extensor indicis proprius; *FDS*, flexor digitorum superficialis; *EPB*, extensor pollicis brevis; *EPL*, extensor pollicis longus; *FCR*, flexor carpi radialis; *FDP*, flexor digitorum profundus; *FPB*, flexor pollicis brevis; *FPL*, flexor pollicis longus; *MMT*, manual muscle test; *PIN*, posterior interosseus nerve; *PQ*, pronator quadratus; *PT*, pronator teres; *SRN*, superficial radial nerve.

Radial Nerve

The radial nerve innervates the extensor-supinator group of muscles of the forearm, including the brachioradialis, extensor carpi radialis longus, extensor carpi radialis brevis, extensor digitorum communis, extensor digiti minimi, extensor indicis, extensor carpi ulnaris, supinator, abductor pollicis longus, extensor pollicis brevis, and extensor pollicis longus. The sensory distribution of the radial nerve is a strip of the posterior upper arm and the forearm; dorsum of the thumb; and index and middle fingers and radial half of the ring finger to the PIP joints. Sensory loss of the radial nerve does not usually result in dysfunction.

Clinical signs of a high-level radial nerve injury (above the supinator) are pronation of the forearm, wrist flexion, and the thumb held in palmar abduction resulting from the unopposed action of the flexor pollicis brevis and the abductor pollicis brevis.[80] Injury to the posterior interosseous nerve spares the extensor carpi radialis longus and brevis. Posterior interosseous nerve syndrome includes normal sensation and wrist extension with loss of finger and thumb extension. Clinical signs of low-level radial nerve injury include incomplete extension of the MP joints of the fingers and thumb. The interossei extend the interphalangeal (IP) joints of the fingers, but the MP joints rest in about 30 degrees of flexion.

A dynamic splint, applied to the dorsum of the hand, that provides wrist extension, MP extension, and thumb extension should be provided to protect the extensor tendons from overstretching during the healing phase and to position the hand for functional use (Figure 39-6). A dynamic splint is commonly provided.

Median Nerve

The median nerve innervates the flexors of the forearm and hand and is often called the "eyes" of the hands because of its importance in sensory innervation of the volar surface of the thumb, index, and middle fingers. Median nerve loss may result from lacerations, as well as from compression syndromes of the wrist, such as carpal tunnel syndrome.

Motor distribution of the median nerve is to the pronator teres, palmaris longus, flexor carpi radialis, flexor digitorum profundus of the index and middle fingers, flexor digitorum superficialis, flexor pollicis longus, pronator quadratus, abductor pollicis brevis, opponens pollicis, superficial head of the flexor pollicis brevis, and first and second lumbricals.

Sensory distribution of the median nerve is to the volar surface of the thumb, index, and middle fingers; radial half of the ring finger and dorsal surface of the index and middle fingers; and radial half of the ring finger distal to the PIP joints.

Clinical signs of a high-level median nerve injury are ulnar flexion of the wrist caused by loss of the flexor carpi radialis, loss of palmar abduction, and opposition of the thumb. Active pronation is absent, but the client may appear to pronate with the assistance of gravity. In a wrist-level median nerve injury, the thenar eminence appears flat and there is a loss of thumb flexion, palmar abduction, and opposition.[80]

The sensory loss associated with median nerve injury is particularly disabling because there is no sensation to the volar aspects of the thumb and index and middle fingers and the radial side of the ring finger. When blindfolded, the client substitutes pinch to the ring and small fingers to compensate for this loss. An injury in the forearm that involves the anterior interosseous nerve does not result in sensory loss. Motor loss includes paralysis of the flexor pollicis longus, the flexor digitorum profundus of the index and middle fingers, and the pronator quadratus. The pronator teres is not affected. Pinch is affected.

Splints that position the thumb in palmar abduction and slight opposition increase functional use of the hand (Figure 39-7). If clawing of the index and middle fingers is present, a splint should be fabricated to prevent hyperextension of

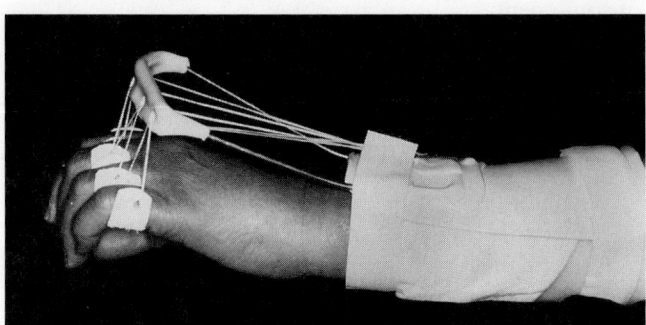

Figure 39-6 Low-profile radial nerve splint is carefully balanced to pull metacarpophalangeal (MP) joints into extension when wrist is flexed and allows the MP joints to fall into slight flexion when wrist is extended, thus preserving normal balance between two joints and preserving joint contracture. (Splint courtesy of Judy C. Colditz, Raleigh Hand Rehabilitation Center.)

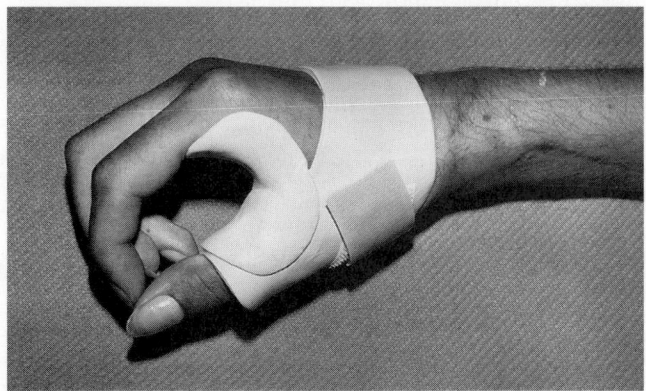

Figure 39-7 Thumb stabilization splint may be used with median nerve injury to protect thumb and to improve functioning by placing thumb in position of pinch. Normal pinch cannot be achieved with median nerve injury because of paralysis of thumb musculature.

the MP joints. Clients report that they avoid use of the hand with a median nerve injury because of lack of sensation rather than because of muscle paralysis. Nevertheless, the weakened or paralyzed muscles should be protected.

Ulnar Nerve

The ulnar nerve in the forearm innervates only the flexor carpi ulnaris and the median half of the flexor digitorum profundus. It travels down the volar forearm through the canal of Guyon, innervating the intrinsic muscles of the hand, including the palmaris brevis, abductor digiti minimi, opponens digiti minimi, flexor digiti minimi, dorsal and volar interossei, third and fourth lumbricals, and medial head of the flexor pollicis brevis. The sensory distribution of the ulnar nerve is the dorsal and volar surfaces of the small finger ray and the ulnar half of the dorsal and volar surface of the ring finger ray.

A high-level ulnar nerve injury results in hyperextension of the MP joints of the ring and small fingers (also called *clawing*) as a response to overaction of the extensor digitorum communis that is not held in check by the third and fourth lumbricals.[82] The IP joints of the ring and small fingers do not demonstrate a great flexion deformity because of the paralysis of the flexor digitorum profundus. The hypothenar muscles and interossei are absent. The wrist assumes a position of radial extension caused by the loss of the flexor carpi ulnaris. In a low-level ulnar nerve injury, the ring and small fingers claw at the MP joints and the IP joints exhibit a greater tendency toward flexion because the flexor digitorum profundus is present. Wrist extension is normal.

Clinical signs of a high-level ulnar nerve injury may include clawhand deformity (as described above) with a loss of the hypothenar and the interosseous muscles. In a low-level ulnar nerve injury, the flexor digitorum profundus and flexor carpi ulnaris are present and unopposed by the intrinsic muscles. There is a positive Froment's sign. Long-standing compression of the ulnar nerve in the canal of Guyon results in a flattening of the hypothenar area and conspicuous atrophy of the first dorsal interosseous muscle.[12]

With a low-level ulnar nerve injury a small splint may be provided to prevent hyperextension of the small and ring fingers without limiting full flexion at the MP joints. Stabilization of the MP joints will allow the extensor digitorum communis to extend the IP joints fully (Figure 39-8).

Sensory loss of the ulnar nerve results in frequent injury, especially burns, to the ulnar side of the hand. Clients must be instructed in visual protection of the anesthetic area.

Postoperative Management After Nerve Repair

After nerve repair the hand is placed in a position that minimizes tension on the nerve. For example, after repair of the median nerve, the wrist is immobilized in a flexed position. Immobilization usually lasts for 2 to 3 weeks, after which protective stretching of the joints may begin. The therapist must exercise great care not to put excessive traction on the

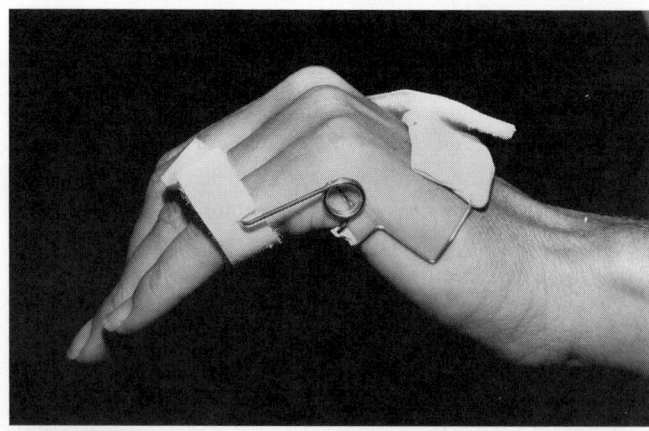

Figure 39-8 Dynamic ulnar nerve splint blocks hyperextension of metacarpophalangeal (MP) joints that occurs with paralysis of ulnar intrinsic muscles and allows MP flexion, which maintains normal range of motion of MP joints. (Splint courtesy of Mary Dimick, University of California-San Diego Hand Rehabilitation Center.)

newly repaired nerve. A repaired digital nerve will also be protected with flexion of the PIP joint.

Correction of a contracture may take 4 to 6 weeks. Active exercise is the preferred method of gaining full extension, although a light dynamic splint may be applied with the surgeon's supervision. Splinting to assist or substitute for weakened musculature may be necessary for an extended period during nerve regeneration. Splints should be removed as soon as possible to allow active exercise of the weakened muscles. It is important to instruct the client in correct patterns of motion, however, so that substitution is minimized.

Intervention is initially directed toward the prevention of deformity and correction of poor positioning during the acute and regenerative stages. Clients must be instructed in visual protection of the anesthetic area. ADLs should be assessed, and new methods or devices may be needed for independence. Use of the hand in the client's work should be assessed, and the client should be returned to employment with any necessary job modifications or adaptations of equipment.

Careful muscle, sensory, and functional testing should be done frequently. As the nerve regenerates, splints may be changed or eliminated. Exercises and activities should be revised to reflect the client's new gains, and adapted equipment should be discarded as soon as possible.

As motor function begins to return to the paralyzed muscles, a careful program of specific exercises should be devised to facilitate the return. Proprioceptive neuromuscular facilitation (PNF) techniques, such as hold-relax, contract-relax, quick stretch, and icing, may assist a fair-strength muscle and increase ROM. Neuromuscular electrical stimulation (NMES) can also provide an external stimulus to help strengthen the newly innervated muscle. When the muscle has reached a good rating, functional activities should be used to complete the return to normal strength.

Sensory reeducation

Assessment of sensibility is described in some detail earlier in this chapter. This information should be used to prepare a program of sensory reeducation after nerve repair.

When a nerve is repaired, regeneration is not perfect and results in fewer and smaller nerve fibers and receptors distal to the repair. The goal of sensory reeducation is to maximize the functional level of sensation or tactile gnosis.

Parry first described sensory reeducation in 1966,[80] and Dellon reported a highly structured sensory reeducation program in 1974.[32] Dellon divided his program into early- and late-phase training, based on vibratory sensation for early phase and perception of moving and constant touch sensation for late-phase reeducation. Localization of stimuli and recognition of objects were used by both Parry and Dellon. Higher cortical integration was achieved by focusing attention on the stimuli through visual clues and by employing memory when vision was occluded. The clients were taught to compensate for sensory deficits by improving specific skills and generalizing them to other sensory stimuli. Daily repetition appears to be a necessary component of reeducation.

Callahan[18] outlined a program of protective sensory reeducation and discriminative sensory reeducation if protective sensation is present and touch sensation has returned to the fingertips. Waylett-Rendall[100] also described a sensory reeducation program using crafts and functional activities, as well as desensitization techniques. All programs emphasize a variety of stimuli used in a repetitive manner to bombard the sensory receptors. A sequence of eyes-closed, eyes-open, eyes-closed is used to provide feedback during the training process. Sessions are limited in length to prevent fatigue and frustration. To prevent further trauma, objects must not be potentially harmful to the insensate areas. A home program should be provided to reinforce learning that occurs in the clinical setting.

Researchers[18,29,100] have found that sensory reeducation can result in improved functional sensibility in motivated clients. Objective measurement of sensation after reeducation must be performed and then accurately compared with initial testing to assess the success of the program.

Tendon transfers

If a motor nerve has not reinnervated its muscle after a minimum period of 1 year after nerve repair, the surgeon may consider tendon transfers to restore a needed motion. The rules of tendon transfer are to evaluate what is absent, what is needed for function, and what is available to transfer.[85]

Some muscles, such as the extensor carpi radialis longus and the flexor digitorum sublimis to the ring finger, are commonly used for transfers because their motions are easily substituted by the extensor carpi radialis brevis and flexor digitorum profundus, respectively, to the ring finger. The pronator teres is often used to restore wrist extension for

radial nerve paralysis. The surgeon may request assistance from the therapist in evaluating motor status to determine the best motor transfer. Therapy before tendon transfer is essential if the motor being used is not of normal strength. A muscle loses a grade of strength when transferred, and a strengthening program of progressive resistive exercises, NMES, and isolated motion will help ensure success of the transfer. There must be full passive ROM of all joints before tendon transfer can be attempted.

After transfer, many clients require instruction to perceive the correct muscle during active use of the transfer. Use of surface EMG-biofeedback, careful instruction, and supervised activity to note any substitution patterns during active use usually help the client to use the transfer correctly. Therapy must be initiated before the client has time to develop incorrect use patterns. NMES may be used to isolate the muscle and strengthen it postoperatively.

TENDON INJURIES

Flexor Tendons

Tendon injuries may be isolated or may occur in conjunction with other injuries, especially fractures or crushes. Flexor tendons injured in the area between the distal palmar crease and the insertion of the flexor digitorum superficialis are considered the most difficult to treat because the tendons lie in their sheaths in this area beneath the fibrous pulley system and any scarring causes adhesions. This area is often referred to as *zone two* or "no-man's-land."

Primary repair of the flexor tendons within zone 2 is most frequently attempted after a clean laceration. Several methods of postoperative management have been proposed with the common goals of promoting gliding of the tendons and minimizing the formation of scar adhesions.

Controlled mobilization of acute flexor tendon injuries: Louisville technique

Dr. Harold Kleinert of the University of Louisville School of Medicine was an early advocate of rubber band traction after repair of flexor tendons in zone two. This technique is often referred to as the *Kleinert technique*. The doctor and therapist do not actively participate in moving the tendon or finger when this protocol is followed as outlined by Kutz.[56]

After surgical repair, rubber bands are attached to the nails of the involved fingers, using a suture through the nail or a hook held in place with cyanoacrylate glue. A dorsal blocking splint is fabricated of low-temperature thermoplastic material, with the MP joints held in about 60 degrees of flexion. The splint is constructed so that the IP joints are able to extend fully to the splint. The rubber bands are passed through a safety pin in the palm and are attached to the distal strap of the splint. The rubber bands should be placed in sufficient tension to hold the PIP joints in 40 to 60 degrees of flexion without tension on the rubber bands. The client

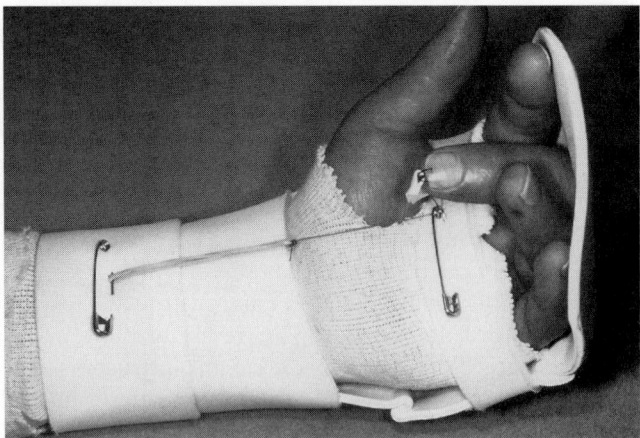

Figure 39-9 After flexor tendon repair, wrist is placed in 30 degrees flexion with traction applied from the nail through a safety pin pulley in the palm and attached to proximal strap of splint. Metacarpophalangeal joints should be maintained in about 70 degrees flexion, allowing full passive interphalangeal joint flexion and active extension.

must be able to fully extend the IP joints actively within the splint, or joint contractures will develop (Figure 39-9).

The client wears the splint 24 hours a day for 3 weeks and is instructed to actively extend the fingers several times a day in the splint, allowing the rubber bands to pull the fingers into flexion. This movement of the tendon through the tendon sheath and pulley system minimizes scar adhesions while enhancing tendon nutrition and blood flow.

The dorsal blocking splint is removed at 3 weeks, and the rubber band is attached to a wristband, which is worn for 1 to 5 additional weeks, depending on the judgment of the surgeon. The primary disadvantage of this technique is that contractures of the PIP joints frequently occur as a result of excessive tension on the rubber band or incomplete IP extension within the splint.

Dynamic extension splinting of the PIP joint can be started at 5 to 6 weeks if a flexion contracture is present. To be successful, this technique requires a motivated client who thoroughly understands the program.

Controlled passive motion: Duran and Houser technique

Duran and Houser[34] suggested the use of controlled passive motion to achieve optimal results after primary repair, allowing 3 to 5 mm of tendon excursion. They found this amount sufficient to prevent adherence of the repaired tendons. On the third postoperative day, the client begins a twice-daily exercise regimen of passive flexion and extension of six to eight motions for each tendon. Care is taken to keep the wrist flexed and the MPs in 70 degrees of flexion during passive exercise. Between exercise periods the hand is wrapped in stockinette. At $4^{1}/2$ weeks, the protective dorsal splint is removed and the rubber band traction is attached to a wristband. Active extension and passive flexion are performed for

an additional week and gradually increased over the next several weeks.

Early active motion

As methods of tendon suturing and the suture materials themselves have evolved, some clinicians have begun to prescribe active movement of the repaired tendon within days of surgery. This technique is usually performed only with the most experienced surgeons and therapists working closely together. The condition of the tendon and the technique of repair must be communicated to the therapist, and the client must be closely monitored. As the rate of rupture decreases with more sophisticated repairs, the results after tendon injury have improved.[90]

There are several well-documented early active motion protocols, but all of the protocols share in common several important factors. First, the tendon repair strength must be sufficient to be able to withstand the forces of active mobilization, and it is generally agreed that a suture strand repair be performed to use this intervention approach. Second, the timing and the initiation of therapy must be considered. It has been suggested that early active motion be initiated between 2 and 4 days after repair to allow inflammation to subside, thus reducing the amount of force on the tendon during active flexion. Third, the client must be able to comprehend and be compliant with the exercise program for the tendon rehabilitation to be successful and to prevent rupture of the tendon by overstressing the repair site. Finally, for this technique to be successful, the therapist and surgeon must be in good communication and be skilled in the rehabilitation of flexor tendons.

Because early active mobilization of newly repaired flexor tendons involves a somewhat higher risk of rupture if managed incorrectly, it is strongly recommended that this approach be used with the full cooperation of the surgeon. Again, this approach should not be used by an inexperienced therapist or with a poorly compliant client.

Immobilization technique

A third postoperative program involves complete immobilization for 3 to 4 weeks after tendon repair. Good results have not been consistently achieved with immobilization, and this technique may increase the risk of tendon rupture after repair because a tendon gains tensile strength when submitted to gentle tension at the repair site. It is still the preferred method when treating young children or with a noncompliant client.[91]

Many practitioners have modified the tendon protocols, using a combination of passive flexion and active extension techniques, on the basis of clinical experience. Protocols are suggested as guidelines, but they vary in actual practice.

Postacute flexor tendon rehabilitation

When active flexion is begun out of the splint after any of the postoperative management techniques described previously,

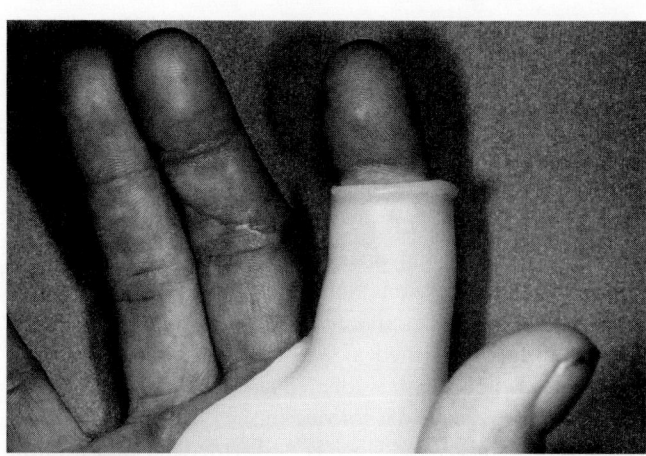

Figure 39-10 Blocking splint can be used to isolate tendon pull-through and joint range of motion by blocking out proximal joints. This splint is being used to facilitate motion at distal interphalangeal joint following repair of flexor digitorum profundus tendon.

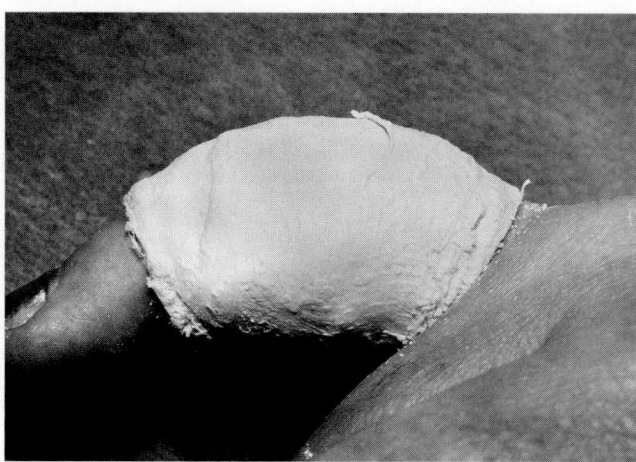

Figure 39-12 Plaster cylindrical splint is used to apply static stretch of proximal interphalangeal joint contracture. It is not removed by client and must be replaced frequently by therapist with careful monitoring of skin condition.

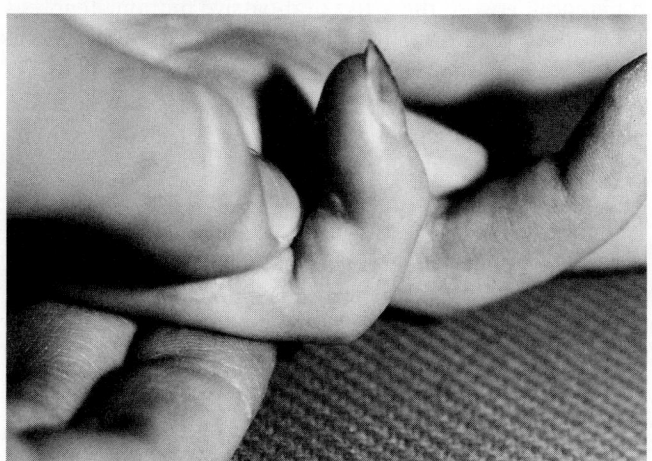

Figure 39-11 Manual blocking of metacarpophalangeal joint during flexion of proximal interphalangeal joint.

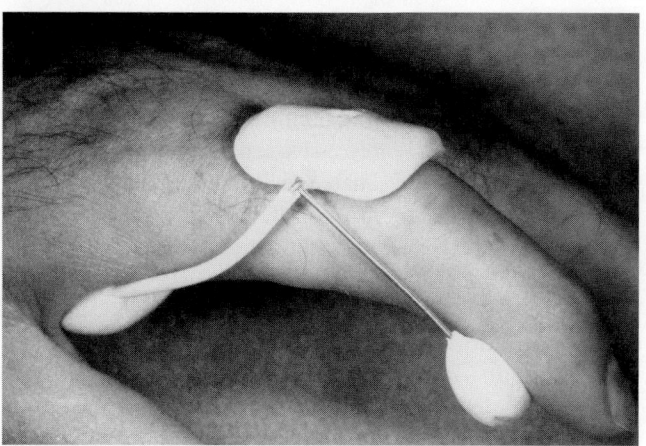

Figure 39-13 This finger splint is used to increase extension of proximal interphalangeal joint. (Splint available from DeRoyal/LMB, DeRoyal Industries, Powell, TN.)

the client should be instructed in exercises to facilitate differential tendon gliding.[102] Wehbe[103] recommends three positions—hook, straight fist, and fist—to maximize isolated gliding of the flexor digitorum superficialis and the flexor digitorum profundus tendons, as well as stretching of the intrinsic musculature and gliding of the extensor mechanism. Tendon gliding exercises should be done for 10 repetitions of each position, two or three times a day.

Isolated exercises to assist tendon gliding may also be performed using a blocking splint (Figure 39-10)[35] or the opposite hand (Figure 39-11). The MP joints should be held in extension during blocking so that the intrinsic muscles that act on it cannot overcome the power of the repaired flexor tendons. Care should be taken not to hyperextend the PIP joints and overstretch the repaired tendons.

After 6 to 8 weeks, passive extension may be started and splinting may be necessary to correct a flexion contracture at the PIP joint. A cylindrical plaster splint may be fabricated to apply constant static pressure on the contracture, as described by Bell-Krotoski (Figure 39-12).[9] Static splinting may be especially effective with a flexion contracture greater than 25 degrees. A finger gutter splint may be made using 1/16-inch (0.16-cm) thermoplastic material for static extension at night, which will help maintain extension gains made during the day. Gentle dynamic traction may be applied using a commercial splint such as a spring finger extension assist (Figure 39-13) or one that is fabricated by the therapist (Figure 39-14). Dynamic flexion splinting may be necessary if the client has difficulty regaining passive flexion.

At about 8 weeks the client may begin light resistive exercises and activities. The hand can now be used for light

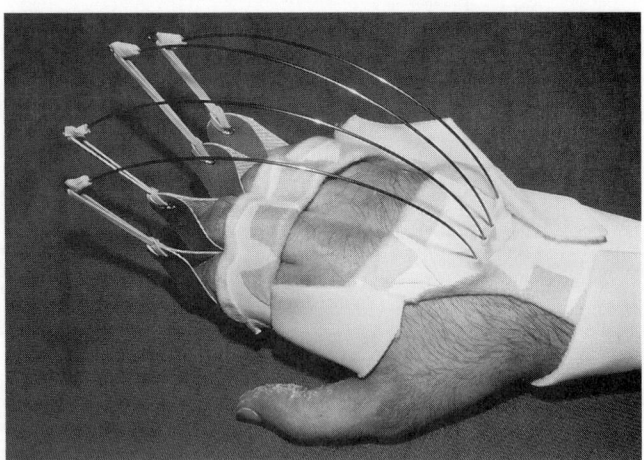

Figure 39-14 Dynamic outrigger splint using spring-steel outriggers with a lumbrical block can be used to assist proximal interphalangeal (PIP) joint extension, stretch against scar adhesions of extrinsic flexors, or reduce PIP joint contractures. Proper fit and tension of rubber bands must be assessed frequently by therapist.

ADLs, but the client should continue to avoid heavy lifting with the affected hand or excessive resistance. Sports activities should be discouraged. Such activities as clay work, woodworking, and macramé are excellent, however. Full resistance and normal work activities can be started 3 months after surgery.

After a hand has sustained a tendon injury, passive versus active limitations of joint motion must be evaluated. Limitations in active motion may indicate joint stiffness, muscle weakness, or scar adhesions.[81] If passive motion is greater than active motion, the therapist should consider that tendons may be caught in the scar tissue. The therapist should be able to determine if a tendon is adhering and causing a flexion contracture or if the tendon is free but the joint itself is stiff. Intervention should be based on this type of evaluation.

ROM, strength, function, and sensibility testing (if digital nerves were also injured) should be performed frequently, with splints and activities geared to progress. Although performance of ADLs is generally not a problem, the therapist should ask the client about any problems he or she may have or anticipate. Disuse and neglect of a finger, especially the index finger, are common and should be prevented.

Gains in flexion and extension may continue to be recorded for 6 months postoperatively. A finger with limber joints and minimal scarring preoperatively will function better after repair than one that is stiff and scarred and has trophic skin changes.[13] Therefore, it is important that all joints, skin, and scars be supple and movable before reconstructive surgery is attempted. A functional to excellent result is obtained if the combined loss of extension is less than 40 degrees in the PIP and DIP joints of the index and

middle fingers and less than 60 degrees in the ring and small fingers[91] and if the finger can flex to the palm.[13]

Flexor tendon reconstruction

If the tendon is damaged as a result of a crush injury or if the laceration cannot be cleaned up enough to allow for a primary repair, staged flexor tendon reconstruction may be performed. At the first operation, a Silastic rod is inserted beneath the pulley system and attached to the distal phalanx. Other reconstructive procedures, such as pulley reconstruction, are performed at the same time. A mesothelial cell–lined pseudosheath is formed about the rod, and a fluid similar to synovial fluid is formed in the postoperative recovery phase.[57] The second stage is performed about 4 months later, when the digit can be moved passively to the palm. A tendon graft is inserted and the Silastic rod removed. The postoperative program is carried out in the same manner as for a primary tendon repair.[45]

After a two-stage tendon reconstruction or primary repair, a tenolysis may be performed if there is a substantial difference between the active and passive motion. Tenolysis is usually not performed for 6 months to 1 year after tendon repair. At the time of tenolysis surgery, scar adhesions are removed from the tendon and gliding of the tendons is assessed. Clients are often asked to move their fingers in the operating room at the time of lysis to determine the extent of scar removal. Active motion is begun within the first 24 hours using bupivacaine (Marcaine) blocks[86] or transcutaneous electrical nerve stimulation (TENS)[19] to control pain.

LaSalle and Strickland[57] have recommended a system for evaluating the results of tenolysis surgery by comparing the preoperative passive IP joint motion with the postoperative IP joint motion. On the basis of this comparison, LaSalle and Strickland found that in one group of clients undergoing tenolysis 40% had an improvement in motion of 50% or better, compared with their preoperative status.

Extensor Tendons

Treatment of extensor tendon injuries requires a thorough knowledge of the extensor anatomy and biomechanics of the hand. The extensor mechanism of the hand is a highly sophisticated and complicated system. It is divided into seven zones for the fingers and five for the thumb. The level of injury will dictate the intervention regimen. Time lines for immobilization, initiation of motion, and resistive exercise depend on the level of injury and the unique healing time frames for the structures in the different zones.

There are four zones distal to the MP joint and three zones starting at the MP joint and proximal. Zones I and II consist of the structures at the DIP joint and middle phalanx, and injuries to this area are treated similarly. Zones III and IV are the areas over the PIP joint and proximal phalanx; again, these zones are treated similarly depending on the structures repaired. Zone V consists of the area over the MP joint, whereas zone VI is the area over the dorsal hand

and zone VII the area over the wrist. In the thumb, zone T1 consists of the area over the DIP joint, T2 the middle phalanx, T3 the MP joint, T4 the proximal phalanx, and T5 the area over the CMC joint and wrist.

Dorsal scar adherence is the most difficult problem after injury to the extensor tendons because of the tendency of the dorsal extensor hood to adhere to the underlying structures and thus limit its normal excursion during flexion and extension. Overstretching the extensor tendon is another common occurrence of the extensor tendon and can result in an extensor lag, or lack of full active extension.

Extensor tendon injuries distal to the MP joint (zones I-IV) generally require a longer period of immobilization, usually 6 weeks. As with flexor tendon injuries, controlled mobilization is being used with increasing frequency for zones III and IV. A protocol developed by Evans called *the Short Arc Motion protocol*, or *SAM protocol*,[36] allows for immediate active flexion of the PIP joint to 30 degrees followed by full passive extension. Complete immobilization for 6 weeks or longer is necessary for injuries in zones I and II.

Several finger abnormal joint changes are associated with injuries distal to the MP joints. An injury to zones I or II, when there is a traumatic disruption of the terminal extensor tendon, is called a *mallet finger*. This joint change is characterized by flexion of the DIP joint and the inability to actively extend this joint. A swan-neck posture is a result of the dorsal displacement of the lateral bands (part of the extensor mechanism) in zone III and results in hyperextension of the PIP joint and flexion of the DIP joint. Another abnormal joint position originating from zone III is known as the *boutonnière deformity*. A boutonnière deformity results when the common extensor tendon is ruptured and the lateral bands sublux volarly. This volar subluxation of the lateral bands results in flexion of the PIP joint and hyperextension of the DIP joint.

Extensor tendons in zones V, VI, and VII (proximal to the MP joints) become adherent because they are encased in paratenon and synovial sheaths and respond to injury in a way similar to flexor tendons, resulting in either incomplete extension, also known as *extensor lag*, or incomplete flexion caused by loss of gliding of the extensor tendon.

Evans[36,37] studied the normal excursion of the extensor digitorum communis in zones V, VI, and VII to suggest guidelines for early passive motion of extensor tendons. She concluded that 5 mm of tendon glide after repair was safe and effective in limiting tendon adhesions and designed a postoperative splint that allows slight active flexion while providing passive extension.[37] The splint is worn for 3 weeks, with the initiation of active motion between the third and fourth weeks. A removable volar splint is used between exercise periods to protect the tendon for 2 additional weeks. Dynamic flexion splinting may be started at 6 weeks after surgery to regain flexion if needed.

Injuries to extensor tendons proximal to the MP joint may be immobilized for 3 weeks. After this period, the

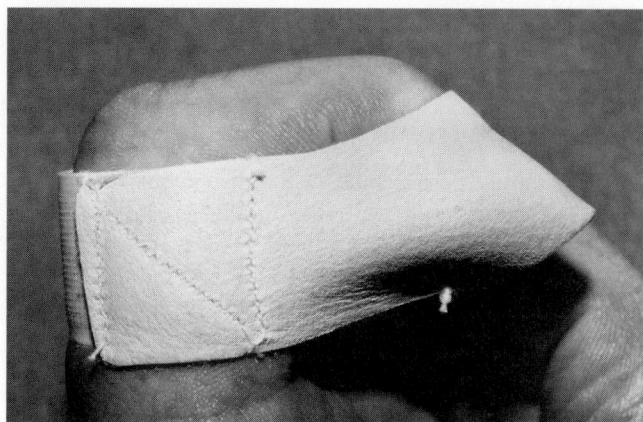

Figure 39-15 Proximal interphalangeal (PIP)-distal interphalangeal (DIP) splint may be used to increase flexion of both PIP and DIP joints. Tension can be adjusted with Velcro closure. Wearing time should be determined by therapist.

finger may be placed in a removable volar splint that is worn between exercise periods for an additional 2 weeks. Progressive ROM is begun at 3 weeks, and if full flexion is not regained rapidly, dynamic flexion may be started at 6 weeks.

Dynamic splints may include a PIP-DIP splint, first described by Hollis and now available commercially (Figure 39-15),* a web strap made of lamp wick or elastic, a fingernail hook with rubber band traction, a traction glove, or another splint.

If a lysis of scar tissue is required because of persistent scar adhesion, the surgeon may place a thin sheet of Silastic between the tendon and bone at the time of surgery to reduce further scar adherence. The client begins exercising within the first 24 hours, and splints are applied as needed. Active exercise is essential, and the client must be carefully instructed in a home program. The client is encouraged to use the hand for all activities except those requiring heavy resistance. After 4 to 6 weeks, the Silastic sheet is removed and ROM should be maintained.

Total Active Motion and Total Passive Motion

Total active motion (TAM) and total passive motion (TPM) are methods of recording joint ROM that are used to compare tendon excursion (active) and joint mobility (passive). It is the measure of flexion minus extensor lag of three joints. The American Society for Surgery of the Hand has recommended TAM and TPM for use in reporting joint motion.[4]

TAM is computed by adding the sum of the angles formed by the MP, PIP, and DIP joints in flexion, minus incomplete active extension at each of the three joints.

*DeRoyal/LMB, DeRoyal Industries, Powell, TN.

For example, MP joint flexion is 85 degrees with full extension, PIP is 100 degrees and lacks 15 degrees extension, and DIP is 65 degrees with full extension; therefore,

$$TAM = 85 + 100 + 65 - 15 = 235 \text{ degrees.}$$

TAM should be measured while the client makes a fist. It is used for a single digit and should be compared with the same digit of the opposite hand or subsequent measurements of the same digit. It should not be used to compute a percentage of loss of impairment. TPM is calculated in the same manner but measures only passive motion.

COMPLEX INJURIES

Complex injuries to the hand or injuries to multiple anatomical structures of the hand are some of the most challenging injuries for the therapist to treat. Complex injuries to the hand differ from other types of hand injuries because they involve trauma to multiple anatomical systems of the hand, resulting in a varied clinical picture. Injuries to these anatomic systems include skin, nerve, tendon, skeletal, and vascular injuries. Because of the complex nature of these injuries and because each injured structure has a unique healing time frame, precaution, and treatment approach, there is no set protocol to follow in treating these injuries.

Many of the treatment precautions established for any one of the aforementioned injuries contradict one another. Therefore, the therapist's challenge is to determine when it is safe for the client to move forward with treatment without risking injury to healing structures. "The therapist must have a thorough knowledge of anatomy, wound healing, biomechanics, and treatment guidelines of various traumatic injuries"[21] as well as a "thorough understanding of the injuries and types of repairs performed. That understanding should include location and quality of repair, types of sutures used, associated injuries, and any structures that were injured but not repaired."[21] Consequently, the therapist must maintain close communication with the treating surgeon. Types of complex hand injuries include crush injuries, amputations with or without replantation, and avulsion injuries and may be caused by motor vehicle accidents, explosions, gunshots, and machinery accidents. Gerry, the client discussed in the case study at the beginning of this chapter, sustained a complex injury to his hand. All of the anatomical structures of his hand were affected by the saw injury; his intervention plan needed to take into account the unique healing time frames and precautions for each of these anatomical structures.

Generally, and in the case of Gerry, the rehabilitation process for these types of injuries is divided into three stages: early or protective stage (first 5-10 days), intermediate or mobilization stage (1-8 weeks after surgery), and late or strengthening stage (6-8 weeks after surgery). The therapist and surgeon must be skilled and experienced in the rehabilitation of these injuries.

 ETHICAL CONSIDERATIONS

EDEMA

Although edema is a normal consequence of trauma, it must be quickly and aggressively treated to prevent permanent stiffness and disability. Within hours of trauma, vasodilatation and local edema occur, with an increase in white blood cells in the damaged area.[38] The inflammatory response to the injury results in a decrease in bacteria to control infection.

Early control of edema should be achieved through elevation, massage, compression, and active ROM. The client is instructed at the time of injury to keep the hand elevated, and a compressive dressing is used to reduce early swelling. Pitting edema appears early and can be recognized as a bloated swelling that creates a pitted appearance when pressed. Pitting may be more pronounced on the dorsal surface, where the venous and lymphatic systems provide return of fluid to the heart. Active motion is especially important to produce retrograde venous and lymphatic flow.

If the swelling continues, a serofibrinous exudate invades the area. Fibrin is deposited in the spaces surrounding the joints, tendons, and ligaments, resulting in reduced mobility, flattening of the arches of the hand, tissue atrophy, and further disuse.[33] Normal gliding of the tissues is eliminated, and a stiff, often painful hand is the result. Scar adhesions form and further limit tissue mobility. If untreated, these losses may become permanent.

Early recognition of persistent edema through observation and volume and circumference measurement is important. It may be necessary to use several of the suggested edema control techniques.

Elevation

Early elevation with the hand above the heart is essential. Slings tend to reduce blood flow and should be avoided. Resting the hand on pillows while seated or lying down is effective. Resting the hand on top of the head or using devices that elevate the hand with the elbow in extension has been suggested.

The client should use the hand for ADLs, within the limitations of resistance prescribed by the physician. Light ADLs that can be accomplished while the hand is in the dressing are permitted.

Contrast Baths

Alternating soaks of cold and warm water that is 66° and 96° F (18.9° and 35.6° C) are generally preferred over warm water soaks or whirlpool baths. The contrast baths can be done for 20 minutes, alternating the hand between cool water for 1 minute and warm water for 1 minute, starting and ending with cool water. A sponge can be placed in each tub so that the hand is moving (gentle squeezing of the sponge) during the soaking period. The tubs should be placed as high as possible to provide elevation of the extremity. The alternating warm and cool water cause vasodilatation and vasoconstriction, resulting in a pumping action on the edema. Combined with elevation and active motion, edema may be reduced and pain is often alleviated by this technique.

Manual Edema Mobilization

Manual edema mobilization (MEM) is a method of edema reduction based on methods to activate the lymphatic system. These methods include the principles of manual lymphedema treatment (MLT) massage, medical compression bandaging, exercise, and external compression adapted to meet the specific needs of subacute and chronic post-surgical and poststroke UE edema. The goals are to stimulate the initial lymphatics to absorb excessive fluid and large molecules from the interstitium and to move this lymph centrally. "MEM is not indicated for all hand clients but can be highly effective in cases of recalcitrant subacute or chronic edema. MEM is used to prevent or reduce subacute or chronic high-protein edema as seen in postsurgical, trauma, or post-cerebrovascular accident (CVA) hand edema."[6]

MEM is an advanced skill that requires specialized training of the practitioner.

An overview is provided below to acquaint the reader with the techniques involved in MEM.[6]

- Provide light, stroking massage of the involved area. It has been shown that more than 40 mm Hg pressure will cause collapse of the lymphatic pathways.
- Incorporate exercise before and after massage in a specific sequence, following the recommended guidelines.
- Massage, done in segments, is proximal to distal, then distal to proximal, always following movement of the therapist's hand in the proximal direction.
- Massage follows the flow of lymphatic pathways.
- Massage reroutes around the incision area.
- Method does not cause additional inflammation.
- Include a client home self-massage program.
- Guide intervention to avoid increased edema from other intervention techniques.
- Incorporate low stretch compression bandaging and warmth to soften hardened tissues, especially at night.

Active Range of Motion

Normal blood flow is dependent on muscle activity. Active motion does not mean wiggling the fingers; instead, it means

maximal available ROM, performed firmly. Casts and splints must allow mobility of uninjured parts while protecting newly injured structures. The shoulder and elbow should be moved through full available ROM several times a day. The importance of active ROM for edema control, tendon gliding, and tissue nutrition cannot be overemphasized.

Compression

Light compression using Coban wraps* of the affected area (Figure 39-16) or light compressive garments such as those made by Aris† or Jobst[47] (Figure 39-17) will help to control swelling, especially at night.

WOUND HEALING AND SCAR REMODELING

The basis of hand therapy is the histology of wound healing. Acute intervention must be planned using the foundation

---

*Coban (available from Smith & Nephew, Inc, Germantown, WI).
†Aris Isotoner gloves (available from North Coast Medical, Morgan Hill, CA).

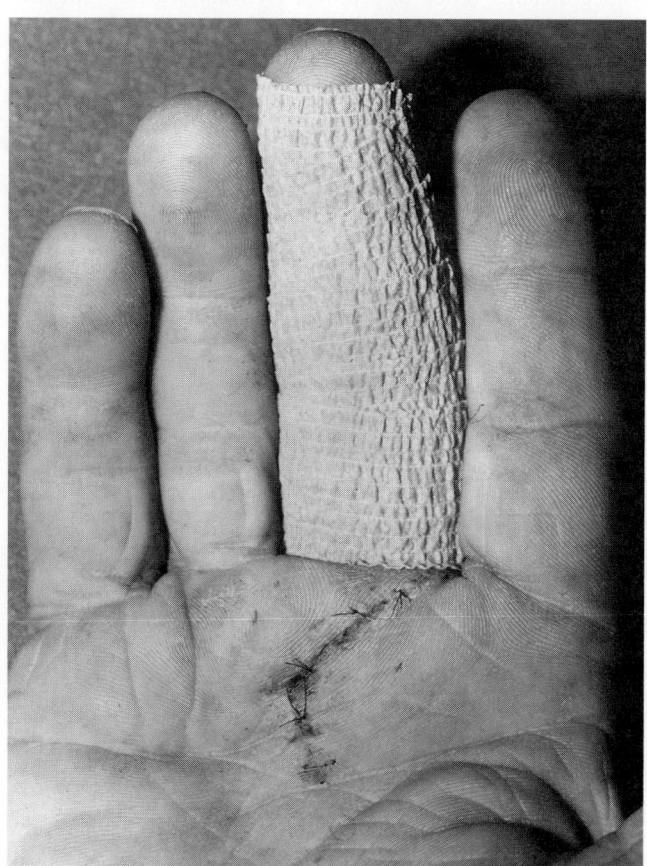

Figure 39-16 One-inch Coban is wrapped with minimal pressure from distal end to proximal crease of digit. Client is instructed to be aware of vascular compression or tingling. Coban may be worn several hours a day to reduce edema. (Product available from Medical Products Division/3M, St. Paul, MN.)

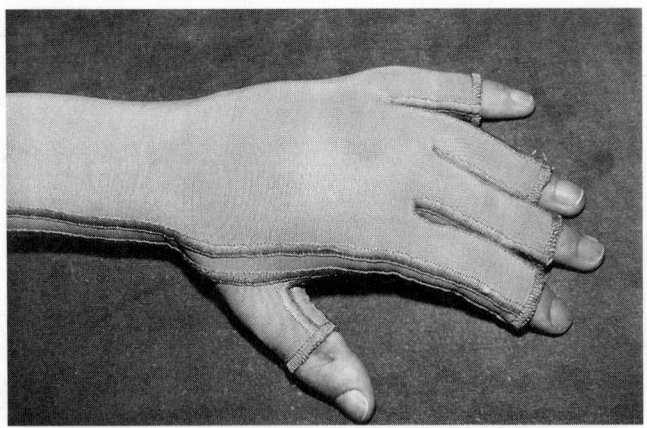

Figure 39-17 Custom-fit Jobst garment may be used to reduce edema and reduce and prevent hypertrophic scar formation after burns or trauma. Inserts may be used with garment to increase pressure over natural curves, such as dorsum of wrist.

of tissue healing as a guide. Bones, tendons, nerves, and skin follow a progression of healing phases. Intervention must respect healing tissue to promote recovery and prevent further damage. The therapist must take care to do no harm, and that can be accomplished only with a thorough understanding of the physiology of healing.

The first phase of wound healing, the acute inflammatory phase, is initiated within hours, when the tissues are disrupted through injury or surgery, causing vasodilatation, local edema, and migration of white blood cells and phagocytic cells to the area. The phagocytes remove tissue fragments and foreign bodies and are critical to healing. The inflammatory process can subside or persist indefinitely, depending on the degree of bacterial contamination.[38]

Fibroblasts, in combination with associated capillaries, begin to invade the wound within the first 72 hours and gradually replace the phagocytes, leading to the second phase: the collagen or granulation phase, between the fifth and fourteenth days. Collagen fiber formation follows the invasion by fibroblasts, so that by the end of the second week the wound is rich with fibroblasts, a capillary network, and early collagen fibers. This increased vascularization results in the erythema (redness) of the new scar.

During the third to sixth weeks, fibroblasts are slowly replaced with scar collagen fibers, and the wound becomes stronger and more able to withstand progressive stresses, leading to the last phase of scar maturation. Tissue strength continues to increase for 3 months or longer. The collagen metabolizes and synthesizes during this period, so that new collagen replaces old while the wound remains relatively stable. Covalent bonding between collagen molecules leads to dense scar adhesions and the formation of whorl-like patterns of collagen deposits, which may be altered as the scar architecture and collagen fiber organization within the wound change over time.[33]

Myofibroblasts, which are fibroblasts with properties similar to smooth muscle cells, are contractile and cause a shortening of the wound.

Tissues that have restored gliding have different scar architecture from those that do not develop the ability to glide. With gliding, the scar resembles the state of the tissues before injury, whereas the nongliding scar remains fixed on surrounding structures. Controlled tension on the scar has been shown to facilitate remodeling. Scar formation is also influenced by age and the quantity of scar deposited.[38]

Wound Care and Dressings

Wounds may be described using a "three-color concept" of red, yellow, or black wounds.[38] This system simplifies wound description and intervention. Guidelines for treating the three wound types help the therapist choose the proper method of cleansing and dressing wounds. The reader is encouraged to review this material and obtain advanced education before treating wounds.

Topical intervention such as antimicrobials may be used to control bacteria. There are a variety of dressings that can be placed on a wound, including gauze that has been impregnated with petroleum, such as Xeroform gauze or Adaptic. Ointments such as Polysporin are also commonly applied. N-Terface* is a dry mesh fabric that looks and feels like the interfacing used in sewing. Because it is nonadherent, it can be used directly over wounds. Sterile dressings can be applied directly over the N-Terface without ointments or gels. The selection of materials depends on the amount of exudate and the goal of the dressing (which may include removing debris, absorbing exudate, or protecting new cells).

Spenco Second Skin† is an inert gel sheeting made from 96% water and 4% polyethylene oxide. It removes friction between two moving surfaces and is said to clean wounds by absorbing secretions. It comes in sterile and nonsterile packs and is encased in a light plastic covering. It is especially effective with abrasions or areas of skin loss because it is cool and reduces itching. It can be used after burns.

Spenco Dermal Pads* are artificial fat pads that can be used to prevent pressure sores or can be cut to size to use around an existing pressure sore or wound to allow it to heal. Dermal pads are $^1/8$ inch thick (0.32 cm) and will adhere to the skin when the protective film is removed. The pad can be held in place with a dressing or pressure garment. It also can be washed without reducing its adherence. Dermal pads can be cut and placed around a healing wound to protect it under a splint or dressing. They are generally not needed after the wound is healed.

The wound can be cleaned with a solution of hydrogen peroxide and sterile saline, with dead tissue then being gently removed with sterile swabs. Sterile saline solution can be

---

*N-Terface, made by Winfield Laboratories (available from North Coast Medical, Morgan Hill, CA).
†Spenco Medical Corp, Waco, TX.

used to soak off adherent bandages rather than pulling them off the client. The therapist should pour a very small amount of saline on the area that is sticking, wait a few moments, and gently pry the dressing off. Dead skin can be debrided using iris scissors and pickups. Soft surgical scrub sponges may be used for cleaning and desensitization of the wound once it is healed and the stitches have been removed. The client also can do this procedure at home. Sterile whirlpool baths may be used for debridement, especially if the wound is infected.

Pressure

A hypertrophic scar or a scar that is randomly laid down and thickened is reduced by the application of pressure, often by means of pressure garments.[49]* Use of an insert of neoprene† fabric or molds made from Silastic elastomer[64]‡ under the pressure garment increases the conformity of the garment. Pressure should be applied for most of the 24-hour period, and with a hypertrophic burn scar this intervention should continue for 6 months to 1 year after the injury. Silicone Gel Sheets§ have been found to reduce hypertrophic scarring when worn on a regular basis for 12 to 24 hours a day.

Massage

Gentle to firm massage of the scarred area using a thick ointment rapidly softens scar tissue and should be followed immediately with active hand use so that tendons glide against the softened scar.[28] Vibration to the area with a small, low-intensity vibrator will have a similar effect.[28,48] Active exercise, using facilitation techniques and against resistance, or functional activity, should follow vibration. Massage and vibration may be started 4 weeks after injury.

Thermal heat in the form of paraffin dips, hot packs, or fluidotherapy, immediately followed by stretching while the tissue cools, provides stretch to the scar tissue. Wrapping the scarred or stiff digit into flexion with Coban during the application of heat often increases mobility in the area. Heat should not be used on insensate areas or if swelling persists.[49]

Active Range of Motion and Electrical Stimulation

Active ROM provides an internal stretch against resistant scar, and its use cannot be overemphasized. If the client is unable to achieve active motion because of scar adhesions or weakness, use of a battery-operated NMES may augment the motion.[104] Stimulation may be performed by the client for several hours at home and has been shown to increase ROM and tendon excursion.[72]

Many hand therapists use high-voltage direct current as a intervention to increase motor activity, and it may be used for scar remodeling.[2] Ultrasound interventions are often prescribed but may be more effective if done within the first few months after trauma. A continuous passive motion (CPM) device may be used at home to maintain passive ROM and promote tendon gliding. It should be used for several hours a day for maximal benefit.

PAIN SYNDROMES

Pain, the subjective manifestation of trauma transmitted by the sympathetic nervous system, may interfere with normal functioning. Because pain leads to overprotection of the affected part and disuse of the extremity, it should be treated early.

Desensitization

Stimulation of the large afferent A nerve fibers leads to a reduction of pain by decreasing summation in the slowly adapting, small, unmyelineated C fibers, which carry pain sensation. The A-axons can be stimulated mechanically with pressure, rubbing, vibration, TENS, percussion, and active motion. Desensitization techniques are based on the amplification of inhibitory mechanisms.

Yerxa[106] has described a desensitization program that "employs short periods of contact with three sensory modalities: dowel textures, immersion or contact particles, and vibration." This program allows the client to rank 10 dowel textures and 10 immersion textures on the degree of irritation produced by the stimulus. Intervention begins with a stimulus that is irritating but tolerable. The stimulus is applied for 10 minutes, three or four times a day. The vibration hierarchy is predetermined and based on cycles per second of vibration, the placement of the vibrator, and the duration of the intervention. Complete instructions for assembling the Downey Hand Center desensitization kit can be found in the literature in the references. The Downey Hand Center Hand Sensitivity Test can be used to establish a desensitization intervention program and measure progress in decreasing hypersensitivity.[7,106]

Neuromas

Neuromas are a complication of nerve suture or amputation. A traumatic neuroma is an unorganized mass of nerve fibers that results from accidental or surgical cutting of the nerve. A neuroma in continuity occurs on a nerve that is intact.[94] Neuromas may be clinically identified by a specific, sharp pain. Stimulation of a neuroma usually causes the client to pull the hand away quickly; many clients report a burning pain that radiates up the forearm. Neuromas are disabling because any stimulation causes intense pain and the client avoids the sensitive area.

A generalized desensitization program may not work because the client never develops a tolerance for stimulation

---

*Bio-Concepts, Phoenix, AZ. Cica-Care Silicone Gel Sheets (available from Smith & Nephew, Germantown, WI).

†Neoprene (available from Benik Corp, Silverdale, WA).

‡Silicone elastomers (available from Smith & Nephew, Germantown, WI).

§Cica-Care Silicone Gel Sheets (available from Smith & Nephew, Germantown, WI).

of the neuroma. Injection of cortisone acetate may help break up the neuroma, making desensitization techniques more effective. Surgically excising the neuroma or burying the nerve endings deeper may be necessary.

Complex Regional Pain Syndrome

Complex regional pain syndrome (CRPS) is the term that replaced "reflex sympathetic dystrophy (RSD)" to describe a group of disorders that "involve pain and dysfunction of severity or duration out of proportion to those expected from the initiating event."[105]

Complex denotes the complex nature of the pain response, which may include inflammation and autonomic, cutaneous, motor, and dystrophic changes. *Regional* refers to the wide distribution of symptoms beyond the area of the original lesion. *Pain* is the primary characteristic of this syndrome. It includes spontaneous pain, thermal changes, and at times burning pain. CRPS, type I, corresponds to RSD. Type II corresponds to causalgia, a severe, burning pain first described during the Civil War.

Diagnostic criteria for CRPS must include spontaneous pain beyond the territory of a single peripheral nerve and disproportionate to the inciting event. There is generally edema, skin blood-flow abnormality, or abnormal sudomotor activity in the area of the pain. The diagnosis is excluded by the existence of conditions that would otherwise account for the pain. The hallmarks of CRPS are pain; edema; blotchy-looking, shiny skin; and coolness of the extremity. Sensory changes may occur. Excessive sweating or dryness may occur if there is associated sympathetic dysfunction. The degree of trauma does not correlate with the severity of the pain and may occur after any injury. CRPS, type I may be triggered by a cycle of vasospasm and vasodilatation after an injury. Abnormal edema and constrictive dressings or casts may be a factor in initiating the vasospasm. A vasospasm "causes tissue anoxia and edema and therefore more pain, which continues the abnormal cycle."[79] Circulation is decreased, which causes the extremity to become cool and pale.

Fibrosis after tissue anoxia and the presence of protein-rich exudates result in joint stiffness. The client may cradle the hand and prefer to keep it wrapped. There may be an exaggerated reaction to touch, especially light touch. Osteoporosis may be apparent on X-ray films by 8 weeks after trauma after active use of the hand. Burning pain associated with causalgia (CRPS, type II) is a symptom that may be alleviated by interruption of the sympathetic nerve pathways.

There are three stages of CRPS. Stage I (traumatic stage) may last up to 3 months; it is characterized by pain, pitting edema, and discoloration. Stage II (dystrophic stage) may last an additional 6 to 9 months. Pain, brawny edema, stiffness, redness, heat, and bony demineralization are usually found in this stage. The hand usually has a glossy appearance. Stage III (atrophic stage) may last several years or indefinitely. Pain usually peaks in stage II and decreases in stage III.

Thickening around the joints occurs, and fixed contractures may be present. If swelling is present, it is hard and not responsive to techniques such as elevation. The hand may be pale, dry, and cool. There may be substantial dysfunction of the limb.

CRPS is treated by decreasing sympathetic stimulation. It is most responsive in stage I. The first goal of intervention is reduction of the pain and hypersensitivity to light touch. This goal may be accomplished with application of warm (not hot), moist heat; fluidotherapy; gentle handling of the hand; acupressure; desensitization; and TENS before active ROM. Intervention that increases pain (such as passive ROM) should be avoided. Many clients respond well to gentle manual edema mobilization,[6] which reduces the edema and reintroduces touching of the hand. Stellate ganglion blocks to eliminate the pain are effective early. They should be coordinated with therapy so that the client can perform active ROM and functional activities during the pain-free period after the blocks. Active ROM is crucial. Gravity-eliminated exercise, either in water or on a tabletop, may be more easily tolerated.

A variety of drugs may be used, including sympatholytic drugs[55] that reduce the vasoconstrictive action of the peripheral vessels. Neurontin is often effective in reducing pain and increasing temperature in the extremity. Calcium channel blockers are also effective. Carefully monitored use of narcotics may interrupt the pain cycle and allow active use of the hand. A stress-loading program that has been used effectively to reduce symptoms of RSD (CRPS, type I) has been described.[99] It can easily be adapted for home use.

Edema control techniques should be started immediately. Elevation, manual edema mobilization, contrast baths, and high-voltage direct current in water have been found to be effective. Surface EMG-biofeedback training for relaxation may help muscle spasms and increase blood flow, in addition to reducing anxiety.

CRPS frequently triggers shoulder pain and stiffness, resulting in shoulder-hand syndrome or adhesive capsulitis of the shoulder ("frozen shoulder"). Therefore, active ROM and functional activities should include the entire upper quadrant. Use of skateboard exercises is helpful in the early stages for active-assisted exercise of the shoulder. Splints that reduce joint stiffness should be used as tolerated. Splints must not cause pain or increase swelling. Reliance on immobilization splinting should be avoided because clients with CRPS prefer not to move the affected part, which ultimately makes their symptoms worse.

A tendency to develop CRPS should be suspected in any client who seems to complain excessively about pain, appears anxious, and complains of profuse sweating and temperature changes in the hand. Some clients report nausea associated with touching the hand. Clients tend to overprotect the hand. Early intervention with a structured therapy program of functional activities, group interaction, and exercises that include the hand and shoulder may prevent the occurrence of a fully developed CRPS. This problem is best recognized early and treated with tempered aggressiveness and empathy.

Transcutaneous Electrical Nerve Stimulation

TENS is an intervention technique that is thought to stimulate the afferent A nerve fibers in the high-frequency mode and stimulate the release of morphine like neural hormones, the enkephalins, in the low-frequency mode. Its efficacy as an intervention for pain control is well documented in medical literature. As with other electrical modalities that may be used by occupational therapists, TENS should be correlated with functional use of the hand.

TENS should be used for intervention periods not to exceed 60 minutes at a time to achieve pain control.[51] A TENS diary should be used to record the level of pain on a scale of 1 to 10 before and after intervention, as well as activities that exacerbate the pain. To prevent overuse, TENS may be tapered as the pain-free periods increase. Intervention can be continued as long as necessary to provide pain control.

JOINT STIFFNESS

Joint stiffness has been discussed in other sections of this chapter because it is seen after almost any hand trauma or disease. In the acute phase it may also result from "internal splinting" done unconsciously by the client to avoid pain. It may be prevented by early mobilization, pain control, reduction of edema, active and passive ROM, use of a CPM device, and appropriate splinting techniques. Grades I and II joint mobilization are especially helpful in preparing for passive and active motion and providing pain relief.

Treatment of established joint stiffness is more difficult. Thermal modalities, joint mobilization, ultrasound and electrical stimulation, dynamic splinting, serial casting, and active and passive motion in preparation for functional use should all be included in the intervention regimen.

CUMULATIVE TRAUMA DISORDERS

A number of terms are used throughout the world to describe injuries to the musculoskeletal system, including overuse syndromes, repetitive strain injuries, cervical-brachial disorders, repetitive motion injuries, and in the United States, **cumulative trauma disorders** (CTDs). There were 281,800 cases of CTDs reported in private industry in the United States in 1992.[53] According to statistics reported by the U.S. Department of Labor in 2001, the cases of musculoskeletal disorders of the neck, shoulder, and upper extremities declined to 202,398 cases (http://www.bls.gov). This decline in reported CTDs may be associated with recognition of the need for early prevention, ergonomic intervention, and proper work station or tool modifications. Women account for about two thirds of work-related repetitive motion injuries.

The term *cumulative trauma disorder* should be viewed as a description of the mechanism of injury and not a diagnosis. Even when the presenting symptoms are confusing, attempts to define a specific diagnosis are necessary because "each disorder has a different cause, intervention, and prognosis."[83] Diagnoses associated with cumulative trauma usually fall into one of three categories: tendinitis (such as lateral epicondylitis—tennis elbow or de Quervain's tenosynovitis), nerve compression syndromes (such as carpal tunnel syndrome or cubital tunnel syndrome), or myofascial pain.

Cumulative trauma occurs when force is applied to the same muscle or muscle group, causing an inflammatory response in the tendon or muscle.[83] Muscle fatigue is an important aspect of cumulative trauma. Excessive use of the muscle or body system (overuse or overexertion) is experienced as a muscle cramp. Acute overuse is relieved by rest, but chronic fatigue is not relieved by rest. The amount of fatigue is related to the amount of force and the duration of force application.

Fatigue occurs more quickly with high force. If force is maintained, repetitions must be reduced to allow recovery. Therefore, if the force is decreased while repetitions are maintained and recovery time is adequate, harm is less likely to occur. The combination of repetitions without adequate recovery time and high force establishes an environment that is likely to lead to injury. Byl[17] found that repetitive hand opening and closing may lead to motor control problems and the development of focal hand dystonias through a degradation of the cortical representation. Applying this research may help therapists develop more effective intervention programs for cumulative trauma and chronic pain.

Intervention may be divided into phases. Acute-phase intervention is geared toward decreasing the inflammation through dynamic rest. Splints are used for immobilization. Splinting alone may relieve symptoms; splinting is often combined with cortisone injections to reduce inflammation. Icing, contrast baths, ultrasound phonophoresis, iontophoresis (the movement of ions through biological material under the influence of an electric current), and interferential and high-voltage electrical stimulation have all been found to be effective in reducing pain and decreasing inflammation. Nonsteroidal antiinflammatory drugs are also frequently used. When splints are used, they should be removed three times a day for stretching of the affected musculature (e.g., the extensor group with lateral epicondylitis) to maintain or increase muscle length and to prevent joint stiffness. Painful activities should be avoided during the dynamic rest phase. Vibration is contraindicated because vibration may contribute to inflammatory problems.

As the acute symptoms decrease, the client begins the exercise phase of intervention. After warmup of the muscles by slow stretching, the client begins controlled progressive exercise. Resistance should be given at the end of range when progressive resistive exercise is performed. A tennis-elbow armband (for lateral epicondylitis) can be worn over the extensor muscle bellies to limit full excursion of the muscle during active use of the arm. Resistance should be increased slowly and should not cause an increase in pain.

Clients are instructed to continue stretching three times a day, especially before activity, for an indefinite time. Proper body mechanics are critical in the long-term control of inflammatory problems, so clients must become aware of what triggers their symptoms and learn early intervention if symptoms reappear. Icing, splints, stretching, and modified activities combined with correct body mechanics are usually effective. The key is that the clients learn self-management techniques and take an active role in their intervention.

Work-related risk factors for CTDs include the following[5]:
- Repetition
- High force
- Awkward joint posture
- Direct pressure
- Vibration
- Prolonged static positioning

An assessment of the job site, tools used, and hand position during work activities may be indicated with the client whose symptoms are related to job demands. Modification of the equipment used and strengthening of the dominant muscle groups and their antagonist muscles may permit continued employment and control the inflammatory problem.

Tendinitis (inflammation of the tendon) and tenosynovitis (inflammation of the tendon sheath) are frequently seen in cumulative trauma. The cycle of overuse leading to microtrauma, swelling, pain, and limitations in movement is followed by rest, disuse, and weakness. Normal activity is resumed, and the cycle begins again.

Clients usually have a combination of localized pain, swelling, pain with resisted motion of the affected musculotendinous unit, limitations in motion, weakness, and crepitation of the tendons. Symptoms are reproduced with activity or work simulation. Using functional grades to describe the associated symptoms assists in evaluation, as well as in monitoring of improvement (Table 39-5).[50] Although isometric grip strength may be normal, wrist and forearm strength are often decreased and out of balance. Dynamic grip strength may be more limited because tendon gliding is more likely to increase inflammation and pain. Muscle imbalance leads to positioning and substitution patterns that may result in worsening or spreading of symptoms.

Nerve compression syndromes, especially carpal tunnel syndrome, are frequently seen.[59] Carpal tunnel syndrome is caused by pressure on the median nerve as it travels beneath the transverse carpal ligament at the volar surface of the wrist.[40] The syndrome is associated with increased pressure in the carpal canal because of trauma, edema, retention of fluids as a result of pregnancy, flexor tenosynovitis, repetitive wrist motions, or static loading of the wrist.

TABLE 39-5   Functional Grading of Cumulative Trauma Disorders

Grade	Description
Grade I	Pain after activity; resolves quickly with rest
	No decrease in amount or speed of work
	Objective findings usually absent
Grade II	Pain in one site while working
	Pain consistent while working but resolves when activity stops
	Productivity sometimes mildly affected
	May have objective findings
Grade III	Pain in one or more sites while working
	Persistent pain after cessation of activity
	Productivity affected and multiple breaks sometimes necessary to continue working
	May affect other activities away from work
	May have weakness, loss of control and dexterity, tingling, numbness, and other objective findings
	May have latent or active trigger points
Grade IV	All common uses of hand and upper extremity resulting in pain, which is present 50% to 75% of the time
	May be unable to work or works in limited capacity
	May have weakness, loss of control and dexterity, tingling, numbness, trigger points, and other objective findings
Grade V	Loss of capacity to use upper extremities because of chronic, unrelenting pain
	Usually unable to work
	Symptoms sometimes of indefinite duration

From Kasch MC: Therapist's evaluation and treatment of upper extremity trauma disorders. In Mackin EJ, et al, editors: *Rehabilitation of the hand and upper extremity*, ed 5, St Louis, 2002, Mosby.

Symptoms are night pain that is severe enough to waken the client; tingling in the thumb and index and middle fingers; and, if advanced, wasting of the thenar musculature caused by pressure on the motor branch of the nerve. Early carpal tunnel syndrome may be recognized during a thorough nerve evaluation.

Conservative intervention is usually attempted first and includes splinting of the wrist in no more than 20 degrees extension, contrast baths to reduce edema, wearing of Isotoner gloves, and activity analysis. A semiflexible or neoprene splint rather than a completely rigid splint may be used to provide support while allowing a small amount of flexion and extension for greater functional use in carpal tunnel syndrome.

Ultrasound phonophoresis and iontophoresis may be used to reduce inflammation, and icing techniques are beneficial. Specific strengthening exercises of the wrist, fingers, and thumb should be given when the pain and inflammation have been controlled.

In 1988, 35,000 carpal tunnel releases were performed in the United States. In 2002, this number climbed to over 200,000.[88] Most clients report a relief of numbness, but many have persistent pain. Therapy is often provided after surgical release and may include a combination of ultrasound to the scar, massage, manual edema mobilization, desensitization, dexterity activities, and strengthening.

Myofascial pain and fibrositis are also conditions of pain elicited by activation of trigger points within the muscles and resulting in pain referred to a distal area; these are frequently encountered conditions. Travell[96] has studied myofascial pain and mapped out the traditional trigger points and their referral patterns. Poor posture and positioning of the body out of normal alignment are often the mechanisms of injury in myofascial pain, so careful examination of the client and his or her normal daily activities is indicated. The therapist should observe the client performing the activity rather than rely on a verbal description.

Myofascial pain should be considered if direct intervention of the painful area does not relieve the pain. Evaluation for trigger points must be done meticulously, and mapping of the trigger points and the referral areas must be documented. Because the pain is referred, the trigger point must be treated, not the referral area. The interventions used for other inflammatory problems, such as ice and ultrasound phonophoresis, can be used. In addition, specific interventions for the trigger points, such as friction massage and TENS, may relieve the pain. Activity analysis is an essential part of intervention to relieve the stresses on the affected tissues.

Kinesio Taping

First developed in Japan in the 1970s, Kinesio Taping* has become increasingly popular with therapists in the intervention of CTDs in the United States since its introduction here in 1994. Kinesio Taping is a taping technique that uses a special elastic tape called *Kinesio Flex tape*. Unlike athletic taping, which is restrictive and is used to provide stability and restrict joint motion, Kinesio Flex tape is elastic and designed to "mimic the elastic properties of muscle, skin, and fascia."[24] When properly applied, the elasticity of the Kinesio tape does not restrict the movement of soft tissue but provides support to weakened muscles and allows for full movement of the joints.

There are many variations in Kinesio taping techniques. Depending on the problem being addressed, the tape is anchored at either the origin or insertion of a muscle and then gently stretched and taped over or around either a shortened or elongated muscle, after which time the muscle is placed back in a neutral position. The tape is believed to affect the peripheral somatosensory receptors located in the superficial skin, which in turn affects the skin and lymphatic

system, as well as muscle and joint function, as they relate to pain, proprioception, and motor control.[23]

Goals and concepts of Kinesio Taping include the following[23,24]:

- Decrease pain by increasing the somatosensory system.
- Reduce inflammation and edema by stimulating the lymphatic system.
- Normalize muscle tone by reducing overstretching and overcontraction of muscles.
- Reduce muscle fatigue by supporting and enhancing the contraction of weakened muscles.
- Improve ROM by relieving pain.
- Provide support and alignment to joints by supporting weakened ligaments.
- Prevent injuries during ADLs by providing support to muscles and ligaments.

STRENGTHENING ACTIVITIES

Acute care is followed by a gradual return of motion, sensibility, and preparation to return to normal ADL and IADL routines.

The client usually cannot strengthen the injured and neglected extremity at home because of the fear of further injury and pain. Because every hand clinic has its own armamentarium of strengthening exercises and media, only a few suggestions are provided here.

Computerized Evaluation and Exercise Equipment

Baltimore Therapeutic Equipment (BTE) has made available the BTE Work Simulator (Figure 39-18),[27] an electromechanical device that has more than 20 interchangeable tool handles and can be used for both work evaluation and UE strengthening. Resistance can vary from no resistance to complete static resistance, with tool height and angle also adjustable. When the device is used for strengthening, the resistance is usually set low and gradually increased. Length of exercise is increased when a base level of strength has been achieved. The BTE Work Simulator allows for close simulation of real-world tasks that are easily translatable into physical demands common to manual work.

Other computerized evaluation equipment allows the therapist to record the results of assessment and print a report. Percentage of impairment can also be determined electronically. Portable systems are being developed that allow the therapist to record daily intervention and download the information into a computerized network. Outcome data from many sources can then be compared. The advancement of technology in rehabilitation will allow the therapist to be more efficient and also capture important information that is not available through traditional means.

Many practitioners use real occupation-based interventions that simulate the actual work done, either in the clinic or at the work site. These methods are the most in keeping with the Occupational Therapy Practice Framework.

---

*Kinesio Tape (available from North Coast Medical, Morgan Hill, CA.)

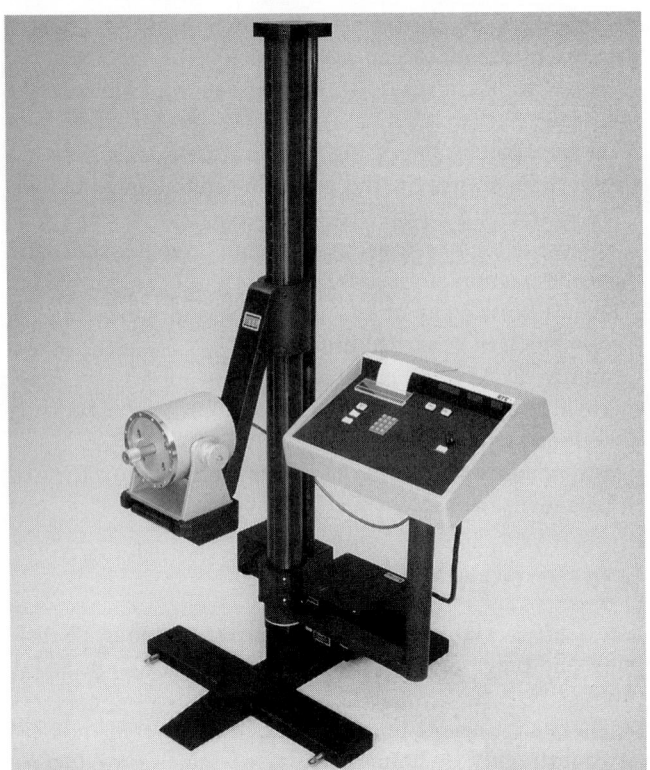

Figure 39-18 BTE Work Simulator is an electromechanical device used to simulate real-life tasks for upper extremity evaluation and strengthening. Client's progress is monitored through computerized print-out, and program can be modified to increase resistance and endurance.

Weight Well

The Weight Well[7] was developed at the Downey Community Hospital Hand Center in Downey, California, and is available commercially.* Rods with a variety of handle shapes are placed through holes in the box and have weights suspended. The rods are turned against resistance throughout the ROM to encourage full grasp and release of the injured hand, wrist flexion and extension, pinch, and pronation and supination patterns. The Weight Well can be graded for resistance and repetitions and is an excellent tool for progressive resistive exercise.

Theraband

Theraband[†] is a 6-inch (15.2-cm) wide rubber sheet that is available by the yard and is color coded by degrees of resistance. It can be cut into any length required and used for resistive exercise for the UE. Use of Theraband is limited only by the therapist's imagination, and it can be adapted to diagonal patterns of motion, wrist exercises, follow-up

*Upper Extremity Technology Weight Well (available from Upper Extremity Technology, Glenwood Springs, CO).
[†]Theraband (available from Smith & Nephew, Germantown, WI).

intervention of tennis elbow, and other uses. The Theraband can be combined with dowel rods and other equipment to provide resistance throughout the ROM. It is inexpensive and easy to incorporate into a home intervention program.

Hand-Strengthening Equipment

Hand grips of graded resistance are available from rehabilitation supply companies and sporting goods stores. They can be purchased with various resistance levels and can be used for progressive resistive hand exercises.

The therapist is cautioned against using overly resistive spring-loaded grippers often sold in sporting goods stores. These devices may be beneficial to the seasoned athlete but are usually too resistive for the recently injured.

Therapy putty can be purchased in bulk, and the amount given to the client is geared to hand size and strength. Putty is also available in grades of resistance, and some provide chips that can be added to progressively increase resistance. It can be adapted to most finger motions and is easily incorporated into a home program.

Household items such as spring-type clothespins have been used to increase strength of grasp and pinch. Imaginative use of common objects should present a challenge to the hand therapist.

PURPOSEFUL AND OCCUPATION-BASED ACTIVITY

Purposeful and occupation-based activities are an integral part of rehabilitation of the hand. Purposeful and occupation-based activities include crafts, games, dexterity activities, ADLs, and work samples. Several studies have shown that clients are more likely to choose occupationally embedded exercise and performed better using this type of exercise over rote exercise.[77,107] Many of the intervention techniques described previously are used as preparatory methods for the hand in preparation for purposeful activity.

Activities should be started as soon as possible at whatever level the client can perform them with adaptations to compensate for limited ROM and strength. They should be used in conjunction with other interventions. The occupational therapist must continually assess the client's functional capacities and initiate changes in the intervention plan to incorporate activities as soon as possible in the restorative phase.

Vocational and leisure goals should be established at the time of initial evaluation and taken into account when devising the intervention plan. The needs of a brick mason may be quite different from those of a mother with small children, and the environmental needs of the client must not be neglected.

Crafts should be graded from light resistance to heavy resistance and from gross dexterity to fine dexterity. Crafts that have been found to work extremely well with hand injuries include macramé, Turkish knot weaving, clay molding, leather tooling, and woodworking. All of these crafts can be adapted and graded to the client's capabilities and have been found to have a high level of client acceptance. When integrated into a program of total hand rehabilitation, they are viewed as another milestone of achievement and not as a diversion to fill up empty hours. For example, the pride of accomplishment for Gerry, who was able to complete his first simple woodworking project, is evidence that the purposeful activity of crafts belongs in hand rehabilitation.

Activities that do not have an end product but provide practice in dexterity and ADL skills also fit into the category of purposeful activities. Developmental games and activities that require pinch or grasp and release may be graded and timed to increase difficulty. ADL boards that have a variety of opening and closing devices provide practice for use of the hand at home and increase self-confidence. String and finger games are challenging coordination activities that can be done in pairs and are fun to do.

A hobby can often be adapted for use in the clinic. Fly-tying is a difficult dexterity activity but one that is frequently enjoyed by an avid fisherman. Golf clubs and fishing poles can be adapted in the clinic; in the case of Gerry, therapy with these tools allowed early return to a favorite form of relaxation.

Humor and interaction with the therapists and the other clients are vital but intangible benefits of hand therapy intervention. The intervention should be planned to promote both.

FUNCTIONAL CAPACITY EVALUATION

The ultimate goal of therapy for an injured worker is to return to full employment. Many weeks or months may have elapsed between the time of the injury and the point at which the physician believes that a return to work is appropriate from a medical standpoint. Despite the fact that X-ray examinations may show full healing and restored ROM, many clients do not feel that they have the strength, dexterity, or endurance to return to their former jobs. Pain may continue to be a limiting factor, especially with heavy activities. Light duty or part-time positions may not be available, and the physician, therapist, industrial insurance carrier, and especially the client are frustrated by the lack of an objective method of evaluating an individual's physical capacity for work. Occupational therapists with training in evaluation, kinesiology, and adaptation of environmental factors coupled with a functional approach to the client may play a key role in **functional capacity evaluation.**

A renewed interest in evaluation of prevocational factors has brought the profession of OT full circle (see Chapter 13). Although regarded as one of the cornerstones of the profession in its early years, prevocational evaluation was neglected in many centers during the 1960s and 1970s. Since the early 1980s, however, occupational therapists have rediscovered a need that the profession is in a unique position to provide.

The term "prevocational evaluation" ambiguously implied that occupational therapists were involved in assessing the vocational needs of clients they treated. The terms *functional capacity evaluation (FCE)* and *work tolerance screening (WTS)*, however, more clearly describe the process of measuring an individual's ability to perform the physical demands of work.

The results of the FCE allow the therapist, worker, physician, and vocational counselor to establish a specific, attainable employment goal using reliable data. This approach relieves the physician of the responsibility of returning the client to work without objective information about the client's ability to do a job. It also allows the client to test his or her own abilities and may result in increased self-confidence about returning to work.

Many techniques for performing a functional capacity evaluation have been proposed.[8,43,65,66,87] Some basic steps may be followed regardless of the specific technique adopted. The client should be evaluated for grip and pinch strength, sensation, and ROM. Edema and pain must also be assessed and reassessed during the course of the evaluation.

The GULHEMP (general physique, UE, lower extremity, hearing, eyesight, mentality, and personality) Work Capacity Evaluation Worksheet[65] may be used as a general method of determining functional abilities. The GULHEMP Physical Development Analysis Worksheet[65] may be used to evaluate the job.

Job analysis may also be provided by a rehabilitation counselor and through information provided by the client. The therapist should consult the *Dictionary of Occupational Titles* (DOT)[97] to obtain information about the worker traits required for the expected job. This dictionary contains 12,900 job descriptions and 20,000 job titles. If sufficient information about the job is not available through these methods, an on-site job analysis by the therapist may be necessary. Once the physical demand characteristics of work have been documented, it is possible to evaluate the client's ability to perform them. The U.S. Department of Labor sponsors the Occupational Information Network online (http://online.onetcenter.org), which includes job titles, job accommodations, and the ability to search for job information using several criteria.

Schultz-Johnson[87] described an FCE adapted for UE injuries based on the physical demands established by the U.S. Department of Labor. After evaluation, the therapist may recommend a work therapy program.[87] Work therapy can include simulated job tasks to increase job performance.

Matheson[65,66] has written several manuals and articles that describe work capacity evaluation (WCE). This 8- to 10-day work assessment includes evaluation of the client's feasibility for employment (worker characteristics, such as safety and dependability), employability, work tolerances (e.g., strength, endurance, and the effect of pain on work performance), the physical demand characteristics of the job, and the worker's ability to "dependably sustain performance in response to broadly defined work demands."[66]

Tests with well-accepted reliability, such as the Purdue Pegboard Test,[95] the Crawford Small Parts Dexterity Test,[25] the Minnesota Manual Dexterity Test,[73] and the Jebsen Hand Dexterity Test,[46] may be administered as a screening process. These tests will give the therapist valuable information through observation, whether the normal tables are used or the test is adapted to an individual worker.

Many assessments and job simulation devices are available and should be reviewed before a physical capacity evaluation program is established. To choose appropriate work samples, the therapist should determine the job market in a specific area. This can be done by consulting rehabilitation counselors and representatives from vocational schools and employment agencies in the area.

Work samples, available through Jewish Employment and Vocational Service,[98] Singer,* VALPAR, and Work Evaluation Systems Technology (WEST),† may be used to test specific skills. The therapist may also develop job samples by using information on jobs in the local area. Discarded electronic assembly boards, a lawn mower motor, an automobile engine, or other items from the local hardware store may provide valuable information about the worker's ability.

Work simulation using job samples or the BTE Work Simulator assesses the worker's specific physical capacities, as well as endurance and symptoms that become cumulative with prolonged use of the injured part (called *symptom response to activity,* or *SRA*). Monitoring the client's SRA may prevent loss of time and money expended in training for an inappropriate vocational goal.

A combination of "normed" tests, job samples, job simulation, and WCE devices may provide the therapist with the best information about a worker's physical capacity. For more information about vocational evaluation and rehabilitation, the reader is encouraged to visit the Web site for the University of Wisconsin-Stout at http://www.rtc. uwstout.edu/.‡

WORK HARDENING

Work hardening is the progressive use of simulated work samples to increase endurance, strength, productivity, and often feasibility. Work hardening may be performed for a period of weeks, and the progressive ongoing nature of the work usually results in improvements in physical capacity. It is an important contribution to return to work.

Because FCE is also performed over time, it may be difficult to identify the difference between FCE and work hardening. An FCE is generally done when the client has stopped improving with traditional therapy methods and may have

been released from acute medical care. The client may be unable to return to his or her former employment, or the client's ability to do the former work may be in doubt. An FCE may be initiated by a physician, rehabilitation counselor, insurance adjustor, or attorney.

Work hardening or work conditioning may be initiated earlier in the rehabilitation process, perhaps by the treating physician or therapist who recognizes that an individual may have difficulty returning to the former employment. It is performed before the end of medical care and may serve as a final checkout before discontinuing intervention.

Standards for work hardening services have been developed by the Commission on Accreditation of Rehabilitation Facilities (CARF)[22] to ensure that injured workers are offered high-quality programs that are maximally effective in returning them to gainful employment. The Employment and Rehabilitation Institute of California (ERIC)[35] offers many publications and resources to therapists interested in establishing WCE, work tolerance screening, or work hardening services. A publications and equipment list is available on request.

FCE and work hardening are adjuncts to the vocational rehabilitation process. Occupational therapists are trained to observe behavior and have the skills necessary to translate that observation into useful data. FCE and work hardening should not compete with the work of rehabilitation or vocational counselors; instead, they should provide critical information about a worker's physical functioning and foster reentry into the job market.

CONSULTATION WITH INDUSTRY

Occupational therapists may be asked to visit the job site to make recommendations for **ergonomic** adaptations, including tool modification, ergonomic furniture and accessories, and training of workers in proper positioning to reduce the incidence of CTDs. Because prevention substantially reduces the costs to industry, occupational therapists have a unique opportunity to apply their training in activity analysis and adaptation of the environment in a new setting. The Americans with Disabilities Act (ADA) mandates reasonable accommodations for workers with disabilities (see Chapter 14). Many occupational therapists have become active in helping companies comply with the requirements of the ADA. The American Occupational Therapy Association is an excellent resource for information about the ways in which therapists can be involved in these efforts in their communities.[3]

PSYCHOSOCIAL EFFECTS OF HAND INJURIES

After a hand injury, a number of psychosocial reactions may occur, including changed body-image and self-image, depression, anxiety, and decreased self-worth (as experienced by Gerry, the cabinet maker with the amputated fingers and

---

*Singer Education Division, Career Systems, Rochester, NY.
†Work Evaluation Systems Technology, Fort Bragg, CA.
‡Materials Development Center, Stout Vocational Rehabilitation Institute, University of Wisconsin-Stout, Menomonie, WI.

surgical replantation in the case study), to name but a few. For traumatic hand injuries, acute stress disorder and post-traumatic stress disorder are not uncommon and can be problematic for the client, especially if they are not addressed promptly. The hand therapist is often the primary contact for the client after injury and may see the client several times per week on a one-to-one basis. The hand therapist, therefore, plays a "very important role in helping the client return to pre-injury physical and emotional functioning."[15] Not only do occupational therapists who specialize in hand therapy provide emotional support for the client; they are also critical in recognizing psychosocial issues that the client may be having; are educated in evaluating and providing intervention for these; and, when necessary, because of the severity of the problem, facilitating referral to an appropriate mental health professional.

SUMMARY

This chapter provides an overview of intervention of the UE. Evaluation procedures are discussed, as well as the basic intervention techniques. Management of both acute injuries and cumulative trauma is included, as well as information on strengthening and

programs for industrial injuries. Most occupational therapists working in physical disabilities should be familiar with the basic intervention approaches described for the UE because they work with clients who have some limitation in the UEs. Specialization in hand therapy requires both advanced academic study and clinical experience. Therapists who specialize in this area of practice and who meet minimum requirements may choose to take the Hand Therapy Certification Examination and become a Certified Hand Therapist (CHT). Both levels of expertise are needed in the profession. For more information on becoming a CHT, contact the Hand Therapy Certification Commission (www.htcc.org).[42] Links to educational resources are also available on this Web site.

Although much of UE rehabilitation involves the use of preparatory methods such as exercise, splinting, and physical agent modalities, these interventions should be used in preparation for purposeful or occupation-based activities. The goal is always for the client to be as independent as possible and to use these preparatory methods to achieve the client's occupation-based performance goals. Purposeful activity is used whenever feasible in the hand clinic according to space and time constraints, and clients are encouraged to use their new skills in their own home or work contexts and bring back to the clinic information about the obstacles that they experience in achieving their performance goals.

 **THREADED CASE STUDY: GERRY, PART 2**

The case study presented at the beginning of this chapter described Gerry, a 32-year-old cabinetmaker with an acute, complex hand injury involving amputation and surgical replantation of three digits. Gerry progressed through all phases of rehabilitation over the course of 15 months, from the acute hospital stay to return to work and play activities. Based on the case presented, how would the intervention plan change over the course of Gerry's recovery, and what specific intervention approaches could be used by his occupational therapist?

During the acute phase, one of the therapist's goals was to promote and maintain the health of the client's unaffected joints that were vulnerable to becoming stiff from protective posturing. Another goal during the acute phase was to prevent further injury or abnormal joint changes to the left hand. ROM exercises were administered to maintain the healthy function of the client's unaffected joints such as the shoulder and elbow and a protective splint was fabricated positioning Gerry in a protective and functional position of mild wrist flexion, MP flexion and IP extension. During this phase of recovery, education was an important component of the client's intervention plan. Gerry was taught appropriate postoperative precautions and splint wear and care; his family was received education on wound care, dressing changes, and signs of infection. Written material was given to Gerry regarding this home program.

During the intermediate phase of his recovery, the intervention approach was to *restore* active and passive ROM, strength, and coordination to Gerry's hand so that he could return to his previous occupations (specifically, cabinetry, golf, and softball). The ROM activities were graded, and motion was progressively added as the tendons, nerves, and vessels healed. Strengthening exercises were added during the late phase of recovery, and at this point Gerry could safely attempt to return to his previous activities. It was at this time that purposeful and occupation-based activities were added to Gerry's therapy regimen. In addition, Gerry's areas of occupation had to be modified for the loss of mobility, strength, and coordination of the hand. One-handed ADLs were taught to Gerry during the acute phase of recovery so that he could be self-sufficient until he regained the use of his left hand. Modifications to his activity demands were also implemented, such as enlarging the handles of his golf clubs to compensate for lack of full finger ROM during the intermediate to late phases of recovery. Finally, Gerry was taught to prevent further injury to his hand through visual compensation techniques for loss of sensation, to monitor for signs of infection, and to undertake post-surgical precautions during the acute phase of his injury.

Throughout Gerry's intervention, his performance skills were reviewed to identify barriers to performance using a variety of

Continued

THREADED CASE STUDY: GERRY, PART 2—cont'd

assessment tools. A grip dynamometer, pinch meter, and manual muscle tests were used to assess grip, pinch, and muscle strength. A goniometer was used to assess ROM, and Semmes-Weinstein monofilaments were used to assess sensation. A volumeter and circumferential measurements were used to assess edema, and the Jebson Test of Hand Function was used to assess functional use of Gerry's hand in a standardized format. The evaluation data were then interpreted and the intervention plan modified to achieve the targeted outcomes.

Once the intervention plan was established, various preparatory methods and purposeful activities were chosen to achieve Gerry's occupational goals. For the occupational performance goal of golfing, splints were used as a preparatory method during the intermediate phase of recovery to gain passive ROM of stiff joints and to increase overall flexion of the replanted digits so that Gerry could eventually hold a golf club. Physical agent modalities such as paraffin and ultrasound were applied before performance of purposeful activity during the intermediate and late phases of recovery. Purposeful activities such as swinging a golf club in the clinic, simulating a golf swing on

the BTE work simulator, and gradually increasing the physical resistive demands of this golf swing were performed. Gerry also practiced putting in the clinic with special "flexion gloves" early on so that he could hold the golf club; later, he progressed to wearing no glove but instead enlarging the handle of the golf club to facilitate a secure grip.

To address Gerry's occupational goal of returning to work as a cabinetmaker, a volunteer opportunity was arranged for him to participate in the purposeful activity of making "wooden sliding/transfer boards" and other assistive devices for the acute rehabilitation clients. Not only was this activity goal-directed and directly related to his work occupation, but it also fulfilled Gerry's desire to use his talents in carpentry to help other clients in the hospital; this contributed to improving his feelings of decreased self-worth. During the late phase of Gerry's recovery, additional occupation-based activity was initiated to address his avocational interests. During the actual performance of golfing and softball outside of the clinic, it was found that Gerry was hyper-sensitive in the palm over the scars. Desensitization techniques were performed as part of his home program, and he purchased gloves with gel inserts to absorb the shock of hitting the ball.

Review Questions

1. A client is seen for a hand problem and found to have limited or painful ROM of the shoulder. List three tests that should be performed.

2. Discuss three approaches to postoperative care of flexor tendon injuries, and describe how the differences among the methods would influence the initiation of OT.

3. To what does *joint dysfunction* refer? What are its causes?

4. Discuss the three classifications of nerve injury.

5. Define the area referred to as "no-man's land." What distinguishes injury to this area?

6. What techniques are used to evaluate the physical demand characteristics of work?

7. List three methods of applying pressure to a hypertrophic scar.

8. Which functional activities could be used for restoration of hand function following laceration and repair of the extrinsic finger flexors?

9. Which assessments should be included in a functional capacity evaluation?

10. List five tests used to assess joint integrity in the hand.

11. List three objectives of splinting as they relate to injury of the radial, median, and ulnar nerves.

12. What are the characteristics of complex regional pain syndrome, type I? What are the intervention goals?

13. Define work hardening. How can work hardening be incorporated into OT?

14. How is the presence of edema evaluated? List three methods used to reduce edema.

15. What are the primary work-related risk factors associated with cumulative trauma? How can the occupational therapist intervene to prevent the development of cumulative trauma?

REFERENCES

1. Adson A, Coffey J: Cervical rib: a method of anterior approach for relief of symptoms by division of scalenus anticus, *Ann Surg* 85:834, 1927.

2. Alon G: *High voltage stimulation*, Chattanooga, TN, 1984, Chattanooga.

3. American Occupational Therapy Association, ADA Network, and Practice Division: 4720 Montgomery Lane, PO Box 31220, Bethesda, MD 20824-1220.

4. American Society for Surgery of the Hand: *The hand examination and diagnosis*, ed 3, New York, 1990, Churchill Livingstone.

5. Armstrong TJ: Cumulative trauma disorders of the upper limb and identification of work-related factors. In Millender LH, Louis DS, Simmons BP, editors: *Occupational disorders of the upper extremity*, New York, 1992, Churchill Livingstone.

6. Atrzberger SM: Manual edema mobilization: treatment for edema in the subacute hand. In Mackin EJ, et al, editors: *Rehabilitation of the hand and upper extremity*, ed 5, St Louis, 2002, Mosby.

7. Barber LM: Occupational therapy for the treatment of reflex sympathetic dystrophy and post-traumatic hypersensitivity of the injured hand. In Fredericks S, Brody G, editors:

Symposium on the neurologic aspects of plastic surgery, St Louis, 1978, Mosby.

8. Baxter-Petralia P, Bruening L, Blackmore S: The work tolerance program of the Hand Rehabilitation Center in Philadelphia. In Hunter JM, et al, editors: *Rehabilitation of the hand*, ed 3, St Louis, 1990, Mosby.

9. Bell-Krotoski JA: Plaster cylinder casting for contractures of the interphalangeal joints. In Mackin EJ, et al, editors: *Rehabilitation of the hand and upper extremity*, ed 5, St Louis, 2002, Mosby.

10. Bell-Krotoski JA: Sensibility testing with the Semmes-Weinstein monofilaments. In Mackin EJ, et al, editors: *Rehabilitation of the hand and upper extremity*, ed 5, St Louis, 2002, Mosby.

11. Bennett G: *Hand-tool dexterity test*, New York, 1981, Harcourt, Brace, Jovanovich.

12. Boyes JH: *Bunnell's surgery of the hand*, ed 5, Philadelphia, 1970, JB Lippincott.

13. Boyes JH, Stark HH: Flexor-tendon grafts in the fingers and thumb, *J Bone Joint Surg Am* 53(7):1332, 1971.

14. Brand PW, Hollister A: *Clinical mechanics of the hand*, ed 3, St Louis, 1999, Mosby.

15. Brown PW: Psychologically based hand disorders. In Mackin EJ, et al, editors: *Rehabilitation of the hand and upper extremity*, ed 5, St Louis, 2002, Mosby.

16. Butler D: *Mobilisation of the nervous system*, New York, 1991, Churchill Livingstone.

17. Byl N, Melnick M: The neural consequences of repetition: clinical implications of a learning hypothesis, *J Hand Ther* 10(2):160, 1997.

18. Callahan AD: Sensibility assessment for nerve lesion-in-continuity and nerve lacerations. In Mackin EJ, et al, editors: *Rehabilitation of the hand and upper extremity*, ed 5, St Louis, 2002, Mosby.

19. Cannon N, et al: Control of immediate postoperative pain following tenolysis and capsulectomies of the hand with TENS, *J Hand Surg Am* 8:625, 1983.

20. Carroll D: A quantitative test of upper extremity function, *J Chronic Dis* 18:479, 1965.

21. Chan SW, LaStayo P: Hand therapy management following mutilating hand injuries, *Hand Clin* 19(1):133, 2003.

22. Commission on Accreditation of Rehabilitation Facilities (CARF): 2500 N. Pantano Rd., Tucson, AZ 85715.

23. Coopee RA: Kinesio taping. In Mackin EJ, et al, editors: *Rehabilitation of the hand and upper extremity*, ed 5, St Louis, 2002, Mosby.

24. Coopee RA: Taping techniques. In Jacobs A, Austin N: *Splinting the hand and upper extremity*, Baltimore, 2003, Lippincott Williams & Wilkins.

25. Crawford J, Crawford D: *Crawford small parts dexterity test manual*, New York, 1981, Harcourt, Brace, Jovanovich.

26. Creelman G: Volumeters Unlimited, Idyllwild, CA.

27. Curtis RM, Engalitcheff J: A work simulator for rehabilitating the upper extremity: preliminary report, *J Hand Surg* 6(5):499, 1981.

28. Cyriax J: Clinical applications of massage. In Basmajian JV, editor: *Manipulation, traction and massage*, ed 3, Baltimore, 1985, Williams & Wilkins.

29. Dellon AL: Clinical use of vibratory stimuli to evaluate peripheral nerve injury and compression neuropathy, *Plast Reconstr Surg* 65(4):466, 1980.

30. Dellon AL: Evaluation of sensibility and reeducation of sensation in the hand, Baltimore, 1981, Williams & Wilkins.

31. Dellon AL: The vibrometer, *Plast Reconstr Surg* 71(3):427, 1983.

32. Dellon AL, Curtis RM, Edgerton MT: Reeducation of sensation in the hand after nerve injury and repair, *Plast Reconstr Surg* 53(3):297, 1974.

33. Donatelli R, Owens-Burkhart H: Effects of immobilization on the extensibility of periarticular connective tissue, *J Orthop Sports Phys Ther* 3:67, 1981.

34. Duran R, et al: Management of flexor tendon lacerations in zone 2 using controlled passive motion postoperatively. In Hunter JM, et al, editors: *Rehabilitation of the hand*, ed 3, St Louis, 1990, Mosby.

35. Employment and Rehabilitation Institute of California (ERIC): 1160 N Gilbert St., Anaheim, CA, 92801.

36. Evans RB: Clinical management of extensor tendon injuries. In Mackin EJ, et al, editors: *Rehabilitation of the hand and upper extremity*, ed 5, St Louis, 2002, Mosby.

37. Evans RB, Burkhalter WE: A study of the dynamic anatomy of extensor tendons and implications for treatment, *J Hand Surg* 11(5):774, 1986.

38. Evans RB, McAuliffe JA: Wound classification and management. In Mackin EJ, et al, editors: *Rehabilitation of the hand and upper extremity*, ed 5, St Louis, 2002, Mosby.

39. Fess E, Moran C: *Clinical assessment recommendations*, Indianapolis, 1981, American Society of Hand Therapists.

40. Gelberman RH, et al: The carpal tunnel syndrome: a study of carpal canal pressures, *J Bone Joint Surg* 63(3):380, 1981.

41. Gelberman RH, et al: Sensibility testing in peripheral-nerve compression syndromes: an experimental study in humans, *J Bone Joint Surg* 65(5):632, 1983.

42. Hand Therapy Certification Commission: 11160 Sun Center Drive, Rancho Cordova, CA.

43. Harrand G: *The Harrand guide for developing physical capacity evaluations*, Menomonie, WI, 1982, Stout Vocational Rehabilitation Institute.

44. Hawkins R, Kennedy J: Impingement syndrome in athletes, *Am J Sports Med* 8(3):151, 1980.

45. Hunter JM: *Staged flexor tendon reconstruction*, Part I. In Mackin EJ, et al, editors: *Rehabilitation of the hand and upper extremity*, ed 5, St Louis, 2002, Mosby.

46. Jebsen RH, Taylor N, Trieschmann RB, et al: An objective and standardized test of hand function, *Arch Phys Med Rehabil* 50(6):311, 1969.

47. Jobst Institute: PO Box 653, Toledo, OH 43694.

48. Kamenetz H: Mechanical devices of massage. In Basmajian JV, editor: *Manipulation, traction and massage*, ed 3, Baltimore, 1985, Williams & Wilkins.

49. Kasch MC: Clinical management of scar tissue, *OT in Health Care* 4:37, 1987.

50. Kasch MC: Therapist's evaluation and treatment of upper extremity cumulative trauma disorders. In Mackin EJ, et al, editors: *Rehabilitation of the hand and upper extremity*, ed 5, St Louis, 2002, Mosby.

51. Kasch MC, Hester L: Low-frequency TENS and the release of endorphins, *J Hand Surg* 8:626, 1983.

52. Kellor M, et al: *Technical manual of hand strength and dexterity test*, Minneapolis, 1971, Sister Kenney Rehabilitation Institute.

53. Kelsey JL, et al: *Upper extremity disorders: frequency, impact and cost*, New York, 1997, Churchill Livingstone.

54. Kessler RM, Hertling D: Joint mobilization techniques. In Kessler RM, Hertling D, editors: *Management of common musculoskeletal disorders*, New York, 1983, Harper & Row.

55. Koman LA, Smith BP, Smith TL: Reflex sympathetic dystrophy (complex regional pain syndromes—types 1 and 2). In Mackin EJ, et al, editors: *Rehabilitation of the hand and upper extremity*, ed 5, St Louis, 2002, Mosby.

56. Kutz JE: Controlled mobilization of acute flexor tendon injuries: Louisville technique. In Hunter JM, Schneider LH, Mackin EJ, editors: *Tendon surgery in the hand*, St Louis, 1987, Mosby.

57. LaSalle WB, Strickland JW: An evaluation of the two-stage flexor tendon reconstruction technique, *J Hand Surg* 8(3):263, 1983.

58. Louis DS, et al: Evaluation of normal values for stationary and moving two-point discrimination in the hand, *J Hand Surg* 9(4):552, 1984.

59. Lublin JS: Unions and firms focus on hand disorder that can be caused by repetitive tasks, *The Wall Street Journal*, January 14, 1983.

60. Lundborg G, et al: Digital vibrogram: a new diagnostic tool for sensory testing in compression neuropathy, *J Hand Surg* 11(5):693, 1986.

61. Mackinnon SE, Dellon AL: Two-point discrimination tester, *J Hand Surg* 19(6 pt 1):906, 1985.

62. Magee DJ: *Orthopedic physical assessment*, ed 3, Philadelphia, 1997, WB Saunders.

63. Maitland G: *Peripheral manipulation*, Boston, 1977, Butterworth.

64. Malick MH, Carr JA: Flexible elastomer molds in burn scar control, *Am J Occup Ther* 34(9):603, 1980.

65. Matheson LN: *Work capacity evaluation: a training manual for occupational therapists*, Trabuco Canyon, CA, 1982, Rehabilitation Institute of Southern California.

66. Matheson LN, Ogden LD: *Work tolerance screening*, Trabuco Canyon, CA, 1983, Rehabilitation Institute of Southern California.

67. Mathiowetz V, et al: Grip and pinch strength: normative data for adults, *Arch Phys Med Rehabil* 66(2):69, 1985.

68. Mathiowetz V, et al: Reliability and validity of grip and pinch strength evaluations, *J Hand Surg* 9(2):222, 1984.

69. Melvin J: *Rheumatic disease occupational therapy and rehabilitation*, ed 3, Philadelphia, 1989, FA Davis.

70. Mennell JM: *Joint pain*, Boston, 1964, Little, Brown.

71. Mennell JM, Zohn DA: *Musculoskeletal pain: diagnosis and physical treatment*, Boston, 1976, Little, Brown.

72. Michlovitz SL: Ultrasound and selected physical agent modalities in upper extremity rehabilitation. In Mackin EJ, et al, editors: *Rehabilitation of the hand and upper extremity*, ed 5, St Louis, 2002, Mosby.

73. Minnesota Manual Dexterity Test: Available from Lafayette Instrument Co, PO Box 5729, Lafayette, IN 47903.

74. Moberg E: Objective methods of determining functional value of sensibility in the hand, *J Bone Joint Surg* 40A:454, 1958.

75. Muenzen PA, et al: A new practice analysis of hand therapy, *J Hand Ther* 15(3):215, 2002.

76. Neer C, Welch R: The shoulder in sports, *Orthop Clin North Am* 8(3):583, 1977.

77. Nelson DL, et al: The effects of occupationally embedded exercise on bilaterally assisted supination in persons with hemiplegia, *Am J Occup Ther* 50(8):639, 1996.

78. O'Riain S: New and simple test of nerve function in the hand, *Br Med J* 3:615, 1973.

79. Omer G: Management of pain syndromes in the upper extremity. In Hunter JM, et al, editors: *Rehabilitation of the hand*, ed 3, St Louis, 1990, Mosby.

80. Parry C: *Rehabilitation of the hand*, ed 4, London, 1984, Butterworth.

81. Peacock EE, Madden JW, Trier WC: Postoperative recovery of flexor tendon function, *Am J Surg* 122(5):686, 1971.

82. Post M: *Physical examination of the musculoskeletal system*, Chicago, 1987, Book Medical Publisher.

83. Rempel DM: Work-related cumulative trauma disorders of the upper extremity, *JAMA* 267(6):838, 1992.

84. Roos D: Congenital anomalies associated with thoracic outlet syndrome, *Am J Surg* 132(6):771, 1976.

85. Schneider LH: Tendon transfers an overview. In Mackin EJ, et al, editors: *Rehabilitation of the hand and upper extremity*, ed 5, St Louis, 2002, Mosby.

86. Schneider L, Hunter J: Flexor tenolysis. In Hunter JM, et al, editors: *AAOS: symposium on tendon surgery in the hand*, St Louis, 1975, Mosby.

87. Schultz-Johnson K: Upper extremity functional capacity evaluation. In Mackin EJ, et al, editors: *Rehabilitation of the hand and upper extremity*, ed 5, St Louis, 2002, Mosby.

88. Simon H: Carpal tunnel syndrome, 2004.

89. Smith P: *Lister's the hand: diagnosis and indications*, ed 4, New York, 2002, Churchill Livingstone.

90. Strickland JW: Biologic rationale, clinical application, and results of early motion following flexor tendon repair, *J Hand Ther* 2:71, 1989.

91. Strickland JW, Glogovac SV: Digital function following flexor tendon repair in zone II: a comparison of immobilization and controlled passive motion techniques, *J Hand Surg* 5(6):537, 1980.

92. Szabo RM, et al: Vibratory sensory testing in acute peripheral nerve compression, *J Hand Surg* 9A(1):104, 1984.

93. Tetro A, et al: A new provocative test for carpal tunnel syndrome: assessment of wrist flexion and nerve compression, *J Bone Joint Surg Br* 80(3):493, 1998.

94. Thomas CL, editor: *Taber's cyclopedic medical dictionary*, ed 14, Philadelphia, 1981, FA Davis.

95. Tiffin J: *Purdue pegboard examiner manual*, Chicago, 1968, Science Research Associates.

96. Travell J, Simons D: *Myofascial pain and dysfunction: the trigger point manual*, ed 2, Baltimore, 1992, Williams & Wilkins.

97. U.S. Department of Labor Employment and Training Administration: *Dictionary of occupational titles*, ed 4, Washington, DC, 1991, U.S. Government Printing Office.

98. Vocational Research Institute, Jewish Employment and Vocational Service (JEVS): Philadelphia.

99. Watson HK, Carlson L: Treatment of reflex sympathetic dystrophy of the hand with an active "stress loading" program, *J Hand Surg* 12(5 pt 1):779, 1987.

100. Waylett-Rendall J: Sensibility evaluation and rehabilitation, *Orthop Clin North Am* 19(1):43, 1988.

101. Waylett-Rendall J, Seibly D: A study of the accuracy of a commercially available volumeter, *J Hand Ther* 4:10, 1991.

102. Wehbe MA: Tendon gliding exercises, *Am J Occup Ther* 41(3):164, 1987.

103. Wehbe MA, Hunter JM: Flexor tendon gliding in the hand. II: Differential gliding, *J Hand Surg* 10(4):575, 1985.

104. Wolf SL: *Electrotherapy*, New York, 1981, Churchill Livingstone.

105. Wong GY, Wilson PR: Classification of complex regional pain syndromes, *Hand Clin* 13(3):319, 1997.

106. Yerxa EJ, et al: Development of a hand sensitivity test for the hypersensitive hand, *Am J Occup Ther* 37(3):176, 1983.

107. Zimmerer-Branum S, Nelson DL: Occupationally embedded exercise versus rote exercise: a choice between occupational forms by elderly nursing home residents, *Am J Occup Ther* 49(5):397, 1995.

40

Hip Fractures and Lower Extremity Joint Replacement

SONIA LAWSON

KEY TERMS

Spica cast
Osteoporosis
Open reduction and internal
fixation

Weight-bearing restrictions
Arthroplasty
Avascular necrosis

Anterolateral approach
Posterolateral approach
Hip precautions

Minimally invasive technique
Knee immobilizer
Leg lifter

LEARNING OBJECTIVES

After studying this chapter the student or practitioner will be able to do the following:

1. Describe the etiology of hip fractures and joint replacements and how these problems limit participation in daily activities.
2. Describe the medical management for these conditions.
3. Identify the medical precautions associated with hip fractures and joint replacements.
4. Identify occupational therapy intervention goals.
5. Identify and discuss areas of intervention for occupational therapy.
6. Discuss appropriate treatment techniques that address all areas of occupational performance.
7. Discuss the impact of hip fractures and joint replacement on occupational performance and performance patterns.

CHAPTER OUTLINE

General medical management of fractures
  Etiology of fractures
  Medical management
Hip fractures
  Types of hip fractures and medical management
Hip joint replacement
  Etiology
Knee joint replacement
  Etiology and medical management
General considerations for lower extremity joint replacements
Psychological factors

Rehabilitation
Role of occupational therapy
  Evaluation and intervention
  Client education
  Specific training techniques
  Training procedures for persons with hip surgery
  Training procedures for persons with total knee replacement
  General considerations and evidence for occupational therapy
    intervention
  Special equipment
Summary

THREADED CASE STUDY: MRS. HERNANDEZ, PART 1

Mrs. Hernandez, a 70-year-old Hispanic grandmother to three small children, has been experiencing increasing right hip pain over the last few years. Mrs. Hernandez is usually very active, attending swimming classes twice a week, helping her daughter care for her three children, and heading two committees at her parish church. Mrs. Hernandez has been a widow for 5 years and lives alone in an apartment with elevator access. However, her daughter and her family live only 15 minutes away and often visit and involve her in many of their family activities.

At this point, her hip pain has increased so much that it is keeping her from attending the swimming classes she enjoys so much. Climbing in and out of the pool is simply too painful. Driving has also become difficult at times because her hip "catches," causing her to worry that she will lose control of the car. Her participation in activities with her grandchildren has been greatly affected. She had looked forward to being a very involved grandparent, especially after her husband died. However, now she can no longer get on the floor with them or go on trips that include a great deal of walking (e.g., an amusement park). She has resorted to using a cane when walking to help reduce the pressure on her right leg. She has been relying on her church friends and daughter to bring her to church each week but has cut back on attending the meetings for the committees to which she belongs.

Her doctor tells her that the pain is a result of degenerative joint disease and that her hip joint is essentially wearing out. He recommends a total hip replacement and tells her that after she recovers from surgery, she will be able to go back to doing all of the things she enjoyed before her hip pain limited her participation.

Critical Thinking Questions

1. Describe the supporting and non-supporting contextual factors affecting Mrs. Hernandez.
2. How would you prioritize the problems Mrs. Hernandez has as a result of her hip pain? What is your rationale for prioritizing the problems in this way?
3. How would Mrs. Hernandez's life be affected if she continues with the hip pain and does not have the hip replacement?
4. What does it seem that Mrs. Hernandez values in her life?

Hip fractures and lower extremity (LE) joint replacements are two orthopedic conditions that occur with a relatively high frequency. Persons who have been involved in sports or occupations that put great amounts of stress on the knee or hip joints may experience joint pain and degeneration as they get older. In addition, older individuals are more likely to have orthopedic problems such as osteoporosis and degenerative joint changes as a part of the aging process. Medical advances have made the treatment of hip fractures and LE joint problems safer and easier to manage. LE joint problems can lead to temporary or more long-lasting disability. In both hip and knee conditions, a large weight-bearing joint is unstable for a period of time, which limits an individual's participation in meaningful daily occupations. For example, Mrs. Hernandez discontinued swimming and limited her physical activities with her grandchildren because of her hip pain. Both of these occupations were valued aspects of her life in which she now feels unable to participate.

The elderly population is most at risk for hip fractures. Reduced mobility and the presence of osteoporosis are two specific risk factors. Elderly women, in particular, develop osteoporosis to a greater degree than men and thus tend to have more hip fractures when they fall.[3]

Mobility is compromised in the elderly population because of decreased flexibility, diminished strength, reduced vision, slowed reaction time, and the use of assistive ambulatory aids such as canes and walkers. Many elderly people become more cautious when moving about and are fearful of falling. In some cases, individuals trip over a cane or walker, which causes a fall. Not seeing a step or threshold is also a common cause for falling.

Individuals with a history of arthritis or other joint disease are primary candidates for LE joint replacement. Individuals who elect to undergo this surgical procedure usually have been living with increasing pain in their joints for many months or years and are already limited in their ability to perform daily tasks. By having the painful joint replaced, they hope to return to a more active and satisfying lifestyle.

Occupational therapy (OT) plays a key role in identifying and remediating the many functional problems imposed by these acute and chronic orthopedic conditions, thus sharing in the goal of returning the orthopedic client to optimal performance of safe, independent, and meaningful occupations. For example, OT can help Mrs. Hernandez identify alternative ways of participating in her daily occupations safely; the therapist must make sure to address all of the occupations that the client identifies as important.

This chapter discusses hip fractures and LE joint replacements, their medical and surgical management, the psychological implications of hospitalization and disability, the healthcare team approach in both the acute hospital and rehabilitation settings, and the specific OT evaluation and intervention strategies appropriate for people with these diagnoses.

GENERAL MEDICAL MANAGEMENT OF FRACTURES

 OT PRACTICE NOTE

It is important for the occupational therapist working with clients who have orthopedic problems or diagnoses to have a good understanding of the site, type, and cause of the fracture before starting treatment. A basic understanding of fracture healing and medical management is also necessary to appreciate risks, precautions, and complications involved. The occupational therapist is advised to consult an orthopedic manual for specific information regarding the specifics of the fracture healing process.

In general, a fracture occurs when the bone's ability to absorb tension, compression, or shearing forces is exceeded.[4] The healing process begins after the fracture. Osteoblasts, cells that form bone, multiply to mend the fractured area. A good blood supply is necessary to supply the cells with oxygen for proper healing. The fracture site is protected during the healing process by pins, plates, and wires. In rare cases in which extra protection is needed, a **spica cast** may be used for the hip. A spica cast extends around the pelvis and down the thigh of the fractured hip. Other types of casts may be used for fractures at other parts of the LE. Several months may be needed for a bone fracture to heal completely. The time needed varies with the age and health of the client, the site and configuration of the fracture, initial displacement of the bone, and the blood supply to the fragments.

ETIOLOGY OF FRACTURES

Trauma is the major cause of fractures. In most cases, the trauma occurs as a result of falling. Poor lighting, throw rugs, and unmarked steps are particular hazards that can lead to a fall. **Osteoporosis** is a common bone disease affecting people as they get older. It results in decreased bone density, most commonly in the vertebral bodies, the neck of the femur, the humerus, and the distal end of the radius. Because the bone becomes porous and therefore fragile, the affected bones are prone to fracture during a fall or other traumatic event. A pathological fracture can occur in a bone weakened by disease or tumor, as with osteomyelitis and cancers that have metastasized to the bone.[4]

MEDICAL MANAGEMENT

The goals of fracture treatment are to relieve pain, maintain good position of the bone, allow fracture healing, and restore optimal function to the client. *Reduction of a fracture*

refers to restoring the bone fragments to normal alignment.[4] This can be done by a closed procedure (manipulation) or by an open procedure (surgery). The physician performs a closed reduction by applying force to the displaced bone, opposite to the force that produced the fracture. Depending on the nature of the fracture, the reduction is maintained in a cast, brace, traction, or skeletal fixation. With open reduction, the fracture site is exposed surgically so that the bone fragments can be aligned. The fragments are held in place with internal fixation by pins, screws, a plate, nails, or a rod. Further immobilization by a cast or a brace may be necessary. Because an **open reduction and internal fixation (ORIF)** usually must be protected from excessive forces, **weight-bearing restrictions** are indicated.[4]

There are several levels of weight-bearing restrictions. The physician indicates at which level the client should be placed and changes the restrictions as the fracture site heals and becomes stronger. The levels of weight-bearing restrictions are listed in Box 40-1.[6]

HIP FRACTURES

TYPES OF HIP FRACTURES AND MEDICAL MANAGEMENT

Knowledge of hip anatomy is necessary for understanding medical management of hip fractures. An anatomy and physiology reference text should be consulted for details. See Figure 40-1 for an illustration of the normal hip joint.

The typical levels of fracture lines are shown in Figure 40-2. The names of the fractures generally reflect the site and severity of injury and may signal the form of medical treatment

---

| BOX **40-1** | WEIGHT-BEARING RESTRICTIONS |

NWB (non–weight bearing) indicates that no weight at all can be placed on the extremity involved.

TTWB (toe-touch weight bearing) indicates that only the toe can be placed on the ground to provide some balance while standing—90% of the weight is still on the unaffected leg. In toe-touch weight bearing, clients are instructed to imagine that an egg is under their foot.

PWB (partial weight bearing) indicates that only 50% of the person's body weight can be placed on the affected leg.

WBAT (weight bearing at tolerance) indicates that clients are allowed to judge how much weight they are able to put on the affected leg without causing too much pain.

FWB (full weight bearing) indicates that clients should be able to put 100% of their weight on the affected leg without causing damage to the fracture site.

From Early MB: *Physical dysfunction: practical skills for the occupational therapy assistant,* St Louis, 1998, Mosby.

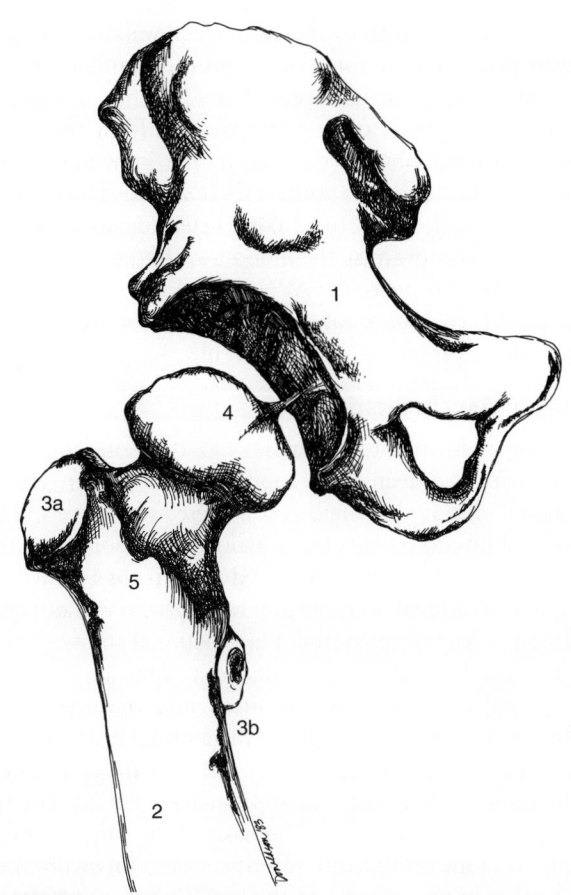

Figure 40-1   Normal hip anatomy. *1*, Acetabulum. *2*, Femur. *3a*, Greater trochanter. *3b*, Lesser trochanter. *4*, Ligamentum teres. *5*, Intertrochanteric crest. (Modified from Croch JE: *Functional human anatomy*, ed 3, Philadelphia, 1978, Lea & Febiger; Grant LC: *Grant's atlas of anatomy*, ed 6, Baltimore, 1972, Williams & Wilkins.)

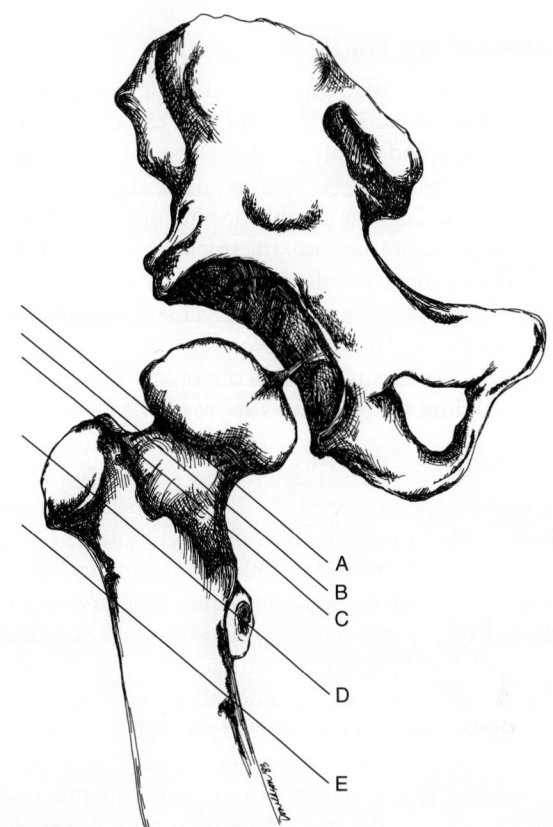

Figure 40-2   Levels of femoral fracture. **A,** Subcapital. **B,** Transcervical. **C,** Basilar. **D,** Intertrochanteric. **E,** Subtrochanteric. (Modified from Crow I: Fracture of the hip: a self study, *ONA J* 5:12, 1978.)

that will be used. For example, a femoral neck fracture will be treated with femoral neck stabilization.[11]

Femoral Neck Fractures

Femoral neck fractures, which include subcapital, transcervical, and basilar fractures, are common in adults over 60 years old and occur more frequently in women. If the bone is osteoporotic, fracture may result from even a slight trauma or rotational force.[7] Treatment of a displaced fracture in this area is complicated by poor blood supply, osteoporotic bone that is not suited to hold metallic fixation, and a thin periosteum covering the bone. The type of surgical treatment used is based on the amount of displacement and the circulation in the femoral head.

The age and health of the client are considered in deciding on the surgical procedure. Generally, hip pinning (application of a compression screw and plate) is used when displacement is minimal to moderate and blood supply is intact. With a physician's approval, a client is usually able to

begin limited out-of-bed activities 1 to 3 days after surgery. Per physician's orders, weight-bearing restrictions may be necessary, with the aid of a walker or crutches for at least 6 to 8 weeks while the fracture is healing. Weight bearing may be limited beyond this time if precautions are not observed or if delayed union occurs.[11]

With severe displacement or in the case of a femoral head with poor blood supply (avascular) or nonunion (a poorly healing fracture site where new bone does not form) and degenerative joint disease, the femoral head is surgically removed and replaced by an endoprosthesis. This joint replacement is referred to as a *hemipolar* or *bipolar arthroplasty.*[8,11] This surgical procedure may be documented as a *hemiarthroplasty.* Several types of metal prostheses can be used; each has its own shape and advantages. Weight-bearing restrictions are sometimes indicated. Depending on the surgical procedure used (posterolateral or anterolateral approach), specific precautions for positioning the hip must be observed to prevent dislocation. These precautions are the same as for a total hip replacement, which will be outlined later in this chapter. Clients who have had a prosthesis implanted can usually begin limited out-of-bed activity, with a physician's approval, about 1 to 3 days after surgery.[8,11]

Intertrochanteric Fractures

...es between the greater and lesser trochanter are ...psular, or outside the articular capsule of the hip ...d the blood supply is not affected. Like femoral neck ...s, intertrochanteric fractures occur mostly in women but in a slightly older age group. The fracture is usually caused by direct trauma or force over the trochanter, as in a fall. The preferred treatment for these fractures is ORIF. A nail or compression screw with a sideplate is used. Weight-bearing restrictions must be observed for up to 4 to 6 months during ambulation. The client is allowed out of bed 1 to 3 days after surgery, pending the physician's approval.[11]

Subtrochanteric Fractures

Subtrochanteric fractures 1 to 2 inches below the lesser trochanter usually occur because of direct trauma, as in falls, motor vehicle accidents, or any other situation in which there is a direct blow to the hip area. These fractures are most often seen in persons younger than 60 years old. Skeletal traction followed by ORIF is the usual treatment. A nail with a long sideplate or an intramedullary rod is used. An intramedullary rod is a rod inserted through the central part of the shaft of bone to help maintain proper alignment for bone healing.[4] In all types of hip fractures, the practitioner should be aware of the co-existing conditions of soft-tissue trauma, edema, and bruising that occur around the fracture site.[4,8,11] These conditions can greatly affect the amount of pain and discomfort that a client may experience.

HIP JOINT REPLACEMENT

ETIOLOGY

Restoration of joint motion and treatment of pain by total hip replacement, or **arthroplasty,** is sometimes indicated, primarily in osteoarthritis and rheumatoid arthritis and occasionally in other disease processes. Osteoarthritis or degenerative joint disease may develop spontaneously in middle age and progress as the normal aging process of joints is accelerated. Degenerative changes may also develop as the result of trauma, congenital deformity, or a disease that damages articular cartilage. Weight-bearing joints such as the hip, knee, and lumbar spine are usually affected. In the hip there is a loss of cartilage centrally on the joint surface and formation of osteophytes on the periphery of the acetabulum, producing joint incongruity. Pain originates from the bone, synovial membrane, or fibrous capsule and from muscle spasm. When movement of the hip causes pain and limited mobility, the muscles shorten, which can result in a hip position of flexion, adduction, and internal rotation that causes a painful limp.[10]

The "catching" that Mrs. Hernandez experienced was a result of the loss of cartilage around the femoral head and acetabulum in her hip. Because the joint surfaces were uneven, she experienced a great deal of pain when walking. Using the cane helped to relieve some of the pressure on her hip.

Rheumatoid arthritis (see Chapter 38) may involve the hip joint. Surgery is often performed early in the disease process to limit fibrotic damage to the joint and tendon structures.[4] Other disease processes (e.g., lupus and cancer) and some medications (e.g., corticosteroids such as prednisone) can compromise the blood flow to the hip joint and lead to **avascular necrosis** (AVN, a condition in which bone cells die because of poor blood supply) or osteoporosis; either condition results in a painful hip.[10]

Medical Management

When other forms of treatment (e.g., cortisone injections) for the pain and decreased mobility have not been successful, a total joint replacement is considered to restore an individual's ability to participate in daily occupations. The total joint replacement is not considered for persons who will not comply with a rehabilitation program or who will not experience significant improvement in functional ability.[8,9] There are two mechanical components to a "total hip." A high-density polyethylene socket is fitted into the acetabulum, and a metallic prosthesis replaces the femoral head and neck. Methylmethacrylate or acrylic cement fixes the components to the bone. Various surgical approaches are used. The specific approach is selected on the basis of the surgical skill or technique of the orthopedist, severity of the joint involvement, and history of past surgery to the hip. With an **anterolateral approach,** the client will be unstable in external rotation, adduction, and extension of the operated hip and usually must observe precautions to prevent these movements for 6 to 12 weeks. If a **posterolateral approach** is used, the client must be cautioned not to move the operated hip past specific ranges of flexion (usually 60 degrees to 90 degrees) and not to internally rotate or adduct the leg. Failure to maintain these **hip precautions** during muscle and soft-tissue healing may result in hip dislocation (Box 40-2).

Box **40-2**   Hip Precautions

POSTEROLATERAL APPROACH

- No hip flexion greater than 90 degrees
- No internal rotation
- No adduction (crossing legs or feet)

ANTEROLATERAL APPROACH

- No external rotation
- No adduction (crossing legs or feet)
- No extension

From Early MB: *Physical dysfunction: practical skills for the occupational therapy assistant*, St Louis, 1998, Mosby.

Most surgeons do not restrict weight bearing postoperatively when cement fixation is used. However, one of the major problems with total hip replacement is the loss of fixation at the prosthesis interface. The use of biological fixation, wherein bony in-growth, instead of cement, secures the prosthesis, can improve fixation at the prosthesis interface. In other words, new bone grows into openings in the prosthesis, and this secures the prosthesis to the bone (Figure 40-3). The precautions following the surgery are identical to those of the anterior or posterior hip replacements, with an additional restriction on weight bearing for 6 to 8 weeks. The restrictions on weight bearing vary in terms of amount of pressure and length of time. A walking aid, usually a walker or crutches, is necessary for at least the first month while the hip is healing and muscles are becoming stronger. Clients with total joint replacements usually begin out-of-bed activity 1 to 3 days after surgery.[8]

Recently, orthopedic surgeons have used a technique to perform the posterolateral approach. This technique, which is called a **minimally invasive technique,** reduces the amount of trauma to the tissues and allows for faster recovery.

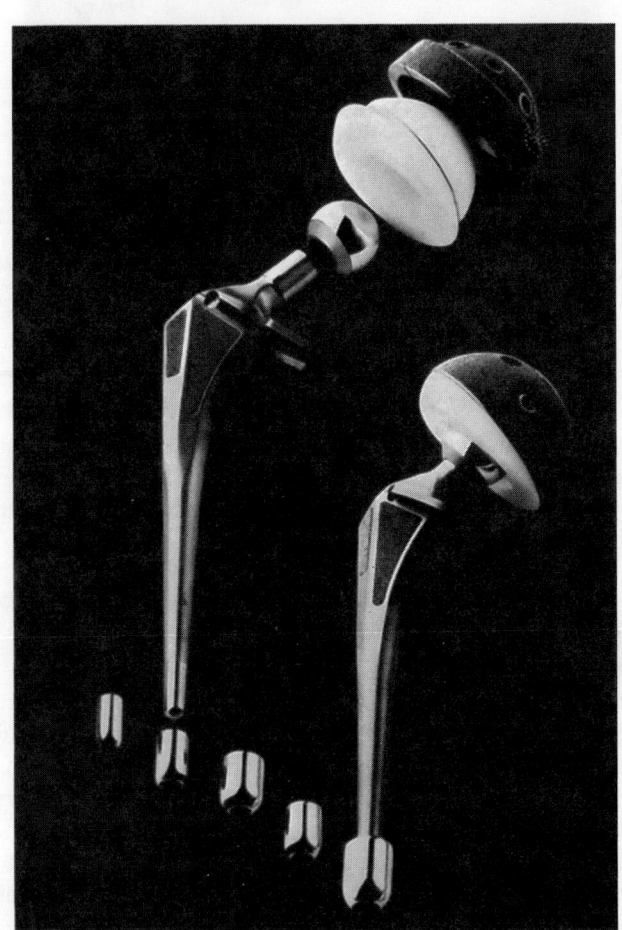

Figure 40-3   Modular total hip prosthesis designed for bony ingrowth. (From Kottke FJ: *Krusen's handbook of physical medicine and rehabilitation,* ed 4, Philadelphia, 1990, WB Saunders.)

The traditional surgical technique requires that a long (about 10 inches) incision be made and muscles detached to get to the hip joint. In the minimally invasive technique, two incisions of approximately 2 inches are needed and no detachment of muscles is required. Because no muscles are detached, the hip is more likely to remain in a stable position during the healing process. This technique is not appropriate for all total hip arthroplasties. Persons with severe damage to the hip joint will require the traditional surgical method. Hip precautions that are identified for the posterolateral approach are indicated for persons receiving the minimally invasive technique.[12]

To reinforce proper hip precautions and guide treatment intervention and discharge planning, the occupational therapist must know the type of surgical procedure that was performed. For example, someone with a hip replacement in which the minimally invasive technique was used may tolerate more activity after surgery than someone who underwent the traditional surgical technique.

Total joint surface replacements, which are rarely used, are a variation of the total hip replacement.[10] The surface of the femur is capped by a metallic shell, and the acetabular cavity receives a plastic cup. Both are held in place by methylmethacrylate (acrylic cement). This technique preserves the femoral head and neck. With this technique, no weight-bearing restrictions apply.[10]

In Mrs. Hernandez's case, the orthopedic surgeon decided to perform the total hip replacement using the traditional surgical technique because of the severity of the damage to Mrs. Hernandez's hip.

KNEE JOINT REPLACEMENT

ETIOLOGY AND MEDICAL MANAGEMENT

The reason for a total knee replacement is similar to that for the total hip replacement, except that the degenerative changes occur in the knee joint. Total knee replacement, or total knee arthroplasty (TKA), is designed to alleviate pain, increase motion, and maintain alignment and stability of the knee joint. The process involves cutting away the damaged bone (as little bone as possible) and attaching a prosthesis for the new joint. There are various types of prostheses. The type used depends on the severity of joint damage (Figures 40-4 and 40-5). The prosthesis can be cemented to the bone with acrylic cement or not cemented. With a cemented prosthesis, clients are usually able to bear weight at tolerance on the operated leg. With a noncemented prosthesis, weight bearing is usually avoided initially. Clients may start out-of-bed activities 1 to 3 days after surgery, pending the physician's orders. Clients may use a **knee immobilizer** (Figure 40-6) to provide support to the knee when moving in and out of the bed and ambulating. The client should avoid any rotation at the knee for up to 12 weeks after surgery. There is usually no restriction on bending the knee.

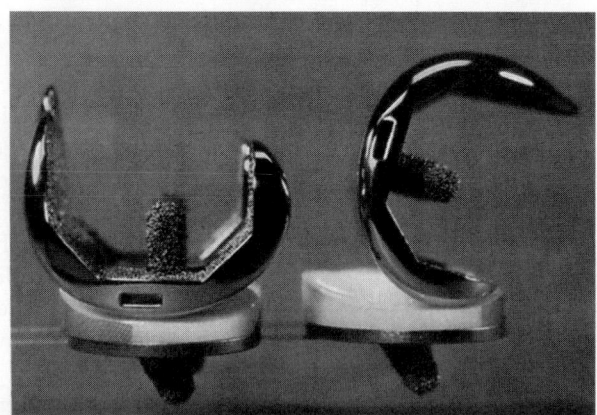

Figure 40-4 Porous-coated total knee prosthesis. Note resurfacing features of components and beaded surfaces for biological fixation. (From Kottke FJ: *Krusen's handbook of physical medicine and rehabilitation*, ed 4, Philadelphia, 1990, WB Saunders.)

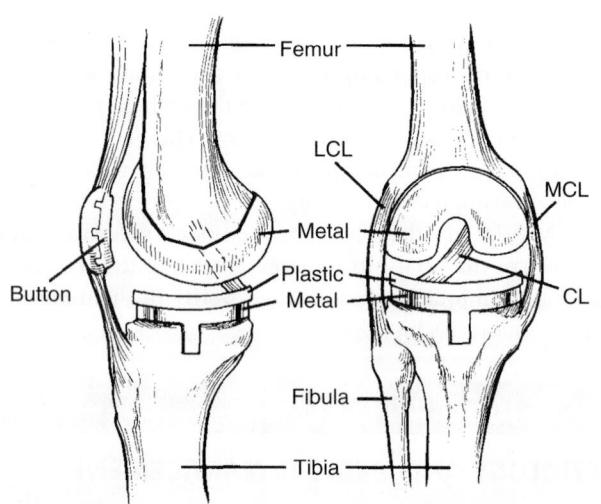

Figure 40-5 Total knee replacement. The metal aspects of the prosthesis cover the distal portion of the femur and the end of the tibia. There is a polyethylene plastic-bearing surface (*plastic*) between the metallic aspects of the two surfaces. The patella is replaced by a polyethylene button. The medial collateral ligament (*MCL*), lateral collateral ligament (*LCL*), and cruciate ligaments (*CL*) are retained. (From Early MB: *Physical dysfunction: practical skills for the occupational therapy assistant*, St Louis, 1998, Mosby; modified from Calliet R: *Knee pain and instability*, ed 3, Philadelphia, 1992, FA Davis.)

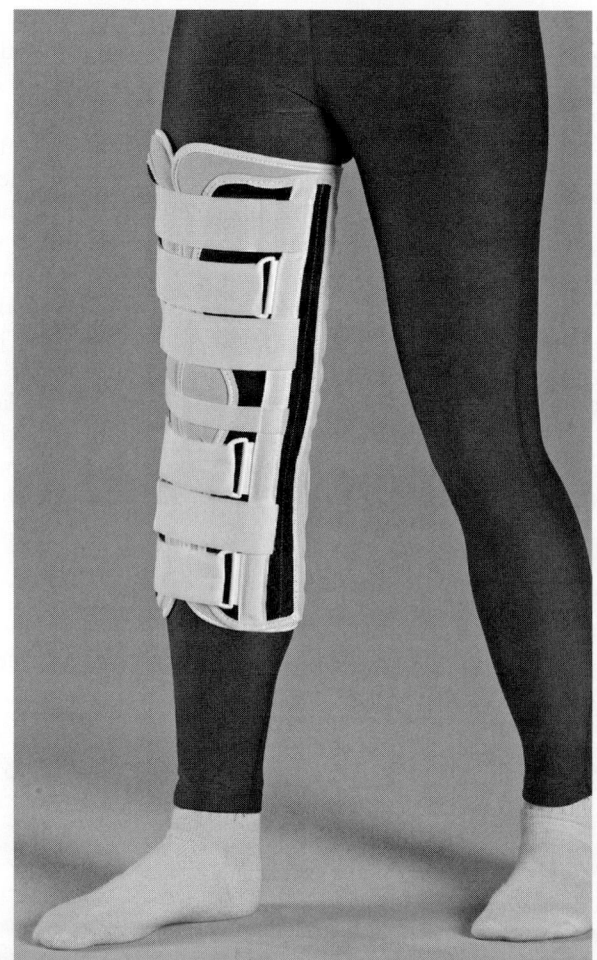

Figure 40-6 A knee immobilizer is used to support and stabilize the knee joint during mobility. (Courtesy DeRoyal, Powell, Tenn.)

In fact, maintaining the mobility of the knee is important to ensure adequate mobility during healing.[2,8,11]

As with the hip replacement, a minimally invasive technique has been developed for knee replacements. Proponents of this technique report that clients can achieve greater knee flexion (up to 90 degrees) a couple of days after surgery. In addition, because fewer ligaments are cut, increased lateral and medial stability is obtained immediately, eliminating the need for a knee immobilizer.[14] To determine whether to reinforce the use of a knee immobilizer and encourage an appropriate amount of knee flexion, the occupational therapist should be aware of the surgical technique that was used for the procedure.

GENERAL CONSIDERATIONS FOR LOWER EXTREMITY JOINT REPLACEMENTS

Individuals with joint changes that result in increasing pain may have multiple joint involvement (i.e., both knees or hips). Some clients opt to have both joints replaced during the same hospitalization, either during the same surgery or with procedures 1 week apart. This can complicate the rehabilitation process because the client will not be able to rely on the stronger leg when walking and performing daily occupations.

It is important to be aware of complications or special procedures that occurred during surgery and to inquire about additional precautions and risks. Common complications include dislocation, wearing out of parts, fracture of bone next to implanted parts, and loosening of parts. A special procedure for individuals at high risk for a dislocation involves using a spica cast to immobilize the hip joint.[4]

Emphasis in rehabilitation is on maintaining or increasing joint motion, slowly increasing the strength of surrounding musculature, decreasing swelling, and increasing the client's independence in activities of daily living (ADLs). The occupational therapist's role in this process is primarily in educating the client who has undergone joint replacement about adaptive techniques for ADLs and instrumental activities of daily living (IADLs) with limited mobility.

PSYCHOLOGICAL FACTORS

Psychological issues are critical in the overall treatment of the orthopedic client. Many clients in this population are faced with a chronic disability (e.g., rheumatoid arthritis), a life-threatening disease (e.g., cancer), or consequences of the aging process. The loss or potential loss of mobility and physical ability that limits participation in daily activities is a major concern for most of these clients. Adjusting to loss is stressful, requiring an enormous amount of physical and emotional energy.[7] An awareness of and a sensitivity toward the psychosocial challenges of the person with an orthopedic problem are critical for the delivery of optimal client care.

Clients with a chronic orthopedic disability often experience one or all of the following: disease of a body part, fear, anxiety, change in body image, decreased functional ability, joint deformity, and pain. Treatment of a client with a chronic orthopedic disability must address these issues and provide the support needed for the grieving process to take place. Without an opportunity to confront these issues, the client is likely to become depressed, filled with guilt and anxiety, and paralyzed with fear. These emotions inhibit the client's progress and further damage the client's self-image. OT clinicians can help clients acknowledge and express some of these feelings, an experience that ultimately enhances the treatment process. One way to ease anxiety and fear is to make sure that the client understands the treatment and procedures he or she is receiving. Taking time to answer questions and provide additional information can be crucial for successful adjustment.

The elderly client experiencing disability deals with additional issues specific to the aging process: fear of dependence and relocation trauma. With the onset of a disability late in life, the client may be forced to let go of independence and self-sufficiency.[7] This can be a devastating experience for some clients, and prolonged grieving may be necessary before adjustment. Others may use dependence for secondary gain, remaining in the hospital for extra attention or manipulating their support systems to avoid taking responsibility for themselves and others. When individuals are removed from their familiar environment, confusion, disorientation, and emotional lability may result. Decorating the client's room with familiar items and using a calendar can be helpful in reducing the traumatic effects of relocation.

Learning to cope and adjust to the changes resulting from chronic disability or the aging process is a critical aspect of recovery. Practitioners must realize that the client has relinquished a great deal of functional independence as a result of disease or disability. The occupational therapist must address the psychosocial issues resulting from this loss while focusing on increasing the client's functional level of independence.[7]

Mrs. Hernandez may be experiencing all or many of the aforementioned feelings and issues. The occupational therapist must provide her with educational resources and opportunities to ask questions regarding her problems and recovery. Mrs. Hernandez may be unaware of the adaptive aids available that would improve her performance skills. Access to these resources may provide the impetus for a more positive perspective on aging and remaining active and independent. It is important for the occupational therapist to help Mrs. Hernandez develop strategies and coping skills to deal with the psychosocial aspects of having hip surgery. Individual or group intervention should provide Mrs. Hernandez with the opportunity to share her feelings and explore ways to resume her occupational routines; these might include interacting with her grandchildren, swimming, and participating in church activities. The occupational therapist can assist Mrs. Hernandez in finding a more accessible pool (e.g., one with ramp access) for swimming and alternative transportation to get to church so that she need not rely on her friends and family.

An important area of ADLs that is often overlooked is sexual activity. Persons with a hip fracture or LE joint replacement will have difficulty performing sexual activities in their usual manner (see Chapter 12). It is recommended that such persons refrain from sexual activity for 6 weeks so that they maintain the movement precautions applicable to their condition.[8] Clients of all ages and both genders may have questions regarding the level of sexual activity that is allowed. The occupational therapist must create an environment in which the client feels comfortable enough to ask personal questions. The therapist can do this by being open-minded and realizing that sexual activity is important and meaningful. The therapist may need to suggest ways for the client to position the operated leg during sexual activity to maintain precautions. Side-lying on the nonoperated side is one option. Abduction precautions can be maintained via pillows between the knees. To prevent excessive external rotation at the hips while in the supine position, the client can place pillows under the knees. Clients with knee replacements or weight-bearing precautions should refrain from kneeling.[8] Written information with diagrams can be helpful when addressing such a personal issue. The client can read it privately or with his or her partner at another time.

REHABILITATION

Good communication and clear role delineation among members of the healthcare team are essential for an efficient and smooth therapy program. The healthcare team usually consists of a primary physician, nursing staff, an occupational therapist and/or assistant, a physical therapist and/or assistant, a nutritionist, a pharmacist, and a case coordinator. Many facilities have a protocol or critical pathway that outlines each team member's responsibilities and a time frame for accomplishing assigned tasks related to the client's rehabilitation. Regular team meetings to discuss each client's ongoing treatment, progress, and discharge plans are necessary for coordinating individual treatment programs. Members from each service usually attend each meeting to provide information and consultation.

The role of the physician is to inform the team of the client's medical status. This includes information regarding previous medical history, diagnosis of the present problem, and a complete account of the surgical procedure performed. Information provided may include the type of appliance inserted, the anatomical approach, and any movement or weight-bearing precautions that could endanger the client. The physician is also responsible for ordering specific medications and therapies. Any change or progression in therapy or change in the client's medication regimen should be approved by the physician.

The nursing staff is responsible for the physical care of the client during hospitalization. The orthopedic nurse must have a thorough understanding of the surgical procedures and movement precautions for each client. Proper positioning using pillows and wedges is carried out by the nurse, especially in the first few days after surgery. As the client's therapy program progresses, the client starts to take more responsibility for proper positioning and physical care. The nurse works closely with the occupational and physical therapists to carry through self-care and mobility skills that the client has already learned in therapy.

The physical therapist is responsible for evaluation and treatment in the areas of musculoskeletal status, sensation, pain, skin integrity, and mobility (especially gait). In many cases involving total joint replacement and surgical repair of hip fracture, physical therapy is initiated on the first day after surgery. Adhering to the prescribed precautions of protocol, the physical therapist obtains baseline information, including range of motion (ROM), strength of all extremities, muscle tone, and mobility. A treatment program that includes therapeutic exercises, ROM activities, transfer training, and progressive gait activities is established. The physical therapist is responsible for recommending the appropriate assistive device to be used during ambulation. As the client's ambulation status advances, instruction in stair climbing, managing curbs, and outside ambulation is given.[8]

The nutritionist consults with each client to ensure that adequate and appropriate nutrition is received to aid the healing process. The pharmacist monitors the client's drug therapy and provides information and assistance with pain management.

The role of the case coordinator is to ensure that each client is being discharged to the appropriate living situation or facility. The case coordinator is usually a registered nurse or social worker with a thorough knowledge of available community resources and nursing care facilities. However, occupational therapists have served in the position of case coordinator. Occupational therapists typically have access to community resources for equipment and living accommodations because those are areas that are addressed in the occupational therapy intervention plan. With input from the healthcare team, the case coordinator makes the arrangements for ongoing therapy after hospitalization, for admission to a rehabilitation facility for further intensive therapy, or for nursing home care if necessary. The case coordinator works closely with the healthcare team and is instrumental in coordinating the program after the client's discharge from the hospital.

ROLE OF OCCUPATIONAL THERAPY

After a total joint replacement or surgical repair of a fractured hip, OT typically begins when the client is ready to start getting out of bed, usually 1 to 3 days after surgery. The actual time varies, depending on the age and general health of the client and on surgical events or medical complications involved. Before any physical assessment, it is important to introduce and explain the role of OT and complete an occupational profile. This profile involves gathering information regarding the client's occupational history, prior functional status in ADLs and IADLs, descriptions of performance contexts (e.g., home environment and social support available), and the client's goals. The goal of OT is for the client to maximize performance in daily occupations, with all movement precautions observed during activities. The role of the occupational therapist and assistant is to teach the client ways and means of performing daily occupations safely.[7]

EVALUATION AND INTERVENTION

The role of the occupational therapist and OT assistant can be clearly defined with cases of total joint replacement and hip fractures. The occupational therapist is responsible for performing any necessary assessments. In addition to an occupational profile, an assessment of the psychosocial issues related to the surgery and the surgery's impact on the client's lifestyle is completed via interview. A baseline physical evaluation is necessary for determining whether any physical limitations not related to surgery might prevent functional independence. Performance skills such as upper extremity (UE) ROM, muscle strength, sensation, and coordination and status of mental functions are assessed before a functional evaluation is made. The certified occupational therapy assistant can participate in the ADL evaluation. During evaluation it is also important to observe any signs of pain and fear at rest or during movement.

OT involves an intervention program of functional activities that gradually enables a person to regain abilities and skills that allow for greater participation in identified areas of occupation. The therapist introduces and trains clients in the use of assistive devices, proper transfer techniques, and ADL and IADL techniques while maintaining hip precautions. Specific training techniques are discussed later in the chapter. An OT assistant may play a large role in this training. Both the occupational therapist and the OT assistant are involved in treatment planning, documentation, and discharge planning (including the recommendation of equipment and home exercise programs).

CLIENT EDUCATION

Although hip fractures are never a planned occurrence, total joint replacements are usually preplanned and scheduled to be performed on a specific date. Occupational therapists provide education classes for individuals at risk for fractures and those planning joint replacement. For the person who may be at risk for falling, attending a class on fall prevention is a wise recommendation. Topics may include home modifications (e.g., removal of throw rugs, telephone cords, and clutter), safe transfer techniques, use of public transportation, and community mobility tips. The person who is having an elective total joint replacement may

benefit from a class offered before surgery that explains the procedures, introduces assistive devices, and describes therapy procedures.

SPECIFIC TRAINING TECHNIQUES

Some common assistive devices are useful for many people with hip fractures or joint replacements (Figure 40-7). Helpful assistive devices or adaptive aids include a dressing stick, sock aid, long-handled sponge, long-handled shoe horn, reacher, elastic shoe laces, elevated toilet or commode seat, leg lifter, and shower chair or bench. Walker bags are helpful for people using walkers who need to carry small items from one place to another. The OT clinic should have samples of these devices and should be able to issue them to clients for use during the training process.

TRAINING PROCEDURES FOR PERSONS WITH HIP SURGERY

The training procedures outlined below apply to hip fractures and both types of hip joint replacement (posterolateral and anterolateral) unless otherwise noted. The positions of hip instability for both types of surgical procedures for hip replacement are important to remember. For the posterolateral approach, positions of instability include adduction, internal rotation, and flexion greater than precautions. For the anterolateral approach, positions of instability include adduction, external rotation, and excessive hyperextension.

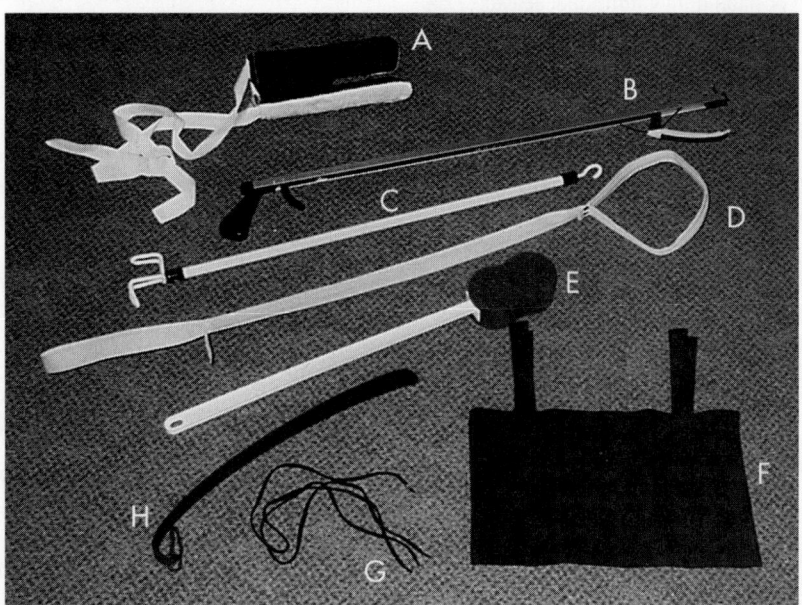

Figure 40-7 Assistive devices for ADLs. **A,** Sock aid. **B,** Reacher. **C,** Dressing stick. **D,** Leg lifter. **E,** Long-handled sponge. **F,** Walker bag. **G,** Elastic shoe laces. **H,** Long-handled shoe horn. (From Early MB: *Physical dysfunction: practical skills for the occupational therapy assistant,* St Louis, 1998, Mosby.)

Bed Mobility

The supine position with the appropriate wedge or pillow in place is recommended. If a client sleeps in the side-lying position, sleeping on the operated side is recommended if tolerable. When sleeping on the nonoperated side, the client must keep the legs abducted with the wedge or larger pillows and the operated leg supported to prevent rotation. The client is instructed in getting out of bed on both sides, although initially it may be easier to observe precautions by moving toward the nonoperated leg. Careful instruction is given to avoid adduction past midline. It is important to determine the type and height of the client's bed at home. When getting in and out of bed initially, the client may use a **leg lifter** to help the operated leg move from one surface to another. Some clients have an overhead trapeze placed on the bed to assist with bed mobility. It is important to wean the client away from using this device because he or she will most likely not have one at home.

Transfers

It is always helpful for the client to observe the proper technique for transfers before attempting the movement.

 OT PRACTICE NOTE

A helpful hint for therapists to understand the impact of maintaining the proper hip position during the healing process is for the therapist to tape a goniometer to his or her own hip when positioned at 90 degrees and attempt to do the transfers listed below. Therapists will soon discover the difficulty of maintaining the proper hip position during functional activities!

Chair

A firmly based chair with armrests is recommended. The client is instructed to extend the operated leg forward, reach back for the armrests, and sit slowly. For the person with a posterolateral approach, care should be taken not to lean forward when sitting down (Figure 40-8). To stand, the client extends the operated leg and pushes off from the armrests. Because of the hip flexion precaution for the posterolateral approach, the client should sit on the front part of the chair and lean back (see Figure 40-8, *C*). Firm cushions or blankets may be used to increase the height of chairs and may be especially helpful if the client is tall. Low chairs, soft chairs, reclining chairs, and rocking chairs should be avoided.[1]

Commode chair

Three-in-one commode chairs with armrests can be used in the hospital and at home. For the person with a posterolateral approach, the height and angle can be adjusted so that the front legs are one notch lower than the back legs; thus, with the client seated, the precautionary hip angle of flexion is not exceeded. A person with an anterolateral approach may have enough hip mobility to use a standard toilet seat safely at the time of discharge. All clients should wipe between the legs in a sitting position or from behind in a standing position and use caution to avoid rotation of the hip. The client is to stand up and step to turn to face the toilet to flush.[1]

Shower stall

Nonskid strips or stickers are recommended in all shower stalls and tubs. When the client is entering, the walker or crutches go first, then the operated leg, and then the nonoperated leg. A shower chair with adjustable legs or a stool and grab bars should be installed if balance is a problem or if weight-bearing precautions are present.

Shower-over-tub (without shower doors)

The client is instructed to stand parallel to the tub facing the shower fixtures. Using the walker, crutches, or grab bars for support, the client is to transfer in sideways by bending at the knees, not at the hips. For clients with weight-bearing precautions or poor balance, purchase of a tub bench may be considered; this device allows the client to sit on the edge of the bench and then swing the legs over the tub while observing flexion precautions. Sponge bathing at the sink is an alternative activity.[1]

Car

Bucket seats in small cars should be avoided. Bench-type seats are recommended. The client is instructed to back up to the front passenger seat, hold onto a stable part of the car, extend the operated leg, and slowly sit in the car. Remembering to lean back, the client then slides the buttocks toward the driver's seat. The upper body and LEs move as one unit to turn to face the forward direction. It is helpful to have the seat moved back and reclined to accommodate the hip flexion precaution. Pillows in the seat may be necessary to increase the height of the seat. Prolonged sitting in the car should be avoided. If transferring to the front passenger seat is a problem, transferring to the back seat of a four-door car is an alternative. The client backs to the seat, extends the operated leg, and slowly sits in the car. Then he or she slides back so that the operated leg is resting on the seat fully supported.

Lower Body Dressing

The client is instructed to sit in a chair with arms or on the edge of the bed for dressing activities. The client is instructed to avoid adduction and rotation or crossing the legs to dress. The client must refrain from crossing the operated extremity over the nonoperated extremity at either the ankles or the knees. Assistive devices may be necessary for observing precautions (see Figure 40-7). To maintain hip precautions, the client uses a reacher or dressing stick to don and remove

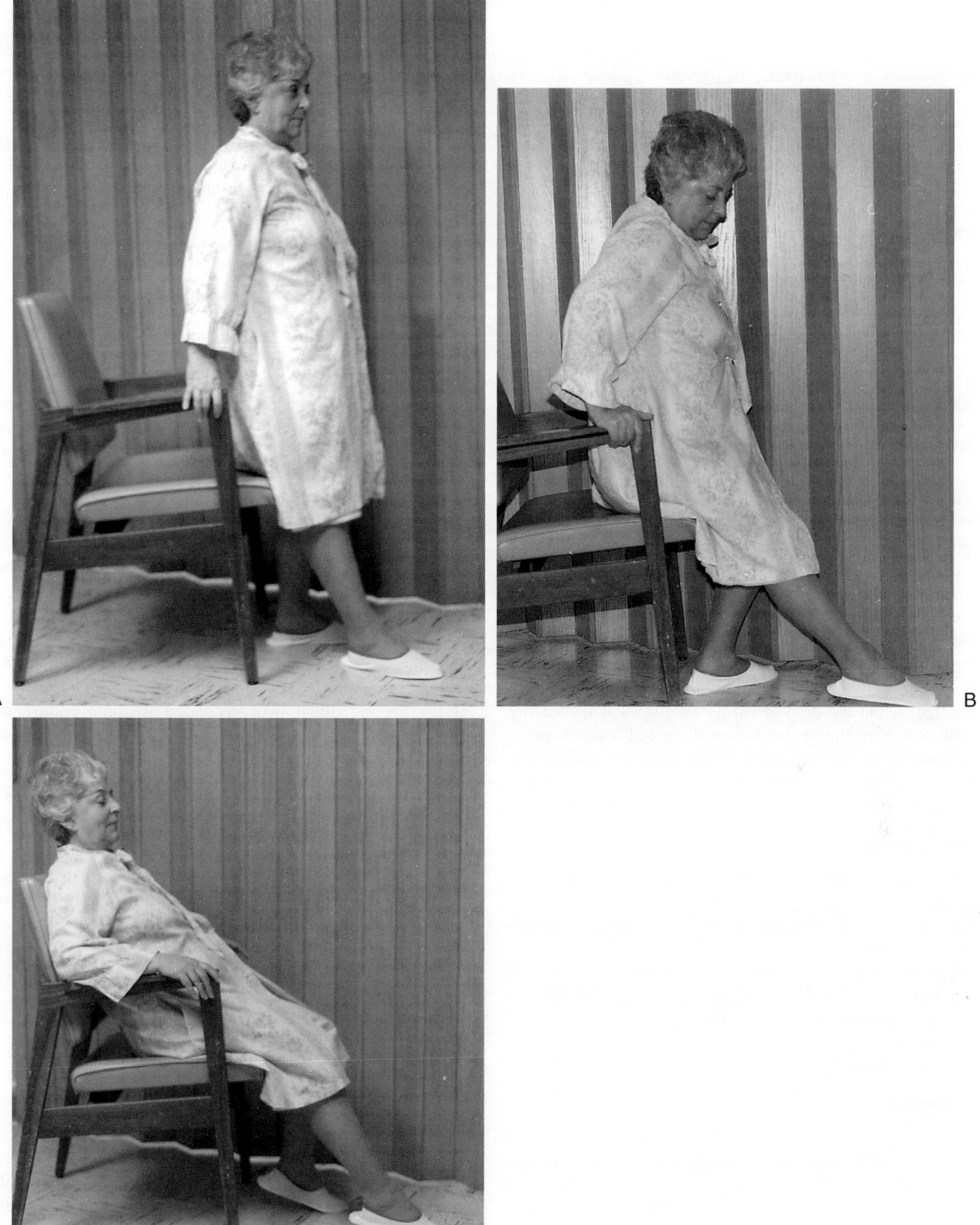

Figure 40-8 Chair transfer technique. **A,** Client extends operated leg and reaches for armrests. **B** and **C,** Bearing some weight on arms, the client sits down slowly, maintaining some extension of the operated leg.

pants and shoes. For pants, the operated leg is dressed first by using the reacher or dressing stick to bring the pants over the foot and up to the knee. A sock aid is used to don socks or knee-high nylons, and a reacher or dressing stick is used to doff them. A reacher, elastic laces, and a long-handled shoehorn can also be provided.[1]

Lower Body Bathing

The section on transfers describes the proper method of getting in and out of the shower or tub. Sponge bathing at the sink is indicated until the physician indicates that it is safe for the client to shower. A long-handled bath sponge or back brush is used to reach the lower legs and feet safely. Soap-on-a-rope is used to prevent the soap from dropping, and a towel is wrapped on a reacher to dry the lower legs.[1]

Hair Shampoo

Until able to shower, the client is instructed to obtain assistance for shampooing hair. The client can have a helper wash the hair while the client is supine, using pillows for back support and a bucket or bowl to catch the water poured from a pitcher to rinse the hair. Another method involves having the client sit in a chair with the back to the sink. The client leans backward to position the head over the sink while the helper washes the hair. The client can also visit a hair salon until he or she is able to perform hair washing independently. If unable to obtain any assistance, the client may shampoo the hair while standing or sitting on a stool at the kitchen sink, observing hip precautions at all times. Because bending forward at the kitchen sink does not require much hip flexion, most clients can observe the proper hip precautions using this method.

Homemaking

The client should initially refrain from heavy housework, such as vacuuming, lifting, and bed making. Kitchen activities are practiced, with suggestions made to keep commonly used items at countertop level. The client can carry items by using an apron with large pockets, sliding items along the counter top, using a utility cart, attaching a small basket or bag to a walker, or wearing a fanny pack around the waist. Reachers are provided to grasp items in low cupboards or retrieve items from the floor.

Caregiver Training

A family member, friend, or caregiver should be present for at least one OT treatment session so that any questions may be answered. Appropriate supervision recommendations and instruction regarding activity precautions are given at this time. So that they fully understand the impact of following the hip precautions, caregivers should be encouraged to practice doing the adapted activities as well. Instructional booklets on hip fractures and total hip and knee surgery may be purchased from the American Occupational Therapy Association to supplement training.[1]

TRAINING PROCEDURES FOR PERSONS WITH TOTAL KNEE REPLACEMENT

Procedures for ADL and IADL training for persons with total knee replacement are described in the following paragraphs. Many of the techniques used with a hip replacement can be used for someone with a knee replacement. Positions of knee instability include internal and external rotation at the hip and knee flexion greater than ROM permits.

Bed Mobility

The supine position is recommended, with the entire leg slightly elevated via balanced suspension or pillows, with or without a knee immobilizer. This will help to reduce edema and prevent knee flexion contractures. It is recommended that a person not sleep on the operated side. As in hip replacement, a pillow or wedge can be placed between the legs if this is necessary for side-lying and if the person lies on the nonoperated side.

Transfers

In general, the client can bend at the hip as much as he or she is able. Because of decreased knee flexion, the client may need to use the same techniques for commode and car transfers as have been described for hip replacements. Use of grab bars or a shower chair or bench is recommended, especially for transferring to the shower over the tub, as well as for the individual with decreased standing endurance or inability to bend the knee enough to sit on the bottom of the tub.

Lower Extremity Dressing

The dressing of lower extremities presents a problem only if the client is unable to reach his or her toes. In such a case, techniques described for the hip replacement can be used. The client should practice donning and doffing the knee immobilizer. The client should be cautioned to prevent torque or rotation at the knee joint when dressing by not twisting the body or leg while bearing weight on the operated leg.

Homemaking and caregiver training is the same as that for hip replacement.

GENERAL CONSIDERATIONS AND EVIDENCE FOR OCCUPATIONAL THERAPY INTERVENTION

In addition to the ADL and IADL strategies previously specified, the occupational therapist should be sure to address all areas of occupation that may be difficult for the client as well as those that may pose a safety risk. Occupations such as care of a pet, navigating through a cafeteria for meals, traveling in vehicles other than cars, and attending religious activities that require transfer to a church pew are all examples of activities that may be part of a client's typical performance pattern and should be addressed by OT. The occupational therapist can assist the client in approaching meaningful occupations safely, observing any movement precautions that are required and suggesting and demonstrating alternative methods and assistive devices.

A limited number of studies have examined OT intervention for LE joint replacements and hip fractures. According to a small Swedish study of clients who had incurred hip fractures, clients reported a significant decline in their ability to perform hobbies and social activities that they had participated in before their hip fracture. These activities were cited by these clients as more important than self-care–type activities.[13] Another study supports the idea that hip fractures affected social interaction the most.[5] By designing an intervention that targets the client's prior performance patterns and psychosocial needs, the occupational therapist can play a key role in contributing to the client's satisfactory psychosocial adjustment to physical limitations and helping the client return to full participation in meaningful activities.

For Mrs. Hernandez, in addition to ADL and IADL training, OT intervention will include car transfers, ways to sit safely in a church pew, and methods for engaging in activities with her grandchildren without damaging her newly replaced hip. The occupational therapist will also discuss community mobility and recommend that Mrs. Hernandez obtain clearance from her surgeon before returning to driving. Because Mrs. Hernandez's daughter lives nearby and is very involved in her mother's life, she should be provided with caregiver training so that she can help reinforce safe mobility and hip precautions.

SPECIAL EQUIPMENT

The OT practitioner should be familiar with the following equipment that is commonly used in the treatment of hip fracture and total hip replacement.

Hemovac: During surgery a plastic drainage tube is inserted at the surgical site to assist with postoperative drainage of blood. It has an area for collection of drainage and may be connected to a portable suction machine. The unit should *not* be disconnected for any activity because this may create a blockage in the system. The Hemovac is usually left in place for 2 days after surgery.

Abduction wedge: Large and small triangular foam wedges (Figure 40-9) are used when the client is supine to maintain the LEs in the abducted position.

Balanced suspension: This is fabricated and set up by an orthopedic technician and can be used for about 3 days after surgery. Its purpose is to support the affected LE in the first few postoperative days. The client's leg can be taken out of the device for exercise only.[11]

Reclining wheelchair: A wheelchair with an adjustable backrest that allows a reclining position is used for clients who have hip flexion precautions while sitting.

Commode chairs: The use of a commode chair instead of the regular toilet aids in safe transfers and allows the client to observe necessary hip flexion precautions.

Sequential compression devices (SCDs): SCDs are used postoperatively to reduce the risk of deep vein thrombosis. They are inflatable, external leggings that provide intermittent pneumatic compression of the legs.[4]

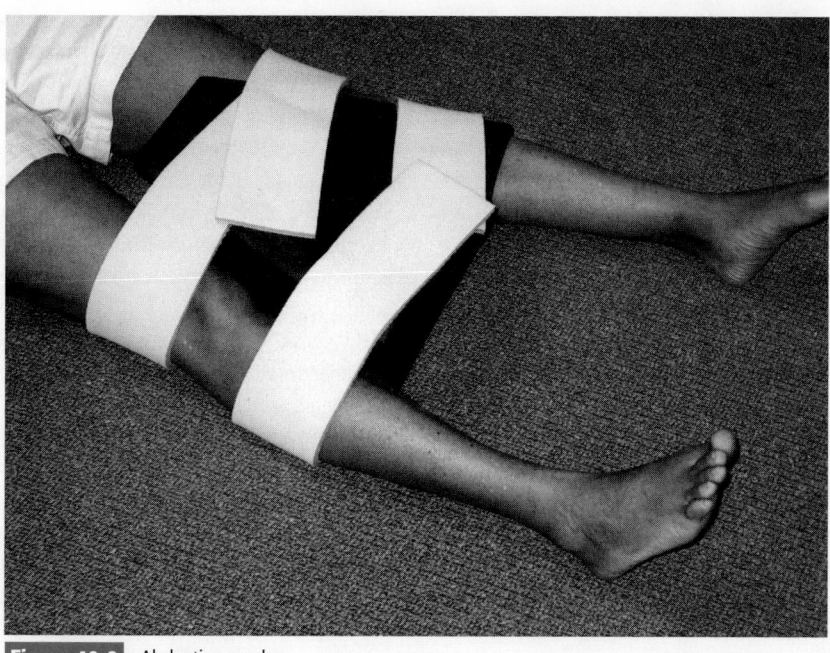

Figure 40-9 Abduction wedge.

Antiembolus hose: These are thigh-high hosiery that are worn 24 hours a day and removed only during bathing. Their purpose is to assist circulation, prevent edema, and thus reduce the risk of deep-vein thrombosis.[4]

Client-controlled administration (PCA) IV: The amount of medication is predetermined and programmed by the physician and nursing staff to allow the client to self-administer pain medication by pushing a button.

Incentive spirometer: This portable breathing apparatus is used to encourage deep breathing and prevent the development of postoperative pneumonia.

SUMMARY

Hip fractures and LE joint replacement are orthopedic conditions in which OT intervention may speed the client's return to optimal participation in daily activities safely and comfortably. OT intervention begins with obtaining the client's occupational profile and an assessment of the psychosocial issues related to the surgery and the surgery's potential impact on the client's lifestyle. Awareness of and a sensitivity toward the psychosocial challenges of the person with an orthopedic problem are critical for the delivery of optimal occupational therapy.

The protocol for other areas of OT intervention is determined by the surgical procedure performed and by the precautions prescribed by the physician. Clients who have weight-bearing precautions must be trained to observe these during all ADL and IADL routines. A simulation of the home environment or a home assessment is helpful in preparing the client for potential problems that may arise after discharge. Areas to assess include the entry, stairs, bathroom, bedroom, sitting surfaces, and kitchen. Recommendations to remove throw rugs and slippery floor coverings and obstacles are made because the client will most likely be going home using an assistive device for ambulation. A kitchen stool or utility cart may be indicated. It is important to assess and instruct the client and caregiver regarding ADLs and IADLs with adaptive equipment, as well as any movement precautions. Home therapy may be indicated after a hospital stay to ensure safety and independence in daily occupations if these goals were not met during hospitalization.

Preoperative teaching programs are invaluable in aiding client adjustment. The class familiarizes the client with the hospital, nursing, physical therapy, OT, and discharge planning. Procedures and equipment, concerns regarding hospitalization and discharge, and therapy are addressed. Participation in this type of class has been shown to relieve anxiety and fear, empower the client during the hospitalization, and decrease the hospital length of stay.

THREADED CASE STUDY: MRS. HERNANDEZ, PART 2

After reading the chapter, the occupational therapist can plan an effective treatment intervention. Mrs. Hernandez's occupational profile reveals that she has many roles that she finds meaningful: grandmother, church member, and swimmer. She also seems to value being independent: She not only does things with her daughter and her family but also has interests and activities in which she participates on her own. Supporting contextual factors include an accessible home, a daughter nearby who involves her in many activities with her children, church friends who can offer some assistance, and strong spiritual beliefs that can help her through recovery from surgery. Non-supportive contextual factors include an inaccessible swimming pool and the fact that she lives alone.

Her problems center on her inability to participate in meaningful occupations. They can be prioritized as follows: not being able to drive, participate in activities with her grandchildren, swim, and attend church meetings. Because driving allows her to get to the swimming classes, church meetings, and her daughter's home, this is placed as first in the list of problems. There is also a safety factor involved. She is at risk for having an accident if her hip "catches" at the wrong time. Because she lost part of her family when she lost her husband, spending time with her daughter and grandchildren is

placed as the next important issue to address; Mrs. Hernandez obviously values her family, and it provides a source of support. Swimming and attending church are placed toward the end of the list. She is still able to attend church, which is very meaningful to her, but cannot attend all of the meetings. All of these problems should be addressed through occupational therapy.

An implied but not directly stated problem is that she may have a great deal of difficulty completing her self-care activities, especially in the morning when her joints are stiffer. Because she lives alone, she needs to be able to complete all of her ADLs and IADLs independently. The therapist should be sure to question Mrs. Hernandez about these types of occupations as well. If her problems are not addressed by either surgery or adaptations (or both), she may begin to suffer from depression and other health problems, such as pneumonia and worsening arthritis. These problems would result from inactivity and little contact with those people whom she loves and whose company she enjoys.

By using the ADL and IADL strategies presented in the chapter and reinforcing healthful behaviors such as joint protection, Mrs. Hernandez can return to optimal participation in occupations that she finds meaningful.

Review Questions

1. Explain the difference in precautions for the anterolateral and posterolateral approaches for a hip replacement.
2. When a client is being transferred from one surface to another, what is the general procedure to follow to ensure safety and protection of the involved side?
3. List the most common items of adaptive equipment used during rehabilitation of hip fractures and LE joint replacements, and describe their purpose.
4. Describe how the case coordinator and occupational therapist can work together on similar issues.
5. List two specific suggestions for performing sexual activities for someone with a hip replacement.
6. What information should be obtained when completing the occupational profile?
7. Identify two factors that affect fracture healing.
8. What is the difference between closed and open reduction procedures?
9. Why are weight-bearing precautions observed with an ORIF?
10. Compare rehabilitation techniques between clients with a hip replacement and clients with a knee replacement.
11. What are the benefits of conducting client education preoperative classes for persons who are at risk for falls or who are planning a joint replacement?
12. How might a person's rehabilitation program be affected by bilateral joint replacements?

REFERENCES

1. American Occupational Therapy Association: *After your hip surgery: a guide to daily activities,* rev ed, Rockville, Md, 2001, the Association.
2. Calliet R: *Knee pain and disability,* ed 3, Philadelphia, 1992, FA Davis.
3. Crandell T, Crandell C, editors: *Human development,* ed 7, Boston, 2000, McGraw Hill.
4. Delisa J, Gans B: *Rehabilitation medicine: principles and practice,* ed 2, Philadelphia, 1993, JB Lippincott.
5. Elinge E, et al: A group learning programme for old people with hip fracture: a randomized study, *Scand J Occup Ther* 10:27, 2003.
6. Gray H: *Gray's anatomy,* Philadelphia, 1974, Running Press.
7. Larson K, et al: *Role of occupational therapy with the elderly,* Bethesda, Md, 1996, American Occupational Therapy Association.
8. Melvin J, Gall V: *Rheumatic rehabilitation series: surgical rehabilitation,* vol 5, Bethesda, Md, 1999, American Occupational Therapy Association.
9. Melvin J, Jensen G: *Rheumatic rehabilitation series: assessment and management,* vol 1, Bethesda, Md, 1998, American Occupational Therapy Association.
10. Opitz J: Reconstructive surgery of the extremities. In Kottle F, Lehmann J, editors: *Krusen's handbook of physical medicine and rehabilitation,* ed 4, Philadelphia, 1990, WB Saunders.
11. Richardson JK, Iglarsh ZA: *Clinical orthopaedic physical therapy,* Philadelphia, 1994, WB Saunders.
12. Sherry E, et al: Minimal invasive surgery for hip replacement: a new technique using the NILNAV hip system, *ANZ J Surg* 73:157, 2003.
13. Sirkka M, Branholm I: Consequences of a hip fracture in activity performance and life satisfaction in an elderly Swedish clientele, *Scand J Occup Ther* 10:34, 2003.
14. Tsai C, Chen C, Liu T: Lateral approach with ligament release in total knee arthroplasty: new concepts in the surgical technique, *Artificial Organs* 25(8):638, 2001.

41 LOW BACK PAIN

LUELLA GRANGAARD

KEY TERMS

Dynamic lumbar stabilization   Golfer's lift   Energy conservation
Neutral spine   Body mechanics   Pacing

LEARNING OBJECTIVES

After studying this chapter the student or practitioner will be able to do the following:

1. Define *neutral spine*.
2. Demonstrate how neutral spine is integrated into a variety of activities of daily living (ADLs) and instrumental activities of daily living (IADLs).
3 Demonstrate the use of "golfer's lift" in an ADL.
4. Identify the basic concepts of body mechanics.
5. Demonstrate the relationship between anatomy and body mechanics.
6. Articulate normal back anatomy in terms that a client can comprehend.
7. Identify the occupational therapist's role in evaluation and intervention.
8. Recognize the psychosocial effect of low back pain (LBP).

CHAPTER OUTLINE

Spinal anatomy
  Vertebral column
Incidence of low back pain
Rehabilitation
  Physician
  Physical therapy
  Occupational therapy
Occupational therapy interventions
  Client education
  Back stabilization and neutral spine
  Body mechanics
  Adaptive equipment
  Ergonomics
  Energy conservation
  Occupations to increase strength and endurance
  Strategies for stress reduction and coping
Analysis of occupations
Activities of daily living and instrumental activities of daily living

Bathing
Dressing
Functional mobility
Personal hygiene
Sexual activity
Sleep
Toileting
Childcare
Computer use
Driving
Home establishment and management
Shopping
Work
Leisure
Surgical intervention
  Postoperative occupational therapy evaluation and intervention
  Postoperative activities of daily living
Summary

THREADED CASE STUDY: PILAR, PART 1

Pilar is 45 years old. She lives with her husband and four children, ages 4, 6, 10, and 14. She is a homemaker. She complains of lower back pain primarily on the right side. Her pain increases as she does housework and cooks. Pilar was referred to occupational therapy for pain reduction during activities. During her occupational profile, pain is noted during activities requiring bending, such as removing clothing from the washing machine and dryer, cleaning the bathtub, making the bed, and taking items from the oven. As a result, she often asks her husband and children to help at home. She avoids preparing any meals that require baking and no longer makes cookies or brownies for her children. She is very concerned that she not being a good mother or wife because it is difficult to cook and care for her family.

The initial analysis of her occupational performance in a kitchen setting indicates that she bends at the waist repeatedly while retrieving items from the refrigerator, lower cabinets, and dishwasher. While performing these occupations, she reports an increase of pain from 2 to 7 on a scale of 10. Activities that require reaching, such as reaching into the washer and dryer, resulted in reports of increased pain. It was also noted that she was bending at the waist when she reached into the dryer. When her self-care activities were assessed, it was found that she had pain while donning socks, shoes, and pants. In addition, she experiences pain while washing her face and brushing her teeth. While performing all of the self-care activities for which she reported pain, she demonstrated bending at the waist.

Pilar's occupational therapy intervention plan will focus on client education. Education will include incorporation of information obtained from physical therapy with respect to pelvic positioning during activities and using that information in daily activities. Education will also employ demonstration of daily activities incorporating various movement techniques, positioning, and body mechanics to decrease lower back pain. All of Pilar's newly learned back safety strategies must become habitual so that she may transfer them into future occupations.

Critical Thinking Questions

1. How is back anatomy and physiology related to Pilar's motor performance?
2. Can the evaluator identify movement patterns that result in pain during performance of daily occupations?
3. How can Pilar's movements be modified through interventions for pain-free occupations?

Low back pain (LBP) is a complaint that often causes the afflicted individual to seek help from the medical system. Four out of five adults will experience significant LBP sometime during their lives. After the common cold, LBP is the most frequent cause of lost workdays among adults younger than 45 years of age. Most cases of LBP are not serious and respond to simple treatments such as rest or antiinflammatory drugs. Common causes of LBP include poor conditioning, improper use of the back, obesity, smoking, age, and simple wear and tear over time. Osteoporosis, arthritis, fractures of the spine, and protruding discs are the most common causes of structural problems with the low back. Before consulting a physician or occupational therapist, patients often seek help from chiropractors, massage therapists, acupuncturists, and proponents of the latest fads (e.g., magnets) to reduce the pain.

SPINAL ANATOMY

The occupational therapist must understand both the normal anatomy and the pathology for numerous back problems. To educate the patient regarding the rationale for proper body mechanics, the occupational therapist must also understand how the anatomy and pathology are related to movement and daily occupations. Furthermore, the occupational therapist must be able to convey this information in a way that is accessible to clients with varying degrees of knowledge about anatomy and back pathology.

VERTEBRAL COLUMN

The structures that compose the vertebral column are vertebrae and intervertebral discs. Each vertebra comprises the vertebral body, which is the weight-bearing component, and the vertebral arch, which arises from the back of the vertebral body (Figure 41-1). The vertebral arch is composed of two pedicles (one on each side) that extend into the lamina. The laminae join together to form the vertebral foramina, which form the vertebral canal in which the spinal cord resides. From the pedicle and joining of lamina are three bony projections called *processes*. These lateral processes join to form joints with adjacent vertebrae superiorly and inferiorly (Figure 41-2). Between the joint of these adjacent vertebrae is the intervertebral foramen, from which the spinal nerves enter and exit. At the back of the spinal arch is the spinous process, where muscles attach. The low back is composed of five lumbar vertebra.

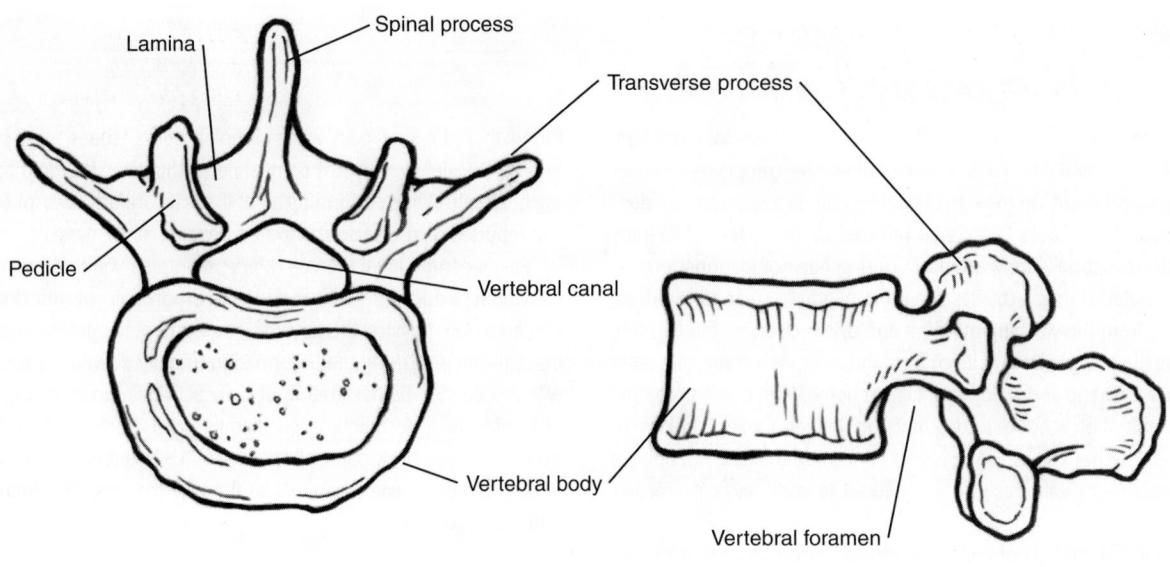

Vertebra side view

Figure 41-1 Vertebra from above and side view.

Between the vertebrae are intervertebral discs. The intervertebral discs are composed of fibrocartilage and a central mass of pulpy tissue, the nucleus pulposus (Figure 41-3).

Under pressure, the disc bulges. The discs work as shock absorbers and are relieved of pressure only when the body is supine. Being the nonrigid part of the column, they provide flexibility for movement. When a person is standing with a neutral spine, the disc is under uniform pressure. Movements such as bending, twisting, and reaching result in extension of the spine, and the pressure on the disc may increase in one part of the back, whereas in another part of the back it may be under a stretch (Figure 41-4).

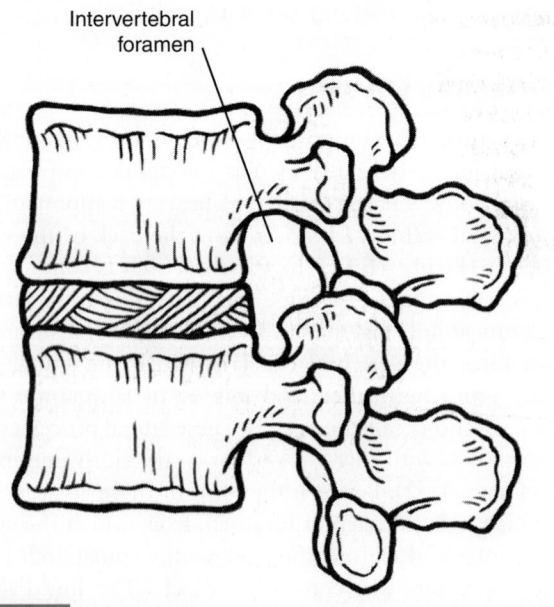

Figure 41-2 Two vertebrae in articulation. The spinal nerve exits via the intervertebral foramen.

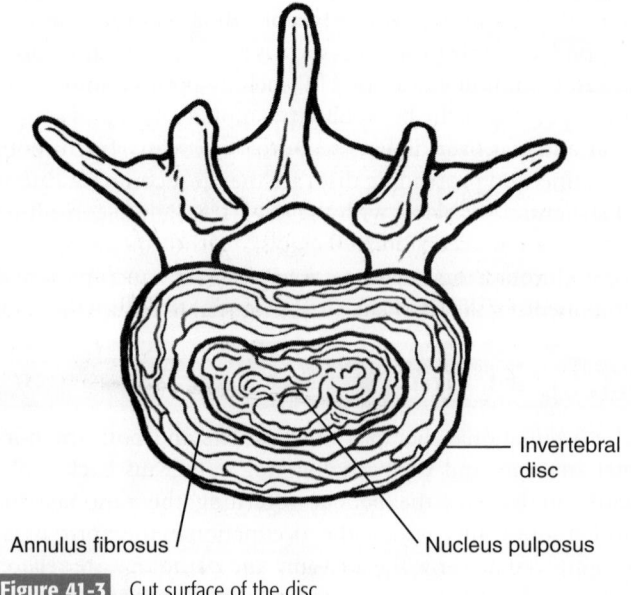

Figure 41-3 Cut surface of the disc.

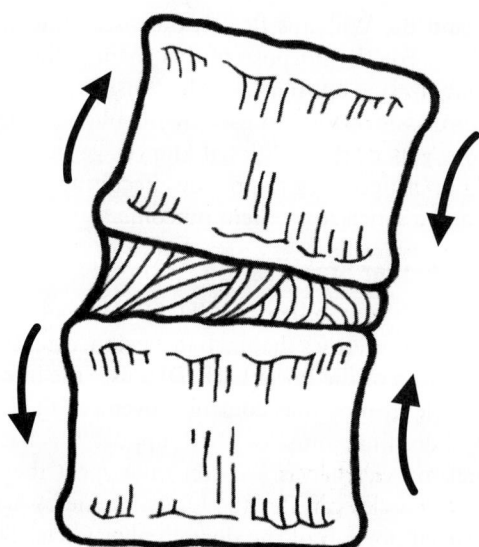

Figure 41-4 The same disk may be under compression and extension at the same time.

There is an anterior and posterior longitudinal ligament that extends the length of the vertebral column and is attached to vertebral bodies and intervertebral discs. These ligaments check excessive movement of the column. The sacrum is the lower fused portion of the vertebral column. The sacrum is attached to the pelvis. Movement of the pelvis changes the lordosis, or curve of the lower spine.

Muscles of the lumbar spine include the intertransversarri and interspinalis, which are small intersegmental muscles that connect transverse process to spinous process of adjacent vertebrae. The lumbar multifidus, lumbar longissimus, and iliocostalis make up the lumbar muscles. These muscles are primarily extensors for the spine, but the lumbar longissimus and iliocostalis can also assist in lateral flexion. In addition, muscles of the abdominal wall contribute to the stabilization of the spine, including the transversus abdominis and the oblique internus abdominis by providing a corseting effect. For further information on the interaction of the back and abdominal muscles on specific movements, the reader is advised to do additional reading in this area.

INCIDENCE OF LOW BACK PAIN

LBP resolves within 6 weeks for 90% of clients. It resolves in 12 weeks for another 5%.[1] "Less than 1% of back pain is due to 'serious' spinal disease (e.g., tumor, infection). Less than 1% of back pain stems from inflammatory disease, and less than 5% is true nerve root pain."[1] Typically, back pain is a result of poor physical fitness, obesity, reduced muscle strength and endurance, or use of poor body mechanics.

Actual changes in structure or mechanics of the lower back may result in problems, including the following:

- Sciatic (nerve root) pain: The nerve is entrapped by disc herniation.
- Spinal stensosis: Narrowing of the intervertebral foramen decreases the space where the spinal nerve exits or enters the spine.
- Facet joint pain: This is inflammation or joint changes of the spinal joints.
- Spondyloysis: This is a stress fracture of the dorsal to the transverse process.
- Spondylolisthesis: There is a slippage of one vertebra on another.
- Herniated nucleus pulposus: Stress may tear fibers of the disc, resulting in outward bulge of the enclosed nucleus pulposus. This bulge may press on spinal nerves and cause various symptoms, including nerve entrapment.

REHABILITATION

The best intervention for the client with LBP is a team approach using the skills not only of an occupational therapist but also those of a physician, physical therapist, caseworker, and psychologist. Depending on the circumstances of the client, other team members, such as the vocational counselor, social worker, discharge planner, nutritionist, and nurse, could be vital to successful intervention outcomes. These members may be part of the rehabilitation team, pain team, managed care group, and so forth.

The main member of this team, however, is the client. The client's goals and desired outcome should direct the way in which the team approaches care. Each member must be aware of the context or contexts that will influence the client's performance. This will affect the way that the client may or may not participate or take responsibility for his or her performance outcome.

Much has been written about workers and the effects of job satisfaction and limitations resulting from back pain. However, Waddell "asserts upon extensive review of the literature that 'social class' is probably the strongest personal predictor of incurring back trouble. This is in part due to heavy manual labor and in past due to 'social disadvantages' such as poor health care or lifestyle."[4] People who experience more anxiety with loss of work and the resulting financial implications frequently require the assistance of a psychologist. However, both of these issues—decreased job satisfaction and anxiety—may surface during the patient's occupational profile and should be addressed by all members of the team.

PHYSICIAN

The physician is responsible for the initial workup (or evaluation) of the client. Although the evaluation process varies according to the type of physician, the examination usually includes a thorough medical history, current symptoms and complaints, functional limitations, posture, gait, strength, reflexes and sensation, and past interventions for this problem. A diagnosis is usually made at this time, or the physician may order additional tests, such as nerve conduction tests, computed tomography (CT) scans, magnetic resonance imaging (MRI), and blood work. After arriving at a diagnosis, the physician often prescribes medication and determines activity restrictions and exercise guidelines. To reevaluate progress or lack thereof, the physician will typically see the patient in 1 or 2 weeks for a follow-up visit. If the symptoms have not decreased by that time, the client may be referred to physical therapy.

 OT PRACTICE NOTE

Unfortunately, intervention with clients with low back pain is often not regarded or recognized as an appropriate role for occupational therapy because of the medical focus being on physical symptoms rather than on performance outcomes. Working with and educating physicians and physical therapists in the ways that occupational therapy can assist these clients is vital not only for quality intervention for the client but also for program development in this area of practice.

During the client's course of treatment, the skilled services of psychology, vocational counseling, and social work may be required. A low back injury may significantly affect many areas of the client's life, including personal interactions, work, and finances; these consequences can increase the client's stress and affect the outcome of treatment.

PHYSICAL THERAPY

The client is usually referred to physical therapy (PT) to address pain, spasms, limited flexibility, and posture. The PT evaluation usually includes a review of the mechanism of injury, date of injury, progression of symptoms, medical history, recent tests and procedures, medications, past treatment history, prior level of functioning, and the client's goal for therapy. A subjective history of activities of daily living (ADLs) and sleep disturbances is reviewed. An objective examination will include analysis of posture, gait, active range of motion (ROM) of spine, active ROM of extremities, pelvic symmetry, nerve tension signs, strength, reflexes and sensation, leg length, and palpation of soft tissue. On the basis of the collected data, the physical therapist develops a treatment plan that includes pain and spasm control, exercises, determination of pelvic basis for daily activities, and patient education. The goals of physical therapy are to reduce symptoms and increase strength and flexibility to achieve a functional pain-free outcome for the client.

A number of different theories are used by physical therapists. Two popular approaches are the McKenzie extension exercises and the Williams flexion exercises,[1] but there are many others. For the purpose of this chapter, the dynamic lumbar stabilization approach will be considered. Regardless of the approach or program used by the physical therapists with whom you work, additional knowledge of the theory and program is necessary to provide effective team communication and a satisfactory client outcome.[3]

Dynamic Lumbar Stabilization

Dynamic lumbar stabilization (DLS) incorporates many physical therapy theories that include flexion, extension, and body mechanics of the lower back. DLS uses the integration of the muscle groups that control movement of the spine and the abdominal muscles that support the back. The abdominal muscles act as a corset to support the lumbar area. These muscles can flex the lumbar spine by acting on the superficial portion of the dorsolumbar fascia. They can also extend the lumbar spine by acting on the deep portions of the fascia, which form the interspinal ligaments. Control of lordosis in flexion and extension is extremely important. Because repetitive loads applied to the lumbar intervertebral joint can lead to progressive tearing, fatigue, and progressive disc prolapse, the client must learn to balance muscular function and flexibility to control the stresses involved in movement.

Each client must be able to identify his or her own "neutral position." **Neutral spine** does not mean an absence, or no lordosis or curve, of the lower spine, but rather refers to the most comfortable spinal position for the individual to complete movement patterns and then integrate this neutral position into daily occupations. The neutral position for each client is the condition under which the vertebrae and discs are under equal pressure.

To find the neutral position (called "finding neutral"), the client should stand with knees slightly bent and weight distributed evenly. Using the abdominal muscles to tilt the pelvis, the client should flex and extend the lumbar spine until attaining the balanced position of optimal function and stability (Figure 41-5). The abdominal muscles should be contracted to maintain this position, much as a corset would. This position or stabilization should be maintained and integrated into the performance of the client's occupations. Some individuals experience no pain while in a greater degree of extension, or with a greater curve in the lower back, whereas others prefer a neutral position of flexion, displaying more of a flattened abdomen.

Clients who prefer a neutral position in extension find extension of the back is beneficial for pain generated from flexion, which is a result of impingement of the nerve from narrowing of the foramen by arthritis or a disc problem. The focus is on extension exercises and positioning of the low back with a greater low back curve. This takes the pressure off the disc and places it on the facet joints, allowing the nucleus pulposus to migrate anteriorly away from the area of impingement. The neutral with flexion position is most

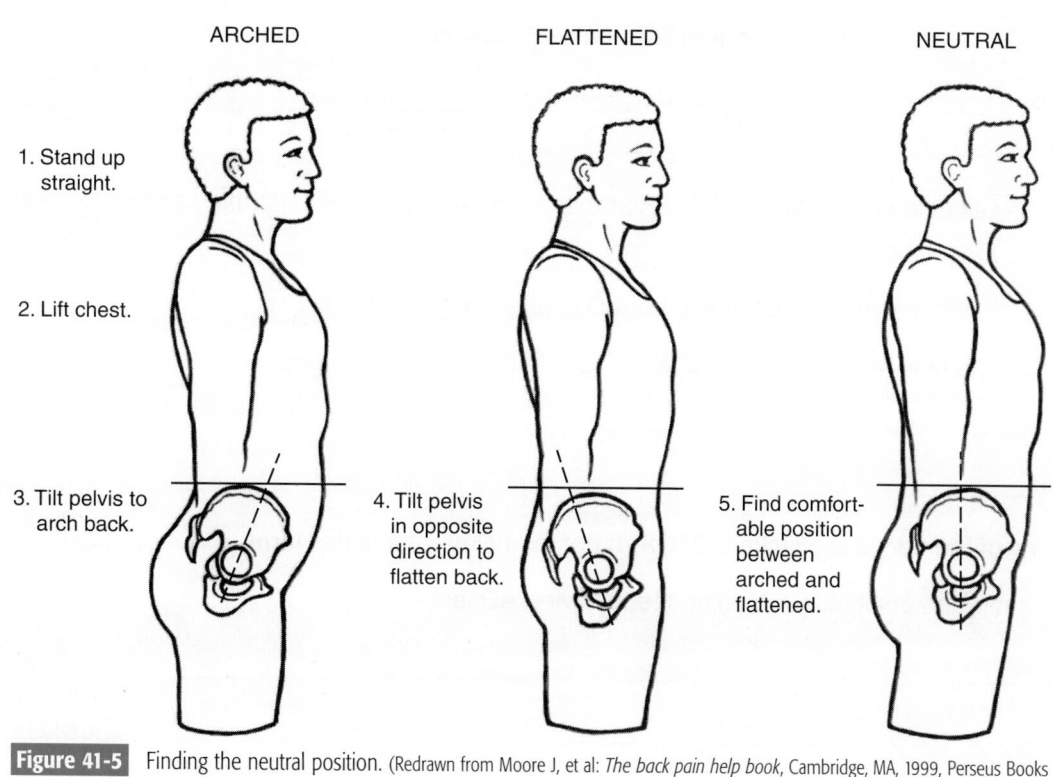

ARCHED   FLATTENED   NEUTRAL

1. Stand up straight.

2. Lift chest.

3. Tilt pelvis to arch back.

4. Tilt pelvis in opposite direction to flatten back.

5. Find comfortable position between arched and flattened.

Figure 41-5   Finding the neutral position. (Redrawn from Moore J, et al: *The back pain help book*, Cambridge, MA, 1999, Perseus Books Group.)

commonly used with patients who have a posterior spine problem such as facet pain. Positioning the spine in flexion acts to reduce facet joint compression and places the pressure on the disc and vertebra body.

As a team member, the physical therapist will communicate the appropriate pelvic position for the client to the rest of the team. On the basis of the physical therapist's recommendations for pelvic positioning, the occupational therapist will work with the client to incorporate the proper movement into daily occupations (Figure 41-6).

OCCUPATIONAL THERAPY

The occupational therapist will work with the client to develop an occupational profile. This is achieved by using an occupational self-report questionnaire and interview process. Filling out a questionnaire before the actual interview allows the client to begin to identify problem areas of occupation and stimulates conversation during the occupational profile. However, depending on the treatment setting, the client may regard the use of a questionnaire and subsequent review of the same material with the therapist as redundant and a waste of time. Development of a thorough occupational profile should identify performance areas that have been affected by back pain. Analysis of occupational performance can best be determined by actual performance. To structure

the evaluation within the clinic setting, an obstacle course consisting of various ADLs and instrumental activities of daily living (IADLs) may be used to assess various performance skills within predetermined occupations (Figure 41-7). In addition, occupations identified as problematic during the interview should be assessed in the same way.

Assessment of performance in specific problematic areas of occupation will help formulate the intervention plan and outcomes. A combination of intervention methods will provide the best outcomes for the client. For the intervention plan to succeed, the therapist should discuss with the client anatomy, pathology, back stabilization, ergonomics, body mechanics, and pacing. The plan must incorporate education and demonstration of back protection techniques while the client is engaged in actual occupations. The most important part of this process is to have the client understand, practice, demonstrate, and then incorporate the learned information into current and new occupations. The education received and incorporated into performance of occupations by the client must become a habit to ensure pain-free living. The client's outcomes will include reduction of pain, use of back stabilization techniques, use of adaptive equipment, and incorporation of body mechanics, and ergonomics into client-specific areas of occupation, as well as the ability to adapt this learning to new occupations to prevent future problems.

Back Client ADL Referral/Follow-up

Name: _____ Phone: _____

Dx: _____ Onset Date: _____

☐ Client is very familiar with back stabilization concepts, demonstrating excellent body mechanics.

☐ Client has had ADL training from OT within the past 2 years.

☐ Client is not appropriate for an ADL evaluation. If so, explain:

_____

P.T. _____

If any of the above is checked, STOP. If not, complete rest of this form.

Recommend emphasis in training the following ADLs:

_____

_____

Symptom irritability: ☐ Minimal/none   ☐ Moderate   ☐ Severe

MUST avoid the following lumbar positions: ☐ Flexion   ☐ Extension

                                                  ☐ Both   ☐ No precaution

Ability to squat: ☐ Full   ☐ ¾   ☐ ½   ☐ ¼   ☐ Unable

Knee pathology?   ☐ Yes ☐ No

If yes, explain: _____

Hamstring flexibility: ☐ <45°   ☐ <45°-70°   ☐ >70°

ADL training: ☐ Indoor   ☐ Outdoor

Comments: _____

_____

Figure 41-6 Back client ADL referral/follow-up form. (Courtesy of Eisenhower Medical Center, Rehabilitation Services, Rancho Mirage, CA.)

OCCUPATIONAL THERAPY INTERVENTIONS

On the basis of the client's evaluation, the therapist develops an intervention plan that may use any or all of the following:

- Education regarding normal back anatomy and the physiology of back movement as they relate to performance of occupations
- Use of neutral spine back stabilization in occupational performance to reduce pain
- Education in basic body mechanics
- Training in use of adaptive equipment to modify tasks
- Task analysis and use of ergonomic design to modify the environment
- Training in use of energy conservation to maintain participation in occupation

BACK STABILIZATION ADL PERFORMANCE

Initial Pain Level _____   Pretest   Posttest

Level I		Correct	Incorrect	Correct	Incorrect
1. Getting in bed					
2. Demo sleep position					
3. Up from bed					
4. Don/doff shoes					
5. Use sheet to make bed					
6. Pick up pencil off floor					
7. Brush teeth					
8. Reach small item from low cabinet					
9. Move clothes from washer to dryer					
10. Remove clothes from dryer					
11. Dishes in and out of dishwasher					
12. Remove container from top shelf					
13.					
14.					
15.					
Pain level					
Level II Indoor					
16. Lift 5-lb box					
17. Vacuum					
18. Sweep/mop					
19. Reach/remove 5-lb box overhead					
20.					
21.					
Pain Level					
Level II Outdoor					
22. Lift 10-lb box					
23. Spade/rake					
24. Reach into trunk/under hood					
25. Reach/remove 10-lb. box overhead					
26.					
27.					
Pain Level					

Demonstrate:
 Neutral spine
 Squat
 Diagonal lift
 Golfer's lift

Patient is able to verbalize and demonstrate the relationship between back stabilization education and ADLs   ☐ Yes   ☐ No

Equipment recommended:

Comments:

_____OTR

Figure 41-7   Back stabilization ADL performance form. (Courtesy of Eisenhower Medical Center, Rehabilitation Services, Rancho Mirage, CA.)

- Use of occupations to increase strength and endurance
- Education in strategies for pain management, stress reduction, and coping.

CLIENT EDUCATION

As described and reiterated throughout this chapter, client education seems to be the key to success for the client with LBP. Knowledge of basic anatomy and physiology helps the client understand what is occurring when movement while engaging in an occupation results in pain. This knowledge is the foundation upon which to build the rest of the intervention plan and ultimately select the appropriate interventions. Education can be provided in both a group and an individual setting.

 OT PRACTICE NOTE

> Information individualized to each client's needs is ideal. There are many books, videos, card systems, and computerized educational systems available from vendors. Also, charts and models of anatomy are available to assist the client in understanding anatomy and physiology.

BACK STABILIZATION AND NEUTRAL SPINE

Before starting each activity, the occupational therapist should work with the client to identify the proper position for his or her lower back. It is important to monitor and cue the client as needed during the activity to maintain the proper position (see Figure 41-5).

In addition to neutral spine, there are a number of positions that the client will need to learn and integrate into activities to help with lifting and movement. These include the squat, diagonal lift, and **golfer's lift.** The client's ability to perform the squat requires an absence of any knee or hip pathology. While performing a squat, the client keeps the back straight while maintaining neutral spine (Figure 41-8, A). The diagonal lift requires the lift to be performed with one foot in front of the other and the legs shoulder length apart (see Figure 41-8, B). The golfer's lift requires bending at the hips while raising one leg behind (see Figure 41-8, C). Using a team method, the physical therapist identifies the client's ability to squat as well as the type of neutral spine. Proper analysis of specific ADLs and the best position for the commencement of activities requires a thorough understanding of the client's particular type of neutral spine, either flexion or extension.

BODY MECHANICS

The client's thorough knowledge of the concepts of **body mechanics** is critical to the use of back stabilization. These concepts include maintaining a straight back, bending from the hip, avoiding twisting, maintaining good posture, carrying objects close to the body, lifting with legs to promote safe performance, and using a wide base of support. Another key concept that is incorporated into activities is reducing back stress while standing. Using a small stool or opening a cabinet door and resting the foot inside the cabinet base usually accomplishes this goal. Instruction in avoiding any twisting of the back during activities is also essential, as will be noted in many habitual activities, such as flushing the toilet. In these instances, the client must be instructed to turn as a unit while maintaining a neutral spine.

ADAPTIVE EQUIPMENT

Adaptive equipment is often useful. The most frequently recommended pieces of equipment for persons with LBP include long-handled sponges or brushes, reachers, long-handled shoehorns, sock aids, elevated commodes or toilet seats, hand-held shower sprayers, and footstools.

ERGONOMICS

Much has been done to create environments that better fit the individual needs of the person with LBP. For example, office chairs that allow height, back angle, and back height adjustments allow the user to fit the chair. A chair for desktop work must provide back support and maintain the hips and knees at 90 degrees with the feet flat on the floor or a footrest. The back of the chair should not be so far back that it cuts into the back of the legs or causes forward bending of the back and straining with the arms. The rest of the body position should allow the client to complete the desktop activity with proper positioning of the neck and upper extremities.

An analysis of the client's work tasks should be completed and modifications made. In addition, the worker needs to change positions and take breaks. The AOTA offers a screensaver that reminds workers to take stretch breaks. Occupational therapists and other specialists in ergonomics are available to provide consultation, and work-site assessment and recommendations to employers or to give the client information that allows him or her to complete a task analysis independently in the relevant environment. The Internet and office supply companies offer a great deal of information, as well as products for the consumer.

ENERGY CONSERVATION

Given their busy lives, clients may not realize that vacuuming, dusting, cleaning bathrooms, and preparing dinner for guests may be more than they—or their backs—can tolerate. Teaching clients the principles of **energy conservation** can help alleviate or minimize problems in this area. These principles include planning ahead, pacing oneself, setting priorities, eliminating unnecessary tasks, balancing activity with rest, and learning one's activity tolerance.

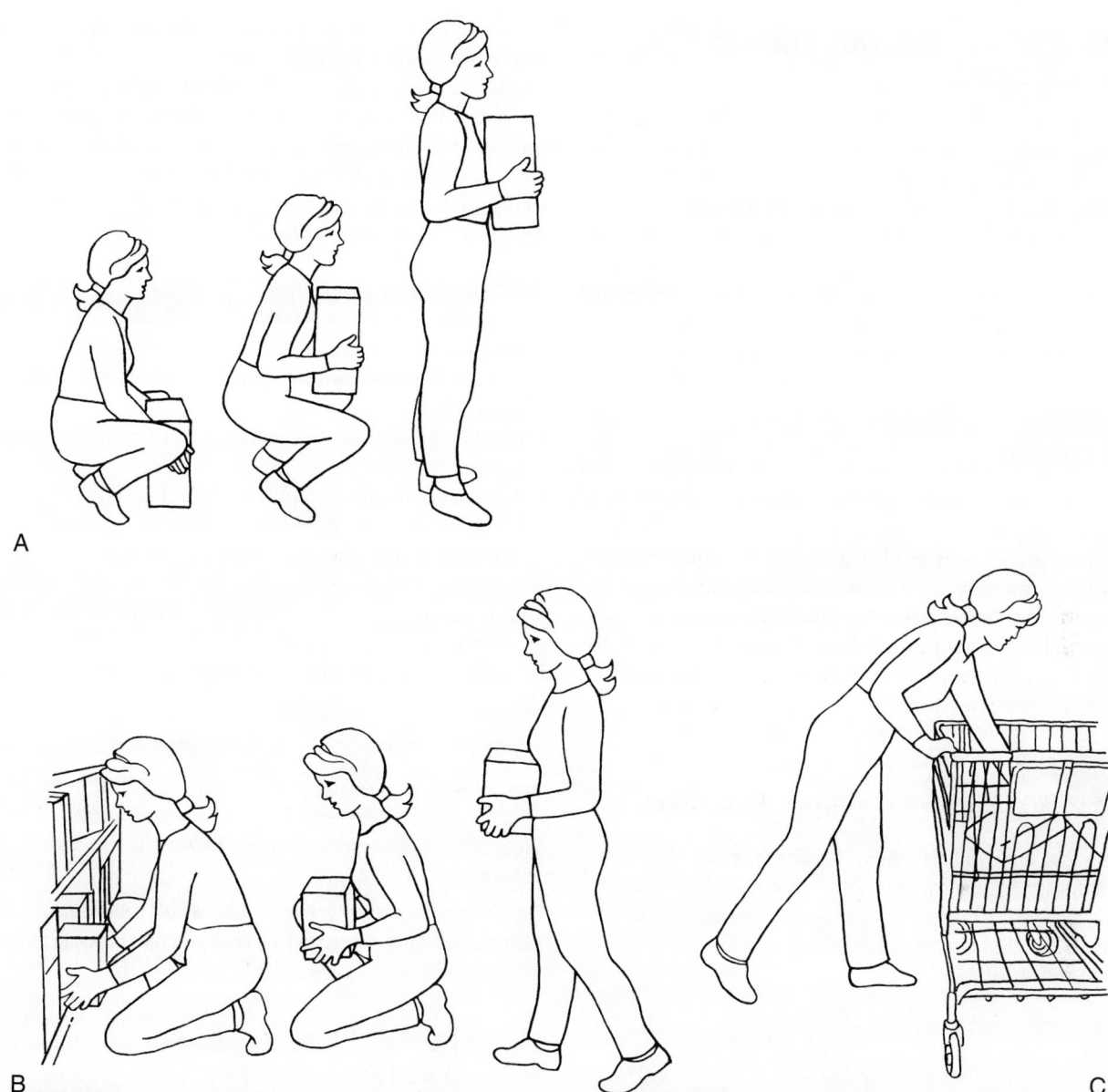

Figure 41-8   **A,** Squat. Squat and lift with both arms held against upper trunk. Tighten stomach muscles without holding breath. Use smooth movements to avoid jerking. **B,** Diagonal lift. Squat down and bring item close to lift. **C,** Golfer's lift. When reaching into cart, lift opposite leg to keep back straight.

Planning ahead, for example, might involve preparing portions of a meal ahead of time for company and freezing them so that they may be reheated. **Pacing** requires examination of the required task, the time frame for completion, and the individual's ability to complete the task without resulting dysfunction. An example of pacing might include the recommendation that the client finish dusting a room in the morning and then vacuum in the afternoon instead of completing both tasks in one session. The principle of setting priorities might be illustrated by the client going out to dinner with company rather than preparing a large meal (cooking, serving, and cleaning); the former affords the client a greater opportunity to enjoy the evening.

The principle of eliminating unnecessary tasks might involve using paper towels for guests instead of cloth towels that create extra laundry. One example of balancing rest with an activity is to use a stool and sit while preparing food, thus resting the back while completing a task. Similarly, the therapist might suggest that the client complete grocery shopping in the morning and read in the afternoon to rest after the morning task. The key to success in incorporating energy conservation into one's daily occupational life is for the client to be aware of his or her individual activity tolerance, including specific knowledge regarding triggers of fatigue and the amount lof rest necessary for recovery.

OCCUPATIONS TO INCREASE STRENGTH AND ENDURANCE

Once the principles of energy conservation have been taught and incorporated into several of the client's occupations, it is important to build upon that knowledge and enable the client to increase strength and endurance for engagement in more favored occupations. Given the opportunity to prepare a meal nightly, the client can soon develop the endurance to prepare a meal for guests. Sitting at a computer to write a letter while maintaining neutral spine strengthens the abdominal muscles; it also increases the ability to sit in the car for a ride.

STRATEGIES FOR STRESS REDUCTION AND COPING

Numerous methods can be used to promote stress reduction and coping, including relaxation techniques, deep breathing, meditation, prayer, and guided imagery. Avoiding frustration, managing angry feelings and negative thoughts, and, most important, participating in meaningful daily occupations can help the client avoid stress that results in pain. In addition to the services provided by occupational therapists and other professionals, the local bookstore offers many self-help books addressing LBP.

The following sections describe specific areas of occupation, which may be identified during the occupational profile, and identify the type of back position that can be used to reduce back stress. It is important to begin by analyzing each occupation using an approach such as the one described in the next section.

ANALYSIS OF OCCUPATIONS

- After the client has completed the occupational profile and identified specific problem areas, ask yourself the following questions:
- What is the normal movement in this activity? Analyze the activity.
- What separate movements make up this activity?
- Which movements could trigger pain in this client?

    Now plan for the way that this intervention will be provided:
- How can this activity be properly performed to avoid the position that causes pain?
- Could the environment be changed or adapted?

 **THREADED CASE STUDY: PILAR, PART 2**

While observing Pilar obtaining vegetables from the refrigerator, the therapist notices that once Pilar opens the refrigerator, she bends at the waist, reaching and pulling open the vegetable drawer with one arm, then reaches into the drawer to grab a bag of carrots (Figure 41-9, *A*).

What is the Normal Movement in the Activity for Most Individuals?

From observation, you note that most individuals bend at the waist to reach the vegetable drawer and then pull the drawer open to remove the vegetables.

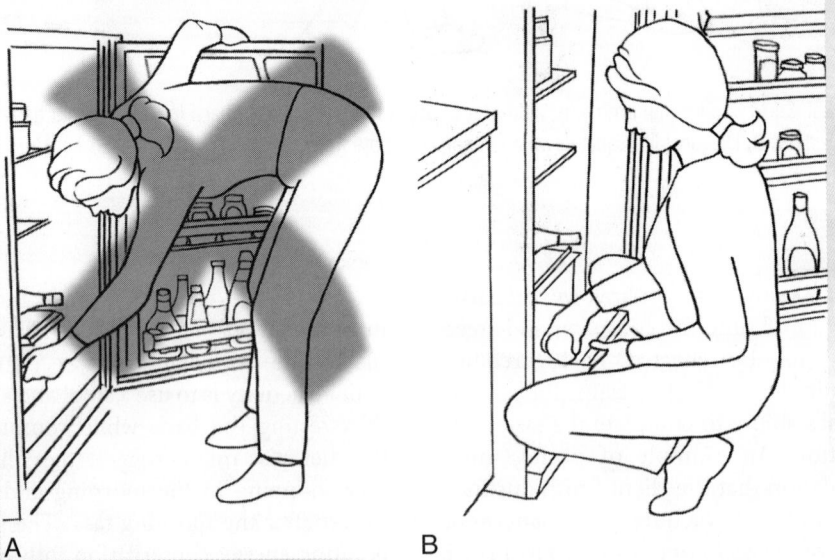

A   B

Figure 41-9   **A,** Incorrect way to reach into drawer. **B,** Squat with knees apart to reach lower shelves and drawers.

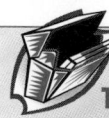

THREADED CASE STUDY: PILAR, PART 2—cont'd

What Separate Movements Occur During this Activity?

Bending, reaching, pulling, and pushing.

What Movements Could Position this Client for Pain?

Bending, reaching, pulling, and pushing with the arms while the back is in a bent position could result in pain. We know, however, based on normal anatomy, that bending at the waist increases pressure at the anterior portion of the vertebral body and disc, with increased stretch at the back of the disc. As the arms extend and reach forward, more weight is pulling forward on an already compressed anterior portion of the disc.

How Can this Activity Be Properly Performed to Avoid the Position that Causes Pain?

Pilar should squat, keeping a straight back while positioned close to the drawer. Next, she should pull open the drawer, remove the carrots, and hold them close to the body. During all of these movements, the structures in the back remain in a neutral spine position (Figure 41-9, *B*).

Could the Environment Be Changed or Adapted?

The carrots could be placed on a higher shelf. Pilar might also consider purchasing one of the newer refrigerator models that have the least used portion—the freezer—positioned on the bottom, thus reducing the frequency of the need to bend.

The interventions described may sound as if they require many more movements, but in reality the movements are the same, just done properly. With practice the new movement patterns will become a habit, replacing the old painful movements.

ACTIVITIES OF DAILY LIVING AND INSTRUMENTAL ACTIVITIES OF DAILY LIVING

This section reviews specific areas of occupation that may be identified during the occupational profile and the type of back position that can be used to reduce back stress.

BATHING

For a person with LBP, a shower is usually better than a bath because it is easier to maintain neutral spine while standing. It is also more difficult to get in and out of the tub safely.

OT PRACTICE NOTE

Back schools have been developed (by the various healthcare professionals mentioned) over the years to deliver information similar to that presented in this chapter. This is a cost-effective way to deliver these services. Many HMOs or therapy groups deliver services this way to decrease costs and prevent overuse and possible duplication of services. The theory is that this type of information can meet the client's needs when delivered in a group setting. One therapist for six clients per hour is more cost effective than 1 hour per each client and the accompanying paperwork. The group teaching session offers the added advantage of peer support and opportunities for discussions that might not occur during an individual session. However, with an individualized program, the therapist can better determine the unique occupational needs of the client and more closely assess the learning that has occurred.

One tip to make showering easier on the back is to keep all items within easy reach in the shower. Many types of racks that allow the client to place items below the showerhead are available for purchase. Long-handled scrub brushes or sponges allow washing of the back, legs, and feet without bending and twisting. A hand-held shower attachment also allows control of the water flow and decreases unnecessary movements. With significant back pain, a shower chair can be used. A simple plastic lawn chair outfitted with nonskid safety feet will work well. If a client must use a tub, he or she could sit in a plastic chair and use a hand-held shower attachment. When sitting in the tub, the client should always use a bath mat to reduce the chance of slipping and drain the water before attempting to get out.

DRESSING

The client should sit while dressing, keeping the back straight, or lie flat on the bed while pulling clothing up. Clients should refrain from getting dressed while bending forward. To don and doff socks and shoes, the client should sit and bring the foot to rest on the knee. Clients who do not have good external rotation of the hip may place their feet on a stool while donning and doffing socks and shoes (Figure 41-10). Slip-on shoes are easier to use than lace-up shoes. A long-handled shoehorn is useful to assist with donning shoes that require tying. Similarly, the client can thread a belt through the belt loops before donning slacks to keep from twisting the back. Loose-fitting clothing is easier to put on than tight clothing. Back protection techniques should be used for both dressing and undressing.

FUNCTIONAL MOBILITY

The use of a "logroll" to roll in bed requires movement of the body as a whole unit (Figure 41-11, *A*). To sit up or

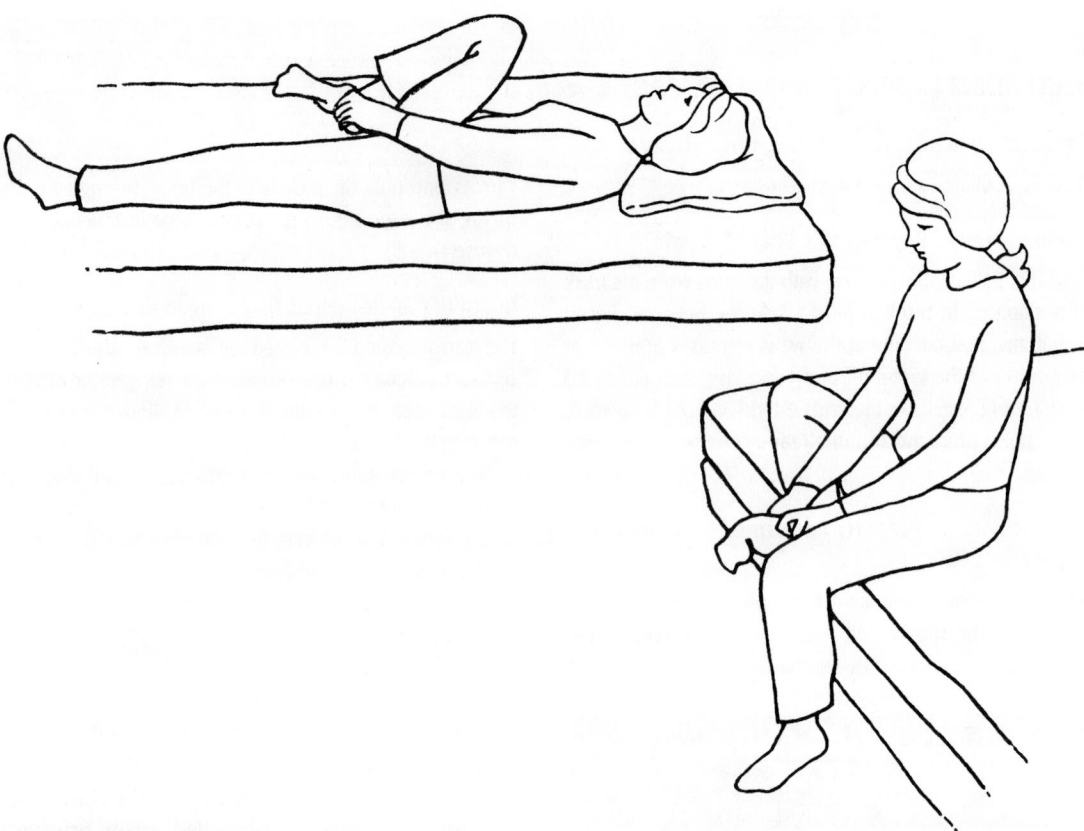

Figure 41-10   Dressing. Lie on back to place socks or slacks over feet, or bend leg up while keeping back straight.

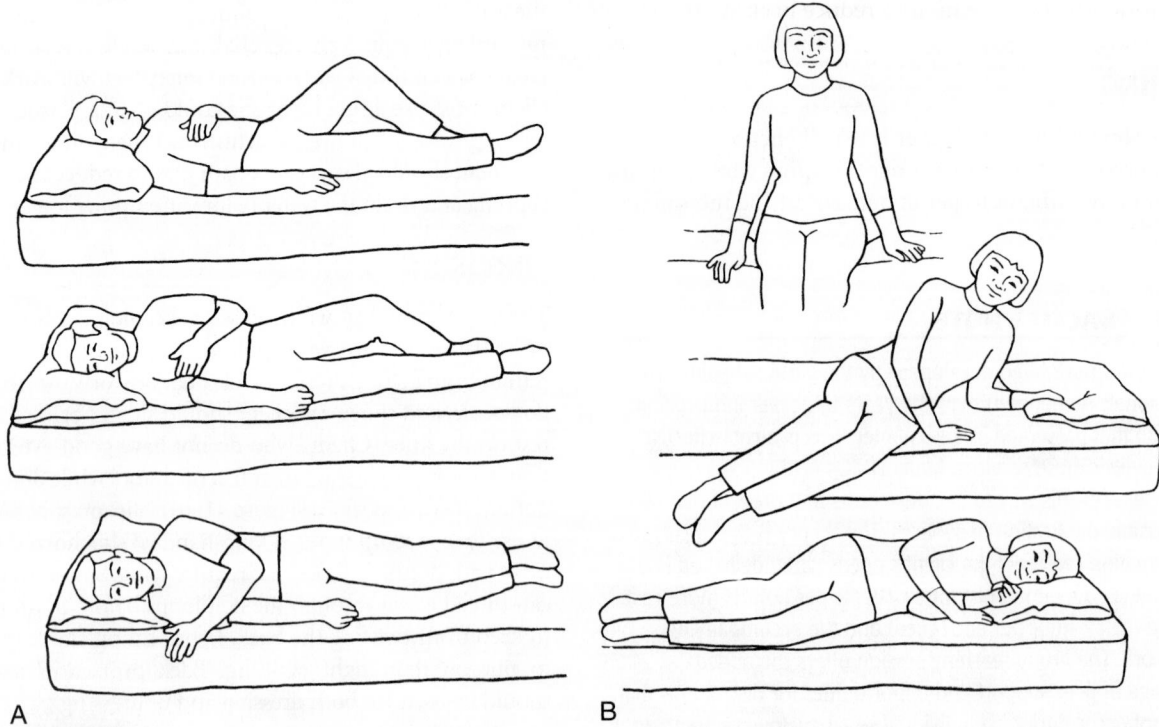

A   B

Figure 41-11   **A,** Logroll. Lying on back, bend left knee and place left arm across chest. Roll all in one movement to right. Reverse for rolling to left. Always move as one unit. **B,** Movement in and out of bed. Lower body to lie down on one side by raising legs and lowering head at the same time. Use arms to assist in moving without twisting. Bend both knees to roll onto back if desired. To sit up, start by lying on side, and use the same movements in reverse. Keep trunk aligned with legs.

lie down, the client bends the knees and pushes up with the arms while coming to a sitting position (see Figure 41-11, *B*). To lie down, the client brings the legs up and uses the arms to lower the body to the bedside. For both movements, the client is instructed to lie down and bring the legs up while using the arms to lower the body to the bedside. During both movements, the client must keep the back straight and tighten the abdominal muscles to support the back.

When getting on and off a toilet, the client must lower the body while maintaining a straight back and neutral spine. Supporting the hands on the thighs is helpful. Grab bars at the side of the toilet are also useful. However, grab bars must be secured properly and designed exclusively for this purpose; clients sometimes jeopardize their safety by using towel bars or tissue holders, which may cause further injury. In addition, clients sometimes grab a countertop on one side and the tub on the other, resulting in twisting of the back or lateral flexion.

It is recommended that the client use a firm-armed chair that is supportive and not too low (rather than a soft couch). The client can use the chair arms to push up to a standing position (Figure 41-12). To reduce stiffness, the client should not sit longer than 15 or 20 minutes.

PERSONAL HYGIENE

Activities at a bathroom sink can be difficult due to the fact that most sinks are designed to accommodate both children and adults; this low positioning forces most adults to bend forward, putting increased stress on the back structures. While brushing teeth, shaving, or washing the face, the client should place a foot inside the base cabinet to reduce strain on the lower back and bend from the hips, keeping the back straight (Figure 41-13). Alternatively, the client may bend forward, bearing his or her weight through one knee while extending a straight leg back for balance and support and

maintaining a neutral spine position. To apply cosmetics, the client should use a hand-held mirror or a mirror that attaches to the wall so that the height can be adjusted.

SEXUAL ACTIVITY

Sexual activities require positions that place the lower back in the neutral position. Clients with back pain may be most comfortable taking a passive position on their back. Positioning pillows under the buttocks or upper back may help reduce arching of the back. A rolled towel under the lower back may also help maintain a neutral back position. In addition, the client is advised to start slowly and gradually work up to more vigorous movements. Stretching and warming up muscles may enable greater activity. Taking a warm shower or bath before sexual activity may also relax muscles and help reduce pain. A bit of planning will allow for enjoyment of sexual relations (Figure 41-14).

SLEEP

We spend a third of our lives in bed, so it is important to consider the effects that being supine has on our backs. A firm, supportive mattress is important. The pillow should support the neck and head without causing the neck to flex. Many types of formed foam pillows are helpful. While sleeping on the back, the client should place a pillow under the knees to reduce the strain on the lower back and help maintain a balanced lower back position (Figure 41-15, *A*). While lying on the side, the client should place a pillow between the knees to keep the top leg from moving out of alignment and twisting the lower back (see Figure 41-15, *B*).

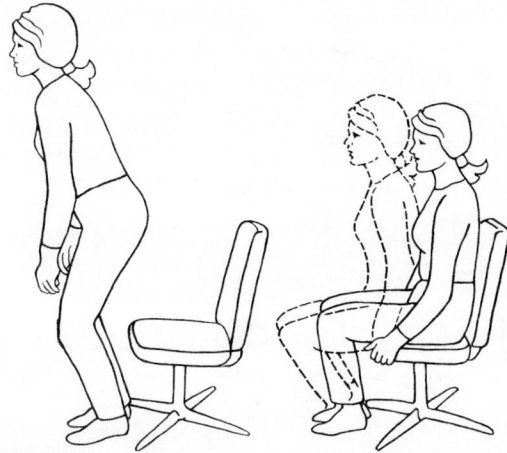

Figure 41-12 Stand to sit and sit to stand. To sit: Bend knees to lower body onto front edge of chair, then scoot back on seat. To stand: Reverse sequence by placing one foot forward, and scoot to front of seat. Use rocking motion to stand up.

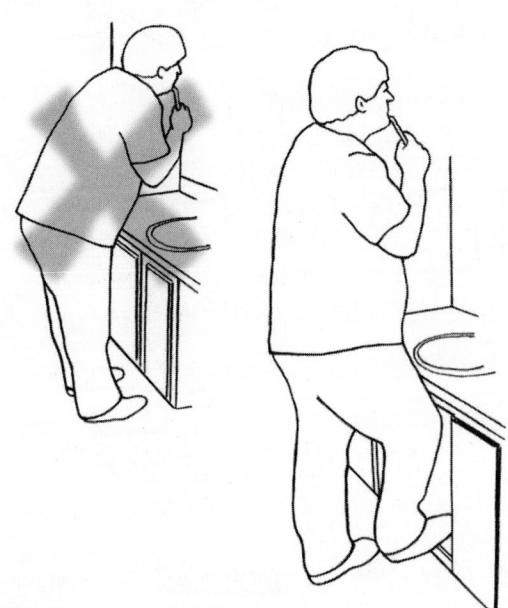

Figure 41-13 Shaving. Stay upright with one foot on ledge of cabinet under sink. (Courtesy of Visual Health Information, Tacoma, WA.)

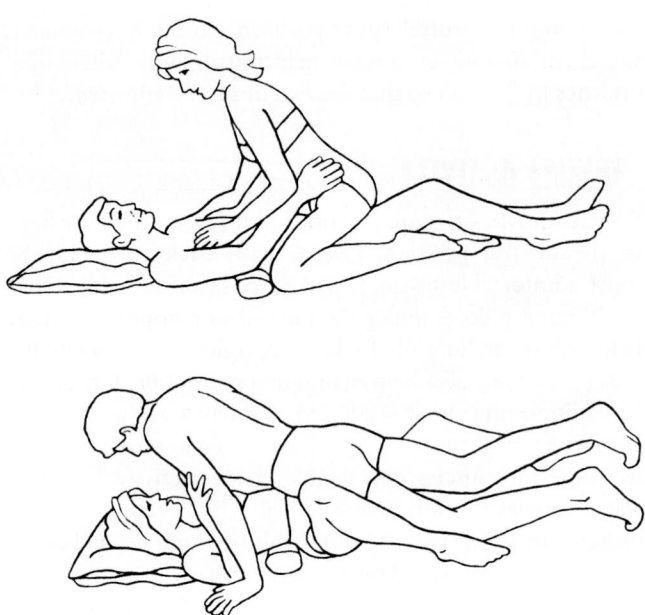

Figure 41-14 Sex positions. Communicate with your partner to find the position that is most comfortable for you. Plan ahead, and use pillows and rolls for support as needed.

For some individuals, sleeping on the stomach is appropriate (see Figure 41-15, *C*). In this position, pillows would not be appropriate and a small pillow under the feet to bend the ankles and knees will take stress off the lower back.[2]

TOILETING

When cleaning after toileting, the client should reach between the legs to avoid twisting the back. When turning to flush the toilet, the client should turn all the way around and face the toilet to flush it rather than twisting and reaching. During an acute episode of back pain, a toilet can be used by straddling the seat and facing the back of the toilet. This affords a wider base of support and also provides use of the toilet tank when coming to a stand.

CHILDCARE

Handling children requires special precautions for individuals with back pain. Sudden movements can increase the client's pain and interfere with the ability to handle the child safely. Clients should use a changing table or elevated surface when dressing the child. Bathing can be performed in a kitchen sink or in a portable tub on an elevated surface. Many contemporary cribs have drop-down rails so that the client does not need to extend his or her arms to lift the child over the crib.

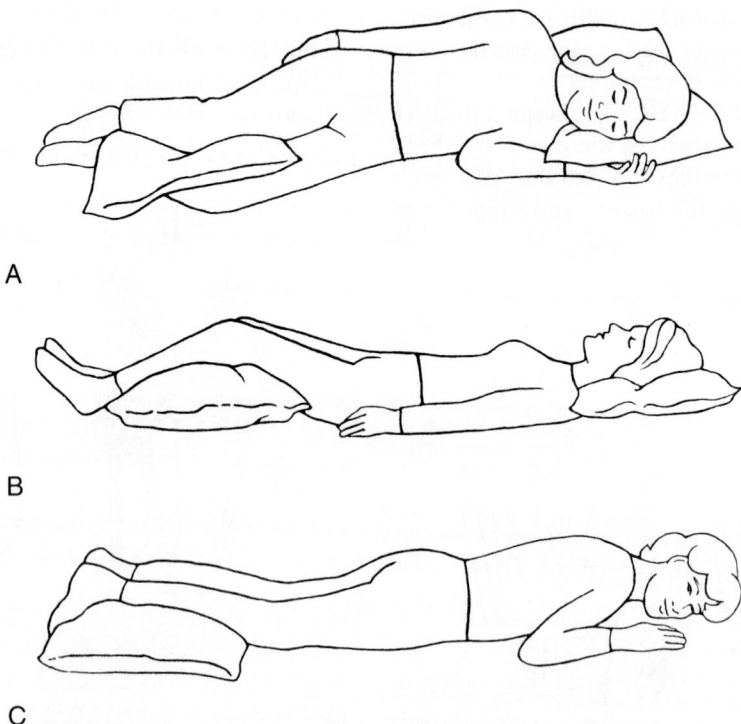

A

B

C

Figure 41-15 **A,** Sleeping on side. Place pillow between knees. Use cervical support under neck and a roll around waist as needed. **B,** Sleeping on back. Place pillow under knees. A pillow with cervical support and a roll around waist are also helpful. **C,** Sleeping on stomach. If this is the only desirable sleep position, place pillow under lower legs and under stomach or chest as needed.

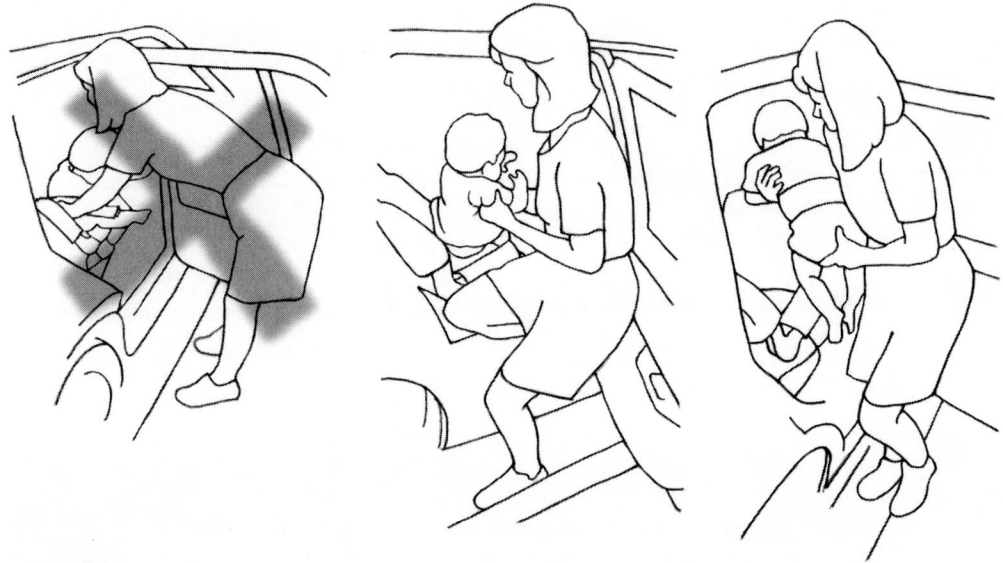

Figure 41-16   Childcare, in and out of car. Stand close, and keep back straight. Bend knees to put baby in or take baby out of car seat.

Always remind the client to bend at the hips and keep the back straight during all of these tasks. To lift a child from the ground, the client should squat down and bring the child close before standing up. As the child gets older, the client should ask the child to stand or sit on a chair or couch before being lifted. This decreases the distance the child must be lifted and eliminates the client's need to bend forward. To place a child in a car seat, the client should stand close to the car seat and keep the back straight (Figure 41-16).

COMPUTER USE

Much has been written about the use of computers and their effect on the body. It is important to position work so that the client is facing forward and ensure that the body is in good alignment. The keyboard and monitor should be directly in front of the client. The top of the monitor should be approximately at eye level. Clients are instructed to use a proper work height and seat height with feet flat on floor, wrists in a neutral position with forearms parallel with the floor, and elbows at a 90-degree angle. If the client is using a laptop computer, the same guidelines should be used. Clients are taught to look at the screen by lowering their eyes rather than flexing their necks. In addition, clients are encouraged to stretch, take breaks, and change positions often. Document holders can assist with proper placement to prevent the need to twist the body. (See the previous section on ergonomics and Chapter 13 for additional information on seating.)

DRIVING

When getting in and out of a car, the client should sit on the seat and turn the body as a unit to keep from twisting.

In some cars, this may require adjusting the seat to get in and out; the client should sit with the knees no higher than the hips. A small, rolled-up towel positioned in the lumbar area may be helpful. Most cars now allow adjustments of the seat height, seat angle, seat position, and steering wheel angle. When riding for extended periods of time, the client should schedule rest breaks to change positions. For drivers with back pain, use of cruise control allows more frequent changes of position.

HOME ESTABLISHMENT AND MANAGEMENT

The client should organize all workspaces so that the equipment and materials needed for specific tasks are within the work area. For example, if the client is planning to bake cookies, flour, sugar, baking spices, bowls, and measuring cups should all be within reach. The mixer (if used regularly) should be on the counter to obviate the need for lifting and reaching. Work areas should allow flexion in the elbows and no bending or straining in the lower back. Routinely used items in cabinets should be at reach overhead, and the client should not be required to extend the back or neck to retrieve them. Items in lower cabinets should allow easy access with a partial squat. Cabinets can be modified with slide out shelves/drawers that allow easier access. Items that are used less frequently can be stored in hard-to-reach cabinets. To prepare meals, the client must work at a proper workspace. The ideal height for most individuals allows comfortable work with the elbows bent at 90 degrees, above and below extension of the arms without extension of the back and neck or bending. The kitchen setup should feature work areas in which the items needed for a particular task are within easy reach.

To remove clothing from the washer when doing laundry, the client should use a golfer's lift to reach inside the

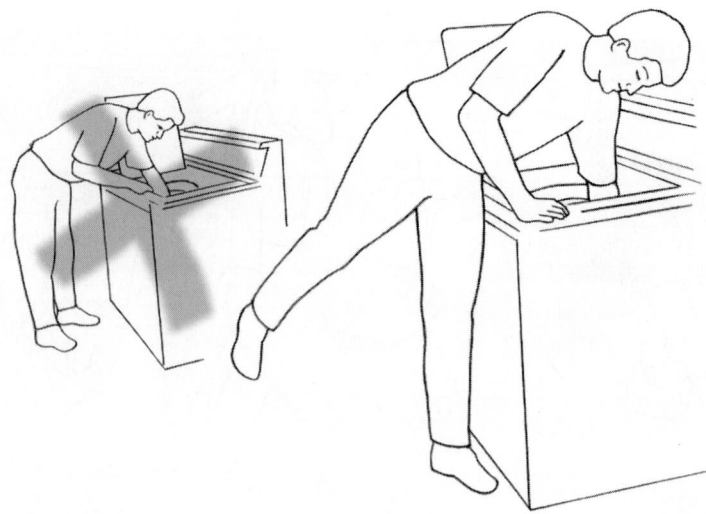

Figure 41-17   Laundry, unloading wash. To unload small items at bottom of washer, lift leg opposite to arm used to reach.

machine (Figure 41-17). To place clothes in the dryer, the client is instructed to squat down and then load the dryer. To retrieve clothes, the client repeats the squat, removes the clothes, and places the clothes in a basket that is positioned nearby. When carrying the basket, the client should hold it close to the body; the same is true while lifting the basket when coming from a squat to a standing position.

For ironing, it is recommended that the client raise the ironing board to the proper height, thus allowing the client to have the elbow flexed at 90 degrees as well as providing adequate extension of the elbow to avoid twisting of the lower back. While ironing, the client is instructed to rest one foot on a low stool to help reduce low back strain. Ironing can also be completed while sitting if the ironing board is lowered beforehand. Because of the adjustability of an ironing board, this surface can be used for many other activities, such as folding clothes and wrapping packages.

A long-handled brush or sponge is recommended to clean the bottom of a tub. Using a hand-held sprayer and a spray cleaner is easier than scrubbing and rinsing the surfaces. While vacuuming, clients should move their feet and legs rather then reach or bend forward. They are also cautioned to avoid twisting; when vacuuming under a table or chair, they should bend at the hips and knees to keep the back in a balanced position.

When mowing the lawn, the client should face forward and align the hips with the mower. Keeping the back straight, the spine in a neutral position, and the abdominal muscles tight, the client should take frequent breaks and refrain from twisting. While using a shovel, the client should bend at the hips and knees, rather than at the waist, and keep the shovel and its load close to the body. The preferred method for emptying the shovel is to turn the entire body, keeping

the hips and shoulders in alignment while maintaining the load close to the body and facing the location to unload the shovel. None of these household activities should be attempted when the client is in an unstable condition with acute pain.

SHOPPING

When retrieving items from a lower shelf, the client should squat or go down on one knee while keeping the back straight. The shelf should be used as support when returning to a stand. When items are located overhead, the client should get as close as possible and use one hand for support on the shelf. To use a shopping cart, the client should find his or her neutral spine position, which should cause the abdominal muscles to tighten. The client should stand up straight, pushing the cart with the elbows at the side. The force to move the cart should come from the legs and body, not the back. Use of the cart is preferable to carrying a basket, even for small loads. Clients can place items in the child's portion of the cart rather than carry a basket in one hand, which puts an uneven stress on the back. When unloading the cart, the client should use the golfer's lift to obtain items from the bottom. While carrying packages, the client should evenly distribute the weight between both arms, reducing uneven lateral bend on one side. Or better yet, the client can carry packages close to the body and use both arms.

WORK

The demands of jobs vary considerably. Many employers now have someone on staff to assess workstations and determine whether modifications can be made (see Chapter 13).

In many cases, however, it is up to the individual worker to modify his or her work situation. Many improvements can be made by simply using correct lifting techniques, using the proper equipment for the job, pacing the activity, and asking for help.

LEISURE

When reading, clients should sit in a supported chair, not curl up on a sofa. Tabletop hobbies such as sewing and building models require attention to the table height, the chair position, and the positioning of the work items for the upper extremities; these positioning recommendations resemble those for computers. All of these modifications will reduce uneven pulling and twisting of the body.

When traveling, the client should use a pull-type suitcase on wheels, which is easier on the back. Backpacks and fanny packs with light loads can also be used. Travelers are encouraged to pack lightly and take only what is needed for the trip. Checking luggage and having someone else carry the load instead of trying to lift items overhead are also recommended.

Gardening can be challenging for clients with back problems. Raised garden beds and container gardening are good options to reduce back strain. There are many carts or moving seats on the market that allow safer back positioning when working at ground level. Knee pads make gardening in a kneeling position more comfortable. The gardener is cautioned to work only within his or her immediate reach to avoid bending forward or twisting.

Only a few of the many possible interventions have been described here. Each client and each occupation must be analyzed, and an individual intervention should be developed for each client. ADL body mechanics cards from Visual Health Information can be used to customize each program. This is a card file system from which cards can be selected and copied to develop interventions for each client according to his or her individual needs. Also available are many preprinted booklets and computer programs that may assist in client instruction. It is important to remember that most insurance companies do not cover adaptive equipment, and hospitals typically have large markups on vended equipment. Consequently, many clinics offer sample equipment for clients to try and provide community resources for equipment or consumer catalogs from vendors such as Sammons/Preston/Rolyan or North Coast Medical. Consumers should be made aware that many items once considered adaptive therapy equipment or ergonomic items are frequently available at a lower cost in discount stores.

SURGICAL INTERVENTION

Recently, the surgical treatment of back problems has undergone many advances. Current interventions include laminectomies, fusions, decompression of the nerve, and disc dissection. The surgical interventions are divided into two basic types: surgery that decompresses the nerve or stabilization of the spine to reduce pain. Surgeries that decompress the nerve open the transverse foramen and increase the space for the spinal nerve exit and entrance to the spinal cord. Some surgeries may remove a structure, such as part of a disc or an osteophyte, which may create pressure on the nerve root. Stabilization can include the use of various pieces of hardware, such as screw, wires, rods, and bone grafts, to increase stability of the bony structures of the spine.

 OT PRACTICE NOTE

It is very important that the therapist understand what each of these surgeries involves and be able to articulate this information to the client. As part of the occupational therapy intervention in the hospital, education regarding the surgical procedure enables the client to understand the reason that certain precautions are required during the rehabilitation phase and to maintain a healthy back.

Client precautions must be identified. Therapists should work with the physician to develop protocols or standards of care for specific surgeries. It is also important to identify the types of braces, corsets, and other equipment that may be used for a specific surgery by a specific physician so that the occupational therapist can provide the expected instructions and precautions for use of the equipment in daily occupations. For example, one physician may allow a client to put the corset on while sitting at bedside, whereas another physician may require the client to logroll into the brace and complete donning the brace before coming to a seated position.

POSTOPERATIVE OCCUPATIONAL THERAPY EVALUATION AND INTERVENTION

When seeing a client for the first time postoperatively, the occupational therapist should obtain the client's history and occupational profile as well as a description of his or her home environment to ascertain types of modifications required for safety. During the occupational profile, ADL and IADL issues should be identified. As part of the home assessment, education in work simplification techniques, in conjunction with directive questions, helps the client identify further needs. Home modifications may include picking up rugs to prevent falls, increasing awareness of pets, and selecting a type of chair that is easy to get in and out of and that provides good support and fits the client. The therapist should also determine whether the home contains a standard toilet and shower and whether modifications are required.

Next, the therapist must educate the client in the required performance precautions for daily occupations; this should take place before even attempting to have the client get out of bed. This evaluation is somewhat contrary to customary practice in occupational therapy. In this situation, the therapist does not want to observe performance before the intervention. Instead, the primary focus is to educate and then cue the client through the process to avoid any improper positions or posture that creates stress on the surgical area. The outcome of occupational therapy intervention is to maintain a straight back, avoid twisting, and perform ADLs while safely incorporating back safety techniques and using adaptive equipment.

POSTOPERATIVE ACTIVITIES OF DAILY LIVING

While in the hospital, the most basic ADLs must be addressed initially. It is important to educate the client regarding proper positions for sleeping and have the client demonstrate the correct positions. The client will need to use the logroll for functional mobility in the bed. Proper methods are also taught for getting in and out of bed, in and out of a chair, and on and off a toilet; brushing teeth; washing the face; shaving; and dressing using the back protection techniques discussed earlier in this chapter. Clients are instructed to use adaptive equipment to prevent back stress in daily activities, including getting in and out of an automobile.

The hospital stay for these clients can be between 24 hours and 3 to 5 days, depending on the procedure and the prior level of function. Most clients are discharged home. Because the client's stay is so short, it is good to provide them with resources to help them should specific occupations be overlooked during the hospital stay. Some facilities develop educational materials that include basic body mechanics information, hints on ADLs, and anatomy and surgical information. Various publications include post-surgical back "dos and don'ts." Many hospitals have computerized education programs, which allow the provider to issue information on the surgical procedure and the resulting back precautions. Most insurance plans do not cover adaptive equipment such as reachers and long-handled sponges; however, this equipment is necessary to ensure a successful postoperative outcome. Raised commodes and shower chairs are usually not covered, but many clients purchase these items and have them delivered to their homes before discharge. To prepare the client for home and occupation modifications, many hospitals provide preoperative education classes.

SUMMARY

Providing effective occupational therapy intervention for the client with LBP requires a good understanding of back anatomy and physiology. The ability to analyze daily occupations and determine how back positions are affected by the occupation is crucial to providing a successful outcome. Good communication between all team members is important to provide both reduction of symptoms and integration of knowledge to support the performance of meaningful occupations.

THREADED CASE STUDY: PILAR, PART 3

When reexamining our case study, we note that Pilar has problems with bending over while performing her daily activities. Because bending over causes increased pain, it is apparent that she is bending through her lumbar area. We know from our review of anatomy that, when bending from the waist, pressure will increase on the anterior portion of the vertebra and disc and could cause impingement on the nerve root, resulting in pain. The activities that Pilar has identified as painful will be the focus of intervention for education with respect to anatomy and the probable cause of her pain as a result of bending at the waist.

Once she understands how her movement affects her pain, introduction of neutral spine will ensure even pressure on the vertebrae and discs. Her knowledge and use of proper body mechanics in maintaining a straight back will ensure even pressure on the lumbar structures. Learning the relationship between both mechanically correct and incorrect movement patterns and her pain will help her develop pain-free movement patterns. As Pilar is able to demonstrate correct movements and reduction of pain, she should be able to assimilate this information into other activities not identified and be in control of her pain, positively affecting her engagement in daily occupations.

Review Questions

1. List four causes of LBP.
2. Identify the major components of the spine.
3. Explain the ways that back movements affect the spinal components while the client engages in an occupation.
4. Define *neutral spine*.
5. Identify the interventions used for patients with LBP.
6. Identify the interventions used for post-surgical patients.

REFERENCES

1. Brotzman SB, Wilk K: *Clinical orthopaedic rehabilitation*, ed 2, St Louis, 2003, Mosby.
2. Melnik MS, Saunders R, Saunders HD: *Self-help manual managing back pain*, Bloomington, MN, 1989, Educational Opportunities.
3. Nelson DL, Ciriani DJ, Thomas JJ: Physical therapy and occupational therapy partners in rehabilitation for persons with movement impairments, *Occup Ther Health Care* 17:34, 2001.
4. Waddell G: *The back pain revolution*, New York, 1998, Churchill Livingstone.

SUGGESTED READINGS

Cole AJ, Herring SA: *The low back pain handbook: a practical guide for the primary care clinician*, Philadelphia, 1997, Hanley and Belfus.

Larson BA: *Occupational therapy practice guidelines for adults with low back pain*, Bethesda, MD, 1996, American Occupational Therapy Association.

Maxey L, Magnusson J: *Rehabilitation for the postsurgical orthopedic patient*, St. Louis, 2001, Mosby.

Moore J, et al: *The back pain help book*, Cambridge, MA, 1999, Perseus Books Group.

RESOURCES

WORKBOOK

San Francisco Spine Institute at Seton Medical Center, 1989.
Body Mechanics Resource Library
Visual Health Information
P.O. Box 44646
Tacoma, WA 98444
206-536-4922

42 Burns and Burn Rehabilitation[1]

SANDRA UTLEY REEVES

KEY TERMS

Dermis

Epidermis

Superficial burn

Superficial partial-thickness burns

Deep partial-thickness burn

Full-thickness burn

Subdermal burns

Hypertrophic scar

Keloid scar

Compartment syndrome

Ischemia

Escharotomy

Xenograft

Allograft

Autograft

Eschar

Scar maturation

Heterotopic ossification

LEARNING OBJECTIVES

After studying this chapter the student or practitioner will be able to do the following:

1. Recognize and understand the characteristics of the different types of burn injury and the clinical techniques for determining wound depth and severity.
2. Understand the anatomy of the skin and its functional significance on performance skills and on both external and internal contexts.
3. Describe the phases of recovery and focus of occupational therapy (OT) intervention for each phase.
4. Identify factors that increase potential for scar hypertrophy and contracture.

5. Comprehend the impact of ongoing patient and caregiver education on long-term compliance with treatment.
6. Understand the impact of early involvement of burn patients in their own self-care activities of daily living (ADLs) on the resumption of role and performance patterns.
7. Acknowledge and anticipate complications characteristic of a severe burn.
8. Appreciate the impact that a severe burn has on the performance patterns, life roles, self-image, and valued context of the patient.

CHAPTER OUTLINE

Incidence of burn injuries and burn-related deaths

Skin anatomy

Skin function

Mechanism of injury and burn depth

Percent total body surface area involved

Severity of injury

Phases of wound healing

  Inflammatory phase

  Proliferation phase

  Maturation phase

  Scar formation

Initial medical management

  Fluid resuscitation and edema

  Respiratory management

  Wound care and infection control

Associated problems and complications

  Stress

Pain

Psychosocial factors

Burn rehabilitation

  The team

  Goals of rehabilitation

  Phases of recovery

Occupational therapy intervention

  Acute-care phase

  Surgical and postoperative phase

  Rehabilitation phase: inpatient

  Rehabilitation phase: outpatient

Burn-related complications

  Heterotopic ossification

  Neuromuscular complications

  Facial disfigurement

Summary

---

[1]In this chapter, the terms *patient* and *client* are both used, with *client* used in occupational therapy contexts.

THREADED CASE STUDY: STEVEN, KENJII, PATRICE, PART 1

Steven

Steven, a 38-year-old Caucasian father, was a truck driver when he received 25% total body surface area (TBSA) battery acid burns in a rollover automobile accident in which he was pinned under his vehicle. As a result of the spilled battery acid, he sustained deep burns to his upper chest, upper back, right arm extending from the anterior fold of his axilla, circumferential upper arm, forearm, dorsal hand, and right index finger. He also suffered serious battery acid burns of his neck and face. Other injuries included skin lacerations of his forehead, fracture of his coccyx, right elbow sprain, and chest trauma resulting in a lacerated spleen, and a collapsed upper lobe of his right lung. His medical history was significant only for sleep apnea and psoriasis on both lower legs. He was right-hand dominant and independent in all ADLs and IADLs before this injury.

At the time of his injury, Steven lived alone in a mobile home but shared custody of his 3-year-old son, who stayed with him on alternate weekends. He has a high-school education and had worked for 18 years as a truck driver until the time of his accident. He had also worked part time at night as a bouncer at a local bar, a job he enjoyed because he was "paid to hang out with my friends." His leisure interests included fishing, working out at the gym, and competitive power lifting. He had been capable of lifting 325 pounds and had won three trophies at regional weight-lifting competitions the year before his injury.

Kenjii

Kenjii, a 22-year-old male rock musician of Asian descent, received severe burn injuries when a canister of stage pyrotechnic gunpowder caught fire. The gunpowder had been stored in the band's dressing room where someone apparently mistook the canister for a trash can and flipped a cigarette into it. As the gunpowder burned, it superheated the room, and Kenjii barely escaped by crawling out of the room on his hands and knees. His long hair, cotton blue jeans, t-shirt, and boots helped to protect much of his body, but his unprotected arms, hands, and face became severely burned. Because of the depth of the burns on his hands, he developed severe deformities on most of his fingers, and his interphalangeal joints had to be fused, leaving only active movement in his metacarpophalangeal joints. Because of a genetic predisposition for scarring and the locations of his initial injury, he developed severe scarring and disfigurement of much of his face, arms, and hands. Even surgical and skin graft donor sites scarred severely.

The distortion of Kenjii's facial appearance and impairment of hand function resulted in the loss of both his personal identity and the dexterity skills he had used to play flute, guitar, and piano. Kenjii lost the factors on which he based his livelihood and personal identity. He lost his autonomy when he became financially dependent on his parents, who had not approved of his career choice as a musician.

Patrice

Patrice, an African-American child, was scalded when she was 7 days old by her schizophrenic biological mother during a psychotic episode. Her burns were located on her face, the top of her head, her left thigh, her abdomen, her left forearm, and the back of her left hand. Because of her young age, her burns had to be treated conservatively and allowed to heal initially without surgical intervention. Her hand was too tiny and her skull bones not developed enough for use of conventional scar prevention techniques. As a consequence, she developed tight scars that distorted her facial features and the growth of her hand. Her hand burn was serious but did not involve her fingers. However, in spite of frequent therapy sessions and the excellent care provided by a devoted foster mother, the longitudinal force of the hand scar prevented the natural growth of the bones in her middle, ring, and little fingers. There was so little growth in the bones of her little finger that, as the rest of her hand continued to grow, the little finger gradually receded into her hand and essentially disappeared.

Critical Thinking Questions

1. The upper extremities and faces of each of these three clients were seriously injured. Which specific areas of occupation (including ADLs; IADLs; and education, work, play, leisure, and social participation) will be affected for each of them?

2. When planning OT intervention for these clients, how will understanding their pre-injury occupational life and contexts influence the establishment of treatment priorities?

3. Both of the adults lost the performance skills on which they relied for their livelihood. The facial appearance of all three was distorted, a condition that would affect their self-perception and personal identity. How and when should the occupational therapist address the emotional impact of these losses?

4. As you read through the chapter, also reflect on the information presented on burn rehabilitation. How did OT intervention affect the client factors, performance skills, performance patterns, long-term performance in areas of occupations, and final contexts of each of the three clients portrayed in the case scenarios?

Increasing numbers of individuals are surviving burn injuries that in the past would have proved fatal. Over the past 40 years, advances in burn management, such as resuscitation, early excision and grafting, and surgical critical care, have dramatically improved the percentage of survivors of severe burn injuries.[11] With this improvement in survival comes the increased need for comprehensive burn rehabilitation so that when a life is saved, the quality of lifestyle and participation in meaningful occupation are also preserved.

INCIDENCE OF BURN INJURIES AND BURN-RELATED DEATHS

Globally an estimated 6 million people sustain burns each year, with many requiring hospitalization in specialized burn units.[13] It has been estimated that over 1 million burn injuries occur each year in the United States alone. However, in the United States there has been a significant decline in the incidence of burn injury since the early 1960s, when an estimated 2 million injuries occurred annually.[3] The total for fire- and burn-related deaths is currently estimated at 4500 per year. This total includes an estimated 3750 deaths from both fires and smoke inhalation poisoning and 750 from other sources of burn injury, including motor vehicle and aircraft crashes and contact with electricity, hot liquids, chemicals, and other caustic substances.

Fire- and burn-related deaths in the United States declined about 50% from 1971 to 1998. Given that the U.S. population grew by 25% during that period, the decline in the death rate was actually over 60%.[3] Burn prevention and fire safety measures have also reduced the incidence of severe burn injury to the extent that burn centers are now admitting greater numbers of patients with less severe burns and fewer large, deep burns.[77]

Since the early 1970s, advances in the medical, surgical, and rehabilitative management of individuals who sustain burns have expanded the focus of burn care professionals from simply ensuring patient survival to include regaining the quality of life and previous life context after a burn injury. Although functional recovery may be a long and arduous process, most burn survivors can expect to resume their roles, function at a level that is comparatively close to their pre-injury level of independence, and continue engagement in occupation for satisfactory participation in life. However, from the date of injury through the outpatient phase of care, a multidisciplinary team approach is necessary to effectively manage the medical, functional, and psychosocial problems encountered during recovery.

SKIN ANATOMY

The skin is the largest organ of the body. It varies greatly in thickness, flexibility, presence and amount of hair, degree of pigmentation, vascularity, nerve supply and sensitivity, amount of keratin, and types of glands present in different locations. Keratin is the tough protein substance present in the skin that also makes up hair, nails, and callused areas of skin on the hands or feet. Most of the body is covered with thin, hairy skin. However, thicker, tougher, hairless skin, known as *glabrous skin*, covers the soles of the feet and the palmar surfaces of the hand and fingers.

Anatomically the skin consists primarily of two layers: the dermis and the epidermis (Figure 42-1). The **dermis,** or corium, is composed of fibrous connective tissue made of collagen and elastin and contains numerous capillaries, lymphatic and nerve endings. In it are the hair follicles and their smooth muscle fibers, sebaceous glands, and sweat glands and their ducts. [88]

The **epidermis** is the outermost layer of epithelium that also lines the nail beds and the skin appendages, which are pockets of epithelium that extend down into the dermis and contain the hair follicles, sweat glands, and sebaceous glands. The epidermis consists of four or five layers, depending on the location and type of skin. The innermost layer of the epidermis is the stratum germinativum, where the keratinocytes that synthesize keratin are formed. Above this lies the stratum spinosum, in which the progressive stages of keratinization occur. The keratinocytes in this layer have a well-developed capacity for phagocytosis, which helps control infections by ingesting and breaking down bacteria and particulate debris. Melanin granules, which give the skin and hair their colors, are present in the cytoplasm of certain cells in the stratum spinosum. In the next layer, the stratum granulosum, the cells making their way toward the surface become flattened and accumulate many large keratin granules, termed *keratohyalin*. In this layer, cells lose their nucleus, change from viable to nonviable, and become

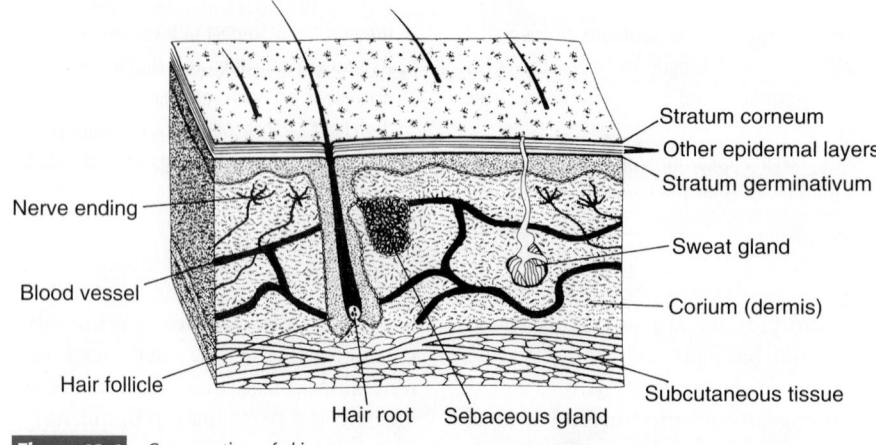

Figure 42-1   Cross section of skin. (From Iles RL: *Wound care: the skin,* 1988, Marion Laboratories.)

a cornified layer composed chiefly of keratin filaments. Above this layer is the stratum lucidum, seen best in glabrous skin, which is thicker. The outermost layer, the stratum corneum, is composed of tightly packed dead keratinocytes known as *squames* that become the cornified, flattened skin cells that eventually separate from one another and detach from the surface of the epidermis. The time for a newly formed keratinocyte to pass from the deepest layer to the surface to be shed is estimated to take 45 to 75 days. This is the natural manner in which the epidermis continually renews itself.[88]

SKIN FUNCTION

The skin serves as an environmental barrier that protects against ultraviolet rays, chemical contamination, and bacterial invasion. It also serves as a moisture barrier to prevent excessive moisture absorption or evaporative loss. Temperature regulation is also a function of the skin, with hair to insulate and perspiration to cool the body. The skin perceives injury or infection through tactile sensory receptors located in the dermis layer of the skin. These receptors heighten environmental awareness through perceived touch, pressure, pain, and temperature. When the skin is damaged, various systemic, physiological, and functional problems can occur. A burn injury causes destruction of the protective environmental barrier, resulting in exposed nerve endings, loss of body heat, seepage of body fluids, and exposure to bacterial invasion.

The skin also influences the development of an individual's body image and personal identity and enhances nonverbal social interaction. Along with age, gender, body type, and voice, the skin's scent, texture, coloration, and the appearance of facial features contribute strongly to a person's external context (physical) and self-concept–related internal contexts (e.g., body image, self-regard, sense of social and cultural acceptance). Because of all these factors, a large burn injury is considered to be one of the most physically and psychologically painful forms of trauma.

After a burn injury, many factors are taken into consideration in determining the severity of injury, potential for functional recovery, and treatment needs. Primary considerations for burn wound evaluation are the mechanism of injury, the depth and extent of the burn, specific body areas burned, and associated or concurrent injuries such as an inhalation injury or fractures. The individual's age, medical history, pre-injury health, and previous life context are of equal importance in determining the impact of a serious burn injury on future occupational performance.

MECHANISM OF INJURY AND BURN DEPTH

Burns can be thermal, chemical, or electrical in nature and can be caused by flame, steam, hot liquids, hot surfaces, and radiation.[24] The severity of the injury depends on the area of the body exposed and the duration and intensity of thermal exposure. Burn wounds are classified by depth, which is determined by clinical assessment of the appearance, sensitivity, and pliability of the wound.[93] Burn injuries were traditionally classified as *first, second,* and *third degree.* They are now classified as *superficial, superficial partial-thickness, deep partial-thickness, full thickness,* and *subdermal.*[29, 41] The depth of injury is established by clinical determination according to which of the anatomic layers of the skin are involved.[85]

Superficial burns, sometimes referred to as *first-degree burns,* involve only the upper layers of the epidermis. Damage through the epidermis and upper third of the dermis is referred to as **superficial partial-thickness burns.** The term **deep partial-thickness burn** describes damage to the epidermis and upper two thirds of the dermis, and **full-thickness burn** describes an injury that extends down through the entire dermis. **Subdermal burns** involve burns to the fatty layer, fascia, muscle, tendon, bone, or other subdermal tissues (e.g., those seen in electrical injuries; Table 42-1).

Superficial burns are usually caused by sun exposure or brief contact with rapidly cooling, nonviscous, hot fluids or surfaces (e.g., spilled coffee and a hot pan). Superficial partial-thickness burns are usually caused by prolonged sun exposure, contact with flames, or brief contact with viscous hot liquids (Figure 42-2, *A*). Deep partial-thickness burns are caused by longer exposure to intense heat, such as immersion in hot water or contact of the skin with flaming materials. Full-thickness burns usually result from prolonged immersion scalds, contact with flaming or high-temperature viscous materials such as hot grease or melted tar, extended exposure to chemical agents, and contact with electrical current (Figure 42-2, *B*).

Superficial partial-thickness and deep partial-thickness burns usually heal without surgical intervention. However, once healed, they tend to be excessively dry, itchy, and subsequently susceptible to excoriation (i.e., abrasion or tearing of the skin surface) caused by shear forces from rubbing, scratching, and other trauma. These shear forces can cause blisters and compromise long-term skin integrity as a result of the repetitive reopening of the wound. Partial-thickness and full-thickness burns usually lead to uneven pigmentation of the healed scar. Deep partial- and full-thickness burns have a greater potential for thick, hypertrophic scar and contracture formation because of the prolonged healing period. This is especially true if a burn converts from partial-thickness to full-thickness because of infection or repeated trauma. Most full-thickness wounds require surgical intervention or skin grafting for wound closure. Skin graft donor sites usually heal in the same manner that superficial partial-thickness burns heal, with less scarring but uneven pigmentation. In all three of the case studies, the majority of the patients' burns were deep partial-thickness injuries but with serious posthealing scar development.

TABLE **42-1** **Burn Wound Characteristics**

Burn Depth	Common Causes	Tissue Depth	Clinical Findings	Healing Time	Scar Potential
Superficial (first-degree)	Sunburn, brief flash burns, brief exposure to hot liquids or chemicals	Superficial epidermis	Erythema, dry, no blisters, short-term moderate pain	3-7 days	No potential for hypertrophic scar or contractures
Superficial partial-thickness (superficial second-degree) and donor sites	Severe sunburn or radiation burns, prolonged exposure to hot liquids, brief contact with hot metal objects	Epidermis, upper dermis	Erythema, wet, blisters; significant pain	Less than 2 weeks	Minimal potential for hypertrophy or contractures if healing is not delayed by secondary infection or further trauma
Deep partial-thickness (deep second-degree)	Flames; firm or prolonged contact with hot metal objects; prolonged contact with hot, viscous liquids	Epidermis and much of dermis nonviable, but survival of skin appendages from which skin may regenerate	Erythema; larger, usually broken blisters on skin with hair; on glabrous skin of palms and soles of feet, large, possibly intact blisters over beefy red dermis; severe pain to even light touch	Greater than 2 weeks, may convert to full thickness with onset of infection	High potential for hypertrophic scarring and contractures across joints, web spaces, and facial contours; high risk for boutonnière deformities if dorsal fingers involved
Full-thickness (third-degree)	Extreme heat or prolonged exposure to heat, hot objects, or chemicals for extended periods	Epidermis and dermis: nonviable skin appendages and nerve endings	Pale, nonblanching, dry, coagulated capillaries possible; no sensation to light touch except at deep partial-thickness borders	Surgical intervention required for wound closure in larger areas; possible for smaller areas to heal in from borders over extended period of time	Extremely high potential for hypertrophic scarring or contractures depending on the method used for wound closure
Subdermal	Electrical burns and severe long-duration burns (e.g., house fires, entrapment in or under a burning motor vehicle or hot exhaust system, smoking in bed or alcohol- related burns)	Full-thickness burn with damage to underlying tissues	Possible charring of nonviable surface, or, with exposed fat, possible presence of small external wounds on tendons, muscles; with electrical injuries, possibility for small external wounds with significant secondary subdermal tissue loss and peripheral nerve damage	Requires surgical intervention for wound closure; may require amputation or significant reconstruction	Similar to full-thickness burns except when amputation removes the burn site

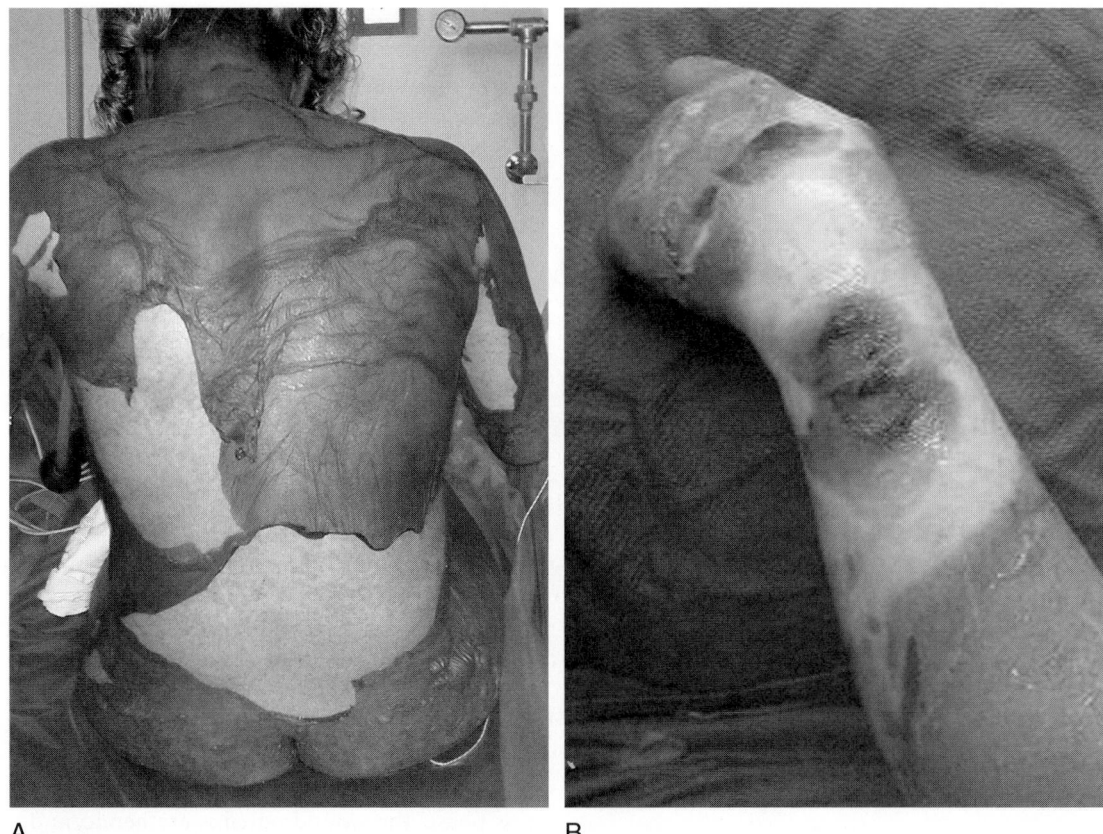

A   B

Figure 42-2 **A,** Superficial partial-thickness burns are wet, painful, with peeling epidermal blisters. **B,** The different depths of burns can be seen in the "target" appearance of this electrical burn with superficial partial-thickness at the periphery, deep-partial and parchment-white full thickness leading into charred subdermal burns in the center. (Courtesy of Edward Vergara, Gainesville, FL.)

PERCENT TOTAL BODY SURFACE AREA INVOLVED

The extent of a burn is classified as a percentage of the total body surface area (%TBSA) burned. The two most common methods for estimating %TBSA are the "rule of nines" and the Lund and Browder chart.[83] The rule of nines divides the body surface into areas comprising 9%, or multiples of 9%, with the perineum making up the final 1%. The head and neck area is 9%, each upper extremity (UE) is 9%, each lower extremity (LE) is 18%, and the front and back of the trunk are each 18%. The rule of nines is simple to use; however, it applies only to adults. Body proportions vary with children depending on their age, especially in the head and legs[17] (Figure 42-3). The Lund and Browder chart[54] provides a more accurate estimate of the total body surface area[68] and is used in most burn centers. This chart assigns a percentage of surface area to body segments (Figure 42-4), with adjusted calculations for different age groups. For smaller %TBSA injuries, the therapist can obtain a quick, rough estimate using the size of the patient's palm (i.e., the hand excluding the fingers) to equal approximately 1% of the individual's total body surface area. Steven's burns included his right arm and hand (8%), upper chest and back (13%), anterior neck (1%), and face (3%), totaling 25% TBSA. Kenjii's burns included both circumferential arms and dorsal hands (9% each) and his face and neck (5%), totaling 23% TBSA. Neither Steven's nor Kenjii's TBSA estimates included their skin graft donor sites, which added to their total injured body surface area.

SEVERITY OF INJURY

The %TBSA and depth of burn are primary indicators of the severity of injury. A burned surface area of 20% or greater was once the determining criterion for admission to a burn intensive care unit. However, depending on the patient's age and pre-injury health, partial- or full-thickness burn wounds of less than 10% TBSA can be considered serious enough to warrant admission.

A survey of 28 burn centers found that the average size of a burn injury on admission is about 14% TBSA. Since 1965,

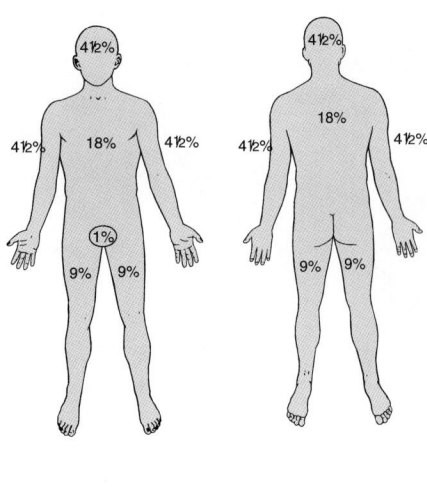

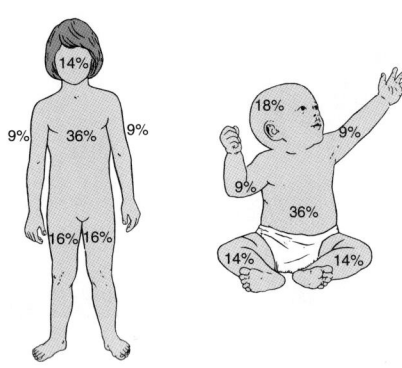

Figure 42-3   Rule of nines. Proportions for adult/adolescent, child, and infant. Note the relatively greater surface area of the head and slightly lesser surface area of the lower extremities in young children when compared with adults. (From *Mosby's medical, nursing & allied health dictionary*, ed 6, St Louis, 2002, Mosby.)

the number of people admitted to burn centers with burns of 10% TBSA or less has more than doubled, from 26% to 54% of total admissions, whereas large burns (60% TBSA or greater) have declined from 10% to less than 4% of total admissions. This trend reflects both a decrease in the number of large burn injuries and an increased recognition of the importance of specialized burn care experience and facilities for treating significant burn injuries, regardless of size.

Deep partial- and full-thickness burns of greater than 30% TBSA usually require a prolonged period to achieve wound closure and intensive rehabilitation for functional recovery. However, even burn injuries with limited %TBSA may be classified as severe and warrant admission to a burn center. Because of the complexity of medical treatment and rehabilitation, the severity of an injury is greater if there is an inhalation injury or if deep partial- or full-thickness burns involve the hands, face, or perineum.[93]

PHASES OF WOUND HEALING

Wound healing takes place in three overlapping phases: the inflammatory phase, the proliferation phase, and the maturation phase.

INFLAMMATORY PHASE

The inflammatory phase usually lasts 3 to 10 days after onset. During this phase, there is a vascular and cellular response, with neutrophils and monocytes migrating to the wound to attack bacteria, debride the wound, and initiate the healing process. The wound typically is painful, warm, and erythematous (red) and develops edema.

PROLIFERATION PHASE

The proliferation phase begins by the third day after the injury and lasts until the wound heals. It is during this phase that revascularization, reepithelialization, and contraction of the burn wound take place. Endothelial cells bud at the end of capillaries, causing them to grow and creating a vascular bed for new skin growth. Epithelial cells migrate over the vascular bed to form a new skin layer. Fibroblasts deposit collagen fibers, which contract to reduce wound size. During this phase, the wound remains erythemic, and raised, rigid scars may develop. The tensile strength of the newly healed scars is poor and easily excoriated or injured.

MATURATION PHASE

The maturation phase usually begins by the third week after initial healing and may last 2 or more years after the initial burn injury or the date of the last reconstructive surgical procedure performed. During this phase, the fibroblasts leave and collagen remodeling takes place. Erythema fades, and the scar softens and flattens. Tensile strength of the scars increases but never recovers more than 80% of the original tensile strength of the unburned skin.

SCAR FORMATION

After initial healing, most burn wounds have an erythematous, flat appearance. As the healing process continues, the wound's appearance may change as a result of scar hypertrophy and contraction. The long-term quality of a mature burn scar can be affected by numerous factors, some of which occur during the early phases of burn care.[37,51] The amount of time needed to achieve wound closure is a strong determinant. Bacterial infections in the wound increase the inflammatory response, which can delay wound healing and contribute to scar formation.[44] However, any factor that delays healing will increase the potential for scarring.

Hypertrophic scars are thick, rigid, erythematous scars that become apparent 6 to 8 weeks after wound closure.[1]

Modified Lund and Browder Chart

Area	Age (Years)					% Partial-thickness	% Full-thickness	% Total
	0-1	1-4	5-9	10-15	Adult			
Head	19	17	13	10	7			
Neck	2	2	2	2	2			
Ant. trunk	13	13	13	13	13			
Post. trunk	13	13	13	13	13			
R. buttock	2.5	2.5	2.5	2.5	2.5			
L. buttock	2.5	2.5	2.5	2.5	2.5			
Genitalia	1	1	1	1	1			
R. U. arm	4	4	4	4	4			
L. U. arm	4	4	4	4	4			
R. L. arm	3	3	3	3	3			
L. L. arm	3	3	3	3	3			
R. hand	2.5	2.5	2.5	2.5	2.5			
L. hand	2.5	2.5	2.5	2.5	2.5			
R. thigh	5.5	6.5	8.5	8.5	9.5			
L. thigh	5.5	6.5	8.5	8.5	9.5			
R. leg	5	5	5.5	6	7			
L. leg	5	5	5.5	6	7			
R. foot	3.5	3.5	3.5	3.5	3.5			
L. foot	3.5	3.5	3.5	3.5	3.5			
					Total			

Figure 42-4   Modified Lund and Browder chart. Burns size can be determined most accurately in children by using the Lund and Browder chart, which accounts for changes in the size of body parts that occur with growth. (Modified from Lund CC, Browder NC: The estimation of areas of burns, *Surg Gynecol Obstet* 79:352, 1944.)

Histologically, these immature scars have increased vascularity, fibroblasts, myofibroblasts, mast cells, and collagen fibers arranged in whorls or nodules that make the scar raised and rigid.[8,67] Biochemical investigations have discovered increased synthesis of collagen fibers and connective tissue in hypertrophic scars. As hypertrophic scars mature, capillaries, fibroblasts, and myofibroblasts decrease significantly, collagen fibers relax into parallel bands, and the scar becomes flatter and more pliable, especially if the scar is treated with compression throughout the maturation phase. The time needed for scars to mature differs markedly among individuals depending on genetics (as with Kenjii, who has a genetic predisposition to hypertrophic scarring), the age of the patient, the location and depth of the original burn wound, the presence of chronic inflammation, wound contamination, and other factors that have been reported to influence hypertrophic scarring.[23,84] Superficial burns that heal in less than 2 weeks generally will not form a hypertrophic scar. Deeper burns that take longer than 2 weeks

to heal have a greater potential to form hypertrophic scars. Although most hypertrophic scars mature in 12 to 24 months,[51] excessive scar formation, such as a **keloid scar,** may take up to 3 years to mature (Figure 42-5). All three subjects in the case studies were of different age groups and ethnic/genetic background and had different occupational therapy (OT) interventions. Nevertheless, they all experienced serious scarring as a result of their burns.

All scars initially have an increased vascularity and a red appearance. Scars that remain erythematous for longer than 2 months are more likely to develop into hypertrophic scars. They become progressively firmer and thicker, rising above the original surface level of the skin. There is a marked increase in production of fibroblasts, myofibroblasts, collagen, and interstitial material, all with contractile properties that help draw together the borders of a wound but can also cause scar tightness. Pain and skin tightness cause most patients to become less active. These patients prefer to rest in a flexed, adducted position for comfort. This allows the new

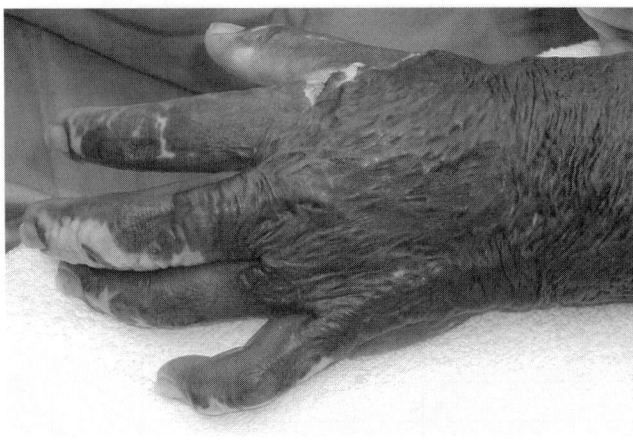
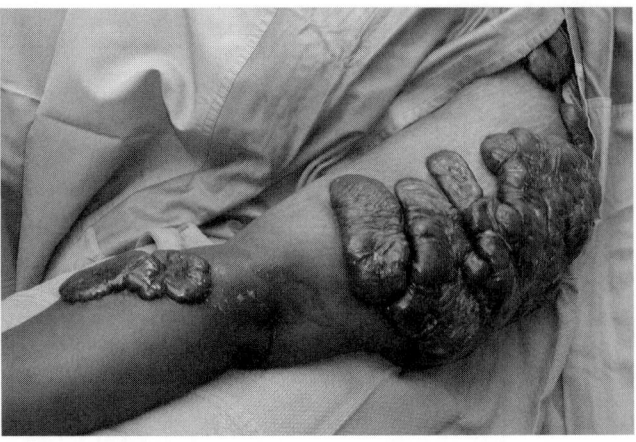

A   B

Figure 42-5 **A,** Thick hypertrophic dorsal hand and wrist scars impair the flexibility necessary for functional grasp. **B,** Severe keloid scars usually require surgical removal and aggressive compression therapy to help prevent recurrence. (Courtesy of Edward Vergara, Gainesville, FL.)

collagen fibers in the wound to link and fuse together in the contracted position. The fibers become progressively more compact, coiling up into the whorls and nodules that give the scar surface the textured appearance that often leads to disfigurement. If the scar extends over one or more joints, the progressive tightness leads to a scar contracture and loss of active motion. Fortunately, collagen linkage is less stable in new scars, and the restructuring of an immature hypertrophic scar contracture can be influenced by sustained mechanical forces such as proper positioning, exercise, splinting, and compression.

INITIAL MEDICAL MANAGEMENT

FLUID RESUSCITATION AND EDEMA

Immediately after a burn injury, during the inflammatory phase, the permeability of blood vessels increases. This causes rapid leakage of protein-rich intravascular fluid into surrounding extravascular tissues.[62] In larger burns, extensive intravascular fluid loss can result in hypovolemia or burn shock because of decreased plasma and blood volumes with reduced cardiac output.[34] Fluid resuscitation with an intravenous fluid such as lactated Ringer's solution is essential for promptly replacing venous fluid and electrolytes. The fluid volume required is determined by various formulas, such as the Parkland and modified Brook formulas,[5] and is based on the extent of the burn and the weight of the patient. The rate of fluid infusion is determined by monitoring pulse rate, central venous pressure, hematocrit, and urinary output.

The lymphatic system, which normally carries away excess tissue fluid, often becomes overloaded, causing subcutaneous edema. With circumferential full-thickness burns, loss of

burned skin elasticity combined with increased edema can cause **compartment syndrome,** a condition in which the interstitial pressure becomes severe enough to compress blood vessels, tendons, or nerves, which could result in secondary tissue damage. When blood vessels are compressed, **ischemia,** or restriction of circulation, could result in tissue death to the areas of compromised circulation or even the entire distal extremity.[24] Tight burned tissue can also restrict chest expansion during respiration. **Escharotomy,** or incision through the necrotic burned tissue, is performed to release the binding effect of the tight eschar (adherent dead tissue that forms on skin with deep partial- or full-thickness burns), relieve the interstitial pressure, and restore distal circulation (Figure 42-6, *A*). In deeper wounds, an incision down to and through the muscle fascia, or fasciotomy, may be required to achieve adequate pressure relief (Figure 42-6, *B*).

RESPIRATORY MANAGEMENT

A smoke inhalation injury is a common secondary diagnosis with thermal injury and can significantly increase mortality in patients with burn injuries. When the face is burned, when the burn was caused by a fire in an enclosed space, or when there is other objective evidence of a possible inhalation injury, bronchoscopy, arterial blood gas readings, and chest X-ray examinations are used to confirm the diagnosis. Intubation and mechanical ventilatory support may be required in addition to vigorous respiratory therapy. A tracheostomy is performed if the airway is difficult to maintain or if ventilatory support is prolonged.[94] This procedure, which involves surgical incision through the trachea and relocation of the ventilation tube to the neck, is more comfortable for the patient, allows for oral care, and helps

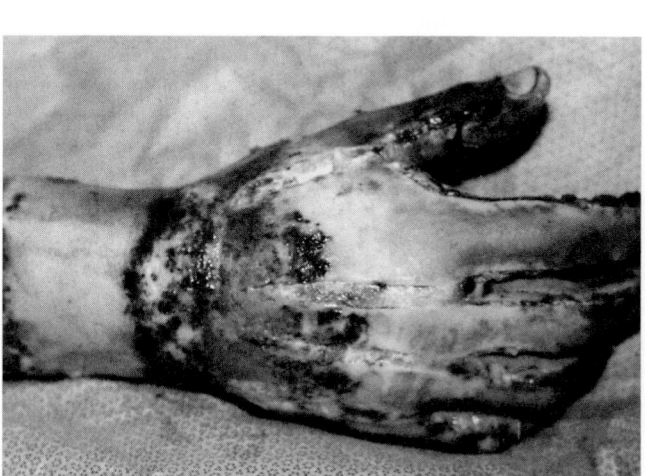
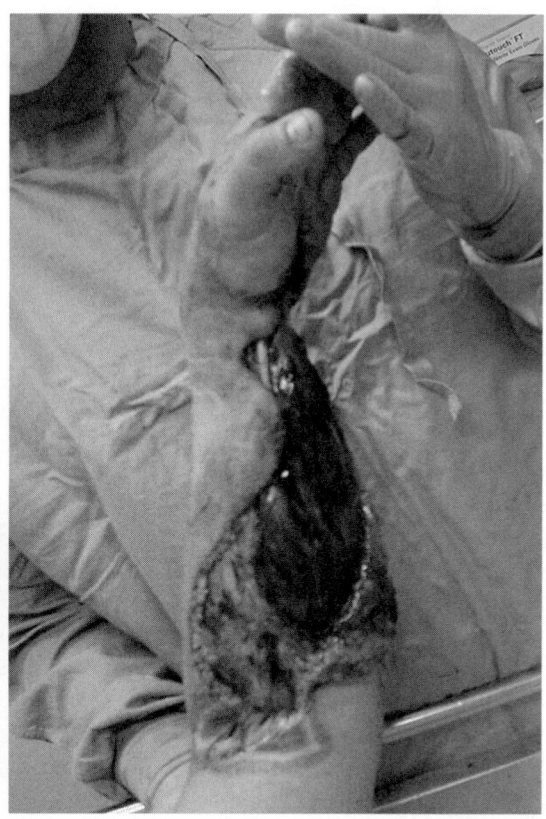

A   B

Figure 42-6 **A,** Escharotomies performed on the dorsal surface of a hand with full-thickness burns. **B,** Electrical injury requiring an escharotomy/faciotomy, which will allow the forearm muscle belly to expand and prevent loss of blood flow to the hand. Note the distances between the edges of the incisions and the exposed tendon. (Courtesy of Edward Vergara, Gainesville, FL.)

prevent permanent damage to the larynx or vocal cords, which may occur with extended oral intubation.

WOUND CARE AND INFECTION CONTROL

After a patent airway and fluid resuscitation have been established, attention is directed to wound care. A burn wound is dynamic, and improper treatment (e.g., lack of proper wound-care, edema formation, lack of resuscitation) may actually increase the size and depth of the wound.

Wound treatment may involve a combination of surgical and nonsurgical treatments.[43] Nonsurgical treatment involves the use of products to promote healing in a partial-thickness wound. These products are usually in the form of topical antibiotics, biological dressings, and nonbiological skin substitute dressings.

Topical Antibiotics

Topical antimicrobial agents have been shown to decrease wound-related infections and morbidity in burn wounds when used appropriately. The goal of topical antimicrobial therapy is to control microbial colonization, thus preventing development of invasive infections.

There are an ever-increasing variety of topical antimicrobials used for burn wound care.[92] Neomycin/polymixin B/bacitracin antibiotic ointments are often used for facial and superficial burns. The ointment is applied, and the burn wound is left open. Silver sulfadiazine (Silvadene® cream, Hoechst/Marion Roussel, Inc.) is a commonly used antibacterial cream applied heavily over larger burns and held in place with layers of gauze dressings. Mafenide acetate (Sulfamylon®, Bertex Pharmaceuticals) and papain/urea (Accuzyme®) topical solution and creams are used to loosen eschar and facilitate debridement through enzymatic digestion.[65] Mafenide HCl cream is hyperosmolar and can be painful when applied to larger areas. However, it is often used on the ears, where it can penetrate eschar to prevent chondritis, the inflammation of the ear cartilage. Mupirocin (Bactroban®, SmithKline Beecham) is an agent used to treat wounds infected with methicillin-resistant *Staphylococcus aureus* (MRSA) and *Staphlococcus pyogenes*.[86] A modified Dakin's solution is a highly diluted, neutral antiseptic solution consisting of 0.025% sodium hypochlorite (household bleach [NaOCl]) and boric acid to neutralize the alkalinity. Its solvent action on dead cells hastens the separation of eschar from living tissue. Nystatin (Nilstat®, Lederle Laboratories) may be used in combination with other topical agents against fungal infections caused by secondary immunosuppression. These fungal infections are often caused by long-term antibacterial use, usually originate in the gastrointestinal tract, and can be life-threatening if they infect large surface area burns or invade the bloodstream.

With the improved resuscitation measures for burns developed in the 1960s, infection became the predominant cause of morbidity and mortality. Silver salts and other chemically active silver compounds have been used in various forms because of their potent antimicrobial properties and ability to reduce burn wound infection. These substances have included silver colloidal solution, which was later replaced by silver nitrate solution, and silver sulfadiazine. Silver sulfadiazine is a water-soluble cream that is usually applied twice a day to the wound surface, as opposed to the continuous soaking required of silver nitrate. Over the past 40 years, silver sulfadiazine has become the preferred option for silver therapy antimicrobial treatment of burns.[22]

Recent major technological advances have resulted in the ability to crystallize silver in a nanocrystal form, which can release pure silver onto a wound surface in large quantities. This silver nanocrystalline delivery system is a three-ply dressing that may consist of an inner rayon/polyester core between two layers of silver-coated mesh.[10,98] The ionic silver and silver radicals are released in high concentrations when exposed to water. A layer between the wound and silver membrane maintains moisture for healing and decreases exudate formation.[22] The dressings, applied directly to the wound surface, promote healing by stimulating cellular de-differentiation, followed by cellular proliferation. The dressings also have antibacterial, antifungal, and analgesic properties. These dressings have been found to be highly microbicidal against aerobic and anaerobic bacteria (including antibiotic-resistant strains), yeasts, and filamentous fungi[10] and can remain active and in place for up to 7 days instead of having to be changed every 12 to 24 hours.

Biological Dressings

Biological dressings serve as temporary coverings to close a wound, prevent contamination, reduce fluid loss, and alleviate pain.[57] Theoretically, biologic products may deliver growth factors to a wound as well.

Traditional biological adressings, such as xenografts (porcine skin) and allografts (human cadaver skin), are still widely used in burn care. Although allograft is generally used with full-thickness burns, it has compared favorably in studies with silver sulfadiazine in partial-thickness burns, almost doubling the number of patients healed at 21 days (76% versus 40%).[50,51] Similar results have been seen when xenograft was used on partial-thickness burns.[53] Xenografts may adhere to the superficial surface film of partial-thickness burns and facilitate eschar debridement. Human amnion has also been used as a biological burn dressing, especially in developing countries.[52]

Biosynthetic Products

Biosynthetic products have been widely used in burn care. Closure of wounds with these dressings may lead to less pain, faster skin regrowth, and therefore less scarring. They are used until the wound is healed over, usually in 10 to 14 days, then the dressing peels off.

Biobrane®, a biosynthetic skin substitute wound-dressing sheet (Bertek Pharmaceuticals, Morgantown, WV), has been used extensively. It is constructed of an outer silicone film (the epidermal analog) with a nylon fabric partially imbedded into the film collagen. The nylon components bind to the wound surface fibrin and collagen, resulting in the initial adherence (dermal analog). Small pores are present in the structure to allow for drainage of exudates and increase the permeability to topical antibiotics. However, if used improperly, the dressing can enclose dead tissue in the wound, providing a medium for bacterial overgrowth and invasive wound infection.[55]

TransCyte®, a human fibroblast–derived temporary skin substitute (Smith & Nephew, Largo, FL) has also been used on mid-dermal burns after debridement and has shown faster healing with less pain in two prospective trials.[56,59]

Hydrotherapy

Once the patient's condition is sufficiently stable, hydrotherapy is usually performed at least once a day to remove loose debris and "stale" topical antibiotics. It provides a thorough cleansing of both the wound and the uninvolved areas. This is usually accomplished by placing the patient on a "shower trolley" covered with a sterile plastic sheet and washing and showering the wounds for 20 to 30 minutes. This nonsubmersive showering method of hydrotherapy has become the preferred method of cleansing burn wounds to prevent cross contamination of wounds between patients, replacing the traditional whirlpool form of hydrotherapy.[2,27] Fresh topical agents are then reapplied to delay colonization of organisms and reduce bacterial counts in the burn wounds.[34] During hydrotherapy the patient has usually received some form of analgesics and is unencumbered by dressings. Therefore, hydrotherapy provides an excellent opportunity for the therapist to perform assessments and range of motion (ROM) exercises.

Sepsis

Burn wound colonization begins at the moment of injury, with gram-negative organisms replacing normal bacterial flora. Wound cultures and biopsies are performed to monitor this growth when there are signs of possible serious infection. A severe infection can result in sepsis, in which the infection spreads from the original site through the bloodstream, a condition known as *septicemia*. Septicemia initiates a systemic response that affects the flow of blood to the vital organs. Bacterial infections are the most common source of sepsis but can also result from fungal, parasitic, and mycobacterial infections, especially if the patient is immunocompromised. Broad-spectrum antibiotic therapy is usually initiated. However, if host defenses continue to be overwhelmed, the bacterial by-products or endotoxins accumulate in the bloodstream, a condition known as *toxemia,* which eventually leads to septic shock, a cardiovascular response that impedes blood flow to the organ systems and generalized circulatory collapse. Septic shock may be characterized by ischemia, diminished urine output, tachycardia, hypotension, tachypnea, hypothermia, disorientation, and coma. Septicemia and septic shock often require multisystem supportive measures for recovery, such as use of cardiovascular medications, hemodialysis, and mechanical ventilation.

Surgical Intervention

Although all burn wounds are treated with some type of topical antibacterial agent, when the depth and extent of the wound require more than 2 weeks for healing, surgical intervention is indicated to decrease burn morbidity and mortality. Surgical treatment for burns usually consists of excision of the nonviable burned tissue, or eschar, and placement of biological or synthetic skin grafts.

There are essentially three types of biological grafts. A **xenograft,** or heterograft, is processed pigskin. A homograft, or **allograft,** is processed human cadaver skin. These are used as biological dressings to provide temporary wound coverage and pain relief. An **autograft** is a permanent surgical transplantation of the upper layers or split-thickness skin graft (STSG) of the person's own skin with that taken from an unburned donor site. The STSG is applied to the clean, excised tissues of the burn wound graft site. Skin grafts placed as a sheet have superior appearance and quality, but to cover large surface areas rapidly, the graft may be "meshed" in order to allow a single sheet of skin to be expanded to cover a larger surface area (Figure 42-7). The meshed graft attaches to the burn surface in the same manner as a sheet graft, but the interstices, or openings in the meshed skin, must heal by re-epithelializing over granulation tissue. This leads to more scarring and a permanent mesh pattern on the skin.

Now that the size of a survivable burn has increased, the amount of available donor sites for autografting has conversely decreased. For this reason, alternatives to autografts have been developed. Examples of such alternatives are epidermal cultured skin substitutes[33] and cultured epidermal autograft (CEA).[7,18] A wound may be limited in size, but the defect may be so deep that bone or tendon survival is at risk. In these instances, split-thickness skin graft adherence is difficult to obtain, and a full-thickness skin graft or microvascular skin flap may be indicated.

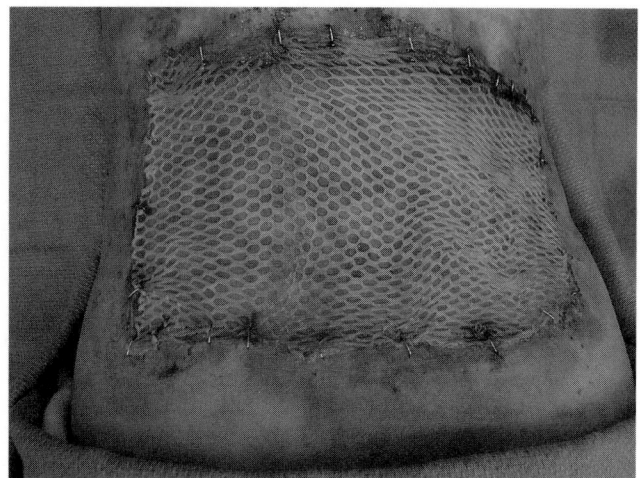

Figure 42-7   Meshed skin grafts expand to cover a larger surface area but heal with more scarring, leaving a permanent mesh pattern on the skin. (Courtesy of Edward Vergara, Gainesville, FL.)

Vacuum-Assisted Closure

Negative pressure wound therapy, also known as *vacuum-assisted closure (VAC),* is a treatment in which a sealed dressing and controlled negative pressure are used to provide evacuation of wound fluid, stimulate growth of granulation tissue, and decrease bacterial colonization, especially in deeper wounds.[58] Since their introduction, VAC (VAC® Therapy™; KCI Concepts, San Antonio, TX) dressings have been used in a number of surgical specialties, including burn care. By assisting in the debridement of necrotic tissue and the removal of soluble inflammatory substances, VAC therapy reduces the number of dressing changes required and shortens the time interval between debridement and wound closure. This has been shown to facilitate the growth of granulation tissue even in deep wounds, making graft uptake adherence more successful.[79]

Using a VAC device to secure a skin graft prevents fluid collection beneath the graft, ensures full contact between the bed and the transplanted skin, and distributes an even amount of pressure over the entire surface, regardless of the irregularity of the recipient bed. However, movement of the recipient surface could compromise the graft if it is not immobilized by proper positioning or splinting.[81] During treatment the therapist must be attentive to the VAC dressings and avoid activities with the patient that could disrupt the seal around the dressing and cause an air leak.

Nutrition

Adequate nutrition is essential during wound healing because the metabolic rate of the patient with a burn injury greatly increases with corresponding increases in protein, vitamin, mineral, and calorie needs.[34,56] Protein is especially important for wound healing and must be provided in substantial amounts. Nutritional requirements are calculated on the basis of the %TBSA and the patient's admission weight.

Calorie counts and the patient's weight are closely monitored to ensure adequate nutrition. If the patient is unable to meet individual requirements through the diet, high-protein and calorie supplements are given either orally or through a nasogastric or gastric tube. If the gastrointestinal tract is compromised, intravenous hyperalimentation is frequently necessary with severe burns of extensive %TBSA. This solution contains sufficient amino acids, glucose, fatty acids, electrolytes, vitamins, and minerals to sustain life, maintain normal growth and development, and foster needed tissue repair. It is often infused through a central line catheter into the superior vena cava of the heart. Later, as wound closure is achieved and normal feeding resumes, nutritional demands decrease and the individual's eating habits must be normalized to prevent excessive weight gain.

ASSOCIATED PROBLEMS AND COMPLICATIONS

STRESS

Traumatic events associated with severe burns include natural and intentional disasters such as tornadoes, lightning, house fires, motor vehicle accidents, acts of war or terrorism, physical or sexual assault, and the sudden death of loved ones or friends. Burn treatment further traumatizes the patient with associated painful medical procedures (e.g., wound care, limb amputations, multiple surgical procedures, and painful therapies). Mental health professionals are increasing their understanding of the factors associated with increased psychiatric risk and the ways in which burn patients, especially children, cope with the stress and pain triggered by traumatic events. Responses to major stress often include reliving the event, avoidance, and hypervigilance; these responses may continue long after the precipitating event. Post-traumatic stress disorder (PTSD) is a common psychiatric disorder after traumatic experiences, including physical injuries such as burns.[25,26] Mood, anxiety, sleep, conduct, learning, and attention problems are often comorbid conditions, especially in children. Treatment involves pain assessment followed by specific interventions, such as pain management, psychiatric consultation, and crisis intervention initiated promptly after the traumatic event. Intervention should also involve the burn survivor's family.[15]

PAIN

Pain Assessment

Some of the most commonly used pain assessment tools include the visual analog, color scales, word and faces scales, and the adjective scale. A 1998 study indicates that patients prefer the faces and color scales over commonly used visual analog and adjective scales.[32] Pain levels should be assessed during a quiet time and again immediately after any painful activity.

Pain Management

Because pain has adverse physiological and emotional effects, pain management is an important factor for better outcomes. Developmentally appropriate and culturally sensitive pain assessment, pain relief, and reevaluation are essential in treatment. Pain control guidelines should address both background and procedural pain and associated anxiety. The occupational therapist should assist nursing staff with focused surveillance of burn pain and its successful treatment.[60]

Pharmacological treatment is primary, strengthened by new concepts from neurobiology, clinical science, and the introduction of more effective drugs offering fewer adverse side effects and decreased toxicity. Opiates remain the most common form of analgesic therapy for patients with burns, but because these patients require increased opiate dosages, optimal relief of burn pain can be difficult. Alternative pain control methods include acetaminophen as a useful analgesic in minor burns. Nonsteroidal antiinflammatory drugs (NSAIDs) and benzodiazepines are often combined with opiates. Antidepressants appear to enhance opiate-induced analgesia, whereas anticonvulsants are useful in the treatment of sympathetically maintained pain following burns. Ketamine has been extensively used during burn dressing changes, but its psychological side effects, such as delirium and hallucinations, have limited its use.[64]

Nonpharmacological intervention using various hypnotic, cognitive, behavioral, and sensory treatment methods is becoming more accepted. Transcutaneous electrical nerve stimulation (TENS), topical and systemic local anesthetics, and psychological techniques are also useful adjuncts.[8] Hypnosis may be a very useful alternative when opioid pain medication proves to be dangerous or ineffective; it has received strong anecdotal support from case reports.[63] The mechanisms behind hypnotic analgesia for burn pain are poorly understood; however, patients with burn injuries are more receptive to hypnosis than the general population, possibly because of increased motivation, dissociation, and regressive behaviors.[66] Other methods of nonpharmaceutical pain reduction may be helpful. Relaxation techniques that may be of benefit include progressive relaxation, breathing exercises, guided imagery, aromatherapy, music therapy, and teaching of individualized coping strategies. As with hypnosis, distraction and relaxation techniques work best with alert, motivated patients.[61]

Patients with a severe burn injury naturally respond to pain by resisting painful motions or activities. Behavioral regression is also a normal response among most children (and many adults). When this regression occurs, the therapist should be supportive, continually explaining beforehand what needs to be done and why in terms that the patient can understand.

Most patients are usually more interested in whether the procedure will hurt and how long it will last than in lengthy explanations or technical information. Coordinating treatments with scheduled pain medications is often helpful and highly recommended, especially if active participation is necessary. The therapist should be aware of and use techniques to minimize preventable pain (e.g., applying adequate vascular support to the lower extremities before standing or ambulation). The therapist must also inform the nursing staff about any noted side effects from pain medication as well as the observed effectiveness of the currently used pain management regimen. The need for short-term breakthrough pain relief should be coordinated with nursing staff to reduce discomfort and stress during intensive therapy procedures. If a patient's anxiety or pain is disproportionate to the treatment, antianxiety medication may be indicated both to relieve anxiety and to increase the effectiveness of pain medication. Time limits on painful treatment sessions should be predetermined with all patients who are cognizant and capable of participation. The therapist should consistently adhere to these time limits to foster trust and a sense of control for the patient. By reducing the patient's anxiety, the therapist reduces the fear factor that can exacerbate perceived pain.[71] As the wound heals, the amount of narcotic analgesia is gradually decreased, and patients usually require minimal pain medication by discharge.

PSYCHOSOCIAL FACTORS

After a burn injury, there is a potential for psychological reactions, including depression; withdrawal reactions caused by disfigurement; behavioral regression; and anxiety over the ability to resume work, family, community, and leisure roles.[30] The way in which a person copes with burn trauma is strongly influenced by his or her psychological status before the injury and whether the injury was a result of arson, assault, or a suicide attempt. The psychological ramifications can include anxiety, depression, regression, increased hostility, and existential crisis.[61] In the case of permanent loss of function and deformity, the patient may experience severe grief as a result of decreased physical abilities, changes in personal appearance and identity, loss of vocation, or loss of loved ones who were killed in the same accident. In the case of facial disfigurement and amputations, the patent's previous support system may also be reduced or lost as a result of abandonment by friends or significant others who cannot adjust to the physical changes in the patient.

Whether the permanent loss is social or physical, the patient may need to move through stages of grief similar to the five stages of grief of patients with a terminal diagnosis as described by Dr. Kubler-Ross in her book *On Death and Dying*.[48] The stages include the following:

- *Denial and isolation:* "I can't believe this happened to me ... it will be okay ... just go away!"
- *Anger:* The patient may express anger toward others, self, or the circumstances and be belligerent and uncooperative.

- *Bargaining:* Typically, this is the stage of procrastination (e.g., "I'll exercise tomorrow"). Children and teenagers are particularly adept at procrastination because they do not always understand the long-range effects of the burns.
- *Depression:* The patient grieves for loss of lifestyle and personal appearance and may experience guilt about surviving when a loved one did not.
- *Acceptance:* The patient learns to accept a new body image, physical and social limitations, and other losses. At this stage, it is important to help the patient focus on remaining abilities, develop new skills, and expand or replace social support systems.

If the patient does not reach the stage of acceptance, the rehabilitation process could be severely impaired. Providing emotional support and education and helping the patient develop coping mechanisms and self-direction can promote the psychological adjustment of patients with burn injuries. However, a severe burn injury occasionally results in a reassessment of personal values and relationships or a renewed appreciation of life. The complex interactions among premorbid personality style, extent of injury, and social and environmental contexts should be considered when determining how patients will adjust psychologically to a severe burn injury.[61]

 OT PRACTICE NOTE

OT intervention must address the psychological aspects from the initial assessment and onset of OT intervention and continue through discharge from OT services at the end of the rehabilitation phase. Even after discharge from rehabilitation, the client may continue to need psychosocial OT intervention as he or she attempts to become actively involved in the community, resume social activities and relationships, and return or enter the paid work force.

BURN REHABILITATION

THE TEAM

Successful care and rehabilitation of burn survivors require a multidisciplinary team approach that begins immediately after the patient's admission to the hospital and continues through and beyond hospitalization.[5,74] Ideally, the burn care team includes physicians, nurses, physical and occupational therapists, respiratory therapists, nutritionists, social workers, psychiatrists and psychologists, speech and language pathologists, orthotists and prosthetists, child care and recreational therapists, pastoral caregivers or clergy, interpreters or cultural support personnel, and vocational counselors. The most important members of the team, however, are the client and the client's family or support system.[51,78,82]

OT PRACTICE NOTES

All healthcare professionals must continue to update their knowledge and professional competencies, keeping abreast of the rapidly changing treatments and therapies available for treating burn patients.[82] Recommended ways to continue professional development include the following:

- Review of professional journals such as *Journal of Burn Care and Rehabilitation, Burns, Journal of Wound Care, Journal of Trauma,* and *Journal of Burns.*
- Obtain membership in burn care associations such as the American Burn Association and the International Society of Burn Injuries.
- Attend local, regional, and national association meetings. Visit regional burn centers to confer with other burn therapists.
- Visit online websites of professional burn associations, and participate in online discussions with other burn care professionals.

GOALS OF REHABILITATION

The entire burn team is involved in some aspect of burn rehabilitation, whether for providing verbal support, preparing the patient for self-care tasks, reinforcing the importance of active motion, or providing patient education. The long-term goals of OT are quite similar to the long-term goals of the entire burn team. Although specific goals may be the responsibility of various team members, everyone's efforts are focused on the same outcome. OT treatment goals should therefore be compatible with all other treatment regimens and established in collaboration with the patient, family, and the entire rehabilitation team. Inherent in this concept is the need for close communication and cooperation of all burn team members. Role delineation between different disciplines, especially OT and physical therapy, differs among burn care facilities and may be determined by insurance reimbursement rather than by traditional roles or the specialized skills of the individual therapist. Therefore, it is especially important that all disciplines work closely together with ongoing communication, so that patients benefit from the skills and viewpoints of all areas of specialization. Occupational, physical, and speech therapists who specialize in burn rehabilitation increasingly use co-treatments that promote independence with both mobility and activities of daily living (ADLs).

PHASES OF RECOVERY

Rehabilitation management of burn survivors can be divided into three overlapping phases to aid in categorizing and determining effective intervention goals. These phases of recovery are the acute-care phase, the surgical and postoperative phase, and the inpatient and outpatient rehabilitation phase.[51]

The acute-care phase is usually the first 72 hours after a major burn injury. However, if the burn is superficial partial thickness and heals spontaneously in less than 2 weeks without surgical intervention, the time from injury until epithelial healing is also considered as an acute-care phase.[73]

The surgical and postoperative phase follows the acute phase and continues for varying lengths of time, depending on the size of the burn injury and presence of associated medical complications. During this period, vulnerability to wound infection, sepsis, and septic shock is especially great, and medical treatment is focused on promoting healing and minimizing infection.

The rehabilitation phase covers both inpatient and outpatient care and can extend for an indeterminate length of time. This phase follows the postgrafting period, when the patient is medically stable and most open wounds are healed. The quality of wound healing, scar formation, and need for aggressive rehabilitation make this the most challenging phase for burn patients, their families, and their therapists.

Acute-Care Phase

During the acute-care phase, medical management is of utmost importance for survival of the patient, and the goal of OT is primarily preventive. As the patient recovers and wound closure progresses, the nature of OT also changes, with treatment directed at restoring function. Initially, however, when the wounds are deep partial or full thickness, the acute-care rehabilitation goals are as follows:

- Provide cognitive reorientation and psychological support.
- Reduce edema.
- Prevent loss of joint and skin mobility.
- Prevent loss of strength and activity tolerance.
- Promote occupational performance, such as independence with self-care skills.
- Provide patient and caregiver education.

Surgical and Postoperative Phase

Rehabilitation goals during the surgical and postoperative phase are focused on preserving or enhancing performance skills and patterns while supporting surgical objectives. Excision and grafting procedures usually require periods of immobilization of the areas treated to allow for graft adherence. The preferred position and length of immobilization will vary by physician prerogative and burn center protocol, with the average period of immobilization being between 2 and 7 days.[14,35,39,54,80] The most advantageous postoperative position usually maintains the grafted area in the position that maximizes the surface area of the grafted site. For example, a hand with a dorsal burn should be splinted with the wrist in neutral or flexed position, the metacarpophalangeal joints flexed, and the thumb abducted and in opposition to the fifth digit to stretch the dorsal surface of the hand before application of the skin grafted.

During this phase the goals of therapy include the following:

- Promote cognitive awareness by providing orientation activities when necessary, and continue psychological support.
- Protect and preserve graft and donor sites by fabricating splints and establishing positioning techniques that support the surgeon's postoperative care orders.
- Prevent muscular atrophy and loss of activity tolerance, and reduce thrombophlebitis risk by providing exercise for areas that are not immobilized.
- Increase self-care independence by teaching alternative techniques and providing adaptive equipment as needed.
- Educate and reassure the patient and family members regarding this phase of recovery.

Rehabilitation Phase

The third phase of recovery is the rehabilitation phase, which begins as wound closure occurs. Individuals with large %TBSA burns frequently enter this phase needing further surgery. However, the majority of their wounds are closed, and scar maturation is commencing. The focus of intervention during this phase is on maximizing self-care, promoting physical and emotional independence, and managing scar formation to prevent deformity and contracture formation. Patient and family education is especially important for developing competence in wound care and therapy programs in preparation for discharge.

The rehabilitation phase extends past hospital discharge and continues until maturation of all burn wounds and surgical sites is complete. Before discharge from the hospital, emphasis is on independence and education. Once the client is home, emotional support and intervention must continue to help sustain the client's confidence, self-esteem, and motivation, qualities that the client needs to cope with the physical, social, and emotional consequences of a severe burn injury.

Intervention goals for this phase can be exhaustive, considering the potentially disabling effects of burn scar.[51] Moreover, it is also important for the therapist to incorporate the patient's personal goals from the very beginning of the rehabilitation process.

Treatment goals for the rehabilitation phase are expanded to include the following:

- Continue to provide psychological support as the patient progresses toward physical and emotional independence.
- Improve joint mobility and reduce contractures by using correct positioning, sustained passive stretching exercises, and splinting as needed.
- Restore muscle strength, coordination, and activity tolerance.
- Initiate a compression therapy and scar management program using vascular support garments, custom scar compression garments, and pressure adapters to minimize scar hypertrophy, contractures, and disfigurement.[51]
- Promote independent self-care skills, including appropriate positioning, exercise, and skin care. Provide instruction and

opportunities to practice instrumental activities of daily living (IADLs), including vocational and home-care activities.
- Continue to provide instruction regarding scar development, including potential sensory and cosmetic changes, scar management techniques, and related safety precautions.
- Guide the implementation of a postdischarge plan that supports resumption of school, work, social, and leisure occupations.

Occupational Therapy Evaluation

Although medical status issues are a primary concern during acute care, whenever possible the occupational therapist should complete an initial evaluation within the first 24 to 48 hours after hospital admission. The burn etiology, medical history, and any secondary diagnoses are obtained from the medical record and team. The wounds are then visually assessed to determine the extent and depth of injury. Any areas affecting future occupational performance and context are noted and documented.

Whenever possible, both the client and the family are interviewed to establish rapport and to obtain the history of the client's previous occupational performance. This history should include pre-injury body structures and body functions (i.e., hand dominance, previous injuries, and performance-limiting illnesses or conditions) and specific information regarding past performance skills and patterns, daily routines, and activities (including professional, educational, and domestic responsibilities). Obtaining data concerning pre-injury personality traits and psychological status is equally important. With this information, the therapist can monitor for changes in the client's behavior and cognition functioning and can choose the most appropriate interactive approach to encourage the client's involvement in goal setting and the rehabilitation process. In the case of a severe burn requiring intubation and mechanical ventilation, this information must be obtained from family members and significant others to verify and supplement what the patient may relay nonverbally.

OT PRACTICE NOTE

Ideally, the client's history of occupational performance would be obtained before assessment of current client factors.
However, the acuity of the injury, time constraints, and the need to coordinate physical assessment with pain medications, wound dressing changes, and other medical procedures may supersede completion of a detailed performance history.

Only after a baseline assessment of pre-injury and current performance skills is ascertained can an intervention plan be established.[51] Involved and uninvolved areas should be evaluated for joint mobility, strength, sensation, and functional use. However, before beginning this evaluation, the therapist should explain the purpose of OT and what the client should expect during the assessment, including the potential for discomfort. Pre-assessment instruction and ongoing encouragement help reassure patients and decrease anxiety, allowing clients to perform at their best. Emphasis is placed on the ultimate long-term goal of resuming engagement in meaningful occupation and participation in life contexts.

The initial evaluation should address all areas of potential OT intervention. They include assessment of wound severity, presence and severity of edema, passive range of motion (PROM) and active range of motion (AROM), muscle strength, gross and fine motor coordination, changes in sensation, and level of cognitive awareness. Ideally, the initial OT wound, ROM, strength, and sensory assessment should take place during a dressing change or hydrotherapy, when the depth and exact location of the burns can be directly examined and accurately documented.

During the initial evaluation, distinctions are made among superficial, superficial-partial, and deep partial-thickness burns, as well as full-thickness burns, on the basis of appearance and presence of sensation. The therapist must view the wounds as soon as possible after the injury, before the development of burn eschar. **Eschar** causes deep partial-thickness burns to closely resemble full-thickness burns and makes accurate evaluation of depth difficult. Attention should also be directed to burned joint surface areas and the presence of any circumferential burns. An active or active assistive ROM assessment should be performed without dressings to evaluate joint mobility and general strength before significant edema develops or restrictive dressings are applied.

Instructing the client regarding the types of movements and the number of repetitions expected while gently guiding the individual through the specific motion can help ensure achievement of full range. When possible, a goniometer should be used for assessing ROM to accurately document baseline deficits and future changes in recorded measurements. If pain, edema, tight eschar, or bulky dressings limit full ROM, such information should also be documented. Preexisting conditions that may alter expected AROM should be investigated during the patient and family interview. Although AROM is preferred, PROM should be measured if a client is unresponsive or unable to sufficiently move the extremity. When using PROM, care must be taken not to apply excessive force, especially with older clients who have degenerative joint disease or small children with hypermobile joints.

With deeper partial or full-thickness dorsal hand burns, boutonnière precautions should be initiated until the integrity of the hand's extensor hood mechanisms can be verified. Boutonnière precautions involve the avoidance of composite active or passive flexion of the fingers. Instead, isolated metacarpophalangeal (MP) flexion is combined with interphalangeal (IP) joint extension to prevent stress and possible damage to a compromised extensor tendon mechanism. All passive proximal interphalangeal (PIP) flexion is avoided, and protective splinting is promptly initiated to maintain the PIP joints in extension.

A gross sensory screening that includes all sensory distribution areas should be performed without dressings. This is especially important in the case of electrical injury or history of long-standing diabetes in which peripheral neuropathies may be present.

If the client possessed normal functional muscle strength before injury, an initial test of gross muscle strength may not be needed if the AROM assessment revealed adequate strength to work against gravity. Manual muscle testing of major muscle groups is indicated if the burn resulted from an electrical contact injury, if the presence of severe edema might cause a compartment syndrome, or if other musculoskeletal or neurological injuries are suspected.[97] If the hand is unburned or if the burn is superficial partial thickness, a dynamometer and pinch gauge provide objective baseline measurements of grip and pinch strength.

ADL assessment begins by interviewing the client or the family to obtain the client's pre-injury level of physical, cognitive, and social performance skills and patterns. When the burn injury is severe, the ADL assessment is postponed until the client is medically stable and able to participate in the pursuit of more advanced occupational goals. Clients with less severe burns and those who are not mechanically ventilated should be assessed for basic ADL skills, such as the ability to feed oneself, basic grooming skills, and donning and doffing of hospital gowns. Any compensatory actions or awkward movements used to complete the activity should be noted. Any abnormal patterns should be investigated and discussed to determine whether they were present before the burn injury.

After completion of an initial evaluation (Table 42-2), short- and long-term goals should be established with the client's collaboration. The client's previous context and lifestyle, personal long-term goals, and current priorities should be taken into account when establishing OT intervention goals. All short-term goals should be specific and realistic and have an established time frame for completion. After goals are agreed upon, the intervention plan can be formulated. The OT intervention plan should be practical and should complement and support the goals of the other team members.

Two fundamental principles must be kept in mind when working in burn rehabilitation: (1) The main factor hindering postburn functional recovery is the formation of scar contractures and hypertrophic scarring, and (2) severe scars and contractures are often preventable with prompt therapeutic intervention.[72] Therefore, most burn rehabilitation intervention techniques and objectives are directed at prevention as well as restoration.

OCCUPATIONAL THERAPY INTERVENTION

ACUTE CARE PHASE
Preventive Positioning

The purpose of preventive positioning is to reduce edema and to maintain involved extremities in an antideformity position (Table 42-3). Proper positioning is critical because

TABLE **42-2** **Burn Rehabilitation Evaluation Components**

Initial	Inpatient Rehabilitation	Outpatient Rehabilitation
Burn cause	Graft adherence	
%TBSA, depth of burn	Skin or scar condition	Skin or scar condition
Area(s) involved	Contracture concerns	Compression garment fit
Age, hand dominance	Edema (if present)	Volumetrics if needed
Functional status	ADL performance level	ADL performance level
Occupation	Work skills	Work skills
ROM and strength	Active and passive ROM, TAM	Active and passive ROM, TAM
Mobility and activity tolerance	Strength and activity tolerance	Strength and activity tolerance
Developmental level (child)	Developmental level (child)	Developmental level (child)
Psychological status	Psychological status	Psychological status
Social support	Social support	Social support
Leisure activities	Leisure activities	Leisure activities
	Compression garment needs	Compression garment needs
	Home management	Home management
		Home care understanding
		Return to work capacity
		Return to school potential and need for reentry program

ADLs, Activities of daily living; *ROM*, range of motion; *TAM*, total active motion; *TBSA*, total body surface area.

TABLE **42-3** **Antideformity Positioning for Specific Body Areas Following Burn Injury**

Body Area	Antideformity Position	Equipment and Technique
Neck	Neutral to slight extension	No pillow; soft collar, neck conformer, or triple-component neck splint
Chest and abdomen	Trunk extension, shoulder retraction	Lower top of bed, towel roll beneath thoracic spine, clavicle straps
Axilla	Shoulder abduction 90 to 100 degrees	Armboards, airplane splint, clavicle straps, overhead traction
Elbow and forearm	Elbow extension, forearm neutral	Pillows, armboards, conformer splints, dynamic splints
Wrist and hand	Wrist extension 30 degrees, thumb abducted and extended, MP flexion 50 to 70 degrees, IP extension	Elevate with pillows, volar burn hand splint
Hip and thigh	Neutral extension, hips 10 to 15 degrees abduction	Trochanter rolls, pillow between knees, wedges
Knee and lower leg	Knee extension; anterior burn: slight flexion	Knee conformer, casts, elevation when sitting, dynamic splints
Ankle and foot	Neutral to 0 to 5 degrees dorsiflexion	Custom splint, cast, AFO
Ears and face	Prevent pressure	No pillows; headgear[32]

IP, Interphalangeal; *MP*, metacarpophalangeal; *AFO*, ankle-foot orthosis.

the position of greatest comfort for the patient is usually the position of contracture.[49,51] The typical position of comfort consists of adduction and flexion of the UEs, flexion of the hips and knees, and plantar flexion of the ankles. Toes are typically pulled dorsally. Acutely burned hands are held by edema in a dysfunctional position consisting of wrist flexion, MP extension, IP flexion, and thumb adduction. This position, often called the "claw hand" position, can lead to severe dysfunction if it is not prevented during active scar formation.

During the initial wound assessment, positioning needs are determined by evaluating the surface areas burned and the presence of edema, considering the posture the individual tends to assume, and assessing whether that posture would limit function if allowed. For example, if the burn injury involves the shoulder, chest, and axillae, the client's UEs should be elevated and positioned in approximately 90 degrees of shoulder abduction, 45 degrees of external rotation, and 60 degrees of horizontal adduction, using pillow inclines and arm boards or supporting the arms using

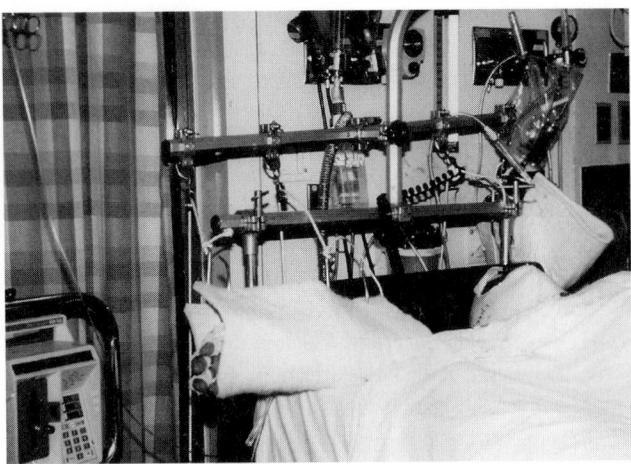

Figure 42-8 Shoulder positioning using slings and overhead traction rigging. Light-weight loads allow for active movement but encourage abduction as the patient relaxes.

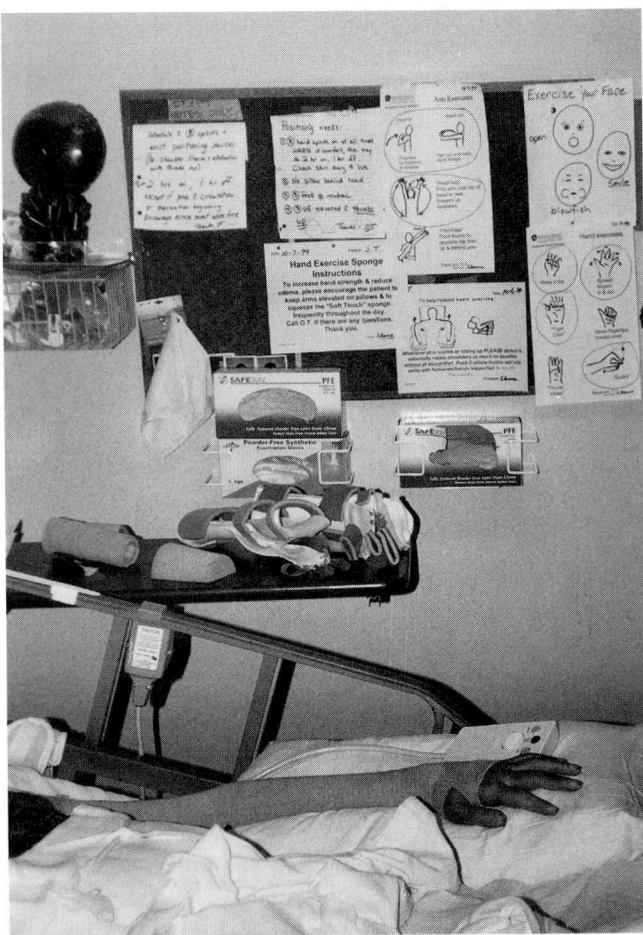

Figure 42-9 Highly visible bedside posters are beneficial as reminders to the client, staff, and visitors regarding positioning, exercises, and splinting instructions.

sheepskin slings suspended from an overhead traction rig (Figure 42-8). Achieving full shoulder flexion and abduction with frequent exercise and activity is critical to preventing axillary web contractures and subsequent loss of overhead reach as wound healing progresses. Once positioning needs are determined, illustrated guidelines should be posted at bedside so that the nursing staff and the team can assist with ongoing correct positioning (Figure 42-9).

After admission, positioning is initiated primarily to reduce edema formation.[70] Elevation of the entire extremity above heart level can reduce the severity of distal edema formation, especially when paired with AROM exercises. As edema decreases and wound closure progresses, positioning goals should be directed toward prevention of skin tightness over joint surfaces (see Table 42-3).[51]

Splinting

Splinting is initiated to maintain correct positioning and protect compromised tissues. It is *not* necessary for splints to be worn at all times to prevent contractures. When a splint is used during the acute phase, it is generally static in design and applied when at rest, with activity and exercise emphasized during waking hours. Volar hand splints are indicated if a burned hand has chronic edema, active motion is limited, or unsupervised movement is contraindicated because of deep dorsal burns or other traumatic injury. The typical volar hand splint provides approximately 30 degrees of wrist extension, 50 to 70 degrees of MP joint flexion, full IP joint extension, and combined thumb abduction and extension (Figure 42-10).[51] Elbows or knees should be splinted at approximately 5 degrees of flexion to avoid joint hyperextension and subsequent pain.

When checking the fit of any splint, the therapist should consider potential pressure points and ensure correct placement. Splints fabricated shortly after injury require daily

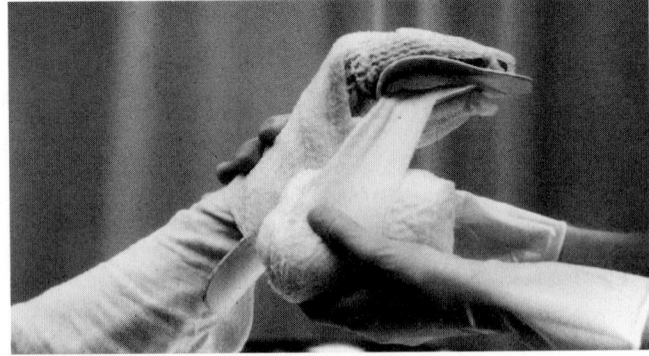

Figure 42-10 A postburn hand splint secured over compression bandages using a figure-8 pattern to apply the wraps.

assessment and may require alterations to accommodate any significant changes in edema. Hand splints are secured in place with a figure 8 wrap of gauze bandage and elastic wraps, with fingertips exposed so that circulation can be monitored. Folded 4×4-inch gauze sponges are used over the proximal phalanges and under the wrap to keep the fingers extended and secured in the splint. Detachable straps, although convenient for later use, may be inappropriate for use on acute burn splints because of infection control concerns and the potential for constriction during fluctuations in distal edema.

When there is a partial- or full-thickness burn to the external ear, protection is desirable to prevent further damage caused by pressure from pillows, dressings, or endotracheal tubing. An ear protection splint should be fitted at the earliest opportunity and worn until the external ear burns have healed. The splint can be fabricated of two thermoplastic ear cups or cushioned oxygen masks secured in place by a dressing or a three-point stabilizing strapping technique.[21, 46]

Activities of Daily Living

A client's ability to perform self-care is often limited during the acute-care phase because of his or her current medical condition. The need for artificial ventilation, multiple lines, catheters, and other supportive equipment interferes with independence with ADLs, and clients are dependent on nursing staff for self-care.

While the client is on the ventilator and orally intubated, ADL activity may be limited to self-suctioning of the oral cavity and, if there are no facial burns, basic facial hygiene. After extubation, oral care is often the next ADL attempted. When the client is medically cleared to take fluid or food by mouth, the occupational therapist should assess self-feeding abilities. Airway damage, accompanied by compromised speech and swallowing abilities, often results from an extended period of intubation or direct damage during the burn injury. In these cases, the occupational therapist works in concert with the speech pathologist on common goals that promote effective communication skills and independent self-feeding. Burns of the UEs and associated pain, dressings, and edema may interfere with self-feeding motions, making temporary use of adaptive equipment necessary. This equipment may include use of built-up or extended handles on utensils, a plate guard, or an insulated travel mug with a lid and straw. Hair grooming and shaving are other self-care activities to initiate early, depending on the client's strength and activity tolerance.

In the acute phase, ADL tasks should be selected that are valued by the client and have a high probability of success even though temporary adaptations may be necessary. Modifications to the client's environment, equipment, or previous performance patterns may be necessary to support independence. However, the eventual discontinuation of adaptive techniques and devices is a long-term goal of therapy and should be presented to the client as a sign of progress during the course of therapy. A goal, shared by both the client and therapist alike, should be independence with all ADLs, using previous performance patterns, completed within an appropriate length of time and with minimal adaptations.

Therapeutic Exercise and Activity Tolerance

Sitting tolerance, transfers, and ambulation activities are initiated as soon as the client is medically cleared to get out of bed and bear weight on his or her LEs. If the client has burns of the LEs, elastic wraps should be applied before the client sits up and the feet become dependent. A figure-eight pattern should be used from the base of the toes, over and including the heel, to at least the knees, and up to the groin as needed. When the client is sitting in a chair, the LEs should be kept elevated. Any time spent dangling the feet or static standing should be limited to prevent distal venous congestion and unnecessary discomfort.

In addition to functional activities, active exercise is a primary component in every burn treatment plan. Exercise techniques used during acute care are not unique to the injury.[51] Active, active-assisted, or passive exercises are used, depending on the client's condition. The focus of exercise in acute care is to preserve ROM and functional strength, build cardiopulmonary endurance, and decrease edema.

Strengthening activities are introduced into the acute-care intervention program as soon as the patient's condition allows. These activities range from simple active movement to resistive activities, as tolerated, to counteract the deconditioning effects of hospitalization.[52] Exercise after a severe burn injury was once thought to overstress an already hypermetabolic client. However, research and experience have shown that graded, progressive exercise is beneficial in acute burn recovery.[40]

Client Education

Although client education is the responsibility of all burn team members, the success of the OT intervention program depends on the client's recognition of long-term activity demands, contextual needs, and role responsibilities. Initial educational objectives should focus on developing an understanding of the stages of burn recovery, the need for and importance of independent activity and motion, and pain- and stress-management techniques. Meeting these goals promotes the motivation, compliance, and engagement in occupation that are so essential for successful treatment outcomes.[31]

SURGICAL AND POSTOPERATIVE PHASE

Positioning and Postoperative Splinting

Excision and grafting procedures usually require a period of postoperative immobilization to allow adherence and vascularization of the grafted skin.[21] It is beneficial for the occupational therapist to discuss postoperative positioning needs with the surgeon before surgery so that splints and positioning devices can be prefabricated and applied in the operating room immediately after the surgical procedure. A wide variety of materials and protocols are available. All have the common purposes of immobilizing the grafted area, preventing edema, and assisting wound healing.[73]

Postoperative positioning may follow standard positioning techniques or may be unique, designed exclusively for the specific surgical procedure. Although standard burn splints position the extremity in the antideformity position, preoperative or postoperative splints should hold the extremity in the position that promotes the greatest surface area for graft placement. For dorsal hand grafts, the wrist is positioned in neutral, the MP joints in flexion, and the thumb in abduction to maximize the dorsal grafted surface area. Another example is that in which an axillary advancement flap is performed; the shoulder is abducted only 45 degrees. Gaining prior knowledge of the surgical procedure and determining potential postoperative complications enable the therapist to establish effective positioning and splinting procedures.

Although postoperative immobilization is often achieved through the use of bulky restrictive dressings and standard positioning equipment, splints are often needed to maintain the position. Most splints are typically made using plaster bandages or thermoplastics (Figure 42-11). If a wet dressing will cover the graft site, a perforated or open-weave splinting material may be preferred to permit continuous drainage and prevent graft maceration.[21] In some instances, movement of adjacent joints may disrupt graft adherence even though the graft does not cover the joint surface. In these cases, the splint design should incorporate immobilization of those joints in a functional position. A postoperative thermoplastic splint generally can be made by using a drape-and-trim technique.[21] Most postoperative splints are molded into positions for temporary use and are discontinued once graft adherence is ensured. However, if the splints are made of thermoplastics, they can later be remolded into the antideformity position.

Therapeutic Exercise and Activity

Throughout the postoperative phase of care, active and resistive exercise of the uninvolved extremities should be

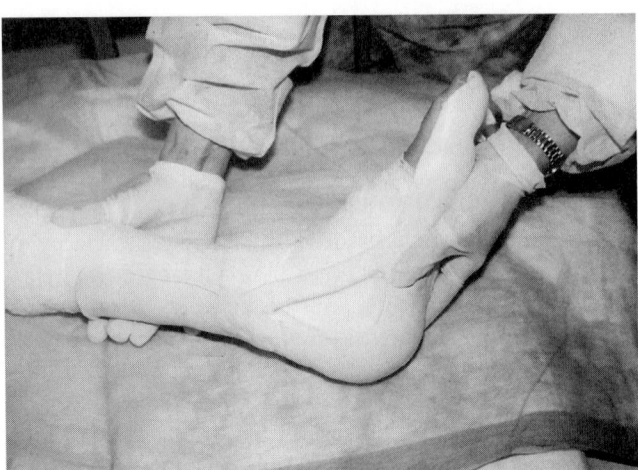

Figure 42-11 A thermoplastic total-contact ankle dorsiflexion splint to prevent a plantar flexion contracture.

continued when possible to prevent loss of ROM and strength. Immediately after excision and grafting procedures, exercises for adjacent body areas are usually discontinued for a short time. Although the time varies among burn centers, the average period of immobilization is 3 to 5 days for most STSGs and 7 to 10 days for cultured epithelium grafts.[14,31,39] Exercises can be resumed as soon as graft adherence is confirmed. Before resuming exercises, the occupational therapist should view the grafts and adjacent areas to determine graft integrity and whether there are any exposed tendons or compromised subcutaneous tissues.

Gentle active ROM is the treatment choice to avoid shearing of the new grafts. If the client exhibited normal ROM before surgery and was immobilized for only 3 to 5 days, baseline ROM should be expected within 3 days after resumption of activity. Active exercise of a body area with a donor site is generally permitted after 2 to 3 days if there is no active bleeding. Donor sites on the LEs are treated similarly to burns of the LEs; therefore, standard treatment involves elevation and wrapping with elastic bandage.

Ambulation following excision and grafting of the LEs is usually not resumed until 5 to 7 days after surgery. With the physician's consent, the client is encouraged and assisted to ambulate for short distances and then slowly increase the distance. Before ambulation, double elastic bandage wraps should be applied over a fluff gauze dressing to prevent graft shearing or vascular pooling. Use of an elastic bandage, elevation, and a stance that discourages static are particularly important for protecting grafts of the LEs. When the client is able to walk, exercise on a stationary cycle ergometer is beneficial for increasing activity tolerance.

Activities of Daily Living and Client Education

Self-care and leisure-promoting activities should be continued and increased in a way that is commensurate with the demands of the activity, the client's physical abilities, and the client's activity tolerance. Self-care is often difficult during this phase because of the immobilization positions necessary to ensure graft adherence. If an upper extremity is immobilized, creative ADL adaptations may be needed to allow clients continued involvement in their care and control over their environment. Although only temporary, simple techniques such as universal cuffs strapped over splints or extended-handle utensils help preserve newly reacquired independence and foster confidence and feelings of self-actualization. Continued psychosocial support and burn care education are also essential to insure understanding of postsurgical precautions and procedures.

REHABILITATION PHASE: INPATIENT

The rehabilitation phase generally begins when a severely burned patient no longer needs the intensive wound care provided on the burn unit. Most of the wounds are now closed, and the patient may move to a step-down unit or transfer to a rehabilitation setting. Here patients are expected to assume a more active role in establishing treatment goals, demonstrate more independence in their care, and fully participate in their therapy. An upgraded exercise program, a variety of self-help and rehabilitation equipment, and new techniques are introduced to help increase ROM, strength, activity tolerance, and independence with higher level ADLs and IADLs. Intervention and patient education focuses on work, recreation, and self-care skills necessary to help prepare clients for returning to normal daily activity routines, including the resumption of previous performance patterns and roles. Potential roadblocks to resuming participation in occupation in prior personal contexts, including community reentry concerns and psychological adjustments, are anticipated and addressed during this phase.

Reassessment and Intervention Goals

As wound closure occurs, scar formation develops, resulting in frequent reports from clients of increased skin tightness that restricts certain functional movements and inhibits completion of ADLs. Intervention techniques to counteract the effects of scar development include skin conditioning, scar massage, compression therapy, and therapeutic exercise preceded by slow, gentle sustained stretching.

During the inpatient rehabilitation phase, OT evaluation should emphasize a thorough ongoing assessment of performance skills. Active and passive goniometric measurements should be taken to document any limitations caused by joint restrictions or scar tightness. Joint-specific measurements can be used to document individual joint restriction, but if skin tightness affects several joints in the same extremity, the total active motion (TAM) measurements or the total passive motion (TPM) measurements of all the joints in combined movement pattern should be documented. If the injury is unilateral, measurements taken from the unaffected side can be used to establish normal values for the injured extremity. Muscle strength can be measured using manual muscle testing (MMT). However, when MMT is used, caution is required when the therapist applies resistance, so as not to shear newly healed skin. Other components of the evaluation should include muscular and cardiopulmonary endurance, performance of self-care and home management activities, skin integrity, presence of edema, and scar development that indicates the need for scar compression garments (see Table 42-2).

Treatment goals during inpatient rehabilitation are to increase ROM, strength, and activity tolerance to achieve independence with self-care; begin skin conditioning; aid psychological adjustment; and provide patient and caregiver education, including familiarizing the client with the care necessary for discharge from the hospital. Although these goals are continued and progressively increased during the outpatient rehabilitation phase, other goals are added as the client prepares for reintegration into the home and community.

Skin Conditioning

Skin conditioning techniques are used to improve scar integrity and durability against minor trauma caused by pressure or shearing forces of garments; decrease hypersensitivity; and moisturize dry, newly healed skin. These techniques should be used with any burned areas or surgical sites that took longer than 2 weeks to heal. Lubrication and massage with a water-based cream or lotion should be performed three to four times a day or whenever the skin feels excessively dry, tight, or itchy. This action provides needed lubrication for skin that is dry because of damaged sweat and sebaceous glands. Massage is beneficial for desensitizing well-healed but hypersensitive grafted areas or burn scars and for softening tight scar bands during sustained stretching exercises. When massaging a scar band, the therapist should be sure that the scar is fully stretched and premoisturized to reduce shearing forces and prevent splitting of immature or unstable, problematic scar tissue. Massage should be performed using a circular motion, with more pressure applied gradually as tolerated over time. Because of damaged or lost skin pigment, burn survivors are at a greater risk for sunburn. Precautions, including use of sunblock and avoidance of prolonged sun exposure, are taught before the client is discharged.

Compression Therapy

Compression therapy should be initiated early in the inpatient rehabilitation phase, as soon as most of the larger wounds are closed. Temporary interim pressure bandages or garments assist with general skin desensitization, edema control, and early scar compression. The type of compression chosen and the degree of compression gradient applied depend on how much pressure and shear force the client's newly healed skin can initially tolerate; both are upgraded as the integrity of the skin improves. The type of interim compression bandage or garments is chosen on the basis of the degree and consistency of pressure that it applies, the ease of application, and the potential for damage from shear forces during application.[12] Elastic bandage wraps, self-adherent elastic wraps, tubular elastic support bandages, presized elastic pressure garments, and commercial or custom-made elastic garments are all commonly employed (Figure 42-12).[4,59] Approximately 5 to 7 days after removal of postoperative dressings, temporary compression dressings or garments can usually be applied. Tubular elastic bandages, presized or ready-made temporary elastic garments, Spandex® "bicycle pants," and Isotoner®-style gloves can be worn over light dressings. When patients have small open areas requiring minimal gauze dressings, a standard knee- or thigh-high nylon stocking can be applied over the dressings before the donning of tubular bandages or garments to reduce shearing forces and prevent displacement of the dressings. Temporary compression dressings and garments are taken off only for bathing, dressing changes, skin care, and garment laundering.

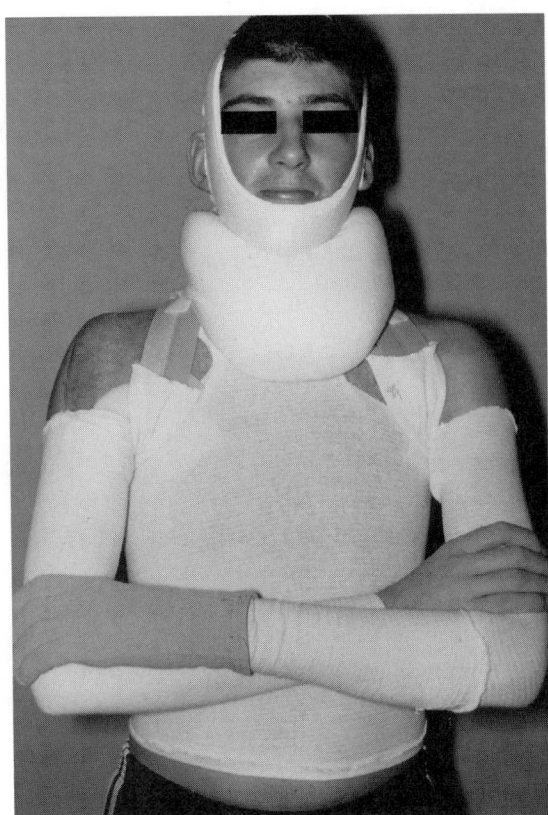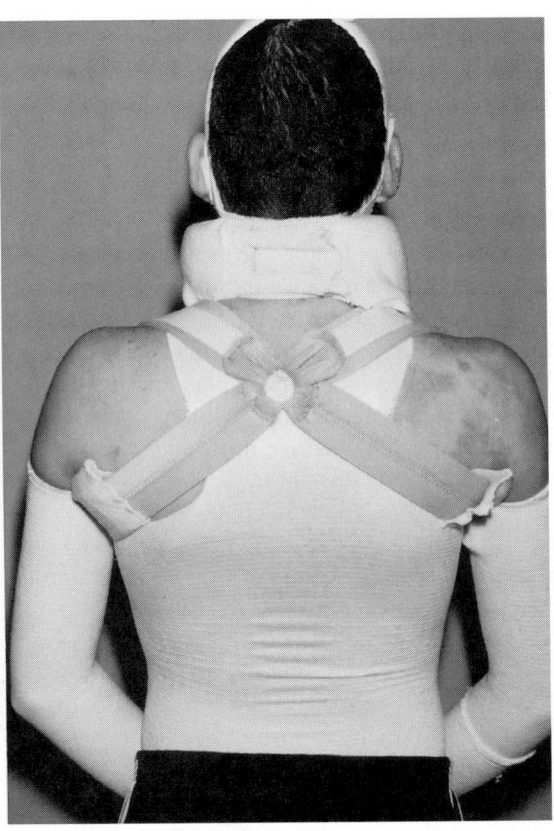

Figure 42-12 Early compression techniques: tubular elastic dressings, ready-made gloves and chin strap, custom-fabricated foam collar, and padded clavicular strap to preserve neck and axillary contours.

Independent donning and doffing of interim garments are incorporated into the client's ADL training.

Therapeutic Exercise and Activity

Newly healed skin tends to blister as a result of shearing forces or split as a result of overstretching, especially when the skin is dry. Every therapy session should therefore begin with massage of the scars using a moisturizing lotion to prepare the dry or tight skin for increased motion. Whenever possible, clients should learn to perform their own skin care independently before their scheduled therapy. Once the scars are moisturized and lubricated, stretching is performed to increase flexibility and fluidity of movement.[53] Stretches should be slow and sustained, and forceful dynamic stretch should be avoided, with attention given to the position of adjacent joints during the stretching motion. Massage with additional moisturizers during stretch exercises helps relieve itching and discomfort. Stretching in front of a mirror provides positive visual feedback for the patient and is helpful for correcting abnormal posturing.

AROM exercises, strengthening, and tasks to increase activity tolerance should follow stretching exercises. During the rehabilitation phase, emphasis is placed on flexibility exercises using complex motions that require movement of several joints simultaneously. An activity that requires hand manipulation skills while reaching overhead is an example of a complex motion for a burn injury that involves the shoulder, elbow, and hand. Most ADLs require complex motions, and exercise programs should emphasize not just individual joint ROM but combined joint mobility in functional patterns of movement (Figure 42-13).

For clients recovering from severe hand and UE burns, intervention activities may involve a variety of exercise and activity treatment media. Strengthening activities may involve the use of cuff weights or dumbbells, the WEST II,[96] or the BTE Work Simulator.[6] The Valpar Full Body ROM Sample provides full body range, as well as finger manipulation.[90] Activities for hand strengthening and coordination may include using exercise putty, hand manipulation boards, the BTE Work Simulator,[6] Valpar Work Samples,[90] and crafts; typing on a computer; dialing a cell phone; and playing cards or board games with visitors, as well as other activities.

Edema Management

During the rehabilitation phase, edema often continues because of decreased function, dependent positioning without adequate external compression, or circumferential scarring of the extremity with associated lymphatic damage. When edema is present, motion is limited and painful; if the edema becomes chronic, it may lead to fibrosis.[52] To treat

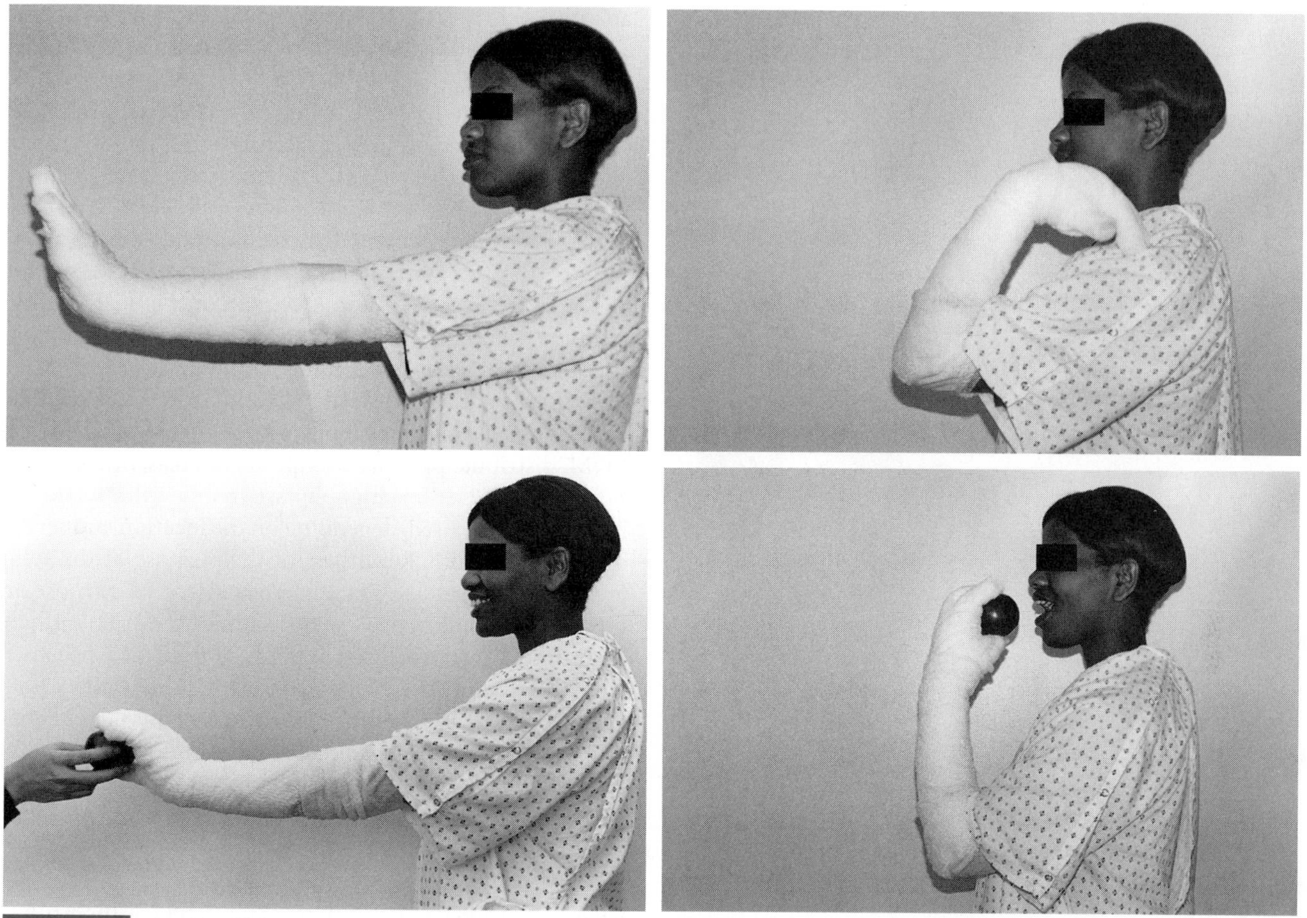

Figure 42-13 Combined joint motions used to obtain the greatest total active motion are often the same functional patterns of movement used when performing ADLs.

extremity edema, elevation, progressive compression, and activity are recommended.

Self-adherent elastic bandage material (Coban or Cowrap) is often used as an early form of compression dressing for the digits, hands, and feet. It is applied in a spiral fashion, from distal to proximal, overlapping the previous lap by one half overlap starting on each digit and continuing in this manner across the hand or foot and onto the wrist or ankle. Strips are also applied to each web space (Figure 42-14). The distal tips of digits are left open to monitor color, which should be rosy and not blanched or bluish. The rest of the extremity is wrapped with an elastic bandage or other forms of temporary compression garments. The wrapped hand should be used during ADLs and other functional motions and elevated just above heart level when the client is resting. For edema of the LEs, use of a double layer of elastic wraps when ambulating, elevation when resting, active ankle exercises, and avoidance of static standing are recommended. Intermittent compression pump therapy is often used to treat chronic edema of the distal extremities. Whenever compression therapy is used to treat edema of the hands or feet, before-and-after circumferential or volumetric

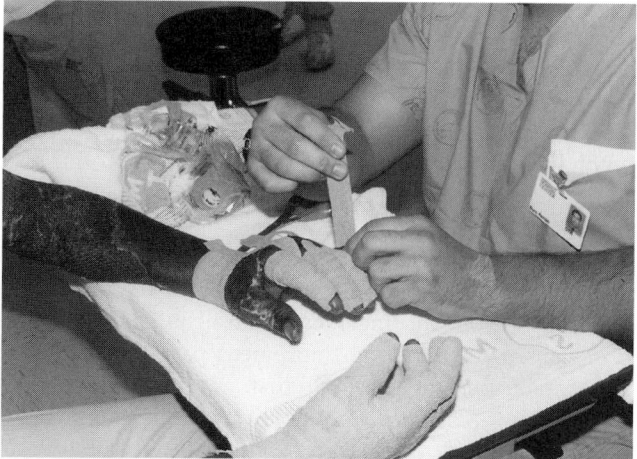

Figure 41-14 Application of self-adherent elastic wrap (such as Coban) to newly healed hands and feet provides external compression for treatment of edema and early scarring.

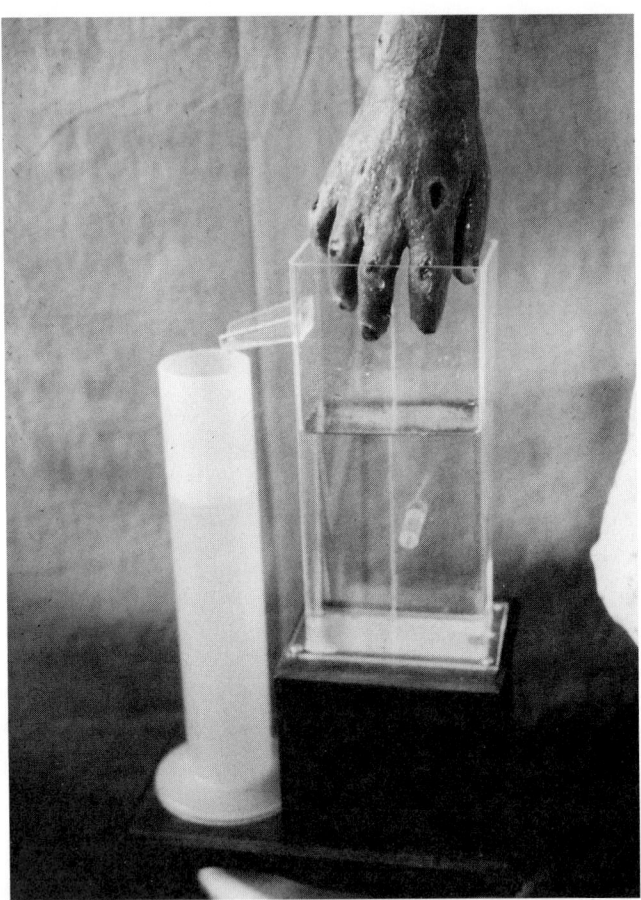

Figure 41-15   In the treatment of extremity edema, sequential circumferences and volumetric measurements are methods to monitor and document treatment efficacy.

measurements are recommended to monitor the effectiveness of the treatment (Figure 42-15).

Activities of Daily Living

As patients approach discharge from the hospital, the therapist must stress the importance of independent self-care. Eating, dressing, grooming, and bathing skills should be emphasized as part of the normal daily routine to increase independence and activity tolerance. When problems occur, the therapist must determine whether the dysfunction originates from a physical limitation, scar contracture, pain, edema, or an assumed abnormal postural reaction. Early identification of abnormal movements helps patients understand and relearn normal movement patterns before the abnormal patterns become habitual.

Practicing ADLs with personal care items and supplies from home helps to foster self-confidence regarding functional performance skills before hospital discharge. Clients with major burn injuries initially may require adaptations to support independence. However, when assessing the need for adaptive self-care, the therapist should differentiate between a physical limitation that can be rehabilitated and a permanent loss of function.

In addition to basic ADL and self-care tasks, IADL tasks, such as home management responsibilities, should be practiced before discharge. Fears of items associated with the injury, such as hot water, the stove, or an electric iron, can hinder functional recovery. For clients injured during a home activity, the therapist should arrange counseling, support, and practice of the skills or activity in the clinic. Prevention techniques taught as part of the inpatient treatment program should also be part of the home program.[99]

Splinting at this stage is used to limit or reverse potentially disabling or disfiguring contracture formations, increase ROM, distribute pressure over problem areas, or assist function (Figure 42-16). Static splints, dynamic splints, and casting[9,45,73] may be used, depending on the location and severity of the contracture. Regardless of the purpose of the splint, every effort should be made to ensure that its purpose and method of application are fully understood. Splinting at nighttime and during rest periods is preferred because it allows functional use of the extremity during waking hours and provides treatment of contractures while the client is unoccupied. However, splints must fit comfortably, and corrective splinting should not cause discomfort that interferes with the client's rest.

Client Education

Client and caregiver education becomes increasingly important during the predischarge phase to aid the transition from hospital to home. Increased understanding is needed in the areas of wound healing, the importance of preserving independence in ADLs and IADLs, the need for continued activity and exercise, the causes and effects of scar contracture, and scar management techniques and principles. Before discharge from the hospital or transfer to an inpatient rehabilitation facility, the client and family should receive a comprehensive home care education review (Table 42-4).[42,47] To reinforce learning, information should be presented and reinforced through a variety of methods, such as verbal instruction, printed handouts, demonstrations, and educational videos. Most important, opportunities should be provided for the client and caregivers to practice wound care, garment and splint application, and all exercises under staff supervision in the weeks preceding discharge. Only with a detailed understanding of home care techniques and potential outcomes can clients be expected to assume responsibility for their own care and recovery.[99]

REHABILITATION PHASE: OUTPATIENT

Reassessment

Reassessment procedures take on greater significance after discharge. ROM, strength, activity tolerance, ADLs and IADLs, and skin and scar status must be assessed frequently

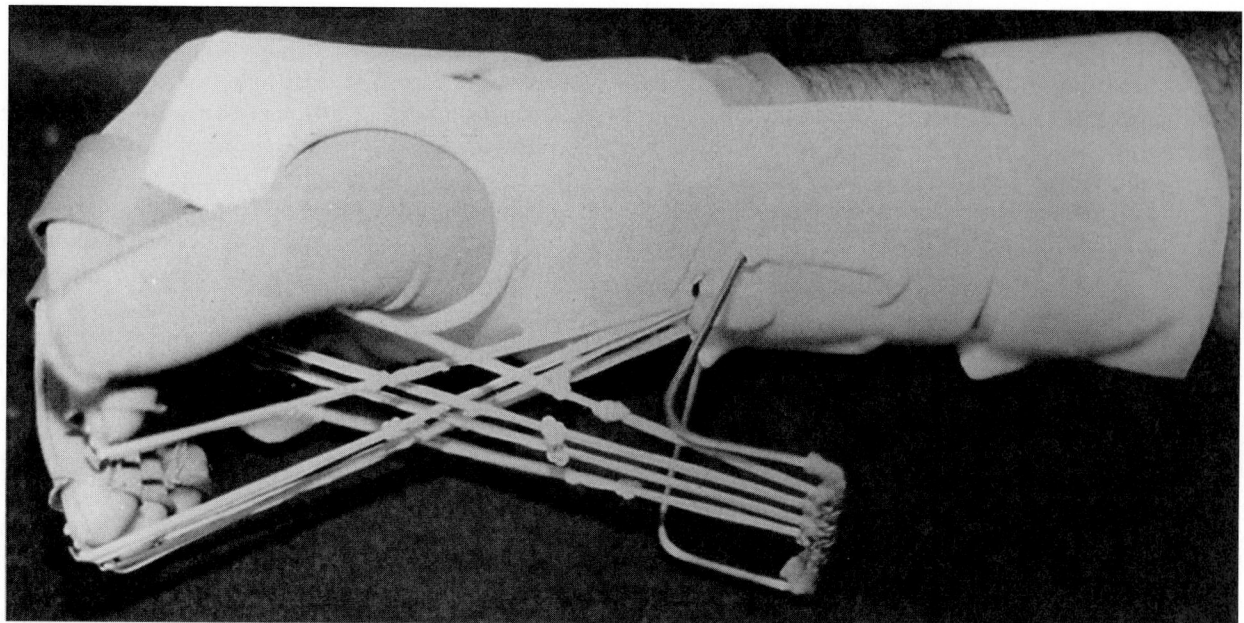

Figure 42-16 A bivalved dynamic splint is used over a presized intermediate scar compression glove. The splint is worn part time to facilitate increased MP and proximal interphalangeal joint flexion.

TABLE 42-4 **Home Program Outline**

Item	Information Needed
Wound care, positioning	Dressing change technique, precautions, elevation
Skin and scar care	Lubricant frequency, sun protection, and trauma precautions
Self-care	Techniques and equipment needed
Splints and orthotics	Donning techniques, schedule, precautions
*Pressure garments	Purpose, washing, reordering, donning techniques
Exercises	Frequency, techniques for specific areas

*Custom-made garments are available from Jobst Institute, Charlotte, NC (800) 221-7573; Barton Carey, Perrysburg, OH (800) 421-0444; Bio-Concepts, Phoenix, AZ (800) 421-5647; Medical-Z, Seattle, WA (800) 368-7478.

to ensure early identification of specific problem areas. In addition to these rehabilitation components, the effectiveness of compression garments, the fit and need for continuation of certain splints, home care activities, emotional coping skills, and resumption of engagement in preburn occupation to support participation in contexts or life situations should also be closely monitored.

Activity tolerance and work skills reassessment are indicated to help determine whether clients are ready to return to school or work or be referred for vocational rehabilitation. Driving evaluation and prevocational assessment, using simulated work activities or work sample testing, may also

be indicated for the more severely injured burn survivor. Vocational counseling and exploration should be undertaken in the later stages of recovery if residual dysfunction necessitates a change in work environment or vocational role.

Therapeutic Exercise and Activity

Inpatient rehabilitation techniques, equipment, and therapeutic activities continue to be appropriate during outpatient therapy. However, progressive grading of exercise and activity frequency, intensity, and duration is necessary to successfully regain or improve the client's strength, activity tolerance, and performance skills and patterns, as well as abilities in performance in areas of occupation. Sequencing the order of intervention activities is necessary to prevent injury, minimize client discomfort, and prevent excessive fatigue. Skin lubrication, massage, and stretching should precede progressive strengthening exercises and activities.[53] Before being discharged, clients should learn how to prepare for exercise and activity by performing their own skin lubrication, massage, and stretching. Doing their own pretreatment skin care and stretching will allow outpatients to maximize actual therapy time and develop habits that promote compliance with their home activities and independent exercise program.

Scar Management

A primary objective of most burn rehabilitation techniques is the prevention or treatment of hypertrophic scars and scar contractures. For effective treatment of scar problems, scar characteristics must be monitored to recognize when maturation occurs. Active scars have been described as erythematous, raised, and rigid.[42] As they mature, scars become less vascular in color, with flatter and more pliable contours and a smoother texture. **Scar maturation** usually takes from 12 to 18 months after injury, depending on the length of time that the original burn takes to heal. However, it is important to remember that each patient heals differently. Some scars mature in less than 1 year, whereas others may take more than 2 years.[74]

A rating scale has been designed that allows serial assessment of scar pigment, vascularity, pliability, and height.[87] Although the ratings are somewhat subjective and time consuming, the scale is a useful clinical tool. However, use of digital photography or high-quality Polaroid® photos is a time-efficient and objective method of documenting changes in scar appearance; copies of the images can be easily inserted into the medical record.

Wearing intermediate pressure garments prepares the skin for the later fitting of custom-made compression garments. Use of compression garments is indicated for all donor sites, graft sites, and burn wounds that take more than 2 weeks to heal spontaneously.[16,19,54] The occupational therapist is often responsible for the measurement, ordering, and fitting of these garments. The occupational therapist must often make special on-the-spot modifications during a clinic visit or fabricate underlying conformers to ensure uniform pressure. All custom-made garments are measured and ordered according to the specific instructions of the manufacturer. Most compression garment manufacturers offer a variety of design options, including special zippers or Velcro closures, custom inserts, and assorted colors.

Clients should be fitted with custom-made compression garments no later than 3 weeks after wound healing; otherwise, the wearing of interim garments is continued until custom garments can be applied. It may be necessary to order garments on a piecemeal basis because different areas of the client may be ready for compression treatment at different points in time. Custom-made compression garments are constructed to provide gradient pressure, starting with 35 mm Hg pressure distally (Figure 42-17). They should be worn 23 hours a day, being removed only for bathing, massage, skin care, or sexual activity. Face masks and gloves also may be removed for meals. Compression therapy should be applied to the burned area for approximately 12 to 18 months or until scar maturation is complete. Donor sites may also require compression garments, depending on the thickness of the donor skin taken and whether healing occurred in less than 2 weeks.

Once proper fit is established, it is recommended that the client possess a minimum of two sets of garments at any one time to allow for both around-the-clock compression therapy and laundering. Because of the elastic construction of the fabric, clients should hand wash the garments with mild soap and allow them to air dry unless otherwise advised by the manufacturer,. To prolong the life of the garments, washing machines, dryers, direct heat, strong detergents, or bleach should not be used. If they are properly cared for, most garments will last approximately 2 to 3 months before replacements are needed. Children may need replacements more frequently as a result of their growth and active lifestyle. Toddlers undergoing toilet training and incontinent adults may need extra garments and design options that make independent toileting easier. Adults employed indoors are able to return to work and previous activities without interference from the garments. However, some individuals who work outside in warmer climates may find compression garments too hot in summer months and may need to change their work setting until compression therapy is no longer required.

To be effective, compression garments must exert equal pressure over the entire burn surface area. Because of body contours, bony prominences, and postural adjustments, flexible inserts or pressure-adapting conformers are often needed under the garments to distribute the pressure more evenly. Areas commonly requiring pressure adapters are the supraclavicular region of the upper chest; the areas between and under the breasts of women or obese men; the nasolabial folds; the midface and chin; the areas between the scapulae and over the axillary folds, gluteal fold, and perineum; the web spaces of the hands and feet; and the perineum.

Pressure inserts and conformers are now made from a variety of materials; the choice is based on the area to be treated and the need for flexibility when applied. As with the garments, the fit of a conformer should be monitored at regular intervals for effectiveness and signs of deterioration and replaced as needed to maintain exact contouring. Silicone gel pads, Silastic® elastomer, Otoform-K®, Plastazote®, and Velfoam® are useful for hand scars. One-sixteenth-inch Aquaplast® and Silastic® elastomer work well on face scars; closed cell foams, prosthetic foam elastomer, silicone gel pads, Plastazote®, Otoform-K®, and Velfoam® are also useful for other body areas. Velfoam and silicone gel pads are also effective at the flexion

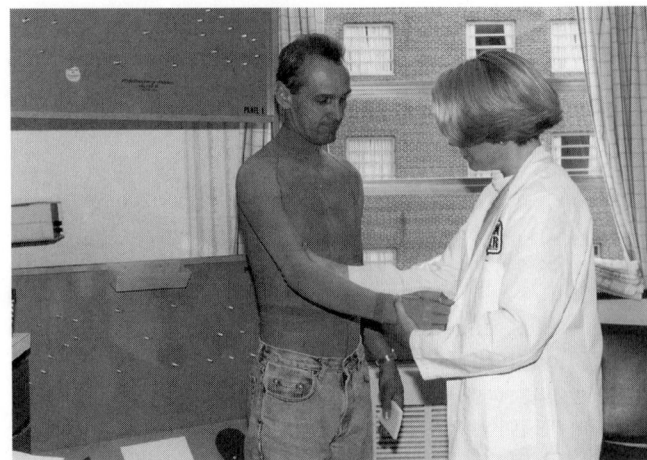

Figure 42-17   The fit of custom-made compression garments must be regularly reassessed to ensure adequate compression for effective scar management.

creases of the knees, elbows, and anterior ankle to equalize pressure and prevent discomfort during activities.

Activities of Daily Living

In addition to continued exercise, skin care, and scar management, the outpatient intervention plan should be directed at increasing independence with home care while also emphasizing resumption of past life roles and context. This includes returning to previous work, school, social, and leisure activities. Scar contracture is often the primary cause of dysfunction (Figure 42-18). Therefore activities performed in therapy should not only promote strength, activity tolerance, and functional ROM to counteract the effects of scarring but also preserve independence in performance of occupation related to clients' personal contexts and interests.

Community Reentry

Returning to school or work becomes a primary objective during outpatient rehabilitation. However, most recovering burn survivors are capable of resuming normal daily routines and performance patterns long before their scars completely mature.

Returning to previous community settings (e.g., school, work, and social settings) and becoming reacquainted with friends and co-workers can be a difficult process for burn survivors who have cosmetic disfigurement, loss of functional performance, or activity restrictions. A community reentry program should be implemented before the client's return to school or work. Correspondence sent to the community setting before the client's return helps to educate employers, teachers, and peers about burn injuries and what the client has experienced. This correspondence should explain the purpose of compression garments, splints, exercise, and skin care precautions. The goal of a reentry program is to reduce restrictions to the client's activities and ease the transition of returning to previous areas of occupation.[53]

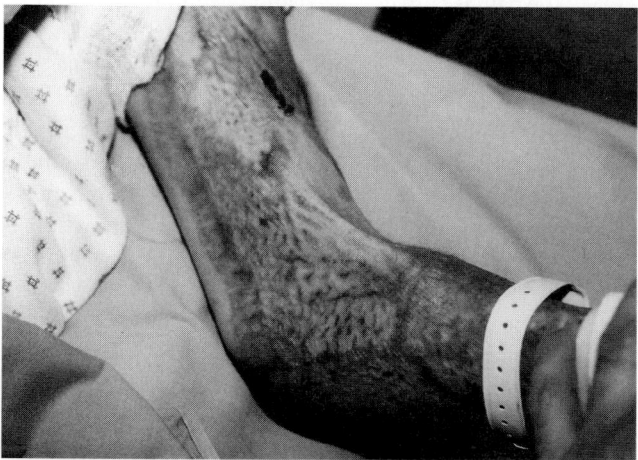

Figure 42-18 A scar contracture occurs when tight scars limit the free extension of a joint.

Children may have a more difficult time reintegrating into their previous roles as students and playmates. Many burn centers offer school reentry programs to assist children with the emotional and physical challenges of returning to their school environment.[53] With prior parental permission, predischarge plans are made to send written information to the child's teacher, classmates, and (when available) a community-based therapist working in the school system to acquaint them with the child's changed appearance and special needs. A videotaped message recorded by the child to his or her classmates explaining what happened can be very effective, especially when delivered by a family member or healthcare professional who can then answer the children's questions. The tape can show the child both with and, if appropriate, without compression garments to help satisfy classmates' curiosity and concerns before the burned child returns to the classroom. Such preparations ease the resumption of the student role for the child and can help improve acceptance by other children, who may misunderstand the cause of the disfigurement and the need for splints, adapted equipment, and scar-compression garments. Informed classmates often serve as advocates for the burned child, passing information to students in other grades or on the bus and providing support when misinformed students reveal their ignorance or fear by teasing or taunting the burned child. Regional burn summer camps, often sponsored by local firefighter organizations or burn centers, also help children adjust by placing them in settings where they can socialize with peers who also have been burned.

Preparing a burn patient for return to work does not have to be a long-term process. Burn rehabilitation and work skills training have many similarities; therefore, it is possible to design treatment activities that simulate not only functional activities but also various work skills. Strength, activity tolerance, and flexibility, often identified as work tolerances, are obvious goals of burn rehabilitation.[50] Physical demands of jobs, as described in the *Dictionary of Occupational Titles*,[89] are also components of functional skills; lifting, stooping, pushing, pulling, handling, and manipulating are a few examples. A job analysis interview, as part of the activity needs analysis, will provide the type of information needed to integrate activities into the intervention plan that should not only improve functional ability but also provide reconditioning for returning to work.

Preparing the client for community reentry after burn injury also requires attention to two other types of tolerance: skin and temperature. Most clients will still need to wear compression garments and inserts, avoid prolonged sun exposure, and perform skin care while they are at school or work. Skin-conditioning activities and exercises performed while wearing garments will improve skin tolerance for friction and shear force demands (Figure 42-19). Education regarding the body's response to temperature variations and precautions for dealing with extremes of temperature are necessary for the patient to plan for anticipated temperature tolerance problems.

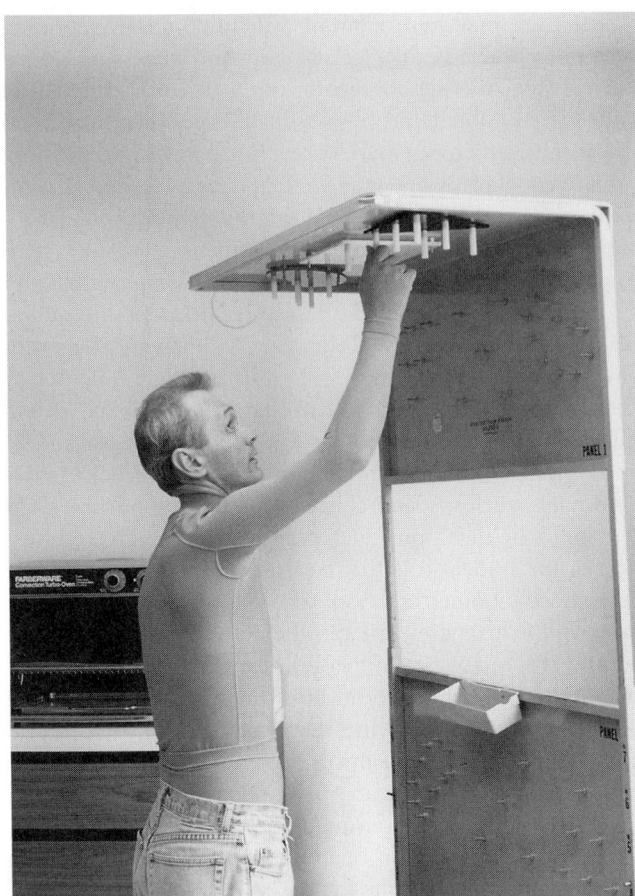

Figure 42-19　Valpar Whole Body range of motion (ROM) equipment is useful to increase strength and active ROM of the upper extremities as well as improving activity tolerance.

Psychological Adjustment

During outpatient rehabilitation, clients may undergo numerous physical and emotional changes. Once discharged from the hospital, they must face the overwhelming task of becoming responsible and self-reliant while dealing with the stress associated with developing scars and a changing self image. They may not participate fully in therapy or adequately follow through with home care activities because of the physical and emotional effects of the injury.[44] Apathy, avoidance of pain, scar tightness, and hypersensitivity all contribute to noncompliance and subsequent dysfunction after injury. Clients may experience symptoms of post-traumatic stress disorder, nightmares, and appetite changes with subsequent weight gain or loss. They may become reclusive or disengage from previous relationships. Depression may occur even before discharge.[69]

In addition to established treatments such as counseling, support, training in pain management, and relaxation techniques, visits from a recovered burn survivor to a new inpatient are often of great benefit before the patient is discharged. After discharge, attending a burn support group can also help the burn survivor with psychological adjustment.

Research has shown that burn survivors at different stages of recovery tend to provide positive support to one another. Group discussions among burn survivors promote acceptance of what they have already experienced and realistic expectations of what they still need to accomplish.[44]

Discharge from Treatment

The outpatient therapy program should be reevaluated periodically to determine whether the frequency of treatment, program progression, or professional or educational status should be changed (e.g., a return to work or school).[53] When clients have resumed their pre-injury activities, outpatient therapy may be discontinued. Because burn scar maturation may take more than 18 months, a schedule of follow-up care, with appointments every 2 to 3 months, is needed until the wearing of compression garments is discontinued. However, for children, annual burn clinic visits are recommended, even after discontinuation of compression garments, until full physical maturity is reached to ensure that growth is not impeded by scar inflexibility (see this chapter's case study).

BURN-RELATED COMPLICATIONS

HETEROTOPIC OSSIFICATION

Heterotopic ossification (HO) is formation of bone in locations that normally do not contain bone tissue.[28,91] The underlying cause of heterotopic ossification is not yet fully understood. It typically develops either in the soft tissue around the joint or in the joint capsule and ligaments, and it often forms a bony bridge across the joint, resulting in a fused joint.[38] Although HO is frequently found in the posterior aspect of the elbow, it may occur in other joint areas, such as the shoulder, wrist, hand, hip, knee, and ankle. It may occur in either extremity or bilaterally, even if the extremities were not burned. Signs that HO may be present usually appear during the latter stages of hospitalization, with the patient experiencing increased pain at a certain point in the joint's ROM. The pain is fairly localized and severe, and loss of ROM is usually rapid, with development of a hard, unyielding feel at the joint's end of available ROM. Inflammatory signs, such as redness or swelling, are not easily discernible within healing burn wounds. Once HO has been detected, frequent AROM exercise of the joint should be carried out within the pain-free range to preserve as much joint motion as possible.[20] Use of dynamic splints or forceful passive stretching of the involved joint should be discontinued. If the condition does not resolve itself with time, eventual surgical intervention may be necessary to release fused joints, followed by therapy to preserve the regained ROM.

NEUROMUSCULAR COMPLICATIONS

Peripheral neuropathic conditions are the most common neurological disorder observed in burn patients. They usually occur in high-voltage electrical burns or burns of greater than 20% TBSA.[36] Peripheral nerve damage may be caused by infections, metabolic abnormalities, or neurotoxicities. A peripheral neuropathic condition is generally demonstrated with symmetrical distal weakness, with or without sensory symptoms. Most conditions improve with time; however, patients often complain of fatigue and decreased activity tolerance that may last for months.[36]

In addition to peripheral neuropathic conditions, localized compression or stretch injuries to nerves are encountered during burn recovery. Causes of localized nerve injury include improper or prolonged positioning in bed or on the operating room table, tourniquet injury, and extreme edema. Common injury sites are the brachial plexus and ulnar and peroneal nerves. Prolonged frog-leg positioning can cause a stretch injury, whereas prolonged side lying can cause a compression injury to the peroneal nerve.[36] The ulnar nerve is subject to a compression injury if the client rests on a firm surface with the elbows flexed and the forearms pronated. The brachial plexus is subject to stretch or compression injury if inappropriate shoulder positioning techniques are used. To implement more effective prevention and intervention techniques, therapists should be aware of the causes of various nerve injuries.

Contact with high-voltage electrical current often produces permanent damage to peripheral nerves as a result of thermal damage at the entrance and exit sites of the electrical current. Damage also occurs to peripheral nerves because of secondary compression of the blood supply caused by swelling of surrounding tissues. Delayed neurological complications are caused by direct thermal damage, resulting in demyelination and subsequent nerve cell death, or vascular compromise to the brain or spinal cord. This generalized damage may be manifested by paralysis, cognitive impairment, aphasia, seizures, balance problems, or other neurological symptoms. The therapist should be attentive to developing symptoms of sensory or motor dysfunction in a client who was initially neurologically intact.[95]

FACIAL DISFIGUREMENT

Facial scars can be devastating, both functionally and psychologically. Tight or hypertrophic scars not only distort the smooth contours of the cheeks and forehead but also can flatten the nasal contours, evert eyelids and lips, and constrict optic and oral commissures. Vision, speech, feeding, and dental hygiene can be adversely affected by oral and eye contractures. Facial disfigurement is also damaging to an individual's self-image and inhibits social reentry. A significant amount of communication and social interaction depends on nonverbal facial expressions and eye contact. Severe facial burn scars not only distort the face and restrict expression but also damage the patient's self-esteem when they are met by social rejection.

Two main compression therapy methods are used to prevent or manage hypertrophic facial scars. An elastic face mask can be worn with underlying flexible thermoplastic conformers. The other option is a rigid, total-contact transparent facial orthosis.[75] Each has advantages and disadvantages.

Because face masks are made of elastic fabric, usually enclose the entire head and neck, and use flexible conformers, they provide uniform multidirectional compression during movement or changes in position. However, because they occlude the face, they are cosmetically and socially less acceptable. Effectiveness of the compression is based on subjective feedback from the patient and observations made by the therapist during outpatient clinic visits. Most underlying conformers are easy to modify or replace to provide effective pressure distribution over facial concavities and contours.

Conventional fabrication of a transparent, rigid facial orthosis is an involved and often expensive process. First, a cast is made of the patient's face using dental alginate over the surface of the face, and then the alginate is reinforced with a layer of fast-setting plaster strips. The patient must lie still and breathe through straws or small openings left in the alginate, which can be difficult for claustrophobic adults or small children. For this reason, some patients are unable to cooperate with this procedure unless they are under anesthesia. After the cast is removed from the patient, the breathing and neck openings are closed with more plaster strips and the facial cast is filled with plaster of Paris. The resulting exact duplicate plaster model is polished smooth of scars and defects by hand. Additional plaster is carved off as needed to increase pressure to specific scarred areas of the face. Clear, high-temperature thermoplastic is then heated, stretched over the model, and either vacuum-molded to the model or manually stretched and molded by hand. The edges are finished, elastic straps are applied, and the orthosis is fitted to the patient.[44] Because the material is clear, the rigid face mask has the advantage of allowing the therapist to view the face and objectively evaluate the amount of pressure exerted on the scars. By noting the presence of scar blanching under the clear mask, precise adjustments can be made as needed. The clear mask allows the face to be seen but has the disadvantage of exerting primarily unilateral compression, which may be compromised by speech, facial expressions, or side-lying positions. The mask does not allow perspiration to evaporate and must be removed and wiped clean regularly, especially in warmer climates.

Recently, computer-aided design and manufacturing systems have been developed to efficiently and economically fabricate transparent face masks.[76] A software system integrates shape capture, mask design, and model fabrication with a linear scan noncontact laser imager used for facial topography acquisition. The computer then integrates with a milling machine to fabricate a positive model out of urethane foam. The foam model is modified through use of the computer program and lined with a layer of polypropylene to smooth the foam texture. The model is then sprayed with silicone mold release and used basically in the same manner as the plaster model described previously. The rest of the

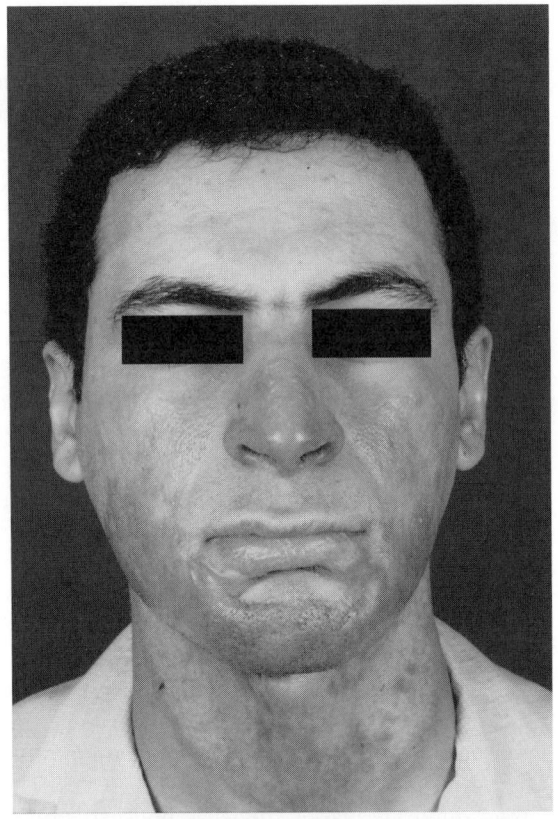

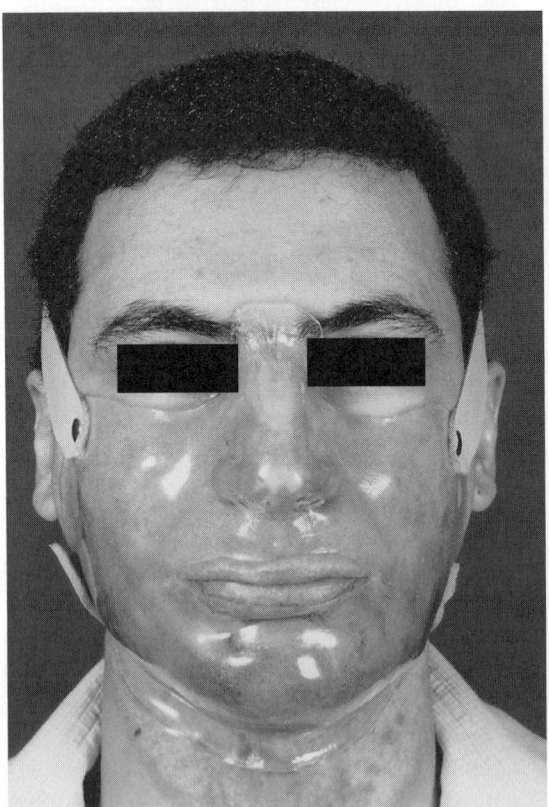

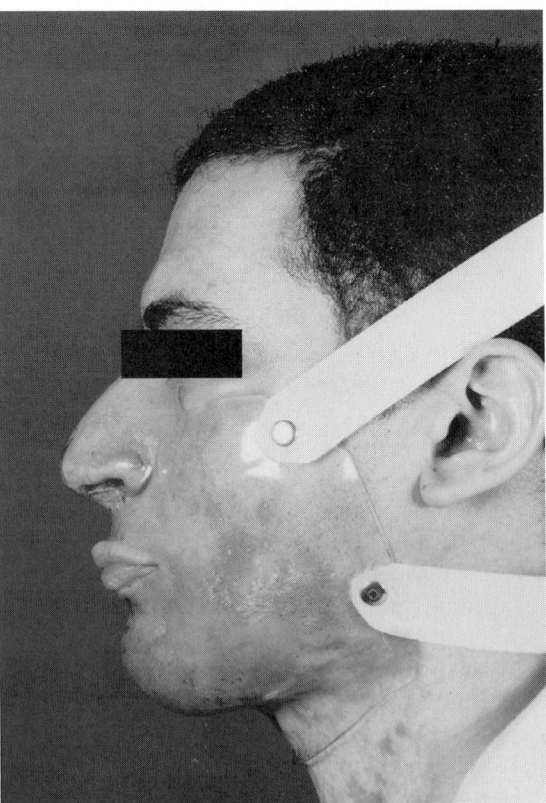

Figure 42-20   A close-up view of a transparent rigid facial orthosis. The mask contours and strap system are modified to adjust the amount of pressure over specific scarred areas (note the blanching of the scars on the lower lip and lateral chin).

fabrication process also works in a similar way. The advantage of computerized imaging and model fabrication is the speed of model fabrication and the ability to obtain a model without having to take a direct cast of the patient's face.

With either method, frequent alterations are necessary to achieve and maintain adequate compression of all facial scars (Figure 42-20). The choice of method is based on the preferences of the patient and physician. However, a combination of both types may be advantageous: The patient wears a clear, rigid face mask in social settings and the fabric mask with conformers at nighttime and at home. Appropriate skin care education is also important. Massage with lotion twice a day will aid in scar desensitization and provide necessary lubrication. Facial massage and exercises are performed at least four times a day to help stretch tight facial skin, maintain eyelid and mouth flexibility, and maintain nostril openings.

Just as with any compression therapy technique, patient compliance is essential to the effectiveness of the treatment. The patient is instructed to wear the face mask at all times, except while eating, bathing, or engaging in sexual activity. The patient should carry written verification from the burn physician verifying the medical necessity for the mask.

Regardless, patients should always remove their masks before entering any public facility so as not to provoke the suspicion that they are prepared to commit robbery or violence. This is especially important when entering banks, convenience stores, or government facilities, even if the patient is well known to employees.

Individuals wearing either type of mask will initially experience acute feelings of self-consciousness and may avoid going out in public. Parents may have difficulty putting the mask on their children and may experience feelings of guilt if the child rebels. Supportive intervention from family members and therapists is an important way to successfully manage these social and personal issues.

Compliance is especially critical in preventing or correcting facial scarring and disfigurement. Before applying the mask, the therapist must provide early education, ongoing encouragement, and continual support to ensure the client's compliance with wearing a facial orthosis. Once the scars are mature and compression therapy is no longer needed, the client should be instructed in the use of special camouflaging cosmetics such as Covermark® by Lydia O'Leary® that will cover minor texture flaws and correct uneven pigmentation.

THREADED CASE STUDY: STEVEN, PART 2

Interventions and Final Outcome

Steven's airway and respiration were compromised because of facial swelling, pharyngeal edema, and pulmonary contusions to his right lung from the crush injury, with subsequent intubation, mechanical ventilation, and tracheostomy to maintain a patent airway. He required mesh STSG to the right upper extremity and sheet STSG to his face with donor sites from his anterior thighs and upper chest. He was extubated on the nineteenth day after the injury, and his tracheostomy was removed 6 days later. He was discharged to home 28 days after his injury. At discharge, Steven was eating a regular diet but still had unhealed areas on his face and lips.

Evaluation and Goals

Because of the emergent nature of his injuries, Steven required intubation, mechanical ventilation, and heavily sedating medications for pain management. The initial absence of his family further delayed determination of his occupational profile, context, and personal priorities until well after his initial evaluation. His original evaluation instead concentrated on body functions and structures, including assessment of burn severity and location of burned surface areas; cognitive and emotional status; communication abilities; active ROM, strength, and coordination; presence and degree of edema; and screening for changes in neurological function or sensation.

Steven's performance skills were initially impaired by an acute decline in mental status and by significant edema of the face and UEs. As Steven became more alert and able to participate in treatment, OT reassessment noted peripheral nerve damage to his right median nerve, with a subsequent decrease in his right hand strength and sensation. After Steven became cognizant, treatment goals were discussed and prioritized according to his pre-injury life context and personal preferences.

Acute phase treatment goals were as follows:
- Reduce facial and extremity edema.
- Improve cognitive awareness, involve the client in goal setting, and promote engagement in occupation.
- Preserve functional mobility, strength and coordination of the neck, and both UEs.
- Regain independence with basic ADLs.

A goal was added during the postoperative phase:
- Protect and immobilize surgical graft sites to maximize graft take.

Goals of increased focus in the rehabilitation phase were as follows:
- Minimize hypertrophic scarring and disfigurement.
- Preserve facial function (i.e., prevent ectropion of the eyes, oral microstomia, loss of nasal passages).
- Regain independence with ADLs, and increase activity tolerance.

Continued

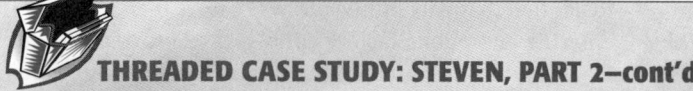

THREADED CASE STUDY: STEVEN, PART 2—cont'd

- Develop coping strategies to address pain and facial disfigurement (added later after irreversible facial scarring occurred) and to prevent social isolation. The long-term goals of treatment were to return Steven's performance skills and patterns and performance in ADLs and other areas of occupation to his pre-injury level of independence by 4 months after the injury. Acceptance of permanent losses (e.g., vocations, physical identity, abandonment by previous friends unable to cope with his change in personal appearance) and establishment of a new set of personal contexts incorporating these changes would typically take a year or longer.

Treatment interventions initiated in the acute-care phase:

- Positioning guidelines were established with the head of the patient's bed elevated 20 degrees or more; bilateral upper extremities elevated on pillow inclines with right UE abducted to 90 degrees. Illustrated positioning recommendations were posted at Steven's bedside. As wounds healed, retrograde massage was provided to assist with edema reduction in the hands.

- Cognitive reorientation and client education activities were integrated into Steven's earliest treatment sessions. Emotional support was provided as he became more aware of the severity of his injuries, and nonpharmaceutical methods of pain management were incorporated into exercise and activity treatment sessions as needed to reduce anxiety and discomfort.

- PROM exercises were provided when Steven was not alert enough to participate. Later, as he became more cognizant, an active assistive exercise program was provided to promote edema reduction and return of functional use of the extremities and face. His exercise program was posted bedside and included right arm and facial stretching exercises. Therapeutic activities of interest were encouraged to increase motivation, activity tolerance, and fine motor coordination. Steven particularly enjoyed working out on the stationary bicycle.

- After he was fully cognizant, extubated, and allowed food by mouth, he began to practice basic oral and facial ADLs, sitting supported in bed or in a bedside chair. Sponge handles were initially applied to his eating utensils and toothbrush and removed after hand edema subsided and his right grip strength improved. Safety-related training was practiced to prevent further injury to asensate areas of his right hand.

Treatment interventions begun in the postoperative phase:

- A right postoperative elbow extension splint was fabricated and worn over dressings full time postoperatively for 5 days until his grafts adhered. Then the splint was worn part time at night until full AROM was regained.

Treatment interventions initiated during the rehabilitation phase:

- After Steven was orally extubated, he was measured and fitted with a microstomia prevention appliance (MPA) mouth splint that he wore initially when sleeping, but MPA use was later increased to include daytime periods because of increased oral tightness. He was measured for a manufactured elastic face mask, chin strap, and sleeve. A temporary right compressive sleeve was fabricated and applied. Upon arrival, the garments were fitted and underlying conformers provided to be worn under the elastic face mask and sleeve. Fabrication of a clear acrylic face mask was initiated before discharge and applied on an outpatient basis. After discharge, Steven continued to receive OT services for right UE exercise program, scar management, and monitoring of the fit of compression garments and acrylic face mask.

- Because of the severity of the acid burns and a genetic predisposition for scarring, his scars continued to contract, resulting in anterior axilla web tightness and facial distortion. The tight anterior axilla was treated with moist heat; manual massage; and slow, sustained stretching. Facial exercises were intensified, with an emphasis on client participation. Horizontal stretch exercises to the healed eyelids and midface were performed by Steven using skin traction. Oral stretch exercises, initiated by the therapist during the acute phase using plastic thermometer covers, were continued. However, in this phase the mouth exercises were performed more aggressively using acrylic straws for horizontal oral commissure stretch and stacked tongue depressor sticks between the teeth for vertical stretch of cheek and jaw tightness.[28]

- Practice of ADLs was continued, progressing with performance of self-care tasks, sitting on the edge of the bed and later standing at the sink in order to increase general strength and activity tolerance while becoming more independent with self-care tasks.

- Relaxation techniques were taught to help Steven cope with discomfort during therapy. Emotional support was provided to help with grief over loss of facial appearance, employment, and previous social contacts. OT staff assisted with coping strategies and community reentry planning. Steven was also referred for professional counseling while still an inpatient.

Outcomes

In spite of compression therapy, mouth splinting, and facial exercises, Steven's facial scars continued to contract, causing eye, nasal, and oral constriction; lip eversion; eyelid ectropion; and flattening of his facial features. About 2 months after discharge, Steven abandoned the use of the acrylic face mask because the frequent long-distance trips for adjustments to the mask could not keep pace with the rapidly changing facial contours. Instead, Steven preferred using the elastic fabric face masks and flexible conformers. He continued nighttime use of his MPA for approximately 1 year after discharge to prevent further constriction of his mouth, but he continued to have webbing at each oral commissure. Steven's right arm graft sites and burn scars responded well to exercise and the consistent use of elastic compression sleeves, with resulting full AROM; a supple, flattened texture; and an appearance that was acceptable to him. The scars on his upper shoulders did not receive compression therapy because of his preference to use a sleeve rather a full vest, but these scars, while having a slightly raised texture, were also acceptable to him. He continued to use sunblock lotion to protect his scars from sunburn and hyperpigmentation, especially after he began to work outside.

THREADED CASE STUDY: STEVEN, PART 2—cont'd

Over the next 6 years, Steven had 21 surgical revisions for treatment of recurrent facial and neck contractures caused by the severe acid burn scarring and an unusually extended period to obtain facial scar maturation (over 3 years). He eventually regained full right-hand strength, but the impaired sensation in his thumb and forefinger required approximately 38 months to completely resolve. Although he could never return to competitive lifting, Steven returned to working out and could lift up to 280 pounds; however, he continued to experience chronic low back pain. He was referred to a pain clinic, where he was diagnosed with degenerative disc disease in the L4 and L5 vertebrae, and had to further restrict his lifting activities.

Because of limited field of vision caused by distorted eyelids and right eye blurring, Steven could not return to working as a professional truck driver. To support himself, he started a part-time business providing lawn-care services for private homes and local businesses. In the winter months, he expanded his business to provide pressure-washing services for sidewalks and trailers. After living with his sister's family for 3 years, Steven was financially able to return to his own home.

Although multiple surgical procedures and the use of facial compression therapy provided some improvement, Steven's facial appearance still remained unacceptable according to the social standards of the general public. His attempts to reenter previous social circles resulted in mixed responses, and in some instances led to physical altercations. Steven and his 3-year-old son had maintained contact by telephone throughout his hospitalization. During OT treatment sessions before discharge, the child had been gradually introduced to Steven's changed facial features, first with photos, then with the elastic or the clear face mask in place, and later without either mask. His son continues to remain fully accepting of his father despite his altered appearance; at age 10, Steven's son still takes personal offense when people ridicule his father.

Steven's Personal Long-Term Goals

"Because of my eyes, I'll never be able to work as a truck driver again, and because of my back, I can't power lift anymore, but I'd like to build up my lawn service. I'm still going to outpatient therapy near home. My skin is still so fragile and sometimes splits when bumped because it's thin and tight.

"Emotionally, I'm doing okay. I have my ups and downs. I can go out to eat at a restaurant now because I've learned to accept how I look. Sometimes, my appearance startles people, but usually if people see that I'm comfortable with myself, that makes them more comfortable, too. I don't like it when people stare at me and then look away without giving me a chance to nod or speak. It's rude. Children are more honest. They're just being curious. If I wave or smile, they're usually okay and wave back. My son's classmates accept me. I even go on field trips with them. I'd really like to be able to breathe better through my nose, and I wish my eyes didn't water so much. It makes me look like I'm crying. The doctors want me to come back in for a procedure to fix the tight skin on my neck."

However, after 6 years, Steven says, "I'm taking a break from surgery for a while."

THREADED CASE STUDY: KENJII, PART 2

Interventions and Final Outcome

OT interventions included the following:

- *Prevention and reduction of scar contractures and promotion of strength, mobility, and coordination, especially in his hands and face:* This involved use of exercise, splinting, and massage to stretch out developing scar contractures. Scar management techniques were used, such as fitting and modifying compression garments and conformers for his hypertrophic burn and donor site scars on his face, UEs, and torso.
- *Teaching of relaxation techniques and other nonpharmaceutical methods of pain management*
- *Building of activity tolerance with therapeutic activities and independence with ADLs by teaching alternate methods of accomplishing tasks and by providing adapted aids as needed:* Initially learning to perform self-care tasks with adaptive aids, he eventually required only adaptive techniques to perform most tasks without the use of adaptive aids (except for using a button hook to fasten tight blue jeans, a performance routine of value to him).
- *Exploration of new performance skills and occupations incorporating past values and current interests through therapeutic activities and promotion of the development of a new life context:* Various adaptive techniques explored to pursue alternate outlets for his musical interests resulted in poor satisfaction for Kenjii, who was unable to resolve his decreased performance in an area in which he had once excelled. During exploration of alternate interests, Jing was noted to be skilled in creative art media and had a talent for mathematics.
- *Psychological support to assist with the grieving process and promote the eventual acceptance of permanently lost skills, body image, and lifestyle:* During his extended stay, Kenjii voiced his

Continued

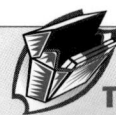

THREADED CASE STUDY: KENJII, PART 2—cont'd

grief to the extent of expressing suicidal ideation. He received counseling, but the occupational therapist also offered support and tried to develop and emphasize retained skills and talents that survived his burn injury.

Final Outcome

Almost 30 years after his burn injury, contact was made with Kenjii via the Internet to find him teaching mathematics at a university. He was completing work toward a doctorate degree and happily married to someone he described as his "soul mate." Kenjii said that he did not attempt to resume playing any of the musical instruments on which he was once was so proficient. "I knew I would never play as I once did, and the perfectionist in me could not accept less, so I chose to

leave that part of my life behind." However, the creative skills that he demonstrated so many years ago in OT activities have been well combined with his desire for perfection. In spite of permanent ROM limitations in his hands, he has become an accomplished artist in a variety of media. He had undergone numerous reconstructive surgeries in the years immediately after his burn injury, but he no longer seeks to change his appearance. He states that he long ago came to accept his appearance. He is very comfortable with his public role as an educator and is very popular with his students. He often relays his burn experience in class—initially to satisfy his students' curiosity but also to share his journey to acceptance and renewed life satisfaction. He still credits OT for "empowering" him and helping him to "survive the tough times by offering hope."

THREADED CASE STUDY: PATRICE, PART 2

Interventions and Final Outcome

Patrice required long-term therapy and multiple surgeries to counteract the effects of the restricting scars that continued to cause problems as she grew. After the fontanel of her skull closed, she was fitted with an elastic face mask and underlying conformer in an attempt to reduce the hypertrophic scarring and contracting scars that were pulling her nose to the side. However, neither she nor her adoptive mother (her previous foster mother) could tolerate the mask. Therefore, a series of acrylic face masks were fabricated until her scars matured. She eventually required surgical intervention to release a scar that was causing facial asymmetry and nasal distortion. As an adolescent, Patrice required a surgical release of the abdominal scar to allow for unrestricted growth of her left breast.

To prevent hypertrophic scarring, her hand was initially placed in a "sandwich" splint consisting of dorsal and volar thermoplastic splinting material lined with a thick layer of conforming padding. The splint provided compression to the scars and prevented the development of thick scarring and dorsal contractures of the fingers. However, this measure did not affect the longitudinal constricting force of the scar. In spite of frequent therapy sessions and the excellent care provided by her devoted mother, the scar could not stretch fast enough to keep pace with the rapid growth of her hand. A skin graft was eventually applied to the dorsum of Patrice's hand, but the graft also could not stretch fast enough. As mentioned previously, this binding effect of the scar resulted in restriction of the natural growth of her fingers. This same scarring required ongoing therapy to preserve the function of the index, long, and ring fingers.

Although the bones of Patrice's little finger did not develop, the skin of this finger grew, resulting in a button of accumulated skin tissue where the finger should have been. The scar on the back of her hand continued to restrict MP flexion and use of her long and middle digits. When Patrice was a toddler, the tight scar on her dorsal hand was excised; the resulting defect was repaired using skin from the extra fifth digit, which was filleted and transposed onto the dorsal hand as a skin flap. The volar, glabrous skin had an unusual appearance on her dorsal hand but was able to keep pace with the growth of her hand, allowing for unimpaired hand development and improved function.

Twenty years later, Patrice related how her life has been affected by serious burns received at such an early age:

"I can remember some of the surgeries to my face and hand. I remember how I hated the face masks, but I liked the glove because the therapist always let me pick the colors.

"I still can't use any of the fingers of my left hand except my thumb and index finger, but I don't feel like I'm handicapped. I'm right-handed, of course. I can do anything I really want to now, but in elementary school, I couldn't play on the monkey bars because I couldn't hold on with my left hand. I remember that this was something that I really wanted to do, and it made me feel left out. Because I had to stay out of the sun, I wasn't allowed to go to recess outside or gym until middle school.

"I finished high school with a grade point average of 3.5. I went to college for 2 years on a grant with plans to go to medical school, but now I'm working at Walmart. I'd like to return to college later this year, but I don't know exactly what degree I want to go for—something

THREADED CASE STUDY: PATRICE, PART 2—cont'd

in the medical profession, maybe a nurse or EMT. When I'm not working, I like to go out with my friends, go jogging, type on my computer, read, and watch TV; I also like to draw.

"The bald areas on my head don't bother me too much. My doctor wanted to do surgery to stretch my scalp and cut out some of the bald skin, but I didn't want to. The rest of my hair is very thick, and I can pull it back into a ponytail and hide most of the bald spots. I like wigs. I just bought a new blonde one. I don't wear them because of the bald areas; I just do it for fun.

"I'm a little quiet and shy around new people, but after I get to know someone, I'm not a bit shy anymore. I have a boyfriend now. We met at work. We've been dating a few months now.

"My face is OK. The appearance of my hand bothers me more than my face. People seem to notice it more. Sometimes I feel like I'm being watched. People stare; I guess they're curious. I wish they would just ask me instead of staring, but I just ignore it. I don't address it directly. If they ask, then I'll tell them about being burned.

"I still wonder—I guess I always will—why this happened to me ...."

SUMMARY

A serious thermal injury is one of the most devastating physical and psychological injuries that a person can endure, especially if appropriate treatment is not received in a timely and comprehensive manner. Successful burn care requires a coordinated, multidisciplinary team approach beginning from the date of injury and continuing until wound maturation is complete.

Advancements in medical and surgical burn care have made it possible to expect not only self-care independence but also early resumption of occupation, including return to school, work, leisure, and social activities. Even when functional recovery is possible, pain, disfigurement, and adverse psychological reactions (e.g., noncompliance, apathy, and depression) can contribute to postinjury dysfunction. In addition to progressive physical rehabilitation, ongoing client education is crucial. A comprehensive OT program that includes client education must be initiated early, incorporating information about the physical, psychological, and social components of burn injury to facilitate the client's cooperation and adjustment to the injury. Frequent reassessments of the client's physical abilities, abilities to engage in areas of occupation, emotional status, and social needs are also required to ensure effective intervention and the client's optimal recovery.

The occupational therapist is an integral member of the burn team, providing intervention activities such as preventive positioning, therapeutic exercise and activity, training in ADLs and other areas of occupation, preventive and corrective splinting, skin conditioning and scar management techniques, client and family education, and emotional support to promote psychosocial adjustment. A basic OT concept that is crucial in burn care, or when working with any diagnosis, is the importance of holistic treatment, or treatment of the whole person. As a profession, OT has not only focused on the recovery of functional performance skills and patterns but has also always recognized the primacy of engagement in occupation and the need to preserve the client's participation in various contexts to support a meaningful lifestyle.

Review Questions

1. Name the two layers of the skin. In which layer are the nerves and sebaceous glands?
2. Which factors are considered in determining burn severity?
3. What is an escharotomy, and why is it performed? How does it differ from a fasciotomy?
4. Describe two factors that affect the quality of burn wound healing and promote excessive scar formation.
5. During the acute care phase, which factors may limit full ROM?
6. What is a boutonnière deformity, and what are boutonnière precautions?
7. What are the two basic principles underlying most burn rehabilitation treatment techniques?
8. What is the primary objective for positioning during acute care?
9. What are the indications for initiating splints during the acute-care phase?
10. When a splint is indicated, what is the preferred wearing schedule and why?
11. When should client education about burn injury and rehabilitation begin?
12. What would cause a patient to require temporary adaptations for self-care during the acute-care phase?
13. Why are patients immobilized postoperatively? On average, how soon after grafting can gentle AROM exercises be resumed?
14. How soon postoperatively should an intermediate compression dressing or garment be applied?
15. What are the two main compression therapy options for facial scar treatment?
16. Why are skin conditioning activities used in burn rehabilitation? What are examples of skin conditioning techniques?
17. What is the average length of time required for scar maturation?
18. What are possible causes of limitations in ADLs during the rehabilitation phase?
19. What information should be included in predischarge education and home program review?
20. What is the primary cause of dysfunction after a burn injury?

REFERENCES

1. Abston S: Scar reaction after thermal injury and prevention of scars and contractures. In Boswick JA, editor: *The art and science of burn care*, Rockville, MD, 1987, Aspen.

2. Akin S, Ozcan M: Using a plastic sheet to prevent the risk of contamination of the burn wound during the shower, *Burns* 29(3):280, 2003.

3. American Burn Association: Burn Incidence and Treatment in the US: 2000 Fact Sheet Downloaded 11/12/04 http://www.ameriburn.org/pub/BurnIncidenceFactSheet.htm

4. Apfel LM, et al: Computer-drafted pressure support gloves, *J Burn Care Rehabil* 9(2):165, 1988.

5. Artz CP, Moncrief JA, Pruitt BA: *Burns: a team approach*, Philadelphia, 1979, WB Saunders.

6. Baltimore Therapeutic Equipment Co, 1201 Bernard Dr., Baltimore, MD, 21223.

7. Bariollo DJ, Nangle ME, Farrell K: Preliminary experience with cultured epidermal autograft in a community hospital burn unit, *J Burn Care Rehabil* 13(1):158, 1992.

8. Baur PS, et al: Wound contractions, scar contractures and myofibroblasts: a classical case study, *J Trauma* 18(1):8, 1978.

9. Bennett GB, et al: Serial casting: a method for treating burn contracture, *J Burn Care Rehabil* 10(6):543, 1989.

10. Bowler PG, et al: Microbicidal properties of a silver-containing Hydrofiber® dressing against a variety of burn wound pathogens, *J Burn Care Rehabil* 25(2):192, 2004.

11. Brigham PA, McLoughlin E: Burn incidence and medical care use in the United States: estimates, trends, and data sources, *J Burn Care Rehabil* 17(2):95, 1996.

12. Bruster J, Pullium G: Gradient pressure, *Am J Occup Ther* 37(7): 485, 1983.

13. Burn Survivors Online, http://www.burnsurvivorsonline.com/ Downloaded 11/12/04

14. Burnsworth B, Krob MJ, Langer-Schnepp M: Immediate ambulation of patients with lower extremity grafts, *J Burn Care Rehabil* 13(1):89, 1992.

15. Caffo E, Belaise C. Psychological aspects of traumatic injury in children and adolescents, *Child Adolesc Psychiatr Clin North Am* 12(3):493, 2003.

16. Carr-Collins JA: Pressure techniques for the prevention of hypertrophic scar. In Salisbury RE, editor: *Clinics in plastic surgery: burn rehabilitation and reconstruction*, Philadelphia, 1992, WB Saunders.

17. Carvajal HF: Resuscitation of the burned child. In Carvajal HF, Parks DH, editors: *Burns in children: pediatric burn management*, Chicago, 1988, Year Book Medical Publishers.

18. Clark JA, Burt AM, Eldad A: Culture epithelium as a skin substitute, *Burns Incl Therm Inj* 13(3):173, 1987.

19. Covey MH: Occupational therapy. In Boswick JA, editor: *The art and science of burn care*, Rockville, MD, 1987, Aspen.

20. Crawford CM, et al: Heterotopic ossification: are range of motion exercises contraindicated? *J Burn Care Rehabil* 7(4):323, 1986.

21. Daugherty MB, Carr-Collins JA: Splinting techniques for the burn patient. In Richard RL, Staley MJ, editors: *Burn care and rehabilitation: principles and practice*, Philadelphia, 1994, FA Davis.

22. Demling RH, DeSanti L: How can silver be delivered to the burn wound? In *The beneficial effects of a nanocrystalline silver delivery system for management of wounds: part II section III*. Downloaded 3/6 from http://www.burnsurgery.com/Modules/nano/sec3.htm Copyright 2002, Burnsurgery.org.

23. Dietch EA, et al: Hypertrophic burn scars: analysis of variables, *J Trauma* 23(10):895, 1983.

24. Dyer C: Burn care in the emergent period, *J Emerg Nurs* 6(1):9, 1980.

25. Ehde DM, et al: Post-traumatic stress symptoms and distress following acute burn injury, *Burns* 25(7):587, 1999.

26. El Hamaoui Y, et al: Post-traumatic stress disorder in burned patients, *Burns* 28(7):647, 2002.

27. Embil JM, et al: An outbreak of methicillin resistant *Staphylococcus aureus* on a burn unit: potential role of contaminated hydrotherapy equipment, *Burns* 27(7):681, 2001.

28. Evans EB: Heterotopic bone formation in thermal burns, *Clinical Orthopedics* 263:94, 1991.

29. Feller I, Archambeault C: *Nursing the burned patient*, Ann Arbor, MI, 1973, Institute for Burn Medicine.

30. Fleet J: The psychological effects of burn injuries: a literature review, *Brit J Occup Ther* 55(5):198, 1992.

31. Giuliani CA, Perry GA: Factors to consider in the rehabilitation aspect of burn care, *Phys Ther* 65(5):619, 1985.

32. Gordon M, et al: Use of pain assessment tools: is there a preference? *J Burn Care Rehabil Institute* 19(5):451, 1998.

33. Hansbrough JF: Current status of skin replacements for coverage of extensive burn wounds, *J Trauma* 30(suppl 12):S155, 1990.

34. Hartford C: Surgical management. In Fisher S, Helm P: *Comprehensive rehabilitation of burns*, Baltimore, 1984, Williams & Wilkins.

35. Heimbach DM, Engrav LH: *Surgical management of the burn wound*, New York, 1984, Raven Press.

36. Helm PA: Neuromuscular considerations. In Fisher SV, Helm PA, editors: *Comprehensive rehabilitation of burns*, Baltimore, 1984, Williams & Wilkins.

37. Helm PA, Fisher SV: Rehabilitation of the patient with burns. In Delisa J, Currie D, Gans B, editors: *Rehabilitation medicine: principles and practice*, Philadelphia, 1988, JB Lippincott.

38. Hoffer MM, Brody G, Ferlic F: Excision of heterotopic ossification about elbows in patients with thermal injury, *J Trauma* 18(9):667, 1978.

39. Howell JW: Management of the acutely burned hand for the nonspecialized clinician, *Phys Ther* 69(12):1077, 1989.

40. Humphrey C, Richard RL, Staley MJ: Soft tissue management and exercise. In Richard RL, Staley MJ, editors: *Burn care and rehabilitation: principles and practice*, Philadelphia, 1994, FA Davis.

41. Johnson C: Pathologic manifestation of burn injury. In Richard RL, Staley MJ, editors: *Burn care and rehabilitation: principles and practice*, Philadelphia, 1994, FA Davis.

42. Johnson CL: Physical therapists as scar modifiers, *Phys Ther* 64(9):1381, 1984.

43. Johnson RM, Richard R: Partial-thickness burns: identification and management, *Advances in Skin & Wound Care* 16(4):178, 2003.

44. Jordan CL, Allely RA, Gallagher J: Self-care strategies following severe burns. In Christiansen C, editor: *Ways of living: self-care strategies for special needs*, Rockville, MD, 1994, American Occupational Therapy Association.

45. Jordan MH, et al: Dynamic plaster casting for burn scar contracture, *Proc Am Burn Assoc* 16:17, 1984.

46. Jordan MH, et al: A pressure prevention device for burned ears, *J Burn Care Rehabil* 13(1):673, 1992.

47. Kaplan SH: Patient education techniques used at burn centers, *Am J Occup Ther* 39(1):655, 1985.

48. Kubler-Ross E: *Death and dying*, New York, 1997, Simon & Schuster.

49. Larson DL, et al: Techniques for decreasing scar formation and contracture in the burned patient, *J Trauma* 11(10):807, 1971.

50. Leman CH: An approach to work hardening in burn rehabilitation, *Top Acute Care Trauma Rehabil* 1(4):62, 1987.

51. Leman CJ: Burn rehabilitation. In Hopkins HL, Smith HD, editors: *Willard & Spackman's occupational therapy*, ed 8, Philadelphia, 1993, JB Lippincott.

52. Leman CJ, et al: Exercise physiology in the acute burn patient: do we really know what we're doing? *Proc Am Burn Assoc* 24:91, 1992.

53. Leman CJ, Ricks N: Discharge planning and follow-up burn care. In Richard RL, Staley MJ, editors: *Burn care and rehabilitation: principles and practice*, Philadelphia, 1994, FA Davis.

54. Linares HA: Hypertrophic healing: controversies and etiopathogenic review. In Carvajal HF, Parks DH, editors: *Burns in children: pediatric burn management*, Chicago, 1988, Year Book Medical Publishers.

55. Lund C, Browder N: The estimation of area of burns, *Surg Gynecol Obstet* 79:352, 1944.

56. Mahon LM, Neufeld N: The effect of informational feedback on food intake of adult burn patients, *Appl Behav Annal* 17(3):391, 1984.

57. May SR: The effects of biological wound dressings on the healing process, *Clin Mater* 8(3-4):243, 1991.

58. Mendez-Eastman S: Negative pressure wound therapy, *Plastic Surg Nurs* 18(1):27, 1998.

59. Miles WK, Grigsby L: Remodeling of scar tissue in the burned hand. In Hunter JM, et al, editors: *Rehabilitation of the hand*, St Louis, 1990, Mosby.

60. Montgomery RK: Pain management in burn injury, *Crit Care Nurs Clin North Am* 16(1):39, 2004.

61. Moss BF, Everett JJ, Patterson DR: Psychologic support and pain management of the burn patient. In Richard RL, Staley MJ, editors: *Burn care and rehabilitation: principles and practice*, Philadelphia, 1994, FA Davis.

62. Nolan WB: Acute management of thermal injury, *Ann Plast Surg* 7(3):243, 1981.

63. Ohrbach R, et al: Hypnosis after an adverse response to opioids in an ICU burn patient, *Clin J Pain* 14(2):167, 1998.

64. Pal SK, Cortiella J, Herndon D: Adjunctive methods of pain control in burns, *Burns* 23(5):404, 1997.

65. Palmieri TL, Greenhalgh DG: Topical treatment of pediatric patients with burns: a practical guide, *Am J Clin Dermatol* 3(8):529, 2002.

66. Patterson DR, Adcock RJ, Bombardier CH: Factors predicting hypnotic analgesia in clinical burn pain, *Int J Clin Exp Hypn* 45(4):377, 1997.

67. Peacock EE Jr: *Wound repair*, ed 3, Philadelphia, 1984, WB Saunders.

68. Pietsch J: Care of the child with burns. In Hazinski MF, editor: *Manual of pediatric critical care*, St Louis, 1999, Mosby.

69. Ptacek JT, Patterson DR, Heimbach DM: Inpatient depression in persons with burns, *J Burn Care Rehabil* 23(1):1, 2002.

70. Pullium G: Splinting and positioning. In Fisher SV, Helm PA, editors: *Comprehensive rehabilitation of burns*, Baltimore, 1984, Williams & Wilkins.

71. Reeves SU: Adaptive strategies after severe burns. In Christiansen CH, Matuska KM, editors: *Ways of living: adaptive strategies for special needs*, ed 3, Bethesda, MD, 2004, AOTA.

72. Richard RL, Staley MJ: Burn patient evaluation and treatment planning. In Richard RL, Staley MJ, editors: *Burn care and rehabilitation: principles and practice*, Philadelphia, 1994, FA Davis Co.

73. Rivers EA: Rehabilitation management of the burn patient, *Advances in Clin Rehabil* 1:177, 1978.

74. Rivers EA, Fisher SV: Rehabilitation for burn patients. In Kottke FJ, Lehmann JF, editors: *Krusen's handbook of physical medicine and rehabilitation*, ed 4, Philadelphia, 1990, WB Saunders.

75. Rivers EA, Strate R, Solem L: The transparent face mask, *Am J Occup Ther* 33(2):108, 1979.

76. Rogers B, et al: Computerized manufacturing or transparent face masks for the treatment of facial scarring, *J Burn Care Rehabil* 24(2):91, 2003.

77. Saffle JR: The 2002 Presidential Address: NPDGB and other surgical sayings, *J Burn Care Rehabil* 23(6):375, 2002.

78. Salisbury RE, Petro JA: Rehabilitation of burn patients. In Boswick JA, editor: *The art and science of burn care*, Rockville, MD, 1987, Aspen.

79. Scherer LA, et al: The vacuum assisted closure device: a method of securing skin grafts and improving graft survival, *Arch Surg* 137(8):930, 2002.

80. Schmitt MA, French L, Kalil ET: How soon is safe? Ambulation of the patient with burns after lower-extremity skin grafting, *J Burn Care Rehabil* 12(1):33, 1991.

81. Schneider AM, Morykwas MJ, Argenta LC: A new and reliable method of securing skin grafts to the difficult recipient bed, *J Plastic Reconstr Surg* 102(4):1195, 1998.

82. Simons M, King S, Edgar D, Occupational therapy and physiotherapy for the patient with burns: principles and management guidelines, *J Burn Care Rehabil* 24(5):323, 2003.

83. Solem L: Classification. In Fisher S, Helm P, editors: *Comprehensive rehabilitation of burns*, Baltimore, 1984, Williams & Wilkins.

84. Staley MJ, Richard RL: Scar management. In Richard RL, Staley MJ, editors: *Burn care and rehabilitation: principles and practice*, Philadelphia, 1994, FA Davis.

85. Staley MJ, Richard RL, Falkel JE: Burns. In O'Sullivan SB, Schmitz TJ, editors: *Physical rehabilitation: assessment and treatment*, ed 3, Philadelphia, 1994, FA Davis.

86. Strock LL, et al: Topical Bactroban (mupirocin): efficacy in treating burn wounds infected with methicillin-resistant staphylococci, *J Burn Care Rehabil* 11(5):454, 1990.

87. Sullivan T, et al: Rating the burn scar, *J Burn Care Rehabil* 11(3):256, 1990.

88. Thomas CL, editor: *Taber's cyclopedic medical dictionary*, ed 18, Philadelphia, 1993, FA Davis.

89. United States Department of Labor: *Dictionary of occupational titles*, ed 4, Washington, DC, 1977, US Government Printing Office.

90. Valpar Component Work Samples, Valpar International Corporation, PO Box 5767, Tucson, Ariz.

91. Varghese G: Musculoskeletal conditions. In Fisher SV, Helm PA, editors: *Comprehensive rehabilitation of burns*, Baltimore, 1984, Williams & Wilkins.

92. Vu H, et al: Burn wound infection susceptibilities to topical agents: the Nathan's agar well diffusion technique, *P&T* 27(8): 390, 2002.

93. Wachtel T: Epidemiology, classification, initial care, and administrative considerations for critically burned patients. In Wachtel T: *Critical care clinics*, Philadelphia, 1985, WB Saunders.

94. Weil R, et al: Smoke inhalation injury, *Ann Plast Surg* 4(2):121, 1980.

95. Whittman ML: Electrical and chemical burns. In Richard RL, Staley MJ, editors: *Burn care and rehabilitation: principles and practice*, Philadelphia, 1994, FA Davis.

96. Work Evaluation Systems Technology (WEST), PO Box 2477, Fort Bragg, CA 95437.

97. Wright PC: Fundamentals of acute burn care and physical therapy management, *Phys Ther* 64(8):1217, 1984.

98. Yin HQ, Langford R, Burrell RE: Comparative evaluation of the antimicrobial activity of Acticoat antimicrobial barrier dressing, *J Burn Care Rehabil* 20(3):195, 1999.

99. Yurko L, Fratianne R: Evaluation of burn discharge teaching, *J Burn Care Rehabil* 9(6):643, 1988.

RESOURCES

American Burn Association
www.ameriburn.org/

Burn Survivors Online
www.burnsurvivorsonline.com/

Cool the Burn
www.cooltheburn.com/home.html

Covermark Cosmetics
A vender of special camouflaging cosmetics for burn patients.
Veterans Dr., Suite D,
Northvale, NJ 07647
(800) 524-1120157
www.covermark.com/

The Phoenix Society for Burn Survivors
phoenix-society.org/

43 Amputations and Prosthetics

DENISE D. KEENAN

JENNIFER S. GLOVER

KEY TERMS

Preprosthetic phase	Neuroma	Myoelectric prosthesis	Residual limb support
Prosthetic phase	Phantom limb	Hybrid prosthesis	Pylon
Residual limb	Phantom sensations	Above-knee amputation	
Postprosthetic phase	Terminal device	Below-knee amputation	
Socket	Separation of controls	Syme's amputation	

LEARNING OBJECTIVES

After studying this chapter the student or practitioner will be able to do the following:

1. List the common reasons for amputation.
2. Discuss the occupational therapist's role in rehabilitation after amputation.
3. List the goals of amputation surgery.
4. Name two types of surgical procedures.
5. Name four factors that can interfere with prosthetic training.
6. Define *neuroma, phantom limb*, and *phantom pain*.
7. Describe the typical psychological consequences of amputation surgery.
8. Describe how the occupational therapist facilitates adjustment to amputation.
9. Describe the role of the occupational therapist in the rehabilitation of the individual with an upper extremity (UE) amputation.
10. Discuss the impact of the residual limb status on the success of fitting and operating a UE prosthesis.
11. Name the five components common to all body-powered prostheses.
12. List the motions used to operate the body-powered prosthesis.
13. Describe at least two techniques for donning the body-powered prosthesis.
14. Describe the importance of prepositioning the terminal device.
15. List the two phases of training in the use of a UE prosthesis.
16. Explain why it is necessary to introduce postprosthetic training in three levels.
17. Describe the basic operation of an electric prosthesis.
18. Discuss the primary function of any prosthesis in different daily tasks.
19. List the types and causes of lower extremity (LE) amputation.
20. Describe the types of equipment that may be used by a person who has had an LE amputation.
21. Describe how LE amputation may affect a person's occupational performance.
22. Identify the effects that LE amputation may have on client factors, performance skills, and performance patterns.
23. Discuss the potential psychosocial repercussions of LE amputation.
24. Describe the role of the occupational therapist in working with a person who has had an LE amputation.
25. Explain how context and activity demands can be altered to improve a client's ability to participate in a given occupation.
26. Discuss additional concerns that may be present for an older person who has had an LE amputation.

CHAPTER OUTLINE

Section 1: General Considerations of Upper and Lower Extremity Amputations

Causes and incidence of amputation
Surgical management
Client social, cultural, personal, and spiritual contexts
  Psychosocial contexts influencing adjustment to amputation

Post-surgical physical client factors and performance skills
  Skin
  Sensation
  Bone
  Wound healing

SECTION 1: GENERAL CONSIDERATIONS OF UPPER AND LOWER EXTREMITY AMPUTATIONS

Denise D. Keenan

Limb loss can result from disease, injury, or congenital causes. Individuals born with congenital limb deficiencies or whose amputations occur early in life usually grow and develop sensorimotor skills and self-images without the limb. The individual who undergoes an amputation in adolescence or adulthood is confronted with the task of adjusting to the loss of a well-integrated part of the body scheme and self-image. These two types of client populations present different problems for the rehabilitation worker.[6,64,65]

The occupational therapist's primary responsibility in the rehabilitation program is the formulation and execution of the preprosthetic program and prosthetic training. During the **preprosthetic phase,** the treatment plan involves preparing the limb for a prosthesis; during the **prosthetic phase,** treatment involves increasing tolerance and functional use of the prosthesis. The rehabilitation program involves an individualized intervention plan that helps the client with physical and psychological adjustments. This program is designed so that the client may learn to accept the new body image and function as independently as possible.[6,64,65]

CAUSES AND INCIDENCE OF AMPUTATION

The majority of amputations result from trauma; peripheral vascular disease (PVD); peripheral vasospastic diseases; chronic infection; chemical, thermal, or electrical injuries; and malignant tumor. Elective upper extremity (UE) amputations may occur as a result of a severe or complete brachial plexus injury.[9]

Each year an estimated 50,000 Americans lose a limb. Between 4000 and 5500 lose a hand or arm. This ratio of upper limb loss to lower limb loss is 1 of every 11. The incidence of amputation remains fairly constant between the ages of 1 and 15. From 15 to 54 years of age, however, there is a gradual increase in incidence because of work-related injuries and highway accidents. Approximately 75% of UE amputations in adults are caused by trauma,[1,34,43] as was the case for Roberto.

The major cause of lower extremity (LE) amputation is PVD, often associated with smoking and diabetes.[36,39,56] Between 1988 and 1996, 82% of all lower limb amputations occurred as a result of vascular problems.[15] Despite major improvements in noninvasive diagnosis, revascularization, and wound-healing techniques, 2% to 5% of individuals without diabetes but with PVD and 6% to 25% of those with both PVD and diabetes undergo amputation.[28,29,41,45,68] Perioperative mortality rates of persons with LE amputation have been variously reported as between 7% and 13% and are usually associated with other medical problems, such as cardiac disease and stroke.[22,28,29]

The second leading cause of LE amputation, accounting for approximately 17% of amputations, is trauma,[15] usually the result of motor vehicle accidents or gunshots. Individuals with traumatic amputations are usually young adults and more frequently men.[20,27] Improved imaging techniques, more effective chemotherapy, and better limb salvage procedures have reduced the incidence of amputation from osteogenic sarcoma. Tumor resection followed by limb reconstruction frequently provides an extremity that is as functional as a prosthesis and does not appear to affect the 5-year survival rate.[30,38,61,67,75]

SURGICAL MANAGEMENT

The surgeon is an important team member. Before performing surgery, the surgeon should consult with the healthcare team to maximize the functional outcome. The surgeon attempts to preserve as much length as possible and provide a **residual limb** that has good skin coverage and vascularization. Conservation of residual limb length and uncomplicated wound healing are important. During and after surgery, the primary goal is to form a residual limb that maintains maximal function of the remaining tissue and allows maximal use of the prosthesis.[6,34,64]

Blood vessels and nerves are severed and allowed to retract so that residual limb pain is minimized during prosthetic use. Bone beveling is a surgical procedure that smooths the rough edges and prevents the development of spurs (small projections of bone beyond the natural surface) on the remaining bone. Muscles are sutured to the bones distally by a surgical process called *myodesis*. The muscles involved in the function of the amputated limb are correspondingly affected by the loss.[51]

Surgical techniques vary with the level and cause of amputation.[63,64] A closed or open surgical procedure may be performed. The open method allows drainage as the surgical site heals and minimizes the possibility of infection. The closed method reduces the period of hospitalization but also reduces free drainage and increases the risk of infection.[64] The specific type of amputation performed is at the discretion of the surgeon and is often determined by the status of the extremity at the time of amputation. The surgery may be ablative (removal of devitalized tissues) only or reconstructive. In either case, the surgeon must remove the part of the limb that has to be eliminated and allow for primary or secondary wound healing. When the surgeon reconstructs a residual limb (sometimes referred to as a *stump*), it is for optimal prosthetic fitting and function. The residual limb that results should be strong and resilient.[64]

CLIENT SOCIAL, CULTURAL, PERSONAL, AND SPIRITUAL CONTEXTS

Profound psychological shock and disbelief are likely to accompany amputation, particularly for those who experience a sudden trauma that causes or necessitates amputation.[17,32,34] Seeing the residual limb for the first time can cause shock, panic, despair, self-pity, suicidal impulses, and even rage.[49] Subsequently, there can be feelings of hopelessness, despondency, bitterness, and anger. Some individuals may mourn not only the lost limb but also the possible loss of a job or the ability to participate in favorite sports or activities.

The person may feel lonely, isolated, and an object of pity. Concerns about the future, body image and function, the responses of family and friends, and employment all affect the person's emotional status.[49] Reactions to amputation may be less severe in individuals who have had a chance to adjust before the surgery.[17,32,34] Older persons may demonstrate postoperative confusion, whereas younger persons may have a sense of mutilation, emasculation, or castration.[17,32]

The person's personality; age; cultural background; and psychological, social, economic, and vocational resources influence the reaction to amputation. Ultimately, the individual must come to terms with the consequences of limb loss and the perception of diminished attractiveness. The person confronts discomfort, inconvenience, economic expense, loss of function, increased energy expenditure, and possible curtailment of favorite occupations. He or she may need to change employment because of social discrimination and cope with resultant medical problems.[17] Roberto expressed a strong desire to return to work. He recognized that his work capabilities had always been in the manual labor category. Roberto accepted consultation with a vocational counselor to assist him in the goal of returning to gainful employment as quickly as possible. He accepted the fact that the jobs identified by the counselor may be unfamiliar to him.

Cultural factors are important in the reaction to amputation. In some social, cultural, or religious groups, the amputation may be considered a means of punishment or atonement. Such beliefs and society's general aversion to amputation can cause the affected person to adopt the same viewpoint or perpetuate his or her own preexisting viewpoint. Similar attitudes can result in self-hatred and self-deprecation, which may affect the person's reaction and adjustment to the disability.[17]

Depression and a sense of futility are considered a normal part of the adjustment process.[17] If depression is severe and prolonged, psychological or psychiatric referral is indicated. Medication may be necessary to reduce depression.[17] The preexisting personality of the client determines the severity and duration of the reaction and ultimately the adjustment to the amputation and to prosthetic use.[16,17] Roberto acknowledged his depression, reported that it was decreasing (6 months after the amputation), and said that he was actively involved in planning his life and attaining his goals for the future.

PSYCHOSOCIAL CONTEXTS INFLUENCING ADJUSTMENT TO AMPUTATION

Psychosocial adjustment depends on various factors: the individual's character and essence, the quality of the social support systems available, and sociocultural reactions to amputation and the team's management of the rehabilitation.[17] Social, personal, and spiritual contexts may be significantly altered for those who have experienced amputation. Through the interview with Roberto, the therapist identifies successful adaptation and coping strategies already in place and does not note a significant change in his spiritual self.

The process of adjustment to amputations is analogous to the grieving process. The client experiences identifiable stages of denial, anger, depression, coping, and acceptance.[17] Some clients move through these stages and ultimately adapt to the loss. The cause of the amputation may contribute significantly to the client's response. For example, if the amputation was caused by negligence on the part of the affected person or others, there might be accompanying self-blame, guilt, or anger at others.

During any phase, clients may react with hostility toward themselves and the medical team. Often, overt solicitousness and friendliness may mask such hostility. Caregivers should make allowances for such behavior rather than respond in kind. Positive reinforcement through involvement in the rehabilitation process and contact with people who experienced similar amputations help the client solve the problem of returning to former life roles.[17]

The client may be afraid to return to family, social, vocational, and sexual roles. Frequent discussions of fears and solutions to real or imagined problems (if possible, with a similar, successfully rehabilitated client) are important for facilitating adjustment.[17]

After a mourning period, the client may minimize the significance of the amputation and actually joke about it. When this phase of adjustment has subsided, the client begins seriously to consider the future. At this point, the therapist may discuss social, vocational, and educational plans with the client.[17]

Loss of a body part necessitates a revision and acceptance of the body image. Problems with the acceptance of the change in body image may cause difficulties in prosthetic training.[64,65] Fostering acceptance of the prosthesis is a crucial way to promote the client's adjustment. Establishing a training program that presents the prosthesis in a manner that meets the client's needs and goals has a beneficial effect in integrating the prosthesis into the body scheme. The prosthesis must become part of the self before it can be used most effectively. The prosthesis contributes to what society regards as a normal appearance, which may in turn help the client continue to identify with able-bodied individuals. Thus, the client may reconnect more quickly with his or her former image, leaving the door open for reconfiguration of that image to include the newly changed body.[17,64,65]

Long-term adjustment depends on the client's basic personality structure; sense of accomplishment; and place in the family, community, and world. Generally, individuals who have had an amputation may dream of themselves as not being amputated. This image may be so vivid that persons with LE amputation fall as they get up at night and attempt to walk to the bathroom without a prosthesis.[49]

The rehabilitation team members can help the client understand the importance of the prosthetic training program.

The use of new prosthetic technology that addresses different lifestyles promotes participation in meaningful occupation and enhances normal appearance. The client's preferred body image should be stressed.

OT PRACTICE NOTE

The client needs to receive reassurance and understanding from the entire rehabilitation team, with the focus of occupational therapy intervention on facilitation of engagement in occupation to increase participation in contexts.[49]

POST-SURGICAL PHYSICAL CLIENT FACTORS AND PERFORMANCE SKILLS

Several factors and potential problems can affect the outcome of rehabilitation. Length of the residual limb, skin integrity, edema, sensation, the time for healing, infection, and allergic reaction to the prosthesis are among the physical factors that affect rehabilitation potential.[37]

SKIN

Skin complications account for most post-surgical problems. These complications occur in either the preprosthetic or the prosthetic phase. Delayed healing and extensive skin grafting are complications in the preprosthetic phase. Skin breakdown, ulcers, infected sebaceous cysts, and allergic reactions can occur in the prosthetic phase. Residual limb edema can occur in either phase. Delayed healing of the incision site is one of the earliest preprosthetic complications resulting in postponed prosthetic fitting. Necrotic areas may develop, requiring surgical intervention.[7]

To achieve a residual limb length suitable for prosthetic use, the surgeon may perform extensive skin grafting. If the skin graft adheres to bone, the area may ulcerate and require medical attention.[7] Daily gentle massages by the individual, family members, or the therapist decrease the likelihood of skin graft adherence to bone and the associated complications.

Immediately after surgery, the residual limb is normally edematous as a result of fluid that collects within the soft tissues, especially in its distal portion. Compression wrapping or a rigid dressing helps decrease the edema.[8,23,34]

During the **postprosthetic phase,** an ill-fitting **socket** or wrinkles in the prosthetic sock may cause skin breakdown or scar adhesions.[24] Residual limb ulceration is associated with ischemia and pressure exerted by the prosthesis on the limb. The physician should see the client in this case, and the prosthesis should not be worn until the area heals. The prosthetist should also examine the prosthesis to determine whether the socket requires adjustment. If problems persist, surgical revision of the limb may be necessary before rehabilitation can continue.[51]

The torque forces between the socket and the residual limb cause a predisposition to the development of sebaceous cysts. Treatment involves the application of moist heat. When the cyst becomes infected, drainage ensues and enucleation of the cyst wall may be required.[7]

The development of residual limb edema during the postprosthetic phase usually indicates an ill-fitting socket. Proximal tightness of the socket may result in distal edema, which may require a new, well-fitted socket.[7]

SENSATION

The loss of sensory feedback from the amputated limb is a major problem for clients. This loss of sensation is especially significant for the person with a UE amputation because sensory feedback from the hand, so essential for function, is lost. Residual limb hyperesthesia, neuroma, and phantom sensations are problems that may interfere with the functional use of the limb either with or without the prosthesis.

Residual limb hyperesthesia, or an overly sensitive limb, limits functional use and causes discomfort. Desensitization consists of tapping and massage, which help decrease the discomfort.[6,24] Sympathetic nerve blocks may be used medically to manage residual limb hypersensitivity.[55]

The residual limb may have areas of absent or impaired sensation that require special attention and education when the prosthesis is worn. The client must rely on visual and proprioceptive feedback because sensation is functionally lost when the prosthesis is on the residual limb. The client must adjust to new sensations, such as the pressure of the residual limb inside the socket and the feel of the harness system, if used.[64]

Neuroma

Severed peripheral nerves form neuromas in the residual limb.[39,44] A **neuroma** is a small ball of nerve tissue that develops when growing axons attempt to reach the distal end of the residual limb. As the axons grow, they turn back on themselves, producing a ball of nerve tissue. If the neuroma adheres to scar tissue or skin subject to repetitive pressure, it can be painful when pressed. Diagnosis is made by palpating the neuroma.[8] Most neuromas occur 1 to 2 inches (2.5 to 5 cm) proximal to the end of the residual limb and are not troublesome.[7]

So that pain will not interfere with prosthetic wear, the neuroma must be well surrounded by soft tissue. During surgery, the surgeon identifies the major nerves, pulls them down under some tension, cuts them clearly and sharply, and allows them to retract into soft tissue of the residual limb. Neuromas that form close to scar tissue or bone generally cause pain.[39,44]

Treatment for painful neuromas involves local anesthetic injections or ultrasound. Both treatments should be followed

by massage and stretching. Surgical intervention may be necessary. The surgical options are to (1) redirect the nerve more proximally into a padded area, (2) tie the nerve ending into a proximal wound bed to protect it, or (3) tie two nerve ends to each other to prevent neuroma development. In addition, the residual limb socket may be fabricated or modified to accommodate the neuroma.[6,71,72]

Phantom Limb

Most clients who have had an amputation experience **phantom limb.** In its simplest form, the phantom is the sensation of the limb that is no longer there. The phantom usually occurs initially immediately after surgery. The distal part of the extremity is most frequently felt, although sometimes the person feels the whole extremity. The sensation is influenced by external stimuli such as bandaging or rigid dressing. It may dissipate over time, or the person may experience the phantom sensation throughout life. Phantom sensation does not usually interfere with prosthetic rehabilitation. The client should be assured that the feeling is quite normal.[63,72]

Education, supportive counseling, and early use of the residual limb with a preparatory or permanent prosthesis are effective measures for dealing with phantom limb.[64] In many cases it is best not to dwell on the discussion of phantom limb but rather to focus on prosthetic training and the return to a former lifestyle.

Phantom Sensation

Phantom sensations are different from phantom limb in that they are detailed sensations of the limb. Individuals may describe these as cramping, squeezing, relaxed, numb, tingling, painful, moving, stuck, shooting, burning, cold, hot, or achy. Phantom sensations are described as being constant or intermittent. Some clients report a variety of sensations occurring simultaneously, especially in the hand itself. For example, they may feel the second through fifth digits cramped tightly into flexion and describe the absence of a thumb sensation, as was the case with Roberto. Alternatively, an individual may describe a painful wrist that feels stuck in one position although the phantom forearm rotates easily without any pain. Pain is one phantom sensation. The therapist must be careful when describing or questioning the client about phantom sensations to avoid using the term *phantom pain.* This phrase is most often interpreted by clients as the absence of true pain; their psychological responses to this concept may be fear, anger, distrust in the practitioner's knowledge or support, or confusion. The pain may diminish over time or become a permanent and sometimes disabling condition.

No treatment protocol has been established for the pain associated with phantom sensation. Isometric exercises of the phantom and residual limb initiated 5 to 7 days after the amputation and performed several times throughout the day may help minimize pain. Active movement of the muscles associated with the phantom limb can be beneficial, especially when the sensations are described as stuck, cramped, or tight. Biofeedback, transcutaneous electrical nerve stimulation (TENS), ultrasound, progressive relaxation exercises, and controlled breathing exercises may reduce the pain. Activities such as massaging, tapping, and applying pressure to the residual limb may be beneficial. A physician may treat the pain by prescribing oral medications, injecting anesthetics into a specific soft tissue area, or performing sympathetic nerve blocks. Surgical revision of the residual limb is sometimes necessary to alleviate the pain.[6,13,71] An individual may take nonpharmaceutical oral supplements to decrease the pain. A client's excessive concern with phantom sensation requires the intervention of the team. The therapist can allay the client's fears about these phenomena by offering support, information, reassurance, and contact with other prosthesis wearers.

BONE

The formation of bone spurs is another complication that may occur during the preprosthetic phase. Because most bone spurs are not palpable, an X-ray examination is necessary to confirm their presence or absence. Bone spurs that cause pain or result in persistent drainage require surgical excision.

WOUND HEALING

For clients with LE amputations, delayed wound healing and excessive skin grafting are potential complications during the preprosthetic phase.

Many factors may affect normal wound healing. Postoperative infection from external or internal sources is a major concern. Clients with wounds contaminated from injury, infected foot ulcers, or wounds with other causes are at greater risk for infection. Research indicates that smoking is a major deterrent to wound healing because it diminishes or restricts circulation to the distal extremities. One study reported that individuals who smoke are approximately 2.5 times more likely to have a higher rate of infection and reamputation than nonsmokers.[15,37] There is some indication that failure of limb revascularization may negatively influence healing at below-knee levels. Other factors that influence wound healing are the severity of the vascular problems, diabetes, renal disease, and other medical conditions such as cardiac disease.[14,39,68,70]

SECTION 2: UPPER EXTREMITY AMPUTATIONS

Denise D. Keenan

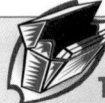

THREADED CASE STUDY: ROBERTO, PART 1

Roberto is 41 years old and married. He has three children and lives at home in a small community. He sustained a transhumeral amputation of his nondominant left upper extremity (UE) as the result of an automobile injury 6 months ago. The residual limb is well healed, with good shrinkage. He does not describe pain in the residual limb. There have been no postoperative medical complications. Roberto reports that he is performing most of his activities of daily living (ADLs) independently, using the sound right arm, except for bilateral activities such as cutting meat, buttoning his shirt, picking up his 2-year-old child, applying deodorant, carrying large objects, and tying his shoes. He is observed to have difficulty problem solving and identifying different strategies that would be beneficial if he is trying to complete an activity using two hands. There are several instrumental activities of daily living (IADLs) that challenge him, including home maintenance, car maintenance, and safely caring for his children on his own. Roberto expresses sadness about the change in his body and how it will affect his ability to work. He is concerned that his 14-year-old son will be embarrassed by his visibly weakened body or that his daughter will be less interested in sitting with him and showing him affection. He knows that he and his wife will cope with this change, but he is worried about their financial security.

Roberto has lived in poverty all his life. His previous jobs included work as a janitor and as a field hand. Roberto says that it is important to him to return to work but that he does not feel that he can perform the types of jobs in which he engaged before the injury. He identifies primarily with the role of caretaker for his family. Because his formal education concluded at the sixth-grade level and his process and communication skills have always been limited, Roberto feels that he is capable of performing only manual labor jobs. He reads basic vocabulary necessary for everyday life at home, at work, and in the community (e.g., signs and newspaper headlines). He wants to be able to provide for his family financially, and the ability to work is important to him. There is no hesitation in his declaration that he will find work and do it well, but he becomes tearful when he discusses this subject and states that he fears failing in this capacity. When employed, Roberto describes himself as a strong and steady worker. His avocational interests are watching television, playing cards, woodcarving, and playing with his children.

Roberto is currently receiving state aid and a prosthesis was funded through this source. Occupational therapy services have been authorized for him. He was referred to occupational therapy for prosthetic training and vocational evaluation.

THREADED CASE STUDY: ROBERTO, PART 1—cont'd

At initial occupational therapy evaluation, Roberto states that he is accepting the prosthesis and that his depression about the loss of his arm is decreasing. He wants to wear the prosthesis and return to some type of employment. Motor skills were treated with progressive resistive exercises to increase the strength of the shoulder rotators and adductors and manual resistive exercises to strengthen the control movements. The names and functions of all parts of the prosthesis were reviewed, and Roberto practiced putting on and removing the prosthesis smoothly and efficiently to increase his process skills. Control training included practice in elbow flexion, elbow locking, elbow and wrist rotation, and terminal device (TD) opening and closing in sequence. Training in grasp and release of objects of various weights, textures, sizes, and shapes in a variety of positions (cans, wood cylinders, pencils, cabinet handles, doorknobs) was completed. Roberto describes phantom sensations in the residual arm that are not painful but are difficult to ignore. He has difficulty opening the TD because he perceives that the flexor muscle group is cramped. The ADL bilateral activities that were addressed included the following: fastening trousers, handling a wallet, tying shoes, cleaning fingernails, applying deodorant, tying a necktie, buttoning a shirt, using the phone, cutting food, planting seeds in a pot, and playing cards. Work simulation activities included cleaning the floor, emptying trash, assembling electronic parts, and using hand tools.

At the completion of five occupational therapy treatment sessions, Roberto tolerates the prosthesis throughout full daytime hours. He has worn it for 90% of his community and social outings. He is incorporating it automatically into 85% of his bilateral ADL tasks. He does become physically fatigued with constant use that lasts more than 2 hours and must take a brief respite. Roberto is pleased with the simple household maintenance activities that he has been able to perform with the help of the prosthesis. He is anxious to return to gainful employment and has met with a vocational counselor twice. The results of his occupational therapy evaluation and treatments were shared with the state vocational rehabilitation counselor assigned to him. He is scheduled for prevocational testing, and three potential jobs have been identified as possibilities for him. Future occupational therapy visits will address job simulation activities and training for the job identified to facilitate his success at the performance requirements.

Critical Thinking Questions

1. Why is Roberto currently unable to work?
2. What are the performance skills that would be appropriately addressed in occupational therapy treatment to increase Roberto's function?
3. What specific interventions would be most effective for increasing Roberto's skills in functioning with the prosthesis?

BODY-POWERED PROSTHESES

CANDIDATES FOR PROSTHESES

Information regarding prostheses and the rehabilitation program should be provided before the amputation, if possible, because subsequent pain medication and anxiety may interfere with the client's ability to process new information. Team discussion that includes the client is vital for determining whether to generate a prosthetic prescription and, if so, which components to include, or, alternatively, whether a prosthesis is inappropriate. The client's age, medical status, amputation level, skin coverage, skin condition, cognitive status, and desire for a prosthesis are important factors in making the decision.

LEVELS OF AMPUTATION AND FUNCTIONAL LOSSES IN THE UPPER EXTREMITY

The higher the level of amputation, the greater the functional loss of the arm. Greater functional loss necessitates a more complex prosthesis and more extensive training in operation and use of the prosthesis (Figure 43-1).[27] Table 43-1 provides an outline of progressively higher UE amputations, associated loss of function, and appropriate components

required for a functional body-powered prosthesis.[22,27] Partial hand amputations are commonly seen. When surgical replantation is not feasible, the focus is placed on reconstruction of the remaining hand. Successful fit of a partial hand prosthesis can preserve the general function of the hand or provide improved cosmesis (Figure 43-2).

COMPONENT PARTS OF THE UPPER EXTREMITY BODY-POWERED PROSTHESIS

Various prosthetic components are available for each level of amputation (Figure 43-3). Each prosthesis is prescribed according to the client's needs and lifestyle and is custom made and individually fitted. The prosthesis can be either a functional prosthesis or a passive prosthesis. *Passive* does not mean nonfunctional; the prosthesis provides postural balance and can assist the client in securing items for the functional limb.

The first five prosthetic components described in the following sections are common to all body-powered prostheses prescribed for wrist disarticulation and higher levels. They are the socket, harness, cable, terminal device (TD), and wrist unit. Many people with UE amputations wear a prosthetic sock between the residual limb and the prosthesis.[62]

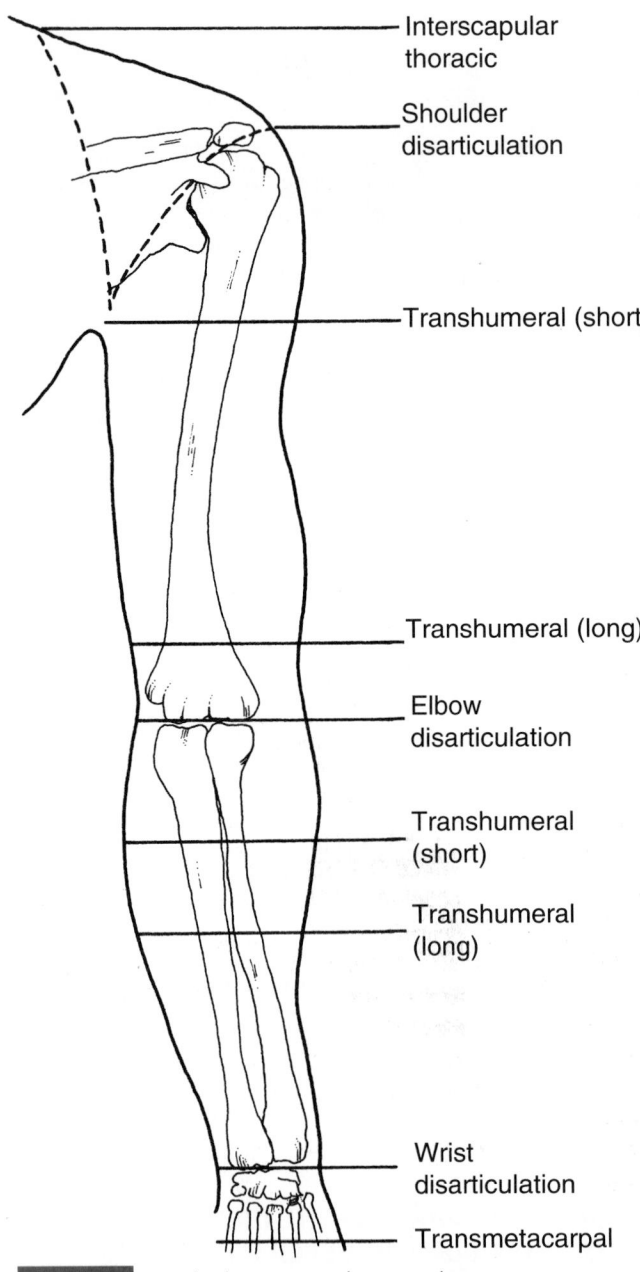

Figure 43-1 Levels of upper extremity amputation.

Labels in figure:
- Interscapular thoracic
- Shoulder disarticulation
- Transhumeral (short)
- Transhumeral (long)
- Elbow disarticulation
- Transhumeral (short)
- Transhumeral (long)
- Wrist disarticulation
- Transmetacarpal

Prosthetic Sock

A prosthetic sock of knit wool, cotton, or Orlon-Lycra is worn between the prosthesis and the limb (Figure 43-4). Silipos makes Silo-Line, which assists in minimizing hypertrophic scarring and may be worn as the prosthetic sock or covered with an additional sock. The function of the prosthetic sock is to absorb perspiration and protect against irritation that can result from direct contact of the skin with the socket. The sock compensates for volume change in the residual limb and contributes to fit and comfort in the socket.[62,74]

Socket

The socket is the fundamental component to which the remaining components are attached. A cast molding of the residual limb is used to construct the socket to optimize fit, comfort, and function. It fits snugly over the limb and extends as far as the wrist unit with a below-elbow (BE) prosthesis or to the elbow unit with an above-elbow (AE) prosthesis. It should cover enough of the residual limb to be stable but not so much that it unnecessarily restricts movement. Uneven pressure distribution may lead to skin problems.[62,72]

The length of the residual limb determines whether a socket is of single- or double-wall construction. The single wall is most commonly used with a wrist disarticulation or elbow disarticulation level of amputation. The single-wall socket requires no shaping over the residual limb. Most sockets have a double wall. This construction involves an inner socket with an outer shape created in foam or wax, covered with an outer shell that is laminated to it. The two shells, inner and outer, become one. The outer wall provides a structurally cosmetic surface. The inner wall maintains total contact with the residual limb's skin surface to distribute the socket pressure evenly. Recently, flexible frame-type sockets have been favored. The inner socket is flexible and is covered with a rigid outer frame that carries the hardware. This type of socket allows for volume and contour changes that occur when muscles contract and relax. Wearers report that this type of socket is cooler than conventional alternatives.[3] The Utah Dynamic Socket is a unique socket design that provides mediolateral and rotational stability through shaping of the shoulder region.[3]

Harness and Control System

The prosthetic control system functions through the interaction of a Dacron harness and stainless-steel cable. The figure-eight harness is commonly used, although others are available. The harness is worn across the back and shoulders or around the chest and fastens to the socket to secure the prosthesis. When the amputation level is higher, the harnessing system becomes more complex.

Loss of muscle power and range of motion (ROM) may necessitate variations in the harness design. A properly fitted harness is important for both comfort and function.[58,62,72]

A flexible stainless-steel cable, contained in a Teflon housing, attaches to the harness on one end via a T-bar or hanger fitting and attaches to a functional component of the prosthesis on the other end. Spectra fiber, an extremely strong material, has been used recently instead of the stainless-steel cable because it glides through the housing with less friction. A BE prosthesis uses one cable to operate the TD, which is connected by a ball swivel. An AE prosthesis uses a second cable to lock and unlock the elbow unit. Specific upper body movements create tension on the cables, thereby operating the prosthesis. A properly fitted control system maximizes prosthetic control while minimizing body movements and exertion.[2,58,72]

TABLE **43-1** **Amputation Levels, Functional Losses, and Suggested Prosthetic Components**

Level of Amputation	Loss of Function	Suggested Functional Prosthetic Components
Partial hand	Some or all grip functions	Dependent on cosmesis and functional loss
Wrist disarticulation	Hand and wrist function; about 50% of pronation and supination	Harness, control cable, socket, flexible elbow hinges
Long transradial	Hand and wrist function; most pronation and supination	Same as for wrist disarticulation but circular wrist unit
Short transradial	Hand and wrist function; all pronation and supination; impaired elbow flexion and extension	Harness, control cable, socket, rigid elbow hinges, biceps half cuff, wrist unit, and terminal device
Elbow disarticulation	Hand and wrist function; all pronation and supination; elbow flexion and extension	Harness, dual-control cables, socket, externally locking elbow, forearm shell, wrist unit, and terminal device
Long transhumeral	Hand and wrist function; all pronation and supination; elbow flexion and extension	Harness, dual-control cables, socket, internally locking elbow, lift assist, turntable, forearm shell, wrist unit, and terminal device
Short transhumeral	All of the above; shoulder internal and external rotation	Same as for long transhumeral, but socket may partially cover shoulder, restricting its function
Shoulder disarticulation	Loss of all arm and hand functions	Same as for long transhumeral, but socket covers shoulder; chest strap; shoulder unit; upper arm shell; chin-operated nudge control for elbow unit
Interscapular thoracic	Loss of all arm and hand functions; partial or complete loss of clavicle and scapula	May be same as above but with lightweight materials; when minimal function is attainable, endoskeletal cosmetic prosthesis sometimes preferred
Bilateral amputation	Dependent on levels of amputation	Appropriate to level of amputation, plus wrist flexion unit and cable-operated wrist rotator

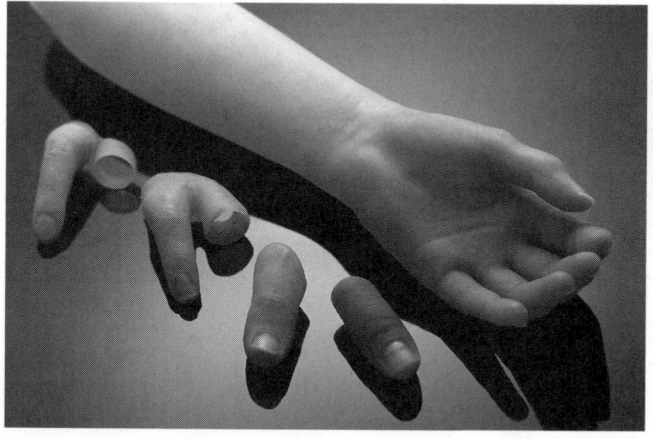
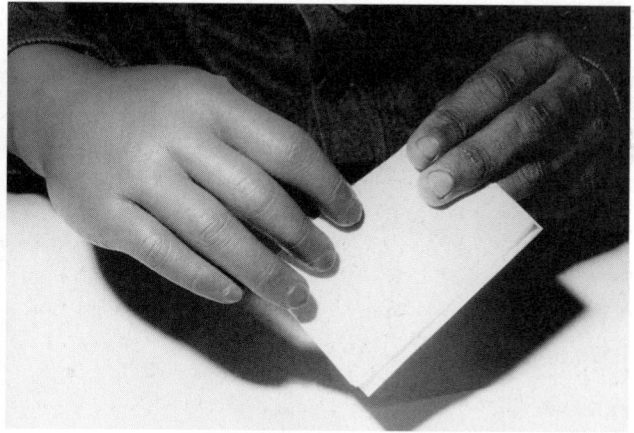

A   B

Figure 43-2 Prostheses for a partial hand amputation. (*A:* Courtesy Otto Bock HealthCare, Minneapolis, MN; *B:* from Boscheinen-Morrin J, Conolly WB: *The hand: fundamentals of therapy*, ed 3, Oxford, 2001, Butterworth-Heinemann.)

Terminal Device

The **terminal device,** the most distal component, functions to grasp and hold an object. When choosing the most appropriate TD for a prosthesis, team members consider the client's age and life roles.

Two styles of TDs are commonly prescribed: the hook and the hand. Many TDs and prosthetic hands have the same shaft size at their base, which allows them to be interchangeable. Hooks are of two basic designs: canted or lyre shaped.[18] They may be either voluntary opening (VO) or voluntary closing (VC).[46]

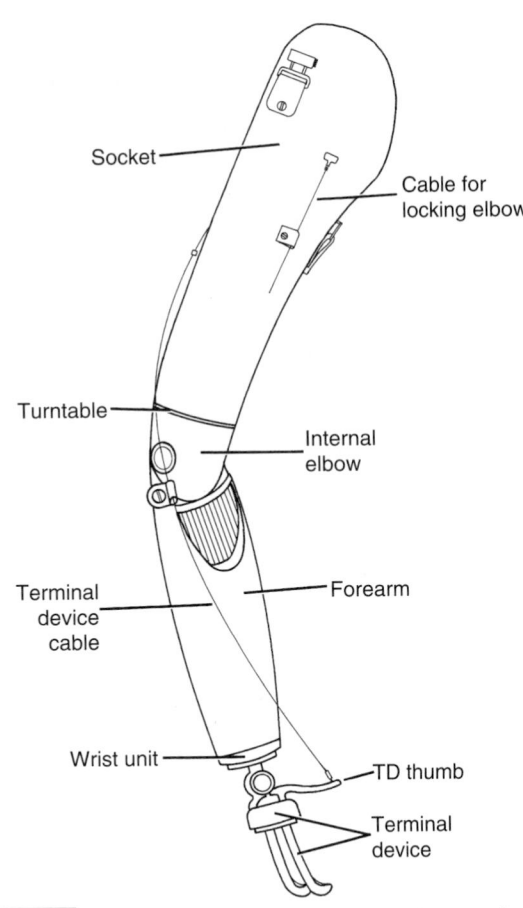

Figure 43-3 Component parts of standard above-elbow prosthesis.

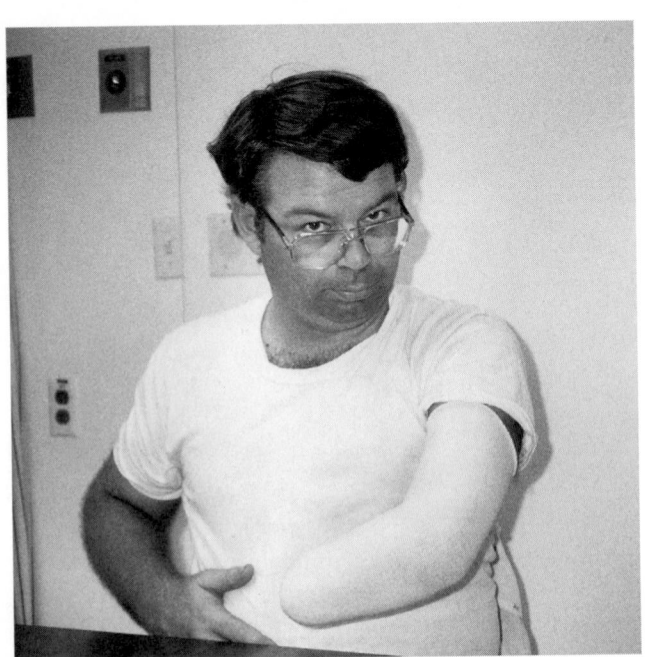

Figure 43-4 Prosthetic sock worn under the prosthesis.

The VO TD opens when the wearer exerts tension on the control cable that connects to the "thumb" of the TD. When tension is released, rubber bands or springs close the fingers of the TD. The number of rubber bands or springs determines the holding force of the TD.

VC TDs close by tension applied to the control cable. The tension may also lock the TD and maintain the grasp on the object. The VC TD automatically opens by spring operation when the cable is relaxed. The VO TD was commonly prescribed in the past. Since World War II, more modern alternatives have become available (Figure 43-5).[2,3,10]

VO TDs have several options to better suit the wearer's lifestyle. The option chosen depends on the desired durability, weight, or grip of the TD.

Stainless-steel TDs are prescribed for activities requiring a durable TD, such as yard work or construction. Aluminum TDs are recommended for lighter work and to reduce the total weight of the prosthesis for a person with a higher-level amputation. Most TDs have either a neoprene lining or a serrated grid between their fingers. The neoprene lining increases the holding friction and minimizes damage when holding objects. Neoprene is a high-density rubber that wears out faster than the stainless-steel grid and disintegrates if it comes in excessive contact with some chemical solutions. The TD must be sent back to the manufacturer for neoprene replacement.

A variation of the standard VO TD is the heavy-duty model. This model is made of stainless steel and has a serrated grid between its fingers. The heavy-duty model is designed to hold tools, nails, and long-handled instruments such as a broom or shovel.

A prosthetic hand is also available as a TD. It attaches to the wrist unit and is either passively operated or cable operated. The passive hand has cosmetic and lightweight appeal, but it is also functional because it is used to push, pull, and stabilize objects. The same control cable that operates the

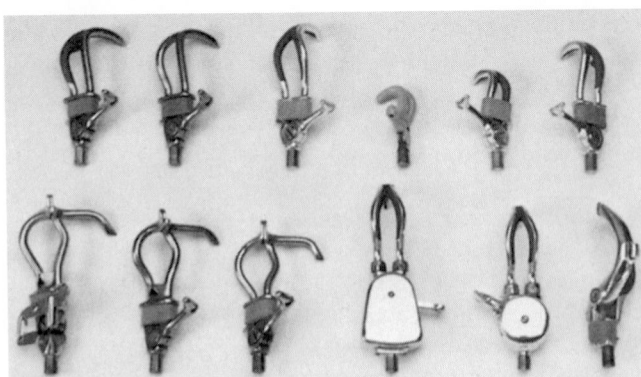

Figure 43-5 The Hosmer-Dorrance hook terminal devices are available in a variety of materials, shapes, and sizes that can be matched to the particular functional needs of a child or adult. (Courtesy Hosmer-Dorrance Corp., Campbell, CA.)

hook activates the functional prosthetic hand. It comes in VO and VC styles. Like the hook-style TD, the VO hand is preferred and prescribed more often than the VC hand. A flesh-colored rubber glove fits over the prosthetic hand for protection and a more realistic appearance.[62]

The client's lifestyle and activities determine the most appropriate TDs. It is important to provide the wearer with certain information regarding the differences between hook- and hand-style TDs. The hook TD is lighter and provides better visibility when grasping objects. It is more durable and functional than prosthetic hands. The hook VO TDs are mechanically simpler than both the VC TDs and functional prosthetic hands. Prosthetic hands are more cosmetically appealing than the prosthetic hook TDs. However, the cosmetic glove that covers the hand stains easily, wears out quickly, and disintegrates if it comes in contact with certain cleaning solutions and chemicals. Many clients with amputations choose an interchangeable hand for social occasions in addition to a hook TD for manual work.[18]

Wrist Unit

The wrist unit connects the TD to the forearm socket and serves as the unit to interchange and to pronate and supinate the TD for prepositioning purposes. The wearer rotates the TD by turning it with the sound hand, by pushing the TD against an object or a surface, or by stabilizing the TD between the knees and using the arm to rotate it. With bilateral amputations, TD rotation in the wrist unit may be accomplished by cable operation. There are five basic types of wrist units selected according to their ability to meet the person's needs in daily living and vocational activities: the friction-held unit, the locking unit, the wrist flexion unit, the oval unit, and the ball-and-socket unit.

The friction-held wrist units hold the TD in place by friction provided by a rubber washer or setscrews. Tightening the washer or screws increases the friction. There is sufficient friction to hold the TD against moderate loads. The friction-held units are mechanically simple but not as strong as locking units.

The locking wrist unit allows the TD to be manually positioned and locked into place. The quick-disconnect locking wrist unit is most common. An adapter is permanently attached to the base of the TD. The unit has a button on its side that locks, unlocks, and ejects the TD. Inserting the TD into the wrist unit locks it into place. Another style of TD with the same adapter type on its base may be locked into place. The friction and locking wrist units allow the TD to be rotated up and down but not deviated in toward the body.

The wrist flexion unit allows the TD to be manually flexed and locked into position. It is generally used on the dominant side of a person with bilateral amputations for facilitating midline activities close to the body, such as dressing and toileting.[2,46,62,72,74]

The oval unit, which conforms to the shape of the wrist, is used on the wrist disarticulation prosthesis. It is thinner than the other wrist units, so the prosthesis may more closely match the length of the sound arm.

A ball-and-socket wrist unit is also available (Figure 43-6). This unit is unique in that it allows prepositioning in multiple wrist positions. It has constant friction, and the magnitude of the loading is adjustable.[18]

The socket, harness, control system, TD, and wrist unit are components common to all body-powered prostheses. The remaining body-powered prosthetic components maximize function at specific levels of amputation. These components are the elbow hinges for BE prostheses, elbow units for AE prostheses, and shoulder units designed for shoulder prostheses.

Below-elbow hinges

A BE prosthesis employs two hinges, one on each side of the elbow, that attach to the socket below the elbow and to a pad or cuff above the elbow. The hinges stabilize and align the BE prosthesis on the residual limb. When properly aligned, the hinges help distribute the stress of the prosthesis on the limb.

Two hinge styles, flexible and rigid, are available for a BE prosthesis. Flexible hinges are used on wrist amputation and long BE prostheses. They are usually made of Dacron and connect the socket to a triceps pad positioned over the triceps muscle. The flexibility permits some forearm rotation, decreasing the need to rotate the TD manually in the wrist.

Medium-to-short BE prostheses have a socket that covers most of the residual limb below the elbow and rigid hinges to provide stability. Rigid hinges are usually made of steel and attached to a laminated Dacron biceps half-cuff positioned behind the arm, which is sturdier and provides more support than the triceps pad. Team members consider the

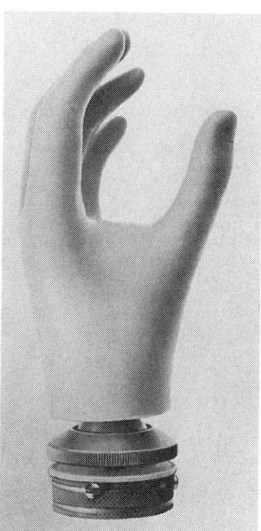

Figure 43-6 Ball-and-socket wrist unit. (Courtesy Otto Bock HealthCare, Minneapolis, MN.)

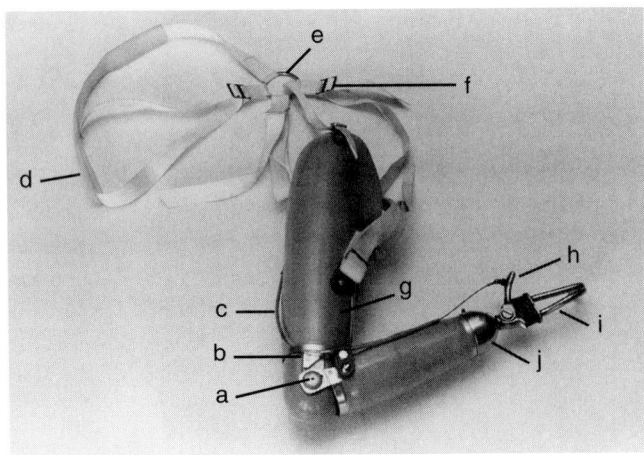

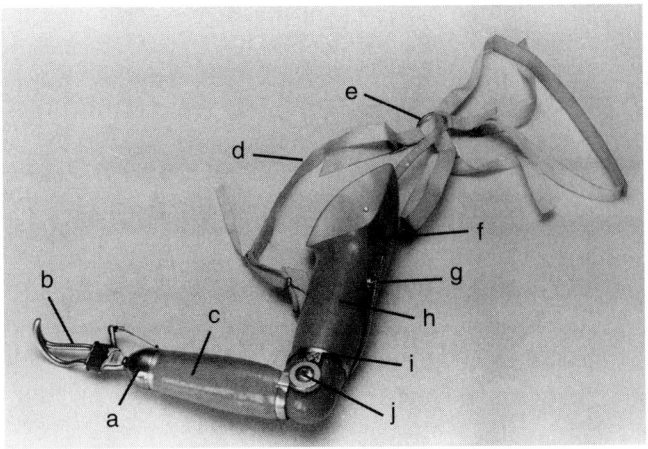

A

B

Figure 43-7 **A,** Lateral side of above-elbow prosthesis: *a,* elbow unit; *b,* turntable; *c,* control cable; *d,* adjustable axilla loop; *e,* harness ring; *f,* figure-of-eight harness; *g,* elbow lock cable; *h,* terminal device (TD) thumb; *i,* hook TD; *j,* wrist flexion unit. **B,** Medial side of AE prosthesis: *a,* wrist unit; *b,* hook TD; *c,* forearm; *d,* harness; *e,* harness ring; *f,* control cable; *g,* baseplate and retainer; *h,* socket; *i,* turntable; *j,* spring-loading device.

amount of residual function and the limb's length when choosing the appropriate style hinge for the BE prosthesis.[46]

Elbow units for above-elbow prostheses

A prosthetic elbow unit is prescribed for the person who has had an amputation through the level of the elbow or higher. The elbow unit allows 5 to 135 degrees of elbow flexion and locks in various positions. The two main types of elbow units are the internally and externally locking units. The more durable internally locking unit is prescribed for a person who has had an amputation 2 inches or more above the elbow. The unit connects the AE socket to the prosthetic forearm. The locking mechanism is contained within the unit and attaches to a control cable. A lift assist, which consists of a tightly coiled spring attached to the elbow unit and forearm shell, helps reduce the amount of energy required to lift the forearm shell. The lift assist also allows a slight bounce in the forearm when walking with the elbow unlocked, which increases the appearance of a natural arm swing.

Correspondingly, the externally locking elbow unit is prescribed for a person who has an elbow disarticulation or an amputation within 2 inches above the elbow. This unit, which consists of a pair of hinges positioned on either side of the prosthesis, attaches the socket to the forearm. The cable attaches to one of the hinges, which locks and unlocks the unit.

A friction-held turntable positioned on top of the elbow unit allows the prosthetic forearm to be rotated manually toward or away from the body. The lateral and medial aspects of a transhumeral prosthesis are shown in Figure 43-7. The internally locking unit is 2 inches long and therefore does not fit on a person who has had an amputation close to the elbow.

Shoulder units

A person with an amputation at the shoulder requires a prosthesis with a shoulder unit in addition to the TD, wrist unit, forearm shell, elbow unit, socket, harness, and cables. Because of the high level of amputation, however, shoulder and back movements are not sufficient to use a cable-operated shoulder unit. Thus, most shoulder units are manually operated and friction held. The TD and elbow units may still be cable operated.

Two shoulder unit styles that are often prescribed are the flexion-abduction unit and the locking shoulder joint. The flexion-abduction (or double-axis) unit provides manual prosthetic positioning in flexion and abduction and is friction held (Figure 43-8).[18] The locking unit allows the prosthesis to be locked in various degrees of shoulder flexion. This feature is helpful because the prosthesis is heavy and the friction style may not be strong enough.

With an interscapular thoracic amputation, all or a portion of the scapula and clavicle is removed with the arm. If standard prosthetic components were used, the prosthesis might be too heavy for practical use. Therefore, an endoskeletal prosthesis, made from lightweight materials such as a single aluminum alloy surrounded by a soft foam shape, is often prescribed to decrease its weight. The system provides its own style of prosthetic joints, which will not withstand heavy-duty usage. The endoskeletal prosthesis is commonly prescribed as an aesthetic prosthesis with limited functional value.

UPPER-EXTREMITY PREPROSTHETIC PROGRAM

The preprosthetic program begins when the decision to perform an amputation is made or when a client is evaluated after a traumatic amputation.[34] Education regarding prosthesis

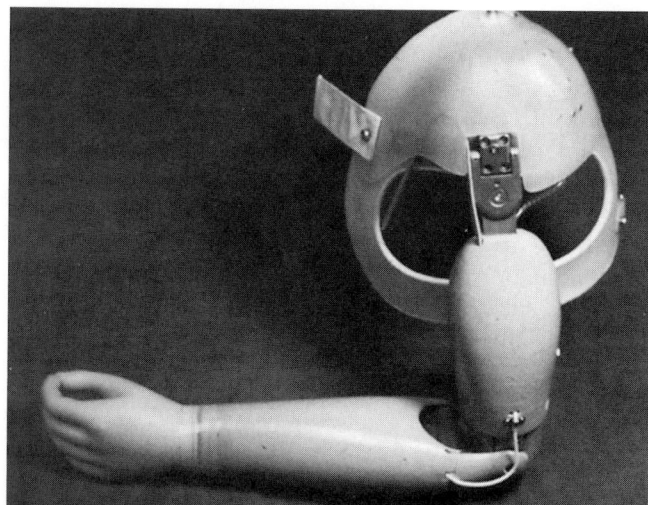

Figure 43-8 Hosmer-Dorrance "Flexion/Abduction Shoulder Joint," shown attached to a shoulder disarticulation-type prosthesis, provides passive mechanical range of motion in flexion to 90 degrees and abduction to 135 degrees. An extension stop is provided to restrict extension. (From Hunter JM, Mackin EJ, Callahan AD: *Rehabilitation of the hand: surgery and therapy*, ed 4, St Louis, 1995, Mosby.)

options, relaxation techniques, and general strengthening may begin in some cases before the surgical amputation. During the period between the amputation and the fitting of the prosthesis, the client participates in a program designed to prepare the residual limb for a prosthesis, facilitate adjustment to his or her loss, and achieve maximal independence in self-care.[50,72] The occupational therapist is the primary person who will be coordinating this program. It is also important for the team to assist the client in securing the financial resources necessary to complete rehabilitation and obtain a prosthesis if desired.

Preprosthetic Evaluation

To establish an individualized intervention plan, the therapist must complete a thorough evaluation. The evaluation includes assessments of the client's medical history; body functions (mental, sensory, movement, skin); motor skills (posture, coordination, strength and effort, energy); process skills (adaptation, organizing space and objects); activities of daily living (ADLs); instrumental activities of daily living (IADLs); education; work; leisure; and social participation.[1] A statement of the client's goals is important for orienting the treatment toward meeting the goals and for determining the client's understanding of the program and the prosthesis.[6] The interview portion of Roberto's evaluation was essential in establishing his desires, goals, and concerns and is necessary in developing the most appropriate intervention for him.

Preprosthetic Treatment

The intervention plan is based on evaluation results. Most plans include the interventions for body functions,

body structures, and performance skills that are listed in Box 43-1.

Depending on the level of amputation, medical conditions, and ADL status, the decision is made whether to complete the preprosthetic program on an inpatient or outpatient basis. In most cases in which the client has undergone a unilateral amputation, therapy services are offered on an outpatient basis. When an individual loses a dominant hand, which is often the case with unilateral amputation, minimal training in one-handed activity completion may take place. The focus of this training is on problem-solving approaches to task completion with new hand dominance and on encouraging the client to practice completing activities independently. Some clients who lose the dominant extremity choose to remain dominant with their prosthetic side. A person with bilateral amputations may need to be admitted to a facility because of the significant amount of therapy and assistance required. In the case of bilateral UE limb loss, the client has significant issues with functional independence to address as well as emotional issues related to a severe life change that affects emotions, finances, life goals, body image, and relationships. The complexity of the issues is best addressed in an inpatient setting. A client who has had both upper limbs amputated will appreciate being introduced to other persons using one or two prostheses to function. The team closely monitors the residual limb and reports problems to the physician. If the client is followed on an outpatient basis, frequent medical visits may be necessary to monitor progress. Early fit of a prosthesis has been shown to significantly increase functional prosthetic use.[53] Fitting clients with a preparatory prosthesis before they become "one-handed" facilitates their success with prosthetic function.

Body image, self-image, psychosocial adjustment

Facilitating the client's return to developmentally appropriate activities and resuming family, occupational, and social

---

Box **43-1** INTERVENTIONS FOR BODY FUNCTIONS, BODY STRUCTURES, AND PERFORMANCE SKILLS
Improve body image, self-image, psychosocial adjustment.
Promote independent function during ADLs and IADLs.
Promote wound healing.
Improve desensitization of the limb.
Establish pain management practices.
Promote residual limb shaping and shrinking.
Promote proper skin hygiene.
Promote care of insensate skin.
Maintain and restore passive and active range of motion.
Maintain and restore upper body strength and endurance.
Improve understanding of prosthetic components and options.
Recommend appropriate prosthetic components.

roles is a primary focus of occupational therapy intervention. The therapist helps the client integrate the physical loss into his or her life. It is essential that the therapist validate the client's right to be in control of his or her life. Roberto's strong work ethic and goal of returning to work as quickly as possible to fulfill his role identity must be honored. It is not uncommon for individuals who have undergone an amputation to experience a physical shock to their body as well as an emotional shock to their spirit. Fear, confusion, anger or frustration, emotional swings, introspectiveness, and dependence are common responses following loss. Allow the client to experience and express these feelings during therapy, and educate family members and the client in the common nature of these feelings.[1]

Assist the client in describing which of his or her features are pleasing. Encourage the client to continue with useful habits to maintain a normal routine. Give positive feedback for every accomplishment reported or observed.

Once the client's level of social participation before the amputation is explored, facilitate opportunities to engage in similar events. The client may be encouraged to participate in one event monthly or weekly, initially in the company of a family member or friend. Introduce the client to others who have suffered a similar limb loss to allow communication with a peer. Provide adaptive equipment that allows the client to resume leisure activities and increase his or her quality of life. Some clients are uncomfortable with the changes in fashion and clothing style that are recommended to ease the dressing process. Recommend a tailoring service, or help the client identify a family member, friend, or neighbor who would be willing to modify some of the client's clothing.

Activities of daily living

During the preprosthetic period, the client with a unilateral amputation should be encouraged to use the sound arm to perform ADLs. If the dominant arm was amputated, training may be required for the nondominant limb to assume the dominant role. In the author's experience, most clients change dominance to the sound extremity automatically as a result of the adaptive process, and minimal intervention is necessary for this to occur. Some clients need support and a few sessions of practice engaging in meaningful activities with the nondominant hand to understand and accept their ability to perform this way. Rather, the focus of training is on problem-solving techniques and adaptations that will allow clients to modify multiple activities in their daily lives. Some adaptive equipment is appropriate for increasing independence with bilateral activities. Practice in writing and activities requiring dexterity and coordination may be helpful in the retraining process.[50,62,72] The importance of early fitting of a prosthesis cannot be minimized. Early fit programs are very successful in helping the client with an amputation to incorporate the new extremity more rapidly into their daily activities.[2]

In the case of a bilateral amputation, adaptive equipment should be introduced as soon as possible to increase the client's level of independence. The equipment may include a utensil cuff secured by elastic or Velcro to the residual limb to aid in eating, writing, and hygiene; a dressing tree, with hooks to hold articles of clothing in a position conducive to donning them, to improve dressing independence; and loops added to items such as socks and towels. Clients with a bilateral amputation can also learn to complete activities using foot skills, such as holding items between the toes in a functional pinch for dressing, eating, and turning pages, or using the toes to push buttons on a keyboard or telephone pad.

Wound healing

When the surgical dressing is removed, the residual limb is massaged to discourage scar adhesions, increase circulation, aid in desensitization, and reduce swelling. Massage of the limb also helps the client overcome fear of touching or moving the residual limb. Massage over the incision site begins once the incision has stabilized.[6] Initially, light massage over healed areas is performed, followed by deeper pressures, as tolerated by the client. If skin grafts have been placed, the therapist must confer with the surgeon to determine tissue status before performing scar massage.

Desensitization

The residual limb may be hypersensitive after surgery and require a technique known as *desensitization.* By overstimulating a hypersensitive peripheral area with nonharmful stimuli, the central nervous system learns to accept these stimuli as nonharmful and minimize the aversive responses to them. Massage is one method of desensitization. Other methods are tapping, vibration, constant pressure, and the rubbing of various textures on the limb, such as terry cloth, silk, and cotton. The therapist introduces the tissue to soft, lightweight, smooth textures and progresses to rough, hard, uneven, heavier textures as the client is able to tolerate them. A therapist with a thorough understanding of nerve anatomy and hierarchy of response to stimuli should be consulted, and the intervening therapist must understand this information before subjecting the client's tissues to a desensitization program. As the techniques are performed, the therapist teaches them to the client and his or her family members or caregivers to facilitate completion of a home program basis.[6,24]

Wrapping

Shrinking and shaping the residual limb are necessary to form a tapered limb that will tolerate a prosthesis and fit closely. Compression using an elastic bandage, a tubular bandage, or a shrinker sock applied to the residual limb aids in the shrinking and shaping process. When an elastic bandage is applied to the limb, a figure-eight method (Figure 43-9) is used, not a circumferential method in which the bandage is wrapped around the limb spirally. Care must be taken to apply the bandage smoothly, evenly, and not too tightly from

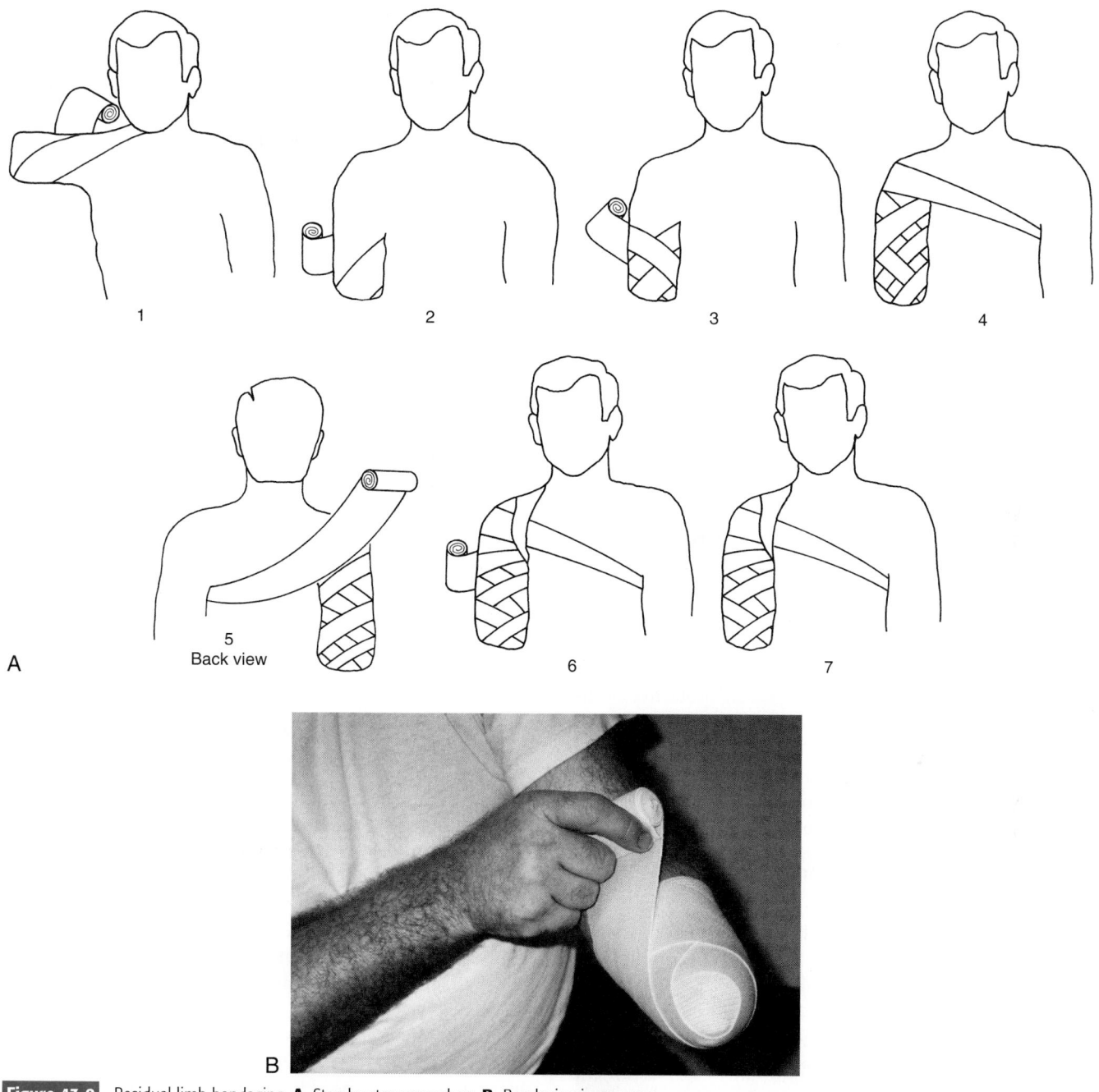

Figure 43-9 Residual limb bandaging. **A,** Step-by-step procedure. **B,** Bandaging in progress.

the distal to the proximal end of the residual limb. Care must also be taken to avoid wrapping skin-grafted areas too tightly or without an inner nonadherent dressing applied, so that the graft is not compromised. A limb that is wrapped incorrectly may not be able to be fitted with a prosthesis or may take longer to shrink and shape. A limb with a transradial amputation should be wrapped up to or above the elbow. A limb with a transhumeral amputation should be wrapped up to or above the shoulder. Short transhumeral amputations usually must be wrapped around the chest to help stabilize

the wrap.[62,72] The elastic bandage should be changed several times a day and the skin checked between wrappings. Several compression wraps are required so that the limb can be wrapped in a clean bandage at all times, except when bathing. The wraps should be washed often with a mild soap, rinsed well, and allowed to dry thoroughly while lying flat. For longer life, the bandages should not be wrung out after washing.[6]

Shrinker socks are generally preferred over elastic bandage wrapping because the client can more independently don the sock and because changing the sock is much quicker than changing the wrap. Compression tubing sewed closed or with a knot tied at one end is commonly used. The tubing may be attached to a chest strap if necessary.

Circumference measurements

The residual limb's circumference measurements are taken often and in the same area to determine when the person is ready to be casted for a prosthesis. The therapist uses a tape measure to establish baseline and subsequent measurements (Figure 43-10). When the edema is gone and the circumference measurements have stabilized, the limb is ready to be casted.

Skin hygiene

Instruction in proper residual limb hygiene is an important aspect of the preprosthetic program. The limb should be washed daily using a mild soap, rinsed thoroughly, and patted dry. The limb should dry completely before the wrap or sock is reapplied.[5]

Insensate skin

The client with a UE amputation requires instruction regarding the care and safety of a residual limb that lacks all or partial sensation. The client is taught to inspect the limb when removing the wrap and washing the limb. Problems should be reported to the therapist or physician. The client should also learn to visually track a sensory-impaired residual limb when completing activities, such as wearing protective clothing while engaged in yard work or recreational activities or adjusting the position of the limb when seated in a chair and reading to prevent stretch or compression injury to the tissues, and to refrain from using the limb for sensory input, such as testing water temperature.

Upper extremity range of motion, strength, and endurance

After medical approval, the client begins exercises designed to maintain and increase ROM and strengthen upper quadrant

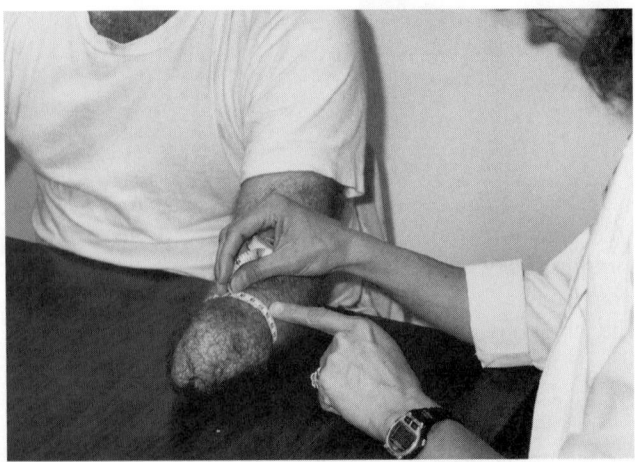

Figure 43-10 Measuring residual limb circumference.

and trunk muscles. Depending on the level of amputation, the therapist instructs the client to complete specific exercises that mimic the movements required to operate the prosthesis. The therapist manually positions and holds the residual limb in the desired posture and asks the client to resist the hold, facilitating increased strength of the appropriate muscles. In the case of a transradial amputation, it is important to strengthen the muscles of the shoulder, elbow, and scapula. Pronation and supination movements are also important for long transradial amputations. Transhumeral amputation strengthening may include a movement combining shoulder depression, extension, and abduction that mimics the operation of the body-powered prosthesis. Isometric exercises enable the client to engage in a strengthening program without equipment. Exercises may also be completed with rubber tubing, elastic band, or strap-on weights. It may be appropriate to guide the client in the modified use of home or gym equipment to complete exercises. Chest expansion capability is important for higher-level amputations and when the harness wraps around the chest. A tape measure positioned around the chest helps in the documentation of increased chest expansion.

A home program containing exercises for general strengthening and body conditioning, as well as the specific movements taught during therapy, should be provided (Figure 43-11).

PROSTHETIC INFORMATION AND PRESCRIPTION

During the preprosthetic period, the client should receive information about the benefits and limitations of a variety of prostheses. The prosthetist generally provides information regarding specific prosthetic options, and the therapist promotes the client's understanding of the options as well as facilitates the client's goal acquisition. The therapist must be aware of what the amputation and the prosthesis mean to the client at this stage and what the client's future goals are. Roberto verbalized his desires for return to gainful and fulfilling employment to provide for his family. In selecting prosthetic components, the therapist must consider whether the client's primary need is function or cosmesis and which style is most appropriate to the client's needs and choices. Prosthetic components can be introduced in several ways: through slides, videotapes, photographs, interaction with a person with a similar amputation wearing a prosthesis, practice in handling a prosthesis, and a joint visit to the prosthetist.

PROSTHETIC PROGRAM

The amount of training each person needs depends on how quickly he or she is able to understand the body mechanics required to operate the prosthesis, the person's problem-solving skills and motivation, the cueing needed to include

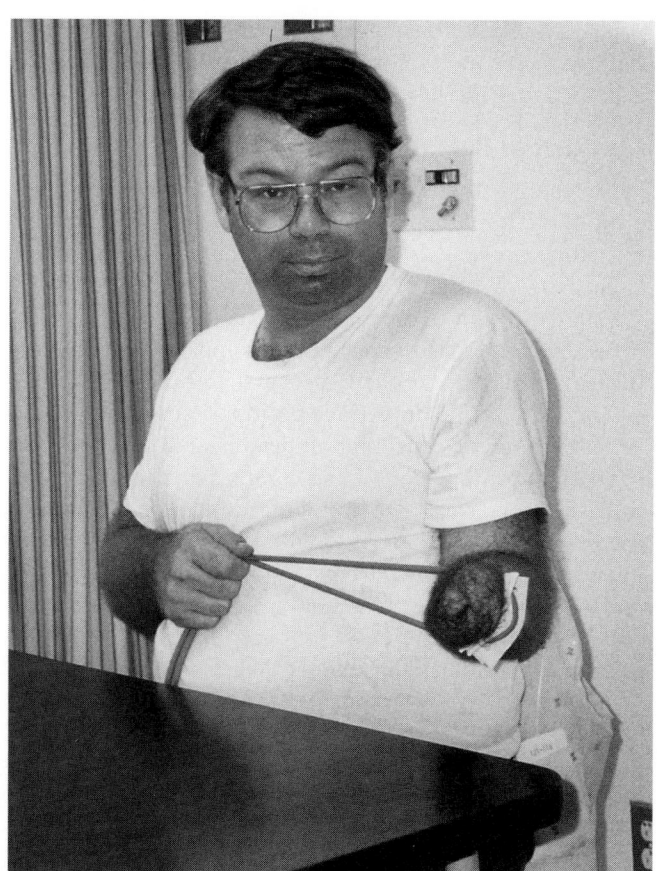

Figure 43-11 Home program of upper extremity strengthening to prepare arm for prosthesis. Thera-tubing is being used for resistive exercise.

the prosthesis in an activity, and the carryover between activities. When a long period has elapsed between the amputation and receipt of the prosthesis, the client may require more cueing because he or she has become adept at one-handed activities. Some clients arrive at therapy already able to operate the prosthesis, whereas others require extensive training.

Ideally, the prosthetist and therapist coordinate the final fitting of the prosthesis and the initial training session. The therapist may arrange to be present for the final fitting. Communication between the wearer, therapist, and prosthetist is essential to ensure that the prosthesis fits and functions optimally. The therapist should be aware of the possible need for adjustment of the prosthesis and consultation with the prosthetist if this need becomes evident.

The prosthesis will not be as functional as a normal arm, and training for the client with a unilateral amputation should stress that the prosthesis functions primarily as an assist or helper to the sound arm. If the prosthesis is presented in this manner, the wearer may experience less difficulty when incorporating it into daily function. In training the person with a bilateral amputation to function with prostheses, the likelihood of success with one prosthesis is strong as the wearer instantly recognizes the benefit of the prosthesis to independent function.

The prosthetic program begins after the final fitting of the prosthesis. This final fitting may be with a preparatory prosthesis rather than a definitive prosthesis, incomplete in its cosmetic form. Although a treatment plan focuses on the wearer's prosthetic goals, some educational information and initial training points are common to all prosthetic intervention plans. These include the following:

- Promote positive body image and self-image
- Establish successful adaptation and problem-solving skills
- Promote proper residual limb and prosthetic sock hygiene
- Promote recognition of prosthesis terminology and function
- Promote proper care of the prosthesis
- Establish a prosthesis-wearing schedule
- Promote control of the prosthesis (control training)
- Promote use of the prosthesis in activity (use training)
- Promote independent ADL and IADL function with the prosthesis (Functional Training)
- Promote driving modifications and ability
- Establish a home activity program
- Maintain UE muscles necessary for operation of the prosthesis
- Prevent repetitive use injury of the sound arm
- Promote vocational re-entry
- Establish follow-up care
- Promote social routines and community integration

The prosthesis checkout, control training, use, and functional training are individualized according to the client's level of amputation.

Body Image and Self-Image

The interview process reveals the client's lifestyle, primary role, and personal relationships. The occupational therapist is the professional who investigates and responds to the spiritual essence of the client. Expanding the interview with questions about the client's interests, social activities, style of dress and appearance, and self-concept is necessary to establish the client's pre-injury behaviors and skills. The therapist observes the client's body language. Is the residual limb hidden? Does the client use the hand and arm to communicate? Is the client visually attentive and engaged in the interview or intervention? What does this tell you about the client's self-image and body image? Provide opportunities for the client to focus on his or her accomplishments and skills. Assist the client to enhance those parts of the body with which he or she is most pleased. Prioritize interventions to facilitate the client's ability to style hair, apply jewelry, fasten a tie, apply makeup, resume general physical activity and recreation, drive independently, and manage a briefcase and personal electronic equipment.

Residual Limb and Prosthetic Sock Hygiene

The client is instructed in residual limb hygiene and care of the prosthetic sock in the early phase of prosthetic training.

The residual limb and armpit should be inspected, washed, and patted dry, and deodorant should be applied daily. If the client chooses to wear a prosthetic sock, he or she should own several so that a clean one may be worn daily to decrease chances of skin problems. The socks should be hand washed, gently squeezed, and placed on a flat surface to dry in their original dimensions. Wearing an undergarment under the harness is often recommended because it will absorb perspiration and protect the axilla and back from irritation. It may be necessary to change prosthetic socks and undergarments twice a day in hot weather.[72,74] To minimize sweating, educate the client in the application of deodorant to the portion of the extremity within the socket.

Prosthesis Terminology and Function

The wearer should learn the terminology and function of each prosthetic component. This task allows the client to communicate with the rehabilitation team, using terminology understood by all, regarding operation of the prosthesis and difficulties with or repairs needed to the prosthesis.[5,72,74]

Care of the Prosthesis

Instructions regarding care of the prosthesis are provided and reviewed. Generally, the prosthetist educates the person in this area and the therapist reviews the information with the wearer. The socket should be cleaned daily with a soft cloth and mild soap and rinsed thoroughly with warm water. Cleaning at night is recommended to allow the prosthesis to dry completely. Wearing the prosthesis when the socket is wet may lead to skin problems. Components should be cleaned and maintained according to the manufacturer's or prosthetist's specifications. Daily inspection of the prosthesis will help prevent unnecessary problems.[5]

Prosthesis-Wearing Schedule

A prosthesis-wearing schedule is established and reviewed during the first training session. The client initially wears the prosthesis 15 to 30 minutes three times a day. The skin must be closely monitored, and wearing time is increased only if the skin remains in good condition. If there are no skin problems, the three scheduled wearing periods may be increased by 30 minutes each day. By the end of the first week, the client may be wearing the prosthesis all day, as was the case with Roberto. If skin problems occur, the therapist, prosthetist, or physician must be notified. The prosthesis should not be worn until the skin problem has cleared. Restarting the initial wearing schedule may be necessary to decrease the risk of more skin problems.[5]

As the person's wearing tolerance increases, the number of rubber bands on the TD can be increased. Each rubber band added to the TD increases the pinch force by approximately 1 pound. It is best to wait several days after adding one rubber band before adding another to allow the residual limb's skin and strength to acclimate. If the addition of a rubber band substantially increases limb pain or skin irritation, it should be removed until the pain diminishes and skin tolerance increases.

Checkout of the Prosthesis

When the prosthesis is received, team members check it to ensure that it meets prescription requirements, is functioning efficiently, and is mechanically sound. The prosthesis is checked for fit and function against specific mechanical standards developed from actual tests on prostheses worn by individuals. Tests performed are comparative ROM with the prosthesis on and off; control system function and efficiency; TD opening in various positions; amount of socket slippage on the residual limb under various degrees of load or tension; compression fit and comfort; and force required to flex the forearm.[2,58,72] Communication among the wearer, therapist, and prosthetist is essential to ensure an efficiently operating and comfortable prosthesis. The following methods and standards for the prosthesis checkout were adapted primarily from Wellerson.[72] Step-by-step instructions for the prosthetic checkout are available in Wellerson[72] and Santschi.[58]

Below-Elbow Prosthesis

The therapist measures elbow flexion with the BE prosthesis on and off the wearer. The ROM should not differ by more than 10 degrees, except when there are joint or muscle limitations. Pronation and supination of a wrist disarticulation or long transradial residual limb with the prosthesis on should not be less than 50% of the rotation possible without the prosthesis.

With the elbow flexed at 90 degrees, the client should be able to open the TD fully. The TD is also opened near the mouth (elbow fully flexed) and again near the zipper of the trousers (elbow extended). From 70% to 100% of TD opening should be achieved in these two positions.

Above-Elbow and Shoulder Prosthesis

With the AE prosthesis on and the elbow locked, the client is instructed to move the residual limb (humerus) into shoulder flexion, extension, abduction, and internal and external rotation. The ROM of each of these is measured. Minimal standards for shoulder ROM with the prosthesis on are as follows: 90-degree flexion, 30-degree extension, 90-degree abduction, and 45-degree rotation. The previous part of the checkout is not applicable for the shoulder prosthesis.

With the elbow unlocked, the client is instructed to flex the shoulder slowly, which flexes the mechanical elbow. The elbow ROM should be about 10 to 135 degrees. The therapist measures the amount of shoulder flexion, which should not exceed 45 degrees, that is required to fully flex the mechanical elbow. The client should also be able to abduct the prosthesis to 60 degrees without locking of the elbow.

The client flexes the elbow to 90 degrees, locks the elbow, and then activates the TD. Full TD opening should be attained in this position. The TD is then opened in full elbow flexion with elbow locked (Figure 43-12) and extension with elbow locked (TD at fly of trousers). At least 50% of full TD opening should be obtained.

With the elbow unlocked, the client is asked to walk and practice swinging the prosthesis without locking the elbow. This action mimics a normal arm swing during gait.

The client flexes the elbow to 90 degrees, locks the elbow, abducts the residual limb to 60 degrees, and then rotates the humerus. The client should be able to control the prosthesis during this motion. The socket should not slip around the residual limb, and the client should not feel pain or discomfort during these maneuvers. When the prosthesis is removed, the residual limb should not appear discolored or irritated.

The prosthesis checkout also includes a technical inspection of the prosthesis to determine correct length, fit, and mechanical function of all parts. Various forms have been devised to record all information for the complete checkout of the prosthesis. The initial checkout is performed before prosthetic training begins, and the final checkout is done after prosthetic revisions and adjustments and either during or after training.[5,58]

Donning and Doffing the Prosthesis

The two common methods of donning and doffing the body-powered prosthesis are the coat method and the sweater method. Either method can be used with unilateral or bilateral amputations. The method used depends on the client's ease of use. Whichever the method, the harness and cables must not be kinked or twisted around the prosthesis before starting.

When the prosthesis is removed, it should be placed on a surface so that it is ready for the client to don again.

Coat method

The coat method is similar to placing one arm in the coat sleeve and manipulating the coat to a position where the other arm can reach the sleeve. The coat method has two variants. In the first method, the client places the prosthesis on a table or bed and pushes the residual limb between the control cable and the Y-strap from the medial side into the socket. By raising the residual limb or leaning sideways, the client places the harness across the shoulder on the amputated side and dangles the harness down the back. The sound hand reaches around the back and slips into the axilla loop. The client then slips into the harness as if putting on a coat. The shoulders are shrugged to shift the harness forward and into the correct position.

The second method works by placing the axilla loop of the harness on the sound arm first. For example, if the client has a transhumeral amputation, it might be easier to lock the elbow at 90 degrees; position the axilla loop on the sound arm above the elbow; grasp the prosthetic forearm; and raise the prosthesis over the head, allowing the harness to position itself across the back. By raising the residual limb, the client positions it in the socket (Figure 43-13).

To remove the prosthesis, the client uses the TD to slip the axilla loop off the sound side and then slips the shoulder strap off the amputated side. The harness is then slipped off like a coat.[2,58,72]

The client with bilateral amputations can use the coat method by placing the prostheses face up on a surface, placing the longer residual limb into the socket, and elevating the

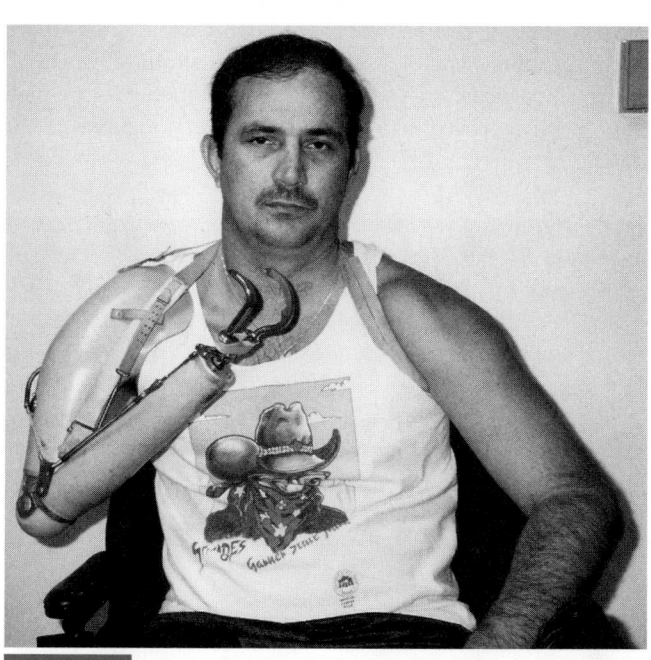

Figure 43-12 Above-elbow prosthesis checkout: opening terminal device at mouth with elbow locked in full flexion.

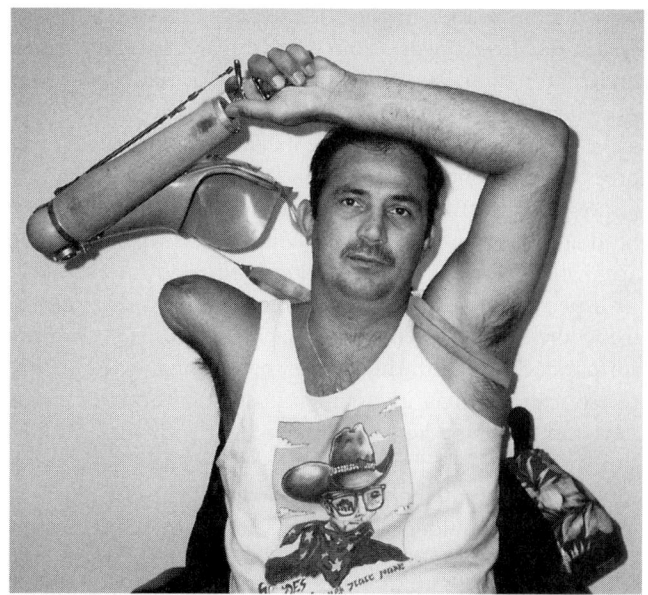

Figure 43-13 Coat method of donning prosthesis.

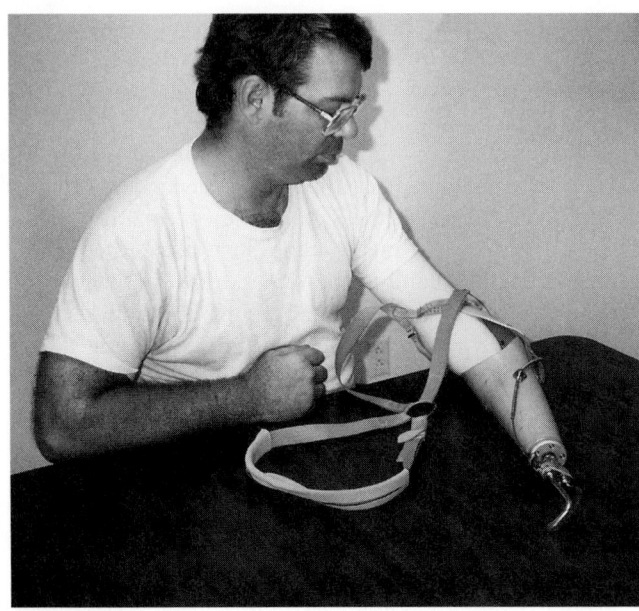

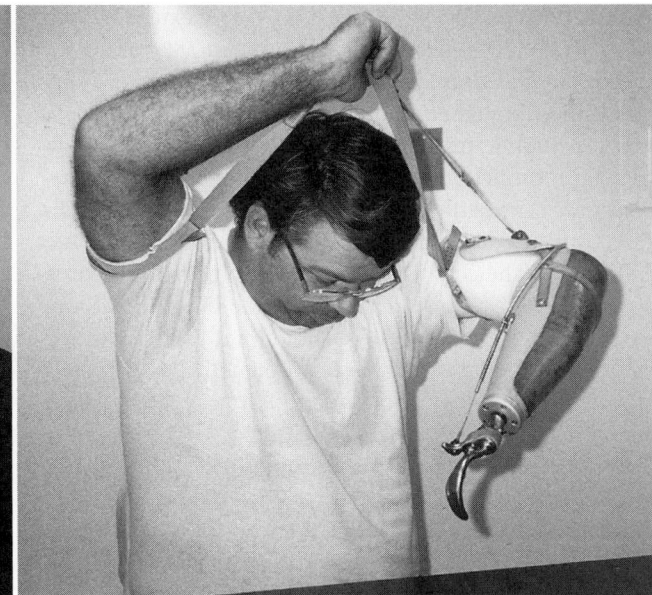

A   B

Figure 43-14 Sweater method of donning prosthesis.

prosthesis, allowing the other prosthesis to hang across the back. The client then leans to the side and places the shorter limb in the prosthesis.[58,74] To remove the prosthesis, the client shrugs the harness off the shoulders and removes the prosthesis from the shorter side first. Before removing the prosthesis on the longer side, the client should position the prostheses somewhere convenient for the next donning.

Sweater method

The sweater method (Figure 43-14) is equivalent to entering both sleeves at the same time and then raising both arms up, out, and up to don the sweater. To apply a unilateral prosthesis using the sweater method, the client places the prosthesis on a surface face up, positions the residual limb in the socket under the Y-strap, and places the opposite arm in the harness. The client then raises both arms above the head, allowing the axilla loop to slide down to the axilla and the harness to be properly positioned across the back and on the shoulders. To remove the prosthesis, the client raises both arms above the head and grasps and removes the prosthesis with the sound arm, while allowing the axilla loop to slide off the arm.[58]

A person with bilateral amputations dons the prostheses using the sweater method by placing the prostheses on a surface, face up. With the longer limb stabilizing the socket, the shorter residual limb is then positioned under the harness and in the socket. The longer limb is then positioned similarly under the harness in the socket, and the arms are raised, allowing the harness to flip over the head and across the back and shoulders. The client removes the prostheses by shrugging the shoulders to bring the harness up, grasping it with the TD, and pulling it over the head while allowing the residual limbs to come out of their sockets.

Control Training

Control training is best accomplished in front of a mirror to help the client learn the minimal motions necessary to operate the prosthesis while maintaining proper body mechanics (Figure 43-15).

Acquiring skill in the operation of the prosthesis is emphasized in control training. The therapist educates the wearer in the importance of the practice drills that will ensure more successful function with the prosthesis in daily activities. Joint protection, energy conservation, and work simplification principles and techniques should be stressed during this phase of training. Each prosthetic component should be reviewed separately and understood before the

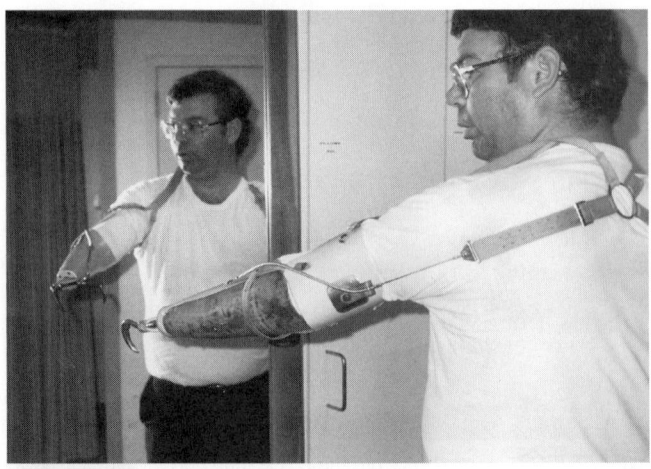

Figure 43-15 Control training in front of mirror.

components are combined into functional activities. Such movements as elbow flexion and TD opening are cable operated. Other movements, such as TD or elbow rotation, are passively positioned using the sound hand or an item in the environment. Emphasizing external assists from the environment is an important part of this training process. A client preparing to cut vegetables at the counter may be instructed to use the countertop to rotate the TD in the best position to stabilize the vegetable while the sound hand holds a knife.

Control training for the unilateral below-elbow prosthesis

Terminal device control

Scapula abduction and glenohumeral flexion are the motions necessary to open and close the TD. The client is instructed to operate the TD first, by flexing the humerus on the amputated side, then by scapula abduction while the humerus remains at the body's side. The therapist instructs the client to operate the TD with the arm in various positions in space, such as overhead and leaning over toward the floor.[74]

Pronation and supination

If the residual limb is long enough for flexible hinges to be prescribed on the prosthesis, pronation and supination should be practiced. The therapist asks the client to stabilize the elbow at 90 degrees and to pronate and supinate the forearm. If rigid hinges were prescribed, the TD is manually rotated in the wrist unit to achieve pronation and supination. Using the opposite hand or stabilizing the TD between the knees and turning the forearm or shoulder accomplishes manual TD rotation.

Exchanging terminal devices

The client learns to exchange the TD in the wrist unit if more than one TD is prescribed. Cable slack is necessary to release the cable from the TD. To obtain enough slack in the cable, it may be necessary to place an item between the fingers of the hook or hand. The TD is then removed according to the specifications of the prescribed wrist unit. When the TD has been removed, another TD style may then be positioned in the wrist unit and the cable attached to it.

To complete control training with a BE prosthesis, the therapist instructs the client to repeat the motions required to position and operate the TD until they are performed in one continuous smooth and natural sequence in both sitting and standing positions.[72] Once control training is completed, use training may begin to improve the client's application of the prosthesis in a variety of the person's customary daily occupations.

Control training for the unilateral above-elbow prosthesis

Most AE prostheses operate through the use of a dual-control cable system. When tension is applied on the cable attached to the elbow unit, it locks and unlocks. When the elbow unit is unlocked, tension on the second cable attached to the TD raises the prosthetic forearm (flexes the elbow). A spring assist helps reduce the amount of effort required to raise the forearm, and gravity assists in lowering it. When the elbow unit is locked, tension on the second cable is used to operate the TD. The client learns to operate each component separately.

Internal and external rotation

Many internally locking elbow units have a manually operated turntable located between the elbow unit and the socket that allows internal and external forearm rotation. The client operates the turntable, first with the elbow at 90 degrees by manually rotating the forearm medially (toward the body) or laterally (away from the body).

Elbow flexion and extension

Flexion and extension of the mechanical elbow are the next steps in the training process. The therapist should protect the client's face when teaching elbow flexion control. This precaution is important because initially the client may have poor control over elbow flexion, which could cause the TD to hit the face.[2]

The therapist makes sure that the elbow unit is unlocked. Then the therapist asks the client to flex the humerus slowly and simultaneously abduct the scapula to accomplish elbow flexion and slowly extend the shoulder to achieve elbow extension. This movement is repeated until the client gains sufficient control to accomplish elbow flexion and extension smoothly and easily.[2,74]

Elbow locking

The elbow unit operation has an audible two-click cycle. Both clicks must be heard each time the unit is locked or unlocked. The same body movement both locks and unlocks the unit. The client is instructed to operate the elbow unit by moving the shoulder into a combination of hyperextension, abduction, and scapula depression. This movement places tension on the cable that attaches the harness to the elbow unit and may be difficult to master. The reminder "down, out, and away" may be repeated until the client develops a proprioceptive memory. The client is then asked to practice locking and unlocking the elbow in various ranges of elbow flexion and extension (Figure 43-16).[2,5,74]

Terminal device control

The same motions of shoulder flexion and scapula abduction that flex the forearm with the elbow unlocked also control the TD when the elbow is locked. The person is instructed to lock the elbow, first at 90 degrees, and perform the motions to operate the TD. Care must be taken not to unlock the elbow by placing tension on the cable that operates the elbow unit. The sequence of elbow positioning, elbow locking, TD operation, elbow unlocking, elbow repositioning, and locking is repeated at various points in the elbow ROM from full extension to full flexion.[2,74]

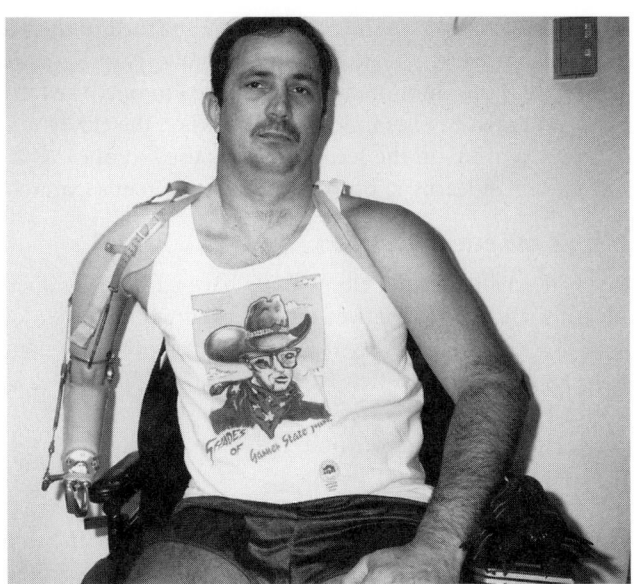

Figure 43-16   "Down, out, and away" movement used to unlock the elbow unit.

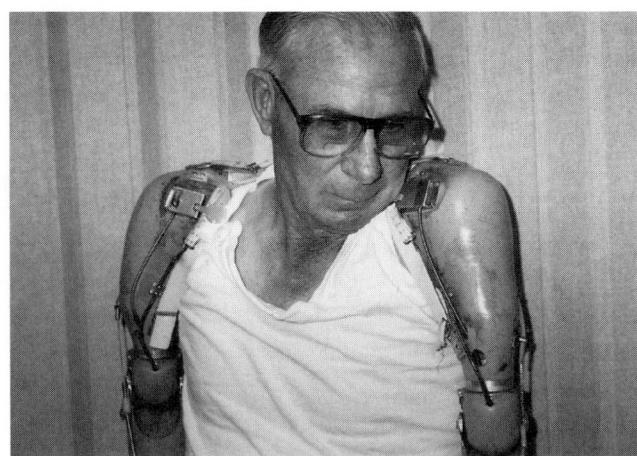

Figure 43-17   Nudge control used to operate the elbow unit for shoulder disarticulation prosthesis.

The person then learns how to rotate the TD manually in the wrist unit and to exchange TDs in the same manner as described previously for the BE prosthesis. Once the AE prosthesis controls are performed in a smooth manner, use training begins.

Control training for the shoulder disarticulation prosthesis

A prosthesis prescribed for a client with a shoulder disarticulation may have different components and methods of operation than those of the AE prosthesis. The prosthesis may have a manually operated, friction-held shoulder unit that the client prepositions using the sound arm or a table's edge. A chin-operated nudge control may be used to operate the elbow unit if the client does not have the shoulder movements needed to lock and unlock the elbow (Figure 43-17). A cable connects the nudge control to the elbow unit. The client still learns the two-click cycle and dual-cable system of operation described previously for the AE prosthesis. The elbow turntable is also available for a shoulder prosthesis.

A chest harness may be needed to secure the prosthesis on the client. It can also assist TD operation by using chest expansion to increase tension on the TD cable. Shoulder flexion and scapula abduction on the opposite side also assist in TD operation. Wrist operation is the same as explained for the BE prosthesis.

Control training for bilateral prostheses

A client with bilateral amputations usually receives two prostheses that are attached to one harness (Figure 43-18, *A*). Operating one of the prostheses may transmit tension through the harness to the other prosthesis, causing it to operate also. The client must learn to operate each prosthetic component

without affecting the components on either side. This skill is called **separation of controls,** and the client may need extensive practice to master it. Each prosthesis operates according to the level of amputation as described in the previous sections, with special attention given to relaxing the opposite side (Figure 43-18, *B*).

Two components not generally used on unilateral prostheses may be prescribed on bilateral prostheses to improve the client's independence. These components are the wrist flexion unit and a cable-operated wrist rotation unit. The wrist flexion unit assists in the completion of midline activities and is prescribed either for both prostheses or for the dominant side. The ability to achieve midline is important for completing activities such as dressing, grooming, and eating. Depressing the unit's control button and creating tension on the TD cable operate the flexion unit. The opposite TD, a surface edge, the knee, or another surface can depress the button. The TD cable must be medial to the flexion axis of the unit to pull the TD into flexion. A spring in the flexion unit repositions the TD in extension when the button is depressed and slack is provided in the TD cable.

Wrist rotation may be achieved in several ways. One is by using the wrist units mentioned earlier and rotating the TD by placing it between the knees or by pulling on the thumb of one hook with the other. Another method is use of a button on the medial side of the forearm, which controls a cable attached inside the forearm to a wrist-locking device. The wrist is locked and unlocked by pressing the button against the side of the body. When the wrist is unlocked, tension on the TD cable rotates the TD to the desired position.

Use Training

Use training begins after the client understands how to operate and control the prosthetic components. This training applies the mechanics of operation to activities. Repetition is important for the wearer to gain an understanding of how to

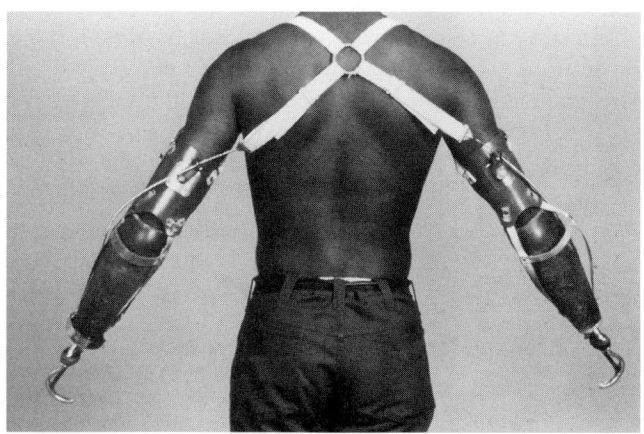

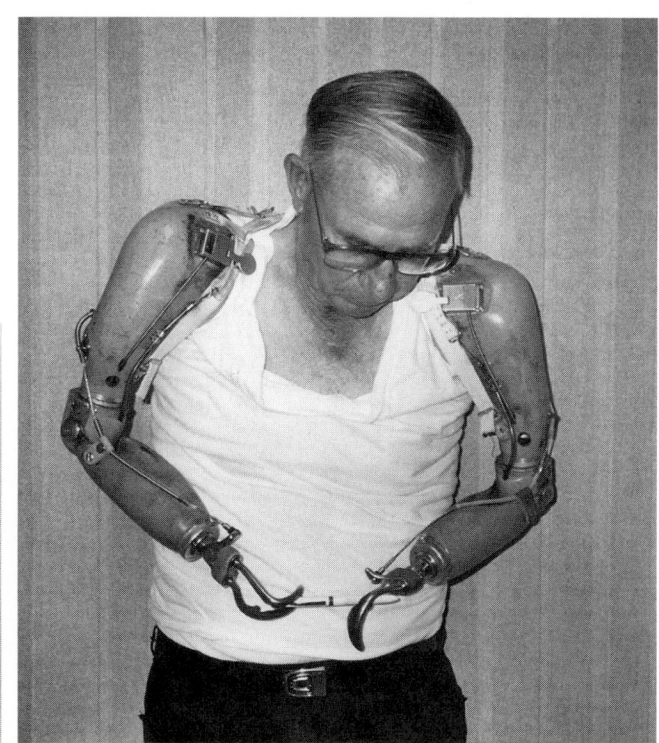

A   B

Figure 43-18   **A,** Single harness for bilateral prostheses. **B,** Passing a pen from one prosthesis to the other to practice separation of controls.

preposition the prosthesis and the objects and how to use the environment to help preposition them. Along with prepositioning, prehension training begins.

Prepositioning

Prepositioning involves moving the prosthetic units in their optimal position to grasp an object or perform a given activity. All prosthetic components must be prepositioned in a proximal-to-distal order. Thus, the client with the BE prosthesis rotates the TD into the desired degree of pronation or supination to accomplish an activity. With an AE prosthesis, the client flexes and locks the elbow and rotates the turntable before prepositioning the TD. The client with a shoulder disarticulation prepositions the shoulder unit before the elbow and wrist components. The client with bilateral prostheses must still preposition all components in the same fashion. The goal of prepositioning is to allow the person to approach the object or activity as one would with a normal hand and thereby avoid awkward body movements used to compensate for poor prepositioning.[58]

Prehension training

The prosthesis should be regarded as an assistive arm and not as the dominant arm.[72] Training objects are used to allow the wearer to practice TD control. The person should first use large, hard objects such as blocks, cans, and jars and progress to soft, then to crushable objects, such as rubber

balls, sponges, paper boxes, cones, and paper cups. These objects should be placed in positions that require elbow and TD prepositioning and TD operation at various heights. The hook TD has a nonmovable and a movable finger. If a hook is used to pick up objects, the person is taught to stabilize the item with the nonmovable finger and then release the tension on the movable finger to secure the object. Prehension training should be completed using all prescribed TDs.[72,74]

Use training for bilateral prostheses

After the client understands how the components operate, he or she gains control of the prostheses by practicing passing items such as a ruler or a piece of paper back and forth between the TDs without dropping them (see Figure 43-18, *B*). Another activity that helps the client learn separation of controls is holding an object in one prosthesis without dropping it while completing an activity with the other prosthesis.

Functional Training

Functional training applies the concepts of control and use of the prosthesis to functional activities. The prosthesis wearer is now introduced to completion of specific tasks important to him or her. Prehension training and methods to complete ADLs and IADLs, including vocational, leisure, and driving skills, are addressed in this phase. The key to successful functional training is teaching the wearer a problem-solving approach with respect to the activity being performed.

Prehension training

Prehension training teaches the client to use all prescribed TDs in a meaningful manner, such as using the heavy-duty TD with tools and the hand to eat. Items such as a pencil sharpener, lock and key, jar and lid, and bottle opener may be used to allow practice.[2,72] In bilateral activities, the person should be encouraged to determine the best position and appropriate use for the prosthesis and their sound arm. For details, the therapist is referred to Santschi's work on prosthetic training.[58] Movements become less cognitive and more automatic during this phase, and prepositioning occurs naturally.

Activities of daily living

Functional training should progress to the performance of necessary ADLs and IADLs. Activities should be introduced in a simple-to-complex order. Self-care activities are performed first. The therapist should also ask the client what activities are important for him or her to accomplish. It is not unusual to begin the training process with clients who indicate that there are multiple tasks that they have not tried since their amputation. The client is encouraged to analyze and perform the activities of eating, hygiene and grooming, toileting, dressing, meal preparation, care of pets, shopping, financial management, job performance, play, leisure participation, and community participation as independently as possible. Roberto was confident of his goals and ready to progress with the prosthesis to accomplish them. Frequently, individuals find it difficult to identify what they want to accomplish because of the fear that they may not be able to perform adequately with the prosthesis to accomplish their goals. When appropriate, home management skills and child care should be included as part of the client's training.[62] The therapist may help the client analyze and accomplish a task or achieve it by means of adaptive equipment or by encouraging repetitive practice to reach maximal speed and skill. The sound arm or longer prosthesis should complete most of the work while the opposite side acts as a stabilizer or assist.[72]

Adaptation and problem solving

There is no specific manner or technique to accomplish most tasks. Each person must learn to approach an activity in a manner that will lead him or her to successful completion. When Roberto was asked to button his trousers, plant seeds in a pot, and clean the floor, he was allowed to approach the task in a manner that made sense to him. The therapist offers guidance and recommendations to enable completion of activities in an efficient manner. Some clients consistently approach activities with the prosthetic arm as the dominant arm and confront limitations in coordination, sensation, and mobilization. With guidance and practice, they can accomplish the activity with their sound arm as the dominant arm and use the prosthesis to assist. Prepositioning of the prosthesis helps the client complete an activity at a more natural and rapid pace. As previously mentioned, if the client wears the prosthesis often, more practice with daily activities is experienced and the better the functional outcome. After two or three trials with a grooming activity, the approach to completion becomes automatic and successful.

Work-related activities

Prevocational evaluation may be included in the rehabilitation program. The therapist assesses the client's potential for returning to a former occupation or a possible change of vocation. A visit to the worksite may be necessary to make recommendations that will enable the client to return to work in a safe and efficient environment. It may also be necessary to restrict work activities, such as restricting the amount of weight that the client may lift and carry or restricting work on ladders. Initially, the client may be able to work only part time, improving work endurance gradually. Training and education for new jobs may be necessary (see Chapter 13).

Social routines and community integration

Incorporating the prosthesis into one's lifestyle includes being in the community and participating in one's usual social events. Clients may require encouragement to don the prosthesis when going to the grocery store or taking a walk with their young children. Roberto reported wearing his prosthesis for 90% of his social outings, although many people are uncomfortable wearing the prosthesis out of their immediate home or work settings.

Driver training

The ability to drive increases independence and may enhance vocational opportunities. The client may be referred to an adaptive driving program where he or she can be evaluated and trained in using assistive devices such as a driving ring or a steering knob (Figure 43-19). The controls of the car, such as the ignition switch and turn signals, can be modified to improve safety and comfort. The amount of training and

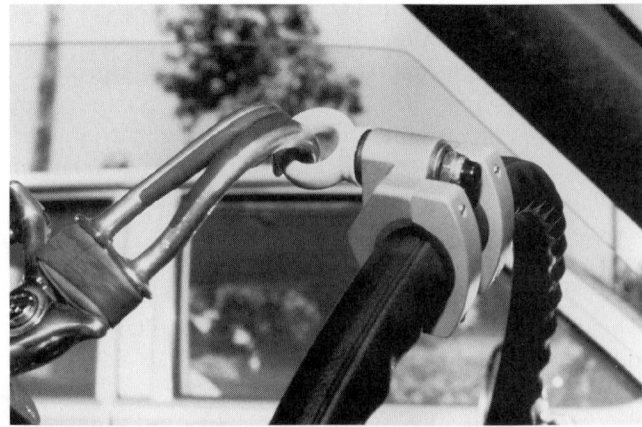

Figure 43-19 Steering ring used for driving with a prosthesis.

extent of modifications will vary, depending on the level of amputation.

The occupational therapist is responsible for assessing predriving skills. A predriving evaluation may consist of an assessment of visual acuity, traffic signal recognition, color vision, glare recovery, night vision, peripheral vision, depth perception, reaction time, and UE function. When necessary, additional cognitive, visual, and perceptual skills are evaluated. (See Chapter 11 for more information on driving.)

After completing the predriving evaluation, the therapist is responsible for making driving recommendations. These may include treatment for deficits, referral to a driver education center for training, and installation of assistive devices. The therapist's evaluation should include a statement regarding the client's potential for safe driving. If the client is unable to drive, alternative methods of transportation should be explored.

In some states, any change in physical health status must be reported to the motor vehicle department and to the person's insurance company. Failure to do so may result in a loss of automobile insurance.

Leisure activities

The rehabilitation program should include information and training regarding leisure interests. With the client's and the rehabilitation team's joint effort and motivation, the client should be able to return to a meaningful and productive life. A wide variety of specialized prosthetic devices are available for many sports and recreational hobbies. Texas Assistive Devices and Therapeutic Recreational Systems (TRS) provide prosthetic devices designed to improve the wearer's ability to participate in such activities as photography, ball games, pool, guitar playing, fishing, and skiing.[5]

Duration of training

The average adult with a unilateral transradial amputation who is otherwise healthy and well adjusted will require approximately 8 hours of training (five to eight treatment sessions) to master control and use of the prosthesis for daily living. The person with a unilateral transhumeral amputation under the same conditions will require approximately 12 hours of training. About 15 hours will be required for bilateral transhumeral prosthetic training, whereas about 20 hours is required for bilateral transhumeral prosthetic training. The initial training session should be about 1 hour long, and subsequent sessions may be briefer, increasing in duration commensurate with the wearer's increased prosthesis tolerance and physical endurance.[5,34,72]

SUMMARY

Acquired UE amputations can occur as a result of trauma, infections, neoplasms, and vascular diseases. Occupational therapists play an essential role in the rehabilitation process by addressing residual limb conditioning and care, preprosthetic exercise, and prosthetic training. The desired outcomes

of occupational therapy include the client's adaptation to his or her altered body; independent management of ADLs; satisfaction with independent function; resumption of work, social, and leisure roles; and acceptable quality of life.

Working with a client who has an amputation can be a real challenge. Careful assessment of the client's needs, a creative approach to therapeutic intervention, an emphasis on problem solving, and close communication with the team can make the challenge rewarding and successful.

Roberto was able to operate the body-powered prosthesis successfully early in his rehabilitation. He is considered a functional user of a prosthesis, successfully incorporating it into his lifestyle. The state insurance system provided him with the customary body-powered prosthesis, which was also the least expensive type. The therapist documented his successful operation of the prosthesis and explored the advantages and disadvantages of an electric prosthesis with Roberto, in conjunction with the prosthetist. For some clients, the electric prosthesis offers more control and success with activity completion.

ELECTRIC-POWERED PROSTHESES

Externally powered electric UE prostheses have opened a new world of freedom and function for persons with UE amputations. The advent of electronic microminiaturization has allowed the development of prosthetic devices with totally self-contained services of power, motor units, and electrodes.[25] Powered prostheses have existed for decades, but it was not until the 1960s that myoelectrically controlled prostheses were clinically introduced. The activities of the Otto Bock Company in Duderstadt, Germany, began this process by aiming for the development of an electromechanically driven prosthetic hand that would match both the technical and cosmetic demands of a human hand.[47]

The clinical use of the electric devices began in Europe because of government-supported healthcare systems and a large client population of persons with congenital (postthalidomide) amputations. By the late 1970s and early 1980s, clinicians in North America had an increasing but limited experience with myoelectric prostheses.[12] When funding permits, hundreds of myoelectric prostheses are prescribed for children and adults throughout the United States.

The term **myoelectric prosthesis** is often used interchangeably with *electric prosthesis*. A myoelectric prosthesis uses muscle surface electricity to control the prosthetic hand function. The muscle membrane generates an electric potential at the time of contraction. The myoelectric signal is sensed, amplified, and processed by a control unit that generates a motor, which in turn drives a terminal device.[12] This terminal device is often an electromechanical hand (Figure 43-20).[10] There are several different types of myoelectric hands available. The myoelectric control can be a digital control or a dynamic mode control (proportional control). Digital systems are operated at only one speed, allowing them

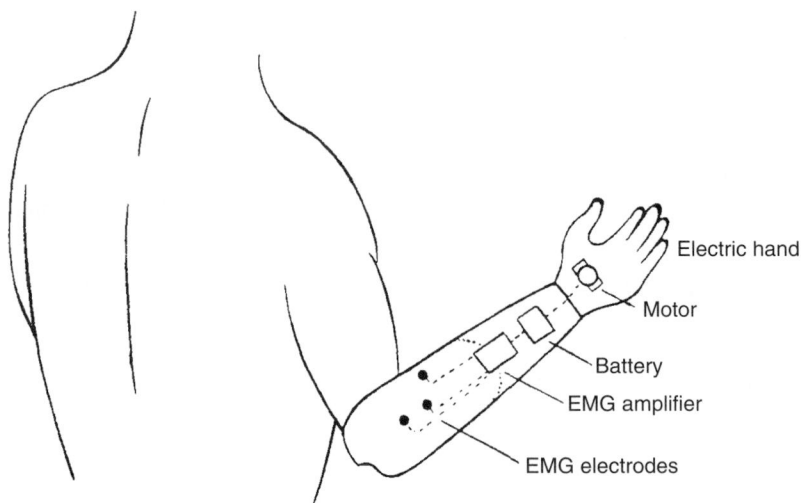

Figure 43-20 A typical electric-powered myoelectrically controlled, below-elbow prosthesis with an electromechanical hand terminal device activated by electromyographic potentials. (From Billock JN: Upper limb prosthetic terminal devices: hands versus hooks, *Clin Prosthet Orthot* 10(2):59, 1986.)

to either turn on or turn off. Proportional control means that the myoelectric signal (power) to the hand is proportional to the level of muscle signal that the wearer generates, so the wearer's effort directly controls the speed of the hand.[3] A SensorHand™, which provides automatic grasping when the object in the hand is slipping and its center of gravity is changing, is now available (Figure 43-21). The motor automatically increases the pressure applied to the object being held to prevent dropping of the object.

Myoelectric controls require minimal physical effort for operation and rarely require adjustment. The muscle groups in the BE area are used according to their physiological function—that is, the wrist extensor muscles are used for hand opening and the wrist flexor muscles for hand closing. Surface electrodes recessed within the wall of the prosthetic socket (Figure 43-22) detect muscular contractions.

CANDIDATES FOR PROSTHESES

An electric prosthesis might be chosen because of the combination of a natural appearance and the functions of high pinch force without a high level of effort. Also, a myoelectric prosthesis requires no cables for control, so the harnessing can be much more comfortable. The client's work,

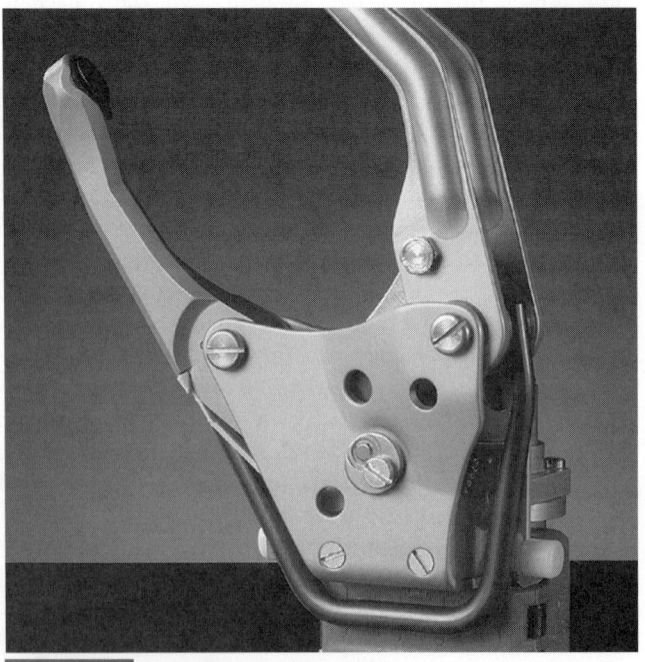

Figure 43-21 The Sensor Hand® Speed. (Courtesy Otto Bock HealthCare, Minneapolis, MN.)

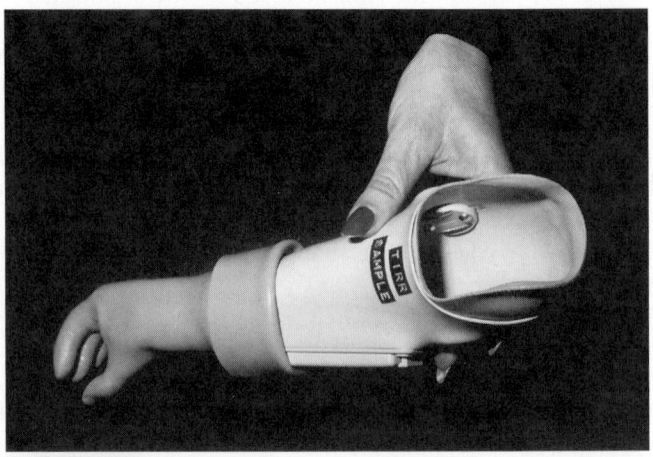

Figure 43-22 Surface electrodes, recessed within the wall of the myoelectric socket, detect muscle contractions.

home, and recreational needs and activities must all be considered. Previous experience with other prostheses may also be relevant.

In the past, the transradial amputation has been the most common condition for which these prostheses were prescribed. For amputation levels above the elbow, the complexity of function and the power level required to accomplish functional movement increase considerably. At the same time, the capability of the client to operate a prosthesis by harnessing body movement via straps and cables, in the traditional body-powered manner, decreases considerably.[60] More recently, with advances in technology, myoelectric prostheses for persons with higher levels of amputations are increasingly prescribed because their functional possibilities are greater.[3]

The Utah Arm 3, released in 2004, introduced microprocessor technology into the prosthetic arm with a computer interface that allows the prosthetist to fine-tune the adjustments in maximize the wearer's performance. It offers simultaneous elbow and hand control because it has two microprocessors. Roberto may experience the common difficulties in unlocking the elbow unit efficiently or in operating the TD with the same control quality of the elbow unit, which individuals with transhumeral amputations frequently experience using an electric prosthesis. This design minimizes the separateness of elbow and hand control and may be appropriate for Roberto.

The task of training a client with a very short transhumeral amputation or shoulder disarticulation to operate and function with a body-powered prosthesis is substantially more challenging than training with an electric-powered prosthesis.

Before a myoelectric prosthesis is prescribed, the client should have adequate strength and an ability to contract muscles independently. A minimum signal of 5 microvolts will operate the most sensitive system. The candidate with this minimum signal should be capable of developing stronger signals for longer-term use of the prosthesis. Independent contraction of each muscle is important to produce smooth and controllable prosthetic function. As a general guideline, the prosthesis can be operated with a 10-microvolt difference, but the wearer will use the prosthesis more easily if a 20- to 30-microvolt difference can be controlled. The surface electric signals are amplified by a miniature electrode and led to the relay system. The relay is responsible for the energy supply to the battery-operated motor in the electric hand. When the alternating contractions of extensor and flexor muscles take place, the direction of the current changes in the electric motor and the hand opens and closes accordingly.[47]

Some rehabilitation professionals who work with clients who have UE amputations believe that electric components may be the only appropriate alternative for high-level unilateral or high-level bilateral amputations. Conversely, some rehabilitation professionals believe that body-powered prostheses are the most functional and appropriate type of prosthesis for most clients, despite the level of amputation. There are many schools of thought regarding the advantages and disadvantages of myoelectric prostheses. Box 43-2 describes some of the points that differentiate the myoelectric prosthesis from a body-powered, cable-controlled, hook-type TD.

HYBRID PROSTHESES

A **hybrid prosthesis** is one that combines body power with electrical power. These designs have been created and used more and more in the past several years. Hybrid prostheses, using various components and control methods from various systems, can in many cases result in a prosthesis that is more functional and more acceptable to the individual.[10] The improved technology of electric hands has increased the cost of myoelectric prostheses. The hybrid design decreases the overall cost of the prosthesis. Some hybrid designs eliminate the cable and harness, thereby eliminating pressure on the sound side when the prosthesis is operated. One hybrid design involves the use of a body-powered elbow flexion device with a myoelectric hand.[10] Another configuration might be the use of a cable elbow and hook TD with an electric wrist rotator. For a person with bilateral amputations, a powered elbow combined with a cable-hook TD offers a quick elbow motion and less overall bulk of the prosthesis and dedicates all excursion of the cable to the TD. A hybrid prosthesis can decrease the overall weight of a prosthesis. It can be less expensive and less complex. All excursion of

---

Box 43-2 ADVANTAGES AND DISADVANTAGES OF A MYOELECTRIC PROSTHESIS

ADVANTAGES

1. Improved cosmesis
2. Increased grip force (approximately 25 lb in an adult myoelectric hand)
3. Minimal or no harnessing
4. Ability to use overhead
5. Minimal effort needed to control
6. Control more closely corresponding to human physiological control

DISADVANTAGES

1. Cost of prosthesis
2. Frequency of maintenance and repair
3. Fragile nature of glove and necessity of frequent replacements
4. Lack of sensory feedback (a body-powered prosthesis has some sense of proprioceptive feedback)
5. Slowness in responsiveness of electric hand
6. Increased weight

the existing cable is dedicated to one component, as opposed to multiple components. This feature requires less overall force on the part of the wearer for operating the prosthesis.

PREPROSTHETIC THERAPY

Awareness of postoperative and subsequent preprosthetic principles of care is crucial for the successful management of the client who has sustained traumatic limb loss.

 ETHICAL CONSIDERATIONS

The client has little control over what is happening and must depend on the healthcare team to provide the best treatment possible.[6]

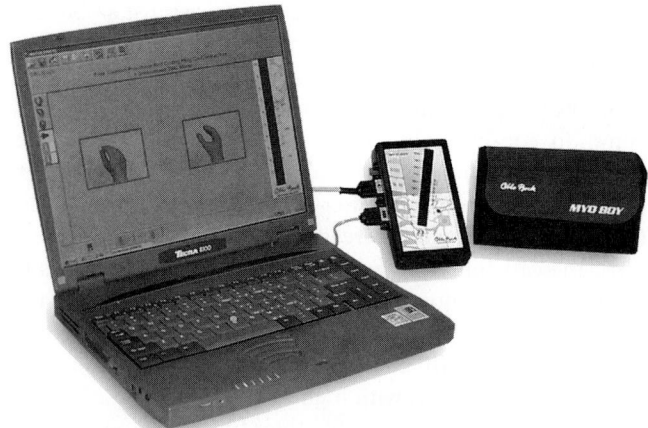

Figure 43-23 Otto Bock MyoBoy system used to determine magnitude of muscle contraction. (Courtesy Otto Bock HealthCare, Minneapolis, MN.)

The rehabilitation team, which ideally includes the physician, nurse, occupational therapist, physical therapist, social worker, insurance representative, and client, addresses goals previously described in the first section of this chapter. With an electric prosthesis, additional treatment goals are as follows:

- Identify or test potential muscle sites for prosthesis control.
- Improve muscle site control and strength (once identified).
- Obtain adequate financial sponsorship for the prosthesis and training.[42]

Identify Potential Muscle Sites

A myoelectric prosthesis functions by detecting electromyographic (EMG) signals produced by muscles. Locating appropriate superficial muscle sites is the most important aspect of the successful operation of a myoelectric prosthesis. Physical examination of a person's arm can often reveal sufficient strength in natural agonist-antagonist pairs, such as the wrist extensor and wrist flexor muscles in the person with a transradial amputation and the biceps and triceps muscles in the person with a transhumeral amputation. Individuals with a short transhumeral amputation often have an effective pectoralis or deltoid site anteriorly and an infraspinatus or trapezius site posteriorly. It is more difficult to identify proximal muscle sites that are both adequate in signal and allow the prosthetist to position the electrodes within the socket and hold them securely against the skin. On occasion, trauma or nerve injuries do not allow the choice of a natural pair. If a particular site could cause tissue breakdown under the pressure of an electrode, it must be avoided. Often, healed skin or muscle grafts can tolerate the pressure well. Consult the physician when dealing with repaired tissue. If the best muscle site contractions are weak during the physical examination, the therapist and prosthetist will require a biofeedback system or myotester to identify the amount of signal generated by the muscle (Figure 43-23). When surface potentials are being measured with electrodes and a myotester, it is important that all electrodes have good contact with the skin and be aligned along the general direction of the muscle fibers. Moistening the skin slightly with water may improve the EMG signal by lowering skin resistance. EMG testing begins with the most distal portion of the remnant muscle.

The goal of this testing is to identify two muscle sites that would fit appropriately within the socket with the greatest microvolt difference between them, not necessarily the two strongest muscle site signals. The selection can be considered complete when the client can tolerate a 1-hour training session with the biofeedback system and is consistently generating sufficient signals to operate a prosthesis in basic functions such as opening and closing of the TD. The therapist should check with the prosthetist for the minimum signal required for operating the myoelectric system chosen for the client.[48]

Muscle Site Control Training

The more proximal the level of the client's amputation, the more challenging it is for the prosthetist to fit the prosthesis and for the therapist to train the person to function with the prosthesis. For the client to understand a desired muscle contraction, the therapist instructs the client to imitate the desired contraction or movement with both arms. The therapist should ask the client to raise the sound hand at the wrist (wrist extension) and imagine this motion with the phantom hand on the amputated side (Figure 43-24). A therapist can often palpate the wrist flexors and extensors on the residual limb during this exercise. The person is instructed to contract and relax each muscle group separately and on command. For this step, a myoelectric tester is particularly useful because it indicates the magnitude of the EMG signal as the client contracts the muscle as well as the decrease in signal as the client relaxes the muscle. Many clients have difficulty relaxing a muscle completely, which causes a decrease in muscle signal separation.

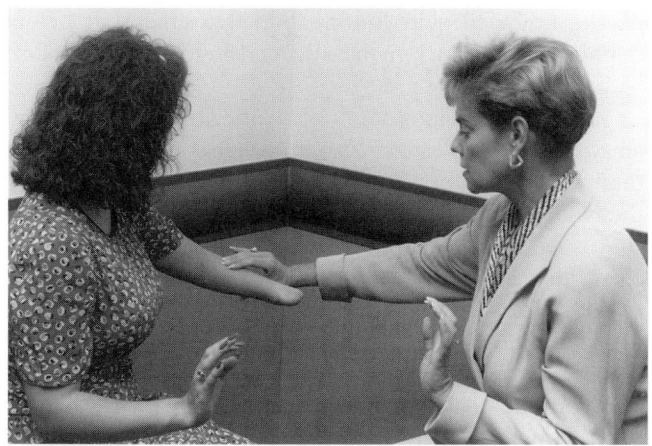

Figure 43-24 Therapist instructs client to imitate desired muscle contraction on both sides.

The myoelectric tester can be used to train the muscles with both visual and auditory feedback. Various models are available to therapists (Figure 43-25). The goals of training at this point are to increase muscle strength and to isolate muscle contractions. As confidence and accuracy improve, the visual or auditory feedback should be removed. Practicing muscle contractions without feedback teaches the client to internalize the feeling of each control movement. The advantage of creating this internalized awareness of proper muscle control is that control and strengthening practice can be continued between treatment sessions without the feedback equipment.[66] The therapist must learn to recognize muscle fatigue, which is frequently a side effect in

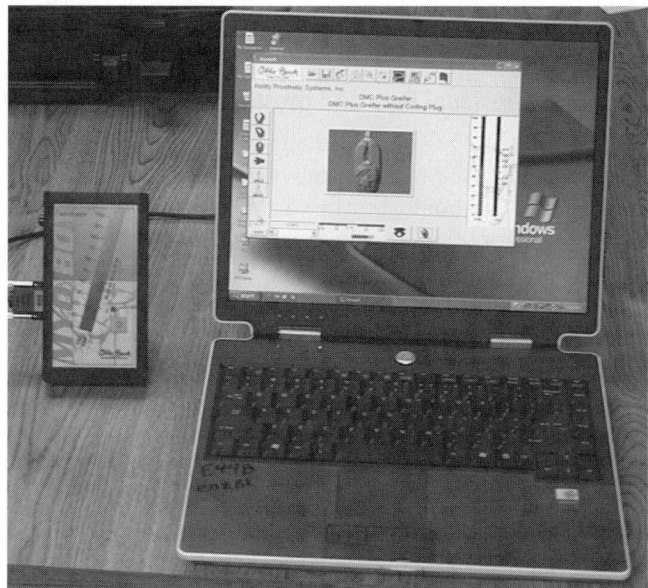

Figure 43-25 Myotester used for training purposes.

this process, and allow sufficient time for that muscle to recover during the treatment session.

Ideally, the client with an amputation receives adequate training and practice in initiating these muscle contractions before receiving the completed myoelectric prosthesis from the prosthetist. Prosthetists commonly engage a client in muscle site training with the preparatory socket and prosthesis fitting. This training, which usually occurs as prosthetists strive for optimal electrode placement and socket fit, is not adequate for most clients. Anxiety and frustration often accompany training in use of a myoelectric prosthesis, and the development of a team approach to training by the therapist and prosthetist can minimize these responses. The client's success and effectiveness in using the prosthesis are closely related to the quality of the preprosthetic training.

PROSTHETIC PROGRAM

Orientation in what the prosthesis realistically can and cannot do is an important aspect of a prosthetic training program. If clients harbor unrealistic expectations about the usefulness of the prosthesis as a replacement arm, they may become dissatisfied with the ultimate functioning of the prosthesis and reject it altogether. It is imperative that the therapist be honest and positive about the function of the prosthesis. If the client understands the functional potential and limitations of the prosthesis, success can be more realistically achieved.[4]

Orientation and Education

Training with a prosthesis should begin as soon as the prosthesis is received, preferably the same day. The textbook *Comprehensive Management of the Upper Limb Amputee* is an excellent resource in the training process of a client with a myoelectric hand.[6]

Important areas to review during the initial visits are orientation to prosthesis terminology and operation, independence in donning and doffing the prosthesis, orientation to a prosthesis-wearing schedule, and care of the residual limb and prosthesis.

Orientation to prosthesis terminology

Considering that the prosthesis is a natural extension of the client's body, it is particularly important to know the function and names of its major parts, such as the electrodes, battery, glove, and electric hand. The initial visit is an appropriate time to review the battery-charging procedure with the client.

The batteries are energy-storing devices, and most are rechargeable. Some control systems use a 9-volt disposable battery. The prosthetist supplying the prosthesis will instruct the client in proper installation and recharging. Rechargers are plugged into a standard electrical outlet. Most manufacturers' rechargers have some type of indicator, which alerts the client when the battery is fully charged. Some rechargers require 12 hours of charging time, whereas others may take as long as 24 hours. A fast charger, which requires only 1 or 2 hours of charging time, may be available. For best results, the batteries should be just about completely drained before recharging. The prosthesis will begin to operate more slowly when the battery is low, and some unexpected control problems could occur. Therefore, the first troubleshooting step is always to make certain that the battery is freshly installed.[48]

Although the myoelectric hand is the most commonly prescribed electric terminal device, a specially designed gripping device, or Greifer, is frequently recommended. Designed by the Otto Bock Company, the Greifer is a universal working tool designed to handle various specialized tasks. It can be used for heavy work in industry or farming and in mechanical activities at work or home because it allows for quick handling and precise manipulation of small objects. Features of the Greifer include a 38-lb grasp, as well as parallel gripping surfaces and a manually controlled flexion joint for dorsal and volar flexion (Figure 43-26).[47]

Instruction manuals from the manufacturer for the battery charger and the prosthesis are often provided for the client's reference, and they are excellent tools for the occupational therapist to use for review and education.

Independence in donning and doffing the prosthesis

The client should be able to put on and remove the prosthesis independently. With proper instruction and the help of the prosthetist in suspension design, the wearer will be successful. Donning the prosthesis should be performed with the electronic components in the off position to prevent any uncontrolled movements. A client with a transradial amputation usually has the advantage of not requiring a harness and control cables because a supracondylar suspension at the elbow is often used. The wearer can place the residual limb directly into the socket. A pull sock is sometimes used to facilitate an intimate interface between the arm and the socket.

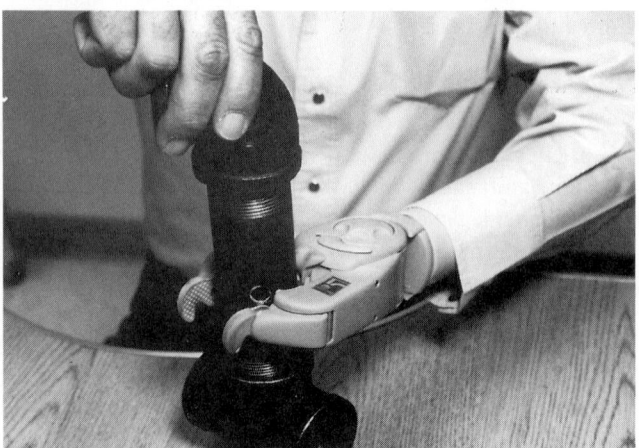

Figure 43-26   The myoelectric Greifer is designed as a universal working tool with parallel gripping force of up to 38 pounds.

A silicone-based skin lotion applied to the skin before donning the pull sock enables the person to pull the sock off with less effort.

Suspension designs for the client with a transhumeral amputation usually require a pull sock for donning the prosthesis. The sock is applied to the residual limb, and the prosthesis socket is pulled over it. A weighted cord from the pull sock is fed through a hole in the bottom of the socket. The client then pulls the sock off the arm and through the hole in the socket, creating very close contact of the prosthesis with the limb. This is a successful application, particularly for very short residual limbs. The wearer must be sure not to start with the stocking too high on the residual limb because this will increase friction during pulling and make it harder to pull the sock out of the bottom of the socket. It may be necessary to experiment with different sock materials, powder on the skin, and various donning techniques until the most successful materials and techniques are identified.

Good electrical contact is achieved after approximately 1 minute of donning. A wearer can also moisten the skin at the electrode sites to eliminate the waiting period for perspiration to occur. The prosthetic arm should be stored in the off position with the batteries removed. The hand should be fully opened when stored to keep the thumb web space stretched.

Prosthesis-wearing schedule

Initial wearing periods should be no longer than 15 to 30 minutes. This limit is particularly important if scarring or insensate areas are present on the residual limb. If redness persists for more than 20 minutes in a particular area after removal of the prosthesis, the client should return the prosthesis to the prosthetist for adjustments. If no skin problems exist, the wearing periods can be increased in 30-minute increments two to three times a day. Some clients have difficulty tolerating the weight of the prosthesis or the heat generated by its application. By the end of a week, full-time wearing should be achieved.

Care of the residual limb and prosthesis

Appropriate care of the skin is vitally important. The residual limb should be washed daily with mild soap and lukewarm water. It should be rinsed thoroughly and dried by using patting motions with a towel, so as not to irritate sensitive or scar tissue.

The prosthesis may be cleaned with soap and water by using a damp cloth. Rubbing alcohol may be used to clean the inside of the socket if an odor develops. The cosmetic glove stains easily; special care must be taken to avoid contact with ink, newsprint, mustard, carrots, grease, and dirt. Wiping with soap and water or a glove-cleansing cream obtained from the prosthetist will remove general soil but not stains. The average life of a glove is approximately 6 months. Polyvinylchloride (PVC) plastic gloves are the least expensive, most flexible, and toughest. Silicone gloves are being used more frequently because the new silicone formulas are tougher and less susceptible to the yellowing and brittleness that frequently set in with age; they also allow the greatest cosmesis.[10] The prosthesis itself should never be immersed in water because this will seriously damage the internal electronic components. Additionally, it is important to advise myoelectric wearers against excess vibration, sand, dirt, and the extremes of heat and cold. These, too, can seriously impair the electronic components.

The prosthesis should be checked occasionally for loose screws and harness attachments, and these should be brought to the attention of the prosthetist. The covers of the prosthesis should not be opened unless the prosthetist instructs the wearer or therapist to do so.

Control Training

The first function to master is opening and closing the TD. The client now understands the muscle contractions required to perform these actions. Simple opening and closing of the terminal are practiced. The muscles should contract as independently as possible. Next, the client practices opening the hand halfway, then stopping and relaxing so the hand does not move. If a proportional control system is used, the client can also practice opening and closing quickly and slowly. The client will improve in accuracy and speed with practice. Often, the therapist will design a home program of specific patterns of terminal device action that the person performs in order to offer more practice. The control of the prosthesis continues to improve throughout the other phases of training.

Use Training

The repetitive grasp and release of objects is introduced after control training. Simple approach, grasp, and release activities are practiced with objects of various shapes, sizes, and densities. Objects that may be presented include paper or plastic cups, blocks, cubes of sponge, empty plastic containers, small weights, large bolts, empty glass jars of various sizes, and ping-pong balls. It is important for the individual first to visualize how the object should be approached and grasped, then to preposition the myoelectric hand. Prepositioning involves placing the TD in the optimal position to approach an object. In approaching a glass, the hand should face in toward the midline to grasp the glass as a normal hand would (Figure 43-27). The fingers of the hand should not be positioned downward because a normal hand does not approach a glass in this position.

Another important goal of training a client to grasp an object is mastering pressure control or the gripping force of the TD. This skill involves close visual attention to grade the muscle contraction for a specific result in the myoelectric hand. The client must learn how to pick up the object without crushing it. Too strong a grasp crushes the object being held (Figure 43-28). Good grasp control through training with foam, cotton balls, or wet sponges will help develop the control necessary to handle paper cups, eggs, potato chips, lotion bottles, and sandwiches or even to hold someone's hand.[66]

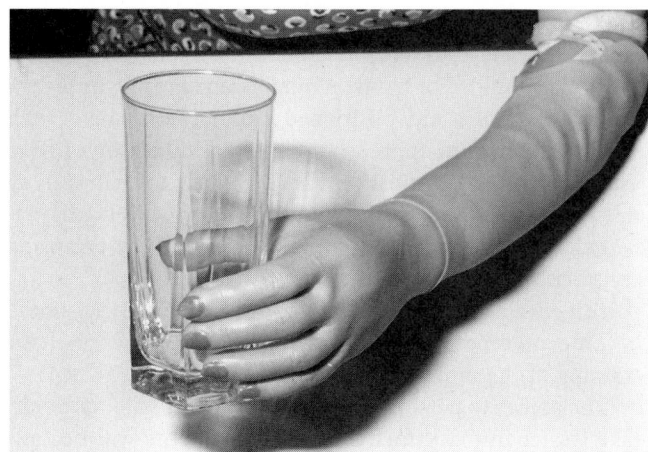

Figure 43-27 When approaching the glass, the hand is prepositioned in midline to grasp the glass as a normal hand.

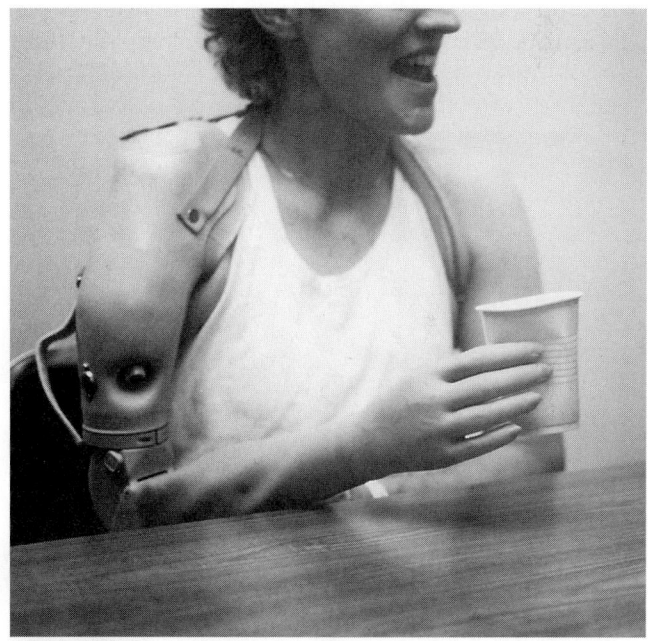

Figure 43-28 Above-elbow amputee demonstrates how excessive grasp crushes the object (plastic cup) being held.

Working on approach, grasp, and release in multiple arm positions then follows. The client will grasp objects at counter height, table height, overhead, on the floor, cupboard height, alongside the body, and behind the body. The client with a transhumeral amputation who uses a body-powered or electric elbow should ensure that the position of the terminal hand and angle of elbow flexion are appropriate to complete the grasp in a natural manner. Often, the client automatically adjusts the body using compensatory body motions (e.g., bending forward rather than adjusting the elbow position or prepositioning the hand). It is important to discourage this adjustment because it looks unnatural, becomes habitual, and may lead to secondary musculoskeletal problems in the neck, shoulder, or trunk. A mirror can help clients see the way their bodies are positioned and visualize how their sound arms would approach a particular object or activity. The therapist often must remind the client to maintain an upright posture and avoid extraneous body movements.

Release is accomplished by visualizing a wrist extension contraction or a quick "hand up" or "fingers open" in the person with a transradial amputation. This response should become automatic if there has been good preprosthetic training of the muscles.

The ability to perform specific movements will eventually take less cognitive effort, and the movements will become automatic. The wearer now has muscle endurance and prosthesis tolerance sufficient for 1-hour therapy sessions. Next, functional activities are introduced into the therapy program.

Functional Training

The prosthesis is used as a functional assist in most bilateral activities. Therefore, most ADLs are accomplished with the uninvolved arm and hand. Other than perhaps for practice, it is not appropriate to train a person with a unilateral amputation to eat holding a spoon, write, or brush his or her teeth using the myoelectric hand. In almost all cases, the sound hand becomes the dominant extremity and performs these tasks. Occasionally, if the right arm was dominant and is amputated and if the client is fitted with a myoelectric hand in a timely manner, he or she may prefer to use the myoelectric hand for some of these activities. The critically important component of sensory feedback is often the determining factor in deciding which hand to use. A client with an amputation almost always chooses to perform activities with a hand that has feeling. A myoelectric hand lacks this sensory feedback. Feedback is provided more proximally with the action of muscle contraction, yet responding to this stimulus is difficult for the wearer.

The therapist should review a list of bilateral ADLs with the client to determine which tasks are most important for him or her to accomplish. The therapist should focus on these activities during training, stressing throughout that the myoelectric hand is used as an assist and a stabilizer (Figure 43-29).

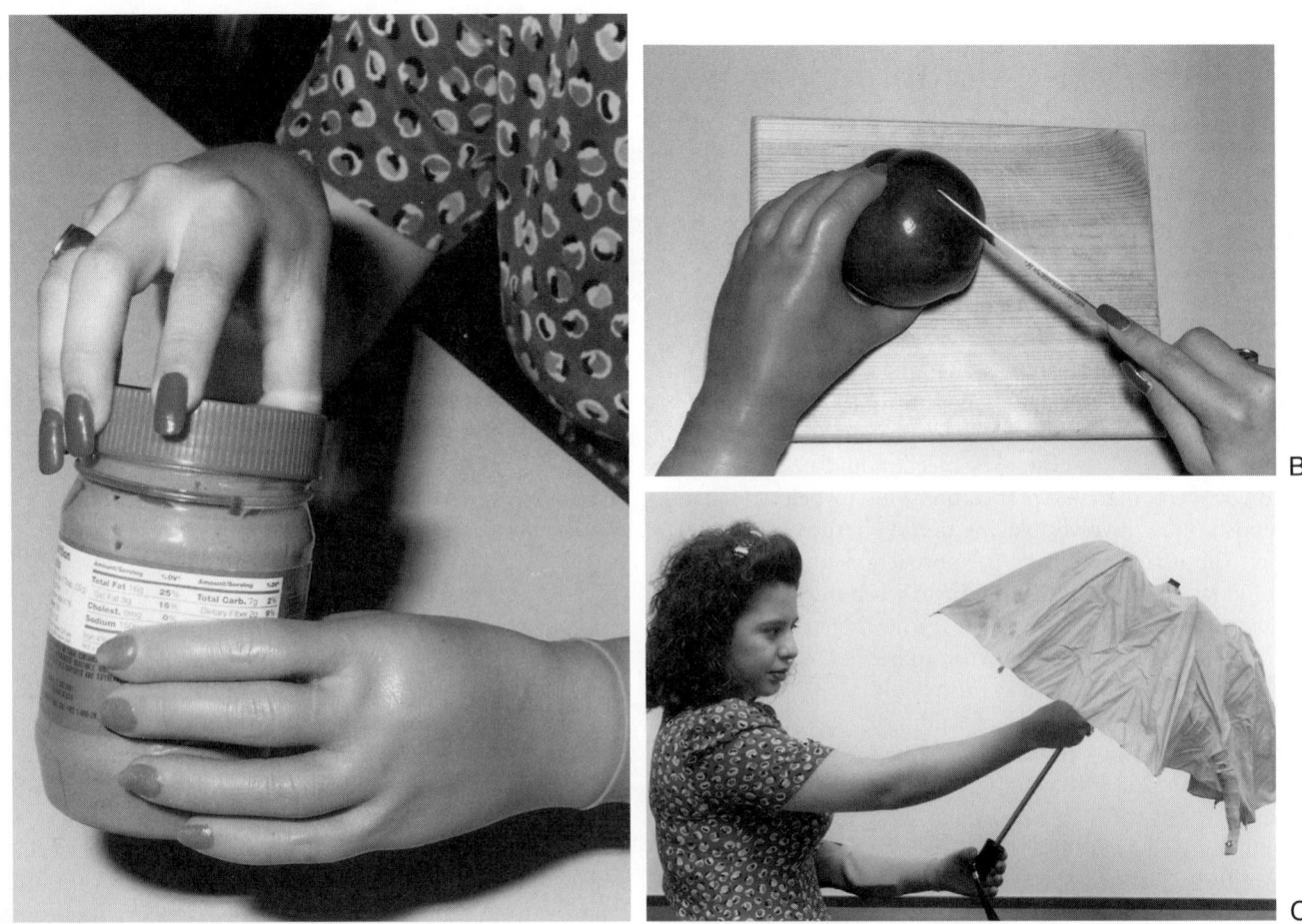

Figure 43-29 Activities of daily living. **A,** Opening a jar is accomplished with the myoelectric hand holding the jar and the sound hand turning the lid. **B,** Cutting an apple is accomplished with the myoelectric hand holding the apple while the sound hand holds the knife to cut. **C,** Opening an umbrella is accomplished by holding the base knob of the umbrella with the myoelectric hand and using the sound hand to open as normal.

TABLE **43-2** **Roles of Myoelectric Hand and Sound Hand in Bilateral Activities of Daily Living**

Activity	Myoelectric Hand	Sound Hand
Cutting meat	Hold the fork with prongs facing downward; hold the knife as grip strength increases.	Hold knife. Hold fork.
Opening a jar (see Figure 43-30, *A*)	Hold the jar.	Turn the lid.
Opening a tube of toothpaste	Hold the tube.	Turn the cap.
Stirring something in a bowl	Hold the bowl with a strong grip.	Hold the mixing spoon or fork.
Cutting fruit or vegetables (see Figure 43-30, *B*)	Hold the fruit or vegetable firmly.	Hold the knife to cut.
Using scissors to cut paper	Hold the paper to be cut.	Use scissors in normal fashion.
Buckling a belt	Hold the buckle end of belt to keep stable.	Manipulate long end of belt into buckle.
Zipping a jacket from bottom up	Hold anchor tab.	Manipulate pull tab at base, and pull upward.
Applying socks	Hold one side of socks.	Hold other side of socks, and pull upward.
Opening an umbrella (see Figure 43-30, *C*)	Hold base knob of umbrella.	Open as normal.

If unilateral tasks are presented to the client, his or her need to operate the prosthesis is minimized or absent. These tasks should be avoided for the purpose of training. The bilateral activities listed in Table 43-2 are good examples to practice.

With practice, these activities and many others will become easier to perform, occurring almost automatically. It is important to reinforce and emphasize the fact that bathing, grooming, and hygiene skills involving water must be done without a myoelectric TD or with a myoelectric TD that is water resistant because of the damaging effects of water on the electric motor and battery.

Vocational and leisure activities

As training proceeds and a sense of the person's self-acceptance and comfort with the amputation is achieved, the therapist should address the subject of return to work. Ideally, the therapist makes an on-site visit. If possible, the various job requirements can be discussed and then practiced in a simulated, step-by-step process. If changes and adjustments to the work environment are necessary, the therapist will advise in these modifications. This intervention can often be enhanced by collaboration with the vocational counselor. In Roberto's case, the occupational therapist was instrumental in describing to the counselor what skills and abilities could be safe and reasonable to attempt with the body-powered and electric prostheses. This improves the match of the individual to the occupation identified. (See Chapters 13 and 14 for additional information.)

Recreational activities are also critically important to discuss at this time because these activities contribute not only to physical well-being but also to psychological well-being. The TDs used for sports and recreational activities are not generally myoelectric. If the activity is something that requires fine motor skills, an electric TD may be beneficial. The author worked with an individual with bilateral amputations who was fitted with bilateral electric prostheses and who was able to successfully resume his fly-tying business. As discussed in the first section of this chapter, Therapeutic Recreation Systems (TRS) offers a number of excellent TD adaptation components, including an Amputee Golf Grip (Figure 43-30, *A*) and a Super Sports TD (Figure 43-30, *B*). Clients are encouraged to continue engagement in any recreational activities that they performed before the loss of their extremity.

Self-management instruction

During training and during the review that takes place at the conclusion of training, information regarding a wearing schedule, care instructions, and additional tasks to practice should be shared with the wearer and his or her family members. A follow-up appointment should be made at this time, as well as a list of the rehabilitation team members and their telephone numbers, so that the client may contact the appropriate person when problems arise.

SUMMARY

The rehabilitation process for clients with upper limb loss can be challenging and rewarding. In the case of a transhumeral amputation, shoulder disarticulation amputation, or bilateral limb loss, training and expertise on the part of the therapist is essential. There are several resources that the therapist can review to increase his or her knowledge in this area of occupational therapy intervention.

The potential of individuals with amputation is limitless; they often are able to accomplish activities that no one ever would have predicted. The success of rehabilitation does not rest solely on the quality of training in the use of the prosthesis. Rather, success depends on such complex factors as the quality of medical management, the type and fit of the prosthesis, the client's interest in learning to use the prosthesis, and conscientious follow-up once the rehabilitation phase is complete. Follow-up is critically important and often overlooked.

Perhaps the most important aspect of a successful rehabilitation program is the client's desire to become more independent. All team members should cultivate and reinforce this desire, which is a pivotal ingredient of successful intervention. The effect of the occupational therapist during this important process will remain with the client for life.

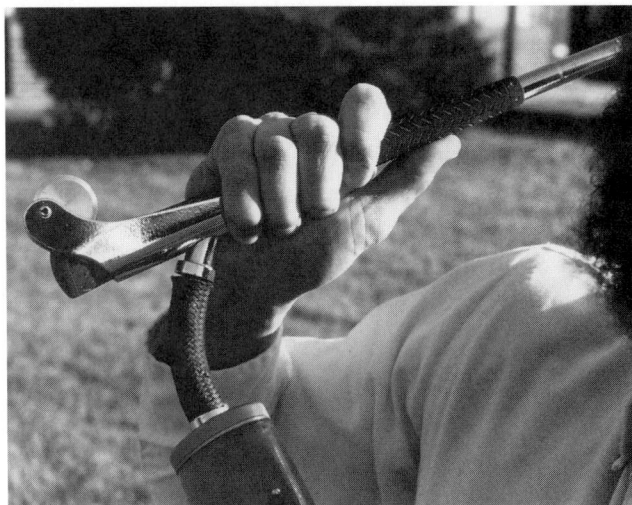

A

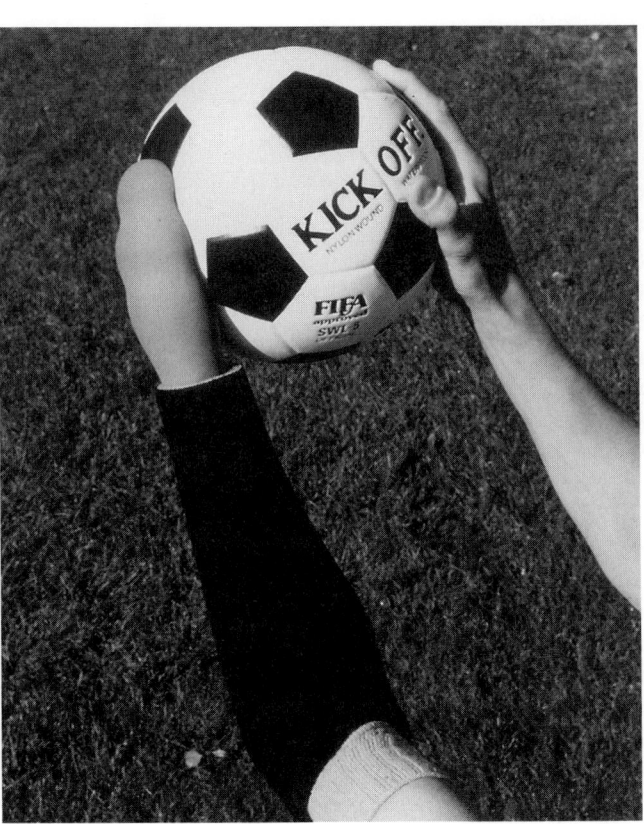

B

Figure 43-30 TD adaptation components. **A,** Amputee Golf Grip is a high-performance prosthetic golf accessory that allows smooth swings and complete follow through. **B,** Super Sports terminal device is a highly flexible, strong, prosthetic sports accessory for volleyball, soccer, football, floor exercise gymnastics, or any activity in which shock absorption, safety, and bilateral control are important.

THREADED CASE STUDY: ROBERTO, PART 2

Roberto's inability to work is based on his inability to function with the prosthesis in bilateral activities. Roberto's cultural, physical, social, and personal contexts affect his rehabilitation, and the occupational therapist must address each of these to facilitate his successful adaptation in ADLs and work. His belief in his role as the sole financial provider for his family means that the therapist must address his return to work as a vital component of his rehabilitation.

The therapist must clearly document the benefits of an electric-powered prosthesis over a body-powered prosthesis if the former facilitates Roberto's return to successful gainful employment and ADL independence.

Because Roberto's involvement with his children is important to him, the therapist must promote his ability to function comfortably in social settings. Roberto's performance skills of temporal organization, adaptation, and organization of space and objects are addressed in occupational therapy intervention to facilitate greater function with his prosthesis in usual activities, especially those that involve bilateral function. The therapist presents the following activities to Roberto that allow him to practice the skills of prepositioning of the prosthesis, recognizing the role of the prosthesis as an assist, and developing problem-solving strategies when approaching activities: drying dishes, folding clothes, shuffling cards, washing car or house windows, pushing a lawn mower, sweeping with a broom, using hand-held tools to repair something, taking money in and out of his wallet, emptying trash at home and in the clinic, and assembling electronic or mechanical parts.

Communication of the results of the occupational therapy evaluation and Roberto's performance in treatment to the vocational evaluator and vocational rehabilitation counselor is essential in the coordination of Roberto's care and return to successful employment.

THREADED CASE STUDY: ROBERTO, PART 2—cont'd

Roberto's satisfactions with function, level of ADL independence, and return to gainful employment are the outcome measures used to assess the efficacy of the occupational therapy intervention. He was highly motivated to meet the goal of returning to work that he identified at the initial occupational therapy interview and was successful in meeting this goal. Roberto participated in the vocational counseling and testing program offered through his state agency. He secured a position as a full-time janitor in a public elementary school.

Future occupational therapy interventions will focus on recommending a work schedule that gradually increases his endurance and function, educating him about a home exercise program of strengthening and stretching, and practicing job activities (simulation and actual) with the prosthesis and the residual arm, especially those tasks that remain challenging: lifting heavy items, using mops and brooms, climbing ladders, and carrying supplies.

SECTION 3: LOWER EXTREMITY AMPUTATIONS

Jennifer S. Glover

THREADED CASE STUDY: LENA, PART 1

Lena is a 72-year-old woman who lives by herself in a one-story house near downtown. She was widowed 5 years ago and has two adult children who also live in town. Lena has adult-onset diabetes as well as chronic obstructive pulmonary disease (COPD). She worked part-time as a clerk at a department store until her 50s, when she retired because she could no longer stand comfortably for long periods of time. After retirement, Lena would drive for shopping and appointments and would walk the short distance to church. The circulation in Lena's legs got progressively worse over the years, and she began to spend increasing amounts of time at home. Lena's day usually involved watching television, birdwatching through the window, and occasionally painting ceramic figurines.

At 62, Lena stubbed her toe on her left foot, cutting it. The circulation in her foot was not sufficient for it to heal, and the toe was amputated. She had another toe amputated 2 years later, and 2 weeks ago she had a below-knee amputation of her left leg because of wounds that wouldn't heal.

Lena has just been transferred to a skilled nursing facility in her hometown. The occupational therapist met with Lena for her initial evaluation today, after which the two set goals for Lena's course of treatment.

Critical Thinking Questions

1. What is an area of occupation that will make Lena feel like herself again?
2. What treatment activities can be used to best address challenges presented by Lena's amputation and help her return to participation in her chosen occupations?
3. How can the occupational therapist help Lena prepare not only to return home but also to reduce her risk of rehospitalization?

LEVELS OF LOWER EXTREMITY AMPUTATION

LE amputations are typically discussed as being above-knee or below-knee; however, variability exists even within these categories (Figure 43-31). Generally, the more proximal an amputation is, the greater the functional challenge presented to the person with the amputation. Proximal LE amputations include hemipelvectomy and hip disarticulation amputations, resulting in the loss of the entire lower extremity; such severe amputations are typically performed in cases of trauma or malignancy. Wound healing from such proximal amputations is typically slow, and skin grafting may be required for full healing. In cases of hemipelvectomy, a muscle flap will cover the internal organs.

A transfemoral or **above-knee amputation** (AKA) results in loss of the knee and everything distal to it. The residual limb length from an AKA typically varies from 10 to 12 inches (5.4 to 30.5 cm) from the greater trochanter[7]; transfemoral amputations can also be classified as *upper, middle,* or *lower third,* indicating the amputation distance from the ischium. A through-the-knee (disarticulation) amputation does result in loss of knee joint function, but it also allows for a high level of prosthetic control and mobility.

A transtibial or **below-knee amputation** (BKA) preserves the knee and thus eliminates the necessity for a mechanical knee joint in the prosthesis. The residual limb from a BKA typically varies from 4 to 6 inches (10.1 to 15.2 cm) in length from the tibial plateau.[7] A **Syme's amputation,** or ankle disarticulation, results in loss of both ankle and foot function and is typically performed in cases of trauma or infection. A transmetatarsal amputation results in severing the foot through the metatarsal bones, but the ankle remains intact. Clients may also experience amputation of toes; although amputation of the first toe impairs ambulation by preventing toe off (which is the end of the stance or support phase of gait), loss of the small toes does not usually result in impaired ambulation. In Lena's case, because her left leg was amputated approximately 5 inches below the tibial plateau, the amputation is considered a BKA.

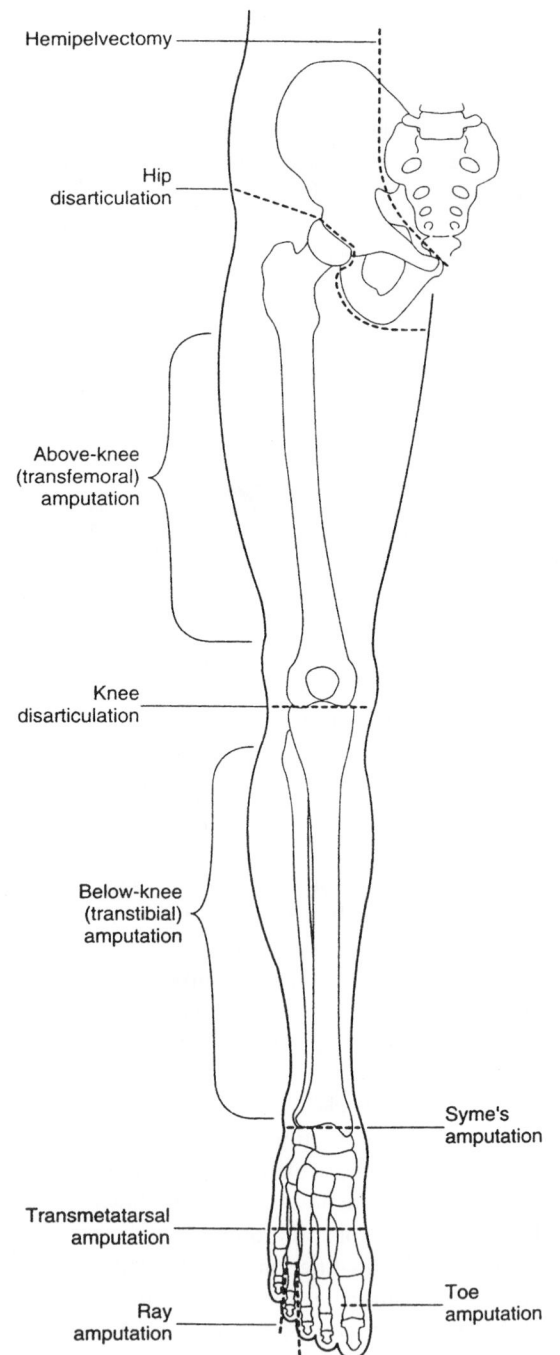

Hemipelvectomy

Hip
disarticulation

Above-knee
(transfemoral)
amputation

Knee
disarticulation

Below-knee
(transtibial)
amputation

Syme's
amputation

Transmetatarsal
amputation

Toe
amputation

Ray
amputation

Figure 43-31   Levels of lower extremity amputation. (From Paz JC, West MP: *Acute care handbook for physical therapists*, ed 2, Oxford, 2002, Butterworth-Heinemann.)

CAUSES OF LOWER EXTREMITY AMPUTATION

In the United States, 95% of LE amputations are performed as a result of complications of PVD[26]; ultimately, 25% to 50% of these cases are due to diabetes mellitus.[54] Trauma is the second most common cause of amputation in the United States, but because of land mines and other environmental hazards, it is the leading cause in developing countries.[54] An amputation may also be performed in cases of malignancy in an effort to prevent it from spreading to other sites or systems in the body.

In Lena's case, diabetes mellitus and PVD resulted in poor circulation in her LEs. Because of this complication, blood flow to her left foot and leg was not adequate for her limb to heal, even from what initially appeared to be a small wound. Therefore, she was obliged to undergo progressive amputations of her left LE, eventually leading to her recent BKA.

POST-SURGERY RESIDUAL LIMB CARE

Skin care and positioning are extremely important throughout the course of rehabilitation, especially immediately after surgery. Once the surgical wound has begun to heal, some form of specialized post-surgical dressing will be used to help prevent swelling and to shape the residual limb for ease of future prosthetic use. Wrapping with an elastic bandage, such as an Ace wrap, is a common method to control edema after surgery. However, smooth wrapping does require skilled and consistent technique, which is necessary to prevent poor shaping of the residual limb. A series of gradually smaller residual limb shrinkers can be worn, as an alternative to elastic bandage wrapping, to encourage constant, even shrinkage of the residual limb for fit with a final prosthesis. Both elastic bandages and shrinkers can be used early after surgery, even if the client's surgical wound still has a dressing on it. In such a case, a nylon stocking would first be applied to prevent the bandage or shrinker from dislodging the dressing. Once the final prosthesis is made and adjusted, the client will frequently continue to wear a shrinker during the day when he or she is not wearing the prosthesis, as well as at night. This shrinking and shaping process can take up to 3 months or more in some cases, depending on the client's condition.

If the client (or his or her caregiver) is unable to demonstrate proper technique with wrapping or shrinker use, a Jobst compression pump may be used. The pump is an air-filled sleeve that surrounds the residual limb, placing constant, equal pressure on all sides, quickly shrinking and shaping the residual limb. A rigid dressing, or cast, is frequently used for active clients after surgery. The end of the cast is made to work with a simple training prosthesis so that the client can begin training for standing and walking immediately. Scar massage may also be necessary later in the healing to prevent adhesions and increase comfort around the surgical site, and this massage technique can be taught to the client. The Ace wrap bandaging of Lena's residual limb was performed by the nurses in the hospital. After Lena's arrival at the skilled nursing facility, the nursing staff consulted the occupational therapist to determine whether Lena had the cognitive and visual function, as well as the necessary motor skills, to learn how to apply her own wrap or shrinker and perform her own scar massage.

LOWER EXTREMITY EQUIPMENT AND PROSTHESES

Movement and time out of bed are typically reduced immediately after LE amputation. The surgery itself can make movement uncomfortable, and many persons who have undergone amputation surgery also have preexisting conditions that may further reduce mobility. For these reasons, clients may require the use of bed rails or a metal trapeze bar hanging over the bed to help reposition themselves in bed and to transition between supine and sitting. Wheelchairs also present a challenge because the client is no longer able to support the affected limb by resting the now absent foot on the floor or on the footrest of the wheelchair. A **residual limb support** is basically a padded board that is placed on the seat of the wheelchair, which has an extended component on the side of the affected limb that projects forward from the seat of the chair (Figure 43-32). This extension provides a surface for the residual limb to rest on, thus placing the limb in a nondependent position and reducing the stresses placed on the hip joint. A person with a BKA is often at risk for developing a flexion contracture of the knee joint, and the residual limb support can also facilitate extension of the knee joint in sitting, thus helping to prevent both edema in the residual limb and contracture of the knee joint.[73] A residual limb support is sometimes still referred to, in less acceptable terminology, as a *stump support*. For a person with bilateral LE amputations, the large wheels on the wheelchair must be placed farther back to accommodate the change in body weight distribution. Antitippers, commercially available wheelchair accessories, can also be used on the back

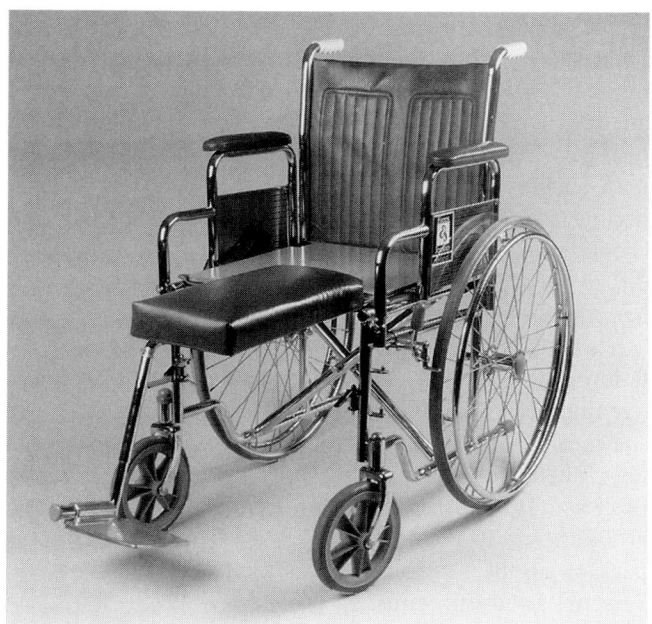

Figure 43-32 Wheelchair with support for residual limb.

of the chair to reduce the likelihood of tipping backward during weight shifting.

Most clients will use a walker during at least the initial phases of their rehabilitation. Some clients with LE amputations will go on to use a walker at all times for ambulation. Both four-footed (standard) and two-wheeled (rolling) walkers may be used, depending on the client's individual characteristics and needs. It has been suggested that using a two-wheeled walker may allow those using prosthetic limbs to ambulate more quickly and with less interruption,[69] but walker choice should always be made on the basis of a total assessment of the client's abilities and needs.

There are many types of prostheses for the LE, and technology is improving daily. For all prostheses, comfort, ease of application, appearance, and function of a prosthesis, including the client's ability to perform ADLs and IADLs with use of the affected extremity, correlate significantly with the client's walking distance and also with his or her perceived quality of life after a LE amputation.[40] It is very important for the rehabilitation team to keep this in mind during a client's fitting for and training with a prosthesis.

The main components of an LE prosthesis are the socket, a sock or gel liner, a suspension system, a pylon, and a terminal device. For some prostheses, an articulating joint is also necessary. The socket is the direct connection between the residual limb and the prosthesis. A person's residual limb may change in volume during the day and over the course of time, presenting challenges for maintaining an adequate fit within the socket. This challenge is frequently addressed by adding to, or removing socks from, the residual limb in order to adapt to its volume changes. Smart variable geometry socket (SVGS) technology was recently developed to help reduce this challenge.[21] SVGS adds and removes liquid from the intrasocket environment on the basis of intrasocket pressure during wear, continuously accommodating for residual limb volume changes and thus maintaining the fit of the socket without having to remove the prosthesis. Static elastomeric liners are also used for the prosthesis socket, and the choice of liner is based on variables such as fit, comfort, friction tolerance, and price.[57] There are various suspension mechanisms used to attach the socket to the residual limb, including belts, straps, wedges, or suction; sometimes mechanisms are combined to ensure appropriate fit.

The **pylon** is the structure that attaches the socket to the TD (Figure 43-33). Vertical shock pylons function as shock absorbers for LE prostheses. Many clients who have had an LE amputation express a preference for walking with these devices.[19] Such shock absorption is especially beneficial during high-impact activities, such as running, and for other activities that are part of daily life for many clients, such as descending curbs and stairs. A pylon can be a basic, static device that provides minimal cosmetic benefits; it can also be a dynamic device, such as that outlined in the preceding paragraph, and can be modified to provide a close cosmetic match to the client's unaffected limb.

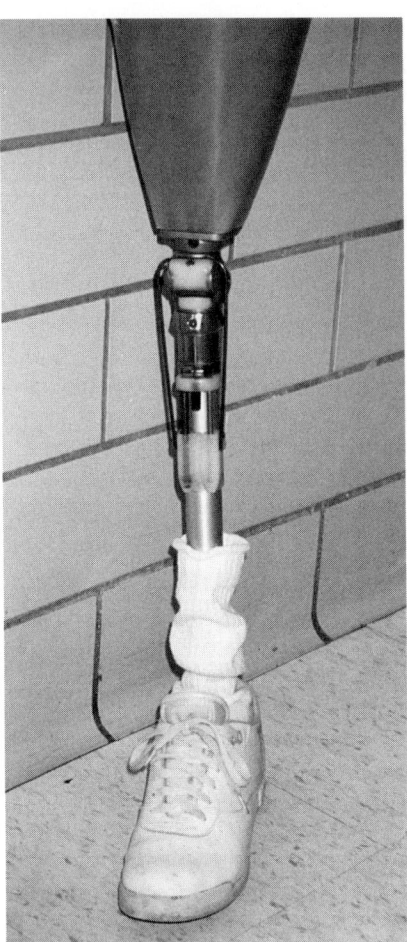

Figure 43-33   A typical pylon.

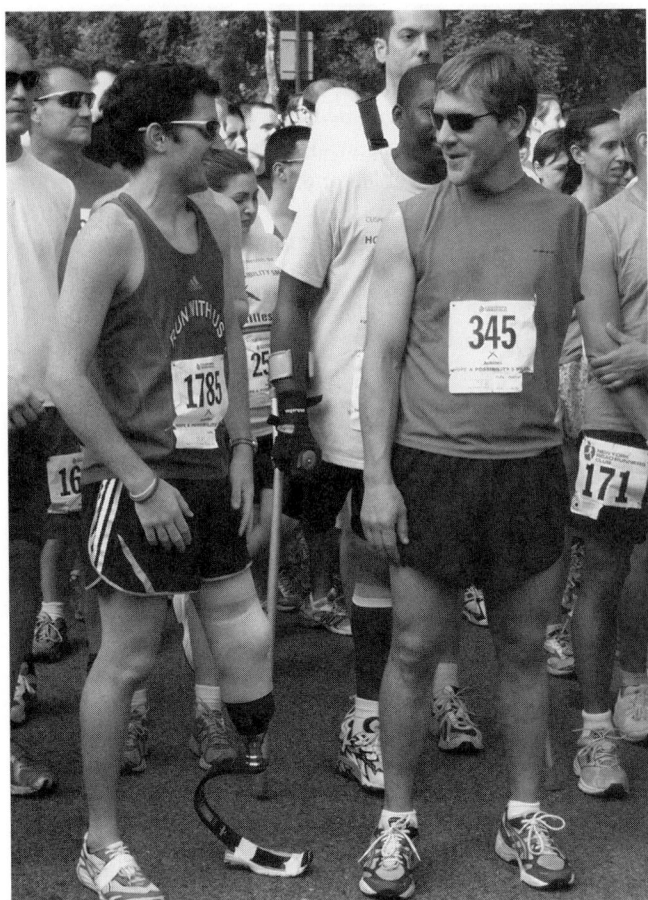

Figure 43-34   An athlete with a specialized running prosthesis at the start of a race. (From Chalufour M: Reasons to run: unexpected perspectives, *Running Times* 330:35, 2005.)

The TD is the prosthetic foot, which provides a stable weight-bearing surface and can itself function as a shock absorber. The many types of available TDs provide varying degrees of mechanical ankle movement and dynamic response, according to the needs and abilities of the client. There are also specialized TDs— indeed, entire LE prostheses—designed to accommodate the challenges presented by various sports and activities (Figure 43-34). To help select the best prosthesis, Lena's prosthetist consulted with her occupational therapist to explore the activities and lifestyle to which Lena wished to return.

PARTICIPATION IN AREAS OF OCCUPATION

 OT PRACTICE NOTE

A thorough occupational history along with evaluation and analysis of occupational performance, obtained during the initial evaluation, will help the occupational therapist to identify areas of strength and of challenge for the client who has undergone an amputation.

For some clients, particularly ones who underwent a traumatic amputation, the activities to which they wish to return are ones that they engaged in right up to the point of injury or illness. However, given the nature of PVD and diabetes, many clients with LE amputations experience a progressive decline in function over the course of several years. For these clients, amputation and subsequent rehabilitation, although difficult, may allow a return to fulfilling occupations that had been absent from the clients' repertoire for quite some time.

Participation in most ADLs will be affected by LE amputation. Although a client with an LE amputation will be learning new mobility techniques in physical therapy, he or she must also participate in occupational therapy to learn new functional mobility techniques with which to accomplish familiar tasks. Bathing, dressing, personal hygiene, grooming, and toileting will likely need to be addressed as part of an occupational therapy intervention program. Personal device care must be addressed if the client is using an LE prosthesis. Participation in IADLs will also be affected. Particular attention should be paid to care of others, care of pets, child rearing, community mobility, health management and maintenance, home management, meal preparation and cleanup, safety procedures and emergency responses, and shopping.

Participation in educational, professional, and leisure activities is usually affected by LE amputation and should be addressed during occupational therapy, as should social participation. Although intervention often assumes a greater role with these areas of occupation later in the rehabilitation process, they can still be addressed even during the acute rehabilitation phase, thus reinforcing to the client that these are areas of occupation in which a return to active participation is indeed possible. It is essential that the occupational therapist help clients to explore all of the avenues of occupation in which they may wish to participate, ensuring that even activities that had been abandoned in the past are possible again.[33] As a result of changes in function after amputation, clients may not be able to return to participation in prior work or leisure activities or to participation at the level to which they were accustomed. In such cases, the occupational therapist should help clients explore other opportunities that they might find fulfilling through identification of interests, skills, and opportunities.

Early in her course of occupational therapy at the skilled nursing facility, Lena spoke with her therapist about how much she missed walking to her church and helping to bake pies for its annual autumn festival. Lena said that she stopped doing this about 10 years ago because it became so difficult; she then discussed feelings of isolation and uselessness. Lena said that she had been known throughout her town for her pies, and she proudly recounted how each year people would tell her that she should open her own restaurant. Although Lena and her occupational therapist had initially set her long-term goals for independence with self-care and basic home management, they decided to add a goal for community re-entry that focused on being able to re-engage in this occupation.

CLIENT FACTORS

Structures related to movement, as well as skin and related structures, are always altered by an LE amputation. The status of other body structures must also be assessed, however, to determine the level of support or challenge that these structures might present during the rehabilitation process.

Neuromuscular and movement-related functions will be altered by LE amputation and will affect occupational performance after surgery. This alteration of function may occur not only in the affected limb but also in other parts of the body. Because of the changes in the affected limb, greater stresses will be placed on the rest of the body; the unaffected leg as well as the arms will experience increased weight bearing during many functional activities, and surgical wound healing, as well as increased time in bed, will place greater demand on skin functions.

Of particular importance is attention to sensations of pain. Up to 84% of persons who have had an LE amputation have experienced phantom limb pain.[11] In such an instance, the client may experience sensations in the part of the extremity that has been removed, such as feelings of cramping, squeezing, shooting, or burning pain. In these cases, the therapist can use desensitization techniques (such as massage of the residual limb), exercise, hot and cold therapy, or electrical stimulation[54] to help decrease these sensations and allow the client to more easily and comfortably participate in chosen occupations.

Clients with PVD already have compromised cardiovascular function, and care must be taken to determine how much activity can safely be tolerated during therapy. A client's mental and sensory functions will affect the way in which therapy, including education, is delivered; it will also affect what types of prosthesis and equipment are used.[31] Some clients may be able to incorporate new techniques quickly, recalling information from one session or even from reading material, and may be able to independently apply this learning to new situations. However, other clients will require adaptation of training and may require prolonged treatment to turn the new techniques that they have learned into habits.

The occupational therapist found that Lena would need to increase her upper body strength to help support herself during transfers and ambulation with the walker. She also needed to improve her post-surgical standing balance to participate in her chosen occupations. Lena was experiencing pain and sensitivity of her residual limb. However, Lena's cognitive function was found to be a strength, and her vision and sensation in her hands, although slightly diminished, were assessed at a level sufficient to support her desired functional activities.

PERFORMANCE SKILLS

The most overt effects of LE amputation will be evident in the area of motor skills. Posture, mobility, coordination, strength and effort, and energy are all altered after surgery, and the client must address each of these skills in therapy to return to a full balance of occupations. The client's level of process skills (such as knowledge and adaptation) and communication/interaction skills will also affect his or her participation in treatment and the therapist's choice of treatment methods.

Lena's occupational therapist found that, as she expected, Lena exhibited impairment in stabilization, alignment, positioning, walking, reaching, bending, moving, transporting, lifting while standing, and endurance. The therapist also found that knowledge, temporal organization, organization of space and objects, physicality during interaction, and information exchange were all at functional levels for Lena. However, Lena did exhibit difficulty with adaptation as she began attempting to perform activities with a changed body structure and in different positions. The therapist also noticed that Lena was having difficulty with relations, exhibiting trouble focusing, relating, and collaborating during many occupations. The therapist would need to address these areas in therapy to help Lena return to her optimal level of participation in occupation.

PERFORMANCE PATTERNS

Whatever a client's performance patterns were before the amputation, they are likely to be altered after the amputation. The client may already have useful habits, routines, and roles that can be drawn upon in therapy to facilitate his or her return to prior levels of occupational performance. However, for many clients, the occupational history will reveal prior impoverished habits and lack of, or maladaptive, routines that may present challenges to the rehabilitative process. Although Lena's diabetes and PVD placed her at increased risk for poor wound healing, she had never developed the habit of routinely checking her feet and legs for cuts or infections. This impoverished habit led to three amputations on her left leg. Lena's morning routine in her kitchen also involved crossing the room many times and carrying multiple items in her hands at once. In conversations with her occupational therapist, Lena did indicate that she had already begun to drop things during this routine, that she had nearly fallen a few times, and that she worried about being able to safely make her own breakfast at home.

PSYCHOSOCIAL REPERCUSSIONS

Amputation of a limb represents a loss and therefore involves a grief process. This process involves dealing with one's feelings regarding change in body structure, functional abilities, and participation in occupations. It can also involve anger, acknowledgment of unpleasant realities regarding one's health status, and fears about one's functional and financial future. Social acceptance and community function are also significant concerns for a person who has undergone an amputation. These are all areas that can be addressed by an interdisciplinary rehabilitation team in an effort to help the client adapt and should also inform all aspects of occupational therapy intervention.

The occupational therapist may use several techniques to help a person adapt to his or her amputation and create a new sense of self. The therapeutic relationship and the therapeutic use of self can provide a safe environment and catalyst for the client to discuss feelings of loss, thoughts regarding body changes, and fears for the future. The therapist can teach the client coping skills for dealing with anxiety and depression as well as techniques for improving post-surgical body image.[52] The therapeutic use of occupation that has been graded to the client's current abilities provides opportunities to master skills and experience success.

The therapist's encouragement during such sessions not only fosters development and provides support but also provides evidence to the client that recovery of function and return to participation in chosen occupations are indeed possible[52]; this knowledge fosters hope and a vision of the future.

It is important to recognize that an outside observer's rating of a person's adaptation to an LE amputation may not be the same as that person's self-rating. A surgeon may rate success on the basis of the healing of the surgical wound, a prosthetist on the fit between residual limb and prosthesis, a physical therapist on the client's ability to ambulate, and an occupational therapist on the client's ability to participate in areas of occupation. However, clients may place greater emphasis on other criteria in their determination of successful adaptation to an LE amputation. Some related variables that appear of primary concern to clients include feeling comfortable being active in the presence of strangers, not feeling like a burden to one's family, being able to care for others, and being able to exercise recreationally.[40]

CONTEXT AND ACTIVITY DEMANDS

An understanding of the client's context and the demands of daily activities will help the therapist design a treatment program that will best help the client re-engage in chosen occupations within his or her natural environment. It will also help the therapist adapt the activity demands of the client's chosen occupations to facilitate greater independence and development of proficiency. Lena's occupational therapist took a detailed floor plan of the setup of Lena's bedroom and was able to move the furniture in her room in the SNF so as to closely approximate her bedroom setup at home. When Lena performed her morning and evening ADLs within the room, she was then doing so in a more natural environment. Lena's therapist initially made significant adaptations to Lena's morning routine demands, wheeling Lena up to the sink in the bathroom for sponge-bathing and bringing her clothes to her in the bathroom, where she would stand with the help of a grab bar so that the therapist could pull Lena's pants up. Over the course of time, as Lena improved her performance skills, improved her performance patterns, and incorporated new ADL techniques taught during therapy into her routine, her occupational therapist was able to decrease the adaptation of activity demands and Lena progressed to independence with routines that she would be able to sustain at home.

ADDITIONAL CONSIDERATIONS FOR ELDERLY CLIENTS

Although LE amputation may be performed to preserve function or to save the client's life, it does carry an increased mortality risk as the age of the client increases. One study of older persons who underwent a BKA found the survival probability after BKA to be 77% at 1 year, 57% at 3 years, and 28% at 7½ years.[35] Because this increased mortality risk is related not only to the amputation surgery but also to preexisting health and environment factors, attention to the overall health status of the client is of the utmost importance.

Many body structures and functions are already compromised in elderly clients, making the rehabilitation process longer and more delicate. An elderly person may take more time to recover from the effects of anesthesia after surgery,

including effects on cognition and the respiratory system. For unilateral amputees, leg balance on the unaffected limb is a significant predictor for prosthetic use.[59] Because balance may already be decreased, elderly clients learning to use a prosthetic limb may present a greater challenge, as can declining cognition. Elderly clients have already experienced many losses, which may include loss of family and friends, home, health, and function; the psychological sequelae of amputation can be all the more traumatic when layered over these previous losses.

THREADED CASE STUDY: LENA, PART 2

Amputation of a lower extremity has a significant functional impact on a person, but a return to an active and fulfilling life is still possible. Lena required extensive assistance to take care of herself when she entered the skilled nursing facility, but her goal was to return home, independently able to take care of herself and her home. During the course of occupational therapy, Lena also realized that she had been slowly decreasing her participation in the very activities that helped her feel active and vital and helped her define who she was. She then decided to work with her therapist toward being able to reclaim these activities, particularly going back to her church and helping to bake pies for its upcoming autumn festival.

During the course of her occupational therapy, Lena's therapist presented her with activities that addressed the areas that Lena needed to improve to reach her goals. These goals, which Lena had identified as of interest to her, were adapted to provide an appropriate level of challenge. Because Lena liked to watch birds and had enjoyed decorative painting in the past, her occupational therapy sessions included building and painting birdhouses. This increased Lena's upper body strength and provided progressive challenges to her sitting and eventually standing balance, facilitating her return to independence with ambulatory tasks and providing an activity that Lena could perform at home and a product that she could donate to her church's fall festival.

As Lena's stay at the skilled nursing facility neared its end, she also participated in community re-entry sessions with her occupational therapist. Because Lena had mentioned her desire to help bake pies with the congregation for the festival, she and her occupational therapist visited the church together during a community re-entry

session; this gave Lena a chance to interact with some of the members of the baking committee so that they could see Lena's capable self, allaying their fears about interacting with a person with a disability and setting the expectation that Lena would be involved. Through supported engagement in this social community occupation, Lena also gained confidence that she is still an accepted and desired member of her community. Together, Lena and her occupational therapist identified potential challenges presented by the layout of the kitchen. Lena engaged in trials and problem-solving strategies with her therapist to determine methods to allow safe participation in the baking. In preparation for her return to the church as a member of the baking team, Lena then perfected these techniques in the occupational therapy kitchen back at the facility.

Lena's occupational therapist also worked with Lena to discuss the ways in which some of her prehospitalization habits and routines had contributed to high-risk situations and to identify strategies to help reduce her risks of rehospitalization. Lena learned how to perform her own lower body skin checks and was performing them regularly by the end of her stay. She went home with a daily routine that would help her stay active throughout the day but also incorporated techniques that minimized periods of prolonged standing and reduced the amount of energy required to accomplish tasks. Lena's family then reorganized items in her kitchen, according to recommendations determined by Lena in collaboration with her occupational therapist, so that her environment placed less strain on her during daily activities. Lena went home independent with her daily activities, able to engage in individual and social occupations that made her feel happy and vital, and reclaimed a role that had long been abandoned.

Review Questions

1. Define the following abbreviations: AE, TD, BE, AKA, and BKA.
2. List six reasons for amputation.
3. What are the four main reasons for LE amputation?
4. What are the primary goals of amputation surgery?
5. Name the two types of surgical procedures that can be performed, and list the advantages of each.
6. Name at least four post-surgical factors that can interfere with prosthetic training and rehabilitation. How is each solved?
7. Define *neuroma*. How does it affect the wearing of the prosthesis?
8. What is the difference between *phantom limb* and *phantom pain*?

9. What are some of the typical and expected psychosocial consequences of limb loss?

10. How can members of the rehabilitation team facilitate adjustment to amputation and prosthesis wear?

11. Which arm function is lost and which functions are maintained in a long transradial amputation?

12. What is the purpose of the preprosthetic program?

13. Describe activities and exercises suitable for the preprosthetic period.

14. Before the TD on an AE prosthesis can be operated, what must the wearer do?

15. How does the prosthesis wearer preposition the TD?

16. Name two types of electric TDs.

17. How is functional training graded?

18. What is the source of power that activates the electric-powered prosthesis?

19. What are some advantages of the electric-powered prosthesis?

20. What is a hybrid prosthesis?

21. What does *muscle site control training* mean?

22. Describe the relative roles of a prosthesis and a sound arm and hand in the following activities: cutting meat, opening a jar, using scissors, buckling a belt, using an eggbeater, and hammering a nail.

23. Name two significant concerns for the residual limb immediately after surgery.

24. What is the purpose of a shrinker?

25. What should be done with the wheelchair to accommodate the residual limb? To accommodate a person with bilateral AKAs?

26. Name the main components of an LE prosthesis.

27. What is the purpose of using a sock on the residual limb?

28. How will LE amputation affect other parts of the body?

29. How might LE amputation affect an individual's participation in areas of occupation?

30. Which performance skills are most likely to be affected after LE amputation?

31. How can preexisting performance patterns affect a client's participation in occupations after the amputation?

32. What are the potential psychosocial repercussions of LE amputation?

33. How can ADL activity demands be adapted to foster greater independence after LE amputation?

34. What additional considerations does LE amputation present for elderly clients?

REFERENCES

1. American Occupational Therapy Association: Occupational therapy practice framework: domain and process, *Am J Occup Ther* 56(6):609, 2002.

2. Anderson MH, Bechtol CO, Sollars RE: *Clinical prosthetics for physicians and therapists*, Springfield, IL, 1959, Charles C Thomas.

3. Andrew JT: Prosthetic principles. In Bowker JH, Michael JW, editors: *Atlas of limb prosthetics: surgical, prosthetic, and rehabilitation principles*, ed 2, St Louis, 1992, Mosby.

4. Atkins DJ: Adult myoelectric upper-limb prosthetic training. In Atkins DJ, Meier RH, editors: *Comprehensive management of the upper limb amputee*, New York, 1989, Springer-Verlag.

5. Atkins DJ: Adult upper limb prosthetic training. In Atkins DJ, Meier RH, editors: *Comprehensive management of the upper-limb amputee*, New York, 1989, Springer-Verlag.

6. Atkins DJ: Postoperative and preprosthetic therapy programs. In Atkins DJ, Meier RH, editors: *Comprehensive management of the upper-limb amputee*, New York, 1989, Springer-Verlag.

7. Banerjee SJ: *Rehabilitation management of amputees*, Baltimore, 1982, Williams & Wilkins.

8. Bennett JB, Alexander CB: Amputation levels and surgical techniques. In Atkins DJ, Meier RH, editors: *Comprehensive management of the upper-limb amputee*, New York, 1989, Springer-Verlag.

9. Bennett JB, Gartsman GM: Surgical options for brachial plexus and stroke patients. In Atkins DJ, Meier RH, editors: *Comprehensive management of the upper-limb amputee*, New York, 1989, Springer-Verlag.

10. Billock JN: Prosthetic management of complete hand and arm deficiencies. In Hunter JM, Mackin EJ, Callahan AD, editors: *Rehabilitation of the hand: surgery and therapy*, ed 4, St Louis, 1995, Mosby.

11. Czerniecki JM, Ehde DM: Chronic pain after lower extremity amputation, *Critical Review Phys Med Rehabil* 15:309, 2003.

12. Dalsey R, et al: Myoelectric prosthetic replacement in the upper extremity amputee, *Orthop Rev* 18(6):697, 1989.

13. DiMartine C: Capturing the phantom, *inMotion* 10(5):7, 2000.

14. Evans WE, Hayes JP, Vermillion BO: Effect of a failed distal reconstruction on the level of amputation, *Am J Surg* 160(2):217, 1990.

15. Fan T, Fedder DO: *Smoking gun: the impact of smoking on amputees*, Baltimore, MD, 2003, Pharmaceutical Health Service Research Program, University of Maryland, Baltimore. Accessed September, 13, 2005 at http://www.amputee-coalition.org/related_articles/smoking_gun.html.

16. Friedman LW: Rehabilitation of the amputee. In Goodgold J, editor: *Rehabilitation medicine*, St Louis, 1988, Mosby.

17. Friedman LW: *The psychological rehabilitation of the amputee*, Springfield, IL, 1978, Charles C Thomas.

18. Fryer CM, Michael JW: Body-powered components. In Bowker JH, Michael JW, editors: *Atlas of limb prosthetics: surgical, prosthetic, and rehabilitation principles*, ed 2, St Louis, 1992, Mosby.

19. Gard SA, Childress DS: A study to determine the biomechanical effects of shock-absorbing pylons, *Rehabil R&D Progress Reports* 35:18, 1998.

20. Glattly HW: A statistical study of 12,000 new amputees, *South Med J* 57:1373, 1964.

21. Greenwald RM, Dean RC, Board WJ: Volume management: smart variable geometry socket (SVGS) technology for lower-limb prostheses, *J Prosthetics Orthotics* 15:107, 2003.

22. Harris KA, et al: Rehabilitation potential of elderly patients with major amputations, *J Cardiovasc Surg (Torino)* 32(5):648, 1991.

23. Hill SL: Interventions for the elderly amputee, *Rehabil Nurs* 10(3):23, 1985.

24. Hirschberg G, Lewis L, Thomas D: *Rehabilitation*, Philadelphia, 1964, JB Lippincott.

25. Jacobsen SC, et al: Development of the Utah Artificial Arm, *IEEE Trans Biomed Eng* 29(4):249, 1982.

26. Jelic M, Eldar R: Rehabilitation following major traumatic amputation of lower limbs: a review, *Critical Review Phys Rehabil Med* 15:235, 2003.

27. Kay HW, Newman JD: Relative incidence of new amputations: statistical comparisons of 6,000 new amputees, *Orthot Prosthet* 59:109, 1978.

28. Knighton DR, et al: Amputation prevention in an independently reviewed at-risk diabetic population using a comprehensive wound care protocol, *Am J Surg* 160(5):466, 1990.

29. Krajewski LP, Olin JW: Atherosclerosis of the aorta and lower extremities arteries. In Young JR, et al, editors: *Peripheral vascular diseases*, St Louis, 1991, Mosby.

30. Lane JM, Kroll MA, Rossbach P: New advances and concepts in amputee management after treatment for bone and soft tissue sarcomas, *Clin Orthop* Jul(256):280, 1990.

31. Larner S, vanRoss E, Hale C: Do psychological measures predict the ability of lower limb amputees to learn to use a prosthesis, *Clinical Rehabil* 17:493, 2003.

32. Larson CB, Gould M: *Orthopedic nursing*, ed 8, St Louis, 1974, Mosby.

33. Legro MW, et al: Recreational activities of lower-limb amputees with prostheses, *J Rehabil Res Development* 38:319, 2001.

34. Leonard JA, Meier RH: Prosthetics. In DeLisa JA, editor: *Rehabilitation medicine principles and practice*, Philadelphia, 1988, JB Lippincott.

35. Levin AZ: Functional outcome following amputation, *Topics Geriatr Rehabil* 20:253, 2004.

36. Levy LA: Smoking and peripheral vascular disease, *Clin Podiatr Med Surg* 9(1):165, 1992.

37. Lind J, Kramhhaft M, Badtker S: The influence of smoking on complications after primary amputations of the lower extremity, *Clin Orthop* 267:211, 1992.

38. Link MP, et al: Adjuvant chemotherapy of high grade osteosarcoma of the extremity, *Clin Orthop* 270:8, 1991.

39. Malone JM, Goldstone J: Lower extremity amputation. In Moore WS, editor: *Vascular surgery: a comprehensive review*, New York, 1984, Grune & Stratton.

40. Matsen SL, Malchow D, Matsen FA: Correlations with patients' perspectives of the result of lower-extremity amputation, *J Bone Joint Surg* 82A:1089, 2000.

41. McIntyre KE Jr: The diabetic foot and management of infectious gangrene. In Moore WS, Malone JHM, editors: *Lower extremity amputation*, Philadelphia, 1989, WB Saunders.

42. Meier RH: Amputations and prosthetic fitting. In Fisher S, editor: *Comprehensive rehabilitation of burns*, Baltimore, 1984, Williams & Wilkins.

43. Meier RH, Atkins DJ: Preface. In Atkins DJ, Meier RH, editors: *Comprehensive management of the upper-limb amputee*, New York, 1989, Springer-Verlag.

44. Michaels JA: The selection of amputation level: an approach using decision analysis, *Eur J Vasc Surg* 5(4):451, 1991.

45. Moss SE, Klein R, Klein BE: The prevalence and incidence of lower extremity amputation in a diabetic population, *Arch Intern Med* 152(3):610, 1992.

46. Muilenburg AL, LeBlanc MA: Body-powered upper-limb components. In Atkins DJ, Meier RH, editors: *Comprehensive management of the upper-limb amputee*, New York, 1989, Springer-Verlag.

47. Nader M, Ing EH: The artificial substitution of missing hands with myoelectric prostheses, *Clin Orthop* 258:9, 1990.

48. NovaCare: *Motion control: training the client with an electric arm prosthesis*, King of Prussia, PA, 1997, NovaCare (videotape).

49. Novotny MP: Psychosocial issues affecting rehabilitation, *Phys Med Rehabil Clin North Am* 2:273, 1991.

50. Olivett BL: Management and prosthetic training of the adult amputee. In Hunter JM, editor: *Rehabilitation of the hand*, St Louis, 1984, Mosby.

51. O'Sullivan S, Cullen K, Schmitz T: *Physical rehabilitation: evaluation and treatment procedures*, Philadelphia, 1981, FA Davis.

52. Pendleton HM, Schultz-Krohn W: Psychosocial issues in physical disability. In Cara E, MacRae A, editors: *Psychosocial occupational therapy: a clinical practice*, Clifton Park, NY, 2005, Thomson Delmar Learning.

53. Pinzur MS, et al: Functional outcome following traumatic upper limb amputation and prosthetic limb fitting, *JHS* 19A(5):836, 1994.

54. Rand JD, Paz JC: Amputation. In Paz JC, West MP, editors: *Acute care handbook for physical therapists*, Woburn, MA, 2002, Butterworth-Heinemann.

55. Raney R, Brashear H: *Shands' handbook of orthopaedic surgery*, ed 8, St Louis, 1971, Mosby.

56. Ritz G, Friedman S, Osbourne A: Diabetes and peripheral vascular disease, *Clin Podiatr Med Surg* 9(1):125, 1992.

57. Sanders JE, et al: Testing of elastomeric liners used in limb prosthetics: classification of 15 products by mechanical performance, *J Rehabil Res Development* 41:175, 2004.

58. Santschi WR, editor: *Manual of upper extremity prosthetics*, ed 2, Los Angeles, 1958, University of California Press.

59. Schoppen T, et al: Physical, mental and social predictors of functional outcome in unilateral lower-limb amputees, *Arch Phys Med Rehabil* 84:803, 2003.

60. Scott RN, Parker PA: Myoelectric prostheses: state of the art, *J Med Eng Technol* 12(4):143, 1988.

61. Simon M: Limb salvage for osteosarcoma in the 1980s, *Clin Orthop* 270:264, 1990.

62. Spencer EA: Amputation and prosthetic replacement. In Hopkins HL, Smith HD, editors: *Willard & Spackman's occupational therapy*, ed 8, Philadelphia, 1993, JB Lippincott.

63. Spencer EA: Amputations. In Hopkins HL, Smith HD, editors: *Willard & Spackman's occupational therapy*, ed 5, Philadelphia, 1978, JB Lippincott.

64. Spencer EA: Functional restoration. III: Amputation and prosthetic replacement. In Hopkins HL, Smith HD, editors: *Willard & Spackman's occupational therapy*, ed 8, Philadelphia, 1993, JB Lippincott.

65. Spencer EA: Musculoskeletal dysfunction in adults. In Neistadt ME, Crepeau EB, editors: *Willard & Spackman's occupational therapy*, ed 9, Philadelphia, 1998, JB Lippincott.

66. Spiegal SR: Adult myoelectric upper-limb prosthetic training. In Atkins DJ, Meier RH, editors: *Comprehensive management of the upper-limb amputee*, New York, 1989, Springer-Verlag.

67. Springfield DS: Introduction to limb-salvage surgery for sarcoma, *Orthop Clin North Am* 22(1):1, 1991.

68. Taylor LM, et al: Limb salvage versus amputation for critical ischemia, *Arch Surg* 126(10):1251, 1991.

69. Tsai HA, et al: Aided gait of people with lower-limb amputations: comparison of 4-footed and 2-wheeled walkers, *Arch Phys Med Rehabil* 84:584, 2003.

70. Tsang GM, et al: Failed femorocrural reconstruction does not prejudice amputation level, *Br J Surg* 78(12):1479, 1991.

71. Walsh NE, et al: Treatment of the patient with chronic pain. In DeLisa JA, editor: *Rehabilitation medicine principles and practice*, Philadelphia, 1988, JB Lippincott.

72. Wellerson TL: *A manual for occupational therapists on the rehabilitation of upper extremity amputees*, Dubuque, IA, 1958, William C. Brown.

73. White EA: Wheelchair stump boards and their use with lower limb amputees, *Br J Occup Ther* 55:174, 1992.

74. Wright G: *Controls training for the upper extremity amputee* (film), San Jose, CA, Instructional Resources Center, San Jose State University.

75. Yaw KM, Wurtz LD: Resection and reconstruction for bone tumor in proximal tibia, *Orthop Clin North Am* 22(1):133, 1991.

RESOURCES

ALPS Skin Lotion
ALPS Corporate Offices
2895 42nd Ave. North
St. Petersburg, FL 33714
800-574-5426

Texas Assistive Devices, LLC
9483 County Road 628
Brazonia, TX 77422
800-532-6840

Therapeutic Recreation Systems, Inc.
3090 Sterling Co. Studio A
Boulder, CO 80301
800-279-1865

44

CARDIAC AND PULMONARY DISEASE

MAUREEN MICHELE MATTHEWS

KEY TERMS

Heart rate	Rate pressure product	Pursed-lip breathing
Blood pressure	Chronic obstructive pulmonary disease	Diaphragmatic breathing
Ischemic heart disease	Pack year history	
Myocardial infarction	Pulmonary rehabilitation	

LEARNING OBJECTIVES

After studying this chapter the student or practitioner will be able to do the following:

1. Briefly describe the cardiovascular system and its function.
2. Identify the significance of ischemic heart disease and valvular diseases of the heart.
3. Differentiate between modifiable and nonmodifiable risk factors.
4. Identify signs and symptoms of cardiac distress.
5. Describe the course of action that should be taken if signs and symptoms of cardiac distress exist.
6. List the psychosocial considerations for persons with cardiovascular or pulmonary disease.
7. Describe methods for taking heart rate and blood pressure.
8. Determine rate pressure product, given heart rate and blood pressure.

9. Give a brief overview of the respiratory system, and identify its primary function.
10. Define *chronic obstructive pulmonary disease (COPD)*.
11. Identify pulmonary risk factors and psychosocial considerations.
12. Describe dyspnea control postures, pursed-lip breathing, and diaphragmatic breathing.
13. Describe a relaxation technique, and explain its purpose.
14. List interview questions that will help the clinician know what the patient understands about intervention.
15. List the principles of energy conservation.
16. Explain the significance of an MET chart in the progression of activity, and describe how to use it.

CHAPTER OUTLINE

Cardiovascular system
  Anatomy and circulation
  What causes the heart to contract?
  Cardiac cycle
Pathology of cardiac disease
  Ischemic heart disease
  Valvular disease
  Cardiac risk factors
  Medical management
Pulmonary system

Anatomy and physiology of respiration
Innervation of the respiratory system
Chronic lung disease
Pulmonary risk factors
Medical management
Occupational therapy evaluation and intervention: cardiopulmonary dysfunction
  Evaluation
  Intervention
Summary

In this chapter the term patient is used instead of client reflecting the practice setting and the acute nature of the diagnoses to the individuals described in the case studies.

THREADED CASE STUDY: FRANKLIN, PART 1

Franklin is a 48-year-old auto mechanic who experienced substernal chest pain of 10/10 on a pain scale, accompanied by nausea and shortness of breath while working under an automobile 2 days ago. He had been working 60 hours per week and had not taken any time off, despite feeling "under the weather" for a few weeks before these most recent severe symptoms. He was given a diagnosis of an acute anterolateral myocardial infarction (MI) complicated by subsequent congestive heart failure (CHF). He is married and the father of three children, ages 9, 5, and 4. His wife works full time and was unable to manage his care at home, so he was placed temporarily in a skilled nursing facility.

During the initial occupational therapy (OT) evaluation, the occupational profile revealed that Franklin is anxious and expresses concern that he will die in the facility, just as his father did. He inherited the auto repair shop from his father and wants to be able to hand it off to his 9-year-old son when he retires. He reports that his wife "is a very desirable woman and a hardworking mother." He wants to return to his home and return to work. He is able to safely walk to the bathroom, according to physical therapy findings. Besides playing catch with his son and attending little league games, Franklin's typical day is spent working and watching TV, seven days a week.

The OT evaluation also indicates that Franklin, although anxious, was cooperative and motivated to participate in therapy. Although not formally tested, the client factors of strength, range of motion, and perceptual and cognitive ability were grossly functional during a routine activities of daily living (ADLs) assessment of 2.5-basal metabolic equivalent (MET measurement is described elsewhere in the chapter) seated sponge bathing and dressing. Vital signs were appropriate during the evaluation, except that blood pressure (BP) fell 20 mm Hg in recovery (3 minutes after completion of bathing), and Franklin became symptomatic (experiencing nausea and shortness of breath). Symptoms and vital signs stabilized after 5 minutes of rest. Franklin needed frequent cues to pace the activity and demonstrated little knowledge about signs and symptoms of cardiac distress. His risk factors include male gender, family history, smoking, and a sedentary lifestyle.

Franklin is concerned that he be able to do everything for himself if he is discharged home.

Critical Thinking Questions

1. What probative questions might the occupational therapist ask to clarify what Franklin means by "able to do everything for himself"?
2. What skills must Franklin acquire to reduce his risk of another cardiac event?
3. What areas of occupation might the therapist choose for the next intervention session and, based on Franklin's occupational profile, what goals might be included in his OT intervention plan?

Individuals with disorders of the cardiovascular or pulmonary system may be severely limited in endurance and performance in areas of occupation, including activities of daily living (ADLs) and instrumental activities of daily living (IADLs). Occupational therapy (OT) services may benefit such individuals and are available throughout the continuum of healthcare. An understanding of the normal function of the cardiopulmonary system, the pathology of cardiopulmonary disease, common risk factors, clinical terminology, medical interventions, precautions, and standard treatment techniques will guide the occupational therapist in providing effective care and promoting recovery of function in clients with compromised cardiovascular or pulmonary systems.

Every living cell of the body has three major requirements for life: (1) a constant supply of nutrients and oxygen, (2) continual removal of carbon dioxide and other waste products, and (3) a relatively constant temperature. The cardiovascular and pulmonary systems play key roles in meeting these requirements.

CARDIOVASCULAR SYSTEM[13,18,22]

ANATOMY AND CIRCULATION

The heart and blood vessels work together to maintain a constant flow of blood throughout the body. The heart, located between the lungs, is pear shaped and about the size of a fist. It functions as a two-sided pump. The right side pumps blood from the body to the lungs; the left side simultaneously pumps blood from the lungs to the body. Each side of the heart has two chambers: an upper atrium and a lower ventricle.

Blood flows to the heart from the venous system. The blood enters the right atrium, which contracts and squeezes the blood into the right ventricle. Next, the right ventricle contracts and ejects the blood into the lungs, where carbon dioxide is exchanged for oxygen. Oxygen-rich blood flows from the lungs to the left atrium. As the left atrium contracts, it forces blood into the left ventricle, which then contracts and ejects its contents into the aorta for systemic circulation (Figure 44-1). Blood travels from the aorta to the arteries and through progressively smaller blood vessels to networks of very tiny capillaries. In the capillaries, blood cells exchange their oxygen for carbon dioxide.

Each of the ventricles has two valves: an input valve and an output valve. The valves open and close as the heart muscle (myocardium) contracts and relaxes. These valves control the direction and flow of blood. The input valves are the mitral, or bicuspid, valve (between the left atrium and ventricle) and the tricuspid valve (between the right atrium and ventricle). The output valves comprise the aortic and pulmonary valves.

The heart is living tissue and requires a blood supply (through an arterial and venous system of its own), or it will die. Coronary arteries cross over the myocardium to supply it with oxygen-rich blood. The coronary arteries are named for their location on the myocardium (Figure 44-2). Cardiologists generally refer to these arteries by abbreviations, such as "LAD" for "left anterior descending" and "RCA" for "right coronary artery." The LAD is on the left, anterior portion of the heart and runs in a downward direction, supplying part of the left ventricle. A blockage of this coronary artery will interrupt the blood supply to the left ventricle. Because the left ventricle supplies the body and brain with blood, a heart attack caused by LAD blockage can have serious consequences.

WHAT CAUSES THE HEART TO CONTRACT?

In addition to the ordinary muscle tissue of the heart, the myocardium is composed of two other types of tissue: nodal and Purkinje. These tissues are part of a specialized electrical conduction system that causes the heart to contract and relax (Figure 44-3). An electrical impulse usually originates in the right atrium at a site called the sinoatrial (SA) node. The impulse travels along internodal pathways to the atrioventricular (AV) node, through the bundle of His, to the left and right bundle branches, and then to the Purkinje fibers. Nerve impulses normally travel this pathway 60 to 100 times every minute, first causing both atria to contract, pushing blood into the ventricles, and then provoking the ventricles to contract. The electrical impulse created by the heart's conduction system can easily be studied. Electrodes placed on a person's limbs and chest can pick up the heart's electrical impulse, which can be translated to paper via an electrocardiogram (ECG). The resulting ECG tracing is frequently used to help diagnose cardiac disease.

The SA node responds to vagal and sympathetic nervous system input.[18] This is why **heart rate** (HR) increases in response to exercise and anxiety and decreases in response to relaxation techniques, such as deep breathing and meditation. Each cell within the electrical conduction system of the

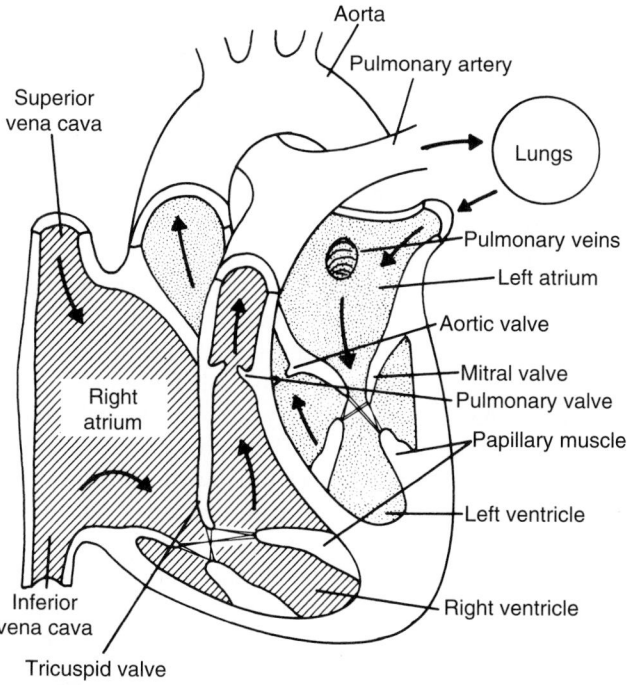

Figure 44-1 Anatomy of the heart. (Modified from Guyton AC: *Textbook of medical physiology*, ed 11, 2005, WB Saunders.)

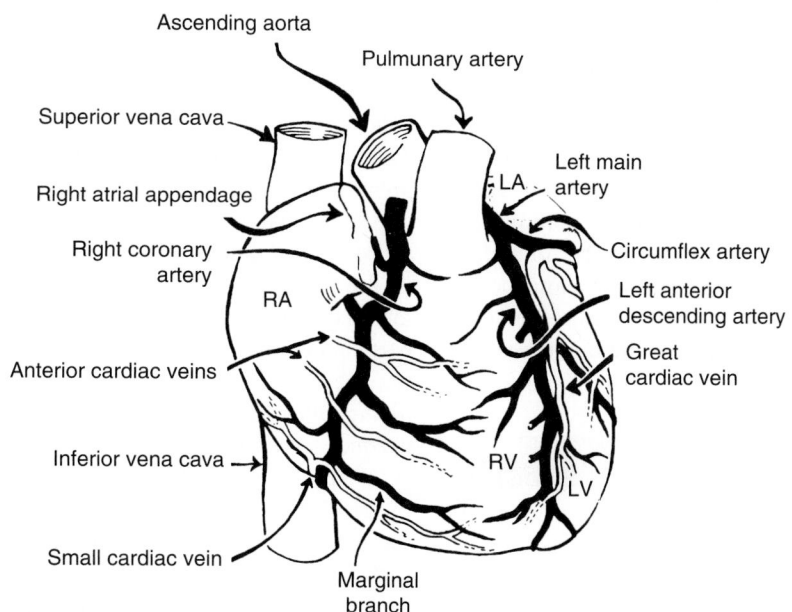

Figure 44-2 Coronary circulation. (From Underhill SL et al, editors: *Cardiac nursing*, Philadelphia, 1982, JB Lippincott.)

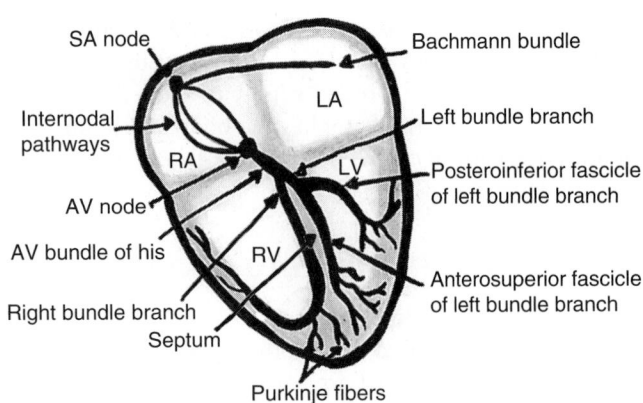

Figure 44-3   Cardiac conduction. (Modified from Andreoli KG, et al: *Comprehensive cardiac care: a text for nurses, physicians, and other health practitioners,* St Louis, 1983, Mosby.)

heart can respond to, conduct, resist for a brief period, and generate an electrical impulse. Because of this capacity, electrical impulses causing the heart muscle to contract can be generated from anywhere along the electrical conduction system. This is desirable when part of the conduction system has been damaged and is unable do its job, but it is undesirable when life-threatening conduction irregularities develop.

CARDIAC CYCLE

HR and **blood pressure** (BP) determine cardiac output, the amount of blood ejected by the heart each minute. The cardiac cycle occurs in two phases: input (diastole) and output (systole).

During the input phase, blood flows through the atria and into the ventricles. The atria contract, pushing more blood into the ventricles. Once the pressure inside the ventricles is equal to the pressure in the atria, the input valves (tricuspid in the right ventricle and mitral [or bicuspid] in the left ventricle) close. The ventricles then contract, resulting in rapidly increasing ventricular pressure. When the pressure inside the ventricles exceeds the pressure in the blood vessels beyond, the output valves (pulmonary in the right and aortic in the left) open, and the diastolic BP is attained.

The ventricles continue to contract, squeezing blood under greater and greater pressure into the pulmonary and body circulation. Systolic BP is attained when pressures in the emptying ventricles fall below pressure in the blood vessels beyond, causing the output valves to close.

PATHOLOGY OF CARDIAC DISEASE

ISCHEMIC HEART DISEASE

Ischemic heart disease (ischemia) occurs when a part of the heart is temporarily deprived of sufficient oxygen to meet its demand. The most common cause of cardiac ischemia is

coronary artery disease (CAD). CAD usually develops over a period of many years without causing symptoms. The internal wall of an artery can become injured by years of cigarette smoking or high BP. Once the wall is damaged, it becomes irregular in shape and more prone to collect plaque (fatty deposits such as cholesterol). Platelets also gather along the arterial wall and clog the artery, creating a lesion in the same manner in which rust can clog a pipe. The artery gradually narrows, allowing a smaller volume of blood to pass through it. This disease process is called *atherosclerosis.*

If a coronary artery is partially or completely blocked, the part of the heart supplied by that artery may not receive sufficient oxygen to meet its needs. Persons with partial blockage of a coronary artery may be free of symptoms at rest but have angina, a type of chest pain, with eating, exercise, exertion, or exposure to cold. Angina varies from individual to individual and has been described as squeezing, tightness, fullness, pressure, or a sharp pain in the chest. The pain may also radiate to other parts of the body, usually the arm, back, neck, or jaw. Angina has also been confused with indigestion. Rest or medication (or both) will frequently relieve angina. Usually, no permanent heart damage will result. Angina is a warning sign that should not be ignored. It is a sign that CAD is present— that the individual may be a candidate for a heart attack. Chest pain that is not relieved by rest or nitroglycerin indicates a **myocardial infarction** (MI), or heart attack. The patient who has this type of pain should be evaluated promptly by a physician. In the case of Franklin, his substernal chest pain was a warning sign that one or more of his coronary arteries were blocked. The blood flow to the heart muscle was interrupted, and, starved of the necessary oxygen, Franklin's heart began to die.

MI is significant because part of the heart muscle dies as a result of lack of oxygen. If a substantial section of the heart is damaged, it will stop pumping (cardiac arrest). Activity restrictions are prescribed for the first 6 weeks after a heart attack because newly damaged heart muscle, like any injured body tissue, is easily reinjured. During the heart attack, metabolic waste products accumulate in the damaged myocardium, making it irritable and prone to electrical irregularities such as premature ventricular contractions (PVCs). A delicate balance of rest and activity must be maintained to allow the damaged area of myocardium to heal while also maintaining the strength of the healthy part of the heart. OT is frequently recommended to guide the patient toward a safe level of activity, or participation in occupation, during this acute period of recovery. Franklin requires guidance from the therapist in recognizing signs of fatigue, determining when rest breaks are needed, and choosing activities that can be performed safely.

At approximately 6 weeks after MI, scar tissue forms and the risk of extending the MI decreases. The scarred part of the heart muscle is not elastic and does not contract with each heartbeat. Therefore, the heart does not pump as well. A graded exercise program will help strengthen the healthy part of the myocardium and improve cardiac output.

Congestive heart failure (CHF) occurs when the heart is unable to pump effectively, causing fluid to back up into the lungs or the body. Fluid overload is serious because it puts a greater workload on the heart as the heart strains while attempting to clear the excess fluid. This may result in further congestion. Heart size is often enlarged in persons with CHF because the heart muscle thickens (hypertrophy) from working so hard. Diuretics can be prescribed for persons with CHF to promote fluid loss through the urinary system. Low-sodium diets and fluid restrictions reduce the overall amount of fluid in the body. CHF can usually be controlled with diet, medications, and rest.

Once an acute exacerbation of CHF is controlled, a gradual resumption of activity will promote improved function. If activity is resumed too quickly, another acute episode may follow. Patients who have difficulty resuming their former level of activity may self-limit their recovery. OT can guide clients with acute CHF toward an optimal level of function through graded self-care tasks. Some individuals ultimately eliminate their tendency to develop CHF altogether, whereas others develop severe heart failure.

Table 44-1 delineates the four functional classifications of heart disease. OT can be of great benefit to persons with stage 3 and 4 heart disease.

TABLE **44-1** **A Comparison of Three Methods of Assessing Cardiovascular Disability**

Class	New York Association Functional Classification	Canadian Cardiovascular Society Functional Classification	Specific Activity Scale
I	This category includes patients with cardiac disease but without resulting limitations of physical activity. Ordinary physical activity does not cause undue fatigue, palpitations, dyspnea, or anginal pain.	Ordinary physical activity, such as walking and climbing stairs, does not cause angina. Angina occurs with strenuous, rapid, or prolonged exertion during work or recreation.	Patient can perform to completion any activity requiring ≤ 7 METs (e.g., can carry objects that weigh 80 lb; do outdoor work [shovel snow, spade soil]; do recreational activities [skiing, basketball, squash, handball, job/walk 5 mph]).
II	This category includes patients with cardiac disease resulting in slight limitations of physical activity. They are comfortable at rest. Less than ordinary physical activity causes fatigue, palpitations, dyspnea, or anginal pain.	Ordinary activity is somewhat limited. This includes walking or climbing stairs rapidly; walking uphill; and walking or climbing stairs after meals, in cold, in wind, when under emotional stress, or only during the few hours after waking. This also includes walking more than two blocks on a level surface and climbing more than one flight of stairs at a normal pace and in normal conditions.	Patient can perform to completion any activity requiring ≤ 5 METs (e.g., have sexual intercourse without stopping, garden, rake, weed, roller skate, dance the foxtrot, walk at 4 mph on level ground) but cannot and does not perform to completion activities requiring ≥ 7 METs.
III	This category includes patients with cardiac disease resulting in marked limitation in physical activity. They are comfortable at rest. Less than ordinary physical activity causes fatigue, palpitation, dyspnea, or anginal pain.	Ordinary physical activity is significantly limited. This includes walking one to two blocks on a level surface and climbing more than one flight in normal conditions.	Patient can perform to completion any activity requiring ≤ 2 METs (e.g., shower without stopping, strip and make bed, clean windows, walk 2.5 miles, bowl, play golf, dress without stopping) but cannot and does not perform to completion activities requiring ≥ 5 METs.
IV	This category includes patients with cardiac disease resulting in inability to carry on any physical activity without discomfort. Symptoms of cardiac insufficiency or of the anginal syndrome may be present even at rest. If any physical activity is undertaken, discomfort is increased.	Patient is unable to carry on any physical activity without discomfort; anginal syndrome may be present at rest.	Patient cannot perform to completion any activity requiring ≥ 2 METs and cannot carry out activities listed above (Specific Activity Scale, Class III).

From Goldman L, Hashimoto B, Cook EF, et al: Comparative reproducibility and validity of systems for assessing cardiovascular functional class: advantages of a new specific activity scale, *Circulation* 64:1227, 1981.

VALVULAR DISEASE

The heart valves, which are responsible for controlling the direction and flow of the blood through the heart, may become damaged through disease or infection. Two complications result from valvular disease: volume overload and pressure overload. A fibrous mitral valve will fail to close properly. Blood will be regurgitated back to the atria when the left ventricle contracts. Volume overload results when fluid accumulates in the lungs, causing shortness of breath. Volume overload increases the potential for atrial fibrillation, which causes irregular and ineffective contractions in both atria. Blood flow through the heart slows, and blood clots (emboli) may develop in the ventricles. Many cerebrovascular accidents are caused when emboli ejected from the left ventricle enter the circulatory system of the brain.

If the aortic valve fails to close properly (aortic insufficiency), CHF or ischemia may result. Another disorder of the aortic valve is aortic stenosis (narrowing), which results in pressure overload. The left ventricle, which must work harder to open the sticky valve, becomes enlarged, and cardiac output decreases. Ventricular arrhythmia (irregular rhythm of heartbeats), cerebral insufficiency, confusion, syncope (fainting), and even sudden death may result from aortic stenosis. Surgery to repair or replace the damaged valves is frequently recommended.

CARDIAC RISK FACTORS

There have been many scientific studies to determine the causes of heart disease. The most famous of these studies, the Framingham study,[9] helped identify many factors that put an individual at risk for atherosclerosis. Risk factors are divided into three major categories: those that cannot be changed (heredity, male gender, and age); those that can be changed (high blood pressure, cigarette smoking, cholesterol levels, and an inactive lifestyle); and contributing factors (diabetes, stress, and obesity). The more risk factors that an individual has, the greater is the individual's risk of CAD. All team members—the physician, nurse, physical therapist, case manager, social worker, nutritionist, and occupational therapist—should support the patient's attempts to reduce risk factors.

MEDICAL MANAGEMENT

Patients who have suffered a heart attack are initially managed in a coronary care unit, where they are closely observed for complications. Approximately 90% of persons who have had an MI will have arrhythmia.[4] Heart failure, the development of blood clots (thrombosis and emboli), aneurysms, ruptures of part of the heart muscle, inflammation of the sac around the heart (pericarditis), and even death are potential outcomes of an MI. Close medical management is imperative.

Generally, patients are managed for 2 to 3 days after MI in an intensive care unit. Once their condition is stabilized, they graduate to a monitored hospital bed. Patients typically stay 4 to 6 days in the hospital after an acute MI. Vital signs are closely monitored while activity is gradually increased. OT personnel may be called upon to monitor the patient's response to activity and educate the patient about the disease process, risk factors, and lifestyle modification.

Should the patient not respond well to increased activity, surgical intervention may be necessary. Various surgical procedures can correct circulatory problems associated with CAD. Balloon angioplasty, also called *percutaneous transluminal coronary angioplasty (PTCA)*, and *coronary artery bypass graft (CABG)* are most common. During a PTCA, a wire mesh tube, called a *stent*, may be implanted into the coronary artery to keep the artery open.[8]

In a PTCA, a catheter is inserted into the femoral artery and guided through the circulatory system into the coronary arteries. Radioactive dye is injected into the arteries, and the site of the lesion is pinpointed. A balloon is then inflated at the site of the lesion to push plaque against the arterial wall. When the balloon is deflated and the catheter removed, improved circulation to the myocardium usually results. Ensuring that the patient rests in bed for 8 hours after the PTCA helps prevent hemorrhage from the femoral artery.

If a lesion is too diffuse or if an artery reoccludes after a PTCA, a CABG may be performed. The diseased section of the coronary arteries is bypassed with healthy blood vessels (taken from other parts of the body), thus improving coronary circulation. In performing a CABG, the surgeon usually opens the chest wall by cracking the sternum and spreading the ribs to gain access to the heart. Post-surgical precautions to prevent trauma to the new graft sites, incisions, and sternum generally last about 8 weeks after surgery and include the following: avoiding Valsalva maneuvers (e.g., straining during a bowel movement); avoiding rapid movement of the upper body; adhering to a 10-pound lifting restriction; wearing compressive hose; refraining from driving (which creates problems because of upper body torque); and traveling in a seat without an airbag when riding in a car.

When the heart's pumping ability has become too compromised by CHF or cardiomyopathy, a heart transplant or heart-lung transplant may be considered. After the healthy tissue of a recently deceased person is harvested, the patient's diseased organ (or organs) are removed, and the harvested tissue is transplanted into the patient's body. Transplant patients are typically maintained on special medication to decrease the risk of organ rejection. If the surgery is successful, the patient can generally be rehabilitated to a level of function significantly higher than in the months before surgery.

Cardiac Medications

Knowledge of the purpose and side effects of cardiac medication promotes understanding of the patient's response to activity. Table 44-2 lists common cardiac medications.

TABLE 44-2 **Common Cardiac Medications**

Category	Common Names	Purpose and Uses	Side Effects
Diuretics	Lasix (furosemide) Dyazide HCTZ	Lowers BP; decreases edema	Orthostatic HTN; dehydration; muscle spasms
Vasodilators	Hydralazine Captopril	Lowers BP; controls CHF	Tachycardia; palpitations; orthostatic HTN
Cardiac glycosides	Digoxin Lanoxin	Lowers heart rate; controls ventricular heart rate	Anorexia; nausea; arrhythmia; heart block
Anticoagulants	Coumadin (warfarin) Heparin Aspirin Persantine	Prevents blood clots	Hemorrhage; nausea and vomiting; abdominal cramps
Antiarrhythmics	Procainamide Amiodarone Sotalol	Corrects irregular heartbeat; slow and overactive heart	Can aggravate ventricular arrhythmias; bradycardia
Beta blockers	Propranolol (Inderal); atenolol (Tenormin); other drugs ending in "-olol"	Lowers blood pressure; manages angina, controls CHF	Impotence; weakness; heart failure; bradycardia
Calcium channel blockers	Diltiazem (Cardizem); verapamil (Isoptin, Calan)	To control high blood pressure; angina; dilates blood vessels and may slow heart rate	Orthostatic HTN; sinus pause; AV block; heart failure
Nitrates	NTG sublingual Nitropaste Isordil	Relaxes blood vessels; improves blood and oxygen supply to the heart; decreases cardiac workload	Orthostatic HTN; headache
Cholesterol-lowering drugs	Atorvastatin (Lipitor); simvastatin (Zocor)	Reduces low density lipoprotein	Liver failure; rhabdomyolysis

HCTZ, Hydrochlorothiazide; *NTG,* nitroglycerin; *BP,* blood pressure; *CHF,* congestive heart failure; *LDL,* low-density lipoprotein; *HTN,* hypotension; *AV,* atrioventricular.

Psychosocial Considerations

Persons who have experienced MI pass through a number of phases of adjustment to disability. Fear and anxiety develop initially, as patients confront their mortality. Sedatives may be prescribed to reduce stress and allow rest so that the cardiovascular system can begin to heal. Once stabilized, patients must confront the reality of their physical limitations. Education and supportive communication will greatly reduce anxiety.[13]

As patients begin to resume more normal activities, such as self-care and walking around the ward, feelings of helplessness may begin to subside. Patients feel more secure when familiar coping mechanisms allow them to respond to the stress, but some former coping mechanisms (e.g., smoking, drinking, consuming fatty foods) are harmful and should be discouraged and replaced by newly learned coping strategies, often those taught by the occupational therapist and other members of the intervention team. Typically, the nutritionist directs the patient toward healthy food choices, the physical therapist provides guidance toward exercise, and the nurse oversees medication management.

Denial is common among patients with cardiac disease. Patients in denial must be closely monitored during the acute phase of recovery. Persons in denial may ignore all precautions and could stress and further damage their cardiovascular systems.

Depression is common 3 to 6 days after MI and may last many months.[3] Forced inactivity during the recovery phase can compromise coping for a person who has previously dealt with stress by exercising until exhaustion. The patient's family must be included in the education so that their misconceptions and anxieties do not compound the patient's fears. In Franklin's case, his fear of dying in the facility, as did his father before him, could influence him to resist any activity.

Cardiac Rehabilitation

During the first 1 to 3 days after MI, stabilization of the patient's medical condition is usually attained. This acute phase is followed by a period of early mobilization. Phase one of treatment, inpatient cardiac rehabilitation, includes monitored low-level physical activity, including self-care; reinforcement of cardiac and post-surgical precautions; instruction in energy conservation and graded activity; and establishment of guidelines for appropriate activity levels at discharge. Through monitored activity, the ill effects of prolonged inactivity can be averted while medical problems, poor responses to medications, and atypical chest pain can be addressed.

Phase two of treatment, outpatient cardiac rehabilitation, usually begins at discharge. During this phase, exercise can be advanced while the patient is closely monitored on an outpatient basis. Community-based exercise programs follow in phase three. Some individuals require treatment in their place of residence because they are not strong enough to tolerate outpatient therapy.

Healthcare costs can be significantly reduced, and positive health effects can result from comprehensive cardiac rehabilitation.[20] Additional research indicates reduced mortality among selected patients who have had cardiac rehabilitation after acute MI.[25] Cardiac rehabilitation has also been found to benefit patients with left ventricular dysfunction by improving physical work capacity.[16] Patients who acquire skills in relaxation and breathing control after MI have been found to require fewer hospitalizations and less expensive medical management even 5 years after the MI.[29]

Early and accurate identification of the signs and symptoms of cardiac distress and modification of treatment to remedy distress are imperative to the well-being of the patient. If the clinician observes any of the signs of cardiac distress (Table 44-3) during treatment, the proper response is to stop the activity, allow the patient to rest, seek emergency medical help if the symptoms do not resolve, report the symptoms to the team, and modify future activity to decrease the workload on the heart.

Box 44-1, the Borg Rate of Perceived Exertion Scale, is a tool used to measure the perceived exertion. The patient is shown the scale before an activity and instructed that a rating of "6" means no exertion at all and a "19" indicates extremely strenuous activity, equal to the most strenuous activity the patient has ever performed. After the activity has been completed, the patient is asked to appraise his or her feelings of exertion as accurately as possible and give a rating to the activity.

Monitoring Response to Activity

When the patient's response to an activity is being assessed, symptoms provide one indication that the patient is or is not tolerating the activity. HR, BP, rate pressure product (RPP), and ECG readings are other measures that may be used to evaluate the cardiovascular system's response to work.

Heart rate

HR, the number of beats per minute, can be monitored by feeling the patient's pulse at the radial, brachial, or carotid sites. The radial pulse is located on the volar surface of the wrist, just lateral to the head of the radius. The brachial pulse is found in the antecubital fossa, slightly medial to the midline of the forearm. The carotid pulse, located on the neck

TABLE 44-3 Signs and Symptoms of Cardiac Distress

Sign/Symptom	What to Look For
Angina	Look for chest pain that may be described as squeezing, tightness, aching, burning, or choking. Pain is generally substernal and may radiate to the arms, jaw, neck, or back. More intense or longer-lasting pain forewarns of greater ischemia.
Dyspnea	Look for shortness of breath with activity or at rest. Note the activity that brought on the dyspnea and the amount of time that it takes to resolve. Dyspnea at rest, and with resting respiratory rate over 30 breaths per minute, is a sign of acute CHF. The patient may require emergency medical help.
Orthopnea	Look for dyspnea brought on by lying supine. Count the number of pillows that the patient needs to breathe comfortably during sleep (1, 2, 3, or 4 pillows needed to relieve orthopnea).
Nausea/emesis	Look for vomiting or signs that the patient feels sick to the stomach.
Diaphoresis	Look for a cold, clammy sweat.
Fatigue	Look for a generalized feeling of exhaustion. The Borg rate of perceived exertion (RPE) scale is a tool used to grade fatigue (see Box 44-1).
Cerebral signs	Ataxia, dizziness, confusion, and fainting (syncope) are all signs that the brain is not getting enough oxygen.
Orthostatic	Look for a drop in systolic blood pressure hypotension of greater than 10 mm Hg with change of position from supine to sitting or sitting to standing.

lateral to the Adam's apple, should be palpated gently; if overstimulated, it can cause the HR to drop below 60 beats per minute (bradycardia). To determine the HR, the clinician applies the second and third fingers (flat, not with the tips) to the pulse site. If the pulse is even (regular), the clinician counts the number of beats in 10 seconds and multiplies the finding by 6. The thumb should never be used to take a pulse because it has its own pulse.

All clinicians who assess HR, as well as patients, should be able to note the evenness (regularity) of the heartbeat. HR can be regular or irregular. An irregular heartbeat may be described as regularly irregular, meaning there is a consistent irregular pattern (e.g., every third beat is premature). It may be described as irregularly irregular, meaning that there is no pattern to premature or skipped beats. HR irregularities include skipped beats, delayed beats, premature beats, and beats originating from outside the normal conduction pathway

During the work we want you to rate your perception of exertion (i.e., how heavy and strenuous the exercise feels to you and how tired you are). The perception of exertion is mainly felt as strain and fatigue in your muscles and as breathlessness, or aches in the chest. All work requires some effort, even if this is only minimal. This is true also if you only move a little (e.g., walking slowly).

Use this scale from 6 to 20, with **6** meaning "No exertion at all" and **20** meaning "maximal exertion."

6 "No exertion at all," means that you don't feel any exertion whatsoever (e.g., no muscle fatigue, no breathlessness, or difficulties breathing).

9 "Very light" exertion, such as taking a shorter walk at your own pace.

13 A "Somewhat hard" work, but it still feels OK to continue.

15 It is "hard" and tiring, but continuing isn't terribly difficult.

17 "Very hard." This is very strenuous work. You can still go on, but you really have to push yourself and you are very tired.

19 An "extremely" strenuous level. For most people this is the most strenuous work they have ever experienced.

Try to appraise your feeling of exertion and fatigue as spontaneously and as honestly as possible, without thinking about what the actual physical load is. Try not to underestimate and not to overestimate your exertion. It's your own feeling of effort and exertion that is important, not how this compares with other people's. Look at the scale and the expressions and then give a number. Use any number you like on the scale, not just one of those with an explanation behind it.

---

in the heart. Although an irregular HR is not normal, many individuals function quite well with an irregular rate. Clinicians should note the client's normal rate pattern as well as any variations. A sudden change in HR from regular to irregular should be reported to the physician. An ECG or other diagnostic test may be ordered on the basis of such findings. When the HR is irregular, the number of beats should be counted for a full minute. Patients can be taught to take their own pulse and monitor the response of HR to activity. As a general rule, HR should rise in response to activity.

Blood pressure

BP is the pressure that the blood exerts against the walls of any vessel as the heart beats. It is highest in the left ventricle during systole and decreases in the arterial system with distance from the heart.[30] A stethoscope and BP cuff (sphygmomanometer) are used to indirectly determine BP. The BP cuff is placed snugly (but not tightly) around the patient's upper arm just above the elbow, with the bladder of the cuff centered above the brachial artery. The examiner inflates the cuff while palpating the brachial artery to 20 mm Hg above the point at which the brachial pulse is last felt. With the earpieces of the stethoscope angled forward in the examiner's ears, the dome of the stethoscope is placed over the patient's brachial artery. Supporting the patient's arm in extension with the pulse point of the brachial artery and the gauge of the stethoscope at the patient's heart level, the examiner deflates the cuff at a rate of approximately 2 mm Hg per second. Listening is imperative when taking BP. The first two sounds heard correspond to the systolic BP. The examiner continues to listen until the last pulse is heard and the diastolic BP is attained.

Physicians usually indicate treatment parameters for the HR and BP of patients in medical facilities. Parameters are frequently written in abbreviations, such as "Call HO if SBP > 150 < 90; DBP > 90 < 60; HR > 120 < 60." (In other words, "Call the house office or physician on call if systolic BP is greater than 150 or less than 90; if diastolic BP is greater than 90 or less than 60; and if HR is greater than 120 or less than 60.").

HR and BP will fluctuate in response to activity; cardiac output is affected by both HR and BP. **Rate pressure product** (RPP) measurement can give a more accurate indication of how well the heart is pumping. RPP is the product of HR and systolic BP ($RPP = HR \times SBP$). It is usually a five-digit number but is reported in three digits by dropping the last two digits (for example, HR 100 × SBP 120 = 12,000 = RPP 120). During any activity, RPP should rise at peak and return to baseline in recovery (after 5 to 10 minutes of rest).

The correct reading and interpretation of ECG is a skill that requires hours of learning and practice for proficiency. Electrocardiography is not available in most nonacute settings. The reader is referred to Dubin's *Rapid Interpretation of EKG*,[10] which is an excellent resource for persons unfamiliar with the subject.

There are many similarities in the evaluation and treatment of persons with cardiac disease and those with pulmonary dysfunction. A review of the pulmonary system and its disease processes follows.

PULMONARY SYSTEM

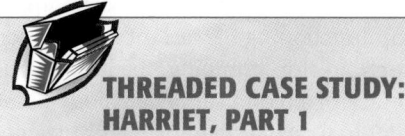

THREADED CASE STUDY: HARRIET, PART 1

Harriet is a 64-year-old widow and mother of an adult daughter. She retired 3 years ago from her housekeeping job because of fatigue and shortness of breath. She was diagnosed with chronic obstructive pulmonary disease (COPD) at that time. She has been smoking cigarettes since the age of 20 and currently smokes one

Continued

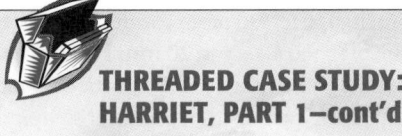

THREADED CASE STUDY: HARRIET, PART 1–cont'd

pack per day. She shares a small one-bedroom apartment with her terrier, Sir Filo. There is a first-floor laundry room in her building. Harriet's daughter lives three blocks away and checks on her mother daily. Harriet's baseline level of function 4 weeks ago consisted of walking the dog around the block slowly, fixing meals, doing laundry, and performing activities of daily living (ADLs) independently. She also enjoys playing bingo on Tuesday nights at her local church and cards with her widowers-and-widows group. Her daughter assists her with grocery shopping and cleaning.

Harriet was released from the acute care hospital 3 days ago, her condition having been stabilized after an acute exacerbationof COPD. Since her recent discharge, her daughter empties Harriet's bedside commode, shops for groceries, and fixes dinner for Harriet and Sir Filo. Results of the occupational therapy evaluation indicated that Harriet became short of breath when combing her hair. She was unable to pace activity, to coordinate pursed-lip breathing with activity, or to assume dyspnea control postures when needed. She was receiving 2 liters of oxygen by nasal cannula at all times. Harriet wants to be able to feed Sir Filo herself, stating that dogs become attached to people who feed them. She does not want her daughter to empty her dirty commode, and she wants to be able to prepare dinner for herself. She does not want to be a burden to her daughter but rather to enjoy visiting with her.

Critical Thinking Questions

1. What goals may Harriet find relevant in her therapy?
2. What safety concerns might arise?
3. Do Harriet's goals appear realistic given her baseline level of function?

ANATOMY AND PHYSIOLOGY OF RESPIRATION[4,22]

While the heart provides oxygen-rich blood to the body and transports carbon dioxide and other waste products to the lungs, the respiratory system exchanges oxygen for carbon dioxide. The cardiac and pulmonary systems are interdependent. If no oxygen were delivered to the bloodstream, the heart would soon stop functioning for lack of oxygen; conversely, if the heart were to stop pumping, the lungs would cease functioning for lack of a blood supply. All body tissues depend on the cardiopulmonary system for their nutrients.

The respiratory system supplies oxygen to the blood and removes waste products, primarily carbon dioxide, from the blood. Air enters the body via the nose and mouth and travels through the nasopharynx to the larynx or voice box. From there, the air continues downward into the lungs by way of the trachea or windpipe. The trachea consists of a ribbed cartilage approximately 10 cm long. The cartilage is lined with a mucous layer and cilia to help to filter out dust. When the trachea or pharynx becomes blocked, a small incision may be made into the trachea to allow air to pass freely into the lungs. This procedure is called a *tracheotomy*.

Two main bronchi branch off from the trachea, carrying air into the left and right lungs. The bronchi continue to branch off into smaller tubes, called *bronchioles*. Bronchioles are segmented into smaller passages called the *alveolar ducts*. Each alveolar duct is divided and leads into three or more alveolar sacs. The entire respiratory passageway from bronchi to alveolar ducts is often referred to as "the pulmonary tree" because its structure is much like that of an upside-down tree, with the alveolar sacs representing the leaves.

Each alveolar sac contains more than 10 alveoli. A very fine, semipermeable membrane separates the alveolus from the capillary network. Across this membrane, oxygen is transported and exchanged for carbon dioxide. Carbon dioxide is exhaled into the air after traveling upward through the "pulmonary tree" (Figure 44-4).

The musculature of the thorax is responsible for inspiration and expiration. Inspiration, the muscle power for breathing air into the lungs, is provided primarily by the diaphragm. Originating from the sternum, ribs, lumbar vertebrae, and lumbocostal arches, the diaphragm forms the inferior border of the thorax. The muscle fibers of the diaphragm insert into a central tendon. Innervated by the left and right phrenic nerves, the diaphragm contracts and domes downward when it is stimulated. This downward doming of the diaphragm enlarges the volume of the thorax and causes a drop in pressure in the lungs relative to the air in the environment. Air then enters the lungs to equalize inside and outside pressures. Accessory muscles, the intercostals and scalenes, are also active during inspiration. The intercostals maintain the alignment of the ribs, and the scalene helps elevate the rib cage.

At rest, expiration is primarily a passive relaxation of the inspiratory musculature. The lungs help to draw the thorax inward as the inspiratory muscles relax. Forced expiration requires active contraction of the abdominal muscles to compress the viscera and squeeze the diaphragm upward in the thorax. Expiration can be further forced by flexing the torso forward and pressing with the arms on the chest or abdomen. As the volume of the thorax decreases, air is forced out of the lungs.

INNERVATION OF THE RESPIRATORY SYSTEM

Breathing is mostly involuntary. A person does not have to think to take a breath. The autonomic nervous system has control over breathing. With anxiety and increased activity, the sympathetic nervous system will automatically increase the depth and rate of inspiration.

Inspiration and expiration have a volitional component. This volitional control allows us to control our breathing as we swim and to play the harmonica. Additionally, receptors within and outside the lungs can, when stimulated, cause changes in the depth and rate of breathing. Although the pons, medulla, and other parts of the brain provide the central

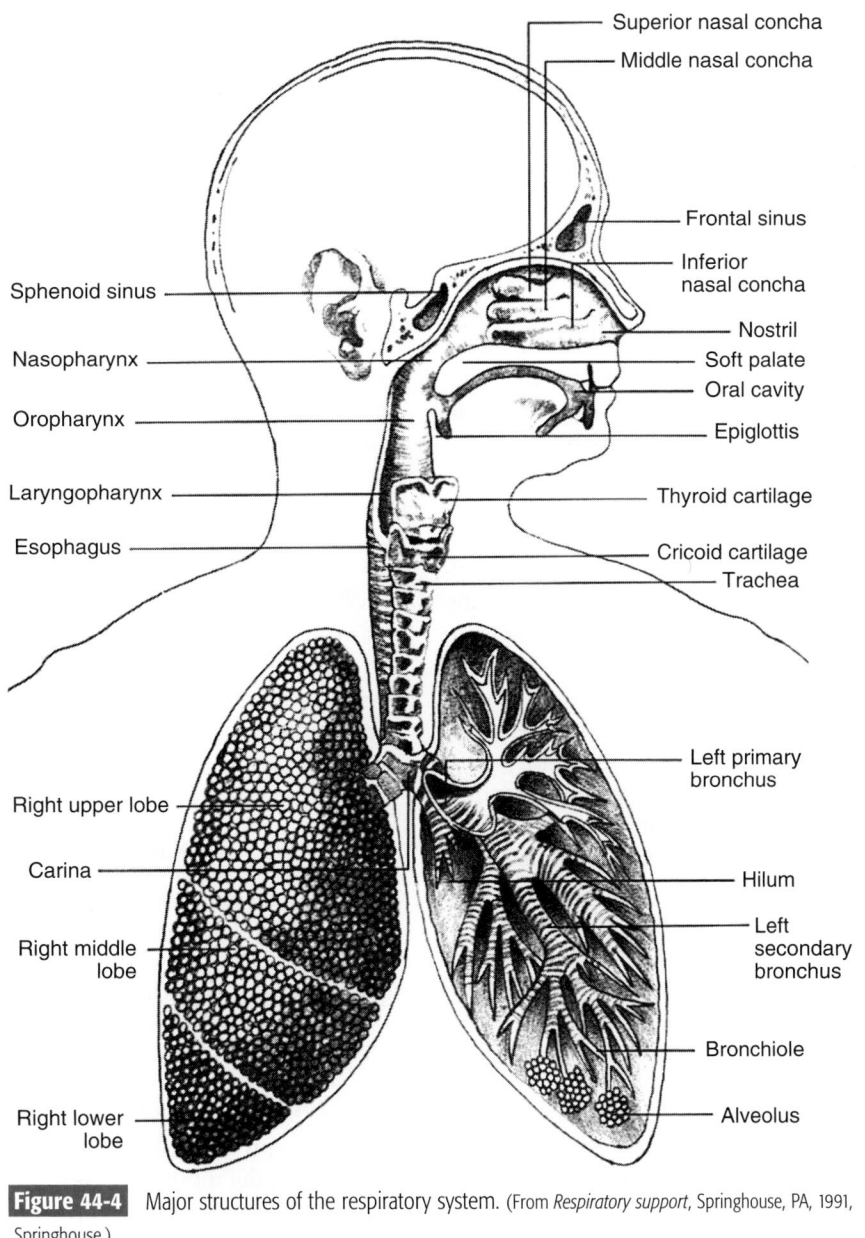

Figure 44-4   Major structures of the respiratory system. (From *Respiratory support*, Springhouse, PA, 1991, Springhouse.)

control for breathing, they adjust their response to input from receptors in the lungs, the aorta, and the carotid artery.

CHRONIC LUNG DISEASE[2,4]

Common chronic disorders of the lungs for which pulmonary rehabilitation is typically prescribed include **chronic obstructive pulmonary disease** (COPD) and asthma.[4] COPD is characterized by "damage to the alveolar wall and inflammation of the conducting airways"[2] and includes emphysema, peripheral airway disease, and chronic bronchitis. COPD has been diagnosed in more than 15 million Americans, including Harriet.

Emphysema is a condition in which the alveoli become enlarged or ruptured, usually because of a restriction during expiration or a decrease in the elasticity of the lungs.[30] Chronic

emphysema is most prevalent in men between the ages of 45 and 65 who have a history of chronic bronchitis; smoking; working in areas with high levels of air pollution; or exposure to cold, damp environments. Persons with chronic bronchitis experience shortness of breath (dyspnea) on exertion, and as the disease progresses, dyspnea occurs at rest.

Inflammation, fibrosis (thickening of the connective tissue), and narrowing of the terminal airways of the lungs are the physiological changes that occur with peripheral airway disease. Smoking and other environmental pollutants irritate the airways, leading to the development of abnormal terminal airways. Coughing and spitting up mucus from the lungs are common clinical manifestations of this disorder. The disease process may never progress beyond this initial phase, or it may evolve into emphysema and full-fledged COPD.

Chronic bronchitis is diagnosed after a 2-year period of repeated episodes, greater than 3 months in length, of mucus-producing cough of unknown origin. A direct relationship exists between the development of chronic bronchitis and a history of cigarette smoking. Clinical manifestations of the disease increase as the package-year history increases. **Pack-year history** is calculated by multiplying the number of packs of cigarettes consumed per day by the number of years of smoking. Harriet began smoking at the age of 20. She is 64 years old now. Therefore, her pack-year history is 64 − 20 = 44 × 1 pack/year = 44 package years. As with other forms of COPD, the onset of physical disability is typically gradual, with dyspnea on exertion representing the initial phases of disability and devolving to shortness of breath at rest.

Asthma is characterized by irritability of the bronchotracheal tree and is typically episodic in its onset. Persons suffering from asthma experience wheezing and shortness of breath that may resolve spontaneously or may necessitate the use of medication for calming the airway. Persons with asthma may be free of symptoms for periods of time between the episodes of wheezing and dyspnea. Some individuals appear to have a genetic predisposition to asthma. Allergenic causes of asthma may include pollens and respiratory irritants such as perfume, dust, pollen, and cleaning agents. Bronchospasms occurring with exposure to cold air or induced by exercise are sometimes the first clinical manifestations of asthma. Irritation of the airway leads to a narrowing of air passages and interferes with ventilation of the alveolar sacs. If the obstruction of the airway is significant enough, a reduction in the oxygen levels in the bloodstream will result in hypoxemia.[12] If left untreated, a severe asthmatic episode may result in death.

PULMONARY RISK FACTORS

Cigarette smoking is the primary cause of COPD, and smoking cessation will slow the progression of disability in persons with COPD.[23] Because cigarette smoke is a pulmonary irritant, it may also be a causative agent in asthmatic episodes. Other environmental irritants, such as air pollution and chemical exposure, are contributory risk factors in the development of COPD and asthma.

MEDICAL MANAGEMENT

COPD is a progressive, chronic disease. The onset of the disease is insidious. When patients initially seek medical attention, they are frequently seen in a physician's clinic rather than at a medical center. Besides evaluating the patient's medical history and symptoms and performing a physical examination, the physician will assess the patient's history of smoking and occupational exposure to respiratory irritants. Blood work and an X-ray examination will be performed to further assess the patient's clinical status. Medications prescribed for persons with pulmonary disease include antiinflammatory agents (e.g., steroids and cromolyn sodium), bronchodilators (e.g., albuterol and theophylline) that help open the airway, and expectorants (e.g., iodides and guaifenesin) to help loosen and clear mucus. Oxygen therapy may also be prescribed at a specific flow rate. Occasionally, persons receiving oxygen therapy may be tempted to increase the liter-per-minute flow, erroneously thinking that more is better. This can result in carbon dioxide retention and lead to failure of the right side of the heart.

Persons with acute respiratory distress may initially be managed with a ventilator before being weaned to oxygen. Ventilators provide a mechanical assist to the process of inspiration and do not increase the number of healthy alveolar sacs. Ventilators will not slow the end-stage disease process of COPD. Mechanical ventilation is frequently prescribed for persons with an acute exacerbation of the disease process caused by pneumonia, influenza, or CHF.

When a patient's endurance decreases sufficiently enough to impair performance of ADLs, the physician may refer the patient to OT. Regrettably, the client is not likely to be seen by an occupational therapist or receive an assessment of occupational lifestyle as the first line of defense.

 OT PRACTICE NOTE

Frequently, the occupational therapist's role in treating clients with COPD involves salvage rather than the prevention of the disease process. Earlier intervention by an occupational therapist is critical to disease prevention.

Signs and Symptoms of Respiratory Distress

Dyspnea is probably the most obvious sign of a breathing difficulty. In the most severe form of dyspnea, the patient is short of breath even at rest. Clients with this level of dyspnea are unable to utter a short phrase without gasping for air. When reporting that a client has dyspnea, the practitioner should note the precipitating factors and associated circumstances; for example, "Harriet becomes short of breath when washing her face while seated in front of the sink."

Other signs that the body is not getting enough oxygen include extreme fatigue, a nonproductive cough, confusion, impaired judgment, and cyanosis (bluish skin color caused by insufficient oxygen in the blood).

Psychosocial Considerations

Because COPD is a progressive and debilitating physical illness, it is not surprising that the psychosocial effects of the disease are considerable. Depression and anxiety are common; persons with anxiety and depression are more inclined to experience relapses after initial emergency department visits,[7] and 96% of patients with COPD have reported having disabling anxiety.[1] Other patients with COPD complain of faintness or difficulty concentrating.[11] Training in progressive muscle relaxation can be a successful tool for controlling dyspnea and anxiety and for lowering HR.[26]

Most cardiac and respiratory disease processes are preventable. Individuals with these diseases may lack basic skills in coping and setting limits with themselves or with others. The therapist's role includes encouraging the patient to engage in activities that will develop his or her skills and in promoting resumption of occupations, which bring value, meaning, and participation back into the patient's life. With these skills, the patient begins to see himself or herself as a person actively making choices to get better. By working with Harriet on ways to engage with her dog when she does not have the endurance to take a walk, the occupational therapist not only teaches energy conservation but also conveys this information in a meaningful manner to the patient.

Most persons with end-stage COPD realize that they will die as a result of their disease. Fear of death from suffocation is misplaced. Persons with such concerns should be referred to their physician, who can reassure them that individuals with CO_2 retention die peacefully in their sleep.[17]

Pulmonary Rehabilitation

The goal of **pulmonary rehabilitation** is to stabilize or reverse the disease process and return the patient's function and participation in activity/occupation to his or her highest capacity. A multidisciplinary rehabilitation team working with the patient can design an individualized intervention program to meet this end. Accurate diagnosis, medical management, therapy, education, and emotional support are components of a pulmonary rehabilitation program. OT personnel are frequently part of the patient's team, which is headed by the patient and also includes the physician, nurse, and patient's family and social supports. Respiratory therapists, dietitians, physical therapists, social workers, and psychologists may also be team members. Roles of team members vary slightly among facilities. Knowledge of specialized pulmonary treatment techniques is imperative for each team member when treating persons with pulmonary disease.

Intervention techniques

Dyspnea control postures

Adopting certain postures can reduce breathlessness. In a seated position, the patient bends forward slightly at the waist while supporting the upper body by leaning the forearms on the table or thighs. In a standing position, relief may be obtained by leaning forward and propping oneself on a counter or shopping cart.

Pursed-lip breathing

Pursed-lip breathing (PLB) is thought to prevent tightness in the airway by providing resistance to expiration. This technique has been shown to increase use of the diaphragm and decrease accessory muscle recruitment.[5] Persons with COPD sometimes instinctively adopt this technique, whereas others may need to be taught it. Instructions for PLB are as follows:

1. Purse the lips as if to whistle.
2. Slowly exhale through pursed lips. Some resistance should be felt.
3. Inhale deeply through the nose.
4. It should take twice as long to exhale as it does to inhale.

Diaphragmatic breathing

Another breathing pattern, which calls for increased use of the diaphragm to improve chest volume, is **diaphragmatic breathing.** Many persons learn this technique by placing a small paperback novel on the abdomen just below the xiphoid process (base of the sternum or breastbone). The novel provides a visual cue for diaphragmatic movement. The patient lies supine and is instructed to inhale slowly and make the book rise. Exhalation through pursed lips should cause the book to fall.

Relaxation

Progressive muscle relaxation in conjunction with breathing exercises can be effective in decreasing anxiety and controlling shortness of breath. One technique involves tensing muscle groups while slowly inhaling, then relaxing the muscle groups when exhaling twice as slowly through pursed lips. It is helpful to teach the patient a sequence of muscle groups to tense and relax. One common sequence involves tensing and relaxing first the face; followed by the face and the neck; then the face, neck, and shoulders; and so on, down the body to the toes. A calm, quiet, and comfortable environment is important for the novice in learning any relaxation technique. Biofeedback in conjunction with relaxation therapy promotes a more timely mastery of relaxation skills.[15]

Other treatments and considerations

Physical therapists are generally called on to instruct the patient in chest expansion exercises, a series of exercises intended to increase the flexibility of the chest. Percussion and postural drainage use gravity and gentle drumming on the patient's back to loosen secretions and help drain the secretions from the lungs. By isometrically contracting his or her arms and hands while they are placed on the patient's thorax, the therapist may transmit vibration to the patient. Vibration is performed during the expiratory phase of breathing and helps to loosen secretions. Percussion and postural drainage may be contraindicated in acutely ill patients and those who are medically unstable.

Humidity, pollution, extremes of temperature, and stagnant air have deleterious effects on persons with respiratory ailments. The therapist and patient should take these factors into consideration when planning activity.

OCCUPATIONAL THERAPY EVALUATION AND INTERVENTION: CARDIOPULMONARY DYSFUNCTION

Individuals with chronic respiratory or cardiovascular limitations are frequently limited in their ability to perform ADLs. OT intervention can promote improvements in the client's life-management skills and quality of life.

EVALUATION

Review of the Medical Record

A review of the medical record will identify the patient's medical history (diagnosis, severity, associated conditions, and secondary diagnoses), social history, test results, medications, and precautions.

Patient Interview

It is common courtesy and good medical practice to begin every encounter with a patient by introducing oneself and explaining the purpose of the evaluation or intervention. Good interviewing skills, including asking the right questions, listening to the patient's response, and observing the patient as he or she responds, are all considered integral aspects of the therapeutic use of self. Thoughtful, probing questions will help the patient and therapist identify areas of concern and lay the groundwork for establishing mutually agreeable goals. The therapist should observe the patient for signs of anxiety, shortness of breath, confusion, difficulty comprehending, fatigue, abnormal posture, reduced endurance, reduced ability to move, and stressful family dynamics. Interview questions should not only seek clarification of information that was unclear in the medical record but also clarify the patient's understanding of his or her condition and treatment.

A patient with a history of angina should be asked to describe what the angina feels like. If the patient has also had an MI, the patient should be asked if he or she can differentiate between the angina and the MI chest pain. Clarification of symptoms before treatment can prove invaluable should symptoms arise.

Asking patients to describe a typical day, to identify activities that bring on shortness of breath or angina, and to tell how their physical limitations interfere with the activities or occupations they need to do or most enjoy doing will reveal problems that are meaningful and relevant to the patient.

Clinical Evaluation

The purpose of the clinical assessment is to establish the patient's present functional ability and limitations. The content of an occupational therapist's clinical evaluation will vary from patient to patient and setting to setting. Clients with impairments of the cardiovascular system will require monitoring of HR, BP, signs and symptoms of cardiac distress, and possibly ECG readings during an assessment of tolerance to postural changes and during a functional task. Table 44-4 provides a summary of appropriate versus inappropriate responses to activity. Individuals with disorders of the respiratory system should be closely monitored for signs and symptoms of respiratory distress. If an oxygen saturation monitor is available, the patient's range of motion, strength, and sensation may be grossly assessed within the context of the ADL assessment. The patient's cognitive and psychosocial status will become apparent to the skilled clinician via interview and observation.

After completing the evaluation, the clinician has sufficient information to formulate an intervention plan. In establishing the intervention goals and objectives, the clinician verifies that the patient agrees with the intervention plans and projected outcome.

INTERVENTION

Client goals, present clinical status, recent occupational performance history, response to current activities and occupations, and prognosis all help to guide progression of intervention for persons with cardiovascular or respiratory impairment. Clients with significant cardiac or pulmonary impairment, limited recent ability to participate in occupation, inappropriate responses to activities and occupations or orthostatic change, and a poor prognosis will progress very slowly. Individuals with little impairment of the heart

TABLE 44-4 **Cardiovascular Response to Activity**

	Appropriate	Inappropriate
Heart rate (HR)	Increases with activity, to no more than 20 beats/min above resting heart rate	HR more than beats/min above resting heart rate (RHR) with activity, RHR ≥ 120, HR drops or does not rise with activity
Blood pressure (BP)	Systolic blood pressure (SBP) rises with activity	SBP ≥ 220 mm Hg; postural hypotension (≥ 10-20 mm Hg drop in SBP); decrease in SBP with activity
Signs and symptoms	Absence of adverse symptoms	Excessive shortness of breath; angina; nausea and vomiting; excessive sweating; extreme fatigue (RPE ≥ 15); cerebral symptoms

RPE, Rate of perceived exertion

or lungs, a recent history of normal occupational performance, appropriate responses to orthostatic change and activities and occupations, and a good prognosis will progress rapidly by comparison.

Progression and Energy Costs

The energy costs of an activity or occupation and the factors that influence energy costs can further guide the clinician in the safe progression of activity or participation in occupation. Oxygen consumption suggests how hard the heart and lungs are working, indicating the amount of energy needed to complete a task. Resting quietly in bed requires the lowest amount of oxygen per kilogram of body weight, roughly 3.5 ml O_2 per kg of body weight. This can also be expressed as 1 basal metabolic equivalent (MET). As activity increases, more oxygen is needed to meet the demands of the task. For instance, dressing requires 2.5 METs, or roughly twice the amount of energy that lying in bed requires (Table 44-5). Franklin had a 2.5 MET for seated bathing and dressing. Guided by an MET table, the patient's response to activity or occupation, the prognosis, and the patient's goals, the occupational therapist will be able to determine a logical intervention progression. As a general rule, once a patient tolerates an activity (e.g., seated sponge bathing) with appropriate responses, the patient may progress to the next higher MET-level activity (e.g., standing sponge bath).

The duration of sustained physical activity must be taken into account when activity guidelines are being determined. Obviously, persons who have difficulty performing a 2-MET activity must still use a commode (3.6 METs) or bedpan (4.7 METs) for their bowel management. This is possible because a person can perform at a higher-than-usual MET level for brief periods without adverse effects.

At 5 METs, sexual activity is frequently a grave concern to persons with impaired cardiovascular function and to their partners. Sexual intercourse is intermittent in its peak demands for energy. Patients are frequently able to return to sexual intercourse once they can climb up and down two flights of steps in 1 minute with appropriate cardiovascular responses.[28] Providing the patient with information about when it is safe to resume sexual activity can reduce anxiety surrounding the resumption of sexual intercourse. Anxiety may be further decreased through discussion of sexual activity guidelines with the patient and partner and identification of various forms of romantic intimacy, such as hand holding and kissing, when intercourse is not feasible. Besides instructing the patient to monitor HR and symptoms of cardiac distress before and after intercourse, the therapist should inform the patient and partner that cardiac medications might affect the patient's libido. The patient should be encouraged to inform the physician of problems related to sexual activity. In many cases, the physician can adjust the patient's medications to control symptoms (see Chapter 12 for additional appropriate clinical interventions).

Energy Conservation

When patients are taught methods to conserve their energy resources, they will be able to perform at a higher functional level without expending more energy. The principles of energy conservation and work simplification are based on knowledge of the ways in which specific factors cause various cardiovascular responses. Ogden[24] identified six variables that will increase oxygen demand: increased rate, increased resistance, increased use of large muscles, increased involvement of trunk musculature, raising one's arms, and isometric work (straining). Upper extremity activity has also been shown to require a greater cardiovascular output than lower extremity activity, and standing activity requires more energy than seated activity. Extremes of temperature, high humidity, and pollution make the heart work harder. By applying

TABLE **44-5** **Basal Metabolic Equivalent Table of Self-Care and Homemaking Tasks**

MET Level	Activities of Daily Living	Instrumental Activities of Daily Living, Work, Play, and Leisure
1-2	Eating, seated[21]; transfers, bed to chair; washing face and hands; brushing hair[21]; walking 1 mph	Hand sewing[6]; machine sewing; sweeping floors[6]; driving automatic car, drawing, knitting[27]
2-3	Seated sponge bath[27]; standing sponge bath[27]; dressing and undressing[19]; seated warm shower[27]; walk 2-3 mph; wheelchair propulsion 1.2 mph	Dusting[21]; kneading dough[6]; hand washing small items[6]; using electric vacuum[21]; preparing a meal[19]; washing dishes[27]; golf[27]
3-4	Standing shower, warm[19]; bowel movement on toilet[6]; climbing stairs at 24 ft/min[27]	Making a bed[19]; sweeping, mopping, gardening[27]
4-5	Hot shower[19]; bowel movement on bedpan[19]; sexual intercourse[27]	Changing bed linens[21]; garden, rake, weed; rollerskate[14]; swim 20 yards/min[27]
5-6	Sexual intercourse[27]; walking up stairs at 30 feet/min[27]	Biking 10 mph on level ground[27]
6-7	Walk with braces and crutches	Swim breaststroke[27]; ski, play basketball, walk 5 mph, shovel snow, spade soil[27]

this information, a skilled clinician can suggest activity modifications that will decrease the amount of energy needed for the task.

Energy conservation training should be individualized for each patient. Time management is an invaluable tool for energy conservation. Time management involves learning to plan one's activity or participation in occupation so that tasks requiring high energy expenditure are interspersed with lighter tasks and so that rest breaks are scheduled throughout the day, especially after meals. The most important part of educating the client is incorporating his or her active involvement in planning the day. Client involvement increases the likelihood of realistic goal attainment. Rather than prescribing how Harriet might sequence her ADLs, IADLs, and rest breaks throughout her typical day, the therapist might engage her in a conversation about what works or does not work well for her in her current performance patterns. The therapist would then ask probing questions, such as "Have you tried taking your shower at a different time of day?" and "Would laying your clothes out the night before help your morning go more smoothly?" Such a client-centered approach engages the patient in the process of designing realistic performance patterns that incorporate principles of energy conservation according to his or her own circumstances and values. Through this collaboration, the therapist demonstrates respect for the patient's needs and increases the likelihood that changes will be successfully implemented.

Written material may augment energy conservation instruction. However, until the patient has successfully applied energy conservation principles to activity, the therapist should expect little follow-through with energy conservation recommendations. Practice and practical application of skills are critical to changing behavior.

The specific pulmonary rehabilitation intervention techniques of PLB, diaphragmatic breathing, dyspnea control postures, and relaxation techniques are discussed earlier in this chapter. Exhaling with exertion is another breathing principle for persons with compromised cardiac or pulmonary function. Franklin might be taught to exhale when having a bowel movement rather than holding his breath and straining. Harriet might be taught to exhale when lifting or lowering her pet's water bowl. This technique is more energy efficient and helps control systolic BP responses to activity. It is important for the patient to practice these skills during treatment. Therapeutic support is often critical in learning.

Lifestyle Modification

Lifestyle modification is a key component in improving cardiovascular health. Exercise education should include the benefits of exercise; a graded program of increased activity and participation in occupation; stretching, strengthening, and aerobic activity; guidelines for monitoring HR, BP, and rate of perceived exertion; cool down; safety issues related to clothing, environmental factors, and warning signs; a plan for resuming exercise if it is skipped for a period of time; and

emergency guidelines. Although the physical therapist typically designs and oversees the exercise program, the occupational therapist can provide valuable insight into forms of exercise that might be meaningful to the patient. Modification of diet may be addressed by the dietitian but can be readily reinforced during meal preparation activities. To stop smoking, refrain from excessive alcohol consumption, and stop abusing drugs are challenging goals for clients who have developed these habits. Support groups, counseling, and medical management play key roles in successful cessation or modification of these risk factors. Occupational therapists believe that enabling the client's participation in rounds of personally meaningful and healthy occupations can also play a key role in supporting health and controlling such risk factors.

Patient and Family Education

As members of the healthcare team, occupational therapists share the responsibility for patient and family education. The team must instruct the patient and family members in cardiac or pulmonary anatomy, the disease process, symptom management, risk factors, diet, exercise, and energy conservation and must reinforce the teaching. The inclusion of family members in an education program provides support indirectly to the client, through the family unit. Such support is critical when the client depends on the assistance of a family member to accomplish everyday tasks.

SUMMARY

Healthy persons are able to meet the varying demands of their bodies for oxygen because their heart and respiratory rates adjust to meet oxygen demand. When either the cardiovascular or the pulmonary system (or both) is compromised, the ability to perform normal activities or occupations declines. This chapter is intended to guide the occupational therapist in the treatment of clients with impairment of the heart or lungs and in designing programs to maximize clients' independent performance in areas of occupation to support participation in context. The two case studies presented in this chapter and related information portray the range of problems with client factors, contextual issues, performance skills, and performance patterns that typically interfere with the client's ability to perform customary activities and occupations.

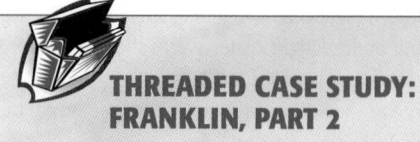

THREADED CASE STUDY: FRANKLIN, PART 2

Reflecting on the case of Franklin, who had just experienced his first myocardial infarction (MI) at the age of 48, the reader should consider the importance of really listening to the patient and following up with probative questions to develop more client-centered and, thus, more relevant goals. The first question the

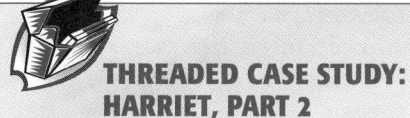

THREADED CASE STUDY:
FRANKLIN, PART 2—cont'd

reader was asked to consider while reading the chapter was "What probative questions might the occupational therapist ask to clarify what Franklin means by being 'able to do everything for himself'"? Franklin provided some clues in his occupational profile that readily yield themselves to further exploration. Besides independence in activities of daily living (ADLs), identification of potential concerns in his role as father, husband, and provider might be addressed more thoroughly by (1) asking if he assists his children with homework and sporting activities and participates in other childcare responsibilities; (2) asking if he and his wife would like to discuss safe resumption of sexual activities; and (3) clarifying the job-specific tasks that are most relevant for him to return to work.

With regard to the second question, there are numerous skills and strategies Franklin might benefit from learning and applying to his participation in daily life and meaningful occupations so that he can reduce his risk of another cardiac episode. These include the following: (1) recognizing the signs and symptoms of cardiac distress; (2) monitoring his heart rate; (3) grading his ADLs and modifying participation in other meaningful occupations according to his comfort level; (4) using relaxation techniques when stressed or anxious; (5) implementing emergency measures; and (6) modifying or redesigning his lifestyle, including stopping smoking and instituting exercise and healthy eating routines.

Finally, the reader was asked to consider what areas of occupation might the therapist choose for the next intervention session and, depending on Franklin's occupational profile, what goals might be included in his occupational therapy intervention plan. Repeating the seated sponge bathing task or combining energy conservation techniques with seated showering would be a good choice of activities for the next therapy session. Franklin's initial response to seated sponge bathing was inappropriate. By incorporating practice in safely pacing the activity and self-monitoring heart rate, his therapist will begin practical application of skills essential to safe management of his cardiac condition. Occupational therapy intervention will most likely end before Franklin returns to work. It is critical that he understand how he might apply energy conservation principles to his work in the auto shop. The occupational therapist intervenes by using education to engage Franklin in a conversation about ways that he might adapt these principles to his work. Thus, the therapist sets the groundwork for carryover of principles into that setting. Franklin is asked questions such as "Where might you place your tools to decrease the number of trips across the room?" and "How might you apply the principle of exhale on exertion when changing an oil filter?"

THREADED CASE STUDY:
HARRIET, PART 2

When considering the case of Harriet, the reader was asked what goals she might find relevant in her therapy. Harriet identified several meaningful goals during the initial occupational therapy evaluation, including feeding her dog, Mr. Filo; preparing her own dinner; and being able to empty her bedside commode herself. Another question involved the safety concerns that might arise in treating Harriet. Additional goals relevant to her safety include learning to pace her activity, coordinating her breathing with function, increasing her ability to assume dyspnea control postures when needed, and increasing her safety with oxygen. The oxygen line not only poses a potential trip hazard but also presents a fire hazard, given her meal preparation goals and smoking habit. Smoking cessation is a goal that can be explored but will only be meaningful if Harriet wants to quit. Finally, the reader was asked to determine what goals appear realistic given Harriet's baseline level of function. Given her baseline level of function, all the goals she identified appear realistic.

Review Questions

1. Describe the heart, including its size, anatomy, and functional parts.
2. Name the heart valves, and give their locations and functions.
3. Discuss the relationship between the coronary arteries and the health of the heart.
4. List and describe the symptoms of cardiac distress.
5. What are the typical psychosocial responses to a diagnosis of heart disease?
6. How is cardiac response to activity monitored? How does the therapist know that a change in activity level is warranted?
7. Describe the functional parts of the pulmonary system.
8. What is COPD, and what is its significance for occupational performance?
9. What can the OT practitioner do to help prevent or reduce the incidence of COPD?
10. Demonstrate the recommended dyspnea control postures.
11. Compare pursed-lip breathing with diaphragmatic breathing. When should one be used rather than the other?
12. Describe appropriate evaluation content and approach for patients with cardiac and pulmonary problems.
13. What is an MET, and what is the clinical value of an MET table for occupational therapists?
14. How would you teach energy conservation techniques to the following individuals, all of whom have received diagnoses of cardiac or pulmonary disease?
    - A 40-year-old female marathon runner
    - A 50-year-old homemaker and adoptive mother of eight (including three children under the age of 6)

- A 60-year-old air conditioner repairman
- A 72-year-old man who says his main pleasures are riding Thoroughbreds, drinking good Kentucky bourbon, smoking cigars, and enjoying the company of lovely women

REFERENCES

1. Agle DP, Baum GL: Psychological aspects of chronic obstructive pulmonary disease, *Med Clin North Am* 61(4):744, 1977.

2. American Thoracic Society: Definitions and classifications of chronic bronchitis, asthma, and pulmonary emphysema, *Am Rev Respir Dis* 85:762, 1962.

3. Bragg TL: Psychological response to myocardial infarction, *Nurs Forum* 14(4):383, 1975.

4. Brannon FJ, et al: *Cardiopulmonary rehabilitation: basic theory and application*, ed 3, Philadelphia, 1997, FA Davis.

5. Breslin EH: The pattern of respiratory muscle recruitment during pursed-lip breathing, *Chest* 101(1):75, 1992.

6. Colorado Heart Association: *Exercise equivalent* (pamphlet), Boston, 1970, Cardiac Reconditioning & Work Evaluation Unit, Spaulding Rehabilitation Center.

7. Dahlén I, Janson C: Anxiety and depression are related to the outcome of emergency treatment in patients with obstructive pulmonary disease, *Chest* 122:1933, 2002.

8. Dangas G, Kuepper F: Cardiology patient age, restenosis: repeat narrowing of a coronary artery: prevention and treatment, *Circulation* 105(22):2586, 2002.

9. Dawber TR: The Framingham study, the epidemiology of atherosclerotic disease, Cambridge, MA, 1980, Harvard University Press.

10. Dubin D: *Rapid interpretation of EKGs*, ed 6, Tampa, FL, 2000, Cover Publishing.

11. Dudley DL, et al: Psychosocial concomitants to rehabilitation in chronic obstructive pulmonary disease. Part 2: Psychosocial treatment, *Chest* 77(4):544, 1980.

12. Farzan S: *A concise handbook of respiratory diseases*, ed 4, Reston, VA, 1997, Reston Publishing.

13. Goldberger E: *Essentials of clinical cardiology*, Philadelphia, 1990, JB Lippincott.

14. Goldman L, et al: Comparative reproducibility and validity of systems for assessing cardiovascular functional class: advantages of a new specific activity scale, *Circulation* 64:1227, 1981.

15. Green E: Biofeedback techniques for deep relaxation, *Psychophysiology* 6(3):371, 1969.

16. Greenland P: Efficacy of supervised cardiac rehabilitation programs for coronary patients: update 1986-1990, *Cardiopulmonary Rehab* 11:190, 1991.

17. Hodgkin JE, Celli BR, Connors GL: *Pulmonary rehabilitation guidelines to success*, ed 3, Philadelphia, 2000, Lippincott Williams & Wilkins.

18. Kinney M: *Andreoli's comprehensive cardiac care*, ed 8, St Louis, 1995, Mosby.

19. Kottke FJ: Common cardiovascular problems in rehabilitation. In Krusen FH, Kottke FJ, Elwood PM, editors: *Handbook of physical medicine and rehabilitation*, Philadelphia, 1971, WB Saunders.

20. Levin LA, Perk J, Hedback B: Cardiac rehabilitation: a cost analysis, *J Intern Med* 230(5):427, 1991.

21. Maloney FP, Moss K: *Energy requirements for selected activities*, Denver, 1974, Department of Physical Medicine, National Jewish Hospital (Unpublished).

22. Mythos for SoftKey: *BodyWorks 4.0: human anatomy leaps to life*, Cambridge, MA, 1993-1995, SoftKey International.

23. Nemery B, et al: Changes in lung function after smoking cessation: an assessment from a cross-sectional survey, *Am Rev Respir Dis* 125(1):122, 1982.

24. Ogden LD: *Guidelines for analysis and testing of activities of daily living with cardiac patients*, Downey, CA, 1981, Cardiac Rehabilitation Resources.

25. Oldridge NB, et al: Cardiac rehabilitation after myocardial infarction, *JAMA* 260(7):945, 1988.

26. Renfroe KL: Effect of progressive relaxation on dyspnea and state anxiety in patients with chronic obstructive pulmonary disease, *Heart Lung* 17(4):408, 1988.

27. Santa Clara Valley Medical Center: *Graded activity sheets*, San Jose, CA, 1994, The Center.

28. Scalzi C, Burke L: Myocardial infarction: behavioral responses of patient and spouses. In Underhill SL, et al, editors: *Cardiac nursing*, Philadelphia, 1982, JB Lippincott.

29. van Dixhoorn JJ, Duivenvoorden HJ: Effect of relaxation therapy on cardiac events after myocardial infarction: a 5-year follow-up study, *J Cardiopulmonary Rehabil* 19(3):178, 1999.

30. Venes D, Thomas CL, Taber CW: *Taber's cyclopedic medical dictionary*, ed 19, Philadelphia, 2001, FA Davis.

45

ONCOLOGY

ANN BURKHARDT

KEY TERMS

Cancer	Chemotherapy	Edema	Palliative
Metastases	Radiation	Hospice	Lymphedema
Surgery	Oncology		

LEARNING OBJECTIVES

After studying this chapter the student or practitioner will be able to do the following:

1. Describe cancer and its diagnosis and medical and surgical treatments.
2. Identify common psychological conditions associated with life-threatening illness and loss.
3. Identify strategies for helping patients cope with the side effects of the treatments for cancer.
4. Identify common physical dysfunction issues resulting primarily from the cancer and secondarily from the treatment.
5. Identify techniques used in addressing a variety of occupational therapy goals with cancer patients, according to practice setting.
6. Identify problems that may arise as a result of the disease process or the sequelae of disease that could affect a person's occupational roles, activities of importance to those roles, and task performance; identify possible solutions to the problems.

CHAPTER OUTLINE

Prevention
Early postdiagnosis phase
Postoperative phase
Chemotherapy
Radiation therapy
Rehabilitative phase
Palliative care
Psychological and emotional aspects of living with cancer
Long-term and special chronic disease issues
Disease progression
Summary

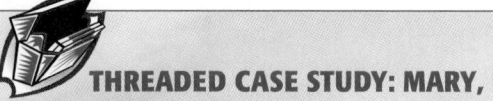

THREADED CASE STUDY: MARY, PART 1

Mary is a 35-year-old married woman and mother of three small children. She has recently received a diagnosis of Hodgkin's lymphoma. Her doctor noticed a lump on palpation of her neck during a routine physical examination. Mary has had chemotherapy and is receiving radiation to the mantle region of the right side of her chest. After the second week of 4 weeks of planned radiation treatment, Mary has been experiencing edema and a glovelike distribution of numbness in her right hand (irradiated side). She has received a diagnosis of lymphedema and radiation-induced brachial plexopathy. Mary is a teacher and uses her right hand to write on the board. In her role as a wife and mother, she does all of the shopping, cooking, and cleaning for her family. Mary is also a "soccer mom" and prides herself on the fact that she hasn't missed one of her children's soccer games in 3 years.

On administration of the Canadian Occupational Performance Measure (COPM), Mary voiced concern about being able to drive, interact with families (because she can no longer shake hands), and write on the blackboard. Mary is also concerned about being able to do her basic and instrumental (higher-level) activities of daily living. She states that she expects her husband will assist with grocery shopping, but she wants to be able to do the laundry, lay out soccer uniforms and clothing for her children, drive, cook, and perform light housekeeping.

The Assessment of Motor and Process Skills (AMPS) suggested that Mary needs some assistance to problem solve and implement strategies to compensate for the functional loss in her arm and hand. She is at risk for injuring her arm and hand because of the sensory loss. She could also benefit from training in energy conservation and work simplification. Because Mary is driving primarily with one hand, she could benefit from adaptations to her car that would increase her safety while driving. The table below provides an analysis of Mary's situation.

Occupation	Impairment	Activity Barrier	Participation Barrier
Housewife Wife Mother	Loss of bimanual function	Inability to use arm in tasks requiring use of both hands: hand washing clothes Shopping and carrying bags home on public transportation	Lacks access to technology that could assist her to do task efficiently by herself; lacks funding to purchase a vehicle (social/environ-mental factors) for community mobility and instrumental ADL use (e.g., shopping, yard work, infant/childcare, and cooking adaptations)
Work: teacher	Mobility and sensory impairment	Cannot sustain closed chain activity of holding chalk in her hand and writing concepts, diagrams, etc on the blackboard	Needs access to technology to allow her to project images instead of writing at a blackboard Workstation modification needed: sit to lecture versus stand Needs assistance to determine how to advocate for her needs within the workplace (social justice issue)
Soccer enthusiast	Fatigue Mobility and sensory impairment	Cannot sit in the bleachers for an entire soccer game Lacks enough access and postural support to comfortably remain at the game	Needs assistance from others to set up a supportive, comfortable chair on the ground adjacent to bleachers Needs a lightweight megaphone so her child can hear her cheers

At the end of treatment, Mary has returned to work. She uses a high stool to teach the class so that she conserves her energy for activities that she will need to do later in the day with her family. Mary has further adapted her workstation (i.e., classroom) by asking her employer to obtain a specialized overhead projector. She now writes on overheads instead of the blackboard. The students like Mary's class—she always uses colors to write and teaches with fun overheads with comics. Mary has explained to the students that she had an injury that prevents her from using her arm and hand but that she is trying to do all that she did before, using the new adaptations. Mary has received lots of support from the students and the community.

At home, Mary's husband, Tom, has been doing the shopping and vacuuming. Mary is able to prepare meals, load the dishwasher, and lift her children into her lap from a seated position. She dresses herself independently and needs only occasional help to put on a necklace or a bracelet when she goes out. Mary has learned to take rest breaks and "power naps." She has joined a SHARE support group and reports that she is so grateful for having found new friends and inspiration from the group.

Mary's doctor has informed her that her cancer is now in remission. She will need to see the doctor every 3 months for the next year. She will need to be watched closely for recurrence for the next 5 years, but the doctor is very positive about her response to treatment.

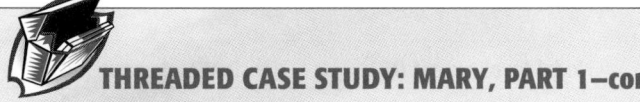

Mary's lymphedema has been contained at a minimal level. She performs self-massage and wears a gradient compression bandage daily. Although she has permanent nerve damage that prevents the return of functional use of her hand, Mary states that people are very supportive and comment less and less on her condition. She says that her lymphedema has become "the least of my problems." Mary recognizes the signs of infection and monitors the measurements of her arm weekly, increasing her self-awareness of any changes in the condition. She seems pleased that the edema has become a background issue in her daily life.

Mary states that she continues to be a "soccer mom." Her second child is now playing in a junior league. She says that her participation in occupational therapy has given her a new lease on life. She is grateful to feel in charge of the things that give her life meaning. Although she is sad about the function she has lost, she looks forward to seeing her children grow and spending years to come with her best friend, her husband.

Critical Thinking Questions

1. What occupational performance difficulties would you anticipate from the sensory disturbance in her right hand?
2. What occupational roles may have to be modified, and what changes would you recommend?
3. What additional assessments may be helpful when developing an intervention plan for Mary?
4. How would you decide which approach to use with Mary, and when would you reassess or potentially alter this approach depending on the disease process? What types of information or clues from her health and medical disease management would require you to reframe your intervention and approach to care?
5. Can you give some examples of how occupational therapy may be helpful to Mary throughout her disease and recovery process? How will Mary potentially benefit across her lifespan from periodic reassessment and intervention from an occupational therapist?

Cancer is a broad grouping of diseases, all of which are linked by the presence of malignant tumor cells in the body. Cancers are described by the type of tissue in which they arise: carcinoma (within an organ), sarcoma (connective tissue), chondroma (cartilage), lymphoma (lymphatic tissue), or leukemia (blood-forming tissue). Malignancies can be low grade (slowly developing) or high grade (rapidly developing) and can adapt within and spread throughout the body (metastasizing). **Metastases** are pieces of tumor that have broken off from the main tumor, traveled in the circulatory system, and reseeded themselves in new organs or tissues in the body. When biopsy of a metastatic lesion is performed (the lesion is sampled to observe its histology or tissue type), the lesion cells appear similar to the cells in the tumor of origin. For example, breast cancer that metastasizes to the lung is breast cancer, not lung cancer, at the cellular level. Tumors occupy space within an organ system and interrupt the function of that organ. For example, liver tumors or lesions can cause the affected person to have abnormal liver function, observed on a blood test or through a clinical sign such as jaundice.

Tumor cells sometimes secrete hormonelike substances. These pseudohormones disrupt the function of organs. The clinical picture may appear as something unrelated to cancer; there is often no tumor mass, just freely circulating tumor cells, resulting in a paraneoplastic syndrome. For example, lung cancer can cause a paraneoplastic syndrome that looks like quadriparesis. Paraneoplastic syndrome is often considered in a differential diagnosis when polyneuropathy or dermatomyositis is seen. The presence of acute onset quadriparesis without evident physical trauma suggests

that lung cancer may be an underlying cause. Blood tests will detect tumor markers, and the cancer can be diagnosed. Once the cancer diagnosis is known, chemotherapy or procedures that can filter the neoplastic cells from the blood (e.g., photophoresis) can rapidly change and possibly improve the functional clinical picture. Cancers are "staged," or classified, in an effort to predict prognosis and identify appropriate intervention (Table 45-1).

PREVENTION

At a number of levels of cancer care, it is appropriate for an occupational therapist to work with the person with cancer. Probably the most valuable, yet often overlooked, time for an occupational therapist to intervene is at the level of cancer prevention. For example, influencing a person's choice of and ability to change habits and behaviors that negatively influence health is a starting point. Occupational therapists can give positive health messages to all the people with whom they are in contact. Children and adolescents may not start smoking if they hear a positive smoking prevention message or if they are involved as role models in an education project focused on communication with their peers or siblings.

Occupational therapists can also intervene by helping smokers quit smoking. In 1998, the Representative Assembly (RA) of the American Occupational Therapy Association (AOTA) voted to support the Clinical Practice Guideline of the Agency for Healthcare Policy Research.[1] This action supports the role occupational therapists may play in helping their patients set health improvement goals to prevent chronic

TABLE 45-1   **Cancer Staging: TNM Definition**

Stage	Primary Tumor (T)	Nodal Involvement (N)	Distant Metastasis (M)
I	Tumor 5 cm or less in size; no invasion of adjacent tissues	No regional positive nodes	No (known) distant metastasis
II	Tumor greater than 5 cm in size; no invasion of adjacent tissues	No regional positive nodes	No (known) distant metastasis
III	Tumor outside organ in fat and surrounding soft tissues	No regional positive nodes	No (known) distant metastasis
	Tumor 5 cm or less in size; no invasion of adjacent tissues, or tumor greater than 5 cm in size; no invasion of adjacent tissues	Positive regional nodes	No (known) distant metastasis
IV	Tumor outside organ in fat and surrounding soft tissues, or tumor invading adjacent organs	Positive regional nodes	No (known) distant metastasis
	Tumor 5 cm or less in size; no invasion of adjacent tissues; Tumor 5 cm or less in size; no invasion of adjacent tissues; tumor outside organ in fat and surrounding soft tissues; or tumor invading adjacent organs	No regional positive nodes or positive regional nodes	Distant metastasis present

Data from Norton JA, Le HN: Adrenal tumors. In DeVita VT Jr, Hellman S, Rosenberg SA, editors: *Cancer: principles and practice of oncology*, ed 6, p. 1770, Philadelphia, 2001, Lippincott Williams & Wilkins.

disease and disability. Smoking cessation initiatives are one example of a cancer prevention intervention. Smoking cessation interventions may be individual, group, or population based and geared to reach any age group across the life span. Other prevention efforts may focus on self-examination and follow-up in scheduling and going for cancer detection tests (e.g., breast self-examinations, mammograms, Pap smears, and colonoscopies).

OT PRACTICE NOTE

Because the focus in occupational therapy (OT) is on helping people achieve a balanced lifestyle that supports a balance between self-care, work, play and leisure, and rest, occupational therapists are a natural group of professionals to be involved in cancer prevention initiatives.

EARLY POSTDIAGNOSIS PHASE

The occupational therapist also plays an important role in working with persons with cancer who are recovering from such invasive procedures as surgery, chemotherapy, and radiation therapy. This level of occupational therapy (OT) intervention may occur in a hospital, home health, or community health setting. People who experience a change in their functional status and have difficulty participating in daily activities such as self-care, work, play, and leisure activities, or with the ability to rest, may benefit from OT. The prevention of long-term disability, the restoration of normal function, and the support of function through rehabilitative means or through provision of palliative (comfort) care are all appropriate reasons for an OT referral. Mary voiced concerns

regarding her ability to perform meaningful roles within her family. These concerns should be addressed throughout the OT intervention program.

The initial intervention for cancer may involve a series of treatments including surgery, chemotherapy, radiation therapy, or immunotherapy. Each of these treatments has side effects. **Surgery** may include removal of a mass, more resection of tissue in addition to the mass (for staging of the disease or for complete removal of tumor-invaded tissue), reconstructive surgery to correct cosmetic or functional defects or the surgical resection, or amputation. Before surgery, the therapist can be involved in patient education and training—preparing the patient for what to expect after the surgery. Some researchers believe that training the patient preoperatively may improve functional outcomes and reduce the rehabilitation needed in the postoperative recovery phase.

POSTOPERATIVE PHASE

In the early postoperative stage, the occupational therapist may work with clients to encourage them and enable them to participate safely in daily occupations and goal-directed activities. Patients may be frightened to move and may need guidance concerning how much is safe to attempt and which movements they need to avoid until healing occurs. Pulling of the incision commonly occurs when patients' bodies are used dynamically in activities. This pulling sensation may be threatening to people who are uncertain about how much movement is too much or too little. The therapist often receives special movement precautions from the surgeon in the early postoperative phase of OT referral and intervention. Postoperative precautions and protocols vary from surgeon to surgeon and facility to facility and must be verified at the time of the referral.

Several types of surgery are used to treat tumors. An en bloc resection is removal of the tumor and surrounding or involved tissues in one block or piece. An en bloc resection can be done when the nerves and vascular structures are patent, unobstructed by tumor growth. Radical surgery, including amputation, is a wide surgical resection. The diseased tissue is removed along with surrounding lymphatic tissue and other soft tissue (skin, nerve, muscle, or bone). If the neurovascular bundle to the limb is involved, the limb has to be amputated.

Amputation is a life-altering event resulting in the loss of a limb or part of a limb (e.g., arm or leg) or of a body part (e.g., breast). The loss always causes a visible change in physical appearance. One difference between amputation as a result of cancer diagnosis and a traumatic amputation in an accident or necessitated by complications of a disease (e.g., diabetes) is that cancer requires further medical management beyond traditional wound care and preprosthetic or prosthetic training. Life span and survival rates and the person's perception of the relative value of such an investment vary and may affect the person's decision about whether to purchase an artificial limb. For example, someone who has a postamputation life expectancy of 2 years or less may decline a prosthesis because of the expense and the time that must be invested in a training regimen. He or she may have other plans for the money or time that are more meaningful to quality of life.

When adapted equipment or techniques are indicated, the therapist may also provide them and train the patient to use them to compensate for motion that is lost or compromised after surgery. If the surgery causes a temporary functional change, the use of adaptation may be only for the immediate, subacute phase of healing. If surgery has caused muscle or bone loss, the functional changes and adaptations may be strategies that will be used for the remainder of life.

CHEMOTHERAPY

Chemotherapy is the use of a variety of toxic chemical substances to kill cancer cells within the body. Each form of chemotherapy has its own pattern of possible side effects. Some of the most common side effects that occupational therapists encounter are alopecia (hair loss), peripheral neuropathy, thrombocytopenia (diminished platelet levels and slow clotting time of the blood), fatigue (associated with such factors as impaired liver function), changes in the red blood cell composition of the blood (e.g., anemia), and function-limiting anxiety and fear.

Chemotherapy-induced neuropathy usually causes wrist-drop and foot-drop, which are transient. Neuropathy can also cause burning, tingling pain. Neuropathic pain can severely limit function because afflicted people are reluctant to hold on to objects or to stand on their feet when pain is serious.

Many people who are receiving chemotherapy contract opportunistic infections because chemotherapy causes immunosuppression. One infection, cytomegalovirus (CMV), can cause blindness, as well as hepatitis. People who have low vision or blindness and chemoneuropathy have a severe handicapping situation because they cannot use one sensory system (tactile) to substitute for another (vision) functionally. Another infection, a yeast *(Candida albicans)* infection, can cause dysphagia, an inability to swallow safely. The affected person may have to stop eating by mouth or eat a restricted-consistency diet until the infection resolves.

In the acute phase of hospitalization, clients receiving chemotherapy may be referred to OT because they have been on prolonged bed rest and may have stopped initiating or participating in their self-care. Also, fatigue may limit their level of participation because a person who is fatigued may not be able or sufficiently motivated to participate in daily occupations.

Peripheral neuropathy causes weakness and sensory changes in the hands and feet. Often, people cannot hold on to objects adequately to use them as intended. Hyperesthesia (tingling, numbness, or burning) and loss of grasp and fine motor hand function can interfere with the ability to do daily tasks and activities; the person may drop objects or experience pain when trying to use common objects such as a comb or a brush.

The client who has decreased platelet levels may bleed easily and may have to forgo some normal daily activities for a few days until blood levels improve. When someone's platelet level is below 45,000/mm^3, for example, the individual may have excessive bleeding of the gums when brushing teeth. While the platelet level is low, using a sponge toothette or a glycerine swab may be all the individual can tolerate until blood levels normalize. Blood levels generally improve as the person's body metabolizes the chemotherapy, in the first few days after a treatment.

Hormone therapy and immunotherapy are also used as forms of chemotherapy. For example, some tumors thrive on estrogens. Hormones such as Lupron or tamoxifen can be used to block estrogen receptors or to prevent the body from producing estrogens. These hormones often have the side effect of inducing menopause. Women may complain about mood swings and hot flashes. Immunotherapy is the use of substances that block the response of the immune system or that heighten the response. For instance, white blood cells phagocytose (ingest) cancer cells and carry them through the lymphatic system to other areas of the body. This response can spread cancer in the local region or carry the cancer cells to other places in the body. Interferon is an immunotherapeutic agent that can be used to fight this spread. People who receive interferon treatment may have a tendency toward hyperactive skin responses, such as forms of eczema. If these individuals are scratched, welts may easily develop. These are normal responses to the drug and should not generate fear or anxiety in the patients who use these substances.

RADIATION THERAPY

Another method of treatment that people may undergo in the acute phase of cancer intervention is radiation therapy. **Radiation** is the use of radioactive materials directly in tumors or the surrounding tissue to kill cancer cells. Radiation is effective when the cancer cells are sensitive to its effects. Radioactive seeds (small pieces or pellets of material) can be directly implanted for a short time in the body (radioactive seed implantation). Seeds are sometimes placed in flexible tubing that is run through the tumor bed (brachytherapy). Another approach involves directing a beam of radioactivity to a generalized area of the body via a linear accelerator machine. The beam can cover a broad area of a quadrant of the body (wide-beam) or be directed to a more focused area (coned down). An occupational therapist may work collaboratively in some settings with the radiation **oncology** staff to mold body positioners from thermoplastic (splinting) materials. These devices are used to help the patient remain in the position needed for the duration of the radiation treatment. Radiation may also be used in late disease as a form of palliative treatment, particularly to reduce pain.

Burns are a possible side effect of radiation treatment. The topical ointments used to treat a burn caused by radiation are different from those used for burns of other causes. The skin absorbs moisturizing agents. These agents can change the surface composition of the skin and result in an enhancement of the burn at the next radiation treatment. Many interventional radiologists recommend water-based ointments (e.g., Aquaphor) for their patients. Others allow their patients to use silicone gel pads to cover the burn and manage the burn-related pain and discomfort. When people have burns resulting from radiation, they should avoid movement that stretches or pulls the burned area. People may need assistance with range of motion to prevent such complications as frozen shoulder.

REHABILITATIVE PHASE

Therapists who work with people who have cancer in the acute care phase of treatment are generally working toward the goal of getting the patient ready to go home or be transferred to an inpatient rehabilitation setting, a subacute center, long-term care, or a hospice setting (at home or in a facility).

Clients who have completed their initial cancer treatment may be well enough to participate in aggressive rehabilitation programs. Patients are sometimes admitted to a rehabilitation unit on a trial therapy basis to test their ability to tolerate 3 hours of therapy per day. After initial healing of a surgery and after or during chemotherapy regimens, clients who have cancer may be able to tolerate this intensive type of rehabilitation program. On a rehabilitation unit, goals for cancer patients generally involve restoration and support of function within a rehabilitative model of care—learning to live with an acquired handicap. The goal of therapy in a function-based treatment setting is to restore the ability of clients to participate in goal-directed activities that give their lives meaning. Some of the pertinent areas for OT assessment and intervention are analyzed in Table 45-2.

Cancer and cancer treatment can cause a number of functional problems that result in physical disability and handicapping situations. One of the most important issues associated with cancer is impaired mobility. Community mobility—leaving home, crossing the street, getting around the neighborhood, and getting to and from business or medical appointments—is basic to daily life. A number of factors can contribute to mobility impairments.

Weakness is probably the most common impairment causing disability and restricted activity participation in people with cancer. Weakness leads to a lack of endurance needed for navigating distances and decreased tolerance for sitting or being upright for prolonged periods. Weakness may also limit customary movement within homes or public buildings

TABLE **45-2** **Areas of OT Assessment and Intervention**

Cancer Involvement (Body Structure/ Body Function)	Impairment	Activity Restriction	Participation Issues (Personal and Environmental Factors)
Brain	Motor	Mobility	Access
			Architectural barriers
			Adaptation
	Sensory	Safety/pain	Safety: need for supervision or a helper
			Pain: intolerance of participation in activities that exacerbate pain to level of intolerance
			Pain medicine: blurring senses, inability to drive or operate heavy machinery
	Cognitive	Planning	Inability to lead
		Sequencing	Lack of ability to plan or implement change
		Memory	Social inappropriateness/stigma

TABLE **45-2** **Areas of OT Assessment and Intervention—cont'd**

Cancer Involvement (Body Structure/ Body Function)	Impairment	Activity Restriction	Participation Issues (Personal and Environmental Factors)
Brain—cont'd		Insight Safety	Loss of occupational roles: work roles, family roles, ability to participate in leisure or sport activities
	Neurobehavioral Visual impairment: hemianopsia, neglect, low vision, cortical blindness, loss of spatial relations perception. Motor planning	Interference with ADLs/self-care and instrumental activities	Inability to be independently involved in daily occupations
	Communication	Speaking Reading Writing	Loss or major change in socialization and sharing ideas Severity of participation restriction dependent on individual interests and roles
Bone	Loss of motion Pain Impaired mobility Risk of re-injury of affected part	ADLs (basic and instrumental)	Ability to dress, bathe, toilet in context Need for adaptation of environment or presence of a caregiver Decreased ability to get around Possible effect on employment Severity of participation restriction dependent on individual interests and roles
Breast	Loss of motion Pain Impaired mobility Risk of re-injury of affected part	ADLs (basic and instrumental) Shoulder mobility restrictions: sports, etc.	Temporary or long-term disruption in ability to do housework, job, leisure activities Risk of injury because of lymphatic compromise; impact on sexuality
Lung	Shoulder mobility impairment (Pancoast tumor; post-thoracotomy) Impaired respiratory status Fatigue	ADLs (basic and instrumental) Shoulder mobility restrictions: sports, etc. Respiratory tolerance	Mobility issues respiratory tolerance and distance navigated Temporary or long-term disruption in ability to do housework, job, leisure activities Risk of injury because of respiratory compromise Need for oxygen or nebulizing equipment
Colon	Change in way that bowels are managed (toileting-colostomy) Change in way body is washed (stomal issues) Chemoneuropathy impairment potential Fatigue	ADLs (basic and instrumental) Fatigue Social stigma of stoma (odor, bag ruptures, etc.) Fine motor impairment related to chemotherapy	Socially stigmatizing in community relationships
Prostate	Urinary continence Inability to perform sexually	ADLs (basic and instrumental)	Loss of sense of self as a sexual being Stigma associated with incontinence
Head and neck	Inability to swallow/eat Loss of voice Neck and shoulder decrease in range of motion; loss of scapular stability	ADLs (feeding and eating; swallowing) Respiratory: management of oral secretions Bimanual overhead mobility activities Intimacy issues	Socially stigmatizing in community relationships Need to change contributory habits (smoking)

if there are architectural barriers, such as flights of stairs. The inability to get around presents a person with a handicapping situation because he or she does not have access to the venues needed to fulfill occupational roles.

THREADED CASE STUDY: MARY, PART 2

Mary had cone-down external beam radiation to her right supraclavicular and clavicular region (mantle). When the initial radiation is given, a wide beam is used, and in Mary's case, this beam also radiated her shoulder joint capsule. Mary experienced stiffness and pain when trying to use her right shoulder with rotation in the joint. She had to stretch her arm several times throughout the day to be able to prepare to use her arm in activity.

Edema may result from a number of causes. When a tumor invades the tissues near a limb (or limbs) or when lymph nodes adjacent to a body part are resected or irradiated, a person may develop lymphedema. Lymphedema, an inflammatory response of the body, is caused by a shifting of protein-rich white blood cells flooding the area where the cancer has spread, or where there is scar tissue forming. Lymph nodes and vessels usually assist in the transit of white blood cells. When they are impaired, the fluid may accumulate and cause local swelling in the limb. The edema is a colloid. Colloids initially are fluidlike in presentation. Over time, colloids may change to be more gelatinous or firm (brawny). Specially trained therapists use techniques known as manual decongestive therapy or manual lymph massage. The massage targets the lymphatic structures and pathway of lymphatic flow. Often, the limb is bandaged with support bandaging that is later alternated with the use of gradient compression support garments (stockings and sleeves). Education is also usually given concerning skin and wound precautions and exercises that may assist to decongest, or clear, the edema from the involved limb (or limbs). If the limb becomes engorged, reddened, and acutely painful, the patient may have cellulitis, an acute infection of connective tissue. Before the therapist can treat the edema, cellulitis requires antibiotic therapy.

Edema may also result from organ system failure. This type of edema tends to be protein poor and more liquidlike in its presentation. When it is present only in the limbs (such as in pedal edema), this may be somewhat less serious than when the edema is present throughout the trunk and limbs, a condition called *anasarca*. Compression bandaging or support garments may be of some help, as long as treating the limbs does not put undue stress on the organs that are experiencing failure (e.g., the heart, lungs, and kidneys).

Having edema is uncomfortable, and patients who suffer from this condition may complain of soreness or achy pain

in their limbs. The presence of edema also may limit the person's ability to ambulate distances required for community mobility, for example. Also, persons with edema may find it difficult to wear their normal clothing and accessories if use of these items causes circulatory restriction.

THREADED CASE STUDY: MARY, PART 3

Mary's lymphedema was mild. She was initially taught to do her own lymphatic massage, and she wears a compression sleeve and glove during the day when she is using her arm in resistive tasks. She also wears the sleeve and glove when she flies in an airplane, so the edema is not exacerbated by the change in cabin pressure. Mary also knows how to recognize an infection in her arm (the signs of cellulitis) and is aware of steps she can take to prevent infection when a situation arises that could lead to an infection or a lymphedema flare-up (e.g., cuts, bug bites, pricks from sharp objects, and burns).

Impaired sensation predisposes people to injury from heat sources or sharp tools. If the sensory impairment is hyperesthetic (intensifying sensation), burning pain can decrease the ability to hold objects, to modulate grasp or pinch to manipulate objects enough to use them, or to tolerate wearing of socks or shoes. The physically disabling condition creates an inability to carry out all of the self-care and other daily activities that involve hand function or foot function.[2]

Impaired cognition is disabling because an affected person may not be able to initiate or follow through on tasks. With memory impairment, a patient may forget what he or she is doing or why he or she is doing it. Impaired judgment, if sufficiently grave, means that a person cannot be left alone. The potential risk of injury or elopement from familiar surroundings may be too great a risk to allow any independence. Impaired cognition may be permanent or transient. If the impairment is associated with a central nervous system structural abnormality, the person may recover only rudimentary cognitive skill and may benefit most from the development of cueing systems to complete daily activities. If the person has a cognitive impairment associated with metabolism of an anesthetic or the introduction of a new pain medication (opiates such as morphine have this property), cognitive abilities may return to normal baseline when the drug is metabolized by the body. Because the liver's ability to metabolize drugs and anesthesia slows with age, many older persons who undergo major surgery experience this phenomenon. Although the acquired cognitive impairments from anesthesia resolve within weeks of surgery, many people need constant supervision during this recovery phase.

Impaired vision is sometimes associated with brain tumors or a CMV infection. Impaired vision of recent onset in a sighted person can be very disorienting. Most sighted people cannot easily orient themselves to daily activities if visual impairment or blindness develops suddenly. The degree of functional impairment will be associated with the daily activities a person enjoys or needs to complete. For example, a person may not be able to resume driving a vehicle. This limits community mobility. A person may not be able to sign or write checks. Participation skills and abilities in other basic and instrumental activities of daily living (ADLs) may be lost as a result of vision loss.

Diminished hearing may result from use of metal-based chemotherapy drugs (e.g., cisplatin). These chemotherapy drugs are toxic to auditory nerves. Severe hearing loss or deafness may develop following treatment. Children who receive these drugs may not develop language skills. Adults may have difficulty with social interactions and the use of standard communication devices (e.g., telephones). People who are caregivers for others may have to relinquish their responsibilities or may require training and adapted devices to modify the way they perform essential tasks. People who rely on hearing to work, such as musicians, may need assistance from a therapist to find a new role that is less dependent on hearing.

Chronic fatigue results from a variety of factors after cancer treatment. Chronic fatigue may eventually resolve as factors causing the condition resolve and as the body heals after cancer diagnosis and treatment. However, management of chronic fatigue is necessary for coping during the disease and treatment process. Participation in living can instill hope and the perception that some things can change or be positively managed to give the patient a sense of being able to control his or her own life. Both emotionally and psychologically, hope is crucial to recovery.

Strategies that occupational therapists can use to assist patients who have chronic fatigue include energy conservation and work simplification, as well as scheduling intervals of rest between periods of work or activity. When fatigue is severely disabling, an occupational therapist can help the patient and caregivers prioritize the tasks and activities that the patient wants to do, balancing these with the tasks or activities that must be done. Sometimes, recognizing the need for help allows people the opportunity to choose the truly important and meaningful occupations that define who they are as people and contributing members of society.

PALLIATIVE CARE

When patients have received diagnoses of advanced cancer and are not expected to recover, their physicians can declare or certify them as terminally ill. This legal certification entitles these patients to have access to hospice services. **Hospice** is a form of palliative care. There are several models of hospice care. Home care hospice occurs in the home of the dying person or of a significant other who is caring for the dying person in the final stages of life. Inpatient facilities

may be obtained either through skilled nursing facilities or through dedicated inpatient hospice settings. The money to cover inpatient care is part of Medicare part A services and therefore often part of a bundled reimbursement charge. Some hospices provide additional, extended services through philanthropic funding. The services in hospices with private funding may provide expanded service options that have a greater emphasis on quality of life programming, such as services offered during the off hours (evenings and weekends). **Palliative care** is directed toward achieving comfort and ease of participation in activity. Occupational therapists involved in hospice care may intervene directly with the person who is dying or indirectly with families, volunteers, and caregivers as educators, trainers, and intermediaries to improve the quality of life for the person who is dying and those around them.[5] Some examples of this role are to adapt the environment, train caregivers to assist with daily life tasks, counsel for psychological or emotional issues related to the disease process, and provide assistance with issues concerning death and dying.

OT PRACTICE NOTE

Occupational therapists may work with the patient on activities that help the patient plan for death. Reminiscence activities, such as creating memory scrap books, making video "cards," writing letters, making phone calls, and arranging visits are examples of creative tasks that can help the dying person revisit relationships and review life.

One OT qualitative research study was conducted using the doing-being-becoming framework.[3] The experiences of 23 (13 male and 10 female) day hospice participants were investigated through use of (1) a combination of focus groups, (2) individual interviews, and (3) participant observation. The data were interpreted using constant comparison, coding, and theme-building methodology. Experiences of doing were evident in accounts of losing and maintaining valued occupations and striving to preserve physical and mental functioning. A sense of being through occupational engagement arose in social relationships and self-exploration that enhanced feelings of self-worth. Occupation promoted the experience of becoming by providing fresh learning opportunities and a sense of contributing to others' welfare.

In palliative care, the occupational therapist may assist with promoting positioning for comfort, providing treatment to prevent or relieve pain, promoting engagement in activity that is physically tolerable, and creating an opportunity to engage in a full occupational life review as part of the process of planning for death. For the client involved in the active process of dying, having an opportunity to resolve life issues is critical. Creativity still plays a role. When people create and give back something to others, they live in hope.

Hope is essential in all phases of life, even in the process of dying, because it motivates us to live each day to the fullest, despite illness and disease.

PSYCHOLOGICAL AND EMOTIONAL ASPECTS OF LIVING WITH CANCER

People with cancer may have social, psychological, and emotional issues that affect their ability to function. Acquaintances may avoid the patient with cancer, not knowing how to respond to the news of a life-threatening illness. Some people mistakenly assume that they can catch cancer from the person. Many people, regardless of the stage of their disease, automatically assume they are dying. In reality, more and more people are surviving with diagnoses of cancer for longer and longer periods.

Coping mechanisms are essential for dealing with the stress of having a cancer diagnosis, as well as for facing the inevitability of treatments necessary for seeking control or cure of the cancer. The emotional side effects of the progression of cancer include fear and anticipation of pain, which produces anxiety and stress. Surgery is usually painful. Chemotherapy can cause painful neuropathies. Burns from radiation are painful. Metastatic lesions on bone, muscle, or nerve are painful. Some positive coping mechanisms for dealing with a rational fear of pain are self-hypnosis, meditation, and other relaxation techniques (see Chapter 27).

People who are anxious by temperament often have heightened anxiety when they are trying to cope with cancer diagnoses and treatment. People with anxiety disorders can become overly focused on signs or symptoms that they experience. They may not be able to sleep. They may be unable to take part in their normal activities, losing perspective on their situation. They may find it difficult to concentrate on normal life tasks. Treatment for an anxiety disorder includes supportive counseling and pharmacological intervention. Once the anxiety is controlled and the fears that underlie the anxiety are addressed, coping behaviors can be developed and improve the person's ability to engage in the rehabilitative process.

Many people living with a diagnosis of cancer experience depression. Depression may be reactive or organic in origin. Depression may also have an organic cause, such as medications, the disease process, or a hereditary predisposition. Depression is characterized by feelings of helplessness and hopelessness. People adjusting to disease or disability go through a normal grieving process. During this time, they may experience a number of feelings or stages. The stages of adjustment generally encountered are anger, denial, bargaining, and acceptance. These stages tend to be experienced in combination. Depressed people generally have to be able to see something hopeful concerning their personal circumstances for change to occur and for the effects of the depression to lessen.

Participation in support groups may be helpful for some people. Even people with advanced cancer have been found to benefit from support groups. Women with stage IV breast cancer who participated in support groups lived better and longer than those who did not participate in a support group.[4] Although the exact mechanism is not clear, the experience of knowing that others share what you are feeling and that others care about you can have a positive impact on the immune system. Recent studies have shown that even avoidance of pessimism supports health and well-being.

LONG-TERM AND SPECIAL CHRONIC DISEASE ISSUES

Lymphedema is edema (enlargement of one or more limbs) that results from impaired lymphatic circulation. Lymphatic circulation can be impaired by lymph node dissection, radiation of the lymphatics, or a tumor that has spread into the lymphatic vessels or nodes. Lymphedema is protein-rich edema and is inflammatory in nature. Lymphedema can occur throughout the body but is commonly seen by therapists when it impairs function in a limb by changing the mobility of the extremity or by producing pain in the involved limb. Lymphedema in the arm, in particular, produces a social impairment. A normal approach to social interaction in our society includes extending a hand to shake hands. When a person has lymphedema in an arm and hand, people may react negatively to the appearance of the limb. As discussed previously, publicly sharing knowledge of a diagnosis of cancer can be socially stigmatizing and lead to social rejection.

Self-treatment for lymphedema usually involves following guidelines and education in skin care and wound precautions. The limb is fitted with a compressive garment or wrap. Compliance with the use of garments may be challenging for some people. The pressure against the skin by support garments should feel good to the person. Some people report having difficulty tolerating the squeezing sensation of the support garment at work. Light compression can be provided by a tubular support bandage or toning gloves or garments. Moderate (20 to 30 mm Hg) to firm (30 to 40, or 40 to 60 mm Hg) compression can be achieved by using a high-gradient garment (e.g., Jobst, Juzo, Medi, or Sigvarus). Manual lymphatic therapy (massage) can be performed by a professional or by the trained patient or caregiver to correct the lymphedema. Bandaging with cotton-based support bandages often follows massage treatment. A person can be taught self-massage to improve carryover of the treatment program. Also, pneumatic compression pumps may help reduce edema in the limbs.

Someone who has lymphedema generally self-monitors the condition and may require treatment that continues over a period of time. When the limb is in an inflammatory state, treatment must be ongoing and aggressive to maximally reduce the size of the limb. In time, and if the person avoids repeat injury, the frequency of treatment may lessen. People with lymphedema must be consistent in their management of the condition. Cellulitis (infection in the subcutaneous tissues of the lymphatically impaired limb) may occur; the person should be taught to recognize the urgent need for antibiotic treatment and reassessment with the therapist. Untreated cellulitis can lead rapidly to a systemic infection. Once infection becomes systemic, the person will require hospitalization and intravenous antibiotic treatment. As a prophylactic measure, physicians who treat people with cancer routinely give their patients antibiotic prescriptions for rapid self-treatment when a crisis occurs.

DISEASE PROGRESSION

One long-term condition that can develop as a result of spread of disease or as an aftereffect of radiation treatment is brachial plexopathy. The most common complaint associated with the development of brachial plexopathy is progressive loss of function in the arm. Patients complain of clumsiness, inability to hold on to objects, and lack of coordination. Brachial plexopathy associated with cancer treatment or disease progression is irreversible. A person with the condition will lose function and mobility of the arm. The extremity can become flail. When mobility and strength remain, adapted techniques can preserve function for as long as possible. Some patients benefit from functional splinting to preserve function; for example, tenodesis splinting (see Chapter 41 for this concept) may be helpful when a patient is motivated to use a splint to support function. When the limb is flail, positioning for protection is crucial. Sensory loss may develop in addition to the motor loss, including loss of protective sensation. Reinforcing safety issues during activity participation can support safe participation in daily tasks and activities.

SUMMARY

OT is beneficial for many people who have cancer. Occupational therapists may encounter patients with cancer in inpatient settings, home care, outpatient settings, community-based settings, work settings, and school or early intervention. This area of OT practice is closely aligned with the medical model, given that many people who have cancer-related rehabilitation diagnoses have medical qualifiers that affect their participation in OT treatment. Other OT models are also important in addressing quality of life issues.

The most important tools that we have as OT practitioners are (1) our ability to work with our patients beyond the impairment level of disability and (2) our skills as holistic practitioners that allow us to be effective in intervening with people at the activity and participation levels of their occupational abilities. Given the potential side effects of participation in activities, our knowledge of the medical model will enable us in the future to further develop creative and needed interventions for this population—a

population for which we must document and produce intervention outcome data.

Review Questions

1. Contrast the role of the OT practitioner in cancer care during the early postdiagnosis phase versus that in the postoperative phase.
2. List and describe side effects of chemotherapy and radiation therapy.
3. Describe how chemotherapy and radiation therapy may affect occupational performance.
4. What are the causes and effects of impaired sensation and cognition during cancer treatment?
5. What are the psychological and social consequences of a diagnosis of cancer? To what extent do you think these can be affected by the patient's attitude and by social support? How can the occupational therapist assist the patient in facing and managing psychological and social challenges?
6. Describe the protocol for managing lymphedema.

REFERENCES

1. Agency for Health Care Policy and Research: Smoking cessation clinical practice guideline, *JAMA* 275(16):1270, 1996.
2. Burkhardt A, Joachim J: Cancers of the bone. In *A therapist's guide to oncology: medical issues affecting management,* San Antonio, TX, 1996, Therapy Skill Builders.
3. Lyons M, et al: Doing-being-becoming: occupational experiences of persons with life-threatening illnesses, *Am J Occup Ther* 56(3):285, 2002.
4. Spiegel D: Effect of psychosocial treatment on survival of patients with metastatic breast cancer, *Lancet* 2(8668):888, 1989.
5. Trump S: The role of occupational therapy in hospice, *Home Community Health Special Interest Section Quarterly* 7:1, 2000.

SUGGESTED READING

Bates SE, Longo DL: Use of serum tumor markers in cancer diagnosis and management, *Semin Oncol* 14:102, 1997.
Calibrisi P, Schein PS: *Medical oncology,* New York, 1993, McGraw-Hill.
Dewys WD, Hall TC: Paraneoplastic syndromes. In Rubin P, editor: *Clinical oncology: a multidisciplinary approach for physicians and students,* Philadelphia, 1993, WB Saunders.
Dimeo F, et al: Correlation between physical performance and fatigue in cancer patients, *Ann Oncol* 8(12):1251, 1997.

RESOURCES FOR CANCER INFORMATION

National Cancer Institute (NCI)
1-800-4-CANCER
www.nci.nih.gov

American Cancer Society
1-800-ACS-2345
www.cancer.org

American Lung Association
1-800-LUNG-USA
www.lungusa.org

Cancer Care, Inc.
1-800-813-HOPE
www.cancercare.org

Cancer Hope Network
1-877-HOPENET
email: info@cancerhopenetwork.org
(on-line cancer support groups)
www.cancerhopenetwork.org/

Coping with Cancer Magazine
615-790-2400
Copingmag@aol.com
www.copingmag.com/

Leukemia Society of America
1-800-955-4LSA
www.leukemia.org

National Brain Tumor Foundation
1-800-934-CURE
www.braintumor.org

46

SPECIAL NEEDS OF THE OLDER ADULT

CAROLYN GLOGOSKI

MICHAEL W.K. CHAN

KEY TERMS

Frail elders	Gerontologists	Young-old	Age-related changes
Geriatric specialists	Older adult	Old-old	Memory

LEARNING OBJECTIVES

After studying this chapter the student or practitioner will be able to do the following:

1. Describe the aging population of the future in demographic terms.
2. Identify typical patterns of age-related physical and cognitive changes.
3. Identify typical cognitive impairments of an older adult with vascular dementia.
4. Describe at least one style of problem solving that may be common to older adults as they cope with aging.
5. Identify common psychiatric conditions of later life.
6. Analyze personal biases in working with aging clients.

7. Identify performance areas, performance skills, client factors, and activity patterns important in the evaluation of the aging adult with an identified physical disorder.
8. Describe the ways in which context affects decisions regarding the focus of intervention.
9. Identify ways in which the focus of an entry-level occupational therapist during evaluation and intervention might differ from that of a more experienced colleague.
10. Describe how the learning needs and styles of older adults may differ from those of younger persons.

CHAPTER OUTLINE

THREADED CASE STUDY: MR. LEE, PART 1

Lee Kam Gai (Mr. Lee) is an 82-year-old retired restaurant owner of Chinese descent. He immigrated to San Francisco in 1968 from a small village in southern China with the help of relatives already living in the U.S. (In 1965, the New Immigration Act was passed, and persons with kin already in the U.S. were favored for immigration.[121]) He had decided to make a fresh start in the U.S. after the accidental deaths of his wife and two sons in China in 1965. After 5 years in the U.S., Mr. Lee was lonely; in 1973, he made arrangements to bring over a bride from China. Mei-Ling was 14 years younger than Mr. Lee. They lived a very traditional Chinese life on the outskirts of the bustling Chinatown in San Francisco and had two sons, now 31 and 25.

Mr. Lee started as a waiter in his uncle's restaurant and eventually purchased the restaurant with two other friends 10 years after his second marriage. During the occupational profile interview, he reported that he has always been a good provider to his second wife and sons and that Mrs. Lee was very diligent in attending to Mr. Lee's every need.

About 4 years ago, Mr. Lee experienced a right generalized cerebrovascular accident (CVA) that resulted in his being incapacitated for several weeks. This event created considerable consternation for Mr. and Mrs. Lee because they worried that Mr. Lee might need to remain in a nursing home for an extended period of recuperation. His wife was slight of build and had rheumatoid arthritis, which prevented her from providing the necessary physical care. However, after 6 weeks of intensive occupational and physical therapy, Mr. Lee regained moderate motor control of his left side, was walking with a pronounced limp, and required only minimal physical assistance performing his activities of daily living (ADLs). He returned home. At the time of discharge, the occupational therapist reported mild to moderate residual problems in client factors, particularly mental functions of cognition and, especially, short-term memory affecting functional and community mobility areas.

In the intervening years since the first stroke, Mrs. Lee reported that they had become quite active at the local Chinese senior center. Mr. Lee had become increasingly demanding of Mrs. Lee and had begun aggressively flirting with other women at the senior center. These behaviors seemed to worsen as Mrs. Lee took over more of the home management activities. Her main worry was that her husband's flirtatious behavior would lead to infidelity and possibly infection with the human immunodeficiency virus (HIV). Mr. Lee's loss of traditional gender roles, such as major home purchases, outside maintenance, and car maintenance, was the cause of frequent arguments and aggressive behavior by Mr. Lee. Mrs. Lee actually feared for her health and safety as a result of Mr. Lee's behavior. Mr. Lee, she explained, was completely oblivious to her concerns and had actually begun accusing her of having affairs with other men because she was less interested in intimate relationships and often away from the home on account of household errands. Over the intervening 2 years,

Mr. Lee experienced a number of episodes of mild confusion, as well as difficulty finding things; poor judgment; lack of self-monitoring; poor insight; and sporadic, increased hemiparesis on the left side. He also developed cataracts, for which he refused surgery, believing that this "mild problem seeing" might resolve on its own. He had become extremely hard of hearing (HOH) since his last hospitalization.

After a recent incident of weakness and confusion, Mr. Lee was taken to the emergency room and briefly hospitalized. The magnetic resonance imaging (MRI) scan ordered by the emergency room physician revealed several small strokes in the posterior cerebral artery and a very recent stroke of moderate size. A referral was made for home care to follow hospital discharge. At the time of discharge, Mr. Lee has fluctuating dynamic standing balance, limited endurance, and unreliable use of his left extremities because of hemiparesis. Subsequently, he was prescribed a rolling walker. Cognitive impairments included mild difficulty attending to tasks, fair to poor concentration, and progressive problems with short-term memory (e.g., forgetting appointments, important recent past events, and the names of friends and asking the same questions repeatedly). His wife finds him to be even more argumentative, demanding, and suspicious. Mrs. Lee has taken over all of the instrumental activities of daily living (IADLs) except for banking, which Mr. Lee refuses to relinquish, although she stands by while he performs each money management task and takes him to the bank. Mr. Lee now requires minimal physical assistance with grooming and moderate physical assistance with minimal verbal cues while showering, toileting, and ambulating.

Mr. Lee's goal is to be more independent in mobility without use of aids, especially outside of the home. His long-term goal is to get back to driving so that he can attend the local Buddhist temple for worship. Another, more immediate goal is to resume his role as the man of the house and "the one in charge." A third goal is to return to the senior center so that he can visit with friends and engage in the card games that he enjoys with others at the center. He has limited insight into the deficits that he is experiencing. He does not seem to grasp that his sons are seriously considering seeking control over the family finances and placing him in a setting with more care because they believe that he has become too difficult for Mrs. Lee to manage at home alone.

Critical Thinking Questions

1. What are some of the concerns for the occupational therapist addressing the multiplicity of factors in this case of the older adult involving age-associated changes?
2. What should be the primary focus of the occupational therapy evaluation and intervention process?
3. What contextual conditions are most relevant to this case, and what contextual conditions require further exploration and modification?
4. What activity performance patterns are of highest priority?

The growth rate of the population of older adults (OAs) in the U.S. surpassed the growth rate of the total U.S. population during the twentieth century.[54] From 1900 to 1997, the number of persons in the U.S. who were over the age of 65 increased by a factor of 11, although the total population only tripled. The segment of the OA population that has seen the most rapid expansion in numbers is the old-old (i.e., persons 80 years of age or older) adult population; this is true both in the United States and in many parts of the world. The growth rate of OAs is an unprecedented social phenomenon, one never before seen in the history of the world. The pattern of growth of the old-old is therefore of vital concern and poses substantial challenges to public policy makers. This success story—low mortality resulting from better education, nutrition, health, and healthcare—has obvious implications for the practice of occupational therapy (OT). Our mission is to promote the occupational performance of the elderly, including the old-old, despite the many challenges presented.

Members of this rapidly expanding segment of the older population have multiple, complex needs, which entail significantly greater social responsibilities. OAs use a substantial percentage of healthcare resources. How can OT respond to this new social phenomenon and its impact on healthcare? The purpose of this chapter is to help OT practitioners understand and respond to the often complex needs of OAs. Because the oldest-old and **frail elders** (i.e., persons 65 or older with significant physical and cognitive health problems)[54] frequently suffer from numerous health problems and exhibit multiple symptoms that interact in complex ways, performance dysfunction occurs in several occupational performance areas.

OT helps OAs continue or resume participation in everyday activities, to compensate when possible, or to develop new occupations as the need arises. This approach seeks to preserve quality of life and foster greater well-being for OAs by helping them to achieve a satisfactory level of engagement in their chosen areas of occupation within their own relevant and appropriate contexts.[4] Providing high-quality care to an OA will be one of the most rewarding and challenging practice areas for occupational therapists in the coming decade and beyond.

Occupational therapists who work primarily with OAs may be identified as **geriatric specialists.** Many are also considered **gerontologists** (i.e., they have completed further study in gerontology). OT practitioners with the geriatric population as well as students of gerontology must identify relevant frames of reference and conceptual models of practice[57] in building their own therapeutic frame of reference. A developmental frame of reference should be the foundation of practice in geriatrics. Occupational therapists with a specialty in geriatrics focus on disruptions in the normal maturational processes of OAs in the physical, cognitive, psychological, and social realms. The goal of intervention is to restore desired occupational performance and performance skills. When restoration is not possible, occupational therapists help OAs adapt to the pathological condition by way of various client factors that interfere with and underlie occupational performance. An understanding of normal human development and concepts such as the life course and the developmental tasks that relate to age-appropriate life roles, living situations, and occupations is a prerequisite for therapists working in this area. It is important to remember that development across the life span does not occur in distinct, hierarchical stages; rather, it is a dynamic and cyclical process. With a life course perspective, the emphasis is on the social pathways of human lives, their sequence of events, transitions, and social roles resulting in the creation of each OA's unique tapestry of life. This unique tapestry accounts for the great variation and richness of persons who comprise this population.

The clinical reasoning for OT practice in geriatrics is the focus of this chapter. The first section of the chapter illustrates the clinical reasoning process[97] through the case study of Mr. Lee. The second section provides information about the OA, aging demographics, age-related health changes, pathological conditions, and psychological adaptation; this review aims to prepare the reader for diagnostic[89] and procedural reasoning.[33] Therapists are encouraged to elicit the OA's personal story in developing therapeutic relationships and to use narrative reasoning.[73] Pragmatic reasoning[98] is highlighted so that the reader can better understand the practical realities of service delivery with OAs. The goal of this chapter is to help all OT practitioners, both novice and expert, better appreciate the complexities involved in working with OAs. It is hoped that readers will broaden their perspectives and employ better clinical reasoning and a multidimensional intervention approach to address the OA's physical, cognitive, psychological, and occupational performance needs.

OLDER ADULTS AND OCCUPATIONAL THERAPY

The growth of the OA population in the next few decades is expected to have an unprecedented effect on our society as a whole—on politics, economics, family life, and the health and human services industry. A better understanding of how to categorize or think about this population will be helpful because the increased number of OAs will change the practice of OT in the twenty-first century.

WHO IS THE OLDER ADULT?

Chronological age, or time since birth, is one method of categorizing the OA population. The term **older adult,** for comparative purposes, is defined as an individual 55 years of age or older (for labor force data collection).[54] Typically, though, persons 65 years of age or older are considered to be OAs. The population is further divided into categories of

young-old, composed of individuals age 65 to 74 years, and **old-old,** composed of individuals over 80 years of age. Concerns about the aged population that will directly and indirectly affect OT practice include the following:

- Greater life expectancy and increased numbers of OAs surviving longer with illness and disease
- Demographics related to gender, income, institutionalization, and living arrangements
- Increasing diversity within the aging population
- Higher prevalence of chronic conditions
- Greater numbers of limitations in performance of activities of daily living (ADLs) and instrumental activities of daily living (IADLs) as well as other areas of occupation
- Higher incidence of cognitive impairment
- Psychosocial issues that are compounded by age-associated changes and contextual features
- Greater demands for healthcare services
- More demands for alternative supported living and care facilities
- Need for more social supports
- Higher healthcare costs
- Increased demands for public funding
- Increased out-of-pocket health expenses
- Complex clinical presentations involving the interaction of age-associated changes, various clinical conditions, numerous medications, and many contextual and role changes

DEMOGRAPHIC FACTORS AND IMPLICATIONS FOR OCCUPATIONAL THERAPY

The number of OAs will continue to increase in the next three decades. Currently, the older population accounts for a little less than 13% of the total U.S. population but is expected to reach 20% in the year 2030.[31,54,113] At the present time, OAs use over a third of the nation's healthcare dollars, account for over a third of all hospital stays, and spend three times more of their total personal expenditures on healthcare than do consumers younger than age 65. Surprisingly, health expenditures peak for OAs in the 75- to 79-year-old age grouping and decline thereafter until old-old age, just before death, when expenditures markedly increase.[81]

There are more old-old women than men. Old-old women typically are widowed, live alone, and have lower income, especially after age 85.[109] Many OAs, especially women who are childless or whose children are not available, require support services and are more likely to be institutionalized when they reach the age of 80 or beyond. On average, OAs, especially those who are non-Caucasian, have a lower yearly income than all other adult groups. Older men, however, are twice as likely to be married or, if widowed, to remarry. Being married or living with family in later life is associated with higher household income, assistance with ADLs, social support, and reduced risk of institutionalization. It is projected that modernization and urbanization may begin to change the traditional family structures of cultures that typically have extended family households, especially in more developed Asian countries.[123] Assuming that they can afford it, OAs in the most developed countries tend to choose independent dwellings while maintaining close contact with family members, who provide support.[39]

The living arrangement needs of the OA population are expected to change in the second and third decades of the twenty-first century. Parents of current baby boomers are likely to live with or near their families and get support from children when they are very old.[32,47] However, as baby boomers reach old-old age, they may want or need more individualized care services. They are likely to wield more political power, expect more social services, and opt for more independence. They are likely to seek more supported housing alternatives or environmental adaptations to help them live independently at home.[17] Some suggest that institutionalization will become a less viable option.[54]

The institutionalization of OAs continues to remain stable at 5%.[54] Only a relatively small number of OAs live in institutions at any point in their lives; however, 25% to 30% of persons who reach the age of 65 can expect to spend some time in an institution before dying. Greater use is being made of residential care facilities, especially medical residential care. There has been a shift toward a mix of institutional long-term care and home-based care for the old-old.

The OA population is becoming more racially and ethnically diverse, requiring culturally competent therapists, healthcare professionals, and service agencies. According to 1998 data from the U.S. Bureau of the Census, minorities make up 15.7% of the 65+ population.[110] The smallest group is Native Alaskans or American Indians, followed by Asian-Americans and Hispanics; African-Americans make up the largest segment of this group. The number of OAs of minority race and ethnicity is expected to double by the year 2030. Future consumers of OT services are much more likely to be ethnically different from the OT practitioner providing intervention. Elders from minority racial and ethnic groups have higher rates of poverty compared with their Caucasian counterparts.[111] Poverty is often a barrier to obtaining quality healthcare, including OT.

The following factors are relevant in appreciating the diversity of the OA population:

- Each OA is unique as a result of varied life experiences and contexts.
- The degree to which a particular OA may identify with an ethnic group and the cultural traditions of that group (acculturation) is highly variable.
- Particular historical events that occurred during specific age periods in the OA's lifetime can be very influential.[121]

Elders of a particular ethnic group may share similar experiences with other same-age elders of that ethnic group (cohort of interest) but differ greatly from elders who have the same ethnicity but are 10 years younger or 10 years older. Sensitivity to these factors can help the therapist better understand the types of discrimination that the OA may have experienced and how history, race, and ethnicity can affect health beliefs, values, illness behaviors, self-image, and the degree of trust in and expectations of healthcare providers.[119] The OA must at all times be seen as a unique and worthy individual, a person who has a special "story of life" and configuration of occupations to share. A web-based resource for clinicians who work with OAs whose cultures and religions are different from their own, entitled *Diversity, Healing, and Health Care* (www.gasi.org/diversity), was developed by Bonnie Napier-Tibere, PhD, OTR/L, and co-sponsored by the Stanford Geriatric Education Center and On-Lok Senior Health. This helpful resource offers information on cohort life events, religious beliefs, and healing practices, as well as scenarios and useful definitions for the healthcare professional.

THREADED CASE STUDY: MR. LEE, PART 2

The Occupational Therapy Practice Framework is used to briefly discuss how Mr. Lee compares with other older adults living in the United States in terms of the cultural, physical, social, personal, and temporal aspects of context.[4] Mr. Lee, at the age of 83, belongs to the old-old age group. He fulfills many of the characteristics describing the old-old discussed in the previous section. As a Chinese-American man of 83 years he is in the minority, according to statistics on gender and ethnicity. Consistent with other demographic factors about OAs is that (1) Mr. Lee is remarried, (2) he lives with his wife, (3) his children are involved in his daily life and are living nearby, (4) he has assistance with ADLs, (5) he makes significant use of the healthcare system, (6) his income allows him to live independent of his children, (7) and he has been at low risk for institutionalization until recently. He is very traditional in terms of gender roles, which is consistent with his ethnicity, cohort group, and time of immigration. He values a patriarchical, traditional family structure that includes personal control and male independence and decision making as to home management. However, he embraces some degree of acculturation as it applies to medical intervention, preferring Western medicine over more traditional forms of health intervention.

HEALTH IN LATER LIFE

Improvements in sanitation, standards of living, medical care, technology, and access to healthcare have contributed to a longer lifespan. The price of this longevity has been a higher incidence of chronic medical conditions and associated limitations in daily activities, primarily for the old-old individual.[112] Functional limitations caused by chronic conditions increase with age. More than one third of persons 65 years of age and older identify a chronic condition that imposes some limitation in everyday living, but only 10% report that the limitation affects a major activity. The four most frequently reported medical conditions in later life are arthritis, heart disease, hearing impairments, and orthopedic impairments. Three fourths of the old-old identify one disability; more than half identify two or more disabling conditions. Old-old adults have twice as many problems with ADLs as do young-old adults. Of the old-old, 40% also have problems with IADLs.[112] Despite chronic medical conditions, OAs are generally able to adapt and maintain function until very late in life. Some researchers suggest that future estimates for disease burden vastly underestimate neuropsychiatric disorders as major and increasing sources of disease burden in the years to come.[77,78]

THEORY OF AGE-RELATED CHANGES

The process of aging is complex and inescapable, with an increased prevalence of degenerative diseases and a physiological decline in several body systems. Researchers question the extent to which decline is a normal part of aging. Most biological theories can be roughly grouped according to two major suppositions.[18,32,76] Some researchers believe that aging is the result of preprogrammed genes, which contain a master plan that triggers various mechanisms to cause cells to die.[44,106] Other theorists believe that aging is the result of accumulated cell damage. A number of accidental events occur, involving free-radical damage to genetic material and damage to cell components.[26,82,83] Immune system malfunction may cause cell damage and death.[10,115] Most experts agree that aging-related pathology involves both programmed genetic changes and accidental events.[93] Some of this aging-related pathology can be attenuated by environmental and lifestyle changes.

Age-Associated Physical Changes in Client Factors

Age-related changes, especially in organ systems, varies. A genetic component is partially responsible; other issues include progressive disease processes, environmental factors (e.g., environmental toxins and poverty), and lifestyle behaviors (e.g., smoking, lack of exercise, and poor nutrition) that can be changed or modified. The dietary restriction model suggests that dietary restriction (reduced calories) affects lifespan and extends life by decreasing metabolic rate. This decrease in metabolism can prolong life and modulate bone loss and the production of free radicals.[18] The ability to adapt to changes in the body system and the effect of those changes on everyday activity greatly depend on the OA's cognitive state, emotional state, social support systems, and basic physiology (e.g., client factors and context). Some of the changes identified in the following paragraphs have functional implications affecting occupational performance areas, but it is important to remember that the degree of change and the effect on function vary greatly for each OA.[32,66,70]

Sensory losses, especially with vision and hearing, are common. The effects can include problems with safety, self-image, relationships, and quality of life.[46,96] Asking about the OA's use of hearing aids and eyeglasses is recommended. Vision disturbances include less visual acuity under low light conditions, decreased accommodation speed in focusing, presbyopia (farsightedness), poorer color discrimination, cataract formation (with sensitivity to glare and blurring), and age-related macular degeneration (AMD).[79] These changes can negatively affect performance areas of driving, leisure performance, functional and community mobility, and many other IADLs and ADLs.

 OT PRACTICE NOTE

Surveys and other brief evaluations or screening of vision and hearing are always recommended before evaluating and carrying out interventions with older adults in any therapy setting.

Hearing discrimination is reduced, especially for high-frequency sounds and when distinguishing words in the presence of competing background noise. Hearing loss may be due to poor conduction (excess ear wax, calcifying ossicles, dislocated bones), sensorineural loss (damaged cochlea or auditory nerve), or presbycusis (damaged cochlea or deterioration in central auditory pathways). Hearing impairment affects several performance skills, negatively influencing the ability to interact with the environment and communicate effectively with others. This can lead to increased social isolation, depression, helplessness, paranoid thoughts, and cognitive decline.

Decreased efficiency of the kidneys in filtering wastes leads to lower thresholds for drug toxicity.[32,118] Less lean body mass, higher percentages of fat, and less water in the body all can alter the distribution of drugs in the body of OAs, leading to high blood concentration and excessive effects of medications. Therapists should be alert to the increased potential for drug toxicity in OAs and bring this information to the attention of the primary physician or nurse case manager.

Lungs become less elastic and efficient in the exchange of gases, and the diaphragm and intercostal muscles are weaker, therefore making the work of breathing more difficult. Decreased cardiovascular capacity on exertion affects endurance for demanding activity.[32,66] It can be difficult at times to determine whether such changes are due to the normal aging process or to physical deconditioning, underlying disease, or an associated response to medication interventions.[20] An appropriately designed exercise and training program, at less than maximal intensities, can positively affect quality of life and promote greater functional independence. Biological aging and disease and functional changes in the

OA's lifestyle can affect strength, flexibility, posture, gait, and pain levels.[70] As we age, more cross linkages occur, producing changes in the main supportive protein known as *collagen*. Muscle, skin, and tendons become less flexible because of changes in collagen and through decreased movement and activity. OAs experience decreased bone density and muscle mass in varying degrees, decreased muscular strength, and less joint flexibility, which can impede movement and mobility. Skin integrity is compromised because of decreased elasticity, leading to more wrinkles and thinning skin and increasing the risk of skin breakdown, tearing, and infection. A functional range of motion (ROM) and manual muscle test screening and a quick check of skin integrity are suggested.

Changes in the central nervous system (CNS) brain pathology, often seen at autopsy or on radiographic scans, include fewer neurons in select areas of the brain, a decreased number of dendrites, an increased number of amyloid deposits, more plaques, more neurofibrillary tangles, and reduced levels of certain neurotransmitters. These CNS changes in healthy OAs are puzzling, because many of these changes are also seen to a greater degree in dementia. An overall slowing of response time is common. Mild somatosensory changes occur in somatic receptors, in smell, in taste, and in the vestibular system; these can affect sensitivity thresholds and increase the risk of food poisoning, thermal and mechanical injuries, and falls. Asking OAs whether they have noticed any changes in these areas is prudent. Minimal age-associated changes also occur in the gastrointestinal system and the immune system.

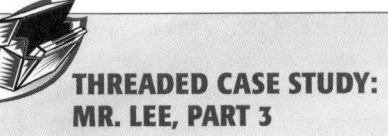 **THREADED CASE STUDY: MR. LEE, PART 3**

Mr. Lee, like many older adults, has experienced some age-associated physical changes in client factors of sensation. He is hard of hearing, which interferes with his performance skill of communication; information exchange; and relations with his wife, sons, and others in his social circle. It may also contribute to the ongoing stress in his marriage, his suspicions about his wife, and his role as a husband. He has established some dominating habits in his performance patterns related to suspicious thoughts concerning his wife. The interrelated client factor of decline in mental functions (discussed in the next section) increases the complexity of the effects of the physical changes experienced by Mr. Lee. As a result of cognitive changes and the decreased visual acuity from cataracts, left-sided weakness, and balance problems, compounded by age-related loss of muscle mass and less flexibility, Mr. Lee is at a high risk for falls and for other safety hazards, especially those involving the performance areas of functional and community mobility.

Age-Associated Cognitive Changes in Client Factors Mental Function

Changes in cognition, a client factor of mental function, often affect the ability to function because information processing and problem solving are so vital to safety and independence in ADLs. Actual cognitive decline can be a major threat to quality of life, and this threat is compounded when physical function, especially sensation, is impaired as well.[64] Many of these cognitive changes are related to treatable, temporary, or manageable medical problems. Some of the more important considerations when working with an OA include medication side effects; alcohol and nonprescription drug use; vision and hearing deficits; nutritional deficiencies; stress; sleep dysfunction; depression; and medical illnesses, such as diabetes, high cholesterol, and high blood pressure. These conditions may also be predictive of functional decline.[27] Cognitive decline becomes more substantial with each new medical condition that develops.

Occupational therapists find that cognitive capacity greatly affects the client's ability to benefit from rehabilitation. A more detailed discussion of cognitive aging can be found in other sources.[63,64,67] Cognition as a mental function is also discussed in Chapter 25. Age-associated differences exist in almost all aspects of cognition in healthy OAs, but this difference is usually minor, requiring more time and more extensive processing; it usually is not disabling, although it may be annoying. Age-associated differences in cognition usually do not present serious implications for ADLs and IADLs.[64,80] Researchers have found that cognitive processing efficiency, especially for working memory, information processing, and reaction time, is 1.5 times slower in OAs than in middle-aged or young adults.[51] Generally, OAs can, with effort and training, remember details with the same accuracy as younger persons.

Loss of memory is a concern for many OAs. **Memory** involves the retention, storage, and retrieval of information. Memory requires adequate attention to sensory-perceptual cues at the initial stages of reception and encoding.[65,104] Age differences have been found in working memory—one component of short-term memory. OAs exhibit poorer function in complex deliberate processing (i.e., simultaneously performing a cognitive task while trying to remember the information for a later task) than they do in automatic processing (i.e., remembering how to do a performed activity).[51,104] OAs also exhibit a decreased ability to inhibit thoughts that are irrelevant to the task.[65] Age-related deficits have been found in the recall of information, when information is retrieved from secondary (storage) memory levels, and this deficit worsens with advancing age.[25,63,64] However, the overall effects of age-related differences or changes in memory on daily function are minimal. Most healthy OAs are able to compensate for reduced processing resources by using the relevant context of situations, targeting environmental cues, providing environmental supports, rehearsing with elaboration, and developing new skills built on personal associations. Another area of aging-related effects is seen with impairments in recent episodic memories that are being retrieved. Often, rehabilitation services rely on the OA's use of this type of information, and it is important to develop these episodic memory skills until they become automatic and a part of procedural memory in long-term memory stores.[64]

When impaired cognition (especially memory) interferes with relationships, diminishes daily function, or affects quality of life, the causes should be explored because many of them are potentially treatable. Milder forms of memory loss are present in significant numbers of OAs. The *Diagnostic and Statistical Manual of Mental Disorders IV-TR* (DSM-IV-TR)[5] includes a classification of aging-associated cognitive change as "age-related cognitive decline" or age-associated memory impairment (AAMI), a part of normal aging affecting as many as 90% of OAs.[64] This is not a psychiatric disorder. Among the criteria for these cognitive changes is a decline in memory that is sufficient to worry the OA but not in excess of normal age function, as seen in dementia. The decline must be within normal limits when the client is compared, through psychometric testing, with others who are the same age. OAs who are tired, under stress, sick, or distracted are more likely to experience slower thinking and recall, experience more difficulty attending to and organizing information, and have difficulty recalling information, especially names, the placement of objects, and tasks requiring multiple actions, according to Levy.[64]

Memory loss that falls outside of normal limits by one standard deviation on test scores, with more severe memory lapses evident in recent memory that are persistent and begin to interfere with work and social activity (not ADLs), is identified as mild cognitive impairment (MCI).[5,84] In 50% of individuals with MCI, dementia develops within 3 years, although symptoms may have been evident for up to 7 years prior.[64,84] When cognitive impairment becomes so severe that it affects daily function, particularly a significant decline resulting in dependence in ADLs, a diagnosis of dementia is often made.

Therapists working with OA clients will encounter varying degrees of cognitive decline, and it is essential that they screen for cognitive impairments and consider cognition as a major factor when planning the intervention approach and carrying out interventions. Levy[64] suggests that occupational therapists can make an important contribution in the early detection and monitoring of cognitive decline by regularly assessing mental status on an informal basis during intervention and formally screening during the initial evaluation and periodically thereafter. Assessments such as the Mini Mental Status Exam,[34] with scoring adjusted for age, culture, and educational level, are helpful as screening tools.[1] An assessment tool such as the Functional Activities Questionnaire (FAQ)[85] has been used to assess functional abilities in IADLs to distinguish OAs who are experiencing more severe cognitive impairment from those who are experiencing MCI.[1,108]

Pathological Mental Conditions

Pathological or disease-related conditions may occur in OAs but are not part of normal aging. Dementia of the Alzheimer's type is a slowly developing, progressive, degenerative disease process involving short-term memory deficits (especially for recent events), noticeable decline in IADLs and ADLs, and a lack of awareness of functional decline that occurs with increasing frequency in some OAs as they age (see the discussion of Alzheimer's disease in Chapter 35). It is important to note that dementia of the Alzheimer's type is not an accelerated form of cognitive aging.[64] With an increased number of OAs attaining old-old status, occupational therapists can expect to see greater numbers of OA clients with dementia or other significant impairments in cognitive processing. Cognitive changes that emerge abruptly could be due to a medical condition such as a stroke. Sudden changes are often caused by delirium, the result of a more acute medical condition or toxic event that requires medical intervention. Therapists must learn to recognize cognitive decline. Training programs for clients can be designed to reverse AAMI. In the case of conditions that cause more severe impairments, occupational therapists can help clients and families manage the performance context and train caregivers to compensate for more severe information-processing deficits. These interventions may allow clients to remain in less restrictive settings longer and to have a better quality of life.[69]

Mr. Lee is experiencing noticeable and progressive deficits in short-term memory, especially for recent episodic events. He has difficulty attending, concentrating, and finding things. He also exhibits poor judgment, lack of self-monitoring, and poor insight according to the inpatient occupational therapist. Many of these deficits represent impaired executive functions. He continues to experience a significant change in his social and occupational functioning. Certainly, depending on the results of further evaluation, an MCI disorder or dementia, either vascular or of the Alzheimer's type, should be considered.

Psychological Adaptation

A new model postulates that successful aging is contingent on three elements: avoiding disease and disability, sustaining high cognitive and physical function, and engaging with life.[92] Most people are able to adapt successfully and manage the many transitions occurring in later life. Some of the positive aspects of later life include special relationships with grandchildren, an increased amount of free time to pursue one's own interests, and respect for one's wisdom and life experiences. Researchers and clinicians view OAs as proactive individuals who are able to cope with restrictions and prevail over challenging circumstances by continuously developing, taking action, recreating themselves, engaging in greater acceptance, and re-appraising priorities as needed.[94]

Stressors for OAs can be categorized as (1) major stressors, such as the death of family or friends or loss of identity after retirement; (2) persistent stressors, such as financial limitations and decreasing physical abilities; and (3) everyday hassles, such as intense arguments or other episodic conflicts. Persistent stressors are associated with a higher incidence of depression, and an increased number of everyday stressors is predictive of poorer reported health in the elderly.[56,116] According to research reviewed by Ruth and Coleman,[94] most OAs rate life events encountered in later years as no more stressful than events experienced earlier. The stresses of previous life events do not seem to have a cumulatively negative effect. The majority of OAs seems able to draw on personal and social resources to cope. Interestingly, their coping strategies (e.g., sublimation, suppression, and humor) are often more successful than the strategies used by younger adults.[24]

OAs use coping strategies such as considering themselves to be better off than OAs who may be doing less well, changing their priorities from goals that seem less attainable to those that are more realistic, and attributing failure to sources outside of themselves.[29,45] OAs also generally cope with threats of illness by using more positive strategies.[53,90] Experiencing quality of life and well-being is linked to the ability to engage in affect management—regulating feeling states, being proactive, and using self-management strategies to influence affective change; such techniques are especially useful when applied in a person's social realm.[19,59] In general, OAs seem to experience less anger as they age.[41,71,74] This decrease is consistent with a reduced need to effect change in the environment, a greater acceptance of secondary control, and the tendency to avoid strain in important interpersonal relationships. With positive adaptation to aging may come the ability to modulate negative emotions more effectively and to regulate the self rather than the environment.[72]

The occupational therapist assessing the relative coping abilities of an OA should consider whether the client's emotional stability and information-processing skills match his or her demands and resources. Problem-solving skills may be affected by four elements. The first element is the presence of antecedents such as the following:

- Health (both objective and subjective)
- Basic cognitive ability
- Personality characteristics, such as flexibility versus rigidity

The second element involves the client's approach to the problem and the nature of the problem to be solved. Do clients use an active or a passive individual approach? Can clients clearly identify problems and solutions? Is the problem itself well-structured or ill-structured? The third element affecting problem solving is the presence of contextual demands. Is the sociocultural and physical environment rich and supportive? The fourth element is related to whether the individual is likely to experience satisfaction and a sense of well-being when the problem is resolved.[117]

When antecedents are not optimal (e.g., diminished cognition or avoidance and high anxiety), when the problem is poorly structured, or when the environment lacks resources, problem solving with an OA can present challenges. In many cases, the problem-solving approaches used by OAs involve quick decision making and the use of solutions that are low in energy demand to achieve a quick resolution and reduce anxiety. This type of problem solving typically involves a very limited information search; uses fewer pieces of information; and emphasizes personalized, episodic knowledge about medical problems.[117] This frequently used approach relies almost exclusively on the extensive knowledge and past experience of the client, with limited or no search for new information.[103] This emphasis on the client's knowledge may mean that little attention is paid to gathering new data or more objective information.

In general, to reduce the distress and anxiety caused by the threat of illness, OAs generally are more vigilant about health problems, respond more quickly to health concerns, and make decisions more quickly than middle-aged adults.[62] OT practitioners can show respect for their clients as they carefully collaborate with them during each phase of the OT process, soliciting their beliefs and opinions during the clinical encounter and influencing the ways in which clients perceive health and solve problems.[120] OT practitioners should devote attention to eliciting from OAs and care providers their perspectives on health, health behaviors, experiences of illness, causes of illness, potential consequences of illness, and possible intervention strategies (Box 46-1). The practitioner can follow up on information from the client by using the LEARN (Berlin) mnemonic strategies (Box 46-2).

Not enough is known about the coping skills of frail elders. As people age, they may become more vulnerable to loss of perceived control and may acquire "learned helplessness."[102] This response in turn may make them more susceptible to illness.[91] The use of direct coping strategies, greater impulse control, positive appraisal of conflict situations, and optimism has been linked to better physical and psychological health, greater responsibility for managing personal health, and cushioning of the ill effects of stress.[28,87,101] The use of direct control strategies works well for many OAs in adapting to changes in later life. Sometimes, OAs find themselves in uncontrollable situations (e.g., eviction from their homes, chronic illness, or loss of driving privileges). In these circumstances, OAs might benefit from using coping mechanisms that render such situations more palatable and reduce internal dissonance. The old-old adult may actually adapt best by accepting change, accommodating to negative events, and framing events in a more positive way.

Occupational therapists who work in geriatric settings are encouraged to work collaboratively, empowering their OA clients to be active problem solvers, to attempt to reframe challenges, to see the potential of positive outcomes, and to consider several perspectives when framing problems. Clark and colleagues have identified several domains of interest and adaptive strategies focused on the concept of fostering occupational performance by OAs.[22] Well-elderly lifestyle redesign programming based on these life domains

---

Box 46-1 | **KEY QUESTIONS FOR CLIENT-PRACTITIONER DIALOGUE**

1. How would you describe the problem that has brought you to me?
2. What do you think is wrong, or what is causing your problem?
3. Why do you think this problem happened to you?
4. Why do you think this problem started when it did?
5. What do you think your sickness does to you? How does it work?
6. How bad (severe) do you think your illness is? Do you think it will last a long time, or do you think it will get better soon?
7. Why did you decide to come to me for treatment?
8. Apart from me, who else do you think can help you get better?
9. What do you think will help clear up your problem?
10. What are the most important results that you hope to get from treatment?
11. Are there things that make you feel better or give you relief that the doctors don't know about?
12. Has anyone else helped you with this problem?
    A. What did that person say was wrong with you?
    B. What did that person say you should do for this problem?
    C. Do you agree?
    D. Did you try it?
13. What are the chief problems that your illness has caused you?
14. Does it cause problems for your family?
15. What worries you most about your sickness?
16. Is there anyone else that you would like me to talk to about your problem?
17. Is there anything else that you would like to discuss?

Data from Harwood E: Rationale, psychology, philosophy and reason for recreational activities for the frail aged, *Aust Nurses J* 10(7):38, 1981; Kleinman A, Eisenberg L, Good B: Culture, illness, and care, *Ann Intern Med* 88:251, 1978.

Box 46-2 | **LEARN MNEMONIC**

L   *Listen* with sympathy and understanding to the client's perceptions.

E   *Explain* your perception of the problem.

A   *Acknowledge* and discuss the differences and similarities.

R   *Recommend* treatment.

N   *Negotiate* agreement.

From Berlin EA for Stanford University Division of Family Medicine and the South Bay Area Health Education Center, DHHS Grant Number 5-UOI-PE-00053-04 (date unknown).

has resulted in lower healthcare expenditures and improved health outcomes.[21] Occupational therapists are in a unique position to help OA clients take some measure of personal control over their everyday lives by collaboratively constructing meaningful routines that can reduce the health risks of older adulthood. OT offers opportunities to take risks, confront obstacles, achieve personal control, and improve self-efficacy. Through therapeutic use of self and other psychosocial interventions, therapists can facilitate clients' management of dissonant or disturbing thoughts and feelings.

THREADED CASE STUDY:
MR. LEE, PART 4

Mr. Lee is struggling to adapt psychologically to situations over which he has little control, such as changed physical and mental status and the loss of highly valued roles and occupations (e.g., traditional role of husband, control over home matters, and activities of daily living, especially community mobility and driving). He responds by becoming more demanding and critical of his wife's attempts at assistance. He has become increasingly suspicious of her absences from the home when she does errands without him. He shows limited ability to adapt to negative events; has difficulty framing events in a positive light; and shows an attitude of fatalism about things that he can change, such as cataract surgery. The coping mechanisms are less effective at reducing the internal dissonance that he is experiencing, leaving him feeling angry and blaming things outside of himself. These emotions result in behavior that threatens his personal and social relationships and his potential for more positive rehabilitation outcomes.

Mr. Lee's ability to constructively problem solve is impeded by several elements. First, he is in poor to fair health, has notable deficits in cognition related to memory and executive function, and tends to display some rigid personality characteristics. Second, while he generally has used an active approach to problem solving, he is having difficulty accurately identifying problems, the problems are ill-structured, and solutions are frequently viewed as externally situated. Third, the context has several social and cultural factors that support Mr. Lee's particular view of reality, offers a willing caregiving partner, and an adaptable physical environment with necessary financial resources. Fourth, it is unclear whether Mr. Lee will experience satisfaction at the resolution of problems that he considers to be less important but that are identified as important on the basis of the demands of his current environment and context.

Psychiatric disorders

Approximately 22% of individuals who are 65 years of age or older meet the diagnostic criteria for a mental disorder.[50,107] It is important to remember that even if prevalence rates of mental disorders in the OA population stay the same, the number of OAs with mental disorders will rise as the crude number of adults surviving into old age across the world also increases.[38] Mental disorders in OAs may occur because of one of the following scenarios:

- A continuation or recurrence of a condition that first emerged earlier in the person's life
- A first appearance of a disorder that was already present in a latent form (e.g., a mental health liability from the past that has been exacerbated in old adulthood, as when developmental issues remain unresolved)
- A new mental disorder occurring in later life

Pathological mental conditions often occur in older adulthood because of physiologically based changes in brain function or brain disorders. Less frequently, the cause is an inability to adapt to changes, losses, and transitions, or these factors may exacerbate an existing condition. OAs who have adjusted poorly to previous stressors, who are overwhelmed by multiple simultaneous stressors, or who have little social support are particularly vulnerable. Anxiety is the most common mental disorder of OAs (11.5%), followed by severe cognitive disorders (6.6%; discussed previously in this chapter) and depressive disorders (4.4%).[107] Alcohol abuse and personality disorders are less common but are still cause for concern because they further complicate the clinical picture.

Alcohol abuse

Alcohol abuse may be considered a hidden disease in later life because many OAs who drink alcohol, particularly men, do so at home.[68,107] Symptoms of alcohol abuse include an increased tolerance to the effects of the substance and increased consumption over time.

OAs are more susceptible to the effects of alcohol, even when they consume less of it, because of age-related changes such as decreased liver and kidney function and reduced water content and body mass. Many OAs are taking medications, and the concurrent use of alcohol and use or abuse of medications can lead to greater risk of intoxication or toxicity. Substance abuse leads to increased accidents, a greater risk of falls, poor nutrition, poor hygiene, increased mental health problems (e.g., depression, delirium, dementia, and psychosis), a higher suicide rate, higher risk of disease (e.g., liver disease, cancer, cardiovascular problems, and diabetes), and increased mortality. Physicians may not regularly question OA clients about their drinking habits; moreover, if the client does disclose that he or she drinks alcohol, the physician may minimize the severity and consequences. Generally, heavy drinking is defined as 12 to 21 drinks per week.[107] The CAGE questionnaire is useful for screening for alcohol abuse.[30] Effective interventions include self-help groups such as Alcoholics Anonymous (AA), counseling, psychotherapy, and medications. Occupational therapists may ask OAs questions from the CAGE questionnaire. It is anticipated that alcohol abuse will increase among OAs as baby boomers age because this cohort has a greater history of alcohol abuse than the current cohort of older adults.[107]

Depression

The rate of major depression is relatively low—about 5% or less in OAs,[42] using the DSM criteria of depressed mood and loss of interest or pleasure in activities, significant weight loss or gain, sleep disturbance, psychomotor agitation or retardation, fatigue, feelings of worthlessness, loss of concentration, and recurrent thoughts of death or suicide.

OAs are less likely to report dysphoric symptoms or express hopelessness, both benchmarks for a diagnosis of major depression. The presence of depressive symptoms notwithstanding, a type of subclinical depression seems to increase with advancing age, especially in women and when symptom-based assessments are used. Depressive symptoms and syndromes have been identified in 8% to 20% of older community residents.[2,35] The symptoms (associated with depression) most frequently reported by OAs are fatigue, difficulty in waking in the early morning, difficulty in going back to sleep, and memory complaints. These complaints are less likely to include sadness (e.g., hopelessness, worthlessness, thoughts of death, wanting to die, and suicide), but this pattern of complaints leaves the OA at increased risk for subsequent functional impairment, cognitive impairment, psychological distress, and death.[36]

Suicide is a major risk in late-life depression. Caucasian men between the ages of 60 and 85 years have an increased risk of suicide, especially if they are 85 and older, have a medical illness, or live alone. Many saw their physician within 1 month of the suicide.[107] Mortality from other diseases, such as heart disease and cancer, has been linked to depression.

The incidence of depression in OAs may be higher than reported because of underreporting or lack of recognition.[61] Many healthcare providers focus on somatic symptoms, linking patient complaints to a succession of physical problems without screening for depression. Risk factors for late-life depression include persistent insomnia; unresolved, untreated grief after the death of a loved one; and structural neuroanatomical changes (e.g., enlarged lateral ventricles, cortical atrophy, increased white matter, decreased caudate size, and vascular lesions in the caudate nucleus).[107]

Depression may increase the degree of disability associated with several medical conditions and negatively affect rehabilitation outcomes. Depression also may complicate the clinical picture of dementia or cause complaints and symptoms that are confused with dementia.[86] Depression can have a major influence on the engagement of an OA in occupational performance areas, including ADLs, IADLs, and social participation. OAs are not likely to seek intervention for depressive symptoms, perhaps because myths about aging create the mistaken belief that depression is inevitable and justifiable. Other barriers to intervention are lack of access to care or the need to be stoic. Occupational therapists in all geriatric settings should screen for depressive symptoms in OAs if this is not being done by other healthcare professionals. Screening measures include the Geriatric Depression Scale (GDS)[122] and the Beck Depression Inventory (BDI).[7]

Theories abound as to the causes of depression. One theory proposes that depression is biologically caused and may result from medications (toxicity) and certain somatic illnesses. A second theory suggests that depression is really a reaction to the stress of illness or disability. Depression can be treated successfully with medications in most cases. Clients can return to previous energy levels and again take pleasure in life. OT can help clients regain lost occupations, develop pleasurable and health-promoting routines, learn how to reframe events, change habits of nonproductive thinking, develop social contacts, and experience success.

Anxiety disorders are also very common in OAs, but these conditions have received much less attention. Anxiety usually begins earlier in life and infrequently in late life, the most common disorder being a phobic anxiety disorder.[107] Anxiety disorders may take various forms:

- Recurring, sudden episodes of intense apprehension with shortness of breath and chest pain (panic disorders)
- Fear and the disproportionate avoidance of a perceived danger (phobic disorder)
- Chronic, persistent, and excessive anxiety (generalized anxiety disorder)[37]

Biologically based explanations for age-related anxiety suggest that it may be associated with changes in neurotransmitters, decreased noradrenergic function, side effects of some medications, and anxiety-like symptoms of medical conditions (e.g., myocardial infarct or pulmonary embolism). Worry or "nervous tension," rather than specific anxiety syndromes, may be more important in OAs. Anxiety symptoms that do not fulfill the criteria for specific syndromes are reported in up to 17% of older men and 21% of older women.[107] From a psychological perspective, OAs may in fact have a realistic basis for their anxiety.[37] It is not uncommon for anxiety to coexist with depression and other mental disorders.[107] Anxiety may be related to concerns about pain, safety, memory loss, fear of the unknown, finances, or caregivers. Anxiety may be crippling when it interferes with attention, memory, enjoyment of pleasurable events, social skills, and the ability to begin or follow through with the therapy program.

In addition, some anxiety disorders that have received less study in OAs, such as post-traumatic stress disorder (PTSD), may become more important in the near future. PTSD is expected to assume increasing importance as Vietnam veterans age and as more individuals are exposed to catastrophic events. Vietnam-era veterans have been found to have a PTSD prevalence of 15% 19 years after exposure to combat.[75,107] Therapists should routinely assess the client's level of anxiety and determine the degree to which anxiety may affect function. Le Barge provides a scale to evaluate anxiety in clients with mild cognitive impairments.[60]

Personality disorders

Personality disorders (PDs) are lifelong, enduring, inflexible, and pervasive tendencies that interfere with the client's functioning and may cause distress. They are characterized by distorted perception, obliviousness to the reaction of others, inappropriate emotional outbursts, and difficulty controlling impulsive behaviors.[5] Although PDs do not develop in later life, they may not be noticed until that point, when an initially vulnerable individual becomes increasingly less adaptive.[95] OAs with PDs can be found in all areas of adult practice and provide an interesting challenge. Clients with certain PDs make some of the greatest demands on the therapist's time and patience and can disrupt the therapist's emotional equilibrium. Therapists who find themselves feeling frustrated, confused, and guilty (or avoiding particular clients) should consult with a knowledgeable colleague and explore their feelings about the client-therapist relationship. Butin provides a useful description of several characterological types and offers some helpful suggestions to OT practitioners.[16]

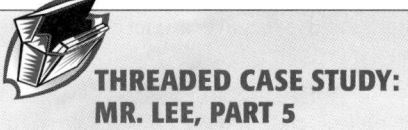

THREADED CASE STUDY: MR. LEE, PART 5

Mr. Lee is experiencing several depressive symptoms, including decreased interest in previously enjoyable activities, increased irritability, fatigue, difficulty waking in the early morning and trouble returning to sleep, decreased appetite, and feelings of worthlessness. He also expresses passive suicidal thoughts ("I would be better off dead") without outlining a specific plan or means. He reports that others are better off than he is, he is not satisfied with his life, he often gets bored, he is afraid something bad is going to happen to him, he feels his life is empty, he would rather stay at home than do new things, he has more problems with memory than most, he feels his situation is hopeless, it is not wonderful to be alive now, and he feels helpless. He scored 10 out of 15 on the GDS, a score indicating moderate depression.

STEREOTYPES OF OLDER ADULTS

Many of the attitudes and values associated with practice in geriatrics are based on stereotypes and personal experiences. Some stereotypes are negative, and others are positive (Table 46-1). Taken to extremes, stereotypes can influence the clinical reasoning of all members of the healthcare team. Because the therapeutic relationship is such a powerful agent for change, OT practitioners must assess their various motives for choosing geriatric practice and then assess the effects of these motives, attitudes, and values on the client, the therapeutic relationship, and the OT process.

The preceding information should frame the discussion that follows regarding the OT process in geriatric practice.

OCCUPATIONAL THERAPY PROCESS

The remainder of this chapter considers the evaluation and intervention process for the OA with a complex clinical presentation. Evaluation and intervention are discussed from the perspectives of both the entry-level and the experienced clinician. We believe that effective interventions with OAs require the therapist to consider multiple perspectives and a range of variables concurrently. Hence, the clinician must possess abundant common sense and a fair amount of experience and must use the OTPF, focusing on the categories that contribute to the OA's engagement in meaningful occupations for maximal participation in the contexts of their lives.

EVALUATION PROCESS

The OTPF guides the evaluation process. Using the occupational profile, the occupational therapist engages in a client-centered process to determine why the OA is seeking OT services. The therapist, working collaboratively with the OA and significant others, helps determine what occupations and activities are successful and which are problematic. The performance context of the OA is evaluated to ascertain barriers and supports. The OA's occupational history is obtained, his or her priorities are established, and outcomes for therapy are determined and agreed upon.

Consider the referral information for the case study of Mr. Lee. An occupational therapist would begin by interviewing Mr. Lee to determine his perception of his ability to function, valued roles, routines and habits, areas of interest, activities in which he has been involved (areas of occupation and performance patterns), his prior level of functioning, and his current level of functioning. An evaluation or standardized assessment of current functioning and of the occupational performance contexts would follow. The therapist would also interview the family about their perceptions of his ability to function and his needs. The therapist would encourage family members to express their concerns.

ANALYSIS OF OCCUPATIONAL PERFORMANCE

EVALUATION

The therapist will want to determine the importance that the client places on the seven different areas of occupation: ADLs, IADLs, education, work, play, leisure, and social participation.[4] Methods of evaluation may include interviews and performance-based observations and assessments. Both the OA and any significant others should, at some point, participate in the interview. The roles of each person and his

TABLE **46-1**   **Stereotypes About Older Adults**

Myth	Reactions of Care Providers	Facts About Aging
Old people are all alike.	Providers may come to the initial evaluation with preconceptions about older adults that can influence observations and data collected and lower expectations for treatment results.	Older adults demonstrate greater heterogeneity than in any other age group; their collection of experiences and different lifestyles make them a very diverse group.
Old people are lonely and ignored by their family.	Providers might not collaborate with the family in the therapy process. They may not explore the older adult's role in the family. They may ignore the client's desire for more limited socialization and may make plans for the client out of pity or a sense that the therapist knows best.	Older adults are generally more satisfied than other groups. Most are in close contact with their families. Most are cared for by their family when possible, rather than institutionalized; if they live alone, it is usually by choice.
Old people are senile. Old people can't learn new things.	Providers may use overly simple words and condescend to the older adult. Providers may talk to the caregiver or adult children instead of allowing older adults to make decisions for themselves. Providers may expect older adults to prove their competence and may act as if older adults cannot give an accurate history. Providers may not make efforts to use educational or teaching methods.	Older adults show slower cognitive response time than younger adults. Confusion and significant memory loss are not a normal part of aging and should be investigated for such causes as dementia, depression, medication toxicity, and other medical problems.
Most older adults are sickly and end up in nursing homes.	Providers may emphasize illness without considering strengths as well. Providers may have lowered expectations for recovery, may not make the therapy situation challenging enough, and may not provide instruction in wellness, prevention, and maintenance.	Only 5% of older adults are institutionalized at any one time. The risk for institutionalization increases with age. Most older adults do not suffer from activity restrictions despite having at least one chronic medical problem when young-old. Most elders report their health to be good when compared with others their age.
Older people are rigid, don't like change, and live in the past.	Providers may negate the usefulness of reminiscing and stop listening. They may stop planning for new activities and stop active planning for the future, may stop providing older adults with information and talk to their children or others instead, and may negate the experiences of older adults as old-fashioned and unscientific.	Most likely, rigid older adults were also rigid when they were younger. Personality characteristics tend to remain stable over time. Older adults have a tendency to conserve cognitive energy when making decisions and may give greater credence to experience at the expense of new information for decisions.
Older people are not attractive or sexy.	Providers may view sexual interest as abnormal. They may expect that desire for sex will stop in late life. They may minimize the importance of grooming and dressing attractively. Providers may make no provisions for privacy for sexual activity and may joke about sexual activity or flirtations from older adults.	Desire and ability for sexual functioning change, but with good health, sex can remain satisfying and people can remain active into the tenth decade of life.

Adapted from Ferrini AF, Ferrini RL: *Health in the later years*, ed 3, Boston, 2000, McGraw-Hill.

or her interrelationships with the occupational performance areas must be considered.

Performance-based evaluations may involve both a standardized assessment and informal or more structured observation. A standardized assessment will permit comparing the client's results with an objective standard. The validity of each assessment should be considered as it applies to norms for an older population. Among the many resources for assessments are Asher's *Annotated Index of Occupational Therapy Evaluation*

Tools,[6] Hinojosa and colleagues' *Evaluation*,[48] and Larson and colleagues' *Role of Occupational Therapy and the Elderly*.[58]

Optimally, the evaluation is completed in the same context (i.e., same time of day and physical environment) in which the OA will be functioning. A familiar context allows the OA to use environmental cues to facilitate performance. This familiarity is particularly important for OAs with cognitive, perceptual, or sensory deficits. Such individuals typically develop compensatory strategies within their living environment that allow them to function independently. When removed from their living environment, they become more dependent.

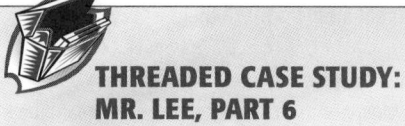

THREADED CASE STUDY:
MR. LEE, PART 6

During the analysis of occupational performance, the occupational therapist, after synthesizing information from the occupational profile, would observe performance in the areas that involve functional and community mobility because these were Mr. Lee's priority. A secondary focus, as the therapy progresses, would be on the area of social participation as it relates to his family and eventually to his relationships at the senior center. The therapist chooses to observe mobility outside and around the home and observe the activities of daily living that involved functional mobility as it related to bathing and showering and toileting; she used the Functional Independence Measure (FIM), the BERG balance scale to assess functional balance,[8] the GDS to assess mood,[122] the MMSE to assess basic mental status in cognition,[34] and the Caregiver Strain Questionnaire to elicit family concerns and burdens.[88]

Mr. Lee scored 92/126 on the FIM scale, indicating problems with independence that will require some form of supervision (less for physical assistance and more for safety reasons related to Mr. Lee's impulsivity and poor problem-solving skills). His score of 33/56 on the Berg balance scale suggests that his mobility is severely affected and he is often at risk for falls—a major problem. He would probably be able to achieve functional ambulation in the home because he is familiar with the surroundings. However, he will be less functional when out in the community, where there are more novel and unpredictable challenges. He will require constant supervision when ambulating in the community. On the MMSE he scored a total of 20 out of 30, below average for his age and educational level, with mild deficits in orientation to time and place, moderate deficits in initial and delayed recall in short-term memory, poor concentration, difficulties with calculations, poor repetition, poor comprehension, and mild problems with praxis. His GDS score of 10/15 indicates moderate depression.

This evaluation strategy was consistent with Mr. Lee's desire for more independence in mobility inside and outside the home. His desire to be more independent in daily occupations reflects his wish to exert more personal control and competence in his daily life. This therapeutic perspective involved viewing Mr. Lee's occupational performance through the lens of contextual issues that included cultural traditions and male dominance in the home and in his relationships. These factors were very important motivations for him.

Another approach, rather than identifying specific neuropsychological functions, would involve the therapist's choice to use the Cognitive Performance Test (CPT)[11-15,52] or the Allen Diagnostic Module craft project (or both).[3]

This method of assessing functional performance identifies information-processing capabilities influencing occupational performance.[64] It would be an alternative strategy, given the degree of cognitive disability present in this case. The CPT, being performance based, is useful in determining the ways in which executive dysfunction influences functional performance. Executive abilities can also be determined through direct and systematic observation of ADLs, especially in naturalistic settings.[40,99,100]

Activities of Daily Living

The initial evaluation of ADLs must consider the mental and physical fatigue of the client, as well as time constraints placed on the therapist, and therefore may not include all aspects of self-care. It is not unusual for an entry-level therapist to attempt to evaluate all aspects of ADLs, perhaps following a checklist from top to bottom without regard for the client's needs. The experienced clinician is able to select a few key ADLs from the checklist or a key standardized assessment that efficiently covers an array of tasks. The information gathered from a performance evaluation produces data concerning functional activities and abilities and limitations in performance skills. Consider the information gathered from the initial evaluation for Mr. Lee, summarized in the subsequent paragraphs.

During the initial portion of the home visit, while evaluating functional mobility, the OT observed that Mr. Lee walked with a rolling walker with a pronounced list to the right. He had difficulty negotiating changes in walking surfaces and getting around some obstacles in the living room, kitchen, and bathroom. He seemed surprised by these difficulties when they were brought to his attention and quickly blamed his wife and the walker for impairments in his mobility. He displayed visual and perceptual deficits, poor motor planning, and poor problem-solving ability when adapting to changing environments. His performance improved when he was able to rely on tactful verbal cues from his wife. He had great difficulty getting up the stairs, and the couple reported that their sons come over once a week to provide maximal physical assistance to get up the stairs. He receives a sponge bath from his wife in the downstairs bathroom during the week.

During evaluation of his showering abilities in the second-floor bathroom, Mr. Lee was asked to demonstrate how he got in and out of the shower stall. Just before entering the bathroom, he left his walker at the door, instead using the wall and fixtures for support. He grasped the towel rack for balance when entering and exiting the shower stall. No rubber mats or tub bench were present. He entered the shower stall without first turning on the water and testing the temperature. He was breathing heavily and obviously fatigued after standing in the shower and was unable to complete the demonstration of his showering and drying routine during a 4-minute interval. During the drying simulation, he had difficulty managing the large bath towel effectively, nearly losing his balance on several occasions. He began yelling at his wife, demanding that she help him. He promptly quit the activity when the therapist asked his wife to step back for a few moments. Mrs. Lee reports that she often physically assists him during the showering process, helping him in and out of the shower and assisting him with washing, rinsing, and drying. Mr. Lee used the wall-mounted vanity to assist with lowering and rising from the low toilet. He was observed dropping to the toilet seat from a distance of 12 inches. He had difficulty maintaining his balance when toileting involved bowel hygiene and clothes fastening because he could not use his left upper extremity for stabilization.

The last occupational performance ADL evaluated was Mr. Lee's ability to get in and out of the car and safely ambulate from the car to his destination. Mr. Lee was observed ambulating from the house to the car. He descended the two stairs to the garage by using the wall for support while his wife carried his walker. He impatiently told her to hurry up with his walker. He first attempted to go down the steps using alternate legs per step, and he almost fell. He had to resort to taking one step at a time because of the weakness in his legs. Similar difficulties were observed when he attempted to go down two steps from the entrance of his home to the street. He demonstrated poor problem-solving ability, failing to anticipate the consequences of his most recent stroke and the resultant changes in his abilities. He lacked the ability to self-monitor and self-correct for his errors in judgment and required cueing from the therapist to prevent a fall. It was apparent that he did not remember the stair training that he received as an inpatient 5 days earlier from his physical therapist. He failed to use his walker when attempting to ambulate 6 feet from the stairs to the car and relied on items such as the lawn-mower for support, retorting that his wife was too slow in bringing the walker to him. While stepping into the car, he failed to position his body correctly, hit his head against the roof of the car, and neglected to use the car for support. When exiting the car, he did not wait for his wife to bring the walker to him and started to walk while holding on to the body of the car.

The evaluation approach for analyzing occupational performance requires clinical judgment as to the best way to develop rapport with the client. Starting the evaluation with an assessment of performance skills (e.g., motor, process, and communication) while explaining the relationship of results to function may be most acceptable to a client who is reticent about his personal life and who is very task-oriented. On the other hand, beginning with an open-ended question, such as "Tell me what a typical day is like for you" or "Please tell me how this illness has affected you and your family," may be more effective for other clients. For example, a client who is uncomfortable being touched, who dislikes the feeling of being "tested," or who has a different cultural perspective might be more comfortable with self-report or interview-based assessment than with an initial evaluation of performance skills. The skillful OT practitioner considers performance in all areas of occupation but uses seasoned observation skills to determine which key performance skills should be evaluated in light of their effects on areas of occupation.

Prior Level of Function

When working with a younger client with a newly acquired physical disability, the occupational therapist may assume that the client was independent, active, and healthy before the injury or illness; often, the therapist will adopt an approach based on biomechanical evaluation and intervention. The typical OA will have a more complex clinical picture, sometimes with multiple chronic conditions (multichronicity) in addition to the main diagnosis. Therefore, a rehabilitation approach might be more appropriate than a biomechanical one, even though restoration of prior motor skill is the ideal goal. The entry-level clinician may focus on the newly acquired disability and not consider the ways in which other age-related changes, pathological conditions, or performance contexts affect function. The more experienced clinician evaluates for age-related changes, gathers pertinent history of prior pathological conditions, and considers the potential effect. An objective evaluation, in conjunction with a medical history and interview with the client and significant others, will provide the clinician with the most accurate information about the OA's previous functional level.

Therapists must guard against stereotypical thinking that may lead to erroneous beliefs. For example, a lengthy medical history with multiple diagnoses may conjure visions of an OA with severe limitations when, in fact, the person is quite active. Conversely, the OA client with a newly acquired physical disability, no prior medical history, and minor age-related changes may provide a history that is more limited in the scope of activities than the therapist might anticipate.

Performance Context

During the evaluation process the occupational therapist must take into consideration the client's performance contexts (cultural, physical, social, personal, spiritual, temporal, and virtual).[4] The OA's social, cultural, and physical context affects the degree and type of involvement in areas of occupation.

Social and cultural context

A person's perception of the aging process, disease, and disability is filtered through the lenses of social and cultural expectations and beliefs. Fortunately, elders are respected in the traditional Chinese culture; members of the community still consult Mr. Lee about many matters, especially financial and business issues. This form of respect extends to a patriarchical role for the eldest man in the family, whose decisions are interpreted as law for the rest of the family. For example, the therapist observed that Mr. Lee was sitting and having his wife wait on him rather than helping himself. By talking with Mr. Lee, the therapist learned that his mother had cared for his father after his father had experienced several episodes of myocardial infarctions, and this caregiver role was expected. Mr. Lee's father had progressively declined and was dependent on family members. Even though Mr. Lee, unlike his father, is recovering and improving with intervention, cultural traditions are a powerful contextual factor. Mr. Lee has the potential to be independent, according to the perspective of the therapist, but he has a longstanding history of expecting certain subservient behaviors from his wife. The occupational therapist must be sensitive when working with Mr. Lee, respecting his role as a male elder in his community while still helping him see the progress that he is making. It may be useful to help him identify with other OAs of his acquaintance who have also recovered from a serious illness. The senior center, a place that Mr. Lee values, may offer such resources. Mr. Lee's cognitive impairment and emotional distress are affecting his judgment and relationships with his family. Other aspects for the therapist to consider are the sudden demands that he is placing on Mrs. Lee for personal assistance and accountability for her whereabouts, his blaming behavior, and his overall aggressiveness when relating to her.

The OT practitioner must cautiously examine the notion of independence, which is interpreted differently depending on culture. The practitioner must consider how to frame the intervention approach so as to best collaborate with the client and family members and incorporate their cultural beliefs into the intervention plan. This initially involves listening closely to the family's beliefs and concerns and may involve educating the family members about the client's condition and teaching them ways in which they can assist the older client more effectively.

During the interview, the occupational therapist asks questions to elicit the OA's views of disability (see Box 46-1). Asking open-ended questions demonstrates respect and allows the client to express concerns, ideas, and beliefs; in turn, this gives the therapist a clearer sense of the client's knowledge, values, stereotypes, and motivations. Mr. Lee, like many Chinese-born persons of the same age, has a fatalistic view of illness. This perspective is reflected in his resigned attitude about his visual impairment and in his expectations that his wife will take care of things that he is no longer able to do. His cultural perspective hampers his motivation to regain functional independence in several areas of personal care, but it fuels his desire for competence in functional and community mobility that involves "keeping face" in the public eye. Cultural and social expectations are particularly evident in ADLs. Examples of respectful consideration include awareness of the client's need for privacy, because culture may dictate issues (gender or age restrictions) regarding private functions, and respecting the client's selection of the family members who are allowed to assist with dressing or bathing. The therapist should also be aware of the client's religious or cultural dietary restrictions and traditions for food preparation and consumption, such as vegetarianism or adherence to kosher practices.

A fine balance must be maintained in evaluating and considering cultural and social values with people of diverse backgrounds. The therapist must refrain from ethnocentrism and stereotyping. The OT practitioner must be sensitive to each client's degree of acculturation. Even with awareness of cultural diversity, the practitioner must also be sensitive to the uniqueness and the particular value system of each client and social or cultural context.

Spiritual, personal, and temporal context

Spiritual needs and personal factors may affect the OA's intervention goals and motivation. Mr. Lee is Buddhist. Attendance at the Buddhist temple and ancestor worship at home require brief periods of kneeling and frequent changing of position. The occupational therapist worked with the physical therapist, Mr. Lee's sons, and the Buddhist monk at the temple to help Mr. Lee see that respectful worship was still possible without kneeling at this time. With the inclusion of his sons and the support of the Buddhist monk, Mr. Lee came to accept that worship and attendance at temple were priorities over the ritual of kneeling. The occupational therapist was then able to shift the intervention focus to safe functional mobility as it related to engaging in worship at home and identifying suitable transportation to worship at the Buddhist temple.

At 82, Mr. Lee is in the retirement phase of life. He has several investment properties and is still a restaurant owner. He has done exceptionally well for a person who did not receive a high-school education. He is insured with Medi-Care, parts A and B, and the recently implemented part D prescription coverage. In addition, he has sufficient gap insurance, which allows him to finance his medical needs. He owns his home and is financially secure and able to fund additional in-home services and durable medical equipment (DME).

Physical and virtual context

For many OAs, access to computers and other technology can help to facilitate occupations and social and business relationships. This access can be especially important to persons with limited mobility caused by dysfunction, disability status, or geographical and social isolation. Mr. Lee has expressed no interest in developing his virtual context. He reports that he relies on service professionals (e.g., lawyers, accountants) and family members in this area and that he believes the telephone to be more than adequate for his communication needs.

The appropriate physical context may significantly improve the OA's functioning. The evaluation should elicit information about the environment to which the OA will be discharged. If possible, the occupational therapist may complete a predischarge home evaluation. In many cases, this evaluation is not a reimbursable service, so the occupational therapist must work closely with family members to explore potential obstacles in the home environment and determine needed equipment or modifications by interview rather than direct observation. Home evaluations entail consideration not only of the newly acquired physical disability but also of existing and predicted age-related changes.[105] Given the OA's deficits in neuromusculoskeletal, sensory, and mental body functions and skills in motor, process, and communication, the evaluation should consider safety and home modifications to promote independent functioning and prevent falls.

Entry-level clinicians tend to focus primarily on current problems and may not consider the interaction of age-related problems, preexisting deficits, and current problems with regard to the OA's function in the discharge environment. The more experienced clinician consistently attempts to consider age-associated factors and all of the relevant factors in the client's performance contexts when determining the effect of OT recommendations on both the client and the family. A more sophisticated approach is to help the family prioritize the list of recommendations for home and environmental modifications.

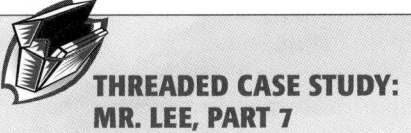

THREADED CASE STUDY:
MR. LEE, PART 7

Mr. and Mrs. Lee live in a bi-level condominium in the Nob Hill area of San Francisco, on the outskirts of Chinatown. They have access to the two-car garage by way of two steps down from the first floor of their home. The stairs lack a railing and direct lighting. The first floor contains a large kitchen, full dining room, living room, family room, a small study, and a half bathroom. Their condominium has four bedrooms and two bathrooms upstairs. Since the most recent exacerbation of his cerebrovascular disease, they have converted the study on the main floor for use as his bedroom. Their eldest son has discussed the feasibility of installing a stair lift to the second floor, suggesting that his parents have plenty of resources to fund such a project. Mr. and Mrs. Lee are not enthusiastic about this idea, believing that it could reduce the property value of their home.

The entire condominium is carpeted with plush carpeting and large oriental rugs, making it difficult for Mr. Lee to maneuver his walker. Mr. Lee insists on wearing Chinese slippers and a long bathrobe and has fallen several times since discharge from the hospital. There are several pieces of bulky mahogany furniture with low seating surfaces, several large statues, and big potted plants in the living room, family room, dining room, and study/bedroom. The half bathroom is rather large, containing a wall-mounted sink and a low European-style toilet, but it lacks any adaptive equipment. The kitchen is also large, with a breakfast nook, a central cooking island, and sufficient room for Mr. Lee to maneuver his walker. Mr. Lee prefers to eat in the kitchen but does no cooking and expects his wife to make and serve his meals. The study/bedroom on the first floor accommodates a twin-size bed and seating area with two deep chairs and an entertainment center.

Occupational Performance Interventions

In providing OT intervention for OAs, the occupational therapist is primarily guided by the OTPF process and by consideration of age-associated changes and issues that could be unique when intervening with an OA population. The following sections address the probative questions that pertain to the case study at the beginning of the chapter.

Determining client's prognosis (potential)

What are some of the concerns for the occupational therapist to consider when addressing the multiplicity of factors in the case of the OA involving age-associated changes?

Before setting realistic goals in collaboration with the client, the occupational therapist must estimate the client's potential to benefit from OT intervention. The process of determining a client's potential is complex and requires consideration of many factors, including the therapist's knowledge base and previous clinical experience, results of the OA's evaluation, and input from other health professionals treating the client. The occupational therapist compares the identified deficits with the client's past level of function, considering the client's level of motivation; performance contexts; severity of deficits; history of recovery; and motor, processing, and communication or interaction skill deficits. If the potential cannot be determined immediately, the therapist provides a trial of therapy to determine whether the OA is able to make progress. The therapist is then better able to project what the client's status will be at the end of a given length of intervention and can justify ongoing intervention.

Determining potential is a complex process. The therapist must consider the OA's learning potential, determine the degree of motivation as affected by the performance context, and judge the severity of the performance skill deficits in relation to functional deficits in performance areas. All these are considered within the larger context of age-related changes that are expected to occur in the future.

Consider again the case of Mr. Lee. The following questions may be helpful in determining his potential for improvement:

- Will he be able to use a front-wheeled walker with minimal or no supervision around the house? In the community?
- Will he be able to safely use a reverse lock rolling walker with a seat?
- Will he learn to consistently anticipate and negotiate barriers in his environment with functional and community mobility?
- To what extent can he improve his balance?
- Can he improve or compensate for his limitations in upper and lower extremity strength, endurance, and cognition for more independent showering and toileting?
- Will he be able to safely negotiate stairs and transfer to the family car or taxi for community mobility?

- Are his depressive symptoms a chronic condition, and do they interfere (and to what extent) with optimal functional performance?
- Will he be able to improve his psychological adaptation and develop improved problem-solving skills?
- Will he be able to develop more appropriate relationships, in terms of respect and social conformity within his desired roles and occupations?
- Will he be able to cope with future age- or disease-related physical and mental health changes?
- Does he recognize the ways in which his life story has changed, and can he develop a new life story as he continues to age and experience changing abilities?
- Have he and his family discussed both the near and far future in terms of his functioning, care, and living situation within the family home?

Mr. Lee exhibits moderate motivation for change. His wife wants to bring him home and continue to provide assistance to him in ADLs. His short-term memory problems are becoming slightly worse with each successive stroke and are further complicated by sensory deficits and a pattern of suspiciousness. It is unclear to what degree depression is contributing to his cognitive deficits and whether he may experience better function after pharmacological intervention for his depression takes effect. This matter requires further evaluation and a trial of intervention to evaluate progress.

The occupational therapist may share evaluation results with other professionals to gain a broader perspective. In Mr. Lee's case, the occupational therapist may speak to the inpatient physical therapist regarding the client's potential to improve his ambulation with the walker. The occupational therapist will confer with the inpatient occupational therapist to determine the extent to which Mr. Lee is able to learn and the ways in which his cognitive deficits affected safety and function while he was an inpatient. Consultation with the inpatient therapist revealed that, just before discharge, Mr. Lee exhibited selective motion throughout his affected left upper and lower extremities, which were slightly weaker than his dominant right side. His active ROM (AROM) and passive ROM (PROM) were all within functional limits (WFL) throughout both UEs. His endurance has been a major limiting factor for functional mobility within the home. Although he was able to ambulate more than 50 feet, he has difficulties with the stairs. He is able to stand for 8 minutes without the need for rest but has difficulties standing for the length of time necessary for showering. It was the OT's opinion that Mr. Lee's poor endurance would severely limit his participation in his preferred community outings at this time.

The complexity of such a case makes determination of a client's potential a cumbersome task for the entry-level therapist, who may need to consider each goal carefully and review methodically whether the client has the potential to attain it. The entry-level therapist may attempt to treat every problem even when improvement may not be possible.

The experienced clinician is more skilled in weighing multiple factors and has a repertoire of previous successful clinical interventions against which such complex cases may be compared. To the entry-level therapist, the experienced therapist may seem to work on an intuitive level, pulling together all of the performance issues and client factors that affect the client's rehabilitation potential. In fact, what appears to be intuition is actually a series of clinical reasoning decisions based on evidence from evaluation, previous cases, and reports from the literature. Decisions are made as the evaluation is in progress.

Goal setting

During evaluation, the therapist identifies problems that may be improved. Goal setting is always accomplished in collaboration with the OA and family or partner or with the care providers. Client-centered practice and collaborative goal setting are the cornerstones of OT practice and essential in motivating a client.[4] Hoppes's survey found that clients will accomplish set goals if they know specifically what those goals are.[49] He also found that clients frequently feel that they are not involved in choosing therapy goals, although the therapist has reported involving the client. The following suggestions may help increase the client's perceived control:

- Make sure that the goals are focused on outcomes that the client wants to achieve and feels capable of achieving.
- Provide specific written goals using guidelines such as the RUMBA (Relevant, Understandable, Measurable, Behavioral, Achievable) rule.[23]
- Design challenging goals.
- Make sure that the client remembers the goals. Goals with measurable outcomes offer evidence of success.

The therapist must involve family members in goal setting because they are essential components of the performance context and will be responsible for supervision and follow-through at home. Families may feel overwhelmed with this responsibility, but after providing some input into the intervention plan, they are frequently willing to develop the skills necessary to care for their family member. The entry-level clinician may be tempted to inform the OA of the intervention goals, but the experienced clinician will collaborate with OAs and their families in establishing goals. The experienced clinician will be able to articulate the differences and the similarities between the client's and the therapist's goals and will negotiate agreement with the client. The entry-level clinician may have difficulty accepting a client's refusal to work on some intervention goals. The experienced clinician accepts these differences in cultural and social values and focuses on the goals that the client feels are pertinent.

Intervention

What should be the primary focus of the occupational therapy evaluation and intervention process?

The first area to address would be that of safety, for Mr. Lee as well as Mrs. Lee. Home modifications (e.g., installation of grab bars and stair railings) and the prescription of assistive devices (e.g., a raised toilet seat, shower bench) must be carried out as soon as possible. This intervention is certainly feasible; all are relatively simple tasks. Mrs. Lee will be taught proper body mechanics when physically assisting Mr. Lee. The second area would involve teaching adaptive techniques to Mr. Lee so that he can be more independent in his ADLs and less reliant on Mrs. Lee in general. Some form of family therapy would be appropriate to delineate the role changes that have occurred. Clearly, some of Mr. Lee's impatience and anger toward Mrs. Lee is in response to the loss of his roles and habits after his cerebrovascular accidents.

The approach used as part of the OT intervention would be to restore some of Mr. Lee's performance skills, performance patterns, and client factors to the greatest degree possible. However, the primary focus of the intervention would entail modifying the performance context, modifying activity demands, and modifying performance patterns to help Mr. Lee and his family attain their goals and support his occupational performance in the community.

The intervention process involves teaching and learning. Adults have specific learning needs. Integrating the learning needs of the adult into the intervention will increase the effectiveness of the teaching session. Some of the assumptions in the following list are related to adult learning and are pertinent to OT intervention:

- Adults need to understand the reasoning behind the learning.
- The adult learner brings a breadth of experience and knowledge to learning situations.
- Adults are willing and ready to learn whatever is necessary.
- Adults are typically pragmatic and willing to learn those things that will help them with day-to-day experiences.
- The greatest motivators are internal pressures.

In addition to the preceding principles, it is important to remember the following when working with older adults[65]:

- The processing of information takes longer than it does with younger adults.
- Elaboration of information involves making connections between the new information and building on, or making additional associations to, existing knowledge.
- Strategies that group information in an organized way promote effective storage.
- Attending to the internal and external contextual factors during the learning process and recreating those contextual factors for later retrieval significantly improve remembering.
- Using stored information repeatedly strengthens the pattern of connections by rehearsing, using, and practicing.
- Providing cues that offer opportunities for recognition or matching information with previously learned information is more effective than not providing external associational cues and expecting free recall of information.

Knowles also recommends an environment of mutual trust, respect, and acceptance of differences.[55] During initial contacts with the OA, the therapist must take the time to listen to and get to know the client. By the time intervention begins, the occupational therapist will have an understanding of the client's learning style, deficits that may require specific types of teaching, and any cognitive or perceptual deficits that should be considered. The pace and style of the intervention will be individualized to suit the client's learning needs.

Restore performance skills and client factors

Consider Mr. Lee's case and the relevant circumstances in these areas. He has sensory deficits that include moderate visual impairment, and he is hard of hearing. His cognitive deficits include difficulties in concentration and memory impairments, especially for episodic events. To help Mr. Lee become more independent and increase his safety during personal mobility, the occupational therapist must ensure that the learning environment and methods of encoding and storing information are effective for Mr. Lee. Mr. Lee has already identified as an important goal greater independence in mobility and some ADLs. Training in safe mobility and transfers in the environment in which they will naturally occur, his own home, provides many of the contextual cues that will be beneficial to Mr. Lee. When speaking to Mr. Lee, the therapist should look at him to make sure he is hearing any instructions. So that Mr. Lee can better hear and concentrate, mobility and transfer training should occur in a quiet environment. The therapist should organize and group information according to the methods or techniques to be used and build on these methods during Mr. Lee's inpatient stay. The therapist should review methods and procedures from previous interventions at the beginning of each new intervention session to create continuity and reinforce skills. More repetition will enhance learning and develop memory for these procedures. A few examples were provided here but much more can be done in this area of intervention.

What contextual conditions are most relevant to this case, and what contextual conditions require further exploration and modification? What activity performance patterns are of highest priority?

Involvement of family members is important because they will ultimately be responsible for the daily care and performance of the client. Training family members to use the same techniques as those used by the therapist in interventions with Mr. Lee will improve contextual continuity, follow through, and compliance. The therapist, whom Mr. Lee regards as an expert who is helping him with something that he considers important, can support Mrs. Lee in her efforts in providing care by training her in the techniques used during the home visits.

Recommendations for modifying the physical context in the home require planning and direct input from the OA and family members. Changes in the context, such as modifying the bathroom, buying a shower seat, or hiring part-time help if the OA will need 24-hour supervision, are disruptive and sometimes costly solutions. The OA may have a partner or spouse who is also older and has his or her own medical condition and set of functional problems. The occupational therapist may indirectly evaluate the caregiver's ability to learn and cope with new and complex situations; this helps determine the degree to which the caregiver will be able to assist the client physically. During family training, the occupational therapist must keep in mind the learning needs of the caregiver, who may require repetition and practice of new skills. Teaching the caregiver a little more during each home visit can keep the caregiver from feeling overwhelmed and help her or him retain what is taught.

Modifying context

In the case of Mr. Lee, many modifications in the physical context were recommended. After the initial home visit and evaluation, the therapist suggested that sturdy railings be installed for the stairs from the house down to the garage and for the stairs from the front door to the street level. The use of nonslip material on the stairs, with bright contrast for the edges of the stairs, was recommended to decrease the likelihood of falls. Another recommendation was to increase lighting to the garage and the brightness of lights from the front door to street.

To increase safety in the bathroom, the therapist recommended the installation of grab bars in each bathroom: a set by the sink and another at the entrance to the shower. The therapist also suggested that additional shower bars be installed inside the shower stall itself. Also recommended were a shower bench, soap mitt, long-handled shower brush, and nonslip shower floor lining. A raised toilet seat with a flip-away toilet grab bar frame was suggested for the commode because Mrs. Lee did not want to replace her European-style toilet.

For the common living areas, the therapist suggested that the oriental rugs from the first floor be removed and low-pile carpeting installed throughout the first floor. Rearrangement of furniture, statuary, and plants for ease of travel throughout the house was negotiated with Mr. and Mrs. Lee's approval. Other suggestions included replacement of cushions of the existing chairs in each room with firmer, thicker cushions and the purchase of new chairs with armrests to facilitate ease and safety in getting in and out of chairs. For the main floor bedroom and study, the therapist suggested that a floor-to-ceiling transfer pole be installed next to the bed and higher wattage, nonglare bulbs be used to increase lighting in the bedroom and throughout the house. Mr. Lee was strongly encouraged to abandon his traditional Chinese slippers for sturdier footwear to be worn indoors and outdoors, with special attention paid to hem lengths on his robe and pants.

As Mr. Lee's safety awareness, motor planning, and endurance for community mobility improved, the therapist discussed future modifications and adaptive equipment purchases with Mr. and Mrs. Lee, including a reverse lock and a rolling walker with a built-in seat. They also discussed enlarging the first floor bathroom and study to incorporate the half bath into a master bath with a walk-in shower, rubberized coated flooring, and a drain in the bathroom floor. Turning the study into a larger master bedroom in view of future age-associated changes in function was an idea embraced eagerly by Mr. and Mrs. Lee. These changes could enable the Lees to age in place and remain in their home much longer.

Providing caregiver training to Mrs. Lee in her own home is an example of modifying the social context and modifying activity demands and performance patterns as they relate to occupational performance for Mr. Lee. Family caregiver training allows the occupational therapist to model for the family ways to supervise and provide varying degrees of assistance. For example, the occupational therapist will include Mrs. Lee in sessions on safe transfer down stairs, in and out of the car, and to the shower. The occupational therapist can model ways to assist the client, minimally cueing for safety when transferring, positioning the walker within reach, using grab bars and rails, safely removing or fastening clothes, and entering the car or tub. The therapist models assistance with showering by making sure that the items Mr. Lee needs (e.g., shampoo, long-handled sponge, shower hose, liquid soap with shower mitt, shower seat) are within reach. Mr. Lee will also be able to demonstrate the compensatory techniques that he has learned to wash his hair and body, using the shower bench, shower hose, and shower mitts and remaining on the shower bench to dry himself with a towel. During the next intervention session, the occupational therapist may step back and observe Mrs. Lee providing minimal assistance with bathing. Transfer training, safety, and types of additional bathroom equipment may also be reviewed. The establishment of new routines and patterns of performance is crucial. Suggestions for a regular schedule for showering and other activities each week are made, including the use of a calendar to mark upcoming and past events and to elicit cooperation with Mr. Lee's sons. This approach takes into account the adult learning and OT principles promoting client collaboration and principles for improving and supporting short-term memory. The caregiver and client are able to provide input into their learning experiences and make any modifications in structuring problems and making plans while consulting with the therapist in their own home. The occupational therapist eventually steps out of the role of authority and allows the caregiver and client to solve problems independently.

During family training sessions, the occupational therapist may note problems with the caregiver's ability to cope and learn and with communication or interaction skills. These problems may complicate home care discharge plans and the client's future safety and well-being. At such a point, the occupational therapist should alert the social worker, nurse, and other team members to the potential problems and obtain additional resources if needed.

Reevaluation and modification

Intervention requires ongoing reevaluation and modification of the original intervention plan. The experienced clinician recognizes this necessity and modifies the plan accordingly. At some point in the intervention continuum, the occupational therapist must determine if and how the OA will be able to solve problems in unique situations. It is important to see whether the client can function in a less predictable physical or social environment. The therapist may modify the physical or social environment to challenge the client and aid in the transfer of newly learned compensatory strategies and skills to a variety of settings.

Discharge planning from home care

Discharge planning requires a team effort, with forethought given to the needs of the OA and family members. Discharge planning begins at the first meeting with the client. The occupational therapist has many opportunities to develop goals collaboratively with the OA and family and to discuss the frequency and duration of intervention and plans for discharge. Discharge planning may include recommending home health aide assistance or the services of another healthcare professional. The therapist can clarify for the client those circumstances that might warrant additional services. The discharging occupational therapist makes sure that a discharge summary is sent to the next occupational therapist or healthcare professional to document previous intervention and progress.

Discharge planning should include referral to other community resources. Community resources aid in the transition from one level of care to another and often provide the support that families need to continue to care for the OA at home. Typically, various members of the healthcare team recommend community resources according to the type of service that each team member provides. The social worker or discharge planner may provide information about in-home meals and home health aide services. The physical therapist may refer the client to a community-based exercise class. The occupational therapist may encourage the client to attend the local senior center and may provide information on equipment loan closets. Caregivers often are unaware of the many resources available. It is up to the healthcare team to provide OAs and their families with resource information and teach them how to obtain those services.

SUMMARY

The OA population continues to grow at a rapid pace. Many OAs will need rehabilitative services and the skills of occupational therapists. Occupational therapists who specialize in geriatric practice must do a great deal, perhaps more than therapists in any other area of practice. Occupational therapists who specialize in geriatrics not only must have the basic knowledge and skills to address occupation and performance but also must have advanced clinical reasoning skills to address the complex, multidimensional issues that encompass occupational performance for the OA client. Collaborating with OA clients and their caregivers is essential in understanding the client's unique circumstances. Defining problems, framing those problems, and determining what aspects of occupational performance to address depend on several key factors. These include the knowledge, experience, and attitudes of the therapist; the type of care setting and limitations imposed by the reimbursement source; and the particular life experiences, health status, illness experience, personal circumstances, and occupations of the client.

Clinical reasoning that primarily addresses the client's pathological condition or that addresses only limited aspects of occupational performance is inadequate and ineffective in addressing the multidimensional problems of an OA adjusting to age-related changes and struggling with the onset of new disabilities. A more integrated approach to the evaluation and intervention of OAs has been presented here.

Review Questions

1. What will be the demographic characteristics of a typical geriatric client seeking occupational therapy services in the year 2010?
2. List seven age-related physical changes that a therapist would consider in a client who is 85 years of age and who has had an inactive lifestyle.
3. Name three cognitive changes associated with aging, and provide three strategies to enhance encoding or learning of new information.
4. What are some risk factors for suicide in an older adult?
5. List five specific client factors that you would immediately observe or screen for when meeting an OA client for the first time.
6. What other aspects of Mr. Lee's performance areas, skills, context, patterns, or activity demands might merit further consideration?

REFERENCES

1. Agency for Health Care Policy and Research: *Recognition and initial assessment of Alzheimer's disease and related dementias: clinical practice guideline*, No. 19, 1996, P. H. S. U.S. Department of Health and Human Services, Agency for Health Care Policy and Research. AHCPR Publication No. 97-0702.
2. Alexopoulos GS, et al: Vascular depression hypothesis, *Arch Gen Psychiatry* 54(10):915, 1997.
3. Allen CK, Earhart CA, Blue T: *Occupational therapy treatment goals for the physically and cognitively disabled*, Rockville, MD, 1992, American Occupational Therapy Association.
4. American Occupational Therapy Association: Occupational therapy practice framework: domain and process, *Am J Occup Ther* 56(6):609, 2002.
5. American Psychiatric Association: *Diagnostic and statistical manual of mental disorders: DSM-IV-TR*, Washington, DC, 2000, American Psychiatric Association.
6. Asher I: *Occupational therapy assessment tools: an annotated index*, ed 2, Bethesda, MD, 1996, American Occupational Therapy Association.
7. Beck A, Steer R: *Beck depression inventory manual*, San Antonio, TX, 1987, The Psychological Corp.

8. Berg K, et al: Measuring balance in the elderly: preliminary development of an instrument, *Physiother Can* 41:304, 1989.

9. Berlin E: *Guidelines for health practitioners* (DHHS Grant No. 5-UO1-PE-00053-04). Date Unknown, Stanford University Division of Family Medicine and the South Bay Area Health Education Center.

10. Burns E, Goodwin J: Immunodeficiency of aging, *Drugs Aging* 11(5):374, 1997.

11. Burns T: *Cognitive performance test (CPT)*, Minneapolis, 2002, Geriatric Research, Education and Clinical Center, Minneapolis Veterans Affairs Medical Center.

12. Burns T: *Cognitive performance test (CPT)*, Pequannock, NJ, 2004, Ableware, Maddak Inc.

13. Burns T: *Cognitive performance test (CPT): a measure of cognitive capacity for the performance of routine tasks*, Minneapolis, 1991, Geriatric Research, Education and Clinical Center, Minneapolis Veterans Affairs Medical Center.

14. Burns T: The cognitive performance test: an approach to cognitive level assessment in Alzheimer's disease. In Allen CK, Earhart CA, Blue T: *Occupational therapy treatment goals for the physically and cognitively disabled*, Rockville, MD, 1992, American Occupational Therapy Association.

15. Burns T, Mortimer JA, Merchak P: Cognitive performance test: a new approach to functional assessment in Alzheimer's disease, *J Geriatr Psychiatry Neurol* 7(1):46, 1994.

16. Butin DN: *Psychosocial and psychological components*, ed 2, Bethesda, MD, 1996, American Occupational Therapy Association.

17. Cantor M: Family and community: changing roles in an aging society, *Gerontologist* 31(3):337, 1991.

18. Carlson JC, Riley JC: A consideration of some notable aging theories, *Exp Gerontol* 33(1-2):127, 1998.

19. Carstensen LL: Evidence for a life span theory of socioemotional selectivity, *Current Directions Psychological Science* 4:151, 1995.

20. Certo C: Cardiopulmonary rehabilitation of the geriatric patient and client. In Lewis CB: *Aging: the health care challenge*, ed 4, Philadelphia, 2002, FA Davis.

21. Clark F, et al: Occupational therapy for independent living older adults, *JAMA* 278(16):1321, 1997.

22. Clark F, et al: Life domains and adaptive strategy of a group of low-income, well older adults, *Am J Occup Ther* 50(2):106, 1996.

23. College of St. Catherines: *Goal writing: documenting outcomes* (hand-out), St Paul, MN, 2001, College of St Catherine's.

24. Costa P, McCrae R: Psychological stress and coping in old age. In Breznitz LGS, editor: *Handbook of stress: theoretical and clinical aspects*, New York, 1993, Free Press.

25. Craik F, Jennings J: Human memory. In Craik FC, Salthouse TA, editors: *The handbook of aging and cognition*, Hillsdale, NJ, 1992, Erlbaum.

26. Cristofala V: The destiny of cells: mechanisms and implications of senescence, *Gerontologist* 25:577, 1985.

27. Deeg D, Kardaun J, Fozard J: Health, behavior and aging. In Birren JE, Schaie KW, editors: *Handbook of the psychology of aging*, ed 4, San Diego, CA, 1996, Academic Press.

28. Diehl M, Coyle N, Labouvie-Vief: Age and sex differences in coping and defense across the life span, *Psychol Aging* 11(1):127, 1996.

29. Dittmann-Kohli F: The construction of meaning in old age: possibilities and constraints, *Aging and Society* 10:279, 1990.

30. Ewing J: Detecting alcoholism: the CAGE questionnaire, *JAMA* 252(14):1905, 1984.

31. *Federal Interagency on Age-Related Statistics*, 2004, Washington DC. http://www.agingstats.gov/, accessed 11/01/2005.

32. Ferrini AF, Ferrini RL: *Health in the later years*, ed 3, Boston, 2000, McGraw-Hill.

33. Fleming M: Procedural reasoning: addressing functional limitations. In Mattingly C, Fleming MH, editors: *Clinical reasoning: forms of inquiry in a therapeutic practice*, Philadelphia, 1994, FA Davis.

34. Folstein MF, Folstein MF, McHugh PR: Mini-Mental State: a practical method for grading the cognitive state of patients for the clinician, *J Psychiatr Res* 12(3):189, 1975.

35. Gallo JJ, Lebowitz BD: The epidemiology of common late-life mental disorders in the community: themes for a new century, *Psychiatr Serv* 50(9):1158, 1999.

36. Gallo JJ, et al: Depression without sadness: functional outcomes of nondysphoric depression in later life, *J Am Geriatr Soc* 45(5):570, 1997.

37. Gatz M, Kasl-Godley J, Karel M: Aging and mental disorders. In Birren JE, Schaie KW, editors: *Handbook of the psychology of aging*, ed 4, San Diego, CA, 1996, Academic Press.

38. Gatz M, Smyer M: Mental health and aging at the onset of the twenty-first century. In Birren JE, Schaie KW, editors: *Handbook of the psychology of aging*, ed 5, San Diego, CA, 2001, Academic Press.

39. Gierveld JDJ: *Gender and well being: the elderly in the industrialized world*. Seminar on Population Ageing in the Industrialized Countries: Challenges and Responses, Tokyo, 2001, International Union for the Scientific Study of Population.

40. Giovannetti T, et al: Naturalistic action impairments in dementia, *Neuropsychologia* 40(8):1220, 2002.

41. Gross JJ, et al: Emotion and aging: experience, expression and control, *Psychol Aging* 12(4):590, 1997.

42. Gurland BJ, Cross PS, Katz E: Epidemiological perspectives on opportunities for treatment of depression, *Am J Geriatr Psychiatry* 4(Suppl 1):S7, 1996.

43. Harman D: Extending functional life span, *Exp Gerontol* 33(1-2):95, 1998.

44. Hayflick L: New approaches to old age, *Nature* 403:365, 2000.

45. Heidrich S, Ryff C: The role of social comparisons processes in the psychological adaptation of elderly adults, *J Gerontol* 48(3):P127, 1993.

46. Hill G: *The changing realm of the senses*, Philadelphia, 2002, FA Davis.

47. Himes C: Future caregivers: projected family structures of older people, *J Gerontol* 47(1):S23, 1992.

48. Hinojosa J, Kramer P, Crist P, editors: *Evaluation: obtaining and interpreting data*, Bethesda, MD, 2005, American Occupational Therapy Association Press.

49. Hoppes S: Motivating clients through goal setting, *OT Practice,* June 1997, p. 22.

50. Jeste DV, et al: Consensus statement on the upcoming crisis in geriatric mental health: research agenda for the next 2 decades, *Arch Gen Psychiatry* 56(9):848, 1999.

51. Kausler DH: *Learning and memory in normal aging,* San Diego, 1994, Academic Press.

52. Kehrberg K: Part II: The large ACL. In Allen CK, Earhart CA, Blue T: *Occupational therapy treatment goals for the physically and cognitively disabled,* Rockville, MD, 1992, American Occupational Therapy Association.

53. Keller M, Leventhal E, Larson B: Aging: the lived experience, *Int J Aging Hum Dev* 29(1):67, 1989.

54. Kinsella K, Vicotira V: *An aging world: 2001,* Washington DC, 2001, U.S. Census Bureau, U.S. Government Printing Office.

55. Knowles M: *The adult learner: a neglected species,* Houston, TX, 1984, Gulf Publishing.

56. Kraus N: Life stress as a correlate of depression among older adults, *Psychiatry Research* 18(3):227, 1986.

57. Larson KO: *Conceptual models of practice and frames of reference,* ed 2, Bethesda, MD, 1996, American Occupational Therapy Association.

58. Larson KO, et al, editors: *Role of occupational therapy with the elderly,* ed 2, Bethesda, MD, 1996, American Occupational Therapy Association.

59. Lawton MP: Quality of life and affect in later life. In Magai C, McFadden SH: *Handbook of emotion, adult development and aging,* San Diego, 1996, Academic Press.

60. LeBarge E: A preliminary scale to measure degree of worry among mildly demented Alzheimer's disease patients, *Phys Occup Ther Geriatr* 11:43, 1993.

61. Lebowitz B, Pearson J, Schneider L: Diagnosis and treatment of depression in late life: consensus statement update, *JAMA* 278(14):1186, 1997.

62. Leventhal H, Leventhal E, Schaeffer P: Vigilant coping and health behaviors. In Ory MG, Abeles RP, Lipman PD, editors: *Aging, health and behavior,* Newbury Park, CA, 1992, Sage.

63. Levy L: *Cognition and the aging adult,* ed 2, Bethesda, MD, 1996, American Occupational Therapy Association.

64. Levy L: Cognitive aging in perspective: implications for occupational therapy practitioners. In Katz N: *Cognition and occupation across the life span: Models for intervention in occupational therapy,* ed 2, Bethesda, MD, 2005, American Occupational Therapy Association.

65. Levy L: Cognitive aging in perspective: information processing, cognition and memory. In Katz N: *Cognition and occupation across the life span: Models for intervention in occupational therapy,* ed 2, Bethesda, MD, 2005, American Occupational Therapy Association.

66. Levy L: *Health and impairment: the performance component,* Bethesda, MD, 1996, American Occupational Therapy Association.

67. Levy L: Information processing and dementia. II: Cognitive disability in perspective, *OT Practice* December 4(10):CE-1, 1999.

68. Levy L: *Mental disorders in aging adults,* ed 2, Bethesda, MD, 1996, American Occupational Therapy Association.

69. Levy LL, Burns T: Cognitive disabilities reconsidered: rehabilitation of older adults with dementia. In Katz N: *Cognition and occupation across the life span: Models for intervention in occupational therapy,* ed 2, Bethesda, MD, 2005, American Occupational Therapy Association.

70. Lewis CB, Kellems S: Musculoskeletal changes with age: clinical implications. In Lewis CB, editor: *Aging: The health care challenge,* ed 4, Philadelphia, 2002, FA Davis Company.

71. Magai C: Personality change in adulthood: loci of change and the role of interpersonal process, *Int J Aging Hum Dev* 49(4):339, 1999.

72. Magai C: Emotions over the life span. In Birren JE, Schaie KW, editors: *Handbook of the psychology of aging,* ed 5, San Diego, CA, 2001, Academic Press.

73. Mattingly C: The narrative nature of clinical reasoning. In Mattingly C, Fleming MH, editors: *Clinical reasoning: forms of inquiry in a therapeutic practice,* Philadelphia, 1994, FA Davis.

74. McConatha JT, Huba HM: Primary, secondary, and emotional control across adulthood, *Current Psychology: Developmental, Learning, Personality, Social* 18:164-170, 1999.

75. McFarlane AC: Resilience, vulnerability, and the course of posttraumatic reactions. In van der Kolk BA, McFarlane AC, Weisath L, editors: *Traumatic stress: the effects of overwhelming experience on mind, body and society,* New York, 1996, Guilford Press.

76. Miller B: Theories of aging. In Lewis CB, editor: *Aging: The health care challenge,* ed 4, Philadelphia, 2002, FA Davis.

77. Murray C, Lopez A: *The global burden of disease,* Cambridge, 1996, Harvard School of Public Health.

78. Murray CJ, Lopez AD: Global mortality, disability and the contribution of risk factors: global burden of disease study, *Lancet* 349(9063):1436, 1997.

79. National Eye Institute: *Age related macular degeneration: what you should know,* Washington DC, 2005, United States Department of Health and Human Services.

80. National Research Council: Structure of the aging mind. In National Research Council: *The aging mind: opportunities for cognitive research,* Washington DC, 2003, National Academy Press.

81. Office of Employment and Community Development: *Maintaining prosperity in an ageing society,* Paris, 1998.

82. Orgel L: The maintenance of the accuracy of protein synthesis and its relevancy to aging, *Proc Natl Acad Sci USA* 49:517, 1963.

83. Orgel L: The maintenance of the accuracy of protein synthesis and its relevancy to aging, *Proc Natl Acad Sci* 67:1496, 1973.

84. Petersen RC, et al: Mild cognitive impairment: clinical characterization and outcome, *Arch Neurol* 56(3):303, 1999.

85. Pfeffer RI, et al: Measurement of functional activities in older adults in the community, *J Gerontol* 37(3):323, 1982.

86. Reifler B: Detection and treatment of mixed cognitive and affective symptoms in the elderly: is it dementia, depression or both? *Clin Geriatr* 6:17, 1998.

87. Reyff CD, Kwan CML, Singer BH: Personality and aging: flourishing agendas and future challenges. In Birren JE, Schaie KW, editors: *Handbook of the psychology of aging*, ed 5, San Diego, CA, 2001, Academic Press.

88. Robinson BC: Validation of caregiver strain index, *J Gerontol* 38(3):344, 1983.

89. Rogers J, Holm M: Occupational therapy diagnostic reasoning: a component of clinical reasoning, *Am J Occup Ther* 45(11):1045, 1991.

90. Rott C, Thomae H: Coping in longitudinal perspective: findings from the Bonn Longitudinal Study on Aging, *J Cross-Cultural Gerontol* 6:23, 1991.

91. Rowe J, Kahn R: Human aging: usual and successful, *Science* 237(4811):143, 1987.

92. Rowe J, Kahn R: Successful aging, *Gerontologist* 37(4):433, 1997.

93. Rusting R: Why do we age? *Sci Am* 267(6):130, 1987.

94. Ruth JE, Coleman P: Personality and aging: coping and management of the self in later life. In Birren JE, Schaie KW, editors: *Handbook of the psychology of aging*, San Diego, CA, 1996, Academic Press.

95. Sadavoy J, Fogel F: Personality disorders in old age. In Birren JE, Sloane RB, Cohen GD, editors: *Handbook of mental health and aging*, San Diego, CA, 1992, Academic Press.

96. Scheiman M: *Understanding and managing vision deficits: a guide for occupational therapists*, Thorofare, NJ, 2002, Slack.

97. Schell BAB: Clinical reasoning: the basis of practice. In Crepeau E, Cohn ES, Schell BAB: *Willard and Spackman's occupational therapy*, ed 10, Philadelphia, 2003, Lippincott Williams & Wilkins.

98. Schell B, Cervero R: Clinical reasoning in occupational therapy: an integrative review, *Am J Occup Ther* 47(7):605, 1993.

99. Schwartz M: Re-examining the role of executive functions in routine action production. In Grafman J, Holyoak K, Boller F, editors: *Annals of New York Academy of Sciences. Vol 769. Structure and function of the human prefrontal cortex*, New York, 1995, New York Academy of Sciences.

100. Schwartz MF, et al: Cognitive theory and the study of everyday action disorders after brain damage, *J Head Trauma Rehabil* 8(1):59, 1993.

101. Segerstrom SC, et al: Optimism is associated with mood, coping, and immune change in response to stress, *J Pers Soc Psychol* 74(6):1646, 1998.

102. Seligman M: *Helplessness: on depression, development and death*, San Francisco, 1975, Freeman.

103. Sinnott J: A model for solution of ill-structured problems: implications for everyday and abstract problem solving. In Sinnott JD, editor: *Everyday problem solving: theory and applications*, New York, 1989, Praeger.

104. Smith A, editor: *Memory*, San Diego, 1996, Academic Press.

105. Stark S: Home modifications that enable occupational performance. In Letts L, Rigby P, Steward D: *Using environments to enable occupational performance*, Thorofare, NJ, 2003, Slack.

106. Strehler B: A new age for aging, *Natural History* 2:8, 1973.

107. Surgeon General: *Older adults and mental health*, Washington DC, 1999.

108. Tabert MH, et al: Functional deficits in patients with mild cognitive impairment: prediction of AD, *Neurology* 58(5):758, 2002.

109. United States Bureau of the Census: Household and family characteristics, *Current Population Reports*, March 1998, PPL-20-515.

110. United States Bureau of the Census: Population projections of the United States by age, sex, race and Hispanic origin: 1995-2050, *Current Population Reports*, 1998, P25-1130.

111. United States Bureau of the Census: Poverty in the United States: 1998, *Current Population Reports*, September 1999, P60-207.

112. United States Bureau of the Census: Sex by age by types of disability for the civilian non-institutionalized population 5 years and over, *Current Population Reports*, 2000.

113. United States Bureau of the Census: U.S. Interim projection by age, sex, race and Hispanic origin, *Current Population Reports*, 2004.

114. Vaillant G: *Adaptation to life*, Boston, 1977, Little, Brown.

115. Walford R: The clinical promise of diet restriction, *Geriatrics* 45(4):81, 1990.

116. Weinberger M, Hiner SL, Tierney WM: In support of hassles as a measure of stress in predicting health outcomes, *J Behav Med* 10(1):19, 1987.

117. Willis S: Everyday problem solving. In Birren JE, Schaie KW, editors: *Handbook of the psychology of aging*, San Diego, CA, 1996, Academic Press.

118. Yee B, Williams B: Medication management and appropriate substance use for elderly individuals. In Lewis CB: *Aging: the health care challenge*, ed 4, Philadelphia, 2002, FA Davis.

119. Yeo G: The need for culturally competent models of long term care. In Stanford Geriatric Education Center: *AARP series on ethnicity and long term care*, 1997, Stanford Geriatric Education Center.

120. Yeo G, et al: *Core curriculum in ethnogeriatrics* (Curriculum guide—Bureau of Health Professions Health Resources and Services Administration and U.S. Department of Health and Human Services Grant Report No. 97-0260), Stanford, CA, 1999, Stanford Geriatric Education Center.

121. Yeo G, et al: *Cohort analysis as a tool in ethnogeriatrics: historical profiles of elders from eight ethnic populations in the United States*, ed 2, Stanford, CA, 1998, Stanford Geriatric Education Center.

122. Yesavage JA, et al: Development and validation of a geriatric depression scale: a preliminary report, *J Psychiatr Res* 17(1):37, 1982-1983.

123. Zhou Y: Will China's current population policy change its kinship system? *Research Paper Series*, Tokyo, 2000, Nihon University Population Research Institute.

SUGGESTED READING

Bonder B: *Growing old in the U.S.*, Philadelphia, 2001, FA Davis.

47

HIV Infection and AIDS[1]

MICHAEL A. PIZZI

KEY TERMS

Human immunodeficiency
  virus (HIV)
Acquired immunodeficiency
  syndrome (AIDS)

Highly active antiretroviral
  therapy (HAART)
Positive prevention

Primary prevention
Secondary prevention
Tertiary prevention

LEARNING OBJECTIVES

After studying this chapter the student or practitioner will be able to do the following:

1. Understand the stages of HIV and AIDS.
2. Discuss the impact of medical interventions on HIV.
3. Assess a person with HIV or AIDS holistically.
4. Design an intervention program directed toward optimizing health and occupational participation.

5. Understand the importance of a health promotion and prevention perspective in occupational therapy services for people with HIV and AIDS.

CHAPTER OUTLINE

Transmission, signs, and symptoms
Pharmacology
Positive prevention

Assessment
Intervention
Summary

---

[1]This chapter was designed to address primarily the issues facing adults with HIV and AIDS. Most of the interventions and considerations for therapists can apply to children, adolescents, and adults. Assessment questions can be addressed to caregivers of children with HIV in conjunction with pediatric assessments.

THREADED CASE STUDY: BILLY, PART 1

Billy is a lawyer and internal medicine physician living with Tom, his partner of 15 years. He was married for 6 years and has two grown children, Alexis (24 years old) and Charlie (22 years old). After his divorce, both children were raised by Billy and Tom. While married, Billy had two male lovers with whom he had occasional unprotected sex, and his wife was using injectable drugs to no one's knowledge. The mode of infection for Billy is unknown, and he has lived for over 20 years with a diagnosis of HIV. Billy's former wife died before the children reached adolescence.

Billy has been practicing medicine successfully, as well as doing pro bono work as a legal advocate for people with HIV and AIDS. Recently, he developed his first opportunistic infection. He was hospitalized for 4 days, placed on a drug regimen, and was sent home. He became fatigued, depressed, and anxious about this change in his health status. He has a tremendous social support network, but this does not seem to help his anxiety and concerns about living life fully. To complicate matters, Billy also began to experience slight changes in his memory. This deficit became his greatest concern because of his pride in having what he calls a "mind like a steel trap."

As a health professional, Billy possesses the knowledge required to care for his own health and well-being; however, he does not apply this knowledge to his own daily life. His partner, while supportive, is becoming increasingly angry, irritable, and concerned, and these emotions appear to have impaired his own occupational performance in work, home, and leisure occupations.

As of December 2003, the following are the trends of the **human immunodeficiency virus (HIV)** pandemic:

- At the global level, the number of people living with HIV continues to grow—from 35 million in 2001 to 38 million in 2003.
- An estimated 5 million people acquired HIV in 2003, the greatest number in any one year since the beginning of the epidemic.

- In 2003, almost three million were killed by AIDS; over 20 million have died since the first cases of AIDS were identified in 1981.[3]

HIV is a retrovirus that replicates within the human body and infects the white blood cells of the immune system. HIV causes the **acquired immunodeficiency virus (AIDS),** which was first discovered in 1981. This triggered a Centers for Disease Control (CDC) investigation that led to the eventual discovery of HIV as a virus that does not discriminate between gender (Table 47-1), race (Table 47-2), culture, sexual orientation, or age (Tables 47-3 and 47-4). HIV affects all of humanity. It affects not only the people who are infected with the virus but also their parents, siblings, friends, lovers, children, and coworkers. After being diagnosed as HIV positive, an individual can be immobilized and drastically alter his or her occupational performance and participation in society or the individual can treat the diagnosis as an impetus to act in positive, life-transforming ways.

This chapter is dedicated to explaining the effect of HIV on the human body and society and the challenges that it poses to the occupational therapist and occupational therapy (OT) assistant. Readers will be knowledgeable about assessments and interventions that can make a powerful difference in the quality of life and participation in favored and meaningful occupations for people with HIV and AIDS.

TRANSMISSION, SIGNS, AND SYMPTOMS

HIV is transmitted via unprotected sex with an infected partner, contact with infected blood via transfusions (currently, that risk is very small risk thanks to heat treatment and much more careful screening of blood before transfusion), sharing of a needle with someone infected with HIV, and transmission from infected mother to newborn. Health professionals are at a very low risk of infection.[9]

In 1993, the CDC revised the categories that determined one's HIV or AIDS status.[4] They include the following:

- Category 1 (C1): CD4+ cell counts of 500 or more cells per microliter of blood
- Category 2 (C2): counts from 200 to 499 CD4+ cells

TABLE **47-1** **Cases by Exposure Category**

Following is the distribution of the estimated number of diagnoses of AIDS among adults and adolescents by exposure category, through 2003. A breakdown by sex is provided where appropriate.

Exposure Category	Male	Female	Total
Male-to-male sexual contact	440,887	-	440,887
Injection drug use	175,988	70,558	246,546
Male-to-male sexual contact and intravenous drug use	62,418	-	62,418
Heterosexual contact	56,403	93,586	149,989
Other (includes hemophilia, blood transfusion, perinatal, and risk not reported or not identified)	14,191	6,535	20,726

From Centers for Disease Control: *Basic statistics*, 2004. Retrieved July 1, 2005, from http://www.cdc.gov/hiv/stats.htm#cumaids.

TABLE **47-2**   **Cumulative Cases by Race/Ethnicity**

Estimated numbers of diagnoses of AIDS by race or ethnicity:

Race or Ethnicity	# of Cumulative AIDS Cases Through 2003
White, not Hispanic	376,834
Black, not Hispanic	368,169
Hispanic	172,993
Asian/Pacific Islander	7,166
American Indian/Alaska Native	3,026

From Centers for Disease Control: *Basic statistics*, 2004. Retrieved July 1, 2005, from http://www.cdc.gov/hiv/stats.htm#cumaids.

TABLE **47-3**   **Cumulative Cases by Age**

Of the estimated number of AIDS cases, person's age at time of diagnosis was distributed as follows:

Age	# of Cumulative AIDS Cases Through 2003
Under 13	9419
Ages 13 to 14	891
Ages 15 to 24	37,599
Ages 25 to 34	311,137
Ages 35 to 44	365,432
Ages 45 to 54	148,347
Ages 55 to 64	43,451
Ages 65 or older	13,711

From Centers for Disease Control: *Basic statistics*, 2004. Retrieved July 1, 2005, from http://www.cdc.gov/hiv/stats.htm#cumaids.

- Category 3 (C3): counts below 200 CD4+ cells

The second set of categories relates to the expression of HIV from a clinical perspective:

- Category A: individuals who have been asymptomatic except for persistent, generalized lymphadenopathy sero-conversion syndrome. This includes the initial acute onset of HIV exposure
- Category B: individuals who have never had an AIDS-defining illness but have had some symptoms of HIV infection, such as candidiasis, fever, persistent diarrhea, oral hairy leukoplakia, herpes zoster, idiopathic thrombo-cytopenic purpura, peripheral neuropathy, cervical dysplasia, or pelvic inflammatory disease
- Category C: individuals who have or have had one or more of the AIDS-defining illnesses

An individual is determined to have HIV infection if one category from each set applies. For example, an individual would be diagnosed with AIDS if the person is designated C3 (has fewer than 200 CD4+ cells) and has had at least one AIDS-defining illness. Categories 1 and 2 and A and B are considered HIV positive (a less grave condition), whereas

TABLE **47-4**   **The Distribution of the Estimated Number of Diagnoses of AIDS Among Children* by Exposure Categories**

Exposure Category	# of AIDS Cases through 2003
Mother with or at risk for HIV infection	8,749
Hemophilia/coagulation disorder, receipt of blood transfusion, blood components, or tissue	670
Other/risk not reported or identified	

*The term *children* refers to persons under age 13 at the time of diagnosis.
From Centers for Disease Control: *Basic statistics*, 2004. Retrieved July 1, 2005, from http://www.cdc.gov/hiv/stats.htm#cumaids.

categories 3 and C are defined as AIDS. These categories are used primarily to pinpoint an individual's placement along the continuum of HIV infection.[8]

Occupational therapists and OT assistants have the opportunity to positively affect the daily lives of people with HIV and AIDS in all of these stages of illness. Promoting health, quality of life, and well-being is one focus of OT intervention.[1]

People with HIV are living longer and healthier lives as a result of improvements in medications, health education, and behavioral changes. However, medications are costly and often provided only to those who can afford them or have other access to them. Thus, people with HIV who are not privy to information on community resources or whose accessibility is otherwise limited experience numerous opportunistic infections (infections resulting from a compromised immune system), such as *Pneumocystis carinii* pneuomonia or Kaposi's sarcoma (the latter being less common).

OT practitioners may see a diverse population of people with AIDS, with numerous occupational deficits. Many physical and psychosocial factors indicate the need for OT. Factors experienced by people with HIV and AIDS include, but are not limited to, the following:

- Fatigue and shortness of breath
- Impairment of the central nervous system (CNS)
- Impairment of the peripheral nervous system
- Visual deficits
- Sensory deficits (including painful neuropathies)
- Cardiac problems
- Muscle atrophy
- Altered ability to cope with and adapt to the changes that illness creates
- Depression
- Anxiety
- Guilt
- Anger
- Preoccupation with illness versus wellness

All of these factors affect one's occupational performance in meaningful, health-promoting daily occupations. OT can benefit all people with HIV and AIDS who experience any one of the aforementioned problems.

THREADED CASE STUDY: BILLY, PART 2

Billy appears to have more mental health issues surrounding his illness than physical concerns at this time. He does experience fatigue and slight memory problems. The occupational therapist may ask the following questions:

1. Is the fatigue experienced related to the medical condition or the mental health issues that Billy is experiencing?

In this case, the fatigue that Billy reports could certainly be related to both physical and mental health issues. He could be experiencing AIDS dementia complex (ADC), which manifests itself, in the context of occupational performance, as altered cognitive processing and impaired memory, among other conditions. ADC appears to be related to the destruction of subcortical structures in the CNS and is estimated to be present in more than half of the individuals diagnosed with AIDS.[5] Having an awareness of this disease could lead to increased anxiety and fear and possible depression, especially with regard to the impact on the worker role. Billy should be encouraged to discuss these fears in the context of his daily living occupational performance.

Billy's ability to use effective habits and routines in the workplace might serve to reduce his anxiety about his diminished memory. Devices such as electronic organizers and calendars may be helpful to Billy as memory aids. A conversation about these issues would involve Billy's knowledge of his life situation, thus making the OT sessions very client centered.

2. If Billy is preoccupied with his change of health status, how does he function in his work, home, community, and other contexts?

Using specifically guided questions, the therapist might examine the contexts in which Billy engages to elicit information that might have been unknown to him before OT interventions. He would benefit from an assessment such as the PWHA described later in this case study.

3. Are there mental and physical health issues that can be incorporated into a prevention and health promotion occupational therapy program?

Billy could engage in a reality-checking exercise in which he explores the positive aspects and strengths in his life (e.g., good social support, advanced knowledge in the area of healthcare). These strengths can help him maintain a positive sense of self and engage in more health-promoting behaviors on a physical level, such as a regular exercise program.

PHARMACOLOGY

After a quarter century of the HIV epidemic, there is still no cure. Over the years, researchers have made extraordinary progress in the development of medications to alter the course of the disease. These medications have helped to promote healthier functioning for people with HIV and AIDS, which assists in facilitating continued occupational participation.

The types of medications in current use include the following[2]:

- Nonnucleoside reverse transcriptase inhibitor (NNRTI): This class of drugs blocks reverse transcriptase, an enzyme that HIV needs to make more copies of itself.
- Fusion inhibitors: These work by blocking the HIV virus from entering human cells.
- Nucleoside reverse transcriptase inhibitor (NRTI): This class of drugs blocks reverse transcriptase, an enzyme (protein that helps chemical reactions) that HIV needs to make more copies of itself.
- Protease inhibitors (PIs): PIs act by blocking protease, a protein that HIV needs to make more copies of itself.

The combination of protease inhibitors with two other drugs called *reverse transcriptase inhibitors* is called **highly active antiretroviral therapy (HAART).** HAART has been an effective medical intervention that has significantly altered the landscape of HIV, creating improved health and well-being for tens of thousands of infected individuals. HAART produces nearly undetectable levels of HIV; however, once a person is infected with HIV, that person is always able to transmit the virus. Unfortunately, access to affordable healthcare is limited or nonexistent for millions of people worldwide, and efforts are under way to make these important medications more accessible. Karon et al[7] stated that it was HAART, not behavioral change, that was primarily responsible for dramatic declines in AIDS-related deaths; however, the declines did not continue after 1997, and HIV continues to spread among men who have sex with men (MSM), people who have sex with intravenous drug users (IDUs), and heterosexuals.

From 1990 to 1999, the number of living persons diagnosed with AIDS increased fourfold, to 312,000 persons. Increasing proportions of persons with AIDS are women, African-Americans or Hispanics, IDUs, heterosexuals, and residents of the South, reflecting earlier trends in HIV transmission, differences in testing behaviors, and differential effects of HAART. Synthesis of surveillance data also shows that the poor are disproportionately affected and that HIV incidence rates are especially high among African-Americans with high-risk behavior, and it suggests that HIV incidence has not declined since the early 1990s.[7] (Karon et al, 2001, Discussion, 1)

Despite best practice in medicine, the cure for AIDS remains elusive. However, thanks to medical advances, people continue to live full and productive lives while coping with the daily issues of living with HIV. Unfortunately, these life-enhancing medical regimens are associated with myriad side effects, many of which clients receiving OT services will experience. Understanding these side effects is important because they affect occupational performance. These side effects include CNS disorders, peripheral polyneuropathy, gastrointestinal disorders, hepatotoxicity, anemia, pancreatitis, osteopenia and osteoarthritis, lipodystrophy, diabetes, and hyperglycemia. Because of the many pharmacological side effects, many people with HIV have great difficulty in deciding the appropriate time to begin a drug regimen.[6]

OT PRACTICE NOTE

It is essential that occupational therapists and OT assistants understand the importance of their contributions in improving the health and well-being of people with HIV and AIDS at all stages of illness, and understand the psychosocial, physical, contextual, and emotional impacts of all areas of living with HIV.

POSITIVE PREVENTION

Reflecting the changing needs of people with HIV and in consideration of the improved drugs to combat the disease and its secondary conditions, the term **positive prevention** has been developed and used by the CDC.3 The Serostatus Approach to Fighting the Epidemic (SAFE) helps reduce the risk of transmission to supplement current risk reduction programs. Several action steps are recommended that focus on diagnosing HIV, linking infected persons to appropriate preventive services, helping them adhere to treatment regimens, and providing support to develop healthy habits for sustaining behavior that reduces the risk of HIV. It is one of the first programs to dovetail traditional infectious disease control with behavioral interventions. Although occupational therapists may primarily intervene with people who have already been infected, prevention can still be integrated into a holistic program of care.

Prevention and health promotion can be a primary area of intervention in OT. In **primary prevention,** the practitioner may develop and implement health education and risk reduction strategies to help individuals and communities understand the impact of reducing risk on occupational participation. An OT primary prevention strategy could be development of a developmentally appropriate lecture or workshop on abstinence and safe sex for schools, church groups, and community centers. These workshops could incorporate mental health strategies, culturally relevant information, and interpersonal skill-building exercises in which OT practitioners are well educated.

Secondary prevention, wherein OT services are provided for people who are already infected with the virus, would include activities that create and promote healthy lifestyles and thereby prevent future opportunistic infections and promote balance and well-being. OT intervention focused on providing secondary prevention can significantly affect communities that have large number of people who are infected with the HIV virus. An emphasis on establishing and maintaining the habits and routines that support engagement in occupations would be appropriate for secondary prevention programs.

Tertiary prevention is provided when clients suffer from a disability that is secondary to the disease. Tertiary prevention includes a strong emphasis on rehabilitation; health promotion programming can also be included to positively affect a person's lifestyle and provide hope for continued and healthful functioning. Strategies that support continued participation in occupations, even if the occupation has been modified, would be addressed in tertiary prevention programs. An example would be the use of adaptive equipment to support continued engagement in a desired occupation (e.g., woodworking, cooking) when muscular weakness or peripheral nerve damage compromises occupational performance.

ASSESSMENT

Pizzi[11] has developed two assessments that focus on enhancing health and well-being (see Chapter 5): One is for general use, and the other is for use with people who have an HIV infection. The one related to HIV specifically is the Pizzi Assessment of Productive Living for Adults with HIV Infection and AIDS (PAPL; Figure 47-1).

One of the first assessments in OT specifically designed as a client-centered and subjective health promotion tool is the Pizzi Holistic Wellness Assessment (PHWA).[11] An occupational history format is used. The emphasis of the PHWA is to explore an individual's self-perception of health and strategies for self-responsibility. It is vital that practitioners incorporate the goals, beliefs, values, attitudes, and occupational meanings identified by the client being served. Reductionistic interventions (e.g., range of motion, strengthening, cognitive retraining) are incorporated into meaningful occupations and not addressed separately.

The PHWA is a self-assessment tool that incorporates both a qualitative and a quantitative component. Clients self-assess eight areas of health on a scale of 1 through 10. They then address each area with the help of the practitioner in terms of their self-perceptions of occupational participation in the respective area. This dialog helps clients become aware of important health issues affecting their daily occupational performance. In each area of health, the client explores strategies to optimize health and determines which strategies could be used to promote health and well-being.

Even when it appears that a specific intervention positively changes occupational performance, the person experiences wellness through the self-discovery of how to best manage his or her being. After self-discovery, the therapy process unfolds collaboratively between the client and therapist.[11] (p. 57)

Pizzi Assessment of Productive Living for Adults with HIV Infection and AIDS (PAPL)

Demographics

Name_____Age_____

Sex_____Lives with (relationship)_____

Identified caregiver_____

Race _____Culture_____Religion_____

Practicing?_____How does spirituality play a role in your life, if

any?_____

Primary occupational roles:

_____

Primary diagnosis:

_____

Secondary diagnosis:

_____

Stage of HIV_____

Past Medical History:

_____

Medications:

_____

Activities of Daily Living (use ADL performance assessment)
Are you doing these now?

_____

Do you perform homemaking tasks?

_____

(For areas of difficulty) Would you like to be able to do these again like you did

before?_____ Which ones? _____

Work

Job _____When last worked_____

Describe type of activity_____

Work environment _____

If not working, would you like to be able to?_____

Figure 47-1 Pizzi Assessment of Productive Living for Adults with HIV Infection and AIDS (PAPL). *STG*, short-term goals; *LTG*, long-term goals. (Courtesy of Michael Pizzi© 1991.)

Do you miss being productive?_____

Types of activity engaged in_____

If not, would you like to?_____Which ones?_____

Would you like to try other things as well?_____

Is it important to be independent in daily living activities?_____

Play/Leisure (interests and current participation)_____

_____

Sleep issues (habits, patterns)_____

Physical Function

Active and Passive range of motion:

Strength:

Sensation:

Coordination (gross and fine motor or dexterity):

Visual-perceptual:

Hearing:

Balance (sit and stand):

Ambulation, Transfers, and Mobility:

Activity tolerance/endurance:

Physical pain:

Location:

_____

Does it interfere with doing important activities?_____

Sexual function:

Cognition

(Attention span, problem solving, memory, orientation, judgment, reasoning, decision making, safety awareness)

Time Organization

Former daily routine (before diagnosis)

Figure 47-1, cont'd

Continued

Has this changed since diagnosis?_____

If so, how? _____

Are there certain times of day that are better for you to carry out daily tasks?

_____

Do you consider yourself regimented in organizing time and activity or pretty

flexible? _____

What would you change, if anything, in how your day is set up?

_____

Body image and self-image

In the last 6 months, has there been a recent change in your physical body and how it

looks?_____How do you feel about this?_____

_____

Social environment (Describe support available and utilized by patient)

Physical environment (Describe environments where patient performs daily tasks and

level of support or impediment for function)

Stressors

What are some things, people, or situations that are/were stressful?_____

_____

What are some current ways you manage stress?_____

_____

Situational Coping

How do you feel you are dealing with:

a) your diagnosis

_____

_____

b) changes in the ability to do things important to you?

_____

_____

c) other psychosocial observations

_____

_____

Figure 47-1, cont'd

Occupational Questions

What do you feel to be important to you right now?

_____

Do you feel you can do things important to you now? In the future?

_____

Do you deal well with change?

_____

What are your hopes, dreams, aspirations? What are some of your goals?

_____

Have these changed since you were diagnosed? How?

_____

Do you feel in control of your life at this time?

_____

What do you wish to accomplish with the rest of your life?

_____

Plan:

STG:

LTG:

Frequency:

Duration:

Therapist:

Figure 47-1, cont'd

Immediate and meaningful occupational areas are identified through this assessment. A holistic view of the client is inherent in the assessment, guided by the principles of health promotion and the values of OT.

PAPL; (see Figure 47-1) is a holistic assessment for therapists to gather data on the physical, psychosocial, emotional, and spiritual aspects of the client's life. The resultant data is synthesized using the practitioner's clinical reasoning skills, producing a collaborative intervention that is client centered. All areas of occupational performance are addressed.

Holistic assessments are useful for practitioners as they address the multitude of issues and problem areas experienced by people with HIV and AIDS. The clinical reasoning of practitioners will then be challenged to integrate knowledge and skill in all areas of OT to best serve the clients' needs.

INTERVENTION

"'Engagement in occupation' is viewed as the overarching outcome of the occupational therapy process."[1] OT practitioners engage and facilitate engagement in meaningful and productive daily life occupations through a variety of techniques, strategies, and inventive programming. Promotion of healthy lifestyles while living with the disease is crucial for all clients experiencing HIV. Interventions are individually tailored to meet the many physical, psychosocial, and contextual issues of people with HIV and AIDS. Because of the diverse features of HIV and AIDS, there are many considerations for practitioners when developing plans and goals. These considerations, listed below, also incorporate several occupational interventions that can be implemented[10]:

1. Use of universal precautions should be employed as appropriate. Check with clinic or departmental policies

(for updated universal precautions, go to http://www.cdc.gov/ncidod/hip/BLOOD/UNIVERSA.HTM).

2. Subtle cognitive and physical status changes can occur rapidly, and reassessment is indicated informally each visit.

3. Most adults with HIV have experienced perceived or real discrimination. Having a nonjudgmental, open, caring, and honest attitude and approach can make the difference in a therapy program.

4. More unique psychosocial aspects of HIV rehabilitation are present than in most other physical or psychosocial cases. Many people with HIV have lost numerous friends to the same disease for which they are receiving therapy; have undergone losses of work and family as a result of discrimination, rejection, or physical inabilities; and may have lost life partners to the same disease. For many clients, all these losses can occur before the age of 40. Women with HIV experience the aforementioned losses but must also frequently cope with poverty and homelessness; women are often underrecognized in the epidemic.

5. There is no known cure or vaccine for HIV to date, although the research is promising. This is a major consideration as a stressor of daily living.

6. Most clients with symptomatic HIV and AIDS have an altered worker role. Specific interventions regarding alternatives to work and productive living are necessary if work is a valued role. Physical as well as psychosocial work assessment for holistic work hardening programming is vital.

7. Fatigue and generalized weakness and deconditioning are primary physical manifestations of HIV. Energy conservation, work simplification, and occupational adaptations are used to enhance productivity and participation.

8. Adaptive equipment and positioning are used to assist in return to independent performance of activities of daily living (ADLs), work, and leisure occupations. Often, people with HIV may reject such equipment even though it can benefit them. This rejection signals the rejection of the sick role and sometimes denial of diminished abilities. This attitude must be respected until the time when the person chooses, if at all, to use the equipment.

9. Habit training and adaptation of the routine of daily living are essential interventions and include performance of favored occupations, with respect to physical and cognitive status; level at which the person feels comfortable adapting routines; and times of day, contexts, and with whom the person chooses to perform the occupations. Whenever possible, clients must be given choices of scheduling within their own personal routines and not those that fit the health professionals' schedule.

10. Control and choices of daily living options must be provided as much as possible. Often, people with HIV feel a sense of loss of control as the virus slowly invades bodily systems and manifests itself by further limitations in occupational performance. Providing choices can prove beneficial to clients when control in life is compromised by the virus.

11. Short- and long-term goals must be readily adapted and changed as needed.

12. Complementary therapies must be considered as interventions before and during occupational performance. These can include progressive relaxation, biofeedback, prayer, therapeutic touch, traditional Chinese medicine techniques, myofascial release, craniosacral therapy, imagery, and visualization.

13. Proper nutrition is vital for people with HIV and AIDS and can be incorporated into the OT program through homemaking occupations and health education.

These are several areas of intervention to help maintain and restore occupational performance and prevent secondary conditions and impairments from emerging.

OT PRACTICE NOTE

OCCUPATIONAL THERAPY GOALS

The goals of the OT program are to address such quality-of-life issues as pain and stress; to maintain strength, flexibility, mobility, and endurance; to maintain and increase independence in ADLs; to improve lifestyle and coping mechanisms through counseling and education; to provide support and education to the family; and to facilitate the client's adjustment to diagnosis.

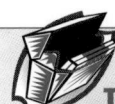

THREADED CASE STUDY: BILLY, PART 3

Billy required several types of OT interventions to strengthen mind, body, and spirit. Promotion of the therapeutic use of self, with a nonjudgmental and caring, compassionate attitude, will help Billy relax during OT sessions and engage him in discovering the best ways to establish balance and well-being in his life. As a result of his apparent depression and fatigue, he may be experiencing altered occupational role performance. Fatigue and depression can also impair cognition. Understanding exactly how these roles are compromised and the underlying body function impairments will help the therapy process unfold, with specific interventions being implemented as appropriate. Billy, as determined through an occupational profile, is a habit-oriented man. Helping him to explore his daily habits and routines, understanding where he senses an impairment (along with OT evaluation data), and encouraging him to adapt to change can help him in restoring both his emotional health and his physical well-being.

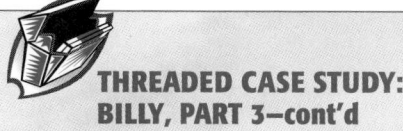

THREADED CASE STUDY:
BILLY, PART 3—cont'd

Using an occupation- and client-centered approach and understanding the disease process afford the occupational therapist unique insight into the best ways to assess and treat people with HIV and AIDS. Promoting health and well-being will also establish a higher quality of life. The focus of OT is always to enable participation in meaningful life occupations that support life satisfaction and quality of life.

SUMMARY

It is essential that OT practitioners engage in open, honest, caring, and compassionate practice at all times; this is especially crucial when serving people with HIV and AIDS. For client-centered treatment, practitioners must holistically examine the needs, values, beliefs, and wishes of those being served. A focus on occupational participation in life can be achieved through a compassionate view of the client's difficulties and struggles. This compassion can only strengthen the bond of the practitioner and client, providing hope and wellness when hope seems illusory.

Review Questions

1. What is the difference between HIV infection and AIDS?
2. What are the routes of transmission of HIV?
3. Name three side effects of the drug regimen that affect the quality of life for persons who have HIV or AIDS.
4. Differentiate primary, secondary, and tertiary prevention programs.
5. Identify one potential neurological, physical, and psychosocial problem seen in clients who have HIV or AIDS.
6. Why might a client be hesitant to accept the use of adaptive equipment to engage in occupation?
7. What are at least three health promotion and prevention goals for a client with HIV? For a client with AIDS?
8. How might you address caregiver concerns regarding sexuality issues when both partners are in their sexual prime?
9. If a client with AIDS came to you about the perception of prejudice from other healthcare personnel, how might you respond?
10. List and discuss at least four strategies to promote the health and well-being of Billy and his partner, Tom.

REFERENCES

1. American Occupational Therapy Association: Occupational therapy practice framework: domain and process, *Am J Occup Ther* 56(6):609, 2002.
2. Centers for Disease Control: *AIDSinfo: drug details*, 2004. Retrieved September 16, 2004, from http://aidsinfo.nih.gov/drugs/drugsdetail.asp?rec_id=17.
3. Centers for Disease Control: CDC National Prevention Information Network (NPIN), 2004. Retrieved February 15, 2005, from http://www.cdcnpin.org/scripts/hiv/programs.asp.
4. Centers for Disease Control: 1993 Revised classification system for HIV infection and expanded surveillance case definition for AIDS among adolescents and adults, *MMWR* 41:RR, 1992.
5. Galantino M: Human immunodeficiency virus (HIV) infection: living with a chronic illness. In Umphred D, editor: *Neurological rehabilitation*, ed 4, St Louis, 2001, Mosby.
6. Hoffman C, Kamps BS: *HIV Medicine 2003*. Retrieved September 18, 2004, from http://www.hivmedicine.com/pdf/hivmedicine2003.pdf.
7. Karon JM et al: *HIV in the United States at the turn of the century: an epidemic in transition*, 2001. Retrieved September 10, 2004, from http://www.cdc.gov/hiv/pubs/ovid/epidemic-in-transition.htm.
8. McGovern T, Smith R: Case definition of AIDS. In McGovern T, Smith R: *Encyclopedia of AIDS: a social, political, cultural and scientific record of the HIV epidemic*, Chicago, 1998, Fitzroy Dearborn Publishers.
9. National Institute of Allergy and Infectious Diseases: *HIV infection and AIDS: an overview*, 2003. Retrieved September 18, 2004, from http://www.niaid.nih.gov/factsheets/hivinf.htm.
10. Pizzi M: HIV Infection and AIDS. In Helen Hopkins H, Smith H, editors: *Willard and Spackman's occupational therapy*, ed 8, Philadelphia, 1993, Lippincott Williams & Wilkins.
11. Pizzi M: The Pizzi Holistic Wellness Assessment. In Velde B, Wittman P, editors: *Occupational therapy in health care* (special issue on community based practice) 13(3/4):51, Binghamton, NY, 2001, Haworth Press.

SUGGESTED READING

Janssen RS et al: The serostatus approach to fighting the HIV epidemic: prevention strategies for infected individuals, *Am J Public Health* 91(7):1019, 2001.

GLOSSARY

Above-knee amputation
Amputation that results in loss of the knee and everything distal to it; transfemoral amputation.

Abstract thinking
Thought process that enables a person to see relationships between objects, events, or ideas; to discriminate relevant from irrelevant detail; and to recognize absurdities.

Accessibility audit
A review of the access and inclusion practices of a place of pubic accommodation from a physical and policy perspective.

Accessibility
Ability or convenience of use.

Acquired immunodeficiency syndrome (AIDS)
An HIV infection with fewer than 200 CD4+ cells.

Action processes
Specific behavioral steps involved in implementing thinking processes.

Active exercise
Exercise to maintain joint motion and flexibility performed solely by the individual.

Active occupation
Activities in which people engage as part of their life's roles, including personal care; the constructional tasks that involve the use of hand and mechanical tools; technological activities involving such tools as calculators, computers, and electronics; games of various sorts; and vocational skills.

Active range of motion
The amount of movement that is possible when the muscles that act on a particular joint work to move the joint.

Activities
Tasks or actions completed by an individual.

Activities of daily living
Tasks that include self-care, functional mobility, sexual activity, and sleep/rest.

Activity demands
The requirements needed to engage in a specific activity.

Acute care
Inpatient setting in which the client has suffered a decline in health and is exhibiting new symptoms requiring treatment.

Acute pain
Pain with a well-defined onset; the purpose of directing attention to injury, irritation, or disease and signaling the need for immobilization and protection of a body part; amenable to pain medication.

Acute rehabilitation
Inpatient rehabilitation for acute-care patients who are medically stable and able to tolerate 3 hours of combined therapy services for 5 to 6 days a week.

Adaptive approaches
Training in daily living behaviors to facilitate adaptation to the client's unique contextual environment.

Adaptive occupation
The use of education and consultation in combination with the provision of technical aides and assistive technology, teaching the client alternative ways of doing, and modification of the task or the physical or social environment.

Adjunctive modalities
Modalities including therapeutic exercise, orthotics, sensory stimulation, and physical agent modalities.

Against gravity
Movements away from the floor or in the gravity-minimized plane (parallel to the floor) if moving against gravity is not possible.

Age-related changes
Changes to the mind, body, social systems, and so forth that result as part of aging.

Agnosia
Impairment in the ability to identify objects via visual input caused by lesions in the right occipital lobe or posterior multimodal association area.

Agraphesthesia
The inability to recognize numbers, letters, or forms written on the skin.

Allograft
Surgical burn intervention using human cadaver skin.

Alzheimer's disease
Progressive neurological disorder resulting in dementia and noticeable impairment in social and occupational functioning caused by progressive and diffuse neuronal loss in the cerebral cortex and the hippocampus.

Ambulation aids
Tools, such as canes, crutches, and walkers, used to compensate for deficits in balance and strength.

Americans with Disabilities Act
A landmark bill banning discrimination against the disabled; includes public transportation jurisdiction.

Amyotrophic lateral sclerosis
A group of progressive, degenerative neuromuscular diseases that involve destruction of the motor neurons within the spinal cord, brainstem, and motor cortex.

Anosognosia

Lack of knowledge or denial about deficits or disease process and the implications of the deficit.

Anterolateral approach

Surgical approach to replacement of the hip joint that exposes the joint by dissecting between the gluteus medius and the tensor fascia.

Antiseptic

Chemical used to prevent the growth of microorganisms.

Aphasia

A language disorder that results from neurological impairment that can affect auditory comprehension, reading comprehension (alexia), oral expression, written expression (agraphia), and the ability to interpret gestures.

Approximation

Pushing on a joint creating a compression of joint surfaces.

Apraxia

Motor perception disorder that affects motor planning; can result from damage to either side of the brain or to the corpus callosum or left hemisphere damage.

Areas of occupation

All activities required to fully participate in life, ranging from basic daily activities, work, leisure, play, education, and interacting with one's environment.

Arterial monitoring line (A line)

Catheter that is inserted into an artery to continuously and accurately measure blood pressure or to obtain blood samples without repeated needle punctures.

Arthritis

Rheumatic disease characterized by joint inflammation, chronic pain, and progressive physical impairment of joints and soft tissues.

Arthroplasty

Total hip replacement.

Arts and Crafts movement

Early movement in occupational therapy based on the belief that craftwork can improve physical and mental health through exercise and the satisfaction gained from creating a useful or decorative article with one's own hands.

Aspiration

Entry of food or material into the airway below the level of the true vocal folds.

Assessment

The tools, instruments, or interactions used during the evaluation process.

Assistive technology

Technologies that assist a person with a disability in performing tasks.

Astereognosis

A deficit in stereognosis; inability to recognize a common object through tactile perception without visual aid.

Asymmetrical patterns

Paired extremities performing movements toward one side of the body at the same time facilitating trunk movement.

Augmentative and alternative communications

Systems that supplement or replace communication by voice or gestures among people.

Autoclave

Machine used to sterilize items by steam under pressure.

Autograft

Permanent surgical transplantation of the upper layers or split-thickness skin graft (STSG) of the person's own skin "shaved" from an unburned donor site.

Autonomic dysreflexia

Overactivity of the autonomic nervous system common to individuals with spinal cord injury at or above the fifth thoracic vertebra.

Autonomic dysreflexia

Reflex action of the autonomic nervous system in response to some stimulus, such as a distended bladder, fecal mass, bladder irritation, rectal manipulation, thermal or pain stimuli, or visceral distention seen in persons with injuries above the T4 to T6 level.

Auxiliary aides

Aides such as qualified interpreters, assistive listening devices, closed caption decoders on televisions, materials in braille, and taped texts to assist individuals with disabilities.

Avascular necrosis

A condition in which bone cells die because of poor blood supply.

Axis of motion

A stable line that does not move when the bones of a joint move in relation to one another.

Backward chaining

Method in which the therapist assists the client until the last step of the process and then allows the client to perform this step independently; after the client has mastered the final step, the therapist assists until the second to last step and so on until the client has mastered all steps of the task.

Below-knee amputation

Amputation that preserves the knee and thus eliminates the necessity for a mechanical knee joint in the prosthesis; transtibial amputation.

Binocular vision

The ability of the central nervous system to receive two separate visual images and perceive them as a single image.

Biopsychosocial model

Treatment model that addresses the multilayered nature of pain by emphasizing the interactions among an individual's body, mind, and environment.

Blocked practice

Practice of a single task until mastery is achieved.

Blood pressure
Measurement of the pressure of the blood flowing into and out of the heart.

Body functions
Natural functions of the human body systems.

Body mechanics
Proper positioning and movement of the body, such as maintaining a straight back, bending from the hip, avoiding twisting, maintaining good posture, carrying objects close to body, lifting with legs to promote safe performance, and using a wide base of support.

Body scheme
A person's sense of his or her body's shape, position, and capacity.

Bolus
Cohesive mass or ball of food particles.

Brachial plexus
The nerves from C5 through T1.

Brain plasticity
The ability of the brain to reorganize and develop new pathways.

Cancer
A broad grouping of diseases characterized by the presence of malignant tumor cells in the body.

Cardiopulmonary resuscitation
A procedure used to massage the heart and provide artificial respiration to maintain blood flow and oxygenation.

Catheter
Plastic tubing used to remove urine from the bladder when the client is unable to satisfactorily control retention or release.

Centers for Disease Control and Prevention
One of the units under the Department of Health and Human Services, which is the principal agency in the United States government for protecting the health and safety of all Americans; one of its main tasks is to control the spread of infectious disease.

Central executive
The ability to process new information using selected and divided attention mechanisms.

Cerebral hypertonia
Patterns of muscle flexion or extension causing the limb to be pulled in one direction.

Chemoreceptors
Nerves that respond to cell injury or damage and are stimulated by substances that the injured cells release.

Chemotherapy
The use of a variety of toxic chemical substances to kill cancer cells within the body.

Chorea
Rapid, involuntary, irregular movements.

Chronic obstructive pulmonary disease
Disease of the lungs characterized by damaged alveoli and inflamed bronchi; includes emphysema, peripheral airway disease, and chronic bronchitis.

Chronic pain
Pain that endures beyond the point at which an underlying pathological condition can be identified and not amenable to pain medication.

Client factors
Two categories, body functions and body structures, used to assess functioning, disability, and health in persons with disabilities.

Client-centered approach
Occupational therapy process that focuses on the client's priorities and fosters an active participation toward the outcome.

Client-centered assessment
An evaluation in which the occupational therapist scores the quality of the person's motor and process skills in the context of performance of client-chosen tasks.

Client-centered care
A health promotion perspective focusing on the primacy of people, empowerment, and enablement.

Client-centered goals
Clearly stated, measurable objectives that focus on the client's engagement in occupations and activities to support participation in life.

Clinical assessment
A screening or pre-driving evaluation.

Clinical observation
The monitoring and recording of events in a clinical setting.

Clinical reasoning
Skills used to properly and effectively document, plan, direct, perform, and reflect on client care; this process is used to understand the client's occupational needs and make decisions about intervention services.

Clonus
A specific type of spasticity; repetitive contractions in the antagonistic muscles in response to rapid stretch.

Cocontraction
Also referred to as *coinnervation;* muscle pattern that provides the foundation of postural control through the simultaneous contraction of the agonist muscle and antagonist muscle.

Coeffect
The interaction of one or more forces upon the other force(s), suggesting a state or condition of active interdependence.

Cognition
The acquisition and use of knowledge involving a number of mental components.

Color agnosia
Inability to remember and recognize the specific colors of common objects in the environment.

Color anomia
Inability to name the color of objects.

Communication/interaction skills
Observable, only in the context of a social task, goal-directed actions that a person carries out one-by-one during naturalistic and relevant daily life task performances.

Community mobility
The action of moving one's self in the community, including driving and the use of public or private transportation.

Community-based settings
The client's natural physical, social, and cultural environments.

Compartment syndrome
Condition in which the interstitial pressure becomes severe enough to compress blood vessels, tendons, or nerves, which could result in secondary tissue damage.

Compensatory model
Model that maintains the repair of damaged brain tissue either has occurred to its full extent or cannot occur, leaving the individual unable to perform lost functions without external assistance.

Complex regional pain syndrome
A group of disorders in which spontaneous pain, thermal changes, and at times burning pain occur in a wide area of distribution from the original lesion; characterized by edema, skin blood-flow abnormality, or abnormal sudomotor activity in the area of the pain.

Concrete thinking
The interpretation of events literally.

Conditional reasoning
The process concerned with the contexts in which interventions occur, the contexts in which the client performs occupations, and the ways in which various factors might affect the outcomes and direction of therapy.

Consensual realm
Occupational therapists' comprehensive knowledge of the effects of society and social interactions on individual and group performance.

Constraint-induced therapy
Approach in which clients suffering from strokes learn to use the stronger, or less involved, arm for daily activities.

Constructional disorder
The inability to organize or assemble parts into a whole, as in putting together block designs (three-dimensional) or drawings (two-dimensional).

Contexts
The circumstances or events that influence the client's occupational performance and form the environment within which engagement in occupation takes place.

Contextual interference
Factors in the learning environment that increase the difficulty of initial learning.

Contract-relax
Passive motion to the point of limitation in movement patterns, followed by an isotonic contraction of the antagonist pattern against maximal resistance, with only the rotational component of the diagonal movement allowed, followed by relaxation, then by further passive movement into the agonistic pattern.

Convergence insufficiency
A condition in which the client is unable to obtain or sustain convergence of the eyes.

Convergent thinking
Thought process that enables a person to arrive at a central idea.

Coordination
The ability to produce accurate, controlled movement.

Crepitus
An audible or palpable crunching or popping in the joint caused by irregularity of opposing cartilage surfaces.

Cumulative trauma disorders
Group of injuries caused when force is applied to the same muscle or muscle group, causing an inflammatory response in the tendon or muscle.

Decerebrate rigidity
Rigidity in both the upper and lower extremities as a result of damage to the brainstem and extrapyramidal tracts.

Declarative learning
The process of creating knowledge that can be cognitively recalled.

Decorticate rigidity
Flexion hypertonus in the upper extremities and as extension tone in the lower extremities.

Decorticate rigidity
Rigidity in the extremities resulting from damage to the cerebral hemispheres (particularly the internal capsules), causing an interruption in the corticospinal tracts.

Decubitus ulcer
Pressure sores, typically on the ischial, trochanteric, and sacral bony prominences.

Deductive reasoning
A thinking process that begins with a theory and reduces the theory to its parts, which are then verified or discounted through examination.

Deep partial-thickness burn
Burn that causes damage to the epidermis and upper two thirds of the dermis.

Deglutition
The normal consumption of solids or liquids.

Dermis

Layer of skin composed of fibrous connective tissue made of collagen and elastin; contains numerous capillaries, lymphatic structures, and nerve endings.

Descriptive note

A method used to relay important information about the client not otherwise included in the patient's notes.

Desensitization

A form of treatment that aims to elicit habituation for hypersensitivity.

Devaluation

Negative psychological effects of being labeled a "disabled individual."

Diaphragmatic breathing

Breathing pattern that calls for increased use of the diaphragm to improve chest volume.

Diffuse axonal injury (DAI)

Prototypical lesion of the brain as a result of rapid deceleration; degree of injury varies from primary axonotomy, with complete disruption of the nerve, to axonal dysfunction, wherein the structural integrity of the nerve remains but there is loss of ability to transmit normally along neuronal pathways.

Diplopia

Perception of a double image.

Direct threat

A significant risk of substantial harm to the health or safety of the individual or others that cannot be eliminated or reduced to less than a significant risk by reasonable accommodation.

Disability prevention

Prevention of possible occupational performance impediments for persons with or without disability.

Disability rights movement

A paradigm that put the individual with disability at the center of the treatment model as the expert in knowing what it was like to have a disability, in contrast to the physician-centered medical model.

Discharge goal

Also known as the *long-term goal;* the ultimate purpose of the client's therapy.

Discharge report

Statement of functional performance from the initial evaluation to the discharge used to demonstrate progress, summarize the skilled interventions, and enumerate discharge recommendations.

Divergent thinking

Thought process aimed at generating alternatives.

Documentation

The creation of a permanent record of what occurred with the client.

Domain

Concept embodying the work done by occupational therapists.

Dressing apraxia

Inability to carry out the motor act of dressing on verbal command or imitation.

Driver competence

The ability to operate a motor vehicle safely.

Driving

The physical act of operating a motor vehicle.

Driving retirement

The transition from driver to nondriver.

Durable medical equipment

Items such as wheelchairs and seating systems.

Dynamic lumbar stabilization

Incorporation of many physical therapy theories that include flexion, extension, and body mechanics of the lower back to control movement of the spine and the abdominals that support the back.

Dynamic splint

Splint designed to increase passive motion, to augment active motion by assisting a joint through its range, or to substitute for lost motion; usually includes compounds of elastics, rubber bands, or springs.

Dynamic systems theory

Theory that motor behavior is a dynamic interaction between client factors (e.g., sensorimotor, cognitive, perceptual, and psychosocial), the context (e.g., physical, cultural, spiritual, social, temporal, personal, and virtual), and the occupations that must be performed to enact the client's roles.

Dysarthria

Paralysis and incoordination of the organs of speech, causing the speech to sound thick, slurred, and sluggish resulting from dysfunction of the central nervous system mechanisms that control speech musculature.

Dyscalculia

A deficit in the reasoning ability used to perform simple calculations.

Dysphagia

Difficulty with swallowing or the inability to swallow.

Dyspnea control postures

Positions used to reduce breathlessness in clients in respiratory distress.

Eating

Also known as *deglutition;* refers to the ability to manipulate and swallow food and liquids.

Edema

An abnormal accumulation of fluid in the body spaces as a consequence of trauma, impaired lymph flow, or organ failure.

Egocentric realm

The occupational therapist's refined knowledge of what contributes to a client's performance in all aspects of the mind and body; such factors include motor, neurological, perceptual-cognitive, and emotional skills.

Electronic aids to daily living

Devices that can be used to control electrical devices in the client's environment.

Emasculation

Feeling of loss of perceived male characteristics.

Empowerment

The development of autonomy and self-control.

Enablement

The ability of people to identify their own needs and solve their own problems in the manner that best suits the individual.

End-feel

The normal resistance to further joint motion because of stretching of soft tissue, stretching of ligaments and joint capsule, approximation of soft tissue, and bone contacting bone.

Endotracheal tube

A catheter inserted through the nose or mouth into the trachea usually used to deliver gas by the ventilator.

Energy conservation

Principles designed to reduce stress on the body, such as planning ahead, pacing oneself, setting priorities, eliminating unnecessary tasks, balancing activity with rest, and learning one's activity tolerance.

Environmental interventions

Altering objects or other environmental features to facilitate appropriate behaviors, inhibit unwanted behaviors, and maintain individual safety.

Epidermis

The outermost layer of epithelium, consisting of four to five layers.

Episodic memory

Recall of events that have been personally experienced and are connected to a particular place and time and relevant factual information.

Ergonomic evaluation

Assessment used to eliminate those factors in the work environment that contributed to the injury in the first place.

Ergonomics

Human performance and well-being in relation to one's job, equipment, tools, and environment.

Erogenous

Areas of the body associated with sexual stimulation.

Eschar

Adherent dead tissue that forms on skin with deep partial- or full-thickness burns.

Escharotomy

Incision through the necrotic burned tissue performed to release the binding effect of the tight eschar, relieve the interstitial pressure, and restore distal circulation.

Essential job functions

Those job duties fundamental to the position the individual holds.

Essential tasks

Those job duties fundamental to the position the individual holds.

Ethical dilemmas

Situations that present morally difficult choices regarding the care of a patient.

Ethical reasoning

Thought process by which the therapist determines the most appropriate therapy intervention to address the client's occupational performance needs.

Ethics

Moral principles guiding treatment and care of patients.

Evaluation

The process of obtaining and interpreting data necessary to understand the individual and initiate appropriate treatment.

Evidence

Data that are generated by positivist, experimental-type inquiry, or the full range of methods that can generate useful evidence.

Evidence-based practice

Practice models that integrate multiple methods of inquiry into all domains of professional practice.

Exacerbation

An episode in the progression of multiple sclerosis as minor as fatigue and sensory loss or as extensive as total paralysis in all extremities and loss of bladder control.

Executive functions

The functions needed for volition to take action; planning and organizing steps; implementing a plan; and ensuring effective performance by monitoring, self-correcting, and regulating aspects of the performance to achieve success.

Exocentric realm

Knowledge of the effects of society and social interactions on individual and group performance.

Expert-centered

Approach that comes from therapists without inclusion of clients or their caregivers.

Explicit memory

The conscious process whereby information is recalled.

Extrinsic feedback

Information provided from an outside source.

Fasciculations

Twitching of the muscle fascicles at rest.

Feeding pump
System that will administer fluids and nutrients at a preselected, constant flow rate.

Feeding
The ability of the client to bring food or fluids to the mouth.

Fiberoptic endoscopy
Technique employing a flexible fiberoptic nasopharyngolaryngoscope used to visualize and assess bolus formation, tongue movement, swallowing action, and aspiration, if it occurs.

Figure-ground discrimination
Ability to perceive the foreground from the background in a visual array.

Finger agnosia
The inability to discriminate the fingers of the hand.

Fixed route
Public transportation that relies on defined routes with predetermined stops that runs on a published schedule.

Flaccidity
The absence of muscle tone.

Flare
Arthritis exacerbation characterized by acute pain.

Follow-up services
Steps taken to guarantee that an adapted vehicle is meeting quality assurance and safety measures.

Force
A measure of stress, friction, or torque; as it relates to splinting, *force* describes the effect materials and dynamic components have on bone and tissue.

Form constancy
The recognition of various forms, shapes, and objects, regardless of their position, location, or size.

Fowler's position
Positioning of the bed so that the upper portion is raised 45 to 60 degrees; facilitates lung expansion, improves breathing, and decreases cardiac workload.

Frail elders
Persons 65 years of age or older with significant physical and cognitive health problems.

Frame of reference
A narrowly focused way to structure intervention and think about intervention progressions.

Friction
The result when one surface impedes or prevents gliding of a surface on another.

Full-thickness burn
Burn that causes an injury that extends down through the entire dermis.

Functional activity
Activity consistent with an individual's life roles and life environments.

Functional activity limitation
Activity that prevents an individual from fully participating in activities consistent with the individual's life roles and life environments.

Functional ambulation
A term used to describe the way a person walks while achieving a goal, such as carrying a plate to the table or carrying groceries from the car to the house.

Functional capacity evaluation
An objective assessment of an individual's ability to perform work-related activity.

Functional motion assessment
A gross assessment of joint mobility and muscle strength associated with functional tasks.

Functional range of motion
The amount of joint range necessary to perform essential activities of daily living and instrumental activities of daily living without the use of special equipment.

Gait training
Rehabilitation of disorders of the complex interactions among neuromuscular and structural elements of the body involved in walking.

Gastrostomy tube
G tube; non-oral feeding device inserted through a hole made in the stomach.

Gelling
Morning stiffness (of less than 30 minutes' duration) and stiffness after periods of inactivity.

General vocational evaluation
A comprehensive assessment to evaluate a person's potential to do any type of work.

Generalizability
Activities that provide approximation of real-life context and increase treatment effectiveness.

Geriatric specialist
An occupational therapist who works primarily with older adults.

Gerontologist
A geriatric specialist who has completed further study and coursework in gerontology.

Goal
A vision statement about future desires that is delimited by the need that it addresses.

Golfer's lift
Motion in which one bends at the hips while raising one leg behind.

Goniometer
Angle-measuring device consisting of a body, a stationary (proximal) bar, and a movable (distal) bar.

Grading activity
Pacing an activity appropriately and modifying it for the client's maximal performance.

Graphesthesia
The ability to recognize numbers, letters, or forms written on the skin.

Graphical communication
All forms of communication that are mediated by graphic symbols.

Gravity-minimized
Test performed in a horizontal plane (i.e., parallel to the floor) to reduce the resistance of gravity on muscle power.

Guillain-Barré syndrome
An acute inflammatory condition involving the spinal nerve roots, peripheral nerves, and, in some cases, selected cranial nerves.

Habituation
A decrease in neuron response following repeated benign stimulus.

Health Insurance Portability and Accountability Act (HIPAA)
The expectations of healthcare professionals in issues of confidentiality, privacy, and security standards to protect confidential medical information of patients.

Health promotion
Any group of actions conducive to promotion of health in individuals, groups, or communities.

Health protection
Control of infectious diseases, immunizations, protection from occupational hazards, and governmental standards for the regulation of clean air and water, sanitation, and food and drug safety, among other things.

Heart rate
The number of times that the heart contracts in 1 minute.

Heavy work
Postural pattern in which the proximal muscles contract and move, whereas the distal segment is fixed.

Hemi-inattention
Visual search deficits associated with right hemisphere injury characterized by avoidance in searching the left half of the visual space.

Heterarchical model
Model in which each component (e.g., client, environment, and occupational performance) is viewed as critical in a dynamic interaction supporting the client's ability to engage in occupation.

Heterotopic ossification
Bone that develops in abnormal anatomical locations.

Hierarchical model
Model in which higher centers in the central nervous system have control over the subordinate lower centers.

Higher-level cognition
The synthesis of awareness and executive functions in an individual.

Highly active anti-retroviral therapy (HAART)
Therapy that combines the use of protease inhibitors with two other drugs called *reverse transcriptase inhibitors.*

Hip precautions
Limits set to the range of motion a patient can use after hip replacement surgery to ensure proper muscle and soft tissue healing as well as prevent dislocation.

Hold-relax
Isometric contraction (no movement allowed) of the antagonist, followed by relaxation and then active movement into the agonistic pattern.

Home assessment
Evaluation of client's home environment used to measure maximal independence in the living environment.

Hospice
A form of palliative care used mainly to treat the terminally ill.

Human immunodeficiency virus (HIV)
Retrovirus that replicates within the human body and infects the white blood cells of the immune system and causes acquired immunodeficiency virus (AIDS).

Human interface assessment (HIA) model
A detailed look at the skills and abilities of the human in the skill areas of motor, process, and communication/interaction, as well as the demands of an activity.

Humor
The skill of making others laugh.

Huntington's disease
A fatal, degenerative neurological disorder transmitted in an autosomal dominant pattern; caused by deterioration of the corpus striatum.

Hybrid prosthesis
Prosthesis that combines body power with electrical power.

Hyperalimentation
Infusion of large amounts of nutrients needed to promote tissue growth.

Hypertonic stretch reflexes
Increased muscle tone producing stiffness in movement upon quick stretch to the muscle; occurs primarily in the flexor muscles of the upper and lower extremities.

Hypertonus
Increased muscle tone characterized by muscle inflexibility and tension.

Hypertrophic scar
Thick, rigid, erythemic scars that become apparent 6 to 8 weeks after wound closure.

Hypotonus
A decrease of normal muscle tone in which deep tendon reflexes are diminished or absent.

Ideation
The goal of the movement.

Ideational apraxia
Conceptual deficit seen as an inability to use real objects appropriately.

Ideomotor apraxia
Inability to carry out a motor act on verbal command or imitation.

Immobilization splint
Splint designed to provide protection to prevent injury, for rest to reduce inflammation or pain, or for positioning to facilitate proper healing after surgery; eliminates joint movement.

Impaired initiation
The inability to initiate activities without assistance.

Impairments
Any problem resulting from injury or disability that disrupts the proper functioning of systems used for effective movement strategies.

Implicit memory
The automatic recall of information.

Independent living movement
A model that proposed that individuals with disability were the best experts on disability, were best served through holistic treatment programs, and should be integrated into the community through social and environmental changes.

Individual activity analysis
Observing a client perform selected tasks to diagnose the occupational performance problems of that client.

Individual with a disability
A person suffering from a physical ailment, disfiguration, or mental disorder that severely limits participation in daily living functions.

Individualized functional outcomes
Achievable, reimbursable, functional activities consistent with a client's life roles, support systems, medical condition, life environments, and physical limitations resulting from cerebrovascular accident.

Inductive reasoning
A thinking process whereby one begins with seemingly unrelated data and links these data together by discovering relationships and principles within the data set, enables a person to draw generalizations from specific experiences.

Industrial rehabilitation
Range of services provided to injured workers, including functional capacity evaluation, vocational evaluation, job demands analysis, worksite evaluation, pre-employment screening, work hardening/conditioning, on-site rehabilitation, modified/transitional employment, education, ergonomics, wellness, and preventive services.

Ineffective movement strategies
Compensatory movement strategies used by an individual when all components of movement required for a planned activity are not available.

Information flow
The hierarchy of thought processes that contribute to conscious movement.

Inhibitory techniques
The use of neutral warmth, slow stroking, light joint compression, and rocking in developmental patterns to affect muscle tone and nerve stimulation.

Inpatient setting
Settings in which the client receives nursing and other healthcare services while staying overnight.

Instrumental activities of daily living
Tasks that include communication device use, health management and maintenance, financial management, meal preparation and cleanup, and community mobility.

Instrumental assessment
Important techniques for assessing a client's swallowing technique.

Interactive interventions
Approaches that the staff and caregivers use to interact with the individual.

Interactive reasoning
Form of reasoning used to engage with, to understand, and to motivate the client throughout the care process.

International Classification of Functioning, Disability and Health
World Health Organization (WHO) definition that viewed physical disability as a continuum in conjunction with its effects on body functions and structures, activities, and participation.

Intervention plan
Steps taken to effectively deliver treatment to a patient.

Intrathecal baclofen pump
Surgically implanted pump that enables baclofen to enter the body at the spinal level and avoids the centrally mediated side effects of oral baclofen.

Intravenous (IV) lines
Needles or catheters placed in the superficial veins.

Intravenous feeding
Infusion of large amounts of nutrients needed to promote tissue growth.

Intrinsic feedback
Information generated by an individual's sensory systems.

Inversion
The use of inverted positions to alter muscle tone in selected muscles.

Ischemia
Restriction of circulation.

Ischemic heart disease
Disease that occurs when a part of the heart is temporarily deprived of sufficient oxygen to meet its demand.

Isolation systems
Enclosures designed to protect a person or object from becoming contaminated or infected by transmissible pathogens.

Isometric exercise
Exercise in which the muscle length does not change and that is performed through an exertion of effort against a resistant force.

Isotonic exercise
Exercise in which equal muscle tension at both the beginning and end of the range of motion is used to strengthen the muscle.

Job demands analysis
Assessment used to define the actual demands of the job.

Joint laxity
Instability of individual joints in medial/lateral and anterior/posterior directions.

Joint measurement
An assessment tool used for physical disabilities that cause limited joint motion.

Keloid scar
Large, irregular-shaped scar caused by excessive collagen formation.

Knee immobilizer
Prosthesis used to provide no range of motion in the knee following surgery.

Learned nonuse
Phenomenon in which an individual effectively forgets to use the affected, or involved, extremity because of the extreme difficulty coordinating movement after the onset of a stroke.

Leg lifter
Devices used to lift the leg of a patient when moving from one surface to another after surgery.

Leisure
Activities performed outside of the time required for work, sleep, or self-care.

Leisure exploration
Identifying the activities one might enjoy performing outside of the time required for work, sleep, or self-care.

Leisure participation
Actively performing activities of leisure.

Levels of independence
Performance of activity or activities divided into six categories: independent, supervised, minimal assistance, moderate assistance, maximal assistance, and dependent.

Liminality
The observation that people with disability have the social experience of pervasive exclusion from ordinary life, the denial of full humanity, and a lack of full societal membership.

Long-term memory
An unlimited permanent storage component of information processing used for retrieval at a later time.

Lower motor neuron system
The cell bodies in the anterior horn of the spinal cord and their axons and the nuclei of cranial nerves III through X and their axons.

Lower motor neurons
Neurons directly innervate the skeletal muscles.

Lymphedema
An inflammatory response of the body that is caused by a shifting of protein-rich white blood cells flooding the area where the cancer has spread or where there is scar tissue forming.

Major life activities
Daily living functions such as caring for oneself, performing manual tasks, talking, seeing, hearing, speaking, learning, and working.

Manual contacts
Strategy in which the client is taught to feel movement patterns that are coordinated and balanced via the tactile input supplied through the therapist's guiding and reinforcing the desired response.

Manual cues
Physical handling of key points of control to gain access to missing components of movement.

Manual muscle test
Means of evaluating the maximal contraction of a muscle or muscle group.

Mass movement patterns
The developmental sequencing of movement and the balanced interplay between agonist and antagonist in producing volitional movement, which are diagonal in nature for the limbs and trunk.

Maximal resistance
Procedure in which the greatest amount of resistance that can be applied to an active contraction while allowing full range of motion to occur, or to an isometric contraction without defeating or breaking the client's hold, takes place.

Mechanoreceptors
Nerves that respond to touch, pressure, stretch, and vibration and are stimulated by mechanical deformation.

Medical model
Viewing disability and providing treatment from the perspective of biological deficit that could be ameliorated with professional treatment; placed physician at the center of treatment and the patient at the periphery.

Medical necessity
Anything required for the rehabilitation and successful treatment of a client, used especially in cases of billing justification and so forth.

Memory
The retention, storage, and retrieval of information.

Message composition system
System that allows the user to construct messages to be communicated to others.

Message transmission system
System that allows the communication partner to receive the message from the user.

Metacognition
Knowledge and regulation of personal cognitive processes and capacities.

Meta-emotion
The conceptualization and study of the interactions or coeffects between emotions, the body, and occupation.

Metamorphopsia
The visual distortion of objects, such as the physical properties of size and weight.

Metastases
Pieces of tumor that have broken off from the main tumor, traveled in the circulatory system, and reseeded themselves in new organs or tissues in the body.

Minimally invasive technique
Surgical technique used for hip replacement in which two approximately 2-inch incisions are needed and no detachment of muscles is required.

Missing components of movement
The building blocks of movement used in effective movement strategies that are lost as a result of injury or disability.

Mobile arm support
Mechanical devices that support the weight of the arm and provide assistance to shoulder and elbow motions through a linkage of ball-bearing joints.

Mobilization splint
Splint designed to increase limited range of motion or to restore or augment function.

Modeling
Teaching method in which the client tries to copy or reproduce the action or behavior of the therapist.

Moral treatment
Early movement in occupational therapy that included a respect for human individuality, acceptance of the unity of mind and body, and belief that a humane approach using daily routine and occupation could lead to recovery.

Motivational urge
The impulse to act.

Motor control
The outcome of motor learning involving the ability to produce purposeful movements of the extremities and postural adjustments in response to activity and environmental demands.

Motor learning
The acquisition and/or modification of learned movement patterns over time.

Motor program
The procedure or the spatiotemporal order of muscle activation that is needed for smooth and accurate motor performance.

Motor skills
The observable, goal-directed actions that a person carries out one-by-one during naturalistic and relevant daily life task performances as the person interacts with and moves task objects and moves around the task environment.

Motor unit
The basic functional unit of the peripheral nervous system consisting of four elements: the cell body of the motor neuron in the anterior horn of the spinal cord; the axon of the motor neuron, which travels via spinal nerves and peripheral nerves to muscle; the neuromuscular junction; and the muscle fibers innervated by the neuron.

Movement strategy
The programming that best achieves the goal of the movement.

Multiple sclerosis
A progressive neurological disease that damages the myelin sheath in the central nervous system.

Muscle coordination
The smooth, rhythmic interaction of muscle function.

Muscle endurance
The number of times the muscle can contract at its maximal level and resist fatigue.

Muscle grades
System of ranking severity of muscle weakness ranging from mild (G range) to moderate (F to F+) or severe (P to 0).

Muscular dystrophy
Group of diseases characterized by progressive degeneration of muscle fibers while the neuronal innervation to muscle and sensation remain intact.

Myasthenia gravis
Weakness and fatigability of skeletal muscles caused by an autoimmune response in which antibodies are produced that block, alter, or destroy the nicotinic acetylcholine receptors on the postsynaptic membrane and interfere with synaptic transmission at the nerve-muscle junction.

Myocardial infarction
A heart attack.

Myoelectric prosthesis
Prosthesis that uses muscle surface electricity to control the prosthetic hand function.

Narrative note
Format of notes used to document daily client performance and usually organized in the following subsections: problem, program, results/progress, and plan.

Narrative reasoning
The therapist's use of information gained through interviews of the client to evaluate the meaning that occupational performance limitations might have to the client.

Nasogastric tube
Abbreviated as NG tube; non-oral feeding tube inserted through the nasal passages terminating in the client's stomach.

Neck cocontraction
Position to promote neck stability and extraocular control; pattern elicits the tonic labyrinthine righting reaction when the face is perpendicular to the floor.

Need statement
A systematic, evidence-based claim, linked to all or part of a problem, that specifies what conditions and actions are necessary to resolve the part of the problem to be addressed.

Nerve blocks
Injections of a chemical agent to diminish or obliterate tone.

Neurobehavioral deficits
Functional impairments characterized by defective skill performance resulting from neurological processing dysfunction that affects performance components.

Neuro-Developmental Treatment (NDT)
The use of manual cues for recovering functional use of components of movement.

Neuroma
A small ball of nerve tissue that develops when growing axons attempt to reach the distal end of the residual limb.

Neuromuscular re-education
Retraining the neuromuscular components to produce smooth, coordinated movement.

Neuropathy
Dysfunction of the peripheral nervous system.

Neuroplasticity
The ability of the central nervous system to shape or renew itself (or both) in response to practiced activities.

Neutral spine
The most comfortable spinal position for the individual to complete movement patterns.

New body
Perception of the body after disability or during progressive disability.

Nociceptors
Subset of sensory neurons that sense pain when stimulated.

Nodes
Bony enlargements indicative of cartilage damage from osteoarthritis.

Nodules
Soft tissue masses commonly found over the extensor surface of the proximal ulna or at the olecranon.

Nosocomial infection
Hospital-acquired infection.

Objective activity analysis
Analysis of sensorimotor requirements of activities of daily living.

Objective
Statements about both how to reach a goal and how to determine whether all or part of the goal has been reached.

Occupation
Dynamic and action-oriented activities that support full participation in life.

Occupational genesis
Interactions among physical and mental capacities, the tangible world, and the roles people play in their worlds and the impact it has on the activities in which people engage throughout their lives.

Occupational justice
Providing people equitable opportunities to meet their fullest potential and achieve a state of well-being.

Occupational Safety and Health Administration
Organization that issues regulations to protect the employees of healthcare facilities.

Occupational therapist
Professional skilled in the science and delivery of occupational therapy.

Occupational therapy aide
Professional whose job is to provide to clients supportive services related to occupational therapy but always under the supervision of a professional therapist.

Occupational Therapy Practice Framework
A tool to more clearly articulate and enhance the understanding of what occupational therapy practitioners do and how they do it.

Occupational therapy practitioner
Professional skilled in the science and delivery of occupational therapy.

Occupation-based functional motion assessment
A way of assessing range of motion, strength, and motor control available for task performance by observing the client during performance of functional occupations, instrumental activities of daily living, work, or leisure activities in varied contexts.

Oculomotor control
Eye movements completed quickly and accurately to ensure perceptual stability.

Older adult
An individual 55 years of age or older.

Old-old
Individuals 80 years of age or older.

Oncology
Medical specialty that focuses on the treatment of cancer.

On-road evaluation
Examination given to determine whether a person is capable of safely operating a motor vehicle on streets with traffic.

Ontogenetic patterns
Movement patterns following a developmental progression.

Open reduction and internal fixation
Procedure in which the fracture site is exposed surgically so that the bone fragments can be aligned; the fragments are held in place by pins, screws, a plate, nails, or a rod.

Orientation
An individual's ongoing attentiveness to situations, the environment, and the passage of time.

Orthosis
Splints and suspension arm devices used to compensate for bone deformity or bone-deforming forces.

Osteoarthritis
The most common rheumatic disease, also referred to as *degenerative joint disease*, that causes the breakdown of cartilage in joints, leading to joint pain and stiffness.

Osteoporosis
A common bone disease that results in decreased bone density, most commonly in the vertebral bodies, the neck of the femur, humerus, and distal end of the radius.

Outcome objective
The criteria that must occur or exist to determine that all or part of the goal has been reached.

Pacing
Process in which the therapist helps the individual examine the required tasks, time frame for completion, and the individual's ability to complete without resulting dysfunction.

Package-year history
Calculation of the number of packs of cigarettes smoked per year (number of packs of cigarettes consumed per day multiplied by the numbers of years of smoking).

Pain
An unpleasant sensory and emotional experience associated with actual or potential tissue damage or described in terms of such damage.

Pain evaluation
Method involving the use of pain self-evaluation and clinical evaluation to assess the existence and intensity of pain.

Pain intervention
Multifaceted method of treatment with a focus on increasing physical capacities, productive and satisfying performance of life tasks and roles, mastery of self and environment through activities, and education.

Palliative
Treatment directed toward achieving comfort and ease of participation in activity.

Palpation
Use of the hands to feel beneath the surface of the skin in order to better diagnose a condition.

Paralytic strabismus
Condition in which the eye is unable to move in the direction of cranial nerve–controlled muscles that have been weakened or paralyzed; the eye may be unable to maintain a central position in the eye socket.

Paraplegia
Paralysis of the lower extremities with some involvement of the trunk, depending on the level of the lesion.

Paratransit
Public transportation that uses a demand-response service within a prescribed geographical area.

Paresis
Slight or incomplete paralysis or weakness.

Parkinson's disease
One of the more common adult-onset, degenerative neurological disorders, characterized by neurodegeneration found in the pars compacta substantia nigra.

Participation
Taking part in life activities within the natural context of daily life.

Part-task practice
Approach that emphasizes the parts of the task that the client is unable to perform independently so as to create habit patterns that occur automatically without voluntary effort.

Passive exercise
Activity used for performing passive range of motion exercise performed by an outside force such as the therapist or a device.

Passive range of motion
The amount of movement that is possible when an outside force, such as the therapist, moves a joint.

Pathogen
Infectious microorganism.

Pattern recognition
Identifying the salient features of an object and using these features to distinguish the object from its surroundings.

Pelvic alignment
Alignment of hips and trunk in a proper seated position.

Pelvic tilt
The angle of the pelvis relative to the spine and legs.

Perception
The mechanism by which the brain interprets sensory information received from the environment.

Performance analysis
An evaluation of the quality of the smallest units of occupation that the occupational therapist can directly observe as a person engages in the performance of a daily life task.

Performance patterns
Observable patterns of behavior that support or constrain the client's engagement in occupation.

Performance skills
Small units of observable action that are linked together in the process of executing a daily life task performance. Three components required for successful engagement in occupation or occupational performance: motor skills, process skills, and communication/interaction skills.

Peripheral nerve injuries
Injuries to the axillary nerve, brachial plexus, and long thoracic nerve.

Peripheral neuropathies
Lesions of the lower motor neuron system.

Person-first language
The use of language that acknowledges the individual's status as a human being before that of someone with a disability.

Phantom limb
The sensation of the limb that is no longer there; usually initially occurs immediately after surgery.

Phantom sensation
Sensations of the limb that may include cramping, squeezing, relaxed, numb, tingling, painful, moving, stuck, shooting, burning, cold, hot, or achy; different from phantom limb in that these are detailed sensations.

Physical agent modalities
Therapies to aid the development of the individual's ability to perform purposeful occupation; traditionally associated with physical therapy but increasingly used in the realm of occupational therapy.

Pivot prone
Position associated with the labyrinthine righting reaction of the head that demands a full range of extension of the neck, shoulders, trunk, and lower extremities; plays an important role in preparation for stability of the extensor muscles in the upright position.

Places of public accommodation
Privately owned entities in which business of some kind is transacted or affected.

Plasticity
Motor relearning through the use of existing neural pathways or through the development of new neural connections.

Play
Activities that suggest fun often associated with laughter.

PLISSIT
A progressive approach to guide the therapist in helping the client deal with sexual information (permission, limited information, specific suggestion, and intensive therapy).

Pointing system
System in which the user is able to make selections by pointing to a region of a graphical keyboard and performing a selection action.

Poliomyelitis
Highly contagious viral disease that infects the motor neurons of the anterior horn and brain stem.

Positioning mass
The client's center of gravity relative to that of the therapist's.

Positive prevention
Steps used to prevent the transmission of human immunodeficiency virus (HIV), such as a focus on diagnosing HIV, linking infected persons to appropriate preventive services, helping them adhere to treatment regimens, and providing support to develop healthy habits for sustaining HIV risk–reduction behavior.

Posterolateral approach
Approach from the side toward the posterior region; includes surgical approaches.

Postpolio syndrome
New muscle weakness or paralysis resulting from prior infection with polio.

Postprosthetic phase
The treatment plan involved in preparing the limb for a prosthesis.

Posttraumatic amnesia (PTA)
The length of time from the injury to the moment when the individual regains ongoing memory of daily events.

Postural control
Ability to control muscles associated with maintaining a standing or seated position.

Postural deficits
A result of an imbalance in muscle tone throughout the body causing abnormal posture.

Postural mechanism
Automatic movements that provide an appropriate level of stability and mobility.

Power switching
Control of the electrical supply for devices in a room.

Practice setting
The environment in which occupational therapy intervention occurs, including the physical facility or structure along with the social, economic, cultural, and political contexts.

Pragmatic reasoning
Form of reasoning that integrates the demands of the intervention setting, the therapist's competence, the client's social and financial resources, and the client's potential discharge environment.

Praxis
The ability to plan and perform purposeful movement.

PRECEDE-PROCEED model
A two-phase, 9-stage model encompassing (1) a comprehensive needs assessment and (2) an evaluation of the intervention, including process, impact, and outcome measures

needed for a successful health promotion intervention within a population.

Preprosthetic phase
The treatment plan involved in preparing the limb for a prosthesis.

Prevention
Reducing the risk or possible occurrence of a health-threatening event.

Primary controls
Those devices that control the steering, accelerator, and braking of a vehicle.

Primary memory
The amount of information that can be attended to and held in short-term memory.

Primary prevention
Development and implementation of health education and risk reduction strategies to help individuals and communities understand the impact of reducing risk on occupational participation.

Principles of management
Concepts to guide intervention for clients.

Private transportation
Privately owned, on-demand, 24-hour–available transportation service with immediate origin-to-destination travel offering flexibility to modify travel plans.

Problem mapping
A method whereby one expands a problem statement beyond its initial conceptualization by asking two questions repeatedly: (1) What caused the problem? and (2) What are the consequences of the problem?

Problem solving
An approach that allows for dynamic decision making.

Problem statement
As a specific claim of what is not desired or of what should be changed.

Problem-oriented medical record (POMR)
A numbered list of the client's problems (as opposed to his or her diagnosis) that becomes part of the permanent medical record.

Procedural learning
Performing tasks that are typically done automatically, without attention or conscious thought, such as many motor and perceptual skills.

Procedural memory
Memory for skill performance; a blend of cognitive, motor, and perceptual skills involved in performance-based information that through repetition becomes automatic.

Procedural reasoning
The process of medical problem solving used in accomplishing the client's therapy.

Process
Concept embodying the ways in which occupational therapists do their work.

Process objective
Concrete steps necessary to attain a goal; interventions or services that will be provided or structured by the occupational therapy practitioner.

Process skills
Motor skill actions performed as the person selects, interacts with, and uses task tools and materials; carries out individual actions and steps; and modifies performance when problems are encountered.

Progress report
Document that states the client's improvement, demonstrates the skilled therapy provided, and provides updated goals.

Proprioception
The awareness of joint position.

Proprioceptive neuromuscular facilitation
Philosophy of intervention used to address the client factors of posture, mobility, strength, effort, and coordination based on mass movement patterns that are spiral and diagonal in nature and that resemble movement seen in functional activities.

Proprioceptive stimulation
The use of sensory input to improve movement of body parts by the facilitation of muscle spindles, Golgi tendon organs, joint receptors, and the vestibular apparatus.

Prosopagnosia
Inability to recognize and identify familiar faces caused by lesions to the right posterior hemisphere.

Prosthetic phase
Treatment plan involved in increasing prosthesis-wearing tolerance and functional use.

Provocative tests
Tests used to assess ligament, capsule, and joint instability.

Pulmonary rehabilitation
Rehabilitation process used to stabilize or reverse the disease process of the respiratory system and return the patient's function and participation in activity or occupation to his or her highest capacity.

Purposeful occupation and activity
An occupation or activity with an autonomous or inherent goal beyond the motor function required to perform the task; a goal rather than a process-oriented task.

Pursed-lip breathing
Breathing technique believed to prevent tightness in the airway by providing resistance to expiration.

Pylon
The structure that attaches the socket to the terminal device of a prosthesis.

Pyriform sinuses
Pear-shaped sinuses.

Qualified person with a disability
A person with disability who meets the basic job requirements and can perform the essential functions of the job with reasonable accommodations.

Quality of life
An individual's judgment of self as measured by factors such as health, satisfaction, self-concept, and socioeconomic measures.

Radiation
The use of radioactive materials directly in tumors or the surrounding tissue to kill cancer cells.

Random practice
Attempting multiple tasks or variations of a task before mastering any one of the tasks.

Range of motion
The amount of movement that is possible at a joint.

Rate pressure product
The product of heart rate and systolic blood pressure ($RPP = HR \times SBP$)

Reasonable accommodations
Any change in the work environment or in the way work is customarily performed that enables an individual with a disability to enjoy equal employment opportunity.

Reciprocal inhibition
Early mobility pattern that serves a protective function; phasic (quick) type of movement that requires contraction of the agonist muscle as the antagonist muscle relaxes.

Reciprocal patterns
Paired extremities moving in opposite directions simultaneously, either in the same diagonal or in combined diagonals.

Referral
Recommendation of occupational therapy for a patient.

Reflex and hierarchical models
Model stating that reflexes are motor responses that occur in response to specific sensory stimuli and that the central nervous system has a specific organizational structure and both motor development and function depend on that structure.

Reflexogenic erection
Stiffening of the penis through tactile stimulation.

Rehabilitation model
Interdisciplinary approach to occupational therapy composed of medical, (including occupational and physical therapy), psychological, social, and vocational therapies for the chronically disabled.

Rehabilitation technology
Technologies that are intended to restore an individual to a previous level of function following the onset of pathology.

Rehabilitation technology supplier
Skilled member of the rehabilitation team responsible for insurance billing, repairs, and reordering of wheelchair and seating system for clients.

Rehabilitative model
Therapy model that relies on the body and brain's ability to repair or reorganize its neural pathways that had been lost as a result of neural damage sustained in the accident.

Remedial approaches
Training designed to cause some change in central nervous system functions.

Remission
An episode in the progression of multiple sclerosis that may involve a total resolution of the symptoms, may result in a short plateau, or may result in some loss of function.

Repeated contractions
Procedure in which the client's voluntary movement is repeated in conjunction with stretch and resistance to develop strength, range of motion, and endurance.

Residual limb
Part of a limb not removed during surgery that maintains good skin coverage and vascularization.

Residual limb support
A padded board placed on the seat of the wheelchair that provides a surface on which the residual limb can rest.

Resistance
Application of force given to the test motions to obtain a gross estimate of strength.

Resistive exercise
Exercises that use isotonic muscle contraction against a specific amount of weight to move the load through a certain range of motion.

Restorative occupation
The use of education and consultation in combination with the engagement of the client in occupations that can gradually be graded or modified so as to develop or restore performance skills.

Restriction splint
Splint designed to limit joint range of motion but not completely stop joint motion.

Rheumatoid arthritis
A chronic, systemic inflammatory condition characterized by an autoimmune inflammatory response in the joint lining of a genetically predisposed host.

Rhythmic initiation
Technique that involves voluntary relaxation, passive movement, and repeated isotonic contractions of the agonistic pattern; is used to improve the ability to initiate movement.

Rhythmic rotation
Technique in which the therapist passively moves the body part in the desired pattern: When tightness or restriction of movement is felt, the therapist rotates the body part slowly and rhythmically in both directions; after relaxation is felt, the therapist continues to move the body part into the newly available range.

Rhythmic stabilization
Simultaneous isometric contractions of antagonistic muscle groups.

Right-left discrimination
The ability to accurately use the concepts of right and left.

Rigidity
The stiffness within a muscle that impedes smooth movement.

Risk factors
Human characteristics or behaviors, circumstances, or conditions that increase the likelihood or predispose an individual or community to manifest certain health problems.

Rollover
Mobility pattern used for individuals who are dominated by tonic reflex patterns in the supine position; activates the extremities and lateral trunk musculature.

RUMBA
An acronym identifying something that the therapist should keep in mind when documenting the therapeutic process (Relevant, Understandable, Measurable, Behavioral, Achievable).

Scar maturation
Process in which scars become less vascular in color with more pliable, flatter contours and a smoother texture.

Scientific management
Theory recommending a scientific approach to therapy emphasizing efficiency and a mechanistic approach to medical care.

Scientific reasoning
The therapist's use of scientific knowledge to understand the client's impairments, disabilities, and performance contexts and to determine how these might influence occupational performance.

Screening
An initial assessment of the patient's suitability for occupational therapy.

Screening test
Evaluation used for observing areas of strength and weakness and for determining which areas require specific manual muscle testing.

Search
Organized and thorough scanning of the visual array.

Secondary conditions
Health conditions that arise as a result of existing impairments in individuals with disabilities.

Secondary controls
Devices used in the operation of a motor vehicle not necessary for its locomotion, such as turn-signal indicators, horn, dimmer, and windshield wipers.

Secondary prevention
The goal of arresting the disease progression and preventing complications and disability in persons at risk or in the early stages of disease.

Self-awareness
The ability to perceive the self in relative objectivity while still maintaining a subjective sense of self through one's thoughts and feelings.

Self-perception
Awareness and judgment of one's own person.

Semantic memory
Memory for words and factual information that builds on new information using prior knowledge.

Sensorimotor system
The structures of the brain that control movement through feedback regarding the accuracy of movement provided by exteroceptors and proprioceptors.

Sensory fusion
The process of combining two visual images into one.

Sensory regulation
Intervention used to increase level of awareness by trying to increase arousal with controlled sensory input, thereby increasing neurological signals to the reticular activation system.

Sensory stimulation
The use of slow rolling, neutral warmth, deep pressure, tapping, and prolonged stretch applied to muscles and joints to elicit a specific motor response.

Sensory threshold
The least stimulus needed to elicit response in a neuron.

Sensory-perceptual component
The registration of sensory information from the environment (taste, smell, touch, sound, sight) and internal stimuli that affect the sensory receptors.

Sensuality
The state of desire for pleasures of the senses.

Separation of controls
The act of operating each prosthetic component without affecting the components on either side.

Serial casting
Inhibitive casting or splinting done sequentially.

Serial static splint
Splint designed to achieve a slow, progressive increase in range of motion by repeated remolding of the splint or cast; has no movable or resilient components.

Sexual abuse
Exploitation of a person for the purpose of sexual activity.

Sexual harassment
Inappropriate sexual advances.

Sexual history
Documenting information about how a person thinks and feels about sex and bodily functions.

Sexual values
How a person thinks and feels about sex and bodily functions.

Sexuality
Interest in sexual activity.

Sexually transmitted diseases
Diseases spread through sexual contact.

Shaping
Behavioral techniques that approach a desired motor outcome in small, successive increments allowing subjects to experience successful gains in performance with relatively small amounts of motor improvement.

Short-term memory
Information held in simple storage (the primary memory) and then processed by reflecting and thinking about the information in a working space (working memory).

Simulated or enabling activity
Creating appropriate active occupation activities by adapting the environment or activity to meet the client's needs and retain his or her interest.

Simultagnosia
Inability to recognize and interpret a visual array as a whole caused by lesions to the right hemisphere of the brain.

Skill
The highest level of motor control; combines the effort of mobility and stability.

Skilled interventions
Skilled therapy services requiring the unique skills of an occupational therapist.

Skilled nursing facility
Institution that meets Medicare or Medicaid criteria for skilled nursing care, including rehabilitation services for subacute patients.

Skin breakdown
Skin lesions caused by pressure, heat, moisture, and shearing.

Slow reversal
An isotonic contraction (against resistance) of the antagonist followed by an isotonic contraction (against resistance) of the agonist.

Slow reversal-hold-relax
Technique that begins with an isotonic contraction, followed by an isometric contraction, relaxation of the antagonistic pattern, and then active movement of the agonistic pattern; used in clients able to move agonist actively.

SOAP note
A method of charting notes addressing a client's problems (Subjective, Objective, Assessment, and Plan).

Social model
A model proposing that disability was created because of environmental factors that prevented individuals from being fully functioning members of society as a result of environmental factors such as physical, political, social, and legal stigma associated with disability.

Socket
The part of the prosthesis that receives the residual limb.

Somatic marker
The collection of feelings or emotional tone of a person at any given time in a learned response to a given situation.

Somatosensory instruction
The use of tactile, proprioceptive, and kinesthetic cues to help guide the speed and direction of a movement.

Spasticity
An involuntary muscle contraction below the level of injury that results from lack of inhibition from the brain.

Spatial relations
The relative orientation of a shape or object to the self.

Specific vocational evaluation
An assessment to evaluate a person's readiness to return to a particular occupation.

Specificity
Relevance of the process objective and outcome objective to the patient.

Spica cast
A cast that extends around the pelvis and down the thigh of the fractured hip.

Spinal hypertonia
Pattern of muscle flexion or extension in which affected extremities first develop flexor and adductor tone, then extensor tone develops and becomes predominant in the lower extremities.

Splinting
Application of an immobilizing device.

Spread
How the presence of disability or an atypical physique serves as a stimulus to inferences, assumptions, or expectations about the person who has disability.

Stabilizing reversals
Alternating isotonic contractions opposed by enough resistance to prevent motion.

Standard precautions
Isolation of all bodily secretions and fluids, mucous membranes, and nonintact skin; used with all clients, not just those identified as infected.

Static progressive splint
Splint designed to be repositioned at end range without the need to remold the splint; includes a static mechanism that adjusts the amount or angle of traction acting on a part.

Static splint
Splint fabricated to rest or protect, to reduce pain, or to prevent muscle shortening or contracture; usually composed of no movable components.

Stepwise procedures
Approach in which performance of each part of the task is improved by combining practice with appropriate sensory cues and techniques of facilitation.

Stereognosis

Also known as *tactile gnosis,* the perceptual skill that enables an individual to identify common objects and geometric shapes through tactile perception without the aid of vision.

Stereopsis

The inability to perceive depth in relation to the self or various objects in the environment.

Stereotactic surgery

Surgery in which specific lesions are made in neurological structures to decrease the severity of Parkinson's disease symptoms.

Stereotype

Part of the stigmatization process, applied to those perceived to exhibit certain unvarying qualities.

Stigma

The social discrediting process in strained relations between disabled and nondisabled people that reduces the life chances of people with disability or other differences.

Strategies

An organized plan or sets of rules that guide action in a variety of situations.

Subacute rehabilitation

Inpatient rehabilitation for clients not requiring acute care.

Subdermal burn

Burns to the fatty layer, fascia, muscle, tendon, bone, or other subdermal tissues such as those seen in electrical injuries.

Subluxation

Any degree of malalignment in which articular structures are only in partial contact; characterized by volar or dorsal displacement of joints.

Substitution

Muscle or muscle group that attempts to compensate for the function of a weaker muscle to accomplish a movement.

Sulcus

Part of the oral cavity between the jaw and cheek.

Superficial burn

Burn involving only the upper layers of the epidermis.

Superficial partial-thickness burn

Burn that causes damage through the epidermis and upper third of the dermis.

Supine withdrawal

Protective position requiring flexion of the neck and the crossing of the arms and legs to protect the anterior surface of the body; total flexion response toward the vertebral level of T10.

Surgery

Procedures performed to treat cancer, including removal of a mass, more resection of tissue in addition to the mass, reconstructive surgery to correct cosmetic or functional defects or the surgical resection, or amputation.

Suspension arm device

Device suspended from above the head, generally on an overhead suspension rod that is most often attached to a wheelchair designed to support the shoulder and forearm, encourage motion of weakened proximal musculature, prevent disuse atrophy, prevent loss of range of motion, provide pain relief, provide proximal support for distal function, and enable occupational performance.

Syme's amputation

Amputation that results in loss of both ankle and foot function; ankle disarticulation surgery.

Symmetrical patterns

Paired extremities performing similar movements at the same time.

Synovitis

Inflammation of the synovial membrane that lines the joint capsule of diarthrodial joints.

System theory

Looking at worker performance via the interactions of all aspects of the domain of occupational therapy.

Systematic occupational therapy practice

The integration of critical, analytic, and scientific thinking and action processes throughout all phases and domains of occupational therapy practice.

Systemic

Affecting the entire body.

Task

The unit of action that will be done once the person is finished performing.

Task-oriented approach

Treatment method in which occupational performance and motor recovery occur from a dynamic interaction of the person, the environment, and the occupations that they are performing.

Tendon injuries

Injuries to the dense fibrous connective tissue that attaches muscle to bones.

Tenodesis

The action of wrist extension producing finger flexion and wrist flexion and resulting in finger extension.

Tenosynovitis

Inflammation of the tendon sheath.

Terminal device

The most distal component of a prosthesis; functions to grasp and hold an object.

Tertiary prevention

Therapy provided when patients exhibit disability secondary to disease; includes a strong emphasis on rehabilitation.

Tetraplegia
Any degree of paralysis of the four limbs and trunk musculature.

Thermoreceptors
Nerves that respond to the stimulation of heating or cooling.

Thinking processes
Selection of a theoretical framework in which the occupational therapy practitioner plans the steps necessary to assess problems, evaluate intervention, specify desired outcomes, and plan a strategy to determine and systematically demonstrate the degree to which client-centered outcomes were met for an individual receiving occupational therapy services.

Top-down approach to assessment
An assessment that focuses on the evaluation of performance areas.

Torque
A measure of the force that results in rotation of a lever around an axis.

Total parenteral nutrition
Infusion of large amounts of nutrients needed to promote tissue growth.

Tracheostomy
A tube inserted into the trachea to assist breathing.

Traction
Pulling on a joint that creates a separation of the joint surfaces.

Transfer of learning
The ability of a patient to spontaneously perform the necessary skills or tasks in different environments.

Transient ischemic attack
Perfusion failure of the cerebrovasculature that is characterized by mild, isolated, or repetitive neurological symptoms that develop suddenly, last from a few minutes to several hours but not longer than 24 hours, and clear completely.

Translational force
The force that results from an approach angle of less than or greater than 90 degrees; results in translation of some rotational force away from producing joint extension and directs the force into joint compression or joint distraction.

Transmission-based precautions
Guidelines for patients with highly transmissible pathogens or pathogens of epidemiological interest requiring additional precautions beyond the standard precautions.

Transtheoretical model
The premise that change occurs in stages: precontemplation, contemplation, preparation, action, maintenance, and termination.

Traumatic brain injury (TBI)
Damage to brain tissue caused by an external mechanical force with resultant loss of consciousness, post-traumatic amnesia (PTA), skull fracture, or objective neurological findings that can be attributed to the traumatic event by radiological findings or physical or mental status examination.

Undue hardship
Any accommodation that would be unduly costly, extensive, substantial, or disruptive or that would fundamentally alter the nature or operation of the business.

Unilateral neglect
Perceptual deficit in which the individual has lost the ability to integrate perceptions from one side of the body or environment; commonly caused by a lesion to the right parietal lobe but also can occur as a result of frontal and occipital lobe damage.

Universal design
Devices designed with the needs of people with a wide range of abilities.

Universal precautions
Infection control procedures designed to interrupt or establish barriers to the infection cycle used to prevent the spread of disease and infection among clients, healthcare workers, and others.

Upper motor neurons
The motor neurons located in the motor cortex and brain stem.

Upper quadrant
Area of the body that includes the scapula, shoulder, and arm.

User control system
System that allows the user to generate messages and control the device.

Vaginal atrophy
A condition of gradually declining tissue activity in the female reproductive tract.

Velopharyngeal port
Opening into the nasal cavity from the back of the mouth and throat composed of the velum and the pharynx.

Velum
The soft palate of the mouth.

Verbal commands
Tone of voice used to affect the quality of a client's motor performance.

Verbal instruction
Conveying information using spoken cues.

Verbal mediation
Strategy in which clients are taught to say aloud the steps required to perform a task safely and independently.

Vestibular stimulation
Facilitatory or inhibitory stimulation caused by linear acceleration and deceleration in horizontal and vertical planes and during angular acceleration and deceleration, such as spinning, rolling, and swinging.

Videofluoroscopy
Radiographic procedure using a modified barium swallow recorded on videotape that allows the therapist to assess the stages of the swallowing technique and the ability of the client to swallow various consistencies of food textures, see the client's jaw and tongue movement, measure the transit times of the oral and pharyngeal stages, observe the swallowing technique, note any residue in the valleculae and the pyriform sinuses, and check for any aspiration.

Visual acuity
The accurate visual information sent to the central nervous system.

Visual attention
Thought given to any novel object moving or suddenly appearing in the peripheral visual field.

Visual cognition
The ability to manipulate and integrate visual input with other sensory information to gain knowledge, solve problems, formulate plans, and make decisions.

Visual field deficit
The results of damage to the receptor cells in the retina or to the optic pathway that relays retinal information to the central nervous system for processing.

Visual fields
The visual scene for which the central nervous system receives complete visual information.

Visual instruction
The process of demonstrating an activity while the client observes the therapist and follows the therapist's example.

Visual memory
The ability to create and retain a picture of the object in the mind's eye.

Visual neglect
Creation of severe inattention to the visual field caused by the combination of hemi-inattention and left visual field deficit.

Visual perception
The process that integrates vision with other sensory input for adaptation and survival.

Visual perceptual hierarchy
The processes of visual cognition, visual memory, pattern recognition, visual scanning, and visual attention.

Visual scanning
Organized and thorough scanning of the visual array.

Visual-spatial perception
The capacity to appreciate the spatial arrangement of one's body, objects in relationship to oneself, and relationships between objects in space.

Vital capacity
Thoracic cavity volume.

Vocational evaluation
Assessment of work habits, work behaviors, physical and cognitive abilities, psychosocial skills, and work skills in relation to the client's interests, motivation, age, and educational level to determine a reasonable occupation for the client to pursue.

Weight bearing
The act of supporting one's weight.

Weight-bearing restrictions
The amount or level of weight that a patient is allowed to place on fracture sites.

Wellness
The state of mental and physical balance and fitness.

Whole-task practice
Approach in which a whole task is learned to be completed automatically without voluntary effort through repetitive practice of its component skills.

Work conditioning
Replicating the physical demands of the job through physical conditioning alone, which covers strength, aerobic fitness, flexibility, coordination, and endurance.

Work hardening
Formal multidisciplinary programs for rehabilitating the injured worker.

Work readiness program
Program designed to help individuals who desire to work identify vocational options that match their interests, skills, and abilities.

Working memory
Information stored in a holding area of the mind so that the information can be further processed.

Work-related musculoskeletal disorder
A class of soft injuries affecting the muscles, tendons, and nerves.

Worksite evaluation
On-the-job assessments to determine whether an individual can return to work after onset of a disability or whether a person can benefit from reasonable accommodations to maintain employment.

Xenograft
Surgical burn intervention using processed porcine skin.

Young-old
Individuals 65 to 74 years of age.